Rutter's Child and Adolescent Psychiatry

Rutter's Child and Adolescent Psychiatry

Sixth Edition

Edited By

Anita Thapar   and

Professor of Child and Adolescent Psychiatry, Child and
Adolescent Psychiatry Section, Institute of Psychological
Medicine and Clinical Neurosciences, Cardiff University
School of Medicine, Cardiff, UK

Daniel S. Pine

Chief, Section on Development and Affective Neuroscience,
National Institute of Mental Health Intramural Research
Program, Bethesda, MD, USA

James F. Leckman

Neison Harris Professor, Child Study Center and the Departments of Psychiatry, Pediatrics and Psychology, Yale University, New Haven, CT, USA

Stephen Scott

Professor of Child Health and Behavior, Institute of Psychiatry, Psychology and Neuroscience, King's College London, London, UK;
Head, National Conduct Problems and National Adoption and Fostering Services, Maudsley Hospital, London, UK

Margaret J. Snowling

President, St. John's College and Professor of Psychology, Department of Experimental Psychology, University of Oxford, Oxford, UK

Eric Taylor

Emeritus Professor of Child and Adolescent Psychiatry, Department of Child and Adolescent Psychiatry, Institute of Psychiatry, Psychology and
Neuroscience, King's College London, London, UK

WILEY Blackwell

Registered Office
John Wiley & Sons Ltd, The Atrium, Southern Gate, Chichester, West Sussex, PO19 8SQ, UK

Editorial Office
9600 Garsington Road, Oxford, OX4 2DQ, UK

For details of our global editorial offices, customer services, and more information about Wiley products visit us at
www.wiley.com.

Wiley also publishes its books in a variety of electronic formats and by print-on-demand. Some content that appears in
standard print versions of this book may not be available in other formats.

Library of Congress Cataloging-in-Publication Data
Rutter's child and adolescent psychiatry / edited by Anita Thapar and Daniel S. Pine, James F. Leckman, Stephen Scott,
Margaret J. Snowling, Eric Taylor. – Sixth edition.
       p. ; cm.
   Child and adolescent psychiatry
   Preceded by: Rutter's child and adolescent psychiatry / edited by Michael Rutter ... [et al.]. 5th ed. 2008.
   Includes bibliographical references and index.
   ISBN 978-1-118-38196-0 (cloth) 978-1-118-38188-5 (paper)
   I. Thapar, Anita, editor. II. Title: Child and adolescent psychiatry.
   [DNLM: 1. Mental Disorders. 2. Adolescent Behavior. 3. Adolescent. 4. Child. 5. Developmental Disabilities. WS 350]
   RJ499
   618.92′89–dc23
                                                                                      2014032477

Cover design: Wiley
Cover images: (Brain) © skodonnell/Gettyimages; (Ethnic Kids) GlobalStock/Gettyimages;
(DNA Abstract) © kirstypargeter/Gettyimages

Set in 9.5/12pt MinionPro by SPi Global, Chennai, India
Printed and bound by CPI Group (UK) Ltd, Croydon CR0 4YY

C000422_080322

Contents

List of contributors

Annah N. Abrams MD
Chief, Child and Adolescent Psychiatry Consultation Service, Massachusetts General Hospital, Boston, MA, USA

Louise Arseneault PhD
Professor of Developmental Psychology, Institute of Psychiatry, Psychology and Neuroscience, King's College London, London, UK

Camilla Azis-Clauson BSc
Research Psychologist, Institute of Psychiatry, Psychology and Neuroscience, King's College London, London, UK

Marian J. Bakermans-Kranenburg PhD
Professor, Center for Child and Family Studies, Leiden University, Leiden, The Netherlands

Rachael Bedford PhD
Sir Henry Wellcome Postdoctoral Fellow, Department of Biostatistics, Institute of Psychiatry, Psychology and Neuroscience, London, UK

Kristin Bernard PhD
Assistant Professor of Clinical Psychology, Department of Psychology, Stony Brook University, Stony Brook, NY, USA

Theresa S. Betancourt ScD, MA
Associate Professor and Director, Department of Global Health and Population, Harvard School of Public Health, Harvard University, Boston, MA, USA

Michael H. Bloch MD
Assistant Professor, Child Study Center and the Department of Psychiatry, Yale University, New Haven, CT, USA

David Brent MD, MS Hyg
Endowed Chair in Suicide Studies and Professor of Psychiatry, Pediatrics, Epidemiology, and Clinical and Translational Science, Western Psychiatric Institute, University of Pittsburgh, Pittsburgh, PA, USA

Maggie Bruck PhD
Professor, School of Medicine, Johns Hopkins University, Baltimore, MD, USA

Rachel Bryant-Waugh BSc, MSc, DPhil
Consultant Clinical Psychologist, Lead for Feeding Disorders Team, Joint Head of Feeding and Eating Disorders Service, Department of Child and Adolescent Mental Health, Great Ormond Street Hospital for Children NHS Foundation Trust, London, UK

Stephen J. Ceci PhD
Helen L. Carr Professor of Developmental Psychology, Department of Human Development, Cornell University, New York, USA

Tony Charman MA, Msc, PhD
Professor of Clinical Child Psychology, Department of Psychology, Institute of Psychiatry, Psychology & Neuroscience, King's College London, London, UK

Erica M. Chin PhD
Assistant Professor, Division of Child and Adolescent Psychiatry, New York Presbyterian Hospital, Columbia University Medical Center, New York, NY, USA

Richard Church MB, BChir, MRCPsych, DCH, AKC
Consultant Psychiatrist, South London and Maudsley NHS Foundation Trust, London, UK

Nancy J. Cohen PhD, CPsych
Professor of Child and Adolescent Psychiatry, Department of Psychiatry, University of Toronto, Toronto, Ontario, Canada
Director of Research, Hincks-Dellcrest Center, Gail Appel Institute, Toronto, Ontario, Canada

Stephan Collishaw DPhil
Senior Lecturer, Institute of Psychological Medicine and Clinical Neurosciences, Cardiff University School of Medicine, Cardiff, UK

Michael Crowley PhD
Assistant Professor, Child Study Center Program for Anxiety Disorders; Associate Director, Developmental Electrophysiology Laboratory, Yale University School of Medicine, New Haven, CT, USA

Thomas J. Crowley MD
Professor, Department of Psychiatry, University of Colorado School of Medicine, Aurora, CO, USA

Colleen M. Cummings PhD
Child, Pediatric and Adolescent Psychologist, Department of Psychology, Temple University, Philadelphia, PA, USA

Naomi Dale MA, PhD, CPsychol
Consultant Clinical Psychologist, Head of Psychology (Neurodisability), The Wolfson Neurodisability Service, Great Ormond Street Hospital, NHS Foundation Trust, London, UK

Andrea Danese MD PhD
Clinical Senior Lecturer and Consultant, Child and Adolescent Psychiatrist, Institute of Psychiatry, Psychology & Neuroscience, King's College London, London, UK
National and Specialist Clinic for Child Traumatic Stress and Anxiety Disorders, South London and Maudsley NHS Foundation Trust, London, UK

Daniel P. Dickstein MD
Director, PediMIND Program, Associate Director of Research, Bradley Hospital, East Providence, RI, USA
Division of Child Psychiatry, Department of Psychiatry and Human Behavior, Alpert Medical School of Brown University, Providence, RI, USA

Mary Dozier
Amy E DuPont Chair of Child Development, Professor, Department of Psychological and Brain Sciences, University of Delaware, Newark, DE, USA

Lindsey Edwards PhD
Consultant Clinical Psychologist, Cochlear Implant Programme, Great Ormond Street Hospital, NHS Foundation Trust, London, UK

Ivan Eisler MA, PhD, FAcSS, FAED
Emeritus Professor of Family Psychology and Family Therapy, Institute of Psychiatry, Psychology and Neuroscience, King's College London, London, UK

Sara Evans-Lacko PhD
Lecturer, Institute of Psychiatry, Psychology and Neuroscience, King's College London, UK

Fataneh Farnia PhD
Assistant Professor, Department of Psychiatry, University of Toronto, Toronto, Ontario, Canada
Hincks-Dellcrest Centre, Gail Appel Institute, Toronto, Ontario, Canada

Mina Fazel MB BCh, MRCPsych, DM
Research Fellow, Department of Psychiatry, University of Oxford, Oxford, UK

Prudence W. Fisher PhD
Assistant Professor, Division of Child and Adolescent Psychiatry, Columbia University and New York State Psychiatric Institute, New York, NY USA

Tamsin Ford PhD, FRCPsych
Professor of Child and Adolescent Psychiatry, Institute of Health Research, University of Exeter Medical School, Exeter, UK

Jane Fortin LLB, Solicitor
Emeritus Professor, Sussex Law School, University of Sussex, Brighton, UK

Nathan A. Fox PhD
Distinguished University Professor and Interim Chair, Department of Human Development and Quantitative Methodology, University of Maryland, College Park, MD, USA

Frances Gardner MPhil, DPhil
Professor of Child and Family Psychology, Centre for Evidence-Based Intervention, Department of Social Policy and Intervention, University of Oxford, Oxford, UK

M. Elena Garralda MD, MPhil, FRCPsych, FRCPCH DPM
Emeritus Professor, Academic Unit of Child and Adolescent Psychiatry, Imperial College London, London, UK

Danya Glaser MB, DCH, FRCPsych, Hon FRCPCH
Honorary Consultant Child and Adolescent Psychiatrist, Great Ormond Street Hospital for Children NHS Foundation Trust, London, UK

Robert Goodman PhD FRCPsych
Professor of Brain and Behavioral Medicine, Institute of Psychiatry, Psychology and Neuroscience, King's College London, UK

Jonathan Green MA, MBBS, FRCPsych, DCH
Professor of Child and Adolescent Psychiatry, Institute of Brain, Behavior and Mental Health, University of Manchester and Manchester Academic Health Sciences Centre; Honorable Consultant, Royal Manchester Children's Hospital, Manchester, UK

Mark T. Greenberg PhD
Bennett Chair in Prevention Research Center for the Promotion of Human Development, Pennsylvania State University, University Park, PA, USA

David J. Grelotti MD
Assistant Professor, Department of Psychiatry, University of California San Diego School of Medicine, La Jolla, CA, USA
Staff Psychiatrist, Owen HIV Clinic, University of California San Diego Health System, San Diego, CA, USA

Brenda Hale DBE, PC, MA (Cantab), FRCPsych (Hon), LL.D (Hon), DUniv (Hon), FBA
Deputy President, Supreme Court of the United Kingdom, London, UK

Nathan B. Hansen PhD
Associate Professor and Department Head, Department of Health Promotion and Behavior, College of Public Health, University of Georgia, Athens, GA, USA

Gordon Harold BSc, MSc, PhD
Director and Andrew and Virginia Rudd Chair in Psychology, Rudd Centre for Adoption Research and Practice, School of Psychology, University of Sussex, Brighton, UK

Allison G. Harvey PhD
Professor of Psychology, Department of Psychology, University of California, Berkeley, CA, USA

Keith Hawton FMedSci DSc FRCPsych
Director, Centre for Suicide Research, University Department of Psychiatry, Warneford Hospital, Oxford, UK

Isobel Heyman MBBS PhD FRCPsych
Consultant Child and Adolescent Psychiatrist, Psychological Medicine, Great Ormond Street Hospital for Children, London, UK
Honorary Professor, Institute of Child Health, UCL School of Life and Medical Sciences, University College London, London, UK

Jonathan Hill BA, MBBChir, MRCP, FRCPsych
Professor of Child and Adolescent Psychiatry, School of Psychology and Clinical Language Sciences, University of Reading, Reading, UK

Chris Hollis PhD MRCPsych
Professor of Child and Adolescent Psychiatry, Division of Psychiatry and Applied Psychology, Institute of Mental Health, University of Nottingham, UK

Jane Hood BSc, MSc, PGCE, DEdPsy, C. Psychol
Consultant Pediatric Neuropsychologist and Educational Psychologist, Centre for Developmental Neuropsychology, Oxon, UK

Patricia Howlin BA, MSc, PhD, FBPS

Emeritus Professor of Clinical Child Psychology, Department of Psychology, Institute of Psychiatry, Psychology and Neuroscience, King's College London, London, UK; Professor of Developmental Disability, Faculty of Health Sciences, University of Sydney, New South Wales, Australia

Charles Hulme MA, DPhil, FBPsS

Professor of Psychology, Division of Psychology and Language Sciences, University College London, London, UK

Marinus H. van IJzendoorn PhD

Professor of Child and Family Studies, Centre for Child and Family Studies, Leiden University, Leiden, The Netherlands

Anthony James MB, BS, MRCP, MRCPsych, MPhil, MA(Oxon)

Consultant Child and Adolescent Psychiatrist, Department of Psychiatry, University of Oxford, Oxford, UK

Jennifer Jenkins PhD

Atkinson Chair of Early Child Development and Education, Applied Psychology and Human Development, University of Toronto, Ontario, Canada

Mark H. Johnson PhD FBA

Director, Centre for Brain and Cognitive Development, School of Psychology, Birkbeck College, University of London, London, UK

Philip C. Kendall PhD, ABPP

Distinguished University Professor and Laura H. Carnell Professor of Psychology, Department of Psychology, Temple University, Philadelphia, PA, USA

Christian Kieling MD, PhD

Lecturer, Department of Psychiatry, School of Medicine, Universidade Federal do Rio Grande do Sul, Porto Alegre, Brazil

Rachel G. Klein PhD

Fascitelli Family Professor The Child Study Center at New York University Langone Medical Center Department of Child and Adolescent Psychiatry, New York University School of Medicine, NY, USA

Martin Knapp PhD

Professor of Social Policy, Department of Social Policy, London School of Economics and Political Science, London, UK

Helena Chmura Kraemer PhD

Professor of Biostatistics in Psychiatry (Emerita), Stanford University, Stanford, CA, USA

Adjunct, Department of Psychiatry, School of Medicine, University of Pittsburgh, Pittsburgh, USA

Tami Kramer MBBCh, MRCPsych

Consultant Child and Adolescent Psychiatrist, and Senior Clinical Research Fellow, Academic Unit of Child and Adolescent Psychiatry, Imperial College London, London, UK

Judith Lask BA, MSc, ADFT, CQSW

Family and Systemic Psychotherapist, University of Exeter, Exeter, UK

Nancy Lau AM

PhD Candidate in Clinical Psychology, Department of Psychology, Harvard University, Cambridge, MA, USA

Ann Le Couteur BSc Psychology, MBBS, FRC Psych, FRCPCH

Professor of Child and Adolescent Psychiatry, Institute of Health and Society, Newcastle University, Newcastle upon Tyne, UK and Northumberland, Tyne and Wear NHS Foundation Trust, Newcastle upon Tyne, UK

James F. Leckman MD, PhD

Neison Harris Professor, Child Study Center and the Departments of Psychiatry, Pediatrics and Psychology, Yale University, New Haven, CT, USA

Ellen Leibenluft MD

Senior Investigator and Chief of the Section on Bipolar Spectrum Disorders, Emotion and Development Branch, National Institute of Mental Health, Bethesda, MD, USA

Fadi Maalouf MD

Director, Child and Adolescent Psychiatry Program, Department of Psychiatry, American University of Beirut, Beirut, Lebanon

Sheri Madigan PhD

Post Doctoral Fellow, Applied Psychology and Human Development, University of Toronto, Ontario, Canada

Barbara Maughan PhD

Professor of Developmental Epidemiology, MRC Social, Genetic and Developmental Psychiatry Centre, Institute of Psychiatry, Psychology and Neuroscience, King's College London, London, UK

Eamon McCrory PhD DClinPsy

Professor of Developmental Neuroscience and Psychopathology Division of Psychology and Language Sciences, University College London, London, UK Anna Freud Centre, London, UK

Eleanor L. McGlinchey PhD

Postdoctoral research fellow, Department of Psychology, University of California, Berkeley, CA, USA
New York State Psychiatric Institute, Columbia University Medical Center, New York, NY, USA

Michael J. Meaney CM, CQ, FRSC, PhD

James McGill Professor, Ludmer Centre for Neuroinformatics and Mental Health, Douglas Mental Health University Institute, McGill University, Montreal, Canada
Singapore Institute of Clinical Sciences, A*STAR, Brenner Centre for Molecular Medicine, Singapore

Monica Melby-Lervåg PhD

Professor, Deputy Dean for Research, Department of Special Needs Education, University of Oslo, Oslo, Norway

Sally N Merry FRANZCP CCAP

Professor, Department of Psychological Medicine, Auckland School of Medicine, University of Auckland, Auckland, New Zealand

Stephanie Moor MRCPsych
Child and Adolescent Psychiatrist and Senior Lecturer, Department of
Psychological Medicine, Christchurch School of Medicine, University of Otago,
Christchurch, New Zealand

Mei Yi Ng AM
Ph.D. Candidate in Clinical Psychology, Department of Psychology, Harvard
University, Cambridge, MA, USA

Courtenay Frazier Norbury DPhil
Professor, Department of Psychology, Royal Holloway, University of London,
Surrey, UK

Rory C. O'Connor PhD, CPsychol, AFBPsS, FAcSS
Professor of Health Psychology, Suicidal Behaviour Research Laboratory,
Institute of Health and Wellbeing, University of Glasgow, Glasgow, UK

Kieran J. O'Donnell PhD
Postdoctoral Fellow, Ludmer Centre for Neuroinformatics and Mental Health,
Douglas Mental Health University Institute, McGill University, Montreal,
Canada

Lena Palaniyappan PhD MRCPsych
Clinical Associate Professor, Division of Psychiatry and Applied Psychology,
Institute of Mental Health, University of Nottingham, Nottingham, UK

Rhea Paul Ph, CCC-SLP
Professor and Chair, Department of Speech-Language Pathology, College of
Health Professions, Sacred Heart University, Fairfield, CT, USA

Kevin Pelphrey PhD
Harris Professor, Child Study Center and Department of Psychology, Yale
University, New Haven, CT, USA

Jeremy S. Peterman MA
PhD Student, Clinical Psychology, Child and Adolescent Anxiety Disorders
Clinic (CAADC), Department of Psychology, Temple University, Philadelphia,
PA, USA

Andrew Pickles PhD
Chair in Biostatistics, Department of Biostatistics, Institute of Psychiatry,
Psychology and Neuroscience, King's College London, London, UK

Daniel S. Pine MD
Chief, Section on Development and Affective Neuroscience, National Institute
of Mental Health (NIMH) Intramural Research Program, Bethesda,
MD, USA

Elizabeth Pinsky MD
Clinical Fellow in Psychiatry, Child and Adolescent Psychiatry Consultation
Service, Massachusetts General Hospital, Boston, MA, USA

Kaija Puura MD, PhD
Associate Professor, Department of Child Psychiatry, University of Tampere and
Tampere University Hospital, Tampere, Finland

Atif Rahman MRCPsych, PhD
Professor of Child Psychiatry, Institute of Psychology, Health and Society,
University of Liverpool, Liverpool, UK

Judith L. Rapoport MD
Chief, Section on Childhood Neuropsychiatric Disorders, Child Psychiatry
Branch, National Institute of Mental Health, Bethesda, MD, USA

Charlotte Ulrikka Rask MD, PhD
Consultant, Senior Researcher, Research Clinic for Functional Disorders and
Psychosomatics, Aarhus University Hospital, Aarhus, Denmark
Clinical Associate Professor, Regional Centre for Child and Adolescent
Psychiatry, Aarhus University Hospital, Aarhus, Denmark

Paula K. Rauch MD
Director, Marjorie E. Korff, PACT (Parenting At a Challenging Time)
Program, Child and Adolescent Psychiatry Consultation Service and MGH
Cancer Center Parenting Program, Massachusetts General Hospital,
Boston, MA, USA

Ruth Reed MB BChir, MRCPsych, MRCPCH
Specialty Registrar, Department of Psychiatry, University of Oxford, Oxford, UK

Nathaniel R. Riggs PhD
Associate Professor of Human Development and Family Studies, Department of
Human Development and Family Studies, Colorado State University, Fort
Collins, CO, USA

Michael Rutter CBE, MD, FRCP, FRCPsych, FRS, FMedSci, FBA
Professor of Developmental Psychopathology, Social, Genetic and
Developmental Psychiatry (SGDP) Research Centre, Institute of Psychiatry,
Psychology and Neuroscience, King's College London, London, UK

Joseph T. Sakai MD
Associate Professor, Department of Psychiatry, University of Colorado School of
Medicine, Aurora, CO, USA

Kate E.A. Saunders BMBCh, MA, MRCPsych
Honorary Consultant Psychiatrist, Department of Psychiatry, University of
Oxford, Oxford, UK

Stephen Scott FRCP, FRCPsych
Professor of Child Health and Behavior, Director of National Academy for
Parenting Research, Institute of Psychiatry, Psychology and Neuroscience,
Kings's College London, London, UK; Head, National Conduct Problems and
National Adoption and Fostering Services, Maudsley Hospital, London, UK

Michael C. Seto PhD
Director of Forensic Rehabilitation Research, Royal Ottawa Health Care Group,
Integrated Forensic Program, Brockville, Canada

Philip Shaw BM, BCh, PhD
Investigator, Social and Behavioral Research Branch, and Head,
Neurobehavioral Clinical Research Section, National Human Genome Research
Institute, Bethesda, MD, USA

Emily Simonoff MD, FRCPsych
Professor of Child and Adolescent Psychiatry, Department of Child and Adolescent Psychiatry, Institute of Psychiatry, Psychology and Neuroscience, King's College London, London, UK and NIHR Biomedical Research Centre for Mental Health, King's College London, London, UK

David Skuse MD, FRCP, FRCPsych, FRCPCH
Chair of Behavioral and Brain Sciences, Institute of Child Health, UCL School of Life and Medical Sciences, University College London, London, UK

Patrick Smith PhD
Senior Lecturer and Honorary Consultant Clinical Psychologist, Institute of Psychiatry, Psychology and Neuroscience, Kings's College London, London, UK

Anna T. Smyke PhD
Clinical Associate Professor of Psychiatry and Behavioral Sciences, Department of Psychiatry and Behavioral Sciences, Tulane University School of Medicine, New Orleans, LA, USA

Margaret J. Snowling PhD, Dip Clin Psych, FBA, F Med Sci, FBPsS
President, St John's College and Professor of Psychology, Department of Experimental Psychology, University of Oxford, Oxford, UK

Edmund J.S. Sonuga-Barke PhD
Professor of Psychology, Developmental Psychopathology and Director, Developmental Brain-Behavior Laboratory, Department of Psychology, University of Southampton, Southampton, UK
Guest Professor, Department of Experimental Clinical and Health Psychology, Ghent University, Ghent, Belgium

Matthew W. State MD, PhD
Oberndorf Family Distinguished Professor of Psychiatry; Chair, Department of Psychiatry; Director, Langley Porter Psychiatric Institute, University of California, San Francisco, CA, USA

Alan Stein MB, BCh, MA, FRCPsych
Head of Section, Child and Adolescent Psychiatry, Department of Psychiatry, University of Oxford, Oxford, UK

Argyris Stringaris MD, MRCPsych, PhD
Senior Lecturer, Head of Mood and Development Laboratory, Wellcome Trust Fellow, Department of Child and Adolescent Psychiatry, Institute of Psychiatry, Psychology and Neuroscience, King's College London, London, UK
Consultant Psychiatrist, Maudsley Hospital, London, UK

Peter Szatmari MD, MSc, FRCP
Chief of the Child and Youth Mental Health Collaborative, Hospital for Sick Children, Centre for Addiction and Mental Health, Director of the Division of Child and Adolescent Psychiatry, University of Toronto, Ontario, Canada.

Tuula Tamminen MD, PhD
Professor of Child Psychiatry, Department of Child Psychiatry, University of Tampere and Tampere University Hospital, Tampere, Finland

Eric Taylor MA, MB, FRCP, FRCPsych, FMedSci
Emeritus Professor of Child and Adolescent Psychiatry, Department of Child and Adolescent Psychiatry, Institute of Psychiatry, Psychology and Neuroscience, King's College London, London, UK

Anita Thapar MBBCH, FRCPsych, PhD, FMedSci
Professor of Child and Adolescent Psychiatry, Child and Adolescent Psychiatry Section, Institute of Psychological Medicine and Clinical Neurosciences, Cardiff University School of Medicine, Cardiff, UK

Kenneth E. Towbin MD
Chief, Clinical Child and Adolescent Psychiatry, Emotion and Development Branch, National Institute of Mental Health, Intramural Research Program, Bethesda, MD, USA
Clinical Professor of Psychiatry and Behavioral Sciences and Pediatrics, Psychiatry and Behavioral Health, The George Washington University School of Medicine, Washington, DC, USA

Hilary B. Vidair PhD
Co-Director of Clinical Training, Clinical Psychology Doctoral Program, Assistant Professor of Psychology, Department of Psychology, Long Island University, Post Campus, Brookville, NY, USA

Essi Viding PhD
Professor of Developmental Psychopathology, Faculty of Brain Sciences, University College London, London, UK
Professor of Cognitive Neuroscience, Institute of Psychiatry, Psychology and Neurosciences, King's College London, London, UK

Olga L. Walker PhD
Research Associate, Department of Human Development and Quantitative Methodology, University of Maryland, College Park MD, USA

Beth Watkins PhD
Clinical Psychologist, Feeding and Eating Disorders Service, Department of Child and Adolescent Mental Health, Great Ormond Street Hospital for Children NHS Foundation Trust, London, UK

John R. Weisz PhD, ABPP
Professor, Department of Psychology, Harvard University, Cambridge, MA, USA

Miranda Wolpert MA, PsychD
Director, Evidence Based Practice Unit, University College London; Anna Freud Centre; and Director of Child Outcomes Research Consortium, London, UK

Anne Worrall-Davies MB, ChB (Hons), MMedSc, MRCPsych, MD
Consultant Child and Adolescent Psychiatrist, Adolescent Inpatient Service, Leeds Community Healthcare NHS Foundation Trust, Leeds, UK

Brent Vander Wyk PhD
Assistant Professor, Child Study Center, Yale University, New Haven, CT, USA

Susan Young BSc, DClinPsy, PhD, AFBPS, CPsychol
Clinical Senior Lecturer in Forensic Clinical Psychology, Centre for Mental Health, Imperial College London, London, UK

William Yule MA, DipPsychol, PhD, FBPsS, C. Psychol
Emeritus Professor of Applied Child Psychology, Institute of Psychiatry, Psychology and Neuroscience, Kings's College London, London, UK

Charles H. Zeanah MD
Sellars Polchow Chair in Psychiatry Vice Chair, Child and Adolescent Psychiatry, Department of Psychiatry and Behavioral Sciences, Tulane University School of Medicine, New Orleans, LA, USA

Kenneth J. Zucker PhD
Clinical Lead, Gender Identity Clinic, Child, Youth and Family Services, Centre for Addiction and Mental Health, Toronto, Ontario, Canada
Professor, Department of Psychiatry, University of Toronto, Totonto, Ontario, Canada

Foreword

In the first edition of this textbook in 1976 the preface quoted the words of Sir Aubrey Lewis with respect to the need for psychiatrists to acquire "reasoning and understanding" and enable the combination of what he called "the scientific and humane temper" in his studies. That aspiration has been a continuous theme across the six editions of the textbook. That is, although a key part of what the textbook has provided has been current knowledge on empirical findings, it has given at least as much weight to the concepts involved so that readers are in a better position to deal with new findings and new ideas as they come along. That typifies this sixth edition as much as it did the previous five. The chapters seek to provide an appropriate balance between the questioning approach that is essential in both science and clinical work and a positive style that provides useful guidance on how to proceed in clinical practice. I am delighted with the skilful way in which the new team of editors has succeeded in this task.

In planning how they would deal with this new sixth edition, the editors will have wanted to think about some of the changes that have taken place over time. Some of these preceded the last edition but were not fully recognized at that time but all have increased in importance since then. First, there has been the evidence that there is much more overlap among diagnostic categories than used to be appreciated. This is noted in the chapter on classification. Second, there have been numerous important developments in genetics – including the discovery of rare genetic mutations, the role of copy number variations, the multiple clinical pictures associated with any of the single genes that have been found, and the importance of gene–environment interactions. These are well covered in the chapter on genetics. Third, there is the appreciation that not only are most risk factors dimensional in their operation but so, too, most disorders are also dimensional. The field has struggled somewhat in knowing how to deal with dimensions as well as categories but the topic crops up in many of the chapters throughout the volume. Fourth, the new edition of the American Psychiatric Association's (APA) Diagnostic and Statistical Manual (DSM-5) has been published. It provides some worthwhile advances over the last edition, but overall it has to be said that it is disappointing in not dealing adequately with many of the challenges. Thus, the huge number of diagnostic categories remains and so does the overlap among them. The field of personality disorders and that of addictions are particularly poorly dealt with, as discussed in the relevant chapters of the new edition. Brain imaging remains a crucially important research tool but, with respect to looking at interconnectivity among brain regions, there is evidence of the artifacts that may derive from motion during the scanning. This is discussed in the chapter on imaging. Finally, there has been a proliferation in the guidelines produced by the National Institute of Health and Care Excellence (NICE) that are relevant to child and adolescent psychiatry. These are noted in the relevant chapters of clinical disorders.

While retaining the strengths of previous editions, the editors have been creative in introducing several new topics. Thus, there is a chapter on systems neuroscience that is highly informative, but which treats neuroscience as a way of providing an understanding on clinical issues, rather than a field of knowledge that is separate from that. Animal models have come up from time to time in previous editions but this time the editors were surely right to recognize that so much use is now being made of animal models (some sound and some not quite so sound) that what can and cannot be achieved through their use deserved fuller discussion (as in Chapter 12) in this new edition. It is particularly good that animal models are treated not as a separate topic but rather as part of broader research strategies.

From the outset, the textbook has sought to provide guidance on how to move from statistical associations to causal inferences and this has become a major topic in the field. As in the previous edition, there is a very informative chapter on what clinicians need to know about statistical issues and methods. In addition, however, there is a new chapter on evaluating interventions. This deals with the statistical challenges but does so in a way that is focused on the concepts that clinicians need to appreciate when reading accounts of randomized controlled trials.

Through several editions, there has been attention to cultural variations and to national differences in service provision and the time was clearly ripe to bring this together in a new chapter on global psychiatry. Psychosocial researchers have, on the whole, been rather reluctant to consider biological implications of the psychosocial environment, but the empirical findings across what is now quite a broad literature indicate that this is mistaken. The new chapter on biological aspects of environmental effects seeks to bring all of this together – pointing to its relevance for certain key clinical issues.

The topic of epigenetics has become somewhat of a flavor of the moment but there is extensive evidence now that epigenetic effects are observable across a broad range of species and that they may matter in terms of the effects of experiences. The new chapter dedicated to considering this topic in its own right succeeds admirably in outlining what is involved in a way that is readily understandable to those who work outside of the laboratory.

Resilience had a clear place in the last edition of the textbook but the findings have grown over the years and the new chapter seeks to bring together the concepts, findings, and clinical implications of what might be involved in the mechanisms that underlie the huge individual differences in children's responses to all manner of adversities.

The clinical chapters and the chapters on treatments all provide updating on what is known but two new chapters are worth comment. There is no longer a chapter on psychodynamic treatments because, as the chapter on this topic in the last edition indicated, psychodynamic approaches are now reflected in a wide range of treatments and, to a substantial extent, relationship-based treatments are the natural successor to psychodynamic treatments. The new chapter on this topic discusses what these involve and also indicates the ways in which they may be employed clinically. School-based mental health interventions are dealt with in another new chapter.

Again, they played a part in earlier editions but the time was ripe to consider them more fully on their own.

I greatly welcome this new edition as providing both a continuity with the past and a substantial, and extremely helpful, new look. As with previous editions, the breadth and strength of the editorial team has meant that all chapters have been peer reviewed by several, usually all, editors. This was the case last time and it remains a distinctive feature of the textbook. Not only do the editors provide a wide and varied range of clinical expertise but they provide scientific excellence. For example, most are active members of the relevant national scientific academies. I have been generously invited to contribute some chapters, but I have been happy to step aside from involvement in the editorship because I had such confidence that the new team of editors would do a great job, and clearly they have. I was pleased with the last edition but I think that readers will see that the quality of the sixth edition is actually superior to that of its predecessor.

Michael Rutter

Preface

Rutter's Child and Adolescent Psychiatry is an internationally leading textbook in our field. We have felt enormously privileged to have been entrusted with the role of lead editors for this new edition. It has been an exciting, instructive, and, sometimes challenging journey that has led us to the final version of this edition. We have been very fortunate that throughout the process we have had unfailing support and advice from Michael Rutter. We are very grateful to him for his help and have strongly appreciated his commitment and confidence in us.

Michael Rutter initiated a rigorous editing approach for the last edition that involves all chapters including initial outlines being peer-reviewed by the editors. The chapters cover a huge breadth of topics, and this process simply could not have been achieved without a team of skilled international editors. We have worked as part of a wonderful editorial team: James Leckman, Stephen Scott, Maggie Snowling, and Eric Taylor, who have a breadth of diverse interests, backgrounds, and experiences.

This textbook has relied on contributions from internationally outstanding experts. We are extremely grateful to all the contributors who have so readily engaged with the editorial team. It has been a pleasure to work with the authors of the chapters.

We have sought to maintain the very high standard set by the earlier editions, retain the conceptual and developmental aspects of the book as well as the strong clinical chapters, but also introduce some important changes. New chapters include those on systems neuroscience, using experimental models in humans and animals to study causal hypotheses and evaluating interventions, global psychiatry, epigenetics, resilience, relationship-based treatments, and school-based mental health interventions. The timing of the textbook means that Diagnostic and Statistical Manual of Mental Disorders, Fifth Edition (DSM-5) changes are also covered.

Finally, we thank Caroline Warren at Cwm Taf University Health Board, who has worked with all the editors, overseen the organization, and provided all the administrative support for this book. We have been tremendously grateful for her commitment, hard work, and organization.

Anita Thapar and Daniel S. Pine

CHAPTER 1

Development and psychopathology: a life course perspective

Barbara Maughan[1] and Stephan Collishaw[2]

[1] MRC Social, Genetic and Developmental Psychiatry Centre, Institute of Psychiatry, Psychology and Neuroscience, King's College London, UK
[2] Institute of Psychological Medicine and Clinical Neurosciences, Cardiff University School of Medicine, UK

Introduction

A life course perspective is central to developmental psychopathology. Michael Rutter and Alan Sroufe, founding fathers of the discipline, argued this need from the outset (Sroufe & Rutter, 1984; Rutter & Sroufe, 2000), and the intervening decades have amply confirmed their view. Longitudinal research has consistently demonstrated that most adult disorders have roots in childhood difficulties, and most childhood disorders have sequelae that persist to adult life. In mapping these long-term linkages, developmental findings have challenged etiological assumptions, highlighted unexpected connections across the life course, and raised key questions about the mechanisms—biological, psychological, and social—that underlie continuity and change.

Numerous insights have flowed from adopting a life course view. It is now clear, for example, that the burden of psychiatric disorders begins early in development. Disorder onsets fall into distinctive groupings (Angold & Egger, 2007), but most occur in childhood and adolescence. Some—such as the neurodevelopmental disorders—emerge very early in childhood; some—such as depression—show a sharp rise in the teens; and some—schizophrenia being the most obvious example—though typically emerging later in development have clear precursors in the childhood years. These differing onset profiles point to differences in underlying mechanisms. Developmental neuroscience is beginning to map the delays and perturbations in brain development characteristic of specific childhood disorders (Shaw et al., 2010); to clarify the effects of stress exposure at different stages in the life course (Lupien et al., 2009); and to highlight how both the pre- and postnatal environments affect epigenetic programming, with the potential for pervasive influences on the developing brain (Kofink et al., 2013).

Long-term studies have also documented the strikingly high cumulative prevalence of mental health problems in the first two decades of life. Cross-sectional surveys identify around 10–12% of young people as disordered at any particular point in time; repeated longitudinal assessments, by contrast, suggest that well over 50% of young people will meet criteria for at least one psychiatric disorder by age 21 (see e.g. Copeland et al., 2011). Looking backwards from adulthood, early vulnerability to adult disorder is equally clear; one follow-back study found that half of those with treated mental health problems in early adulthood had first met criteria for disorder by age 15 (Kim-Cohen et al., 2003). Underlying these general linkages, developmental findings reveal a complex mix of continuities and discontinuities, and evidence of both *homotypic* prediction—the persistence or recurrence of the same disorder in different developmental periods—and apparently *heterotypic* transitions, where earlier and later vulnerabilities differ in form. Early emotional and behavioral difficulties also foreshadow a broad spectrum of problems in adult social functioning; poor physical health and health-related behaviors; poor economic circumstances (Goodman et al., 2011); and, in some instances at least, an increased risk of early death (Jokela et al., 2009).

Identifying the processes that underlie these differing pathways is central to the developmental psychopathology approach (Sroufe & Rutter, 1984). This chapter draws together evidence of this kind, using findings on selected disorders and early risks to highlight current issues in the field. Because tracing long-term developmental linkages poses particular methodological challenges, we begin with a brief overview of methodological issues, highlighting the strengths and limitations of differing research designs in identifying life course pathways, and the new techniques now available to investigators to delineate developmental mechanisms in longitudinal research.

Rutter's Child and Adolescent Psychiatry, Sixth Edition.
Edited by Anita Thapar and Daniel S. Pine, James F. Leckman, Stephen Scott, Margaret J. Snowling, Eric Taylor.
© 2015 John Wiley & Sons Ltd. Published 2018 by John Wiley & Sons Ltd.

Methodological considerations

Research designs

Optimal research designs vary with the question of interest. Robins' classic study of child guidance patients (Robins, 1966) is a landmark example of a "catch-up" study, designed to examine long-term outcomes of childhood conduct problems. Identifying her sample from child guidance records, Robins traced and interviewed prior clinic attenders in adulthood, gaining a broad picture of strengths as well as difficulties in their later lives. She used a general population sample from the same geographical area as a comparison group, and also paid attention to differences in outcomes within the treated group. The findings proved hugely influential: diagnostic criteria for Antisocial Personality Disorder were largely shaped by her findings, and the study generated numerous other developmental hypotheses that have stood the test of time.

Prospective studies of non-referred samples provide for a variety of extensions to this approach. First, they can include research-based assessments from the outset, allowing more nuanced tests of the early features most important in influencing later outcomes. Second, because they can include multiple assessment waves, they allow better tests of the timing and patterning of difficulties as they unfold over time. And third, they offer better opportunities to test hypotheses about possible causal mechanisms. Numerous studies have now used strategies of this kind; to take just one example, Laub and Sampson's (2003) long-term follow-up (to age 70) of the Gluecks' juvenile delinquency sample has been especially informative on the role of adult experiences, showing how both negative and positive experiences continue to shape developmental trajectories well into adult life.

Prospective studies of non-referred, population-based cohorts share many of these advantages, but have additional strengths: they are unaffected by referral biases; they can examine effects of environmental risk exposures; and they can also be used to study outcomes of dimensionally-defined behaviors or traits. Follow-back analyses tracing the childhood histories of individuals with particular later outcomes can also be derived from epidemiological/longitudinal data. Alongside these strengths, there are, of course, potential limitations. Some level of attrition is almost inevitable in long-term follow-ups, and may affect the representativeness of the retained samples; in addition, changes in diagnostic criteria may mean that study definitions devised in one era do not map precisely to more recent conceptualizations of disorder. The strengths of this design are, however, well attested by the extensive insights that continue to emerge from key epidemiological/longitudinal studies, including the Dunedin (http://dunedinstudy.otago.ac.nz/) and Christchurch (http://www.otago.ac.nz/christchurch/research/healthdevelopment/) studies in New Zealand, the Great Smoky Mountains Study in the United States (http://devepi.duhs.duke.edu/gsms.html/) and the Avon Longitudinal Study of Parents and Children (ALSPAC) in the United Kingdom (http://www.bristol.ac.uk/alspac). Biomarkers are now frequently collected in longitudinal studies of this kind; prenatal influences are being investigated in studies beginning in pregnancy; and longitudinal twin studies are increasingly being used to document stability and change in genetic influences across development.

For some research questions, other designs are valuable. Studies of the very early precursors of disorder, for example, can capitalize on high-risk designs, tracking children selected on the basis of family or genetic risk. Lyytinen et al.'s (2008) prospective study of babies in families with dyslexia, for example, obtained detailed cognitive and neurophysiological measures from very early in development, identifying hypothesized precursor deficits well before children were exposed to the demands of learning to read. High-risk designs can also be used to assess long-term outcomes of early adversities such as maltreatment or early institutional deprivation, allowing both for tests of environmental risk mediation and contributors to variations in outcome within high risk groups.

Retrospective and prospective measures

In general, "prospective," contemporaneous measures of childhood behaviors or experiences are almost always preferable to retrospective reports of childhood collected in adult life. People are much better at remembering *whether* something happened than exactly *when* it occurred, and memories of the temporal ordering of events or behaviors—often required to test causal hypotheses—are especially open to bias. Retrospective reports of the age of onset of anxiety disorders, for example, seem heavily influenced by the age at which respondents are questioned (Beesdo et al., 2009), and estimates of the lifetime prevalence of a number of common disorders are markedly higher when calculated from prospective rather than retrospective reports (Moffitt et al., 2010). For memorable, easily defined events such as parental divorce or the timing of menarche, retrospective recall seems unlikely to be problematic (Hardt & Rutter, 2004). Deliberate falsifications are probably uncommon, and the main source of bias seems to arise from individuals who are functioning well in adulthood forgetting or underreporting early risk exposures, rather than those with poor outcomes exaggerating early adversities. Some events—such as early exposure to sexual or physical abuse—cannot usually be assessed in non-referred samples in childhood on ethical grounds, so much of what we know about their long-term implications is inevitably based on retrospective reports. Where comparisons with prospective data have been feasible, some have found very similar associations with risk for later disorder (Scott et al., 2012), while others have not (Widom et al., 2007); other evidence suggests that measurement errors in retrospective reports of child maltreatment have a quite limited influence on associations with later mental health (Fergusson et al., 2011). As a result, although prospective data are to be preferred whenever feasible, it is important not to exaggerate the problems of retrospective reporting, and to appreciate that there are circumstances where it is the only strategy realistically available. Finally, it is of course worth remembering that most "prospective" studies actually involve an element of retrospective reporting, reflecting events or behaviors occurring between study assessments.

Statistical methods for longitudinal research

Many long-term studies now include multiple assessments spanning long periods of the life course. To optimize the value of these rich resources, a range of specific statistical techniques has been developed (see Chapter 15). Some (such as multiple imputation) are designed to deal with problems of attrition; some (such as latent variable models) provide approaches to handling the complexity of both environmental and genetic risks for child mental health; and some (including structural equation modeling and cross-lagged panel analyses) provide tests of hypothesized mediating mechanisms and bidirectional effects. Arguably the most prominent recent developments, however, are methods that explicitly model patterns of stability and change over development, including group-based trajectory modeling, used to identify sub groups within the population that differ in their developmental course (Nagin & Odgers, 2010). First widely used in longitudinal studies of antisocial behavior, group-based modeling of this kind has since been applied to a wide range of phenomena, from pathways in early reading development (Lyytinen *et al.*, 2006) to trajectories of common mental health symptoms across the life course (Colman *et al.*, 2007). Trajectory modeling provides a direct means of testing etiological influences on sub groups with distinct developmental profiles, and can also be used to evaluate variations in intervention response.

Childhood–adulthood continuities

We turn now to examine life course findings in selected disorder groups. Detailed discussions of these disorders are presented in later chapters. Our aim here is to use emerging findings to illustrate more general developmental issues, focusing in particular on patterns of childhood–adulthood continuity. To begin, we focus on homotypic continuities in four selected disorder groupings (antisocial behaviors, depression, anxiety and exemplar neurodevelopmental disorders), chosen to reflect differing patterns of disorder onset and course. Following this, we explore the more complex heterotypic continuities identified in so much longitudinal research.

Antisocial behavior

Antisocial behaviors and delinquency were among the first aspects of child behavior to attract attention from longitudinal researchers; as a result, a good deal is now known about their basic developmental profiles and course (see Chapter 65).

Many indicators of antisocial behavior show highly distinctive age-related trends: physical aggression, for example, is at its peak very early in childhood (Tremblay, 2010), while delinquency rises sharply across the teens, declining gradually in the early adult years. In addition, longitudinal data consistently highlight the paradox that while most severely antisocial adults were antisocial children, only perhaps half of antisocial children go on to show marked antisocial behavior in adult life (Robins, 1966).

These findings point to heterogeneity in the antisocial population, and a number of approaches to subtyping have been proposed (Lahey & Waldman, 2012). Moffitt's (1993) developmental taxonomy highlights age at onset as the core distinguishing feature; other well-established markers of heterogeneity include comorbidity with ADHD, distinctions between physically aggressive and non-aggressive behaviors, and the presence of associated callous-unemotional (CU) traits (see Chapter 68). Considered individually, each of these features predicts long-term continuities in antisocial behavior; investigators are still working to clarify whether they constitute different facets of a single high-risk sub group or separable associated risks.

A further striking feature of longitudinal findings in the antisocial field is the wide spectrum of adverse outcomes faced by young people with disruptive behavior problems later in their lives. Fergusson *et al.* (2004), for example, found that (in addition to continuities in antisocial behavior), childhood conduct problems were associated with poor educational and occupational achievements; problems in sexual and partner relationships; early parenthood; and elevated rates of substance use, mood and anxiety disorders, and suicidal acts. Subsequent studies have documented associations with poor health-related behaviors and markers of chronic disease early in adulthood (Odgers *et al.*, 2008) and later—in representative as well as high risk samples—with increased risk of premature death (Maughan *et al.*, 2014).

What accounts for this broad spectrum of adverse outcomes? First, genetic liabilities are almost certain to play some part. Longitudinal twin studies point to genetic continuity in general antisocial phenotypes from late childhood to early adulthood, along with new genetic (and environmental) influences in adolescence (Wichers *et al.*, 2013). In addition, early onset conduct problems, physical aggression, and CU traits—all of which carry high risks of persistence—are all strongly heritable. At the same time, child conduct problems are also strongly associated with adverse environmental conditions. Studies of gene–environment interplay highlight the complex ways in which genetic and environmental factors combine to impact risk for the persistence of disorder over time. On the one hand, genetic factors may *moderate susceptibility* to individual and family-based risks (see Chapter 24). In the Christchurch longitudinal study, for example, variations in the *MAOA* genotype interacted with factors as varied as maternal smoking in pregnancy, material deprivation, maltreatment, and lack of school-leaving qualifications to influence risk for adolescent and early adult offending (Fergusson *et al.*, 2012).

On the other, genetically influenced traits may affect *exposure* to adverse environments. It has long been known, for example, that aspects of children's temperament and behavior can evoke negative reinforcing responses from parents. Evidence is now emerging that similar processes occur with peers: as early as the kindergarten years, genetically-influenced hyperactive and disruptive behaviors can evoke peer victimization and rejection (Boivin *et al.*, 2013), while later in development, genetic factors contribute to affiliations with deviant peers (Kendler *et al.*, 2007). Across development, cumulating consequences of this kind can function to stabilize maladaptive behaviors, selecting antisocial young people into risk-prone environments, and restricting their opportunities for involvement in more positive relationships and roles.

For children with early onset conduct problems, developmental "cascades" of this kind seem likely to contribute in important ways to the persistence of antisocial behavior over time. Where adolescent onset problems persist, substance abuse has been highlighted as one especially salient "snare" that can hinder desistance from offending (Hussong *et al.*, 2004). In addition, antisocial young people may vary in the extent to which they have access to, or can benefit from, later positive experiences. Sweeten *et al.* (2013), for example, identified changes in antisocial peer affiliations and peer influence as among the strongest correlates of reductions in offending among adjudicated offenders, while Laub and Sampson (2003) highlighted the role of adult "turning point" experiences, including social attachments to work, and supportive marital relationships, in promoting desistance from crime. The great majority of offenders eventually desist; these findings point to intervention targets that may accelerate that process and help to break—or at least interrupt—chains of risk.

Depression

Developmental findings have also been salient in relation to depressive disorders, markedly changing conceptualization of depression over time. Before the 1980s many viewed depression as a predominantly adult disorder: pre-pubertal children were thought too immature to experience depressive disorders, and adolescent low mood was assumed to reflect normative teenage mood swings. A wealth of evidence from clinical and epidemiological studies has changed these views. It is now clear that, though uncommon (1–2%), depressive disorders do occur in pre-pubertal children, and that depressive-like phenomena are also observed in some children as early as the preschool years (Angold & Egger, 2007).

Despite these early manifestations, adolescence is now recognized as a particularly important life stage in the development of depression. First, rates of depression increase markedly across the adolescent years, with median 12-month prevalence estimates equivalent to those for adults (4–5%), and a cumulative prevalence as high as 20% across the teens. New onsets of major depressive disorder continue across the life course, but for many sufferers the disorder begins in the adolescent years.

Second, unlike childhood depression, adolescent depression shows strong continuity to adulthood; in referred young people, initial remission is followed by a recurrence in around 50–70% of patients within 5 years (Thapar *et al.*, 2012). And third, the female preponderance typical of adult depression becomes clearly established in the teens. The emergent sex difference seems more closely linked to pubertal stage than chronological age, pointing to the likely role of hormonal factors (Angold *et al.*, 1999); sex differences in adolescent brain development and in the cognitive processing of stressful experiences may also contribute to rising rates of depression in girls (Hyde *et al.*, 2008).

Depressive disorders in childhood, adolescence, and adulthood are typically defined by the same underlying features; despite this, it remains unclear whether depression at these different ages does indeed reflect a single homogenous disorder or common etiology. Childhood depression differs from adolescent and adult depression in a number of important ways: the prevalence is lower, there is no marked gender difference, and continuity with adult depression is low. There are also important etiological differences, with twin studies demonstrating consistently lower heritability for depression in children than in adolescents or adults. Distinctions between adolescent and adult depression are less clear. Studies comparing the psychosocial risk profiles of "juvenile"- and adult-onset depression suggest that early adversity, parental neglect, and problematic peer relationships are more strongly associated with early-onset depression (Jaffee *et al.*, 2002). Others have argued, however, that such findings reflect recency of risk exposure, and that developmentally-salient stressors are associated with depression at all stages of the life-course (Shanahan *et al.*, 2011). Treatment responses also show developmental variation, with tricyclic antidepressants effective in adult but not in child or adolescent depression (Hazell *et al.*, 2002). It remains unclear whether these differences in risk correlates and treatment response reflect maturation of relevant neurobiological systems, heterogeneity in the underlying nature of depression, or stage of illness factors.

Given the high rates of recurrence in depression, studies of the mechanisms underlying continuity across developmental periods are especially important. Heritable factors clearly play a part here, contributing to stability in depressive symptoms in both adolescence and adulthood (Lau & Eley, 2006). In addition, extensive evidence suggests that—as with antisocial behavior—genes act in concert with environmental influences to increase both *susceptibility* to psychosocial stressors (gene–environment interaction) and *exposure* to stressful environments (gene–environment correlation). Maladaptive coping styles such as rumination, depressogenic cognitive biases, and difficulties in interpersonal relationships are both predictors and outcomes of depression, forming further contributors to recurrence risk (Abramson *et al.*, 2002). And finally, vulnerability to relapse and illness severity appear to increase across the course of depressive illness, becoming increasingly autonomous from severe precipitants as the number of episodes increases (Kendler *et al.*, 2000). Often referred to as "kindling," processes of this kind suggest that depression itself may increase sensitivity to stress, so that in time even relatively minor everyday stressors can trigger a recurrence (Post, 2010; but see also Monroe & Harkness, 2005).

As these findings suggest, developmental studies have provided important insights into influences on both onset and recurrence of depression. More evidence is now needed on factors that distinguish young people with more and less benign courses of early illness, to maximize the contribution of developmentally-sensitive findings for prevention and treatment.

Anxiety disorders

Different issues arise in relation to anxiety disorders, stemming in large part from the complexities of current nosology, where numerous different anxiety diagnoses are defined. Debate continues over the utility of this approach, and whether other distinctions—derived, for example, from neuroscience frameworks—could provide a more appropriate basis for classification (Pine, 2007). Developmental findings can contribute to these debates.

Beginning with age at onset, it is now clear that there is meaningful heterogeneity in onset patterns among anxiety diagnoses: some typically onset in childhood, some in early adolescence, and some in late adolescence/early adulthood. Separation anxiety and specific phobias have the earliest onset ages; in the German Early Developmental Stages of Psychopathology (EDSP) study, 50% of these disorders had begun by ages 5 and 8 years respectively, and almost all cases had emerged by age 12 (Beesdo-Baum & Knappe, 2012). Rates of social phobia and OCD (obsessive compulsive disorder) rose sharply in early adolescence, while agoraphobia, panic disorder, and GAD (generalized anxiety disorder) became more common later in adolescence and early adulthood. These later onset disorders lack the circumscribed fears seen in childhood onset disorders, possibly indexing a developmental shift in the expression of anxiety with age, and raising intriguing questions about the mechanisms involved.

Much less diagnostic specificity is evident in findings on developmental course. Retrospective studies point to the persistence of early anxiety disorders and suggest a relatively chronic or recurrent course (see e.g. Kessler et al., 2012). Prospective findings paint a rather different picture; while they confirm above-chance levels of homotypic continuity, they also report quite low rates of stability in specific anxiety diagnoses and—especially in younger age groups—a tendency for anxiety symptoms to wax and wane over time (Bittner et al., 2007; Beesdo-Baum & Knappe, 2012). Onset of a first ("pure") anxiety disorder is often followed by the development of other anxieties in adolescence/early adulthood; in its turn, this "load" of anxiety predicts other adverse outcomes including depression, substance use, and suicidality, along with psychosocial difficulties and poor health and relationship functioning (Copeland et al., 2014).

Follow-back findings from the Dunedin study (Gregory et al., 2007) are broadly consistent with this view, with little specificity in the childhood–adulthood linkages involved; specific phobias in adulthood had a significant history of juvenile phobias, but other adult anxiety disorders were likely to have been preceded by a range of anxiety diagnoses. Alone among DSM-IV adult anxiety diagnoses, PTSD stood out in having a history of behavioral as well as emotional difficulties earlier in development (Koenen, 2010); in conjunction with other individual and family factors, these early influences appeared to play a key role in shaping both exposure and responses to trauma later in life. Finally, we note that recent evidence is providing empirical support for one pattern of childhood–adult continuity of longstanding clinical interest: the possibility that separation anxiety in childhood may be a precursor to panic disorder later in life. Rates of separation anxiety fall sharply in the early teens, but a recent meta-analysis has identified a significant association with later panic (Kossowsky et al., 2013), and longitudinal twin study findings have identified a common genetic diathesis between separation anxiety disorder and panic attacks (Roberson-Nay et al., 2012).

Relatively little is known about the mechanisms that contribute to the persistence or recurrence of anxiety across development. Twin studies point to genetic influences on stability, but also highlight more "developmentally dynamic" patterns, with attenuation of the genetic effects on some late childhood anxiety phenotypes by early adulthood, along with the emergence of new genetic influences later in development (McGrath et al., 2012). In a follow-up of social anxiety disorders from adolescence to early adulthood, Beesdo-Baum and colleagues (2012) identified earlier age at onset, severity of avoidance, impairment, and a high number of catastrophic cognitions as associated with persistence and diagnostic stability. Established risk factors for the onset of anxiety disorders, including both behavioral inhibition and a family history of social phobia or depression, also signaled a poorer prognosis.

Behavioral inhibition is a strong risk factor for the development of anxiety disorders, and social anxiety in particular (Clauss & Blackford, 2012; see Chapter 8). A variety of environmental factors have also been implicated, including maternal personality, aspects of the mother–child relationship, and an oversolicitous, intrusive, or controlling parenting style (Degnan et al., 2010). Evidence is now emerging that parenting can moderate temperamental vulnerabilities, with risks for anxiety disorders especially marked when behavioral inhibition occurs in the context of parental over control. Biased attention-orienting to threat—a well-established concomitant of many anxiety disorders—also appears to modulate associations between inhibition and disorder (Shechner et al., 2012). In addition, aspects of the peer context may moderate, maintain, and possibly exacerbate temperamental influences (Degnan et al., 2010). Inhibited children tend to be less socially competent than their peers; as a result, they are more likely to be excluded from peer groups, and may be targets of bullying—both factors known to increase risk of anxiety disorders. To date, interpersonal processes of this kind have primarily been documented in early and middle childhood. We must await further evidence to determine how far similar relational processes occur later in the life course, amplifying the effects of early temperamental characteristics and increasing vulnerability to the persistence of anxiety beyond the childhood years.

Neurodevelopmental disorders

We conclude with a brief overview of the rather different issues raised by current findings on outcomes in some of the earliest onset disorders of childhood: the neurodevelopmental disorders. As discussed in Chapter 3, and in the individual disorder chapters, extensive effort continues to be devoted to improving our understanding of the etiology of these complex difficulties. Evidence on later outcomes is much more sparse, but current findings leave little doubt that neurodevelopmental disorders are lifelong conditions. In general, some diminution in core symptoms seems typical with age, but alongside this it is also clear that broader functional impairments persist at least to adolescence, and often to adult life. We focus here on findings in just two areas—autism spectrum disorders (ASDs) and ADHD—to illustrate some of the issues that arise.

Beginning with autism, a recent review of follow-ups to early adulthood (Howlin & Moss, 2012) concluded that although the severity of symptoms tends to decrease with age, adult outcome is very mixed, including for individuals with normal IQ. One of the longest-term follow-ups to date (Howlin et al., 2013) found some improvements in core symptoms and language skills by middle adulthood, but psychosocial outcomes were often poor, and in some instances appeared to have deteriorated over time. Over half in this sample had never worked, or were long-term unemployed; the majority had little autonomy in terms of daily living; and most had no close friend. The samples studied to date were, of course, diagnosed some decades ago, before early interventions and specialist educational supports were generally available, and when only more severely affected children were likely to receive a diagnosis. Outcomes for young people with ASDs today may be more promising; current findings can still, however, provide important pointers to factors that underlie variations in long-term outcomes. Early difficulties in reciprocal social interaction appear to be important here (Howlin et al., 2013), along with the extent and severity of core symptoms, the extent of cognitive impairment, and the presence of co-occurring psychopathology. Environmental supports may also be crucial; indeed, some reports suggest that lack of appropriate support in adulthood can have a more deleterious effect on outcomes than factors such as IQ. The transition to adulthood raises new and potentially difficult psychosocial challenges for many individuals with ASDs, yet appropriate support services in adulthood are often severely lacking. Recent years have seen major advances in the development of comprehensive diagnostic and intervention services for young children with autism; findings from long-term studies point to the need for equally effective interventions across the life span.

Evidence on adult outcomes of ADHD is more extensive, though again few studies have tracked samples beyond the early adult years. Most children with ADHD show persistence of symptoms in adolescence and adulthood, with inattentiveness slower to decline with age than hyperactivity/impulsivity. A meta-analysis of follow-up findings (Faraone et al., 2006) showed that although only around 15% met full criteria for disorder in early adulthood, a further 50% continued to face impairments associated with residual symptoms. In addition, follow-up studies highlight a strong persistence of earlier conduct problems in children with ADHD, as well as new onsets of antisocial behavior and substance misuse in adolescence (Langley et al., 2010a); heightened risks for health risk behaviors in adulthood (Olazagasti et al., 2013); and a range of negative educational, occupational, and psychosocial outcomes that appear to persist at least to mid life (Klein et al., 2012). Even when ADHD is diagnosed and treated, only a minority of individuals subsequently exhibit full functional and symptomatic recovery.

The persistence of symptoms and later impairments seems especially marked in those with co-occurring conduct disorder/antisocial behavior; in addition, initial severity, IQ, and poor childhood school and social functioning have also been found to predict persistence, as have parental psychopathology and family conflict (Cherkasova et al., 2013). Despite continuing needs, clinical recognition and service provision in adulthood remains limited, and individuals with ADHD are often reported to become disengaged from services and treatment. Increasing awareness of the lifelong consequences of ADHD, improved transitions from child to adult mental health services, and continued support in adulthood are all increasingly underlined as important priorities (Young et al., 2011).

As these brief overviews suggest, evidence from differing neuro-developmental disorders highlights that adult outcomes for affected individuals are often poor. The stability of core symptoms varies, and may indeed show some improvements with age; alongside this, however, effects on psychosocial functioning may be more marked in face of the more complex demands of adolescence and adult life. Current evidence points to the benefits of supportive social contexts in adulthood, and the crucial need for continuing, appropriate services for many individuals with neurodevelopmental conditions.

Heterotypic transitions and psychopathological progressions

In addition to these "homotypic" continuities, developmental studies also make clear that more complex, "heterotypic" transitions among apparently distinct disorders are far from uncommon. Because multiple disorders often co-occur, some of these observed associations may be "epiphenomenal"—the product (at least statistically) of associations among other disorders. As a result, the strongest basis for identifying "independent" heterotypic transitions among disorders comes from prospective, population-based studies that assess multiple disorders over time.

Copeland et al. (2013a) have recently reported findings of this kind, bringing together data from three major long-term studies to examine diagnostic transitions in common disorders from childhood to adolescence, and from adolescence to early adult life. Overall, continuities across developmental periods were strong, and bivariate analyses highlighted numerous heterotypic as well as homotypic links. Once prior "comorbidities" were controlled, heterotypic linkages were less common, but still clearly emerged. Between childhood and adolescence, the most robust transitions were from ADHD to ODD (oppositional defiant disorder), and from both CD (conduct disorder) and depression to later substance use. Between adolescence and adulthood, depression, and anxiety cross-predicted; adolescent substance use predicted early adult depression; and both CD and ADHD were associated with increased risks of later substance disorders. Predictions from CD to internalizing disorders were not supported in adjusted analyses; predictions from adolescent ODD to early adult depression fell just short of significance. Copeland et al. (2013a) were not able to examine transitions within the years of childhood, or between more common disorders and either neurodevelopmental problems or schizophrenia. From other evidence, however, it seems likely that early transitions from ADHD to CD, associations between schizophrenia and earlier emotional/behavioral difficulties, and the emergence of emotional/behavioral difficulties in children with specific learning problems should be added to this list of "independent" heterotypic progressions.

How might patterns of this kind arise? Two broad types of explanation have been put forward: that heterotypic continuities reflect age-varying expressions of the same underlying liability, or that one disorder or its associated impairments constitute risk factors for a second, distinct condition. In practice, elements of both processes may often be involved and shared genetic vulnerabilities implicated. Behavior genetic analyses have consistently identified shared genetic influences on pairs of disorders; more recently, multivariate genetic studies have highlighted more widespread genetic pleiotropy, suggesting that most common forms of child psychopathology share some genetic liabilities (see e.g. Lahey et al., 2011). It is also becoming clear that specific molecular genetic risk factors operate across different disorders (Owen et al., 2011; see Chapter 24). From a developmental perspective, findings of this kind may suggest that the same genetically-based vulnerabilities are manifest in different ways at different stages in development, in part, perhaps, as a result of interactions with normative maturational processes or changes in young people's social worlds. Investigators are now beginning to identify heritable neurobehavioral vulnerabilities that may contribute to processes of this kind. In relation to progressions from childhood anxiety to adolescent depression, for example, changes in sensitivity to social evaluative threats around the time of puberty may constitute intermediate

phenotypes of this kind (Silk et al., 2012). Emerging evidence suggests that the brain systems involved in responding to social information may become more sensitive or active during puberty—a time when peer and romantic relationships are also growing in importance, and when social evaluations become increasingly salient. If confirmed, models of this kind not only move us closer to understanding how genetically-based vulnerabilities may contribute to transitions among disorders, but may also suggest new targets for intervention.

The value of examining pathways of this kind has also emerged in studies of progressions from ADHD to conduct problems. Here, replicated evidence has shown that the *COMT* val158met variant high-activity genotype is associated with increased risk for antisocial behavior specifically in the presence of ADHD (Caspi et al., 2008). This gene variant has well-established associations with executive functioning, and also with problems in social cognition—both known correlates of antisocial behavior, and both thus plausible intermediate phenotypes. Langley et al. (2010b) tested both as potential mediators in the ALSPAC cohort; problems in social understanding were on the pathway from genotype to antisocial outcomes in children with ADHD, while measures of executive control were not. Once again, these findings may have clinical as well as theoretical significance, suggesting that interventions to improve social understanding in ADHD may reduce risks of the development of aggression and conduct problems.

Conduct problems figure prominently in reports of heterotypic continuity; indeed, follow-back analyses of early adult disorders in the Dunedin cohort showed that CD/ODD was part of the developmental history of *all* the young adult disorders assessed, including manic episodes and schizophreniform disorders (Kim-Cohen et al., 2003). Progressions from CD to substance use are among the best-established associations, likely reflecting shared, genetically-based personality features. Here, however, associations are not simply unidirectional: CD predicts adolescent substance use, but early adolescent alcohol and cannabis use also predict subsequent delinquency. Mediating mechanisms appear to vary at different stages of substance use, with, for example, shared environmental influences most important for transitions to early alcohol use, but shared genetic liability the dominant influence on links between antisocial behavior and later alcohol dependence (Malone et al., 2004). Once established, substance problems may affect persistence in antisocial behavior through a variety of pathways including neurobiological effects on disinhibition, peer influences, adverse effects on family relationships, and the need for money to support drink and drug habits.

In addition to progressions to other "behavioral" disorders, child and adolescent conduct problems have also frequently been associated with increased risk for depression. To date, progressions of this kind have largely been assumed to reflect "down stream" effects of conduct problems, whether via selection into stress-prone environments, the development of negative self-cognitions, or, in some instances, the pharmacological effects of substance use. Recently, however, studies have begun to highlight the possibility of shared temperamental influences centering on irritability. Longitudinal findings suggest that ODD, rather than CD, may be the more salient predictor of depression risk (Copeland *et al.*, 2009), with irritable mood a key element in this progression; adolescent irritability has also been found to predict suicidality later in adulthood (Pickles *et al.*, 2010), and twin studies point to common genetic underpinnings with low mood (Stringaris *et al.*, 2012; see Chapter 5).

As these examples suggest, many developmental associations among apparently distinct disorders may in part at least reflect expressions of the same underlying liability. Some, however, do seem likely to reflect *psychopathological progressions*, whereby the experience of one disorder contributes, directly or indirectly, to risk for another. Though evidence is still limited, some emotional/behavioral concomitants of specific learning difficulties may be of this kind; links between reading difficulties and anxiety, for example, show no clear evidence of shared genetic influence in the twin samples studied to date (e.g. Whitehouse *et al.*, 2009), suggesting that reading problems may constitute a direct risk for the development of anxiety in some children. Associations between substance use and later depression provide a second, quite different, example. Links between these disorders are strong, raising important questions over both the likely direction of effects and the causal processes involved. In the case of alcohol abuse disorders, a recent review and meta-analysis concluded that links with depression could not be attributed to confounders; that evidence was strongest for an effect of alcohol abuse on depression; and that potential mechanisms include neurophysiological and metabolic changes resulting from alcohol exposure (Boden & Fergusson, 2011).

Long-term effects of early experience

We conclude by examining a different aspect of childhood–adult "continuity": links between adverse experiences early in development and risk for psychopathology later in life. The shorter-term sequelae of childhood adversities are examined in detail in Chapter 26. We focus here on evidence for their persisting impact beyond the childhood years; on issues involved in interpreting evidence on such long-term links; and on some of the intervening mechanisms that are likely to be involved.

There is by now extensive, well-replicated evidence of associations between exposure to early adversity and risk for both psychiatric disorder and poor physical health later in life. Both chronic stress and severe acute experiences seem implicated, spanning exposures as varied as maltreatment and neglect, maladaptive family relationships, parental psychopathology, depriving institutional rearing, bullying victimization, and socioeconomic disadvantage (Odgers & Jaffee, 2013).

Retrospective evidence for associations with adult outcomes comes from large-scale epidemiological surveys such as the Adverse Childhood Experiences (ACE) study (Dube *et al.*, 2001), where information on adult disease is linked to respondents' recollections of childhood. Studies of this kind have shown strong links between childhood adversity and adverse health sequelae across the adult years (Odgers & Jaffee, 2013). Long-term prospective follow-ups of both high-risk and epidemiological samples are now confirming these findings in an increasing range of areas. Prospectively-reported childhood family adversities, extra familial adversities such as bullying, and follow-ups of abused and neglected children all show substantial predictive associations with psychiatric disorder in adult life (e.g. Copeland *et al.*, 2013b; Horwitz *et al.*, 2001).

The consistency of these findings is compelling; nonetheless, some caution is required in interpreting their meaning. Statistical associations do not, of course, necessarily imply causation. Shared genetic liabilities may contribute to children's vulnerability to adverse experiences, but also to their exposure to them; as a result, associations between psychopathology and adversity may reflect reverse causation, or reciprocal influences that play out in complex ways over time (Sameroff & Mackenzie, 2003).

As discussed in Chapter 12, increasingly sophisticated analytic methods are now being applied to tease these differing possibilities apart. In some instances, evidence for causal influences has proved limited, once shared genetic and environmental confounders are taken into account. In others, correlated adversities may form elements in a causal chain, with, for example, the effects of distal risk factors such as poverty or parental divorce mediated via more proximal aspects of family functioning (Conger *et al.*, 1994). Early adversities rarely occur in isolation, and the clustering of adversities makes it difficult to identify unique risk effects. Traditionally, identifying specific influences has relied on multivariate statistical techniques, but these have inherent limitations; where possible, evidence from intervention studies, genetically sensitive designs and other quasi-experimental approaches provides for more powerful tests (see Chapter 12). Such approaches already provide evidence of the likely causal effects of a range of adversities on psychopathology in childhood; though currently more limited, genetically sensitive studies are also beginning to point to long-term causal influences (see e.g. Kendler & Gardner, 2001).

Studies are also clarifying other aspects of adversity-outcome associations. First, contrary to some early assumptions, most early adversities appear to show relatively nonspecific predictions to a broad range of later psychopathology (Gershon *et al.*, 2013), as well as impacts on cognitive development, educational, and occupational functioning, social relationships, and health (Odgers & Jaffee, 2013). Second, the effects of exposure to multiple adversities are cumulative. Childhood adversities often cluster, and negative adult outcomes are most common in those who experience multiple risks. In the ACE study, for example, the risk of suicide attempt was elevated 2–5 fold when individual childhood adversities were examined separately, but increased up to 30-fold when the cumulative burden of adverse early experience was taken into account (Dube *et al.*, 2001).

Third, in relation to timing, it has been proposed that exposure to stress at critical periods of brain development may carry especially high risk for later psychopathology (Heim & Binder, 2012). In observational studies, however, it is difficult to identify discrete sensitive periods because so many risk exposures are chronic or recurring. At present there is little support for the notion that the risk effects of adversity are *confined* to particular sensitive periods, though there is evidence for developmental variation in risk effects. Studies of Romanian children adopted from extremely depriving institutions, for example, highlight not only that very early privation can have persistent deleterious effects on development, but also that age at placement is an important determinant of the degree of later impairment and post adoption catch-up (Rutter *et al.*, 2012).

Progress has also been made in identifying the range of mechanisms that may underlie the long-term effects of early adversity. Evidence on the biological embedding of early experience—how early adversity "gets under the skin"—is reviewed in detail in Chapter 23. Negative impacts may also be mediated via effects on cognitive, affective, and psychological development. Exposure to maltreatment, for example, has been shown to influence children's emerging capacity to regulate emotions; to contribute to deficits and biases in processing affective stimuli; and to lead to problems in social information processing (Dodge, 2006). In addition, problems in close friendships and intimate relationships are also common, depriving individuals of the benefits of supportive relationships, and studies of adult victims of maltreatment highlight increased exposure to further adverse life events (including revictimization) in adult life.

In part, long term risk effects may also be mediated by effects on early-onset psychopathology, though current evidence suggests that this is unlikely to provide a complete explanation. Data from the Great Smoky Mountains Study, for example, demonstrate that victims of bullying experienced elevated rates of psychiatric disorder in childhood, adolescence, and adulthood; when earlier psychopathology was accounted for, however, associations with adult psychiatric disorder remained (Copeland *et al.*, 2013b).

Finally, a universal finding is that there is substantial heterogeneity in long-term outcome following all kinds of early adversity (Rutter, 2013). Despite exposure to enduring and severe early stressors, many children maintain adaptive trajectories and achieve positive outcomes later in life. Understanding resilience of this kind is important for two reasons: it can cast new light on developmental processes and may also point to additional foci for preventative interventions— "risk buffers"—that can be promoted to mitigate the impact of early trauma and adversity when amelioration or removal of risk is not feasible.

Resilience is an interactive concept, involving the better-than-expected outcomes achieved by some individuals in the face of early adversity (Rutter, 2012; 2013). The processes that explain resilience (see Chapter 27) are likely to be fluid, encompassing varying psychological, social, and biological features at different stages in development. First, evidence of gene-environment interactions highlights that genetic factors play a role in moderating individual responses to stress. Second, psychological and cognitive processes are important; children differ in their perceptions and understanding of stressful and traumatic events, and those who do not attribute blame to themselves when parents separate, or in the context of maltreatment, are more likely to avoid negative psychological sequelae (McGee *et al.*, 2001). In addition, individuals' personal agency, along with their capacity to self-regulate emotions and plan for the future, are consistently associated with mental health and psychosocial outcomes in high-risk groups. Third, resilience studies indicate that the maintenance of positive social relationships, both with family members and with peers, may be especially important in the context of early adversity (Collishaw *et al.*, 2007); and for some individuals, the transition to adulthood can provide opportunities for positive "turning point" experiences—such as marriage—that can disrupt previously maladaptive trajectories (Jaffee *et al.*, 2013). Fourth, there may be important context-specific predictors; for example, enhancing community support and reducing stigma are promising targets for intervention in communities affected by AIDS (Betancourt *et al.*, 2013; see Chapter 46). And finally, although evidence of "steeling" effects in humans is still preliminary (Rutter, 2012), in some circumstances exposure to mild forms of stress may prepare individuals for dealing with more difficult challenges later in life.

Conclusions

As these brief sketches illustrate, although complex, connections across the life course are meaningful and strong, and a life course perspective brings both scientific and practice-oriented insights that would remain hidden in more developmentally "demarcated" research. Over time, developmental studies have contributed to our etiological understanding, highlighted the heterogeneity in pathways (both adaptive and maladaptive) that follow from childhood disorder, and underscored the possibilities for resilience, recovery, and positive turning points that arise throughout development. Though some long-term studies were initiated many years ago, most are of much more recent origin. This "first generation" of longitudinal research has already provided rich rewards, transforming thinking in numerous domains; we can expect equally rich—and equally challenging—insights as results from the next generation of studies begin to emerge.

References

Abramson, L.Y. *et al.* (2002) Cognitive-vulnerability-stress models of depression in a self-regulatory and psychological context. In: *Handbook of Depression*. (eds I.H. Gotlib & C.L. Hammen). Guilford, New York.

Angold, A. & Egger, H.L. (2007) Preschool psychopathology: lessons for the lifespan. *Journal of Child Psychology and Psychiatry* **48**, 961–966.

Angold, A. *et al.* (1999) Pubertal changes in hormone levels and depression in girls. *Psychological Medicine* **29**, 1043–1053.

Beesdo, K. *et al.* (2009) Anxiety and anxiety disorders in children and adolescents: developmental issues and implications for DSM-V. *Psychiatric Clinics of North America* **32**, 483–524.

Beesdo-Baum, K. & Knappe, S. (2012) Developmental epidemiology of anxiety disorders. *Child and Adolescent Psychiatric Clinics of North America* **21**, 457–478.

Beesdo-Baum, K. *et al.* (2012) The natural course of social anxiety disorder among adolescents and young adults. *Acta Psychiatrica Scandinavica* **126**, 411–425.

Betancourt, T.S. *et al.* (2013) Annual Research Review: mental health and resilience in HIV/AIDS-affected children—a review of the literature and recommendations for future research. *Journal of Child Psychology and Psychiatry* **54**, 423–444.

Bittner, A. *et al.* (2007) What do childhood anxiety disorders predict? *Journal of Child Psychology and Psychiatry* **48**, 1174–1183.

Boden, J.M. & Fergusson, D.M. (2011) Alcohol and depression. *Addiction* **106**, 906–914.

Boivin, M. *et al.* (2013) Evidence of gene-environment correlation for peer difficulties: disruptive behaviors predict early peer relation difficulties in school through genetic effects. *Development and Psychopathology* **25**, 79–92.

Caspi, A. *et al.* (2008) A replicated molecular genetic basis for subtyping antisocial behavior in children with attention-deficit/hyperactivity disorder. *Archives of General Psychiatry* **65**, 203–210.

Cherkasova, M. *et al.* (2013) Developmental course of attention deficit hyperactivity disorder and its predictors. *Journal of the Canadian Academy of Child and Adolescent Psychiatry* **22**, 47–54.

Clauss, J.A. & Blackford, J.U. (2012) Behavioral inhibition and risk for developing social anxiety disorder: a meta-analytic study. *Journal of the American Academy of Child and Adolescent Psychiatry* **51**, 1066–1075.

Collishaw, S. *et al.* (2007) Resilience to adult psychopathology following childhood maltreatment: evidence from a community sample. *Child Abuse and Neglect* **31**, 211–229.

Colman, I. *et al.* (2007) A longitudinal typology of symptoms of depression and anxiety over the life course. *Biological Psychiatry* **62**, 1265–1271.

Conger, R.D. *et al.* (1994) Economic stress, coercive family process, and developmental problems of adolescents. *Child Development* **65**, 541–561.

Copeland, W.E. *et al.* (2009) Childhood and adolescent psychiatric disorders as predictors of young adult disorders. *Archives of General Psychiatry* **66**, 764–772.

Copeland, W.E. *et al.* (2011) Cumulative prevalence of psychiatric disorders by young adulthood: a prospective cohort analysis from the Great Smoky Mountains Study. *Journal of the American Academy of Child and Adolescent Psychiatry* **50**, 252–261.

Copeland, W.E. *et al.* (2013a) Diagnostic transitions from childhood to adolescence to early adulthood. *Journal of Child Psychology and Psychiatry* **54**, 791–799.

Copeland, W.E. *et al.* (2013b) Adult psychiatric outcomes of bullying and being bullied by peers in childhood and adolescence. *JAMA Psychiatry* **70**, 419–426.

Copeland, W.E. *et al.* (2014) Longitudinal patterns of anxiety from childhood to adulthood: the Great Smoky Mountains Study. *Journal of the American Academy of Child and Adolescent Psychiatry* **53**, 21–33.

Degnan, K.A. *et al.* (2010) Temperament and the environment in the etiology of childhood anxiety. *Journal of Child Psychology and Psychiatry* **51**, 497–517.

Dodge, K.A. (2006) Translational science in action: hostile attributional style and the development of aggressive behavior problems. *Development and Psychopathology* **18**, 791–814.

Dube, S.R. *et al.* (2001) Childhood abuse, household dysfunction, and the risk of attempted suicide throughout the lifespan: findings from the Adverse Childhood Experiences Study. *JAMA* **286**, 3089–3096.

Faraone, S.V. *et al.* (2006) The age-dependent decline of attention deficit hyperactivity disorder: a meta-analysis of follow-up studies. *Psychological Medicine* **36**, 159–165.

Fergusson, D.M. *et al.* (2004) Show me the child at seven: the consequences of conduct problems in childhood for psychosocial functioning in adulthood. *Journal of Child Psychology and Psychiatry* **45**, 1–13.

Fergusson, D.M. *et al.* (2011) Structural equation modeling of repeated retrospective reports of childhood maltreatment. *International Journal of Methods in Psychiatric Research* **20**, 93–104.

Fergusson, D.M. *et al.* (2012) Moderating role of the *MAOA* genotype in antisocial behaviour. *British Journal of Psychiatry* **200**, 116–123.

Gershon, A. *et al.* (2013) The long-term impact of early adversity on late-life psychiatric disorder. *Current Psychiatry Reports* **15**, Article No. 352.

Goodman, A. *et al.* (2011) The long shadow cast by childhood physical and mental problems in adult life. *Proceedings of the National Academy of Sciences* **108**, 6032–6037.

Gregory, A.M. *et al.* (2007) Juvenile mental health histories of adults with anxiety disorders. *American Journal of Psychiatry* **164**, 301–308.

Hardt, J. & Rutter, M. (2004) Validity of adult retrospective reports of adverse childhood experiences: review of the evidence. *Journal of Child Psychology and Psychiatry* **45**, 260–273.

Hazell, P. *et al.* (2002) Tricyclic drugs for depression in children and adolescents. *Cochrane Database of Systematic Reviews* CD002317.

Heim, C. & Binder, E.B. (2012) Current research trends in early life stress and depression: review of human studies on sensitive periods, gene-environment interactions, and epigenetics. *Experimental Neurology* **233**, 102–111.

Horwitz, A.V. *et al.* (2001) The impact of childhood abuse and neglect on adult mental health: a prospective study. *Journal of Health and Social Behavior* **42**, 184–201.

Howlin, P. & Moss, P. (2012) Adults with autism spectrum disorders. *Canadian Journal of Psychiatry* **57**, 275–283.

Howlin, P. *et al.* (2013) Social outcomes in mid- to later adulthood among individuals diagnosed with autism and average nonverbal IQ as children. *Journal of the American Academy of Child and Adolescent Psychiatry* **52**, 572–581.

Hussong, A.M. *et al.* (2004) Substance abuse hinders desistance in young adults' antisocial behavior. *Development and Psychopathology* **16**, 1029–1046.

Hyde, J.S. *et al.* (2008) The ABCs of depression: integrating affective, biological, and cognitive models to explain the emergence of the gender difference in depression. *Psychological Review* **115**, 291–313.

Jaffee, S.R. *et al.* (2002) Differences in early childhood risk factors for juvenile-onset and adult-onset depression. *Archives of General Psychiatry* **59**, 215–222.

Jaffee, S.R. *et al.* (2013) Using complementary methods to test whether marriage limits men's antisocial behavior. *Development and Psychopathology* **25**, 65–77.

Jokela, M. *et al.* (2009) Childhood problem behaviors and death by midlife: the British National Child Development Study. *Journal of the American Academy of Child and Adolescent Psychiatry* **48**, 19–24.

Kendler, K.S. & Gardner, C.O. (2001) Monozygotic twins discordant for major depression: a preliminary exploration of the role of environmental experiences in the aetiology and course of illness. *Psychological Medicine* **31**, 411–423.

Kendler, K.S. *et al.* (2000) Stressful life events and previous episodes in the etiology of major depression in women: an evaluation of the 'kindling' hypothesis. *American Journal of Psychiatry* **157**, 1243–1251.

Kendler, K.S. *et al.* (2007) Creating a social world—a developmental twin study of peer-group deviance. *Archives of General Psychiatry* **64**, 958–965.

Kessler, R.C. *et al.* (2012) Prevalence, persistence, and sociodemographic correlates of DSM-IV disorders in the National Comorbidity Survey Replication-Adolescent Supplement. *Archives of General Psychiatry* **69**, 372–380.

Kim-Cohen, J. *et al.* (2003) Prior juvenile diagnoses in adults with mental disorder—developmental follow-back of a prospective-longitudinal cohort. *Archives of General Psychiatry* **60**, 709–717.

Klein, R.G. *et al.* (2012) Clinical and functional outcome of childhood attention-deficit/hyperactivity disorder 33 years later. *Archives of General Psychiatry* **69**, 1295–1303.

Koenen, K.C. (2010) Developmental origins of posttraumatic stress disorder. *Depression and Anxiety* **27**, 413–416.

Kofink, D. *et al.* (2013) Epigenetic dynamics in psychiatric disorders: environmental programming of neurodevelopmental processes. *Neuroscience and Biobehavioral Reviews* **37**, 831–845.

Kossowsky, J. *et al.* (2013) The separation anxiety hypothesis of panic disorder revisited: a meta-analysis. *American Journal of Psychiatry* **170**, 768–781.

Lahey, B.B. & Waldman, I.D. (2012) Phenotypic and causal structure of conduct disorder in the broader context of prevalent forms of psychopathology. *Journal of Child Psychology and Psychiatry* **53**, 556–537.

Lahey, B.B. *et al.* (2011) Higher-order genetic and environmental structure of prevalent forms of child and adolescent psychopathology. *Archives of General Psychiatry* **68**, 181–189.

Langley, K. *et al.* (2010a) Adolescent clinical outcomes for young people with attention-deficit hyperactivity disorder. *British Journal of Psychiatry* **196**, 235–240.

Langley, K. *et al.* (2010b) Genotype link with extreme antisocial behavior: the contribution of cognitive pathways. *Archives of General Psychiatry* **67**, 1317–1323.

Lau, J.Y.F. & Eley, T.C. (2006) Changes in genetic and environmental influences on depressive symptoms across adolescence and young adulthood. *British Journal of Psychiatry* **189**, 422–427.

Laub, J.H. & Sampson, R.J. (2003) *Shared Beginnings, Divergent Lives: Delinquent Boys to Age 70.* Harvard University, Cambridge, MA.

Lupien, S.J. *et al.* (2009) Effects of stress throughout the lifespan on the brain, behaviour and cognition. *Nature Reviews Neuroscience* **10**, 434–445.

Lyytinen, H. *et al.* (2006) Trajectories of reading development; a follow-up from birth to school age of children with and without risk for dyslexia. *Merril-Palmer Quarterly* **52**, 514–546.

Lyytinen, H. *et al.* (2008) Early identification and prevention of dyslexia: results from a prospective follow-up study of children at familial risk for dyslexia. In: *The SAGE Handbook of Dyslexia.* (eds G. Reid, *et al.*), pp. 121–146. Sage Publishers.

Malone, S.M. *et al.* (2004) Genetic and environmental influences on antisocial behavior and alcohol dependence from adolescence to early adulthood. *Development and Psychopathology* **16**, 943–966.

Maughan, B. *et al.* (2014) Adolescent conduct problems and premature mortality: follow-up to age 65 years in a national birth cohort. *Psychological Medicine* **44**, 1077–1086.

McGee, R. *et al.* (2001) Multiple maltreatment, attribution of blame, and adjustment among adolescents. *Development and Psychopathology* **13**, 827–846.

McGrath, L.M. *et al.* (2012) Bringing a developmental perspective to anxiety genetics. *Development and Psychopathology* **24**, 11.

Moffitt, T.E. (1993) Adolescence-limited and life-course-persistent antisocial behavior—a developmental taxonomy. *Psychological Review* **100**, 674–701.

Moffitt, T.E. *et al.* (2010) How common are common mental disorders? Evidence that lifetime prevalence rates are doubled by prospective versus retrospective ascertainment. *Psychological Medicine* **40**, 899–909.

Monroe, S.M. & Harkness, K.L. (2005) Life stress, the 'kindling' hypothesis, and the recurrence of depression: considerations from a life stress perspective. *Psychological Review* **112**, 417–445.

Nagin, D.S. & Odgers, C.L. (2010) Group-based trajectory modeling in clinical research. *Annual Review of Clinical Psychology* **6**, 109–138.

Odgers, C.L. & Jaffee, S.R. (2013) Routine versus catastrophic influences on the developing child. *Annual Review of Public Health* **34**, 29–48.

Odgers, C.L. *et al.* (2008) Female and male antisocial trajectories: from childhood origins to adult outcomes. *Development and Psychopathology* **20**, 673–716.

Olazagasti, M.A.R. *et al.* (2013) Does childhood attention-deficit/hyperactivity disorder predict risk-taking and mental illness in adulthood? *Journal of the American Academy of Child and Adolescent Psychiatry* **52**, 153–162.

Owen, M.J. *et al.* (2011) Neurodevelopmental hypothesis of schizophrenia. *British Journal of Psychiatry* **198**, 173–175.

Pickles, A. *et al.* (2010) Predictors of suicidality across the life span: the Isle of Wight study. *Psychological Medicine* **40**, 1453–1466.

Pine, D.S. (2007) Research review: a neuroscience framework for pediatric anxiety disorders. *Journal of Child Psychology and Psychiatry* **48**, 631–648.

Post, R.M. (2010) Mechanisms of illness progression in the recurrent affective disorders. *Neurotoxicity Research* **18**, 256–271.

Roberson-Nay, R. *et al.* (2012) Childhood Separation Anxiety Disorder and adult onset panic attacks share a common genetic diathesis. *Depression and Anxiety* **29**, 320–327.

Robins, L.N. (1966) *Deviant Children Grown Up.* Williams & Wilkins, Baltimore.

Rutter, M. (2012) Resilience as a dynamic concept. *Development and Psychopathology* **24**, 335–344.

Rutter, M. (2013) Annual research review: resilience—clinical implications. *Journal of Child Psychology and Psychiatry* **54**, 474–487.

Rutter, M. & Sroufe, L.A. (2000) Developmental psychopathology: concepts and challenges. *Development and Psychopathology* **12**, 265–296.

Rutter, M. *et al.* (2012) Longitudinal studies using a "natural experiment" design: the case of adoptees from Romanian institutions. *Journal of the American Academy of Child and Adolescent Psychiatry* **51**, 762–770.

Sameroff, A.J. & Mackenzie, M.J. (2003) Research strategies for capturing transactional models of development: the limits of the possible. *Development and Psychopathology* **15**, 613–640.

Scott, K.M. *et al.* (2012) Childhood maltreatment and DSM-IV adult mental disorders: comparison of prospective and retrospective findings. *British Journal of Psychiatry* **200**, 469–475.

Shanahan, L. *et al.* (2011) Child-, adolescent- and young adult-onset depressions: differential risk factors in development? *Psychological Medicine* **41**, 2265–2274.

Shaw, P. *et al.* (2010) Childhood psychiatric disorders as anomalies in neurodevelopmental trajectories. *Human Brain Mapping* **31**, 917–925.

Shechner, T. *et al.* (2012) Attention biases, anxiety, and development: toward or away from threats or rewards? *Depression and Anxiety* **29**, 282–294.

Silk, J.S. *et al.* (2012) Why do anxious children become depressed teenagers? The role of social-evaluative threat and reward processing. *Psychological Medicine* **42**, 2095–2107.

Sroufe, L.A. & Rutter, M. (1984) The domain of developmental psychopathology. *Child Development* **55**, 17–29.

Stringaris, A. *et al.* (2012) Adolescent irritability: phenotypic associations and genetic links with depressed mood. *American Journal of Psychiatry* **169**, 47–54.

Sweeten, G. *et al.* (2013) Age and the explanation of crime, revisited. *Journal of Youth and Adolescence* **42**, 921–938.

Thapar, A. *et al.* (2012) Depression in adolescence. *Lancet* **379**, 1056–1067.

Tremblay, R.E. (2010) Developmental origins of disruptive behaviour problems: the 'original sin' hypothesis, epigenetics and their consequences for prevention. *Journal of Child Psychology and Psychiatry* **51**, 341–367.

Whitehouse, A.J.O. *et al.* (2009) No clear genetic influences on the association between dyslexia and anxiety in a population-based sample of female twins. *Dyslexia* **4**, 282–290.

Wichers, M. *et al.* (2013) Genetic innovation and stability in externalizing problem behavior across development: a multi-informant twin study. *Behavior Genetics* **43**, 191–201.

Widom, C.S. *et al.* (2007) A prospective investigation of major depressive disorder and comorbidity in abused and neglected children grown up. *Archives of General Psychiatry* **64**, 49–56.

Young, S. *et al.* (2011) Avoiding the 'twilight zone': recommendations for the transition of services from adolescence to adulthood for young people with ADHD. *BMC Psychiatry* **11**, 174.

CHAPTER 2

Diagnosis, diagnostic formulations, and classification

Michael Rutter[1] and Daniel S. Pine[2]

[1] Social, Genetic and Developmental Psychiatry (SGDP) Research Center, Institute of Psychiatry, Psychology and Neuroscience, King's College London, UK

[2] Section on Development and Affective Neuroscience, National Institute of Mental Health (NIMH) Intramural Research Program, Bethesda, MD, USA

Introduction

In essence, classification provides a standardized way of describing phenomena and thereby enabling communications about those phenomena to be possible because all concerned will use terms in the same way. However, classification is a multi-faceted endeavor and, therefore, we need to begin with a discussion of those different facets. After defining key terms, the current chapter delineates major questions that have emerged from prior research on these different facets. This is followed by a review of data on validity, as it informs classification. However, current data on validity leave many questions unanswered. As a result, the chapter closes by delineating the nature of these questions and setting an agenda for addressing them in future classifications schemes that go beyond the forthcoming revision of ICD and DSM-5.

Definition

The purpose of diagnosis is to indicate what each disorder, as evidenced in an individual, has in common with a similar disorder shown by other people. Two points need emphasis. First, it refers to a pattern of signs and symptoms, and *not* to people. It is scientifically misleading to suppose that a single designation could summarize all that is important about a person, and it is offensive to use terminology that implies the contrary. Accordingly, it is now preferred to refer to an individual *with* autism (or ADHD) rather than an autistic (or ADHD) person. This constitutes a reminder that it may be possible to relieve the symptoms without requiring that the person as a whole be radically changed. Cure (in the sense of completely eradicating a condition) is rare across the whole of medicine. Consider diabetes, coronary artery disease, and asthma as examples in internal medicine. On the other hand, it may well be possible to restore sound functioning.

A diagnostic formulation is quite different from a diagnosis, in that only the former involves a discussion of the features that are particularly crucial in that person, even though they may not be so in other people. Such features do not just (or even mainly) concern signs and symptoms. Rather the focus may be on the hypothesized causal influences; the existence of protective features; the family and broader social context; and the range of considerations that need to be considered when planning how best to intervene. It should also end with a hypothesized causal nexus and a plan for care/treatment. Most crucially, it should spell out how the individual's response to the intervention can provide guidance on whether or not the postulated explanation was correct (and, if not, how it, and the treatment plan, should be modified). What this clearly means is that any adequate diagnostic formulation must extend well beyond the listing of signs and symptoms. Moreover, the formulation should provide an anticipated prognosis, together with guidance on how both the child and the family should deal with the problems. For these reasons, it has become best practice to provide each individual and family with a written feedback letter (or report), summarizing what was discussed at the assessment. This should include a brief summary of the basis for the decision-making, and the plans for what is to happen next.

Classification is a generic term that provides a standardized approach to communication, either among clinicians or researchers. Thus, classification is intended to ensure that when a clinical or research report states that, for example, the findings refer to a group of patients with, say, autism or ADHD, everyone will understand what this means and will use the diagnostic term in the same way. However, classification goes beyond individual diagnoses to consider how collections of diagnoses should

Rutter's Child and Adolescent Psychiatry, Sixth Edition.
Edited by Anita Thapar and Daniel S. Pine, James F. Leckman, Stephen Scott, Margaret J. Snowling, Eric Taylor.

be grouped together, or placed in a cluster. Similarly, it will specify the extent to which diagnoses should be split into finer subdivisions, or lumped together with other diagnoses to form a larger grouping. Because this clustering is designed to inform decisions, which arise in many diverse contexts, this means that there can be no simple "right" way to construct a classification. Appropriate classification reflects the purpose at hand. For example, what works best at a primary care level may be much simpler than that which is required in a specialized research center. Also, the organization that is best for clinical purposes (such as for prognosis or planning treatment) may differ from that which is mainly intended to guide biological studies.

Clinical and research classifications

In that connection, there are fundamental differences between a clinical classification and a research classification. First, the aim of a clinical system should be the diagnosis of all disorders, whereas a research system may be constructed on a more restricted basis to fit in with a supposedly "purer," more homogenous, group of disorders. It will not matter that this means that a substantial proportion of disorders are left out, often those with some different associated psychopathology. Second, in order to ensure that all participants in a study have their disorders diagnosed in the same way, it is now standard practice to specify both the diagnostic instruments to be used and the number of specified features that must be present. By sharp contrast, clinical systems need to start with the *concept* of each disorder, moving on to guidelines on the specific features that should be used to assess the concept. So far as possible, these should include detail on differential diagnosis and differentiation from normality—as well represented in the ICD-11 clinical guidelines. The aim is to ensure that all clinicians apply the guidelines in the same way but without the rigidity inherent in requiring particular instruments to be used and in having strict rules on the number of items required to fulfill the diagnostic requirements.

Of course, it is essential that there is a clear and understandable pathway between clinical and research classifications. Nevertheless, they are sufficiently different for it to be a major problem that the DSM has a classification that is intended to meet *both* research and clinical needs. Most especially, the process to develop proposals for DSM-5 started with a consideration of the number of symptoms required in each symptom domain *before* considering the clinical concept that was to be assessed. The proposals for ICD-11, by contrast, have started with the clinical guidelines before turning attention to the standardized research criteria requirements. Both of us are clinicians and researchers and, therefore, are firmly committed to the needs for both types of classification. However, our strong preference is for the ICD approach that separates classifications for clinical use and for research purposes, with a starting point in the concept and the guidelines for its use.

Biomarkers and neural signatures

Since the seminal article by Robins and Guze (1970) on validation of diagnostic categories, there has been a strong interest in the possibility that there might be the discovery of neural activation patterns or structural differences that could indicate, not only that the patient had a mental disorder, but *which* disorder was present (Gillihan & Parens, 2011). Similar questions have been posed more recently with respect to plans for DSM-5 (Hyman, 2007) and for the ICD-11 (Uher & Rutter, 2012a). This is a new approach; up to now, psychiatric classifications have placed a far greater emphasis on diagnostic reliability than biological meaning or validity (Andreasen, 2007). The hope recently has been that psychiatric disorders might be reconceptualized as disorders of brain circuitry, and that findings from cognitive neuroscience, genetics, and experimental laboratory studies might be brought together for the purpose of classification (Insel *et al.*, 2010). However, it remains unclear if or when this could be realized.

The possibilities have been reviewed in relation to neuroimaging (Gillihan & Parens, 2011) and in relation to a wider range of technologies (Uher & Rutter, 2012a). Similar issues with respect to broader perspectives on biomarkers have also been considered (Rutter, 2014). Much of the research has been conducted with supernormal control groups, without much attention to the need to consider differentiation among diagnostic groups. The lack of good evidence on diagnostic specificity is a problem because neuroimaging technologies may tend to identify general psychopathology rather than individual diagnostic features (Insel & Wang, 2010). In addition, extensive within-group heterogeneity has usually been evident. Genetic findings are similarly inconclusive. There is some meaningful diagnostic specificity but these instances emerge against a background of much nonspecificity (Uher & Rutter, 2012a) and great pleiotropy (Lahey *et al.*, 2011). Thus, copy number variations have been found to be associated with autism, ADHD, schizophrenia and intellectual disability (see Rutter, 2013). The same applies to other identified genetic risk factors.

As has now been widely accepted, there is not yet the evidence required for a scientific classification based on brain findings. Opinions differ on whether technological advances might make it possible in the future. Certainly, it is highly desirable, and probably achievable, for future classifications to be more strongly reflective of scientific knowledge, but the key question is whether this could ever replace clinical classifications. Two slightly different issues need to be considered. First, research strongly suggests that many disorders involve more than one biological pathway (Rutter, 1994, 2006). That need not constitute an obstacle if there is a common endpoint that defines the pathophysiology and that might prove to be the case. But what would be the biological findings in the very common situation of co-occurring disorders? That leads on to the second issue of whether clinical needs could be met by a purely neuroscience classification. Clinicians have to deal with psychopathological syndromes, and any adequate classification would have to reflect these. Thus, gene-environment interactions (G × E) findings indicate that the neural reflections of G × E concern processes that are found in individuals without mental disorder (Meyer-Lindenberg & Weinberger, 2006; Hyde *et al.*, 2011). The clinician will nevertheless need to know whether there is a meaningful mental disorder. G × E findings also suggest that the genetic and the environmental pathways are closely associated. In other words, the fact that a disorder has come about through strong environmental influences does not mean that there will be no brain features. After all, there is good evidence that important environmental effects *are* biologically embedded (Rutter, 2012a). Accordingly, we reject the often-made criticism that a focus on the brain neglects the importance of the environment. The workings of the mind (however brought about) have to be based on what is going on in the brain. The more valid reservation concerns practicalities, given current limited understanding of brain function. Namely, future research is likely to reveal cognitive and emotional processes that have a known biological substrate. Nevertheless, it remains unclear how clinically relevant processes can be reducible to what can be measured with respect to brain structure and function in the individual patient.

Dimensions and categories

DSM leaders have urged that DSM-5 should adopt dimensional approaches insofar as that was possible (Regier *et al.*, 2011). There is little agreement on how that might be accomplished, and many questions remain on how many dimensions, what they should assess, and how they might be measured (see Uher & Rutter, 2012a). Several different reasons have led to the consideration of dimensions. First, internal medicine has long used dimensions alongside categorical diagnoses. Thus, pulmonary physicians measure various dimensions of lung function alongside diagnoses such as chronic bronchitis, emphysema, and chronic obstructive lung disease. Similarly, cardiologists use quantitative measures of exercise tolerance, of blood pressure and of degree of coronary artery obstruction together with diagnoses of coronary artery disease, mitral stenosis and hypertension. Note that the diagnoses have the advantage of giving information about the pathophysiology and dimensions have the advantage of assessing severity. Second, dimensions carry statistical advantages with respect to predictive power (because they make use of differences across the entire range), and avoid the errors associated with cut-offs in the middle of a curve rather than at a natural trough separating two distributions (one of which reflects some disorder). Fergusson and Horwood (1995) clearly showed that this applies in the domain of child psychopathology. Third, there is abundant evidence that many mental syndromes, such as depression, conduct disturbance, and ADHD to give just three examples, function dimensionally. That is to say, the meaning of associations between symptoms

and external factors (such as genetics) applies not just at the extremes but across the full range of symptomatic expression. That has been less obvious in the case of autism and schizophrenia but, even with these supposedly qualitatively distinct disorders, the genetic liability extends well beyond the traditional diagnostic category—as evident in the broader autism phenotype (Le Couteur *et al.*, 1996) and schizotypal disorder (Kendler & Gardner, 1997; Kendler *et al.*, 1998). Whether the liability truly extends across the entire range in the general population is not yet known.

Some might look to statistics to resolve the question of dimensions or categories. Are there two distinct curves or just one? The most famous example of this type of dispute is to be found in the competing claims of Platt and Pickering with respect to hypertension (Swales, 1985). The findings clearly showed the difficulties involved in deciding the number of curves. As Zubin (1967) argued years ago, it makes no sense to argue which is correct because it depends on the purpose for which it is intended. All categories can be dimensionalized, and all dimensions can be made into categories. In the psychopathological arena, the most obvious example is provided by intellectual disability. Mild intellectual disability differs from severe (or profound) disability with respect to life expectancy, fecundity, structural brain pathology, and genetics. As shown here, a categorical distinction works best from a biological perspective. On the other hand, if the need is to predict later educational attainments or social functioning, IQ is best used as a continuous dimension.

In relation to clinical usage, categorical distinctions are unavoidable. There have to be decisions on whether or not to use medication, to admit the child to hospital, or take him/her into care. It would make no sense, for example, to vary the dose of antidepressant according to the score of some depression scale. Considerations such as these make it inadvisable to change the whole of classification from categories to dimensions. On the other hand, we see great value in including some dimensions in a mainly categorical classification. Thus, the multi-axial version of ICD-10 for use by child psychiatrists (World Health Organization, 1992) was well accepted and worked very well with dimensions for IQ, and for overall social functioning, for example.

Accordingly, we deplore the bureaucratic decision of WHO that ICD-11 cannot have any dimensions. That is a fundamentally absurd requirement. Thus, with respect to autism spectrum disorders, clinicians need to know the level of language and of intellectual functioning. Neither changes the diagnosis, but they are important for prognostic purposes. Perhaps, the way forward with respect to ICD-11, as with ICD-10, is to have a multi-axial version published by the Mental Health Division rather than WHO itself. In other words, we strongly urge a pragmatic, problem-solving approach.

In that connection, it is important to note that classification has to encompass associated somatic conditions and associated psychosocial circumstances as well as mental disorders. Both are available in the ICD but are *not* provided in the DSM. Nevertheless, there must be a sensible walkway between ICD-11 and DSM-5, however both are organized. Thus, for example, in ICD-11, Rett syndrome will presumably be coded in the neurology section rather than the psychopathology one. The same will probably apply to some sleep disorders (such as narcolepsy).

The supposed separateness of syndromes

Traditionally, diagnoses were conceptualized as syndromes or disorders that were truly distinct and separate from one another. The implication was that mixed or overlapping patterns should be the exception rather than the rule. Ordinarily, there should be, in effect, clear water between diagnostic categories. Clinical and research decision-making would be greatly simplified if this truly were the case, but it is not. Much research has shown, for example, that phenotypic overlap between autism and ADHD is common and that the two disorders (and others) partially show the same genetic liability (Rutter, 2014). Similar issues apply to the connection between bipolar disorder and schizophrenia (Craddock & Owen, 2010). The overlap among diagnoses clearly poses major problems for any classification system; the issues are discussed in Chapter 3. Nevertheless, none of this should be taken to mean that there are no meaningful differences among syndromes. We use, below, a range of possible validating criteria to determine the extent to which there are such differences, but, because of the overlap among syndromes, it cannot be expected that all the criteria will point in the same direction.

Validation of diagnostic categories

For diagnoses to be scientifically meaningful and clinically useful, it is necessary that the diagnostic distinctions be validated. As realized a long time ago (Robins & Guze, 1970; Cantwell, 1975; Rutter, 1978), such validation must be on the basis of criteria that are *external* to the defining signs and symptoms. Such criteria may derive from quite varied sources—such as age and sex trends, response to different forms of treatment, long-term outcome, genetic influences, and psychosocial influences. The expectation cannot be that all of these will validate the diagnosis, but confidence in the validation will increase with the number of sources that show that the diagnostic distinctions hold up. As already noted, a major problem lies in the evidence that diagnoses are not as distinct and separate as was traditionally supposed. However, our initial discussion of validation will be based on what has been found with existing diagnoses. The review here is selective, but it provides guidance on the extent to which there is validating evidence on some of the main diagnoses.

Age trends and sex differences
Age differences were used in the 1960s and 1970s to separate autism and schizophrenia (Rutter, 1972). Up to that time period,

autism had been termed an infantile psychosis and had been regarded as an early manifestation of schizophrenia. However, the data from research by both Kolvin (1971) and Makita (1966) showed that psychoses tended to be either infantile in their first manifestations (suggesting autism) or adolescent in onset (suggesting schizophrenia), with rather few onsets in the intervening years. On this basis, there did not seem to be continuity between autism and schizophrenia. Autism also showed a marked male preponderance (3 or 4 to 1) whereas schizophrenia differed much less in sex ratio.

Later research showed that an onset particularly concentrated in the preschool years picked out a group of disorders, like autism, that involved neurodevelopmental impairment and which were more common in males than females. Thus, this applied to attention deficit hyperactivity disorder (ADHD) (Gershon & Gershon, 2002), dyslexia (Miles *et al.*, 1998), specific language impairment (Bellani *et al.*, 2011), and antisocial behavior with a childhood onset (Moffitt *et al.*, 2001). The disorders where prevalence peaks in adolescence, such as depression and eating disorders, were strikingly different in showing a female preponderance and no particular association with neurodevelopmental impairment (Rutter *et al.*, 2003).

Note that age of onset as such is not as clear a differentiator as might be supposed. Findings from the Dunedin longitudinal study showed that a *majority* of mental disorders requiring treatment in early adult life had already been manifest in childhood or early adolescence (Kim-Cohen *et al.*, 2003, Merikangas *et al.*, 2010). These findings, however, concern first manifestations in the childhood years and *not* onset in infancy.

Familiality and genetics
There is good evidence that autism spectrum disorders (ASD) are associated with a markedly increased family loading for ASD and a somewhat wider range of social and communicative impairments (Rutter & Thapar, 2014). Moreover, twin data indicate that the genetic liability applies across this range (Le Couteur *et al.*, 1996). There is possibly some increase in anxiety disorders but no loading for schizophrenia. Conversely, schizophrenia spectrum disorders (SSD) are associated with an increased familial loading for SSD (including schizotypal disorder) but not for ASD. SSD and bipolar disorder (BD) have a somewhat different set of genetic risk factors, but there is more overlap between SSD and BD than appreciated in the past (Moskvina *et al.*, 2008).

Depressive disorders generally are associated with both an increased familial loading for depressive disorders and with a moderate heritability (Levinson, 2006). However, twin data indicate that there is a strongly shared genetic liability between depression and generalized anxiety disorder (Kendler & Prescott, 2006). The overlap, however, is much less for depression and specific phobic disorders (Franić *et al.*, 2010). Bipolar disorders are associated with an increased family loading for unipolar depressive disorders, but the converse is much less common (McGuffin *et al.*, 2003). That is to say, only a small proportion of the relatives of individuals with a unipolar disorder have a bipolar disorder. The implication would seem to be that the two are meaningfully different. Nevertheless, some relatives of patients with BD will have depression without mania because manic/hypomanic episodes have yet to occur.

Genetic studies indicate some shared genetic liability between obsessive-compulsive disorder (OCD) and tic disorders, including Tourette's syndrome and chronic multiple tics (Leckman *et al.*, 2002). However, there may also be some shared genetic liability between OCD and anxiety disorders (Bolton *et al.*, 2007). There is also good evidence on both the familiality of conduct/dissocial disorder and the fact that to an important extent this reflects genetic influences (Moffitt, 2005). This seems to differ from the findings on emotional disturbance, but there has been rather little study of the possible shared genetic liability between conduct/dissocial disorder and emotional disturbance. Twin and family studies both show the importance of genetic influences on eating disorders that differ from those on other disorders, but the evidence is more contradictory on possible differences between anorexia and bulimia nervosa.

The clearest genetic validation concerns Rett syndrome in which a gene on the X chromosome with a mutation that affects the methyl-CpG-binding protein (MeCP2) is responsible for the disease—this not being found in other autism spectrum disorders.

The subclassification of intellectual disability into severe/profound and mild also has genetic validation in that the former is associated with multiple major genetic mutations (such as that responsible for Down syndrome) whereas that is very much less common in the case of mild intellectual disability. Also, whereas mild disability shares genetic liability with the general population, severe intellectual disability does not.

Both molecular and behavioral genetic findings (Kendler *et al.*, 2003) have shown that misuse of various psychoactive substances share much the same genetic liability. That is, there is very little indication that the misuse of different drugs is associated with different genes.

Within conduct/dissocial disorders, childhood onset is more strongly associated with alcohol/drug problems in one or both parents than it is in adolescent onset (Silberg *et al.*, 2014).

Psychosocial correlates

For the most part, major psychosocial risk factors do not show diagnostic specificity (McMahon *et al.*, 2003) although there is some evidence that this, at least in part, is a consequence of the extensive co-occurrence of disorders (Shanahan *et al.*, 2008). There is some tendency for severe discord and conflict to be particularly associated with conduct disorders (Shanahan *et al.*, 2008) but it also constitutes some risk for other disorders.

The two disorders showing a moderately strong specific association with certain psychosocial features are what used to be called post-traumatic stress disorder (PTSD) and disinhibited

attachment (now social regulation) disorder. PTSD in DSM-IV and ICD-10 was described as a syndrome usually arising soon after some exceptional traumatic event that involved actual or threatened death or serious injury and which included recurrent intrusive recollections of the event, persistent avoidance of stimuli associated with the trauma and increased arousal and hypervigilance. Unfortunately, reports of PTSD have often included a wider range of stress events, and the symptomatology has included rather general features such as irritability and difficulty sleeping. The ICD-11 proposals have argued for four slight but important modifications in order to emphasize the specificity of the disorder. First, a requirement of onset soon after the event (thus eliminating much delayed onset in which the causal connection is less easy to establish); second, a tight restriction to physically threatening or dangerous events; third, an elimination from the diagnostic criteria of features of irritability and insomnia which apply to many forms of mental disorder; and, fourth, a renaming to "hyperarousal/hypervigilance syndrome" in order to avoid its inclusion in a broader range of nonspecific stress related disorders. It is not that the syndrome does not include anxiety or depressive features. To the contrary, they are common, but they are not indicative of the specificity of the syndrome.

The second situation-specific disorder is the "disinhibited social regulation disorder" (previously termed as reactive attachment disorder). Zeanah and Gleason (2011) rightly argued that this should not be classed as an attachment disorder because it was shown by the style of interactions with *strangers* and not by the child's response to separation from and reunion with a caregiver. The syndrome is strongly associated with an early upbringing in profoundly depriving institutions (it is not yet known whether, or how often, it arises following profound deprivation in a family setting or an institutional upbringing that is not globally depriving). Both this syndrome and the "hyperarousal/hypervigilance" syndrome are distinctive in persisting after the risk situation is no longer present.

A third example of a psychosocial validating feature concerns schizophrenia. It differs markedly from the first two examples in that there is no suggestion that schizophrenia usually has a psychosocial origin. Nevertheless, schizophrenia is distinctive by virtue of its association with a prolonged upbringing in an urban environment during the childhood/adolescent years, but apparently not with living in an urban environment only *after* the childhood/adolescent years (see Pedersen & Mortensen, 2001; van Os *et al.*, 2010; Vassos *et al.*, 2012). Schizophrenia is also associated with migration from a developing to a developed country (McGrath *et al.*, 2004; Cantor-Graae & Selten, 2005; Jones & Fung, 2005). Apparently, the risk effect is associated with living in an area in which most of the population does not share the same ethnicity. Some of the key studies have involved migrants from the West Indies to either the UK or Netherlands in which the risk of schizophrenia has been found to exceed that in the island from which they migrated and that in indigenous whites in the countries to which they migrated. Although the main association is with schizophrenia it also applies to a lesser extent to other psychoses.

Whereas mild intellectual disability is much more common in children reared in poverty and social disadvantage, this is not the case with severe intellectual disability.

Poverty is associated with antisocial behavior but not with emotional disturbance to anything like the same extent (see Costello *et al.*, 2003).

Long-term course

Rett syndrome stands out with respect to the downhill course associated with neurological impairment and/or epilepsy. This is not found with any other form of psychopathology in childhood (Neul, 2011). However, autism is also distinctive in terms of the development of epileptic attacks in adolescence/early adult life (Bolton *et al.*, 2011) and with an apparent loss of skills in a minority of individuals, usually associated with both a worsening in behavior and often with epilepsy (which might begin before or after the cognitive loss (Howlin *et al.*, 2014).

Antisocial behavior in adult life is almost always preceded by conduct disorder (CD) in childhood (Robins, 1966, 1978). However, only about two fifths of cases of CD persist into adult life. In DSM-IV and ICD-10, CD was treated as a mental disorder, but antisocial behavior in adult life was treated as a personality disorder, placed on a different axis. In both DSM-5 and ICD-11, the two will be brought together as the same disorder. This is well justified, but it raises the consideration of how to recognize (and code) childhood onset CD/dissocial behavior that does *not* persist into adult life. At the time of writing, no satisfactory empirical solution has been found.

Long-term follow-up studies of patients who suffered from a depressive disorder in childhood have clearly shown a very high rate of recurrence in adult life, associated also with a much increased risk for suicide and attempted suicide (Fombonne *et al.*, 2001a, b). This recurrence rate is relatively specific to depressive and anxiety disorders, unless the depression in childhood is associated with a conduct disorder, in which case the outcome includes a much broader range of psychopathology and of social dysfunction. The risk for suicide is also higher in the group with depression and CD in childhood reflecting the fact that CD, as well as depression, constitutes a risk factor for suicide. The evidence on the frequency of bipolar disorder in adult life is more contradictory. Harrington *et al.* (1990), Fombonne *et al.* (2001a), and Weissman *et al.* (1999) all found that transition from a unipolar depressive episode in childhood to a bipolar disorder in adulthood was quite uncommon, whereas a few others (e.g. Geller *et al.*, 1994) have found it to occur more frequently. Finally, from a classification perspective, it is important to note that the recurrence of further depressive disorders is as high in the case of both dysthymia and minor depression as it is with major depressive disorders (Angst, 2009).

Schizophrenia usually has a profound negative impact on personal development and functioning (Jablensky, 2009). Nevertheless, in about a third of cases, a relatively benign outcome is seen, and yet other cases run an episodic course. The outcome tends to be worse for schizophrenia beginning in childhood, with an insidious onset and much negative symptomatology (Hollis, 2008). About a quarter of patients with schizophrenia followed for many years develop a major depressive disorder. The converse, however, does not apply; only a very small proportion of patients with major depression develop schizophrenic features during a long-term follow-up. Thus, mood disturbances may be considered part of the schizophrenic spectrum, but schizophrenic disturbances are not part of the depression spectrum.

Obsessive-compulsive disorders (OCD) show a strong tendency to persist into adult life but there is waxing and waning of the symptoms, often with associated anxiety and/or depression (Flament & Robaey, 2009). Many cases of OCD also have tics and there is an association with Tourette's syndrome in some cases.

ADHD shows a substantial degree of persistence into adult life (Taylor & Sonuga-Barke, 2008), but the pattern of manifestation changes with increasing age—hyperactivity becomes less frequent, and inattention becomes more prominent (Larsson *et al.*, 2011). In addition, ADHD predisposes to development of conduct disorder. This predisposition is already evident in childhood but, even in cases without CD in childhood, ADHD in early life is associated with an increased risk of antisocial behavior when older (Mannuzza *et al.*, 1998).

CD with an onset in childhood has a substantially greater likelihood of persisting into adult life than CD beginning in adolescence (Silberg *et al.*, 2014).

About half the cases of speech delay that are diagnosable at 4 years of age resolve with little in the way of sequelae but those that do not are followed by a much increased rate of reading disorders, and some increase in emotional and behavioral problems (Rutter, 2008). In cases with a more severe disorder of receptive language, there is also a marked increase in problems in love relationships.

Disinhibited social regulation disorder has been shown to persist long after removal from the depriving circumstances that led to its origin (Bruce *et al.*, 2010; Zeanah & Gleason, 2011), whereas reactive attachment disorder usually remits following a change of circumstances.

Drug response

Given the current views on biological factors in the etiology of mental disorders, it might be supposed that drug responses should be useful in the validation of diagnostic categories. In practice, this has not proved to be the case—primarily because so few drugs have single actions, but also because there are marked individual variations in response to all forms of medication. Thus, prior to Rapoport *et al.*'s (1980) definitive research findings, it was commonly supposed that stimulants had a paradoxical effect in ADHD. She found that, contrary to that supposition, stimulants had much the same qualitative effect of improving attention in everyone. A good response to stimulants in no way validates the diagnosis, and a lack of response does not invalidate it. In adults, tricyclic antidepressants have been widely, and effectively, used in the treatment of depression. However, they have also been shown to bring benefits to individuals with wetting or with ADHD—presumably through different mechanisms. The response of individuals with depression to tricyclic medication does differ, however, between childhood and adult life. In children, unlike in adults, tricyclics bring no benefits for depression (Hazell *et al.*, 1995), whereas selective serotonin reuptake inhibitors (SSRIs) are effective in children (Emslie *et al.*, 2004, March *et al.*, 2004) as well as in adults. This might suggest that depression in childhood/adolescence is different from that in adults, but this would not be supported by other validating criteria.

The nearest approach to a drug response that is diagnostically specific is provided by the use of lithium as an effective prophylactic against the recurrence of bipolar disorder (Tondo *et al.*, 2001; Geddes *et al.*, 2004). However, although not much used in the same way for unipolar depression, there is evidence that it, too, is similarly responsive to lithium (Souza & Goodwin, 1991). In addition, lithium may have useful effects in the treatment of aggressive behavior (Craft *et al.*, 1987; Tyrer, 1994; Einfeld, 2001) and of schizo-affective disorder (Jefferson, 1990). The evidence on these other uses of lithium is much thinner than on its use in the prevention of relapses in bipolar disorder, but a beneficial response to lithium does not validate the diagnosis of bipolar disorder. Thus, even for the strongest potential examples, the data on validation based on therapeutic response do not strongly distinguish specific disorders or even groups of disorders.

The topic may also be considered from the other end. Thus, are there meaningfully different responses to medication in different disorders? The key finding here is that autism is highly unusual in there being little or no effect on core symptoms from any form of medication (Buitelaar, 2003). The implication seems to be that this defines autism as a unique condition. This could mean that it may not involve dysfunction in any of the main neurotransmitter systems. Alternatively, this could mean that any such dysfunction is so fundamental or early-appearing that it remains impervious to current pharmacological approaches.

Cognitive impairments and developmental delay

Beyond the unique response to medications, autism also is distinctive with respect to its associated cognitive profile. Here the disorder exhibits both specific social cognitive features, such as impaired theory of mind and weak central coherence (Frith, 1989; Happé, 1994) and general intellectual disability (Bock & Goode, 2004), as well as unusual talents and savant skills (Happé & Frith, 2010). There is no other diagnosis with this particular pattern of cognitive strengths, limitations, and differences. Baron-Cohen (2002) sought to integrate findings by arguing that autism is associated with high systemizing skills, as well as poor empathizing (Baron-Cohen, 2011). Research by others has raised queries about Baron-Cohen's theory (Morsanyi *et al.*,

2012) and, at least so far, it is not contributory with respect to diagnostic validity.

ADHD has a weaker association with cognitive impairments (as compared with that found with autism), but, at a group level, it is associated with an IQ slightly below 100 and with a variety of executive planning and other deficits (Rutter *et al.*, 1998; Taylor & Sonuga-Barke, 2008; Frick & Nigg, 2012).

Dyslexia is associated with phonological and other related deficits evident in the preschool period (Lyytinen *et al.*, 2006; Snowling & Hulme, 2008). This would seem to be diagnostically distinctive but it has not been studied systematically in other diagnoses.

Schizophrenia is often preceded by mild language and motor impairments in the preschool years and by an IQ below 100 at all ages (Cannon *et al.*, 2002). These associations are not found in anxiety and depressive disorders and are much less evident in bipolar disorders. Thus, there is a substantial degree of diagnostic specificity. On the other hand, the impairments do not follow a recognizable pattern and, therefore, cannot be diagnostically useful at an individual level.

Childhood onset conduct/dissocial disorder is distinctive in its frequent persistence into adult life and lifecourse-persistent antisocial behavior is distinctive in its association with hyperactivity/impulsivity and developmental impairments (Moffitt *et al.*, 2001).

Children with a range of developmental disorders show an increased rate of tics. Thus, Kurlan *et al.* (2001) reported an increase in the prevalence of tic disorders in children in special educational settings. Conversely, children with tics tend to show deficits in visual-motor integration (Schultz *et al.*, 1998; Bloch *et al.*, 2006).

Biology

Severe/profound intellectual disability is the disorder with much the most distinctive biological features (Simonoff *et al.*, 1996). It is associated with a much reduced fecundity, gross neuropathological abnormalities, and with clinical brain disorders (such as cerebral palsy or epilepsy). None of these apply to mild intellectual disability.

Autism is associated with an increased rate of epilepsy (about 20–25%) as compared with the general population, but this does not differ from that found in intellectual disability. However, it does differ with respect to the age of onset of seizures being particularly in adolescence or early adult life (Volkmar & Nelson, 1990; Bolton *et al.*, 2011). Autism is also associated with an increased head size in the preschool years whereas intellectual disability is more often associated with a reduced head size (Woodhouse *et al.*, 1996; Fombonne *et al.*, 2001a).

There is much evidence that other mental disorders are associated with structural and functional brain imaging findings but, whereas these differentiate from normal, there is little or no evidence of diagnostic specificity. Accordingly, they provide little evidence on diagnostic validity. It seems curious to have so few examples of biology providing diagnostic validation. After all, there has been a huge increase in both the quantity and quality of neuroscience (Charney & Nestler, 2011), and this has given rise to many leads on possible biological validators. As already noted, however, most of the research has not included systematic comparisons of different diagnoses.

Validating criteria

Table 2.1 summarizes the findings on the extent to which seven possible criteria support distinctions among diagnostic categories. Three main points need to be made on the findings. First, some of the criteria do not necessarily reflect biological validation. Thus, this is clearly the case with epidemiological findings on age trends/sex differences and the findings on a long-term course. Nevertheless, they are included because they provide data that are likely to have important clinical implications. Second, the research has mainly focussed on categorical distinctions and hence less is known on the validity of the dimensions that have been shown to apply to many multifactorial mental

disorders. Third, the research has largely ignored the evidence on the frequently extensive overlap among diagnoses (as noted earlier in this chapter).

Nevertheless, despite these important limitations, there is quite extensive evidence on validating criteria and, as summarized in Table 2.2, these lead to reasonably robust conclusions. First, there are some nine diagnoses for which there is validating evidence of several different kinds and another half dozen for which there is some validating evidence from at least two different criteria. Second, there are at least half a dozen diagnostic categories for which the evidence suggests a lack of validity. This applies to the subcategorization of personality disorders, of anxiety disorders, of substance abuse disorders, of schizophrenia and of the differences between major depressive disorder and dysthymia, of the diagnosis of adjustment disorder, and of the grouping of nonspecific stress disorders. This lack of validating evidence does not necessarily mean that the diagnoses should be dropped from ICD-11 or DSM-5, but it does mean that the

Table 2.1 Possible validating criteria for different disorders.

	Epidemiology	Familiality	Psychosocial	Drug response	Cognitive impairment	Biology	Long term course
Autism	X	X		X	X	X	X
Schizophrenia	X	X	X		X		X
ADHD	X				X		X
Dyslexia	X				X		X
SLI	X				X		X
Dissocial with childhood onset	X	X					X
Eating disorders	X						
OCD/Tourette	X				X		
Bipolar	X						X
PTSD			X				
Disinhibition			X				
Rett	X					X	X
Substance abuse	X						
Severe intellectual disability	X					X	X
Conduct/dissocial disorder	X		X				X
Anxiety/depression		X					X

Table 2.2 Level of validating evidence for a range of disorders.

Relatively well validated	Some validating evidence	Some evidence suggesting lack of validity
Autism	Disinhibited social regulation	Adjustment disorder
Schizophrenia	Antisocial childhood onset	Subcategories of personality disorder
ADHD	Bipolar disorder	Subcategories of anxiety disorder
Dyslexia	Substance abuse	Differences among substance abuse disorders
Anxiety/depression	Conduct/dissocial disorder	Difference between major depressive disorder and dysthymia
Severe intellectual disability	Early disorders	Subcategories of schizophrenia
Rett		The grouping of non-specific stress disorders
OCD/tourette's		
SLI		

onus has to be placed on those who argue for their retention to demonstrate their utility for either clinical work or research. We return to this question when discussing the changes envisaged for DSM-5 and ICD-11.

"Lumping" or "splitting"

Passionate arguments have often been put in favor of "lumping" diagnoses into broader groupings or "splitting" them up according to many finer distinctions. There can be no single "right" answer on this because all depends on both the purpose of the classification and the type of disorders being considered. Thus, unlike DSM, ICD classifies all medical conditions. These include a large number of infectious and parasitic diseases. Although these share a range of common features, from both biological (scientific) perspectives and clinical usage, there must be much splitting to cover both the specific causative agent and the body organ affected. That does not apply to the multifactorial disorders that constitute most of mental disorders.

However, classifications of psychopathology have usually involved three different levels, and this applies to both ICD-11 and DSM-5. It is often assumed that validation data are strongest at the first broadest level, becoming progressively weaker with increasingly narrow levels. Nevertheless, this assumption is not correct. The first level concerns broad groupings of diagnoses—such as mood disorders and schizophrenia spectrum disorders. In ICD-10 and DSM-IV, these were constrained by the requirement to have only 10 groupings, and some of the clusters were very arbitrary in what they included and excluded. One of the best decisions of WHO, backed by the APA, was to allow more than 10 clusters, and to expect that, so far as possible, these should involve conceptual coherence. This led to the removal of a cluster of childhood onset disorders in view of the evidence that many disorders that largely manifest in adult life (such as schizophrenia) actually show their first manifestations in childhood. It also meant that conduct disorders and antisocial personal disorders were brought together into the same cluster. It has to be accepted that some clusters are less well validated than others. Thus, there are good reasons for having a cluster for obsessive-compulsive and other related disorders, but the evidence that body dysmorphic disorder should be included is less than desirable (Phillips *et al.*, 2010). Similarly, there were practical reasons for combining feeding disorders (such as pica) and eating disorders (such as anorexia nervosa) in the same cluster, despite the paucity of supporting validating evidence (Uher & Rutter, 2012b). Similarly, the grouping together of all elimination disorders is tidy but not well validated. It is evident that the breadth of grouping is not a good index of validity.

The second level is provided by the various specific diagnoses within each cluster. For example, the new cluster of neurodevelopmental disorders has, very reasonably, specific diagnoses for autism spectrum disorders and ADHD. As noted above, some of these are better validated than others. However, the

key concern over the separateness of diagnoses undermines the validity claim. For example, it is clear that both at the phenotypic level and causal influences level there is substantial overlap between ADHD and autism—with the reasons for it still obscure (Rutter, 2013).

The third level is provided by the subcategorization within specific diagnoses. For example, there is a cluster for "disruptive behavior disorders" and, within this cluster, there are separate diagnostic categories for oppositional/defiant disorder (ODD), conduct/dissocial disorder (CDD) and intermittent explosive disorder. At the third level, CDD is subdivided into those with a childhood onset and those in which the onset is in adolescence or adult life. As discussed above, in this case the subcategorization has some supporting validating evidence. The same applies to separation of social regulation disorder from reactive attachment disorder, as well as the split between severe and mild intellectual disability, and the separation of Rett syndrome from the rest of autism spectrum disorders. Some narrow diagnoses do have validating evidence. In other cases, the evidence is largely lacking (see Table 2.2).

In our view, this three level organizational structure provides a good approach and sets a sound agenda for future refinements but questions remain with respect to both the clusters and the individual diagnoses. Perhaps the greatest uncertainties concern the subcategorization. The fields of substance abuse and of personality disorders provide interesting examples of some of the issues at stake. In ICD-10, there is an overall, very large, cluster of mental and behavioral disorders due to psychoactive substance use. That seems appropriate in view of the public health importance of the disorders and the evidence of biological dysfunction. But why does the cluster not include abuse of other substances (such as steroids or antidepressants, which were placed in F55—a quite separate cluster) and why did it not include behavioral addictions (such as pathological gambling, which was coded as habit/impulse disorder, or internet addiction)? Why is the primary coding based on the drug used, rather than the disorder symptom pattern? Clearly, these questions have been asked by others and it appears that the lack of consensus probably reflects both the rigidity of the APA rules and the ideology and the apparent vested interests of some people in the field. In our view, there needs to be a total rethink on how best to deal with this grouping of disorders. It is essential that this is driven by empirical evidence. Hopefully, too, this should lead to a major reduction in the total number of disorders in this cluster.

The field of personality disorder is similar with respect to the need for some such grouping (because of its clinical importance) but it differs in the type of problems. First, there is such a huge frequency of co-occurrence of different personality disorders that it is quite uncommon for only one to be diagnosed. Second, there is a weak evidential basis for many of the separate diagnoses. Third, the approaches in DSM-IV and ICD-10 are rather different with the former using theoretical concepts (such as borderline personality disorder) and the latter mainly using trait features (such as anxious or paranoid). Once again, a total rethink is needed, focussing on empirical research findings—hopefully with a bringing together of the DSM and ICD approaches.

With respect to the overall issue of "lumping" or "splitting," the answer should be to have as many subdivisions as required for either clinical utility or scientific validity, but no more than is needed. In other words, the aim is to have as few subdivisions as essential for the purposes to which the classification is used, but that will vary according to the purpose intended. To take an obvious example, the classification for primary care use will have to have far fewer diagnoses than those used in tertiary care settings because detailed subdivisions will require more data than can be obtained in a brief primary care consultation.

Threshold for diagnosis

There are two rather separate issues with respect to thresholds. First, there is the question of whether or not impaired social functioning should be required. It was in DSM-IV but in ICD-10 it was not. Rather, impairment was coded separately, and the same is likely to apply in DSM-5 and ICD-11. The DSM justification is that certain diagnoses are much too frequent if impairment is not required; the most striking example is provided by phobias. The solution, however, should lie in the specifications for anxiety disorders rather than any overall rule. The ICD justification is that there needs to be a way of recognizing disorders that are well controlled through medication (or other means). Thus, schizophrenia does not cease to exist just because symptoms are well controlled through appropriate psychotropic medication. The parallel might be with well-controlled diabetes. Of course, this is more straightforward if there is some physiological (or other biological) test for the disorder. This would become easier in the field of psychopathology if biomarkers were able to live up to their potential (Rutter, 2014).

The second issue concerns how to deal with sub-syndromal patterns such as the broader autism phenotype and so-called prodromal schizophrenia. There is good evidence that such patterns are reasonably common, that they involve a substantial risk for the development of the traditional syndrome (i.e. autism and schizophrenia in the examples given), and that services are needed to provide interventions and reduce the risk for progression to the traditional syndrome. However, it would not be appropriate to have a diagnosis on the basis of the risk for some mental disorder in the future, particularly since only some are likely to progress to develop the traditional syndrome and by no means all warrant service provision. In our view, it is desirable to include diagnoses for these patterns provided that the criteria are explicit with respect to the severity required and provided the diagnosis is labeled as needing further testing. The latter requirement will be possible in ICD-11 but not in DSM-5 (because disorders needing testing are placed only in an appendix). It needs also to be recognized that there are possible

dangers in such syndromal diagnoses if the interventions used involve serious side-effects (as would be the case with some psychotropic medications). There may also be concerns that pharmaceutical companies will see the opportunity for new marketing that targets those who may not need treatment. It should be added that autism and schizophrenia are by no means the only examples. Closely similar issues apply in the fields of depression and of eating disorders, to which we would apply the same approach—that is, a firm requirement of adequate severity and a clear differentiation of risk profiles from profiles associated with manifest pathology.

For some critics, the provision of new diagnoses implies the medicalization of social problems. ADHD has often been targeted on this basis. However, this is wrong-headed on several different grounds. First, classifications are not restricted to medical diseases. Second, there is abundant evidence that ADHD and even some sub-syndromal problems are accompanied by major suffering that can be alleviated (at least in part) by appropriate treatment. Third, most psychiatric diagnoses are multifactorial and involve psychosocial causal influences to a varying extent. Fourth, there are strong reasons for including diagnoses that are predominantly precipitated by social experiences (as would be the case, for example, with what used to be called PTSD). Fifth, there is substantial evidence showing the biological embedding of psychosocial experiences (Rutter, 2012a).

Separate classifications in different countries

Some countries have wanted to have their own classifications rather than use either DSM or ICD. That would seem to jeopardize the main value of classification for communication among clinicians and researchers. On the other hand, it may be desirable for slight modifications of universal classifications in order to adapt them to fit in with local methods of working. However, when this is done, it is also essential to provide an explicit walkway between the classifications. There might also be a need for a separate classification to deal with supposedly culture-specific syndromes. However, these seem to be decidedly rare and the need is better met by appendices in universal classifications to indicate how to deal with the issue (as was the case in DSM-IV).

Staging or severity of disorders

Throughout medicine it is very common for dimensions to be used to specify either the staging of a disorder or its severity (see, e.g. such usage in the fields of cancer, cardiology and pulmonary medicine). In relation to childhood psychopathology, severity dimensions have been proposed for both language level and intellectual level in the diagnosis of autism spectrum disorders; there are also other examples. We see this as an important and clinically useful application of specifiers and it makes no sense that WHO has issued an edict that dimensions cannot be introduced into ICD-11.

DSM-5 and ICD-11

At the time of writing, while DSM-5 has been published, it will not be known for several years what ICD-11 will look like. Nevertheless, it is appropriate for us to comment on both the process of dealing with the revised classifications and some of the specifics. Regarding the process, it was foolish to prevent any scrutiny or critique of the existing classifications. As one of us has noted (Rutter & Uher, 2012; Rutter, 2012b, c), there are major problems with both ICD-10 and DSM-IV. For example, many diagnoses have rarely, if ever, been used and there are ridiculously high rates of co-occurrence. The way forward ought to have been to consider which inadequacies in the existing classifications required some kind of remedial action—but that is precisely what was forbidden. Second, well after the working groups were established, the APA set up a special committee to examine the scientific validity of new proposals. This was flawed from the start. If diagnoses were not included in DSM-IV in the new form, in most cases validity data were unlikely to be available. In addition, there was the further problem that the special committee was allowed only to comment on the specific working group proposals submitted, which often came piecemeal, preventing any assessment of the diagnostic proposals as a whole. Third, new diagnoses proposed for DSM-5 that required further testing had to be placed outside the main classification in an appendix that effectively prevented their use and, hence, their testing. Fourth, validity was seen as an essential deciding criterion without reference to either clinical usage or public health considerations (although these were added late in the process). Fifth, the DSM field trials were undertaken at a time that *preceded* decision on the diagnoses to be tested. Finally, harmonization between ICD and DSM was not treated as a priority (other than with respect to an early meeting on the clusters to be used).

Despite these serious reservations about the process, we need to go on to ask whether, nevertheless, DSM-5 and ICD-11 will be better than what existed before. The extension of the number of clusters available was certainly a really valuable change. It is also likely that a few anomalies will be corrected. However, at the time of writing, there is little evidence that the problems we have noted will have been dealt with; the number of diagnoses will similarly remain ridiculously large; and extensive co-occurrence of diagnoses will continue. We regret the lack of harmonization between DSM-5 and ICD-11.

As we have tried to explain in this chapter, for all its difficulties, classification is tremendously important, not just to enable effective communication, but because diagnoses constitute a passport to services and shape research approaches. Because both of us have been engaged in ICD-11 and DSM-5 discussions in the past, we have to share the guilt in not succeeding in doing more to make things better. The preparation for classification revisions provided a golden opportunity to move forward in an important

way. We regret, therefore, that, with a few important exceptions, that opportunity was not seized and acted upon.

References

Andreasen, N.C. (2007) DSM and the death of phenomenology in America: an example of unintended consequences. *Schizophrenia Bulletin* **33**, 108–112.

Angst, J. (2009) Course and prognosis of mood disorders. In: *New Oxford Textbook of Psychiatry*. (eds M.G. Gelder, *et al.*), 2nd edn. Oxford University Press, New York.

Baron-Cohen, S. (2002) The extreme male brain theory of autism. *Trends in Cognitive Sciences* **6**, 248–254.

Baron-Cohen, S. (2011) *Zero Degrees of Empathy: A New Theory of Human Cruelty*. Penguin, UK.

Bellani, M. *et al.* (2011) Language disturbances in ADHD. *Epidemiology and Psychiatric Sciences* **20**, 311–315.

Bloch, M.H. *et al.* (2006) Fine-motor skill deficits in childhood predict adulthood tic severity and global psychosocial functioning in Tourette's syndrome. *Journal of Child Psychology and Psychiatry* **47**, 551–559.

Bock, G. & Goode, J.E. (2004) *Autism: Neural Basis and Treatment Possibilities*. John Wiley & Sons, Chichester.

Bolton, P.F. *et al.* (2007) Obsessive-compulsive disorder, tics and anxiety in 6-year-old twins. *Psychological Medicine* **37**, 39–48.

Bolton, P.F. *et al.* (2011) Epilepsy in autism: features and correlates. *British Journal of Psychiatry* **198**, 289–294.

Bruce, J. *et al.* (2010) Disinhibited social behavior among internationally adopted children. *Development and Psychopathology* **21**, 157–171.

Buitelaar, J.K. (2003) Why have drug treatments been so disappointing? In: *Autism: Neural Basis and Treatment Possibilities, No. 251*. Novartis Foundation, John Wiley & Sons, Chichester.

Cannon, M. *et al.* (2002) Evidence for early-childhood, pan-developmental impairment specific to schizophreniform disorder: results from a longitudinal birth cohort. *Archives of General Psychiatry* **59**, 449–456.

Cantor-Graae, E. & Selten, J.P. (2005) Schizophrenia and migration: a meta-analysis and review. *American Journal of Psychiatry* **162**, 12–24.

Cantwell, D. (1975) A model for the investigation of psychiatric disorders of childhood: its application in genetic studies of the hyperkinetic syndrome. In: *Explorations in Child Psychiatry*. (ed E.J. Anthony). Plenum Press, New York.

Charney, D. & Nestler, E.E. (2011) *Neurobiology of Mental Illness*. Oxford University Press, New York.

Costello, E.J. *et al.* (2003) Relationships between poverty and psychopathology: a natural experiment. *JAMA* **290**, 2023–2029.

Craddock, N. & Owen, M.J. (2010) The Kraepelinian dichotomy–going, going … but still not gone. *British Journal of Psychiatry* **196**, 92–95.

Craft, M. *et al.* (1987) Lithium in the treatment of aggression in mentally handicapped patients: a double-blind trial. *British Journal of Psychiatry* **150**, 685–689.

Einfeld, S.L. (2001) Systematic management approach to pharmacotherapy for people with learning disabilities. *Advances in Psychiatric Treatment* **7**, 43–49.

Emslie, G.J. *et al.* (2004) Fluoxetine treatment for prevention of relapse of depression in children and adolescents: a double-blind, placebo-controlled study. *Journal of the American Academy of Child & Adolescent Psychiatry* **43**, 1397–1405.

Fergusson, D.M. & Horwood, L. (1995) Predictive validity of categorically and dimensionally scored measures of disruptive childhood behaviors. *Journal of the American Academy of Child & Adolescent Psychiatry* **34**, 477–487.

Flament, M.F. & Robaey, P. (2009) Obsessive-compulsive disorder and tics in children and adolescents. In: *New Oxford Textbook of Psychiatry.* (eds M.G. Gelder, *et al.*), 2nd edn. Oxford University Press, New York.

Fombonne, E. *et al.* (2001a) The Maudsley long-term follow-up of child and adolescent depression. 1. Psychiatric outcomes in adulthood. *British Journal of Psychiatry* **179**, 210–217.

Fombonne, E. *et al.* (2001b) The Maudsley long-term follow-up of child and adolescent depression. 2. Suicidality, criminality and social dysfunction in adulthood. *British Journal of Psychiatry* **179**, 218–223.

Franić, S. *et al.* (2010) Childhood and adolescent anxiety and depression: beyond heritability. *Journal of the American Academy of Child & Adolescent Psychiatry* **49**, 820–829.

Frick, P.J. & Nigg, J.T. (2012) Current issues in the diagnosis of attention deficit hyperactivity disorder, oppositional defiant disorder, and conduct disorder. *Annual Review of Clinical Psychology* **8**, 77–107.

Frith, U. (1989) *Autism: Explaining the Enigma.* Blackwell Publishing, Malden, Mass.

Geddes, J.R. *et al.* (2004) Long-term lithium therapy for bipolar disorder: systematic review and meta-analysis of randomized controlled trials. *American Journal of Psychiatry* **161**, 217–222.

Geller, B. *et al.* (1994) Rate and predictors of prepubertal bipolarity during follow-up of 6-to 12-year-old depressed children. *Journal of the American Academy of Child & Adolescent Psychiatry* **33**, 461–468.

Gershon, J. & Gershon, J. (2002) A meta-analytic review of gender differences in ADHD. *Journal of Attention Disorders* **5**, 143–154.

Gillihan, S. & Parens, E. (2011) Should we expect 'neural signatures' for DSM diagnoses? *Journal of Clinical Psychiatry* **72**, 1383–1389.

Happé, F. (1994) *Autism: An Introduction to Psychological Theory.* UCL Press Limited, London.

Happé, F. & Frith, U.E. (2010) *Autism and Talent.* Oxford University Press, Oxford.

Harrington, R. *et al.* (1990) Adult outcomes of childhood and adolescent depression. I. Psychiatric status. *Archives of General Psychiatry* **47**, 465–73.

Hazell, P. *et al.* (1995) Efficacy of tricyclic drugs in treating child and adolescent depression: a meta-analysis. *British Medical Journal* **310**, 897–901.

Hollis, C. (2008) Schizophrenia and allied disorders. In: *Rutter's Child and Adolescent Psychiatry.* (eds M. Rutter, *et al.*). Blackwell Publishing Ltd., Malden, Mass, & Oxford.

Howlin, P. *et al.* (2014) Cognitive and language skills in adults with autism: a 40 year follow-up. *Journal of Child and Psychology and Psychiatry* **55**, 49–58.

Hyde, L.W. *et al.* (2011) Understanding risk for psychopathology through imaging gene-environment interactions. *Trends in Cognitive Sciences* **15**, 417–427.

Hyman, S.E. (2007) Can neuroscience be integrated into the DSM-V? *Nature Reviews Neuroscience* **8**, 725–732.

Insel, T.R. & Wang, P.S. (2010) Rethinking mental illness. *JAMA* **303**, 1970–1971.

Insel, T.R. *et al.* (2010) Research domain criteria (RDoC): toward a new classification framework for research on mental disorders. *American Journal of Psychiatry* **167**, 748–751.

Jablensky, A. (2009) Course and outcome of schizophrenia and their prediction. In: *New Oxford Textbook of Psychiatry.* (eds M.G. Gelder, *et al.*), 2nd edn. Oxford University Press, New York.

Jefferson, J. (1990) Lithium: the present and the future. *Journal of Clinical Psychiatry* **51**, 4–8.

Jones, P.B. & Fung, W.L.A. (2005) Ethnicity and mental health: the example of schizophrenia in the African-Caribbean population in Europe. In: *Ethnicity and Causal Mechanisms.* (eds M. Rutter & M. Tienda). Cambridge University Press, New York.

Kendler, K.S. & Gardner, C.O. (1997) The risk for psychiatric disorders in relatives of schizophrenic and control probands: a comparison of three independent studies. *Psychological Medicine* **27**, 411–419.

Kendler, K.S. & Prescott, C.A. (2006) *Genes, Environment, and Psychopathology: Understanding the Causes of Psychiatric and Substance Use Disorders.* Guilford Press, New York.

Kendler, K.S. *et al.* (1998) The structure of psychosis: latent class analysis of probands from the Roscommon Family Study. *Archives of General Psychiatry* **55**, 492–499.

Kendler, K.S. *et al.* (2003) Specificity of genetic and environmental risk factors for use and abuse/dependence of cannabis, cocaine, hallucinogens, sedatives, stimulants, and opiates in male twins. *American Journal of Psychiatry* **160**, 687–695.

Kim-Cohen, J. *et al.* (2003) Prior juvenile diagnoses in adults with mental disorder: developmental follow-back of a prospective-longitudinal cohort. *Archives of General Psychiatry* **60**, 709–717.

Kolvin, I. (1971) Psychoses in childhood—a comparative study. In: *Infantile Autism: Concepts, Characteristics, and Treatment.* (ed M.E. Rutter). Churchill Livingstone, Edinburgh.

Kurlan, R. *et al.* (2001) Prevalence of tics in schoolchildren and association with placement in special education. *Neurology* **57**, 1383–1388.

Lahey, B.B. *et al.* (2011) Higher-order genetic and environmental structure of prevalent forms of child and adolescent psychopathology. *Archives of General Psychiatry* **68**, 181.

Larsson, H. *et al.* (2011) Developmental trajectories of DSM-IV symptoms of attention-deficit/hyperactivity disorder: genetic effects, family risk and associated psychopathology. *Journal of Child Psychology and Psychiatry* **52**, 954–963.

Le Couteur, A. *et al.* (1996) A broader phenotype of autism: the clinical spectrum in twins. *Journal of Child Psychology and Psychiatry* **37**, 785–801.

Leckman, J.F. *et al.* (2002) Obsessive-compulsive symptom dimensions in affected sibling pairs diagnosed with Gilles de la Tourette's syndrome. *American Journal of Medical Genetics Part B: Neuropsychiatric Genetics* **116**, 60–68.

Levinson, D.F. (2006) The genetics of depression: a review. *Biological Psychiatry* **60**, 84–92.

Lyytinen, H. *et al.* (2006) Trajectories of reading development: a follow-up from birth to school age of children with and without risk for dyslexia. *Merrill-Palmer Quarterly* **52**, 514–546.

Makita, K. (1966) The age of onset of childhood schizophrenia. *Psychiatry and Clinical Neurosciences* **20**, 111–121.

Mannuzza, S. *et al.* (1998) Adult psychiatric status of hyperactive boys grown up. *American Journal of Psychiatry* **155**, 493–498.

March, J. *et al.* (2004) Fluoxetine, cognitive-behavioral therapy, and their combination for adolescents with depression: treatment for

Adolescents With Depression Study (TADS) randomized controlled trial. *Journal of American Medical Association* **292**, 807–820.

McGrath, J. *et al.* (2004) A systematic review of the incidence of schizophrenia: the distribution of rates and the influence of sex, urbanicity, migrant status and methodology. *BMC Medicine* **2**, 13.

McGuffin, P. *et al.* (2003) The heritability of bipolar affective disorder and the genetic relationship to unipolar depression. *Archives of General Psychiatry* **60**, 497–502.

McMahon, S.D. *et al.* (2003) Stress and psychopathology in children and adolescents: is there evidence of specificity? *Journal of Child Psychology and Psychiatry* **44**, 107–133.

Merikangas, K.R. *et al.* (2010) Lifetime prevalence of mental disorders in US adolescents: results from the National Comorbidity Study-Adolescent Supplement (NCS-A). *Journal of the American Academy of Child and Adolescent Psychiatry* **49**, 980–989.

Meyer-Lindenberg, A. & Weinberger, D.R. (2006) Intermediate phenotypes and genetic mechanisms of psychiatric disorders. *Nature Reviews Neuroscience* **7**, 818–827.

Miles, T.R. *et al.* (1998) Gender ratio in dyslexia. *Annals of Dyslexia* **48**, 27–55.

Moffitt, T.E. (2005) Genetic and environmental influences on antisocial behaviors: evidence from behavioral–genetic research. *Advances in Genetics* **55**, 41–104.

Moffitt, T.E. *et al.* (2001) *Sex Differences in Antisocial Behaviour: Conduct Disorder, Delinquency, and Violence in the Dunedin Longitudinal Study*. Cambridge University Press, Cambridge.

Morsanyi, K. *et al.* (2012) Are systemizing and autistic traits related to talent and interest in mathematics and engineering? Testing some of the central claims of the empathizing–systemizing theory. *British Journal of Psychology* **103**, 472–496.

Moskvina, V. *et al.* (2008) Gene-wide analyses of genome-wide association data sets: evidence for multiple common risk alleles for schizophrenia and bipolar disorder and for overlap in genetic risk. *Molecular Psychiatry* **14**, 252–260.

Neul, J. (2011) Rett syndrome and MECP2-related disorders. In: *Autism Spectrum Disorders*. (eds D. Amaral, *et al.*). Oxford University Press, New York.

Pedersen, C.B. & Mortensen, P.B. (2001) Evidence of a dose–response relationship between urbanicity during upbringing and schizophrenia risk. *Archives of General Psychiatry* **58**, 1039–1046.

Phillips, K.A. *et al.* (2010) Should an obsessive–compulsive spectrum grouping of disorders be included in DSM-V? *Depression and Anxiety* **27**, 528–555.

Rapoport, J.L. *et al.* (1980) Dextroamphetamine: its cognitive and behavioral effects in normal and hyperactive boys and normal men. *Archives of General Psychiatry* **37**, 933–943.

Regier, D.A. *et al.* (2011) *The Conceptual Evolution of DSM-5*. American Psychiatric Association, Washington, DC.

Robins (1966) *Deviant Children Grown Up: A Sociological and Psychiatric Study of Sociopathic Personality*. Williams & Wilkins, Baltimore.

Robins, L. (1978) Sturdy childhood predictors of adult antisocial behaviour: replications from longitudinal studies. *Psychological Medicine* **8**, 611–622.

Robins, E. & Guze, S.B. (1970) Establishment of diagnostic validity in psychiatric illness: its application to schizophrenia. *American Journal of Psychiatry* **126**, 983–986.

Rutter, M. (1972) Childhood schizophrenia reconsidered. *Journal of Autism and Child Schizophrenia* **2**, 315–337.

Rutter, M. (1978) Diagnostic validity in child psychiatry. *Advances in Biological Psychiatry* **2**, 2–22.

Rutter, M. (1994) Comorbidity: meanings and mechanisms. *Clinical Psychology: Science and Practice* **1**, 100–103.

Rutter, M. (2006) Comorbidity: concepts, claims and choices. *Criminal Behaviour and Mental Health* **7**, 265–285.

Rutter, M. (2008) Autism and specific language impairments: a tantalizing dance. In: *Language Disorders in Children and Adults*. (eds V. Joffee, *et al.*). John Wiley & Sons, Chichester.

Rutter, M. (2012a) Achievements and challenges in the biology of environmental effects. *Proceedings of the National Academy of Sciences* **109**, 17149–17153.

Rutter, M. (2012b) Gene-environment interdependence. *European Journal of Developmental Psychology* **9**, 391–412.

Rutter, M. (2012c) Response to commentaries on discussion paper "gene-environment interdependence". *European Journal of Developmental Psychology* **9**, 426–431.

Rutter, M. (2013) Changing concepts and findings on autism. *Journal of Autism and Developmental Disorders* **43**, 1749–1757.

Rutter, M. (2014) Biomarkers: potential and challenges. In: *BioPrediction of Bad Behavior: Scientific, Ethical and Legal Challenges*. (eds I. Singh, *et al.*). Oxford University Press, Oxford, pp. 188–205.

Rutter, M. & Thapar, A. (2014) Genetics and autism. In: *Handbook of Autism and Pervasive Developmental Disorders. Assessment, Interventions, Policy and Future*. (eds F. Volkmar, *et al.*), 4th edn. John Wiley & Sons, Hoboken, NJ.

Rutter, M. & Uher, R. (2012) Classification issues and challenges in child and adolescent psychopathology. *International Review of Psychiatry* **24**, 514–529.

Rutter, M. *et al.* (1998) *Antisocial Behavior by Young People*. Cambridge University Press, New York.

Rutter, M. *et al.* (2003) Using sex differences in psychopathology to study causal mechanisms: unifying issues and research strategies. *Journal of Child Psychology and Psychiatry* **44**, 1092–1115.

Schultz, R.T. *et al.* (1998) Visual–motor integration functioning in children with Tourette's syndrome. *Neuropsychology* **12**, 134.

Shanahan, L. *et al.* (2008) Specificity of putative psychosocial risk factors for psychiatric disorders in children and adolescents. *Journal of Child Psychology and Psychiatry* **49**, 34–42.

Silberg, J. *et al.* (2014) Age of onset and the subclassification of conduct/dissocial disorder. *Journal of Child Psychology and Psychiatry*.

Simonoff, E. *et al.* (1996) Mental retardation: genetic findings, clinical implications and research agenda. *Journal of Child Psychology and Psychiatry* **37**, 259–280.

Snowling, M.J. & Hulme, C. (2008) Reading and other specific learning difficulties. In: *Rutter's Child and Adolescent Psychiatry*. (eds M. Rutter, *et al.*), 5th edn. Blackwell Press, Oxford.

Souza, F. & Goodwin, G. (1991) Lithium treatment and prophylaxis in unipolar depression: a meta-analysis. *British Journal of Psychiatry* **158**, 666–675.

Swales, J.D. (1985) *Platt Versus Pickering: An Episode in Recent Medical History*. Keynes Press, London.

Taylor, E. & Sonuga-Barke, E. (2008) Disorders of attention and activity. In: *Rutter's Child and Adolescent Psychiatry*. (eds M. Rutter, *et al.*), 5th edn. Blackwell Publishing, Oxford.

Tondo, L. *et al.* (2001) Long-term clinical effectiveness of lithium maintenance treatment in types I and II bipolar disorders. *British Journal of Psychiatry* **178**, s184–s190.

Tyrer, S.P. (1994) Lithium and treatment of aggressive behaviour. *European Neuropsychopharmacology* **4**, 234–236.

Uher, R. & Rutter, M. (2012a) Basing psychiatric classification on scientific foundation: problems and prospects. *International Review of Psychiatry* **24**, 591–605.

Uher, R. & Rutter, M. (2012b) Classification of feeding and eating disorders: review of evidence and proposals for ICD-11. *World Psychiatry* **11**, 80–92.

Van Os, J. *et al.* (2010) The environment and schizophrenia. *Nature* **468**, 203–212.

Vassos, E. *et al.* (2012) Meta-analysis of the association of urbanicity with schizophrenia. *Schizophrenia Bulletin* **38**, 1118–1123.

Volkmar, F.R. & Nelson, D.S. (1990) Seizure disorders in autism. *Journal of the American Academy of Child & Adolescent Psychiatry* **29**, 127–129.

Weissman, M.M. *et al.* (1999) Children with prepubertal-onset major depressive disorder and anxiety grown up. *Archives of General Psychiatry* **56**, 794–801.

Woodhouse, W. *et al.* (1996) Head circumference in autism and other pervasive developmental disorders. *Journal of Child Psychology and Psychiatry* **37**, 665–71.

World Health Organization (1992) *The ICD-10 Classification of Mental and Behavioural Disorders. Clinical Descriptions and Diagnostic Guidelines.* World Health Organization, Geneva.

Zeanah, C.H. & Gleason, M.M. (2011) *Reactive Attachment Disorder: A Review for DSM-V.* American Psychiatric Association, Washington, DC.

Zubin, J. (1967) Classification of the behavior disorders. *Annual Review of Psychology* **18**, 373–406.

CHAPTER 3

Neurodevelopmental disorders

Anita Thapar[1] and Michael Rutter[2]

[1]Child and Adolescent Psychiatry Section, Institute of Psychological Medicine and Clinical Neurosciences, Cardiff University School of Medicine, Cardiff University, UK

[2]Social, Genetic and Developmental Psychiatry (SGDP) Research Centre, Institute of Psychiatry, Psychology and Neuroscience, King's College London, UK

In this chapter we begin by considering what disorders have been classified as neurodevelopmental and why. In DSM-5 and (probably) the forthcoming ICD-11, specific learning disorders (involving reading, writing, and arithmetic), motor disorders, communication disorders, autism spectrum disorder (ASD), attention deficit/hyperactivity disorder (ADHD), intellectual disability (ID) and tic disorders are all placed in a neurodevelopmental cluster. We consider the rationale and discuss both the concept of comorbidity and the hypothesis of "maturational" lag. Detailed descriptions of specific disorders and appropriate interventions are covered in the disorder chapters of this book.

Neurodevelopmental disorders (which show a frequent co-occurrence) can be considered to involve impaired development of cognitive or motor functions manifest from childhood that have a steady course without marked remissions or relapses, but tend to lessen with increasing age. Neurodevelopmental disorders may also involve aberrant functioning. Neurodevelopmental disorders, whilst defined as categories for clinical purposes, can also be viewed as quantitative dimensions (see Chapter 2).

The classification of neurodevelopmental disorders

As discussed by Rutter and Pine in Chapter 2, it is usual in diagnostic classification systems to have several levels of information, and both ICD-11 and DSM-5 are no exception to that. However, there is one very important difference between new classifications and the old. The decision that the overall number of diagnostic groupings or clusters need *not* be restricted to ten means it has been possible to have a more logical conceptualization of each cluster. It is in that spirit that we review the issues and findings with respect to neurodevelopmental disorders.

Rispens *et al.* (1998) have provided a useful historical overview of how neurodevelopmental disorders have been dealt with in classification systems. It was noted that the concept of specific developmental disorders was first used as a generic term that denoted delays in a broad variety of areas of development but that later, disorders such as hyperactivity, enuresis and tics were excluded, with specific developmental disorders being used as a higher order concept uniting impairments in the domains of language, scholastic skills and motor coordination. This group of specific neurodevelopmental disorders was initially put on a separate axis (although that is not the case now) on the grounds that they differed from the general run of psychopathological conditions in three key respects: (1) an onset that is invariably during infancy or childhood; (2) an impairment or delay in the development of functions that are strongly related to biological maturation of the central nervous system; and (3) a steady course that does not involve the remissions and the relapses that tend to be characteristic of many mental disorders. In keeping with these criteria, impairments in most neurodevelopmental disorders tend to lessen as the children grow older, although deficits often continue into adult life.

Harris (1995) has conceptualized neurodevelopmental disorders differently to include single gene disorders such as the Prader–Willi syndrome or disorders deriving from prenatal insults or toxins such as the fetal alcohol syndrome. At first sight, it might be thought that they have much in common with the narrower concept because they usually have neural impairment, involve cognitive deficits of various kinds and are characterized by a steady course without remissions or relapses. However, a grouping based on such a mixed bag of genetic and environmental causes does not seem to be helpful. Accordingly, we have excluded conditions that are not multifactorial in origin because there is a separate category for them in ICD-11 if the distinctive behavioral pattern is *wholly* due to a medical

Rutter's Child and Adolescent Psychiatry, Sixth Edition.
Edited by Anita Thapar and Daniel S. Pine, James F. Leckman, Stephen Scott, Margaret J. Snowling, Eric Taylor.
© 2015 John Wiley & Sons Ltd. Published 2018 by John Wiley & Sons Ltd.

condition classified elsewhere (usually this would be in the neurology section).

In addition to disorders of language, scholastic skills and motor function, the neurodevelopmental cluster in DSM-5 and ICD-11 now includes ID. Intellectual Disability had not been included in earlier concepts because of the importance placed on functioning that was discrepant with mental age. That has not proved a useful approach and therefore it is entirely reasonable to include ID in this cluster. The cluster also includes ASD and ADHD. They differ in not reflecting a straightforward impairment in a development-based skill that is closely related to biological maturation (e.g., motor skills) and both involve deviant functioning as much as impaired functioning. On the other hand, they have been included in this cluster because they share with the other disorders the fact that they are multifactorial in origin, are present from early life, tend to improve with increasing age but are also associated with disordered functioning that extends right into adult life. Both show a marked male preponderance. In addition, they are characterized by neuropsychological impairments of various kinds. They also often co-occur with the specific disorders of language, learning and motor function. It is a matter of judgment, but their placement in the neurodevelopmental cluster is probably more appropriate than elsewhere. It could be argued that ADHD ought to be in a cluster dealing with disruptive behavior but it does not fit well there overall.

It is not quite so obvious that tic disorders belong in this cluster but they show strong associations with other neurodevelopmental disorders (especially ADHD and, to a lesser extent, ASD) and are more common in males. Possibly, too, there may be an overlap in the rare copy number variants associated with ASD and with Tourette's syndrome (Fernandez *et al.*, 2012). Tic disorders tend to wax and wane in severity, may change in nature and can be episodic (see Chapter 56). Accordingly, they are not a really good fit into the cluster of neurodevelopmental disorders but they are probably more satisfactorily placed there than elsewhere.

Finally, neurodevelopmental impairment has been well demonstrated in relation to schizophrenia and, to a lesser extent, it has also been found to be associated with childhood onset conduct disorder. However, both fluctuate over time, they are not particularly associated with biological maturation, and there is more limited co-occurrence with other neurodevelopmental disorders. Accordingly, in our view, it is best for them to be placed elsewhere but with the proviso that the association with neurodevelopmental impairment is recognized as an important aspect of the liability. Thus, schizophrenia is placed in the psychoses cluster and conduct disorder in a disruptive behavior cluster.

Concepts of maturational lag and of plateaus in developmental progress

The concept of maturational lag derives from the extensive evidence that there are huge individual differences in the timing of virtually all developmental functions. This is evident in relation to the timing of the eruption of teeth, the ossification of bones, and the growth spurt associated with puberty. There may well be psychological consequences of unusually early or unusually late maturation but early differences in the tempo of growth are, for the most part, not associated with any differences in outcome (Tanner, 1989). In other words, there is, ultimately, developmental catch-up. There is a similar variation in the age of first acquisition of language (Conti-Ramsden *et al.*, 2012). The question is whether children who are unusually slow to speak can, nevertheless, catch up completely. This has been studied in several different ways.

First, Bishop and Edmundson (1987) undertook a prospective longitudinal study of 87 language-impaired children who were assessed at the ages of 4, 4½, and 5½ years. Excluding those with impaired nonverbal ability, it was found that just over two-fifths showed normal language at 5½ years. These children would seem to have shown maturational lag with a full catch-up. A later follow-up at 15–16 years (Stothard *et al.*, 1998) showed that the children whose language problems had resolved by 5½ did not differ from controls on tests of vocabulary and language comprehension skills. Nevertheless, they performed significantly less well on tests of phonological processing and literary skills—suggesting that the catch-up was by no means fully complete. Those who had still got significant language difficulties at 5½ fell further behind in their language functioning over the follow-up period.

When considering the maturational lag hypothesis more generally in relation to neurodevelopmental impairments, it is clear that, although there is a general tendency for gains in function to be seen with increasing age, nevertheless, delayed early development is not usually followed by later normal functioning (Rutter *et al.*, 2006). Stanovich (1986) suggested that the answer in relation to reading might lie in a so-called "Matthew effect" whereby poor readers get worse and good readers get better as a result of literary experience boosting further language and literacy development. A key paper in that connection is one by Francis *et al.* (1996) who compared individual growth curves of 69 children with a reading disability and 334 without a reading problem. Nine yearly longitudinal assessments showed that both groups tended to plateau at about 13 years of age, with no narrowing or expansion of the gap between the groups. The difference in level, but not in trajectory, runs counter to the Matthew effect. On the other hand, there are circumstances in which an early advantage can lead to learning opportunities that have a lasting impact (Gladwell, 2008); an example is provided by the observation that outstanding sportsmen were disproportionately likely to have been born in the early part of the year. This meant that they were more likely to be selected for special coaching and this intensive special coaching led on to later increased athletic prowess.

Another key study is the Manchester language study undertaken by Conti-Ramsden *et al.* (2012), in which verbal and nonverbal skills were assessed in 242 children with a history of specific language impairment, with later assessments of both types of skills at 7, 8, 11, 14, 16, and 17 years. They found that the developmental trajectories for language skills were generally flat over the age period studied. The nonverbal trajectories showed more individual variation and clear evidence of a slowing down in the growth of nonverbal skills in childhood to adolescence was evident in nearly one-third of the sample.

It may be concluded that the concept of a maturational lag applies to some mild specific language impairments in the preschool years but, even with this group, follow-up has shown that the recovery in some cases was less complete than originally seemed to be the case. By contrast, the concept of maturational lag does not have support with respect to more severe degrees of specific language impairment or reading. Thus, the evidence has not been supportive of a maturational lag with respect to changes after the age of 5 years and was not supportive when the overall picture of functioning was taken into account (including nonverbal as well as verbal skills).

Although the "Matthew effect" may be relevant with respect to highly intensive input, it seems much less likely to be relevant to more ordinary circumstances. The concept of maturational lag stimulated a study documenting changes in cortical thickness over time in children with ADHD, with evidence of normalization in children who had a good outcome, but not in the remainder (Shaw et al., 2006, 2007). Whilst this suggests that some of the brain changes in children with the best outcomes may constitute a maturational lag, that does not apply to the remainder. In addition, however, the normalization could reflect the effects of stimulant medication, or sex differences, or the 35% attrition rate, or the lack of clinical measures in controls (making it impossible to study behavioral change in both groups). Also, the findings on cortical surface area and gyrification provided a somewhat more nuanced picture (Shaw et al., 2012a, b). Furthermore, the ADHD participants were atypical in their high IQ, socially advantaged background and lack of comorbidities (apart from OCD).

Wright and Zecker (2004) have suggested that one possible explanation for the plateauing of functions (with respect to language and literacy problems) stems from the decline in neuroplasticity associated with the onset of puberty. The problem with this explanation is that brain development continues well after the onset of puberty, with higher order association areas maturing only after lower order somatosensory and visual areas (Gogtay et al., 2004, see Chapter 9). Also, as Tanner (1989) pointed out years ago, the timings of development in different functions (such as bone ossification, dental eruption, and growth spurt) are only weakly associated with each other.

In the past, although it was appreciated that neurodevelopmental disorders were not due to some acquired brain lesion, there has been a tendency to suppose that the deficits may reflect something equivalent. Karmiloff-Smith and her colleagues (Karmiloff-Smith et al., 2012; Karmiloff-Smith & Farran, 2012) have argued, on the basis of empirical evidence, that static models of adult brain lesions cannot be used to account for the dynamics of change in neurodevelopmental disorders. So far, there has been rather limited research on age-related changes in the manifestations of neurodevelopmental disorders but

that remains an important task for the future. The changing presentation of neurodevelopmental disorders over time are considered in the chapters on clinical syndromes (see also Chapter 1).

Concept of comorbidity and patterns of co-occurrence within the group of neurodevelopmental disorders

The term "comorbidity" has been very widely used in the literature—both scientific and clinical—but the term is often wrongly used. Comorbidity refers to the situation in which two or more separate and independent disorders are present in the same person. This could be either at the same time or it could be sequential over time. That is not the same as the co-occurrence of different symptom patterns because such co-occurrence may have several other, quite different, meanings (Caron & Rutter, 1991; Rutter, 1997).

Disorders include a diverse mixture of symptoms and many co-occurrences are likely to reflect this diversity. Whilst the neurodevelopmental disorders do not have overlapping diagnostic criteria, apparent comorbidity might arise if disorders that are defined by a main problem or symptom group are artificially subdivided. Thus, for example, both specific language impairment and reading disability comprise disorders of language. The former refers to spoken language and the latter to written language but to consider their co-occurrence in the same person as true comorbidity would not make sense. Also, although reading disability and a mathematical disability differ in important respects and are conceptually distinct, it is relatively common for children to have both (see, e.g., Geary, 1993).

Similar issues apply outside neurodevelopmental disorders, such as the co-occurrence observed among the different anxiety disorders (Kessler et al., 2010) and between the various personality disorders (Lamont & Brunero, 2009). In both cases, co-occurrence across diagnostic categories is extraordinarily frequent. The situation with respect to substance use disorders is even more pronounced. Polydrug use is widespread (Darke & Hall, 1995), yet this has not been recognized adequately in classification systems.

The situation with respect to the co-occurrence of autism and ADHD is a bit different. That there is much more co-occurrence than used to be recognized is clear (see Rutter & Thapar, 2014). This is a situation in which one might want to code both as diagnoses because of the prognostic and therapeutic implications, but the overlap may involve sub threshold disorders in both cases (e.g., Clark et al., 1999; Thede & Coolidge, 2007). One of the basic problems in considering co-occurrence of disorders is that, although there is reasonably good validating evidence for many diagnoses (including autism and ADHD) there is not clear separation of disorders in the way that is supposed to have been the case, for example, in terms of there being distinctive sets of risk factors and correlates (see Chapter 2).

ICD-11 and DSM-5 differ somewhat in their approach to the co-occurrence of disorders. DSM-5 has a few mixed categories when there is good evidence that they both represent a single disorder (e.g., mixed episode of mania and depression). However, the forthcoming ICD-11 has rather more mixed categories. The rationale is that the same disorder commonly gives rise to the particular mixture of symptoms. Nevertheless, the overall placement of the combination category in the classification system carries messages that may be misleading. We doubt whether that is much of a problem in the field of neurodevelopmental disorders.

The big difference between ICD and DSM lies in the approach to mixed symptom patterns that are not covered by a combination category. ICD-11, like its predecessor, implies that a profile recognition or prototypic approach is to be followed. This probably closely approximates ordinary clinical practice that involves making a diagnosis on the basis of pattern recognition but it is quite difficult to make the prototype sufficiently explicit so that they will always be used in the same way. With DSM-5, the mixture of two or more symptom patterns leads to the coding of as many diagnoses as there are patterns. This has the advantage of not requiring hierarchical judgments and of retaining a good deal of information when many patterns are present and no single category would convey them all, but it encourages an unchallenged assumption that the patterns are, indeed, truly independent, and that each can be dealt with in the same way as if there were no other problems. Coexistence of many diagnoses is undoubtedly confusing and works against the key purpose of clarity and an understanding of how the research literature may apply to a particular child. In addition, it is implausible to expect a clinician to review the presence or absence of every possible category and clinicians have been found to vary a good deal in their willingness to record symptom patterns that are not the main presentation (Rutter *et al.*, 1975).

Comorbidity is not specific to neurodevelopmental disorders or psychiatry and is not purely explained by referral bias. It is well recognized in the general medical literature that a substantial proportion of the population, especially those who are more socially disadvantaged, have two or more chronic physical diseases, a phenomenon that is often referred to as "multi-morbidity" (Barnett *et al.*, 2012; Guthrie *et al.*, 2012). The importance and practical implications of multi-morbidities are beginning to be recognized in general medicine because there is emerging evidence that it is common, not simply restricted to older individuals and has an impact on the degree of functional impairment and treatment decisions. For example, when high blood pressure (hypertension) occurs in the presence of diabetes mellitus, it is now recommended that the threshold for treatment is adjusted to a lower level (Barengo & Tuomilehto, 2012). It is being highlighted as a problem that health care organizations and treatment guidelines remain mainly geared toward single disease/disorder approaches when there is a need to explicitly take into account multi-morbidity. The same issues apply to co-morbid neurodevelopmental disorders, although as

yet there are no parallels in terms of adjusted treatment guidelines. It seems plausible however that thresholds for functional impairment and treatment for a given neurodevelopmental disorder might be lowered by the presence of a full-blown or sub-threshold comorbid condition.

There are several different explanatory models of supposed concurrent comorbidity (see Caron & Rutter, 1991) that include the contribution of shared or correlated risk factors to different disorders, as well as there being common or overlapping neural and molecular mechanisms (see Figure 3.1). It is also

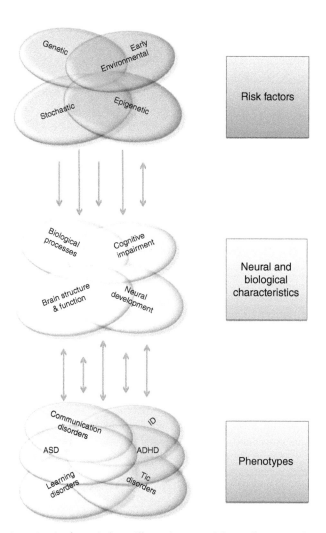

Figure 3.1 A schematic figure illustrating potential contributions to the overlap between different neurodevelopmental disorders. Clinical phenotypes as conceptualized diagnostically overlap with each other. Variation in clinical phenotypes can be conceptualized at a different phenotypic level involving "neural and biological characteristics" (e.g., variation in brain structure and function). These phenotypes can be influenced by genetic and environmental risk factors and stochastic factors that include random occurrences or insults. Epigenetic changes (see Chapter 25) involve biological modifications of the genome that can reflect early environmental exposures, DNA sequence and stochastic factors and can in turn be later modified by later experiences shaped by individual phenotype.

well recognized that neurodevelopmental disorders can be followed by new-onset psychiatric disorders later on in life that include depression and more rarely by serious forms of mental disorder such as schizophrenia and bipolar disorder (e.g., Hutton *et al.*, 2008; Galanter & Leibenluft, 2008). Later antisocial behavior/conduct disorder, criminality and substance misuse appear to be more characteristically associated with ADHD rather than typifying the developmental course of the other neurodevelopmental disorders.

Sequential comorbidity could represent different manifestations of the same underlying disease liability at different ages or represent distinctive disorders that show comorbidity because of shared risks and mechanisms. It could also mean that some subforms of neurodevelopmental disorders in some individuals are actually the early precursors of illness such as schizophrenia and bipolar disorder, especially early onset cases (see disorder chapters). However, most people with neurodevelopmental disorders do not develop such illnesses and the neurodevelopmental problems are also not "replaced" by these second disorders. Links between neurodevelopmental disorders and later onset psychiatric disorders could also arise from psychosocial risks created by specific features of these early neurodevelopmental problems. For example, early neurodevelopmental impairments could create or influence stressors such as peer rejection, social isolation, parental hostility and academic failure that in turn might play a contributory role in unmasking liability for a new later onset psychiatric disorder (see Chapter 12). Evidence on this possibility, however, is mainly lacking.

The co-occurrence of different neurodevelopmental disorders due to shared risks and biological characteristics

Genetics

All of the neurodevelopmental disorders are highly heritable (Thapar *et al.*, 1999; Stromswold, 2001; Deary *et al.*, 2009; O'Rourke *et al.*, 2009; Willcutt *et al.*, 2010; Ronald & Hoekstra, 2011) and shared genetic risks (see Chapter 24) contribute to much of their co-occurrence. Although most of the genetic liability appears to be shared across different neurodevelopmental disorders and traits, there are also disorder-specific influences and the liability extends to disorders outside the neurodevelopmental cluster (Lahey *et al.*, 2011).

For example, the average genetic correlation (meaning the part of the trait correlation that is genetically mediated) between reading and language, reading and mathematics, and language and mathematics is around 0.70 (Haworth & Plomin, 2010). The genetic correlation between ASD and ADHD dimensions is similarly high, estimated at between 0.54 and 0.87 (Ronald *et al.*, 2008; Lichtenstein *et al.*, 2010). It is the inattentive aspects of ADHD that show the most prominent genetic overlap with

reading disability and arithmetic disability (e.g., Paloyelis *et al.*, 2010; Willcutt, *et al.*, 2010; Greven *et al.*, 2011; Greven *et al.*, 2012). Genetic liability for ASD similarly appears to confer broader risks of language and learning impairments in relatives of those affected; what is known as the broader autism phenotype (Rutter & Thapar, 2014). Shared genetic risks again explain much of the covariation between IQ and other neurodevelopmental phenotypes, for example between IQ and ADHD and between IQ and ASD traits (Hoekstra *et al.*, 2010; Ronald & Hoekstra, 2011). In one Scandinavian twin study that simultaneously assessed a broader set of neurodevelopmental categories, shared genetic risks were found to contribute to ADHD, ASD and motor co-ordination problems, as well as tics (Lichtenstein *et al.*, 2010).

Much the same conclusions derive from molecular genetic studies. For example, one variety of genetic mutation, large rare copy number variants (subtle chromosomal deletions and duplications; CNVs), is associated with multiple different types of neurodevelopmental disorders that include ASD, ADHD, and ID (Guilmatre *et al.*, 2009; Williams *et al.*, 2010; Sullivan *et al.*, 2012a, b; Thapar *et al.*, 2013) and also a broader range of disorders outside the neurodevelopmental cluster, notably schizophrenia and epilepsy. Another example of shared genetic risks influencing multiple neurodevelopmental disorders is provided by *CNTNAP2*, a gene that has been implicated in ASD, severe ID and speech and language problems (Peñagarikano & Geschwind, 2012).

The finding that genetic influences are uninformative on the grouping of neurodevelopmental disorders arises from several different considerations. First, most genes are pleiotropic (see Chapter 24). The original notion that each gene affects just one protein with a single effect has proved mistaken. Second, genes affect proteins and not psychiatric categories. There will be effects on disorders, but these are likely to arise from influences on biological pathways that lead to disorder only indirectly. Third, it has been found that different diagnostic categories are not as separate as had once been thought (see Chapter 2; also, Sullivan *et al.*, 2012a, b; Cross-Disorder Group of the Psychiatric Genomics Consortium, 2013; Hamshere *et al.*, 2013a, b; Lahey *et al.*, 2011).

Environmental influences

The same issues, including lack of diagnostic specificity, apply to environmental influences (McMahon *et al.*, 2003). However, there are two disorders that may be considered neurodevelopmental (namely disinhibited disorder of social regulation and quasi-autism) which do show a relatively specific association with institutional deprivation (see Chapter 58). Institutional deprivation that persists beyond the age of 6 months has been found to be associated with a major adverse effect on head growth (and therefore, by implication, brain growth). This applied to institutional deprivation that was unaccompanied by subnutrition, as indexed by body weight

(Sonuga-Barke *et al.*, 2010). Both quasi-autism and disinhibited disorder of social regulation had an association with institutional deprivation that was as strong at 15 years as it had been at 11 years and before that at 6 years and 4 years. Moreover, both disorders showed a strong degree of persistence, with use of professional services, at least up to early adult life.

Shared biological and neural characteristics

There is growing interest in the extent to which early epigenetic changes (see Chapter 25) are involved in the pathogenesis of different neurodevelopmental disorders, given that they are subject to alteration by prenatal and early life exposures (Relton & Davey Smith, 2010), as well as by inherited genes. Epigenetic mechanisms might also help explain how the same sets of risk factors/liabilities result in different clinical features. For example, one genome-wide methylation study of monozygotic twins (who carry the same sets of genetic risk factors) with autism found that patterns of methylation (implying different levels of gene expression) differed between affected and unaffected twins from discordant pairs (Wong *et al.*, 2014).

The cognitive deficits that are common in neurodevelopmental disorders (e.g., Rommelse *et al.*, 2011; Taylor *et al.*, 2012) are observable by early-mid childhood and tend to affect multiple cognitive domains (e.g., executive dysfunction, social cognition) and have often been found to be associated with alterations in brain structure and function (e.g., Cherkasova & Hechtman, 2009; Caylak, 2009; Rykhlevskaia *et al.*, 2009; Anagnostou & Taylor, 2011; Kaufmann *et al.*, 2011; see disorder chapters). Although some cognitive and imaging features are considered to be highly characteristic of one disorder (e.g., impaired theory of mind in ASD or response inhibition in ADHD; Rutter, 2011; Crosbie *et al.*, 2013), there are recognized and prominent overlaps with certain types of deficits crossing diagnostic boundaries (e.g., Rommelse *et al.*, 2011). Cognitive deficits are not however a distinctive feature of neurodevelopmental disorders alone. They characterize many different psychiatric disorders, including the most severe forms of mental illness.

The co-occurrence among neurodevelopmental disorders, shared cognitive and neural features, as well as common genetic risks highlights the possibility of there being overlapping biological processes. Findings from genetic studies have begun to be integrated with knowledge of systems level biology to examine what sorts of shared and unique biological and molecular mechanisms underpin different neurodevelopmental conditions (e.g., Cristino *et al.*, 2014). For example, studies of autism have highlighted genes involved in synapse formation and maintenance and chromatin regulators that are essential for developmental processes, including those involving the brain (Ben-David & Shifman, 2012). The same biological processes have also been implicated as being involved in ID. A number of studies have now highlighted biological commonalities between ASD, ID and ADHD, as well as with schizophrenia.

Important patterns of difference between these disorders are also being observed (e.g., Guilmatre *et al.*, 2009; Cristino *et al.*, 2014). Biological differences between neurodevelopmental disorders would be expected even from already well-established knowledge on medication. Whilst stimulants are effective for ADHD symptoms, they do not help ASD or tics. Antipsychotic medications, although helpful in reducing tics, are not effective in the treatment of core features of ADHD or ASD (see disorder chapters). A recent meta-analysis (Weisman *et al.*, 2013) suggested that alpha-2 agonists were beneficial in treating tics in patients with ADHD but not in those without ADHD.

Sex differences

A striking and consistent feature of neurodevelopmental disorders is that they tend to show a male excess. Specific arithmetical problems may be different in this regard (but see Landerl & Moll, 2010 for a listing of contradictory reports). Whilst the imbalanced gender ratio is more pronounced in those referred to services, it is still evident in population-based studies, and thus not simply explained by an artifact of clinical recognition or referral to services (Lichtenstein *et al.*, 2010). Despite being an established observation, the reasons for a male excess remain unknown (Rutter *et al.*, 2003). What is striking, however, is that male preponderance is mainly a feature of early onset neurodevelopmental disorders, whereas female preponderance is mainly found with adolescent or adult onset emotional or eating disorders. The marked contrast is very likely to have a biological substrate, although what that is remains unidentified.

Three levels of causes have to be considered (Rutter *et al.*, 2003). First, the distal basic starting point has to implicate some aspect of the genetic difference between males and females. Nevertheless, of themselves, the genetic distinctions do not provide an explanation for the sex differences in mental disorders. Is this because genetic variation on a sex chromosome is associated with a risk variable, because of a hormonal effect, or because males are more exposed to, or are more vulnerable to, environmental stressors? These intermediate consequences constitute the second level of causes. There then has to be a third level in which additional proximal risk or protective factors are more directly involved. To explain the sex difference, these proximal features must meet three criteria: (1) evidence that the risk factors do indeed differ between males and females; (2) evidence that within each sex they provide risk for, or protection against, particular disorders; and (3) evidence that when their effect is included in a causal model, they either reduce or eliminate the sex difference. No variables have met all these criteria, but see Moffitt *et al.* (2001) for an approach to this research strategy.

A focus on these different causal levels can be instructive. For example, Angold (2008) showed that the greater underlying liability to depression in females was a function of sex hormone levels but the hormones did not act to provoke the onset of depression. It might be thought that the pubertal surge of male sex hormones would lead to an increased male preponderance of antisocial disorders in adolescence, but, in fact, the rise in adolescence tends to be greater in females (Moffitt *et al.*, 2001).

A polygenic liability threshold model (meaning one based on multiple genes working dimensionally, with disorder manifest only above a certain threshold) provides another framework for considering sex differences (Falconer, 1965). According to this model, gender differences should be explicable on the basis of differing thresholds for males and females and affected females should require a higher polygenic loading to show the disorder if the phenotype occurs less commonly in females. There is some supporting evidence in the case of ADHD and ASD (Hamshere *et al.*, 2013a, b; Rhee and Waldman, 2004; Szatmari *et al.*, 2012). However, the opposite pattern was found with specific language impairment (SLI) (Conti-Ramsden *et al.*, 2007). There are, as yet, too few data for any general conclusions on the validity of polygenic liability threshold models. There has also been a growing interest in the possible contributions of sexually dimorphic patterns of gene expression (see Chapter 25; also Jessen and Auger, 2011) but further evidence is required to consider the possibility.

We urge that systematic research into sex differences in psychopathology should be a priority, and this need extends well beyond neurodevelopmental disorders. An understanding of the causes of the sex differences may provide a crucial understanding of the causal processes for mental disorders within each sex. Of course it cannot be assumed that the mechanisms involved in the difference between groups (in this case the two sexes) will be identical with the mechanisms responsible for individual differences within each group but, equally, it would be foolhardy to assume that this will necessarily be different. Systematic testing of both possibilities is required.

Does neurodevelopmental impairment have the same meaning in all disorders?

In our introduction to this chapter we considered the commonalities among disorders in the neurodevelopmental cluster. We turn now to the opposite question—namely, possible heterogeneity. The first sub grouping comprises learning and language disorders because these constitute the prototype of disorders that are distinctive in being accompanied by cognitive impairments, associated with biological maturation, tending to improve with increasing age, and lacking the remissions and relapses that are a feature of most multifactorial mental disorders. In these disorders, the neurodevelopmental impairment constitutes an intrinsic part of the disorder.

ID is generally classed as a learning disorder but it differs markedly from reading disorder and mathematics disorder in several key respects, although there is great overlap with both. First, there is massive etiological heterogeneity and a meaningful

subdivision between severe and mild disorders in terms of that heterogeneity. Clearly, there is neurodevelopmental impairment in both, but its meaning is likely to be very different, according to the presence/absence of a medical syndrome that constitutes the major cause of ID. Mild ID that is *not* associated with a specific medical condition will involve neurodevelopmental impairment but it will reflect multiple origins, and not just one major cause. ID obviously belongs in the neurodevelopmental cluster but it has more differences than similarities with respect to other disorders in the cluster.

The situation with ADHD and ASD is quite different in that the key core features *do* show remissions and relapses in some cases. The extent to which each condition exhibits neurodevelopmental impairment shows considerable individual variability. When such impairment is present, it seems to constitute an intrinsic feature of the disorder, and not some separate comorbidity. However, the greatest justification for their placement in the neurodevelopmental cluster is that they usually persist into adult life and, when they do, they present considerable problems in service provision because so few adult psychiatrists (or clinical psychologists) have experience in dealing with the clinical problems that derive from the persistence of an early onset neurodevelopmental disorder. Typically, few child professionals are familiar with either manifestations in adult life or the operation of services for adults. As a result, many individuals with either ASD or ADHD receive inadequate care and treatment. Much the same applies to language disorders that persist into adult life.

The situation with both schizophrenia and conduct/dissocial disorder is different yet again. There is good evidence that schizophrenia is often preceded by impairments in either language or motor development or both, and below average IQ scores (Cannon *et al.*, 2002). These impairments are evident at all ages during childhood but it is not known if there is consistency at an individual level. The particular individual cognitive pattern is not diagnostically distinctive and it remains unclear whether the impairments are a function of the genetic liability for schizophrenia (see Chapter 57). Conduct/dissocial disorder is associated with hyperactivity/impulsivity when the onset is in the childhood period (see Chapter 65) but the pattern is not diagnostically distinctive and, as with schizophrenia, the neurodevelopmental impairment is probably a function of the genetic liability to conduct/dissocial disorder. Unlike the situation with ASD and ADHD, the same sort of clinical problem does not tend to be seen in the transition to adult life. For all these reasons, we conclude that, although neurodevelopmental impairment is associated with both disorders, they are probably best grouped outside the neurodevelopmental cluster.

The situation with respect to tics is different yet again. The association with neurodevelopmental impairment is strongest in the case of multiple tics and weakest in the case of simple single tics, but the overall association is both weak and not diagnostically distinctive (see Chapter 56). The meaning of the impairment remains unclear.

Clinical value of neurodevelopmental impairment concepts

There are three main clinical gains from focussing attention on neurodevelopmental impairment. First, it has the practical importance of alerting clinicians to the need to appreciate the importance of paying attention to the challenges in assessment and intervention of the functional deficits associated with neurodevelopment in disorders whose defining features have a different focus (as would be the case with ASD, ADHD, and schizophrenia). Second, with respect to particular individual disorders, it highlights special issues. Thus, in the case of schizophrenia it draws attention to the early risk features in the preschool years of a mental disorder that becomes fully manifest only in early adult life. With respect to CD/dissocial disorder, it underlines the fact that it does not just represent "naughtiness."

Third, it emphasizes the need to broaden research perspectives beyond single disorder specialism in order to determine how risk and protective factors may operate in similar ways across diverse disorders. For example, the strong male preponderance seen with ASD led to the suggestion that autism might represent the extreme male brain (Baron-Cohen, 2003). The observation that ADHD, dyslexia and several other disorders also show both a similar sex difference and neurodevelopmental impairments suggests that there may be causal pathways that span different disorders.

Finally, heterogeneity in the meaning of neurodevelopmental impairment is a reminder that because we give the same name to what is found in autism, schizophrenia and dyslexia should *not* lead us to assume that the same mechanisms apply. Because there is substantial co-occurrence among neurodevelopmental disorders, parents may be puzzled and concerned when different experts give different diagnoses to their child. Thus, when the child's problem concerns a mixture of ADHD and ASD symptoms, experts may vary as to which diagnosis they use, even though, in reality, they do not really differ on the nature of the problem. This is an issue noted years ago in the WHO seminars that gave rise to a multiaxial classification (Rutter *et al.*, 1975). What is new is the appreciation that the issue applies within axes and not just between them. Families need to be helped to understand the implications of the lack of clear water between diagnostic categories.

Acknowledgments

We are extremely grateful to Joanna Martin and Miriam Cooper for their invaluable assistance with the literature search, figure, helpful comments and suggestions.

References

Anagnostou, E. & Taylor, M.J. (2011) Review of neuroimaging in autism spectrum disorders: what have we learned and where we go from here. *Molecular Autism* **2**, 4.

Angold, A. (2008) Sex and developmental psychopathology. In: *Developmental Psychopathology and Wellness: Genetic and Environmental Influences.* (ed J.J. Hudziak), pp. 109–138. American Psychiatric Association, Washington, DC.

Barengo, N.C. & Tuomilehto, J.O. (2012) Blood pressure treatment target in patients with diabetes mellitus - current evidence. *Annals of Medicine* **44**, S36–S42.

Barnett, K. et al. (2012) Epidemiology of multimorbidity and implications for health care, research, and medical education: a cross-sectional study. *Lancet* **380**, 37–43.

Baron-Cohen, S. (2003) *The Essential Difference: Men, Women and the Extreme Male Brain.* Allen Lane, London.

Ben-David, E. & Shifman, S. (2012) Networks of neuronal genes affected by common and rare variants in autism spectrum disorders. *PLoS Genetics* **8**, e1002556.

Bishop, D.V.M. & Edmundson, A. (1987) Language-impaired 4-year-olds: distinguishing transient from persistent impairment. *Journal of Speech and Hearing Disorders* **52**, 156–173.

Cannon, M. et al. (2002) Evidence for early-childhood, pan-developmental impairment specific to schizophreniform disorder: results from a longitudinal birth cohort. *Archives of General Psychiatry* **59**, 449–456.

Caron, C. & Rutter, M. (1991) Comorbidity in child psychopathology: concepts, issues and research strategies. *Journal of Child Psychology and Psychiatry* **32**, 1063–1080.

Caylak, E. (2009) Neurobiological approaches on brains of children with dyslexia: review. *Academic Radiology* **16**, 1003–1024.

Cherkasova, M.V. & Hechtman, L. (2009) Neuroimaging in attention-deficit hyperactivity disorder: beyond the frontostriatal circuitry. *Canadian Journal of Psychiatry* **54**, 651–664.

Clark, T. et al. (1999) Autistic symptoms in children with attention deficit-hyperactivity disorder. *European Child and Adolescent Psychiatry* **8**, 50–5.

Conti-Ramsden, G. et al. (2007) Familial loading in specific language impairment: patterns of differences across proband characteristics, gender and relative type. *Genes, Brain and Behavior* **6**, 216–228.

Conti-Ramsden, G. et al. (2012) Developmental trajectories of verbal and nonverbal skills in individuals with a history of specific language impairment: from childhood to adolescence. *Journal of Speech, Language, and Hearing Research* **55**, 1716–1735.

Cristino, A.S. et al. (2014) Neurodevelopmental and neuropsychiatric disorders represent an interconnected molecular system. *Molecular Psychiatry* **19**, 294–301.

Crosbie, J. et al. (2013) Response inhibition and ADHD traits: correlates and heritability in a community sample. *Journal of Abnormal Child Psychology*, **41**, 497–507.

Cross-Disorder Group of the Psychiatric Genomics Consortium (2013) Identification of risk loci with shared effects on five major psychiatric disorders: a genome-wide analysis. *Lancet* **381**, 1371–1379.

Darke, S. & Hall, W. (1995) Levels and correlates of polydrug use among heroin users and regular amphetamine users. *Drug and Alcohol Dependence* **39**, 231–235.

Deary, I.J. *et al.* (2009) Genetic foundations of human intelligence. *Human Genetics* **126**, 215–232.

Falconer, D.S. (1965) The inheritance of liability to certain diseases, estimated from the incidence among relatives. *Annals of Human Genetics (London)* **29**, 51–76.

Fernandez, T.V. *et al.* (2012) Rare copy number variants in Tourette's syndrome disrupt genes in histaminergic pathways and overlap with autism. *Biological Psychiatry* **71**, 392–402.

Francis, D.J. *et al.* (1996) Developmental lag versus deficit models of reading disability: a longitudinal, individual growth curves analysis. *Journal of Educational Psychology* **88**, 3–17.

Galanter, C.A. & Leibenluft, E. (2008) Frontiers between attention deficit hyperactivity disorder and bipolar disorder. *Child and Adolescent Psychiatric Clinics of North America* **17**, 325–346.

Geary, D.C. (1993) Mathematical disabilities: cognitive, neuropsychological, and genetic components. *Psychological Bulletin* **114**, 345–362.

Gladwell, M. (2008) *Outliers: The Story of Success*. Penguin Books, London.

Gogtay, N. *et al.* (2004) Dynamic mapping of human cortical development during childhood through early adulthood. *Proceedings of the National Academy of Sciences of the United States of America* **101**, 8174–8179.

Greven, C.U. *et al.* (2011) Genetic overlap between ADHD symptoms and reading is largely driven by inattentiveness rather than hyperactivity-impulsivity. *Journal of the Canadian Academy of Child and Adolescent Psychiatry* **20**, 6.

Greven, C.U. *et al.* (2012) A longitudinal twin study on the association between ADHD symptoms and reading. *Journal of Child Psychology and Psychiatry* **53**, 234–242.

Guilmatre, A. *et al.* (2009) Recurrent rearrangements in synaptic and neurodevelopmental genes and shared biologic pathways in schizophrenia, autism, and mental retardation. *Archives of General Psychiatry* **66**, 947.

Guthrie, B. *et al.* (2012) Adapting clinical guidelines to take account of multimorbidity. *British Medical Journal* **4**, 345.

Hamshere, M.L. *et al.* (2013a) Shared polygenic contribution between childhood attention-deficit hyperactivity disorder and adult schizophrenia. *British Journal of Psychiatry* **203**, 107–111.

Hamshere, M.L. *et al.* (2013b) High loading of polygenic risk for ADHD in children with comorbid aggression. *American Journal of Psychiatry* **170**, 909–916.

Harris, J.C. (1995) *Developmental Neuropsychiatry*. Oxford University Press, New York and Oxford.

Haworth, C.M. & Plomin, R. (2010) Quantitative genetics in the era of molecular genetics: learning abilities and disabilities as an example. *Journal of the American Academy of Child and Adolescent Psychiatry* **49**, 783–793.

Hoekstra, R.A. *et al.* (2010) Limited genetic covariance between autistic traits and intelligence: findings from a longitudinal twin study. *American Journal of Medical Genetics Part B: Neuropsychiatric Genetics* **153B**, 994–1007.

Hutton, J. *et al.* (2008) New-onset psychiatric disorders in individuals with autism. *Autism* **12**, 373–390.

Jessen, H.M. & Auger, A.P. (2011) Sex differences in epigenetic mechanisms may underlie risk and resilience for mental health disorders. *Epigenetics* **6**, 857–861.

Karmiloff-Smith, A. & Farran, K. (eds) (2012) *Neurodevelopmental Disorders Across the Lifespan: A Neuro-Constructivist Approach*. Oxford University Press, Oxford.

Karmiloff-Smith, A. *et al.* (2012) Genetic and environmental vulnerabilities in children with neurodevelopmental disorders. *Proceedings of the National Academy of Sciences* **109**, 17261–17265.

Kaufmann, L. *et al.* (2011) Meta-analyses of developmental fMRI studies investigating typical and atypical trajectories of number processing and calculation. *Developmental Neuropsychology* **36**, 763–787.

Kessler, R.C. *et al.* (2010) Epidemiology of anxiety disorders. *Current Topics in Behavioral Neurosciences* **2**, 21–35.

Lahey, B.B. *et al.* (2011) Higher-order genetic and environmental structure of prevalent forms of child and adolescent psychopathology. *Archives of General Psychiatry* **68**, 181–189.

Lamont, S. & Brunero, S. (2009) Personality disorder prevalence and treatment outcomes: a literature review. *Issues in Mental Health Nursing* **30**, 631–637.

Landerl, K. & Moll, K. (2010) Comorbidity of learning disorders: prevalence and familial transmission. *Journal of Child Psychology and Psychiatry* **51**, 287–294.

Lichtenstein, P. *et al.* (2010) The genetics of autism spectrum disorders and related neuropsychiatric disorders in childhood. *American Journal of Psychiatry* **167**, 1357–1363.

McMahon, S.D. *et al.* (2003) Stress and psychopathology in children and adolescents: is there evidence of specificity? *Journal of Child Psychology and Psychiatry* **44**, 107–133.

Moffitt, T.E. *et al.* (2001) *Sex Differences in Antisocial Behaviour: Conduct Disorder, Delinquency, and Violence in the Dunedin Longitudinal Study*. Cambridge University Press, Cambridge.

O'Rourke, J.A. *et al.* (2009) The genetics of Tourette's syndrome: a review. *Journal of Psychosomatic Research* **67**, 533–545.

Paloyelis, Y. *et al.* (2010) The genetic association between ADHD symptoms and reading difficulties: the role of inattentiveness and IQ. *Journal of Abnormal Child Psychology* **38**, 1083–1095.

Peñagarikano, O. & Geschwind, D.H. (2012) What does CNTNAP2 reveal about autism spectrum disorder? *Trends in Molecular Medicine* **18**, 156–163.

Relton, C.L. & Davey Smith, G. (2010) Epigenetic epidemiology of common complex disease: prospects for prediction, prevention, and treatment. *PLoS Medicine* **7**, e1000356.

Rhee, S.H. & Waldman, I.D. (2004) Etiology of sex differences in the prevalence of ADHD: an examination of inattention and hyperactivity–impulsivity. *American Journal of Medical Genetics Part B: Neuropsychiatric Genetics* **127**, 60–64.

Rispens, J. *et al.* (1998) *Perspectives on the classification of specific developmental disorders*. Kluwer Academic Publishers, Dordrecht/Boston/London.

Rommelse, N.N.J. *et al.* (2011) A review on cognitive and brain endophenotypes that may be common in autism spectrum disorder and attention-deficit/hyperactivity disorder and facilitate the search for pleiotropic genes. *Neuroscience and Biobehavioral Reviews* **35**, 1363–1396.

Ronald, A. & Hoekstra, R.A. (2011) Autism spectrum disorders and autistic traits: a decade of new twin studies. *American Journal of Medical Genetics Part B: Neuropsychiatric Genetics* **156**, 255–274.

Ronald, A. *et al.* (2008) Evidence for overlapping genetic influences on autistic and ADHD behaviours in a community twin sample. *Journal of Child Psychology and Psychiatry* **49**, 535–542.

Rutter, M. (1997) Comorbidity: concepts, claims and choices. *Criminal Behaviour and Mental Health* 7, 265–285.

Rutter, M. (2011) Progress in understanding autism: 2007–2010. *Journal of Autism and Developmental Disorders* 41, 395–404.

Rutter, M. & Thapar, A. (2014) Genetics of autism spectrum disorders. In: *Handbook of Autism and Pervasive Developmental Disorders, Assessment, interventions, policy, the future.* (eds R. Volkmar, R. Paul, S.J. Rogers & K.A. Pelphrey), 4th edn. John Wiley & Sons, Hoboken NJ.

Rutter, M. *et al.* (1975) A Multiaxial Classification of Child Psychiatric Disorders. World Health Organization, Geneva, Switzerland.

Rutter, M. *et al.* (2003) Using sex differences in psychopathology to study causal mechanisms: unifying issues and research strategies. *Journal of Child Psychology and Psychiatry* 44, 1092–1115.

Rutter, M. *et al.* (2006) Continuities and discontinuities in psychopathology between childhood and adult life. *Journal of Child Psychology and Psychiatry* 47, 276–295.

Rykhlevskaia, E. *et al.* (2009) Neuroanatomical correlates of developmental dyscalculia: combined evidence from morphometry and tractography. *Frontiers in Human Neuroscience* 3, 51.

Shaw, P. *et al.* (2006) Intellectual ability and cortical development in children and adolescents. *Nature* 30, 676–679.

Shaw, P. *et al.* (2007) Attention-deficit/hyperactivity disorder is characterized by a delay in cortical maturation. *Proceedings of the National Academy of Sciences of the United States of America* 104, 19649–19654.

Shaw, P. *et al.* (2012a) Development of cortical surface area and gyrification in attention-deficit/hyperactivity disorder. *Biological Psychiatry* 72, 191–197.

Shaw, M. *et al.* (2012b) A systematic review and analysis of long-term outcomes in attention deficit hyperactivity disorder: effects of treatment and non-treatment. *BMC Medicine* 10, 99.

Sonuga-Barke *et al.* (2010) vii. Physical growth and maturation following early severe institutional deprivation: do they mediate specific psychopathological effects? *Monographs of the Society for Research in Child Development* 75, 143–166.

Stanovich, K.E. (1986) Matthew effects in reading: some consequences of individual differences in the acquisition of literacy. *Reading Research Quarterly* 21, 360–407.

Stothard, S.E. *et al.* (1998) Language-impaired preschoolers: a follow-up into adolescence. *Journal of Speech, Language, and Hearing Research* 41, 407–418.

Stromswold, K. (2001) The heritability of language: a review and meta-analysis of twin, adoption, and linkage studies. *Language* 77, 647–723.

Sullivan, P.F. *et al.* (2012a) Genetic architectures of psychiatric disorders: the emerging picture and its implications. *Nature Reviews Genetics* 13, 537–551.

Sullivan, P.F. *et al.* (2012b) Family history of schizophrenia and bipolar disorder as risk factors for autism. *Archives of General Psychiatry* 69, 1099–1103.

Szatmari, P. *et al.* (2012) Sex differences in repetitive stereotyped behaviors in autism: implications for genetic liability. *American Journal of Medical Genetics Part B: Neuropsychiatric Genetics* 159B, 5–12.

Tanner, J.M. (1989) *Foetus into Man: Physical Growth from Conception to Maturity*, 2nd edn. Castlemead Publications, Ware, Herts.

Taylor, L.J. *et al.* (2012) Do children with specific language impairment have a cognitive profile reminiscent of autism? A review of the literature. *Journal of Autism and Developmental Disorders* 42, 2067–2083.

Thapar, A. *et al.* (1999) Genetic basis of attention deficit and hyperactivity. *British Journal of Psychiatry* 174, 105–111.

Thapar, A. *et al.* (2013) What have we learnt about the causes of ADHD? *Journal of Child Psychology and Psychiatry* 54, 3–16.

Thede, L.L. & Coolidge, F.L. (2007) Psychological and neurobehavioral comparisons of children with Asperger's Disorder versus High-Functioning Autism. *Journal of Autism and Developmental Disorders* 37, 847–54.

Weisman, H. *et al.* (2013) Systematic review: pharmacological treatment of tic disorders–Efficacy of antipsychotic and alpha-2 adrenergic agonist agents. *Neuroscience & Biobehavioral Reviews* 37, 1162–1171.

Willcutt, E.G. *et al.* (2010) Understanding the complex etiologies of developmental disorders: behavioral and molecular genetic approaches. *Journal of Developmental and Behavioral Pediatrics* 31, 533.

Williams, N.M. *et al.* (2010) Rare chromosomal deletions and duplications in attention-deficit hyperactivity disorder: a genome-wide analysis. *Lancet* 376, 1401–1408.

Wong, C.C. *et al.* (2014) Methylomic analysis of monozygotic twins discordant for autism spectrum disorder and related behavioural traits. *Molecular Psychiatry* 19, 495–503.

Wright, B.A. & Zecker, S.G. (2004) Learning problems, delayed development, and puberty. *Proceedings of the National Academy of Sciences of the United States of America* 101, 9942–9946.

CHAPTER 4

Conceptual issues and empirical challenges in the disruptive behavior disorders

Jonathan Hill[1] and Barbara Maughan[2]

[1]School for Psychology and Clinical Language Sciences, University of Reading, UK

[2]MRC Social, Genetic and Developmental Psychiatry Centre, Institute of Psychiatry, Psychology and Neuroscience, King's College London, UK

The scope of this chapter

The term "disruptive behavior disorders" refers to a broad set of aggressive, disruptive, oppositional, and anger-related behaviors. They are commonly contrasted with "emotional disorders," yet as we shall argue, emotionality is also central to the causes and maintenance of many behavioral problems. A core paradox about childhood disruptive behavior problems is that while they are widely viewed as having social origins, reflecting parental and societal failures, and so readily amenable to social, educational, economic or political solutions, they are also among the most intransigent and harmful of known mental health disorders. A review of conceptual issues has to embrace both sides of this paradox. On the one hand many of these problems represent a failure of socialization in childhood and then in adult life, so that sufferers find themselves in disadvantageous situations, such as social isolation and school exclusion in childhood, youth offender institutions in adolescence and prison in adult life. This socialization process might be altered by changes in social, educational, or economic conditions. On the other hand, children with behavioral problems differ from other children in multiple ways, genetic, temperamental, physiological and social cognitive, and even early in childhood many do not gain from improvements in environmental conditions.

What is the phenotype?

Identifying a phenotype that is both reasonably homogenous and also distinct from other phenotypes is central to understanding the origins, underlying processes, treatment needs, and long-term outcomes of any disorder. The identity of the phenotype in the broad area of disruptive behavior problems is, however, a focus of continuing discussion. This is potentially of value, although it needs to be borne in mind that behavioral phenotypes, however homogenous, may not map precisely on to biological or psychological processes. Furthermore, a common set of processes may underpin diverse behaviors, in which case more purchase may be obtained from a broad characterization of the phenotype.

The American Diagnostic and Statistical Manual (DSM-5; American Psychiatric Association, 2013) distinguishes between oppositional defiant disorder (ODD) and conduct disorder (CD). Behavioral criteria for ODD are: angry and resentful, loses temper, argues with adults, defies and refuses to comply with requests and rules, annoys people, blames others, touchy and easily annoyed, spiteful or vindictive. The criteria for CD are too numerous to list; in contrast to ODD, however, they include aggressive behaviors such as: often bullies, threatens, or intimidates others, and often initiates physical fights, along with rule-breaking behaviors such as lying and stealing, and "serious violations of rules." See Chapter 65.

The ODD/CD distinction is limited as a tool for investigating heterogeneity in disruptive behavior problems because, in contrast to the ODD items, many of the CD criteria are age-dependent, with items such as "has used a weapon that can cause serious harm" or "has forced someone into sexual activity" rarely being encountered before adolescence. Heterogeneity has also been identified, however, using the contrast between "overt" disruptive, oppositional and aggressive behaviors, and "covert" behaviors such as theft and vandalism. Covert behaviors are rarely seen in young children at ages when aggression and opposition are already common, and show increases in later childhood and adolescence. Within overt behaviors, differentiations are often made between aggression, oppositionality, and anger-proneness or irritability; further demarcations of physical aggression differentiate between reactive aggression, which occurs in response to actual or perceived provocation,

Rutter's Child and Adolescent Psychiatry, Sixth Edition.
Edited by Anita Thapar and Daniel S. Pine, James F. Leckman, Stephen Scott, Margaret J. Snowling, Eric Taylor.

and proactive aggression, in which the perpetrator takes the initiative in attacking another.

These characterizations seek to identify heterogeneity in *behaviors*, not in *children*, and indeed in most instances they are highly correlated, for example, overt with covert behaviors (Snyder *et al.*, 2012), and reactive and proactive aggression (Polman *et al.*, 2007). By contrast, the construct of "callous unemotional" traits, characterized by a lack of responsiveness to others' distress, has been used to demarcate subgroups of children (Frick & White, 2008). Studies vary considerably in the ways they characterize disruptive behavior problems, some using broad brush measures such as the aggression scale of the Child Behavior Checklist (which includes aggression, oppositionality, and anger-proneness), others making specific contrasts, for example between overt and covert behaviors, or disruptive children with or without callous unemotional traits. It is extremely unusual to find studies that address more than one of these contrasts in the same analyses.

Finally, we should note that the search for satisfactory phenotypes is not confined to heterogeneity within disruptive behaviors alone. Other emotional and behavioral syndromes, most notably perhaps attention deficit and hyperactivity disorder (ADHD) and depressive disorders, are frequently associated with disruptive behavior disorders. There are a number of much-debated possible explanations for this, including that it reflects true comorbidity (the co-occurrence of different disorders); that there is a broader phenotype extending beyond disruptive behavior problems; or that combinations of disorders are themselves phenotypes, distinct from their component parts.

The starting point: well-replicated findings

The attempt to understand the origins and nature of disruptive behavior problems must start with five well-replicated findings (Table 4.1).

The first and second of these findings—that disruptive behavior problems commonly persist, and that they are associated with criminality and social dysfunction over a broad front—were first described by Lee Robins in her 1960s' follow-up of children seen in child guidance clinics 30 years earlier. In her book "Deviant Children Grown Up" (Robins, 1966), she shows that children with disruptive behavior problems commonly, as adults, showed persistent violence and other illegal behaviors, and that they also had problems that extended well beyond specifically antisocial acts. In particular, they often had unstable lifestyles characterized by brief relationships, job instability, and impulsive, reckless behaviors, summarized in the DSM criteria for Antisocial Personality Disorder in adults.

Subsequent studies of general population cohorts have confirmed that disruptive behavior problems seen in young children commonly persist, and that they are associated with increased risks not only for antisocial and poor interpersonal outcomes, but also for many psychiatric disorders, notably, depression, anxiety disorders, PTSD, and alcohol and drug

Table 4.1 Well-replicated findings for disruptive behavior problems.

1.	Disruptive behavior problems commonly start before age 2 years and may persist over many years
2.	In adult life they are associated with criminality; with the behavioral and social difficulties identified as DSM Antisocial Personality Disorder; and with psychiatric disorders such as substance misuse and depression
3.	Rates of antisocial and delinquent behaviors increase markedly during adolescence and fall in adult life
4.	Between 50% and 70% of children with disruptive behavior problems show improvement during childhood, but some continue to have adjustment problems
5.	Disruptive behavior problems are more common in boys than in girls

misuse (Odgers *et al.*, 2008). Many of these studies have used repeated measurements across childhood to generate developmental trajectories of behavior problems and to assign children to those trajectories (see e.g., Cote *et al.*, 2006). There has been substantial convergence among studies of overt behaviors (either aggressive or oppositional defiant), toward there being a group of children who start high and remain high (Tremblay, 2010). Although the age of onset of this persistent high group is unclear, the first data points in such studies are commonly around 18–24 months, suggesting that children with overt behavior problems manifest them as soon as they have the physical capability to hit or oppose! General population studies have not identified groups of children with new onsets of aggression or oppositional defiant behaviors from toddlerhood up to puberty; however, there may be further groups that can be identified in different samples, for example of clinically referred children. The third well-replicated finding is that rates of antisocial and delinquent behaviors increase dramatically across the teens, then fall back again in early adulthood (Moffitt, 1993). Fourth, the majority of children with early onset disruptive behavior problems (typically estimated at between 50% and 70%) do not show persistence of those problems into adult life, though men in particular may show some isolated difficulties in other domains (Odgers *et al.*, 2008). And finally, most disruptive behavior problems are more common in boys than girls.

What do we need to explain?

It follows from these findings that the search for the causes of childhood disruptive behaviors needs to begin with early life, including pregnancy and infancy, and that we need to explain not only how they are initiated but also why they persist. The question of persistence is especially acute here because we need to be able to explain why problems that are so clearly maladaptive, and attract negative responses from others, are also so apparently resistant to change. We consider four distinct possibilities.

First, maladaptive behaviors have their origins in, and are maintained by, environmental adversities such as physical abuse to which children respond with their own aggression (Kim-Cohen *et al.*, 2006), or there are social rewards for disruptive behaviors (Snyder *et al.*, 2012). Persistence arises either from persistence of the unfavorable environment, from the establishment of inaccurate social cognitive schemas (Dodge *et al.*, 1995) or from consolidation of social learning.

Second, there is an enduring deficit or abnormality, such as a failure of emotional responsiveness to others' expressions of fear, that contributes to indifference to others' distress (Blair, 2008).

Third, disruptive behavior problems are motivated. The child's attempts to find a solution to threats in the environment lead to an adaptation that also creates a vulnerability. Disengaging attention from threat, for example, reduces fear, but may also lead to impoverished monitoring of social interactions, increasing the likelihood of using coercive solutions (Derryberry & Rothbart, 1997). Aggression is then maintained by the child's motivation to solve the problem of being frightened.

Finally, disruptive behaviors arise from the effects of genetic, physiological or behavioral variations and of epigenetic mechanisms (see Chapter 25). Such variations may have been retained in evolution because they are adaptive under some environmental conditions, even though they confer risk under others (Ellis *et al.*, 2011). The paradigm case, the "fetal origins hypothesis," proposes that low birth weight reflects an *in utero* adaptation to an anticipated food-scarce environment, which then creates vulnerability to obesity, hypertension, heart disease, and diabetes in Westernized high calorie environments (Barker, 1998). It seems that several early developmental mechanisms for psychopathology may be associated with biological variations that confer either advantage or risk, depending on the environments encountered. It has been argued that variations in children's susceptibility to the environment may have evolved to ensure that some individuals are not seriously affected if they encounter adverse environments, while others are well placed to take advantage of favorable environments (the differential susceptibility hypothesis, Belsky & Pluess, 2009). Findings based on predictions from fetal programming have not all shown the predicted associations, but associations have been found between low birth weight and adolescent depression (Costello *et al.*, 2007), and prenatal maternal anxiety and disruptive behaviors in offspring (O'Connor *et al.*, 2003, O'Donnell *et al.*, 2014). In a similar way, genetic (Pickles *et al.*, 2013), behavioral (Belsky & Pluess, 2009) and physiological (Obradovic, 2012) reactivity appears to confer advantage or vulnerability in a context-dependent manner.

Unraveling risks for disruptive behavior problems

Numerous risk factors are associated with childhood behavior problems. The list includes parental criminality and psychiatric disorders, prenatal anxiety, smoking in pregnancy, single parent status, marital discord, partner violence, poor parental supervision, harsh parenting, child physical abuse, social deprivation, neighborhood violence, low IQ, language delay, low school achievement, large family size, low family income, antisocial peers, high delinquency-rate schools, and high crime neighborhoods (Murray & Farrington, 2010). Plausible causal mechanisms have been proposed for each, but associations among them are common, and many are likely to be accounted for by third variable effects. For example, there is a widely replicated association between smoking in pregnancy and disruptive behaviors, with plausible causal explanations (Wakschlag, 2002). However, mothers who smoke during pregnancy differ in many respects from mothers who do not; they are more likely to have a history of antisocial behavior, less education, and less income, all of which could explain their children's antisocial behavior. Studies designed to deal with such confounders make use of strategies such as sibling comparisons (where the confounders are the same for each sibling but exposure to smoking varies), and propensity score matching, where smokers and non smokers are matched on risks for smoking, and then the effect of smoking is examined (Jaffee *et al.*, 2012). Family processes such as marital discord and harsh parenting also commonly reflect parental antisocial problems, suggesting that associations between parenting and child disruptive behaviors may in part arise from common genetic effects. Twin and adoption designs can deal with many of the possible genetic confounds (see Chapter 24) and the study of natural experiments has been valuable (see Chapter 12). Asbury *et al.* (2003), for example, showed that differences in the harshness of parenting experienced by identical twins predicted disruptive behaviors, consistent with an environmentally-mediated effect. Independent effects of parental hostility on child behavior problems have also been shown in children conceived by in vitro fertilization (and so genetically unrelated to their parents, Harold *et al.*, 2012), and twin studies have also supported bidirectional effects, with, for example, low child self-control predicting harsh parenting, and harsh parenting predicting disruptive behavior problems, even after accounting for genetic contributions (Cecil *et al.*, 2012). The process of testing alternative explanations for associations of possible risk factors with disruptive behavior problems is crucial to establishing causality (see Chapter 12). These will however remain broad-brush unless more specific hypotheses are developed regarding mechanisms. Here, demarcating contrasting pathways is likely to be key. We will illustrate this by considering three possible pathways, each plausible, each with some supporting evidence, but where in each case the evidence still falls well short of a coherent or complete account. These pathways are illustrated in Figure 4.1.

Anger-proneness in interaction with adverse parenting—a high reactive pathway

We begin with a "high reactive" pathway, in which the vulnerability is created by a combination of temperamental infant anger-proneness and parental negative intrusive behaviors that further increase the negative mood of the child. Marital discord,

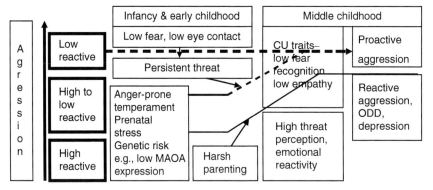

Low reactivity is indicated by the dotted line and high reactivity by the solid line.
Upward direction of a line denotes increasing low or high reactivity

Figure 4.1 Summary of possible pathways to disruptive behavior problems.

partner violence, parental irritability associated with depression, and physical abuse may also contribute to increased emotional dysregulation. Parental negativity may arise both from evocative interactions whereby the infant's intense prolonged displays of anger lead to frustration and parental anger, and shared genetic influences on parent and child negative emotionality. The child may come to respond not only to actual parental threats, but also to perceived threat from apparently innocuous behaviors. Later in childhood, the child's emotional reactivity also leads to conflict with peers and other adults, creating a pervasively hostile environment; those who are able to, avoid contact with the child, leading to social isolation or associations only with children with similar problems. Difficulties in managing social interactions are compounded by low verbal IQ and limitations in flexible adaptive planning associated with prefrontal deficits. The child's aggression is angry and reactive.

Empirical studies in this area vary in the measurement of early temperament, some using the broad characterization of "difficult" temperament, others negative emotionality, and yet others, anger-proneness (see Chapter 8). The available studies are nevertheless consistent in finding an interaction between negative emotionality and parenting during infancy in the prediction of later behavior problems. High negative emotionality in the presence of high parental negativity, or low sensitivity, predicts later disruptive behavior problems (Bradley & Corwyn, 2008; van Aken *et al.*, 2007). However, in line with the differential susceptibility hypothesis, while children with high negative emotionality who received less supportive parenting have the highest rates of disruptive behaviors, those with the most sensitive parents have the lowest levels. It is possible that high negative emotionality creates the conditions in which the skills of emotion regulation are acquired, provided parents are able to respond sensitively. Independent contributions of parental depression (Barker *et al.*, 2012), marital discord (Bornovalova *et al.*, 2014), and physical abuse (Jaffee *et al.*, 2004) to the prediction of disruptive behavior problems have been shown in a range of studies. However, the interplay between parental characteristics, parenting, and temperament has not received much attention. In one of the

few studies to examine temperament, parenting, and marital discord, child anger-proneness in interaction with low parental guidance predicted externalizing symptoms, as did lack of partner support (Smeekens *et al.*, 2007). The model predicts that this developmental pathway should lead specifically to reactive, anger-related aggression. Despite some support for associations between physical abuse, increased threat detection, and reactive aggression (Dodge *et al.*, 1995; Dodge & Pettit, 2003), links between early anger-proneness, parenting and family processes have not yet been described. Indeed it is striking that in spite of the considerable evidence for heterogeneity in disruptive behavior problems, studies of the contributions of early developmental processes rarely move beyond broad-brush assessments of externalizing or oppositional defiance/aggression as outcomes.

Also relevant to this pathway, maternal anxiety and depression during pregnancy have been found to predict childhood behavior problems after controlling for postnatal environmental factors (O'Connor *et al.*, 2003; Barker *et al.*, 2011a), and prenatal maternal anxiety predicts persistence from childhood to adolescence (Barker & Maughan, 2009). These studies have not examined specific mechanisms linking prenatal exposures to behavior problems, but there are good reasons to predict effects on an anger-prone pathway. In animal studies, prenatal stress is associated with emotional and hypothalamic-pituitary-adrenal (HPA) axis hyper-reactivity, and in humans, maternal cortisol during pregnancy predicts infant cortisol reactivity to a stressor (Davis *et al.*, 2011). Prenatal maternal depression predicts infant temperamental negative emotionality (Davis *et al.*, 2007), and this association is modified by postnatal maternal stroking, consistent with effects of tactile stimulation on gene expression in rodents (Sharp *et al.*, 2012). There may also be specific contributions to this pathway from environment-dependent effects of gene variants such as those of MAOA. Several studies have found that a polymorphism of the MAOA gene, associated with low gene expression, predicts antisocial behaviors in adults (Caspi *et al.*, 2002) and behavior problems in children (Kim-Cohen *et al.*, 2006) only among those exposed to maltreatment. Thus far studies have not examined whether

MAOA G×E contributes to specific pathways to disruptive behaviors; however, animal and human studies provide some indications that low MAOA gene expression is likely to be associated with increased negative emotionality (Meyer-Lindenberg & Weinberger, 2006). This is consistent with findings that the MAOA variants interact with life events during pregnancy to predict negative emotionality at 5 weeks (Hill *et al.*, 2013), and with maternal sensitivity at 7 months to predict anger proneness at 14 months (Pickles *et al.*, 2013). These are the first reports of a possible role for MAOA activity status in relation to infant negative emotionality, and replication studies are needed (see Chapter 24).

Lack of responsiveness to others' distress—a low reactive pathway

We turn next to the subgroup of children and adolescents with persistent disruptive behavior problems who are reported by parents and teachers as lacking concern for others' distress, often referred to as showing "callous unemotional" (CU) traits (Frick & White, 2008). (The related concept of psychopathy is covered in Chapter 68). Among adolescents with disruptive behaviors CU traits are predictive of more severe aggression, and more persistent antisocial behavior problems, and there is emerging evidence that this is also the case in children. Individuals with CU traits differ from other disruptive children in multiple ways: they show poorer recognition of sad and fearful faces, lower anxiety levels, superior verbal IQ, and their families have fewer psychosocial risks such as marital discord (Viding *et al.*, 2012). They also show reduced activation of the amygdala in response to viewing fearful faces (Jones *et al.*, 2009), which may contribute to lower empathic responses to others' distress. The prominence of deficits in responding to others' emotional states associated with CU traits poses interesting questions regarding possible overlap with autistic spectrum disorder (ASD). Conceptually, however, there are two major differences. First, CU traits are thought to be associated with lack of responsiveness to sadness or fear, while in the autistic spectrum there are difficulties in understanding emotions in general. Second, the main deficit associated with CU traits is of emotional *responsivity* to distress (affective empathy), while autistic traits are associated with a lack of *understanding* of others feelings—that is, cognitive empathy. This has been examined in a comparison of three groups of clinic-referred boys with ASD, and with conduct disorder with and without CU traits, and a non clinical control group. The children were shown video clips of emotionally loaded situations, and asked how the protagonists felt, why they felt that way, and how they themselves felt watching each video sequence. Children with ASD did less well than others in providing an account of the reasons for the protagonists' feelings, while those in the CU traits group described the lowest levels of emotions on watching the videos (Schwenck *et al.*, 2012).

There are few developmental studies of the infancy origins of CU traits, but several lines of evidence suggest possible elements in the pathway. There appears to be a distinctive genetic contribution to CU traits, which may be stronger than for disruptive behavior problems more generally (Viding *et al.*, 2005). Furthermore, in contrast to other forms of behavior problems, the evidence from most studies is that CU traits are not associated with harsh parenting in community samples in childhood (Frick & Viding, 2009). It is possible therefore that a major contribution to CU traits comes from an inherited vulnerability, for which there are several candidates.

First, vulnerable infants may make less eye contact with parents than other children. Boys with high CU traits show impaired attention to the eye region when viewing standardized emotional faces, but show normal patterns of fear recognition when instructed to focus on the eye region (Dadds *et al.*, 2011), suggesting that the reduced eye contact has a causal role in reduced emotional responsiveness. Boys with high CU traits also show lower eye contact in free play, and lower eye contact is associated with impaired fear recognition and empathy. Dadds and colleagues have proposed that reduced eye contact may lead to less engagement with caregivers and hence fewer opportunities to acquire an understanding of others' emotions.

Second, lack of emotional responsiveness to others' emotions may be increased by temperamental fearlessness because children miss out on the developmental advantages conferred by the experience of fear. Several studies of normally developing children have shown that infant fearfulness is associated with greater evidence of conscience and guilt (Kochanska *et al.*, 2002). Fearlessness may therefore inhibit the development of responsiveness to others' distress. Fearlessness may also be associated with reduced behavioral inhibition. Gray (1987) proposed that the 'Behavioural Inhibition System' is activated by actual or anticipated punishment, leading to anxiety which can be avoided by not behaving in ways that increase the likelihood of being punished. Reduced activation of behavioral inhibition removes a brake on bad behavior, and also makes punishment a less effective means of regulating a child's behavior. Fearlessness may also reduce fear conditioning, such that stimuli that are not inherently aversive come to elicit fear after being paired with unconditioned stimuli. In normal development, the pairing of mild reprimands with strong forms of punishment may lead to the effectiveness of low key adult behaviors in regulating behaviors. This may be impaired in the development of CU traits. Findings of reduced fear conditioning in male antisocial adolescents (Fairchild *et al.*, 2008) are consistent with this possibility, although it remains to be established whether this is specific to CU traits. The infant who experiences fear infrequently or at low levels is also less likely to look to a parent for comfort in the face of threat, and so may experience fewer parent–child attachment sequences, further reducing emotional contact with the parent.

Low eye contact and fear activation may both contribute to lower reinforcement of parental caregiving behaviors and hence lower sensitivity. There is some limited evidence for the link between temperamental fearlessness in infancy and CU traits. In a follow-up of approximately 7000 children to age 13 in the UK

Avon Longitudinal Study of Parents and Children (ALSPAC), females with conduct problems and CU traits (CP/CU) had been reported by parents as showing lower fear at age 2 than those with CP only (Barker *et al.*, 2011b). The interpretation is not however straightforward as the CP/CU group also had been less fearful in infancy than the CU traits only group. Boys in the CP/CU group had been reported as less responsive to punishment in infancy, but not as fearless.

Finally, early physiological under-arousal may contribute to risk for CU traits. Prospective associations between low pulse rate and disruptive and antisocial behavior problems have been replicated across many studies (Raine, 2002). This may reflect autonomic arousal which may in turn contribute to processes such as reduced fear conditioning. Several studies have found that reduced vagal reactivity, indexed by change of respiratory sinus arrhythmia to a stressor, is associated with increased disruptive behavior problems, consistent with an effect of autonomic under-arousal (Calkins *et al.*, 2007). The relationship between autonomic functioning and disruptive behavior problems is, however, complex. Disentangling the contributions of sympathetic and parasympathetic systems is not easy, and, consistent with the earlier review of context-dependent effects of physiological reactivity, may be environment-dependent (Obradovic *et al.*, 2010). Developmental studies from infancy to examine the specificity of physiological under-arousal to CU traits have not yet been conducted.

Adaptations to threat over development—from high reactivity to low reactivity

From Freud's early formulations of the child's attempts to cope with sexual abuse onwards, developmental theorists have understood children as actively regulating their emotional and physiological states to avoid high levels of distress and arousal, and to be able to act effectively in a range of social domains. This can, however, become problematic when a child is faced with chronic threat or maltreatment. As the temperament researchers Derryberry and Rothbart (1997) noted, under these conditions the child "may come to rely upon primarily avoidant strategies, disengaging attention from the threatening situation without attending to sources of relief and available coping options." From an information-processing perspective, the cost of an avoidant strategy may be that the child ceases to attend to the details of a threatening social encounter, or of other social experiences that to a greater or lesser extent resemble it. If the child's attention to the details is diminished, he/she is more likely to work from generalized inaccurate schemas, leading to a limited repertoire of social problem-solving options. Both psychodynamic and information-processing formulations envisage that this coping strategy is used to down-regulate negative emotions. This is likely to have implications for functioning in relationships and for the regulation of aggression. Where an avoidant strategy is used by the child, the negative emotions are not brought into the parent–child relationship, and hence the child is deprived of the experience, and does not practice

the skills, of regulating emotions within close relationships. Down-regulation of fear may inhibit anxious inhibition of antisocial or aggressive behaviors, and reduce fear conditioning. This hypothesis is consistent with the findings of Burgess *et al.* (2003) that the combination of fearlessness at 24 months and avoidant attachment at 14 months predicted behavior problems at 4 years. Avoidant strategies can be assessed in young children using story stem doll play procedures in which children are asked to respond to a range of interpersonal situations. Interpreting interpersonal processes as physical events (adopting the "physical stance") rather than as motivated by emotions, beliefs or desires (adopting the "intentional stance") is one way of avoiding the emotional implications of threat. In a longitudinal study of the children of women with postnatal depression, insecure attachment (mainly avoidant) predicted physical stance responses to a high threat doll play scenario, and this in turn was associated with teacher-reported behavior problems (Hill *et al.*, 2008).

Physiological reactivity to stress may also change over time. Findings that children exposed to major adversities commonly have evidence of increased HPA axis reactivity, while adolescents and adults often show hypoactivity, may be explained by "attenuation" of HPA activity over time (Trickett *et al.*, 2010). The resulting hypoactivity may then contribute to risk of disruptive behaviors via reduced physiological reactivity mediated via corticotrophin-releasing factor (Davies *et al.*, 2007). Overall the evidence linking HPA axis activity to disruptive behavior problems is inconsistent; however, a meta-analysis revealed an association with hyper-reactivity in preschool children, and with hypo activity in school-age children (Alink *et al.*, 2008), consistent with the attenuation hypothesis.

Peer influences

Peer influences are unlikely to be implicated in the earliest stages of the developmental pathways outlined thus far. However, it is well established that aggressive and oppositional children are commonly shunned by most other children, or associate mainly with other children with similar problems. They may therefore lack supportive or enjoyable peer interactions, and also run the risk of having their behaviors maintained or amplified through interactions with deviant peers. Furthermore, while overt behavior problems appear early, covert behaviors, such as stealing, appear later, and may be particularly susceptible to peer influences. There has been a long-standing debate over whether the poor peer relationships of disruptive children are solely a reflection of their problems, or whether they also contribute to them (Hill, 2002). Approaches to this question require prospective designs that examine whether peer processes add to the prediction of disruptive behavior problems after controlling for baseline problems. Several studies have failed to find effects of peer relationships on later antisocial outcomes after accounting for prior behavior problems and associated factors such as family adversities (Tremblay *et al.*, 1995; Woodward & Fergusson, 1999). Recent prospective studies have, however, provided support for a role for peer influences when examining very specific processes, such as deviancy training (the amount of talk between peers about aggression, rule breaking, defiance of authority and property destruction), and the extent to which peers respond positively to such talk. Deviancy training in young school-age children has been associated with the persistence and increase of disruptive, and particularly covert, behaviors over up to 4 years (Snyder *et al.*, 2012).

Sex differences

A conceptual approach to childhood disruptive behaviors also has to attempt to account for their higher prevalence in boys than girls. In their comprehensive review of sex differences in the Dunedin Longitudinal Study, Moffitt and colleagues (Moffitt *et al.*, 2001) concluded that there was no evidence for differences in the *mechanisms* for behavior problems in males and females, and that the difference arose from a higher rate of developmental vulnerabilities in males. This then pushes the question back to: What is the nature of these vulnerabilities? Within the framework outlined earlier we are looking for possible deficits, for evolved variations that may confer risk or advantage depending on context, and for coping strategies. Males are often described as more vulnerable, with elevated rates of developmental disorders such as ADHD and autism cited in support. However that begs the question as to the type of causal process in play. It may be that there is a contribution of higher rates of deficits in males, with, for example, some evidence that the toxic effects of chemicals in utero on cognitive development are greater in males than in females (Horton *et al.*, 2012). Equally, many of the candidates for explaining sex differences are likely to be evolved differences with context-dependent advantages or risks. For example, low pulse rate, an index of under-arousal, is not only a robust predictor of violence in children and adults, it also shows sex differences. Males have a lower resting mean pulse rate than females and this difference is evident in young children, consistent with the early onset of persistent aggression (Raine, 2002). This difference may facilitate sex differences in aggression, seen in the general population, which is probably an evolved functional difference (Glover & Hill, 2012), that at the same time generates a larger number of males than females at the lower end of the normal distribution.

There may also be effects of sex-linked genes. One example is the MAOA gene, which is on the X chromosome. If, as is commonly found, heterozygous females show $G \times E$ patterns similar to the homozygous high activity variants (Hill *et al.*, 2013; Melas *et al.*, 2013), then more males than females are at risk for disruptive behavior problems in the presence of adverse or unsupportive environments.

It may be that mechanisms underpinning the male predominance for disruptive behavior in childhood also contribute to the higher rate of affective disorders in females starting at puberty. The activity of the catechol-O-methyltransferase (COMT) gene, which encodes an enzyme that metabolizes catechol compounds, including dopamine, illustrates the point. COMT's enzyme activity, and the neurochemistry and behavior of COMT knockout mice, are both markedly sexually dimorphic (Tunbridge & Harrison, 2011). In a series of elegant studies Thapar and colleagues have shown that a high activity variant is associated with conduct disorder (CD) comorbid with ADHD, and this finding has been replicated by other investigators (Langley *et al.*, 2010). Whether or not there is a sex difference in the association between COMT and CD in ADHD is not known, but the high activity variant has been associated with lower IQ in boys but not in girls (Barnett *et al.*, 2008). By contrast, the high activity variant is associated, in Caucasians, with panic disorder in females but not in males (Domschke *et al.*, 2007). There are also marked differences between males and females in the rates of neurodevelopmental disorders; the reasons for this are discussed in Chapter 3.

"Comorbidity"

The co-occurrence of disruptive behavior problems with symptoms of apparently different disorders is very common. This is often referred to as "comorbidity"—a term that strictly speaking refers to the co-occurrence of distinct disorders. In this context, however, the term is a misnomer, as in many instances this is unlikely to be the explanation. Nevertheless, consideration of patterns of co-occurrence is central to the investigation of disruptive behavior problems.

As we argued earlier, attempts to build causal models of disruptive behavior problems will flounder either if the phenotype is too broad and heterogeneous, or if it is too narrow. If substantial commonalities could be shown between disruptive behavior problems and other childhood disorders, that could imply that there is a broader phenotype with common underlying mechanisms. We consider this possibility in relation to depressive disorders. Cross-sectionally, links between disruptive and depressive disorders are found across childhood and adolescence, in representative as well as referred samples; a meta-analysis of early epidemiological findings reported a joint odds ratio of over 6, little lower than that for depression-anxiety overlaps (Angold *et al.*, 1999). The two sets of difficulties are also related developmentally: although some studies find that depression predicts disruptive behaviors, by far the most commonly reported sequence is one whereby CD/ODD precedes, and predicts to, subsequent depression. In most early diagnostically-based studies, groups meeting criteria for both CD and ODD were combined. More recently, investigators have begun to examine predictions from these two disorders separately, and found that ODD emerged as the more salient precursor (see e.g., Copeland *et al.*, 2009). It is possible therefore that oppositional defiant and depressive symptoms are manifestations of the same underlying processes. Some of these processes could lie in shared risk exposures. Psychosocial risks for both conduct problems and depression are legion, and undoubtedly overlap; in one study, more than two-thirds of the shared variance between co-occurring conduct disorder and depression in adolescence was attributable to shared risk factors (Fergusson *et al.,* 1996). Shared temperamental features and genetic risks also seem likely to be implicated. Genetically informative studies have pointed to shared genetic and environmental contributions to CD-depression overlaps (see e.g., Subbarao *et al.,* 2008). In addition, investigators are beginning to explore whether effects may be mediated by shared dispositional factors such as negative emotionality (Tackett *et al.,* 2011), or symptoms such as irritable mood (see Chapter 5). As noted above, some studies have found that it is ODD, rather than CD, that presents the stronger risk for subsequent depression. Recent studies have also shown that ODD symptoms include two closely related but separable dimensions: a "headstrong" dimension, related to current and future antisocial behaviors, and an "irritable" dimension, associated with risk for depression. Initial evidence from twin studies suggests that the association between irritability and depression is largely attributable to shared genetic risks (Stringaris *et al.,* 2012). Refining the phenotype may thus entail both narrowing down to specific aspects of disruptive behavior problems—in this case negative emotionality or anger-proneness—and broadening beyond their confines—in this case to depression.

Disruptive behavior problems are also comorbid with ADHD. As described earlier, the high activity variant of the COMT SNP Val158Met is associated with conduct problems among children with ADHD, but not in those without (Langley *et al.,* 2010). This suggests a highly specific developmental pathway, implicating risks for ADHD combined with very specific mechanisms for this subgroup of children with disruptive behavior problems. Promising findings suggest possible mediation between the COMT variant and conduct problems in ADHD by limitations in social understanding (Langley *et al.,* 2010). Thus in this case the identification of a distinctive comorbid subgroup has refined the mapping of heterogeneity in the disruptive domain.

Comorbidity may also arise in other ways that illuminate developmental processes. We return here to the example of depression, where disruptive behaviors may increase risk through repeated experiences of failure at school, in relationships and in other contexts (see e.g., Capaldi, 1992). Associations of this kind have been widely reported, and appear to begin quite early in development; in one study, for example, externalizing problems were associated with increased exposure to stressful life events from early childhood onwards, contributing not only to the persistence of behavioral difficulties but also to increased risk for internalizing problems in both childhood and the teens (Timmermans *et al,* 2010). Given the widespread impact of disruptive behaviors on family and peer relationships, and on school functioning, "developmental cascades" of this kind may be especially important in the disruptive domain, increasing children's vulnerability to associated problems, and also functioning to stabilize underlying behavioral difficulties.

Adolescent onset of disruptive and antisocial behaviors

As we have seen, aggressive and disruptive behaviors are evident from very early in development. Other indicators of antisocial tendencies—most notably, crime and delinquency—follow a quite different developmental course. Across time and cultures, these behaviors show a highly predictable pattern, rising sharply across the teens, then falling back equally clearly in the early adult years. This near-universal phenomenon—the age-crime curve of criminological theory—suggests that new processes relevant to the expression of antisocial tendencies come on stream in adolescence; it may also point to additional sources of heterogeneity.

Building on these observations, Moffitt (1993) proposed a developmental taxonomy whereby the overall "pool" of antisocial young people is made up of two groups, distinguished by age at onset, and differing in both etiology and course. The first, onsetting in childhood, has much in common with the groups discussed thus far, with roots in biologically-based individual differences in temperament and neuropsychological functioning, interacting and transacting with adverse pre- and post natal environments to give rise to early onset behavior problems. The second, emerging in adolescence, owes less to such individual vulnerabilities; instead, Moffitt (1993) argued that the teenage rise in antisocial behavior emerges alongside puberty and is prompted by frustrations attendant on the adolescent maturity gap, cultural and historical contexts influencing adolescence, and social mimicry of behaviorally deviant peers. In relation to longer-term outcomes, Moffitt posited that early onset conduct problems would result in life-course persistent antisocial behavior, while adolescent onset conduct problems would follow a more time-limited course.

In statistical terms, a model of this kind is ideally suited to testing via latent trajectory modeling. A recent review (Jennings & Reingle, 2012) identified over 100 studies using this approach to describe the number and shape of trajectories of violent, aggressive and delinquent behaviors. Despite variability in findings, the authors concluded that results were largely consistent with Moffitt's taxonomy. Over time, however, two relatively well-supported qualifications to the original formulation have emerged. First, as outlined earlier, studies using broad-brush measures of conduct problems have confirmed that by no means all early onset conduct problems persist; indeed, though many children with early onset difficulties do show poor long-term outcomes, a "childhood limited" trajectory has also been detected in numerous studies of this kind. Second, adolescent onset problems have emerged as less transient than first assumed (Odgers *et al.,* 2008). Moffitt's initial discussion noted that adolescent delinquency can result in "snares" such as poor school achievement or substance use that may act to perpetuate antisocial life-styles; subsequent evidence suggests that, for some young people at least, processes of this kind undoubtedly do occur (Hussong *et al.*, 2004).

Many of the etiological factors argued to underlie early onset and persistent conduct problems are, as we have seen, extensively supported by research in childhood samples. Testing for "adolescent-specific" risks is more complex and would ideally require longer-term studies tracking samples prospectively from childhood to the adolescent years. Genetically-informative studies are now beginning to provide evidence of this kind; one recent study found that the genetic factors influencing externalizing behaviors in late childhood still influenced variability in early adulthood, but that new genetic and environmental influences emerged in adolescence (Wichers *et al.*, 2012). Findings from neuroimaging studies are still limited, and predominantly cross-sectional; here, however, current evidence is less consistent with a developmental account, with similar abnormalities in brain structure reported in both early and adolescent onset Conduct Disorder groups (see e.g., Fairchild *et al.*, 2011).

What is now clear, however, is that the onset of puberty is associated with the initiation of a range of neurobiological changes that are likely to be relevant to the overall rise in antisocial behavior in the teens. Much of this research has been designed to explicate the underpinnings of a broader category of risk-taking and the reasons why, across a range of contexts, adolescents appear to take "risky" decisions (Blakemore & Robbins, 2012). Neuroimaging studies have highlighted two features of particular importance here. First, the brain regions involved in cognitive control (including the prefrontal cortex) show protracted structural development that continues throughout adolescence and into early adulthood. At the same time, however, there appear to be heightened brain responses to socially relevant, reward-related cues that are adolescence-specific, prompted by the hormonal changes of puberty (Peper & Dahl, 2013).

In evolutionary terms, such heightened sensitivity to social stimuli should have adaptive advantages, preparing adolescents to meet the new social demands of the adult world. In some contexts, however, it may prove more problematic. Experimental studies have shown, for example, that adolescents are markedly more susceptible to peer influence in risky situations than are adults (Gardner & Steinberg, 2005), suggesting that the presence of peers "primes" motivations to more immediately available, albeit risky, rewards. As much adolescent delinquency is committed in peer contexts, the implications of such findings for antisocial behavior are clear. Peer influences (along with other social-contextual factors) have also been found to moderate hormone-behavior associations in the teens, with evidence, for example, that high testosterone levels are associated with nonaggressive conduct problems in boys with deviant peers, but with indicators of prosocial leadership in those with more conventional friends (Rowe *et al.*, 2004). Finally, early timing of puberty is also associated with increased risk for antisocial

behavior in the teens (Mendle *et al*, 2007; Mendle & Ferrero, 2010). The mechanisms underlying this association are less clear. Though biologically-based influences may be involved, commentators have also proposed a "maturation disparity" hypothesis (whereby the gap between early maturers' physical and psychosocial development puts them at risk of adverse outcomes), or the possibility that pre-existing behavioral difficulties may be accentuated by the new social challenges of adolescence (Ge & Natsuaki, 2009).

Conclusions

Our understanding of disruptive behavior problems has come a long way since Lee Robins (1966) first showed how enduring and impairing they can be. Several key general population longitudinal studies have now provided more detail on how early they start, how they develop over time, and how they arise and are maintained by individual susceptibilities and environmental adversities. Other studies, mainly of clinical samples, have highlighted likely heterogeneity within the disruptive domain, with far-reaching implications for our understanding of early developmental origins. Currently, this is where the evidence becomes sparse. We have many sporadic indicators of the role of genotypic variations, neuroendocrine functioning, and social cognitive processes, in interaction with the child's experiences, but these have not so far been integrated into a coherent model of developmental origins. The aim of this chapter has been threefold: to review what we do know, to highlight what we do not, and to provide indications of what an integrated model of the developmental origins of disruptive behavior problems might look like. This goes beyond the evidence—but that is necessary in framing research hypotheses, just as it is in clinical practice. Informative though it has proved, a broad characterization of disruptive behaviors is a relatively blunt instrument when attempting to formulate a treatment plan. Children and their families differ in many ways, and some respond to current treatment approaches and some do not. The task therefore is to identify differences within the disruptive domain that provide clues to distinctive origins and treatment needs. Developmental histories are the backbone of clinical approaches; a framework of the kind outlined in this chapter, albeit still under construction, can add specificity to the enquiry. This is relevant not only to the clinical formulation, but also to talking with parents and children in ways that convey an understanding of their particular patterns of behaviors and emotions.

References

van Aken, C. *et al.* (2007) The interactive effects of temperament and maternal parenting on toddlers externalizing behaviours. *Infant and Child Development* **16**, 553–572.

Alink, L.R. *et al.* (2008) Cortisol and externalizing behavior in children and adolescents: mixed meta-analytic evidence for the inverse relation of basal cortisol and cortisol reactivity with externalizing behavior. *Developmental Psychobiology* **50**, 427–450.

American Psychiatric Association (2013) *Diagnostic and Statistical Manual of Mental Disorders*, 5th edn. American Psychiatric Association, Washington, DC.

Angold, A. *et al.* (1999) Comorbidity. *Journal of Child Psychology and Psychiatry* **40**, 57–87.

Asbury, K. *et al.* (2003) Nonshared environmental influences on individual differences in early behavioral development: a monozygotic twin differences study. *Child Development* **74**, 933–943.

Barker, D.J.P. (1998) *Mothers, Babies and Health in Later Life*. Churchill Livingstone, Edinburgh.

Barker, E.D. & Maughan, B. (2009) Differentiating early-onset persistent versus childhood-limited conduct problem youth. *American Journal of Psychiatry* **166**, 900–908.

Barker, E.D. *et al.* (2011a) The contribution of prenatal and postnatal maternal anxiety and depression to child maladjustment. *Depression and Anxiety* **28**, 696–702.

Barker, E.D. *et al.* (2011b) The impact of prenatal maternal risk, fearless temperament and early parenting on adolescent callous-unemotional traits: a 14-year longitudinal investigation. *Journal of Child Psychology and Psychiatry* **52**, 878–888.

Barker, E.D. *et al.* (2012) Relative impact of maternal depression and associated risk factors on offspring psychopathology. *British Journal of Psychiatry* **200**, 124–129.

Barnett, J.H. *et al.* (2008) Meta-analysis of the cognitive effects of the catechol-O-methyltransferase gene Val158/108Met polymorphism. *Biological Psychiatry* **64**, 137–144.

Belsky, J. & Pluess, M. (2009) Beyond diathesis stress: differential susceptibility to environmental influences. *Psychological Bulletin* **135**, 885–908.

Blair, R.J. (2008) The amygdala and ventromedial prefrontal cortex: functional contributions and dysfunction in psychopathy. *Philosophical Transactions of the Royal Society of London B Biological Sciences* **363**, 2557–2565.

Blakemore, S.J. & Robbins, T.W. (2012) Decision-making in the adolescent brain. *Nature Neuroscience* **15**, 1184–1191.

Bornovalova, M.A. *et al.* (2014) Understanding the relative contributions of direct environmental effects and passive genotype-environment correlations in the association between familial risk factors and child disruptive behavior disorders. *Psychological Medicine* **44**, 831–844.

Bradley, R.H. & Corwyn, R.F. (2008) Infant temperament, parenting, and externalizing behavior in first grade: a test of the differential susceptibility hypothesis. *Journal of Child Psychology and Psychiatry* **49**, 124–131.

Burgess, K.B. *et al.* (2003) Infant attachment and temperament as predictors of subsequent externalizing problems and cardiac physiology. *Journal of Child Psychology and Psychiatry* **44**, 819–831.

Calkins, S.D. *et al.* (2007) Cardiac vagal regulation differentiates among children at risk for behavior problems. *Biological Psychology* **74**, 144–153.

Capaldi, D.M. (1992) Co-occurrence of conduct problems and depressive symptoms in early adolescent boys. 2. A 2-year follow-up at grade 8. *Development and Psychopathology* **4**, 125–144.

Caspi, A. *et al.* (2002) Role of genotype in the cycle of violence in maltreated children. *Science* **297**, 851–854.

Cecil, C.A. *et al.* (2012) Association between maladaptive parenting and child self-control over time: cross-lagged study using a monozygotic twin difference design. *British Journal of Psychiatry* **201**, 291–297.

Copeland, W.E. *et al.* (2009) Childhood and adolescent psychiatric disorders as predictors of young adult disorders. *Archives of General Psychiatry* **66**, 764–772.

Costello, E.J. *et al.* (2007) Prediction from low birth weight to female adolescent depression: a test of competing hypotheses. *Archives of General Psychiatry* **64**, 338–344.

Cote, S.M. *et al.* (2006) The development of physical aggression from toddlerhood to pre-adolescence: a nation wide longitudinal study of Canadian children. *Journal of Abnormal Psychology* **34**, 71–85.

Dadds, M.R. *et al.* (2011) Impaired attention to the eyes of attachment figures and the developmental origins of psychopathy. *Journal of Child Psychology and Psychiatry* **52**, 238–245.

Davies, P.T. *et al.* (2007) The role of child adrenocortical functioning in pathways between interparental conflict and child maladjustment. *Developmental Psychology* **43**, 918–930.

Davis, E.P. *et al.* (2007) Prenatal exposure to maternal depression and cortisol influences infant temperament. *Journal of the American Academy of Child and Adolescent Psychiatry* **46**, 737–746.

Davis, E.P. *et al.* (2011) Prenatal maternal stress programs infant stress regulation. *Journal of Child Psychology and Psychiatry* **52**, 119–129.

Derryberry, D. & Rothbart, M.K. (1997) Reactive and effortful processes in the organization of temperament. *Development and Psychopathology* **9**, 633–652.

Dodge, K.A. & Pettit, G.S. (2003) A biopsychosocial model of the development of chronic conduct problems in adolescence. *Developmental Psychology* **39**, 349–371.

Dodge, K.A. *et al.* (1995) Social information-processing patterns partially mediate the effect of early physical abuse on later conduct problems. *Journal of Abnormal Psychology* **104**, 632–643.

Domschke, K. *et al.* (2007) Meta-analysis of COMT val158met in panic disorder: ethnic heterogeneity and gender specificity. *American Journal of Medical Genetics B Neuropsychiatric Genetics* **144B**, 667–673.

Ellis, B.J. *et al.* (2011) Differential susceptibility to the environment: an evolutionary–neurodevelopmental theory. *Development and Psychopathology* **23**, 7–28.

Fairchild, G. *et al.* (2008) Fear conditioning and affective modulation of the startle reflex in male adolescents with early-onset or adolescence-onset conduct disorder and healthy control subjects. *Biological Psychiatry* **63**, 279–285.

Fairchild, G. *et al.* (2011) Brain structure abnormalities in early-onset and adolescent-onset Conduct Disorder. *American Journal of Psychiatry* **168**, 624–633.

Fergusson, D.M. *et al.* (1996) Origins of comorbidity between conduct and affective disorders. *Journal of the American Academy of Child and Adolescent Psychiatry* **35**, 451–460.

Frick, P.J. & Viding, E. (2009) Antisocial behavior from a developmental psychopathology perspective. *Development and Psychopathology* **21**, 1111–1131.

Frick, P.J. & White, S.F. (2008) Research review: the importance of callous-unemotional traits for developmental models of aggressive and antisocial behavior. *Journal of Child Psychology and Psychiatry* **49**, 359–375.

Gardner, M. & Steinberg, L. (2005) Peer influence on risk taking, risk preference, and risky decision making in adolescence and adulthood: an experimental study. *Developmental Psychology* **41**, 625–635.

Ge, X. & Natsuaki, M.N. (2009) In search of explanations for early pubertal timing effects on developmental psychopathology. *Current Directions in Psychological Science* **18**, 327–331.

Glover, V. & Hill, J. (2012) Sex differences in the programming effects of prenatal stress on psychopathology and stress responses: an evolutionary perspective. *Physiology and Behavior* **106**, 736–740.

Gray, J.A. (1987) *The Psychology of Fear and Stress*. Cambridge University Press, New York.

Harold, G.T. *et al.* (2012) Interparental conflict, parent psychopathology, hostile parenting, and child antisocial behavior: examining the role of maternal versus paternal influences using a novel genetically sensitive research design. *Development and Psychopathology* **24**, 1283–1295.

Hill, J. (2002) Biological, psychological and social processes in the conduct disorders. *Journal of Child Psychology and Psychiatry* **43**, 133–164.

Hill, J. *et al.* (2008) The dynamics of threat, fear and intentionality in the conduct disorders: longitudinal findings in the children of women with post-natal depression. *Philosophical Transactions of the Royal Society of London B Biological Sciences* **363**, 2529–2541.

Hill, J. *et al.* (2013) Evidence for interplay between genes and maternal stress in utero: monoamine oxidase A polymorphism moderates effects of life events during pregnancy on infant negative emotionality at 5 weeks. *Genes, Brain, and Behavior* **12**, 388–396.

Horton, M.K. *et al.* (2012) Does the home environment and the sex of the child modify the adverse effects of prenatal exposure to chlorpyrifos on child working memory? *Neurotoxicology and Teratology* **34**, 534–541.

Hussong, A.M. *et al.* (2004) Substance abuse hinders desistance in young adults' antisocial behavior. *Development and Psychopathology* **16**, 1029–1046.

Jaffee, S.R. *et al.* (2004) Physical maltreatment victim to antisocial child: evidence of an environmentally mediated process. *Journal of Abnormal Psychology* **113**, 44–55.

Jaffee, S.R. *et al.* (2012) From correlates to causes: can quasi-experimental studies and statistical innovations bring us closer to identifying the causes of antisocial behavior? *Psychological Bulletin* **138**, 272–295.

Jennings, W.G. & Reingle, J.M. (2012) On the number and shape of developmental/life-course violence, aggression, and delinquency trajectories: a state-of-the-art review. *Journal of Criminal Justice* **40**, 472–489.

Jones, A.P. *et al.* (2009) Amygdala hypoactivity to fearful faces in boys with conduct problems and callous-unemotional traits. *American Journal of Psychiatry* **166**, 95–102.

Kim-Cohen, J. *et al.* (2006) MAOA, maltreatment, and gene-environment interaction predicting children's mental health: new evidence and a meta-analysis. *Molecular Psychiatry* **11**, 903–913.

Kochanska, G. *et al.* (2002) Guilt in young children: development, determinants, and relations with a broader system of standards. *Child Development* **73**, 461–482.

Langley, K. *et al.* (2010) Genotype link with extreme antisocial behavior: the contribution of cognitive pathways. *Archives of General Psychiatry* **67**, 1317–1323.

Melas, P.A. *et al.* (2013) Genetic and epigenetic associations of MAOA and NR3C1 with depression and childhood adversities. *International Journal of Neuropsychopharmacology* **16**, 1513–1528.

Mendle, J. & Ferrero, J. (2010) Detrimental psychological outcomes associated with pubertal timing in adolescent boys. *Developmental Review* **32**, 49–66.

Mendle, J. *et al.* (2007) Detrimental psychological outcomes associated with pubertal timing in adolescent girls. *Developmental Review* **21**, 151–171.

Meyer-Lindenberg, A. & Weinberger, D.R. (2006) Intermediate phenotypes and genetic mechanisms of psychiatric disorders. *Nature Reviews Neuroscience* **7**, 818–827.

Moffitt, T.E. (1993) Adolescence-limited and life-course-persistent antisocial behavior—a developmental taxonomy. *Psychological Review* **100**, 674–701.

Moffitt, T.E. *et al.* (2001) *Sex Differences in Antisocial Behaviour*. Cambridge University Press, Cambridge.

Murray, J. & Farrington, D.P. (2010) Risk factors for conduct disorder and delinquency: key findings from longitudinal studies. *Canadian Journal of Psychiatry* **55**, 633–642.

Obradovic, J. (2012) How can the study of physiological reactivity contribute to our understanding of adversity and resilience processes in development? *Development and Psychopathology* **24**, 371–387.

Obradovic, J. *et al.* (2010) Biological sensitivity to context: the interactive effects of stress reactivity and family adversity on socioemotional behavior and school readiness. *Child Development* **81**, 270–289.

O'Connor, T.G. *et al.* (2003) Maternal antenatal anxiety and behavioural/emotional problems in children: a test of a programming hypothesis. *Journal of Child Psychology and Psychiatry* **44**, 1025–1036.

Odgers, C.L. *et al.* (2008) Female and male antisocial trajectories: from childhood origins to adult outcomes. *Development and Psychopathology* **20**, 673–716.

O'Donnell, K.J. *et al.* (2014). The persisting effect of maternal mood in pregnancy on childhood psychopathology. *Development and Psychopathology* **26**, 393–403.

Peper, J.S. & Dahl, R.E. (2013) The teenage brain: surging hormones–brain-behavior interactions during puberty. *Current Directions in Psychological Science* **22**, 134–139.

Pickles, A. *et al.* (2013) Evidence for interplay between genes and parenting on infant temperament in the first year of life: monoamine oxidase A polymorphism moderates effects of maternal sensitivity on infant anger proneness. *Journal of Child Psychology and Psychiatry* **54**, 1308–1317.

Polman, H. *et al.* (2007) A meta-analysis of the distinction between reactive and proactive aggression in children and adolescents. *Journal of Abnormal Child Psychology* **35**, 522–535.

Raine, A. (2002) Annotation: the role of prefrontal deficits, low autonomic arousal, and early health factors in the development of antisocial and aggressive behavior in children. *Journal of Child Psychology and Psychiatry* **43**, 417–434.

Robins, L. (1966) *Deviant Children Grown Up: A Sociological and Psychiatric Study of Sociopathic Personalities*. Williams and Wilkins, Baltimore.

Rowe, R. *et al.* (2004) Testosterone, conduct disorder and social dominance in boys: pubertal development and biosocial interaction. *Biological Psychiatry* **55**, 546–552.

Schwenck, C. *et al.* (2012) Empathy in children with autism and conduct disorder: group-specific profiles and developmental aspects. *Journal of Child Psychology and Psychiatry* **53**, 651–659.

Sharp, H. *et al.* (2012) Frequency of infant stroking reported by mothers moderates the effect of prenatal depression on infant behavioural and physiological outcomes. *PLoS One* **7**, e45446.

Smeekens, S. *et al.* (2007) Multiple determinants of externalizing behavior in 5-year-olds: a longitudinal model. *Journal of Abnormal Child Psychology* **35**, 347–361.

Snyder, J.J. *et al.* (2012) Covert antisocial behavior, peer deviancy training, parenting processes, and sex differences in the development of antisocial behavior during childhood. *Development and Psychopathology* **24**, 1117–1138.

Stringaris, A. *et al.* (2012) Adolescent irritability: phenotypic associations and genetic links with depressed mood. *American Journal of Psychiatry* **169**, 47–54.

Subbarao, A. *et al.* (2008) Common genetic and environmental influences on major depressive disorder and conduct disorder. *Journal of Abnormal Child Psychology* **36**, 433–444.

Tackett, J.L. *et al.* (2011) Shared genetic influences on negative emotionality and major depression/Conduct Disorder comorbidity. *Journal of the American Academy of Child and Adolescent Psychiatry* **50**, 818–827.

Timmermans, M. *et al.* (2010) The role of stressful events in the development of behavioural and emotional problems from early childhood to late adolescence. *Psychological Medicine* **40**, 1659–1668.

Tremblay, R.E. (2010) Developmental origins of disruptive behaviour problems: the 'original sin' hypothesis, epigenetics and their consequences for prevention. *Journal of Child Psychology and Psychiatry* **51**, 341–367.

Tremblay, R.E. *et al.* (1995) A bimodal preventive intervention for disruptive kindergarten boys: its impact through mid-adolescence. *Journal of Consulting and Clinical Psychology* **63**, 560–568.

Trickett, P.K. *et al.* (2010) Attenuation of cortisol across development for victims of sexual abuse. *Development and Psychopathology* **22**, 165–175.

Tunbridge, E.M. & Harrison, P.J. (2011) Importance of the COMT gene for sex differences in brain function and predisposition to psychiatric disorders. *Current Topics in Behavioral Neuroscience* **8**, 119–140.

Viding, E. *et al.* (2005) Evidence for substantial genetic risk for psychopathy in 7-year-olds. *Journal of Child Psychology and Psychiatry* **46**, 592–597.

Viding, E. *et al.* (2012) Antisocial behaviour in children with and without callous-unemotional traits. *Journal of the Royal Society of Medicine* **105**, 195–200.

Wakschlag, L.S. (2002) Maternal smoking during pregnancy and severe antisocial behavior in offspring: a review. *American Journal of Public Health* **92**, 966–974.

Wichers, M. *et al.* (2012) Genetic innovation and stability in externalizing problem behavior across development: a multi-informant twin study. *Behavior Genetics* **43**, 191–201.

Woodward, L.J. & Fergusson, D.M. (1999) Childhood peer relationship problems and psychosocial adjustment in late adolescence. *Journal of Abnormal Child Psychology* **27**, 87–104.

CHAPTER 5

Emotion, emotion regulation and emotional disorders: conceptual issues for clinicians and neuroscientists

Argyris Stringaris

Department of Child and Adolescent Psychiatry, Institute of Psychiatry, Psychology and Neuroscience, King's College London, UK

Terms and definitions

The word emotion is used to describe a wide range of phenomena in humans and animals. Lay people use the term emotion to describe their own feelings or those they observe in others. Clinicians infer their patients' emotions by interviewing and observing them and they diagnose emotional disorders using such descriptive phenomenology. Scientists apply the term emotion to describe a range of phenomena including physiological responses to emotional stimuli, cognitive appraisal of feelings and the way people respond to rewards. As we will see, there is only partial overlap between the various usages of the term emotion, making it impossible to come up with a single satisfactory definition.

An imaginary experiment

The following thought experiment may help map out the various usages of the term emotion. Imagine a teenager with arachnophobia, who has agreed to participate in a large-scale experiment where he is presented with images of spiders. A clinician interviews the patient, cognitive and emotion scientists observe him, a machine monitors his heart rate, and he also has a brain scan, all during the presentation of the spider.

The clinician's approach: description and first-person account

The clinician will rate as an emotion any **valenced** reaction. In this case, the valence will be negative—the patient's unpleasant feelings upon seeing the spider. Similarly, the clinician observes her patient's facial expression, tone of voice, posture and overall communication. This outward display of emotion, the clinician may describe as the young person's affect, which in this case

is negative. The clinician will also easily recognize this as a particular **type of emotion**, namely fear, as opposed to anger or happiness. The teenager himself is likely to describe his **feeling** as fear and may describe its **intensity** as mild, moderate or strong. Similarly, the clinician will rate the **duration** of the response—for example, how long the fear persisted after the image of the spider was no longer on display. The clinician will also have to judge whether the negativity of the experience goes beyond the way the young person usually feels these days. For example, depressed patients will be in a long-lasting state of negative feelings, a **mood**, which could alter their experience of being presented with a spider.

Indeed, valence, type of emotion, intensity, frequency and duration are the building blocks of most interviews and questionnaires used in clinical psychiatry and these are also used to validate the outcomes of most neuroscience research.

A neuroscientist's approach: distinguishing emotions from feelings

This reliance on patients' accounts makes clinicians often use the terms emotion synonymously with **feelings**. However, neuroscientists would argue that emotional reactions can be present even when the patient has no conscious awareness of the emotion-eliciting stimulus. Based on previous findings (Wiens, 2006), they might re-design the experiment to present the spider photographs at such a fast rate that the patient would not know he had seen them. This would show that such subliminal presentation of spiders would make the patient respond as if he had consciously processed the picture. The subliminal presentation could also increase the patient's heart rate and increase neural activity in his amygdala, a brain area implicated in emotion processing. It is argued that because emotional events are relevant to the survival of the organism, they are processed with priority over non-emotional stimuli (Wiens, 2006). Hence, the spider presentation here will lead to the following interconnected events: **biological responses** (such as the increase in heart rate and amygdala activation), **response tendencies** (the actions, such as fight or flight, that result from threat) and the brain states that detect such responses to produce **conscious experience** (Critchley *et al.*, 2004).

More from the neuroscientist: context, and interpretation versus reward and punishment

Other scientists (Barrett, 2011) focus on how **context** and **interpretation** influence the **core affect** and how this may lead to the experience of different emotions. In keeping with this, cognitive scientists would try to show that the way the teenager in this example labels emotion will depend on context; for example, Was he there on his own? Was the environment familiar? Similarly, they would try to show that the young person's **appraisal** of the experience could have an impact on the emotion that will result. Yet others will talk of emotions as **responses to rewards or punishers**. In this experiment, the spider is a stimulus that acts as a punisher, something the person will try to avoid (Rolls, 2007). The principles of this theory are relevant to behavior therapy of emotional disorders as we shall see later on.

More than one way of defining emotions

Each of these ways of defining emotions has its limitations. For example, clinicians rarely distinguish between an emotion—which is meant to be short-lived—and the longer lasting moods. We have also seen that reliance on feelings can miss out important non-conscious processing of emotions. Yet, relying on physiology alone would also be problematic. Increases in heart rate or cortisol are not specific to any emotion and amygdala activation also occurs when people are presented with novel stimuli (Lindquist *et al.*, 2012). Also, while cognitive appraisal and labelling are important, it is sometimes hard to see how they are different from any other nonemotion-related cognitive process. One solution would be to define emotion by combining all this information. However, this is not straightforward—as we shall see further on, there is at best only modest overlap between the various methods and conceptual approaches to emotions. It has even been suggested that new terms should be applied to some of these phenomena and that using the word emotion to describe all of them is confusing (Kagan, 2004). For the time being, it is probably best to resist reifying emotion—it is still a broad concept and it may be either too early or simply wrong to speak of it as if it had clearly-defined material underpinnings.

Basic emotions

In the example above, the psychiatrist refers to fear as a type of emotion and distinguishes it from other negative emotions such as sadness, mirroring the way she would distinguish between anxiety and depressive disorders. Yet, many researchers challenge this common-sense distinction. In this section, I discuss some of the main findings in this area and their clinical implications.

The debate about basic emotions

Our language recognizes a number of different emotions such as anger, sadness and joy. Some authorities claim that a set of emotions exist that are natural kinds (Ekman *et al.*, 2011), but this claim has been disputed (Kagan, 2004). The basic emotion view has certain affinities (Barrett, 2011) with Darwin's project of identifying universal and innate expressions in animals. In Darwin's own words:

> that the chief [emotional] expressive actions are now innate or inherited,—that is, have not been learnt by the individual,—is admitted by everyone. So little has learning or imitation to do with several of them that they are from the earliest days and throughout life quite beyond our control
>
> (Darwin, 1872).

and

> all the chief expressions exhibited by man are the same throughout the world. This fact is interesting as it affords a new argument in favor of the several races being descended from a single parent-stock …
>
> (Darwin, 1872).

Basic emotions are said to be characterized by distinctive universal signals (for example facial expressions), a distinctive physiology, distinctive subjective experience and the fact that they are present in humans as well as other primates (Ekman *et al.*, 2011). Typical examples according to these authors are **anger**, **disgust**, **fear**, **joy**, **surprise**, and **sadness**. However, this notion of basic emotion has been challenged. First, proponents of basic emotion disagree between themselves about how many basic emotions there are. Ortony and Turner (1990) shows that basic emotions range from 6 to 16 according to the author writing about them. Moreover, previous findings about specific relationships between physiological markers and emotions may have been incorrect. It appears that what physiology distinguishes may not be the emotion but the accompanying environmental contingencies: whether one can do something about a challenging situation or not (Frankenhaeuser, 1971). In addition, recent findings challenge the universality of basic emotions. For example, Jack *et al.* (2012) found that Caucasians living in Western countries but not East Asians distinguished between a set of basic emotions. The debate around a recent meta-analysis (Lench *et al.*, 2011) on basic emotions highlights some of the main questions. The authors examined four so-called basic emotions: happiness, sadness, anger and anxiety and found that they can be distinguished from each other with moderate effect sizes and are correlated with changes in behavioral experience and physiology. However, the effect sizes of the differences between emotions of the same valence were very small. A good

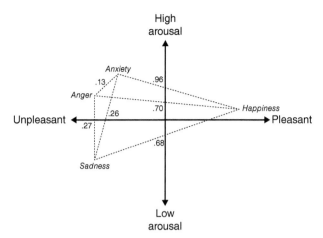

Figure 5.1 The findings of Lench *et al.*'s (2011) pairwise comparisons between emotions can be accounted for by differences in valence and arousal between emotions. Emotion categories are depicted in a circumplex structure based on their average degree of valence and arousal. Average effect sizes for each paired comparison are listed. The largest effect sizes occur for cross-valence comparisons, followed by cross-arousal comparisons. The smallest effect size observed is between anger and anxiety, emotions of the same valence and arousal. *Source:* Lindquist, *et al.* (2013). Reprinted with permission from the American Psychological Association.

example is the distinction between sadness and anger: the best differentiation between these two emotions was through subjective experience ($d = 0.38$, $p < 0.001$); however, neither cognition ($d = 0.12, p > 0.05$) nor behavior ($d = -0.18, p > 0.05$), nor physiology ($d = 0.19, p > 0.05$) distinguished between anger and sadness. In a critique of this meta-analysis, Lindquist *et al.* (2013) suggest that valence and arousal explain most of the differences observed between so-called basic emotions. As shown in Figure 5.1, the strongest effect sizes of the difference are between emotions that differ in valence.

Basic emotions and the brain

Proponents of basic emotion also suggest there are dedicated brain regions subserving each basic emotion. This locationist approach has also come under scrutiny. A recent meta-analysis of brain studies (Lindquist *et al.*, 2012) found little evidence that emotions can be consistently and specifically localized to particular brain areas. Instead, the authors interpreted the evidence as supporting a model according to which emotions emerge out of more basic psychological operations but are not specific to emotions (e.g., such as the detection of salience). The functions of the amygdala are an example that is said to support this view (Lindquist *et al.*, 2012): fear-inducing stimuli fall into a class of uncertain and salient stimuli, all of which can activate the amygdala (Lindquist *et al.*, 2012). However, this constructionist interpretation of emotion processing in the brain has itself come under scrutiny. First, there is at least some evidence for the locationist approach. Perhaps the most characteristic example from the Lindquist *et al.* meta-analysis (Lindquist *et al.*, 2012) is

that the left orbitofrontal cortex (OFC) seemed to be specific to instances of anger. However, brain correlates of anger were not restricted to the OFC but also involved areas of the prefrontal cortex. Second, this meta-analysis may be testing a model that is too simplistic. Current proponents of a locationist approach would propose the existence of a network for basic emotions in the brain rather than specific regions. Third, MRI might still be too crude a method to localize emotions. Experiments with primates show highly specialized subpopulations of neurons within sections of the OFC for the processing of olfactory stimuli (Rolls, 2007). Fourth, this meta-analysis ignores that humans commonly experience feelings that correspond to such discrete emotions. The adolescent in the introduction's imaginary experiment distinguishes between his feeling of fear when faced with the spider and his anger when pushed over in the football pit. It is an important task to explain the conscious experiences that distinguish between such feelings, even if these are not due to localized brain activity but rather interacting networks.

In the introduction, we mentioned that another approach to the young man's emotions was to consider them as states that are elicited by rewards and punishers, so-called instrumental reinforcers (Rolls, 2007). This view, posed by Edmund Rolls, distinguishes between emotions on the basis of whether rewards or punishers have been delivered or omitted.

Emotion regulation

Emotion regulation is defined in various different ways. A broad, yet concise definition is due to Ross Thompson and will provide a useful background for the rest of this chapter:

> Emotion regulation consists of the extrinsic and intrinsic processes responsible for monitoring, evaluating, and modifying emotional reactions, especially their intensive and temporal features, to accomplish one's goals
>
> (Thompson, 1994).

The regulation of emotions has concerned writers at least since the first word of Homer's *Iliad* was scribbled: 'Rage—Goddess, sing the rage of Peleus' son Achilles' (Homer, 1924) to start an account of how a demigod's uncontrolled emotions led to strife, death, and disaster (Harris, 2002). Given the uncertainties about how to define emotion it is no surprise that the compound derivatives 'emotion regulation' or 'emotion dysregulation' are also vaguely defined. Also, the word regulation can give rise to confusion. It is a naïve view that all negative emotion is a bad thing that ought to be regulated. Such a view ignores findings that children prone to negative affect may be more resilient under certain environmental circumstances (deVries, 1984). Similarly, it would ignore that even very intense sadness or fear may be adaptive. Also, regulating an emotion does not necessarily mean suppressing it—for example, sedation is not the same thing as control. I shall return to the issues of boundaries between emotions and normality in the section on psychopathology below.

Distinctions between emotion and emotion regulation

It has been rightly said that emotions are themselves partly defined as a means of evaluating and modifying experience. This suggests that emotions act to regulate emotions in their own right (Cole *et al.*, 2004). For example, the teenager in the introduction's imaginary experiment may experience less fear if he were presented with pleasant emotional stimuli at the same time as he was presented with the spider images. Such an interaction between emotions could be automatic, rather than a deliberate act of regulation. This type of emotion regulation by emotion is rarely studied and therefore much less understood (Moll *et al.*, 2007). Another problem with the distinction between emotion and emotion regulation is methodological. Does the young man of our example in the introduction report intense fear because he has experienced a strong emotional reaction or because he has not been able to regulate his emotion? This challenge may be overcome with physiological measurement, particularly as neuroimaging assesses the temporal relationships between emotion reactions (indexed by limbic activation, see below) and top–down cortical control.

Heterogeneity of emotion regulation

For example, the way infants regulate their anger seems to work far less in regulating their fear responses (Buss *et al.*, 1998). Similarly, a therapist might give different advice to the adolescent in the introduction if his presenting problem were uncontrollable anger towards his schoolmates, rather than fear towards a spider.

Different forms of emotional regulation

A useful classification for developmental scientists is what distinguishes between **intrinsic and extrinsic** emotion regulation (Fox *et al.*, 2003). Intrinsic refers to the ability of a person to regulate one's own emotions and extrinsic is the regulation by others (e.g., one's friend).

One of the most influential ways of classifying emotion regulation is due to James Gross (Gross, 1998), which distinguishes between two major phases of emotion regulation: **antecedent focused** and **response focused**. The first of the antecedent-focused phases is **situation selection**. This refers to approaching or avoiding people, places or objects. In our example from the introduction, the teenager could effectively regulate his emotions by taking precautions to avoid spiders. The second of the antecedent-focused phases of emotion regulation is **situation modification**. The next stage, **attention deployment,** includes **distraction**, **concentration** and **rumination** (Gross, 1998). As we will see below, infants who are better able to distract themselves by shifting their gaze away from distressing stimuli, better regulate their emotion. Similarly, concentrating on pleasant tasks, such as playing a game, may

regulate emotions. Rumination on negative emotions or feelings can have negative emotional consequences (Nolen-Hoeksema *et al.*, 2008). **Cognitive change** refers to how people interpret an emotional experience and it includes cognitive appraisal of a situation. As we will see below, this focus on appraisal has been studied extensively in the emotion regulation literature and is central to cognitive and behavior treatment approaches. **Response modulation** is listed as the only instance of response-focused emotion regulation strategies in Gross's model (Gross, 1998). This is a very wide category and includes taking drugs to decrease physiological responses, as well as exercise and relaxation.

Notwithstanding its heuristic value, this model has a number of shortcomings. First, the boundaries between the phases of emotion regulation are not always clear; for example, cognitive change can involve situation selection and modification and also have attention re-deployment as a consequence. Second, the category of response modulation is quite wide and may obscure important differences between regulation processes as diverse as drug treatment or biofeedback. Third, many important physiological aspects of emotion regulation, such as sleep or food intake, do not fall neatly into any of these categories. Also, exposure and habituation are some of the best-known and clinically-relevant strategies of emotion regulation, which also do not fit well with these distinctions. Because of their relevance for research in practice, I discuss these separately here.

Emotion regulation through **exposure and habituation** involves the activation of a fear through exposure and habituation through successive exposure to such a fear-evoking stimuli (Foa *et al.*, 1986). Habituation simply refers to the decreased response after repeated application of the stimulus (Thompson *et al.*, 1966). The principle is best illustrated through its clinical application in exposure therapy, such as when the teenager of our introduction's example is repeatedly presented with images of the spider; however, it is likely that emotion regulation in everyday life—the warming up in social situations, the improvement of performance by 'facing one's fear'—rely on the same principles. The exposure and habituation experiments also make clear a more general principle relevant to emotion regulation, namely the often reciprocal **relationship between emotions, actions and the environment.** In our example from the introduction, the young man could simply run away—or, if more aggressive and presented with a real spider, he might simply kill it. This is consistent with the definition of emotions as response tendencies and their postulated role in evolution. It is also important, though, to recognize how actions themselves impact on emotions. It is the action of repeated exposure or of avoidance that regulates emotions in different ways.

Linked with the distinction between approach and withdrawal emotion processes is the emotion regulation concept proposed by Davidson (Davidson, 1998). There, distinctions are made between the threshold for emotional reactivity, the amplitude of the response, and two components of 'affective chronometry', namely rise time to peak and the recovery time

(Davidson, 1998). It appears that individual differences in asymmetric prefrontal activation—an electroencephalographic measure—predict differences in components of this emotion-processing system.

I will now discuss some of the mechanisms that may underlie these emotion regulation processes.

The brain in emotion regulation: the generator-regulator model

A distinction most commonly made in brain research on emotion regulation is between a bottom-up process and a top–down regulation. In this model, limbic areas—particularly the amygdala—are involved in **emotion generation and expression**. The amygdala is a phylogenetically old structure involved in learning of emotional associations (Cardinal *et al.*, 2002). If the adolescent in the introduction had suffered damage to his amygdalae, he would probably be unable to experience fear. The amygdala is reciprocally connected with areas of the frontal cortex, such as the medial and inferior prefrontal cortex (mPFC and iPFC respectively) and lateral OFC. These cortical areas are activated during forms of emotion **regulation** such as cognitive appraisal (Ochsner *et al.*, 2012). It has been shown that increases in neural activity in the mPFC, iPFC and OFC are correlated with decreases in neural activity in the amygdala (Banks *et al.*, 2007; Goldin *et al.*, 2008). In our imaginary experiment in the introduction, the young man's ability to decrease his fear would correlate with the cortical dampening of amygdala activity. Such a top–down model (Blackford *et al.*, 2012) based on anatomical connections between prefrontal cortical areas and the amygdala in primates is presented in Figure 5.2 (Ghashghaei *et al* 2007). The regulation of emotion through this vertical integration is said to follow two related principles (Tucker *et al.*, 2000), namely (a) a hierarchical integration of inhibitory control, by which lower circuits are subordinated to more flexible higher networks; (b) by what is called encephalization, where higher, general-purpose brain networks take over functions formerly served by lower, restricted-action circuits (Tucker *et al.*, 2000).

The brain in emotion regulation: recognizing complexity

Brain findings of emotion regulation vary between studies for a number of reasons. A major source of heterogeneity relates to the strategy used in the research. Some forms of regulation such as dyadic regulation (e.g., that between mothers and children that we will discuss later), are difficult to test in a scanning environment and their underlying brain mechanisms remain unknown. However, there are several sources even within one strategy of regulation. In a recent review, Ochsner *et al.* (2012) show that different brain areas and hemispheres are recruited depending on whether a subject is asked to increase a positive emotion or decrease a negative emotion. Another source of heterogeneity relates to the strategy used for reappraisal: reinterpretation of events seems to involve brain regions involved in response selection and inhibition (in the ventrolateral prefrontal cortex,

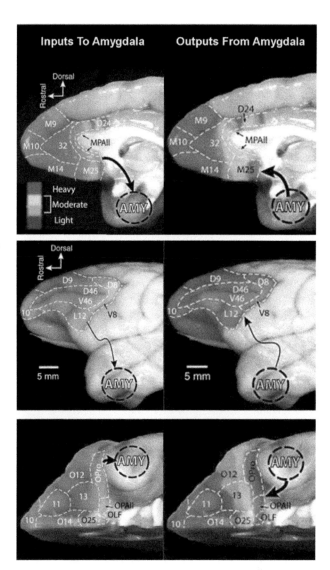

Figure 5.2 Distribution and density of output projections between the prefrontal cortex and the amygdala in the primate brain. Top row, medial aspect of the frontal lobe, middle row, lateral aspect of the frontal lobe, bottom row, orbitofrontal surface of the frontal lobe. AMY = amygdala. *Source:* Ghashghaei HT., Hilgetag CC., and Barbas H. (2007). Reprinted with permission from Elsevier.

vLPFC), whereas distancing recruits regions implicated in perspective taking, such as the parietal cortex (Ochsner *et al.*, 2012). Understanding these sources of heterogeneity is important also when appraising evidence from clinical neuroimaging studies. A recent meta-analysis of functional magnetic resonance imaging (fMRI) studies in depression found that emotional valence had a modulating effect on the comparison between patients and controls (Groenewold *et al.*, 2013). Depressed patients showed stronger activation in the right amygdala, left striatum, and anterior cingulate cortex (ACC) during negative processing; however, the same brain areas show less activation if depressed patients were processing positive stimuli. Also, certain forms of emotion regulation may not involve conscious top–down regulation, but rely on a coordinated network of automated responses. On the basis of research in animals and humans, a brain network has been postulated that involves the striatum (particularly the ventral tegmental area, VTA) in perceiving the pleasure of a stimulus, the VTA and OFC in calculating the reward value of the object of that stimulus (such as food), and the ACC in determining the relative effort required in obtaining such an object (Der-Avakian *et al.*, 2012). As we will see below, such networks may be disrupted in depressive disorder and their restitution may be one of the effects of treatment.

The brain in emotion regulation: the importance of learning and timing

As mentioned in the previous section, exposure and habituation are important forms of emotion regulation. The model used most widely is that of fear conditioning, where what was a neutral stimulus is turned into a *conditioned* stimulus (CS) through pairing with an aversive stimulus (usually called the *unconditioned* stimulus). In our example from the introduction, it would involve presenting the spider paired with a smell or sound that would become the conditioned stimulus. Such conditioning requires the basolateral amygdala, as shown in studies with humans and animals (LeDoux, 2000). Exposure—which typically involves repeated presentation of the CS without the aversive stimulus—leads to extinction or habituation (Phelps *et al.*, 2000). Evidence in animals and humans shows that the mPFC is critical in extinction through its connections with the amygdala (Myers *et al.*, 2007; McNally, 2007). It appears that new protein synthesis is required for extinction in the mPFC, suggesting that this is a process involving **neural plasticity** (Myers *et al.*, 2007)—indeed, it has been suggested that extinction may be better thought of as new learning rather than unlearning (McNally, 2007). A recent interesting finding is that the timing of extinction treatment may determine whether a conditioned memory will be erased or only inhibited. In humans, fear conditioning is extinguished and does not return later in the same context if extinction treatment is done within minutes (as opposed to within hours) (Agren *et al.*, 2012).

Emotion and development

Interest in mechanisms of development has grown in parallel with research efforts in developmental psychopathology (Rutter *et al.*, 2006) and has highlighted challenges to developmental research in this area before appraising the existing evidence.

Emotion and development: challenges to its study

The first challenge concerns the **limits of reporting source** and descriptive phenomenology. Most of the research about mood and emotion in adults relies on self report. Indeed, self-reported emotional states are validating outcomes for most research studies—including imaging and genetics—in adolescence and adults. However, research in newborns, infants, and young children has to rely on parent report or on observation. The correlation between different informants and methods is modest (Achenbach *et al.*, 1987). The use of different informants or different methods of assessment at different age groups limits our ability to judge the continuity of emotional states.

A related challenge is that some experimental paradigms are often **age-specific**. Some, for example the Still Face paradigm which we will discuss below, are particularly suited for early development. Another challenge concerns the technology used to study mood and emotion. For example, fMRI is hard to use in toddlers. Finally, as is the case for most of psychiatric research, it is unclear how best to map findings from different methods and sources onto each other. A particular challenge about research in early development is to map functional findings onto a **changing brain structure** (Giedd *et al.*, 1999).

With these caveats in mind, I will now discuss intra-individual change in emotions in early life, and then present two types of emotion regulation that are developmentally specific and finally discuss some of the challenges relating to transition periods in development.

Emotions and their differentiation in early life

Emotional expression becomes **richer and more differentiated** as children grow. One of the earliest models of emotional development is that of Banham Bridges (Bridges, 1932). It postulates that specific emotions develop from a rather ill-defined initial 'excitement' (Bridges, 1932). Stress and delight appear at 3 months, before the more refined emotions of fear, anger, disgust, distress, and excitement make their appearance. Indeed, studies find the references to feeling states increase as children grow older. A study by Dunn and colleagues (Dunn *et al.*, 1987) shows that the total number of children's references to emotional states (primarily sleepiness, tiredness, hunger, pain, feeling hot or cold, sadness, happiness and pain) increases from 18 to 24 months of age. Studies also show that emotion comprehension improves with age. Pons, Harris and De Rosnay (Pons *et al.*, 2004) show that older children are overall better than younger children at emotion recognition, regulation and ambivalence.

Development and emotion regulation: some examples

Here I will use three examples to highlight influences of development on emotion regulation. One concerns parent–child interactions, the other interaction with peers, and the last one discusses internal capacity for attention allocation.

An important aspect of early emotion regulation is that it can be **dyadic** (in pairs), usually between parent and child, but also with other children or adults. A striking experiment demonstrating this is the Still Face paradigm developed by Tronick (1989). There, infant – mother pairs are observed through three phases: a baseline during which a mother is interacting normally with her child; a still face phase during which the mother follows the instructions to maintain an unresponsive face towards her child; and a reunion phase during which the mother interacts normally again (Mesman *et al.*, 2009). Negative affect increases (with effect sizes around $d = 0.5$) and positive affect decreases (with effect sizes over $d = 0.9$) from baseline to the still face phase. During the reunion, positive affect increases dramatically ($d = 0.75$) but negative affect carries over to the reunion phase ($d = 0.04$). Maternal sensitivity is a significant predictor of the strength of positive affect in infants, while infant's positive affect is positively correlated with quality of attachment at age of one year (Mesman *et al.*, 2009). It also appears that mutual emotion regulation abilities between mother and child are significant predictors of later conduct problems in children: low levels of mutual positive emotion, emotion mismatching and high levels of mutual anger were more common in children with a chronic trajectory of emotional problems (Cole *et al.*, 2003). While these experiments demonstrate mutual emotion regulation in early development, they do not demonstrate causal effects. It remains unclear whether poor dyadic regulation is an indicator of genetically—influenced characteristics of one or both members of the dyad, and whether deficient dyadic regulation has a causal effect on emotion development in its own right.

Another major source of developmental effects on emotion is due to peer influences. The consequences of peer deviance and bullying on the development of behaviour problems are discussed in Chapter 26. Recent work suggests that bullying also has a major and possibly causal effect on the development of emotional problems (Arseneault *et al.*, 2010). Recent experimental work suggests that bullying may have an impact on the regulation of the physiological response to stress. In particular, compared to non-bullied children, those bullied show a blunted response of their hypothalamic-pituitary-adrenal (HPA) axis, as measured using cortisol, following a stress induction experiment (Ouellet-Morin *et al.*, 2011). See also Chapter 29.

Attention allocation is a mechanism that underlines emotion regulation that undergoes developmental changes. For example, when infants are distracted they also express less negative emotion (Harman *et al.*, 1997) and infants with longer attention spans are more likely to show signs of positive emotion (Putnam *et al.*, 2008). A brain indicator of early attention is a frontal negative EEG called the Nc—this is the earliest potential in human development that has been shown to relate to autonomic orientation of attention (Nelson *et al.*, 1996), and probably originates in the anterior cingulate. A recent study has shown that infants who are quicker to show the Nc (lower latencies) and show stronger Nc (higher amplitude) are better able to regulate emotions (Martinos *et al.*, 2012). In other words, infants low on self-regulation are slower to re-orientate attention.

Developmental transitions and emotions

As we have seen, emotional expression develops in childhood without any sharply-demarcated periods of radical change. Indeed, there are no periods that could be considered to be developmentally-sensitive, in the sense this term is being used

in, say, the development of human vision (Thapar *et al.*, 2009). However, a number of changes in emotional expression happen around the vaguely defined period of adolescence and these are worth discussing here.

Two of the most notable changes during adolescence are an **increase in impulsivity** and another is the increase in the **prevalence of depressive disorder** with the emergence of the **2:1 female-to-male** ratio in that disorder.

Impulsivity and emotions during adolescence

The term impulsivity is generally applied to describe a wide range of behaviors that increase during adolescence, including experimentation with alcohol and drugs, conduct problems, and unprotected sex (Casey *et al.*, 2010). It is unclear whether the same sort of impulsivity underlies each of these behaviors as it is unclear whether impulsivity should be seen as an emotional problem. However, the experimental paradigms used to study the possible mechanisms of impulsivity are related to emotion mechanisms as they both implicate reward-related processes. These show that adolescents are better than pre-adolescent children at cognitive tasks that involve response inhibition. However, adolescents find it more difficult to suppress responses to reward-related cues. Some authorities suggest that this increase in impulsivity during adolescence may be best explained by contrasting the curvilinear development of brain areas such as the nucleus accumbens to the linear development of the PFC (prefrontal cortex). For example, Casey and Jones (Casey *et al.*, 2010) challenge the view that behaviors characteristic of adolescence occur because the PFC is not mature enough for top–down control. Adolescence is said to be the time of maximal difference between the subcortical (e.g., nucleus accumbens) structures that mature earlier and the cortical (PFC) structures that only reach full maturity after adolescence (Casey *et al.*, 2010). According to the authors, an acknowledgement of the developmental imbalance between cortical and subcortical systems may provide new insights into the mechanisms mediating adolescent behaviors.

Transitions in emotional disorders

As discussed in Chapter 63, the prevalence of depression increases after puberty and the 2:1 female to male ratio in depression is established. The reasons for this gender difference are unclear and it is plausible that biological, social and cognitive factors interact to increase girls' vulnerability (Hyde *et al.*, 2008). Some of the most convincing evidence from Angold and colleagues (Angold *et al.*, 1999b) shows that pubertal girls with increased levels of sex steroids (testosterone and oestrogen) are more vulnerable to developing depression independently of the timing of pubertal changes or stress levels. The brain mechanisms through which hormones may exert their effects to increase risk for depression remain to be discovered (Blakemore *et al.*, 2006).

Disorders of emotion and emotion regulation: boundaries to normality, relation to basic science, and other challenges

Boundaries to normality

The boundaries between emotional disorder and normality are often unclear. Classification systems typically take the pragmatic approach of using cut-offs that would restrict the prevalence of a disorder to a relatively small proportion of the population. For example, for the recently-introduced category of *Disruptive Mood Dysregulation Disorder (DMDD)*, the criteria stipulate a relatively high *frequency* of temper outbursts as well as irritable mood of long *duration* alongside impairment due to these symptoms. These arbitrary thresholds have meant that the prevalence of DMDD is relatively low, at least in epidemiological samples, and that the associated impairment fits the description of 'disruptive' or 'severe' mood dysregulation. For practicing clinicians, contextual factors, such as the young persons' and the parents' ability to cope with emotional symptoms, are often taken into account before diagnosing. However, such judgements are often problematic as future negative consequences of symptoms are often independent of concurrent impairment (Stringaris *et al.*, 2013). Another approach is to consider whether the emotional reaction is proportional to the stimulus. A typical example is that of the boundaries between bereavement reaction and depression. Such decisions often involve an evaluative judgement about what constitute an appropriate reaction, though in the case of bereavement certain symptoms (e.g., suicidal ideation) are said to predict persistence of depression and impairment (American Psychiatric Association, 2013).

Overlap between basic science and clinical concepts

There are four principle methodological challenges when trying to translate the findings of emotion science to clinical concepts. The first concerns **duration** of the emotion response and the **eliciting object**: laboratory experiments of emotion processing typically focus on short-lived experiences lasting from milliseconds to a few minutes. It would be both ethically questionable and methodologically challenging to induce a long-lasting mood—sadness or irritability that lasts for days—in a laboratory setting. As a result, the brain mechanisms of enduring mood episodes are understudied. Indeed, understanding the difference between emotion and mood may be an important future goal. **Mood** is often defined by the absence of an emotion-eliciting object, such as when the amygdala is electrically stimulated in an animal or when patients are depressed for no apparent reason. It has been argued that mood may in that sense be different from emotion and unique (Rolls, 2007). The other distinction can be made on the basis of the associated **clusters of symptoms** and the heterogeneity within disorders. The adolescent of our imaginary experiment only suffered from a simple phobia. However, clinical syndromes, such as depression, come with a number of other symptoms including anhedonia or low energy. These are hard to elicit and study in isolation. Another distinction can be made on the basis of **intensity** and associated **impairment**. The sadness experienced by patients is often excruciating and certainly impairing (Stringaris *et al.*, 2013), something that is also hard to model in an experimental setup. Finally, there may be other **qualitative distinctions**. It is not at all clear that elation for example – the hallmark of mania – is on the same dimension as ordinary happiness.

One symptom, many disorders

One problem is due to symptoms occurring across different disorders. Irritability and anger are probably the most prominent examples. Emotion theorists would view anger as one of the basic emotions, yet in psychiatric terms anger and irritability are symptoms of both emotional and disruptive disorders. As can be seen in Table 5.1, the symptom of irritability appears in the criteria of at least six different child psychiatric disorders and crosses the boundaries between emotional and disruptive disorders. For nosology, the presence of the same symptom in various disorders can inflate their overlap. The confusion for clinicians is that a motivating behavior (anger) is classified according to its possible consequences—so an angry child has a high chance of being diagnosed with a disruptive behavior disorder (ODD), rather than with an emotional disorder. In this example, the mechanisms underlying anger may be different from those that predispose someone with anger to be antisocial.

Table 5.1 Irritability compared to other common symptoms of child psychiatric disorders.

	Irritability	Worry/ Fear	Sadness	Antisocial behavior
Sep Anx	−	+	−	−
SpPh	+	+	−	−
SoPh	+	+	−	−
PTSD	+	+	−	−
OCD	−	+	−	−
GAD	+	+	−	−
Panic disorder	−	+	−	−
Agoraphobia	−	+	−	−
MDD	+	−	+	−
ADHD	−	−	−	−
ODD	+	−	−	−
CD	−	−	−	+

Sep Anx	separation anxiety
SpPh	specific phobia
SoPh	social phobia
PTSD	post traumatic stress disorder
OCD	obsessive compulsive disorder
GAD	generalized anxiety disorder
MDD	major depressive disorder
ADHD	attention deficit/hyperactivity disorder
ODD	oppositional defiant disorder
CD	conduct disorder

Also, irritability or related symptoms such as mood lability occur with a high frequency in disorders that do not list these symptoms in their criteria (Stringaris *et al.*, 2009c). For example, impairing mood lability occurs at a high rate among children with ADHD (Stringaris *et al.*, 2009c, Taylor, 2009). It remains unclear whether this mood dysregulation is due to ADHD core symptoms, a yet-unrecognized symptom of ADHD, or the manifestation of a dimension of mood dysregulation that cuts across ADHD and other psychiatric disorders (Shaw *et al.*, 2014). Similar questions arise with mood dysregulation in autism spectrum disorders (ASD).

Overlap between emotional and disruptive disorders

Psychiatric disorders overlap considerably: in a study of the UK general population (Maughan *et al.*, 2004) over 10% of children and adolescents with a disruptive disorder had an emotional disorder. Second, emotional and conduct problems share antecedents. For example, temperamental emotionality is a predictor of both emotional and disruptive disorders and seems to be a particularly strong predictor of the comorbidity between the two (Stringaris *et al.*, 2010). Third, emotional and conduct disorders also show sequential comorbidity (Angold *et al.*, 1999a). Indeed, ODD (oppositional defiant disorder) may be one of the most common antecedents of later depression in clinic and community samples (Burke *et al.*, 2005; Copeland *et al.*, 2009). People attempting to explain this overlap between disruptive and emotional disorders have focused on the heterogeneity of oppositional behaviors. Stringaris & Goodman (Stringaris *et al.*, 2009b, d) suggested that oppositional symptoms are made up of three correlated dimensions of irritable, headstrong and hurtful behaviors. Irritability has been shown in various studies to be a relatively specific predictor of later depression and generalized anxiety in up to 20-year follow-up studies (Stringaris *et al.*, 2009a) and an independent predictor of suicidality in a 30-year follow-up (Pickles *et al.*, 2009). Moreover the distinction of irritability from other positional behaviors has been shown in various studies including studies outside Europe or the United States (Krieger *et al.*, 2013). This wide presence of irritability across psychopathology has given rise to two explanatory models that are not mutually exclusive. One holds that irritability may be a cross-cutting dimension in psychopathology, and the other that severe irritability should be classified as a distinct disorder, an approach adopted in the Disruptive Mood Dysregulation Disorder category that has been introduced by the DSM-5 (Leibenluft, 2011; Mikita *et al.*, 2013). Neuroscience research has been helpful in distinguishing between severe irritability and other conditions (notably bipolar disorder, see Chapter 62).

The specificity of emotional disorders

The validity of current distinctions between child psychiatric disorders, then, is questionable (Rutter, 2011). Genetic evidence (Lahey *et al.*, 2011) suggests that there are pleiotropic genetic effects across all psychiatric disorders and that these can be split into two main groups of emotional and disruptive disorders (in their terminology, internalizing and externalizing). Within internalizing disorders, a great proportion of the genetic liability for depression is shared with early anxiety disorders and the personality traits of neuroticism (Kendler *et al.*, 2006). In twin studies, it appears that internalizing disorders have strong genetic overlap, as do externalizing disorders. This has led some researchers to suggest that distinctions between emotional disorders may be redundant and that classification should be reconfigured in accordance with genetic findings (Stringaris, 2013). However, this approach would ignore findings of specificity of some anxiety diagnoses (see Chapter 2). Family and longitudinal and experimental studies seem to distinguish between anxiety disorders such as social phobia and separation anxiety disorder (Pine, 2007). Overall, however, the strong genetic overlap in psychiatric disorders raises the question about what makes them phenotypically distinct. The answer given at the moment is that this may be due to specific environmental circumstances (Eley, 1997).

Understudied emotional symptoms

As a result of the so-called paediatric bipolar disorder (see Chapter 62), researchers have concentrated their efforts on clarifying the role of irritability and understanding the importance of short-lived episodes of mania-like symptoms. Yet, there is far less research into some of the core **mania-like symptoms**, such as euphoria and increases in energy and activity. As a result, several things remain unclear: first, we do not know the developmental origins of such symptoms; second, we do not know whether such symptoms are on a continuum with everyday happiness; third, it is unclear whether such symptoms may be related to aspects of superior adjustment as has been suggested in adults (MacCabe *et al.*, 2010) and more recently adolescents (Stringaris *et al* 2014). We recently found that in the UK general population (Stringaris *et al.*, 2011), episodic, mania-like symptoms are endorsed by a substantial proportion of parents and children. These episodic symptoms of exuberance form a latent factor that is distinct from (yet correlated) with episodic symptoms of undercontrol (such as irritability and disinhibition). Moreover, it seems that such symptoms are not predictive of impairment or comorbid psychopathology, once symptoms of undercontrol have been adjusted for. It remains to be seen whether these symptoms bear any predictive value for future psychopathology in their own right.

Emotions and treatment

Treatments of individual emotional disorders are discussed in the relevant chapters. Here I focus upon two questions about treatment that follow from the discussions above. The first concerns specificity of treatments, the second, whether people's emotional responses influence treatment effects.

Boundaries of treatments and underlying mechanisms

We have seen that the distinctions between categories of emotions are disputed as are the boundaries between the different emotional disorders in psychiatric classification. It is therefore no surprise that treatments for emotional disorders are not specific to any particular condition. The broad term cognitive-behavioral therapy (CBT) is used to describe treatments that have shown to be modestly effective for both depressive and anxiety disorders (see Chapter 38). For example, in children with obsessive-compulsive disorder (OCD) exposure and response prevention treatment appears to be effective for OCD symptoms as well as for depressive symptoms and patient's temper outbursts (Krebs *et al.*, 2013). Similarly, serotonin re-uptake inhibitors (SRIs) are the first-line drugs used to treat emotional disorders, again with rather modest success. Do all these treatments act in the same non-specific way or are there important distinctions? Neuroscience may be helpful in answering these questions. Recent findings suggest that it may be useful to distinguish between cognitive-focused and more activation-focused CBT protocols. Both approaches (Cuijpers *et al.*, 2007; Wiles *et al.*, 2013) seem to be effective at least in adults with depression, yet they may differ in how they achieve this effect. Siegle (Siegle *et al.*, 2012) and his colleagues scanned depressed adults before and after 16–20 sessions of cognitive therapy. They found that patients with the lowest pre-treatment activity in subgenual anterior cingulate cortex (ACC) in response to negative words displayed the most improvement after cognitive therapy. This is particularly interesting given that (as noted earlier) the ACC is known to decrease activity in limbic regions—a top–down form of regulation as one might expect of cognitive therapy. The mechanisms of action of behavioral activation may differ to that of cognitive therapy. An fMRI studied by Dichter *et al.* (2009) suggests that brain areas mediating responses to rewards including the orbitofrontal cortex were modulated by behavioral activation therapy.

Emotion and treatment effects

We have discussed above how a child's difficult temperament might be advantageous under difficult circumstances (deVries, 1984). In recent years, Belsky (Belsky *et al.*, 2009) has proposed that, with supportive parents, infants who score high on negative emotionality may have *better* outcomes than their peers scoring low on negative emotionality. This raises interesting questions about the effects of one's emotions on one's own treatment. It is interesting to examine whether personal characteristics influence response to treatment—put simply, are there patients who benefit in particular or are particularly harmed by certain treatments? Scott and O'Connor (Scott *et al.*, 2010) recently showed that among children with conduct and oppositional problems taking part in a randomized controlled trial, those scoring high on emotional dysregulation were more likely than the rest to respond to a parenting intervention. It has been claimed (Belsky *et al.*, 2009) that plasticity genes (such as 5-HTTLPR, a variant in the promoter region of the gene coding for the serotonin transporter (Uher *et al.*, 2010) may explain emotionality and its effects on treatment. Overall, however, the results for the effects of such

personal characteristics or of genetic prediction or moderation of treatment have been modest. For example, in the pharmacological treatment of depression, no reliable genetic predictor of treatment response to drug treatment has been found (although it does seem that treatment response is modestly influenced by genetic variation) (GENDEP, 2013). Similarly, more evidence is required to understand how genetic variants may influence the outcome of psychological treatments (Lester *et al.*, 2013).

Conclusion and outlook

I wrote this chapter to present the advances in knowledge about emotion and emotional disorders and take on confusing concepts and findings. Some of the problems in the field may be easily overcome if we become aware of the ambiguities and problematic definitions of the terms we use—this applies particularly to the word emotion itself. The same caution is warranted when extending terms used in basic science to clinical concepts and vice versa—as I have shown, a lot more work is needed to translate findings from one into the other. All the challenges discussed in this chapter also need to be tackled by empirical research. Developing new experimental paradigms of emotion regulation—for example to study the effects of activity on emotion—can yield important insights into mechanisms of treatment for emotional disorders. Other challenges will require improvements in technology—reliable longitudinal functional imaging studies that span critical periods of development is a particular example. Some of the most important challenges, such as understanding the relationship between short-lived emotions and the prolonged mood states that clinicians encounter in their patients will require a combination of research approaches and may warrant new terminology to accommodate their implications.

References

Achenbach, T.M. *et al.* (1987) Child/adolescent behavioral and emotional problems: implications of cross-informant correlations for situational specificity. *Psychological Bulletin* **101**, 213–232.

Agren, T. *et al.* (2012) Disruption of reconsolidation erases a fear memory trace in the human amygdala. *Science* **337**, 1550–1552.

American Psychiatric Association (2013) *Diagnostic and Statistical Manual of Mental Disorders*, 5th edn. American Psychiatric Association, Washington, DC.

Angold, A. *et al.* (1999a) Comorbidity. *Journal of Child Psychology and Psychiatry* **40**, 57–87.

Angold, A. *et al.* (1999b) Pubertal changes in hormone levels and depression in girls. *Psychological Medicine* **29**, 1043–53.

Arseneault, L. *et al.* (2010) Bullying victimization in youths and mental health problems: 'much ado about nothing'? *Psychological Medicine* **40**, 717–729.

Banks, S.J. *et al.* (2007) Amygdala–frontal connectivity during emotion regulation. *Social Cognitive and Affective Neuroscience* **2**, 303–312.

Barrett, L.F. (2011) Was Darwin wrong about emotional expressions? *Current Directions in Psychological Science* **20**, 400–406.

Belsky, J. *et al.* (2009) Vulnerability genes or plasticity genes? *Molecular Psychiatry* **14**, 746–754.

Blackford, J.U. *et al.* (2012) Neural substrates of childhood anxiety disorders: a review of neuroimaging findings. *Child and Adolescent Psychiatric Clinics of North America* **21**, 501–525.

Blakemore, S.J. *et al.* (2006) Brain development during puberty: state of the science. *Developmental Science* **9**, 11–14.

Bridges, K.M.B. (1932) Emotional development in early infancy. *Child Development* **3**, 324–341.

Burke, J.D. *et al.* (2005) Developmental transitions among affective and behavioral disorders in adolescent boys. *Journal of Child Psychology and Psychiatry* **46**, 1200–1210.

Buss, K.A. *et al.* (1998) Fear and anger regulation in infancy: effects on the temporal dynamics of affective expression. *Child Development* **69**, 359–374.

Cardinal, R.N. *et al.* (2002) Effects of selective excitotoxic lesions of the nucleus accumbens core, anterior cingulate cortex, and central nucleus of the amygdala on autoshaping performance in rats. *Behavioral Neuroscience* **116**, 553–567.

Casey, B.J. *et al.* (2010) Neurobiology of the adolescent brain and behavior: implications for substance use disorders. *Journal of the American Academy of Child and Adolescent Psychiatry* **49**, 1189–1201.

Cole, P.M. *et al.* (2003) Mutual emotion regulation and the stability of conduct problems between preschool and early school age. *Development and Psychopathology* **15**, 1–18.

Cole, P.M. *et al.* (2004) Emotion regulation as a scientific construct: methodological challenges and directions for child development research. *Child Development* **75**, 317–333.

Copeland, W.E. *et al.* (2009) Childhood and adolescent psychiatric disorders as predictors of young adult disorders. *Archives of General Psychiatry* **66**, 764–772.

Critchley, H.D. *et al.* (2004) Neural systems supporting interoceptive awareness. *Nature Neuroscience* **7**, 189–195.

Cuijpers, P. *et al.* (2007) Behavioral activation treatments of depression: a meta-analysis. *Clinical Psychology Review* **27**, 318–326.

Darwin, C. (1872) *Expression of the Emotions in Man and Animals*. John Murray, London.

Davidson, R.J. (1998) Affective style and affective disorders: perspectives from affective neuroscience. *Cognition & Emotion* **12**, 307–330.

Der-Avakian, A. *et al.* (2012) The neurobiology of anhedonia and other reward-related deficits. *Trends in Neurosciences* **35**, 68–77.

DeVries, M.W. (1984) Temperament and infant mortality among the Masai of East Africa. *American Journal of Psychiatry* **141**, 1189–1194.

Dichter, G.S. *et al.* (2009) The effects of psychotherapy on neural responses to rewards in major depression. *Biological Psychiatry* **66**, 886–897.

Dunn, J. *et al.* (1987) Conversations about feeling states between mothers and their young children. *Developmental Psychology* **23**, 132–139.

Ekman, P. *et al.* (2011) What is meant by calling emotions basic. *Emotion Review* **3**, 364–370.

Eley, T.C. (1997) General genes: a new theme in developmental psychopathology. *Current Directions in Psychological Science* **6**, 90–95.

Foa, E.B. *et al.* (1986) Emotional processing of fear: exposure to corrective information. *Psychological Bulletin* **99**, 20–35.

Fox, N. *et al.* (2003) The development of self-control of emotion: intrinsic and extrinsic influences. *Motivation and Emotion* **27**, 7–26.

Frankenhaeuser, M. (1971) Behavior and circulating catecholamines. *Brain Research* **31**, 241–262.

GENDEP (2013) Common genetic variation and antidepressant efficacy in major depressive disorder: a meta-analysis of three genome-wide pharmacogenetic studies. *American Journal of Psychiatry* **170**, 207–217.

Giedd, J.N. *et al.* (1999) Brain development during childhood and adolescence: a longitudinal MRI study. *Nature Neuroscience* **2**, 861–863.

Goldin, P.R. *et al.* (2008) The neural bases of emotion regulation: reappraisal and suppression of negative emotion. *Biological Psychiatry* **63**, 577–586.

Groenewold, N.A. *et al.* (2013) Emotional valence modulates brain functional abnormalities in depression: evidence from a meta-analysis of fMRI studies. *Neuroscience and Biobehavioral Reviews* **37**, 152–163.

Gross, J.J. (1998) The emerging field of emotion regulation: an integrative review. *Review of General Psychology* **2**, 271–299.

Harman, C. *et al.* (1997) Distress and attention interactions in early infancy. *Motivation and Emotion* **21**, 27–43.

Harris, W.V. (2002) *Restraining Rage: the Ideology of Anger Control in Classical Antiquity*. Harvard University Press, Cambridge, MA.

Homer (1924) *The Iliad*. Harvard University Press, Cambridge, MA.

Hyde, J.S. *et al.* (2008) The ABCs of depression: integrating affective, biological, and cognitive models to explain the emergence of the gender difference in depression. *Psychological Review* **115**, 291–313.

Jack, R.E. *et al.* (2012) Facial expressions of emotion are not culturally universal. *Proceedings of the National Academy of Sciences of the United States of America* **109**, 7241–7244.

Kagan, J. (2004) *What is emotion?* Yale University Press, New Haven, Connecticut.

Kendler, K.S. *et al.* (2006) Toward a comprehensive developmental model for major depression in men. *American Journal of Psychiatry* **163**, 115–124.

Krebs, G. *et al.* (2013) Temper outbursts in paediatric obsessive-compulsive disorder and their association with depressed mood and treatment outcome. *Journal of Child Psychology and Psychiatry* **54**, 313–322.

Krieger, F.V. *et al.* (2013) Dimensions of oppositionality in a Brazilian community sample: testing the DSM-5 proposal and etiological links. *Journal of the American Academy of Child and Adolescent Psychiatry* **52**, 389–400.

Lahey, B.B. *et al.* (2011) Higher-order genetic and environmental structure of prevalent forms of child and adolescent psychopathology. *Archives of General Psychiatry* **68**, 181–189.

Ledoux, J.E. (2000) Emotion circuits in the brain. *Annual Review of Neuroscience* **23**, 155–184.

Leibenluft, E. (2011) Severe mood dysregulation, irritability, and the diagnostic boundaries of bipolar disorder in youths. *American Journal of Psychiatry* **168**, 129–142.

Lench, H.C. *et al.* (2011) Discrete emotions predict changes in cognition, judgment, experience, behavior, and physiology: a meta-analysis of experimental emotion elicitations. *Psychological Bulletin* **137**, 834–855.

Lester, K. *et al.* (2013) Therapygenetics: Using genetic markers to predict response to psychological treatment for mood and anxiety disorders. *Biology of Mood & Anxiety Disorders* **3**, 4.

Lindquist, K.A. *et al.* (2012) The brain basis of emotion: a meta-analytic review. *Behavioral and Brain Sciences* **35**, 121–143.

Lindquist, K.A. *et al.* (2013) The hundred-year emotion war: are emotions natural kinds or psychological constructions? Comment on Lench, Flores, and Bench (2011). *Psychological Bulletin* **139**, 255–263.

MacCabe, J.H. *et al.* (2010) Excellent school performance at age 16 and risk of adult bipolar disorder: national cohort study. *British Journal of Psychiatry* **196**, 109–115.

Martinos, M. *et al.* (2012) Links between infant temperament and neurophysiological measures of attention to happy and fearful faces. *Journal of Child Psychology and Psychiatry* **53**, 1118–1127.

Maughan, B. *et al.* (2004) Conduct disorder and oppositional defiant disorder in a national sample: developmental epidemiology. *Journal of Child Psychology and Psychiatry* **45**, 609–621.

McNally, R.J. (2007) Mechanisms of exposure therapy: how neuroscience can improve psychological treatments for anxiety disorders. *Clinical Psychology Review* **27**, 750–759.

Mesman, J. *et al.* (2009) The many faces of the Still-Face Paradigm: a review and meta-analysis. *Developmental Review* **29**, 120–162.

Mikita, N. *et al.* (2013) Mood dysregulation. *European Child and Adolescent Psychiatry* **22**, 11–16.

Moll, J. *et al.* (2007) Moral judgments, emotions and the utilitarian brain. *Trends in Cognitive Sciences* **11**, 319–321.

Myers, K.M. *et al.* (2007) Mechanisms of fear extinction. *Molecular Psychiatry* **12**, 120–150.

Nelson, C.A. *et al.* (1996) Neural correlates of infants' visual responsiveness to facial expressions of emotion. *Developmental Psychobiology* **29**, 577–595.

Nolen-Hoeksema, S. *et al.* (2008) Rethinking rumination. *Perspectives on Pscyhological Science* **3**, 400–424.

Ochsner, K.N. *et al.* (2012) Functional imaging studies of emotion regulation: a synthetic review and evolving model of the cognitive control of emotion. *Annals of the New York Academy of Sciences* **1251**, E1–E24.

Ortony, A. & Turner, T.J. (1990) What's basic about basic emotions? *Psychological Review* **97**, 315–331.

Ouellet-Morin, I. *et al.* (2011) Blunted cortisol responses to stress signal social and behavioral problems among maltreated/bullied 12-year-old children. *Biological Psychiatry* **70**, 1016–1023.

Phelps, E.A. *et al.* (2000) Performance on indirect measures of race evaluation predicts amygdala activation. *Journal of Cognitive Neuroscience* **12**, 729–738.

Pickles, A. *et al.* (2009) Predictors of suicidality across the life span: the Isle of Wight study. *Psychological Medicine* **40**, 1453–1466.

Pine, D.S. (2007) Research review: a neuroscience framework for pediatric anxiety disorders. *Journal of Child Psychology and Psychiatry* **48**, 631–648.

Pons, F. *et al.* (2004) Emotion comprehension between 3 and 11 years: developmental periods and hierarchical organization. *European Journal of Developmental Psychology* **1**, 127–152.

Putnam, S.P. *et al.* (2008) Homotypic and heterotypic continuity of fine-grained temperament during infancy, toddlerhood, and early childhood. *Infant and Child Development* **17**, 387–405.

Rolls, E.T. (2007) *Emotion Explained.* Oxford University Press, Oxford.

Rutter, M. (2011) Research review: child psychiatric diagnosis and classification: concepts, findings, challenges and potential. *Journal of Child Psychology and Psychiatry* **52**, 647–660.

Rutter, M. *et al.* (2006) Continuities and discontinuities in psychopathology between childhood and adult life. *Journal of Child Psychology and Psychiatry* **47**, 276–295.

Scott, S. *et al.* (2010) Impact of a parenting program in a high-risk, multi-ethnic community: the PALS trial. *Journal of Child Psychology and Psychiatry* **51**, 1331–1341.

Shaw, P. *et al.* (2014) Emotion dysregulation in attention deficit hyperactivity disorder. *American Journal of Psychiatry* **171**, 276–293.

Siegle, G.J. *et al.* (2012) Toward clinically useful neuroimaging in depression treatment: prognostic utility of subgenual cingulate activity for determining depression outcome in cognitive therapy across studies, scanners, and patient characteristics. *Archives of General Psychiatry* **69**, 913–924.

Stringaris, A. (2013) Here/in this issue and there/abstract thinking: gene effects cross the boundaries of psychiatric disorders. *Journal of the American Academy of Child and Adolescent Psychiatry* **52**, 557–558.

Stringaris, A. *et al.* (2009a) Adult outcomes of youth irritability: a 20-year prospective community-based study. *American Journal of Psychiatry* **166**, 1048–1054.

Stringaris, A. *et al.* (2009b) Longitudinal outcome of youth oppositionality: irritable, headstrong, and hurtful behaviors have distinctive predictions. *Journal of the American Academy of Child and Adolescent Psychiatry* **48**, 404–412.

Stringaris, A. *et al.* (2009c) Mood lability and psychopathology in youth. *Psychological Medicine* **39**, 1237–1245.

Stringaris, A. *et al.* (2009d) Three dimensions of oppositionality in youth. *Journal of Child Psychology and Psychiatry* **50**, 216–223.

Stringaris, A. *et al.* (2010) What's in a disruptive disorder: temperamental antecedents of oppositional defiant disorder. *Journal of the American Academy of Child & Adolescent Psychiatry* **49**, 474–483.

Stringaris, A. *et al.* (2011) Dimensions and latent classes of episodic mania-like symptoms in youth: an empirical enquiry. *Journal of Abnormal Child Psychology* **39**, 925–937.

Stringaris, A. *et al.* (2013) The value of measuring impact alongside symptoms in children and adolescents: a longitudinal assessment in a community sample. *Journal of Abnormal Child Psychology* **41**, 1109–1120.

Stringaris, A. *et al.* (2014) Dimensions of manic symptoms in youth: psychosocial impairment and cognitive performance in the IMAGEN sample. *Journal of Child Psychology and Psychiatry* **55**, 1380–1389.

Taylor, E. (2009) Managing bipolar disorders in children and adolescents. *Nature Reviews Neurology* **5**, 484–491.

Thapar, A. *et al.* (2009) Do prenatal risk factors cause psychiatric disorder? Be wary of causal claims. *British Journal of Psychiatry* **195**, 100–101.

Thompson, R.A. (1994) Emotion regulation: a theme in search of definition. *Monographs of the Society for Research in Child Development* **59**, 25–52.

Thompson, R.F. *et al.* (1966) Habituation: a model phenomenon for the study of neuronal substrates of behavior. *Psychological Review* **73**, 16–43.

Tronick, E.Z. (1989) Emotions and emotional communication in infants. *American Psychologist* **44**, 112–119.

Tucker, D.M. *et al.* (2000) Anatomy and physiology of human emotion: vertical integration of brainstem, limbic, and cortical systems. In: *The Neuropsychology of Emotion.* Oxford University Press, New York.

Uher, R. *et al.* (2010) The moderation by the serotonin transporter gene of environmental adversity in the etiology of depression: 2009 update. *Molecular Psychiatry* **15**, 18–22.

Wiens, S. (2006) Subliminal emotion perception in brain imaging: findings, issues, and recommendations. *Progress in Brain Research* **156**, 105–121.

Wiles, N. *et al.* (2013) Cognitive behavioural therapy as an adjunct to pharmacotherapy for primary care based patients with treatment resistant depression: results of the CoBalT randomised controlled trial. *Lancet* **381**, 375–384.

CHAPTER 6

Attachment: normal development, individual differences, and associations with experience

Mary Dozier[1] and Kristin Bernard[2]
[1]Department of Psychological and Brain Sciences, University of Delaware, Newark, DE, USA
[2]Department of Psychology, Stony Brook University, Stony Brook, NY, USA

According to John Bowlby (1969/1982), the attachment system evolved to enhance reproductive fitness. Infants develop attachments to figures who are "older and wiser" than themselves and seek to maintain proximity with these attachment figures under threatening conditions. The infant's behavioral repertoire of crying, smiling, clinging and following represents an organized system, designed to maintain or restore proximity to the caregiver (Sroufe & Waters, 1977a, b; Bowlby, 1988). By the time the infant is capable of crawling or walking, the attachment system has developed fully such that the infant does not want to move far from the parent except when circumstances are familiar (Bretherton, 1985). Under conditions of threat, when proximity is especially important to survival, the need for proximity to the caregiver is intensified (Bowlby, 1969/1982; Rutter *et al.*, 2009). For example, when the infant is fearful of a stranger or a startling sound, the caregiver is sought out for protection, with the response intensified in proportion to the perceived threat. Given the basic evolutionary function of this system, attachments are expected to develop in virtually all ordinary childrearing conditions. Although the attachment system may have special significance for the infant, attachments are thought to remain important for humans throughout life.

Historical context of the development of attachment theory

Attachment theory was developed in response to psychoanalytic and social learning theories of the time, and in the context of observations of the pernicious effects of privation on human and non-human young, and a burgeoning literature on ethology and evolution. John Bowlby articulated what has come to be known as attachment theory. Mary Ainsworth played a critical role as an astute observer of individual differences in attachment, and

on the basis of these observations, in developing a system for classifying infants' attachment quality.

Reaction to psychoanalytic theory

Bowlby was trained as a psychiatrist at a point in time when psychoanalytic thinking dominated the field. While training at the British Psychoanalytic Institute, Bowlby was supervised by Melanie Klein, who, along with many others of the time, believed that the young child's inner fantasy played a much more formative role in development than interactions with his or her real mother. As such, Kleinian psychoanalysts almost entirely ignored the mother's actual behavior in the treatment of young children's emotional needs. This approach very much conflicted with Bowlby's sense of the importance of a child's real caregiving experiences.

Effects of deprivation

Observations of the challenges faced by children who experienced inadequate parental care pushed Bowlby from the base of psychoanalytic thinking. In his first empirical study, Bowlby (1944) documented 44 cases of adolescent thieves. Many of these children were characterized as "affectionless," demonstrating an extreme lack of empathy for others. Through detailed interviews about these children and their histories of caregiving, Bowlby observed that maternal deprivation and separation early in life emerged as a common factor. When he compared these 44 thieves to a sample of emotionally disturbed children who did not steal, Bowlby found that the lack of an important attachment figure in early childhood indeed distinguished the groups.

James Robertson was hired by Bowlby to help him observe hospitalized and institutionalized children who experienced separations from their parents. Robertson carefully observed children at home before they were hospitalized and followed

Rutter's Child and Adolescent Psychiatry, Sixth Edition.
Edited by Anita Thapar and Daniel S. Pine, James F. Leckman, Stephen Scott, Margaret J. Snowling, Eric Taylor.

them into the hospital and home again. Frustrated with his inability to convince professionals of the challenges faced by children undergoing separation, Robertson made the movie, "A Two-Year-Old Goes to Hospital." This film, although initially challenged by many, focused awareness on the consequences for young children of separation from their parents (Robertson & Robertson, 1989; Ainsworth & Bowlby, 1991; Bretherton, 1992).

Bowlby chaired the World Health Organization (WHO) commission on the problems faced by homeless children following World War II and met Spitz (1945) and Goldfarb (1945) who had chronicled the sterility of much institutional care during this period. Ironically, in response to high illness and mortality rates, institutional staff often prescribed minimal contact between staff and children, between children, and certainly between parents and children. What was generally not recognized was that, rather than protecting them from disease, the sterile conditions were making children more vulnerable. In the WHO report, Bowlby (1951) pieced together the different conditions of neglect and deprivation, articulating the importance of the young child's relationship with the parent.

There was much criticism of this early work, with the naturalistic studies of institutional care challenged as not representative, not rigorous, and certainly not experimental (Bowlby & Robertson, 1953; Ainsworth, 1962). Critical to the acceptance of this work were links to Harlow's experimental findings of the effects of deprivation on infant rhesus macaques (Harlow, 1958). Finding that infant macaques became attached to the cloth diaper in their cage even when fed by a wire mesh device made a good case for contact comfort being separate and not driven by "oral needs" (as suggested by psychoanalytic theorists of the time) or reinforcement (as suggested by social learning theorists of the time). Bowlby understood the needs for attachment as deriving from an evolutionarily based system that served to organize responses toward a goal of maintaining proximity to the caregiver (Bowlby, 1969/1982).

Ethology and evolutionary theory
Bowlby was first struck with Lorenz's (1957) findings that goslings became imprinted on their mothers. Lorenz had described goslings' imprinting on the first moving object seen after birth. Usually the first moving object seen is the mother, such that the gosling typically follows the mother, with chances for survival enhanced as a result. Among goslings, this behavior is seen even though goslings are not dependent upon mothers for their food. Based upon these and other observations, Lorenz (1957), Tinbergen (1951), and other developed a theory of ethology, which represented an elaboration of Darwin's theory of evolution. The behaviors described, such as imprinting, were seen as evolutionarily prepared, but dependent on the environmental conditions to elicit them. In nearly all ordinary contexts, the environment could be expected to provide the necessary conditions to elicit the behavioral repertoire.

The influence of ethology on Bowlby's conceptualization was profound (Ainsworth & Bowlby, 1991). Ethology provided a framework for thinking about how the behaviors of the young infant—crying, smiling, clinging, following—all represented early evolutionarily prepared behaviors infants displayed toward the caregiver. The attachment behavioral system, like the imprinting of the gosling, was seen to consist of evolutionarily prepared behaviors. These behaviors are neither instincts (i.e., emerging regardless of environment), nor do they represent secondary reinforcements as the result of pairing with food (i.e., as suggested by both social learning and psychoanalytic theories of the day [e.g., the gosling could feed itself, and the rhesus macaque became attached to cloth "mother"]). Although particular stimuli are needed to elicit such behaviors, an "ordinary" environment would indeed elicit them. Only an environment falling outside that which would promote survival of young (i.e., no mother present) would fail to elicit. Importantly, the behaviors are organized around promoting survival of the individual's genes (Bowlby, 1969/1982). In the case of the gosling and the human, as well as many other mammals, these behaviors are organized around maintaining proximity to caregiver, a goal that enhances survival of the genes.

Ainsworth as methodologist
Mary Ainsworth came to work with Bowlby at the Tavistock Clinic in 1950. As a student, she had worked with William Blatz (1966), who was a proponent of "security theory," (i.e., the theory that children derive security from their parents). Thus, even before working with Bowlby, Ainsworth had come to see parents as providing a secure base for children. In her earliest work with Bowlby, she was responsible for analyzing data from the institutionalized children collected by Robertson. Robertson's intensive observations of the families and children in their natural environments motivated Ainsworth to engage in similarly rich observations in her future work. In 1958, Ainsworth left the Tavistock Clinic for Uganda. With minimal funding, Ainsworth began a study that followed 28 Ganda babies and their 23 families over the first year of life (Ainsworth, 1967). During this period, she carefully observed precursors of attachment behaviors, and attachment behaviors. Ainsworth recognized that the organization of the attachment behaviors was the means by which the attachment develops.

Some years following her Ugandan study, Ainsworth initiated a second observational study, following 26 families in Baltimore, each of which consisted of two middle-class parents and their newborn infant, observing for at least 70 hours in each home throughout the first year of the infant's life. Close to the child's first birthday, parents brought their children in for a laboratory assessment. It is this laboratory assessment of attachment that is among Ainsworth's key legacies. Although previous work had involved extensive hours of observation, she developed a laboratory assessment of attachment that could be conducted in less than 25 minutes. The assessment, the Strange Situation, is a series of separations and reunions between parent and child that provide a compelling context for observing children's behaviors toward the caregiver when distressed. She developed this assessment originally to examine the balance of attachment behaviors and exploratory behaviors in a context of increasing stress (Ainsworth *et al.*, 1978).

Infant attachment quality

Measurement: the strange situation

The Strange Situation that Ainsworth developed has become the gold standard for assessing attachment quality among infants. The Strange Situation consists of eight episodes in which the child is separated from and then reunited with the parent twice (see Table 6.1 for overview of procedure). Of particular relevance for coding attachment is the child's behavior toward the parent during the reunion episodes. This behavior is thought to reflect the child's expectations of caregiver availability when distressed.

Whereas the *presence* of an attachment relationship is essentially universal (except under unusual conditions), there is variability in the *quality* of attachment relationships. Children's behavior during reunion episodes of the Strange Situation highlights these individual differences in attachment patterns (see Table 6.2). Children who turn directly to their parents to be soothed are classified as having secure attachments. Those who turn away are classified as having avoidant attachments. Children who show a combination of proximity seeking and resistance/anger toward the parent are classified as having resistant attachments. These three types of attachment, secure, avoidant, and resistant, are considered organized attachments because they are thought to represent strategies that maximize caregiver availability (Main, 1990). More specifically, secure children are able to move directly to parents, confident that their bids for reassurance will not be rebuffed. Children with avoidant attachments turn away from parents who would rebuff more direct bids for reassurance. Children with resistant attachments are thought to have effective strategies for eliciting responses from inconsistently available parents. Thus, these patterns develop through repeated interactions between children and their parents during which children develop expectations of their parents' availability in times of distress.

For the first decade after Ainsworth *et al.* (1978) published the classification system, researchers used these three categories to classify children's attachment. About a decade later, Main and Solomon (1986, 1990) introduced disorganized attachment as a distinct category. Disorganized attachment was first identified because some children were difficult to classify and/or showed behaviors that fell outside of those characterized in Ainsworth *et al.*'s system. Indeed, about 15% of children in typical samples were difficult to classify using the original criteria for secure, avoidant, and resistant (Main & Solomon, 1986). Disorganized attachment represents a breakdown in attachment strategy, with children appearing to lack a solution for dealing with their distress (Main & Solomon, 1990). Children with disorganized attachment show odd or anomalous behaviors when distressed in their parents' company. Such children do such

Table 6.1 Strange situation overview.

Episode	Participants	Time (min)	Procedure
1	• Mother • Child • Researcher	1	Researcher introduces mother and child to the room and reviews instructions
2	• Mother • Child	3	Mother sits and child plays with toys. Mother can respond if child initiates interaction
3	• Mother • Child • Stranger	3	Stranger enters room and sits quietly for 1 minute, talks to the mother for 1 minute, and engages with child for 1 minute
4	• Child • Stranger	3 (shortened if child is too distressed)	Mother exits the room. Stranger responds to child as needed (picks up crying child, interacts minimally to non-distressed child)
5	• Mother • Child	3	Mother returns and greets child as she normally would. Mother resumes minimal interaction when possible
6	• Child	3 (shortened if child is too distressed)	Mother exits the room. Child is left alone
7	• Child • Stranger	3 (shortened if child is too distressed)	Stranger returns and responds to the child as needed (picks up crying child, interacts minimally to non-distressed child)
8	• Mother • Child	3	Mother returns, greets child, and responds as she normally would

Table 6.2 Overview of strange situation classifications.

SS classification	Percentage[a] (%)	Strange situation behavior	Assumed meaning of behavior
Organized Secure (B)	62	• Acknowledges parent's return upon reunion • Returns to play after soothed • May or may not cry during separation	Confident in parent's availability due to history of sensitive care
Organized Insecure-Avoidant (A)	15	• Fails to acknowledge parent's return—may continue to play, or turn away • Less likely to cry during separation	Not confident in parent's availability due to history of unresponsive or rejecting care
Organized Insecure-Resistant (C)	8	• Mixture of seeking and resisting contact; angry quality • Highly distressed • Difficult to soothe	Not confident in parent's availability due to history of inconsistent care
Disorganized (D)	15	• Odd or anomalous behavior • Contradictory behaviors (e.g., crying while turning away) • Lack of organized strategy	Dysregulated in presence of caregiver due to history of frightening or atypical care (e.g., maltreatment)

[a]Percentages based on meta-analytic findings of middle-class, nonclinical groups in North America (*N* = 2104) from van IJzendoorn *et al.* (1999).

things as freeze or still for a period of time, show contradictory attachment tendencies (distress and avoidance) consecutively or simultaneously, or show apprehension of the parent.

Stability

Evidence for the stability of attachment over time has been mixed, with effect sizes ranging from small to large (e.g., Waters, 1978; Egeland & Farber, 1984; Bar-Haim *et al.*, 2000). Greater instability (e.g., move from secure attachment to insecure or disorganized attachment) has been found for children who experienced more meaningful changes in the family environment, such as changes in caregiving quality or major family events or transitions (Thompson *et al.*, 1982; Vondra *et al.*, 1999).

Cross-cultural

In a meta-analysis of the Strange Situation conducted in eight different countries, van IJzendoorn and Kroonenberg (1988) found that differences within cultures were typically greater than between cultures. However, there were some cross-cultural differences observed. Whereas secure classifications were modal in all countries, there was a greater preponderance of avoidant classifications in Western Europe and resistant classifications in Israel and Japan. Although cross-cultural differences in parenting norms (e.g., infants rarely being separated from mothers in Japan) may play a role in the differences in Strange Situation classification patterns (e.g., Miyake *et al.*, 1985), few studies have examined these questions empirically.

Alternative approaches to measurement

Waters and Deane (1985) developed a Q-sort method of rating attachment security based on observer ratings and on parent ratings in parents' homes. The Q-sort asks the observer to sort descriptors (e.g., "child clearly shows a pattern of using mother as a base from which to explore," "child easily becomes angry at mother") into categories from most to least descriptive of the child, with a forced distribution of items. The resulting Q-sort is then correlated with a prototypical secure sort. Thus, rather than yielding attachment classifications similar to the Strange Situation, the resulting score places children on a secure/insecure continuum. Van IJzendoorn *et al.* (2004) found that the Attachment Q-sort had strong psychometric properties when observers (rather than parents) made the ratings, and spent long periods in the home (i.e., more than 3 hours) prior to making ratings. The Q-sort was moderately associated with attachment quality assessed in the Strange Situation ($r = 0.31$), and was predicted by parental security ($r = 0.39$). Advantages of the Q-sort over the Strange Situation are its ecological validity, and the use with a larger age range than the Strange Situation (van IJzendoorn *et al.*, 2004). Disadvantages include the extensive period of time required for observation, and the lack of assessment of attachment disorganization.

Individual differences

There are a number of factors that contribute to individual differences in the quality of parent–child attachments. We provide an overview of these predictors, beginning with the most proximal—parental behavior—and moving to more distal factors such as parent attachment state of mind, parent psychopathology, and environmental conditions (see Figure 6.1).

Parental behavior

Parental behavior is seen as the critical mechanism by which individual differences in attachment develop. Attachment theory suggests that children will develop secure attachments if

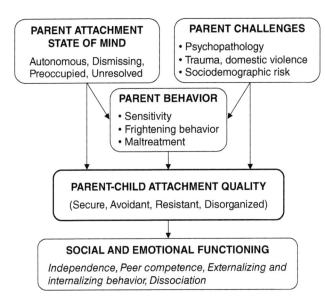

Figure 6.1 Conceptual overview of the predictors of individual differences in parent–child attachment quality and links to later outcomes.

parents are consistently available when they are distressed, and will develop insecure attachments when parents show other patterns of behavior. In her Baltimore study, Ainsworth and colleagues coded maternal behavior on four dimensions (which were highly intercorrelated): sensitivity, acceptance, cooperation, and physical and psychological accessibility. These dimensions strongly predicted infants' attachment classifications, with secure infants having mothers who scored high on all four dimensions (Ainsworth et al., 1978).

Since Ainsworth's seminal work, parental sensitivity has been found to only moderately predict attachment security (De Wolff & van IJzendoorn, 1997). Although there is a range in the length of the observation period, no study of which we are aware has approached Ainsworth's intensive observation schedule. Differences in the context (e.g., play versus distress) may also contribute to the variability in findings. In addition, there are differences in what is defined as sensitive behavior. Recent attempts have been made to tease apart different components of sensitivity, such as responsiveness to children's signal in positive interactions (e.g., synchrony) versus sensitivity to children's cues of distress (McElwain & Booth-LaForce, 2006). Some have argued for a more narrow definition of attachment in which parental protection in the face of threat is the key to the child's sense of security, which most clearly aligns with Bowlby's original definition (Bowlby, 1969/1982; Goldberg et al., 1999).

Odd, anomalous, and/or frightening behavior appears to have effects that are distinct from simply insensitive behaviors. Frightening or frightened parental behavior has been linked specifically to the development of disorganized attachment (Lyons-Ruth et al., 1999; Schuengel et al., 1999; Madigan et al., 2006). Hesse and Main (2006) defined six scales of frightened or frightening (FR) parental behavior, including threatening (e.g., aggressive movements or postures), frightened

(e.g., backing away from distressed infant), dissociative (e.g., stilling, haunted tone of voice), timid/differential (e.g., submissive approach to infant), spousal/romantic (e.g., intimate touch), and disorganized (similar to infant disorganized behaviors). Maternal FR behavior has been linked to children's disorganized attachments (Abrams et al., 2006). Infant attachment disorganization is also predicted by other extreme and atypical behaviors that increase infant arousal, such as negative-intrusive behavior, role confusion, and affective withdrawal (Lyons-Ruth et al., 1999; Madigan et al., 2006).

Not surprisingly, maltreatment is associated with heightened risk for disorganized attachment (Cicchetti et al., 2006). Meta-analyses reveal large effect sizes between maltreatment and insecure and disorganized ($d = 2.10$ and 2.19, respectively) attachments (Cyr et al., 2010).

Attachment state of mind

Attachment state of mind refers to the way in which the parent, or the adult more generally, conceptualizes his or her own attachment experiences. Despite seeming to be less proximal than sensitivity, state of mind is the best-identified predictor of infant attachment (van IJzendoorn, 1995; Pederson et al., 1998). Mary Main and her colleagues deliberately developed the system of assessing attachment state of mind to match children's attachment. That is, commonalities in conceptualizations among parents of children with secure attachments were identified, as were commonalities among parents of children with avoidant, resistant, and disorganized attachment. State of mind was assessed through an interview, the Adult Attachment Interview (AAI; George et al., 1996). The interview asks adults to describe their parents, and to instantiate descriptions with particular examples. Interviewees are asked to recall times from childhood when they were hurt, upset, or rejected, and to think how their adult personality is affected by the way they were raised. Finally, incidences of abuse and loss are recalled. The semi-structured interview is transcribed and coded by reliable coders.

As a group, parents whose children were securely attached to them were called "autonomous" because they appeared able to evaluate attachment experiences freely. Characterizations of attachment figures matched well with specific descriptions for a rich, coherent picture, and attachment was valued. Parents whose children had avoidant attachments were called "dismissive of attachment" because they appeared to devalue attachment experiences. They typically showed a lack of memory with respect to attachment experiences and/or idealization of attachment figures. The parents of children with resistant attachments to them were termed "preoccupied with regard to attachment." These parents were caught up or enmeshed in attachment experiences, as shown by angry involvement and/or rambling discourse. Parents of children with disorganized attachments were most likely to be unresolved with regard to loss or abuse.

Beyond the initial sample of Main's in which the method ensured a good match between parent state of mind and infant attachment, the concordance has been very good.

Van IJzendoorn (1995) conducted a meta-analysis to examine the concordance between state of mind and infant attachment, and found a large combined effect size ($d = 1.06$) and high rate of correspondence (74%) for secure versus insecure concordance. Parent state of mind is moderately associated with parental sensitivity ($r = 0.34$, van IJzendoorn, 1995). Although it was anticipated that sensitivity would mediate the association between parent state of mind and infant attachment, the association between parent state of mind and infant attachment is stronger than the association between sensitivity and attachment, and sensitivity does not fully mediate the association between state of mind and infant attachment (Pederson et al., 1998). It is possible that this is a measurement artifact, however, given that the AAI was developed to relate as closely as possible to infant attachment and/or because sensitivity becomes a less robust measure with shorter or fewer assessments.

Parent challenges

A number of factors can interfere with parents behaving in ways that foster secure attachments. When parents face significant challenges themselves, such as psychiatric disorders, extreme poverty, and their own unresolved issues regarding attachment experiences, it often becomes more difficult to consistently parent in sensitive ways.

Psychopathology

As would be expected, parents with psychiatric disorders, such as depression, borderline personality disorder, and substance abuse, experience particular challenges in parenting. Parental depression, for example, is associated with both withdrawn and intrusive parental behaviors (Goodman & Gotlib, 1999), which would suggest heightened risk for insecure attachments among children. Evidence linking maternal depression with infant attachment quality is mixed, with meta-analyses revealing a small, significant overall association between maternal depression and insecure attachment ($r = 0.18$; Atkinson et al., 2000) and a non-significant association between maternal depression and infant disorganization ($r = 0.06$, $p = 0.06$; van IJzendoorn et al., 1999). Mothers with borderline personality disorder are more likely to interact in intrusive ways and to have infants with disorganized attachments than control mothers without psychopathology (Hobson et al., 2005). In addition to psychiatric disorders being associated with lower quality of parenting, psychiatric disorders are disproportionately associated with non-autonomous states of mind (as will be discussed in more detail later).

Trauma exposure and domestic violence

When parents experience unresolved trauma or domestic violence, it is often difficult for them to effectively buffer children. This failure can be the result of children witnessing violence involving attachment figures, or the result of parents behaving in anomalous ways because of their own trauma experiences (Schuengel et al., 1999). When parents are unresolved with regard to loss or trauma, they are susceptible to behaving with their children in frightening ways and children are at increased risk for disorganized attachments (Schuengel et al., 1999).

Challenging environmental conditions

Living under harsh conditions can also interfere with optimal parenting and threaten the development of secure attachments. Cyr et al. (2010) conducted a meta-analysis of the effect of high-risk conditions on children's attachment. In comparison with samples of children from low-risk backgrounds, high-risk samples had higher proportions of insecure children and disorganized children ($d = 0.48$ and 0.48, respectively). Furthermore, children who were not maltreated but had five or more sociodemographic risk indicators (e.g., low income, parental substance abuse, minority group, single parent, adolescent mother, and low parental education) had similar rates of disorganized attachment as maltreated children (Cyr et al., 2010). Taken together, these studies suggest that adverse environmental conditions can contribute to higher rates of insecure and disorganized attachments.

Other factors: child care and child temperament

The National Institutes of Health in the United States invested enormous resources in assessing the effects of child care on children's development, with a particular focus on attachment relationships (NICHD, 1997). In this study of more than 1300 children, attendance at child care, the quality of child care, and the amount of child care was found to have no direct effects on attachment security. This was at odds with several previous studies (Clarke-Stewart, 1989; Belsky & Rovine, 1988) that had shown effects of the amount of child care on attachment quality. These findings were sustained in assessments of children at the age of 3 (NICHD, 2001).

There has been considerable debate about whether temperament and attachment are overlapping constructs. Temperament refers to individual differences in infant reactivity or regulation across attentional, behavioral, and emotional domains. In general, studies have not found strong evidence for an association between infant temperament and security of attachment (for a review, see Vaughn et al., 2008). Although infant temperament does not determine the likelihood of having a secure or insecure attachment, several studies suggest that temperamental reactivity may influence the type of insecure attachment displayed. For example, infants with higher negative emotionality may be more prone to resistant patterns of insecurity (characterized by high levels of distress), whereas infants with lower negative emotionality may be more prone to avoidant patterns of insecurity (characterized by low levels of distress) (Belsky & Rovine, 1987; Marshall & Fox, 2005).

Links between infant attachment and later outcomes

Attachment quality is predictive of a number of important developmental outcomes, including independence in preschool, peer relations in middle childhood, and internalizing and externalizing behavior problems. Associations are typically stronger among children living in stable environments where conditions stay relatively constant over time than among children living in less stable environments (Weinfield *et al.*, 2000; Vondra *et al.*, 2001). Weinfield *et al.* (2000) have argued that continuity and discontinuity follow lawful patterns, with instability in care predicting discontinuity.

Several large longitudinal studies have studied attachment from infancy through adulthood, including the Minnesota Longitudinal Study (Sroufe *et al.*, 2005), the Bielefeld and Regensburg Projects (Grossman *et al.*, 2005), the London Parent–child Project (Steele & Steele, 2005), the Haifa Longitudinal Study (Sagi-Schwartz & Aviezer, 2005), the Berkeley Longitudinal Study (Main *et al.*, 2005), and the NICHD Study of Early Child Care and Youth Development (NICHD, 1997). The studies have provided both converging and diverging findings regarding how well attachment in infancy predicts subsequent outcomes. Additionally, a number of shorter-term studies that included assessments of attachment in infancy provide important data regarding the prediction of later outcomes.

Social relationships in childhood

Ainsworth (1969) and Bowlby (1969/1982) clearly distinguished attachment from dependency. Although children remain dependent upon their caregivers in a number of ways, secure attachment provides a secure base for exploration, theoretically allowing greater confidence in exploration (Sroufe *et al.*, 1983). Nonetheless, for a number of years, misunderstandings of the two constructs remained. For example, the behavior shown by avoidant children in the Strange Situation (i.e., appearing not to need their parents) led some to question whether, in fact, avoidant children were more independent than secure children. Sroufe *et al.* (1983) assessed this directly by examining preschoolers' dependence on their teachers through observed physical contact seeking and observed guidance, as well as through teacher ratings. Secure children were rated by teachers as more independent than avoidant and resistant children, and sought out contact and guidance less than avoidant and resistant children. These behaviors, although later in development, are in line with similarities observed between children with avoidant and resistant attachments in their home environments (Ainsworth *et al.*, 1978). Consistent with the original attachment theory tenets (Ainsworth, 1969; Bowlby, 1969/1982), these data support the idea that secure attachments in infancy support autonomous functioning in early childhood.

Consistent with these results, infant attachment classification at 15 months predicted social behavior at age 3, controlling for concurrent attachment classifications and maternal sensitivity (McElwain *et al.*, 2003). Specifically, resistant children were less assertive or controlling with a same-sex friend than avoidant children, and avoidant children demonstrated more instrumental aggression than secure and resistant children. Self-reports of social relationships in childhood also show associations with infant classifications. Children classified as resistant report higher loneliness in early childhood relative to children classified as secure (Berlin *et al.*, 1995). In a meta-analysis based on 63 studies, there was a small effect size for the overall association between attachment security and peer relations, $r = 0.20$ (Schneider *et al.*, 2001). Effect sizes were larger in studies of peer relations with close friends compared with peer relations with non-friends (e.g., classmates, acquaintances), and were larger in older childhood relative to early childhood.

Internalizing behavior

Two recent meta-analyses have found a small but significant effect for insecure attachment predicting internalizing behaviors (e.g., depressive symptoms, anxiety), with avoidant attachment most clearly driving the effect (Groh *et al.*, 2012; Madigan *et al.*, 2013). In their meta-analysis of 60 studies, Madigan *et al.* (2013) reported a small to medium effect size ($d = 0.37$) between insecure attachment and internalizing behavior in childhood (age of children across studies ranged from 18 months to 10 years). This effect was moderated by concurrent externalizing behavior, with higher ratings of externalizing behavior strengthening the association between insecure attachment and internalizing behavior. Additionally, studies relying on direct observations of internalizing problems demonstrated larger effect sizes ($d = 0.67$) than studies that used questionnaires, such as the CBCL ($d = 0.34$).

Externalizing behavior

Meta-analytic findings demonstrate that insecure, and most especially disorganized attachment is associated with externalizing behavior during childhood (Fearon *et al.*, 2010). Disorganized children appear most at risk for externalizing behaviors ($d = 0.34$), with smaller effects seen among avoidant ($d = 0.12$) and resistant children ($d = 0.11$). Groh *et al.* (2012) compared the effect sizes for attachment quality predicting externalizing versus internalizing symptoms. Both insecure and disorganized attachment predicted externalizing symptoms more strongly than internalizing symptoms, $d = 0.31$ versus $d = 0.15$ for effects of insecure attachment on externalizing versus internalizing symptoms, and $d = 0.34$ to $d = 0.08$ for effects of disorganized attachment on externalizing versus internalizing symptoms respectively (Groh *et al.*, 2010).

Dissociation

Disorganized attachment has been found to be predictive of later dissociative symptoms such as disruptions in memory and confusion of identity. Carlson (1998) found that disorganized attachment predicted teacher-reported dissociative symptoms in middle childhood and adolescence, and self-reported dissociative symptoms on the Schedule for Affective Disorders and Schizophrenia (K-SADS) at age 17 years and on a questionnaire at 19 years. The theoretical links between disorganized attachment and later dissociative symptoms are strong, but there are fewer empirical studies than with regard to externalizing or internalizing symptoms. Main and Hesse (1990) suggested that disorganized attachment reflects the infant's experiencing an unsolvable dilemma because the child is frightened of the parent from whom he or she must seek protection, resulting in a mini-dissociative episode that can be observed in the child's behavior in the Strange Situation.

Assessments of attachment beyond infancy

Although attachment to a caregiver has particular salience in infancy and early childhood, attachments remain important throughout life. Bowlby (1988) talked of the importance of attachment "from the cradle to the grave" (p. 62). The form that these attachments take changes across development, with children increasingly able to represent attachment figures internally over time (Main et al., 2005).

Preschool

A preschool version of the Strange Situation was developed by Cassidy et al. (1992). This Strange Situation is similar to the infant Strange Situation, but with the stranger episodes eliminated under the assumption that strangers are not as threatening to preschoolers as they are to infants, and with longer separations sometimes used. Categories of attachment generally parallel infant categories. An exception is that controlling behavior is seen to a greater extent than disorganized behavior and is considered the outgrowth of disorganized attachment. That is, children become controlling of parents as a way to cope with feelings of disorganization (Main & Cassidy, 1988). The preschool Strange Situation has been used much less than the infant Strange Situation, and with generally less robust effects. Moss and colleagues have published the strongest findings with the preschool Strange Situation, showing moderate stability over time (Moss et al., 2005).

Move to the level of representation

In infancy, the organization of the child's behavioral system is the essence of attachment, with measurement of attachment based on behavioral observations (e.g., Ainsworth, 1967). Even in infancy, though, these behaviors reflect the child's expectations of the parent's availability, and hence representations of attachment figures. Increasingly, the "move to the level of

representation" becomes more pronounced (Main et al., 2005). With time, it is thought that children develop internal working models of self and caregivers based on their experiences of attachment-relevant events (Bowlby 1969/1982; Bretherton, 1992), with these internal working models providing rules that guide behavior, organize attention, and permit or limit access to memory (Main et al., 1985). A number of measures have been developed to assess attachment at the level of representation in childhood and adulthood.

Story stems and narratives

Semi-projective measures have been used with young children to assess their attachment representations, such as the Separation Anxiety Test (Main et al., 1985) and the Attachment Story Completion Task (Bretherton et al., 1990). In the Separation Anxiety Test, children are asked how they would feel and what they would do in response to a range of separation scenarios (e.g., parents leaving for 2 weeks); in the Attachment Story Completion Task, children are asked to describe "what happens next" in a series of story stems (e.g., a child getting hurt). Coding of children's responses has taken several forms, with some paralleling the Ainsworth classification system, and others defining broader scales of security or related constructs. Although more work is needed to validate these measures with behavioral observations of children's attachment behavior, these representational measures relate to children's behavior in separation paradigms (e.g., Slough & Greenberg, 1990) and predict children's socioemotional functioning (e.g., Easterbrooks & Abeles, 2000).

Child attachment interview

The Child Attachment Interview (Target et al., 2003) is an interview for children and adolescents modeled on the Adult Attachment Interview. Like the AAI, the Child Attachment Interview asks children to generate adjectives to describe parents and to instantiate those adjectives, as well as describe incidents of distress, among other things. Scott et al. (2011) found that attachment representations were related to observed parenting behaviors, and made distinct contributions to predictions of behavior problems. Further, children appear able to modify their narratives and presumably their representations when caregiving changes (Joseph et al., 2014).

Adult attachment interview

The Adult Attachment Interview (AAI; George et al., 1996), described earlier in this chapter, is the assessment of attachment state of mind used among adolescents and adults. As predicted by theory, attachment state of mind is associated with relations with peers and parents in adolescence (Allen et al., 2003), and with adult functioning in romantic relationships (Bouthillier et al., 2002). For example, partners' AAI classifications predict proactive emotion regulation during a problem-solving discussion (Bouthillier et al., 2002), and psychophysiological activity during conflict discussions (Roisman, 2007).

Adults with serious psychiatric disorders are disproportionately characterized by non-autonomous states of mind (for a review, see Dozier *et al.*, 2008). Some psychiatric disorders are associated with dismissing state of mind (i.e., characterized by idealizing of attachment figures and/or lack of memory), whereas others are associated with preoccupied state of mind (i.e., characterized by angry involvement and/or rambling discourse). More specifically, disorders involving an externalizing focus such as antisocial personality disorder are often associated with a dismissing state of mind, and disorders that involve more self-focus such as borderline personality disorder are often associated with preoccupied state of mind (e.g., Fonagy *et al.*, 1996). Nonetheless, as Rutter *et al.* (2009) emphasize, attachment state of mind does not provide an explanation for the disorder in any of these cases.

Self-report assessments

Self-report assessments of attachment have been used extensively and many types of self-report assessments have been developed. Self-reports are very easy to administer relative to the Adult Attachment Interview, but relate weakly or not at all to Adult Attachment Interview assessments (Roisman *et al.*, 2007). In a meta-analysis, Roisman *et al.* (2007) found that the AAI was very weakly related to attachment style (mean $r = 0.09$). Nonetheless, the instruments often relate to variables of interest in meaningful ways (Roisman *et al.*, 2007).

Attachment and neurobiology

Non-human primate and rodent studies have provided compelling evidence for the effects of maternal care on the developing infant's neurobiology. Hofer (1994) has argued that specific maternal behaviors or processes serve as "hidden regulators" for the infant. The mother helps the infant regulate temperature, heart rate, and glucocorticoid production, for example. Hofer suggested that behavioral-sensorimotor processes, involving aspects of mother—infant attunement and synchrony, appeared particularly important to behavioral and neurobiological regulation. Not surprisingly, then, children show different physiological responses depending on caregiving quality and attachment quality.

Avoidance in the strange situation

In the Strange Situation, the apparent indifference shown by avoidant children in reunions with their parents belies their underlying anxiety about parental availability (Ainsworth *et al.*, 1978). These children often turn away from their parents, appearing to distract themselves with toys. If they are effectively distracted, as suggested by their behavior, their heart rates should decelerate; if on the other hand, they are avoiding contact with the parent and only appearing to be distracted by the toys, their heart rates should stay constant or even accelerate. Indeed, Sroufe and Waters (1977a, b) found that children showed increased heart rate regardless of attachment classification, supporting the idea that avoidant children are not effectively engaged with the toys.

Avoidance in the adult attachment interview

Adolescents and adults with dismissive states of mind minimize the importance of attachment-related experiences, indicating that they cannot recall times in their childhood when they were hurt or rejected or denying that these experiences have an impact on their development. If these individuals are truly unaffected about such issues, their skin conductance (i.e., the amount they sweated) should not increase when queried; if however, they are actively avoiding issues, their skin conductance should increase. Paralleling the Sroufe and Waters (1977a, b) findings showing increased heart rate in avoidant children, young North American adults with dismissive attachments showed increases in skin conductance when asked about being rejected, upset, and hurt as children (Dozier & Kobak, 1992).

Cortisol reactivity in the strange situation

The Strange Situation is designed to be stressful to all children. However, Gunnar *et al.* (2006) have argued that, in the presence of supportive caregivers, most young children do not show a cortisol response under ordinary stressful conditions. This buffering function is important in protecting the developing brain from high levels of circulating glucocorticoids. Indeed, children with secure attachments to their parents have not shown increases in cortisol in the Strange Situation in three studies (Spangler & Grossmann, 1993; Bernard *et al.*, 2010); only children with disorganized and/or insecure attachment showed increases in cortisol. These results point to the importance of attachment in helping children to regulate physiologically as well as behaviorally.

Attachment among fathers

Increasing attention has been paid to the role that fathers play in children's development and to father—child attachment relationships (Lamb & Lewis, 2004). The association between paternal sensitivity and infant—father attachment security is weaker than the association between maternal sensitivity and infant—mother attachment security (for meta-analysis, see van IJzendoorn & de Wolff, 1997). As would be predicted given that attachment is considered to be relationship-specific (Sroufe, 1985), infants' attachment to fathers and to mothers is relatively orthogonal. Van IJzendoorn and de Wolff (1997) found only a modest association between infants' attachment to mothers and fathers. Fathers' state of mind is less predictive of infants' attachments to their fathers than mothers' state of mind is to infants' attachments to their mothers (van IJzendoorn, 1995).

Attachment among atypical populations

Attachment among children in foster care

Children in foster care experience disruptions in care at a point when developing and maintaining attachments is a key developmental task. Stovall-McClough and Dozier (2004) studied the development of children's attachment behaviors in their new homes over time. They found that after about 12 months of age, children required a substantial period of time before they appeared to show consistent attachment behaviors and/or to develop a secure relationship. Ultimately, though, foster children placed with autonomous foster parents usually developed secure attachments (Dozier *et al.*, 2001), whereas children placed with foster parents with non-autonomous states of mind usually developed disorganized attachments. Consistent with Bowlby's (1951) observations, disruptions in care are problematic for children, but the quality of surrogate care is important in how they adapt.

Attachment in kibbutz

Kibbutz conditions likely represent the most benign group care conditions possible. Sleep-away kibbutzim existed in Israel for much of the 20th century (Aviezer *et al.*, 2002), with the model driven by an ideological belief in collective living and by practical needs. Care for children was excellent in terms of resources, activities, and time with caregivers other than the parents. Time with parents was limited, and most especially, children slept in groups away from their parents. In two studies, children reared in sleep-away kibbutz showed lower rates of security than seen among usual low-risk children. Sagi *et al.* (1994) found that 48% of children in communally sleeping conditions developed secure attachments, compared with 80% of children in family-based sleeping arrangements.

Attachment and interventions

Infants and toddlers

There are several attachment-based interventions for parents of infants and young children with emerging evidence bases. The interventions range from those that focus more on changing parents' behaviors to those that focus more on changing parents' representations of their own attachment experiences.

Attachment and biobehavioral catch-up

The Attachment and Biobehavioral Catch-up (ABC; Dozier *et al.*, 2012) intervention targets three issues known to affect children's attachment security and self-regulatory capabilities. First, parents are helped to behave in nurturing ways when children are distressed because nurturing behavior is associated with secure attachment (Ainsworth *et al.*, 1978). Second, parents are helped to follow children's lead, which has been demonstrated to enhance children's regulatory capabilities (Raver, 1996). Third, parents are helped to behave in ways that are

not frightening because frightening behavior is associated with disorganized attachment (e.g., Schuengel *et al.*, 1999). These issues are targeted through 10 sessions implemented in families' homes with parents and children present. Although the content is manualized, parent coaches are expected to make frequent "in the moment" comments regarding targeted behaviors. For example, when a parent is observed nurturing her distressed child, comments would focus on: specifically identifying the observed behavior, (e.g., "he fell, and you said, right away, "sweetie, are you ok?"); linking the behavior to the intervention target (e.g., "that's such a good example of nurturing him when he needs you"); and linking to child outcomes (e.g., "that's the kind of thing that will help him to know that he can come to you, no matter what").

The ABC intervention has been shown to be effective in randomized clinical trials in enhancing child attachment security (Bernard *et al.*, 2012). Relative to children randomly assigned to a control intervention, children at high risk for neglect randomly assigned to the ABC showed secure attachments at a higher rate (33% vs 52%, respectively), and disorganized attachment at a lower rate (57% vs 32% respectively). Positive outcomes for the children from the ABC intervention group have also been seen in the areas of diurnal cortisol production (Bernard *et al.*, 2012), emotion regulation (Lind *et al.*, 2014), and executive functioning (Lewis-Morrarty *et al.*, 2012). Further, mothers who received the intervention showed different brain activity (i.e., event-related potentials) when viewing pictures of crying, laughing, and neutral infant faces (Bernard *et al.*, 2013). These effects were observed as long as 3 years after the intervention, suggesting that the intervention helps parents change in fundamental, long-term ways.

Circle of Security

Circle of Security (Hoffman *et al.*, 2006) is a group intervention designed to help parents identify the issues that interfere with parenting the most. Attachment issues are considered to represent a "circle of security," with parents providing a safe haven when children are distressed, and a secure base when children feel prepared to explore the world. Parents are asked to think about whether their own issues (their "shark music," Hoffman *et al.*, 2006) interfere more when they are welcoming the child back for reassurance or allowing the child to move away to explore. Two versions of Circle of Security exist, including a more intensive 20-session format, that is dependent on expertise to assess attachment, and a brief 8-session CD-based version that is not tailored as individually as the longer version. The longer version has been tested in a pre-post-intervention blinded design, and was shown to enhance attachment security (Hoffman *et al.*, 2006). At this point, randomized clinical trials have not been completed but are under way.

Child–parent psychotherapy

Child–parent Psychotherapy focuses on traumatized parents' challenges in behaving in sensitive, nurturing ways with their young children. The intervention grew from Selma Fraiberg's (1980) psychoanalytic approach that considered the parent's "ghosts from the nursery," or challenges from the past. Alicia Lieberman adapted this intervention to be broader and manualized (Lieberman *et al.*, 2006). Child–parent Psychotherapy is designed to help parents understand how their previous experiences affect parenting in a very real way. The relatively intensive, long-term intervention is intended to provide a safe, playful context. Through randomized clinical trials, Child–parent Psychotherapy has been shown to reduce disorganized attachment (Cicchetti *et al.*, 2006) and reduce children's negative self-representations (Toth *et al.*, 2002).

Preschoolers

Several interventions for older children incorporate attachment concepts with social learning principles to greater or lesser extents. Included among these are Video-feedback Intervention to promote Positive Parenting and Sensitive Discipline (VIPP-SD: Juffer *et al.*, 2008), Incredible Years (Webster-Stratton *et al.*, 2001), Parent–child Interaction Therapy (Eyberg *et al.*, 2001), and others. The most explicitly attachment-based of these interventions is the VIPP-SD, which has been shown in a randomized clinical trial to increase mothers' use of more sensitive discipline strategies (van Zeijl *et al.*, 2006).

Children and adolescents

Fewer interventions are explicitly attachment-based for older children and adolescents than for younger children, although many interventions nonetheless are relevant to attachment issues. Attachment-Based Family Therapy (Diamond *et al.*, 2002) is one of the few interventions that very directly targets attachment issues for this older age group. The treatment focuses on both family and individual processes that can help build trust between the adolescent and parents, and directs attention toward enhancing a relationship in which the parent can effectively protect the child.

Future directions

Clinical implications

Bowlby had strong clinical interests and approached attachment theory from this perspective. Ainsworth, however, was primarily a developmental psychologist. Her role as developmental methodologist focused the field on developmental research for the first several decades of attachment research. More recently, in the last several decades, attachment has been increasingly studied in clinical settings, and attachment-based interventions have been developed. Still, the field of attachment-based interventions is fledgling at this point. This is likely to be a rich area for future development.

Cross-cutting research

Attachment research has been characterized by cross-cutting theoretical and methodological approaches since its earliest days. Bowlby borrowed from multiple disciplines in articulating his vision of attachment research, most especially considering ethology and evolutionary theory. Thus, connections across human, non-human primate, and rodent research have been made since Bowlby's first conceptualization of the theory. Linkages to physiology have been made by Sroufe in 1977, and by others since. Nonetheless, recent developments in neurobiology and epigenetics and in translational research more generally, make this an especially important focus of research.

Studying extreme conditions

Links between extreme conditions (e.g., orphanage care and maltreatment among humans, separation among non-human primates) and attachment-related outcomes were of interest to Bowlby in his formulation of attachment theory. Such conditions will continue to be important to study in informing what is critical about parenting. These areas represent the historical context and the future for attachment theory and research.

Conclusions

Attachment has emerged as a powerful construct. As Rutter pointed out (2006), much of what Bowlby proposed in the 1950s and 1960s is now accepted within psychology, social work, and even psychiatry. At the time the theory was introduced, though, it was revolutionary. A rich and growing body of empirical work has followed the seminal observational studies of Bowlby and Ainsworth, including significant longitudinal efforts and critical attention to atypical caregiving circumstances. Remarkably, these studies continue to offer strong support for key tenets of attachment theory.

References

Abrams, K.Y. *et al.* (2006) Examining the roles of parental frightened/ frightening subtypes in predicting disorganized attachment within a brief observational procedure. *Development and Psychopathology* **18**, 345–361.

Ainsworth, M.D. (1962) The effects of maternal deprivation: a review of findings and controversy in the context of research strategy. In: *Deprivation of Maternal Care: A Reassessment of its Effects* (Public Health Papers, No. 15), pp. 87–195. World Health Organization, Geneva, Switzerland.

Ainsworth, M.D.S. (1967) *Infancy in Uganda: Infant Care and the Growth of Love.* Johns Hopkins University Press, Baltimore.

Ainsworth, M.D.S. (1969) Object relations, dependency, and attachment: a theoretical review of the infant-mother relationship. *Child Development* **40**, 969–1026.

Ainsworth, M.D.S. & Bowlby, J. (1991) An ethological approach to personality development. *American Psychologist* **46**, 333–341.

Ainsworth, M.D.S. *et al.* (1978) *Patterns of Attachment.* Erlbaum, Hillsdale, N.J.

Allen, J.P. *et al.* (2003) A secure base in adolescence: markers of attachment security in the mother–adolescent relationship. *Child Development* **74**, 292–307.

Atkinson, L. *et al.* (2000) Attachment security: a meta-analysis of maternal mental health correlates. *Clinical Psychology Review* **20**, 1019–1040.

Aviezer, O. *et al.* (2002) Balancing the family and the collective in raising children: why communal sleeping in kibbutzim was predestined to end. *Family Process* **41**, 435–454.

Bar-Haim, Y. *et al.* (2000) Stability and change in attachment at 14, 24, and 58 months of age: behavior, representation, and life events. *Journal of Child Psychology and Psychiatry* **41**, 381–388.

Belsky, J. & Rovine, M. (1987) Temperament and attachment security in the strange situation: an empirical rapprochement. *Child Development* **58**, 787–795.

Belsky, J. & Rovine, M. (1988) Nonmaternal care in the first year of life and the security of infant–parent attachment. *Child Development* **59**, 157–167.

Berlin, L.J. *et al.* (1995) Loneliness in young children and infant-mother attachment: a longitudinal study. *Merrill-Palmer Quarterly* **41**, 91–103.

Bernard, K. *et al.* (2010) Cortisol production patterns in young children living with birth parents vs children places in foster care following involvement of Child Protective Services. *Archives of Pediatrics and Adolescent Medicine* **164**, 438–443.

Bernard, K. *et al.* (2012) Enhancing attachment organization among maltreated infants: results of a randomized clinical trial. *Child Development* **83**, 623–636.

Bernard, K. *et al.* (2013) *Neurobiology of Maternal Sensitivity and Delight Among High-Risk Mothers: An Event-Related Potential Study*. University of Delaware, Newark, DE Unpublished manuscript.

Bernard, K. *et al.* (in press) *Effects of an attachment-based intervention on CPS-referred mothers' event-related potentials to children's emotions.* Child Development.

Blatz, W.E. (1966) *Human Security: Some Reflections*. University of Toronto Press, Toronto, Canada.

Bouthillier, D. *et al.* (2002) Predictive validity of adult attachment measures in relation to emotion regulation behaviors in marital interactions. *Journal of Adult Development* **9**, 291–305.

Bowlby, J. (1944) Forty-four juvenile thieves: their characters and their home life. *International Journal of Psychoanalysis* **25**, 19–52.

Bowlby, J. (1951) *Maternal Care and Mental Health (WHO Monograph No. 2)*. World Health Organization, Geneva.

Bowlby, J. (1969/1982) *Attachment and Loss: Vol. 1. Attachment*. Basic Books, New York.

Bowlby, J. (1988) *A Secure Base*. Basic Books, New York.

Bowlby, J. & Robertson, J. (1953) A two-year old goes to hospital. *Proceedings of the Royal Society of Medicine* **46**, 425–427.

Bretherton, I. (1985) Attachment: retrospect and prospect. *Monographs of the Society for Research in Child Development* **50**, 3–35.

Bretherton, I. (1992) The origins of attachment theory: John Bowlby and Mary Ainsworth. *Developmental Psychology* **28**, 759–775.

Bretherton, I. *et al.* (1990) Assessing internal working models of the attachment relationship: an attachment story completion task for 3-year-olds. In: *Attachment in the Preschool Years*. (eds M.T. Greenberg, D. Cicchetti & E.M. Cummings), pp. 273–308. University of Chicago Press, Chicago.

Carlson, E.A. (1998) A prospective longitudinal study if attachment disorganization/disorientation. *Child Development* **69**, 1107–1128.

Cassidy, J. *et al.* (1992) *Attachment Organization in Preschool Children: Coding Guidelines*, 4th edn. University of Virginia Unpublished manuscript.

Cicchetti, D. *et al.* (2006) Fostering secure attachment in infants in maltreating families through preventive interventions. *Development and Psychopathology* **18**, 623–649.

Clarke-Stewart, K.A. (1989) Infant day-care: maligned or malignant? *American Psychologist* **44**, 266–273.

Cyr, C. *et al.* (2010) Attachment security and disorganization in maltreating and high-risk families: a series of meta-analyses. *Development and Psychopathology* **22**, 87–108.

De Wolff, M. & van IJzendoorn, M.H. (1997) Sensitivity and attachment: a meta-analysis on parental antecedents of infant attachment. *Child Development* **68**, 571–591.

Diamond, G.S. *et al.* (2002) Attachment-based family therapy for depressed adolescents: a treatment development study. *Journal of the Academy of Child & Adolescent Psychiatry* **41**, 1190–1196.

Dozier, M. & Kobak, R. (1992) Psychophysiology in attachment interviews: converging evidence for deactivating strategies. *Child Development* **63**, 1473–1480.

Dozier, M. & the Infant Caregiver Project Lab (2012) *Attachment and Biobehavioral Catch-up*. University of Delaware Unpublished document.

Dozier, M. *et al.* (2001) Attachment for infants in foster care: the role of caregiver state of mind. *Child Development* **72**, 1467–1477.

Dozier, M. *et al.* (2008) Attachment and psychopathology in adulthood. In: *Handbook of Attachment: Theory, Research, and Clinical Implications*. (eds J. Cassidy & P.R. Shaver), 2nd edn, pp. 718–744. Guilford Press, New York.

Easterbrooks, M.A. & Abeles, R. (2000) Windows to the self in 8-year-olds: bridges to attachment representation and behavioral adjustment. *Attachment & Human Development* **2**, 85–106.

Egeland, B. & Farber, E.A. (1984) Infant-mother attachment: factors related to its development and changes over time. *Child Development* **55**, 753–771.

Eyberg, S.M. *et al.* (2001) Parent–child interaction therapy with behavior problems children: one and two year maintenance of treatment effects in the family. *Child and Family Behavior Therapy* **23**, 1–20.

Fearon, R.P. *et al.* (2010) The significance of insecure attachment and disorganization in the development of children's externalizing behavior: a meta-analytic study. *Child Development* **81**, 435–456.

Fonagy, P. *et al.* (1996) The relation of attachment status, psychiatric classification, and response to psychotherapy. *Journal of Consulting and Clinical Psychology* **64**, 22–31.

Fraiberg, S. (1980) *Clinical Studies in Infant Mental Health: The First Year of Life*. Basic Books, New York.

George, C. *et al.* (1996) *Adult Attachment Interview*. University of California, Berkeley Unpublished manuscript.

Goldberg, S. *et al.* (1999) Confidence in protection: arguments for a narrow definition of attachment. *Journal of Family Psychology* **13**, 475–483.

Goldfarb, W. (1945) Psychological privation in infancy and subsequent adjustment. *American Journal of Orthopsychiatry* **15**, 247–255.

Goodman, S.H. & Gotlib, I.H. (1999) Risk for psychopathology in the children of depressed mothers: a developmental model for understanding mechanisms of transmission. *Psychological Review* **106**, 458–490.

Groh, A.M. *et al.* (2012) The significance of insecure and disorganized attachment for children's internalizing symptoms: a meta-analytic study. *Child Development* **83**, 591–610.

Grossman, K. *et al.* (2005) Early care and the roots of attachment and partnership representations: the Bielefeld and Regensburg longitudinal studies. In: *Attachment from Infancy to Adulthood: The Major Longitudinal Studies.* (eds K.E. Grossman, K. Grossman & E. Waters), pp. 98–136. Guilford Press, New York.

Gunnar, M.R. *et al.* (2006) Bringing basic research on early experience and stress neurobiology to bear on preventive interventions for neglected and maltreated children. *Developmental Psychopathology* **18**, 651–677.

Harlow, H.F. (1958) The nature of love. *American Psychologist* **13**, 673–685.

Hesse, E. & Main, M. (2006) Frightened, threatening, and dissociative parental behavior in low-risk samples: description, discussion, and interpretations. *Development and Psychopatholoy* **18**, 309–343.

Hobson, R.P. *et al.* (2005) Personal relatedness and attachment in infants of mothers with borderline personality disorder. *Development and Psychopathology* **17**, 329–347.

Hofer, M. (1994) Hidden regulators in attachment, separation, and loss. *Monographs of the Society for Research in Child Development* **59**, 192–207.

Hoffman, K.T. *et al.* (2006) Changing toddlers' and preschoolers' attachment classifications: the circle of security intervention. *Journal of Consulting and Clinical Psychology* **74**, 1017–1026.

Joseph, M.A. *et al.* (2014) The formation of secure new attachments by children who were maltreated: an observational study of adolescents in foster care. *Development and Psychopathology* **26**, 67–80.

Juffer, F. *et al.* (2008) *Promoting Positive Parenting: An Attachment-Based Intervention.* Lawrence Earlbaum, New York.

Lamb, M.E. & Lewis, C. (2004) Father-child relationships. In: *Handbook of Father Involvement: Multidisciplinary Perspectives.* (eds M.E. Lamb & C. Lewis), 2nd edn, pp. 119–134. Routledge, New York.

Lewis-Morrarty, E. *et al.* (2012) Cognitive flexibility and theory of mind outcomes among foster children: preschool follow-up results of a randomized clinical trial. *Journal of Adolescent Health* **51**, 17–22.

Lieberman, A.F. *et al.* (2006) Child–parent psychotherapy: 6-month follow up of a randomized controlled trial. *Journal of the American Academy of Child and Adolescent Psychiatry* **45**, 913–918.

Lind, T. *et al.* (2014) Intervention effects on negative affect of CPS-referred children: results of a randomized clinical trial. *Child Abuse and Neglect* **38**, 1459–1467.

Lorenz, K. (1957) *Instinctive Behavior.* International Universities Press, New York.

Lyons-Ruth, K. *et al.* (1999) Maternal frightened, frightening, or atypical behavior and disorganized infant attachment patterns. *Monographs of the Society for Research in Child Development* **64**, 67–96.

Madigan, S. *et al.* (2006) Unresolved states of mind, disorganized attachment relationships, and disrupted interactions of adolescent mothers and their infants. *Developmental Psychology* **42**, 293–304.

Madigan, S. *et al.* (2013) Attachment and internalizing behavior in early childhood: a meta-analysis. *Developmental Psychology* **49**, 672–689.

Main, M. (1990) Cross-cultural studies of attachment organization: recent studies, changing methodologies, and the concept of conditional strategies. *Human Development* **33**, 48–61.

Main, M. & Cassidy, J. (1988) Categories of response to reunion with the parent at age six: predictable from infant attachment classifications and stable over a 1-month-period. *Developmental Psychology* **24**, 415–526.

Main, M. & Hesse, E. (1990) Parents' unresolved traumatic experiences are related to infant disorganized attachment status: is frightened and/or frightened parental behavior the linking mechanism? In: *Attachment in the Preschool Years: Theory, Research, and Intervention.* (eds M. Greenberg, D. Cicchetti & E.M. Cummings), pp. 161–182. University of Chicago Press, Chicago.

Main, M. & Solomon, J. (1986) Discovery of a new, insecure-disorganized/disoriented attachment pattern. In: *Affective Development in Infancy.* (eds T.B. Brazelton & M. Yogman), pp. 95–124. Ablex, Norwood, New Jersey.

Main, M. & Solomon, J. (1990) Procedures for identifying infants as disorganized/disoriented during the Ainsworth Strange Situation. In: *Attachment in the Pre-School Years: Theory, Research, and intervention.* (eds M.T. Greenberg, D. Cicchetti & E. Cummings), pp. 161–182. University of Chicago Press, Chicago.

Main, M. *et al.* (1985) Security in infancy, childhood, and adulthood: a move to the level of representation. *Monographs of the Society for Research in Child Development* **50**, 66–104.

Main, M. *et al.* (2005) Predictability of attachment behavior and representational processes at 1, 6, and 19 years of age. In: *Attachment from Infancy to Adulthood: The Major Longitudinal Studies.* (eds K.E. Grossman, K. Grossman & E. Waters), pp. 245–304. Guilford Press, New York.

Marshall, P.J. & Fox, N.A. (2005) Relations between behavioral reactivity at 4 months and attachment classification at 14 months in a selected sample. *Infant Behavior & Development* **28**, 492–502.

McElwain, N.L. & Booth-LaForce, C. (2006) Maternal sensitivity to infant distress and nondistress as predictors of infant-mother attachment security. *Journal of Family Pscyhology* **20**, 247–255.

McElwain, N.L. *et al.* (2003) Differentiating among insecure mother-infant attachment classifications: a focus on child-friend interaction and exploration during solitary play at 36 months. *Attachment & Human Development* **5**, 136–164.

Miyake, K. *et al.* (1985) Infant temperament, mother's mode of interaction, and attachment in Japan: an interim report. *Monographs of the Society for Research in Child Development* **50**, 276–297.

Moss, E. *et al.* (2005) Stability of attachment during the preschool years. *Developmental Psychology* **41**, 773–783.

NICHD Early Child Care Research Network (1997) The effects of infant child care on infant-mother attachment security: results of the NICHD Study of Early Child Care. *Child Development* **68**, 860–879.

NICHD Early Child Care Research Network (2001) Child-care and family predictors of preschool attachment and stability from infancy. *Developmental Psychology* **37**, 847–862.

Pederson, D.R. *et al.* (1998) Maternal attachment representations, maternal sensitivity, and the infant-mother attachment relationship. *Developmental Psychology* **34**, 925–933.

Raver, C. (1996) Relations between social contingency in mother-child interaction and 2-year-olds' social competence. *Developmental Psychology* **32**, 850–859.

Robertson, J. & Robertson, J. (1989) *Separation and the Very Young.* Free Association Books, London.

Roisman, G.I. (2007) The psychophysiology of adult attachment relationships: autonomic reactivity in marital and premarital interactions. *Developmental Psychology* **43**, 39–53.

Roisman, G.I. *et al.* (2007) The Adult Attachment Interview and self-reports of attachment style: an empirical rapprochement. *Journal of Personality and Social Psychology* **92**, 678–697.

Rutter, M. (2006) Review of Attachment from infancy to adulthood. The major longitudinal studies. *Journal of Child Psychology and Psychiatry* **47**, 974–977.

Rutter, M. *et al.* (2009) Emanuel Miller lecture: attachment insecurity, disinhibited attachment, and attachment disorder: where do research findings leave the concepts? *Journal of Child Psychology and Psychiatry* **50**, 529–543.

Sagi, A. *et al.* (1994) Sleeping out of home in kibbutz communal arrangement: it makes a difference for infant-mother attachment. *Child Development* **65**, 992–1004.

Sagi-Schwartz, A. & Aviezer, O. (2005) Correlates of attachment to multiple caregivers in Kibbutz children from birth to emerging adulthood: the Haifa Longitudinal Study. In: *Attachment from Infancy to Adulthood: The Major Longitudinal Studies.* (eds K.E. Grossman, K. Grossman & E. Waters), pp. 165–197. Guilford Press, New York.

Schneider, B.H. *et al.* (2001) Child–parent attachment and children's peer relations: a quantitative review. *Developmental Psychology* **37**, 86–100.

Schuengel, C. *et al.* (1999) Frightening maternal behavior linking unresolved loss and disorganized infant attachment. *Journal of Consulting and Clinical Psychology* **67**, 54–63.

Scott, S. *et al.* (2011) Attachment in adolescence: overlap with parenting and unique prediction of behavioral adjustment. *Journal of Child Psychology and Psychiatry* **52**, 1052–1062.

Slough, N.M. & Greenberg, M.T. (1990) Five-year-olds' representations of separation from parents: responses from the perspective of self and other. *New Directions for Child Development* **48**, 67–84.

Spangler, G. & Grossmann, K.E. (1993) Biobehavioral organization in securely and insecurely attached infants. *Child Development* **64**, 1439–1450.

Spitz, R. (1945) Hospitalism: an inquiry into the genesis of psychiatric conditions in early childhood. *Psychoanalytic Study of the Child* **1**, 53–74.

Sroufe, L.A. (1985) Attachment classification from the perspective of infant-caregiver relationships and infant temperament. *Child Development* **56**, 1–14.

Sroufe, L.A. & Waters, E. (1977a) Heart rate as a convergent measure in clinical and developmental research. *Merrill-Palmer Quarterly* **23**, 3–27.

Sroufe, L.A. & Waters, E. (1977b) Attachment as an organizational construct. *Child Development* **48**, 1184–1199.

Sroufe, L.A. *et al.* (1983) Attachment and dependency in developmental perspective. *Child Development* **54**, 1615–1627.

Sroufe, L.A. *et al.* (2005) *The Development of the Person: The Minnesota Study of Risk and Adaptation from Birth to Adulthood.* Guilford Press, New York.

Steele, H. & Steele, M. (2005) Understanding and resolving emotional conflict: findings from the London Parent–child Project. In: *Attachment from Infancy to Adulthood: The Major Longitudinal Studies.* (eds K.E. Grossman, K. Grossman & E. Waters), pp. 137–164. Guilford Press, New York.

Stovall-McClough, K.C. & Dozier, M. (2004) Forming attachments in foster care: infant attachment behaviors during the first 2 months of placement. *Development and Psychopathology* **16**, 253–271.

Target, M. *et al.* (2003) Attachment representations in school-age children: the development of the Child Attachment Interview. *Journal of Child Psychotherapy* **29**, 171–186.

Thompson, R.A. *et al.* (1982) Stability of infant-mother attachment and its relationship to changing life circumstances in an unselected middle-class sample. *Child Development* **53**, 144–148.

Tinbergen, N. (1951) *The Study of Instinct.* Clarendon Press, Oxford.

Toth, S.L. *et al.* (2002) The relative efficacy of two interventions in altering maltreated preschool children's representational models: implications for attachment theory. *Development and Psychopathology* **14**, 877–908.

van IJzendoorn, M.H. (1995) Adult attachment representations, parental responsiveness, and infant attachment: a meta-analysis on the predictive validity of the adult attachment interview. *Psychological Bulletin* **117**, 387–403.

van IJzendoorn, M.H. & de Wolff, M.S. (1997) In search of the absent father – meta-analysis of infant-father attachment: a rejoinder to our discussants. *Child Development* **68**, 604–609.

van IJzendoorn, M.H. & Kroonenberg, P.M. (1988) Cross-cultural patterns of attachment: a meta-analysis of the Strange Situation. *Child Development* **59**, 147–156.

van IJzendoorn, M.H. *et al.* (1999) Disorganized attachment in early childhood: meta-analysis of precursors, concomitants, and sequelae. *Development and Psychopathology* **11**, 225–249.

van IJzendoorn, M.H. *et al.* (2004) Assessing attachment security with the Attachment Q-Sort: meta-analytic evidence for validity of the Observer AQS. *Child Development* **75**, 1188–1213.

Vaughn, B.E. *et al.* (2008) Attachment and temperament: additive and interactive influences on behavior, affect, and cognition during infancy and childhood. In: *Handbook of Attachment: Theory, Research, and Clinical Implications.* (eds J. Cassidy & P.R. Shaver), 2nd edn, pp. 192–216. Guilford Press, New York.

Vondra, J.I. *et al.* (1999) Stability and change in infant attachment style in a low-income sample. *Monographs of the Society for Research in Child Development* **64**, 119–144.

Vondra, J.I. *et al.* (2001) Attachment stability and emotional and behavioral regulation from infancy to preschool age. *Development and Psychopathology* **13**, 13–33.

Waters, E. (1978) The reliability and stability of individual differences in infant mother attachment. *Child Development* **49**, 483–494.

Waters, E. & Deane, K.E. (1985) Defining and assessing individual differences in attachment relationships: Q-methodology and the organization of behavior in infancy and early childhood. *Monographs of the Society for Research in Child Development* **50**, 41–65.

Webster-Stratton, C. *et al.* (2001) Social skills and problems-solving training for children with early-onset conduct problems: who benefits. *Journal of Child Psychology and Psychiatry* **42**, 943–952.

Weinfield, N.S. *et al.* (2000) Attachment from infancy to early adulthood in a high-risk sample: continuity, discontinuity, and their correlates. *Child Development* **71**, 695–702.

van Zeijl, J. *et al.* (2006) Attachment-based intervention for enhancing sensitive discipline in mothers of 1- to 3-year-old children at risk for externalizing behaviour problems: a randomized clinical trial. *Journal of Consulting and Clinical Psychology* **74**, 994–1005.

CHAPTER 7

Infant/early years mental health

Tuula Tamminen and Kaija Puura

Department of Child Psychiatry, University of Tampere and Tampere University Hospital, Tampere, Finland

Introduction

The concepts of infancy and infant mental health

Infancy can refer to different age groups. In this chapter we focus mainly on the first year but also cover up to the fourth birthday. During infancy, mental health is very strongly connected to the quality of caregiving relationships, especially to the mutual adaptation capacity of an infant and his/her parents (Mäntymaa, 2006, see Chapters 6 and 8). Infant mental health also requires capacities and opportunities for rapid developmental processes (see Chapter 9).

Pregnancy and family perspectives

Pregnancy is a period when both parents undergo the transition to parenthood. Parental perceptions of the future infant and of themselves as parents are based on their own experiences of being parented and their ideals and fears (Raphael-Leff, 2010). Normally, parental expectations of the infant and parenting include both positive and negative aspects, and parents are able to flexibly resolve these. The birth of the first child transforms the couple into a family, with not only dyadic (parent–parent, parent–infant) but also triadic interactions (mother–father–infant). With subsequent births, the number of dyadic relationships in a family increases, and siblings also shape each other's development (Rao & Beidel, 2009).

The development of the central nervous system of the fetus during pregnancy is affected by the health and actions of the mother, and also by the actions of the other parent. In antenatal clinics, attention should be paid to parental well-being, and to supporting abstinence from substance abuse and smoking. Prenatal mental health problems of both parents, most commonly anxiety and depression, should be appropriately treated without delay, as they are linked to postnatal mental health problems and problems in the parent–infant relationship (Luoma *et al.,* 2001; Davis *et al.,* 2004; Kane & Garber, 2004; see Chapter 28).

Aspects of infant's social and emotional development

Mental development has been understood as a continuous process with developmental steps or leaps, when physiological, motor, cognitive, social, and emotional maturation through integration reach a higher reorganizational level. Psychodynamic oriented, often prominently theoretical research, which has concentrated more on the child's subjective experiences, describes these developmental transition points as bio-behavioral shifts.

Empirical neuropsychological research in turn shows mental development as a continual unfolding of the mind (Bale *et al.,* 2010). Research on vision raised the idea of a critical or sensitive period when the maturation of the visual cortex was shown to be dependent on visual stimuli during a certain time frame. Whether or not this is a more general rule of brain maturation is still unclear, but the remarkable plasticity of brain development has become quite evident (see Chapter 9).

Empirical research starting from Darwin (1872, 1965) notes the emergence of human emotions, and the display and range of emotions go from a few to the highly differentiated many, as well as from action patterns to feelings during the first three years (Lewis, 2008). Before the first developmental milestone or bio-behavioral shift, which occurs at 2–3 months, infants show general distress marked by crying and irritability, and pleasure marked by satiation, attention, and responsiveness to the environment. By 3 months an infant becomes more focused and communicative, including social smiling and the emergence of joy. Also, sadness emerges, especially around the withdrawal of positive stimulus events.

Between 7 and 9 months, infants start to understand that human beings have their own individual thoughts and feelings (theory of mind) and that these can be shared in interaction. By this age, infants' emotional behavior reflects the emergence of six early emotions, called primary or basic emotions (joy, sadness, anger, fear, surprise, and disgust) (Izard, 1978).

Rutter's Child and Adolescent Psychiatry, Sixth Edition.
Edited by Anita Thapar and Daniel S. Pine, James F. Leckman, Stephen Scott, Margaret J. Snowling, Eric Taylor.
© 2015 John Wiley & Sons Ltd. Published 2018 by John Wiley & Sons Ltd.

Toward the end of the first and during the second year of life, new cognitive capacities emerge, for example, a qualitative advance in understanding symbols, which has been considered to be the basis for learning to speak. Infants/toddlers now recognize themselves in mirrors and photographs. Simultaneously, "self-conscious emotions," such as embarrassment, envy, and true empathy emerge (Lewis, 2008). Between two and three years of age, cognitive maturation again induces toddlers to learn logical thinking, which greatly increases the communicative options and socioemotional development. The "self-conscious evaluative emotions" emerge, which include pride, shame, and guilt (Lewis, 2008).

After birth, infants' ability to regulate their own physical needs and emotional states is limited and a caregiving adult is responsible for what is called mutual regulation (Tronick *et al.*, 1986) or attunement (Stern, 1985; Field, 1994). When a caregiver is emotionally available and sensitive enough, infants learn step by step to control their own emotions and behavior, which facilitates further social development (Figure 7.1). Infants also learn to control their behavior through mirroring and social referencing, by looking to the caregivers for emotional guidance (Campos & Stenberg, 1981).

Infants from birth act and behave in individual ways. These differences are considered to reflect inborn temperament features. Primary caregiving relationships, especially infants' most important attachment relationships, shape and refine infants' temperamental features, and conversely, an infant's temperament has effects on the quality of parent–infant interaction and their attachment relationships (see Chapter 8).

Play and learning/teaching are important elements of infant–caregiver interaction and influence not only the infant's cognitive but also the emotional and social development. Scaffolding, an adult's ability to provide assistance, and previewing, an adult's ability to be one step ahead of the infant's present abilities, are means of offering increasingly complex new information and thus promote development. Development takes place through ordinary interaction during caretaking (Emde, 1991).

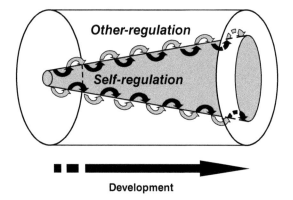

Figure 7.1 Transactional relations between self-regulation and other-regulation (Sameroff, 2010).

Cultural influences in infant mental heath

Children are shaped by culturally regulated customs, child-rearing practices, and belief systems (Harkness & Super, 1995). The first wave of research on culture and parenting focused on minorities versus dominant culture (Super & Harkness, 1997). Cultural discrimination is still a huge problem with multiple socioeconomic and psychological challenges, in particular for parents with young children (Boris, 2006; von Klitzing, 2006). Studies on migration have shown that recurring or prolonged separations, social isolation, and intensive "homesickness" also affect early parenting. Parenthood is inextricably linked to the culture of origin, but the socialization goals of the parents for their child force them to adapt to a new culture. Thus, parenting may become stressful and conflictual (Meléndez, 2005).

The second phase of research concentrated on cross-cultural comparisons. Several studies have identified interesting differences. For instance, Keller and coworkers (2004) revealed that a community with a proximal parenting style during infancy fostered the toddler's interdependency and relatedness, and a community with a distal parenting tradition strengthened independence and autonomy.

The third line of research seeks universal features in parenting practices across different cultures. Referring to these empirical studies, Quinn (2003) stated that different cultures use similar, specific ways in their child-rearing practices, even if these practices may vary according to the parents' cultural values. Three features in parenting practices are common to many cultures: repeating and maintaining the consistency of a child's experience, creating emotional arousal in a child, and giving moral evaluations of a child.

Currently, both parents and professionals need more evidence-based understanding of culture-specific parenting and its impact on early development. Future research might offer a better understanding of ways to integrate the best practices of child rearing around the world (Tamminen, 2006a, b).

Risk and protective factors

Risk factors

Distal risk factors in infancy can be defined as conditions and events rendering caregivers unable to protect the infant from harm, or to care for his/her basic physiological and psychological needs. Such risks may be long-lasting, like poverty, or appear suddenly like natural disasters, accidents, and armed conflicts (see Chapter 26).

All the major risk factors mentioned may disrupt infants' development. An important determinant of the effects of traumatic exposure is the caregivers' ability to restore the sense of safety by successful regulation of infant emotion, sleep, arousal, and attention (Scheeringa & Zeanah, 2001). There is evidence of risk effects being cumulative and further complicated by limited access to health care and education (Walker *et al.*, 2007).

Even outside the most adverse conditions such as institutional rearing (see Chapters 21 and 58) there is now cumulating evidence on how the quality of parenting is a proximal risk factor that may impact mental health in infancy (see Chapter 37). Parental mental and physical health also require consideration as these have an important impact on parenting and the quality of parent care (see Chapter 28). Depression and anxiety are especially common.

Parenthood during adolescence may pose difficult challenges in a phase when adolescents themselves still need psychological, social, and economic support. Adolescent parenting has been associated with poorer adaptation to parental role, poorer social support, increased risk for depression (Reid & Meadows-Oliver, 2007), and adolescent mothers have been shown to be more likely to be insensitive and use more punishment with their infants (Coll *et al.*, 1986). It is likely that the effect of adolescent parenting on child outcome is moderated by coexisting risk and protective factors.

Even in families where there are no apparent risk factors, problems in caregiving may arise if there is a very poor goodness-of-fit between parent and infant (Stern, 1995). A parent who has difficulties in understanding and accepting the behavior and characteristics of the infant may act insensitively in interaction, and also have difficulties in becoming attached to the infant.

Infants' normal psychological development may also be jeopardized by factors directly affecting infant behavior and increasing the perceived burden of parenting. Crying is the infant's main way of communicating distress. In a study of 3259 infants aged 1–6 months, Reijneveld *et al.* (2004) found that 5.6% of parents reported having smothered, slapped or shaken their infant due to crying. Premature infants are often felt to be more difficult to care for, less sociable and parents' attachment to them may vary from normal to avoidant, overprotective or intrusive (Feldman & Eidelman, 2006). Recurrently or chronically sick infants may be at risk for the same reasons, while stressful conditions like poor parenting may increase susceptibility to illness (Mäntymaa *et al.*, 2003). The infant may also be difficult to soothe, show irregularity in biological functions and have difficulties in adapting to new situations, that is, have a difficult temperament, or as a toddler have difficulties with impulse-control (Kochanska *et al.*, 2000), making caregiving more challenging (see Chapter 8).

Protective factors and infant resilience

For infants and young children having a relationship with a responsive, warm, and available caregiver is likely the most important factor for positive outcomes (Rutter, 2013, see Chapters 6 and 27). Children with the capacity to elicit support and positive responses from others by their own positive behavior, for example, smiles, may be at an advantage in this regard (Werner & Smith, 2001, see Chapter 8). Distal protective factors include parents' social network, social security services, and organized health care (Petersen *et al.*, 2010).

Special features in assessing infants

Guidelines for assessment

When assessing infants, clinicians face age-specific challenges. Infants and toddlers are active partners when interacting with others, but limited in their communicative skills compared to older children. Clinicians therefore rely greatly on information from caregivers, and on direct observation of infants. As context and relationships are influential, the variation in infant behavior across settings is highly informative (Clark *et al.*, 2004, see Chapter 32). Rapid development during the first three years requires a developmental perspective to differentiate normality from risk and pathology.

A clinical interview is a cornerstone of assessment. Usually it is easiest to start by discussing the problems and symptoms of the infant with the parents and other caregivers. Parental reports and views on the infant's constitutional characteristics and temperament and on the caregiver–infant relationship and interaction are also important.

Severely disadvantaged life conditions may cause developmental deviance while infant developmental delay may cause problems in early interaction, hence the importance of developmental history starting from the prenatal period. Family functioning and cultural and community patterns are important in assessing the quality of care and parenting, and how this may have affected the infant. Parents' characteristics and health are important, likewise the quality of their partner and co-parenting relationships as these affect caregiving.

Direct observation of an infant and his/her interactions with others is another cornerstone in assessment. Observation may quickly reveal problematic areas in parental caregiving. Also, the infant' s constitutional characteristics and maturation phase, and affective, language, cognitive, motor and sensory patterns need to be assessed by observation, in addition to parental report, to ascertain how challenging his/her caregiving is, and what skills he/she particularly needs to develop or improve.

Assessment of the infant's mental state

Clinicians can also use parental reports on infant development, behavior and characteristics, and psychological testing for assessing the cognitive, social, and emotional state of an infant. Examples are shown in Table 7.1.

Infant and toddler observation methods

Infant observation is an important method for acquiring first-hand information on the development and well-being of the infant and for screening for signs of pathology. Several structured assessment methods based on infant observation are now in use, of which three examples are described here. The Brazelton Neonatal Behavior Assessment Scale (BNBAS, Brazelton, 1973) is meant to examine the integrity of the neonate's central nervous system and to help caregivers to understand and interact with the newborn. The Baby Alarm Distress Scale

Table 7.1 Examples of parental reports used in assessing infants.

Method	Authors	Age range in months	Purpose	Description
Developmental functioning				
Ages and Stages Questionnaire (ASQ)	Bricker *et al.* (1999)	1 to 48 months	Screen for delays in communication and motor and social development	Parental questionnaire
Vineland Adaptive Behavior Scales II	Sparrow *et al.* (2005)	0 to adulthood	Screen for delays in communication, daily skills, socialization, motor skills, maladaptive behaviors	Parental questionnaire
Infant Behavior Questionnaire (IBQ)	Rothbart (1981)	3 to 12 months	Assesses infant temperament and characteristics	Parental questionnaire used mainly for research purposes
Infant Characteristics Questionnaire (ICQ)	Bates *et al.* (1979)	6, 13, and 24 months	Assesses the construct of temperament, subscales for fussiness/difficulties, adaptability, sociability and persistence, high scores indicating more problems with the infant	Parental questionnaire
Infant behavior and symptoms				
Infant-Toddler Social and Emotional Assessment (ITSEA)	Carter & Briggs-Cowan (2006)	12 to 36 months	Comprehensive checklist for evaluating socioemotional and behavioral problems in infants and toddlers	Parental questionnaire
Brief Infant-Toddler Social and Emotional Assessment (BITSEA)	Briggs-Cowan & Carter (2006)	12 to 36 months	Brief parent report for evaluating socioemotional and behavioral problems in infants and toddlers	Parental questionnaire
Child Behavior Checklist (CBCL)	Achenbach & Rescorla (2000)	18 to 60 months	Comprehensive checklist for evaluating socioemotional and behavioral problems in infants and toddlers	Parental questionnaire, parallel version for other caregivers like kindergarten teachers
Behavioral Screening Questionnaire	Richman *et al.* (1975)	From 36 months	Designed to document the occurrence of early behavioral disturbances	Parental questionnaire
Checklist for Autism in Toddlers (CHAT)	Baron-Cohen *et al.* (1992)	18 months	Checklist for detecting autistic symptoms	Checklist administered by health care professional to the parent
Parent interviews				
Mannheim Parent Interview	Esser *et al.* (1989)	3 months–5 years	Research use	Structured interview covering common problems and symptoms in infancy and toddlerhood
European Early Promotion Project (EEPP) Interview	Puura *et al.* (2005a)	From birth to 2 years	Research use	Semi-structured interview based on Isle of Wight family assessment interview, covers demographic information, risk factors, behavioral characteristics, and common problems in infancy
Working Model of the Child-Interview	Zeanah *et al.* (1994)	From birth on	Research and clinical use	Semi-structured interview, assesses caregivers' internal representations of their relationship with the child
Preschool Age Psychiatric Assessment (PAPA)	Egger & Angold (2004)	From 2 to 5 years	Diagnostic interview, research and clinical use	Semi-structured, includes all DSM-IV criteria relevant for children in this age range, all the items in the Diagnostic Classification Zero to Three and additional behaviors and symptoms that may be encountered by toddlers and their families. In addition, assesses the amount of impairment associated with symptoms, family relationships, and environment and life events
Diagnostic Infant and Preschool Assessment Manual (DIPA)	Scheeringa (2004)	From birth to 6 years	Diagnostic interview, research and clinical use	Partly structured and semi-structured interview, includes all DSM-IV criteria relevant for children in this age range

(ADBB, Guedeney & Fermanian 2001) is an observation method for assessing signs of pathology, and was designed to screen for signs of infant social withdrawal reaction as a part of a medical examination in primary care services. The ADBB consists of eight items concerning the behavior and characteristics of the baby (facial expression, eye contact, vocalization, overall level of activity, self-stimulating behavior, briskness of response to stimulation, attraction toward the infant, and relationship between the infant and the observer). The rating is done immediately after observation in a live situation, or on videotape. Higher scores have been found to be associated with insensitive parent–infant interaction and parental mental health problems (e.g., De Rosa *et al.*, 2010; Puura *et al.*, 2013).

An observation scale developed for assessing a particular type of child behavior is the Disruptive Behavior Observation Scale (DB-DOS) for three- to five-year-old children (Wakschlag *et al.*, 2008). The DB-DOS is a 50-min structured observation that is divided into one part with the parent and two parts with the examiner.

Assessment of the parent–infant relationship

Parental reports and observation methods are shown in Table 7.2. Parental reports like the Parenting Stress Index (Abidin, 1997) yield valuable information on how the parent perceives his/her infant, and experiences interaction with the infant.

Table 7.2 Examples of methods for assessing parent–infant interaction and relationship.

Method	Author	Age range	Purpose	Description
Parenting Stress Index (PSI)	Abidin (1997)	0 to adulthood	Assessment of parent–child relationship and parental stress	Parent questionnaire, statements concerning infant characteristics, how the parent feels about the child, and how much stress is caused by child
Infant-Toddler HOME-Inventory	Bradley & Caldwell (1979)	0 to 36 months	Assessment of children's developmental surroundings and parent–child relationship	Semi-structured observation method with an interview, the examiner during a home visit makes observations on the environment of the infant and of parental behavior
Child–Adult Relational Experimental Index (CARE Index)	Crittenden (1981)	0 to 36 months	Assessment of parent–infant interaction in high-risk groups	Observation method, 5 min sequence of videotaped interaction coded for adult sensitivity and child cooperation with the adult
Parent–Child Early Relationship Assessment (PC-ERA)	Clark (1985)	0 months to 7 years	Assessing parent–infant interaction	Observation method, semi- structured procedure with feeding, structured task, free play and separation–reunion sequence videotaped, each 5-min segment of the videotaped scored separately
Global Rating Scales for Mother–Infant Interaction (GRS)	Murray *et al.* (1996)	0 to 4 months	Assessment of parent–infant interaction in clinical groups such as depression and schizophrenia, social adversity and low-risk/- high-risk groups	Observation method, mother and infant videotaped for 5 min in interaction, rated for maternal mood and behavior, infant social behavior and quality of interaction
Emotional Availability Scales; EAS	Biringen *et al.* (1993, 1998); Biringen (2008)	0 to 48 months	Assessing global quality of parent–infant interaction	Observation method, parental sensitivity, structuring, nonintrusiveness and nonhostility are scored, and child responsiveness and child involvement, rated from 20 to 30 min long videotape with both structured tasks and free play, also global rating of the dyadic relationship
PICCOLO	Roggman *et al.* (2013)	0 to 36 months	Assessment and intervention method	Observation method for parental interaction behavior in domains of Affection, Responsiveness, Encouragement and Teaching, coding made in live situation or from 5-min videotaped interaction sequence

Assessment of triadic interaction and coparenting

Lausanne Triadic Play (LTP, Fivaz-Depeursinge and Corboz-Warnery, 1999) was developed to assess how both parents and infant interact and coregulate the interaction in a task where they alternate between dyadic and triadic interaction (Figure 7.2). The parents' ability to negotiate changes and show mutual respect in the interaction indicates how well they can function jointly as parents. Smooth and unproblematic coparenting has been shown to be associated with better child outcome (McHale & Rasmussen, 1998; Schoppe-Sullivan *et al.*, 2009).

Integrating the information from the assessment

The diagnosis and intervention plan is based on appropriate assessment, and entails identifying both strengths and weaknesses of the infant and his/her parents, in the whole family, and in society. Parental reports with data from other caregivers and clinical objective data on the infant's development and behavior

are used to form a comprehensive understanding of the infant and his/her problems. In observed behavior, mutual positive affect, shared pleasure, and mutual engagement between parent and infant are usually seen in nonproblematic interaction, whereas parental flat or negative affect in the interaction, infant withdrawal or avoidant behavior, and slight mutual engagement and pleasure between parent and infant usually indicate problems.

Parental reports and clinical data may yield similar results, for example, when parents have noticed a delay in the development of the infants' skills that is also apparent in observation or in psychological testing. More often than not, there are minor or major discrepancies between parental information and other caregiver reports and clinical observations. A common example is a depressed or exhausted parent who may find the normal needs of an infant or toddler extremely demanding, and report the infant to be difficult or have behavioral problems. The child may also have behavioral problems with one parent but

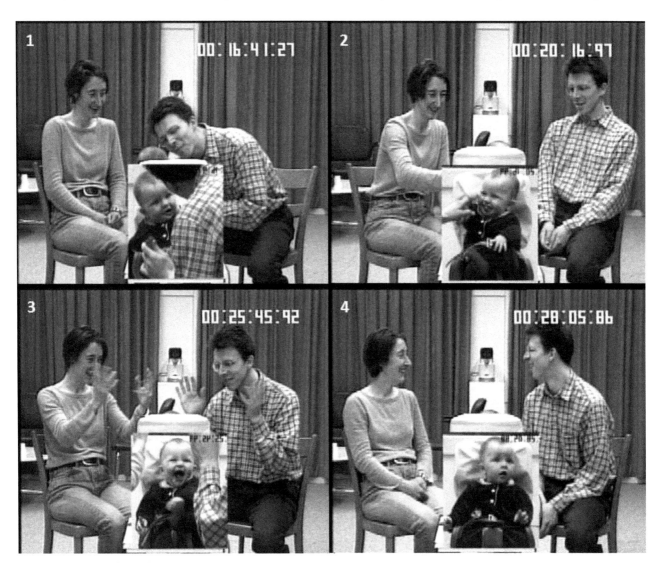

Figure 7.2 Lausanne Trilogue play situation.

not with the other, indicating a problem more likely in that particular relationship or context than in the infant. The parents may also fail to see or report problems in their relationship or in the behavior of the infant, even though these are observable in the assessment. The latter indicates problems in the ability or willingness of the parent to note and respond to the infant's needs.

Common problems versus pathways to psychopathology

What is a problem, a symptom, or a disorder?

Newborn babies are unique individuals who differ greatly. Parents and their life situations also vary. The transition to parenthood and the maturation of biological and psychological regulation mechanisms in caregiving interactions take time; no wonder problems in everyday caretaking and in infant behavior are common, with up to 30% of parents reporting problems (Reijneveld *et al.*, 2001; Crncec *et al.*, 2010).

If the problems are more severe and the buffering capacity of a caregiving relationship is exceeded more permanently, an infant may show more specific symptoms as a sign of general distress, such as withdrawal, irritability, or regulatory difficulties. If these specific symptoms occur in more than one relationship and in different settings, and if there are several symptoms, these should be considered as signs of maladaptive processes or early steps to possible psychopathological trajectories.

In cases of various, serious, and constant symptoms during infancy, the mental health of a young child needs to be properly assessed. Although the empirical evidence of psychiatric disorders in infancy is still quite limited and mostly based on small-sized clinical samples, the possible existence of a mental disorder should be evaluated. If the criteria for a psychiatric disorder (according to ICD-10/11, DSM-5, or The Diagnostic Classification System for Mental Health and Developmental Disorders of Infancy and Early Childhood, DC: 0–3R, 2005) are fulfilled, even an infant is considered to suffer from a disorder. Although the ICD- and DSM-systems take different approaches to diagnostic classification, the main criteria for various disorders are basically quite similar, and the DC: 0–3R-system offers descriptions on how infants and toddlers may exhibit various symptoms. However, it should be noted that the main research gaps in infancy are to be found in the validity of the classification of early disorders and the reliability of diagnostic assessments. Therefore, epidemiological studies on many psychiatric disorders during infancy are still virtually nonexistent.

In the diagnostic assessment of an infant's mental health, both over- and underestimations should be avoided. One should not label problems in young children and in early relationships as medical conditions without strong evidence of diagnostic criteria being met. In addition, the diagnostic processes of infant psychiatric disorders raise specific questions, most notably the need for diagnosis of relationship disorders (Smith Slep & Tamminen, 2013).

Nevertheless, slowly accumulating research findings indicate that mental disorders exist in all ages during the life course. For very early years, this has been shown in an epidemiologically and clinically well-designed birth cohort study in Denmark (Skovgaard *et al.*, 2007). Also, Möricke with his colleagues conducted an analysis of 6330 parents' reports of their 14–15 month old infants' behavior and symptoms in a population-based study. They concluded that even in infancy certain distinct and disorder relevant developmental profiles can be recognized (Möricke *et al.*, 2013).

Young children with psychiatric disorders should receive therapeutic help as early as possible. Many early interventions have demonstrated their effectiveness in treating young children and their parents in separate single studies, but replications of these results and meta-analyses of several studies are sparse. Qualified infant psychiatric services are still globally quite rare but interventions may also be provided by other services and by other professionals working with infants and toddlers.

Problems with sleeping, feeding, and eating

A newborn infant sleeps approximately 16–17 hours per day; by six months of age, sleep often decreases to 13–14 hours with one longer period; and around one year of age, the infant's circadian timing system has developed so that the sleeping–waking cycle has diurnal organization. However, individual variations are wide. Sleep patterns are regulated by both biological and physiological factors (e.g., brain maturation and neurotransmitters involved in the promotion, maintenance, and timing of sleep) and psychological processes (e.g., behavioral and relational aspects and cultural norms).

Parental concerns about infant sleep problems are common during the first three years. Significant sleep difficulties among this age group occur in 15–35%, and most often entail difficulties initiating sleep and waking at night (Crncec *et al.*, 2010).

Various kinds of parent education and behavioral interventions and therapies have been evaluated in controlled experimental studies with quite large treatment effect sizes (Sadeh, 2005; Crncec *et al.*, 2010; see Chapter 70).

Different severity levels of feeding and eating problems occur in approximately 20–40% among normally developing 0- to 3-year-old children and in up to 80% among children with developmental disabilities (Bryant-Waugh *et al.*, 2010). Around 1–3% of infants suffer from severe feeding difficulties associated with poor weight gain (Skovgaard *et al.*, 2007; Chatoor & Macaoay, 2008).

An infant may have difficulties in reaching and maintaining a calm state during feeding and a caregiver may be unable to help the infant. A lack of caregiver–infant reciprocity may also create feeding problems. Young children also have sensory food aversions, so that a child consistently refuses to eat foods with specific tastes, textures, or smells but eats preferred foods without difficulty. Maternal worries about child underweight partially explain the development of negative feeding interactions (Gueron-Sela *et al.*, 2011).

Somatic illnesses and medical conditions may create feeding and eating problems and these may persist even after the medical situation improves. Some young children exhibit food refusals after insertion of nasogastric or endotracheal tubes or suctioning. Other clear insults to the gastrointestinal tract may also trigger intense distress in the infant and lead to severe feeding problems (Arts-Rodas & Benoit, 1998; Chatoor & Macaoay, 2008).

There are also feeding problems with apparently none of these etiological backgrounds, and when the condition is severe enough it has been called infantile anorexia. These feeding problems are serious enough to impede adequate weight gain or produce weight loss and have been suggested to be a psychiatric disorder if they continue at least a month without improvement. Regurgitation or reflux may sometimes be part of the disorder. Persistent eating of nonnutritive substances, so-called pica, is most common in children with intellectual development disorders, but may also occur in maltreated or neglected young children.

Regardless of the etiology, feeding difficulties often affect the infant–caregiver relationship and to successfully treat the problem or disorder, the relational aspects should be considered (see Chapter 71).

Problems in emotion regulation and early mood disorders

Infants have some behaviors to regulate their emotional states (e.g., looking away, self-stimulation, and self-comforting). However, infants' regulation capacities are immature and poorly coordinated, and emotion regulation is dependent on the actions of the caregivers. Throughout their development, children learn and internalize repeated dyadic patterns of emotion regulation.

Both infants and their caretakers share emotional states when interacting. One of the major features of early interaction is how infants and parents constantly attune their gestures, vocalizations, movements, and actions to each other's behavior. This is considered an important part of emotion sharing and regulation. Well-attuned interaction is pleasurable and mis-attunement creates concerns in both partners.

Both infants and their caretakers may have many kinds of problems in emotion regulation and sharing. An infant's difficult temperament or a parent's depressed mood may create difficulties. Also, environmental stressors may affect family atmosphere and disrupt sensitive parent–child interactions. Negative emotions, dissatisfaction, and disappointment are consequently quite normal in new parents; so also are fussing and crying in infants.

Parental psychopathology complicates the dyadic emotion regulation more seriously, and poor quality of attachment relationships or severe traumas may also impair joint emotion regulation and maturation of the child's own affect control. These risk factors may also be cumulative in increasing the

likelihood of a mood disorder in a young child (Guedeney *et al.*, 2013).

If a child has several symptoms occurring most of the day, more days than not, and if these symptoms are generalized across different settings and relationships, and if there is a clear change from the child's earlier mood and behavior, even a young child is considered to have a depression or anxiety disorder. Disorder also entails diminished functional capacities, for example, difficulty focusing attention or concentrating or responding to caregivers, restlessness or loss of energy, and loss of already acquired skills, all of which may impede a child's development.

A very young child can present with depressed or irritable mood or anhedonia, and markedly diminished pleasure or interest in activities such as play or interaction with caregivers. There may be significant weight loss or gain, insomnia or hypersomnia, and psychomotor agitation or retardation. The recurrent and chronic nature of childhood depression underscores the need for early attention to this public health problem (Field *et al.*, 2006; Mathers & Loncar, 2006). Anxiety disorders, notably separation anxiety, can also present in this age group (see Chapter 60).

Problems with behavior regulation and aggression

Children's ability to coordinate and control their own actions and behaviors matures rapidly during the first years of life, and development continues throughout childhood and adolescence. Since emotion regulation is also immature in early childhood, negative behaviors and temper tantrums are frequent. The period after infancy has aptly been called the "terrible twos." Studies on the normative development of externalizing behaviors indicate an increase until the second and third year of life, with a decrease after this age (Tremblay *et al.*, 2004), although considerable individual variations exist.

There are contradictory views on whether it is appropriate to use the term disorder for young children with significant levels of aggressive and disruptive behavior, because intentionality of hostile actions, reduced empathy, guilt, and concern toward others, which are descriptions of core symptoms in these disorders, may not be similar at young ages (Gill & Calkins, 2003). However, in the United States it has been estimated that 1 in 11 preschoolers meets formal DSM criteria for a disruptive behavior disorder, 1 in 14 for an oppositional defiant disorder, and 1 in 30 for a conduct disorder (Egger & Angold, 2006). Early disruptive behavior problems occur in different cultures, exhibit considerable stability, are associated with profound academic and social disability, and increase the risk for later psychopathology and criminality (Copeland *et al.*, 2007; Burke *et al.*, 2010).

Psychosocial treatments focusing on parent–child interaction have demonstrated a large and sustained effect (Comer *et al.*, 2013, see Chapters 37 and 40).

Problems related to adverse experiences and effects of severe trauma

Facing ordinary difficulties and solving everyday problems are considered important promoters of early mental development.

Experiences of surviving adversities and overcoming exceptional challenges may also play a role in the development of resilience.

Severe trauma such as life-threatening injury to the child or family members or chronic child battering or sexual abuse are overwhelming experiences and may lead to posttraumatic stress disorder even in infants and toddlers (Scheeringa & Gaensbauer, 2000).

In posttraumatic stress disorder, the child shows evidence of re-experiencing the traumatic event(s) (e.g., compulsively driven, anxiety-provoking play, recurring nightmares of the traumatic event, flashbacks, and dissociation). The young child also has numbing of responsiveness (e.g., withdrawal and avoidance) and clear developmental problems. After a traumatic event, the child exhibits symptoms of increased arousal. As in all other mental disorders, a young child's functional capacity is also clearly impaired.

Physical and psychological abuse or chronic neglect and deprivation of a very young child by caregivers may also lead to a specific disorder, which in the ICD and DSM systems is described as attachment disorder and in the DC: 0–3R as a deprivation disorder with either an inhibited or indiscriminate pattern (see Chapter 58).

Empirical studies of posttraumatic stress disorder in infants and toddlers have advanced further than that of other disorders in early childhood and findings on the long-lasting consequences of early severe trauma are emerging (Heim *et al.*, 2010). The psychological and biological "footprints" of early trauma are now the focus of intensive research (e.g., negative synaptic circulates, overacting stress reactions, immunological changes) and cumulating evidence indicates traits of pathological development for many somatic and mental disorders (Ladd *et al.*, 2000, see Chapter 23).

Disorders in development and communicating

Variation in the rate of early maturation is wide and slowly developing young children usually grow up normally. The developmental process may also include phases of regression, for example, as a reaction to environmental stress.

However, developmental disorders initiating and manifesting during the first years of life can and should be detected early. Although a developmental disorder is usually obvious, it may at first be difficult to know precisely whether it is intellectual disability, a pervasive developmental disorder, or a reactive attachment disorder. These serious disorders are presented with descriptions also covering infancy and toddlerhood in Chapters 51, 54, and 58.

Special features of interventions in infancy

Goals for treatment

The main treatment goals are improving the developmental environment of the infant so that psychopathology can be prevented and present and future suffering avoided or alleviated. During pregnancy, infant mental health promotion includes adequate health and mental health care of both parents. On a global scale, the provision of adequate nutrition, housing, physical safety, and hygiene are important together with providing each infant with good and sufficient care and emotional interaction with the parents or caregivers. The most common intervention in infancy is sharing the worries of parents and providing guidance or education, both in naturally existing peer or relative relationships, in primary care services, and in the services of nongovernmental organizations. For families with elevated need for support, that is, when the parents or the infant, or their interaction need to be treated for identified severe problems or symptoms, several intervention models and psychotherapeutic techniques have been developed. There is no research on psychotropic medication with infants and toddlers, and no knowledge of their long-term effects on brain development.

Preventive parent–infant programs

The focus of preventive parent–infant programs in infancy is the enhancement of effective, positive parenting, so as to enable children's development and to manage behavioral and emotional problems where necessary (see Chapters 17 and 37). Preventive programs in infancy may include home visiting by nurses on a regular basis from pregnancy until the child's third birthday, be center-based or include both home visits and center-based services. Reported positive results from preventive programs include increased parental sensitivity and emotional support (Love *et al.*, 2005; Puura *et al.*, 2005b), children's better executive functioning and better behavioral adaptation in toddlerhood (Olds *et al.*, 2004), and better mental health in middle childhood and adolescence (Aronen, 1993; Aronen & Kurkela, 1996). However, in studies reporting effect sizes they have been from small to moderate (Davis *et al.*, 2005; Olds *et al.*, 2007), and in many studies the effects favoring intervention families have been limited to subgroups (Olds *et al.*, 2007). Olds *et al.* (2007) examined 16 preventive programs and concluded that the strongest evidence exists for programs with nurse home visiting in high-risk families, focusing on the improvement of prenatal health, the child's health and development, and parents' own economic self-sufficiency.

Parent–infant therapies

When problems are perceived in the interaction and relationship of the infant with one parent or caregiver, parent–infant therapy may be used as the sole treatment or in more complex cases as a part of multimodal treatment. In parent–infant psychotherapy, the focus of the treatment is the parent–infant relationship, not the infant or the parent as individuals (see Chapter 40). The goal of the psychotherapy is to sensitize the parent to the infant's needs by helping him/her to perceive and understand the infant's cues, and to respond to these appropriately. This in turn helps the infant to regulate his/her emotional and physiological states,

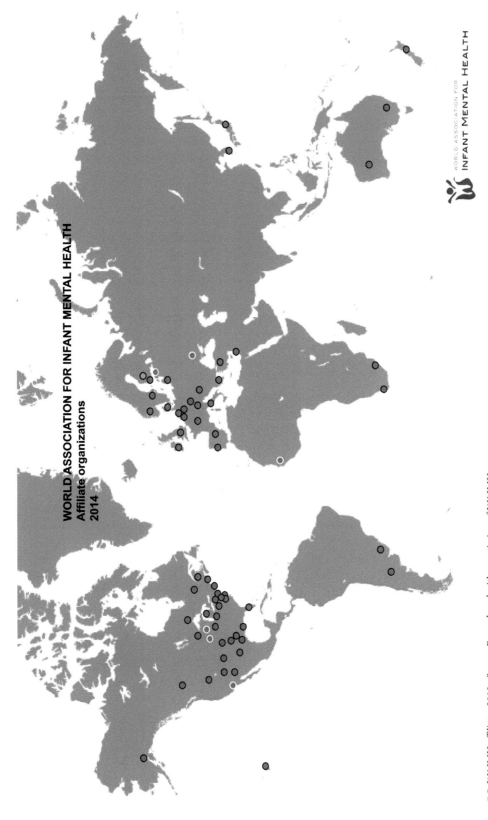

Figure 7.3 WAIMH affiliates 2013. *Source:* Reproduced with permission of WAIMH.

and promotes his/her skills and capacity for initiating and sustaining interaction with the parent, both for learning purposes and for using the relationship as an emotionally secure base.

The approaches used can be divided into psychodynamically oriented parent–infant psychotherapies concentrating on the parent's representations, more behaviorally oriented interactional parent–infant therapies like the Interactional Guidance (McDonough, 2005), and parent–infant therapies integrating elements from both approaches. Some approaches emphasize the infant's active involvement and role as the initiator of interaction, as in Watch, Wait, and Wonder (WWW; Cohen et al., 1999) or Theraplay (Jernberg & Booth, 1998). In the review of Doughty (2007) of three randomized controlled trials, Interaction Guidance resulted in significant improvements in maternal sensitivity and sensitive discipline, and a decrease in the child's overactive behavior in a sample of infants with externalizing disorders. Robert-Tissot et al. (1996) compared Interaction Guidance and psychodynamic therapy for 75 mothers with behaviorally disturbed infants, and found that both interventions reduced infant symptoms, reduced maternal intrusive behavior and negative affect, and increased maternal self-esteem and infant cooperative behavior. Similar results were obtained by Cohen et al. (2002), who divided 67 clinically referred mothers and infants aged 10–30 months to groups receiving WWW or psychodynamic mother–infant therapy. However, research on the efficacy of parent–infant therapies is still scarce.

Family and group interventions

For families where the main concerns are problems of parenting or of the marital relationship, systemic family-centered treatment or family therapy may be an effective way to change dysfunctional interaction patterns. Family therapy may also be offered as the treatment of choice for families with infants and toddlers diagnosed with an illness affecting their development or behavior. Family therapy can be particularly useful for families with infants undergoing a transition, for example, the birth of a sibling or bereavement.

In family therapy, the parents' thoughts and feelings concerning their child and the family situation are elicited to build a therapeutic relationship. Family therapy sessions are then focused on how parents can practice sensitive, coherent coparenting in the presence of the child's disorder or illness. In their meta-analyses of 70 studies, Bakermans-Kranenburg et al. (2003) concluded that the most effective systemic interventions focused on helping mothers develop sensitivity to their infants' cues, involved fathers as well as mothers, and spanned no more than 15 sessions. However, the number of studies on family therapy in infancy is small.

Group therapeutic interventions have also been developed and used in treating parents and infants. According to Barlow and Parsons (2010), group-based parenting programs may be effective in improving the emotional and behavioral adjustment of children under the age of 3. These interventions have usually been used with mothers with psychiatric problems (Pedrina, 2004), but recently also with other high-risk samples. Examples of treatment models for multirisk families include the Circle of Security (Powell et al., 2009) used with delinquent mothers (Cassidy et al., 2010) and psychodynamic group therapy for substance abusing mothers (Belt et al., 2012). Although a number of treatment programs have been developed for multirisk families, there is currently no definite evidence of their efficacy.

Multicomponent interventions for high-risk groups

In families overburdened by parental mental health and substance abuse problems, low social support, unemployment and poverty (Zeanah & Smyke, 2008), a multicomponent strategy including networking with social services, community health services, services for substance abusers, and adult psychiatric services is often necessary. The first task is to assess what services are needed to ensure that the needs of the infant or child are adequately met. The aim is to introduce some stability and predictability into the life of the family. Once this is achieved, parents may be able to engage in working on their parenting with the methods described (Luthar & Walsh, 1995). There is currently no definite evidence of the efficacy of multicomponent interventions.

In the most severe cases, infants have been admitted to residential psychiatric treatment, earlier in adult mental hospitals and nowadays in child psychiatric units. The focus of the treatment in adult mental hospitals has been on the mental health of the mother, and having the infant in the hospital seems to help psychotic mothers to recover more rapidly. The development of infant psychiatric practices has moved toward short, intensive periods of treatment focusing on infant mental health as well as parental mental health (Tamminen & Kaukonen, 1999).

Conclusion

The field of infant mental health is still in its infancy. There are wide gaps in our knowledge. There is still a great need for studies on the validity of diagnostic criteria and the reliability of assessment processes concerning infants and toddlers. However, parents and professionals around the world increasingly recognize the need for and meaningfulness of working with infant mental health problems and disorders (Figure 7.3). Also, there is slowly cumulating research evidence on the effects of early therapeutic interventions, although one should be especially cautious when intervening during this particular life phase.

References

Abidin, R. (1997) Parenting stress index: a measure of the parent–child system. In: *Evaluating Stress: A book of resources.* (eds P.C. Zalaquett & R.J. Wood), pp. 277–291. Scarecrow Education, Lanham, MD, US.

Achenbach, T.M. & Rescorla, L.A. (2000) *Manual for the ASEBA Preschool Forms and Profiles.* University of Vermont, Department of Psychiatry, Burlington.

Aronen, E.T. (1993) The effect of family counseling on the mental health of 10–11-year-old children in low- and high-risk families: a longitudinal approach. *Journal of Child Psychology and Psychiatry* **34**, 155–165.

Aronen, E.T. & Kurkela, S.A. (1996) Long-term effects of an early home-based intervention. *Journal of the American Academy of Child and Adolescent Psychiatry* **35**, 1665–1672.

Arts-Rodas, D. & Benoit, D. (1998) Feeding problems in infancy and early childhood: identification and management. *Paediatrics & Child Health* **3**, 21–27.

Bakermans-Kranenburg, M.J. *et al.* (2003) Less is more: meta-analyses of sensitivity and attachment interventions in early childhood. *Psychological Bulletin* **129**, 195–215.

Bale, T.L. *et al.* (2010) Early life programming and neurodevelopmental disorders. *Biological Psychiatry* **68**, 314–319.

Barlow, J. & Parsons, J. (2010) Group-based parent-training programmes for improving emotional and behavioural adjustment in 0–3 year old children. *Cochrane Database of Systematic Reviews* **2**, CD003680.

Baron-Cohen, S. *et al.* (1992) Can autism be detected at 18 months? The needle, the haystack, and the CHAT. *British Journal of Psychiatry* **161**, 839–843.

Bates, J. *et al.* (1979) Measurement of infant difficultness. *Child Development* **50**, 794–803.

Belt, R. *et al.* (2012) Psychotherapy groups and individual support to enhance mental health and early dyadic interaction among drug abusing mothers. *Infant Mental Health Journal* **33**, 520–534.

Biringen, Z. (2008) *Emotional availability scales, 4th Edition.* Unpublished Manuals for the EAS training (Infancy/Early Childhood/Middle Childhood/Youth versions), [Online], Available: http://www.emotionalavailability.com [21 May 2013].

Biringen, Z. *et al.* (1993, 1998) *Emotional availability scales, 2nd Edition, 3rd Edition.* (Unpublished Manuals for the EAS training), [Online], Available: http://www.emotionalavailability.com [21 May 2013].

Boris, N.W. (2006) Race and research in the southern United States: approaching the elephant in the room. *Infant Mental Health Journal* **27**, 621–624.

Bradley, R. & Caldwell, B. (1979) Home observation for measurement of the environment: a revision of the preschool scale. *American Journal of Mental Deficiency* **84**, 235–244.

Brazelton, T.B. (1973) *Neonatal Behavioral Assessment Scale. Clinics in Developmental Medicine No 50.* Lippincott, Philadelphia.

Bricker, D.D. *et al.* (1999) *The ASQ User's Guide Paul H.* Brookes, Baltimore, MD.

Briggs-Cowan, J. & Carter, A.S. (2006) *The Brief Infant–Toddler Social and Emotional Assessment (BITSEA)* Psychological Corporation. Harcourt Assessment, San Antonio, TX.

Bryant-Waugh, R. *et al.* (2010) Feeding and eating disorders in childhood. *International Journal Eating Disorders* **43**, 98–111.

Burke, J.D. *et al.* (2010) Predictive validity of childhood oppositional defiant disorder and conduct disorder: implications for the DSM-V. *Journal of Abnormal Psychology* **199**, 739–751.

Campos, J.J. & Sternberg, C.R. (1981) Perception, appraisal, and emotions: the onset of social referencing. In: *Infant Social Cognition: Empirical and Theoretical Considerations.* (eds M.E. Lamb & L.R. Sherrod), pp. 273–314. Erlbaum, Hillside, NJ.

Carter, A.S. & Briggs-Cowan, M.J. (2006) *Infant-Toddler Social and Emotional Assessment (ITSEA). Examiner's manual* Harcourt Assessment, San Antonio, TX.

Cassidy, J. *et al.* (2010) Enhancing attachment security in the infants of women in a jail-diversion program. *Attachment and Human Development* **12**, 333–353.

Chatoor, I. & Macaoay, M. (2008) Feeding development and disorders. In: *Encyclopedia of Infant and Early Childhood Development.* (eds M.M. Haith & J.B. Benson), pp. 524–533. Academic Press, New York.

Clark, R. (1985) *The Parent–Child Early Relational Assessment: Instrument and Manual.* University of Wisconsin Medical School, Department of Psychiatry, Madison.

Clark, R. *et al.* (2004) Assessment of parent–child relational disturbances. In: *Handbook of Infant, Toddler, and Preschool Mental Assessment.* (eds R. DelCarmen-Wiggins & A. Carter), pp. 25–60. Oxford University Press, New York.

Cohen, N.J. *et al.* (1999) Watch, wait, and wonder: testing the effectiveness of new approach to mother-infant psychotherapy. *Infant Mental Health Journal* **20**, 429–451.

Cohen, N.J. *et al.* (2002) Six-month follow-up of two mother–infant psychotherapies: convergence of therapeutic outcomes. *Infant Mental Health Journal* **23**, 4361–4380.

Coll, C.M. *et al.* (1986) The effectiveness of early head start for 3-year-old children and their parents: lessons for policy and programs. *Journal of Developmental and Behavioral Pediatrics* **7**, 230–236.

Comer, J.S. *et al.* (2013) Psychosocial treatment efficacy for disruptive behavior problems in very young children: a meta-analytic examination. *Journal of the American Academy of Child & Adolescent Psychiatry* **52**, 26–36.

Copeland, W.E. *et al.* (2007) Childhood psychiatric disorders and young adult crime: a prospective, population-based study. *American Journal of Psychiatry* **164**, 1668–1675.

Crittenden, P.M. (1981) Abusing, neglecting, problematic and adequate dyads: differentiating by patterns of interaction. *Merrill-Palmer Quarterly* **27**, 1–18.

Crncec, R. *et al.* (2010) Infant sleep problems and emotional health: a review of two behavioural approaches. *Journal of Reproductive and Infant Psychology* **28**, 44–54.

Darwin, C. (1965) *The Expression of the Emotions in Man and Animals.* University of Chicago Press, Chicago (Original work published 1872).

Davis, E.P. *et al.* (2004) Prenatal maternal anxiety and depression predict negative behavioral reactivity in infancy. *Infancy* **6**, 319–331.

Davis, E.P. *et al.* (2005) Corticotropin-releasing hormone during pregnancy is associated with infant temperament. *Developmental Neuroscience* **27**, 299–305.

De Rosa, E. *et al.* (2010) Psychometric properties of the Alarm distress baby scale (ADBB) applied to 81 Italian children. Postnatal maternal depression, somatic illness and relational withdrawal in infants. *Devenir* **22**, 209–223.

Doughty, C. (2007) *Effective strategies for promoting attachment between young children and infants* New Zealand Health Technology Assessment (NZHTA). Christchurch, New Zealand.

Egger, H.L. & Angold, A. (2004) The preschool age psychiatric assessment (PAPA): a structured parent interview for diagnosing psychiatric disorders in preschool children. In: *Handbook of Infant, Toddler,* and *Preschool Mental Assessment*. (eds R. DelCarmen-Wiggins & A. Carter), pp. 223–243. Oxford University Press, New York.

Egger, H.L. & Angold, A. (2006) Common emotional and behavioral disorders in preschool children: presentation, nosology, and epidemiology. *Journal of Child Psychology and Psychiatry* **47**, 313–337.

Emde, R.N. (1991) The wonder of our complex enterprises: steps enabled by attachments and the effects of relationships on relationships. *Infant Mental Health Journal* **12**, 163–172.

Esser, G. *et al.* (1989) *Mannheimer Elterninterview* Beltz. Weinheim.

Feldman, R. & Eidelman, A.I. (2006) Neonatal state organization, neuromaturation, mother-infant interaction and cognitive development in small-for-gestational-age premature infants. *Pediatrics* **118**, 869–878.

Field, T. (1994) The effects of mother's physical and emotional unavailability on emotion regulation. *Monographs for the Society for Research in Child Development* **59**, 208–227.

Field, T. *et al.* (2006) Prenatal depression effects on the fetus and newborn: a review. *Infant Behavior and Development* **29**, 445–455.

Fivaz-Depeursinge, E. & Corboz-Warnery, A. (1999) *The Primary Triangle: A Developmental Systems View of Mothers, Fathers and Infants*. Basic Books, New York.

Gill, K.L. & Calkins, S.D. (2003) Do aggressive/destructive toddlers lack concern for others? Behavioral and physiological indicators of empathic responding in 2-year-old children. *Development and Psychopathology* **15**, 55–71.

Guedeney, A. & Fermanian, J. (2001) A validity and reliability study of assessment and screening for sustained withdrawal reaction in infancy: the Alarm Distress Baby Scale. *Infant Mental Health Journal* **22**, 559–575.

Guedeney, A. *et al.* (2013) Social withdrawal behavior in infancy: a history of the concept and a review of published studies using the alarm distress baby scale. *Infant Mental Health Journal* **34**, 516–31.

Gueron-Sela, N. *et al.* (2011) Maternal worries about child underweight mediate and moderate the relationship between child feeding disorders and mother–child feeding interactions. *Journal of Pediatric Psychology* **36**, 827–836.

Harkness, S. & Super, C.M. (1995) Culture and parenting. In: *Handbook of Parenting*. (ed M. Bornstein) Vol. 2, pp. 221–234. Erlbaum, Hillsdale, NJ.

Heim, C. *et al.* (2010) Neurobiological and psychiatric consequences of child abuse and neglect. *Developmental Psychobiology* **52**, 671–690.

Izard, C.E. (1978) Emotions and emotion-cognition relationships. In: *The Genesis of Behavior. The Development of Affect.* (eds M. Lewis & L.A. Rosenblum), vol. **1**, pp. 389–413. Plenum Press, New York.

Jernberg, A.M. & Booth, P.B. (1998) *Theraplay: Helping Parents and Children Build Better Relationships Through Attachment-Based Play*. Jossey-Bass, San Francisco.

Kane, P. & Garber, J. (2004) The relations among fathers, children's psychopathology, and father-child conflict: a meta-analysis. *Clinical Psychology Review* **24**, 339–360.

Keller, H. *et al.* (2004) Developmental consequences of early parenting experiences: self-recognition and self-regulation in three cultural communities. *Child Development* **75**, 1745–1760.

von Klitzing, K. (2006) Cultural influences on early family relationships. *Infant Mental Health Journal* **27**, 618–620.

Kochanska, G. *et al.* (2000) Effortful control in early childhood: continuity and change, antecedants, and implications for social development. *Developmental Psychology* **36**, 220–232.

Ladd, C.O. *et al.* (2000) Long-term behavioral and neuroendocrine adaptations to adverse early experience. *Progress in Brain Research* **122**, 81–103.

Lewis, M. (2008) The emerge of human emotions. In: *Handbook of Emotions* (eds M. Lewis *et al.*), 3rd edn, pp. 304–319. Guilford Press, New York.

Love, J.M. *et al.* (2005) The effectiveness of early head start for 3-year-old children and their parents: lessons for policy and programs. *Developmental Psychology* **41**, 885–901.

Luoma, I. *et al.* (2001) Longitudinal study of maternal depressive symptoms and child well-being. *Journal of the American Academy of Child & Adolescent Psychiatry* **40**, 1367–1374.

Luthar, S. & Walsh, K. (1995) Treatment needs of drug-addicted mothers. Integrated parenting psychotherapy interventions. *Journal of Substance Abuse and Treatment* **5**, 341–348.

Mäntymaa, M. (2006) Early mother-infant interaction: determinants and predictivity. *Acta Universitatis Tamperensis* 1144, Juvenes Print, Tampere.

Mäntymaa, M. *et al.* (2003) Infant-mother interaction as a predictor of child's chronic health problems. *Child Care Health and Development* **29**, 181–191.

Mathers, C.D. & Loncar, D. (2006) Projectors of global mortality and burden of disease from 2002 to 2030. *PLoS Medicine* **2006**, 2011–2030.

McDonough, S.C. (2005) Interaction guidance: understanding and treating early infant-caregiver relationship disturbances. In: *Treating Parent-infant Relationship Problems: Strategies for Intervention.* (eds A. Sameroff, *et al.*), pp. 79–98. Guilford Press, New York.

McHale, J.P. & Rasmussen, J.L. (1998) Coparental and family group-level dynamics during infancy: early family precursors of child and family functioning during preschool. *Development & Psychopathology* **10**, 39–59.

Meléndez, L. (2005) Parental beliefs and practices around early self-regulation. The impact of culture and immigration. *Infants and young children* **18**, 136–146.

Möricke, E. *et al.* (2013) Latent class analysis reveals five homogeneous behavioural and developmental profiles in a large Dutch population sample of infants aged 14–15 months. *European Child & Adolescent Psychiatry* **22**, 103–115.

Murray, L. *et al.* (1996) The impact of postnatal depression and associated adversity on early mother–infant interactions and later infant outcome. *Child Development* **67**, 2512–2526.

Olds, D.L. *et al.* (2004) Effects of home visits by paraprofessionals and by nurses: age 4 follow-up results of a randomised trial. *Pediatrics* **114**, 1560–1568.

Olds, D.L. *et al.* (2007) Programs for parents of infants and toddlers: recent evidence from randomized trials. *Journal of Child Psychology and Psychiatry* **48**, 355–391.

Pedrina, F. (2004) Group therapy with mothers and babies in postpartum crises: preliminary evaluation of a pilot project. *Group Analysis* **37**, 137–151.

Petersen, L. *et al.* (2010) *Promoting Mental Health in Scarce-Resource Context: Emerging Evidence and Practice*. HSRC Press, Cape Town.

Powell *et al.* (2009) The circle of security. In: *Handbook of Infant Mental Health*. (ed C.H. Zeanah), 3rd edn, pp. 450–467. Guilford Press, New York.

Puura, K. *et al.* (2005a) The European early promotion project: description of the service and evaluation study. *International Journal of Mental Health Promotion* **7**, 17–31.

Puura, K. *et al.* (2005b) The outcome of the European early promotion project: mother–child interaction. *International Journal of Mental Health Promotion* **7**, 82–94.

Puura, K. *et al.* (2013) Associations between maternal interaction behavior, maternal perception of infant temperament, and infant social withdrawal. *Infant Mental Health Journal* **34**, 586–93.

Quinn, N. (2003) Cultural selves. *Annals of the New York Academy of Science* **1001**, 145–176.

Rao, P.A. & Beidel, D.C. (2009) The impact of children with high-functioning autism on parental stress, sibling adjustment and family functioning. *Behavior Modification* **33**, 437–451.

Raphael-Leff, J. (2010) Mothers' and fathers' orientations: patterns of pregnancy, parenting and the bonding process. In: *Parenthood and Mental Health: A Bridge between Infant and Adult Psychiatry.* (eds S. Tyano, *et al.*), pp. 9–22. John Wiley & Sons, Chichester.

Reid, V. & Meadows-Oliver, M. (2007) Postpartum depression in adolescent mothers: an integrative review of the literature. *Journal of Pediatric Health Care* **21**, 289–298.

Reijneveld, S.A. *et al.* (2001) Excessive infant crying: the impact of varying definitions. *Pediatrics* **108**, 893–897.

Reijneveld, S.A. *et al.* (2004) Infant crying and abuse. *Lancet* **364**, 1340–1342.

Richman, N. *et al.* (1975) Prevalence of behaviour problems in 3-year-old children: an epidemiological study in a London borough. *Journal of Child Psychology & Psychiatry* **16**, 277–287.

Robert-Tissot, C. *et al.* (1996) Outcome evaluation in brief mother-infant psychotherapies: report on 75 cases. *Infant Mental Health Journal* **17**, 97–114.

Roggman, L.A. *et al.* (2013) Parenting interactions with children: checklist of observations linked to outcomes (PICCOLO) in diverse ethnic groups. *Infant Mental Health Journal* **34**, 290–306.

Rothbart, M.K. (1981) Measurement of temperament in infancy. *Child Development* **52**, 569–578.

Rutter, M. (2013) Annual research review: resilience—clinical implications. *Journal of Child Psychology and Psychiatry* **54**, 474–487.

Sadeh, A. (2005) Cognitive-behavioral treatment for childhood sleep disorders. *Clinical Psychology Review* **25**, 612–628.

Sameroff, A. (2010) A unified theory of development: a dialectic integration of nature and nurture. *Child Development* **81**, 6–22.

Scheeringa, M. (2004) *Diagnostic infant and preschool assessment*, [Online], Available: http://www.infantinstitute.com/MikeSPDF/DIPA_v111710.pdf [21 May 2013].

Scheeringa, M.S. & Gaensbauer, T.J. (2000) Posttraumatic stress disorder. In: *Handbook of Infant Mental Health.* (ed C.H. Zeanah), 2nd edn, pp. 369–381. Guilford Press, New York.

Scheeringa, M.S. & Zeanah, C.H. (2001) A relational perspective on PTSD in early childhood. *Journal of Traumatic Stress* **14**, 799–815.

Schoppe-Sullivan, S.J. *et al.* (2009) Coparenting behavior moderates longitudinal relations between effortful control and preschool children's externalizing behavior. *Journal of Child Psychology & Psychiatry & Allied Disciplines* **50**, 698–706.

Skovgaard, A.M. *et al.* (2007) The prevalence of mental health problems in children 1(1/2) years of age—the Copenhagen Child Cohort 2000. *Journal of Child Psychology & Psychiatry* **48**, 62–70.

Smith Slep, A. & Tamminen, T. (2013) Caregiver–child relational problems: definitions and implications for diagnosis. In: *Family Problems and Family Violence: Reliable Assessment and the ICD-11.* (eds H. Foran, *et al.*), pp. 185–196. Springer, New York.

Sparrow, S.S. *et al.* (2005) *Vineland Adaptive Behavior Scales: (Vineland II), Survey Interview Form/Caregiver Rating form* Pearson Assessments. Livonia, MN.

Stern, D.N. (1985) *The Interpersonal World of the Infant: A View from Psychoanalysis and Developmental Psychology.* Basic Books, New York.

Stern, D.N. (1995) *The Motherhood Constellation: A Unifying View of Parent–Infant Psychotherapies.* Basic Books, New York.

Super, C. & Harkness, S. (1997) The cultural structuring of child development. In: *Cross-Cultural Psychology: Vol. 2. Basic Processes and Human Development.* (eds J.W. Berry, *et al.*), pp. 1–40. Allyn & Bacon, Needham Heights, MA.

Tamminen, T. (2006a) How does culture promote the early development of identity? *Infant Mental Health Journal* **27**, 603–605.

Tamminen, T. (2006b) Infants in the multicultural world. *Infant Mental Health Journal* **27**, 625–626.

Tamminen, T. & Kaukonen, P. (1999) Family ward: a new therapeutic approach. *The Keio Journal of Medicine* **48**, 132–139.

Tremblay, R.E. *et al.* (2004) Physical aggression during early childhood: trajectories and predictors. *Pediatrics* **114**, 43–50.

Tronick, E.Z. *et al.* (1986) The transfer of affect between mothers and infants. In: *Affective Development in Infancy.* (eds T.B. Brazelton & M.W. Young), pp. 11–25. Ablex, Norwood, NJ.

Wakschlag, L.S. *et al.* (2008) Observational assessment of preschool disruptive behavior, Part I: Reliability of the disruptive behavior diagnostic observation schedule (DB-DOS). *American Academy of Child and Adolescent Psychiatry* **47**, 622–641.

Walker, S.P. *et al.* (2007) Child development: risk factors for adverse outcomes in developing countries. *Lancet* **369**, 145–157.

Werner, E.E. & Smith, R.S. (2001) *Journeys from childhood to midlife: risk, resilience and recovery.* Cornell University Press, Ithaca, NY.

Zeanah, C.H. *et al.* (1994) Mothers' representations of their infants are concordant with infant attachment classifications. *Developmental Issues in Psychiatry and Psychology* **1**, 1–14.

Zeanah, C.H. & Smyke, A.T. (2008) Attachment disorders in family and social context *Infant Mental Health Journal* **29**, 219–233.

Zero to Three (2005) *Diagnostic Classification: 0–3R: Diagnostic Classification of Mental Health and Developmental Disorders of Infancy and Early Childhood: revised edition.* Zero to Three Press, Washington, DC.

A: Developmental psychopathology

Temperament: individual differences in reactivity and regulation as antecedent to personality

Nathan A. Fox and Olga L. Walker

Department of Human Development and Quantitative Methodology, University of Maryland, College Park, MD, USA

Introduction

Research on infant temperament has a long history in developmental psychology. With an increased interest in the origins of psychopathology and a renewed appreciation for the influence of individual differences on behavior, considerable recent work has characterized early dispositions and their developmental trajectories. The current chapter is a nonexhaustive review of this vast literature. Interested readers are referred to Chen & Schmidt (2015) for a broader overview of the issues raised here. In the current chapter, we first provide a definition of temperament and contrast it with a definition of personality. We then review a number of the conceptual models used to think about individual differences in temperament and follow that with an overview of assessment methods for studying temperamental behaviors. We briefly review work on the link between genes and individual differences in temperament followed by a broader discussion of the temperament of behavioral inhibition. In the final section of this chapter, we examine the links between temperament and psychological adjustment across age, including the emergence of psychopathology. We end with comments about work examining other types of temperament (exuberance) and suggestions for the future.

Definitions and conceptual distinctions between temperament and personality

Temperament is considered the behavioral style that an infant or young child exhibits in response to a variety of stimuli and across contexts. Chess and Thomas (1986) introduced the concept of temperament to psychology and child psychiatry in the United States; they described temperament as the style of behavior (the "how"). This contrasts with views of personality, which include the content of thought, coping styles, values, and beliefs of an individual (the "what"). Some have argued that temperament is stable across development and could be reflected in personality, though empirical evidence suggests only modest stability (Degnan & Fox, 2007). Personality reflects, as well, patterns of behavior, emotions, and cognition and is focused specifically on aspects of the self (Rothbart, 2011). Though temperament and personality have much in common (see Shiner & Caspi, 2012), they differ in fundamental ways. Temperament is thought to reflect individual differences that are "biological" in origin (whether that be genetic, environmental, or both). Personality is considered to reflect the accruing influences of family, peers, and contexts across development. Temperament is commonly viewed as reflecting "innate, biological" factors. Temperament emerges early in life, evident even in the newborn period, and manifests in other behaviors during the toddler and preschool period that are viewed as "inborn" or maturational (Rothbart, 2011). Personality, on the other hand, emerges later in life to encompass processes learned into adulthood. Temperamental differences exert an influence on cognitive and social development early in life. They form the foundation for personality or perhaps are at its core. Personality traits, on the other hand, deal with issues of self-esteem and self-concept that necessarily involve the child's interactions with multiple contexts and individuals. While those interactions may be initially guided by temperamental style, they are soon modified by ideas of self-worth and self-concept in multiple areas (social, academic, physical) that form the basis of personality.

Given that personality traits increasingly influence behavior across development, one issue is whether temperamental dispositions display continued stability over time. If there is a good deal of overlap between temperament and personality and if personality emerges out of temperament, then measuring unique temperamental dispositions in older children and adults

Rutter's Child and Adolescent Psychiatry, Sixth Edition.
Edited by Anita Thapar and Daniel S. Pine, James F. Leckman, Stephen Scott, Margaret J. Snowling, Eric Taylor.

may be difficult. A related issue is how the same temperamental disposition is expressed at different ages. One way to approach this problem is to assume that the "latent" temperament is manifested in different behaviors over time. For example, at four months of age, infants can be identified with a disposition to react with high intensity motor activity and negative affect to novel or unfamiliar stimuli. Such infants are likely to display behavioral inhibition in the toddler period and social reticence later in childhood (Fox et al., 2005). But the personality trait of neuroticism that may describe the same individual as an adult is the result of complex cognitive processes of self-evaluation. Hence, it may be difficult, if not impossible, to identify constructs that separate at older ages the temperament element in personality.

Approaches to the study of temperament

Alexander Thomas and Stella Chess
One highly influential study in the revival of temperament research was a longitudinal investigation by Thomas, Chess, and colleagues (Thomas et al., 1963). Their New York Longitudinal Study (NYLS) formed the basis of their ideas about temperament, noting patterns of individuality in infant reactivity, including sleep–wake cycle, eating behavior, and response to external stimuli. Their work followed children's development through early childhood. While not widely known, their collaboration with Herbert Birch provided a critical framework. Birch was a colleague of Schneirla, a psychobiologist who wrote about the role of stimulus intensity and approach withdrawal responses in motivated behavior (Schneirla, 1959). With Birch's help, Thomas and Chess organized their observations into nine temperament dimensions that were defined in infancy to form three main temperament groups: (1) easy, (2) difficult, and (3) slow to warm up. Their claim was that these temperament groupings remained fairly stable over time (Thomas et al., 1970).

Thomas and Chess focused on parent–child interactions and coined the phrase "goodness of fit" (Thomas & Chess, 1977), which proposes that positive developmental outcomes are more likely to occur when a match exists between an infant's temperament and environmental characteristics (e.g., parenting). Thus, when nature and nurture harmoniously mesh, adaptive outcomes are most probable. However, when there is conflict or a mismatch between temperament and context (parenting behavior or parent expectations), the child is at heightened risk for behavioral problems. Thomas and Chess were among the first to propose that temperament was critical for understanding child development. They also urged both parents and teachers to recognize these differences and assist children of different temperaments to adapt to various environmental challenges (Thomas et al., 1970).

Mary Rothbart
Temperament has also been conceptualized in motivational terms along an approach-withdrawal-systems framework.

Across species, approach and withdrawal behaviors vary with the intensity of stimuli needed to invoke reactivity, with withdrawal occurring when stimulation is intense and approach occurring when it is more subdued (Schneirla, 1959). Rothbart expanded on these ideas (Rothbart, 1981). First, she adopted a unique conceptual approach to the study of reactivity, as one component of a two-part temperament system. In early infancy, she argued that children primarily differ in their reactivity to sensory stimuli, particularly to novel and intense stimulation. She measured reactivity in the infant by assessing the latency to respond, the intensity of the response, and the duration of that response both behaviorally and physiologically.

While variations in reactivity influence an infant's capability to maintain homeostasis, infants also vary in a second key temperament component, their ability to self-soothe and regulate reactivity, which emerges over the first years of life, with important individual differences. Thus, the self-regulatory aspect of temperament develops over time. Rothbart identified attention as critical, and collaboration with Michael Posner (Rothbart et al. 1990; Posner & Rothbart, 2000) cemented links among temperament, development, and the neural circuitry of attention-based self-regulation. Rothbart (1981) described several temperament features that matured with experience, reflecting a continuous dynamic between reactivity and regulation (Rothbart, 1989). This produced a unique emphasis on regulation, which varies developmentally among children, to modulate the timing and intensity of an individual's reactivity (Rothbart, 1989), particularly through maturation of attentional strategies (Rueda et al., 2004). Over the first months of life, infants switch from a stimulus-driven, externally reactive attention system to a system with more voluntary executive attentional control (Rothbart et al., 1990, 2004). Children are able to resolve conflict more easily, flexibly shift and adapt their response, and inhibit certain dominant responses, thoughts, and emotions to act more appropriately.

Jerome Kagan
Jerome Kagan has for much of his career studied individual differences in infant and child temperament. His longitudinal studies highlighted issues of stability, individual differences, and factors that influence change, with an emphasis on neuroscience (Kagan & Moss, 1962; Kagan, 1971). Perhaps his greatest influence on the field of temperament has been the work on one particular temperament type, known as "behavioral inhibition" (García Coll et al., 1984; Kagan et al., 2007). Initially, Kagan and colleagues identified toddlers who were wary and vigilant to unfamiliar stimuli and contexts. These individual differences appeared to persist into childhood and adolescence and form the core for what personality theorists would call neuroticism. Subsequent to these findings, Kagan described individual differences in reactivity to novelty early in the first year of life, which he claimed reflected the temperament of the child. Infants who displayed high levels of limb movement and distress to novelty had a high reactive temperament and this temperamental disposition served as the basis for subsequent inhibited and shy

behavior. A salient feature of Kagan's approach was not only the identification of high-reactive (typically 15–20% of the sample) infants but the claim that these infants represented a category or temperament type different from less reactive children. The notion is that the confluence of behavioral and physiological reactivity identified this group as unique and a temperament type different from other temperaments. Much as there are physical and biological differences as a function of genetic mutation (e.g., Down syndrome) that set those individuals apart from others without the mutation, so too there are infants with a particular temperament that are different (not just more extreme on some continuum) from others. Although current approaches in temperament research take a more continuous approach to thinking about individual differences in behavior, Kagan's arguments about temperament types continue to influence the field. Kagan's work has considerably shaped the field of temperament over the past two decades for a number of important reasons. His measurement approach has included both behavioral and physiological assessments to characterize this temperament. The pattern of physiology of the high-reactive temperament type is one of heightened autonomic reactivity, elevated stress hormone response, heightened startle, and freezing or avoidant behavior. This "package" of biology and behavior is similar to the pattern of behavior and physiology found in rodent and nonhuman primate models of threat conditioning. Hence, Kagan's work drew great interest from neuroscientists studying the threat system in animal models. As well, the community of biological psychiatry found Kagan's description of this temperament intriguing as it provided a possible basis for understanding at least one origin of anxiety symptoms in adults. The link that has been drawn by others between the temperament of behavioral inhibition and emerging psychopathology has been an important part of the temperament story over the past 20 years.

Assessment of temperament

The two most common methods of measuring temperament are questionnaires and behavioral observations. Age-appropriate questionnaires quantify temperament from parent, teacher, or self-report, with different measures at different ages (e.g., The Infant Behavior Questionnaire—Revised [IBQ-R]; Rothbart, 1981; Garstein & Rothbart, 2003; Toddler Behavior Assessment Questionnaire [TBAQ]; Goldsmith, 1996; The Early Childhood Behavior Questionnaire [ECBQ]; Putnam et al., 2006, The Children's Behavior Questionnaires [CBQ]; Rothbart et al., 2001; Putnam & Rothbart, 2006; Early Adolescent Temperament Questionnaire—Revised [EATQ-R]; Ellis & Rothbart, 2001; Ellis, 2002). Studies examining the validity and reliability of these measures have consistently found three factors: Extraversion/Surgency, Negative Affectivity, and a dimension measuring self-regulation (Orienting/Regulation in the IBQ-R and Effortful Control in the ECBQ, CBQ, and EATQ-R). The latter factor (self-regulation) is conceptualized as emerging over the preschool years, possibly due to developmental shifts in

self-regulation being mainly externally regulated by caregivers during infancy to being internally regulated during early childhood (Garstein & Rothbart, 2003). These three main factors appear to be similar to some dimensions of adult personality (Ahadi & Rothbart, 1994; Rothbart et al., 2004; Rothbart & Bates, 2006). Interestingly, findings with the EATQ-R reported a fourth dimension: Affiliativeness (Ellis & Rothbart, 2001), which is defined as desiring closeness with others, independent of shyness and surgency (Putnam et al., 2001).

Behavioral observations have also been used to measure infant and toddler temperament. Figure 8.1 depicts the context in which such observations are made in infants, toddlers, and school-aged children. As conveyed by these pictures, the contexts of such observations are quite different at different ages. However, at each age, the context is designed to elicit behaviors thought to reflect core aspects of temperament, be it exposure to a novel mobile in infancy, a toy robot in toddlerhood, and novel peers during school age. Various standardized batteries exist for assessing temperament.

The Laboratory Temperament Assessment Battery (LAB-TAB; Goldsmith & Rothbart, 1991) is one such standardized observational measure. The LAB-TAB parallels parent-report questionnaires of Rothbart and colleagues (i.e., IBQ-R and TBAQ). There are two aspects of this battery that make it unique: first is the idea that reactivity and regulation can be measured in part by children's expression of discrete emotions in response to various elicitors. As such, the battery emphasizes the coding of facial expressions of emotion. Second, the battery elicits both reactivity and regulation, with different elicitors for different age groups. Examples of the elicitors include presenting the infant or toddler a toy behind a plastic barrier (to elicit frustration, anger, and approach), or presentation of scary masks (to elicit fear and avoidance).

The Lab-Tab has a manual and a set of behaviors to be coded in response to the various elicitors. Other temperament batteries are similarly structured, having a set of standard elicitors and a set of behaviors to be coded. One such system, described by Kagan et al. (1988) and Fox et al. (2001b) has been used to characterize behavioral inhibition. This system centers on the idea that behavioral inhibition reflects a child's disposition to respond with heightened vigilance, withdrawal and negative affect to novel, uncertain, and unfamiliar stimulus events. The child is exposed to a series of events (an unfamiliar adult approaching and asking the child to play, a toy robot) and behavior is coded for latency to approach, vocalization, and affective response, with ratings combined to create composite scores which rate levels of withdrawal and negative reactivity, reflecting the temperament of behavioral inhibition.

Temperament questionnaires have advantages and disadvantages. One advantage is that parents observe their children in many situations (Kagan & Fox, 2006); another is their ease of use. Disadvantages include their potential for introducing biases, based on parents' individual experiences or misinterpretation of questionnaires (see Kagan, 2000; Kagan, 2003; Kagan & Fox, 2006). Cross-informant correlations are typically low

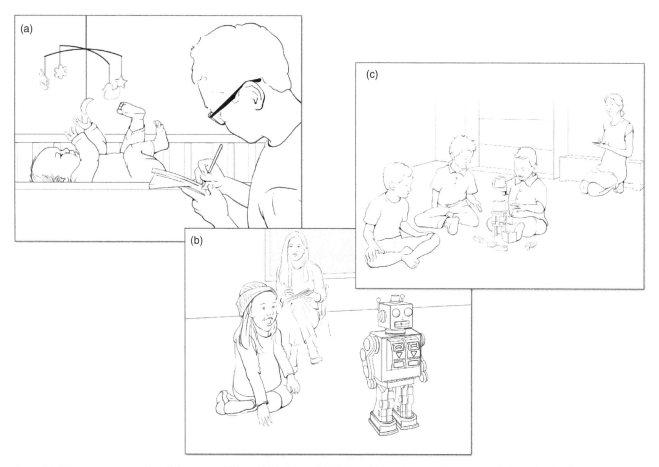

Figure 8.1 Three approaches to identifying young children with behavioral inhibition: (a) reactivity in infancy to novel objects (mobiles); (b) response to unfamiliar objects (a toy robot) in the toddler period; (c) play with unfamiliar same-age peers during preschool age.

to moderate (Rothbart, 1981; Goldsmith 1996; Rothbart *et al.*, 2001; Garstein & Rothbart, 2003). Behavioral assessments are more costly, more labor intensive, which creates other disadvantages (Kagan & Fox, 2006). Moreover, correlations between behavioral observations and parent report of temperament are low to moderate as well (Rothbart *et al.* 2000; Kagan & Fox 2006). Since both measures have advantages and disadvantages, combining the two approaches may more fully capture temperament than relying on either approach alone (Wachs & Bates 2001; Calkins *et al.* 2002; Kagan & Fox 2006; Rothbart & Bates 2006).

Genetic origins of temperament

The idea that temperament is "innate" raises questions about genetics. Research has approached these questions through behavior genetics and, more recently, candidate-gene studies. Behavior genetic approaches comparing monozygotic and dizygotic twins (see Chapter 24) find modest-to-high temperament heritability, particularly for the temperament of fearfulness, (Louisville Twin Study, Matheny, 1989; Colorado Twin Study, Robinson *et al.*, 1992; Smith *et al.*, 2012). A second approach

focuses on molecular genetics, usually adopting the so-called candidate-gene approach, which has been questioned in recent years. This includes studies of the dopamine D4 receptor gene and the serotonin transporter gene. More recently, work with candidate genes has examined the interaction of genes with both positive and negative environments from an approach often called differential susceptibility (Belsky & Pluess, 2009). These particular gene variants (sometimes called plasticity genes) are thought to provide protection and, in fact, result in optimal outcomes in the context of certain supportive or facilitative environments above and beyond what is afforded to noncarriers. Alternatively, in the context of stress or harsh environments, they result in detrimental outcomes. For example, Bakermans-Kranenburg and van IJzendoorn (2006) examined the effects of differences in maternal sensitivity on externalizing behavior amongst children according to carrier status of the 7-repeat allele of a variant in a gene encoding the dopamine D4 receptor. They found that children who carried this allelic variation and whose mothers were insensitive had the highest externalizing behavior, while those with the same gene variant but high in maternal sensitivity had the least externalizing behavior of all. There are now multiple instances of studies like this one with different candidate genes (serotonin transporter [5-HTT]; mono-amine oxidase [MAO-A]) and different types of environmental contexts and obviously different types of child outcomes. The interpretation of candidate-gene studies is discussed in Chapter 24. There remains inconsistency in the findings and questions about the *a priori* or *a posteriori* choice of which genes and which variants in the gene are selected and which environments and which outcomes are examined in certain studies.

There is however, amongst the differential susceptibility approach, a notion compatible with temperament in which individuals are thought to vary in their physiological reactivity. Boyce and Ellis have written about two types of children (i.e., two temperaments), dandelions and orchids, those who can grow anywhere and those who need heightened care and attention in order to flourish (Ellis & Boyce, 2008). Boyce's work focuses specifically on individual differences in autonomic or stress reactivity (via the hypothalamic-pituitary-adrenal [HPA] system) and the role that environments have in leading to either negative or optimal outcomes (Boyce *et al.,* 1995). The closest this work has come to traditional notions of temperament is the work on difficult temperament or negative emotionality, usually measured via caregiver report, and the findings that children with negative or difficult temperaments do more poorly in harsh environments but in some instances thrive and have optimal outcomes under supportive environments. For example, Van Aken *et al.* (2007) showed that 16- to 19-month-old boys with difficult temperament had the lowest levels of externalizing behavior with highly sensitive caregiving but the largest levels with insensitive caregiving. These studies support the differential susceptibility model but the links between those using candidate genes and those examining temperament differences have yet to be established.

Finally, the recent advances in epigenetics (see Chapter 25) provide some promise for understanding how individual differences may be transmitted across generations. Reactivity to specific types of novel stimuli may be a product of the experiences of prior generations and influence subsequent infant reactivity. A recent study by Dias and Ressler (2013) illustrates this epigenetic transmission in a mouse model. Mice were aversively conditioned to an odor and subsequent generations (based apparently on methylation processes at the level of gamete) came to react sensitively to these same odors. This may hold promise for understanding at least some of the variability in individual differences in infant reactivity.

The temperament of behavioral inhibition

As mentioned, Jerome Kagan was the first to describe the temperament of behavioral inhibition, and this work substantively changed the clinical and research approach to temperament, for many reasons. First, Kagan used careful behavioral description, often instead of maternal report, to study temperament. Second, he assessed physiological markers and emphasized

stability of both physiology and behavior. And third, he linked his work to neuroscientific studies of fear, thus providing a basis for thinking about this temperament as a model system for understanding the origins of anxiety. Behavioral inhibition refers to a child's temperamental profile characterized by initial negative emotional and motor reactivity to novelty during infancy (Kagan *et al.* 1984) and tendency in later childhood to display fearful or withdrawn behavior when confronting unfamiliar events, objects, or people (Rothbart & Alansky 1990; Kagan & Snidman 1991; Fox *et al.,* 2005). Behavioral inhibition has an associated physiologic profile, reflected in high heart rate and low-heart rate variability, elevated cortisol secretion, pupil dilation, increased startle response, and right frontal electroencephalographic (EEG) asymmetry (Kagan *et al.,* 1987; Bell & Fox, 1994; Calkins *et al.,* 1996; Lopez *et al.,* 2004; Pérez-Edgar *et al.,* 2008; Reeb-Sutherland *et al.,* 2009). Kagan (2001) proposed that this physiology arose from perturbations in the amygdala, extending work at the time in rodents (Davis, 1986; LeDoux *et al.,* 1988). While this underlying circuitry is undoubtedly complex, interesting cross-species parallels do exist (Pérez-Edgar & Fox, 2005).

There is modest continuity to the temperament of behavioral inhibition. Pérez-Edgar and Fox (2005) report correlations between the ages of 1 and 6 years in the 0.24–0.64 range, with greater stability found among extreme groups. And, across studies children who maintain this disposition are at higher risk for developing an anxiety disorder (Hirshfeld *et al.,* 1992; Turner *et al.,* 1996; Kagan & Snidman, 1999; Prior *et al.,* 2000; Biederman *et al.,* 2001; Chronis-Tuscano *et al.,* 2009). A recent meta-analysis quantifies this association as large in magnitude (Clauss & Blackford, 2012). Nevertheless, half or more of behaviorally inhibited children will not have anxiety disorders in adolescence, suggesting moderation by endogenous and exogenous factors. Degnan and Fox (2007) suggest that these include parenting behaviors and various information-processing functions of the child. One type of parenting style associated with behavioral inhibition is overprotective control or oversolicitous parenting (Rubin *et al.,* 2002). This parenting style is composed of behaviors such as intrusiveness and limiting of the child's opportunity for autonomy (Rubin *et al.,* 1997). For instance, a history of high behavioral inhibition (BI) is associated with symptoms of social anxiety during adolescence, only in the presence of high maternal overcontrol observed during childhood (Lewis-Morrarty *et al.,* 2012).

Peers provide an additional source of socialization, beginning as early as infancy, and continuing as children spend more time at school and in extracurricular activities (see Hay *et al.,* 2009). Indeed, early exposure to different childcare environments during infancy and toddlerhood may have a profound influence on the developmental trajectory of behavioral inhibition. Research has shown that children's relationships with peers can influence the stability of withdrawn or inhibited behavior during the preschool years (Furman *et al.,* 1979), early childhood (Gazelle & Ladd, 2003), and middle childhood (Booth-LaForce &

Oxford, 2008). Fox and colleagues (2001b) found positive effects of childcare on the stability of behavioral inhibition. Children with this temperament placed into peer-oriented day care were less likely to display stable behavioral inhibition over age. This pattern was replicated in an independent sample of infants placed into peer day care. These studies suggest that exposure to peer interactions in childcare settings fosters the development of competent social skills among behaviorally inhibited children. This exposure moderates the temperament of behavioral inhibition and decreases the likelihood of social withdrawal at later ages among this temperament group (Degnan & Fox, 2007).

Temperament and adjustment

Researchers have found that behaviors reflecting different temperamental dispositions such as positive emotionality, irritability, sociability, avoidance, and negative affect are related to adaptive and maladaptive outcomes across development. Positive emotionality, which is a core behavior in the temperament of exuberance, is positively associated with social competence as well as social behavioral problems (Eisenberg et al., 2009; Hayden et al., 2006). Avoidance and negative reactivity, which are core behaviors in the temperament of behavioral inhibition, are related to social reticence and anxious symptoms (Fox et al., 2005).

Studies suggest that heightened motor reactivity and negative affect and behavioral inhibition are associated with, and predictive of, internalizing problems later in childhood and adolescence (Asendorpf, 1991; Fox et al., 2005). Behaviorally inhibited children, as they get older and are exposed to peer situations, may develop anxiety, loneliness, depression, negative self-perceptions of their social competencies, and other internalizing problems (e.g., Coplan et al., 2004; Fox et al., 2005; Kagan et al., 2007). Kagan and colleagues found that adolescents who were high-reactive in toddlerhood displayed higher levels of social anxiety than those who were low-reactive (Schwartz et al., 1999). Chronis-Tuscano et al. (2009) reported that infants and young children who displayed stable behavioral inhibition across early childhood had an increased risk for developing anxiety disorders, particularly social anxiety. And a recent meta-analysis (Clauss & Blackford, 2012) reported a moderate effect size across studies of behavioral inhibition in risk for anxiety disorders. Taken together, several large-scale longitudinal projects have provided convergent evidence that highly reactive and shy-inhibited children are likely to develop internalizing socioemotional problems, such as social anxiety and life dissatisfaction, in adolescence and adulthood. Moreover, these children, particularly boys, tend to experience difficulties in later social relationships and life adjustment (Caspi et al., 2003).

In addition to temperamental behaviors identified in infancy (such as reactivity), behaviors that underlie an individual's ability to regulate their own behavior are both thought of as reflecting temperament and are associated with adjustment later in life. These behaviors, emerging as they do over the preschool period (attention shifting, inhibitory control), are often referred to under the heading of "effortful control." In general, such behaviors facilitate children's ability to behave appropriately across a wide range of contexts (Kochanska et al., 2000; Eisenberg et al., 2009; Rueda, 2012). Longitudinal research suggests that effortful control in early childhood is related to later adjustment (Eisenberg et al. 2009). For example, Eisenberg et al. (2009) found that parent and teacher ratings of low attentional (maintaining or shifting attentional focus according to the task) and low inhibitory (suppressing inappropriate responses) control was associated with externalizing problems in middle childhood. Moreover, low effortful control was associated with an increase in externalizing problems over time.

Caspi and colleagues (2003), with data from the Dunedin study, found that undercontrolled children displayed social and behavioral problems, such as perceived alienation from the world and aggression, in adulthood. Children with undercontrolled temperament were also more likely than well-adjusted children to engage in disordered gambling as adults (Slutske et al., 2012). And Moffitt et al. (2011) described relations between childhood self-control and adulthood health, wealth, and public safety in the Dunedin sample.

Although the broad construct of effortful control has been found to be negatively correlated with negative affect including symptoms of anxiety, when inhibitory control and attention shifting were examined separately, their contribution to the regulation of negative reactivity was distinct from one another. For example, behaviorally inhibited children with high levels of inhibitory control were less socially competent, more socially withdrawn, and reported as being more socially anxious than BI children with low levels of inhibitory control (Fox & Henderson, 2000; Thorell et al., 2004; White et al., 2011). Furthermore, high levels of inhibitory control at age 4 increased the risk for anxiety problems in the preschool years amongst children who were high in behavioral inhibition at age 2, whereas high levels of attention shifting at age 4 decreased the risk for preschool anxiety problems in these children (White et al., 2011).

The paradoxical role of cognitive control in relation to temperamental reactivity is seen best within the literature on error monitoring. Figure 8.2 depicts procedures for monitoring this construct. Error monitoring is often measured by examining response times on trials following an error as compared to response times following correct trials. If inaccurate performance is particularly salient to an individual, more controlled and slower responding in the trial following an error is typically exhibited (Davies et al., 2004). Such behavioral measures can also be supplemented with psychophysiological indices, such as an event-related potential known as the error-related negativity (ERN). The ERN is a specific neural activity pattern associated with cognitive monitoring that is usually observed between 50 and 150 ms post response after the commission of an error and has a centromedial scalp distribution (Falkenstein et al.,

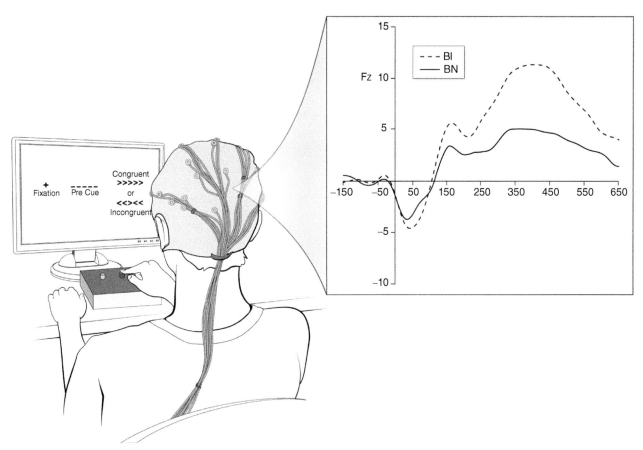

Figure 8.2 Assessment of error monitoring using the Erikson Flanker Task (Eriksen & Eriksen, 1974). The subject's task is to press a button indicating the direction of an arrow in the center of the computer screen. That arrow can be "flanked" by arrows in the same direction or in different directions. During the task, brain electrical activity is recorded and synchronized to the subject's button press. On trials where the subject makes an error an event-related potential (ERP) is generated, called the error-related negativity (ERN).

1991; Gehring et al., 1993; van Veen & Carter, 2002). It appears that error monitoring is heightened in patients with anxiety disorders. Gehring and colleagues (2000) found a heightened ERN in subjects with obsessive compulsive disorder (OCD). Other investigators extended this to other anxious groups (Weinberg *et al.*, 2010; Meyer *et al.*, 2012), as supported in a recent meta-analysis (Moser *et al.*, 2013).

Similar findings manifest in behavioral inhibition (Henderson, 2010). For example, McDermott *et al.* (2009) found the ERN to be larger for adolescents who were characterized with high behavioral inhibition in childhood as compared to adolescents low on childhood behavioral inhibition. In addition, the ERN moderated the relations between early behavioral inhibition and later anxiety disorders during adolescence, such that for those participants high on behavioral inhibition, larger ERNs were related to higher risk of anxiety disorders (McDermott *et al.*, 2009). This pattern of relation between temperament and error monitoring was replicated and extended in an independent sample by Lahat and colleagues (2014). Seven-year-old children who were characterized in infancy with behavioral inhibition were assessed for ERN and symptoms of anxiety were measured via an anxiety scale at age 9. Lahat found first that children

with a history of behavioral inhibition showed heightened ERN amplitudes and, second, that the magnitude of the ERN moderated the link between temperament and anxiety symptoms. Children with the temperament of behavioral inhibition who also had larger ERN amplitude (greater error monitoring) were more likely at age 9 to have more symptoms of anxiety.

Behavioral inhibition: temperament or psychopathology?

Behavioral inhibition may be one of the best and well characterized of child temperaments for understanding the etiology of at least some forms of anxiety. By itself it conveys a heightened risk for anxiety disorders and particularly social anxiety. But that risk is tempered by both the effects of environmental manipulations (caregiving context and behaviors) as well as intrinsic factors such as attention and cognitive control processes. For example, Fox *et al.* (2001b) reported that infants characterized as high-reactive who were placed into peer-oriented day care were less likely to exhibit behavioral inhibition during childhood.

This effect of early caregiving context on temperament was replicated in an independent sample, again demonstrating the effects of environmental manipulations on temperament (Almas *et al.*, 2011).

The interrelations between temperament and psychopathology have led to discussions about the very nature of this temperament and whether the behaviors described as reflecting behavioral inhibition are merely a prodromal manifestation of anxiety. Considerable work examines differences between behavioral inhibition and anxiety (Rapee, 2002; Pérez-Edgar & Fox, 2005). As noted earlier, there are both similarities and differences in these two constructs (see Rapee, 2002; Pérez-Edgar & Fox, 2005). Developmentally, the two constructs appear more distinct than similar. There are a number of reasons to think that this is the case. First, anxiety is usually associated with cognitive rumination, while behavioral inhibition, assessed in infancy and early childhood, is not. Behavioral inhibition is identified early in the first years of life when it is unlikely that ruminative processes are involved. Second, temperamental behavioral inhibition in the early years of life is highly plastic. It is unlikely that anxiety at any period is as malleable. On the other hand, behavioral inhibition is associated with social reticence (observable during the preschool and school years), which is associated with anxious behaviors and cognition such as low self-esteem. Third, perhaps best summarized is the notion that the temperament of behavioral inhibition is reflected in general cautiousness, while anxiety focuses on worry and often specific fears. And fourth, importantly, using self and parent report measures, the overlap between report of behavioral inhibition and anxiety is not high (correlations ranging from 0.3 to 0.6). The most illuminating studies on this topic have been conducted by Rapee (Rapee *et al.,* 2005). He developed a parent-centered intervention for children at risk for anxiety and recruited children with the temperament of behavioral inhibition for such efforts. In one intervention program, behaviorally inhibited preschool children were selected on the basis of maternal report and observations of high levels of inhibition/withdrawal and assigned to either a parent education program or a monitor condition in which they did not receive any intervention (Rapee *et al.*, 2005). Findings indicated that children in the intervention condition showed a decrease in anxiety disorders approximately 12 months after the intervention compared to children in the monitoring condition (Rapee *et al.*, 2005). However, there were no differences between the intervention and control groups on behavioral inhibition one year later. Furthermore, results of a 3-year follow-up indicated that children assigned to the parent education condition during preschool were less likely to develop anxiety disorders or report symptoms of anxiety compared to children in the monitoring condition during middle childhood (Rapee *et al.*, 2010). Again, the intervention continued to have no impact on parent report of the child's temperament, as behavioral inhibition was found to decrease over time regardless of the intervention group (Rapee *et al.*, 2010). These findings suggest that anxiety and the temperament of BI may in fact be separable constructs.

The question before clinicians and parents is whether prevention programs like the one described by Rapee (2013) should be uniformly applied to all children with the temperament of behavioral inhibition. The intervention appears to work and is short in duration. However, most young children with the temperament of behavioral inhibition will not develop anxiety disorders; therefore, administering a prevention/intervention to them may end up being counterproductive. It is the case that many parents of shy reticent children, particularly young boys, are concerned about their child's behavior. Such parents should be provided with information on how to parent their shy reticent child as well as the importance of valuing individual differences in their young children. It may, however, be unnecessary to implement, on a widespread basis, a prevention program for a common temperament, such as behavioral inhibition, that is associated with one type of important individual difference in approaching the world.

Future directions in temperament research

The field of temperament research has brought to the forefront the importance of individual differences when considering the trajectories of social development of young children. There are, no doubt, many different temperament types, each with its unique set of behavioral responses to stimuli in the environment. In particular, there is growing interest in the temperament of exuberance, with research in this area holding great promise.

Temperamental exuberance

Positive reactivity to novelty may be as robust a temperamental construct as avoidance and negative reactivity. There are a number of studies showing associations between individual differences in positive reactions to novelty (approach behavior) in infancy and related to child social-emotional outcomes. Infants who display positive affect and motor reactivity to novel stimuli are more likely to show uninhibited, exuberant, and sociable behavior in infancy (Putnam & Stifter, 2002; Hane *et al.*, 2008) and toddlerhood (Calkins *et al.*, 1996; Park *et al.*, 1997; Fox *et al.*, 2001b; Putnam & Stifter, 2005). In addition, a combination of high positive affect and approach behavior is associated with impulsivity, positivity, and sociability in childhood (Fox *et al.,* 2001a; Pfeifer *et al.*, 2002; Stifter *et al.*, 2008).

In the developmental literature, terms such as positive affectivity, surgency, extraversion, approach reactivity, impulsivity, and sensitivity to reward are often used to describe exuberant temperament (Polak-Toste & Gunnar, 2006; Rothbart & Bates, 2006). Fox and colleagues described a subset of their infant sample as approaching novelty and enjoying social interaction, and suggested links to fearlessness, risk taking, and social competence (Fox *et al.*, 2001a; Hane *et al.*, 2008). Goldsmith and colleagues described their childhood sample in terms of increased positive affect and a heightened, fearless approach to novel stimuli (Pfeifer *et al.*, 2002). In general, positive affect has been posited as the core, distinguishing factor involved in exuberance, surgency, or extraversion (Watson & Clark, 1997; Rothbart *et al.*, 2001; Putnam & Stifter, 2005).

There are clear distinctions between the temperaments of behavioral inhibition and exuberance. For instance, one study examining measures of both behavioral inhibition and exuberance across childhood showed nonlinear relations between them, where high exuberance was predicted by average levels, as opposed to low levels, of behavioral inhibition (Pfeifer *et al.*, 2002). In addition, Putnam and Stifter (2005) described multiple types of behavior, based on levels of approach and positive or negative affect, where low approach combined with negative affect reflected behavioral inhibition and high approach combined with positive affect reflected exuberance. More work is needed to define the underlying neural circuitry and physiological reactions of temperamental exuberance. But it is an area where there is great interest and novel findings are awaited.

Final comments

After the birth of their first child, most parents believe that they can mold or shape that child's behavior as they parent their child toward development. Ask parents after they have had their second child and no doubt they will tell you of the individual differences they see between their first and second child and how their child is as much a determinant of the caregiving environment as their own perceptions and beliefs. Temperament continues to exert its influence across different developmental phases. In childhood, temperament reciprocally shapes individuals' perceptions of their surroundings, including responses to peers and acceptance into the peer group. And no doubt, in adolescence, temperament influences an individual's choice of social network, thus playing an important role in determining the extent and direction of adolescent peer influences and the impact of these on later social and mental health outcomes. Individual variation in response to the environment is what produces the richness and complexity of culture and society. The study of temperament, its underlying biology, and the manner in which it shapes trajectories of development contributes significantly to our understanding of the variation in human behavior.

References

Ahadi, S.A. & Rothbart, M.K. (1994) Temperament, development, and the Big Five. In: *The Developing Structure of Temperament and Personality from Infancy to Adulthood.* (eds C.F. Halverson, *et al.*), pp. 189–207. Erlbaum, Hillsdale, NJ.

van Aken, C. *et al.* (2007) The interactive effects of temperament and maternal parenting on toddlers' externalizing behaviours. *Infant and Child Development* **16**, 553–572.

Almas, A.N. *et al.* (2011) The relations between infant negative reactivity, non-maternal childcare, and children's interactions with familiar and unfamiliar peers. *Social Development* **20**, 718–740.

Asendorpf, J.B. (1991) Development of inhibited children's coping with unfamiliarity. *Child Development* **62**, 1460–1474.

Bakermans-Kranenburg, M. & van IJzendoorn, M.H. (2006) Gene-environment interaction of the dopamine D4 receptor (DRD4) and observed maternal insensitivity predicting externalizing behavior in preschoolers. *Developmental Psychobiology* **48**, 406–409.

Bell, M.A. & Fox, N.A. (1994) Brain development over the first year of life: relations between EEG frequency and coherence and cognitive and affective behaviors. In: *Human Behavior and the Developing Brain.* (eds G. Dawson & K. Fischer), pp. 314–345. Guilford, New York.

Belsky, J. & Pluess, M. (2009) Beyond diathesis stress: differential susceptibility to environmental influences. *Psychological Bulletin* **135**, 885–908.

Biederman, J. *et al.* (2001) Further evidence of association between behavioral inhibition and social anxiety in children. *American Journal of Psychiatry* **158**, 1673–1679.

Booth-LaForce, C. & Oxford, M.L. (2008) Trajectories of social withdrawal from grades 1 to 6: prediction from early parenting, attachment, and temperament. *Developmental Psychology* **44**, 1298–1313.

Boyce, W.T. *et al.* (1995) Psychobiologic reactivity to stress and childhood respiratory illnesses: results of two prospective studies. *Psychosomatic Medicine* **57**, 411–422.

Calkins, S.D. *et al.* (1996) Behavioral and physiological antecedents of inhibited and uninhibited behavior. *Child Development* **67**, 523–540.

Calkins, S.D. *et al.* (2002) Frustration in infancy: implications for emotion regulation, physiological processes, and temperament. *Infancy* **3**, 175–197.

Caspi, A. *et al.* (2003) Influence of life stress on depression: moderation by a polymorphism in the 5-HTT gene. *Science* **5631**, 386–389.

Chen, X. & Schmidt, L. (2015) Temperament and personality development. In: *Handbook of Child Psychology and Developmental Science.* (eds R. Lerner, M. Lamb & C. Garcia-Coll), 7th edn. John Wiley & Sons, Hoboken, NJ.

Chess, S. & Thomas, A. (1986) *Temperament in Clinical Practice.* Guilford Press, New York.

Chronis-Tuscano, A. *et al.* (2009) Stable early maternal report of behavioral inhibition predicts lifetime social anxiety disorder in adolescence. *Journal of the American Academy of Child and Adolescent Psychiatry* **48**, 928–935.

Clauss, J.A. & Blackford, J.U. (2012) Behavioral inhibition and risk for developing social anxiety disorder: a meta-analytic study. *Journal of the American Academy of Child & Adolescent Psychiatry* **51**, 1066–1075.

Coplan, R.J. *et al.* (2004) Do you "want" to play? Distinguishing between conflicted-shyness and social disinterest in early childhood. *Developmental Psychology* **40**, 244–258.

Davies, P.L. *et al.* (2004) Development of response-monitoring ERPs in 7- to 25-year-olds. *Developmental neuropsychology* **25**, 355–376.

Davis, M. (1986) Pharmacological and anatomical analysis of fear conditioning using the fear-potentiated startle paradigm. *Behavioral Neuroscience* **100**, 814.

Degnan, K.A. & Fox, N.A. (2007) Behavioral inhibition and anxiety disorders: multiple levels of a resilience process. *Development and Psychopathology* **19**, 729–746.

Dias, B.G. & Ressler, K.J. (2013) Parental olfactory experience influences behavior and neural structure in subsequent generations. *Nature Neuroscience* **17**, 89–96.

Eisenberg, N. *et al.* (2009) Longitudinal relations of children's effortful control, impulsivity, and negative emotionality to their externalizing, internalizing, and co-occurring behavior problems. *Developmental Psychology* **45**, 988–1008.

Ellis, L. K. (2002) *Individual Differences and Adolescent Psychological Development*. Ph.D. University of Oregon.

Ellis, B.J. & Boyce, W.T. (2008) Biological sensitivity to context. *Current Directions in Psychological Science* **17**, 183–187.

Ellis, L.K. & Rothbart, M.K. (2001) Revision of the Early Adolescent Temperament Questionnaire, poster presented at the Biennial Meeting of the Society for Research in Child Development, Minneapolis, Minnesota.

Eriksen, B.A. & Eriksen, C.W. (1974) Effects of noise letters on the identification of target letters in a non-search task. *Perception and Psychophysics* **16**, 143–149.

Falkenstein, M. *et al.* (1991) Effects of crossmodal divided attention on late ERP components. II. Error processing in choice reaction tasks. *Electroencephalography & Clinical Neurophysiology* **78**, 447–455.

Fox, N.A. & Henderson, H.A. (2000) Temperament, emotion, and executive function: influences on the development of self-regulation. Paper presented at the Annual Meeting of the Cognitive Neuroscience Society, San Francisco.

Fox, N.A. *et al.* (2001a) The biology of temperament: an integrative approach. In: *The Handbook of Developmental Cognitive Neuroscience*. (eds C.A. Nelson & M. Luciana), pp. 631–645. MIT Press, Cambridge, MA.

Fox, N.A. *et al.* (2001b) Continuity and discontinuity of behavioral inhibition and exuberance: psychophysiological and behavioral influences across the first four years of life. *Child Development* **72**, 1–21.

Fox, N.A. *et al.* (2005) Behavioral inhibition: linking biology and behavior within a developmental framework. *Annual Review of Psychology* **56**, 235–262.

Furman, W. *et al.* (1979) Rehabilitation of socially withdrawn preschool children through mixed-age and same-age socialization. *Child Development* **50**, 915–922.

García Coll, C. *et al.* (1984) Behavioral inhibition in young children. *Child Development* **55**, 1005–1019.

Garstein, M.A. & Rothbart, M.K. (2003) Studying infant temperament via the Revised Infant Behavior Questionnaire. *Infant Behavior and Development* **26**, 64–86.

Gazelle, H. & Ladd, G.W. (2003) Anxious solitude and peer exclusion: a diathesis-stress model of internalizing trajectories in childhood. *Child Development* **74**, 257–278.

Gehring, W.J. *et al.* (1993) A neural system for error detection and compensation. *Psychological Science* **4**, 385–390.

Gehring, W.J. *et al.* (2000) Action-monitoring dysfunction in obsessive-compulsive disorder. *Psychological Science* **11**, 1–6.

Goldsmith, H.H. (1996) Studying temperament via construction of the Toddler Behavior Assessment Questionnaire. *Child Development* **67**, 218–235.

Goldsmith, H.H. & Rothbart, M.K. (1991) Contemporary instruments for assessing early temperament by questionnaire and in the laboratory. In: *Explorations in Temperament: International Perspectives on Theory and Measurement*. (eds J. Strelau & A. Angleitner), pp. 249–272. Plenum, New York.

Hane, A.A. *et al.* (2008) Behavioral reactivity and approach-withdrawal bias in infancy. *Developmental Psychology* **44**, 1491–1496.

Hay, D.F. *et al.* (2009) The beginnings of peer relations. In: *Handbook of Peer Interactions, Relationships and Groups*. (eds K.H. Rubin, *et al.*), pp. 121–142. Guilford Press, New York.

Hayden, E.P. *et al.* (2006) Positive emotionality at age 3 predicts cognitive styles in 7-year-old children. *Development and Psychopathology* **18**, 409–423.

Henderson, H.A. (2010) Electrophysiological correlates of cognitive control and the regulation of shyness in children. *Developmental Neuropsychology* **35**, 177–193.

Hirshfeld, D.R. *et al.* (1992) Stable behavioral inhibition and its association with anxiety disorders. *Journal of the American Academy of Child and Adolescent Psychiatry* **21**, 103–111.

Kagan, J. (1971) *Change and Continuity in Infancy*. John Wiley & Sons, Oxford, England.

Kagan, J. (2000) Inhibited and uninhibited temperaments: recent developments. In: *Shyness: Development, Consolidation, and Change*. (ed W.R. Crozier), pp. 22–29. Routledge, New York.

Kagan, J. (2001) Temperamental contributions to affective and behavioral profiles in childhood. In: *From Social Anxiety to Social Phobia: Multiple Perspectives*. (eds S.G. Hoffmann & P.M. Dibartolo), pp. 216–234. Allyn & Bacon, Needham Heights, MA.

Kagan, J. (2003) Behavioral inhibition as a temperamental category. In: *Handbook of Affective Sciences*. (eds R.J. Davidson, *et al.*), pp. 320–331. Oxford University Press, New York.

Kagan, J. & Fox, N.A. (2006) Biology, culture, and temperamental biases. In: *Handbook of Child Psychology: Social, Emotional, and Personality Development*. (eds W. Damon, *et al.*), 6th edn, vol. **3**, pp. 167–225. John Wiley & Sons, Hoboken, NJ.

Kagan, J. & Moss, H.A. (1962) *Birth to Maturity: A Study in Psychological Development*. John Wiley & Sons, New York.

Kagan, J. & Snidman, N. (1991) Infant predictors of inhibited and uninhibited profiles. *Psychological Science* **2**, 40–43.

Kagan, J. & Snidman, N. (1999) Early childhood predictors of adult anxiety disorders. *Society of Biological Psychiatry* **46**, 1536–1541.

Kagan, J. *et al.* (1984) Behavioral inhibition to the unfamiliar. *Child Development* **55**, 2212–2225.

Kagan, J. *et al.* (1987) The physiology and psychology of behavioral inhibition in children. *Child Development* **58**, 1459–1473.

Kagan, J. *et al.* (1988) Childhood derivatives of inhibition and lack of inhibition to the unfamiliar. *Child Development* **59**, 1580–1589.

Kagan, J. *et al.* (2007) The preservation of two infant temperaments into adolescence: III. The current study. *Monographs of the Society for Research in Child Development* **72**, 19–30.

Kochanska, G. *et al.* (2000) Effortful control in early childhood: continuity and change, antecedents, and implications for social development. *Developmental Psychology* **36**, 220–232.

Lahat, A. *et al.* (2014) Early behavioral inhibition and increased error monitoring predict later social phobia symptoms in childhood. *Journal of the American Academy of Child & Adolescent Psychiatry* **53**, 447–455.

LeDoux, J.E. *et al.* (1988) Different projections of the central amygdaloid nucleus mediate autonomic and behavioral correlates of conditioned fear. *Journal of Neuroscience* **8**, 2517–2529.

Lewis-Morrarty, E. *et al.* (2012) Maternal over-control moderates the association between early childhood behavioral inhibition and adolescent social anxiety symptoms. *Journal of Abnormal Child Psychology* **40**, 1363–1373.

Lopez, N.L. *et al.* (2004) An integrative approach to the neurophysiological substrates of social withdrawal and aggression. *Development and Psychopathology* **16**, 69–93.

Matheny, A.P. Jr. (1989) Children's behavioral inhibition over age and across situations. *Journal of Personality* **57**, 215–235.

McDermott, J.M. *et al.* (2009) A history of childhood behavioral inhibition and enhanced response monitoring in adolescence are linked to clinical anxiety. *Biological Psychiatry* **65**, 445–448.

Meyer, A. *et al.* (2012) The development of the error-related negativity (ERN) and its relationship with anxiety: evidence from 8 to 13 year-olds. *Developmental Cognitive Neuroscience* **2**, 152–161.

Moffitt, T.E. *et al.* (2011) A gradient of childhood self-control predicts health, wealth, and public safety. *PNAS Proceedings of the National Academy of Sciences of the United States of America* **108**, 2693–2698.

Moser, J.S. *et al.* (2013) On the relationship between anxiety and error monitoring: a meta-analysis and conceptual framework. *Frontiers of Human Neuroscience* **7**, 466.

Park, S. *et al.* (1997) Infant emotionality, parenting, and 3-year inhibition: exploring stability and lawful discontinuity in a male sample. *Developmental Psychology* **33**, 218–227.

Pérez-Edgar, K. & Fox, N.A. (2005) Temperament and anxiety disorders. *Child and Adolescent Psychiatric Clinics* **14**, 681–706.

Pérez-Edgar, K. *et al.* (2008) Salivary cortisol levels and infant temperament shape developmental trajectories in boys at risk for behavioral maladjustment. *Psychoneuroendocrinology* **33**, 916–925.

Pfeifer, M. *et al.* (2002) Continuity and change in inhibited and uninhibited children. *Child Development* **73**, 1474–1485.

Polak-Toste, C.P. & Gunnar, M.R. (2006) Temperamental exuberance: correlates and consequences. In: *The Development of Social Engagement.* (eds P.J. Marshall & N.A. Fox), pp. 19–45. Oxford University Press, New York.

Posner, M.I. & Rothbart, M.K. (2000) Developing mechanisms of self-regulation. *Development and Psychopathology* **12**, 427–441.

Prior, M. *et al.* (2000) Does shy-inhibited temperament in childhood lead to anxiety problems in adolescence? *Journal of the American Academy of Child and Adolescent Psychiatry* **39**, 461–468.

Putnam, S.P. & Rothbart, M.K. (2006) Development of short and very short forms of the Children's Behavior Questionnaire. *Journal of Personality Assessment* **87**, 102–112.

Putnam, S.P. & Stifter, C.A. (2002) Development of approach and inhibition in the first year: parallel findings from motor behavior, temperament ratings, and directional cardiac response. *Developmental Science* **5**, 441–451.

Putnam, S.P. & Stifter, C.A. (2005) Behavioral approach-inhibition in toddlers: prediction from infancy, positive and negative affective components, and relations with behavior problems. *Child Development* **76**, 212–226.

Putnam, S.P. *et al.* (2001) The structure of temperament from infancy through adolescence. In: *Advances in Research on Temperament.* (eds A. Eliasz & A. Angleitner), pp. 165–182. Pabst Science, Germany.

Putnam, S.P. *et al.* (2006) Measurement of fine-grained aspects of toddler temperament: the Early Childhood Behavior Questionnaire. *Infant Behavior & Development* **29**, 386–401.

Rapee, R.M. (2002) The development and modification of temperamental risk for anxiety disorders: prevention of a lifetime of anxiety? *Biological Psychiatry* **52**, 947–957.

Rapee, R.M. (2013) The preventative effects of a brief, early intervention for preschool-aged children at risk for internalising: follow-up into middle adolescence. *Journal of Child Psychology and Psychiatry* **54**, 780–788.

Rapee, R.M. *et al.* (2005) Prevention and early intervention of anxiety disorders in inhibited preschool children. *Journal of Consulting and Clinical Psychology* **73**, 488–497.

Rapee, R.M. *et al.* (2010) Altering the trajectory of anxiety in at-risk young children. *American Journal of Psychiatry* **167**, 1518–1525.

Reeb-Sutherland, B.C. *et al.* (2009) Startle response in behaviorally inhibited adolescents with a lifetime occurrence of anxiety disorders. *Journal of the American Academy of Child and Adolescent Psychiatry* **48**, 610–617.

Robinson, J.L. *et al.* (1992) The heritability of inhibited and uninhibited behavior: a twin study. *Developmental Psychology* **28**, 1030–1037.

Rothbart, M.K. (1981) Measurement of temperament in infancy. *Child Development* **52**, 569–578.

Rothbart, M.K. (1989) Biological processes of temperament. In: *Temperament in Childhood.* (eds G. Kohnstamm, *et al.*), pp. 77–110. John Wiley & Sons, Chichester.

Rothbart, M.K. (2011) *Becoming Who We Are: Temperament and Personality in Development.* Guilford, New York, NY.

Rothbart, M.K. & Alansky, J.A. (1990) Temperament, behavioral inhibition, and shyness in childhood. In: *Handbook of Social and Evaluation Anxiety.* (ed H. Leitenberg), pp. 139–160. Plenum Press, New York.

Rothbart, M.K. & Bates, J.E. (2006) Temperament. In: *Handbook of Child Psychology. Social, Emotional, and Personality Development.* (eds W. Damon, *et al.*), 6th edn, vol. **3**, pp. 99–166. John Wiley & Sons, New York.

Rothbart, M.K. *et al.* (1990) Regulatory mechanisms in infant development. In: *The Development of Attention: Research and Theory.* (ed J. Enns), pp. 139–160. Elsevier, Amsterdam, Netherlands.

Rothbart, M.K. *et al.* (2000) Stability of temperament in childhood: laboratory infant assessment to parent report at seven years. In: *Temperament and Personality Development Across the Life Span.* (eds V.J. Molfese & D.L. Molfese), pp. 85–119. Erlbaum, Mahweh, NJ.

Rothbart, M.K. *et al.* (2001) Investigations of temperament at three to seven years: the Children's Behavior Questionnaire. *Child Development* **72**, 1394–1408.

Rothbart, M.K. *et al.* (2004) Temperament and self-regulation. In: *Handbook of Self-Regulation: Research, Theory, and Applications.* (eds R.F. Baumeister & K.D. Vohs), pp. 357–370. Guilford Press, New York.

Rubin, K.H. *et al.* (1997) The consistency and concomitants of inhibition: some of the children, all of the time. *Child Development* **68**, 467–483.

Rubin, K.H. *et al.* (2002) Stability and social-behavioral consequences of toddlers' inhibited temperament and parenting behaviors. *Child Development* **73**, 483–495.

Rueda, M.R. (2012) Effortful control. In: *Handbook of Temperament.* (eds M. Zentner & R.L. Shiner), pp. 145–167. Guilford Press, New York.

Rueda, M.R. *et al.* (2004) Attentional control and self-regulation. In: *Handbook of Self-Regulation: Research, Theory, and Applications.* (eds R.F. Baumeister & K.D. Vohs), pp. 283–300. Guildford Press, New York.

Schneirla, T.C. (1959) An evolutionary and developmental theory of biphasic processes underlying approach and withdrawal. In: *Nebraska Symposium on Motivation*. (ed M.R. Jones), pp. 1–42. University of Nebraska Press, Lincoln Nebraska.

Schwartz, C.E. *et al.* (1999) Adolescent social anxiety as an outcome of inhibit temperament in childhood. *Journal of the American Academy of Child & Adolescent Psychiatry* **38**, 1008–1015.

Shiner, R.L. & Caspi, A. (2012) Temperament and the development of personality traits, adaptations, and narratives. In: *Handbook of Temperament*. (eds M. Zentner & R.L. Shiner), pp. 497–516. Guilford Press, New York.

Slutske, W.S. *et al.* (2012) Undercontrolled temperament at age 3 predicts disordered gambling at age 32: a longitudinal study of a complete birth cohort. *Psychological Science* **23**, 510–516.

Smith, A.K. *et al.* (2012) The magnitude of genetic and environmental influences on parental and observations measures of behavioral inhibition and shyness in toddlerhood. *Behavior Genetics* **42**, 764–777.

Stifter, C.A. *et al.* (2008) Exuberant and inhibited toddlers: stability of temperament and risk for problem behavior. *Development and Psychopathology* **20**, 401–421.

Thomas, A. & Chess, S. (1977) *Temperament and Development*. Brunner Mazel, New York.

Thomas, A. *et al.* (1963) *Behavioral Individuality in Early Childhood*. New York University Press, New York.

Thomas, A. *et al.* (1970) The origins of personality. *Scientific American* **223**, 102–109.

Thorell, L. *et al.* (2004) Two types of inhibitory control: predictive relations to social functioning. *International Journal of Behavioral Development* **28**, 193–203.

Turner, S.M. *et al.* (1996) Is behavioral inhibition related to anxiety disorders? *Clinical Psychology Review* **16**, 157–172.

van Veen, V. & Carter, C.S. (2002) The timing of action-monitoring processes in the anterior cingulate cortex. *Journal of Cognitive Neuroscience* **14**, 593–602.

Wachs, T.D. & Bates, J.E. (2001) Temperament. In: *Blackwell Handbook of Infant Development*. (eds J.G. Bremner & A. Fogel), pp. 465–501. Blackwell, Malden, MA.

Watson, D. & Clark, L.A. (1997) Measurement and mismeasurement of mood: recurrent and emergent issues. *Journal of Personality Assessment* **68**, 267–296.

Weinberg, A. *et al.* (2010) Increased error-related brain activity in generalized anxiety disorder. *Biological Psychology* **85**, 472–480.

White, L.K. *et al.* (2011) Behavioral inhibition and anxiety: the moderating roles of inhibitory control and attention shifting. *Journal of Abnormal Child Psychology* **39**, 735–747.

CHAPTER 9

Neurobiological perspectives on developmental psychopathology

Mark H. Johnson

Centre for Brain and Cognitive Development, School of Psychology, Birkbeck College, University of London, UK

Introduction

The brain is an organ of adaptation at multiple time scales. Over evolutionary time, our brain has become adapted in various ways to construct and occupy the niche of our species. In ontogeny (individual development), our brain adapts both to the general features of our environment shared with others, and to the individual circumstances into which we are born. Further, on a scale of days and hours, we can learn and retain information of survival relevance through processes of learning and attention. On the scale of seconds and milliseconds, our neural processes adapt to current sensory input and change state or prepare motor responses. While we can marvel at the complex and dynamic processes that underlie these adaptations, it is not surprising that there are also many different ways for them to go awry.

The brain is also an organ of adaptation at multiple levels of organization. Neuroscience is one of the broadest interdisciplinary fields in biology, spanning from complex molecular interactions, through intra- and intercellular processes, to the emergent computations that result from many thousands of neurons coherently oscillating in their firing patterns. In this chapter I review perspectives on human developmental psychopathology that arise from consideration of theories and evidence from developmental neurobiology. In some respects it seems obvious that the underpinning basic science of the human brain must be relevant to issues in developmental psychopathology. However, in other respects it is less clear that complex mental and behavioral problems can be understood by reducing these phenomena to cellular or neurochemical processes. In what follows we see that the consideration of the underlying neurobiology can benefit developmental psychopathology in several ways. First, assumptions and debates in developmental neurobiology often reflect those at a "higher" level of observable and as such can be informative. Second, the advent of new neuroimaging and genetic methods make a closer integration between the two fields inevitable. Third, it is possible to integrate data from multiple levels of observable in nonreductionist ways that can enhance our understanding of neurocognitive development and the ways that this can go awry in development.

Neurobiology is a broad field that spans multiple levels from molecular and genetic analyses, through cellular level studies, to the study of neural systems and pathways and how these relate to cognitive functions and behavior. We see in what follows that key issues about plasticity, timing, and constraints on development are often reflected in specific debates within the domains of genetics, cellular studies, and neural and cognitive systems.

Key issues in developmental neurobiology

Deterministic versus probabilistic epigenesis

The study of development necessarily implies an interdisciplinary approach in which the relevant pathways from genotype to phenotype are characterized. Gottlieb (1992) distinguished between two different approaches to the study of developmental biology; "deterministic epigenesis" in which it is assumed that there is a unidirectional causal path from genes to structural brain changes to psychological functions, and "probabilistic epigenesis" in which interactions among genes, structural brain changes, and psychological function are viewed as bidirectional, dynamic and emergent. While most would agree with the latter approach when presented in this explicit way, the former view still underpins basic assumptions that remain widespread in our field. For example, it is common in the literature to see claims about particular regions of the human cerebral cortex "coming on-line" at specific ages, with the implication that this is a

Rutter's Child and Adolescent Psychiatry, Sixth Edition.
Edited by Anita Thapar and Daniel S. Pine, James F. Leckman, Stephen Scott, Margaret J. Snowling, Eric Taylor.
© 2015 John Wiley & Sons Ltd. Published 2018 by John Wiley & Sons Ltd.

deterministic process. However, recent advances have revealed how complex context-dependent patterns of expression are the order of the day. In other words, the development of the brain is best viewed as an active self-organizing process involving interactions between genes and their current context, and not as the passive unfolding of a genetic blueprint on a strict maturational timetable.

Mosaic versus regulatory development

In many simpler organisms (such as the nematode *C. elegans*), development proceeds through cell lineages that are largely independent of each other, a process described as "mosaic" (Elman *et al.*, 1996). A cell will divide to yield other more specialized cells along a progression or lineage that is largely uninfluenced by the surrounding context or by other neighboring cells. In contrast, the construction of the brain in vertebrates is better characterized as following a "regulatory" developmental process. In other words, the division of cells to yield more specialized descendants is dependent on the current context, including the presence or absence of other cells of similar or dissimilar types.

These contrasting mechanisms at the cellular developmental level can also inform our thinking about the development of whole brain regions in humans. For nearly two decades, functional imaging studies in human adults were dominated by the search for the specific cortical regions said to be responsible for particular perceptual, cognitive or linguistic functions ("the region for X", where X is a cognitive or perceptual function). In contrast, over the past decade, the view has emerged that the response properties of a particular brain region are largely determined by its patterns of connectivity to other regions as well as by their current activity states (Friston & Price, 2001).

Extending these different approaches to neurodevelopment, it remains a common assumption that the maturational timetable of specific brain regions is largely independent of those of its connectivity neighbours. In contrast to this, at least one domain-general framework for studying human functional brain development (Interactive Specialization (IS), see later section) is based on the opposing assumption that interactions between brain regions are critical for the development of each one, and that networks of regions give rise to emerging functions as a coherent whole.

Static versus dynamic mapping

The assumption that different brain regions are a mosaic of isolated computational units encourages the view that structure–function relations in the brain are static and unchanging. In the context of typical development, this leads to the view that different regions can mature independently of other regions according to their own particular intrinsic timetable, and that developmental disorders could be due to deficits in specific regions. The "static assumption" is partly why it is sometimes considered to be acceptable to study developmental disorders in adulthood and then extrapolate back in time to early development. Contrary to this view, recent evidence suggests

that when a new computation or skill is acquired, there is a reorganization of interactions between different brain structures and regions (Johnson, 2011). This reorganization process may even change how previously acquired cognitive functions are represented in the brain. Thus, different networks of regions can often support the same overt behavior at different ages during development.

Plasticity, epigenetics, and fate maps

The development of biological structures, such as the brain and its constituent parts, is often considered as a process of "restriction of fate." This notion comes from the observation that as development unfolds, increasingly more complex types of cells and specialized structures emerge. However, these are assumed to be just one of the possible outcomes latent in the original stem cells. Indeed, we know this to be the case, as transposing the location of a group of cells within the developing embryo will often cause the cells to form a different structure from that which they would have done originally. The fact that some stem cells can generate multiple different types of tissue is the basis for recent advances in medical science and psychiatry. Underpinning this cellular level plasticity are processes of gene expression (see Chapter 24).

The rapidly evolving field of human genetics has moved from the traditional notion of a "blueprint" that unfolds in a series of predetermined steps, to a view of the human genome as being open to a variety of factors that influence the degree of expression of different genes at different developmental points. For example, we now know that the lifelong expression of genes in individual animals can be regulated by the animal's early environment. For example, maternal behavior toward newborn rats regulates the expression of genes involved in the same rats' responses to stress later in life (Weaver *et al.*, 2004). Thus, early sensory experiences can have lifelong effects through permanent changes in the timing and amount of different proteins expressed by the genes. Work such as this has led to the newly emerging field of "epigenetics" (Chapter 25).

At first sight, the role of epigenetic processes in the construction of a human brain seems under-constrained. Given these deep and powerful mechanisms of latent plasticity, what factors constrain patterns of expression of the genome to give sufficient "stability" in order that the complexity and structure of the human brain results? This key question is currently the focus of much research and a number of factors that constrain the epigenome are beginning to be described. Recent papers have described some of the complexity and dynamics of gene expression derived from developing and adult post mortem human brains (Colantuoni *et al.*, 2011; Kang *et al.*, 2011). Ninety percent of the brain-related genes analyzed were differentially regulated across either different brain regions or points in developmental time. The majority of this differential expression occurred during prenatal development, with patterns of expression tending to become more fixed with increasing age (Kang *et al.*, 2011).

One mechanism that promotes stability within the dynamic epigenome is genomic imprinting. This is a process through which certain genes (less than 1% in mammals) are expressed according to the parent of origin of that variant of the gene. Effectively, genomic imprinting silences the allele from either the mother or the father, leaving the remaining one to be exclusively expressed. These epigenetic marks are present from the outset of an embryo and can be maintained throughout the lifespan. Some developmental disorders, such as Angelman syndrome and Prader–Willi syndrome are associated with deficits in this process (see Chapter 54).

Plasticity in brain development is a phenomenon that has generated much controversy, with several different conceptions and definitions having been presented. Sometimes plasticity is invoked in a specialized series of mechanisms that are activated following brain injury. However, in development we can simply view plasticity as the state of a brain region's structure or function not yet fully specialized. That is, there is still remaining scope for developing more finely tuned neural architecture or responses. By this view the mechanisms of plasticity remain the same throughout the lifespan, but the expression of plasticity is more limited in adulthood because most aspects of brain structure and function have already become specialized, and thus there is less scope for further change. Plasticity is thus the flip side of the coin of "restriction of fate."

The role of time in brain development

The brains of all mammals follow a basic vertebrate brain plan that is found even in species such as salamanders, frogs, and birds. Despite the evolutionary continuity in this basic plan, one of the major differences between these species and higher primates is in the dramatic expansion of the overlying cerebral cortex, together with associated structures such as the basal ganglia. This raises the question of what is unique about the human brain and the developmental processes that give rise to it (and, relatedly, how applicable are studies on other species to our understanding of human brain development).

As a first approximation, across different species, brain size correlates with both body size and the length of developmental time it takes to reach its adult size. As large mammals, primates generally have a much more prolonged timetable for brain development than other mammals. Even between *Homo sapiens* and other primates there is a wide difference in timing. In particular, our species' period of postnatal cortical development is extended by roughly a factor of four compared to most other primates. What is the significance of this extended timetable of brain development?

Finlay and Darlington (1995) compared data on the size of brain structures from 131 mammalian species, and concluded that the relative order of landmarks of brain development is widely conserved. Further, even controlling for overall brain and body size, the time course of these landmarks is related to the relative size of structures of the adult brain in a systematic way and that disproportionately large growth occurs in the later generated structures. From this analysis, the structure most likely to differ in size in the comparatively slowed timetable of neurogenesis in primates is the neocortex.

It seems likely that the increased quantity of cortical tissue in our brains is at least, in part, a by-product of still further slowing down of the overall mammalian time course of brain development (but see Dehay & Kennedy, 2009). This suggests that evidence from other mammals will be highly relevant to the study of human brain development since we are looking at fundamentally the same process, albeit unfolding on a larger scale and a prolonged timetable. In addition to differences in the overall rate of brain development, however, different mammalian species are born at different stages of brain development. In this regard, while humans have the survival disadvantage of being born relatively immature and largely immobile, the highly prolonged period of postnatal development allows much more scope and time for interaction with the social and physical environment of the child to contribute to the tuning and shaping of circuitry. Viewed from this perspective, the high importance of parent–infant bonding and interaction as part of the constructed niche of our species becomes evident (Atzil *et al.,* 2012).

Whether it is just the slowed timing of brain development that produces the unique human brain remains controversial. Subtle differences in the steps of cortical development between primates and rodents are already known, and some reports of possibly species-specific progenitor cells or neurons in humans merit further research (Bystron *et al.*, 2008). It is also clear that sequence differences in the noncoding, regulatory regions of the genome likely account for many of the differences across primate species (Kang *et al.*, 2011).

Human structural brain development

The sequence of events involved in the prenatal development of the human brain closely resembles that of many other vertebrates. After initial divisions of the fertilized cell, a cluster of proliferating cells (called the blastocyst) differentiates into a three-layered structure (the embryonic disk) with each of these layers further differentiating into major organ systems. The outer layer (ectoderm) gives rise to the nervous system through a process known as *neurulation*. Specifically, a portion of the ectoderm begins to fold in on itself to form a hollow cylinder called the *neural tube*, which then differentiates further to give rise to the major subdivisions of the central nervous system, with the forebrain and midbrain arising at one end and the spinal cord at the other. One end differentiates into a series of repeated units or segments to become the spinal cord, while at the other end of the neural tube a series of bulges and convolutions form. Around 5 weeks after conception in humans these bulges can be identified as protoforms for the cortex (telencephalon), the thalamus and hypothalamus (diencephalon), the midbrain (mesencephalon), and others to the cerebellum (metencephalon) and to the medulla (myelencephalon).

Differentiation within these different bulges gives rise to the complex layering patterns and cell types found in the adult brain. Within these bulges, cells *proliferate* (are born), *migrate* (travel), and *differentiate* (change form) into particular types. The vast majority of the cells that will compose the brain are born in the so-called *proliferative zones*. These zones are close to the hollow portion of the neural tube (which subsequently become the ventricles of the brain). The first of these proliferation sites, the *ventricular zone*, may be phylogenetically older (Nowakowski, 1987). The second, the *subventricular zone*, only contributes significantly to phylogenetically recent brain structures such as the neocortex (i.e., "new" cortex). These two zones yield separate glial (support and supply cells) and neuron cell lines and give rise to different forms of migration.

Neurons and glial cells are produced within these zones by division of cells to produce clones (a clone is a group of cells produced by division of a single precursor cell—such a precursor cell is said to give rise to a lineage—see earlier section). *Neuroblasts* produce neurons, and in some cases particular neuroblasts also give rise to specific types of cell. For example, less than a dozen proliferating cells produce all the Purkinje cells of the cerebellar cortex, with each producing around 10,000 cells (Nowakowski, 1987).

A striking new hypothesis is that during evolution nature has capitalized on certain kinds of mutations that occur when cells divide in order to increase the diversity of types of neurons that can be generated (Muotri & Gage, 2006). The argument is that by incorporating somatic mutational mechanisms into development, the variety of different types of neurons that can be produced is much greater. To assess this idea, Evrony *et al.* (2012) developed a method to amplify the genomes of single neurons from human post mortem cerebral cortex and caudate nucleus. In doing so, they found that most neurons lacked the predicted somatic insertions, suggesting that at least one type of mutation is not a major generator of neuronal diversity in typical development. However, this approach remains potentially fruitful for investigating disorders of development at the cellular level, particularly if lack of neuronal diversity is a characteristic of the condition.

After young neurons are born, they *migrate* from the proliferative zones to the particular region where they are located in the mature brain. The first and more common type of migration is *passive cell displacement*. This occurs when cells that have been generated are then simply pushed further away from the proliferative zones by more recently born cells. This form of migration gives rise to an "outside-in" pattern, with the oldest cells being pushed toward the surface of the brain, while the most recently produced cells remain closer to their place of birth. Passive migration gives rise to brain structures such as the thalamus, the dentate gyrus of the hippocampus, and parts of the brain stem.

The second form of migration is more active and involves the young cell moving past previously generated cells to create an "inside-out" pattern. This pattern is found in the cerebral cortex

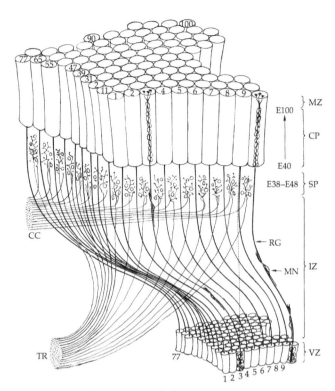

Figure 9.1 The radial unit model of Rakic (1988). Radial glial fibers span from the ventricular zone (VZ) to the cortical plate (CP) via a number of regions: the intermediate zone (IZ) and the subplate zone (SP). RG indicates a radial glial fiber, and MN a migrating neuron. Each MN traverses the IZ and SP zones that contain waiting terminals from the thalamic radiation (TR) and corticocortico (CC) afferents. As described in the text, after entering the cortical plate, the neurons migrate past their predecessors to the marginal zone (MZ). *Source:* Reprinted with permission of Wiley.

and in other areas that have a laminar structure (divided into parallel layers). In the case of the cerebral cortex, a "radial unit model" of neocortical differentiation gives an account of how both the layered and the regional structure of the mammalian cerebral cortex arises (Rakic, 1988). According to the model, the laminar organization of the cerebral cortex is determined by the fact that each proliferative cell (in the subventricular zone) gives rise to approximately 100 neurons. The progeny from each proliferative cell all migrate up the same route, with the latest to be born travelling past their older cousins. The route they take is determined by following a radial glial fiber—a long process that stretches from the top to the bottom of the cortex and originates from a glial cell. These radial glial fibers act like a guidance rope to help ensure that cells produced by one proliferative unit all contribute to one radial column within the cortex (see Figure 9.1).

While the "radial unit model" explains how cortical cells arrange themselves into the (approximately 100 neuron) thickness of the cortex, how does the differentiation into specific layers emerge? While we are far from being able to answer this question definitively at this point, in some cases differentiation into particular cell types occurs *before* each neuron reaches its final location. However, in other cases some of the properties that distinguish among cell types may only form later. For example, the distinctive apical dendrite of pyramidal cells, which often reaches into the upper layer of the cortex (layer 1), is a result of the increasing distance between this layer and other layers resulting from the inside-out pattern of growth (Marin-Padilla, 1990).

It has recently become apparent that not all migration within the cortex follows the radial unit model (Polleux *et al.*, 2002). Interspersed between pyramidal cells are a variety of types of interneurons that help balance excitation and inhibition within the cortex. Several psychiatric disorders, such as autism and schizophrenia, are thought to involve dysregulation of this balance (Le Blanc & Fagiolini, 2011; Lewis *et al.*, 2012), and in some cases this may be due to differences in the molecular mechanisms known to control tangential migration processes (Polleux *et al.*, 2002).

By the time of birth in humans, the vast majority of neurons have been born, migrated to their final locations and have differentiated into recognizable types. The main lobes and sulci of the cortex are also developed. Nevertheless, a considerable portion of human brain development continues into postnatal years.

Key features of postnatal development

As mentioned earlier, key features of human brain development are its comparatively prolonged time schedule, and the relatively immature point on the sequence of development at which we are born. These factors combine to allow for a greatly extended period of postnatal brain development in relation to most other mammals, and a correspondingly large increase in the total volume of the brain from birth to teenage years. Since the formation of neurons and their migration to appropriate brain regions takes place almost entirely within the period of prenatal development in the human, these do not account for the increase in volume. However, there is a dramatic postnatal increase in size and complexity of the dendritic tree of most neurons. While the extent and reach of a cell's dendritic arbor may increase dramatically, its patterns of connectivity with other cells also become more specific. Huttenlocher and colleagues have reported a steady increase in the density of synapses in several regions of the human cerebral cortex (Huttenlocher *et al.*, 1982; Huttenlocher, 1990, 1994). While an increase in synapses (synaptogenesis) begins around the time of birth in humans for all cortical areas studied to date, the most rapid bursts of increase, and the final peak density, occur at different ages in different areas. In the visual cortex there is a rapid burst at 3–4 months, and the maximum density of around 150% of adult level is reached between 4 and 12 months. In contrast, while synaptogenesis starts at the same time in a region of the prefrontal cortex (PFC), density increases much more slowly and does not reach its peak until well after the first year (see Figure 9.2).

Similar "rise and fall" patterns of development have been observed in other measures of human brain development. For example, using PET imaging, Chugani *et al.* (2002) measured overall resting brain metabolism (the uptake of glucose from the blood is essential for cell functioning) in early postnatal development. They observed a sharp increase in glucose uptake followed by a later decline; with a peak approximately 150% above adult levels achieved somewhere around 4–5 years of age for some cortical areas. While this peak occurred somewhat later than that in synaptic density, an adult-like *distribution* of resting activity within and across brain regions was observed by the end of the first year.

While the developmental events discussed so far concern aspects of the structure of the brain, it is important to note that there are also significant changes in the "soft soak" aspects of neural function, molecules involved in the transmission and modulation of neural signals. A number of neurotransmitters in rodents and humans also show the rise and fall developmental pattern (see Benes, 1994, for review). For example, the excitatory intrinsic transmitter glutamate, the intrinsic inhibitory transmitter GABA (Gamma-aminobutyric acid), and the extrinsic transmitter serotonin all show this same developmental trend. Thus, the distinctive "rise and fall" developmental sequence is seen in a number of microscopic and metabolic measures of structural and neurophysiological development in the human cortex.

In contrast to the rise and fall pattern, other aspects of postnatal human brain development such as myelination show a steady increase (Figure 9.2). In the central nervous system, sensory areas tend to myelinate earlier than motor areas. Cortical association areas are known to become myelinated last, with the process continuing into the second decade of life. Because myelination is a prominent feature of postnatal development, there has been much speculation linking it to advances in behavioral and cognitive development. However, while myelination greatly increases the speed and fidelity of transmission of impulses (by as much as 100 times), it is also important to remember that under-myelinated connections in the young human brain are still capable of transmitting signals, and that some connections in the adult brain never myelinate.

Recently, MRI methods have come to the fore in studying the structural development of the brain at a larger scale. MRI reveals brain structure at a more gross scale than neurons and synapses, but sufficient to allow the measurement of gray and white matter in different cortical and subcortical regions. One report described cortical gray matter development in participants from 4 to 21 years (Gogtay *et al.*, 2004). The authors report considerable heterogeneity between different individuals, and between different cortical regions. Nevertheless, they confirmed that cortical gray matter shows the characteristic "rise and fall" pattern described above, and indicates the pruning or elimination of excess connections between neurons. For some cortical regions most of the rise occurs before puberty, and most of the decline after puberty going into early adulthood.

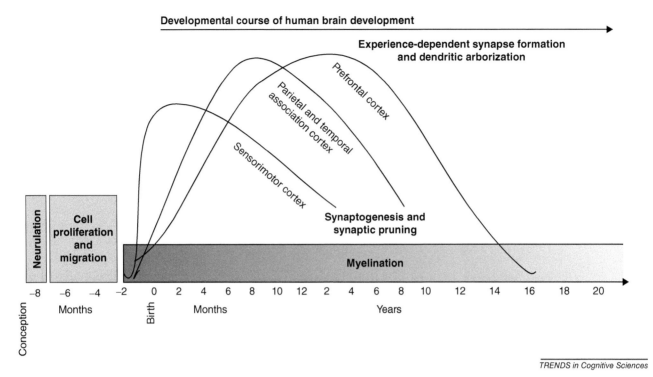

Figure 9.2 An approximate timeline for some of the most important changes in human brain development. *Source:* Reprinted with permission of Elsevier.

Also, broadly consistent with earlier reports based on post mortem neuroanatomical studies, the authors observed that the primary sensory areas of the cortex, along with the frontal and occipital poles, show the fastest growth (and decline) curves.

Most of the remainder of the cortex develops in an approximately back-to-front direction, with the PFC showing the most delayed developmental curve. However, the posterior superior temporal cortex, which is a critical part of the social brain network and integrates information from different sensory modalities, develops last according to this particular measure. Similar MRI data have been collected for the volume of white matter (myelinated fiber bundles), and this shows a general linear increase with age through to early adulthood. The lack of a later decline in this measure may reflect the ongoing life-long myelination of fibers that adds to the overall volume of the brain.

Overall, a number of different measures and laboratories have found the rise and fall pattern for neurons and their local connectivity. However, it should be noted that measures such as synaptic density are but static snapshots of a dynamic process in which both additive and regressive processes are continually in progress. Thus, there are probably not distinct and separate progressive and regressive phases, but a shift in balance between these processes during development. It is also worth noting that for any given cortical region there are often multiple waves of remodeling of synaptic architecture during development. Some of these waves of change in the morphology and density of synapses correspond to sensitive periods in which sensory or

environmental information can have maximum effect on the developing brain (Meredith *et al.*, 2012).

Oscillating rhythms

Even simple nervous systems show spontaneous activity that is only sometimes driven by sensory or motor events. Indeed, recent experiments in which stem cells were cultured *in vitro* to develop into neurons have observed that simple circuits can form with primitive oscillatory firing patterns (Shi *et al.*, 2012), suggesting that oscillatory activity is a fundamental property of nervous systems. In advanced brains, oscillatory activity can occur at multiple different frequencies simultaneously. These frequencies can vary from high (40 Hz or higher, generally characteristic of local circuit activity in cerebral cortex) to low (0.1 Hz or lower generally characteristic of longer range connectivity, or even glial cell activity). Oscillatory activity that is evoked by, or entrained to, sensory events can be studied with ERP or MEG methods (see Chapter 11). Many evoked potentials recorded at the scalp may reflect the entrainment of ongoing oscillatory activity at specific frequencies (Palva & Palva, 2012). In development, some of these spontaneous rhythms may have particular importance in consolidating or weakening structural and functional connections between regions.

From an early stage of prenatal development, interactions between cells are critical, including the transmission of electrical signals between neurons. In one example, patterns of spontaneous firing of cells in the eyes (before they have opened and exposed themselves to light) transmit signals that appear to then help induce the layered structure of the lateral geniculate nucleus (see O'Leary & Nakagawa, 2002; Shatz, 2002). Thus, waves of firing neurons intrinsic to the developing organism may play an important role in specifying aspects of brain structure well before sensory inputs from the external world have any effect.

After birth, when the sensory systems are bombarded with stimulation, the spontaneous oscillations of the brain can become entrained or perturbed by sensory-evoked activity in ways that are still poorly understood (but see Palva & Palva, 2012). Oscillations at different frequencies are not just epiphenomena of patterns of neuron firing, but are likely to "bind" activity states across near and far regions of the brain. Indeed, some have argued that oscillation frequencies characterize distinct functional networks, and keep their information processing distinct from other concurrently active regions (Singer & Gray, 1995).

Scores of studies in developmental psychopathology have focused on differences in specific ERP waveforms assumed to reflect differences in regional patterns of activation, or the time course or degree of the latency jitter of these peaks of voltage change (e.g., Tye et al., 2013). Common findings include less complexity to evoked waveforms and increased variability in their time course (Milne, 2011).

Resting activity and network connectivity

It has been hypothesized that resting state activity in the brain may provide a critical bridge between structural and functional development (Johnson, 2011). This is because resting states can reflect averages of sensory and task-driven activation patterns over a time period, and consolidation of experience-driven co-activation patterns between regions may require the prolonged activation patterns that resting or default states can provide. Specifically, regions that show coherent (in-phase) oscillatory activity may maintain or strengthen structural connections between them. Other regions that may oscillate at similar frequencies, but out of phase, may lose or reduce synaptic connections with the emerging coherent network.

Networks of resting state activity have been used to trace developmental changes in human brain networks and they even provided the basis for a "maturational index" (Schlaggar et al., 2002). While several studies have shown a developmental shift from local to more long-range connectivity (e.g., Fair et al., 2009), these studies are currently under question for methodological reasons associated with greater motion artifact at younger ages (Deen & Pelphrey, 2012). Another change in network structure during development is in the hierarchical structure. Adult networks have a more hierarchical structure that is optimally connected to support top-down relations between one part of the network and another (Supekar

et al., 2009). While hierarchical networks have a number of computational advantages, they are known to be less plastic and more vulnerable to damage or noise in the particular nodes at the top of the hierarchy. Thus, the network arrangement of children may be more adaptable in response to unusual or atypical sensory input or environmental context.

A final aspect of the transition from child brain network to the adult one is the greater connectivity between cortical and subcortical structures seen at younger ages (Supekar et al., 2009), an observation that may be fundamental for our understanding of the emergence of the social brain and memory systems, as it implies that the specialization of some cortical areas may be initially more dominated by structures such as the amygdala and hippocampus.

Determinants of cortical specialization

A long-standing debate among those who study the developmental neurobiology of the cortex concerns the extent to which its structure and function in adults are the result of genetic, molecular and cellular level interactions, as opposed to being the result of the pattern of activity generated by firing of neurons. In the adult primate, most cortical areas can be determined by very detailed differences in their laminar structure, such as the precise thickness of certain layers. Often, however, the borderlines between areas are sometimes indistinct and controversial. It is commonly assumed that these anatomically defined areas have particular unique functions contained within their boundaries. While this has proved to be the case for early sensory and motor areas, there are many cases of *functional* regions that do not neatly correspond to known *neuroanatomical* divisions or borders.

Traditionally, two opposing possibilities have been put forward to account for the division of the cerebral cortex into distinct areas: *Protomap* and *protocortex*. According to the *protomap* (Rakic, 1988) view, differentiation into cortical regions occurs early in the formation of the cortex, and is due to intrinsic molecular factors. The alternative possibility is that different areas of cortex arise out of an undifferentiated *protocortex*. By this view, differentiation occurs later in the development of cortex, and it depends at least partly on extrinsic factors like input from other parts of the brain or sensory systems. The activity of neurons is required for regional differentiation (Killackey, 1990; O'Leary & Nakagawa, 2002). Reviews of the evidence converge on views that are midway between the protomap and protocortex hypotheses (Kingsbury & Finlay, 2001; Pallas, 2001; Ragsdale & Grove, 2001; Bystron et al., 2008). Most agree that graded patterns of gene expression create large-scale regions with combinations of properties that may better suit certain computations (similar to a coarse or imprecise protomap). It is within these large-scale regions that smaller scale functional areas arise through the activity-dependent mechanisms associated with the protocortex view. Kingsbury and Finlay (2001) refer to this as a "hyperdimensional plaid" because the patterning that emerges in a plaid is the result of small changes in many threads. Similarly, O'Leary and colleagues call this the "cooperative concentration" model since some different gradients of gene expression may act as opposing forces in shaping cortical regions (Hamasaki *et al.*, 2002).

Human functional brain development

Relating evidence on the neuroanatomical development of the brain to the remarkable changes in motor, perceptual and cognitive abilities during the first decade or so of human life presents a considerable challenge. To briefly recap on some the earlier conclusions from this chapter, a probabilistic epigenesis view of development assumes interactions between genes, structural brain changes and psychological function are bidirectional, dynamic and emergent, as opposed to there being a unidirectional causal path from genes to structural changes to psychological consequences. We also saw that mammalian neurodevelopment is best characterized as being regulatory, rather than mosaic; the response properties of a cortical area is heavily interdependent upon its connectivity to other regions and their respective activity patterns. Further, with regard to structure-function mappings, the same overt behavioral responses can sometimes be supported by different combinations of regional activity within the brain, thus providing potential mechanisms for adaptation. We also saw how development can be viewed as a "restriction of fate," and how plasticity becomes correspondingly reduced, as the fate of developmental process is restricted through the increase in specialization of cells or circuits.

Building on these foundations, the Interactive Specialization (IS) framework assumes that postnatal functional brain development, at least within the cerebral cortex, involves a process of organizing patterns of inter-regional interactions (Johnson, 2000; 2011), and it focuses on how partial or immature functioning of regions transitions gradually to their adult state. According to IS, the response properties of a given cortical region are partly determined by its patterns of connectivity to other regions, and their respective patterns of activity. During postnatal development, changes in the response properties of cortical regions occur as they interact and compete with each other to acquire their role in new computational abilities. From this perspective, some cortical regions start with poorly defined, general-purpose functions, and consequently are partially activated in a wide range of different stimuli, contexts and tasks. During development, activity-dependent interactions between regions sharpen up their functions such that their activity becomes restricted to a narrower set of circumstances (i.e., a region originally activated by a wide variety of visual objects may come to confine its response to upright human faces). The onset of new behavioral competencies will therefore be associated with changes in network activity over several regions, and not just by the onset of activity in one or more additional region(s).

Although the IS view can account for evidence from a variety of different domains of human cognition (Johnson, 2011), the area in which it has been most extensively tested is in face processing and in studies of the emergent specialization of the Fusiform Face Area (FFA). Several studies have traced the gradual emergence of a high degree of tuning to faces in this region. For example, Scherf *et al.* (2007) used naturalistic movies of faces, objects, buildings and navigation scenes in a passive viewing task with children (5–8 years), adolescents (11–14 years) and adults. They found that the children exhibited patterns of activation of the face processing areas similar to that commonly reported in adults (such as the FFA). However, this activation was not selective for the category of face stimuli; the regions were equally strongly activated by objects and landscapes.

While experiments such as these provide evidence for the increasing specialization (or tuning) of individual regions of the cortex during human postnatal development, it is clear from the IS viewpoint that the next step is to understand how *networks* involving different regions, each with their own different specializations, emerge. Again, face processing is a good test domain as a "core face network" of cortical regions has been well established in adults and activity in this network is modulated by task demands in adults. Cohen Kadosh *et al.* (2010) examined the emergence of the network underlying face processing in younger (7–8 year old) and older (10–11 years old) school-age children as well as young adults, and found that children showed substantially weaker connectivity within the face network. More notably, no evidence was found for the influence of task demands on the effective connectivity within the network in the two child groups. Thus, while both child groups exhibited similar overall network structures, these weaker networks were not influenced by top-down task demands.

Atypical human neurodevelopment

Consideration of two aspects of typical human brain development should inform our thinking about how things can go wrong to result in developmental psychopathologies. On the one hand, we have seen that constructing a typical brain requires an exquisite and complex series of interacting events in which there are many possibilities for specific events, or their timings, to go awry. From this perspective it is almost surprising how often a typical developmental outcome is achieved! On the other hand, we have also described a number of mechanisms of stability and inherent plasticity that constrain and guide the self-organization of the brain. Viewed from this perspective, brain development is an inevitable outcome of a combination of processes, and seems to be well buffered from any minor perturbations. From the latter perspective, one might speculate that in order to achieve significant deviation from the typical developmental trajectory either some fundamental process would have to be disrupted with likely widespread and devastating consequences, or multiple "minor" factors may have to combine, which then prevent processes of adaptation and compensation from occurring.

Many of the key points from typical human neurodevelopment discussed earlier are of direct relevance to our interpretation of atypical developmental pathways. We have seen that development is a process of increased differentiation of cells, neural regions and networks. Although, for a particular environment, a specific trajectory of differentiation or specialization may characterize the majority outcome, we have also seen that apparently the same behaviors can be supported by different patterns of network activity at different ages. Even in the adult end-state, individual differences can be extensive, and recent research that compares groups of typical adult participants raised in different cultures has also shown a surprising degree of differences in the neural substrates of perceptual and cognitive functions (Chiao, 2009). Thus, the pathway of typical neurodevelopment should not be thought of as a single narrow track from which it is easy to deviate, but rather (to use Waddington's metaphor) as a deep and broad valley whose steep sides buffer against escape. Given that typical neurodevelopment is a broad and robust process, how are we to understand developmental psychopathologies?

Much of the neuroimaging work on developmental disorders such as autism and ADHD to date has aimed at identifying gross abnormalities in discrete brain regions, structures or systems. While there have been some specific claims made with regard to such deficits, reviews of the field tend to find instead that evidence is consistent with diffuse damage to widespread networks and regions of the brain (Deb & Thompson 1998; Rumsey & Ernst, 2000). In other words, we are seeing brains that have developed differently, rather than typically developed brains with overt or discrete damage.

This conclusion also extends to many developmental disorders of known genetic etiology such as Fragile-X, Williams Syndrome and Down Syndrome.

For example, Fragile-X involves the *FMR1* gene on the X chromosome. The defect of the gene results in a lack of the particular protein that it codes for: FMR1 protein. One of the knock-on consequences of the reduction of this protein is a disturbance in the neurotransmitter glutamate. However, despite the apparent specificity of this causal pathway, the effects of this defect are widespread and include several different aspects of physical and cognitive development. Thus, although Fragile-X involves only one gene, there are multiple and widespread neurodevelopmental consequences. Some of the broad effects may be the result of processes of adaptation at molecular, cellular and system levels.

Given these considerations, it is perhaps surprising that the vast majority of neuroimaging studies with developmental disordered groups involve participants from middle childhood to adulthood, and that patients are often grouped together over a wide age range (e.g., Kesler *et al.* (2004): Turner syndrome: 7–33 years; Pinter *et al.* (2001): Down's syndrome 5–23 years). For the IS approach, however, age of testing is critical, and it is especially important to study infancy to understand partial causes of subsequent outcomes (Karmiloff-Smith, 1998; Paterson *et al.*, 1999). For this issue to be assessed, there need to be longitudinal imaging studies of clinical groups, or at least cross-sectional studies at different ages.

Risk

Traditionally, risk factors for human brain development were viewed as either intrinsic to the brain itself due to some pre- or perinatal neuroanatomical or neurochemical atypicality, or environmentally caused. More recently, it has become evident that at least for some of the more common developmental disorders, intrinsic and environmental factors may interact (see Chapter 10). Risk, as defined in the context of the robust, adaptative and self-organizing process of brain development, can be defined as the elimination of alternative options that are normally present.

As mentioned, in most developmental disorders we study brains that have developed differently. At the point of diagnosis, the relevant behavioral phenotypes are, by definition, clearly defined and well embedded. It is evident from the preceding discussion of developmental neurobiology that the phenotypic end state will include not only residual signs of the core atypicality but also compounded effects due to atypical intrinsic and environmental interactions and the results of adaptation. While the vast majority of neuroscience imaging work on children and adults with developmental disorders necessarily conflate these factors, Kaiser *et al.* (2010) used fMRI to study patterns of brain activation in children with autism, unaffected siblings of children with autism and controls while they viewed videos of biological motion. These authors found that unaffected siblings of children with autism had some patterns of activation in common with those with autism, but not controls. This "trait" activity was consistent with a "neuroendophenotype" that extends to unaffected family members, and raises the possibility that unaffected siblings actively overcome this atypicality in some way. Encouraging this view was the existence of patterns of activation consistent with "compensatory activity." These areas were not activated in either those with autism or the controls, and had the hallmark of regions whose additional activity allowed children potentially at-risk to achieve a typical outcome.

In considering the difficulty in interpreting neuroscience data from a brain that has undergone considerable postnatal adaptation, several groups have taken a new approach to developmental disorders based on the prospective longitudinal study of infants at-risk (most commonly, infant siblings in families with an older child already diagnosed). Here, the aim is to identify and study the earliest "pure" manifestations of the condition before the establishment of confounding and compensatory factors that result from the subsequent years of atypical development.

Resilience

Indirect evidence from studies of infants at-risk who may possess an endophenotype associated with a developmental disorder suggests that some of them additionally engage processes of neural adaptation or compensation in order to achieve a typical outcome. Given our review of the mechanisms of typical neurodevelopment, this should not be a surprise for several reasons. First, we have seen that the pathway for typical neurodevelopment can be broad and robust in the face of minor disturbances; a typical outcome is inevitable within certain boundaries. Second, we reviewed evidence that typical neurodevelopment is a constructive and autonomous process, which makes it inherently more robust and adaptable than the passive unfolding of a genetic "blueprint." While the brain, viewed as a self-organizing autonomous system, is consistent with the ability to compensate in the face of adversity, can we specify in more detail the neural systems, regions or mechanisms that may underlie this process?

The unique developmental history of the anterior portion of cortex—PFC—results in the beginnings of activity-dependent development of neural connectivity in the absence of thalamic input, and this may bias the region toward processing information based on intercortical connectivity rather than the close connections to sensory input or motor output characteristic of more posterior regions. It is notable that several common developmental disorders have been associated with deficits in the so-called executive functions (EF) that are generally thought to be supported by PFC (see Chapter 10). While EF deficits often co-occur with diagnostic symptoms in these disorders, evidence indicates that they are, to at least some extent, dissociable (Johnson, 2012). One hypothesis is that instead of poor EF skills being part of a core cluster of symptoms of atypicality or impairment in some developmental disorders, having good EF skills allow the brain to compensate, or better adapt to, atypical functioning in other neural systems in individuals at genetic risk (Johnson, 2012). By this view, poor executive function and self-control skills are associated with some developmental disorders as some of the individual children who end up with these diagnoses have less capacity to compensate in the face of other risk factors early in life. In contrast, individual children with strong EF skills have brains that are better able to adapt at a neural systems level, and thus are less likely to end up with a diagnosis. On the other hand, being at the lower end of typical variation in EF skills early in life may be considered to be an additional risk factor, due to less capacity to adapt in response to other perturbations to the typical developmental pathway.

The traditional view of PFC atypicality in developmental disorders is that later developing regions of the brain are more vulnerable to perturbation at earlier stages. However, recent evidence indicates that the PFC is actively involved in the acquisition of new skills and knowledge from very early in life, and, additionally, that it may play a significant role in establishing and organizing functional specialization in posterior regions of the cortex (see Johnson 2011, for a review). On the assumption that PFC can support at least some EF skills from early in life, and that it plays a role in shaping and organizing other cortical networks, it is reasonable to infer that it may have a critical role in the adaptive reorganization of other cortical pathways in the face of nonoptimal functioning elsewhere.

As discussed, some MRI studies are beginning to reveal glimpses of the processes of brain adaptation that may result in typical outcomes from some children born at-risk, and the compensatory mechanisms that often involve parts of PFC. For example, in Kaiser et al. (2010) the compensatory activity regions were right posterior STS (consistent with biological motion processing) and ventromedial PFC. While the adult functions of the latter region remain unclear, it is often assumed to have a role in the regulation of other brain systems and decision-making (Bechara et al., 2000).

Future directions

Developmental neurobiology is an exciting and very rapidly moving field, with new techniques and methods becoming available every few years. However, the allure of obtaining new kinds and quantities of empirical data should not distract us from the key questions and issues around human developmental psychopathology. It seems likely that for many developmental disorders we will need to understand how large-scale networks of neurons are influenced by alterations of their underlying molecular and cellular function. It will be important to remember that different molecular or cellular atypicalities can sometimes give rise to the same functional consequences at an overall neuronal network level. Thus, ultimately it may be at the level of whole neural systems that some developmental disorders are best understood. However, this change in focus requires us to have a better understanding of the temporal and spatial dynamics of multicellular activity in the brain, something that has been hampered by the fact that most current neuroimaging methods have either relatively poor spatial or temporal resolution.

We began this chapter by stating that the brain is primarily an organ of adaptation at multiple different temporal scales and levels of organization. An exciting challenge for the future will be to understand these processes better and ultimately to harness them in ways that may allow us to reduce the number and/or severity of symptoms of children who end up with diagnoses such as autism and ADHD.

Definitions

Differentiation—the process through which cells take on their final (adult) morphology

Endophenotype—an intermediate phenotype often associated with neural processes or systems

Epigenesis—the expression of genes during development

Laminar—refers to the layered structure of cerebral cortex

Migration—the travelling of cells from their location of origin

Myelination—the process of depositing a fatty sheath around neural fibers

Neurogenesis—the process of generating new neurons

Progenitor cells—stem cells that give rise to neurons

Acknowledgements

I acknowledge financial support from the UK Medical Research Council (Program Grant G9715587) and Birkbeck, University of London.

References

Atzil, S. *et al.* (2012) Synchrony and specificity in the maternal and paternal brain: relations to oxytocin and vasopressin. *Journal of the American Academy of Child & Adolescent Psychiatry* **51**, 798–811.

Bechara, A. *et al.* (2000) Characterization of the decision-making deficit of patients with ventromedial prefrontal cortex lesions. *Brain* **123**, 2189–2202.

Benes, F.M. (1994) Development of the corticolimbic system. In: *Human Behavior and the Developing Brain.* (eds G. Dawson & K.W. Fischer), pp. 176–206. Guilford Press, New York.

Bystron, I. *et al.* (2008) Development of the human cerebral cortex: Boulder Committee revisited. *Nature Reviews Neuroscience* **9**, 110–122.

Chiao, J. (2009) *Cultural Neuroscience: Cultural Influences on Brain Function. Progress in Brain Research.* Elsevier Press.

Chugani, H.T. *et al.* (2002) Positron emission tomography study of human brain functional development. In: *Brain Development and Cognition: A Reader.* (eds M.H. Johnson, Y. Munakata & R. Gilmore), 2nd edn, pp. 101–116. Blackwell, Oxford.

Cohen Kadosh, K. *et al.* (2010) Task-dependent activation of face-sensitive cortex: an fMRI adaptation study. *Journal of Cognitive Neuroscience* **22**, 903–917.

Colantuoni, C. *et al.* (2011) Temporal dynamics and genetic control of transcription in the human prefrontal cortex. *Nature* **478**, 519–523.

Deb, S. & Thompson, B. (1998) Neuroimaging in autism. *Journal of Psychiatry* **173**, 299–302.

Deen, B. & Pelphrey, K. (2012) Perspective: brain scans need a rethink. *Nature* **491**, S20.

Dehay, C. & Kennedy, H. (2009) Transcriptional regulation and alternative splicing make for better brains. *Neuron* **62**, 455–457.

Elman, J.L. *et al.* (1996) *Rethinking innateness: a connectionist perspective on development.* MIT Press, Massachusetts.

Evrony, G.D. *et al.* (2012) Single-neuron sequencing analysis of L1 retrotransposition and somatic mutation in the human brain. *Cell* **151**, 483–496.

Fair, D.A. *et al.* (2009) Functional brain networks develop from a "local to distributed" organization. *PLoS Computational Biology* **5**, e1000381.

Finlay, B. & Darlington, R. (1995) Linked regularities in the development and evolution of mammalian brains. *Science* **268**, 1578–1584.

Friston, K.J. & Price, C.J. (2001) Dynamic representation and generative models of brain function. *Brain Research Bulletin* **54**, 275–285.

Gogtay, N. *et al.* (2004) Dynamic mapping of human cortical development during childhood through early adulthood. *Proceedings of the National Academy of Science, USA* **101**, 8174–8179.

Gottlieb, G. (1992) *Individual Development and Evolution: The Genesis of Novel Behavior.* Oxford University Press, New York.

Hamasaki, T. *et al.* (2002) EMX2 regulates sizes and positioning of the primary sensory and motor areas in neocortex by direct specification of cortical progenitors. *Neuron* **3**, 359–372.

Huttenlocher, P.R. (1990) Morphometric study of human cerebral cortex development. *Neuropsychologia* **28**, 517–527.

Huttenlocher, P.R. (1994) Synaptogenesis, synapse elimination, and neural plasticity in human cerebral cortex: threats to optimal development. In: *The Minnesota Symposia on Child Psychology.* (ed C.A. Nelson) 27, pp. 35–54. Lawrence Erlbaum, Hillsdale, NJ.

Huttenlocher, P.R. *et al.* (1982) Synaptogenesis in human visual cortex — evidence for synapse elimination during normal development. *Neuroscience Letters* **33**, 247–252.

Johnson, M.H. (2000) Functional brain development in infants: elements of an interactive specialization framework. *Child Development* **71**, 75–81.

Johnson, M.H. (2011) *Developmental Cognitive Neuroscience*, 3rd edn. John Wiley & Sons, Oxford.

Johnson, M.H. (2012) Executive function and developmental disorders: the flip side of the coin. *Trends in Cognitive Sciences* **16**, 454–457.

Kaiser, M.D. *et al.* (2010) Neural signatures of autism. *Proceedings of the National Academy of Sciences* **107**, 21223–21228.

Kang, H.J. *et al.* (2011) Spatio-temporal transcriptome of the human brain. *Nature* **478**, 483–489.

Karmiloff-Smith, A. (1998) Development itself is the key to understanding developmental disorders. *Trends in Cognitive Sciences* **2**, 389–398.

Kesler, S.R. *et al.* (2004) Amygdala and hippocampal volumes in Turner syndrome: a high-resolution MRI study of X-monosomy. *Neuropsychologia* **42**, 1971–1978.

Killackey, H.P. (1990) Neocortical expansion: an attempt toward relating phylogeny and ontogeny. *Journal of Cognitive Neuroscience* **2**, 1–17.

Kingsbury, M.A. & Finlay, B.L. (2001) The cortex in multidimensional space: where do cortical areas come from? *Developmental Science* **4**, 125–142.

Le Blanc, J.J. & Fagiolini, M. (2011) Autism: a "critical period" disorder? *Neural Plasticity* **2011**, 1–17.

Lewis, D.A. *et al.* (2012) Cortical parvalbumin interneurons and cognitive dysfunction in schizophrenia. *Trends in Neuroscience* **35**, 57–67.

Marin-Padilla, M. (1990) The pyramidal cell and its local-circuit interneurons: a hypothetical unit of the mammalian cerebral cortex. *Journal of Cognitive Neuroscience* **2**, 180–194.

Meredith, R.M. *et al.* (2012) Sensitive time-windows for susceptibility in neurodevelopmental disorders. *Trends in Neurosciences* **35**, 335–344.

Muotri, A.R. & Gage, F.H. (2006) Generation of neuronal variability and complexity. *Nature* **441**, 1087–1093.

Nowakowski, R.S. (1987) Basic concepts of CNS development. *Child Development* **58**, 568–595.

O'Leary, D.D.M. & Nakagawa, Y. (2002) Patterning centers, regulatory genes and extrinsic mechanisms controlling arealization of the neocortex. *Current Opinion in Neurobiology* **12**, 14–25.

Pallas, S.L. (2001) Intrinsic and extrinsic factors shaping cortical identity. *Neurosciences* **24**, 417–423.

Palva, S. & Palva, J.M. (2012) Discovering oscillatory interaction networks with M/EEG: challenges and breakthroughs. *Trends in Cognitive Science* **16**, 219–230.

Paterson, S.J. *et al.* (1999) Cognitive modularity and genetic disorders. *Science* **286**, 2355–2358.

Pinter, J.D. *et al.* (2001) Neuroanatomy of Down's syndrome: a high-resolution MRI study. *American Journal of Psychiatry* **158**, 1659–1665.

Polleux, F. *et al.* (2002) Control of cortical interneuron migration by neurotrophins and P13-kinase signalling. *Development* **129**, 3147–3169.

Ragsdale, C.W. & Grove, E.A. (2001) Patterning in the mammalian cerebral cortex. *Current Opinions in Neurobiology* **11**, 50–58.

Rakic, P. (1988) Specification of cerebral cortical areas. *Science* **241**, 170–176.

Rumsey, J.M. & Ernst, M. (2000) Functional neuroimaging of autistic disorders. *Mental Retardation and Developmental Disabilities Research Reviews* **6**, 171–179.

Scherf, K.S. *et al.* (2007) Visual category-selectivity for faces, places and objects emerges along different developmental trajectories. *Developmental Science* **10**, F15–F30.

Schlaggar, B.L. *et al.* (2002) Functional neuroanatomical differences between adults and school-age children in the processing of single words. *Science* **296**, 1476–1479.

Shatz, C.J. (2002) Emergence of order in visual system development. In: *Brain Development and Cognition: A Reader.* (eds M.H. Johnson, Y. Munakata & R. Gilmore), 2nd edn, pp. 231–244. Blackwell, Oxford.

Shi, Y. *et al.* (2012) A human stem cell model of early Alzheimer's disease pathology in Down syndrome. *Science Translational Medicine* **4**, 24–29.

Singer, W. & Gray, C.M. (1995) Visual feature integration and the temporal correlation hypothesis. *Annual Review of Neuroscience* **18**, 555–586.

Supekar, K. *et al.* (2009) Development of large-scale functional brain networks in children. *PLoS Biology* **7**, e1000157.

Tye, C. *et al.* (2013) Neurophysiological responses to faces and gaze direction differentiate children with ASD, ADHD and ASD+ADHD. *Developmental Cognitive Neuroscience* **5**, 71–85.

Weaver, I.C. *et al.* (2004) Epigenetic programming by maternal behaviour. *Nature Neuroscience* **7**, 847–854.

CHAPTER 10

Systems neuroscience

Daniel S. Pine

Section on Development and Affective Neuroscience, National Institute of Mental Health (NIMH) Intramural Research Program, Bethesda, MD, USA

Introduction

The term "systems neuroscience" refers to research on neural circuits, which represent collections of neurons that coalesce to function as a unit. Systems neuroscience applications in child psychology and psychiatry examine how brain circuits influence behavior, as it changes in typical and atypical development, often assessed through brain imaging.

These applications are only beginning, unfolding at the interface of psychology, psychiatry, information technology, genetics, and other fields. Newly emerging, multidisciplinary fields often undergo considerable changes with time, complicating attempts to define their boundaries. So it is with systems neuroscience. While interesting applications utilize brain imaging, this is not a prerequisite; relevant research also can focus only on behavior, studied where supporting neural systems have been delineated. Similarly, relevant research can link behaviors to genetic factors by again focusing on behaviors tightly linked to underlying neural systems. In such examples, research in children usually extends mechanistic understandings established through research using methods too invasive for applications with children.

Since specific examples illustrates applications, the bulk of this chapter focuses on four examples: cognitive control, fear, attachment-affiliation, and brain development. Given the multidisciplinary nature of these examples, this chapter overlaps with other chapters but has a uniquely integrative focus to illustrate insights that emerge at the interface of allied disciplines. Figure 10.1 charts how an integrative lens can be applied either narrowly or broadly.

Figure 10.1 depicts the multitiered nature of the targeted phenomena, uniting around the shared pursuit of mechanistic understandings of brain–behavior relationships. At its most focused level, depicted in the top row of Figure 10.1, research targets the genome and its effect on function in individual neurons, extending to brain systems that coalesce through connections among a few such individual neurons to form a circuit. This level can be slightly expanded to examine interactions among components of brain circuits and their effects on behavior, as depicted in Figure 10.1 in the transition from the top to the middle row. Of note, evolutionary perspectives on these inquiries even more broadly inform understandings, as discussed in the chapters on genetics. For example, humans' evolutionary divergence from other primates may reflect cross-species differences in genetic regulatory elements related to cross-species differences in behavior and associated brain functions. Advances in neuroscience also inform genetic research, as reflected in the use of pathway analysis in genetics, informed by neuroscience.

Neuroscience advances provide unique opportunities. Great excitement has emerged for optogenetics, which has become a classic tool (Deisseroth, 2012). With this technique, most typically applied to rodents, activity in neural circuits can be precisely manipulated with great spatial and temporal precision so that the corresponding changes in behavior can be charted. At a more macroscopic level, applications to children often use imaging to chart the connections between behaviors expressed in the laboratory and variations in brain function. Figure 10.1 depicts these levels from the middle to the bottom row of the figure. Still more macroscopic applications can focus on these same sets of behaviors, expressed in the laboratory, as they relate to clinical profiles, expressed through thoughts and behaviors in children's daily lives, as depicted in the bottom row of Figure 10.1. This aspect of the figure also shows how features in the environment, depicted in the classroom, also impact on each level shown in the figure. Finally, by linking so many levels, systems neuroscience becomes clinically relevant.

Rutter's Child and Adolescent Psychiatry, Sixth Edition.
Edited by Anita Thapar and Daniel S. Pine, James F. Leckman, Stephen Scott, Margaret J. Snowling, Eric Taylor.
© 2015 John Wiley & Sons Ltd. Published 2018 by John Wiley & Sons Ltd.

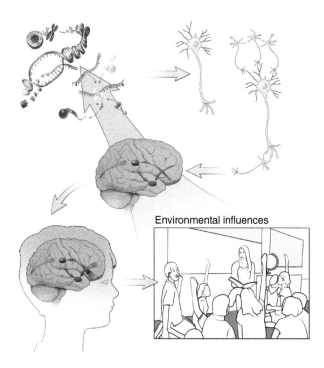

Environmental influences

Figure 10.1 Relationships among constructs targeted in systems neuroscience. The upper left-hand corner depicts molecular-genetic targets in DNA, as they relate to neuron function, depicted toward the right. Individual neuron function can be related to the functions of neural circuits, composed of collections of neurons. This also is depicted in the figure. Finally, these neural circuits can be studied through imaging, in structures that can be assessed in children using brain imaging. With this technique, the functions of the circuit in the child can be related to the functions that children display in their world, as depicted by a frightened child attending school. Finally, it is emphasized how the environment interacts with each level of this multitiered system, extending from the classroom through the molecular-genetic targets displayed in the upper left-hand corner of the figure.

Child psychiatry and systems neuroscience

Understanding systems neuroscience requires mastery of material handled in allied disciplines, particularly material reviewed in the chapters on brain imaging, experimental models, and developmental processes. Readers are encouraged to review these chapters, while referring to Figure 10.1 and searching for mechanistic explanation of specific behaviors as outputs from neural circuits.

Molecular genetics examines the many ways in which deoxyribonucleic acid (DNA) influences neural-circuit function and behavior (Pine *et al.*, 2010). Research in this area links DNA variation to variation in behavior either occurring directly or through interactions with the environment. Chapters in Part II (Influences on Psychopathology) describe core features of the genome that influence behavior. Other sections also relate to systems neuroscience. Because brain imaging research assesses structural and functional variation in neural circuits, this material, appearing in Part I of the textbook, vitally informs

child psychiatry and psychology applications of systems neuroscience. Summaries in these chapters describe key principles emerging from research using methods too invasive for applications to children. Across all of these areas, emphasis is placed on how genes interact with factors in the environment, as is also represented in Figure 10.1.

Chapter 11 provides in-depth descriptions of various techniques, whereas the chapter on development (see Chapter 9) focuses on age variation in brain–behavior relationships. Only small portions of the vast research on imaging, animal models, or developmental psychopathology deeply probe connections between brain systems and specific behaviors with the goal of answering clinically relevant questions. Such a deep probing is the backbone of this chapter, provided through a focus on four specific examples.

While the four examples target distinct areas, they share three features. First, each begins by targeting specific behaviors, ideally ones that can be studied through observation in the laboratory to support cross-species research essential for progress in systems neuroscience. Second, a foundation is laid for expansive research, broadening the field in two opposite directions; one direction focuses on complex behaviors that children display in the world. The second proceeds in the opposite direction, to increasingly narrow contexts. The third and final feature is that for each example, clinically relevant questions are proposed, where answers have not emerged without the tools of systems neuroscience. For illustrative purposes, each example emphasizes one unique contribution, although each example could address many questions.

Finally, emerging systems neuroscience research fails to find clear associations between measures of brain function and psychiatric syndromes as they are currently conceptualized. This may reflect heterogeneity, where children classified as suffering from the same syndrome actually exhibit syndromes that result from distinct pathophysiology. This also may reflect the occurrence of unique clinical profiles from one core form of brain dysfunction, as described in Chapter 24. Given the current state of systems neuroscience research, clinicians can expect the boundaries of mental syndromes to change, much as they do for neoplastic diseases as pathophysiology of cancer is understood in increasing detail.

Cognitive control

Defining specific behaviors

Research on cognitive control usually examines how neural-circuitry function varies during motor-response tasks. In these situations, cognitive control supports two processes: error monitoring and behavioral adjustment (Cohen *et al.*, 2004; Carter, 2005; Carter, 2006; van Veen *et al.*, 2008).

Many tasks engage cognitive-control processes. These include tasks of so-called executive functions, selective attention, delayed motor response, and response reversal. For illustrative

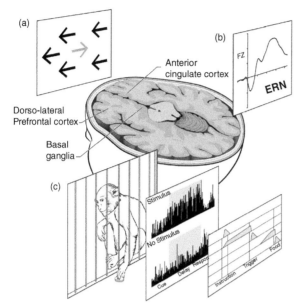

Figure 10.2 Research on cognitive control. (a) The flanker task is displayed on a screen and the corresponding depiction of a child viewing the screen represents brain regions that are engaged when this task is performed in a brain scanner. (b) The error-related negativity (ERN) response, which is recorded from a child's scalp using electroencephalography. (c) Data collected from neurons of a monkey performing a reward task shown in the figure. Over time, individual events with or without a stimulus presented elicit responses that can be plotted in a so-called "raster" diagram. This is shown immediately adjacent to the monkey. These yield characteristic responses in different parts of the cognitive control circuit to instructions, triggers, and food cues, as also is shown in (c).

purposes, Figure 10.2a depicts the format for one such task, the flanker task, which has been used extensively (Nigg, 2007; Geburek *et al.*, 2013). As shown in Figure 10.2a, subjects typically choose one of two responses that are signaled by task stimuli, such as a right-hand or left-hand button press, as indicated by rightward- or leftward-pointing arrows in Figure 10.2a. Difficulty can be adjusted on this task by changing the appearance of arrow targets. For example, on some task trials, target features can be degraded, by making the arrow appear blurry, or a target stimulus can be surrounded by distracters, such as a rightward-pointing target arrow appearing amidst a number of other leftward-pointing arrows. Figure 10.2a presents such a stimulus pattern, with a degraded rightward arrow surrounded by five darker leftward-pointing arrows.

Neural circuit responding has been precisely charted for two specific behaviors that occur on the flanker and similar tasks. One represents the correct execution of a difficult response, such as pushing a right-hand button to a rightward-pointing blurry target arrow in Figure 10.2a that appears among multiple, clear and bright leftward-pointing distracter arrows. Such difficult responses are said to require engagement of cognitive control to minimize probability of errant responding. Another such behavior represents the response to an error, such as a left-hand button response to the trial in Figure 10.2a mentioned earlier,

necessitating a right-hand response. Here, cognitive control initiates a series of behavioral adjustments. In both instances, such behaviors represent the typical targets of systems neuroscience research that maps changes in components of neural circuits that unfold during these events.

Linking the behavior to clinical questions

Systems neuroscience research begins to become clinically relevant when it links precisely delineated behaviors, observed in the laboratory, to clinically relevant behaviors, observed in the world. For cognitive control, research on attention deficit hyperactivity disorder (ADHD) and obsessive compulsive disorder (OCD) demonstrates potential clinical relevance. Both disorders exhibit signs of perturbed cognitive control, as do many other mental illnesses (Carter & Barch, 2007; Hajcak *et al.*, 2008; Geburek *et al.*, 2013), potentially arising from shared involvement of cognitive control deficits (Marsh *et al.*, 2009). Interest on cognitive control research in ADHD and OCD follows from the observation that these two highly comorbid syndromes (Peterson *et al.*, 2001) manifest discrepant signs of cognitive-control perturbations. Thus, ADHD involves reduced cognitive control (Nigg, 2007; Geburek *et al.*, 2013), whereas OCD involves the opposite (Hajcak *et al.*, 2008). Additional information concerning these disorders can be found in Chapters 55 and 61.

Examining the neural circuitry supporting the behavior

While many tasks have been linked to pediatric mental illness, research on cognitive control delineates the underlying neural architecture with particular clarity. Much of this work relies on brain imaging studies in adults and invasive studies in nonhuman primates to show that cognitive control is mediated by a neural circuit connecting four principal structures: the medial prefrontal cortex (mPFC) encompassing the anterior cingulate gyrus, the dorsolateral PFC (DLPFC), the basal ganglia, and the dopaminergic neurons of the ventral tegmental area (VTA) (Schultz, 2001; Cohen *et al.*, 2004; Corbetta *et al.*, 2008). Figure 10.2a also illustrates the architecture of this circuit, where the DLPFC, basal ganglia, and anterior cingulate all are labeled. Moreover, the rudimentary functions of these individual components also have been delineated, though some controversy remains concerning the precise details. The DLPFC is thought to represent stimulus-action rules (Miller & Cohen, 2001), modulating activity throughout the circuit based on these representations, whereas the VTA is thought to generate a prediction error signal, which can train this circuit over time, interacting with the mPFC and the basal ganglia (Schultz, 2001).

Figure 10.2c depicts relevant research. Work on VTA function in monkeys is particularly elegant, where the VTA has been shown to respond to errors in a way that suggests representation of error signaling. Work in rodents extends these studies by further implicating the dopaminergic system in error signaling. Taken together, studies in rodents and nonhuman primates delineate effects on cognitive control with increasing depth and precision, proceeding to the molecular level. For example, the effects of genetic manipulations have been examined (Barnes *et al.*, 2011), which has allowed research in humans to link variations in dopamine genes to variations in brain function and behavior.

Through imaging and electrophysiology, research maps neural correlates of cognitive control perturbations in ADHD and OCD. In both disorders, signs of dysfunction have been detected in mPFC, DLPFC, and the basal ganglia (Hajcak *et al.*, 2008; Cortese *et al.*, 2012; de Wit *et al.*, 2012; Geburek *et al.*, 2013), which are thought also to involve dopaminergic deficits (Barnes *et al.*, 2011). For this chapter, the most relevant findings map differences between ADHD and OCD. In ADHD, the findings suggest a degraded representation of error signals. This is illustrated in research on error-related negativity (ERN), as is also illustrated in Figure 10.2 and appearing in panel 2b. ERN reflects the rapid propagation of a brain signal that occurs in the earliest stage of error commission, before an individual has awareness of the error. This is thought to arise from VTA-to-mPFC signaling (Cohen *et al.*, 2004). In ADHD, reduced error representation manifests for the ERN. In OCD, the opposite manifests, with signs of enhanced ERN.

Extending the current literature

Clearly, this work differentiating ADHD and OCD represents progress, but even greater potential exists for future advances. In this chapter, the four examples illustrate four possible future advances. While each example offers promise for addressing many questions, for illustrative purposes, one specific promising avenue is discussed in each example.

Research on cognitive control shows particular promise in addressing questions on the origins of comorbidity. How can we understand such comorbidity? Despite apparent clinical dissimilarity, does observed comorbidity actually reflect mislabeling of one core, underlying syndrome as two distinct entities? Alternatively, does comorbidity arise from distinct complications of a shared risk factor that ultimately produces over time two distinct syndromes? Finally, is the relationship between the two phenotypes an epiphenomenon, arising due to a superficial resemblance of two syndromes that in reality share very little? These are questions for which systems neuroscience ultimately might provide answers.

In the knowledge of brain–behavior relationships, techniques may advance to the point where neural measures can precisely quantify cognitive control functions in children, using the next generation of measure similar to the ERN. As invasive studies in animals continue to elucidate the causal relationships between brain function and behavior, this knowledge will inform understandings of brain–behavior relationships in children, as quantified with this next generation of measures. The unique patterns currently observed in ADHD and OCD may be increasingly understood, to the point where they will be shown to represent distinct malfunctions. Such a demonstration

will require longitudinal research that charts in tandem changes in brain function and clinical expression.

This could generate findings that resemble those in work on the molecular architecture of cancer, where clinically similar scenarios reflect distinct pathophysiology. Here, distinct types of cancer are identified on the basis of core features of underlying organ system function and genetics. On the other hand, the next generation of cognitive control measures may reveal the unique patterns in ADHD and OCD to reflect strongly shared features, to the point where the two disorders represent alternative manifestations of one process. In this case, distinct late-stage disturbances in the underlying neural architectures would give rise to unique clinical presentation. As brain imaging and electrophysiologic measures advance, these alternative possibilities one day will be adjudicated, allowing clinicians to further subclassify clinical presentations with measures that precisely map pathophysiology.

Fear

Defining specific behaviors

Research on fear shares many features with research on cognitive control. Thus, in both areas, cross-species research maps the underlying neural architecture of specific behaviors that have been conserved across evolution. Perhaps more strongly than in many other areas, this is demonstrated by the remarkable cross-species conservation of brain–behavior relationships as they manifest in fear-related behavior (LeDoux, 2000; Phelps & LeDoux, 2005). Such conservation allows translation of conclusions in one species to another. Moreover, both research on cognitive control and fear target relatively narrow behaviors. However, in other respects, the nature of these behaviors is quite different. Research on cognitive control typically uses difficult motor tasks, whereas applications in research on fear typically expose children to mildly threatening stimuli, such as loud sounds or pictures of angry faces. Some of the most promising research then has mapped responses in two neural circuits, as reflected in two sets of behaviors, illustrated in Figure 10.3.

One set uses fear conditioning, where a neutral conditioned stimulus (CS+) is paired with an aversive unconditioned stimulus (UCS), as depicted in Figure 10.3a, in rodents on the left and humans on the right. In this scenario, children acquire fear of the CS+, as indexed by self-report, behavior, and physiology (Pine *et al.*, 2009). Such fear also can be extinguished by repeatedly presenting the CS+ after conditioning in the absence of the UCS (Quirk & Mueller 2008). The responses expressed by children on these tasks resemble those exhibited by adults and by various other organisms, exposed to comparable procedures. These experiments quantify aspects of learning, where systems neuroscience deeply maps the relevant circuitry.

The second set examines how aversive stimuli capture attention, as illustrated in Figure 10.3b. Because the primate brain is "capacity limited," attention facilitates appropriate evaluation

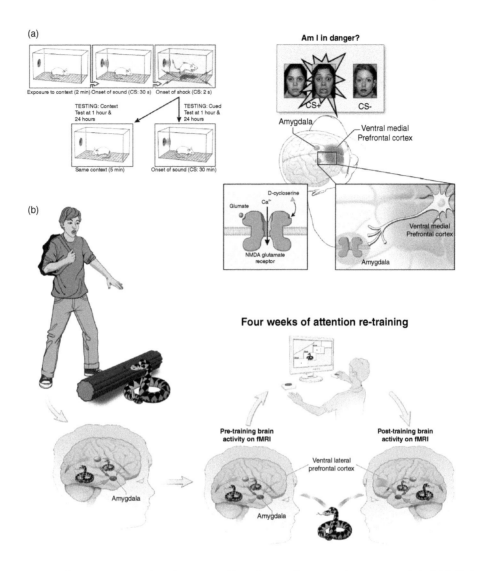

Figure 10.3 Two aspects of research on anxiety that inform therapeutics. (a) Work on conditioning and extinction, with the left half of the figure showing a fear conditioning experiment in rodents and the right half showing circuitry that is thought to be engaged in humans, during extinction. This shows the specific connection between the prefrontal cortex and the amygdala. This includes a depiction of the location where D-cycloserine stimulates the NMDA receptor, which may facilitate extinction and clinical response to cognitive behavioral therapy. (b) Work on attention orienting, as occurs when a threat, such as a snake under a log, is encountered. The circuitry engaged during attention orienting also is shown, as is an apparatus that might be used to provide attention retraining and induce changes in this circuitry.

of the environment by appropriately allocating the brain's limited neural resources (Corbetta *et al.*, 2008). Aversive stimuli receive priority for processing, eliciting attention orienting (LeDoux, 2000; Bar-Haim *et al.*, 2007). This attention response can be quantified using many tasks; one of the most frequently employed procedure uses the "dot-probe" task to present children with two stimuli, before quantifying attention allocation based on eye movements or reaction times. As with conditioning, the relevant circuitry has been mapped with great precision (Pine *et al.*, 2009).

For both areas, many findings extend research in basic science to the clinic by using measures of peripheral physiology, as reviewed in separate chapters on disorder-specific

pathophysiology. For example, considerable research implicates perturbed hypothalamic-pituitary-adrenal (HPA) axis function in both depressive and trauma-related disorders, as reviewed in the chapters on these conditions. Similarly, other research examines relationships between anxiety and measures of autonomic function, as can be captured through assessments of heart rate or skin conductance. Such research emphasizes the need to consider relationships that both brain and mind show with these and other measures of bodily function, as they typically are quantified through measures of peripheral physiology.

Nevertheless, recent systems neuroscience research on psychopathology more frequently relies on brain imaging measures as opposed to such HPA-axis-related or autonomic measures. This is because the most frequently used HPA axis and autonomic physiology measures exhibit relatively weak and inconsistent associations with measures of psychopathology. Some suggest that this reflects the fact that peripheral measures of physiology are influenced by many factors outside of central nervous system function, though work does continue to advance the field using peripheral markers in some areas (Staufenbiel *et al.*, 2013). These suggestions in turn generate interest in acquiring more direct measures of central nervous system function through brain imaging, with the hope of demonstrating stronger relationships between clinical profiles and biological indices.

Behavior, clinical questions, and neural circuitry

Considerable research has studied fear conditioning and extinction in healthy and anxious individuals, as summarized in meta-analysis (Lissek *et al.*, 2005). The ability to acquire fear actually appears similar in children, adolescents, and adults with or without anxiety disorders. The neural architecture of this ability also has been precisely delineated, both in rodents and primates (LeDoux, 2000; Phelps, 2006). This requires changes in a neural circuit encompassing the amygdala, a medial temporal lobe collection of nuclei. Imaging studies also implicate the amygdala in conditioning among children, much as they have done in adults (Lau *et al.*, 2011). While no imaging studies have compared amygdala function in anxious and healthy children during conditioning, one would expect intact amygdala function on conditioning tasks in anxious children, based on data from other conditioning studies. This contrasts with work on amygdala response to innate dangers, where anxious children show enhanced responses relative to healthy children (Beesdo *et al.*, 2009; Pine *et al.*, 2009). Such findings demonstrate the context specificity of amygdala dysfunction in pediatric mental disorders. This dysfunction only manifests in particular contexts, complicating attempts to chart brain–behavior associations.

Conditioning is probably intact in most anxiety disorder patients, but anxious and healthy individuals do have a number of difficulties in other aspects of fear learning. Specifically, anxious individuals more consistently differ from nonanxious individuals in their ability to rapidly learn to make subtle distinction when classifying the boundaries that separate various, similar-appearing threat-related and safe stimuli (Britton *et al.*, 2011). Such distinctions must be made in extinction tasks, where a previously conditioned CS+ stimulus is repeatedly presented in the absence of the UCS, which leads a subject to reclassify the previously dangerous CS+ as an ambiguous threat, one that used to be dangerous but is now safe. This requires a more subtle form of learning than occurs during conditioning, and such learning engages a neural circuit that connects the medial PFC (mPFC) to the basolateral nucleus of the amygdala (Quirk & Mueller, 2008); there is some evidence of perturbed extinction and perturbed mPFC-to-amygdala circuitry dysfunction in anxiety disorders (Greenberg *et al.*, 2013).

While considerable work examines conditioning, an even broader series examines attention orienting (Bar-Haim *et al.*, 2007). In fact, differences in orienting probably represent the most consistent information-processing finding in anxiety. Patients with anxiety disorders consistently show a tendency to orient more strongly to threats than healthy individuals, and this tendency manifests tremendously quickly, even to threats that are presented so rapidly that their occurrence cannot be reported by the patient. Such attention biases have been shown to reflect dysfunction in the same underlying neural circuit that supports attention orienting in the primate (Pine *et al.*, 2009). This circuit connects the amygdala, which is engaged immediately by threat presentation, to the insula and ventrolateral expanse of the PFC, which is engaged more slowly to support attention deployment after threat detection.

Extending the current literature

Research on cognitive control illustrates how systems neuroscience principles inform comorbidity. Research on fear informs therapeutics.

Research on extinction charts the relevant underlying molecular architecture, as depicted in Figure 10.1. This work shows that various chemical manipulations can enhance a rodent's ability to learn the boundaries that separate threat and safety signals. From the clinical perspective, interest has focused on one particular compound, d-cycloserine (DCS), which is an antibiotic that also has effects on the glycine-sensitive site on the N-methyl-D-aspartate (NMDA) glutamate receptor. If patients with anxiety disorders have deficient capacity to learn threat–safety boundaries, this deficit may reflect deficient functioning of the mPFC-amygdala circuit, which relies on the NMDA receptor to facilitate communication in the circuit to support extinction learning. Moreover, if DCS increases functioning in this circuit, specifically at times when threat–safety boundaries are being learned, DCS administered briefly, during exposure therapy sessions that occur in cognitive behavioral therapy (CBT), might enhance the patient's response to CBT. This idea is presented pictorially in Figure 10.3a. Thus, this figure shows the connections between the human amygdala and ventromedial prefrontal cortex that would be engaged by an extinguished CS+, in the form of a picture of a woman. This figure also shows the microscopic connection between a neuron in this frontal region, which synapses in the amygdala, where an NMDA receptor is depicted, with a binding cite for DCS. Of note, other work has pursued different approaches, using knowledge about fear extinction to derive other pharmacological approaches or even nonpharmacological means for diminishing fear through effects on underlying brain circuitry (Pine *et al.*, 2009; Schiller *et al.*, 2010; Agren *et al.*, 2012). While these other approaches have been studied in less depth than approaches relying on DCS, the overall series of research in humans produces novel ideas about treatment for pediatric anxiety disorders.

Findings from randomized controlled trials in both pediatric and adult anxiety disorders provide some preliminary support for the idea that DCS exerts beneficial clinical effects in patients undergoing CBT (Ressler *et al.*, 2004; Storch *et al.*, 2010). That is, in at least a few trials, patients randomized to CBT with DCS show more robust responses than patients randomized to CBT with placebo. Nevertheless, findings are far from clear. As a result, it will be many years before DCS or any similar form of treatment can be recommended for routine clinical use. Regardless, the mode of thinking that led to research on DCS provides an avenue for many other treatments. Such treatments emerge not from the serendipitous clinical observations that have produced most treatments for mental disorders but rather from an understanding of pathophysiology.

In a similar fashion, research on attention orienting also generates novel ideas for new therapies. These ideas extend observations on the underlying neural circuitry that sustains threat-related attention biases in pediatric anxiety disorders. Such biases are thought to reflect perturbed function in a circuit connecting the amygdala to the insula and adjacent ventrolateral PFC. Again, this idea also is presented pictorially in Figure 10.3, specifically in the lower part of the figure as Figure 10.3b. Thus, while extinction involves amygdala-medial-PFC connections shown in Figure 10.3a, attention involves amygdala-lateral-PFC connections shown in Figure 10.3b, demonstrating the key principles of systems neuroscience that link specific behaviors to particular brain circuits (Pine *et al.* 2009). For biases in attention, this perturbed function is considered to be "implicit," because it is expressed very rapidly, so rapidly that patients cannot describe the nature of their attention dysfunction to a therapist; perturbed function even manifests to threats that are presented too rapidly to be reported. In Figure 10.3b, natural threats, such as snakes or angry faces of peers, are thought to very rapidly engage amygdala-based circuitry, more rapidly than in circuitry in the ventral part of the cerebral cortex. This creates the implicit bias in threat-attention interactions. Neuroscience research shows that such implicit biases can be changed more easily and strongly through repeated training than through declarative instruction. Thus, CBT targets biases in attention by instructing patients on the nature of their underlying biases in attention toward threats. Such attempts to change attention in anxious children may be augmented through implicit training procedures that address the underlying rapidly deployed perturbations in brain circuitry.

Attention bias modification training (ABMT) represents an attempt to provide such implicit training of attention. This treatment targets rapidly deployed implicit perturbations through repeated, computer-based training. ABMT can use various procedures, but the most common application repeatedly exposes children to the same types of stimuli used in the dot-probe task, where threat and neutral stimuli are presented side by side. However, in active ABMT, probes repeatedly appear behind the neutral stimulus, which implicitly teaches children to automatically and reflexively avert their attention

for threats. Considerable research uses this technique to reduce threat biases in adult and pediatric anxiety disorders, where preliminary evidence of efficacy has emerged (Hakamata *et al.*, 2010; Eldar *et al.*, 2012). Other work uses alternative ABMT procedures that teach children to attend toward positive stimuli, extending other work linking an avoidance of positive stimuli to anxiety (Waters *et al.*, 2013). Much as in work on extinction and DCS, the major insight to emerge from research on ABMT and threat-related attention bias relates to the process of scientific discovery. The field still remains many years removed from a standard ABMT-like treatment that can be widely applied. However, the process of discovery illustrates a path for future treatment discovery. This path involves the delineation of an underlying behavioral correlate and its neural underpinnings, which then provides knowledge on the most appropriate means for altering the behavior.

Attachment and affiliation

Defining specific behaviors

The third example, attachment and affiliation, considers the neural underpinnings of other specific behaviors that can be isolated and quantified in the laboratory. Work in this area is relatively unique, when contrasted with research on cognitive control or fear. For these first two constructs, the behaviors elicited in humans resemble quite closely the behaviors elicited in rodents and nonhuman primates (see Chapter 6). In fact, many of the paradigms readily translate across species. However, for attachment and affiliation, the differences in rodents, nonhuman primates, and humans force the relevant systems neuroscience research to adopt unique methods in each species. This illustrates a key puzzle that must be solved in all cross-species systems neuroscience research: questions must be addressed in each species at an appropriate level of abstraction, so that species-typical behaviors can be studied in a form that is still applicable to other species. This puzzle has proved relatively easy to solve in work on cognitive control and fear but has been more difficult in research on attachment, given cross-species diversity in attachment and other social behaviors.

Fundamental research on attachment and affiliation probes the behaviors from mothers and their infants that serve to maintain the bond between the two individuals (Carter, 1998). This includes a set of studies targeting behaviors exhibited by the mother and by the offspring that support maintenance of a social bond. Work that appears particularly clinically relevant targets the ways in which mothers and infants respond to particular cues that each partner of the dyad presents to the other. For example, considerable work examines the degree to which the sight, smell, and sound of the infant elicits specific behaviors from the mother, many of which serve to maintain attention orientation and approach behaviors, keeping the infant in close contact with the mother. Similarly, other work examines the unique response elicited in the infant from cues associated with the mother, sometimes presented to the infant within hours of birth. Both sets of studies demonstrate the priority that infant and mother cues receive, when they are presented to each pair of the dyad, amidst a collection of other cues. Recent interest specifically explores the ways in which primate infants respond to their mothers with imitative behaviors, initial signs of emerging processes that might ground future social development (Paukner *et al.*, 2011).

Insights for human attachment behaviors have emerged from cross-species research. This work shows tremendous diversity in the way in which mothers and infants respond to each other, in terms of the specific behaviors and the timing of their expression. Particularly important work compares behaviors among species of voles, rodents common throughout the United States, which generally exhibit great cross-species similarity in physiology and behavior (Insel *et al.* 1993; Carter, 1998). However, two distinct species of vole exhibit markedly different patterns of attachment behavior, emerging against a background of otherwise great similarity in behavior and physiology. In one species, the prairie vole, attachment occurs in a context of rich social behavior among adult male and female voles, which typically are highly social. This pattern contrasts with expression of attachment in the montane vole, where attachment represents an aberration, involving a time when infant voles are raised by their mothers, who typically experience a relatively isolated social existence, including minimal contact with males. Figure 10.4a illustrates these two rodent species, represented as the solitary-appearing montane vole and the social prairie vole. These precise differences in rodent behavior have been used to stimulate other work that has gone on to delineate the underlying neural architecture of attachment in nonhuman primates and humans. This too is illustrated in the distribution of oxytocin receptors in these two species of voles, as is also illustrated in Figure 10.4a. Changes in levels of oxytocin influence breastfeeding and other aspects of maternal behavior. As a result, research linking attachment to central nervous system distributions of this chemical is consistent with the known relationship between oxytocin and maternal behavior. While research on oxytocin focuses most closely on attachment behaviors, this chemical is also relevant to fear-related behaviors described in other sections of this chapter. This may reflect the fact that oxytocin-releasing cells in the brain are in direct contact with hypothalamic neurons that release important regulators of the HPA axis (Feldman, 2012).

Linking the behavior to clinical questions

Like cognitive control, perturbed attachment behavior has been linked to an array of developmental psychopathologies. In fact, a class of mental disorders has been labeled as "attachment disorders" based on the clinical disruption in the parent–child bond. As with the research on cognitive control and fear, studies of attachment behavior conform to a systems neuroscience approach when they adopt a particular approach. This approach must be grounded in precise understandings of brain–behavior

associations, as reflected in functions of dedicated, precisely defined neural circuits. In clinically focused work in child psychiatry and psychology, research on autism spectrum disorders (ASDs) provides one compelling application of systems neuroscience research on attachment. ASDs are recognized as prototypical developmental disorders, which manifest as perturbed maturation of social behavior (see Chapter 51).

A range of paradigms have been used to quantify the social deficits of children with ASDs, with a particularly large number of studies quantifying the responses to faces (Cicchetti *et al.*, 2011). A particularly compelling line of work focuses on attention allocation (Kaiser *et al.*, 2010). Since ASDs are thought to arise within the first year of life, great interest has focused on extending research on social processing to the earliest phases of social development. Here, the best understood process is attachment and affiliation, generating great interest in charting the evolution of attachment behavior in ASDs. Clearly, precise quantification of attachment behaviors in humans is difficult, particularly using the most sophisticated technologies, such as infrared eye-movement cameras. As a result, studies of ASDs have only begun to quantify attachment during infancy with state-of-the-art neuroscience methodology. Nevertheless, emerging work has begun to link disrupted attachment behavior in ASDs to early-life perturbations in attention. This includes a particularly intriguing series of studies examining imitation in ASDs.

Examining the neural circuitry supporting the behavior

Considerable work delineates the underlying neural circuitry that accounts for the unique attachment behaviors in the prairie and montane vole, as depicted in Figure 10.4a. This work illustrates many of the advantages of animal models, where a precise mapping of brain–behavior associations can be achieved in a way that is not approachable with humans. In voles, species typical attachment behaviors reflect aspects of functioning in dopamine systems and in associated components of the ventral striatum mediating reward behaviors for both social and nonsocial stimuli. Moreover, changes in these behaviors following the birth of the infant are mediated by changes in oxytocin, a peptide in hypothalamic neurons that stimulates oxytocin receptors in the striatum.

Research tightly linking oxytocin to attachment behavior in voles has stimulated an extensive series of studies examining the effects of oxytocin in humans. This work suggests that oxytocin administration facilitates a number of social behaviors in humans, as it does in various rodents and nonhuman primates (Meyer-Lindenberg & Tost, 2012). This work is consistent with the long-known role of oxytocin in the facilitation of mother–infant attachment. Controversy remains concerning the nature of these effects in adults, be they related specifically to attachment or to related behaviors, such as dominance. Moreover, based on results from brain imaging studies, interest has also grown in defining the underlying neural circuit through

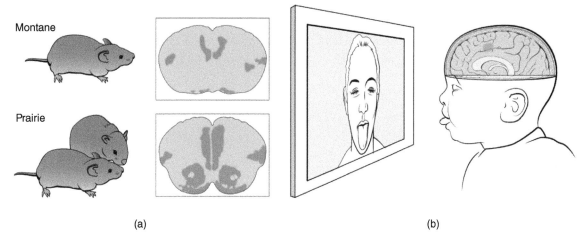

Figure 10.4 Work on aspects of attachment. (a) Two species of voles and associated brain slices depicting differences in the brain chemistry. (b) A task that might be used to engage the mirror neuron system of a child. Using evoked potentials, activity in the medial prefrontal cortex could be mapped, as also shown in (b) in the child's brain activation map.

which such effects unfold in humans. Data in voles focus such interest on the striatum. However, imaging work also implicates the amygdala and cingulate gyrus in oxytocin effects on human attachment behavior (Meyer-Lindenberg & Tost, 2012). This is consistent with a wealth of other research implicating these structures in a range of mammalian social behaviors, including mother–infant attachment.

Extending the current literature

Research on attachment could ultimately generate insights on comorbidity and therapeutics, much like research on cognitive control and fear. In fact, ongoing work considers the degree to which oxytocin might address underlying social deficits in ASDs, demonstrating potential treatment relevance. However, for illustrative purposes, research on attachment is described in a way that might address a distinct set of clinical questions, related to generating insights on risk. Currently, major questions exist on factors that might identify one or another infant as facing a high risk for ASDs. Available imaging data suggest that the underlying neural processes that give rise to ASDs begin to unfold in the first year of life, before a clear diagnosis of ASD can be made solely on clinical grounds (Wolff et al., 2012). As such, understanding the earliest signs of aberrant social development, through careful assessment of the parent–child attachment relationship and associated brain function, may generate insights on risk prediction. Of note, ASDs are recognized to be strongly genetic conditions. Thus, any attempt to identify risk expression in attachment behavior should not be misconstrued as an attempt to identify the causes of autism, which are unlikely to involve a primary causal role for parental behavior. Rather, observations of perturbed attachment might signal the underlying presence of perturbed brain development in the child, instantiated in the brain systems that support social behavior. This shows that the causes of ASDs should be sought in an understanding of neurodevelopment as opposed to parental behavior.

Some of the more exciting research on early ASD risk examines aspects of imitation (Marshall & Shipley 2009; Cicchetti et al., 2011; Marshall & Meltzoff, 2011). Virtually within days of being born, infants show an amazing capacity to imitate the actions of others, a capacity that vanishes after a short period of infant development. Figure 10.4b presents a type of experiment where such imitative behavior can be elicited, by showing an infant a video of an adult protruding the tongue. Interestingly, this ability was once thought to be unique to humans, but emerging evidence suggests that it is shared by at least some other primates. The underlying neural architecture that supports imitative behavior is thought to involve a unique class of neurons, the so-called mirror neuron system, which supports a circuit encompassing the insula cortex as well as the cingulate, a region strongly implicated in social behavior. Technology is emerging for assessing the integrity of the human mirror-neuron system, and there is some preliminary evidence implicating dysfunction in this system in ASDs (Enticott et al., 2012). Typically, in infants, this technology relies on evoked potentials, similar to the technology used to assess the ERN, as discussed in the section on cognitive control. The evoked potential reflecting mirror-neuron function also localizes to the medial area of the brain, as is depicted in Figure 10.4b. Most importantly, it may be possible to monitor the integrity of this system in human infants, before clinical signs of ASDs appear obvious. This would provide a readily quantifiable index of underlying functions in neural systems that might support attachment. As such, research using these methods could generate insights on the earliest signs of aberrant social development, as it manifests in the attachment relationship. Thus, research on attachment in ASDs may answer questions on risk prediction that cannot be addressed with currently available clinical tools.

Brain development

Defining a specific behavior in a clinical context

For this final example, behavior that is quite different from the behaviors addressed in systems neuroscience research on cognitive control, fear, or attachment is presented. For each of these first three examples, research that directly extends results from invasive studies in animal models is described. In each area, specific behaviors are defined, to be quantified in children, after the underlying neural architecture for similar behaviors already has been delineated in rodents, nonhuman primates, and adult humans. Studies in human children thereby extend a wealth of research first conducted in other organisms.

For this final example, the weight of the evidence emerges as much from brain imaging research directly with human children as it does from invasive studies in animal models. As such, research in children informs an expansion of basic research that might map the underlying neural factors that give rise to clinical observations. Moreover, the initial three examples also begin with very precisely defined behaviors already studied in basic research, as is typical in much of systems neuroscience. This final example examines a set of human behaviors that have been charted far less precisely, to illustrate the dual direction in which systems neuroscience can flow. Clearly, major insights have emerged in studies with children that extend findings in animals, as illustrated by the first three examples. However, this final example illustrates the insights that can also emerge in studies with animals that extend findings with children.

Chapter 55 describes the key behaviors of ADHD, one of which is the increased level of activity reported by observers of children with the condition, relative to their healthy peers. Not only do observers report children with ADHD to appear hyperactive, but various objective monitoring devices demonstrate differences in the motor behavior of healthy and ADHD children. Thus, for this final example, neural correlates of ADHD are described, as quantified in mean levels of recorded motor activity. With development, this aspect of ADHD has been shown to change, much as overall levels of activity also change from childhood through adolescence in typically developing children. Overall levels of activity reduce into adolescence, and reports of problematic hyperactivity symptoms in children with ADHD also become less common as these patients develop toward adulthood.

These observations, coupled with similar observations for other aspects of ADHD, have supported a view of the condition as a neurodevelopmental disorder. That is, children with ADHD might exhibit a slowing of the developmental processes that occur in healthy children to support brain development. Due to such slowing, children with ADHD may exhibit behaviors that are maladaptive largely because they are inappropriate for the child of a particular age, even though they may be appropriate for a child of a younger age. This view raises a number of corresponding questions. Does ADHD represent a manifestation of abnormal development, *per se*, or rather, is the condition better characterized as a mere slowing of an otherwise normal developmental process? If ADHD merely represents slowed but normal development, are there factors that predict future acceleration in the pace of development, and might interventions speed this process? Alternatively, if ADHD results from abnormal rather than slowed development, does normalization of hyperactivity represent some form of atypical compensatory response, played out in aspects of brain development? For all of these questions, the neurodevelopmental perspective seeks answers in direct measures of brain development.

Examining the neural circuitry supporting the behavior

With refinements in magnetic resonance imaging (MRI) technology, clinical neuroscience began to widely apply a unique tool in the early 1990s that provided precise quantification of brain structure. While this impacted on systems neuroscience research in broad ways, the impact on child mental health research has been profound. Because MRI is safe and noninvasive, a series of longitudinal MRI investigations began to chart aspects of typical and atypical development. This work has accelerated at an amazing pace, to the point where MRI studies have examined development in thousands of children, assessed with tens of thousands of scans, conducted on the same child passing through various phases of development. Clearly, this research generates rich insights on a range of developmental questions. It has been particularly informative for understandings of ADHD.

Three major conclusions have emerged from quantitative MRI research on typical and atypical development, including ADHD. First, this research shows that brain development is an amazingly complex and slow process. Unique patterns of linear and nonlinear increases and decreases unfold in the brain's architecture. These play out over decades, lasting into the 20s. This supports the now established view of development as a process that extends relatively late in life, a view also reflected in neuroscience data generated prior to widespread application of MRI. Nevertheless, when the first MRI studies began to demonstrate these patterns, the findings were greeted with some level of surprise. Second, cross-sectional associations have been demonstrated between various clinical factors and brain structure. However, few well-replicated findings emerge in large samples, and, when they do, the magnitude of the association is not large. Thus, in the individual child with ADHD or another mental disorder, otherwise free of neurological illness, the measurement of brain structure at any one point in time is unlikely to provide clinically useful information. Finally, longitudinal data uniquely extend data contained in cross-sectional comparisons, even ones made among children of different ages. The defining characteristics of atypical brain development appear less strongly related to brain structure appearance at any specific point in time than to the overall trajectory of changes in the brain, as they play out during development.

Longitudinal research on brain morphometry in ADHD demonstrates a pattern of findings reminiscent of data on developmental changes in hyperactivity (Shaw *et al.*, 2007; Shaw *et al.*, 2010; Shaw *et al.*, 2011). That is, while longitudinal findings are only beginning to appear, thus far, the overall patterns generally appear similar to the pattern that is observed in typical development. Here, brain development in ADHD appears to be a delayed version of brain development for typically developing children. Age-related changes in ADHD occur on a delayed timescale, months after the corresponding changes already have occurred in healthy age-matched peers. This suggests that at least some forms of ADHD may in fact be viewed as a disorder of slowed but normal brain development. Thus, in this group, remission of symptoms might reflect normalization of development. Other forms of ADHD, in contrast, which persist throughout maturation, may exhibit no such slowed but normal patterns of brain development. Finally, considerable work remains to be done; few longitudinal studies exist; and the findings appear relatively complex, in that children with ADHD represent a heterogeneous group. Some children may show typical but slowed patterns of behavioral and brain development, whereas others may show different patterns (Shaw *et al.*, 2006). As such, ADHD likely encompasses multiple disorders, from a systems neuroscience perspective. This may include some variants that represent exaggerated variations on normal development and other variants that represent more distinct expressions of atypical brain development. In the future, these variants may be defined on the basis of measures of brain development.

Extending the current literature

Current findings on brain development and ADHD can be extended through two avenues. One avenue involves an increasingly deep focus on brain–behavior associations in children followed longitudinally. The other avenue involves an increasingly deep focus in experimental animals on the factors that ultimately give rise to patterns of brain development and changes in activity, observed in ADHD and typically developing children. Here again, unlike the first three examples, for research on brain development, findings in children might stimulate a wave of research in experimental animals.

In terms of the first avenue, this will involve an extension of ongoing research. For example, future studies are likely to adopt a continued pursuit of longitudinal research that tracks in tandem changes in brain development and symptomatic expressions of ADHD. These studies also likely will acquire increasingly precise measures of brain function and behavior. This might include both the types of behavior collected in current studies, which focus largely on clinical profiles, as well as future studies that augment these clinical indices with measures more closely linked to systems neuroscience. For example, future studies might rely on paradigms such as the flanker task or other cognitive-control measures. This will allow longitudinal research on clinical-morphometry associations to be referenced more tightly to existing systems neuroscience research. Such a trend is already emerging in existing ADHD morphometry studies, which have begun to augment data on clinical profiles and brain anatomy with data on genetics and other factors known to influence behavior through effects on brain development.

The second avenue will involve increasingly deep research in animals. As discussed in the chapter on brain imaging, the factors that produce changes in brain morphometry observed on MRI remain incompletely understood. Available basic research suggests that the findings are unlikely to reflect neurogenesis or cell death but rather are more likely to arise from refinements in dendritic arborization and axon morphology, including myelinization. However, considerable more work is needed before the underlying brain processes that produce brain–behavior associations in ADHD become clinically relevant. In particular, the pattern of change in morphometry parallels the pattern of change in mean levels of activity in children with ADHD. However, it remains unclear the way in which these two sets of changes relate. This is because basic research has not attempted to reveal the mechanisms that produce these seemingly related trajectories. Invasive, experimental studies in animal models could begin to untangle the underlying neural processes that produce these parallel developmental patterns. Much as in research on extinction, as these processes become increasingly well understood, they will generate novel, clinically relevant ideas potentially pertinent to both outcome prediction and novel therapeutics.

Conclusion

This chapter attempts to accomplish three central goals. First, an introduction to systems neuroscience research is provided, emphasizing the multidisciplinary and newly emerging aspects of the area. Second, the relevance of systems neuroscience for child psychiatry and psychology is reviewed, considering the many other areas in this textbook that inform systems neuroscience thinking. Here the focus is on aspects of systems neuroscience that extend research in other domains, particularly brain imaging. Finally, four specific examples are provided to illustrate the range of clinically relevant questions that might be addressed through research in this area.

References

Agren, T. *et al.* (2012) Disruption of reconsolidation erases a fear memory trace in the human amygdala. *Science* **337** (6101), 1550–1552.

Bar-Haim, Y. *et al.* (2007) Threat-related attentional bias in anxious and nonanxious individuals: a meta-analytic study. *Psychological Bulletin* **133** (1), 1–24.

Barnes, J.J. *et al.* (2011) The molecular genetics of executive function: role of monoamine system genes. *Biological Psychiatry* **69** (12), e127–e143.

Beesdo, K. *et al.* (2009) Common and distinct amygdala-function perturbations in depressed vs anxious adolescents. *Archives of General Psychiatry* **66** (3), 275–285.

Britton, J.C. *et al.* (2011) Development of anxiety: the role of threat appraisal and fear learning. *Depression and Anxiety* **28** (1), 5–17.

Carter, C.S. (1998) Neuroendocrine perspectives on social attachment and love. *Psychoneuroendocrinology* **23** (8), 779–818.

Carter, C.S. (2005) Applying new approaches from cognitive neuroscience to enhance drug development for the treatment of impaired cognition in schizophrenia. *Schizophrenia Bulletin* **31** (4), 810–815.

Carter, C.S. (2006) Re-conceptualizing schizophrenia as a disorder of cognitive and emotional processing: a shot in the arm for translational research. *Biological Psychiatry* **60** (11), 1169–1170.

Carter, C.S. & Barch, D.M. (2007) Cognitive neuroscience-based approaches to measuring and improving treatment effects on cognition in schizophrenia: the CNTRICS initiative. *Schizophrenia Bulletin* **33** (5), 1131–1137.

Cicchetti, D.V. *et al.* (2011) From Bayes through marginal utility to effect sizes: a guide to understanding the clinical and statistical significance of the results of autism research findings. *Journal of Autism and Developmental Disorders* **41** (2), 168–174.

Cohen, J.D. *et al.* (2004) A systems-level perspective on attention and cognitive control: guided activation, adaptive gating, conflict monitoring, and exploitation versus exploration. In: *Cognitive Neuroscience of Attention.* (ed M.I. Posner), pp. 71–90. Guilford Press, New York, NY.

Corbetta, M. *et al.* (2008) The reorienting system of the human brain: from environment to theory of mind. *Neuron* **58** (3), 306–324.

Cortese, S. *et al.* (2012) Toward systems neuroscience of ADHD: a meta-analysis of 55 fMRI studies. *American Journal of Psychiatry* **169** (10), 1038–1055.

Deisseroth, K. (2012) Optogenetics and psychiatry: applications, challenges, and opportunities. *Biological Psychiatry* **71** (12), 1030–1032.

Eldar, S. *et al.* (2012) Attention bias modification treatment for pediatric anxiety disorders: a randomized controlled trial. *American Journal of Psychiatry* **169** (2), 213–220.

Enticott, P.G. *et al.* (2012) Mirror neuron activity associated with social impairments but not age in autism spectrum disorder. *Biological Psychiatry* **71** (5), 427–433.

Feldman, R. (2012) Oxytocin and social affiliation in humans. *Hormones and Behavior* **61** (3), 380–391.

Geburek, A.J. *et al.* (2013) Electrophysiological indices of error monitoring in juvenile and adult attention deficit hyperactivity disorder (ADHD)-A meta-analytic appraisal. *International Journal of Psychophysiology* **87** (3), 349–362.

Greenberg, T. *et al.* (2013) Ventromedial prefrontal cortex reactivity is altered in generalized anxiety disorder during fear generalization. *Depression and Anxiety* **30** (3), 242–250.

Hajcak, G. *et al.* (2008) Increased error-related brain activity in pediatric obsessive-compulsive disorder before and after treatment. *American Journal of Psychiatry* **165** (1), 116–123.

Hakamata, Y. *et al.* (2010) Attention bias modification treatment: a meta-analysis toward the establishment of novel treatment for anxiety. *Biological Psychiatry* **68** (11), 982–990.

Insel, T.R. *et al.* (1993) The role of neurohypophyseal peptides in the central mediation of complex social processes–evidence from comparative studies. *Regulatory Peptides* **45** (1–2), 127–131.

Kaiser, M.D. *et al.* (2010) Neural signatures of autism. *Proceedings of the National Academy of Sciences of the United States of America* **107** (49), 21223–21228.

Lau, J.Y. *et al.* (2011) Distinct neural signatures of threat learning in adolescents and adults. *Proceedings of the National Academy of Sciences of the United States of America* **108** (11), 4500–4505.

LeDoux, J.E. (2000) Emotion circuits in the brain. *Annual Review of Neuroscience* **23**, 155–184.

Lissek, S. *et al.* (2005) Classical fear conditioning in the anxiety disorders: a meta-analysis. *Behaviour Research and Therapy* **43** (11), 1391–424.

Marsh, R. *et al.* (2009) Functional disturbances within frontostriatal circuits across multiple childhood psychopathologies. *American Journal of Psychiatry* **166** (6), 664–674.

Marshall, P.J. & Meltzoff, A.N. (2011) Neural mirroring systems: exploring the EEG mu rhythm in human infancy. *Developmental Cognitive Neuroscience* **1** (2), 110–123.

Marshall, P.J. & Shipley, T.F. (2009) Event-related potentials to point-light displays of human actions in five-month-old infants. *Developmental Neuropsychology* **34** (3), 368–377.

Meyer-Lindenberg, A. & Tost, H. (2012) Neural mechanisms of social risk for psychiatric disorders. *Nature Neuroscience* **15** (5), 663–668.

Miller, E.K. & Cohen, J.D. (2001) An integrative theory of prefrontal cortex function. *Annual Review of Neuroscience* **24**, 167–202.

Nigg, J. (2007) *What Causes ADHD?* Guilford Press, New York.

Paukner, A. *et al.* (2011) Delayed imitation of lipsmacking gestures by infant rhesus macaques (Macaca mulatta). *PLoS One* **6** (12), e28848.

Peterson, B.S. *et al.* (2001) Prospective, longitudinal study of tic, obsessive-compulsive, and attention-deficit/hyperactivity disorders in an epidemiological sample. *Journal of the American Academy of Child and Adolescent Psychiatry* **40** (6), 685–695.

Phelps, E.A. (2006) Emotion and cognition: insights from studies of the human amygdala. *Annual Review of Psychology* **57**, 27–53.

Phelps, E.A. & LeDoux, J.E. (2005) Contributions of the amygdala to emotion processing: from animal models to human behavior. *Neuron* **48** (2), 175–187.

Pine, D.S. *et al.* (2009) Challenges in developing novel treatments for childhood disorders: lessons from research on anxiety. *Neuropsychopharmacology* **34** (1), 213–228.

Pine, D.S. *et al.* (2010) Imaging-genetics applications in child psychiatry. *Journal of the American Academy of Child and Adolescent Psychiatry* **49** (8), 772–782.

Quirk, G.J. & Mueller, D. (2008) Neural mechanisms of extinction learning and retrieval. *Neuropsychopharmacology* **33** (1), 56–72.

Ressler, K.J. *et al.* (2004) Cognitive enhancers as adjuncts to psychotherapy: use of D-cycloserine in phobic individuals to facilitate extinction of fear. *Archives of General Psychiatry* **61** (11), 1136–1144.

Schiller, D. *et al.* (2010) Preventing the return of fear in humans using reconsolidation update mechanisms. *Nature* **463** (7277), 49–53.

Schultz, W. (2001) Reward signaling by dopamine neurons. *Neuroscientist* **7** (4), 293–302.

Shaw, P. *et al.* (2006) Longitudinal mapping of cortical thickness and clinical outcome in children and adolescents with attention-deficit/hyperactivity disorder. *Archives of General Psychiatry* **63** (5), 540–549.

Shaw, P. *et al.* (2007) Attention-deficit/hyperactivity disorder is characterized by a delay in cortical maturation. *Proceedings of the National Academy of Sciences of the United States of America* **104** (49), 19649–19654.

Shaw, P. *et al.* (2010) Childhood psychiatric disorders as anomalies in neurodevelopmental trajectories. *Human Brain Mapping* **31** (6), 917–925.

Shaw, P. *et al.* (2011) Cortical development in typically developing children with symptoms of hyperactivity and impulsivity: support for a dimensional view of attention deficit hyperactivity disorder. *American Journal of Psychiatry* **168** (2), 143–151.

Staufenbiel, S.M. *et al.* (2013) Hair cortisol, stress exposure, and mental health in humans: a systematic review. *Psychoneuroendocrinology* **38** (8), 1220–1235.

Storch, E.A. *et al.* (2010) A preliminary study of D-cycloserine augmentation of cognitive-behavioral therapy in pediatric obsessive-compulsive disorder. *Biological Psychiatry* **68** (11), 1073–1076.

van Veen, V. *et al.* (2008) The neural and computational basis of controlled speed-accuracy tradeoff during task performance. *Journal of Cognitive Neuroscience* **20** (11), 1952–1965.

Waters, A.M. *et al.* (2013) Attention training towards positive stimuli in clinically anxious children. *Developmental Cognitive Neuroscience* **4**, 77–84.

de Wit, S.J. *et al.* (2012) Presupplementary motor area hyperactivity during response inhibition: a candidate endophenotype of obsessive-compulsive disorder. *American Journal of Psychiatry* **169** (10), 1100–1108.

Wolff, J.J. *et al.* (2012) Differences in white matter fiber tract development present from 6 to 24 months in infants with autism. *American Journal of Psychiatry* **169** (6), 589–600.

B: Neurobiology

CHAPTER 11

Neuroimaging in child psychiatry

Kevin Pelphrey, Brent Vander Wyk and Michael Crowley

Child Study Center, Yale University, New Haven, CT, USA

Introduction

Neuroimaging offers an opportunity to better understand psychiatric disorders via investigations of brain structure, function and/or molecular composition, and developmental change. In this chapter, we provide an overview of modern techniques that are currently used for studying the living and developing brain. We illustrate these neuroimaging methods with accessible examples of how the techniques have been used to advance our understanding of childhood psychiatric disorders. More details about specific findings can be found in the chapters devoted to specific disorders; here, we focus on the examples only long enough to bring the different neuroimaging methods to life. Finally, the chapter on systems neuroscience broadly outlines the way in which neuroimaging interfaces with neuroscience to delineate the neural correlates of developmental psychopathology. This provides a conceptual grounding for research on brain–behavior relationships, as can be quantified through imaging.

In its infancy, the study of brain function relied upon recordings of individual neurons grown in petri dishes, invasive electrodes placed in nonhuman animals, and neuropsychological studies of patients with circumscribed lesions. Several neuroimaging approaches, specifically functional magnetic resonance imaging (fMRI), electroencephalography (EEG), and functional near infrared spectroscopy (fNIRS), have emerged over the past 20 years as noninvasive methods by which we can reliably examine the function and structure of the developing human brain across the lifespan. The field can now utilize a "molecules-to-mind" approach, studying key phenomena across multiple levels of analysis including genes, brain, behavior, and the broader environmental context. These neuroimaging techniques are now routinely used to study healthy function, and dysfunction, of the brain during its maturation across development. An increasing proportion of the literature is dedicated to describing results from one neuroimaging method or another, and much of the remaining work is now interpreted in the context of what is known, or thought to be known, about brain function. More and more, those working in the proverbial "trenches" in the field of child and adolescent mental health are expected to be informed and critical consumers of this research.

As with any research or measurement approach, a well-conceptualized research question with clearly defined constructs and operational definitions of those constructs are crucial in maximizing the interpretability and validity of neuroimaging data. But beyond this basic requirement, neuroimaging methods require specialized training and a great deal of expertise to be executed properly. However, training in utilization and interpretation of these techniques and derivative data is not currently part of routine student education and is rare even in psychiatry residency programs. As such, these techniques are most often used by child psychiatrists and psychologists in the context of large multidisciplinary research teams, with associated logistical hurdles.

Two key concepts, *contrast* and *functional resolution*, can be very helpful when evaluating functional neuroimaging approaches (Huettel *et al.*, 2009). Contrast is the intensity difference between the quantities measured by an imaging system (e.g., oxyhemoglobin levels). Contrast is determined mostly by the signal-to-noise ratio, or the magnitude of the intensity difference between quantities divided by the variability in their measurements, and applies to both temporal and spatial properties. The temporal resolution of a system refers to the ability to distinguish two events happening close in time. The spatial contrast of an approach is its ability to distinguish two truly separate effects happening close in space. No technique, neuroimaging, behavioral, or other, is useful in the absence of a valid experimental design. Functional resolution represents the ability of a measurement technique to delineate the relation between underlying neuronal activity and a cognitive or

Rutter's Child and Adolescent Psychiatry, Sixth Edition.
Edited by Anita Thapar and Daniel S. Pine, James F. Leckman, Stephen Scott, Margaret J. Snowling, Eric Taylor.
© 2015 John Wiley & Sons Ltd. Published 2018 by John Wiley & Sons Ltd.

behavioral phenomenon. Functional resolution is determined both by the actual changes that take place in the brain measure and by the ability of the scientist to manipulate experimental features to allow interpretable variation in the phenomenon of interest. Functional resolution of an imaging technique is determined by a consideration of the temporal and spatial resolutions in conjunction with the quality of the experimental design and task selection. Put simply, the selection of tasks in neuroimaging is just as critical as it is with any other method in the psychological sciences. Valid neuroimaging approaches with a high degree of functional resolution can significantly enhance the explanatory power of theories of typical and atypical social, emotional, and cognitive development in four important ways. They can (1) improve models of social, emotional, and cognitive processes via activation-based *dissociations,* that is, when two brain regions or networks show opposite activation patterns in response to the same task; (2) inform understanding of the relative timing and underlying architecture of social, emotional, and cognitive processes; (3) facilitate integration of information from diverse methodologies (e.g., genetics, lesion studies, animal models, and behavioral performance); and (4) help adjudicate between competing psychological theories.

Neuroimaging measures involve several tradeoffs. Most centrally, there is often a tradeoff between invasiveness and the degree of spatial resolution. Another tradeoff exists between temporal and spatial resolution: EEG has excellent temporal but poor spatial resolution, whereas fMRI exhibits the opposite qualities. Different neuroimaging methods provide complementary but somewhat independent measures. That is not to say that the different measures would be uncorrelated. If used to measure the same processes in the same people, especially measured concurrently, we do see convergence for some of the signals acquired across imaging modalities. However, from our perspective, a sensible approach is to triangulate on a particular construct utilizing several different methods, each appropriate to the question of interest and the developmental level of the participant.

Neuroimaging measures also have notable weaknesses, the most salient being threats to data quality and the misinterpretation of results that can follow from inaccurate data. For instance, movement artifacts not only compromise the accuracy of neuroimaging measures, but when unnoticed, they can lead to false, but plausible, conclusions. With these considerations in mind, we review several neuroimaging approaches used with infants, children, and adolescents, their advantages and disadvantages, and the exciting opportunities emerging in the field. We begin by summarizing some of the most commonly used neuroimaging methods, as well as some newer methods. We then discuss some of the critical factors that clinicians and scientists should bear in mind during the analysis and interpretation of neuroimaging research findings. Finally, we discuss the application of neuroimaging to the study of typical brain development and psychiatric disorders, with emphasis on the unique challenges associated with imaging individuals of specific age ranges.

Overview of neuroimaging techniques

Magnetic resonance imaging (MRI)

MRI takes advantage of the way in which protons behave under the influence of a strong magnetic field when bombarded with a specifically tuned radio frequency. The most common MR methods measure signals from protons in water molecules within tissue. The combined effects of the strong magnet in the MR machine and the radio frequency pulses cause protons to emit signals that are picked up by antennae in a head coil. Sophisticated computer algorithms analyze the properties of this signal for use in reconstructing three-dimensional images of the brain.

Structural MRI

In structural MRI the most common targets are the protons in the hydrogen atoms in water molecules. Since different tissues differ in the relative amount of water, the signal intensities will vary, as illustrated in Figure 11.1. This can be performed non-invasively without radiation. The term voxel, derived from "volume pixel," denotes the smallest imageable unit. High-resolution images will have small voxels. In structural imaging, whole brain images with voxels as small as 1 mm³ are routine, and can be acquired in as little as 5–7 min. Higher resolutions are possible with longer scanning protocols. In addition to imaging gross morphological abnormalities, researchers can measure the volume, size, shape, or depth of brain structures.

Functional MRI

Functional MRI (fMRI) is based on principles similar to those of structural MRI. However, instead of measuring water concentration, with fMRI the target is hemoglobin, the oxygen-carrying component of blood. Oxygenated and deoxygenated hemoglobin respond differently in the magnetic field. In this way, the signal generated from any given tissue provides some information about the overall level of blood oxygenation in that tissue. The resulting signal is commonly referred to as the blood-oxygenation-level-dependent signal (BOLD). Since the BOLD signal changes over time as a function of the work being done by neurons in the region, by measuring the *change* in BOLD over time we infer changes in neural activity.

Because neurons do not store reserves of glucose and oxygen, an increase in neuronal activity leads to increased perfusion and

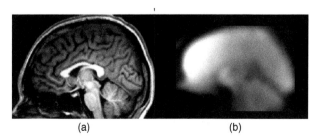

(a)   (b)

Figure 11.1 Structural (a) and functional (b) and MR images.

elevated oxyhemoglobin in active brain areas. Thus, the ratio of oxy:deoxyhemoglobin indirectly reflects brain activity, typically in the surrounding 1–2 mm. As the neurons in specific brain regions "work harder" to perform a specific task, they require more oxygen. Because this hemodynamic response peaks around 4–6 s following the onset of neuronal activity, fMRI has this range of temporal resolution. An accessible review of these, and other issues, appears elsewhere (Huettel *et al.*, 2009). Figure 11.1 depicts a structural and functional image side by side, showing one key property of fMRI: its limited spatial resolution. This reflects unique effects of vascular anatomy and signal-to-noise properties in the two techniques. These factors typically produce fMRI voxels in the 3 mm^3 range, though more advanced techniques can generate finer resolution.

A second key property of fMRI is temporal resolution. The BOLD signal response, reflecting changes in neural activity, is not instantaneous. As shown in Figure 11.2, this response takes approximately 6 s to reach a peak. In turn, the peak may remain elevated for an additional 12–16 seconds and longer if the region remains active. This sluggishness means that observed signals sum many inputs. Thus, the time course of processes commonly examined with fMRI is much more rapid than the 6 or 12–16 s that the BOLD response can take to peak.

Finally, fMRI has other notable limitations. First, research in monkeys suggests that BOLD contrast reflects mainly the inputs to a neuron and the neuron's integrative processing within its body, and less the output firing of neurons. Second, the BOLD signal cannot provide information regarding direction of information flow, be it from feedback and/or feed-forward information flow, that is, when a region is active, fMRI cannot tell us whether the region is active because it is sending a message to another region or because it is receiving information from a region. Similarly, both inhibitory and excitatory inputs contribute to the BOLD signal such that, within a neuron, the inputs might cancel out, leaving a net zero response. In this case, theoretically important brain activity is present, but it is not detected by fMRI. An excellent discussion of these and other related issues appears in Logothetis (2008). Finally, while computing statistics to determine if a contrast is significant, we compare the magnitudes of two sample means relative to their variability. Larger differences in magnitude and lower variability means that it is unlikely the difference could have been observed

by chance. As long as a few assumptions hold, we can assign a probability p to that likelihood. By convention we do not consider a contrast significant unless the likelihood falls under a sufficiently small threshold, say $p < 0.05$. It is important to note that even when a contrast is significant, that is, the difference is not due to chance; there is still a possibility that it is. Incorrectly asserting that a difference, or contrast, is real when it is not, is a called a type I error. If we only make a single comparison, then a type I error is unlikely—it's just the probability p chosen as our threshold. Unfortunately, each time we make another comparison, there is another chance for a type I error. As more and more comparisons are made, the likelihood of a type I error goes from small to certain.

This is the problem with multiple comparisons, and it is ubiquitous in fMRI. The statistical models from which contrast maps are derived can be computed for each voxel in the brain. Specific regions can be interrogated using delineated regions of interest, but most studies are not or cannot be this selective. Since there are tens of thousands of individual voxels in the brain, this means that the analyses will require tens of thousands of statistical contrasts, and consequently tens of thousands of chances to make a type I error. Fortunately, there are a number of methods that researchers can use to correct for multiple comparisons. These methods can be quite technical, but the underlying concepts are fairly straightforward (see Nichols & Hayasaka, 2003; Bennett *et al.*, 2009 for further review and discussion). Uncorrected results, even when published in prominent journals, should be viewed skeptically until they can be replicated.

Notwithstanding these limitations, fMRI does help inform understanding of childhood psychiatric disorders. One set of insights relates to neural correlates of risk. For example, fMRI can measure neural specialization for social information as it relates to risk for autism spectrum disorders (ASD), using biological motion social perception paradigms. Point-light displays track the way in which people move, conveying with a simple stimulus array specific kinds of motion (e.g., walking or dancing). In an fMRI study from our group (Kaiser *et al.*, 2010), 4- to 17-year-olds viewed coherent and scrambled point-light animations of biological motion. Three groups were studied: (i) children with ASD, (ii) unaffected siblings of children with ASD (UAS), and (iii) typically developing children (TD), revealing three kinds of brain activity: (i) perturbed state activity, occurring only in ASD; (ii) perturbed trait activity, occurring in ASD and UAS; and (iii) compensatory activity, where the UAS group differed from the two other groups. Perturbed state activity in this particular task is a correlate of disruption in brain circuitry in ASD, whereas perturbed trait activity could be regarded as an ASD endophenotype (Gottesman & Shields, 1973). Compensatory activity might reflect mechanisms by which UAS overcome risk. In each case, these observations require a direct assessment of brain function, made possible through fMRI, illustrating the power of fMRI and indirectly providing ideas about novel treatments.

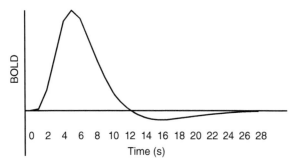

Figure 11.2 Canonical hemodynamic response.

Other fMRI techniques provide more direct clues about treatment. For example, considerable interest focuses on fMRI neurofeedback where much of the research so far has targeted pain. Scheinost and colleagues (2013) extended this technique to target subclinical contamination fears by teaching individuals to reduce their anxiety by altering their BOLD signal patterns. In this study, a region of the orbitofrontal cortex associated with contamination anxiety was targeted, which subjects learned to modulate in a way that simultaneously improved symptoms associated with contamination anxiety and the brain and behavioral changes were correlated. These findings have the potential to support a strong translational connection between research and clinical practice, as they provide an observable marker of treatment working, for whom it works best, and that it can be observed to work at a biological systems level, thereby highlighting the potential for individualized medicine.

Structural and functional connectivity
Diffusion tensor imaging

Since no region of the brain acts in total isolation, it is important to understand how brain areas communicate. To this end, researchers have used both structural MRI and fMRI methods. Diffusion tensor imaging (DTI) is a structural method that measures the momentary diffusion of water through the brain. In unconstrained regions, such as the ventricles, water diffuses isotropically, but in nerve fibers, water diffuses in some directions more than others. By measuring diffusion along such fibers, nerve fiber integrity can be mapped with DTI. However, if axons within a voxel are not traveling along the same path, the average diffusivity will appear isotropic. This "fiber-crossing problem" limits the ability to detect structural connections in less spatially organized areas of white matter.

To illustrate the power of this method, consider the results of a DTI study showing that the developmental trajectory of white matter tracts is different in babies who go on to develop ASD versus those who do not (Wolff *et al.*, 2012). The available evidence suggests that early, overt symptoms of ASD usually emerge late in the first or early in the second year of life. Wolff and colleagues (2012) prospectively traced white matter fiber tract organization from 6 to 24 months in high-risk infants who developed ASD by 24 months. Infant siblings of children with ASD who went on to receive a diagnosis of ASD at 24 months of age had distinct brain patterns at 6 months and abnormal neural development from 6 to 24 months. These results are particularly striking because they demonstrate that aberrant development of white matter pathways may precede the manifestation of autistic symptoms in the first year of life. Biomarkers like these, especially if paired with information from genetic and behavioral screens, could potentially help identify children with ASD before symptoms appear.

Functional connectivity

Two regions are functionally connected if their corresponding BOLD signals correlate in time. The logic is that, all else being equal, if two regions are communicating then such fluctuations will correlate. As with any correlation, functional connectivity may reflect effects of third variables. As an example, upon viewing a face we might observe correlations in the BOLD signal in two brain regions. However, these correlations may be due to communications occurring over connections between the regions, or both regions could be responding to the third variable (the face stimulus). Nevertheless, the ease of assessing resting state functional connectivity has led to widespread use of the technique.

Electrophysiology
Electroencephalography

In contrast to fMRI, EEG and event-related potentials (ERPs) directly measure the firing of groups of cortical neurons. During information processing, neuronal activity creates small electrical currents that can be recorded from noninvasive sensors placed on the scalp, providing precise information about the timing of processing and clarifying brain activity at the millisecond pace at which it unfolds. The high temporal resolution of ERPs complement the high spatial resolution of fMRI. Both have critically informed our understanding of typical and atypical development. FMRI measures have helped identify some of the neural circuitry supporting various psychological processes including social cognition, emotion regulation, face recognition, working memory, and attention. These studies have also provided insight into whether certain regions of the brain are differentially activated at specific points in development. ERP measures inform our understanding of the timing of the stages of psychological processes and help identify the distinct functions that each brain region performs at particular points in time as a psychological task unfolds. For example, several classic fMRI studies independently identified a region of the brain called the "fusiform face area" in the posterior fusiform cortex of the ventral temporal lobe that selectively responds to faces (e.g., Puce *et al.*, 1996; Kanwisher *et al.*, 1997). Electrophysiological measures reveal that this region is engaged in several distinct psychological processes relevant to face processing at different points in time (e.g., Bentin *et al.*, 1996). At approximately 170–200 ms after the appearance of a face, this region exhibits activity supporting the perception of a face as a face, instead of another category of object. Slightly later, at approximately 300–400 ms, another wave of activity that has been linked to the recognition of the face's identity (e.g., a stranger versus a friend or "that is the Queen of England.") is observed. Finally, at 450 ms and beyond, activity supporting the perception of the emotional expression displayed on the face (e.g., anger versus happiness) is observed in the same cortical area. The classic monograph by Luck (2005) is an outstanding introduction to and tutorial about EEG/ERPs.

Examination of the electrical signals captured at the scalp reveals fluctuations or waves called oscillations. These oscillations arise from rhythmic postsynaptic potentials generated by populations of cortical pyramidal neurons. The rhythms underlying the EEG signal can be decomposed into constituent frequencies reflecting various rates of brain oscillation. EEG oscillations are characterized by their frequency in cycles per second (Hertz, Hz). For instance, EEG alpha refers to frequencies typically between 8 Hz and 12 Hz. With an approach called fast Fourier transform (FFT), the proportion of frequencies that make up the signal can describe the EEG signal. Other common EEG frequency bands are labeled delta (1–3 Hz), theta (4–8 Hz), beta (13–24 Hz), and gamma (25–100 Hz). These frequencies coincide with various mental states (e.g., sleep, awake, at rest, etc.), and can also be examined by their patterns (frontal alpha asymmetry), ratios (theta/beta ratio), and changes across contexts (alpha suppression, also known as mu suppression). Oscillatory activity derived from the FFT does not provide information about the timing of neural events, as is the case for ERPs.

ERPs are computed as the average signal across events, locked to a stimulus or action. Thus, tasks designed to acquire ERPs tend to be repetitive, allowing for sufficient numbers of measurements to resolve a reliable ERP. Importantly, ERPs capture the stimulus- or response-driven partial phase alignment, and power increases in the ongoing EEG brought about by the event (Le Van Quyen & Bragin, 2007; Sauseng et al., 2007). Developmental ERP studies are appealing because they are relatively low cost to collect, provide measurement of actual neuronal activity, and are interpretable based on previous cognitive neuroscience studies. The ERP reflects a series of positive- and negative-going peaks thought to reflect stages of sensory and cognitive processing. Different types of experimental tasks are used for eliciting various ERPs; for instance, tasks that require inhibiting a response or tasks that present a novel stimulus among repetitive stimuli. One of the most commonly assessed ERPs is the P300. In ERP nomenclature, the "P" indicates a positive ERP peak and the "300" reflects that the response happens at approximately 300 ms. Other ERPs are labeled for their function, such as the error-related negativity (ERN), which occurs in response to simple cognitive errors, such as responding when a response should be withheld. Although ERPs are not known for their spatial precision, they tend to appear in different regions on the scalp. For instance, faces tend to elicit an N170 response that appears bilaterally in temporal-parietal scalp regions. In psychiatry, ERPs have been used to characterize the neural correlates of information processing and underlying pathophysiology in most neuropsychiatric disorders. They can also be used as indicators of risk or indicators of drug effects and behavioral treatment effects.

ERP measures have revealed subtle differences in processing of social information at the neural level in children at risk for ASD. The lack of reliable indicators of ASD during the first year of life has been a major impediment to early intervention: in the absence of a firm diagnosis until behavioral symptoms emerge, treatment is often delayed for two or more years. Given its strong social components, Elsabbagh et al. (2012) hypothesized that neural sensitivity to eye gaze in early infancy would predict later development of ASD. Notably, there is little behavioral evidence of early disruption in eye gaze processes in infants

later diagnosed with the disorder. The researchers recorded ERP while 6- to 10-month-old high-risk infants (siblings of a child with ASD) viewed faces with dynamic eye gaze directed either toward or away from them. Neural responses to dynamic eye gaze shifts during the first year predicted clinical outcomes at 36 months, despite similar gaze patterns measured by eye tracking. The authors concluded that neural responses to eye gaze in the first year of life reflect disruptions in basic developmental processes linked to the later emergence of ASD.

This finding illustrates that measures of brain function can index developmental and individual differences in underlying processing mechanisms that are otherwise invisible and impervious to study because they do not produce overt behavioral evidence. EEG measures can be leveraged even in very young infants as "neural signatures" of processes that are not available to observation or verbal report. Further, some neural signatures, for example, ERP responses indexing face perception, may be remarkably consistent across the lifespan, allowing researchers to measure certain aspects of socioemotional processing using identical neurophysiological methods even when major developmental changes demand alterations in other measurement strategies (e.g., a shift from behavioral observation to verbal report).

ERPs reflect the aspects of the EEG signal that are in phase (colloquially "in sync"). Any "out of sync" electrical activity tends to be averaged out. ERPs also do not speak directly to which frequencies underlie the brain process in question. In the past 10 years, implementation of advanced signal processing techniques such as short-time Fourier and wavelet transform can investigate the EEG signal in terms of frequency, power, and phase. This approach, broadly conceived as event-related brain dynamics (Makeig et al., 2004), can characterize the EEG signal in terms of frequency, power, and phase (time). Importantly, characterizing oscillatory dynamics in this way probably more closely reflects the activity of underlying neuronal assemblies (Buzsáki, 2006).

Event-time-locked frequency analyses of EEG allow for the measurement changes in EEG power and phase synchrony, across trials, on a millisecond time scale. In particular, event-related spectral perturbations (ERSPs) temporally sensitive indices of the relative change of mean EEG power from baseline associated with stimulus presentation or response execution. Unlike ERPs, ERSPs capture changes in spontaneous EEG activity that occur across several frequency spectra and are sensitive to fluctuations that are temporally stable (Makeig, 1993; Makeig et al., 2004). The value of ERSPs becomes clearer when we view them against the backdrop of a traditional ERP approach. Because ERPs involve signal averaging, we cannot say precisely which frequencies underlie them, only the range of frequencies we started with before averaging. By examining ERSPs we can directly examine which EEG frequencies underlie responses to experimental events, and by extension determine which frequencies underlie ERPs. A well-known example involves the ERN, where Luu et al. (2004) showed that the error-related negativity ERP can be largely accounted for by an increase in evoked (event-related) theta power following an error. Although ERSPs are able to capture induced power changes, not revealed in typically averaged ERPs, they do not reveal details about the synchrony of the event-related EEG signals, discussed next.

The inter trial coherence (ITC) reflects the degree of synchronization of the EEG for events (e.g., stimulus or response) in a task. Analogous to a correlation coefficient, intertrial phase values refer to the degree of association across trials, ranging from 0 to 1. Thus, for a range of frequencies, a larger value indicates greater phase synchrony (more consistent phasic activation) for the frequencies in question. ITC is assessed at a single location or region and thus reflects "temporal coherence," to be distinguished from "spatial coherence," assessed across brain regions. As one example illustrating the value of ITC, on a simple go/no-go task, adolescents with ADHD were found to have comparable ERN ERP responses compared to controls (Groom *et al.*, 2010). However, controls did show greater theta (4–8 Hz) phasic consistency (ITC) in the neural response to errors, which was correlated with a measure of performance (greater d-prime)—ITC was unrelated to performance in the ADHD group. This finding led the authors to suggest that less consistent phasic activation of the neural response to errors might underlie the poorer inhibitory performance (lower d-prime) seen in patients with ADHD, a conclusion that could not be drawn from the ERP data.

Magnetic resonance spectroscopy

Magnetic resonance spectroscopy (MRS) is another imaging modality that relies on the same basic principles of physics used to conduct structural and functional MRI studies. Thus, strong magnets and radiofrequency waves are used to non-invasively assess functional aspects of the brain. The unique feature of MRS relates to the sensitivity of particular chemicals to distinct resonance frequencies that can be detected through MRI. This quantifies the level of one or another chemical in a voxel. However, there are restricted numbers of compounds that can be assessed with MRS, relative to more invasive chemical techniques, like positron emission tomography (PET) (though PET is much too invasive for routine use as a research tool, as discussed later). Typically, these compounds vary in their arrangements of carbon and proton atoms.

Magnetoencephalography

Magnetoencephalography (MEG) is another, less frequently employed, but powerful functional neuroimaging technique. In MEG, brain activity is mapped by recording the magnetic fields resulting from brain electrical activity. MEG is recorded using very sensitive magnetometers. The most common magnetometers are superconducting quantum interference devices (SQUIDs), which are capable of measuring extremely subtle magnetic fields. The signals acquired via MEG resemble those acquired via EEG, in terms of their oscillatory pattern.

Thus, many of the analytic approaches just described for EEG, including signal averaging and oscillatory analyses, can also be done with brain signals acquired through MEG. However, at least for the brain's cortical surface, MEG is able to assess brain activity based on such signals with superior spatial resolution. A comprehensive introduction to MEG can be found in Hansen *et al.* (2010).

Positron emission tomography

Like MRI, PET can produce three-dimensional images of brain structural and function. However, unlike MRI, PET is invasive, as it detects gamma rays emitted from injected radioactive tracers as they decay. Because many neurochemicals can be altered to create radiotracers, PET is particularly well suited for examining functional neurochemistry, provided that an ethical justification exists for such an examination in a child. Thus, while MRS is less invasive than PET, PET can currently quantify a much broader range of chemicals than MRS. Increased metabolic activity, similar to assumptions made in fMRI, is correlated with increased neural activity. Thus, regions in which the tracer concentration is high, measured as locally increased radioactivity, represent highly active regions. In addition to the measure of metabolic activity, some tracers can bind to specific neuroreceptors, such as dopamine receptors (Catafau *et al.*, 2010). Differences in the amount of tracer then indicate differences in the receptor density, which may have profound implications for understanding disease processes in a variety of mental health conditions.

Functional near infrared spectroscopy

fNIRS uses lasers instead of magnetic fields, but like fMRI, it also measures changes in hemoglobin. Similar to a pulse oximeter, fNIRS works via a laser emitting light at one point and a receiver detecting the amount of unabsorbed light at a nearby point. The wavelength of the light is tuned such that the regional oxygenated or deoxygenated blood flow can be inferred from the amount of light absorbed. Although the scalp and skull are opaque to visible light, they are almost transparent to light in the near infrared range (800–2500 nm). Because blood absorbs light photons differently depending upon how much oxygen is present, shining a near infrared light into the head and measuring the intensity of the exiting light can reveal the differential absorption of light as a function of blood oxygenation level, thus providing an indirect measure of brain activity at and just beneath the cortical surface. FNIRS appears to be quite promising for enhancing our understanding of the developing brain particularly in very young children, as well as in older children and adults (Gervain *et al.*, 2011). FNIRS is less sensitive to motion and can be utilized in less-constrained, more ecologically valid experimental paradigms than fMRI and EEG/ERP. Furthermore, by measuring both oxygenated and deoxygenated hemoglobin in brain tissue, fNIRS provides two distinct (but correlated) indicators of neural activity, which allows for absolute measures as opposed to only baseline-relative measures and thus increases its flexibility (Gervain *et al.*, 2011).

A surprisingly large number of studies have used fNIRS to examine social and emotional processes in typically developing neonates to toddlers. Several have focused on the development of face processing. At 4 months, the temporal cortex of infants activates selectively to faces relative to other objects (Csibra *et al.*, 2004; Blasi *et al.*, 2007). At 6 months, infants exhibit increased activity to upright versus inverted faces in the right temporal cortex (Otsuka *et al.*, 2007). At 8 months, activity in temporal regions is observed independent of viewing angle (Nakato *et al.*, 2009). These findings regarding the localization of neural signatures of face processing in infants are unique to fNIRS, particularly the ability to localize activity in infants who are awake and actively attending to visual displays. Researchers investigating responses to dynamic social stimuli such as eye and mouth movements have identified bilateral superior temporal and inferior frontal cortical activations in infants starting as early as 4 months, consistent with activation observed via fMRI in older children, adolescents, and adults in response to the same kinds of stimuli (Grossmann *et al.*, 2008; Lloyd-Fox *et al.*, 2009). See Gervain *et al.* (2011) for a comprehensive review of fNIRS studies of infants.

One might wonder why everyone does not use fNIRS all the time. It is less sensitive to motion and can be utilized in less-constrained, more ecologically valid social paradigms. From the perspective of head motion, the observation is correct. But there are always critical tradeoffs with functional neuroimaging techniques. Even though fNIRS is more resistant to head motion, it only measures activation at the cortical surface. The light used to image brain function does not return to the optodes from deeper cortical areas and, critically, subcortical areas. Many of the key social and emotional brain areas are deep within the cortex or are part of the limbic system, and thus are invisible to fNIRS. Moreover, the more hair on the participant's head, and the thicker the skull, the more difficult it is to use fNIRS; it works best in infants and young children, and aging men.

Imaging genomics

Inspired in part by advances in measurement technologies, developmental scientists are now actively investigating the complex transactions driving developmental changes across multiple levels of organization, including the environment, behavior, cognition and emotion, brain, and genes (Gottlieb, 1992), operating in a transactional bidirectional fashion. Use of *in vivo* pediatric brain imaging techniques in this context offers an additional opportunity for developmental, multilevel analysis across the full lifespan.

Functional neuroimaging offers a potential means by which associations between genetic risk factors and the activity of specific brain circuits, during processing of discrete stimuli or performance of distinct behaviors, can be investigated. There is growing interest in the identification of brain structural and functional changes associated with genetic risks that are being

identified including common allelic risks and high penetrance rare mutations, although there is a need to guard against the possibility of type I errors that arise from multiple testing (see Chapter 24). Replications are required, as with any method. Ideally, associations between gene variants and regional patterns of brain information processing will not only help elucidate the biological mechanisms underlying previously demonstrated gene links with behavior but will also direct attention to new behaviors that are mediated by genetically influenced brain systems and vice versa.

To illustrate, consider a study by Durston and colleagues (2008) on the dopamine transporter (DAT1) gene and attention deficit/hyperactivity disorder (ADHD). Genetic studies had originally suggested a link between the DAT1 gene to ADHD, but findings have been mixed (see section on candidate genes and Chapter 24). Nevertheless, we use this as an illustration. Dopamine transporters are highly expressed in the striatum. In fact, some stimulant medications shown to be effective in ADHD are believed to exert their effects by blocking dopamine transporters in the striatum. The authors investigated the association between one gene variant in the gene encoding DAT1 and brain activation patterns in ADHD. They studied sibling pairs discordant for ADHD and typically developing controls using fMRI and a go/no-go (press a button for "go" stimuli and inhibit a response for "no-go" stimuli) paradigm. The DAT1 genotype was associated with the level of activation in the striatum. As more robust genetic findings are emerging (see Chapter 24), this approach serves as an illustration of the type of research that might be used to assess risk-allele-associated neural signatures.

Despite its promise, the application of imaging genetics to our understanding of typical and atypical development is currently limited by at least three major challenges: (1) most gene variants, with the exception of rare, highly penetrant mutations, have small effects on behavior, and prior imaging studies are likely to have overestimated effect sizes for the brain, due to the challenge of handling multiple testing; (2) imaging genetics remains inherently correlational and suffers from an absence of detailed analysis of mechanisms; (3) all imaging genetic studies to date have focused on cross-sectional samples of adolescents and young adults in racially and culturally homogeneous samples. There is a great need (and opportunity) for longitudinal designs to examine the influence of robust genetic risk variants on developmental trajectories of the social brain and social behavior in diverse populations. If these challenges can be addressed, imaging genetics research could help increase our understanding of how genetic variation interacts with the environment to shape the development of the brain and the corresponding effects on behavior.

Analysis and interpretation of imaging data

Study and experimental design are important points of consideration in any investigation of typical and atypical development.

Brain imaging research is no exception. Indeed, all of the well-known issues that need to be addressed in standard psychological or psychiatric experiments need to be addressed in brain imaging research as well. However, neuroimaging research also imposes unique design constraints discussed in the next section. We consider two issues: the study and the experiment. Conceptually, the study level addresses the question of "who" is being studied, and the experiment level addresses the question of how.

Study level design considerations
Within-subjects designs
Imagine we were interested in whether activation in dorsal lateral prefrontal cortex (DLPFC) is higher during greater cognitive load. To answer this question, we create an experiment where we scan people while they do a task with two levels of difficulty, and compare whether activation in the DLPFC was higher when they were doing the easy level or the hard level. This is a within-subjects design, as is used in many psychiatric brain imaging studies, since each participant receives each condition, and the test is between each person's activation on one condition relative to the other.

Between-subjects designs
Many important questions require between-subjects designs, where not all participants receive all treatments. This includes studies between different groups (autism spectrum disorder versus typical development) or different treatments (cognitive behavior therapy versus waitlist). If the between-group factor is one that is under the experimenter's control, a true experiment, then they can deal with potential group differences using random assignment. For example, in a neuroimaging study of treatments, individuals could be randomly assigned to one treatment or another. So long as the sample sizes are large enough, the logic of random assignment allows the researcher to be confident that group differences should be insignificant. This is true of factors that might impact neuroimaging data. However, it is often the case that studies of interest to psychiatrists are subject to biases from confounds (see Chapter 12). Participants are not assigned to groups by the researcher. For example, we do not assign a child to an anxious group, or to a specific age. The limitations of a design must be considered in the interpretation of neuroimaging results as they are with other studies (see Chapter 12) with particular emphasis on those aspects of group-level differences that impact brain data. A crucial difference between many psychiatric populations and typically developing controls is the ability to comply with instructions that ensure a good quality scan (e.g., remaining still for the duration of an fMRI scan). This point is taken up at length later.

Cross-sectional versus longitudinal studies
Tension between cross-sectional and longitudinal designs exist in neuroimaging as in other areas of developmental research. Cross-sectional studies are quicker and less expensive than longitudinal studies. However, only longitudinal studies map individual developmental trajectories. This approach may be more informative than observed differences in age-specific group averages—especially in a dynamic system such as the developing brain.

Test-retest reliability
An important consideration in evaluating longitudinal fMRI studies is test-retest reliability. Test–retest reliability refers to the ability of a measure to produce systematic results when repeated under similar conditions. If a specific experiment does not generate reliable results across time, its utility as a longitudinal method is limited. Unfortunately, the available studies suggest that while the test–retest reliability of fMRI for adults is quite good, it is poor to fair for younger, school-age children and adolescents (e.g., Koolschijn *et al.*, 2011; van den Bulk *et al.*, 2013).

Experiment level design considerations
Since many of the questions regarding brain function overlap with psychological questions, the experimental paradigms often overlap as well. Many tasks tapping executive functions, language, memory, and so on have been adapted for use in neuroimaging. However, due to the nature of fNIRS and fMRI, particularly the relatively sluggish responses measured, experiments often need significant modification or may not be suitable for neuroimaging.

Block designs
A popular design in fMRI experiments is the block design. In block designs, experimental stimuli are presented, perhaps repeatedly, in a block lasting 12–30 s. For example, a researcher studying the response to emotional facial expressions might present 10 angry faces, each lasting 2 s, in a given block. Repeated presentation of a region's preferred stimulus type can drive activation very strongly, and the long duration allows for the full evolution of the sluggish hemodynamic response. This makes block designs quite powerful from a statistical perspective. However, block designs may not be very naturalistic and designing a blocked version of traditional trial-based psychological experiments may not be feasible in many cases. In addition, different regions of the brain, such as the amygdala, may be more sensitive to habituation than others, and the block design also is sensitive to a number of confounds.

Event-related designs
In event-related designs, individual trials of a given experimental condition are normally presented one by one, making them more analogous to traditional psychological designs and less sensitive to confounds that plague the block design. Individual trials may be brief, so to achieve sufficient power requires a large number of trials. However, even then the spacing between trials must be sufficient to allow for the hemodynamic response to evolve. Researchers differentiate between event-related designs

that use long (16 s or more) and short inter trial intervals (2–8 s). The former, termed slow-event-related designs, permit the BOLD signal to return to a baseline state after the end of stimulation. With the latter, termed fast-event-related designs, the BOLD signal does not necessarily return to baseline between trials. Special analysis strategies must be used with these designs because the observed signal may be driven by contributions from many overlapping trials. The hemodynamic response normally takes 12–16 s after stimulation ends to completely "relax" and return to baseline. If we present stimuli more quickly then every 12–16 s, we have to account for the fact that the hemodynamic response observed at any one point in time may reflect influences from both the current and previous stimulus.

Motion and motion artifacts

Participant motion can compromise analysis. FMRI data for a single volume is acquired over some window of time, usually 2 s, and typically with a predetermined scan slice sequence (i.e., starting at the bottom of the brain and moving up). Participant motion during the acquisition of a single volume can mean that certain brain regions may be missed or imaged more than once. Motion across volumes has the effect that intensity changes as a function of time, which may be driven by changes in the intensity of the underlying structure and not BOLD changes (Figure 11.3). If these changes are correlated with experimental manipulations, spurious "activity" can be observed.

When a participant moves, that motion typically affects all observed voxels, which in turn causes false correlations in the BOLD signal. Since functional connectivity is fundamentally a measure of correlations among BOLD responses, it is particularly susceptible to motion artifacts. Special care needs to be taken to compare motion estimates across different groups in between-subject designs. Different populations may be less able to control their motion in the scanner. Younger children or children with mental health disorders may not be willing or able to stay still over extended periods of time, especially in

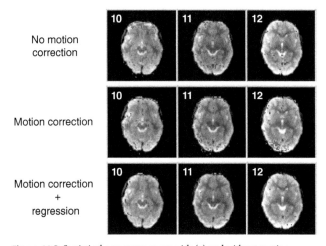

Figure 11.3 Statistical parameter maps with (a) and without motion correction (b).

the context of (boring) psychology experiments. Recognition of this issue in psychiatric neuroimaging has led to an increased interest in developing better methods for dealing with motion differences in statistical models.

Recent work has shown, however, that even tiny movement artifacts (0.004 mm) can lead to insidious biases in fMRI analyses and potentially to false conclusions even without causing noticeably "blurry" images (Power *et al.*, 2012; Van Dijk *et al.*, 2012). The results of two sets of papers representing groundbreaking advances in developmental science illustrate this dilemma. First, via highly innovative, mathematically complex analyses of resting-state functional connectivity data, two papers reported that short-range brain connections are robust in school-age children and weaken into young adulthood, whereas long-range connections begin weak in children and strengthen over time (Fair *et al.*, 2008; Dosenbach *et al.*, 2010). However, recent work demonstrates that these findings actually result from uncontrolled age differences in head motion, with younger children moving more than older children, adolescents, and adults (Power *et al.*, 2012; Van Dijk *et al.*, 2012).

Normalization and group comparisons

Every brain is unique. The specific location, size, and shape of any given anatomical landmark differ from person to person. This poses a challenge for aggregating data across many individuals. Normalization refers to the method of warping a given participant's brain data into a common space or to fit into a common template (Talairach & Tournoux, 1988; Thomason *et al.*, 2013). These routines are usually automated and operate on a high-resolution anatomical scan. Having computed a normalization solution, it is applied to the functional data. Once in a common space, the data can be effectively compared and analyzed across groups.

However, most normalization methods have been developed for application to studies of adults. Automated normalization routines will work best on those brains that are most anatomically like adult brains (older children) and potentially less well on brains that are anatomically different (younger children). Biases introduced by developmental changes in anatomy may mask or exaggerate changes in function. New age-dependent templates are becoming available as larger cohorts of children are entered into databases; however, they are not yet part of standard practice.

Difference maps

Colorful images of patterns on images of brains, often accompanied by descriptions of the activations they represent, are fixtures of both the scientific literature and the lay press. It is important to recognize that many of these images represent areas that show a statistically significant difference between conditions and groups. For example, in Figure 11.3, we see a bright patch in the ventral temporal cortex during a face processing task. It would not be uncommon to have this pattern described as "activation to faces" in support of the argument that this is a face-specific region of the brain. But bearing in mind that these are often difference maps, we could justifiably ask, "activation to faces **relative to what?**" Has this region come from a comparison to fixation, or to some control condition? If there was a control condition, what was it? What was it controlling for? This information should be presented in primary literature, but often is lost in the translation to secondary and tertiary literatures. In this case, the control condition is houses. The region in red on the figure represents a region for which the difference Face − House > 0 is probably true. However, from this result alone a researcher cannot claim that this region does not respond to houses at all.

There are a number of regions in the brain whose characteristic pattern of activation is actually to *deactivate* when external stimuli are presented. This network, sometimes referred to as the task-negative or default mode network, includes the medial prefrontal cortex and the precuneus. These regions are implicated in a number of functions that are of interest to pediatric psychologists and psychiatrists such as mentalization, self-referential processing, reflection, and autobiographical memory. Difference maps for these regions may reflect difference in relative deactivation during the scan.

Conclusions

Neuroimaging is still a new research tool in child psychiatry, though an increasing number of studies will embrace the tool in coming years. A critical consideration is how they relate to observational and verbal report measures of the same or related constructs. Studies that use these new measurement approaches in conjunction with well-understood paradigms and measures are essential to establishing the validity and utility of their empirical findings (e.g., Pfeifer & Peake, 2012). Looking ahead, researchers in child psychiatry are now poised to study directly, in humans, bidirectional transactions among levels of analysis from genes, to brain, to behavior, and the environmental context. Methodological advances provide novel insights into longstanding questions while generating a vast array of new questions.

We are quite optimistic for the future of neuroimaging in child psychiatry. We expect that future research will enable new approaches for studying the neural mechanisms of response to potential behavioral and/or pharmacological treatments. The future will also provide opportunities to assess treatment outcomes at the neural systems level, identify neuroimaging-derived biomarkers that may serve as moderators of treatment response, identify changes in brain mechanisms that may mediate behavioral changes, and determine early efficacy indicators. Work in this area could also inform the ability to predict response to treatment and detect subtle changes that are not yet evident in behavior. As such, neuroimaging studies will contribute to the refinement of efficacious interventions, consistent with the priority of creating individually tailored interventions customized to the behavioral, neural, and genetic characteristics of a given person.

References

Bennett, C.M. *et al.* (2009) The principled control of false positives in neuroimaging. *Social Cognitive and Affective Neuroscience* **4**, 417–422.

Bentin, S. *et al.* (1996) Electrophysiological studies of face perception in humans. *Journal of Cognitive Neuroscience* **8**, 551–565.

Blasi, A. *et al.* (2007) Investigation of depth dependent changes in cerebral haemodynamics during face perception in infants. *Physics in Medicine and Biology* **52**, 6849.

Buzsáki, G. (2006) *Rhythms of the Brain.* Oxford University Press, New York.

Catafau, A.M. *et al.* (2010) Imaging cortical dopamine D1 receptors using 11C NNC112 and ketanserin blockade of the 5-HT 2A receptors. *Journal of Cerebral Blood Flow & Metabolism* **30**, 985–993.

Csibra, G. *et al.* (2004) Near infrared spectroscopy reveals neural activation during face perception in infants and adults. *Journal of Pediatric Neurology* **2**, 85–89.

Dosenbach, N.U. *et al.* (2010) Prediction of individual brain maturity using fMRI. *Science* **329**, 1358–1361.

Durston, S. *et al.* (2008) Dopamine transporter genotype conveys familial risk of attention-deficit/hyperactivity disorder through striatal activation. *Journal of the American Academy of Child and Adolescent Psychiatry* **47**, 61–67.

Elsabbagh, M. *et al.* (2012) Infant neural sensitivity to dynamic eye gaze is associated with later emerging autism. *Current Biology* **22**, 338–342.

Fair, D.A. *et al.* (2008) The maturing architecture of the brain's default network. *Proceedings of the National Academy of Sciences of the USA* **105**, 4028–4032.

Gervain, J. *et al.* (2011) Near-infrared spectroscopy: a report from the McDonnell infant methodology consortium. *Developmental Cognitive Neuroscience* **1**, 22–46.

Gottesman, I.I. & Shields, J. (1973) Genetic theorizing and schizophrenia. *British Journal of Psychiatry.* **122** (566), 15–30.

Gottlieb, G. (1992) *Individual Development and Evolution: The Genesis of Novel Behavior.* Oxford University Press, New York.

Groom, M.J. *et al.* (2010) Electrophysiological indices of abnormal error-processing in adolescents with attention deficit hyperactivity disorder (ADHD). *Journal of Child Psychology and Psychiatry* **51**, 66–76.

Grossmann, T. *et al.* (2008) Early cortical specialization for face-to-face communication in human infants. *Proceedings of the Royal Society B: Biological Sciences* **275**, 2803–2811.

Hansen, P.C. *et al.* (eds) (2010) *MEG: An Introduction to Methods.* Oxford University Press, New York.

Huettel, S.A. *et al.* (2009) *Functional Magnetic Resonance Imaging,* 2nd edn. Sinauer Associates, Sunderland, MA.

Kaiser, M.D. *et al.* (2010) Neural signatures of autism. *Proceedings of the National Academy of Sciences* **107**, 21223–21228.

Kanwisher, N. *et al.* (1997) The fusiform face area: a module in human extrastriate cortex specialized for face perception. *Journal of Neuroscience* **17**, 4302–4311.

Koolschijn, P.C.M. *et al.* (2011) A three-year longitudinal functional magnetic resonance imaging study of performance monitoring and test-retest reliability from childhood to early adulthood. *Journal of Neuroscience* **31**, 4204–4212.

Le Van Quyen, M. & Bragin, A. (2007) Analysis of dynamic brain oscillations: methodological advances. *Trends in Neurosciences* **30**, 365–373.

Lloyd-Fox, S. *et al.* (2009) Social perception in infancy: a near infrared spectroscopy study. *Child Development* **80**, 986–999.

Logothetis, N.K. (2008) What we can do and what we cannot do with fMRI. *Nature* **453**, 869–878.

Luck, S.J. (2005) *An Introduction to the Event-Related Potential Technique.* MIT Press, Massachusetts Institute of Technology.

Luu, P. *et al.* (2004) Frontal midline theta and the error-related negativity: neurophysiological mechanisms of action regulation. *Clinical Neurophysiology* **115**, 1821–1835.

Makeig, S. (1993) Auditory event-related dynamics of the EEG spectrum and effects of exposure to tones. *Electroencephalography & Clinical Neurophysiology* **86**, 283–293.

Makeig, S. *et al.* (2004) Mining event-related brain dynamics. *Trends in Cognitive Sciences* **8**, 204–210.

Nakato, E. *et al.* (2009) When do infants differentiate profile face from frontal face? A near-infrared spectroscopic study. *Human Brain Mapping* **30**, 462–472.

Nichols, T. & Hayasaka, S. (2003) Controlling the familywise error rate in functional neuroimaging: a comparative review. *Statistical Methods in Medical Research* **12** (5), 419–446.

Otsuka, Y. *et al.* (2007) Neural activation to upright and inverted faces in infants measured by near infrared spectroscopy. *NeuroImage* **34**, 399–406.

Pfeifer, J.H. & Peake, S.J. (2012) Self-development: integrating cognitive, socioemotional, and neuroimaging perspectives. *Developmental Cognitive Neuroscience* **2**, 55–69.

Power, J.D. *et al.* (2012) Spurious but systematic correlations in functional connectivity MRI networks arise from subject motion. *NeuroImage* **59**, 2142–2154.

Puce, A. *et al.* (1996) Differential sensitivity of human visual cortex to faces, letterstrings, and textures: a functional magnetic resonance imaging study. *Journal of Neuroscience* **16**, 5205–5215.

Sauseng, P. *et al.* (2007) Are event-related potential components generated by phase resetting of brain oscillations? A critical discussion. *Neuroscience* **146**, 1435–1444.

Scheinost, D. *et al.* (2013) Orbitofrontal cortex neurofeedback produces lasting changes in contamination anxiety and resting-state connectivity. *Translational Psychiatry* **3**, e250.

Talairach, J. & Tournoux, P. (1988) *Co-Planar Stereotaxic Atlas of the Human Brain.3-Dimensional Proportional System: An Approach to Cerebral Imaging.* Thieme Medical Publishers, New York.

Thomason, M.E. *et al.* (2013) Cross-hemispheric functional connectivity in the human fetal brain. *Science: Translational Medicine* **5**, 173ra124.

van den Bulk, B.G. *et al.* (2013) How stable is activation in the amygdala and prefrontal cortex in adolescence? A study of emotional face processing across three measurements. *Developmental Cognitive Neuroscience* **4**, 65–76.

Van Dijk, K.R. *et al.* (2012) The influence of head motion on intrinsic functional connectivity MRI. *NeuroImage* **59**, 431–438.

Wolff, J.J. *et al.* the IBIS Network (2012) Differences in white matter fiber tract development present from 6 to 24 months in infants with autism. *American Journal of Psychiatry* **169**, 589–600.

CHAPTER 12

Using natural experiments and animal models to study causal hypotheses in relation to child mental health problems

Anita Thapar[1] and Michael Rutter[2]

[1]Child and Adolescent Psychiatry Section, Institute of Psychological Medicine and Clinical Neurosciences, Cardiff University School of Medicine, UK

[2]Social, Genetic and Developmental Psychiatry (SGDP) Research Centre, Institute of Psychiatry, Psychology and Neuroscience, King's College London, UK

Introduction

There is enormous scientific and public interest in identifying causes of child mental health problems. However, this pursuit is challenged by multiple factors that threaten the validity of claims about causality. Furthermore, mental health problems and related traits have a complex etiology, as is typical of most common medical disorders. Multiple risk factors contribute and no single risk is necessary or sufficient to cause disorder. Researchers and practitioners need to be aware of these threats and complexities before making causal inferences. As we will discuss, the types of challenges encountered are not simply overcome by the use of ever larger, observational studies, even if they are longitudinal cohorts or through meta-analyses of multiple studies.

We begin this chapter by explaining key terms that are used with respect to the investigation of causal hypotheses. We then describe some of the key problems encountered in the search for causes and explain why natural experiments are useful and what they are. The focus will be on the growing range of different types of natural experiment, with the emphasis on principles and strategy, assumptions and limitations rather than the details of each. We also provide selected illustrative findings. This chapter draws heavily on a report on this topic by the Academy of Medical Sciences (2007) and a series of papers by Michael Rutter (Rutter 2007, 2012; Rutter & Thapar, in press). We then adopt a similar approach to animal models. Interestingly, the major interest in both natural experiments (Campbell & Stanley, 1963) and animal models (Rosenzweig *et al.*, 1962) arose at about the same time in the middle of the last century. Both were concerned about providing rigorous testing of the causal

inference but they faced somewhat different challenges. Natural experiments necessarily involved unusual circumstances and it was necessary to consider the extent to which findings could generalize to more ordinary situations. For example, did special biases arise in the study of adoptees? Animal models had to examine the assumptions involved in the experiments but also had to determine whether the parallels with humans were valid. However, as we discuss, animal models have three main advantages: (1) the ability to study long-term effects (possible because of the much shorter life span of the animals used); (2) the direct testing of the possible causal effect; and (3) the combination of behavioral and brain data providing the ability to investigate the brain processes involved. Accordingly, it is appropriate to consider the two strategies together—as we do here.

The key terms cause, correlate, risk factor, causal risk factor, mediator, and moderator are used ambiguously and this has been comprehensively discussed by Kraemer *et al.* (1997, 2001); these are summarized in Table 12.1. A causal risk factor is one that, if changed, would alter the outcome and the implication is that the burden of disorder would be reduced. As we have already highlighted, there are considerable challenges to identifying true causal risk factors, and no design is perfect. This underpins two key messages of this chapter. It is critical to consider alternative explanatory hypotheses when a risk factor appears to be causal. It is also important to make use of designs that have the potential to disprove hypotheses and not simply focus on repeatedly generating supporting evidence. Any given research design has its own set of assumptions and limitations and faces different threats. Unequivocal proof of causality is difficult if not impossible to generate. Thus, a convergence of findings across different types of natural experiment lends greater confidence toward supporting or refuting causal hypotheses.

Rutter's Child and Adolescent Psychiatry, Sixth Edition.
Edited by Anita Thapar and Daniel S. Pine, James F. Leckman, Stephen Scott, Margaret J. Snowling, Eric Taylor.
© 2015 John Wiley & Sons Ltd. Published 2018 by John Wiley & Sons Ltd.

Table **12.1** Key terms and their conceptual meaning.

Risk	Probability of an outcome in a given population
Risk factor	A measurable exposure or agent that precedes the outcome and is statistically associated with it
Correlate	Meets criteria for risk factor but is measured at the same time or after (thus not known to precede outcome)
Causal risk factor	A risk factor that changes risk of outcome when manipulated
Mediator	A variable via which a causal risk factor exerts its influence on outcome
Moderator	A third variable that influences the association between a risk factor and outcome

Why natural experiments are useful

While the observation of association and identification of risk factors is a start, it is not enough. That is because there are many noncausal explanations for association.

First, there is the problem that risks are not allocated randomly to individuals. Thus, associations with outcomes can simply reflect correlation or association with factors that influence the origins of the risk factor. These can include the effects of social selection and other types of "allocation" bias. Genetic influences on environmental exposure (gene–environment correlation) are also an important consideration. For example, are the higher rates of psychopathology in children born to teenage mothers causally explained by being reared by a young mother or does it reflect something about selection via the attributes of teenagers who become pregnant at this age? Is the elevated rate of antisocial behavior in offspring of mothers who smoke cigarettes in pregnancy because of fetal exposure to the toxic effects of cigarettes during intrauterine life? Or rather, does the association reflect something about selection through the genetic makeup and/or social background of mothers who are unable to quit smoking in pregnancy? We know that mothers who smoke in pregnancy differ on multiple, relevant measured characteristics from non smokers and from those who quit (Pickett et al., 2009).

Another problem lies with assuming that a risk factor is causal when it is in fact a proxy risk; that is, it encompasses some other variable that has the causal risk effect. For example, while "broken homes," on the face of it, appear to be a risk factor for child psychopathology, in the sense that it can temporally precede difficulties, it behaves as a proxy for discordant relationships and impaired parenting, and it is these that explain the link (Brown et al., 1986; Fergusson et al., 1992).

Another problem is one that plagues cross-sectional research and involves associations that arise through reverse causation. That is, where risk factors are brought about by psychopathology or its early manifestations. Many environmental experiences are shaped by individual behavior and perceptions (person–environment correlation). For example, behavior and

behavior problems in children have been shown to affect how adults deal with children even when they are unrelated, as shown in adoption studies, which we discuss later (Ge et al., 1996; O'Connor et al., 1998), or in experimental situations when the adults are not known to them (Anderson et al., 1986). Another example relates to ADHD, which is more common in boys and known to be associated with negative mother–son relationships. While it is theoretically plausible that relationship quality plays a causal role, treatment and longitudinal studies suggest it is the features of ADHD that have contributed to the negative relationships (Schachar et al., 1987; Lifford et al., 2009).

Finally, it is well recognized that spurious associations can arise through confounding where a "third variable" accounts for the link between putative risk factor and outcome. Unfortunately, statistically adjusting for multiple measured confounders using, for example, multivariate methods, does not deal with this for many reasons (Rutter & Thapar, in press). Also, regardless of how well the risk factor, outcome, and confounds are assessed, unmeasured and unknown (the so-called "residual") confounding remains an important problem.

The impossibility of ever being able to completely adjust for selection and confounding through traditional observational epidemiology, coupled with the practical and ethical impossibility of randomly allocating individuals to specific risk exposures, underpins a major motivation for making use of natural experiment and animal models. While randomized controlled trials remain the "gold standard" for testing the effectiveness of treatments and interventions, the mechanisms that mediate treatment effect are not necessarily ones that played an initial causal role.

Natural experiments take advantage of circumstances, whereby links between exposure to the risk factor and other variables are separated by naturally occurring events or situations and the manipulation involved is not undertaken by the researcher. They involve both design and statistical methods that can also be applied to existing data and ongoing studies, including population cohorts and national registries. The types of analyses that have been suggested are more sophisticated than standard multivariate statistical approaches and aim to address the problems of selection and observed and residual confounding.

Natural experiment designs used to test causal hypotheses on environmental risks and that control for genetic contribution

Twin designs

While they are not always acknowledged as such, twin designs do actually represent a natural experiment. These take advantage of the fact that monozygotic (MZ) twins, in principle, share 100% of their genes (meaning DNA sequence), whereas dizygotic (DZ) twins share on average around 50%. The critical assumptions, limitations, and further uses of twin designs are described in greater detail in Chapter 24. The twin design essentially allows for the investigation of the extent to which variation in an observed trait (phenotype) in a given population can be explained by genetic and environmental factors. This partitioning of genetic and environmental contributions (variance) can be undertaken for measured environmental factors (e.g., parenting) as well as for psychopathology. Multivariate twin designs involve examining the association (covariation) between a measured environmental factor and outcome, and decomposing the association or covariation into genetic and environmental components. Ideally, such studies need to be longitudinal. Here, by "controlling" for the genetic contribution it becomes possible to test the extent to which nongenetic influences explain the link between the environmental measure and outcome. The strength of this type of design is that it allows us to test the extent to which observed associations between risk factor and outcome are explained by genetic "confounds." The nongenetic contribution is sometimes referred to as "environmental mediation." However, strictly speaking, it is not possible to distinguish whether there is genuine mediation (see Table 12.1) via environmental mechanisms or whether unmeasured nongenetic factors represent a "third variable" that contributes to both risk measure and outcome.

There is now a large number of published twin studies that have utilized this method. For example, one twin study of antisocial behavior in children (Jaffee *et al.*, 2004) found that the link with corporal punishment was mainly explained by genetic factors. This could arise, for instance, through parental responses to the child's genetically influenced behavior. That was not observed to be the case for physical abuse, where the links were explained by "environmental mediation." However, nevertheless, the use of corporal punishment (perhaps especially if it was severe and frequent) was associated with an environmentally mediated increased likelihood of escalation into abuse. The finding underlines the fact that the origins of a risk factor and its mode of risk mediators are not the same.

Twin studies of depression in children and adolescents (Thapar *et al.*, 1998; Silberg *et al.*, 1999) suggest that while there is a strong genetic contribution to the association between life events and depression, environmental links are still evident but vary with age and the nature of the life event. For example, the relationship between independent life events over which an individual has little control (e.g., death of significant other) and depression seems to be mainly or entirely explained by environment. There is a much stronger genetic contribution to the association of depression with dependent life events. This, in part, appears to be explained by self-selection into risk exposure by those predisposed to depression (Kendler & Gardner, 2010) and that becomes more evident from adolescence on (Silberg *et al.*, 1999; Rice *et al.*, 2003).

These studies are compatible with a causal explanation in relation to links between physical abuse and antisocial behavior. They also suggest that while there is strong association between dependent life events and depression, the causal effects are not of the same effect size indexed by the magnitude of association.

Twin study designs, however, have many assumptions and limitations (Rutter & Thapar, in press). Also, the findings of bivariate twin analyses, even when applied to longitudinal data do not prove causal links. Rather, by modeling genetic contributions that can index selection and unmeasured confounding, they allow investigation of potential threats to causal inferences. This could not be achieved through observational designs that are not genetically informative.

Discordant MZ twin pairs and MZ twin pair differences

This design takes advantage of the fact that MZ twins share 100% of their genes and means that differences in their characteristics or phenotype can be attributed to nongenetic influences (including stochastic—chance—effects and measurement error). This type of design can involve testing whether MZ differences in a trait phenotype (e.g., depression symptom scores) are associated with MZ differences in exposure to an environmental factor (e.g., a quantitative measure of social adversity). An alternative configuration involves examining differences in outcome for MZ twins who are discordant for a specific categorically defined exposure (e.g., a stressful event).

In one longitudinal twin study (Caspi *et al.*, 2004), the association between independently rated measures of hostility and warmth from a recorded 5 minute speech sample from the mother while being asked about the child (expressed emotion), and later teacher-rated behavioral problems was found to be explained by environmental influences (taking into account earlier behavioral symptoms). Another example is provided by a study of MZ twin birth weight differences (Lehn *et al.*, 2007; Groen-Blokhuis *et al.*, 2011). These differences were found to be associated with later MZ differences in ADHD symptom scores, although here the causal inference is more problematic. That is because birth weight is a marker of multiple known and unknown genetic and environmental exposures during the intrauterine period.

Although these designs do control for shared genes, and thus provide some valuable insights, on their own they do not allow us to draw firm conclusions on causality for a number of reasons. The environmental factor could simply be behaving as a proxy risk factor, for example indexing some other environmental risk that impacted on one twin and not the other. Another problem is that discordant MZ twins might be considered as atypical and indeed rare for very highly heritable disorders such as ADHD and autism. These issues raise questions as to why they have been subject to different experiences and whether the risk pathways involved are different in such instances. Also we now know that MZ twins are not 100% genetically identical with respect to gene expression rather than gene sequence, for example through epigenetic differences (see Chapters 24 and 25). Nevertheless, they provide a useful and important contribution by controlling for genetic influences that can be difficult to assess in many other designs.

Discordant DZ and sibling pairs

DZ twins and siblings share on average 50% of their genes; they are not however matched genetically in the way that MZ twins are. Thus, unlike the discordant MZ twin design, these designs can only be used to test family-level (genetic and shared environment) confounds that contribute to differences in phenotypic outcomes. Discordant twin designs cannot be used to examine prenatal exposures because measures of these would be the same for each twin. There has been especial interest in utilizing siblings who are discordant for exposure to prenatal risks.

This type of design has been used extensively to examine siblings who have been discordant for exposure to maternal cigarette smoking during pregnancy. This has enabled investigators to test the relationship between maternal smoking and offspring outcomes. For example, the study conducted by Obel & colleagues (2011) found, in common with most cohort, case control studies and meta-analyses (e.g., Langley et al., 2005), a strong association between maternal smoking in pregnancy and ADHD in the overall sample (odds ratios of over 2). However, the strength of association dropped considerably (to nonsignificant levels of around 1.2) in discordant sibling pairs. That is, the sibling who had been unexposed to smoking in fetal life showed elevated levels of ADHD traits. This was not the case for lower birth weight where the relationship with exposure to cigarette smoke *in utero* remained strong.

Similar findings have been observed in relation to offspring antisocial behavior and substance misuse (D'Onofrio et al., 2012a, b). The findings suggest that selection effects and early unmeasured background confounds are probably contributing to much or all of the observed association between maternal smoking in pregnancy and offspring ADHD and behavioral outcomes.

Gaysina et al. (2013) claimed that three independent genetically sensitive designs showed that, to the contrary, there were real prenatal effects on antisocial behavior. However, that was not the case. One of the three studies used the assisted conception design (see later) but Gaysina et al. excluded it because the sample was too small to be pooled with the other two studies. A second study, the Christchurch study, compared 1088 children reared by biological mothers and 36 reared by nonrelated adoptive mothers. When covariates were included, the effect of maternal smoking became nonsignificant. That left only the Early Growth and Development study of adoptees, in which birth parent data were used to assess maternal smoking and adoptive home data were used only to evaluate child rearing. The initial analysis found a significant effect ($p = 0.007$) of maternal smoking, but the design was not a balanced one, and when confounders were considered the effect of maternal smoking remained but at a reduced significance level ($p = 0.01$). The Gaysina et al. study provides a reminder that the issue is not yet fully resolved but the weight of evidence remains in favor

of a lack of a true causal effect on either ADHD or antisocial behavior but a true effect on birth weight.

Returning to the discordant sibling design which is useful for investigating prenatal risks, again there are assumptions and limitations. Among these, a critical issue is why are mothers behaving differently in different pregnancies? That is certainly important in relation to mothers who are able to quit in one pregnancy versus ones who continue because pregnant mothers who are heavy smokers are characterized by a background of greater psychosocial adversity (Pickett et al., 2009). An additional limitation applies to utilizing DZ twin and sibling discordance to examine postnatal environmental variables. In this situation, the exposed sibling might have an influence on the unexposed sibling outcome. It is also problematic that siblings are born at different times and the risks can change over time for the family unit or at a population level. For example, characteristics of the mother such as being a teenage mother can change (Harden et al., 2007) and creates a potential threat to the interpretation of findings.

Children of twins designs and its extensions

The Children of Twins (CoT) design enables inclusion of genetic contributions to cross-generational links in psychopathology (Silberg & Eaves, 2004; D'Onofrio et al., 2003; see Chapter 28) and to links between parentally influenced risk factors and offspring outcomes. It utilizes the fact that the offspring of MZ and DZ twins are socially cousins but the MZ twin offspring are genetically half siblings (the DZ twins are of course genetically cousins and share around 1/8 of their genes).

For example, this type of design has been used to examine prenatal risks. One study found that in the offspring of alcoholics (Knopik et al., 2006), when genetic influences were included, maternal smoking in pregnancy no longer appeared to be associated with offspring ADHD; a finding similar to that reported in the discordant sibling studies. CoT designs have also been used to examine postnatal adversity. One such study (Lynch et al., 2006) found that harsh physical punishment remained associated with childhood behavioral problems when genetic factors were included, thereby showing convergence with the discordant MZ twin study findings. In an Australian study of twins, their spouses, and offspring, the aim was to assess cross-generational transmission of depression. Here, environmental factors explained the link between parent (twins) and offspring depression even when a history of depression in the spouse of the twin was taken into account (Singh et al., 2011).

An extension to the CoT design (eCoT) involves integrating data from adult twins and their children with data on child twins and their parents. Such designs have also suggested a strong environmental contribution to the cross-generational transmission of depression (Silberg et al., 2010). Interestingly, another investigation that utilized the extended CoT design suggested that while the link between adult antisocial personality disorder and offspring depression was environmental, the association with offspring conduct problems was explained by genetic and environmental factors and the relationship with offspring ADHD was entirely explained by genetic factors (Silberg *et al.*, 2012).

Another variant uses longitudinal data on the adult and child twins (LTaP). Critical limitations of the first two designs include the assumptions that there are no cohort effects and the equivalence of phenotype across generations and ages. Assortative mating (nonrandom selection of partner that is correlated with genetically influenced attributes) is also an important influence that is difficult to control for using measured variables.

Nevertheless, confidence is added by findings from other designs that have different limitations. For example, the environmental contributions to cross-generational links in depression have been observed in two CoT studies (Silberg *et al.*, 2010; Singh *et al.*, 2011) and, as we describe later, an adoption study (Tully *et al.*, 2008) and using an assisted conception design (Lewis *et al.*, 2011). Like all genetically informative designs, while these studies can undertake tests that allow inclusion of genetic contributions, they cannot on their own prove causal hypotheses.

Adoption studies

Adoption studies enable separation of genetic and prenatal influences from postnatal experiences in the adoptive placement. Such studies were originally used to examine genetic contributions to disorders, but they are also an invaluable way of testing postadoption environmental influences. Rearing influences, of the type that are likely to be shaped by genetically influenced parental attributes, would ordinarily be correlated with children's psychopathology but the association could arise from noncausal genetic reasons. This is because of genes shared by parents and their offspring. The strength of adoption studies lies in the removal of this passive gene–environment correlation contribution to postnatal environmental variables, because children are being reared by "biologically independent" adoptive parents. For example, a study of adopted away children (e.g., Ge *et al.*, 1996) showed that negative parenting from the adoptive parent was environmentally linked with their adopted children's antisocial behavior. In addition, adoptive parents' behavior was also associated with their child's biological parental psychiatric problems (substance abuse/dependency or antisocial personality); this association was mainly mediated via the child's hostile/antisocial behavior. These findings are compatible with causal effects of parenting on children's antisocial behavior, and children's genetically influenced antisocial behavior in turn influencing the behaviors of unrelated adoptive parents.

One of the most attractive aspects of adoption designs is that they also allow for testing gene–environment interaction (see Chapter 24); that is, testing whether environmental influences modify the manifestations of genetic liability. For example, one early study found that children who were genetically predisposed to lower cognitive ability (indexed via data on the biological parent) and were reared in more socially advantaged adoptive families showed greater rises in IQ than those reared

in adoptive families of lower social class (Duyme *et al.*, 1999). Another investigation of adoptees identified from national Swedish longitudinal registry data focused on those whose biological parents had died or were hospitalized as a result of suicidal behavior (Wilcox *et al.*, 2012). This alone did not increase risk for adoptee suicidal attempts and neither did exposure to the adoptive mother having a history of psychiatric hospitalization when the adoptee was younger than 18 years. However, the authors reported that in those at genetic risk, exposure to psychiatric hospitalization of the adoptive mother during childhood amplified the risk for a suicidal attempt.

Adoption studies demonstrate the importance of the rearing environment even in those genetically predisposed to developing problems. There are, however, a number of limitations and assumptions to the adoption study design. First, adoption is an unusual and now rare event in many countries. Children who are adopted away are likely to have been exposed to prenatal adversity and carry more risky genes. Thus, while suited to examining contributions of the rearing environment, they are not useful for examining prenatal risks. That is because adoption designs, unlike some of the genetically sensitive designs cannot separate the effects of genes and maternally influenced prenatal environment on offspring satisfactorily as **both** are provided by the biological mother. Another difficulty is that adoptive families tend to be from more advantaged groups, thereby restricting the range of environmental risks and lowering power to detect important risk effects (Stoolmiller, 1999), although as yet that has not been found to be a serious threat. Further, it assumes the absence of selective placement. The timing of adoption is also important. If adoption occurs at birth, that removes the possibility of biologically provided postnatal factors contributing, but this has not always been possible.

Despite these caveats, the adoption strategy provides a very useful means of controlling for genetic factors when examining post adoption environmental influences.

Assisted reproductive technologies

Another design is based on children who have been conceived through assisted reproductive technologies (ART; Thapar *et al.*, 2007). This is especially helpful for separating genetic and intrauterine influences as that cannot be done in twin or adoption studies, although it can also be used for other purposes. Children born through ART differ in the degree of genetic relatedness to the mother. If association between a prenatal factor and outcome is environmentally linked, then the association should be observed regardless of whether the child is genetically related to the woman undergoing the pregnancy (homologous *in vitro* fertilization, sperm donation) or unrelated (egg or embryo donation). This design has been used to investigate associations between maternal smoking in pregnancy and trait measures of ADHD and antisocial behavior (Thapar *et al.*, 2009; Rice *et al.*, 2009). In keeping with previous studies including a meta-analysis undertaken by the authors (Langley *et al.*,

2005), in the total sample, maternal smoking in pregnancy was strongly associated with ADHD and antisocial behavior. However, the association was only observed in genetically related mother–child dyads, suggesting that the contribution of unmeasured genetic confounds accounts for all or much of the association. The sample size was very small, but nevertheless it is interesting that the pattern of findings was different for lower birth weight, in which the results confirmed what was already known about the hazards of smoking during pregnancy. Also, as observed in the discordant sibling studies, including measured confounders was not a substitute for design features.

Investigations of cross-generational transmission and postnatal factors have also been undertaken in this design, as it allows some control (one parent will still be genetically related) of parental genetic factors (passive gene–environment correlation). Using this design, significant environmental links have been observed between maternal and offspring depression (Lewis *et al.*, 2011) and between hostile parenting and offspring antisocial behavior (Harold *et al.*, 2012). There are, however, a number of limitations and assumptions of this design. These include the representativeness of families who have undergone ART treatment, the low prevalence of risks (such as maternal smoking in pregnancy), and the types of measures that have been feasible so far (parent reports and antenatal records). It is of note, however, that there is convergence of findings across different designs in relation to the environmental contribution to cross-generational links in depression as already discussed (Tully *et al.*, 2008; Silberg *et al.*, 2010; Lewis *et al.*, 2011; Singh *et al.*, 2011). The findings on maternal smoking in pregnancy and ADHD and antisocial behavior are also in keeping with those from CoT and discordant sibling studies.

Maternal versus paternal exposure during pregnancy

Another method that has been used to disaggregate intrauterine and genetic or household-level influences is based on examining associations between maternal and paternal exposures during pregnancy and offspring outcomes. Here, if the link between exposure and offspring outcome is via intrauterine effects, a stronger association would be expected in relation to maternal exposure. For example, in a UK population cohort, strong associations have been observed between maternal smoking in pregnancy and shorter birth length (Howe *et al.* 2012) and lower birth weight in offspring (Langley *et al.*, 2012) that were not apparent when exposure to paternal smoking was assessed. However in the same cohort, associations between exposure to smoking in pregnancy and ADHD were as strong for maternal exposures as for fathers, even when paternal smoking was examined in the absence of maternal smoking and the contribution of additional passive smoking was considered (Langley *et al.*, 2012). Limitations of this design include the fact that it can only deal with exposures of the sort that both parents could experience in pregnancy and parents are likely to show

similarities in exposures for genetic (assortative mating) as well as social reasons.

Migration

A very different type of strategy utilizes migration. This has been used to test the contribution of environmental factors while holding group-level genetic ones constant. This design essentially involves investigating rates of disorder in one ethnic group that has migrated to a country with a very different set of environmental exposures and comparing them with rates of disorder in the nonmigrated group based in the country of origin and with nonmigrants in the host country. The best known example here relates to the rate of ischemic heart disease in Japanese who migrated to the United States and became exposed to marked lifestyle changes, for example involving diet. Rates of heart disease rose to levels that were much higher than found in Japan, the country of origin and similar to those found in the host country, that is, the United States. These findings highlighted the important contribution of nongenetic lifestyle factors to ischemic heart disease.

In psychiatry, the best known example is the observed higher prevalence of schizophrenia in migrants of Afro Caribbean origin to the UK and Netherlands (Jones & Fung, 2005; Coid *et al.*, 2008) when compared with the rates of disorder in the Caribbean and among nonmigrants in the host countries. The possibility of the process of migration itself being a key stressor is offset here by the observation that an increased rate was also observed in the subsequent generation. It is not yet known what the key causal environmental risk factors are.

While migration strategies have provided some useful information, there are also important limitations and assumptions. These include potential selection effects in the groups that migrate. Heterogeneous social, economic, and political "push" and "pull" factors lead to migration of some groups and there are potential advantages as well as disadvantages of migration (e.g., better access to health care and educational opportunities in the host country as well as social stresses).

Natural experiment designs that aim to remove or reduce selection or allocation bias in defined populations

We have highlighted that a key challenge to identifying causal environmental influences is that there are important selection and allocation biases including genetic influences that affect exposure. A number of studies have utilized naturally occurring situations whereby risks have been introduced to or removed from an entire population, thereby minimizing such biases.

Universal introduction of risk

Two well-known studies examined the consequences of intrauterine exposure to famine. The 1944–1995 Dutch Hunger Winter (Stein *et al.*, 1975) and the 1959–1961 Chinese famine (St Clair *et al.*, 2005) resulted in essentially universal, time-limited exposure to famine that for some fell around the time of conception or early gestation. Exposed offspring showed around a twofold risk of schizophrenia as well as congenital anomalies of the central nervous system (McClellan *et al.*, 2006). Additional investigation based on imaging a small subsample suggested that those exposed to famine including those with schizophrenia also showed brain abnormalities (Hulshoff Pol *et al.*, 2000). These findings suggest that the observation of elevated rates of schizophrenia is biologically plausible.

Furthermore, in the Dutch study, exposure to famine was found to be associated with later epigenetic dysregulation (Heijmans *et al.*, 2008). A follow-up of those exposed to famine during the Dutch Hunger Winter six decades later found less DNA methylation of the imprinted gene, insulin-like growth factor 2 (*IGF2*), when compared with their same-sex siblings (Heijmans *et al.*, 2008; Tobi *et al.*, 2012). This gene codes for a hormone that plays a major role in fetal growth. The association was specific for periconception exposure. As there was no evidence of selection for risk exposure in both of these famine studies, the findings suggest that extreme prenatal nutritional deficiency in early pregnancy is likely a causal risk factor for schizophrenia. However, whether this has relevance beyond these extreme circumstances is unknown. The findings on brain alterations and the contribution of early life environmental exposures to long-lasting epigenetic changes are intriguing. They also could provide some clues about possible risk mechanisms, although, of course, the exact nature of these requires much more investigation.

Universal removal of risk

The strength of this design is that it removes the influence of personal choice that is a major confound in most observational studies. In one particularly interesting longitudinal epidemiological study of over 1000 children, the investigators took advantage of a naturally occurring situation that arose during the study. This enabled the investigators to examine the effects of family relief from poverty on child mental health (Costello *et al.*, 2003). A quarter of the original study sample consisted of American Indians and halfway through the study, a casino opened on the reserve. This provided a substantial increase to the family income of American Indians that increased every year. Data on child mental health were available before this event and after. The researchers were able to show that the relief of poverty resulted in a decrease in levels of oppositional defiant disorder and conduct disorder. As there was no selection, the findings were consistent with causal effects. The benefits appeared to be mediated via altered parenting that included the provision of increased parental time and supervision. Interestingly, levels of adolescent depression and anxiety were not altered. Further follow-up into early adulthood showed that the family income supplementation provided in childhood continued to be associated with lower rates of total psychopathology, notably alcohol and cannabis abuse and lower rates of convictions for minor

offenses and higher levels of education. There were no links with later nicotine or other drug use, emotional or behavioral disorders (Costello *et al.*, 2010).

Interrupted time series

The interrupted time series design takes advantage of multiple waves of data observation that occur before and after the introduction (or removal) of the putative causal variable, the timing of which is known. This is sometimes used to examine the effects of policy or treatment; for example, the observed drop in deaths from paracetamol overdoses after the introduction of UK legislation to reduce paracetamol package sizes (Hawton *et al.*, 2013). However, this type of design can also take advantage of naturally occurring events and be used to test etiological hypotheses.

One example is provided by investigations of gang membership in relation to delinquent activities. Gang membership is known to be associated with higher rates of delinquency, but it is difficult to know whether this is due to selection effects; that is, whether the observed association is explained by attributes of those who join gangs or arises through the social effects of being in a gang. An early study (Thornberry *et al.*, 1993) contrasted levels of delinquency across different time periods; before boys became gang members against during the time they joined and after they left the gang. Later studies (Thornberry *et al.*, 2003) extended the approach by using more sophisticated analytic approaches to further consider possible biases and retrospectively to examine gang membership prior to the onset of the study. The findings suggested, as might be expected, important selection effects. Boys who joined gangs were more delinquent than those who did not. However, they also showed that gang membership had additional social influences because rates of delinquency dropped once boys left the gang, although not back to the level that they were prior to joining a gang. In this example, it is difficult to rule out reverse causation effects whereby the decision to leave a gang is influenced by a drop in its delinquent activities or to completely rule out a contribution of unmeasured confounders. Also, the designs did not allow for testing the mechanisms by which gangs might have had this effect.

Using changes in policy as natural experiments
China's one child policy

Another quasi-experimental design was provided by China's "one child policy" (Cameron *et al.* 2013) that again was applied to a large population and the timing was known. This allowed a test of the psychological effects of being an only child. In other contexts, being an only child is confounded with multiple factors that influence the decision or likelihood of having only one child, that is, selection or allocation effects. The authors examined children born prior to the introduction of the one child policy in 1979 and compared them to those born after that policy from the same area. They utilized questionnaire measures of personality traits and experimental data generated from standard economic games that were designed to assess altruism, ability to trust others and trustworthiness, risk taking, and competition. This study, based on 421 children, showed that the policy, which behaved as an instrumental variable for being an only child (see later), resulted in individuals who were more pessimistic, more risk averse, less conscientious, less competitive, and less prosocial. The imposed policy meant removal of the usual sorts of selection effects that would be operating and the study dealt effectively with the range of methodological matters needing attention.

Change in legislation on sale of alcohol in Sweden

A different type of study focused on the effects of prenatal alcohol exposure in two regions in Sweden that were exposed to an experimental policy change in the sales of alcohol. The intention had been to shift the population from drinking spirits to drinks with lower alcohol content. However, the policy inadvertently resulted in very marked increases in the consumption of strong beer during a very specific time period. This was especially the case among teenagers due to age restrictions for the purchase of other types of alcohol (Nilsson, 2008). The experimental policy started in 1967 but was terminated abruptly in mid 1968 when it was realized that it had led to a very sharp increase in alcohol consumption. As the experiment was time-limited, it provided the opportunity of comparing the cohort who were *in utero* during this time period to those in adjacent time-unexposed cohorts. As it was geographically restricted, it also provided the opportunity for comparisons of children born in the same cohort from the exposed and unexposed regions. Using Swedish national registry data, it was found that the exposed group who had been *in utero* during the experimental period and were around 30 years, showed greatly reduced educational achievements, lower earnings, and greater welfare dependency than the comparison cohorts. The effects were strongest in males, those exposed for the longest in intrauterine life, and those born to younger mothers. The magnitude, timing, and geographical distribution of the effects suggested that prenatal exposure to alcohol likely had long-lasting consequences on offspring, although the mediating mechanisms are not known. Another problem is that the results are derived from analyses at a group level and there is thus uncertainty about effects on individuals. Nevertheless, this study illustrates how policy changes can provide an opportunity for natural experiments in whole populations. whereby the threats of reverse causation are removed and the problems of selection and contribution of confounders diminished. There are also, however, limitations and assumptions of these types of studies. For example, they rely on inferences rather than direct measures. It is impossible to rule out the contribution of other confounders that operate, for example, postnatally and it is not known how generalizable findings would be outside the quasi-experimental situation.

Radical changes in environment
Adoption following profound institutional deprivation

Another example of a natural experiment that involved change of a different type and that was radical is provided by the English and Romanian Adoptees study (Rutter & Sonuga-Barke, 2010). This involved a longitudinal follow-up investigation of children who were exposed to institutional care from the time of early infancy and extreme deprivation. Many critical selection biases were absent because the children were admitted very early before they may have had an influence on their admission into care, thereby reducing the possibility of reverse causation. Virtually no children left care until the government regime fell in 1989, thereby also removing the possibility of selection as to which children remained in care. These children subsequently experienced a dramatic change in environment after they were adopted into relatively advantaged families in the UK. A natural experiment design was further facilitated by accurate timing of children's removal from this context. The study suggested that institutional care of the type experienced by these children had possible causal effects because there was considerable and major recovery of deficits following removal from that context. The design could not distinguish deprivation effects from benefits attributable to the adoptive home. Nevertheless, variations within the adoptive home environment did not seem to contribute to differences in outcome in the age 15 group. Many tests of alternative explanations were undertaken and, as highlighted at the start of this chapter, this is critical. Overall, these suggested that a causal inference is justified despite some limitations, such as an absence of data on biological parents and the question of the extent to which findings might apply to less severe and more common forms of deprivation. As was the case for the famine studies, sometimes natural experiments have involved extreme and less common forms of environmental risk, thereby raising the issue of generalizability to more typical contexts.

Regression discontinuity

Regression discontinuity (RD) designs were originally put forward as an alternative to randomized controlled trials. They take advantage of situations where an intervention is provided to those who fall beyond a strict cut-point on a specific measure (e.g., level of poverty), rather than where allocation is through randomization. The selection bias here is utilized because it is imposed externally, the bias cannot be caused by the intervention or in nonexperimental settings, the "causal risk."

The slope of a regression line as visualized graphically represents the strength of association between a predictor (e.g., poverty level) and an outcome (e.g., cognition and behavior). Where there is discontinuity in the regression at the cut-point for selection, it suggests a causal effect of intervention on outcome.

This type of design has been used for assessing the effects of experimental interventions, but there is little on its use in relation to testing nonexperimental causal risks. For example, an RD design was used to examine the effects of Head Start, a program for preschool health and social services to poor children aged 3 or 4 years in the United States (Ludwig & Miller, 2005). In 1965, assistance was given to the 300 poorest counties, which led to very marked higher levels of funding and participation in these counties. The RD design involved comparing those just above the cut-point and those just below the cut-point for this assistance. The findings suggested a substantial impact of Head Start on health measures and school graduation but not on noncognitive outcomes. The inference of likely causal effects was strengthened by finding that similar effects were not found in age groups that were unexposed to Head Start or to health outcomes that were not plausibly related to the impact of Head Start. Nevertheless, there are many limitations including a lack of accurate individual level data on exposure (e.g., effects of families moving in and out).

Another example is provided by a study that set out to examine whether cognitive performance in school children was affected by the amount of schooling received versus being older in chronological age (Cahan & Cohen, 1989). This was enabled by a system whereby all children in state-controlled Hebrew language primary/elementary mainstream schools in 1987 were admitted at one time point in December. The authors excluded any children who were under- or over-age in each of the classes studied and those born in November or December. Thus, children at the end of one school year and the beginning of the next would have a one-year difference in schooling received. In any given class, the youngest and oldest would have received the same amount of schooling but differ much more in chronological age. This study showed that the amount of schooling contributed more than older age to nearly all the cognitive measures used.

Using instrumental variables

An instrumental variable is a measured variable that is associated with the predictor (risk factor) being tested but that is not subject to the same social selection effects and confounds including shared genetic influences. Instrumental variables are used as a statistical method to deal with unmeasured confounding in observational and treatment studies, but there are also situations when they can be used as a basis for a natural experiment.

Early puberty provides an example of an instrumental variable in relation to early use and misuse of alcohol. These are behaviors that have been considered as possible causal risks for later alcohol dependence and misuse in adult life. Early puberty is strongly associated with early alcohol use and misuse but is a variable that is not subject to the same selection effects. Three studies find that while early alcohol use and misuse in adolescence is associated with later alcohol related problems, early puberty does not predict adult alcohol problems (Stattin & Magnusson 1990; Caspi & Moffitt, 1991; Pulkkinen et al., 2006). These findings suggest that early alcohol use, rather than being a cause of later alcohol problems, is likely an early manifestation of the same liability.

Mendelian randomization

Mendelian randomization (MR) is a variant of the instrumental variable approach. This method has been proposed to provide another means of testing causal effects when unmeasured confounding is a likely problem. Here, a genotype is used as the instrumental variable for the risk factor in question. It utilizes the fact that there is random assortment of parental genotypes at meiosis and thus, theoretically, genotypes are not subject to the same confounds as the risk factor under consideration. It has perhaps been most successfully used in the realm of cardiovascular disease. For example, MR has recently been used to evaluate the causal risk effects of cholesterol levels on myocardial infarction ("heart attack"). In a very large study (Voight et al., 2012) that utilized two genetic instrumental variables (a composite genetic score and a loss-of-function coding gene variant), the authors found evidence to suggest that increased HDL cholesterol (which is considered the "good type" of cholesterol) does not lower the risk of myocardial infarction. The results suggested that attempts through treatment to increase levels of what has been called a "good" type of cholesterol are not supported. However, there are a number of assumptions of the MR design (e.g., pleiotropy, whereby genes have multiple different effects) that we discuss later.

Another study used risk scores from gene variants in alcohol metabolizing genes as a genetic instrumental variable in a UK birth cohort of several thousand children (Lewis et al., 2012). The authors found that these gene variants were related to lower IQ at age 8 but only in the offspring of mothers who were moderate drinkers of alcohol during pregnancy, not those whose mothers abstained from alcohol.

While an elegant design, there are a number of critical assumptions that require systematic evaluation when MR is applied (Glymour et al., 2012), some of which are especially problematic in relation to mental health phenotypes. For example, there is a need for genetic variants that have a strong and robust association with the risk factor in question. If the genotype (instrument) has pleiotropic effects and has multiple effects on different phenotypes, which seems common in relation to mental health (see Chapter 24), or influences another intermediate phenotype, this creates problems. If that intermediate phenotype affects the clinical outcome or influences a confounding factor, key assumptions are violated.

Statistical methods to reduce selection biases and confounders

We do not provide a detailed description of statistical methods but rather flag up that there are many such analytic techniques. These methods attempt to address selection differences between groups exposed and unexposed to the risk factor in question and take into account measured confounders. While these have been useful developments, because they allow for less biased estimates of association, residual confounding remains a problem. Propensity scores can be used for statistical matching of the group exposed to the risk factor in question (or intervention) to the one that is unexposed. It utilizes the covariates that predict exposure to the risk (or receipt of intervention) that will include variables that preceded the exposure. Thus, it requires observed, measured predictors typically derived from regression analyses and is still limited by the problem of residual confounding and selection effects that are not captured by measured predictors. Inverse probability to treatment weighting involves using propensity scores as weights to create more representative samples (Rutter & Thapar, in press).

A propensity score matching method was used by Kendler and colleagues (2010) to test the likely causal effects of dependent life events on major depression and was strengthened by combining it with a design involving MZ twins who were discordant for exposure to dependent life events. They found a substantial proportion of the association appeared to be due to noncausal effects, but the complementary designs were consistent with life events having a modest causal risk effect.

Other analytic approaches involve statistical modeling that utilizes data from multiple data points. These include structural equation modeling (SEM) and latent growth curve modeling. Where multiple measures and ideally longitudinal data are available, SEM allows for simultaneously testing relationships between hypothesized risk and outcome variables across and within time and for incorporating measured confounders of risk exposure into the statistical model. Latent growth curve modeling requires repeated observations of the same data over time. It moves beyond group-level analyses and allows testing for individual-level change as a function of time. Risk exposures during a certain time can be examined in relation to alterations in growth curves. These methods can also be used to test potential mediating mechanisms. These, however, are statistical methods rather than designs. They rely on *a priori* specification of the causal model and infer causal links by assessing fit of the model according to statistical criteria and the use of measured confounders. Explanatory models and mediating mechanisms that are statistically satisfactory are not necessarily correct. They provide a platform from which to test alternative explanations ideally through different designs.

Experimental manipulation in humans

As a bridge between natural experiments and animal models, it is appropriate to mention the use of human experiments, for example, assessing hyperventilation and anxious behavior in response to a carbon dioxide challenge, because the same strategy may be able to be used in animals as well as humans (Battaglia *et al.*, 2014). Their uses in studying gene–environment interaction by examining how individuals respond to stimuli in an experimental situation are considered in Chapter 23. For example, the use of an experimental induction of emotion showed how a specific genotype (5HTT transporter gene

variant) altered an intermediate brain imaging phenotype in response to the emotional stimulus, with the brain functional changes lying on the same biological pathway as that leading to psychiatric disorder.

Animal models to test environmental influences

Most of the best animal models dealing with environmental effects that are relevant to clinical practice had their origins in clinical observations or theories that were supposed to deal with the clinical features. For example, the Nobel prize winning work by Hubel and Wiesel examining the effects of binocular visual input to the growth of the visual cortex was prompted in part by the observations of Von Senden (1960) that children with congenital cataracts have substantial, and often permanent, visual deficits after removal of the cataracts. Riesen's research with animals provided similar observations (Riesen, 1961). Hubel and Wiesel undertook various experimental manipulations but the one that is prototypical is the suturing of the eyelids of one eye in order to determine the effects on the brain. In keeping with the best of animal models, they examined the possibility that the cortical effects were related more to competition between the eyes than to simple disuse (finding that they were). Also, they went on to examine in much more detail the changes in the visual cortex (Hubel & Wiesel, 2005). In short, the basic science findings in the animal model led on to further studies of what was happening in the brain. The findings from the animal model were important also in indicating the need to intervene early in life to deal with strabismus in young children.

Somewhat similar lessons derive from the research by Rosenzweig and Bennett and their colleagues (Rosenzweig *et al.*, 1962). Their starting point was the observation that laboratory rats that were given formal problem-solving training had neurochemical changes in the cerebral cortex. This led on to experimental studies of deprivation and enrichment. In brief, rats reared in single cages (deprived conditions) were compared with those reared in a large cage containing 10–12 animals, with a variety of stimulus objects that was changed daily (enriched conditions) (see Chapter 23). In the early experiments, the study was done on juvenile animals on the grounds that the effects should only be found at a time of maximal brain growth. Later studies compared juveniles and adults, with the striking finding that effects were broadly similar in adults as in juveniles, although the effects were greater in the young (Rosenzweig & Bennett, 1996). In line with later human studies, it was evident that adult experiences could change brain structure (see Chapter 23).

The work of Levine, undertaken at much the same time, had its basis in Freud's theory that early life stress contributed to the development of subsequent emotional instability. Contrary to expectation, Levine *et al.* (1956) found that rats exposed to intermittent foot shocks actually had a diminished susceptibility to later stress and this explosure also affected the neuroendocrine system (Levine, 1957, 1962). It was typical of a good use of an animal model that the failure to confirm the original expectation led on to further exploration of the "steeling" (strengthening) effect. Thirty years later, Lyons and colleagues, working in the laboratory that Levine founded, began to investigate the long-term effects of brief, intermittent mother–infant separations in squirrel monkeys (Lyons *et al.*, 2010). Socially housed squirrel monkeys were randomized to either brief intermittent separations or a nonseparated control condition at 17 weeks of age. For each of the separations, one monkey was removed from the rearing group for a one-hour session. The aim was to determine whether the intermittent separations (which were designed to mimic those that normally occurred in the wild) provided a form of stress inoculation that enhanced arousal regulation and resilience (Lyons *et al.*, 2009). The findings showed both diminution in anxiety and increased exploration of novel situations but also biological effects in the neuroendocrine system and the brain. In conjunction with other findings, it has been concluded that exposure to challenge and manageable stress can enhance resilience in humans (Rutter, 2013).

Harlow's classic experimental studies with rhesus monkeys showed the profound effects of social isolation. The original motivation for the studies lay in the human studies (such as those by Goldfarb), but Harlow was also influenced by what he saw as the narrowness of classical conditioning such as undertaken by Skinner. His aim was to test the extent to which loving contact was shaped only by the reward of food. The experimental design involved the so-called "cloth" and "wire" mothers, each of which could be made to provide, or not provide, nourishment. The findings were clear cut in showing that the babies sought the comfort of contact irrespective of feeding (Harlow, 1958, 1963). Not only were there immediate differences in behavior but social isolation was also found to have long-lasting effects (Harlow & Suomi, 1971) that were quite difficult to reverse completely (Novak & Harlow, 1975). Harlow's research made a huge impact on the field and the findings were taken up by Bowlby in his writings on attachment. However, the studies dealt with quite extreme conditions and the later studies by Harlow have been generally regarded as unnecessarily cruel and ethically unacceptable (Blum, 2002).

Hinde's research, also dealing with rhesus macaque monkeys, was quite different in focusing on a more normal range of situations and in concentrating on the influences on individual differences (Hinde & Spencer-Booth, 1970; Hinde & Mcginnis, 1977). Three main findings were particularly important with respect to human implications. First, they found that the infant's distress following separation was a function of both the preseparation and contemporaneous mother–infant relationship. Second, changes in the mother–infant interaction largely depended on the mother and, third, the infant showed much less post separation distress and more normal mother–infant interaction when they themselves were removed to a strange place for 13 days and then restored to their mother than when

the mothers were removed to a strange place for a similar period. Hinde has argued convincingly that post separation distress was more a consequence of disturbance in maternal behavior than in the direct effects of the separation itself. These studies are a model of careful, rigorous comparisons that were well designed to test hypotheses, of great potential relevance for humans. The work of Harlow and Hinde are good examples of what can be achieved by animal models and it is important to note that a far wider range of investigators dealt with similar issues (Rutter, 1981; Blum, 2002).

Harlow and Suomi (1974) worked together to develop peer-rearing as an important risk experience for later development. For over a dozen years now, Suomi has run a randomized controlled trial contrasting mother-reared rhesus monkeys, peer-reared rhesus monkeys, and surrogate-peer-reared rhesus monkeys (Conti *et al.*, 2012). Numerous studies have consistently shown the detrimental long-term effects on health associated with peer rearing. The use of animal models by Suomi's group has provided major advances in two respects. First, experimental conditions are randomly allocated (which, perhaps surprisingly, has not been true of many animal models); and, secondly, the outcomes have been examined, not only with respect to cerebrospinal fluid differences during life but also epigenetic findings using postmortem hippocampal tissue. The results were used, amongst other things, to examine gene × environment interactions (G × E) (Lindell *et al.*, 2012). It was found that differential rearing led to differential DNA methylation in both prefrontal cortex and T cells (Provençal *et al.*, 2012). The finding that early life social adversity was associated with modulation of the developing immune system provides confirmation of the human evidence on the same topic (Danese *et al.*, 2008; Danese *et al.*, 2011).

The next example of an animal model concerns Meaney's program of research into the epigenetic effects of the environment on gene expression (see Chapter 25) that represents quite a different form of investigation. Rather than aiming to provide any kind of parallel to human rearing, it sought to examine a mechanism that was likely to operate across species. The research began with the observation that lactating mother rats varied markedly in the extent to which they licked and groomed their offspring and showed associated arch-back nursing (both being *un*associated with the amount of maternal time spent with the pups). These individual differences were associated with neurochemical variations in a particular brain region, as well as individual differences in the pups' behavior and response to stress. A cross-fostering design was used to determine whether the effects were due to biological inheritance or rearing environment—with the findings supporting an effect of rearing. It was then shown that the maternal behavior had altered the endocrine response to stress lastingly via an effect on a specific glucocorticoid receptor gene promoter in the hippocampus. The next question was whether the epigenetic effects could be reversed by using a particular drug to reverse the methylation effect. It was found that reversal could be brought about—providing further confirmation of a causal effect. These initial findings are interesting and important. As ever, replication and further investigations will be needed as complex multifactorial phenotypes such as altered stress response will likely involve different types of epigenetic changes across multiple genomic sites and the rearing environment could also impact on other types of biological mediating mechanisms. Nevertheless, it is no exaggeration to state that the findings from these ingenious, well-controlled experimental studies led to a paradigm shift in the understanding of environmental effects on gene expression.

Fernald and Maruska (2012) also studied epigenetic effects of environmental influences, but did so in relation to experimentally induced changes in social dominance in zebra fish. They first showed that males can rapidly and reversibly switch between dominant and subordinate status, this being accompanied by a dramatic change in body coloration and changes in gene expression in the preoptic area of the brain. They found that visual cues of social encounters were crucial. Two dominant males, differing in size by a factor of 4, were allowed to establish territories out of view of one another because of an opaque barrier. When that was replaced by a transparent barrier, the smaller male suppressed all dominant behavior. Through manipulation of this situation, Fernald and his colleagues were able to induce either a rise or fall in social rank with consequences for gene expression. While the social worlds of zebra fish and humans are very different, social rank is a ubiquitous element in all social systems and an essential organizing principle in understanding social behavior. The experimental control in this animal model provides a good test of causation, with epigenetic findings that are likely to apply widely across species, including humans.

Animal models have also been used to examine the effects of physical toxins and perinatal adversity; most notably, they have been helpful in the study of the effects on the fetus of mother's alcohol consumption during the pregnancy. Once more, the animal models start from a human observation, namely, the identification of the congenital anomalies associated with high levels of alcohol exposure during the first trimester of pregnancy (Jones et al., 1973). Animal studies were informative in showing the same congenital anomaly effects as in humans but were mainly of value in tackling the question as to whether low levels of alcohol exposure might have similar, albeit lesser, effects (Cudd, 2005). This question was important because of the limited relevant data from human studies (see Gray & Henderson, 2006). To date, there have been a rather limited number of studies, using both rats and rhesus monkeys, but these suggest that there may be greater effects from low to moderate levels of alcohol exposure during the pregnancy than had hitherto been supposed (see Gray et al., 2009). Similar approaches have been used to study cigarette and nicotine exposure in utero in rats. The findings have shown a consistent effect, leading to a lower birth weight but not the motor and cognitive changes that might form a parallel with ADHD (LeSage et al., 2006; Winzer-Serhan, 2007). Animal

experimental models have also been used to examine the effects of exposure to perinatal hypoxia. For example, rodents exposed to chronic perinatal hypoxia show cognitive deficits that appear to be related to specific brain and cellular anomalies and that some of these deficits may be ameliorated by environmental enrichment (Vaccarino et al., 2013; Salmaso et al., 2014).

Animal models to study the causal effects of genetic risks

In principle, genetic influences raise the same need for testing of causal inferences. However, at first sight that might seem redundant in the case of diseases due to a single, highly penetrant, mutant gene, such as is the case with Rett syndrome (see, e.g., Zoghbi & Bear, 2012). However, that assumption would be a mistake for three separate reasons. First, the identification of the mutant gene in itself does not identify the causal pathway(s) involved. That was also the case with environmental influences (see discussion of the animal models used by Hinde and by Harlow). Second, there may be more than one mutant gene; for example, tuberous sclerosis is caused by mutation in two distinct genes. Third, often the syndromes involve several rather different features. That is the case, for example, with the fragile X syndrome. Here, we illustrate what may be achieved with animal models of genetic risks by considering Rett syndrome, fragile X, and tuberous sclerosis. In each case, the animal model is created by some variety of engineered deletions of a specific gene or knock-in of a foreign gene. In other words, the aim is *not* to mimic the features of a specific human syndrome but, rather, to directly create an animal with the same relevant mutant gene.

Rett syndrome

Girls with Rett syndrome appear to develop normally up to about 6–18 months but head growth then decelerates leading to microcephaly (Rutter & Thapar, 2014). The children lose purposeful use of their hands and develop stereotypical hand washing movements. Epileptic seizures often start about the age of 4 years but tend to decrease in severity in adult life at a time when there is progressive neurological deterioration. Mutations in the X-linked gene encoding the methyl-CpG-binding protein 2 (MeCP2) have been found to be causal.

Mice lacking functional MeCP2 were created by Chen et al. (2001) and by Guy et al. (2001). There were two surprises in the findings. First, the mutant mice showed a remarkable degree of similarity with the human condition in both course of development (with an initial period of apparently normal development) and behavioral features. Second, despite the devastating neurological features, the brain appeared relatively normal apart from microcephaly, and a decrease in dendritic spine density (see Dani et al., 2005). Thus, what had previously been regarded as a progressive neurodegenerative disorder seemed to involve a disruption of neural networks, but not their destruction (Belichenko et al., 2009). It was found that, at least in the mutant mice, gene reversal led to a reversal of the phenotype (Giacometti et al., 2007; Guy et al., 2007; Tropea et al., 2009). Commentators have generally described this as a reversal of a neurodegenerative disorder but, in our view (Rutter & Thapar, 2014) the relatively normal brain findings combined with reversal or partial reversal suggests instead that the syndrome derives from postnatal malfunction. It remains to be determined whether the same applies in humans, but what is clear is that the genetically based animal model has led to a major rethink on the underlying biology and the causal risk effects of this gene mutation.

Fragile X

The fragile X anomaly was first reported by Lubs (1969), and it was found to be associated with many physical features (such as large testes and large low-set ears), as well as the behavioral features of cognitive impairment, hyperactivity, social anxiety, and autistic-like features. Postmortem studies in humans showed structural abnormalities of the dendritic spines. Fu et al. (1991) and Verkerk et al. (1991) showed that expansions in the fragile X gene (*Fmr1*) caused the syndrome. This evidence provided the means to produce an *Fmr1* knock-out (KO) mouse (Bakker et al., 1994) that has been used in much subsequent research (Dölen et al., 2007) and the suggestion that unchecked mG1uR5 activation might contribute significantly to pathogenesis. *Fmr1* KO mice showed phenotypes similar to the human condition with hyperactivity, repetitive behavior, and seizures. Dolan et al. (2013) used the small molecule PAK inhibitor (FRAX486) to determine whether it could rescue the phenotype. They showed that it both reversed the dendritic spine abnormalities and the behavioral features of hyperactivity and repetitive movement, but it did not impact macroorchidism. Moreover, the reversals were obtained in adult mice as well as in juveniles. Again, the mutant mouse model provided an important lead on the possibility of clinical benefits in humans.

Tuberous sclerosis (TS)

TS is a neurocutaneous, autosomal dominantly inherited multi-system disorder characterized by benign tumors (hamartomas) that occur in many organs including the brain. Because of the gross brain abnormalities it is exceedingly unlikely that reversal could be brought about. Nevertheless, mutant gene rodent models have been produced. It has been found that the immune-suppressive drug rapamycin affects some changes in some phenotypes (see Tsai et al., 2012). In that connection it is relevant that substantial brain dysfunction occurs independently of gross structural brain abnormalities (as in hamartomas) and epilepsy (de Vries, 2010). The mutant mouse model in this instance did not succeed in bringing about a major reversal of the neurodegenerative changes but it did lead to a broadening of the concept of the possible pathophysiological changes that might be involved as a result of specific risk genes and this might ultimately lead to clinical benefits.

These few examples do not cover the long list of mutant models that have been put forward (Robertson & Feng, 2011). Also, it is important to note that even the ones that have not led to major breakthroughs have sometimes helped in drawing attention to processes that had not been previously recognized in the human work. Bowles et al.'s (2012) thoughtful review of gene expression and behavior in mouse models of Huntington's disease provides a good example. Also, mice do not constitute the only source of mutant models (see, e.g., Golzio et al. (2012) on the use of both mice and zebra fish in relation to the role of copy number variations in producing a microcephaly phenotype).

Behavior-based animal models to study causal risks in relation to multifactorial psychiatric disorders

There is a long history of producing animal models based on behavioral similarities to some human disorder of interest. For example, a mouse model of depression has been produced by separation experiences, by forcing the mouse to swim until exhausted, by hanging the mouse upside down by its tail, and many other sources of stress (Cryan & Mombereau, 2004; Cryan & Holmes, 2005; Cryan & Slattery, 2007). The approach follows the recognition that stress and adverse experiences play a substantial role in the genesis of anxiety and depressive disorder in humans (Heim & Nemeroff, 1999). However, depression also involves cognitions such as despair, hopelessness, and self-blame that would be tricky to elicit in mice. Moreover, the stresses used, such as forced swimming, involve a behavior (swimming) not ordinarily used by mice.

A behavioral model of autism raises even greater challenges in that mentalization, skills, and language cannot be assessed in rodents. Nevertheless, Crawley (Crawley, 2007; Yang et al., 2011) has been ingenious in using ultrasonic mouse socialization to index social communication and reciprocal interaction. It may be that this constitutes a useful way forward but it is difficult to see what could be learned from behavior-based models for multifactorial disorders.

It needs to be added that findings have been difficult to replicate in view of strain differences and major social context effects. While it is certainly true that there is huge genetic overlap across species, there are also important differences in the meaning of findings, as illustrated by the occasional examples of findings from animal research leading to wrong conclusions about human applicability (Academy of Medical Sciences, 2006; National Research Council, 2013).

A wide variety of animal species can inform causal research in psychopathology

It is sometimes thought that animal models have to be based on species closely related to humans, but that is not so.

Of course, the validity of findings is crucially dependent on the evolutionary conservation of key functions across species but such conservation seems to be surprisingly strong. Three examples may be given. First, John Sulston chose to use *Caenorhabditis elegans* (a tiny worm about 1 mm long) for sequencing the genome (*C. elegans* Sequencing Consortium, 1998) because it was transparent throughout its life cycle (of about 2 weeks) and it has a limited number of 302 neurons. The research provided the model for sequencing the human genome and it resulted in a Nobel Prize. *C. elegans* has also been used to demonstrate the importance of gene–gene interaction (see Chapter 24). Eric Kandel (2001) chose aplysia, the giant sea snail, because it had only about 2000 neurons and because the cells were so large that investigation of individual neurons was feasible. The research provided findings on learning and memory, which have been extremely informative about human cognitive processes.

The third example provided is the long-established and highly productive field of fruit fly (drosophila) genetics. Hermann Müller won the 1946 Nobel Prize in physiology and medicine for his work showing that radiation exposure produced mutations. Benzer (see Greenspan *et al.*, 2008) went on to use mutagenesis to study the biology of behavior. Fruit fly research has been highly informative in studying circadian rhythms (see Flint *et al.*, 2010 for an excellent fuller discussion of the value of drosophila genetics). We end this section of the chapter by referring to the work of Marla Sokolowski (Osborne *et al.*, 1997), who was responsible for identifying the genes underlying the distinction between fruit fly rovers and sitters. In subsequent work, Burns *et al.* (2012) found a significant gene–environment interaction such that early nutritional adversity in the larval period increased "sitter" but not "rover" exploratory behavior in adult life. There were also effects on the adult reproductive output of "sitters" but not "rovers" indicating a G × E on fitness. These examples demonstrate how animal models across different species can be used to identify causal risks and mechanisms.

Conclusions

The complementary use of natural experiments and animal models has provided some telling examples where generally accepted causes have been challenged and others where causal hypotheses have been strengthened. This has been particularly the case when several different designs have been used and have given rise to similar conclusions. There is an urgent need to identify genuinely causal influences, not only for scientific understanding but also to inform policy and practice. We conclude by restating that neither natural experiments nor animal models constitute a finite list of designs. Rather, they represent a style of thinking about possible causal processes and looking out for new ways in which they may be tested.

References

Academy of Medical Sciences (2006) *The Use of Nonhuman Primates in Research*. Academy of Medical Sciences, London.

Academy of Medical Sciences (2007) *Identifying the Environmental Causes of Disease: How Should we Decide What to Believe and When to Take Action*. Academy of Medical Sciences, London.

Anderson, K.E. *et al.* (1986) Mothers' interactions with normal and conduct-disordered boys: who affects whom? *Developmental Psychology* **22**, 604.

Bakker, C.E. *et al.* (1994) Fmr1 knockout mice: a model to study fragile X mental retardation. *Cell* **78**, 23–33.

Battaglia, M., *et al.* (2014). Early-life risk factors for panic and separation anxiety disorder: insights and outstanding questions arising from human and animal studies of CO2 sensitivity. *Neuroscience and Biobehavioral Reviews*, **46**, 455–464.

Belichenko, P.V. *et al.* (2009) Widespread changes in dendritic and axonal morphology in MeCP2-mutant mouse models of Rett syndrome: evidence for disruption of neuronal networks. *Journal of Comparative Neurology* **514**, 240–258.

Blum, D. (2002) *Love at Goon Park: Harry Harlow and the science of affection*. The Berkley Publishing Group, New York.

Bowles, K. *et al.* (2012) Gene expression and behaviour in mouse models of HD. *Brain Research Bulletin* **88**, 276–284.

Brown, G.W. *et al.* (1986) Long-term effects of early loss of parent. In: *Depression in Young People: Developmental and Clinical Perspectives*. (eds M. Rutter, C. Izard & P. Reed), pp. 251–296. Guilford Press, New York.

Burns, J.G. *et al.* (2012) Gene–environment interplay in Drosophila melanogaster: chronic food deprivation in early life affects adult exploratory and fitness traits. *Proceedings of the National Academy of Sciences* **109**, 17239–17244.

C. elegans Sequencing Consortium (1998) Genome sequence of the nematode C. elegans: a platform for investigating biology. *Science* **282**, 2012–2018.

Cahan, S. & Cohen, N. (1989) Age versus schooling effects on intelligence development. *Child Development* **60**, 1239–1249.

Cameron, L. *et al.* (2013) Little emperors: behavioral impacts of China's one-child policy. *Science* **339**, 953–957.

Campbell, D.T. & Stanley, J.C. (1963) *Experimental and Quasi-Experimental Designs for Research*. Rand McNally, Chicago.

Caspi, A. & Moffitt, T.E. (1991) Individual differences are accentuated during periods of social change: the sample case of girls at puberty. *Journal of Personality and Social Psychology* **61**, 157–168.

Caspi, A. *et al.* (2004) Maternal expressed emotion predicts children's antisocial behavior problems: using monozygotic-twin differences to identify environmental effects on behavioral development. *Developmental Psychology* **40**, 149–161.

Chen, R.Z. *et al.* (2001) Deficiency of methyl-CpG binding protein-2 in CNS neurons results in a Rett-like phenotype in mice. *Nature Genetics* **27**, 327–331.

Coid, J.W. *et al.* (2008) Raised incidence rates of all psychoses among migrant groups: findings from the East London first episode psychosis study. *Archives of General Psychiatry* **65**, 1250–1258.

Conti, G. *et al.* (2012) Primate evidence on the late health effects of early-life adversity. *Proceedings of the National Academy of Sciences* **109**, 8866–8871.

Costello, E.J. *et al.* (2003) Relationships between poverty and psychopathology: a natural experiment. *JAMA* **290**, 2023–2029.

Costello, E.J. *et al.* (2010) Association of family income supplements in adolescence with development of psychiatric and substance use disorders in adulthood among an American Indian population. *JAMA* **303**, 1954–1960.

Crawley, J.N. (2007) Mouse behavioral assays relevant to the symptoms of autism. *Brain Pathology* **17**, 448–459.

Cryan, J.F. & Holmes, A. (2005) The ascent of mouse: advances in modelling human depression and anxiety. *Nature Reviews Drug Discovery* **4**, 775–790.

Cryan, J. & Mombereau, C. (2004) In search of a depressed mouse: utility of models for studying depression-related behavior in genetically modified mice. *Molecular Psychiatry* **9**, 326–357.

Cryan, J.F. & Slattery, D.A. (2007) Animal models of mood disorders: recent developments. *Current Opinion in Psychiatry* **20**, 1–7.

Cudd, T.A. (2005) Animal model systems for the study of alcohol teratology. *Experimental Biology and Medicine* **230**, 389–393.

Danese, A. *et al.* (2008) Elevated inflammation levels in depressed adults with a history of childhood maltreatment. *Archives of General Psychiatry* **65**, 409–415.

Danese, A. *et al.* (2011) Biological embedding of stress through inflammation processes in childhood. *Molecular Psychiatry* **16**, 244–246.

Dani, V.S. *et al.* (2005) Reduced cortical activity due to a shift in the balance between excitation and inhibition in a mouse model of Rett syndrome. *Proceedings of the National Academy of Sciences of the United States of America* **102**, 12560–12565.

De Vries, P.J. (2010) Targeted treatments for cognitive and neurodevelopmental disorders in tuberous sclerosis complex. *Neurotherapeutics* **7**, 275–282.

Dolan, B.M. *et al.* (2013) Rescue of fragile X syndrome phenotypes in Fmr1 KO mice by the small-molecule PAK inhibitor FRAX486. *Proceedings of the National Academy of Sciences* **110**, 5671–5676.

Dölen, G. *et al.* (2007) Correction of fragile X syndrome in mice. *Neuron* **56**, 955–962.

D'Onofrio, B.M. *et al.* (2003) The role of the children of twins design in elucidating causal relations between parent characteristics and child outcomes. *Journal of Child Psychology and Psychiatry* **44**, 1130–1144.

D'Onofrio, B.M. *et al.* (2008) Smoking during pregnancy and offspring externalizing problems: an exploration of genetic and environmental confounds. *Development and Psychopathology* **20**, 139–164.

D'Onofrio, B.M. *et al.* (2012a) Familial confounding of the association between maternal smoking during pregnancy and offspring substance use and problems. *Archives of General Psychiatry* **69**, 1140–1150.

D'Onofrio, B.M. *et al.* (2012b) Is maternal smoking during pregnancy a causal environmental risk factor for adolescent antisocial behaviour? Testing etiological theories and assumptions. *Psychological Medicine* **42**, 1535–1545.

Duyme, M. *et al.* (1999) How can we boost IQs of "dull children"?: a late adoption study. *Proceedings of the National Academy of Sciences of the United States of America* **96**, 8790–8794.

Fergusson, D.M. *et al.* (1992) Family change, parental discord and early offending. *Journal of Child Psychology and Psychiatry* **33**, 1059–1075.

Fernald, R.D. & Maruska, K.P. (2012) Social information changes the brain. *Proceedings of the National Academy of Sciences* **109**, 17194–17199.

Flint, J. *et al.* (2010) *How Genes Influence Behavior.* Oxford University Press, Oxford & New York.

Fu, Y.H. *et al.* (1991) Variation of the CGG repeat at the fragile X site results in genetic instability: resolution of the Sherman paradox. *Cell* **67**, 1047–1058.

Gaysina, D. *et al.* (2013) Maternal smoking during pregnancy and offspring conduct problems: evidence from 3 independent genetically sensitive research designs. *JAMA Psychiatry* **70**, 956–963.

Ge, X. *et al.* (1996) The developmental interface between nature and nurture: a mutual influence model of child antisocial behavior and parent behaviors. *Developmental Psychology* **32**, 574–589.

Giacometti, E. *et al.* (2007) Partial rescue of MeCP2 deficiency by postnatal activation of MeCP2. *Proceedings of the National Academy of Sciences U S A* **104**, 1931–1936.

Glymour, M.M. *et al.* (2012) Credible Mendelian randomization studies: approaches for evaluating the instrumental variable assumptions. *American Journal of Epidemiology* **175**, 332–339.

Golzio, C. *et al.* (2012) KCTD13 is a major driver of mirrored neuroanatomical phenotypes of the 16p11.2 copy number variant. *Nature* **485**, 363–367.

Gray, R. & Henderson, J. (2006) *Review of the Fetal Effects of Prenatal Alcohol Exposure: Report to the Department of Health.* National Perinatal Epidemiology Unit, Oxford.

Gray, R. *et al.* (2009) Alcohol consumption during pregnancy and its effects on neurodevelopment: what is known and what remains uncertain. *Addiction* **104**, 1270–1273.

Greenspan, R.J. *et al.* (2008) Seymour Benzer (1921–2007). *Current Biology* **18**, R106–R110.

Groen-Blokhuis, M.M. *et al.* (2011) Evidence for a causal association of low birth weight and attention problems. *Journal of the American Academy of Child and Adolescent Psychiatry* **50**, 1247–1254.

Guy, J. *et al.* (2001) A mouse MECP2-null mutation causes neurological symptoms that mimic Rett syndrome. *Nature Genetics* **27**, 322–326.

Guy, J. *et al.* (2007) Reversal of neurological defects in a mouse model of Rett syndrome. *Science* **315**, 1143–1147.

Harden, K.P. *et al.* (2007) Marital conflict and conduct problems in children of twins. *Child Development* **78**, 1–18.

Harlow, H.F. (1958) The nature of love. *American Psychologist* **13**, 673–685.

Harlow, H.F. (1963) The maternal affectional system. In: *Determinants of Infant Behavior II.* (ed B.M. Foss), pp. 3–33. Methuen, London.

Harlow, H.F. & Suomi, S.J. (1971) Social recovery by isolation-reared monkeys. *Proceedings of the National Academy of Sciences* **68**, 1534–1538.

Harlow, H.F. & Suomi, S.J. (1974) Induced depression in monkeys. *Behavioral Biology* **12**, 273–296.

Harold, G.T. *et al.* (2012) Interparental conflict, parent psychopathology, hostile parenting, and child antisocial behavior: examining the role of maternal versus paternal influences using a novel genetically sensitive research design. *Development and Psychopathology* **24**, 1283–1295.

Hawton, K. *et al.* (2013) Long term effect of reduced pack sizes of paracetamol on poisoning deaths and liver transplant activity in England and Wales: interrupted time series analyses. *BMJ* **7**, 346.

Heijmans, B.T. *et al.* (2008) Persistent epigenetic differences associated with prenatal exposure to famine in humans. *Proceedings of the National Academy of Sciences of the United States of America* **105**, 17046–17049.

Heim, C. & Nemeroff, C.B. (1999) The impact of early adverse experiences on brain systems involved in the pathophysiology of anxiety and affective disorders. *Biological Psychiatry* **46**, 1509–1522.

Hinde, R. & McGinnis, L. (1977) Some factors influencing the effects of temporary mother-infant separation: some experiments with rhesus monkeys. *Psychological Medicine* **7**, 197–212.

Hinde, R. & Spencer-Booth, Y. (1970) Individual differences in the responses of rhesus monkeys to a period of separation from their mothers. *Journal of Child Psychology and Psychiatry* **11**, 159–176.

Howe, L.D. *et al.* (2012) Maternal smoking during pregnancy and offspring trajectories of height and adiposity: comparing maternal and paternal associations. *International Journal of Epidemiology* **41**, 722–732.

Hubel, D.H. & Wiesel, T.N. (2005) *Brain and Visual Perception: The Story of a 25-Year Collaboration*. Oxford University Press, New York & Oxford.

Hulshoff Pol, H.E. *et al.* (2000) Prenatal exposure to famine and brain morphology in schizophrenia. *American Journal of Psychiatry* **157**, 1170–1172.

Institute of Medicine of the National Academies. (2013) *Improving the Utility and Translation of Animal Models for Nervous System Disorders: Workshop Summary*. The National Academies Press, Washington, DC.

Jaffee, S.R. *et al.* (2004) The limits of child effects: evidence for genetically mediated child effects on corporal punishment but not on physical maltreatment. *Developmental Psychology* **40**, 1047–1058.

Jones, P.B. & Fung, W.L.A. (2005) Ethnicity and mental health: the example of schizophrenia in the African-Caribbean population in Europe. In: *Ethnicity and Causal Mechanisms*. (eds M. Rutter & M. Tienda), pp. 227–261. Cambridge University Press, New York.

Jones, K.L. *et al.* (1973) Pattern of malformation in offspring of chronic alcoholic mothers. *Lancet* **301**, 1267–1271.

Kandel, E.R. (2001) The molecular biology of memory storage: a dialogue between genes and synapses. *Science* **294**, 1030–1038.

Kendler, K.S. & Gardner, C.O. (2010) Dependent stressful life events and prior depressive episodes in the prediction of major depression: the problem of causal inference in psychiatric epidemiology. *Archives of General Psychiatry* **67**, 1120–1127.

Knopik, V.S. *et al.* (2006) Maternal alcohol use disorder and offspring ADHD: disentangling genetic and environmental effects using a children-of-twins design. *Psychological Medicine* **36**, 1461–1472.

Komitova, M. *et al.* (2013) Hypoxia-induced developmental delays of inhibitory interneurons are reversed by environmental enrichment in the postnatal mouse forebrain. *Journal of Neuroscience* **33**, 13375–13387.

Kraemer, H.C. *et al.* (1997) Coming to terms with the terms of risk. *Archives of General Psychiatry* **54**, 337–343.

Kraemer, H.C. *et al.* (2001) How do risk factors work together? Mediators, moderators, and independent, overlapping, and proxy risk factors. *American Journal of Psychiatry* **158**, 848–856.

Langley, K. *et al.* (2005) Maternal smoking during pregnancy as an environmental risk factor for attention deficit hyperactivity disorder behaviour. A review. *Minerva Pediatrica* **57**, 359–371.

Langley, K. *et al.* (2012) Maternal and paternal smoking during pregnancy and risk of ADHD symptoms in offspring: testing for intrauterine effects. *American Journal of Epidemiology* **176**, 261–268.

Lehn, H. *et al.* (2007) Attention problems and attention-deficit/hyperactivity disorder in discordant and concordant monozygotic twins: evidence of environmental mediators. *Journal of the American Academy of Child and Adolescent Psychiatry* **46**, 83–91.

Lesage, M.G. *et al.* (2006) Effects of maternal intravenous nicotine administration on locomotor behavior in pre-weanling rats. *Pharmacology, Biochemistry and Behavior* **85**, 575–583.

Levine, S. (1957) Infantile experience and resistance to physiological stress. *Science* **126**, 405–406.

Levine, S. (1962) The effects of infantile experience on adult behavior. In: *Experimental Foundations of Clinical Psychology*. (ed A.J. Bachrach), pp. 139–169. Basic Books, New York.

Levine, S. *et al.* (1956) The effects of early shock and handling on later avoidance learning. *Journal of Personality* **24**, 475–493.

Lewis, G. *et al.* (2011) Investigating environmental links between parent depression and child depressive/anxiety symptoms using an assisted conception design. *Journal of the American Academy of Child and Adolescent Psychiatry* **50**, 451–459.

Lewis, S.J. *et al.* (2012) Fetal alcohol exposure and IQ at age 8: evidence from a population-based birth-cohort study. *PLoS One* **7**, e49407.

Liang, H. & Eley, T.C. (2005) A monozygotic twin differences study of nonshared environmental influence on adolescent depressive symptoms. *Child Development* **76**, 1247–1260.

Lifford, K.J. *et al.* (2009) Parent-child hostility and child ADHD symptoms: a genetically sensitive and longitudinal analysis. *Journal of Child Psychology and Psychiatry* **50**, 1468–1476.

Lindell, S.G. *et al.* (2012) The serotonin transporter gene is a substrate for age and stress dependent epigenetic regulation in rhesus macaque brain: potential roles in genetic selection and gene × environment interactions. *Development and Psychopathology* **24**, 1391–1400.

Lubs, H.A. (1969) A marker X chromosome. *American Journal of Human Genetics* **21**, 231.

Ludwig, J. & Miller, D.L. (2005) Does Head Start improve children's life chances? Evidence from a regression discontinuity design. *Quarterly Journal of Economics* **122**, 159–208.

Lynch, S.K. *et al.* (2006) A genetically informed study of the association between harsh punishment and offspring behavioral problems. *Journal of Family Psychology* **20**, 190–198.

Lyons, D.M. *et al.* (2009) Developmental cascades linking stress inoculation, arousal regulation, and resilience. *Frontiers in Behavioral Neuroscience* **3** (32).

Lyons, D.M. *et al.* (2010) Animal models of early life stress: implications for understanding resilience. *Developmental Psychobiology* **52**, 616–624.

McClellan, J.M. *et al.* (2006) Maternal famine, de novo mutations, and schizophrenia. *JAMA* **296**, 582–584.

Nilsson, P. (2008) Does a pint a day affect your child's pay. The effect of prenatal alcohol exposure on adult outcomes. The Institute for Fiscal Studies, Dept of Economics, UCL. Cemmap Working Paper CWP22/08.

Novak, M.A. & Harlow, H.F. (1975) Social recovery of monkeys isolated for the first year of life: I. Rehabilitation and therapy. *Developmental Psychology* **11**, 453–465.

Obel, C. *et al.* (2011) Is maternal smoking during pregnancy a risk factor for Hyperkinetic disorder? Findings from a sibling design. *International Journal of Epidemiology* **40**, 338–345.

O'Connor, T.G. *et al.* (1998) Genotype–environment correlations in late childhood and early adolescence: antisocial behavioral problems and coercive parenting. *Developmental Psychology* **34**, 970–981.

Osborne, K.A. *et al.* (1997) Natural behavior polymorphism due to a cGMP-dependent protein kinase of Drosophila. *Science* **277**, 834–836.

Pickett, K.E. *et al.* (2009) The psychosocial context of pregnancy smoking and quitting in the Millennium Cohort Study. *Journal of Epidemiology and Community Health* **63**, 474–480.

Provençal, N. *et al.* (2012) The signature of maternal rearing in the methylome in rhesus macaque prefrontal cortex and T cells. *Journal of Neuroscience* **32**, 15626–15642.

Pulkkinen, L. *et al.* (2006) *Socioemotional Development and Health from Adolescence to Adulthood*. Cambridge University Press, Cambridge.

Rice, F. *et al.* (2003) Negative life events as an account of age-related differences in the genetic aetiology of depression in childhood and adolescence. *Journal of Child Psychology and Psychiatry* **44**, 977–987.

Rice, F. *et al.* (2009) Disentangling prenatal and inherited influences in humans with an experimental design. *Proceedings of the National Academy of Sciences* **106**, 2464–2467.

Riesen, A.H. (1961) Stimulation as a requirement for growth and function in behavioral development. In: *Functions of Varied Experience*. (eds D.W. Fiske & S.R. Maddi). Dorsey Press, Homewood, IL, 50–106.

Robertson, H.R. & Feng, G. (2011) Annual research review: transgenic mouse models of childhood-onset psychiatric disorder. *Journal of Child Psychology and Psychiatry* **52**, 442–475.

Rosenzweig, M.R. & Bennett, E.L. (1996) Psychobiology of plasticity: effects of training and experience on brain and behavior. *Behavioural Brain Research* **78**, 57–65.

Rosenzweig, M.R. *et al.* (1962) Effects of environmental complexity and training on brain chemistry and anatomy: a replication and extension. *Journal of Comparative and Physiological Psychology* **55**, 429–437.

Rutter, M. (1981) *Maternal Deprivation Reassessed*, 2nd edn. Penguin Books Limited, Middlesex, England.

Rutter, M. (2007) Gene-environment interdependence. *Developmental Science* **10**, 12–18.

Rutter, M. (2012) Achievements and challenges in the biology of environmental effects. *Proceedings of the National Academy of Sciences of the United States of America* **109**, 17149–17153.

Rutter, M. (2013) Resilience: clinical implications. *Journal of Child Psychology and Psychiatry* **54**, 474–487.

Rutter, M. & Sonuga-Barke, E.J. (2010) X. Conclusions: Overview of findings from the E.R.A. study, inferences, and research implications. In: *Deprivation-Specific Psychological Patterns: Effects of Institutional Deprivation* Vol. 75, pp. 212–229. Monographs of the Society for Research in Child Development 75, Oxford.

Rutter, M. & Thapar, A. (2014) Genetics of autism spectrum disorders. In: *Handbook of Autism and Pervasive Developmental Disorders: Assessment, Interventions and Policy*. (eds F.R. Volkmar, *et al.*), 4th edn. John Wiley & Sons, Hoboken, NJ.

Rutter, M. & Thapar, A. (in press) Using natural experiments to test environmental mediation hypotheses. In: *Development and Psychopathology*. Volume 1, 3rd edn. (ed. D. Cicchetti). John Wiley & Sons, New York.

Salmaso, N. *et al.* (2014) Neurobiology of premature brain injury. *Nature Neuroscience* **17**, 341–346.

Schachar, R. *et al.* (1987) Changes in family function and relationships in children who respond to methylphenidate. *Journal of the American Academy of Child and Adolescent Psychiatry* **26**, 728–732.

Silberg, J.L. & Eaves, L.J. (2004) Analysing the contributions of genes and parent-child interaction to childhood behavioural and emotional problems: a model for the children of twins. *Psychological Medicine* **34**, 347–356.

Silberg, J. *et al.* (1999) The influence of genetic factors and life stress on depression among adolescent girls. *Archives of General Psychiatry* **56**, 225–232.

Silberg, J.L. *et al.* (2010) Genetic and environmental influences on the transmission of parental depression to children's depression and conduct disturbance: an extended Children of Twins study. *Journal of Child Psychology and Psychiatry* **51**, 734–744.

Silberg, J.L. *et al.* (2012) Unraveling the effect of genes and environment in the transmission of parental antisocial behavior to children's conduct disturbance, depression and hyperactivity. *Journal of Child Psychology and Psychiatry* **53**, 668–677.

Singh, A.L. *et al.* (2011) Parental depression and offspring psychopathology: a children of twins study. *Psychological Medicine* **41**, 1385–1395.

St Clair, D. *et al.* (2005) Rates of adult schizophrenia following prenatal exposure to the Chinese famine of 1959-1961. *Journal of the American Medical Association* **294**, 557–562.

Stattin, H. & Magnusson, D. (1990) *Pubertal Maturation in Female Development* Vol. 2. Lawrence Erlbaum Associates, Inc., Hillsdale, NJ.

Stein, Z.A. *et al.* (1975) *Famine and Human Development: The Dutch Hunger Winter of 1944-1945*. Oxford University Press, New York.

Stoolmiller, M. (1999) Implications of the restricted range of family environments for estimates of heritability and nonshared environment in behavior–genetic adoption studies. *Psychological Bulletin* **125**, 392–409.

Thapar, A. *et al.* (1998) Life events and depressive symptoms in childhood–shared genes or shared adversity? A research note. *Journal of Child Psychology and Psychiatry* **39**, 1153–1158.

Thapar, A. *et al.* (2007) Do intrauterine or genetic influences explain the foetal origins of chronic disease? A novel experimental method for disentangling effects. *BMC Medical Research Methodology* **7**, 25.

Thapar, A. *et al.* (2009) Prenatal smoking might not cause attention-deficit/hyperactivity disorder: evidence from a novel design. *Biological Psychiatry* **66**, 722–727.

Thornberry, T.P. *et al.* (1993) The role of juvenile gangs in facilitating delinquent behavior. *Journal of Research in Crime and Delinquency* **30**, 55–87.

Thornberry, T.P. *et al.* (2003) *Gangs and Delinquency in Developmental Perspective*. Cambridge University Press, New York.

Tobi, E.W. *et al.* (2012) Prenatal famine and genetic variation are Independently and additively associated with DNA methylation at regulatory loci within IGF2/H19. *PLoS One* **7**, e37933.

Tropea, D. *et al.* (2009) Partial reversal of Rett syndrome-like symptoms in MeCP2 mutant mice. *Proceedings of the National Academy of Sciences* **106**, 2029–2034.

Tsai, P.T. *et al.* (2012) Autistic-like behaviour and cerebellar dysfunction in Purkinje cell Tsc1 mutant mice. *Nature* **488**, 647–651.

Verkerk, A. *et al.* (1991) Identification of a gene (FMR-1) containing a CGG repeat coincident with a breakpoint cluster region exhibiting length variation in fragile X syndrome. *Cell* **65**, 905.

Voight, B.F. *et al.* (2012) Plasma HDL cholesterol and risk of myocardial infarction: a mendelian randomisation study. *Lancet* **380**, 572–580.

Von Senden, M. (1960) Space and sight: the perception of space and shape in the congenitally blind before and after operation. *The Free Press*, Glencoe.

Wilcox, H.C. *et al.* (2012) The interaction of parental history of suicidal behaviour and exposure to adoptive parents' psychiatric disorders on adoptee suicide attempt hospitalizations. *American Journal of Psychiatry* **169**, 309–315.

Winzer-Serhan, U.H. (2007) Long-term consequences of maternal smoking and developmental chronic nicotine exposure. *Frontiers in Bioscience: A Journal and Virtual Library* **13**, 636–649.

Yang, M. *et al.* (2011) Behavioral evaluation of genetic mouse models of autism. In: *Autism spectrum Disorders.* (eds D.G. Amaral, *et al.*). Oxford University Press, New York.

Zoghbi, H.Y. & Bear, M.F. (2012) Synaptic dysfunction in neurodevelopmental disorders associated with autism and intellectual disabilities. *Cold Spring Harbor Perspectives in Biology* **4**, 1–22.

CHAPTER 13

Using epidemiology to plan, organize, and evaluate services for children and adolescents with mental health problems

Miranda Wolpert[1] and Tamsin Ford[2]

[1] Evidence Based Practice Unit, University College London; and Anna Freud Centre; and Child Outcomes Research Consortium, London, UK
[2] Child and Adolescent Psychiatry, Institute of Health Research, University of Exeter Medical School, Exeter, UK

Introduction

Epidemiology is the study of who gets what (disorder, risk factor, protective factor, recovery), as well as when, where, how, and why (Evans *et al.*, 2011; Axford & Morpeth, 2013). This chapter explores how service developers, providers, and funders might use epidemiological findings and information to aid the organization, monitoring, and funding for mental health services (Williams & Wright, 1998), and highlights both the challenges and opportunities of using such data in a meaningful way. Our focus throughout is on practical advice for those of us involved in the "swampy lowlands" (Schön, 1987) of real-world practice in relation to service development for young people with problems that range from common behavioral and emotional difficulties to severe and enduring mental illness. We examine these issues in relation to a wide range of service settings across low-, middle-, and high-income countries, including specialist and targeted pediatric and psychiatric services in schools, clinics, and social care settings regardless of funding source.

This chapter does not intend to provide an extensive overview of child psychiatric epidemiological findings, which are covered in relation to particular mental health difficulties in the relevant individual chapters in this edition, nor to consider universal or primary preventions that aim to prevent the development of distress, and/or to improve well-being in children (see Chapter 17).

Why bother?

While we discuss the limitations and complexities of the application of epidemiological data to service planning, organization, evaluation, and funding, we argue that learning from epidemiological studies provides a firmer foundation for services than historical levels of provision or politically determined policy priorities (Flisher *et al.*, 1997; Jenkins, 2001) and may provide insights into routinely gathered outcome data (Ford *et al.*, 2009).

In terms of service **planning**, basing decisions about future provision of services on those currently accessing clinical services may prove misleading. Only a small and atypical group of children currently access services, and these do not necessarily represent those most in need of such input (Angold *et al.*, 1999; Costello *et al.*, 2005; Ford *et al.*, 2008). Without reference to epidemiology, service planning is more likely to be subject to fluctuating political priorities, or skewed by responses to moral panics; whereas using epidemiological findings can aid evidence-based policy making and service planning (Davies *et al.*, 2000; Gray, 2004).

In terms of service **organization**, epidemiological data may have a role to play in focusing on particular difficulties and in holding services to account for meeting the needs of given populations. Ongoing reference to locality-based epidemiological data is essential if services are to meet the needs of groups prioritized for intervention and not overlook the needs of harder to reach communities (Burns *et al.*, 2004). Epidemiological analyses may also inform tracking and decisions in relation to individual cases once within the service. Thus, Lambert (Lambert, 2005; Lambert & Shimokawa, 2011) and others (Duncan *et al.*, 2004) are using trajectory tracking to compare progress for individual clients against anticipated progress based on data for equivalent clinical populations and using this to inform treatment decisions.

Epidemiological information may have a key role to play in terms of service **evaluation**, (Wolpert *et al.*, 2013). There is an increasing interest in the use of epidemiological data to allow meaningful interpretation of the impact of service contact. As Clark *et al.* (2008, 631) note "[i]n the absence of randomization, one has to work very hard to demonstrate that unbalanced patient characteristics or referral practices could not have substantially influenced the treatment outcome comparison." One approach is to use a naturalistic control group drawing on epidemiological data, such as the "added-value" score based on parental report on the Strengths and Difficulties Questionnaire (SDQ: Ford *et al.*, 2009). Using the analogy of height and weight curves, this algorithm compares the follow-up parental SDQ total difficulties score to that predicted from a largely non-treated epidemiological "control group" to estimate the impact of treatment at a group level.

As services across the world strive to find the best ways to use scarce resources to maximize public good, epidemiological data have a role to play in helping inform the development of effective **funding and payment** models and determining appropriate use of scarce resources for best outcomes.

If, however, epidemiological data are to meaningfully contribute to service planning, organization, evaluation, and funding, it is crucial that all involved remain mindful of the methodological limitations and complexities involved as well as the need to draw on other information. Rutter and Stevenson (2008) emphasize the need to consider the effectiveness of interventions, the accessibility and acceptability of services for families, as well as the skills and abilities of potential service providers. While epidemiological data are of vital importance, they should **never** be used as the sole basis for service planning, organization, evaluation, or funding.

We outline here the main methodological issues that need to be considered in epidemiological data, before turning to key findings from the data and then to the way these can be used in terms of service development.

Overview of key methodological issues

Epidemiology in child mental health generally has to rely on human report, whether self or other. There are as yet few medical markers for the vast majority of child mental health issues, so working out who has what is no simple matter. It is vital to be aware of the factors that need to be considered when interpreting epidemiological data; Box 13.1 highlights key questions for a service provider, planner, or commissioner to ask of epidemiological data and the key facts that the data establish for children and adolescents in the United Kingdom (see Box 13.2).

Who was surveyed?
Most epidemiological studies attempt to study the general population, but the method chosen to access participants, such as school or population registers, or the decision to "stratify" samples, to ensure adequate numbers of small or hard to reach groups for study, may influence who eventually participates and, therefore, the findings. Each approach has strengths and weaknesses that need to be considered when applying the findings outside the original study; it is important to ask who might have been excluded by the sampling strategy and how it might influence the findings. This issue is illustrated clearly by

Box 13.1 Key questions to ask of epidemiological data

(a) Which population was studied (cultural context, age groups, socioeconomic status, how sampled, response rate, date, and scope of study)? Is there an adequate sample size for the conclusions drawn? Is there a representative sampling frame? Over what time frame was the sample looked at? How does this population compare with the population I am interested in for my service?

(b) Whose views were canvassed and in what ways (child, teacher, parent, carer, peer, clinician; by interview, survey, observation using what tools and over what period). How reliable are those views? What biases might I expect given the particular viewpoint sampled?

(c) How was categorization made? Using what criteria with what cut off (DSM-IV, ICD 10 or other). Was distress and impairment taken into account as well as other symptoms? Does the categorization used in the study coincide with categorization used in my service? Is the categorization used likely to skew the data in any particular way?

Box 13.2 Key epidemiological and other facts about mental health problems in children and adolescents in the United Kingdom

- Nearly 10% of children and adolescents have a diagnosable mental health disorder, the most prevalent being conduct disorder (6.6%) (Green *et al.*, 2005).
- Yet, less than 5% of current spending on mental health goes to services aimed at children and young people (Kennedy, 2010), and the United Kingdom continues to trail behind other Western industrialized countries on UNICEF's league of childhood well-being.
- The annual cost of crime in England and Wales committed by people with conduct disorder is £22.5 billion.
- Mental illness during childhood and adolescence results in the United Kingdom costs of £11,030 to £59,130 annually per child (Suhrcke *et al.*,

2008). Children with conduct problems cost around 10 times those without conduct problems, and these costs are distributed across many agencies.
- Lifetime costs of a 1-year cohort of children with conduct disorder have been estimated at £5.2 billion. The annual cost of crime attributable to adults who had conduct problems in childhood is estimated at £60 billion in England and Wales, of which £22.5 billion is attributable to conduct disorder and £37.5 billion to sub-threshold conduct disorder (Sainsbury Centre for Mental Health, 2009).

the surprising findings of Kim *et al.*'s (2011) study of the prevalence of autism spectrum disorder among a "low-probability" general school population (1.24%) and "high-probability" disability samples (0.75%)—a discrepancy which may be at least partially explained by large differences in the gender ratio, type of disorder, and proportion with intellectual disability in the two samples recruited.

In general, people who are socioeconomically disadvantaged and in poor mental health are more likely to drop out or decline to participate (Wolke *et al.*, 2009).

Response rate, the proportion of people eligible to participate in a study who are approached and who take part, is often taken as a key indicator of how reliable the findings are, but recent empirical studies have suggested that bias due to nonresponse is not inevitably present (Groves, 2006). There is no absolute cut-point at which a response rate is definitely acceptable, but there has been a consensus that the higher the rate of participation, the less likely it is that systematic factors have influenced participation and therefore by implication, the results. Wherever possible, researchers should present their assessment of background characteristics of those who did not participate and/or those who dropped out, assess the likelihood of selection bias, and consider the potential impact of any differences on their findings.

There are particular challenges in using survey data to understand rare problems, such as psychosis or autism spectrum disorders. For example, the estimated prevalence of pervasive developmental disorders in a large British child mental health survey (7977 school-age children) was 0.9%, or 67 children (Green *et al.*, 2005). Anything other than the simplest of analyses of sociodemographic characteristics among these children is likely to be unreliable because only a few incorrectly categorized children could change or even reverse findings. A tendency to place too great a significance on findings based on very small numbers of individuals, without taking into account imprecision or uncertainty, is a very common error when applying epidemiological techniques to routine clinical practice (Goldstein, 2012). While prevalence is most often the focus of epidemiological surveys, it may also be important to consider incidence, the rate of new cases arising over a particular period of time, which can address questions such as the impact of a particular event (e.g., sudden economic downturn) on mental health, or age at which a particular problem is first likely to occur (e.g., eating disorders, first psychotic episode; c.f. Rutter & Stevenson, 2008). Given the fluctuating pattern and chronic trajectory of most types of psychopathology, it is essential to differentiate between inferences drawn from cross-sectional or longitudinal data (Kim-Cohen *et al.*, 2003). For rare disorders it may be important to supplement information from cross-sectional surveys with information from clinical samples, in particular, where disorders are so severe that clinical contact is almost inevitable, such as early onset psychosis (Boeing *et al.*, 2007). Active surveillance of incident cases across a group of clinicians can be used to gather service-relevant data on incidence and management that avoid the selection bias inherent to case series collected at single centers of excellence (Lynn *et al.*, 2012).

Secular trends in the prevalence of a disorder over time may also be important to service provision and planning, but are often difficult to study. Retrospective reports of lifetime rates of disorder and official statistics for the prescriptions of psychotropic drugs to children, crime, and suicide suggest that the prevalence of psychopathology may have increased in the latter half of the 20th century, but changes in diagnostic criteria, methods of assessment or recording, in addition to biases inherent in retrospective reports provide alternative explanations for these reports (Fombonne, 1998; Collishaw *et al.*, 2004). For example, once the Millennium cohort reached age 7, parent reports of health-professional-assigned diagnoses of autism spectrum disorder (1.7%) were high compared to earlier studies, while reports of attention deficit hyperactivity disorder (ADHD) were low compared to American studies that used the same question (Russell *et al.*, 2013).

The selection of recent studies of populations that resemble the children they plan to serve is particularly important in relation to minority groups, as ethnic identity results from a complex interaction of culture, history, geography, and race.

Whose views were considered?

A key question to ask of any epidemiological data is whose report it is based on. Epidemiologists expect little concordance between different informants, such as children, parents, teachers, or clinicians, in relation to the nature, extent, or progress of difficulties (Verhulst & Van der Ende, 2008). This may relate not just to limitations of measurement but also to real differences in viewpoint or function in different environments. Hawley and Weisz (2005) note no agreement between child, parent, or practitioner about the problems that brought them to seek help, let alone the outcomes of any intervention for 75% of families attending a mental health service in the United States.

Parent/carer reports have often been employed in epidemiological studies, particularly where children are considered too young to provide self-reports (Levitt *et al.*, 2007). Parents' lack of awareness of internalizing difficulties and/or the impact of their own mental health status on their judgments may introduce error (Cornah *et al.*, 2003; Verhulst & Van der Ende, 2008). For children living with surrogate carers, there may be particular issues in using the report of a carer. For example, among children looked after by the state, the response from a given carer may be compromised by the loss of historical information and lack of time to build a relationship (Ford *et al.*, 2007).

Research suggests that teachers may be more sensitive reporters of children's behavioral symptoms; but less sensitive reporters in relation to children's emotional symptoms (e.g., depression, anxiety), perhaps due to the differential salience of these two indices of adjustment within the classroom (Atzaba-Poria *et al.*, 2004).

There are strong moral- and rights-based arguments for the use of child self-reports, wherever possible. However, younger children may be unreliable reporters in that they may be more likely to give socially desirable responses; they may be also less able to understand the language or the concepts used in self-report measures; they typically respond based on "the here and now"; and may be less self-aware of themselves than others around them (Van Roy *et al.*, 2008).

Expert clinical assessment is sometimes used as a key part of epidemiological surveys, but generally this too relies, to at least some extent, on parent or self-report and even clinician judgment may be subject to biases or limitations. For example, there is evidence that clinicians may rate impact differently from parents or children (Bastiaansen *et al.*, 2004) particularly in relation to long-term conditions such as autism where they tend to rate the impact higher than parents.

How was categorization made?

Different categorization systems will lead to different estimates of prevalence, as may cultural differences in perception of severity (Rutter & Stevenson, 2008; Ho *et al.*, 1996). The extent to which impairment is used may have a particularly big impact. Roberts *et al.* (1998) demonstrated that the use of impairment criteria reduced the prevalence estimates to less than half that reported if impairment were not considered, which is highly pertinent to the recent publication of DSM-5, which removes the application of impairment criteria from some diagnoses (American Psychiatric Association, 2013). Common methods to assess impairment applied in studies include scores of below 60 or 70 on the Child Global Assessment Scale (CGAS; Shaffer *et al.*, 1983) and assessments of distress, impact on activities of daily living, and to adults around the child (Roberts *et al.*, 1998). Some children may report impairing psychopathology that does not meet diagnostic criteria, either because the standardized assessment used omits to ask about the type of difficulties that they experience, or because their difficulties do not quite meet the threshold for disorders that are included in the schedule (Costello *et al.*, 2003).

Interpreting epidemiological data

The methodological issues outlined underline the importance for all involved in mental health services for children and their families to have an awareness of the complexities of epidemiological data if these are to be interpreted in meaningful ways (Goldstein, 2012). Initiatives that try to link researchers with providers of mental health services are to be welcomed as one way to encourage greater dialogue between their respective communities, as are initiatives that aim to embed researchers in practice or provide direct training in methodological understanding to service providers, planners, and commissioners. In particular, the emerging field of implementation science is helping to create greater understanding of methodological issues and their use and impact on current service planning and provision (Eccles & Mittman, 2006).

What is need?

The issue of what constitutes need was explored in some depth in an earlier edition of this textbook (Wolpert, 2008). Four overlapping (but not synonymous) populations of children were identified as being referred to as having "mental health needs": (a) those in difficult circumstances, (b) those at risk of developing diagnosable mental health problems, (c) those with diagnosable mental health problems, and (d) those with levels of impairment resulting from mental health issues that make it difficult for them to function in their community or culture (Wolpert, 2008).

Determining the need for each of these groups and planning services accordingly draws on different sets of epidemiological data and raises different issues.

What can epidemiology tell us about levels of need?

There are epidemiological data relevant to each of the groups identified. In terms of those in "difficult circumstances," there is evidence that too many children in the world could be so categorized, and despite government and non-governmental organization (NGO) prioritization of child health and welfare (e.g., Bill Gates Foundation http://www.gates-foundation.org/What-We-Do/Global-Development/Maternal-Neonatal-and-Child-Health, NSPCC http://www.nspcc.org.uk/) world events such as war, famine, and financial meltdown are only likely to swell their numbers. Latest estimates suggest that there are over 14 million AIDS orphans in Africa (World Health Organization, WHO, 2005), 12 million children living below the poverty line in the United States (WHO, 2005), and 3 million girls across the world at risk of suffering genital mutilation every year (WHO, 2008). Not all of these children will have mental health issues and how to best target those who do remains a key challenge.

While some factors related to difficult circumstances may increase the risk of developing diagnosable mental health problems, risk may also be associated with other individual and interpersonal factors such as brain injury, low birth weight, special educational needs, or poor parental mental health (Goodman & Scott, 2005; Rutter & Stevenson, 2008). The number of risk factors included and the level of risk assessed will influence the proportion of children who fall into this category in the general population.

Reviews of epidemiological surveys spanning several countries and over half a century suggest that between 3% and 22% of school-age children can be categorized as having psychiatric disorders (Canino *et al.*, 1995; Offord, 1995; Roberts *et al.*, 1998; Costello *et al.*, 2005). There may be some differences across countries and contexts, with slightly lower rates found in India and Norway, for example (Malhotra *et al.*, 2002; Heiervang *et al.*, 2007), and slightly higher in Brazil, Bangladesh, and Russia (Fleitlich-Bilyk & Goodman, 2004; Mullick & Goodman, 2005). While it is hard to separate out genuine differences from differences arising from methodology, cross-country comparison is more meaningful when the same instruments have been used, linguistic issues aside. Thus, in a predominantly urban municipality in Brazil, researchers identified that prevalence among 7- to 14-year-old school children was 13% using the same instrument (Development and Well-being Assessment; DAWBA) as that employed in the British national survey (Meltzer *et al.*, 2000; Ford *et al.*, 2003), which reported a prevalence of 10% in school-age children. A comparable study of the same age group in a Russian city (Goodman *et al.*, 2005) produced a prevalence of 15.3%, which is very similar to the prevalence of 15% reported among 5- to 10-year-olds in Bangladesh (Mullick & Goodman, 2005).

In the seminal Great Smoky Mountain study, Angold *et al.* (1998) found that half of all children attending a US clinic did not meet diagnostic criteria, but half of these were significantly functionally impaired. High levels of impairment and impact for key difficulties appear to predict later outcomes and potential cost to society. Over half of all adult mental health difficulties start before the age of 15 (Kim-Cohen *et al.*, 2003), and without appropriate intervention can lead to significant long-term impairment. Thus, impairing behavioral disturbance in children has been linked to severe and long-standing outcomes in adult life, including drug abuse, criminal activity, and poor physical health (Broidy *et al.*, 2003). The cost to the state of an unaddressed conduct disorder over a 7-year period in the United States has been estimated to exceed $70,000 largely in costs related to criminal behavior (Foster & Jones, 2005).

What can epidemiology tell us about planning to meet need?

For those exposed to extreme poverty, war, torture, or famine (WHO, 2005), the optimal targeting of limited mental health services is a key challenge that should be tempered by an understanding of the possible iatrogenic effects of misdirected intervention. The demand for specialist mental health provision must be:

> set in the context of other, sometimes competing, "needs" such as the primary need of children to be nourished, sheltered and protected; their need not to be stigmatized or miss education; and their need not to receive inappropriate, ineffective or harmful treatment.
>
> (Wolpert, 2008: 1158).

A focus on mental health at the expense of other provision may be an unhelpful drain on resources. For example, well-intentioned NGO support was provided following a disaster to provide "interventions for post-traumatic stress disorder

(PTSD)" which in fact disrupted and undermined concurrent relief efforts (WHO, 2005).

Where resources permit, it may be advantageous to provide targeted services for these groups to try to promote resilience and forestall the development of later mental health difficulties for those at risk, given the correlation between key risk factors and later psychopathology. Early intervention and support for young people living with parents with severe and enduring mental health issues may be a sensible starting point (Cooklin *et al.*, 2012). Targeted interventions in schools for those at risk of or with mental health problems may help reduce levels of behavioral problems (Wolpert *et al.*, 2011). However, agencies other than mental health services may have a crucial role to play in this kind of provision, such as educational support to manage special educational needs to avoid secondary impacts on mental health, or better housing or other welfare interventions.

The types of disorders identified in epidemiological studies and their relative occurrence are broadly comparable across the world, allowing for cross-country learning and advice, and prevalence does appear to be pretty universally linked to levels of deprivation and other risk factors, suggesting that it is entirely appropriate to target resources on the most deprived groups, provided that interventions are effective in this population.

Service use now

Comparisons of rates of service contact across countries are complex due to variations in the finance and organization of services. Studies vary in how different services are classified; for instance, school counsellors have been conceptualized as a contact with education or mental health services in different studies (Burns *et al.*, 1995; Leaf *et al.*, 1996; Ford *et al.*, 2007). Comparisons between studies about the rates of service use should therefore be made cautiously, but Table 13.1 clearly illustrates that only a small proportion of young people with a psychiatric disorder reach mental health services and that many others are supported by other services, while a large proportion receive no input at all (Ford *et al.*, 2008).

Contact with a service does not necessarily imply that needs are being met, as for some disorders effective interventions have yet to be identified and the small literature on the effectiveness of routine services provides inconsistent evidence of positive outcomes (Harrington *et al.*, 1999; Andrade *et al.*, 2000; Angold *et al.*, 2000; Weisz & Jensen, 2001; Axford & Morpeth, 2013).

What factors predict access?

The presence, severity (including comorbidity), and impact of difficulties are consistently related to contact for mental health problems with all types of services globally (Staghezza-Jaramillo *et al.*, 1995; Zwaanswijk *et al.*, 2003; Ford *et al.*, 2008). Contact with key gatekeepers, such as primary health care and schools,

Table 13.1 Rates of service use for mental health problems in community-based studies among (1) children with impairing psychopathology as defined by individual studies and (2) the population.

Study	Prevalence of impairing psychopathology (%)	Any service use (%)		Specialist mental health (%)		Education (%)		Social services/ Welfare (%)		Acute and community pediatrics (%)		Time period studied	Comment
		1	2	1	2	1	2	1	2	1	2		
Europe–UK													
(Ford et al., 2007)	10	57	20	25	5	25	5	14	3	14	3	Previous 3 years	Nationally representative sample of 2461 British school-age children followed over 3 years
(Haines et al., 2002)	20[d]	58				38		7				Lifetime	5913 4–15 years olds in the Health Survey for England
(North, 2001)	12[e]			14	3							Past year	Cross sectional survey of 1652 9–10 year olds with service use data from administrative records
(Rutter et al., 1970)	7	20		10	1	3						Current	2 phase study of 2199 10 and 11 year old children in the Isle of Wight
Europe–Netherlands													
(Zwaanswijk et al., 2003)	19[a]			8	3							Past year	Cross sectional survey of 1120 Dutch children aged 11–18 years, using Achenbach's Youth Self Report
(Laitinen-Krispijn et al., 1999)	20[f]			14	8							Mean 5 years	Linkage to psychiatric case-register after cross-sectional survey of 2496 Dutch children aged 10-12 followed to 16.
(Verhulst and van der Ende, 1997)	19[g]				4							Past year	Cross sectional survey 2227 Dutch children aged 4–18
Europe–Other													
(Sourander et al., 2001)	Not reported			13	7							8 years	Cohort of 857 children in Finland, aged 16 at time of follow up.
(Gasquet et al., 1999)	10			14								Past year	Self-report questionnaire among 868 French school children aged 14–20 years

Study								Period	Study description
(Gomez-Beneyeto et al., 1994)	22	16	12					Current	2 phase study of 1127 children aged 8, 11 & 15 in Valencia
(Merikangas et al., 2010)	13		50					Past year	National Health And Nutrition Examination Surveys - Cross-sectional survey of 3042 American 8–15 years olds
(Farmer et al., 2003)	Not reported	34		14	24	4	10	3 years	Overlapping cohort design of 1015 9, 11 and 13 year olds in the Great Smoky Mountains
(Sturm et al., 2003)	7 6–9 across States		35	8					National Survey of American Families 1997 +1999; 45,247 children aged 6-17 6 items from Child Behavior Check List
(Kataoka et al., 2002)	5[b]		20–23[c]	6–9[c]				Past year	Secondary analysis of 3 nationally representative studies in America of aged 6–17 in 1996–1997
(Angold et al., 2002)	21	36	13	5	9	1	2	3 months	2 phase cross sectional survey of 3613 children aged 9–17 in North Carolina
(Farmer et al., 1999)	20		21	8	12	1	4	Past year	Overlapping cohort of 1007 9, 11, and 13 year olds from Great Smoky Mountain Study
(Zahner & Daskalakis, 1997)	Not reported			8	19		8	Lifetime	Pooled data on 2519 children aged 6–11 from 2 cross sectional surveys in Connecticut
(Cunningham & Freiman, 1996)	Not reported		5	2				Past year	6216 children aged 6-17 from the USA National Medical Expenditure Survey
(Leaf et al., 1996)	12	37	21	8		2	3	Past year	1 phase study of 1285 children aged 9–17 in four sites in the USA
(Cuffe et al., 1995)	20	56	22					Past year	2 phase school-based study screening for depression, 478 children aged 13–15

USA (country grouping for Merikangas et al., 2010 through Cuffe et al., 1995)

(continued overleaf)

Table 13.1 (*continued*)

Study	Prevalence of impairing psycho-pathology (%)	Any service use (%)		Specialist mental health (%)		Education (%)		Social services/ Welfare (%)		Acute and community pediatrics (%)		Time period studied	Comment
		1	2	1	2	1	2	1	2	1	2		
(Burns et al., 1995)	19	37	16	20	4							3 months	Overlapping cohort design of 1015 9, 11, and 13 year olds in the Great Smoky Mountains
(Zahner et al., 1992)	14–19[c]	51	28	11	5	3	19			13	8	Lifetime	1 phase survey of 822 children aged 6-11 in New Haven
(Cohen et al., 1991)	18			33	11	33	19			6	3	Past year	Cohort of 776 adolescents from New York—results relate to those aged 12–16 (457)
Canada													
(Offord et al., 1987)	18			16[f]								Past 6 months	2 phase study of 3289 children aged 4-16 in Ontario
Australasia													
(Fergusson et al., 1993)	25	21		10								Current	986 children aged 15 in the Christchurch cohort study
(McGee et al., 1990)	22	48										Past 2 years	Cohort of 943 children from Dunedin, aged 15
(Anderson et al., 1987)	18	29										Past 2 years	Cohort of 792 children from Dunedin, aged 11
South America													
(Staghezza-Jaramillo et al., 1995)	18		6	26	6					9	3	Past 6 months	2 phase study of 777 children aged 4–16 in Puerto Rico
(Vicente et al., 2012)	23	42		19		22		<1		6		Past year	Nationally representative stratified multistage cross-sectional survey of 1558 4–18 year olds in Chile

[a] Abnormal range according the Youth self-report version of the Child Behavior Checklist.
[b] Score greater or equal to three on the Mental Health Indicator Screen adapted from the Child Behavior Checklist.
[c] Results reported separately by age and study.
[d] Abnormal or borderline score on the SDQ.
[e] Probable cases as defined by the SDQ.
[f] Abnormal or borderline on the Child Behavior Checklist.
[g] Combines mental health, social services and youth justice.

also strongly predicts service contact across most services (Ford *et al.*, 2008), as does the perception and health literacy of the young person and/or parents and teachers in many, but not all, studies (Garralda & Bailey, 1988; Staghezza-Jaramillo *et al.*, 1995; Zahner & Daskalakis, 1997; Wu *et al.*, 1999; Sourander *et al.*, 2001; Ford *et al.*, 2008). Externalizing symptoms are more strongly associated with service use than internalizing symptoms (Jones *et al.*, 1987; Wu *et al.*, 1999). As Rutter and Stephenson (2008) point out, different communities may be more sensitive to some behaviors than others. In their comparisons between Thailand and the United States, Weisz and Eastman (1995) found that behavioral problems were more likely to lead to clinic referral in the United States than in Thailand, whereas the reverse was true for emotional problems. Referral patterns may also be influenced by the context of what other support is available. Thus, in the United Kingdom, when comparing children who were and were not referred to specialist services from primary care, Garralda and Bailey (1988) found that the nonreferred children had made significantly more primary care visits than the referred children, highlighting the important role of primary care as a provider for these children in this context.

Poor physical health, poor academic performance, nontraditional family structure, parental psychopathology, and adverse life events are all frequently associated with service contact, although they are also strongly associated with the presence of a psychiatric disorder (Jensen *et al.*, 1990; Staghezza-Jaramillo *et al.*, 1995; Verhulst & van der Ende, 1997; Zahner & Daskalakis, 1997; Gasquet *et al.*, 1999; Sourander *et al.*, 2001; Zwaanswijk *et al.*, 2003; Ford *et al.*, 2008). The area where the family resides may influence service contacts, with several authors reporting that service provision does not relate to the level of need across the areas studied (Boyle & Offord, 1988; Thomas & Hargett, 1999; Sturm *et al.*, 2003; Ford *et al.*, 2008).

Most investigators reported no statistical association between service use and socioeconomic status, while equal numbers of studies report significantly more contact from advantaged or disadvantaged groups, which may be partly explained by families of different socioeconomic status accessing different settings, such as middle-class families opting for education-based services (Jensen *et al.*, 1990; Burns *et al.*, 1995; Staghezza-Jaramillo *et al.*, 1995; Zahner & Daskalakis, 1997; Gasquet *et al.*, 1999; Laitinen-Krispijin *et al.*, 1999).

Studies examining ethnicity are equally complex to interpret, and evenly divided between over- and underrepresentation of children from ethnic minorities (Burns *et al.*, 1995; Zahner & Daskalakis, 1997; Wu *et al.*, 1999; Angold *et al.*, 2002; Kataoka *et al.*, 2002; Zwaanswijk *et al.*, 2003).

Using epidemiology to determine organization

Epidemiological surveys can be used to screen for need and target treatment. We would argue against this approach on a number of grounds. Firstly, longitudinal epidemiological data show that many diagnosable mental health problems improve without intervention and rushing to intervene may harm rather than help. Moreover, the dangers of false positives with the potential to distress and stigmatize and the costs of unwarranted assessment and intervention combine to suggest that this approach is unwise and unsafe at this stage in our knowledge.

Different countries have varied service organizations; the only universal finding being that wherever child mental health services are located, boundary issues always arise (Wolpert, 2008). In some areas of Europe, (e.g., Switzerland and Hungary) and in some parts of the United States, most child mental health services are under the auspices of education. This may increase access and reduce stigma, but can make coordination for older adolescents or those with more severe mental illnesses problematic. Learning from epidemiological incidence data that pinpoints late adolescence as a key period of transition and difficulty for many young people, a number of countries have now started to focus on dedicated youth services that stretch from adolescence to early adulthood to encourage flexibility for 18- to 20-year-olds (Hazell, 2005) and development of specialist services for this traditionally underprovided group (Patel *et al.*, 2007). The traditional split between child and adult mental health services places a transition at the peak age of incident severe mental illness, and the study of trajectory into adulthood is complicated by a disjunction in the philosophy and methods of both practitioners and researchers with these populations (Singh *et al.*, 2010).

Constant checking of access against anticipated need for targeted local populations is recommended to ensure equitable access for particularly vulnerable or hard to reach groups. Local services should undertake their own local epidemiological studies to ensure appropriate targeting of need within their area. While we would recommend use of epidemiological data in general, it is important to note in this context that a universal finding in both developing and industrialized countries is the relative lack of services compared to the level of need and that "services everywhere fall well short of even a conservative estimate of requirements" (Rutter & Stevenson, 2008). Thus, attempts to spend time and energy on complicated analysis of local need may not be warranted at this stage, particularly in light of the resources available, as well as the methodological issues discussed. It may be more feasible to use the available epidemiology supplemented by local knowledge where this deviates from the norm.

Using epidemiology to determine funding arrangements

The current financial climate and the resulting restriction in resources have resulted in a particular emphasis on the use of epidemiological data to target service provision. Increasingly, there is an emphasis on service providers agreeing to realistic goals with children and families and working toward these goals in a considered fashion to prevent mission creep as providers get ineffectually caught up in trying to solve multiple complex problems (Weisz *et al.*, 2011; Law, 2012). One suggestion is that a more explicit recognition of what can be achieved and what is realistic to expect be combined with progress tracking against anticipated trajectories of change in order to identify and prevent drop out from "off track" cases (Lambert, 2005) and make the most efficient use of services (Miller *et al.*, 2006).

There are national and international initiatives to find the best and most economic ways of funding child mental health. The proportion of the overall health budget allocated to mental health ranged from 9% in Egypt to 0.01 % in Kenya (WHO, 2005), and the child mental health budget is likely to be a small proportion of that, for example, in the United Kingdom it is less than 5% of the overall mental health spend.

In recent years, there has been an interest in developing prospective, activity-based payment systems, in which providers are paid in advance, on the basis of their likely caseload. These have been referred to as "**casemix,**" or "**payment by results**" systems (http://pbrcamhs.org/). This type of a fee-for-service system applies data (often based on the previous year's caseload) to predict the funding needed for the following year (Mason *et al.*, 2011). Attempts to develop a casemix payment system for mental health provision, which classifies service users according to similarities in presentation (e.g., diagnosis, severity, functioning), are currently under way in Australia, New Zealand, and England but none have yet implemented these. Canada has implemented a casemix payment system for adult inpatient mental health treatment, but this is limited to treatments that are considered "medical" mental-healthcare. The Netherlands has developed a similar system but expanded it to include child and adolescent and "nonmedical" psychiatric care (Mason *et al.*, 2011). In child mental health, the complexities of attempting to develop such a system are compounded by the amount of indirect work done by service providers that is all too often not adequately captured in routine data collection.

Using epidemiological data to understand outcomes of treatment for teams and services

Evaluation of services is increasingly focused on the use of patient-reported outcome measures (PROMs) and/or patient-reported experience measures (PREMs). The use of epidemiological data to inform interpretation of these data involves a decision about what constitutes meaningful (or clinically significant) change, which raises three main issues.

The first issue is whether the change in an outcome measure is greater than is expected by chance variation given the limitations of the measure used. The Reliable Change Index (RCI) aims to assess the amount of change required in an outcome measure to be reasonably confident that the magnitude of change observed is not solely attributable to measurement error and can be calculated in a variety of ways (Jacobson & Truax, 1991). The RCI for the parent SDQ, for example, for a UK population is 7 points, a parent total difficulties score has to move by 7 points to suggest a "reliable change." A more pertinent issue is whether the change recorded is meaningful for the quality of the individual's life. One metric developed for this involves movement from high-symptom scores pretreatment to scores that fall within the nonclinical sample range after treatment. Some have argued that reliable change and movement across the clinical cut-off need to have occurred for clinically significant change to be deemed to have taken place (http://www.iapt.nhs.uk). However, it is not yet clear if this is an appropriate standard to set, and for some conditions, such as autism spectrum disorder, this is probably unrealistic (Wolpert *et al.*, 2013).

It is also important to know whether change might have occurred spontaneously if no intervention had been offered. The SDQ added value score attempts to adjust for regression to the mean, random fluctuation and attenuation and was able to replicate the changes seen in a randomized controlled trial when applied to the intervention and waiting list control arms separately (Ford *et al.*, 2009). The approach taken by CAMHS Outcomes Research Consortium (CORC) is to produce annual reports of aggregated outcomes (both PROMs and PREMs) for teams of clinicians working within the collaboration. These are then compared with aggregated outcomes for consortium members as a whole and any areas of statistically significant difference noted.[1] Members are advised that these should be interpreted in terms of their local knowledge and triangulated with other data. Thus, a series of hypotheses can be tested to explore any differences to check if they are the result of differences in methodology, population being worked with, data entry errors, or genuinely reflect differences in outcomes for similar groups of children and families.

When viewing this sort of data it is important to avoid over-interpretation when datasets are small and what appear to be large variations in outcomes between services may, in fact, reflect normal variation between data points to be expected when small numbers are involved. Using funnel plots to map comparative data to ensure meaningful interpretation may be very helpful in this regard. These plot the statistic of interest, for example, the mean outcome from a service, against a measure of its precision such as the number of children contributing data (Spiegelhalter, 2005). When confidence intervals of the mean (which become narrower as the sample size increases, producing a funnel shape) are applied, it is possible to ascertain which services appear to have unusually good and unusually poor scores.

---

[1] CORC is looking to modify this model further by making comparisons more specific between services in similar contexts and with similar populations of service users.

Conclusion and further directions

Epidemiological data may play a central part in terms of planning, organizing, evaluating, and commissioning services. These data may be key to aid evidence-based policy making and service planning (Davies et al., 2000; Gray, 2004), and have a role to play in helping to determine focus in a particular area and in holding services to account for meeting the needs of given populations. Epidemiological analyses can inform decisions in relation to individual cases once within the service and to overall evaluation of the service. Epidemiological data could inform the development of effective funding and payment models and determine appropriate use of scarce resources for best outcomes.

However, if such data are to meaningfully contribute to any of these aspects, it is crucial that all involved remain mindful of the methodological limitations and complexities involved as well as the need to draw on other relevant information covered in other chapters in this volume, including information as to the effectiveness of interventions, acceptability of services to potential service users and their parents, as well as the skills and abilities of potential service providers. We would argue that while epidemiological data are of vital importance, they should never be used as the sole base for service planning, organization, evaluation, or funding.

Acknowledgments

With thanks to Katy Hopkins for content on funding models and to Thomas Booker for work on references, sourcing content, and formatting. Thanks also to Melanie Jones, Jessica Deighton, and Andrew Fugard for conversations and debates that have contributed to elements of this chapter. All errors and omissions are the authors' own.

References

American Psychiatric Association (2013) *Diagnostic and Statistical Manual of Mental Disorders (DSM-5)*, 5th edn. American Psychiatric Association, Washington, DC.

Anderson, J.C. et al. (1987) DSM-III disorders in preadolescent children. Prevalence in a large sample from the general population. *Archives of General Psychiatry* **44**, 69–76.

Andrade, A.R. et al. (2000) Dose effect in child psychotherapy: outcomes associated with negligible treatment. *Journal of the American Academy of Child and Adolescent Psychiatry* **39**, 161–168.

Angold, A. et al. (1998) Perceived parental burden and service use for child and adolescent psychiatric disorders. *American Journal of Public Health* **88**, 75–80.

Angold, A. et al. (1999) Impaired but undiagnosed. *Journal of the American Academy of Child and Adolescent Psychiatry* **38**, 129–137.

Angold, A. et al. (2000) Effectiveness of nonresidential specialty mental health services for children and adolescents in the "real world". *Journal of the American Academy of Child and Adolescent Psychiatry* **39**, 154–160.

Angold, A. et al. (2002) Psychiatric disorder, impairment, and service use in rural African American and white youth. *Archives of General Psychiatry* **59**, 893–901.

Atzaba-Poria, N. et al. (2004) Internalising and externalising problems in middle childhood: a study of Indian (ethnic minority) and English (ethnic majority) children living in Britain. *International Journal of Behavioral Development* **28**, 449–460.

Axford, N. & Morpeth, L. (2013) Evidence-based programs in children's services: a critical appraisal. *Children and Youth Services Review* **13**, 268–277.

Bastiaansen, D. et al. (2004) Quality of life in children with psychiatric disorders: self-, parent, and clinician report. *Journal of the American Academy of Child and Adolescent Psychiatry* **43**, 221–230.

Boeing, L. et al. (2007) Adolescent-onset psychosis: prevalence, needs and service provision. *British Journal of Psychiatry* **190**, 18–26.

Boyle, M.H. & Offord, D.R. (1988) Prevalence of childhood disorder, perceived need for help, family dysfunction and resource allocation for child welfare and children's mental health services in Ontario. *Canadian Journal of Behavioural Science* **44**, 374–388.

Broidy, L.M. et al. (2003) Developmental trajectories of childhood disruptive behaviors and adolescent delinquency: a six-site, cross-national study. *Developmental Psychology* **39**, 222–245.

Burns, B.J. et al. (1995) Children's mental health service use across service sectors. *Health Affairs (Millwood)* **14**, 147–159.

Burns, B.J. et al. (2004) Mental health need and access to mental health services by youths involved with child welfare: a national survey. *Journal of the American Academy of Child and Adolescent Psychiatry* **43**, 960–970.

Canino, G. et al. (1995) Child psychiatric epidemiology: what have we learned and what we need to learn. *Journal of Methods in Psychiatric Research* **5**, 79–92.

Clark, D.M. et al. (2008) Psychological treatment outcomes in routine NHS services: a commentary on Stiles et al. (2007). *Psychological Medicine* **38**, 629–634.

Cohen, P. et al. (1991) Diagnostic predictors of treatment patterns in a cohort of adolescents. *Journal of the American Academy of Child and Adolescent Psychiatry* **30**, 989–993.

Collishaw, S. et al. (2004) Time trends in adolescent mental health. *Journal of Child Psychology and Psychiatry* **45**, 1350–1362.

Cooklin, A. et al. (2012) *The Kidstime Workshops. A Multi-Family Social Intervention for the Effects of Parental Mental Illness. Manual*. CAMHS Press, London.

Cornah, D. et al. (2003) The impact of maternal mental health and child's behavioural difficulties on attributions about child behaviours. *British Journal of Clinical Psychology* **42**, 69–79.

Costello, E.J. et al. (2003) Prevalence and development of psychiatric disorders in childhood and adolescence. *Archives of General Psychiatry* **60**, 837–844.

Costello, E.J. et al. (2005) 10-year research update review: the epidemiology of child and adolescent psychiatric disorders: I. Methods and public health burden. *Journal of the American Academy of Child and Adolescent Psychiatry* **44**, 972–986.

Cuffe, S.P. et al. (1995) Race and gender differences in the treatment of psychiatric disorders in young adolescents. *Journal of the American Academy of Child and Adolescent Psychiatry* **34**, 1536–1543.

Cunningham, P.J. & Freiman, M.P. (1996) Determinants of ambulatory mental health services use for school-age children and adolescents. *Health Services Research* **31**, 409–427.

Davies, H.T.O. *et al.* (2000) *What Works?: Evidence-Based Policy and Practice in Public Services.* The Policy Press, Bristol.

Duncan, B.L. *et al.* (2004) *The Heroic Client: A Revolutionary Way to Improve Effectiveness Through Client-Directed, Outcome-Informed Therapy.* Jossey-Bass, San Francisco, California [Chichester: John Wiley].

Eccles, M. & Mittman, B. (2006) Welcome to implementation science. *Implementation Science* **1**, 1.

Evans, I. *et al.* (2011) *Testing Treatments; Better Research for Better Healthcare.* Pinter and Martin, London.

Farmer, E.M.Z. *et al.* (1999) Use, persistence and intensity: patterns of care for children's mental health across one year. *Community Mental Health Journal* **35**, 31–46.

Farmer, E.M. *et al.* (2003) Pathways into and through mental health services for children and adolescents. *Psychiatric Services* **54**, 60–66.

Fergusson, D.M. *et al.* (1993) Prevalence and comorbidity of DSM-III-R diagnoses in a birth cohort of 15 year olds. *Journal of the American Academy of Child and Adolescent Psychiatry* **32**, 1127–1134.

Fleitlich-Bilyk, B. & Goodman, R. (2004) Prevalence of child and adolescent psychiatric disorders in southeast Brazil. *Journal of the American Academy of Child and Adolescent Psychiatry* **43**, 727–734.

Flisher, A.J. *et al.* (1997) Correlates of unmet need for mental health services by children and adolescents. *Psychological Medicine* **27**, 1145–1154.

Fombonne, E. (1998) Increased rates of psychosocial disorders in youth. *European Archives of Psychiatry and Clinical Neuroscience* **248**, 14–21.

Ford, T. *et al.* (2003) The British child and adolescent mental health survey 1999: the prevalence of DSM-IV disorders. *Journal of the American Academy of Child and Adolescent Psychiatry* **42**, 1203–1211.

Ford, T. *et al.* (2007) Child mental health is everybody's business: the prevalence of contact with public sector services by type of disorder among British school children in a three-year period. *Child and Adolescent Mental Health* **12**, 13–20.

Ford, T. *et al.* (2008) Five years on: public sector service use related to mental health in young people with ADHD or hyperkinetic disorder five years after diagnosis. *Child and Adolescent Mental Health* **13**, 122–129.

Ford, T. *et al.* (2009) Strengths and difficulties questionnaire added value scores: evaluating effectiveness in child mental health interventions. *British Journal of Psychiatry* **194**, 552–558.

Foster, E.M. & Jones, D.E. (2005) The high costs of aggression: public expenditures resulting from conduct disorder. *American Journal of Public Health* **95**, 1767–1772.

Garralda, M.E. & Bailey, D. (1988) Child and family factors associated with referral to child psychiatrists. *British Journal of Psychiatry* **153**, 81–89.

Gasquet, I. *et al.* (1999) Consultation of mental health professionals by French adolescents with probable psychiatric problems. *Acta Psychiatrica Scandinavica* **99**, 126–134.

Goldstein, H. 2012. *Numerical indigestion: how much data is really good for us. Impact of Social Sciences,* [Online]. Available: http://blogs.lse.ac.uk/impactofsocialsciences/2012/11/27/goldstein-how-much-data-is-good/2013

Gomez-Beneyeto, M. *et al.* (1994) Prevalence of mental disorders among children in Valencia. *Acta Psychiatrica Scandinavia* **89**, 325–357.

Goodman, R. & Scott, S. (2005) *Child Psychiatry.* Blackwell, Oxford.

Goodman, R. *et al.* (2005) Russian child mental health–a cross-sectional study of prevalence and risk factors. *European Child and Adolescent Psychiatry* **14**, 28–33.

Gray, J.A.M. (2004) Evidence based policy making. *British Medical Journal* **329**, 988–989.

Green, H. *et al.* (2005) *Mental Health of Children and Young People in Great Britain, 2004.* Palgrave Macmillan, Basingstoke.

Groves, R.M. (2006) Nonresponse rates and nonresponse bias in household surveys. *Public Opinion Quarterly* **70**, 646–675.

Haines, M.M. *et al.* (2002) Social and demographic predictors of parental consultation for child psychological difficulties. *Journal of Public Health Medicine* **24**, 276–284.

Harrington, R.C. *et al.* (1999) Developing needs led child and adolescent mental health services: issues and prospects. *European Child and Adolescent Psychiatry* **8**, 1–10.

Hawley, K.M. & Weisz, J.R. (2005) Youth versus parent working alliance in usual clinical care: distinctive associations with retention, satisfaction, and treatment outcome. *Journal of Clinical Child and Adolescent Psychology* **34**, 117–128.

Hazell, C. (2005) *Imaginary Groups.* Authorhouse, Bloomington, IN.

Heiervang, E. *et al.* (2007) Psychiatric disorders in Norwegian 8- to 10-year-olds: an epidemiological survey of prevalence, risk factors, and service use. *Journal of the American Academy of Child and Adolescent Psychiatry* **46**, 438–447.

Ho, T.P. *et al.* (1996) Establishing the constructs of childhood behavioural disturbances in a Chinese population: a questionnaire study. *Journal of Abnormal Child Psychology* **24**, 417–431.

Jacobson, N.S. & Truax, P. (1991) Clinical significance: a statistical approach to defining meaningful change in psychotherapy research. *Journal of Consulting and Clinical Psychology* **59**, 12–19.

Jenkins, R. (2001) Making psychiatric epidemiology useful: the contribution of epidemiology to government policy. *Acta Psychiatrica Scandinavica* **103**, 2–14.

Jensen, P.S. *et al.* (1990) Children at risk: II. Risk factors and clinic utilization. *Journal of the American Academy of Child and Adolescent Psychiatry* **29**, 804–812.

Jones, L.R. *et al.* (1987) Inside the hidden mental health network. Examining mental health care delivery of primary care physicians. *General Hospital Psychiatry* **9**, 287–293.

Kataoka, S.H. *et al.* (2002) Unmet need for mental health care among U.S. children: variation by ethnicity and insurance status. *American Journal of Psychiatry* **159**, 1548–1555.

Kennedy, I. (2010). *Getting it right for children and young people. Overcoming cultural barriers in the NHS so as to meet their needs.* Independent review. Crown Copyright.

Kim, Y.S. *et al.* (2011) Prevalence of autism spectrum disorders in a total population sample. *American Journal of Psychiatry* **168**, 904–912.

Kim-Cohen, J. *et al.* (2003) Prior juvenile diagnoses in adults with mental disorder: developmental follow-back of a prospective-longitudinal cohort. *Archives of General Psychiatry* **60**, 709–717.

Laitinen-Krispijin *et al.* (1999) Predicting adolescent mental health service use in a prospective record-linkage survey. *Journal of the American Academy of Child and Adolescent Psychiatry* **38**, 1073–1080.

Lambert, M.J. (2005) JCP special edition: enhancing psychotherapy outcome through feedback. *Journal of Clinical Psychology* **61**, 141–217.

Lambert, M.J. & Shimokawa, K. (2011) Collecting client feedback. *Psychotherapy (Chicago, Ill.)* **48**, 72–79.

Law, D. (2012) *A Practical Guide to Using Service User Feedback & Outcome Tools to Inform Clinical Practice in Child & Adolescent Mental Health Some Initial Guidance from the Children and Young Peoples' Improving Access to Psychological Therapies Outcomes-Oriented Practice (CO-OP) Group*. Department of Health, London.

Leaf, P.J. *et al.* (1996) Mental health service use in the community and schools: results from the four-community MECA Study. Methods for the epidemiology of child and adolescent mental disorders study. *Journal of the American Academy of Child and Adolescent Psychiatry* **35**, 889–897.

Levitt, J.M. *et al.* (2007) Early identification of mental health problems in schools: the status of instrumentation. *Journal of School Psychology* **45**, 163–191.

Lynn, R.M. *et al.* (2012) Ascertainment of early onset eating disorders: a pilot for developing a national child psychiatric surveillance system. *Child and Adolescent Mental Health* **17**, 109–112.

Malhotra, S. *et al.* (2002) Prevalence of psychiatric disorders in school children in Chandigarh, India. *Indian Journal of Medical Research* **116**, 21–28.

Mason, A. *et al.* (2011) Navigating uncharted waters? How international experience can inform the funding of mental health care in England. *Journal of Mental Health* **20**, 234–248.

Mcgee, R. *et al.* (1990) DSM-III disorders in a large sample of adolescents. *Journal of the American Academy of Child and Adolescent Psychiatry* **29**, 611–619.

Meltzer, H. *et al.* (2000) *Mental Health of Children and Adolescents in Great Britain*. The Stationery Office, London.

Merikangas *et al.* (2010) Prevalence and treatment of mental disorders among US children in the 2001–2004 NHANES. *Pediatrics* **125**, 75–81.

Miller, S.D. *et al.* (2006) Using formal client feedback to improve retention and outcome: making ongoing, real-time assessment feasible. *Journal of Brief Therapy* **5**, 5–22.

Mullick, M.S. & Goodman, R. (2005) The prevalence of psychiatric disorders among 5–10 year olds in rural, urban and slum areas in Bangladesh: an exploratory study. *Social Psychiatry and Psychiatric Epidemiology* **40**, 663–671.

North, C. 2001. Psychopathology and service use in 9–10 year old children. *Faculty of Child and Adolescent Psychiatry Annual Residential Meeting 3–5 October.*

Offord, D.R. (1995) Child psychiatric epidemiology: current status and future prospects. *Canadian Journal of Psychiatry* **40**, 284–288.

Offord, D.R. *et al.* (1987) Ontario Child Health Study. II. Six-month prevalence of disorder and rates of service utilization. *Archives of General Psychiatry* **44**, 832–836.

Patel, V. *et al.* (2007) Mental health of young people: a global public-health challenge. *Lancet* **369**, 1302–1313.

Roberts, R. *et al.* (1998) Prevalence of psychopathology among children and adolescents. *American Journal of Psychiatry* **155**, 715–725.

Russell, G. *et al.* (2013) Prevalence of parent-reported ASD and ADHD in the UK: findings from the Millennium Cohort Study. *Journal of Autism and Developmental Disorders* **44**, 31–40.

Rutter, M. & Stevenson, J. (2008) Using epidemiology to plan services: a conceptual approach. In: *Rutter's Child and Adolescent Psychiatry.* (eds M. Rutter, D. Bishop, D.S. Pine, S. Scott, J. Stevenson, E. Taylor & A. Thapar), 5th edn. Blackwell Publishing Ltd, Oxford.

Rutter, M. *et al.* (1970) *Education, Health and Behaviour*. Longmans, London.

Sainsbury Centre For Mental Health (2009) *The Chance of a Lifetime: Preventing Early Conduct Problems and Reducing Crime*. Sainsbury Centre for Mental Health, London.

Schön, D.A. (1987) *Educating the Reflective Practitioner*. Jossey-Bass, San Francisco, CA.

Shaffer, D. *et al.* (1983) A children's global assessment scale (CGAS). *Archives of General Psychiatry* **40**, 1228–1231.

Singh, S.P. *et al.* (2010) Process, outcome and experience of transition from child to adult mental healthcare: multiperspective study. *British Journal of Psychiatry* **197**, 305–312.

Sourander, A. *et al.* (2001) Child and adolescent mental health service use in Finland. *Social Psychiatry and Psychiatric Epidemiology* **36**, 294–298.

Spiegelhalter, D.J. (2005) Funnel plots for comparing institutional performance. *Statistics in Medicine* **24**, 1185–1202.

Staghezza-Jaramillo *et al.* (1995) Mental health service utilisation among Puerto Rican children. *Journal of Child and Family Studies* **4**, 399–418.

Sturm, R. *et al.* (2003) Geographic disparities in children's mental health care. *Pediatrics* **112**, e308–e315.

Suhrcke, M. *et al.* (2008) Economic aspects of mental health in children and adolescents. In: *Social Cohesion for Mental Well-Being Among Adolescents*. WHO Regional Office for Europe, Copenhagen.

Thomas, S.A. & Hargett, T. (1999) Mental health care: a collaborative, holistic approach. *Holistic Nursing Practice* **13**, 78–85.

Van Roy, B. *et al.* (2008) Construct validity of the five-factor Strengths and Difficulties Questionnaire (SDQ) in pre-, early, and late adolescence. *Journal of Child Psychology and Psychiatry* **49**, 1304–1312.

Verhulst, F.C. & Van Der Ende, J. (1997) Factors associated with child mental health service use in the community. *Journal of the American Academy of Child and Adolescent Psychiatry* **36**, 901–909.

Verhulst, F.C. & Van Der Ende, J. (2008) Using rating scales in a clinical context. In: *Rutter's Child and Adolescent Psychiatry.* (eds M. Rutter, D. Bishop, D.S. Pine, S. Scott, J. Stevenson, E. Taylor & A. Thapar), 5th edn. Blackwell Publishing Ltd, Oxford.

Vicente, B. *et al.* (2012) Prevalence of child and adolescent mental disorders in Chile: a community epidemiological study. *Journal of Child Psychology and Psychiatry* **53**, 1026–1035.

Weisz, J.R. & Eastman, K.L. (1995) Cross-national research on child and adolescent psychopathology. In: *The Epidemiology of Child and Adolescent Psychopathology*. (eds F.C. Verhulst & H.M. Koot). Oxford University Press, Oxford.

Weisz, J.R. & Jensen, A.L. (2001) Child and adolescent psychotherapy in research and practice contexts: review of the evidence and suggestions for improving the field. *European Child and Adolescent Psychiatry* **10**, I12–I118.

Weisz, J.R. *et al.* (2011) Youth Top Problems: using idiographic, consumer-guided assessment to identify treatment needs and to track change during psychotherapy. *Journal of Consulting and Clinical Psychology* **79**, 369–380.

Williams, R. & Wright, J. (1998) Epidemiological issues in health needs assessment. *British Medical Journal* **316**, 1379–1382.

Wolke, D. *et al.* (2009) Does selective drop out lead to biased prediction of behaviour disorders. *British Journal of Psychiatry* **195**, 249–256.

Wolpert, M. (2008) Organization of services for children and adolescents with mental health problems. In: *Rutter's Child and Adolescent Psychiatry.* (eds M. Rutter, D. Bishop, D.S. Pine, S. Scott, J. Stevenson, E. Taylor & A. Thapar), 5th edn. Blackwell Publishing Ltd, Oxford.

Wolpert, M. *et al.* (2011) Me and my school: findings from the national evaluation of targeted mental health in schools 2008–2011. In: *Research Report DFE-RR177*. Department for Education, London.

Wolpert, M. *et al.* (2013) Issues in evaluation of psychotherapies. In: *Cognitive Behaviour Therapy for Children and Families*. (eds P. Graham & S. Reynolds), 3rd edn. Cambridge University Press, Cambridge.

World Health Organisation (2005) *The World Health Report 2005: Make Every Mother and Child Count*. World Health Organization, Geneva.

World Health Organisation (2008) *Eliminating Female Genital Mutilation. An interagency statement. OHCHR, UNAIDS, UNDP, UNECA, UNESCO, UNFPA, UNHCR, UNICEF, UNIFEM, WHO*. World Health Organization, Geneva.

Wu, P. *et al.* (1999) Depressive and disruptive disorders and mental health service utilization in children and adolescents. *Journal of the American Academy of Child and Adolescent Psychiatry* **38**, 1081–1090 discussion 1090–2.

Zahner, G.E. & Daskalakis, C. (1997) Factors associated with mental health, general health, and school-based service use for child psychopathology. *American Journal of Public Health* **87**, 1440–1448.

Zahner, G.E. *et al.* (1992) Children's mental health service needs and utilization patterns in an urban community: an epidemiological assessment. *Journal of the American Academy of Child and Adolescent Psychiatry* **31**, 951–960.

Zwaanswijk, M. *et al.* (2003) Help seeking for emotional and behavioural problems in children and adolescents: a review of recent literature. *European Child and Adolescent Psychiatry* **12**, 153–161.

CHAPTER 14

Evaluating interventions

Helena Chmura Kraemer[1,2]
[1] Stanford University (Emerita), Stanford, CA, USA
[2] Department of Psychiatry, School of Medicine, University of Pittsburgh, Pittsburgh, PA, USA

Introduction

"How well will this treatment work for this patient/for me?" is the question to which every patient and his/her clinician wants answers, but one research cannot answer. Yet in absence of research, clinicians can only guess, and patients take the consequences of poor decision making. The question research can answer, however, is "How well will this treatment work for patients *like this* patient?," by taking a sample of patients from a population like this patient, and assessing how well the intervention (T) works for patients in that population. Depending on how well the patient fits within that population, such a result gives the best estimate of the likely impact on the individual patient, the goal of evidence-based medicine. The methodology of evaluating interventions focuses on what must be done to bring that answer as close as possible to accurately and precisely answering the first question.

Many books and papers have been written on this subject. The many ways such research can be conceived, designed, executed, reported, and processed could not possibly be covered here. In what follows, after the basic principles are articulated, the focus is on areas where errors are most likely.

The fundamental principles

The control/comparison groups

How well a treatment works is not answered by simply prescribing T to the patients in the sample and observing the subsequent response. What appears to be a good response to T may actually be no better than what would have occurred had T not been given. In short, one cannot attribute the observed response to the *effect* of T, nor can one judge the *response following T* as beneficial, neutral, or harmful, without comparison with another intervention, a control or comparison intervention (C) that represents what would have happened had T not been

prescribed. C could be absence of any treatment, a placebo, a waiting list, "treatment as usual," standard of care, an active comparator, and so on. What C should be in any particular clinical trial is a contentious question, but the basic principle is that *there must be a control/comparison group* in order to evaluate any intervention.

Measuring the effect of T versus C

Traditionally, what is required in research is to show that there is some difference unlikely due to chance between T and C, a "statistically significant difference." There are long-acknowledged problems with this approach (Shrout, 1997; Hunter, 1997). A better premise: The goal of clinical research comparing T and C is to estimate an effect size showing how much more likely is a clinically preferable response from a patient treated with T than from one treated with C. A number of effect sizes might be used, but here the focus will be success rate difference (SRD), where SRD = Probability (T > C) − Probability (C > T), where "T > C" means that if one randomly sampled a patient treated with T and compared the response with another treated with C, the response of the T-treated patients would be clinically preferable to that of the one treated with C. SRD ranges from +1, when every patient treated with T has a response preferable to every patient treated with C, to −1, when the reverse is true. SRD equal to zero indicates clinical equivalence of T and C.

The traditional goal of showing a "statistically significant effect" is equivalent to showing that SRD is not equal to zero. Instead, we want to estimate SRD (with a confidence interval to show the precision of such estimation), in order to judge, not merely whether SRD equals zero or not, but (1) whether the study is well enough designed to give a reasonably precise estimate of SRD (indicated by the length of the confidence interval), and (2) if so, whether SRD is large enough to be considered clinically significant, large enough to convince patients/clinicians that selecting one intervention over the other is likely to make a real difference to patient outcome.

Rutter's Child and Adolescent Psychiatry, Sixth Edition.
Edited by Anita Thapar and Daniel S. Pine, James F. Leckman, Stephen Scott, Margaret J. Snowling, Eric Taylor.
© 2015 John Wiley & Sons Ltd. Published 2018 by John Wiley & Sons Ltd.

Randomization

To interpret the SRD comparing T versus C, the two samples must obviously be drawn from the *same* population. When, for example, patients who choose T are compared with those who choose C, the two samples may represent different populations, because there are often selection factors (many unknown) that differentiate the two groups. To guarantee that the two samples are drawn from exactly the same population, one sample is drawn from the relevant population, and these patients are *randomly* assigned to T or to C.

It is important to understand that randomization is a systematic, not a haphazard, procedure and that it does not produce two *matched* samples from the population. In fact, 5% of all independent baseline variables would be expected to significantly differentiate the two randomly assigned treatment groups at the 5% significance level. Two treatment groups too well matched at baseline are almost as questionable a situation as two treatment groups differing greatly at baseline. Both suggest that some non-random selection took place.

"Blinding"

Because the assessment of response can easily be colored by knowledge of which intervention was delivered to which patient, some effort must be made to minimize bias resulting from this knowledge. Otherwise, any differences between T and C may be in the eye of the beholder rather than in that of the patients. One such effort is termed "blinding," ensuring that those involved in assessing individual responses should not know which intervention was received.

Analysis by intention to treat

The purpose of randomization is to ensure that the T and C groups are two random samples from the same population. Any removals postrandomization from either treatment group, either by choice of the patient (dropout, noncompliance) or by choice of the clinical researchers (a focus on completers) can reintroduce the selection bias that randomization is designed to preclude. Attrition may reflect the patient's response to treatment, and what factors determine attrition may be different in T and C. Thus, every patient randomized must be included in the final evaluation of the two treatments: analysis by intention to treat.

Ethical issues/clinical equipoise

Patients likely to be harmed by either of the treatments or by the procedures in the study must ethically be excluded from eligibility. Not only must the patient be informed of what the treatments are, of what they are expected to experience during the trial, but of any known ill effects of participation. Ethical considerations mean that a patient cannot be included in a trial without *informed* consent.

Moreover, it is not ethical for a researcher already convinced of the answer to the research question to conduct an RCT: *clinical equipoise*. Ethicists can argue the ethical bases for the necessity for clinical equipoise, but from the point of view

of a biostatistician, the simple fact is that if the researcher is convinced of what the "right" answer is, she/he is prone to biasing all the decisions in designing, conducting, analyzing, and interpreting the results of a study in that direction. Thus, before considering an RCT, the researcher must have rationale and justification for proposing his/her hypothesis, but must also have reasonable doubt as to whether that hypothesis is true or not. Then she/he must design, conduct the trial, analyze the data, and report the results in such a way as to assure that the conclusions are the correct ones, even if they indicate that the researcher's hypothesis was false.

Basic principles of the randomized clinical trial

The basic principles of randomized clinical trials (RCTs) are clinical equipoise, population specification, sampling, randomization to a well-defined T and C, blinding, analysis by intention to treat, fair and unbiased conduct of the trial, and interpretation of trial results. Each of these principles was articulated because earlier trials failed in one way or another, and each is ignored at the risk of incurring failures in future studies. Generally, the RCT is considered the "gold standard" for evaluation of treatments. RCTs are challenging, time-consuming, and costly. Many argue that RCTs are not necessary, that equivalent results can be obtained from other, less rigorous, approaches. Before we consider options available to design valid and powerful RCTs, let us briefly consider certain alternatives.

Alternatives to RCTS?

The pre-post design

Since the primary goal is only to show that T improves treatment response, why not simply assess the clinical status of patients sampled from the relevant population before start of treatment, and then after treatment, and see whether there is/is not an improvement? No need for a control group, randomization, "blinding," and all those messy RCT challenges!

However, even when the clinical status of the patient does not change, one is likely to see what appears to be improvement. Statistical regression to the mean (Campbell & Kenny, 1999) occurs because those who are sampled are assessed to be reasonably highly symptomatic. However, selection of such patients on the basis of a less than perfectly reliable assessment of symptoms means that false positives are included and false negatives excluded from the trial. Subsequent assessment of response will likely correct measurement errors, and the patients as a group will appear to move toward the true value (i.e., appear improved) even in absence of improvement.

Moreover, because assessors know that all patients are given T and expect to see improvement, they often see improvement even when there is none. There may be measurement drift over time, with criteria less stringent at endpoint that at entry. If the patients are not "blinded" to the fact that all are treated, their own expectation effects may produce an appearance of improvement when there is none. Finally, patients may actually improve even without effective treatment, that is, what one sees is not the result of treatment but a natural and inevitable occurrence.

The combination of all of these artifacts means that it is common to see what appears to be improvement when there is none. In many cases, an RCT that results in a "nonstatistically significant result" is misinterpreted as having equally beneficial effects in both T and C because the pre-post change in both groups is found "statistically significant," when all this means is that the same statistical artifacts affected both groups. In short, pre-post trials are not a suitable alternative to RCTs.

Cross-over designs

A more contentious and appealing alternative to RCTs is a cross-over design. In this design, patients are randomly assigned either to T and C in the first time period (a standard RCT). A suitable "wash-out" period follows. Patients assigned to T in the first time period are assigned to C in the second and vice versa. Thus, each patient "serves as his/her own control" in that we can compare each individual patient's response to T and to C directly.

This design has attractive features. It is often easier to recruit patients into such a design, since each patient is assured of getting the "preferred" treatment. It is easier to avoid attrition in the first period, because patients who do not have a good experience may hope that the second period will be better if they persist.

However, the validity of conclusions here depends on complete absence of carry-over effects from the first period to the second, and then crucially on all patients completing both treatment periods. The assumption that all patients have returned to "virgin" status at the end of the wash-out period seldom holds. With drug treatments, the metabolites of the first drug may still be active when the second drug is given, unless the wash-out period is very long, so long that the clinical status of the patient may have changed. It is difficult to imagine that any intervention that involves learning (e.g., psychotherapy or an educational intervention) can ever be "washed out." Moreover, patients who experience benefit in the first period may be reluctant to have that effect "washed out"; patients who experience no benefit in the first period may become discouraged and drop out, particularly if the "wash-out" period is long.

When a cross-over design is used, there must be a careful check for absence of carry-over effects (Brown, 1980; Fleiss *et al.*, 1985). If such effects are detected or strongly suspected, the fallback position is to ignore the second time period and treat the first time period as a simple RCT. However, that will mean wasted time, effort, and resources, and will have put an unnecessary burden on the patients involved in the study.

There is a middle ground that preserves some of the advantages of the cross-over design, but avoids the almost inevitable pitfalls. One might design a standard RCT (the first time period), but offer patients the option, once that period is over, of moving to the alternative treatment, if they so choose. Then there need be no wash-out period, and no necessity for data recruitment and retention is maintained. Patients may choose not to go to the second time period, in which case, whether they accept the burden is their choice, and many will choose not to do so, decreasing waste in time, effort, and resources.

Natural experiments, observational studies, quasi-experimental designs

What if we could not randomize? What if we had access only to nonrandomized samples of patients with T and with C? Could we not compare these groups to draw inferences about the effect of T versus C?

The answer, as many have argued, is that if those samples are representative of the *same* population, of course one can, for, that would then be equivalent to an RCT. Indeed, if we knew what factors relevant to treatment response differentiated the two groups and had good measures of them, there are statistical methods that might remove most or all of the sampling biases (e.g., Rosenbaum & Rubin, 1983; Jo & Stuart, 2009). There are methods designed to bring the credibility of inferences as close to those resulting from RCTs as possible (see Chapter 12).

Effect sizes. Not *P*-values

An effect size is a population parameter that indicates the strength of an effect in a way that can be practically or clinically interpreted (Kraemer & Kupfer, 2006). The most common effect size in RCTs is Cohen's d (Cohen, 1988), the mean difference between the two treatment group means divided by the assumed common standard deviation within the two groups. The problem is that d is meant to compare two normally distributed responses with equal variances. Actual outcome measures often do not satisfy this assumption.

SRD, as defined, can be used with any outcome measure on which responses can be compared, a requirement for any outcome measure in an RCT. If the assumptions underlying Cohen's d hold, then $SRD = 2\Phi(d/\sqrt{2}) - 1$, where $\Phi()$ is the cumulative standard normal distribution. Thus d, when appropriate, is not lost, but simply rescaled.

Another effect size attractive to clinicians, patients, and policy makers is number needed to treat. Since NNT = 1/SRD, NNT is again merely a rescaling of SRD. NNT is the answer to the question: How many patients would have to be treated with T to have one more "success" than if the same number were treated with C. Thus, if NNT = 1, every patient treated with T has response clinically preferable to every patient treated with C (NNT = −1 reverses T and C). Infinite NNT means that the two treatments are clinically equivalent.

Odds ratio is also commonly used as an effect size when the outcome is binary: success/failure. If s1 is the success rate in T and s0 the success rate in C, then odds ratio = s1(1 − s0)/ ((1 − s1)s0), whereas SRD here equals s1 − s0. There is no problem with interpreting odds ratio = 1. This indicates clinical equivalence of T and C and can only occur when SRD = 0. However, what of any other value, say, odds ratio = 25? This can result with s1 = 2.4% and s0 = 0.1%, in which case SRD = 0.023 and NNT = 43, a trivial effect size by usual standards. It can result with s1 = 96.2% and s0 = 50.5%, in which case SRD = 0.457 and NNT = 2.2, a large effect size by usual standards. Such a situation can only confuse the interpretation of RCTs for clinical application.

The difficulty with the odds ratio has to do with division by near-zero numbers. If either s1 or s0 is extreme, very near zero or very near 1, the odds ratio tends to "explode," becoming very large even when the clinical effect may be trivial. When neither s1 nor s0 is extreme, then SRD is approximately equal to $(\sqrt{OR}-1)/(\sqrt{OR}+1)$ (Kraemer & Kupfer, 2006). In general, odds ratio cannot be interpreted as indicating the effect of treatments for clinical decision making and should not be used as an effect size for RCTs (Sackett, 1996; Newcombe, 2006).

There are three different effect sizes of concern in any RCT: the *true effect size* in the population which is never known exactly, the *estimated effect size* after completion of the RCT which provides information about the true effect size and upon which the conclusions of the RCT are based, and the *critical effect size* which is a setting of the threshold of clinical significance upon which power considerations are based before the RCT, and upon which interpretation of the clinical significance of the T versus C choice is based after completion of the RCT.

Cohen, in discussing the role of Cohen's d in power considerations (Cohen, 1988), suggested that $d = 0.2, 0.5, 0.8$ were small, medium, and large effect sizes. These standards, widely used, correspond to SRD = 0.11, 0.28, 0.43 or NNT = 8.9, 3.6, 2.3. However, Cohen rightly warned that any such standards should not be reified. What is clinically significant may change from one situation to another, depending on the severity of the disorder being treated, the consequences of inadequate treatment, the costs and risks of the treatment itself, the vulnerability of the population, and so on, and is determined by perusal of the exploratory materials in the specific context of the research.

Exploratory activities, pilot studies, and RCTS

In Figure 14.1 is an idealized depiction of the scientific method as applied to RCTs. The process begins with exploratory/hypothesis-generating activities: review of the literature, current theories, clinical observations and experience, results from animal models or tissue research, secondary analysis of existing datasets, and so on. In research areas close to the "cutting edge," where there is little in the existing literature, studies specifically designed, to generate hypotheses for testing in future studies (unfortunately derided as "fishing expeditions") might be proposed and executed. From this work, the theoretical rationale and empirical justification for a hypothesis is developed, as well as the information needed to design a valid and powerful RCT to test that hypothesis, and finally an indication of the critical effect size in the context of this hypothesis.

Once the hypothesis is formulated, the focus is on designing a valid and powerful RCT. When that is done, there are often questions about whether certain aspects of the design can be done as proposed in the milieu in which the RCT is to be done. Can one really recruit as many patients per year as proposed? Can T and C be delivered as per protocol? To find out after the RCT is launched, that the study is not feasible, is problematic. Thus, often a pilot study is proposed to test the feasibility of what is proposed, to develop treatment and measurement manuals, to train treatment deliverers and assessment staff, in essence to debug what is proposed in order to guarantee the feasibility of the RCT. Once that is done, the RCT can be executed as designed (i.e., with fidelity), and analyzed as proposed.

It should be noted that pilot studies, so defined, perform a crucial function in ensuring that RCTs are successful, but are not

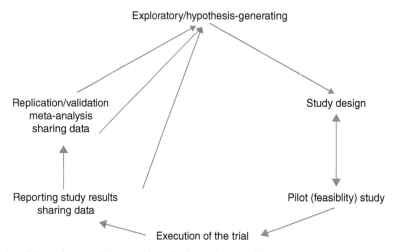

Figure 14.1 An idealized version of the application of the scientific method to evaluation of interventions.

themselves meant to test or to estimate effect sizes. Often the results of a pilot study are not publishable in that they relate to local conditions rather than to scientific questions that generalize across sites or time. It is an unfortunate fact that the term "pilot study" is often preempted to mean a small, badly designed, inadequately powered study, one that cannot provide any trustworthy estimate of the effect size of treatment, either for use in subsequent power calculations or to assure review committees that the RCT will be successful in identifying a viable intervention (Kraemer *et al.*, 2006).

Once the RCT is completed, three things should occur: (1) the conclusions concerning the hypothesis tested are presented; (2) the dataset is explored both to gain a greater understanding of issues related to that hypothesis, and to develop hypotheses that might be important for future research; (3) the dataset is shared with other researchers both to allow a check of the internal validity of the conclusions drawn, and to enrich the resources for exploration in general. In short, the beginning and end of an RCT lie in exploratory data analysis. Without these activities, hypotheses proposed are often weak, the designs used to test the hypotheses lack power, and RCTs are more likely to fail. Let us now focus on the design, execution, and reporting of RCTs.

Formulating the hypothesis

Efficacy versus effectiveness

Efficacy versus effectiveness considerations are crucial to articulating the hypothesis and designing the RCT appropriately (Hoagwood *et al.*, 1995; Weisz *et al.*, 2013). These terms do not refer to two specific types of studies but to a continuum of approaches. An efficacy study asks whether T > C under ideal circumstances, whereas an effectiveness study asks whether T > C under the usual circumstances. The decision as to where on the continuum between "ideal" and "usual" an RCT hypothesis is placed determines all research design decisions.

Population and sampling:

The results of any research study apply to the population represented by the sample. A study sampling a clinic population is unlikely to yield the same results as that sampling a community population. An RCT done at one site does not necessarily yield the same results as exactly the same RCT done at another. An RCT done in 2000 does not necessarily yield the same results as one done in 2010. How, where, and when a research study is done always determines the generalizability of its conclusions.

In an efficacy study, the inclusion/exclusion criteria are usually very narrowly set to include only those patients likely to support the hypothesis. One might exclude those who are too symptomatic or not symptomatic enough, those with comorbidities, children whose parents themselves have psychopathology, or other indications that would presage lack of cooperation, or limited response to treatment. The treatment would be delivered under optimal circumstances, often requiring specially trained

physicians with access to resources not available to ordinary clinicians. Because the true effect size is likely to be large, the sample size necessary for adequate power will tend to be small. Thus, the time and cost of the study will also be low, but generalizability of results limited.

In contrast, in an effectiveness study, only patients one could not ethically include would be excluded, to be as representative as possible of those for whom clinicians might need to make a decision between T and C. The sample randomized would be heterogeneous, compliance might be a problem, and dropout more likely. The clinicians would operate as clinicians are likely to in practice. The sample size then would necessarily be much greater, as would the time, cost, and difficulty. However, the answer would be more relevant to actual clinical decision making (Weisz *et al.*, 2013).

Logically, the very first RCTs comparing a new treatment T against C should probably always be efficacy studies. If T is not substantially better than C in ideal circumstances, it is hardly likely to be better under usual circumstances. However, before dissemination of a treatment, effectiveness studies are badly needed.

Multisite RCTs

It is often difficult to generate a large enough sample size at any one site, the usual argument for a multisite RCT, one in which exactly the same RCT is conducted at more than one site. An even more powerful argument for multisite RCTs stems from the observation that the conclusions of an RCT done at one site do not necessarily generalize to those at other sites. A multisite RCT affords the opportunity to test whether generalization will occur at least to sites represented by those participating in the RCT.

Consequently, in analyzing results, site, choice of treatment, *and* their interaction must be assessed (Kraemer & Robinson, 2005). Testing the site by treatment interaction is a test of the null hypothesis that the effect sizes comparing T and C are the same at all sites, and the main effect of treatment tests whether the *average* within-site effect size over sites is zero. If there is evidence of heterogeneity of treatment effect sizes across sites, the separate effect sizes would need to be reported and possible sources of heterogeneity explored. Otherwise, the pooled within-site effect size and its confidence interval would be reported. The pooled within-site effect size is not generally equal to the overall effect size if site is ignored in the analysis. Many multisite studies in the past have ignored site or site by treatment effects, and thus, in many cases, misreported their conclusions.

Individual versus cluster randomized studies

Generally, in RCTs, T is delivered to each patient individually, and no patient influences another patient's responses. However, there are situations in which T is delivered to groups (therapy groups, classes, families, etc.). Then the unit of randomization and of analysis must be the group, not the individual. For individual interventions, analytic procedures are based on the assumption of independence of responses. When there are between-patient interactions that might affect response, p-values, parameter estimates and confidence intervals based on the usual statistical methods are biased. In such cases, specialized statistical methods must be used to account for the between-patient correlations (Murray, 1998).

Designing the RCT

Choice of control group

What does it mean "if T were not given"? That is the question that should decide the choice of control group, C. In efficacy trials, the choice for C is often an inert placebo, for this gives the easiest challenge to show some effect of T. Otherwise, one might also choose an active placebo, treatment as usual (TAU), standard of care, active comparator, waiting list, and within each of these, variations.

Experience in RCTs suggests that whatever one decides as the appropriate control group, someone will see as the wrong choice. Some researchers, for example, feel strongly that every RCT must have an inert placebo group. Other researchers feel equally strongly that use of an inert placebo group is unethical when known effective treatments already exist, that, in those circumstances, a placebo control group is essentially withholding treatment from patients who need treatment. Some researchers are enthusiastic about a TAU control group since that would be the basis of conveying the message to clinicians that a new treatment T is better than what clinicians are currently generally using. Others point out that TAU would mean heterogeneity of treatments, differently and perhaps inadequately delivered, and no clear indication of which treatments T is better than. Many would prefer a standard of treatment delivered within the study protocol, but which one? Waiting list control also means that treatment is withheld for the duration of the study, but even more troubling, those randomly assigned to the waiting list often seek other treatments and drop out before the waiting period is over, creating major problems with attrition in the analysis. When an active comparator is used, if T ultimately proves preferable to C, that presents a clear message. But if not, whether the two are equally good or equally bad is not clear, in the absence of a separate placebo control group (Leon, 2011). Moreover, if T and C are here two competing drugs from two pharmaceutical companies, it is amazing how often studies conducted by the company producing T find T preferable to C, and vice versa (clinical equipoise?). The arguments go on.

Thus, generally the best one can do is to consider carefully the current situation with regard to T, and what message the study is intended to convey and to whom, and make the most thoughtful choice possible, but without any expectation that choice will avoid criticism.

Randomization

The simplest randomization method involves tossing a fair coin or die to assign each patient to T or C when that patient signs the informed consent form. Every biostatistician, however, can relate some horror story where this was done, only to find, after the RCT was under way or done, that someone gerrymandered assignments. For example, in one RCT, the research assistant, charged with tossing the coin to determine treatment group, when faced with a seriously ill patient who, in his opinion, "really needed T," simply flipped the coin again and again until it dictated assignment to T. After all, he argued, each coin toss was equally random, wasn't it?

Problems stem from lack of "blindness" in recruiting and assigning the patients. When it is known or strongly suspected that the next patient is to be assigned to what the assigner considers a less preferred treatment, she/he can, consciously or not, delay that patient's entry until the prospects are better. Such gerrymandering can be avoided by "blinding" the assigner. For example, one might perform the coin/die tosses *before* the study is started, placing each assignment in a numbered, sealed, envelope, which the assigner must label with the patient's name upon entry to the study *before* opening the envelope. Since the assigner can only know the assignment *after* the patient is signed in on a numbered envelope (which can be checked), this reduces the chance of gerrymandering. Alternatively, a computer program can be set up, into which the patient's identification is entered, upon which the computer delivers the random assignment.

Gerrymandering is only one problem. Another problem is balance. By balance we mean that the proportion of the sample assigned to T matches reasonably well with the proportion the design requires (often equal assignment to two groups). With simple randomization with equal probabilities, if the total sample size is 20, the probability that exactly half end in T is 0.18, and that probability *decreases* as the sample size increases. If the sample size were indeed only 20, there is some chance that the RCT will end with some very uneven split, say 15 in T and 5 in C. Drawing inferences from a sample as small as 5 is risky. If on the other hand, the sample size were 200, 105 in T and 95 in C, a similar imbalance, the situation would not be so uncomfortable because a sample size of 95 remains substantial. Thus, the balance problem is most important when dealing with relatively small sample sizes.

The traditional way of dealing with this problem is blocking. Blocks of 2, 4, 6, 8, and so on, are used with successive block sizes randomly varied within the trial, the size of blocks unknown to any of the researchers. Within each block exactly half are assigned to T, the other half to C. The larger the block, the better is the blinding, and thus the better protection against gerrymandering. At the end of each block, the sample sizes are exactly balanced. However, the larger the block, the more likely the recruitment will end inside a block, sometimes still leaving an unwelcome imbalance.

A better alternative is the Efron procedure (Efron, 1971). As each patient sequentially enters the RCT, the numbers previously assigned to T and C are tracked. If an even split is required, whenever the sample sizes to date are equal, the probability of assignment to T is 0.5. If, however, these numbers are unequal, the probability of assignment to the minority group is slightly higher, say 2/3, and consequently that to the majority group slightly lower, say 1/3. This exerts a constant pressure to keep the group sizes near equal. Yet, it is difficult to predict where the next patient is likely to be assigned, preserving "blindness."

Balancing is one issue, matching yet another. As noted earlier, randomization does not guarantee "matching" between the groups, but produces two random samples from the same population. Thus, the age, gender, initial severity, and so on, of the T and C groups that result would not be expected to have exactly the same means and variances. Many researchers are concerned that the occasional mismatch can compromise the interpretations of any group differences, and try to ensure better matching by a variety of methods including adaptive randomization.

Before considering such options, it should be noted that there are an almost infinite number of baseline variables, but most are irrelevant to treatment outcome. Matching the two groups on an irrelevant variable increases the difficulty of doing the RCT but has no effect on the credibility of conclusions, and may cost power. Moreover, the harder one strives to match groups on one set of baseline variables, the more likely the groups are to end mismatched on others. It all too frequently happens that the variables selected to match the groups are not the variables most important to the outcome, in which case, the results may be more seriously compromised using matching procedures than they would have been without.

In an adaptive randomization, the characteristics of the two groups on a list of crucial variables are tracked as patients enter into the study. If the two groups are matched on these variables, the probability of assignment to T is 0.5; if not, the probability is moved slightly toward assignment to whichever group would bring the characteristics into a better match. This then exerts pressure to keep the two treatment groups matched, at least on the variables selected to be considered.

There are a variety of other randomization tactics designed neither for blinding, balancing, or matching, but to deal with other practical problems often encountered. To take just one: equipoise randomization.

Often eligible patients being recruited to an RCT may not agree to randomization. If such patients are excluded, one may end with an unrepresentative sample from the population of interest. When there are only two treatments in the RCT (the focus so far), say T and C, this does not pose a major problem, for then the conclusions apply to those patients for whom the T versus C choice is possible. Since clinicians are ethically barred from treating patients with a treatment they will not accept, this limitation matters little. However, suppose there were more than two treatments, T1, T2, … Tm?

Traditionally, using the same principle, one should exclude from randomization all patients who would not accept randomization to all m treatments. Quite aside from the fact that this may cause serious problems with access to sufficient sample size, it may also result in a very biased sample from the population of interest. The population, for example, would include many patients who might agree to either T1 or T2, but they would be excluded because they would not agree to T3 or T4.

Equipoise randomization (Lavori *et al.*, 2001) requires that each patient be given the best argument for equipoise among all the m treatments in the informed consent process. If the patient will agree to randomization to at least two of the treatments, that patient is randomized to as many of the m treatments as she/he would accept. Thus, patients who would not accept T3 or T4, but would accept T1 and T2, are included in the sample. Then each pair of treatments is considered separately, on that subsample who would accept that choice and the conclusions from each analysis apply to those patients for whom that particular choice is acceptable.

Choice of outcome measure(s)

In an RCT, outcome measure(s) are specified "*a priori*," should be registered and/or published before the trial is under way, and not modified thereafter (DeAngelis *et al.*, 2005). The question is: Which outcome measure(s)?

Any statistician worth his/her salt will recommend that every RCT have *one* primary outcome measure, and that the RCT be designed to have adequate power to detect T versus C differences on that *one* measure. Then if the RCT shows that there is a clinically significant advantage of T over C, that provides a clear message to clinicians.

Every clinician worth his/her salt will protest that having only one outcome measure can never capture the totality of effects on the patient that should influence clinical decisions between T and C. There are always multiple benefits (hastens remission, minimizes symptoms, improves quality of life, etc.) and multiple harms (increases risk of suicide, weight gain, headaches, etc.)

In response, the statistician will point out that if one tests multiple outcome measures, each with a 5% chance of a result indicating that T > C when there is no difference (a false-positive result), with 2 outcome measures there is a 10% chance, with 3 a 14% chance, with 10 a 40% chance, and so on. Including multiple outcome measures as the basis of clinical decision making proliferates false-positive results unless one adjusts the chance of a false positive so that the overall chance is less than 5%. However such an adjustment is made, it results in a loss of power to detect true treatment effects: the more numerous the outcome measures, the greater the loss of power. Moreover, on some outcomes T will be shown preferable to C, some have T clinically equivalent to C, and some have C preferable to T. What sense any clinician or patient can make of that mixture of recommendations is hard to fathom.

One solution to this problem is emerging: an integrated outcome measure (Kraemer & Frank, 2010; Kraemer *et al.*, 2011; Wallace *et al.*, 2013). The fundamental idea of an integrated outcome measure is that all independent outcome measures of clinical importance are first identified and well and carefully measured in the RCT. Then clinical judgment is used to weigh and balance the cumulative effects of these outcomes on the individual patients.

A simple example was the outcome proposed (but not so used exactly) in the CATIE study evaluating drug treatments for schizophrenia (Lieberman *et al.*, 2005). It was proposed that each patient be clinically tracked over time and the treatment be discontinued for either lack of efficacy or of tolerability based on the clinical judgment of the treating physician "blinded" to treatment. What constituted efficacy (reduction of symptoms, increase in functional status, increase in quality of life, etc.), and what constituted tolerability (increase in weight, tardive dyskinesia symptoms, etc.) and how one would balance one against the other, might vary from patient to patient, and perhaps from clinician to clinician. However, it was left to clinical judgment as to when the total impact of harms exceeded the total impact of benefits on each individual patient. The single outcome measure would be time to treatment failure.

Power and precision

Once all these decisions are made, each of which impacts the sample size, a decision needs to be made as to how large a sample size is needed for adequate power in testing and adequate precision in estimating effect sizes. The classical way is to propose "*a priori*" a significance level, usually 5%, that indicates the minimally acceptable risk of a false-positive result, and then to determine what sample size is needed to have an "*a priori*" level of power, typically 80%, to detect any effect size that would be considered of clinical significance, that is, an effect size greater than the critical effect size. This is the same as the necessary sample size in order that a 95% confidence interval for the effect size does not include zero when the true effect size is greater than the critical effect size, that is, adequate precision for estimation of the effect size. Thus, shifting from consideration of power for a statistical test is tantamount to consideration of precision for estimation of an effect size.

Every decision made, particularly those related to outcome measures, has an impact on the necessary sample size. As a general rule, an outcome measure that is very sensitive to crucial clinical individual differences in response to treatment will yield greater power in testing and greater precision in estimation with smaller sample sizes.

The weakest possible outcome measure is a binary measure: success/failure. For example, if "success" is defined as remission within 1 year, a patient who remits at 1 year + 1 day is considered tied with patients who remit at 2 years, 3 years, or never. A patient who remits at 1 year − 1 day is considered tied with patients who remit at 1 week, 1 month, or 6 months. To choose this outcome measure will require the largest possible sample size for adequate power/precision. The cost of dichotomized outcomes has long been recognized but often ignored (Cohen, 1983).

In this case, we might instead propose to use time to remission (an ordinal variable) as the outcome, and survival methods to test or to estimate an effect size (Kaplan & Meier, 1958). Now the only patients who will be tied are those that remit at the same time, resulting in a major increase in power/precision. But two patients who both remit at the same time may differ radically in their course. One may have experienced a very rapid decrease in symptoms early but then drifted toward remission, while the other may have been highly symptomatic until just shortly before remission. Similarly, two patients may remit at the same time, but one remains symptomatic afterward, while the other completely recovers. Yet these pairs are tied in time to remission.

Instead, we might propose to use repeated measures over time of symptom level (those that define remission), and use a hierarchical linear model (Gibbons *et al.*, 1993) to compare the complete trajectories of response. Now we have an approach sensitive both to the timing of remission and to the course prior to and after remission. To do so will result in a further increase in power/precision, thus reducing the necessary sample size.

The key issues in selecting the outcome measure in an RCT is (a) to consider exactly what responses are crucial in deciding between T and C, no more or fewer than are necessary; (b) to guarantee the reliability and validity of these responses, and to assure maximum sensitivity to crucial individual differences in response among patients, preferably with repeated measures of each over the course of treatment; (c) if necessary, to combine multiple such measures reflecting their importance to clinical decision making. To do this not only increases how clinically informative the results but also increases power/precision and reduces the sample size and hence the difficulty and cost of doing RCTs.

RCT execution/fidelity

The greatest intellectual effort occurs in the process of designing an RCT. All that needs to be done during the RCT is to follow one's own rules. That makes it all the more remarkable how often, once the RCT is under way, the researchers begin to drift from those rules. Inclusion/exclusion criteria become either stricter or looser, measurement procedures are modified, the number and timing of evaluations shifts, and so on. The consequence of any deviations from the original protocol is, at the very least, to introduce extraneous variability into the results, and thus to sacrifice power/precision. At the very most, the validity of the study to test the original hypothesis is compromised. Strict adherence to the research protocol, both in the delivery of the treatments, and in the conduct of the RCT is referred to as "fidelity." Fidelity is often a focus of attention in multisite trials, to ensure that the sites do not end doing different RCTs, precluding combining the results from the different sites, testing generalizability of the results, or estimating a common effect size and its confidence interval. However, fidelity is equally important in a single site RCT. When a well-designed and adequately powered RCT fails, it is most likely due to lack of fidelity.

Primary analysis and presentation of results

In a well-conceived, well-designed RCT, the primary analyses are those specified 'a priori' on which the power calculations determining the sample size of the study were based. Table 1 in any RCT report generally provides descriptive statistics describing the baseline characteristics of the population as estimated in the sample. Often descriptive statistics are provided separately for the T and C groups to document that the randomization produced two similar samples (neither too badly nor too well matched). Often researchers will test the null hypothesis that randomization was done by testing T versus C differences on each baseline variable. This is a puzzling but harmless practice, since the researchers surely know with certainty whether they did or did not randomize!

However, as we've noted, with randomization to two groups, 5% of independent baseline variables should significantly differentiate the two groups at the 5% level. With replication, which variables do so, will vary. However, researchers often respond to finding such differences in an RCT by proposing to "control" these factors by including them as covariates when comparing T and C. Two problems then arise: (a) This is now "post hoc" analysis since the hypothesis being tested was generated by looking at the data to be used in testing that hypothesis and is different from the one originally proposed. (b) Since the variables chosen are those correlated with treatment choice, collinearity is introduced. Both compromise the validity of the testing and estimation. The test done to address the primary research question in the RCT report should still be the analysis proposed "a priori." The CONSORT guidelines (Schulz et al., 2010) provide excellent information on what information needs to be reported from an RCT.

However, after that analysis produces whatever results it does, it would be appropriate, on an exploratory level, to ask whether any baseline variables (whether well matched in the two groups or not) are either nonspecific predictors or moderators of treatment response, with emphasis on effect sizes and their confidence interval, not on statistical tests. If important relationships are thus detected, these findings are then checked against existing literature, and if now there is rationale and justification for hypothesizing a nonspecific predictor or a moderator, this hypothesis would be tested in a *subsequent independent* RCT, with a design better suited to detection of such relationships.

Moving the frontiers: exploration of RCT data

The completion of the primary analysis "as intended" is not the end of the project. There are at least three important strategies that should now be implemented: (a) continued education in RCT methodology; (b) checking the internal validity of the study conclusions; (c) exploratory (hypothesis-generating) studies to set the stage for furthering and deepening the understanding of the results of this RCT, particularly efforts to identify moderators and mediators of treatment response.

There has probably never been an RCT done, that upon completion, the researchers involved could not look back and identify actions they should have taken but did not, actions they did take but need or should not have, actions that might have been improved. Conscious consideration of these actions, a sort of statistical autopsy, is an excellent form of continued education, the less than perfect decisions in one RCT leading to improved methodology in the next. Moreover, it is the investigators' responsibility to identify and to report any challenges they know of to the validity of their findings (internal validity). Statistical autopsy facilitates this process.

Finally, considerable effort should be invested in trying to discover the moderators and mediators of treatment response (Kraemer et al., 2005). A *moderator* of treatment response is a baseline (prerandomization) factor that identifies subgroups of patients within the population sampled who have different effect sizes. Thus, to take a simple example, gender moderates the effect of treatment if the effect size comparing T versus C is different for boys than for girls. In most cases, unrecognized moderators deflate the overall effect size. Indeed, it is possible that the primary analysis demonstrates a zero effect size, but that for girls the effect size is large and positive and for boys large and negative, thus canceling each other out.

Moderators are important since generally no T is uniformly better than C for all in a heterogeneous population. However, without the means to identify which patients would profit more from T and which from C, patients will often be given a treatment ineffective and even sometimes dangerous for them, only because they happen to be in a minority where the majority finds the treatment effective and safe. In recent years, emphasis has been place on personalized medicine (Jain, 2002; Lesko, 2007), efforts to move past this "one size fits all" philosophy.

A *mediator* of treatment response is an event or change that occurs early in treatment before outcome is determined, that differentiates T from C, and that explains some or all of the overall effect size comparing T and C in the population sampled. For example, it may be that a systematic drug treatment (T) for ADHD when compared with TAU leads to an early change in parenting behavior, and that the subsequent change in symptoms posttreatment reflects both the direct pharmacological effect as well as the effect on parenting. In this case, the change in parenting behavior mediates the treatment choice on change in symptoms.

While moderators are important to assigning each patient whichever of T or C is likely to be preferable for him/her, mediators are important to understanding the process by which T produces its effect. Where there are moderators, mediators may be different in subgroups defined by the moderators. Thus, for example, if gender moderates treatment response, the mediators of treatment response may be different for boys and girls. Logically then, the exploration for moderators should precede the exploration for mediators.

Mediators are important to considerations of how treatment might be improved. Finding that the change in parent behavior was a mediator of a drug treatment might suggest either adding components to the drug treatment to amplify this effect on parent behavior, or considering whether focusing on strategies to change parent behavior in absence of the drug treatment might be just as effective, or developing strategies for somehow tying drug dosage decisions to observations of parent behavior.

When moderators and mediators are detected in exploratory analyses post RCT, these are hypotheses to be tested in future independent studies, not conclusions. Considering the sheer number of baseline variables, and the number of different events or changes that might occur early in treatment, such exploratory analysis will generate many false-positive results. Consequently, any potentially important moderation or mediation so detected must first be supported by rationale and justification in the existing literature, and then formally tested in a *new* RCT designed for the purpose.

Completing the cycle: meta-analysis

No single research study ever establishes a scientific fact. That always requires independent validation, either a replication or another study that validates the conclusion. The best method available to establish consensus in multiple studies addressing the same T versus C comparison is meta-analysis.

It is the responsibility of the meta-analyst to identify inclusion/exclusion criteria for the studies to be included. For example, if there are both RCTs and observational studies comparing T versus C, should both be included? If one study samples only women and another a mixed-sex population, should both be included? As inclusion/exclusion criteria for patients in an RCT determine the conclusions to be drawn, so also do the inclusion/exclusion criteria for studies in a meta-analysis determine the conclusions to be drawn there.

Then one effect size from each study (and some measure of the precision of its estimation) is taken from each study, and these effect sizes are tested for homogeneity (i.e., consensus). In the absence of heterogeneity, the effect sizes are then pooled and the confidence interval of the pooled effect size estimated.

There are nine possible configurations of an RCT or a meta-analysis of RCTs (Figure 14.2). If the null effect size is not included in the confidence interval, the result is "statistically significant at the 5% level." Thus, #1,2,3 are all "statistically significant"; #4,5,6 are not. If only effect sizes greater than the critical effect size are included, the result is "clinically significant." If only effect sizes less than the critical effect size are included, the treatments are "clinically equivalent." Thus, #1 shows two

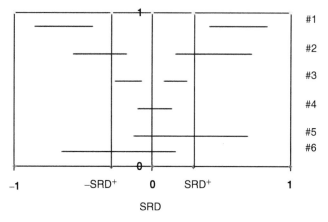

Figure 14.2 Ninety-five percent two-tailed confidence intervals on the effect size comparing T versus C showing the nine possible patterns that might result, where SRD* is the critical effect size.

results (in opposite directions) where the RCT demonstrated both statistical and clinical significance. #2 shows two results where there was statistical significance, but clinical significance remains in doubt, suggesting the necessity for further studies. #3 and #4 both show clinical equivalence, but #3 is statistically significant and #4 is not. #5,6 show failed studies, that is, before these studies, with clinical equipoise, it was not known which of T and C were better, and if so whether the difference was clinically significant. Here, after the studies, no more is known than was known with clinical equipoise before the studies.

After meta-analysis, #1, #3, #4 are conclusive results—consensus has been reached. #2 is promising but not conclusive, perhaps requiring more studies. However, #5,6, would indicate a waste of patient time and effort, time, and resources, for the process of comparing T versus C has not yet truly started.

If the studies included in meta-analysis are all valid and adequately powered to test the same T versus C in the same population on the same outcome, some 3–5 studies in a meta-analysis will likely be conclusive. If, on the other hand, only valid studies but many inadequately powered are included, it may take 10–20 studies to be conclusive. But if the inclusion/exclusion criteria for the meta-analysis are loose enough to include different populations, different outcomes, different versions of T or of C, or studies are included that are not valid, establishing consensus may be an impossible task.

It is not unusual to hear researchers justify a badly designed underpowered study (often erroneously called a "pilot study") by claiming that in itself, such a study may not lead to closure, but in combination with other studies, makes a contribution. Including such studies in meta-analysis not only encourages future such poor studies, but is likely to slow the research process leading to consensus. It is important that meta-analysts do a very complete survey of all studies done on an issue, but they should base their conclusions only on studies that, in their estimation, are both valid and adequately powered.

Discussion

How evaluation of treatment was done in the early 20th century was very different from that in the late, when RCT methodology was introduced and disseminated, and the changes continue. The advent and development of survival methods, the introduction of hierarchical linear models, the development of meta-analysis methods, the recognition of the importance of moderators and mediators of treatment response, and many such methodological advances, changes the way treatments are evaluated. Emphasis on presenting effect sizes and their confidence intervals in addition to p values changes the way results are reported. Changes affect not only analysis of results, but the decision on how and whom to sample, how to design the RCT for maximal validity and power, what outcome measures to use, and so on. The process of change will undoubtedly continue, bringing clinical trials ever closer to realizing the goals of clearly informing clinical decision making.

References

Brown, B.W.J. (1980) The crossover experiment for clinical trials. *Biometrics* **36**, 69–79.

Campbell, D.T. & Kenny, D.A. (1999) *A Primer on Regression Artifacts.* The Guilford Press, New York.

Cohen, J. (1983) The cost of dichotomization. *Applied Psychological Measurement* **7**, 249–253.

Cohen, J. (1988) *Statistical Power Analysis for the Behavioral Sciences.* Lawrence Erlbaum Associates, Hillsdale, NJ.

Deangelis, C.D. *et al.* (2005) Is this clinical trial fully registered? *JAMA* **293**, 2927–2929.

Efron, B. (1971) Forcing a sequential experiment to be balanced. *Biometrika* **58**, 403–417.

Fleiss, J.L. *et al.* (1985) Adjusting for baseline measurement in the two-period crossover study: a cautionary note. *Controlled Clinical Trials* **6**, 192–197.

Gibbons, R.D. *et al.* (1993) Some conceptual and statistical issues in the analysis of longitudinal psychiatric data. *Archives of General Psychiatry* **50**, 739–750.

Hoagwood, K. *et al.* (1995) Introduction to the special section: efficacy and effectiveness in studies of child and adolescent psychotherapy. *Journal of Consulting and Clinical Psychology* **63**, 683–687.

Hunter, J.E. (1997) Needed: a ban on the significance test. *Psychological Science* **8**, 3–7.

Jain, K.K. (2002) Personalized medicine. *Current Opinion in Molecular Therapeutics* **4**, 548–558.

Jo, B. & Stuart, E.E. (2009) On the use of propensity scores in principal causal effect estimation. *Statistics in Medicine* **28**, 2857–2875.

Kaplan, E.L. & Meier, P. (1958) Nonparametric estimation from incomplete observations. *Journal of the American Statistical Association* **53**, 562–563.

Kraemer, H.C. & Frank, E. (2010) Evaluation of comparative treatment trials: assessing the clinical benefits and risks for patients, rather than statistical effects on measures. *JAMA* **304**, 1–2.

Kraemer, H.C. & Kupfer, D.J. (2006) Size of treatment effects and their importance to clinical research and practice. *Biological Psychiatry* **59**, 990–996.

Kraemer, H.C. & Robinson, T.N. (2005) Are certain multicenter randomized clinical trials structures misleading clinical and policy decisions? *Controlled Clinical Trials* **26**, 518–529.

Kraemer, H.C. *et al.* (2005) *To Your Health: How to Understand What Research Tells Us About Risk.* Oxford University Press, Oxford.

Kraemer, H.C. *et al.* (2006) Caution regarding the use of pilot studies to guide power calculations for study proposals. *Archives of General Psychiatry* **63**, 484–489.

Kraemer, H.C. *et al.* (2011) How to assess the clinical impact of treatments on patients, rather than the statistical impact of treatments on measures. *International Journal of Methods in Psychiatric Research* **20**, 63–72.

Lavori, P.W. *et al.* (2001) Strengthening clinical effectiveness trials: equipoise-stratified randomization. *Biological Psychiatry* **50**, 792–801.

Leon, A.C. (2011) Comparative effectiveness clinical trials in psychiatry: superiority, non-inferiority and the role of active comparators. *Journal of Clinical Psychiatry* **72**, 1344–1349.

Lesko, L.J. (2007) Personalized medicine: elusive dream or imminent reality? *Clinical Pharmacology and Therapeutics* **81**, 807–815.

Lieberman, J.A. *et al.* (2005) Effectiveness of antipsychotic drugs in patients with chronic schizophrenia. *New England Journal of Medicine* **353**, 1209–1223.

Murray, D.M. (1998) *Design and Analysis of Group-Randomized Trials.* Oxford University Press, New York.

Newcombe, R.G. (2006) A deficiency of the odds ratio as a measure of effect size. *Statistics in Medicine* **25**, 4235–4240.

Rosenbaum, P.R. & Rubin, D.B. (1983) The central role of the propensity score in observational studies for causal effects. *Biometrika* **70**, 41–55.

Sackett, D.L. (1996) Down with odds ratios!. *Evidence-Based Medicine* **1**, 164–166.

Schulz, K.F. *et al.* (2010) Statement: updated guidelines for reporting parallel group randomised trials. *British Medical Journal* **340**, 698–702.

Shrout, P.E. (1997) Should significance tests be banned? Introduction to a special section exploring the pros and cons. *Psychological Science* **8**, 1–2.

Wallace, M.L. *et al.* (2013) A novel approach for developing and interpreting treatment moderator profiles in randomized clinical trials. *JAMA Psychiatry* **70**, 1241–1247.

Weisz, J.R. *et al.* (2013) Evidence-based youth psychotherapy in the mental health ecosystem. *Journal of clinical Child and Adolescent Psychology* **42**, 274–286.

CHAPTER 15

What clinicians need to know about statistical issues and methods

Andrew Pickles and Rachael Bedford
Department of Biostatistics, Institute of Psychiatry, Psychology and Neuroscience, King's College London, UK

Although as an academic discipline statistics is often associated with mathematics, it has had from its beginnings strong links to science—both in application and in the stimulus for new methodological development. The rationale for the use of statistics is as an objective and efficient operationalization of the scientific method in a context of complex data. Statistical methods should be achieving these aims in several ways: firstly, by requiring precise operational definitions of theories and explicitly specified critical differences or contrasts; secondly, by providing methodology for estimating scientifically meaningful quantities as precisely as possible and freed from as many sources of bias as possible; thirdly, by providing a framework for determining how uncertain our estimates are and whether data are consistent or inconsistent with theory. Some introductory statistics classes and books give the impression that statistics is more concerned with making assumptions; assumptions that appear abstract, derived from probability theory, with little meaning and anyway probably rarely met in practice. This is unfortunate, since in the majority of cases the assumptions correspond to critical scientific simplifications of a kind that most scientists and clinicians could easily comprehend and would have considerable intuition as to whether they are likely to be met or not. Moreover, it is crucial for the quality of the science that it be understood that such assumptions are being made.

For many years there has been a division of approach into experimental and observational/epidemiological studies. Experiments are often seen as strong for determining causation but having weak generalizability, while observational studies are seen as weak on causation but strong on generalization. While trivially apparent from the frequent use of analysis of variance for experiments and regression for observational studies, more profound differences exist. The first, traditionally given great emphasis, is the exploitation of randomization within experiments. The second is the careful pre-specification preceding an experiment. Such differences are amplified by the context of any statistical analysis. In clinical trials of pharmaceutical drugs, the massive financial interest makes the primary role of a statistician a "defensive" one, to prevent false claims of efficacy. In contrast, academic psychology has been more exploratory and theory confirming. Thus, what statistical analysis might be recommended will depend on much more than many introductory texts suggest.

Common misunderstandings, study design, multiple testing, meta-analysis and the natural history of "findings"

There is a common natural history for many "findings." First a small study finds a significant association and persuades an editor of its value. Many small studies fail to replicate the finding, but since everyone knows that small studies have "low power" this comes as no surprise; few, if any, such findings are published. Any small replication studies that do find a significant association are published, apparently confirming the interesting finding. Eventually, a large study fails to replicate the finding, and because of the study's size and the fact this failure is now seen as overturning a received wisdom, the results are published in a prominent journal. Patients then need to be persuaded that something formerly considered effective is now considered ineffective. How does this come about?

One key issue concerns the fact that readers and editors of papers are drawn to reports of significant associations rather than reports of non-significant effects. As a consequence, the p value remains the statistic upon which the success or failure of a study is seen to rest. Every study, regardless of size, has a fixed chance of identifying a significant effect in the sample drawn when there is no such effect in the population. Known as the

Rutter's Child and Adolescent Psychiatry, Sixth Edition.
Edited by Anita Thapar and Daniel S. Pine, James F. Leckman, Stephen Scott, Margaret J. Snowling, Eric Taylor.
© 2015 John Wiley & Sons Ltd. Published 2018 by John Wiley & Sons Ltd.

type 1 error, we usually set this risk as 1 in 20, or 0.05. If we test for the presence of two effects or study the same effect in two samples, then the risk that at least one of these might show a significant finding is now slightly less than 1 in 10. Test for the presence of enough effects or carry out enough studies and some are bound to be falsely significant. This is just the problem that geneticists face when testing for significant associations between a particular disorder and hundreds of thousands of gene single nucleotide polymorphisms (SNPs) or neuroimagers with similar numbers of brain features. The Bonferroni correction can be used to set a meaningful significance criterion when the effects being tested are independent, or alternatively tests can be applied that account for the correlation, for example, permutation and false discovery rate tests (Benjamini & Hochberg, 1995).

Rather than significance, statisticians argue that it is the size of the effect or difference, together with some measure of precision, preferably a confidence interval (CI) that should be reported. The CI gives the opportunity to reflect upon the range of possible values that can be considered as potentially consistent with the data and to assess whether effects of this magnitude would be, say, of clinical importance.

Sample size also needs to be considered when assessing the likely importance of significant effects. It is a common misconception that finding a significant effect in a small study must mean that the effect is substantial. In small studies, the magnitude of the estimate must be large for it to appear as significant—in a small study, all small effect estimates are non significant—and just because the estimate is large does not mean that the true effect is necessarily so. Although both large and small studies have the same chance of falsely identifying one of the many "no-effect" factors as significant (false positive), larger studies have greater power to detect the few true-effect factors as significant. Thus, of the effects found to be significant, a higher proportion of those from a small study will be false and of an exaggerated size as compared to the proportion from a large study.

This is one of the problems that meta-analysis, also known as systematic review, attempts to overcome (Cooper et al., 2009). A systematic review usually consists of four steps. First, assembling an exhaustive list of the potentially relevant published studies; second, selecting against a predefined list of criteria a subset whose design, implementation and clarity of reporting suggest that they are appropriate and of good quality. Where possible this second step should be done blind to authorship and to the actual findings of the study. The third step is to display the findings of these studies in a funnel plot (Light & Pillemer, 1984). Figure 15.1 shows data from several acupuncture studies illustrating the diminution of effect size reported as the sample size increases, to the point where the largest study shows no effect. If the true effect is zero, then the figure also shows evidence of publication bias, since if all little studies were published one would expect their estimates to be scattered symmetrically around the larger studies. Such evidence of publication bias

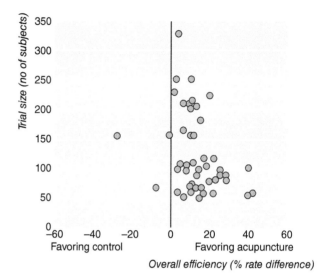

Figure 15.1 Funnel plot showing clear evidence of publication bias. *Source:* From Tang *et al.* (1999). Reproduced with permission of BMJ.

should prompt significant concern and a search for unpublished studies. The final and most technical step in a systematic review is the method used to pool the information to come up with a single overall estimate of the average effect.

A focus on significance, sample size and publication bias are not the only reasons for the natural history of findings with which we began this section. In addition, although there are important exceptions, because large projects cost more and are commonly staffed by more experienced researchers, they tend to be superior on a whole range of methodological measures of quality, such as being prospective rather than retrospective, having blind assessments and being better analyzed and reported. Each of these factors tends to exclude possible biases that can contribute to artifact. Indeed reported effect size does seem to decline as the methodological rigor of the study increases (Schulz *et al.*, 1995).

More recently, some apparently robust findings from epidemiology have been tested in randomized trials, considered by most as the ultimate study design for testing causal effects (see Chapter 14). Results from several high-profile treatments have been not just disappointing, but in the case of hormone replacement therapy (HRT), in contrast to the beneficial effects reported from epidemiological studies (Petitti *et al.*, 1986) the trial finding actually suggested it to be dangerous (Hulley *et al.*, 1998).

A possible explanation for the discrepancy between trials and observational studies may lie in inadequate control of factors such as socioeconomic position (Lawlor *et al.*, 2004). Others have suggested that the discrepancy is resolved if the formal attention to detail in specifying eligibility, treatment and outcome that characterizes an RCT is applied to the epidemiological data (Hernán *et al.*, 2008). Such a proposal, for greater care, clarity and objectivity in the analysis of epidemiological data, we believe to be important and of wide relevance (see Chapters 12 and 14).

Confounding, selection and randomization

Rarely is an outcome of psychiatric interest related to just a single causal factor. In practice, many different processes are and have been at work to give rise to the current mental state of an individual. Moreover, many of the factors of interest in child psychiatry co-occur. Poor families tend to live in poor neighborhoods, with poor educational opportunities and suffer psychosocial risks and stresses that give rise to discord. Thus, a group of children identified by any one of these factors will have an unusually high frequency of the other factors. There are two important aspects of this problem. The first, "independent effects of confounders," relates to the fact that these other factors may have effects which we should attempt to account for. The second, "selection effects," refers to the variation among subjects in their exposure to the factor of interest being correlated with variation in these other factors. In other words, those who are selected to be exposed to one risk factor have commonly experienced and are experiencing these other risks as well. The effect of our factor of interest will be confounded with the effects of these other risks. Broadly speaking, we can attempt to solve our problem if we can deal with either of the two aspects of the problem.

Adjustment for measured confounders: regression and the generalized linear model

One way of dealing with confounding is through standardization, for example, standardizing intelligence scores to remove the effects of age. A large calibration sample is used to translate a raw score into a standardized score that measures the extent of deviation from the norm for a particular raw score at a particular age. Standardization can also take the form of weighting age-specific sample data to correspond to a population with a standard age distribution. However, adjustment for variables about which we know rather less, especially when we have several of them, requires a more generic approach, typically provided by some form of regression model. For continuous outcome measures the familiar regression model is used to combine the effects of several factors. In this model, the expected value of the outcome Y is assumed to be some linear combination of the predictor variables (X_1 and X_2):

$$E(Y) = \alpha + \beta_1 X_1 + \beta_2 X_2$$

and the variance of the outcome around its expected value is assumed to be constant (homoscedasticity). No assumptions are made about the distribution of the X variables, they can be continuous or discrete (binary dummy categorical variables).

Of course, there are many outcomes for which this linear model is not appropriate, and we then often turn to some form of the generalized linear model (GLM; McCullagh & Nelder, 1989). This allows two extensions to the ordinary regression model. Firstly, a choice of link function which transforms the expected value of the response. For example, for a count response a log link would be chosen:

$$\log[E(Y)] = \alpha + \beta_1 X_1 + \beta_2 X_2.$$

This would ensure that all predicted counts are positive. Secondly, a different distribution for the variability of the observed response can be chosen. The key feature of this choice is how the variability in the observed responses might be expected to increase with its expected value. For example, in ordinary regression, no increase is expected while with a Poisson distribution the variance increases with the mean. Poisson regression is often used with count outcomes.

The other commonly used GLM is the logistic regression model suitable for analyzing binary outcomes. This model estimates odds ratios (ORs), a measure of effect that has both desirable and undesirable properties. Desirable is that it is the only measure of association between risk factor and binary outcome that is unaffected by over-sampling risk exposed or by over-sampling outcome cases (but not both at the same time). Thus the odds ratio estimate from a cohort study and a case–control study should be the same. Unfortunately, most readers and, worse still, many authors interpret the odds ratio as a risk ratio, which in psychiatry it approximates only rarely. For example, an odds ratio of 2 does not imply a doubling of the rate unless the outcome is very rare. If the rate in the unexposed group is 2%, then the rate in the risk group does indeed double to $(2 * 0.02/0.98)/(1 + (2 * 0.02/0.98)) = 4\%$. However, with an unexposed group rate of 20%, an OR = 2 implies a rate in the risk group not of 40% but of $(2 * 0.2/0.8)/(1 + (2 * 0.2/0.8)) = 33\%$, and with an unexposed group rate of 80%, then an OR = 2 implies a rate of $(2 * 0.8/0.2)/(1 + (2 * 0.8/0.2)) = 89\%$ in the risk group.

Regression and the more general GLM make adjustment for several covariates straightforward. It is therefore widely applied. However, it should not be considered as a cure-all and should always be accompanied by careful thinking through of the assumptions. A typical example is shown in Figure 15.2 for 167 children from a prospective study of autism (Lord *et al.*, 2006). Initial verbal IQ is associated with initial diagnosis using an observation-based assessment, the Autism Diagnostic Observation Schedule (ADOS; Lord *et al.*, 2000). Verbal IQ significantly relates to autism and autistic spectrum diagnosis but not to pervasive developmental disorder not-otherwise-specified (PDD-NOS) or non autistic spectrum (NS). We might wish to examine how diagnosis made at age 2 is associated with ADOS social-communication score at age 9, taking into account initial verbal IQ. We could do this by covariate adjustment for verbal IQ in an ANOVA where age 2 diagnosis was a between-subjects factor, or equivalently by including both diagnosis and verbal IQ as main effects in a regression. We would obtain the

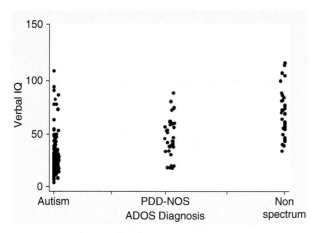

Figure 15.2 Distribution of baseline verbal IQ and diagnostic groups (PDD-NOS = autistic spectrum but not autism).

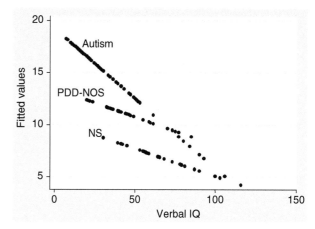

Figure 15.3 Relationship between baseline verbal IQ and follow-up ADOS score by initial diagnosis (NS = non autism spectrum; PDD-NOS = autistic spectrum but not autism).

answer that compared to those initially diagnosed with autism, the PDD-NOS (−2.52; 95% CI −4.69, −0.35) and NS (−4.59; 95% CI −7.20, −1.97) groups score lower on the ADOS at age 9, with each additional verbal IQ point associated with a 0.102 (95% CI 0.144, 0.062) lower ADOS score. But what have we assumed in this adjustment process? We focus here on the assumption of linearity, both within and between groups, which has allowed us to make an adjustment across the whole range of IQ in the sample. A cursory examination of Figure 15.2 shows that most children (71%!) with an initial diagnosis of autism have a verbal IQ below that of the child with the lowest verbal IQ in the NS group. Were we to control for verbal IQ by matching, a non parametric approach that does not assume linearity, these children with autism and low verbal IQ would find no match in the NS group and would be dropped from the analysis. We could restrict our covariance adjustment to the verbal IQ range shared by all three diagnostic groups. The resulting analysis of 78 (previously 167) children gives estimates of outcome differences of −0.92 (CI −4.09, 2.26) and −3.94 (CI −7.37, −0.50), for PDD-NOS and NS respectively, which are smaller and much less precise than the previous estimates. The covariance adjustment using the whole sample may be more powerful, but that power was gained at the expense of a more speculative assumption that the verbal IQ adjustment is correct even though in some areas of the scale the adjustment is being determined solely by children from one diagnostic group.

All these analyses have assumed that the way in which verbal IQ affects outcome is the same within each diagnostic group. Figure 15.3 shows the estimated relationship for each group, obtained from fitting a model that allowed an interaction term between diagnostic group and verbal IQ. Although this term was non significant ($F(2, 161) = 1.65\ p = 0.2$), the figure clearly shows non parallel lines. These imply that the difference in ADOS outcome score depends upon the child's initial verbal IQ, and that the answer obtained from "adjustment" for verbal IQ may represent some sort of average difference that could hide important variation. Unless designed in advance, for example,

by selecting subjects matched on verbal IQ, most studies do not have the power to test effectively for such variation. Unfortunately, designing a study to be powerful in this regard would make it clumsier to analyse for all but the designed contrasts. Moreover, the design would have increased power only with respect to the matched variables, and would exclude important sub-groups of children, in this case the majority of autistic children with low verbal IQs.

There remains the more general question as to what are relevant and suitable control variables. This is not a simple question. Understanding why autism and low verbal IQ are commonly associated, that is whether low verbal IQ increases false-positive autism diagnosis using current instruments, or actually increases risk of autism, or whether autism increases the risk of low verbal IQ, will be important for interpreting results and for deciding whether one should adjust at all.

Mechanisms and statistical interactions and effects scales

The term interaction has distinct substantive and statistical definitions. Since these usually relate to quite different concepts and each may be poorly defined in any particular instance, there is scope for much debate, mostly fruitless. The notion of synergy is often associated with interaction, where risk factors have worse effects when they occur together than when each occurs by itself. The concept may be of special importance within psychiatry where many of the features that are studied as being risk factors may in fact confer risk only in certain contexts. For example, we cannot say that childhood antisocial behavior is universally increased as a result of (1) divorce, since it may be beneficial if the absenting father is antisocial (Jaffee et al., 2003) or (2) high levels of testosterone, since while its association with leadership may confer risk in neighborhoods where deviant peers are common, elsewhere its role may be related to socially valued characteristics (Rowe et al., 2004).

Indeed, many behavioral responses may be adaptive or mal-adaptive depending upon the context. This makes resolving the confusion over interaction all the more pressing.

Where the response variable is continuous, relatively little confusion arises. Thus, as in Figure 15.3, slopes that characterize the relationship of one risk measure to an outcome score may be different in one group compared to another, and this slope variation can be tested for by a test of the interaction term. A group that has a particularly steep slope would be indicative of a form of synergy, though how it was described might also depend upon where the mean levels for the groups lay. More problematic is the circumstance where the outcome is a binary diagnosis or the occurrence of an event. Rothman (1976; Rothman & Greenland, 1986) describes how for causal factors that are relatively uncommon and where no synergism occurs, the combined effect of exposure to two risk factors should be additive. Where synergism occurs, for example, when one factor increases the risk of an individual being in a state of vulnerability, and exposure to the second risk factor increases the risk of occurrence of the final outcome of interest (a two-stage model—cf. Pickles, 1993), then the risk factors will appear to act multiplicatively.

For analyzing binary outcomes, the common models are the log-rate models of survival analysis and the logit model. The routinely applied logistic regression model has many desirable statistical properties, but few users appreciate that in most applications where the pathological outcome is not the majority, this model has closer correspondence to the multiplicative combination of effects (Pickles & De Stavola, 2007). Thus, it may not be appropriate for analyzing additive relationships. Additive main effects on these log-rate and logit scales imply multiplicative effects on the simple rate scale. For these models, the absence of an interaction can be consistent with synergy, and a significant (negative) interaction consistent with no synergy. Simply put, there is no correspondence between the need for a statistical interaction and synergy, since the former depends upon the scale in which the main effects have been combined (Blot & Day, 1979).

Our task should be to fit a parsimonious but adequately fitting model with easily understood and well-behaved parameters, which the logit model is, but then to support the interpretation, particularly the public health interpretation, by examining group-wise predicted outcome rates (see Pickles & De Stavola, 2007).

In treatment research, synergy is referred to as treatment effect moderation. To some extent, research into moderation has been slowed because in RCTs statisticians have regarded it with suspicion, as opening the door to sub-group analysis. Where no overall effect has been found, proponents of a therapy commonly attempt to salvage something by fishing for groups of patients for whom it did appear to work, and doing so with neither the necessary power nor corrections for multiple testing. The more recent enthusiasm for *stratified* or *personalized* medicine has required statisticians to be more sympathetic, for example,

suggesting ways for constructing indices of moderation from a collection of potential moderating variables (Kraemer *et al.*, 2002; Wallace *et al.*, 2013). For psychological therapies, some theoretically important variables, such as the alliance between therapist and patient, are thought to be important moderators of the effect of therapy. However, they represent a substantial statistical challenge as these occur after randomization. Sound methods for such variables are under development (Dunn & Bentall, 2007; Dunn *et al.*, 2013).

Longitudinal data analysis

Longitudinal data arise from repeated observations on one or more variables over time. The nature of this repeated measurement of data makes it expensive to collect both in terms of the number of measurements (at least two for each participant) and the cost of tracking participants over time. However, for addressing questions in development, longitudinal data provide the only real way to examine change over time. Unlike cross-sectional data, which allow only within-time correlations to be examined, longitudinal data enable the ordering of correlations over time to be assessed and thus come closer to addressing questions of causality.

One important issue when thinking about change over time relates to how "change" is measured. One approach is to calculate a simple difference score between time 1 (T1) and time 2 (T2). For example, if we want to look at change in language scores in males and females, we could compute a difference score for both groups separately and compare them. In psychology this is often called an *unconditional analysis*, and it compares the mean change in language scores. Another approach to the question of analyzing change over time is *conditional analysis* or *analysis of covariance (ANCOVA)*, in which T2 language scores are regressed on T1 scores and, typically, a dummy variable for group. This answers the slightly different question of whether, given the same initial language score, the groups have the same expected increase in language scores by T2. ANCOVA allows for regression toward the mean, a term that describes the tendency of the scores of initially high (low) scoring individuals to fall back (rise up) toward the mean of the whole sample. However, ANCOVA assumes that this tendency is shared equally by all groups in the analysis, but evidence is rarely presented to support this assumption. Where groups are formed by random assignment, as in an RCT, this assumption would be expected to hold and ANCOVA is generally recommended as it is more efficient than the change score approach. In other contexts, while the change score might be preferred, some comfort is usually obtained by doing both analyses.

These approaches relate to measuring change for groups, rather than individuals. For small groups and for individuals in particular, it is common for most change in recorded scores to be the result of different measurement errors at the two occasions, a topic to which we now turn.

Measurement error, latent variables and growth models

Psychiatry is one of the few areas of medicine that takes measurement error seriously. Nonetheless, intuitive understanding of its impact on analysis is rarely well developed. Many researchers are familiar with the idea that if a risk factor is measured with error, then in any bivariate regression type model where the measure is used to predict an outcome, the estimated coefficient will be "attenuated" that is, the coefficient magnitude will be lower than if the risk factor had been perfectly measured. It is assumed that this simple attenuation effect carries over to more general settings involving several predictors. In fact, in more practical settings where there are several possibly correlated exposures, with one or more measured with error, such errors can have far more pernicious effects. Measurement error can readily be dealt with in a structural equation modeling framework, which we illustrate with an extended example.

Structural equation modelling

The application of SEM techniques to sociological research questions (Simon, 1954; Blalock, 1964) began over 50 years ago. SEM is a type of multivariate data analysis which can include both observed and latent (unobserved) variables. What a structural equation model is doing, in essence, is dividing the pattern of a variance–covariance matrix among the relationships specified in the model. These relationships can be among the observed variables, among the latent variables and between observed and latent variables (see Figure 15.4 for SEM notation).

The most basic building block of a structural equation model is a regression equation where the error, "e," represents the disagreement between the data and the model, that is, data − model = error. The modelling approach involves both estimating parameters in the model, and assessing the model "goodness of fit," that is, how well the proposed model recreates the variance–covariance structure observed in the data.

Ability scores (percentage of items correct) were collected in 6-, 7-, 9- and 11-year-olds (see Table 15.1) to measure continuity in general ability (Osbourne & Suddick, 1972).

Table 15.1 Summary statistics for the repeated measures of childhood ability (Osbourne & Suddick, 1972).

Age at measurement (years)				
	6	**7**	**9**	**11**
Mean cognitive ability	18.03	25.82	35.26	46.59
Standard deviation	6.37	7.32	7.80	10.39
Correlation matrix		0.809	0.806	0.765
			0.850	0.831
				0.867

A plausible starting model is the first-order autoregressive model (Figure 15.5) where ability at one age, having taken into account ability at the previous measurements, is not associated with any earlier measure. In such a model, an early measure may influence a later measure but only through an intermediate measure. The model consists of three regressions (Y1 on Y2, Y2 on Y3 and Y3 on Y4). In addition to estimating standardized regression coefficients (0.809, 0.850 and 0.867, respectively), as one would do in standard regression modelling, we can assess the model's goodness-of-fit by comparing the observed and expected covariance matrix, from which we would conclude that the autoregressive model had a very poor fit (χ^2 statistic of 61.82 with 3 degrees of freedom[1]). Something is wrong, but what? For many researchers the instinct is to conclude that additional relationships must exist, for example, from Y1 to Y3 and Y2 to Y4. These additional relationships correspond to "sleeper effects," which have no effect on the immediately adjacent measure but yet can influence a subsequent one. There are circumstances where sleeper effects are plausible, for example, if items on a maths test for 7-, 8-, 9-, and 10-year-olds vary in content, with tests at two nonadjacent time points, that is, 7 and 9 years, more similar to one another than those at adjacent time points, that is 7 and 8 years.

---

[1] The degrees of freedom are found from the difference between the 10 observed summary statistics and the seven estimated parameters which are the variances for Y1, E2, E3 and E4 and the three regression coefficients b1, b2 and b3.

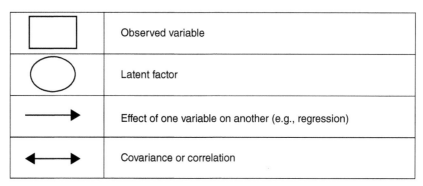

Figure 15.4 Notation for structural equation models.

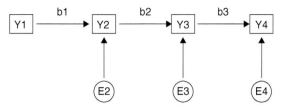

Figure 15.5 An autoregressive model for continuity. Y1–Y4 are observed variables, b1–b3 are regression coefficients, E2–E4 are the residual error terms.

However, before adding additional pathways we should first take the issue of measurement error seriously. In the classical measurement error model, the observed measurement is additively related to a "true variable" F and a measurement error E of constant variance:

$$Y = F + E.$$

We can construct another type of autoregressive model with paths between latent variables, which represent "true" scores, to which the observed measures are related by the addition of measurement error ("E" see Figure 15.6). In order for the model to be estimated, certain constraints, such as, that the measurement error variance remains the same over the four occasions, are required. Though more complex, after imposing these constraints the model involves only one more parameter than the previous model (three regression coefficients between the factors and variances for F1, D2, D3, D4 and the single common measurement error variance for the Es) and yet fits the ability data much better ($\chi^2 = 1.43$ with 2df). Clearly this model has no need of any additional sleeper effect, since it already fits so well. How has this come about? Variability consists of both measurement error and true score variance, of which only the latter can be expected to persist. Thus, in focussing on the apparent continuity in the total variation of a measure, the autoregressive model of Figure 15.5 underestimates the persistence of the true score, and thus the beta coefficients. This underestimation is even greater for temporally distant measures. The continuity

from Y1 to Y4 is given by the product of the standardized regression coefficients b1, b2 and b3 (a 10% underestimation in each coefficient resulting in a $1-0.9 * 0.9 * 0.9 = 27\%$ underestimation of the b1 * b2 * b3 product). Allowing for measurement error corrects each regression coefficient and in so doing removes the gross under-estimation of the model-predicted long-term association.

There are numerous implications from this modest example. The first is that, in general, although measurement error in a covariate X1 may result in systematic underestimation of its relationship with some response, it can also give rise to overestimation of the effects of some other covariate, X2, with which X1 is correlated. Consider the often-repeated finding that current health is not only associated with contemporaneous risk factors but also independently with the same risk factors earlier in childhood. Is this because the risk has its effect through an accumulation of risk exposure, or is it an artifact of measurement error in the contemporaneous or childhood measurements? This latter possibility is rarely properly explored.

A natural alternative model for longitudinal data is a growth curve model in which each child is considered as having a trajectory defined by an initial ability, represented by a latent intercept factor—or random effect—F1, and a latent rate of improvement, represented by a latent slope factor—or random coefficient—F2 (Figures 15.7 and 15.8). The intercept factor "loads," that is, regresses, on all four measurements with a common regression coefficient. The growth or slope factor typically loads on all but the first measurement, with either distinct factor loadings on each path or with constraints such that the loadings vary in proportion with the time since the initial measurement (equivalent to allowing for the linear effects of time to be random). In almost all growth situations, values at the initial starting point are correlated with subsequent growth (i.e. the double-headed arrow linking intercept and slope in Figure 15.7), requiring the two latent factors or random effects to be correlated. Again we can impose restrictions such that the

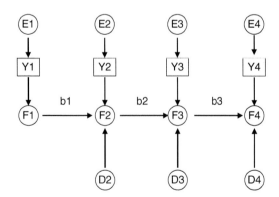

Figure 15.6 A latent variable continuity model. Y1–Y4 are observed variables and E1–E4 are the measurement error terms; F1–F4 are latent variables indicated by the observed variables and D1–D3 are the disturbances or factor residual error terms.

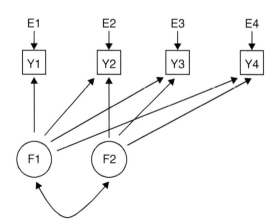

Figure 15.7 Growth curve model with intercept and slope factors or random effects. Y1–Y4 are the observed variables and E1–E4 are the associated error terms. F1 is a latent variable for the random intercept and F2 is the random slope factor.

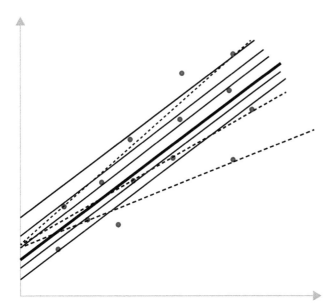

Figure 15.8 Regression line. Thick black line represents typical fixed effects regression line, the thin black lines represent spread of slopes implied by a random intercept factor (F1) and the dashed lines the spread of slopes implied by a random slope factor (F2).

measurement error variances (E1–E4) are constant. This model has one fewer parameter than the model of Figure 15.6 and yet fits these data better ($\chi^2 = 0.92$ with 3df).

Which of the two well-fitting models (Figures 15.6 and 15.7) should we choose? In this case, the choice is likely to rest upon theoretical considerations. The last model has the fewer parameters and in addition has the advantage of cleanly partitioning initial cross-sectional variation from subsequent change. This has appeal, especially were the model extended to allow for the effects of exposures to be associated with both the intercept and slope factors. Where continuous growth or decline are not expected, but instead change may be reversible, then random coefficients can be extended to a quadratic in time (or still higher order terms).

SEM with continuous and discrete variables and interactions: trajectory models

Much theory relates to groups or a categorical typology of individuals. A classic example is Moffitt's (1993) three anti-social behavior groups defined in terms of their longitudinal trajectory; life-course persistent, adolescent limited and never anti-social. Empirically defining these groups may be somewhat arbitrary, so a method that would identify them directly from the data with only general guidance from the researcher is desirable. These ideas may be operationalized within a trajectory model, a form of growth curve model in which the variation in the possible values of the intercept and growth coefficients are restricted to belong, in this case, to just 3 sets of values or "classes." Such a model can be considered as a form of latent class model or a model-based cluster analysis (Curran & Hussong, 2003). We can compare the relative fit of a model with 2 or

4, rather than 3 classes to assess how gross an approximation the restriction to just 3 classes might be. It should not, however, be considered as a tool to identify how many classes actually exist. Two things argue against this. Firstly, the number of classes found as providing the best fit according to some standard information criterion (e.g. Bayesian or Akaike information criteria) varies with the extent of the data available. Secondly, although one can continue to add more classes, both theory and practice (Laird, 1978) have shown that there quickly comes a point where no further improvement in fit occurs, and the additional new class either looks just like an existing class, or is assigned a probability of zero. This set of classes is referred to as the non parametric maximum likelihood (NPML) estimator of the latent growth distribution. Although the NPML estimator is formed of classes it can be shown that it fully characterizes the latent growth distribution even if that distribution is not one of classes but of continuous variability, as in a traditional growth curve model. In other words, even when the data are continuous, a latent class model with only a small number of classes is often a better fit than a model assuming the continuous variability of the "true" model. As a consequence, showing that a latent trajectory class model fits well is merely to say that we can approximate the latent growth distribution, whatever its true discrete or continuous form, by these classes and not that the classes actually exist. Nonetheless, these models allow for an effective summary of the data, helpful for theory building and constructing tests of clinical interest.

Figure 15.9 shows the classes identified from repeated observational assessments on a group of toddlers, showing the observed scores of the individuals assigned to each class, the mean trajectory of their class and how precisely estimated that trajectory is reflected in a confidence envelope. Such models can be estimated in programs such as the SAS procedure TRAJ, the SEM program Mplus (Muthén & Muthén, 2001) or the general Stata procedure gllamm (Rabe-Hesketh et al., 2000).

One of the major limitations of SEM path models is their inability to represent interactions involving latent variables. In fact, this is not a strict limitation, since multiple group methods (models that allow random coefficients, for example, gllamm, Rabe-Hesketh et al., 2003) and a number of other approaches enable such interactions to be considered (Schumacker & Marcoulides, 1998). Nonetheless, few substantive applications have pursued them.

Causal analysis

SEM is often referred to as causal modelling, but although it can provide a framework within which analysis specifically concerned with attempting to isolate evidence for causation can be undertaken, in practice this is rarely done. There is, however, a quite distinct collection of methods that specifically address causal interpretation. We consider two of these, propensity score weighting and instrumental variables.

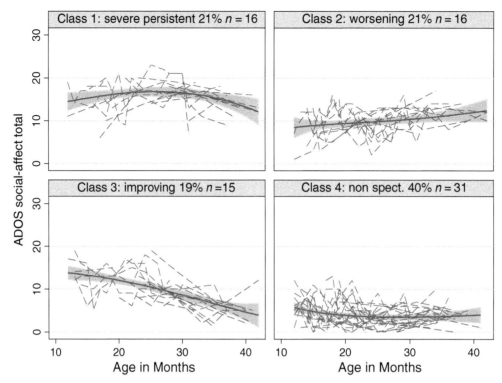

Figure 15.9 Trajectories of early development in ADOS scores (from Lord *et al.*, 2012); (non spect. = non autism spectrum; new algorithm = 2007 scoring of ADOS).

Propensity score approach

Consider the case where, in the population, the effect of X (e.g., smoking) on the outcome Y (e.g., lung cancer) may be confounded only by measured confounders denoted by Z (e.g., socioeconomic status). The propensity score approach allows estimation of the causal effect of X in this circumstance (Rosenbaum & Rubin, 1983). For a binary exposure of interest X, the propensity score for a subject is the conditional probability of exposure given the vector of observed confounders Z. Such a propensity score is usually estimated by logistic regression, with X treated as the response variable and the confounders Z as the predictors. The point estimate of the effect of X from an analysis that also includes the propensity score gives unbiased estimates of the exposure effect under a wider range of conditions than an analysis that covaries for all the variables in Z. For example, if these have greater variability or different patterns of correlation in one exposure group than another, as in Figure 15.3, then direct covariate adjustment would increase the bias or even overcorrect.

An alternative way of using the propensity score idea, proposed by Robins and Rotnitsky (1995), is to weight individuals by the inverse of the probability of experiencing the exposure that they did, that is, 1/propensity score for those that were exposed and 1/(1 − propensity score) for those that were not. In this weighted sample, the exposure of interest is no longer correlated with the possible confounders Z and near standard analysis of such a weighted sample, a so-called marginal structural model (MSM), gives estimates of the effect of X unconfounded with effects of Z.

The analysis thus consists of fitting the usual models for the effects of X on Y, for example, linear or logistic regression, but with subjects' weights $\{w_i\}$. Though a subject may be assigned a weight of two, they nonetheless still possess the variability of response typical of a single individual. Standard errors, and thus p values and confidence intervals, are calculated using the sandwich or robust estimator (Huber, 1967; Binder, 1983) or some other technique (such as bootstrap) that recognizes this.

In a longitudinal study we will commonly be concerned with a time dependent exposure, X_0, X_1, ... , X_k, where we might wish to estimate the effect of a cumulative exposure. With exposures confounded with Z_0, Z_1, ... , Z_k, we can again use weights for the probability of exposure, but now the weight's denominator is the conditional probability that a subject experienced their particular exposure history.

In the single period case, the practical advantage of the MSM approach over more routine covariate adjustment is not obvious. However in the multi-period time-dependent case, the advantage of the MSM approach is clearer. Both approaches attempt adjustment for Z_k, where Z_k is a confounder for later exposure. However, adopting the simpler covariate adjustment approach erroneously controls for the effect that earlier values of the exposure have on Z_k, that is, the value of the confounder during period k. Thus, it would also wrongly partial out causal effects that should be attributed to the exposure. An example is the study of the effect of antiretroviral therapy (the exposure) and CD4 counts (the confounder) on the risk of acquired immunodeficiency syndrome (Cole *et al.*, 2003). In this study, controlling for CD4 leads to the incorrect conclusion that antiretroviral therapy does not work. We have yet to see such methods much used in child psychiatry.

Instrumental variables

The propensity score approach described requires full information on all the confounders of the causal effect of the exposure of interest because these are needed to define the propensity score or the inverse probability weights. But almost always there are numerous possible confounders that we simply have not measured. How then do we proceed?

One way to deal with unmeasured confounding involves having data on a variable R that precedes and is related to exposure but is not directly related to the outcome or the unmeasured confounders (Figure 15.10). A variable with these properties, if it exists, is said to be an "instrument" for the unbiased estimate of the causal effect of the exposure. If all relations are linear, then the instrumental variable estimate of the causal effect is the ratio of the coefficient in the regression of Y on R, and the coefficient in the regression of X on R. With adjustment for measured confounders and multiple instruments the estimation is more complex, though programs are commonly available.

The main problem with this method is that it is rare to identify good instruments. Most examples exploit the occurrence of "natural experiments" (see Chapter 12). Examples include using the Vietnam draft lottery number to examine the effects of traumatic event exposure (Hearst *et al.*, 1986) and geographical variation in treatment provision to assess treatment impact on autism (Lord *et al.*, 2006). More recent novel applications include an example of Mendelian randomization. In this approach, (presumed) functional genes are used as instruments for phenotypes thought to cause certain diseases (Davey-Smith & Ebrahim, 2005).

Of course the most obvious source of an instrument is from deliberate randomization within an actual experiment. In this context, the approach is becoming increasingly popular. The standard intention-to-treat estimator estimates the average effect of the treatment for everyone who was assigned for treatment, ignoring whether anyone actually took any of the treatment to which they were assigned or not. This declines in interest as the proportion of non compliers with treatment increases, and we may want to know what the treatment effect would be on those who would take it if offered. Provided that the effect of being randomized to treatment was to increase exposure to the treatment of interest (and that certain other

assumptions are met; cf. Dunn *et al.*, 2005), then an unbiased effect for this subgroup is estimable using instrumental variable methods; whereas the naïve estimates, such as the so-called the per-protocol effect estimate is biased.

Mediation

A mediation analysis attempts to decompose a causal effect into components that occur along particular causal pathways. It thus falls squarely within the literature of the previous sections, as a topic that has received special attention. Recent work in statistics has attempted to place the more informal early work (Judd & Kenny, 1981; Baron & Kenny, 1986) onto the more formal footing of counter-factual theory, and has attempted to address two problems of mediation research. The problem is that though, in an RCT, the effect of treatment on mediator can be validly estimated, our estimates of the effect of mediator on outcome remain potentially biased due to both confounders and measurement error in the mediator (Dunn & Bentall, 2007; Dunn *et al.*, 2013).

Missing data

Missing data are a common problem and can arise for a variety of reasons ranging from missing questionnaire items to attrition from the study. There are three categories of missing data (Little & Rubin, 1987, 1989): missing completely at random (MCAR), missing at random (MAR) and non ignorable missing. When missing data are completely random, the "missingness" does not depend on the values of either observed or latent variables, and analysis of complete data cases only does not lead to bias. This is the strategy adopted by the majority of research in psychology using list-wise deletion. However, in reality, missing data are rarely unrelated to observed and latent variables, and so this approach is typically biased. MAR assumes that missingness is related to observed, but not latent variables or missing values. For example, if sex influences missingness on a language test, but within males and females separately language ability itself does not relate to the missingness of language test data, then for a model including sex the missing data are MAR, whereas for a model that ignores sex they are not. Though the assumptions of MAR are weaker than MCAR and are more likely to hold in reality, it is not actually possible to test for MAR because the missing data scores are unknown. When missingness is dependent on both observed and unobserved values, missing data are non ignorable, for example, where those with higher depression have more missing data because they were less likely to come in for the study. Such missingness requires more specialist and speculative methods and is probably better thought of as part of a sensitivity analysis testing the robustness of findings (White *et al.*, 2011).

An increasingly popular approach for tackling missing data is multiple imputation (MI; Schafer, 1999). Several datasets that have the same observed data have missing data filled in with values that differ between datasets, the variability depending upon the uncertainty of the missing values. Each dataset is

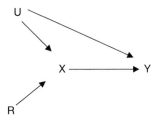

Figure 15.10 Confounding of the causal relationship of X to Y by U and the instrumental variable R.

analyzed and the results pooled using simple formulae (Rubin, 1987) which uses the variability in results from dataset to dataset as the source of the information on how the missing data contributes to uncertainty. In trials, MI for missing baseline data is now common and while the trial outcome data should be included in the imputation step, the general recommendation is that the imputed outcome data be dropped and instead this be accounted for through the usual MAR assumptions of standard maximum likelihood analysis. This is an example of the now common practice of using several different approaches for dealing with different aspects of missing data.

Although MI methods are increasingly common and easy to undertake, mistakes are easy to make, for example, examining sex differences when the imputation model assumed relationships between variables were the same for males and females. Since the MI step is rarely fully described, such mistakes are hard to detect.

Screening, diagnosis and misclassification

As with continuous measures, measurement errors in the form of misclassification of categorical variables can have pernicious effects that lead to widespread misunderstanding. For example, when measuring a category, say present or absent, observers may agree with each other even when simply guessing. Where raters score a category as present just 1% of the time, then the percentage agreement is expected to be 98% even when they score blind to all information. Thus we prefer to use the so-called "chance-corrected" measures of agreement (Dunn, 2000) such as kappa statistics that give credit only for agreement in excess of that obtainable by blind guessing. Where we know the true status then we can also calculate the proportion of true positives that are correctly rated (sensitivity), the proportion of true negatives that are correctly rated (specificity), the positive predictive value (PPV) and the negative predictive power (NPV) and likelihood ratio (LR). Which of the various measures one wants to optimize depends on the purpose of the measure and its context of use.

As part of the impact of "big data" there have been a plethora of claims of high diagnostic validity for an array of biological measures. The multiple testing problem is severe; analysts will inevitably find some features among the hundreds of thousands available, that will by chance discriminate among, say, the 50 children with ADHD and the 50 with depression. While we have developed clever methods to remove bias in estimated classification success, such as leave-one-out cross-validation, these are commonly applied only to the last stages of the study. It is not unusual to start with 50 brain or genetic features suggested by the literature as possible discriminators and then analyse with sound cross-validation methods the available samples, but fail to point out that these same samples had also been used in the preliminary selection of the 50 features. It is also commonplace to report in the context of groups that are 50 : 50 case and non case but then fail to highlight that a seemingly small false-positive rate can make a test useless if the disorder is rare within the population in which the test is to be applied.

Reporting results

Although statistical modelling may be increasingly used as the principal analysis tool, authors should nonetheless be expected to present tables and figures that display the essential features of the raw data. For the reporting of results from trials, guidelines exist (e.g., www.consort-statement.org), while for epidemiologic studies such guidelines are developing (e.g., www.strobe-statement.org). Estimates of effects should be reported in both standard form and in other ways that help interpretation. For example, treatment effects are often reported in terms of both reductions in risk and the number needed to treat in order to cure or avoid one case/death (equal to one over the absolute risk reduction).

In observational studies, where causal interpretation is felt justified, quantities like population attributable fraction (the fraction of cases that could be avoided if the risk exposure could be eliminated) can be helpful. More generally, comparing and describing results based on continuous variables and discrete/group-based analysis is to be encouraged, since these two approaches offer quite different insights and strengths and weaknesses (Pickles & Angold, 2003). As far as possible, results should present both the evidence for and against the principal conclusions. In this respect, we have mentioned how estimates and confidence intervals are preferred to significance levels alone.

A growing problem for the quality of reporting of results is the demand for "hype," whether from the increasing ubiquitous institutional press office, the demand of funders for "impact" or even the competition among editors for a higher journal impact factor. These are corrupting influences, requiring us to be astute and alert for misrepresentation of one's own reports and those of others.

Conclusions

This chapter has highlighted just some of the careful considerations required in undertaking, interpreting and reporting data analysis. The chapter does not provide an exhaustive overview of statistical methods and there are many useful and important tools that we have omitted. The principal message is that statistical science is not a set of recipes, nor a set of hurdles that must be jumped to get to publication, but a set of concepts and principles whose application delivers better science and helps protect us from the fraudulent claims of those with vested interests or merely the well meaning but misguided. Our introduction also contrasted differences between experimental and observational studies, highlighting the different cultures. Those who have undertaken an RCT, especially one with an experienced specialist clinical trials unit, will attest to the unrelenting pre-specification required for all aspects and contingencies of the study. Increasingly, those doing observational studies are rightly being urged to adopt as much as possible of this pre-specified attention to detail so as to avoid often unintended but cumulative biases that have undermined the field. Similarly, more is being demanded of experimentalists, pressing them to answer questions for which randomization alone is not the cure-all (e.g., mediation analysis). As both trends occur, the two cultures are being brought together, hopefully each achieving a more mature understanding as well as greater convergence in findings.

References

Baron, R.M. & Kenny, D.A. (1986) The moderator-mediator variable distinction in social psychological research: conceptual, strategic, and statistical considerations. *Journal of Personality and Social Psychology* **51**, 1173–1182.

Benjamini, Y. & Hochberg, Y. (1995) Controlling the false discovery rate: a practical and powerful approach to multiple testing. *Journal of the Royal Statistical Society B* **57**, 289–300.

Binder, D.A. (1983) On the variance of asymptotically normal estimators from complex surveys. *International Statistical Review* **51**, 279–292.

Blalock, H.M. (1964) *Causal Inferences in Nonexperimental Research.* University of North Carolina, Chapel Hill, NC.

Blot, W.J. & Day, N.E. (1979) Synergism & interaction: are they equivalent. *American Journal of Epidemiology* **110**, 99–100.

Cole, S.R. *et al.* (2003) Effect of highly active antiretroviral therapy on time to acquired immunodeficiency syndrome or death using marginal structural models. *American Journal of Epidemiology* **158**, 687–694.

Cooper, H. *et al.* (2009) *The Handbook of Research Synthesis and Meta-Analysis,* 2nd edn. Russell Sage Foundation, New York.

Curran, P.J. & Hussong, A.M. (2003) The use of latent trajectory models in psychopathology research. *Journal of Abnormal Psychology* **112**, 526–544.

Davey-Smith, G.D. & Ebrahim, S. (2005) What can mendelian randomisation tell us about modifiable behavioural and environmental exposures? *British Medical Journal* **330**, 1076–1079.

Dunn, G. (2000) *Statistics in Psychiatry.* Arnold, London.

Dunn, G. & Bentall, R. (2007) Modelling treatment-effect heterogeneity in randomized controlled trials of complex interventions (psychological treatments). *Statistics in Medicine* **26**, 4719–4745.

Dunn, G. *et al.* (2005) Estimating treatment effects from randomised clinical trials with non-compliance and loss to follow-up: the role of instrumental variables. *Statistical Methods in Medical Research* **14**, 369–395.

Dunn, G. *et al.* (2013) Integrating biomarker information within trials to evaluate treatment mechanisms and efficacy for personalised medicine. *Clinical Trials* **10**, 709–719.

Hearst, N. *et al.* (1986) Delayed effects of military draft on mortality. A randomised natural experiment. *New England Journal of Medicine* **314**, 620–624.

Hernán, M.A. *et al.* (2008) Observational studies analyzed like randomized experiments: an application to postmenopausal hormone therapy and coronary heart disease. *Epidemiology* **19**, 766–779.

Huber, P. (1967) The behaviour of maximum likelihood estimates under non-standard conditions. In: *Proceedings of the Fifth Berkely Symposium on Mathematical Statistics and Probability* **1**, 221–233. University of California Press, Berkeley.

Hulley, S. *et al.* (1998) Randomized trial of estrogen plus progestin for secondary prevention of coronary heart disease in post-menopausal women. Heart and Estrogen/progestin Replacement Study (HERS) Research Group. *JAMA* **280**, 605–613.

Jaffee, S.R. *et al.* (2003) Life with (or without) father: the benefits of living with two biological parents depend on the father's antisocial behavior. *Child Development* **74**, 109–126.

Judd, C.M. & Kenny, D.A. (1981) Process analysis – estimating mediation in treatment evaluations. *Evaluation Review* **5**, 602–619.

Kraemer, H.C. *et al.* (2002) Mediators and moderators of treatment effects in randomized clinical trials. *Archives of General Psychiatry* **59**, 877–883.

Laird, N.M. (1978) Nonparametric maximum likelihood estimation of a mixing distribution. *Journal of the American Statistical Association* **73**, 805–811.

Lawlor, D.A. *et al.* (2004) Socioeconomic position and hormone replacement therapy use: explaining the discrepancy in evidence from observational and randomised controlled trials? *American Journal of Public Health* **94**, 2149–2154.

Light, R.J. & Pillemer, D.B. (1984) *Summing Up. The Science of Reviewing Research.* Harvard University Press, Cambridge, MA.

Little, R.J.A. & Rubin, D.B. (1987) *Statistical Analysis with Missing Data.* John Wiley & Sons, New York.

Little, R.J.A. & Rubin, D.B. (1989) The analysis of social science data with missing values. *Sociological Methods and Research* **18**, 292–326.

Lord, C. *et al.* (2000) The autism diagnostic observation schedule-generic: a standard measure of social and communication deficits associated with the spectrum of autism. *Journal of Autism and Developmental Disorders* **30**, 205–223.

Lord, C. *et al.* (2006) Autism from two to nine. *Archives of General Psychiatry* **63**, 694–701.

Lord, C. *et al.* (2012) Patterns of developmental trajectories in toddlers with autism spectrum disorder. *Journal of Clinical and Consulting Psychology* **80**, 477–489.

McCullagh, P. & Nelder, J.A. (1989) *Generalized Linear Models,* 2nd edn. Chapman and Hall, London.

Moffitt, T.E. (1993) Adolescence-limited and life-course persistent antisocial behavior: a developmental taxonomy. *Psychological Review* **100**, 674–701.

Muthén, L.K. & Muthén, B.O. (2001) *Mplus Users Guide.* Muthen & Muthen, Los Angeles, CA.

Osbourne, R.T. & Suddick, D.E. (1972) A longitudinal investigation of the intellectual differentiation hypothesis. *Journal of Genetic Psychology* **110**, 83–89.

Petitti, D. *et al.* (1986) Postmenopausal estrogen use and heart disease. *New England Journal of Medicine* **315**, 131–132.

Pickles, A. (1993) Stages, precursors and causes in development. In: *Precursors and Causes in Development and Psychopathology.* (eds D.F. Hay & A. Angold), pp. 23–49. John Wiley & Sons, Chichester.

Pickles, A. & Angold, A. (2003) Natural categories or fundamental dimensions: on carving nature at the joints and the re-articulation of psychopathology. *Development and Psychopathology* **15**, 529–551.

Pickles, A. & De Stavola, B. (2007) An overview of models and methods for life course analysis. In: *Methods in Life Course Epidemiology.* (eds A. Pickles, *et al.*), pp. 181–120. Oxford University Press, Oxford.

Rabe-Hesketh, S. *et al.* (2000) Generalised, linear, latent and mixed models. *Stata Technical Bulletin* **53**, 47–57.

Rabe-Hesketh, S. *et al.* (2003) Correcting for measurement error in logistic regression using non-parametric maximum likelihood estimation. *Statistical Modelling* **3**, 215–232.

Robins, J.M. & Rotnitsky, A. (1995) Semiparametric efficiency in multivariate regression models with missing data. *Journal of the American Statistical Association* **90**, 122–129.

Rosenbaum, P.R. & Rubin, D.B. (1983) The central role of the propensity score in observational studies for causal effects. *Biometrika* **70**, 41–55.

Rothman, K.J. (1976) Causes. *American Journal of Epidemiology* **104**, 587–592.

Rothman, K.J. & Greenland, S. (1986) *Modern Epidemiology.* Lippincott-Raven, Philadelphia, PA.

Rowe, R. *et al.* (2004) Testosterone, antisocial behavior, and social dominance in boys: pubertal development and biosocial interaction. *Biological Psychiatry* **5**, 546–552.

Rubin, D.B. (1987) *Multiple Imputation for Nonresponse in Surveys.* John Wiley & Sons, New York.

Schafer, J.L. (1999) Multiple imputation: a primer. *Statistical Methods in Medical Research* **8**, 3–16.

Schulz, K.F. *et al.* (1995) Empirical evidence of bias. Dimensions of methodological quality associated with estimates of treatment effects in controlled trials. *JAMA* **273**, 408–412.

Schumacker, R.E. & Marcoulides, G.A. (1998) *Interaction and Nonlinear Effects in Structural Equation Modeling.* Lawrence Erlbaum Associates Publishers, Mahwah, NJ, US.

Simon, H.A. (1954) Spurious correlation: a causal interpretation. *Journal of the American Statistical Association* **49**, 922–932.

Tang, J.-L. *et al.* (1999) Review of randomized controlled trials of traditional Chinese medicine. *British Medical Journal* **319**, 160–161.

Wallace, M.L. *et al.* (2013) A novel approach for developing and interpreting treatment moderator profiles in randomized clinical trials. *JAMA* **70**, 1241–1247.

White, I.R. *et al.* (2011) Strategy for intention to treat analyses in randomised trials with missing outcome data. *British Medical Journal* **342**, 1–4.

CHAPTER 16

Global psychiatry

Atif Rahman[1] and Christian Kieling[2]

[1] Institute of Psychology, Health and Society, University of Liverpool, UK
[2] Department of Psychiatry, School of Medicine, Universidade Federal do Rio Grande do Sul, Porto Alegre, Brazil

Introduction

Health and disease are universals. The field of child and adolescent psychiatry has undergone significant developments over the last decades, but this progress has not been uniform in all areas of the globe. The growing interconnectedness among nations, and the fact that nine out of ten individuals under the age of 18 years live in low and middle income countries (LMIC), has led to an increased attention to the global aspects of child and adolescent mental health in recent years.

The contemporary concept of global health—the study and practice of improving health and health equity worldwide through international and interdisciplinary collaboration—derives from the fields of public health and international health, which in turn have their origins in tropical medicine (Koplan *et al.*, 2009). Global health can also be understood as health issues that transcend national borders and which may be better addressed from cooperative action (Institute of Medicine, 1997). Other definitions propose that the field: (1) refers to any health issue that affects many countries and is affected by transnational determinants, (2) is more concerned with the scope than with the geography of problems, (3) encompasses the complex inter-actions between societies, (4) uses the resources, knowledge and experiences of different societies to deal with health challenges around the globe, and (5) includes basic sciences, prevention, treatment and rehabilitation (Koplan *et al.*, 2009).

In a way, contemporary conceptualizations of global health are not very distinct from the initial goals established for the World Health Organization (WHO): "the attainment by all peoples of the highest possible level of health." Over the years, however, the global scenario has changed from the reality of 1948, when the WHO was created; there is now a growing interdependence among states, societies and economies, which brings both increases to the number of threats common to several countries and new opportunities for collaboration between nations (Skotheim *et al.*, 2011). The concept of international health, for example, was already used in the late 19th and early 20th centuries, when referring especially to a focus on epidemic control at the borders between nations. The term global health, in turn, implies consideration for the health of all people on the planet, above concerns specific to countries and national boundaries. Both concepts, of course, are not mutually exclusive, sharing many points of overlap (Brown *et al.*, 2006).

Historical context of global health

The boom in international travel, the economic globalization, and the occurrence of pandemics such as the 2009 Influenza A outbreak have magnified awareness of global health issues. Historically, the Age of Exploration, which started early in the 15th century and continued through the 17th century, is regarded as a turning point in global health. In sailing West to reach the Indies by crossing the Atlantic, the Europeans landed on the "new world" and brought on not only the advancement of cultural exchange, but the unification of the microbial world: their arrival in the Americas was accompanied, for example, by the appearance of measles, smallpox, and yellow fever on the continent. It was only in the 19th century, however, that advances in knowledge about the causes of these diseases and the development of effective therapies, along with the recognition of the fundamental rights of all human beings, led to concrete efforts to fight such problems in the international arena (Berlinguer, 1999).

Until recently, the field of global health remained focused on communicable diseases, such as measles, polio, diarrheal diseases, and most significantly HIV infections. The focus on neglected tropical diseases (such as tuberculosis and malaria) strongly dominated the field of global health in the second half of the 20th century. With the increase in life expectancy—especially in the last century, when there was more than half of the gain in number of years lived in the last

Rutter's Child and Adolescent Psychiatry, Sixth Edition.
Edited by Anita Thapar and Daniel S. Pine, James F. Leckman, Stephen Scott, Margaret J. Snowling, Eric Taylor.
© 2015 John Wiley & Sons Ltd. Published 2018 by John Wiley & Sons Ltd.

five millennia—developing nations underwent a demographic transition that led to the so-called "double burden" of disease: the persistence of communicable diseases was accompanied by an increase in chronic conditions.

Mental health in the context of global health

The growing impact of chronic noncommunicable diseases (CNCD) has put this group of diseases in the current focus of attention in the global health discussion (Nugent & Jamison, 2011). CNCD, which include cardiovascular disease, cancer, and diabetes mellitus, are the largest cause of death in the world, being responsible for 63% of deaths worldwide, 80% of them in LMIC. Recognition that schizophrenia, depression, epilepsy, dementia, alcohol dependence, and other mental, neurological, and substance-use (MNS) disorders constitute a large proportion of the global burden of disease has drawn attention to the particular impact of mental health problems on the emerging field of global health.

Global mental health has been defined as the application of the principles of global health to the field of mental health (Patel & Prince, 2010). The neglect of mental health problems at different levels of health care in various countries, both rich and poor, led Arthur Kleinman to describe efforts in global mental health as a "failure of humanity" (Kleinman, 2009). Statistics are now available that show how the impact of mental disorders contrasts with the limited access to care and evidence-based treatments, particularly in resource-poor settings.

It is estimated that 30 million people will try and 1.5 million die from suicide annually by 2020. Even not being among the main direct causes of mortality, MNS already accounted for 12.3% of the global disease burden in 2000, and that proportion is expected to increase to 16.4% in 2030 (Collins et al., 2011). These figures possibly reflect an underestimation of the real impact of mental health problems. Mental disorders increase the risk for communicable and noncommunicable diseases and contribute to intentional and accidental injury (O'Connor et al., 2000). Conversely, many diseases increase the risk for the occurrence and perpetuation of mental disorders, and the presence of comorbidities is also a factor that hinders the search for help, diagnosis and treatment of different diseases (Ickovics et al., 2001). There is no doubt, therefore, that there is no health without mental health (Prince et al., 2007).

Child mental health in the context of global mental health

Initially focused on the so-called common and severe mental disorders, the study of global mental health more recently has also adopted a developmental perspective, prioritizing the care of children and adolescents. The study of mental health of children and adolescents is a relatively new field. The substantial growth that this area has shown, however, has not occurred uniformly across the globe. There has been significant progress in the description of syndromes and disorders, today nosologically better defined; in the early identification of individuals at risk

for developing mental disorders; in the elaboration of preventive and therapeutic evidence-based interventions; and in the implementation of health services that provide such knowledge in various social and cultural contexts. Such advances, however, are not available to the vast majority of the 2.2 billion children and adolescents in the world, particularly in LMIC.

Individuals under the age of 18 years represent almost a third of the entire world's population—and 90% of them live in LMIC, where they constitute up to half of the population in some cases. To a large extent, the enormous burden imposed by mental disorders is attributable to their early incidence in life and to their persistence into adulthood and old age. Prospective data collected from childhood and retrospective studies in adulthood converge to demonstrate that a significant proportion of psychiatric diagnoses among adults have their roots early in life. Additionally, among the major causes of health-related burden for youth aged 10–24 years, three are specific psychiatric diagnoses and the other two are linked to mental health problems: unipolar depressive disorders accounts for 8.2% of all disability-adjusted life years (DALYs) in this age group; road traffic accidents, 5.4%; schizophrenia, 4.1%; bipolar disorder, 3.8%; violence, 3.5% (Gore et al., 2011). Figure 16.1 presents the burden of mental and behavioral disorders according to the 2010 Global Burden of Disease Study (Murray et al., 2012).

The economic case for early investments in global child mental health

It is evident that global child and adolescent mental health is at the center of global mental health—and, subsequently, essential to achieve global health in general. Advances from developmental science indicate that the first years of life represent a window of opportunity to prevent the onset and chronicity of mental health problems. Interventions early in life represent opportunities for long-term health and socioeconomic benefits by reducing the incidence of mental health problems and decreasing their persistence as chronic disorders. This is in accordance with the economic arguments for early investments in the promotion of human capital. The model developed by Heckman and Krueger (2003) proposes that assuming the same investment is made at different points in time over the lifecycle, interventions made in the womb have a higher rate of return than those conducted at later ages: the returns to earlier investments can be reaped over longer time periods, and as capabilities (cognition, physical, and mental health) exhibit both self- and cross-productivity, an early investment has multiple positive effects (Angelucci & DiMaro, 2010). In the absence of longitudinal studies, it is difficult to substantiate the model with hard evidence. One systematic review of 42 effectiveness trials and program assessments of early preventive interventions (e.g., parenting support and education, preprimary or preschool centers, educational media for children), demonstrated that early child development can be improved through these interventions with effects greater for programs of higher quality and for the most vulnerable children, and

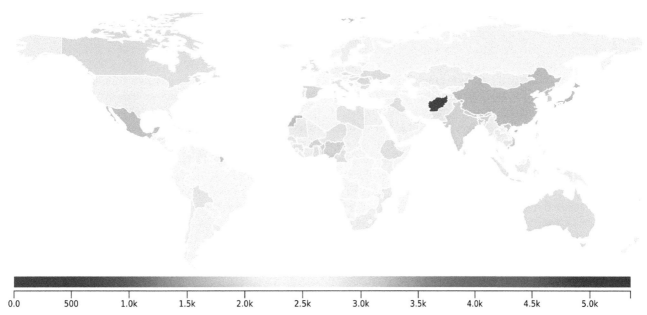

Figure 16.1 The burden of mental and behavioral disorders affecting individuals aged 10–14 years in 2010 (in DALYs/100,000 individuals). *Source:* Extracted from http://viz.healthmetricsandevaluation.org/gbd-compare. Institute for Health Metrics and Evaluation (IHME). GBD Compare Seattle, WA: IHME, University of Washington, 2013. Available from http://vizhub.healthdata.org/gbd-compare/#. Accessed November 26, 2014.

that effective investments in early child development have the potential to reduce inequalities perpetuated by poverty, poor nutrition, and restricted learning opportunities (Engle, 2011). To demonstrate the economic effect of early child development interventions, the authors developed a simulation for one program that focussed on preschool enrollment of children to enhance early cognitive development. This showed a benefit of $10.6 billion for increasing preschool enrollment to 25% in all countries, and $33.7 billion for increasing to 50%, with a benefit-to-cost ratio as large as 17.6–1.

Context heterogeneity

The variety of contexts in which the 2.2 billion children and adolescents in the world live has an impact on their mental health (Kieling *et al.*, 2011). Unfortunately, limited research has been dedicated to systematically study the characteristics of the environment across different countries. For instance, there is a gap in the literature in terms of how cultural heterogeneity affects attitudes towards children. In the absence of operational criteria to classify countries according to multiple environmental factors, the use of economic standards has prevailed in most of the international comparative research.

The most frequently used criterion is the World Bank's classification of economies, a measure that is based on their gross national income (GNI) per capita. The reasons for choosing this index to classify countries include a relative stable correlation with measures of general well-being, such as poverty and infant mortality, and arguments that it would constitute the "best single indicator of economic capacity and progress" (World

Bank, 2013a, b). According to their GNI per capita, economies are classified as low income, middle income (subdivided into lower middle and upper middle), or high income. The GNI of all economies are converted to US dollars using the so-called Atlas conversion factor (to reduce the impact of exchange rate fluctuations in the cross-country comparison). In 2011, the values for each group were the following: low income, $1025 or less; lower middle income, $1026–$4035; upper middle income, $4036–$12,475; and high income, $12,476 or more (World Bank, 2013a, b).

However, owing to the heterogeneity within populations, the GNI per capita method loses precision in nations with larger population sizes, such as China or India, with populations over 1 billion individuals. Moreover, from a global perspective, immediately after these two countries crossed the threshold to the middle-income category a few years ago, the majority of individuals in the world living in poverty (less than $1.25 per day) were classed as living in middle-income countries. An alternative criterion to classify countries according to their development level is the human development index (HDI), a measure based on three indicators: life expectancy at birth; educational level (measured as a combination of the literacy rate and primary, secondary, and tertiary education level enrollment rates); and per capita gross national product (UNDP, 2013). This illustrates the complexity of synthesizing evidence from within LMIC and extrapolating evidence from high income countries (HIC) to LMIC.

Although evidence from both HIC and LMIC converges to associate poverty with emotional, behavioral and developmental problems, other environmental factors have also been identified to negatively affect the mental health of children and adolescents. Knowledge about such factors can be valuable when policy and services are being planned in low resource areas.

Poverty

Research funded by UNICEF (Gordon *et al.*, 2003) to investigate childhood poverty in 46 countries in the developing world showed that over 1 billion children suffer from severe deprivation of basic human needs and over a third lived in absolute poverty. The association between childhood poverty and adverse physical, cognitive, educational, social, and emotional outcomes has been extensively studied, mostly in HIC (Yeung *et al.*, 2002; Engle & Black, 2010). Poverty influences children's developmental outcomes through various pathways. Poor children are more likely to grow up in less stimulating environments, to experience increased psychological distress related to monetary difficulties and to suffer from harsh parenting practices. These negative effects have been found in LMIC, where prevalence rates of poverty are much higher. Fleitlich & Goodman (2001) carried out a cross sectional survey of school children between the ages of 7–14 years in three contrasting neighborhoods in a Brazilian district, a shanty town, a stable urban neighborhood and a rural village and found significant associations of child mental health problems with poverty as well as with maternal mental illness and witnessing family violence.

The project Young Lives is an international collaborative research project about child poverty, involving a large cohort of children from four developing countries, Peru, Vietnam, Ethiopia, and India (Dercon & Krishnan, 2009). Within a cohort of over 4000 12-year-olds, they found that measures of self-efficacy, sense of inclusion, self-esteem, and educational aspirations all correlate with measures of material well-being of the family in which the children were growing up, suggesting a link between economic circumstances and broader dimensions of childhood well-being.

Economic disparity and social inequality between groups living in the same country can be risk factors in their own right (Walker *et al.*, 2011), especially in the context of early child development. The impact of relative poverty and associated psychosocial adversity on child mental health is discussed in Chapter 26.

Malnutrition

Recent success in reducing childhood mortality rates in developing countries has left hundreds of millions of children living in poor conditions with neurodevelopmental delays that receive minimal attention (Susser, 2012). In LMIC, almost a third of all children under the age of 5 are reported to suffer from clinically relevant undernutrition, defined as height-for-age below −2 SD of reference values (UNICEF, 2006). Malnutrition has a clear impact on children's development, including motor, language, and cognitive abilities (Grantham-McGregor, 2007). Controlling for socioeconomic covariates, prospective cohort studies consistently show significant associations between stunting by age 2 or 3 years and later cognitive deficits, school achievement, and dropout (Walker *et al.*, 2007).

Intellectual disability

LMIC have higher rates of intellectual disability (Institute of Medicine, 2001). A recent meta-analysis of 52 population studies published between 1980 and 2009 found a prevalence of intellectual disability of 10.3/1000, with the highest rates in low income countries, where the prevalence/1000 population was 16.41 (Maulik *et al.*, 2011).

Children with intellectual disability also have markedly increased prevalence of psychiatric disorders. A systematic review found prevalence rates between 30% and 50% (Einfeld *et al.*, 2011). In children with intellectual disability, the most commonly associated comorbid psychiatric disorders are autism spectrum disorder, ADHD, and conduct disorder (Matson & Shoemaker, 2009). Emerson and Hatton (2007) found that a significant proportion of the increased risk of psychiatric disorder could be accounted for by the increased risk of psychosocial disadvantage experienced by children with intellectual disability, which has important policy and public health implications for developed and developing countries alike. Furthermore, without intervention, psychopathology tends to persist into adulthood (Einfeld & Emerson, 2008).

Orphans and vulnerable children

Over 140 million children in developing countries—or one in every 13—are orphans (Cluver & Gardner, 2007). In particular, the AIDS epidemic has been a driving force of vulnerability for children, leaving more than 25 million orphans and vulnerable children worldwide (Santa-Ana-Tellez *et al.*, 2011). A review of studies on the mental health of children orphaned by AIDS found that out of 13 studies measuring internalizing problems, 10 reported evidence of increased difficulties, whereas three out of seven found evidence of externalizing behavior difficulties (Cluver & Gardner, 2007).

War and terrorism

War and terrorism expose children to a range of risk factors. Emotional and behavioral consequences include acute stress reactions, post-traumatic stress disorder, anxiety and depressive disorders, regressive behaviors, and sleep and behavior problems (Fremont, 2004). Studies have found that the majority of youth exposed to war/violence experience severe and enduring threats that place them at increased risk for derailment in their developmental trajectory and that the chronicity of the trauma precludes them from recovery (Kletter *et al.*, 2013). War and terrorism also expose children and adolescents to a range of negative situations, such as the risk of dislocation, separation from family and loss of loved ones (Joshi & O'Donnell, 2003) (see Chapter 44). The number of conflict-related traumatic experiences has been shown to correlate positively with the prevalence of mental, behavioral, and emotional problems in children and adolescents living in conflict zones in the Middle East. Prevalence of post-traumatic stress disorder in children and adolescents is estimated to be 5–8% in Israel, 23–70% in Palestine and 10–30% in Iraq (Dimitry, 2012).

In summary, poor children growing up in LMIC encounter several contextual risk factors for mental disorders. Prevention, diagnostic and intervention programs and services focused on LMIC should not simply mirror those in developed countries but need to recognize the specific risk profiles facing these children. Although usually more frequent in LMIC, some contextual risk factors for mental disorders also affect children and adolescents growing up in HIC. In fact, data from HIC suggests that a substantial proportion of young individuals in these countries are also exposed to negative environments. The recent UNICEF Report Card 11 presented data on the well-being of children living in 29 rich countries, focusing on five dimensions of children's lives: material well-being, health and safety, education, behaviors and risks, and housing and environment. The Netherlands was the only country ranked among the top five in all dimensions, also exhibiting the best self-rated scores (when children evaluated their own well-being). The Nordic countries Finland, Iceland, Norway and Sweden occupied the next places in the well-being rank. Although among the four bottom places three were of the poorest countries in the survey (Latvia, Lithuania, and Romania), it was noticeable that the other nation in this group was the United States, suggesting that there was no overall strong relationship between per capita GDP and overall child well-being (Bradshaw et al., 2013; Martorano et al., 2013). A possible explanation for the low well-being estimates in the United States can also be the combination of general economic affluence with high poverty rates among children.

Methods in global child and adolescent psychiatric epidemiology

Population-based surveys from both HIC and LMIC demonstrate the high prevalence of mental disorders affecting children and adolescents in various nations. Despite the wide range of prevalence estimates (discrepancies occur both in HIC and LMIC studies), a large proportion of the surveys estimate that between 10% and 20% of children and adolescents have at least one diagnosable mental disorder according to major diagnostic classifications (the Diagnostic and Statistical Manual of Mental Disorders (DSM) or the International Classification of Diseases (ICD) (Kieling et al., 2011)—Table 16.1.

In addition to the variability in terms of instruments used and data collection strategies, much of the epidemiological research on childhood and adolescence mental disorders has limited methodological rigor. The use of similar instruments, survey strategy and design need to be analogous in order to allow for comparison of data such as prevalence rates. Without such data, limited conclusions can be derived from patterns of occurrence

of both mental disorders and risk factors (such as those covered in the previous section). This reiterates not only the need for conduction of surveys along the lines of the World Mental Health Survey Consortium (Demyttenaere et al., 2004), but with focus on the pediatric population, but also some degree of standardization in terms of measurement of risk and protective factors.

Adaptation of instruments is a process that requires a team composed of multiple experts in order to find balance between literal translation and culturally specific translation, making use of back-translations as a feedback method for the translation of content and intent. Further field-testing in small pilot groups with subsequent larger datasets collection is also essential to qualitatively and quantitatively identify flawed items, establishing reliability, validity, and new norms (Widenfelt et al., 2005). Specifically, cross-cultural studies have frequently assessed the reliability rather than the validity of constructs across different cultural groups (Hollifield et al., 2002; Saxena et al., 2006a, b; Betancourt et al., 2009). In this sense, disentangling methodological and cultural effects that contribute to variability in prevalence estimates has been a continuous challenge in pediatric psychiatric epidemiology (Canino & Alegría, 2008).

Culture can affect the presentation of psychopathology in multiple ways; for instance, by creating and reinforcing specific sources of distress and impairment or by influencing the interpretation of symptoms (Rohde, 2011). Cultural aspects are also relevant to the perception of what represents a mental health problem and how preventive or therapeutic interventions can be implemented in distinct areas of the globe—for example, a desired behavior in one culture can be unacceptable in another.

Diagnostic interviews and questionnaires with more than five studies (each with at least 300 children) from different societies have been assessed in a recent review that described the performance of both categorical and dimensional instruments. This study confirmed the marked disparities in estimates even when using the same diagnostic instrument in different populations: for categorical diagnoses, at least one disorder was present in 1.8% of children and adolescents in India and in 12.7% of young individuals in Brazil when using the Development and Well-Being Assessment (DAWBA) and ranged from 8.8% in New Zealand to 50.6% in areas of the United States and Puerto Rico for the Diagnostic Interview Schedule for Children (DISC) (Achenbach et al., 2012).

Dimensional instruments have also demonstrated to be valuable in the assessment of psychopathology in different contexts, such as the Strengths and Difficulties Questionnaire (SDQ; translated into more than 75 languages and freely available at www.sdqinfo.com), and the Achenbach System of Empirically Based Assessment (the ASEBA set of instruments, including the Child Behavior Checklist [CBCL], and the Teacher Report Form [TRF]; translated into more than 80 languages and commercially available at www.aseba.org). The ASEBA set of

Table 16.1 Studies on the global prevalence of child and adolescent mental disorders in LMIC.

Study	Country	Income (WB)	Sample frame	Diagnostic systems and instruments	Information sources and strategy for combining information	Number of stages	N	Attrition study completion rate %	Age range/mean (SD) (years)	Prevalence rates in % (CI/SE)
Mullick & Goodman, 2005	Bangladesh	Low	Regional community, urban and rural	ICD-10; SDQ & DAWBA	Parents, children (<11 yr) and teachers; best estimate	2	922	75	5–10	15 (11–21)
Anselmi et al., 2010	Brazil	Upper middle	Regional community, urban and rural	DSM-IV/ICD-10; SDQ & DAWBA	Parents and adolescents; best estimate	2	4445	84·7	11 & 12	10·8 (7·1–14·5)
Bilyk & Goodman, 2004	Brazil	Upper middle	Regional school, urban and rural	DSM-IV; DAWBA	Parents, children (<11 yr) and teachers; best estimate	1	519	83	7–14	12·7 (9·8–15·5)
Goodman et al., 2005	Brazil	Upper middle	Regional community, rural	DSM-IV; SDQ & DAWBA	Parents, children (<11 yr) and teachers; best estimate	2	1251	94	5–14	7 (2·3–11·8)
Guan et al., 2010	China	Lower middle	Regional, school, urban and rural	DSM-IV; ISICMD & structured interview designed by authors	Parents	2	9495	NA	5–17	16·22 (15·49–16·97)
Fekadu et al., 2006	Ethiopia	Low	Regional, school, urban	DSM-III-R; DICA	Children	1	528	NA	5–15	12·5 for school children; 20·1 for laborer children;[c] 16·5 combined
Hackett et al., 1999	India	Lower middle	Regional community, rural	ICD-10; Rutter scales A/B & clinical assessment	Parents	2	1403	95	8–12	9·4 (7·9–10·8)
Malhotra et al., 2002	India	Lower middle	Regional school, urban and rural	ICD-10; CPMS/Rutter B scale & clinical interview	Parents, and teachers; best estimate	3	963	91·7	4–11	6·33
Pillai et al., 2008	India	Lower middle	Regional Community, urban and rural	DSM-IV; DAWBA	Adolescent (half sample) and adolescent and parents (half sample)	1	2048	76	12–16	1·81 (1·27–2·48)

Study	Country	Income level	Setting	Criteria/instruments	Informants	Stages	N	Response %	Age range	Prevalence
Srinath et al., 2005	India	Lower middle	Regional community, urban and rural	ICD-10; SCL and VSMS/ CBCL & DISC (4–16 yr) and clinical assessment (0–3 yr)	Parents and children; best estimate	2	2064	90·5	0–16	13·8 (10·6–17) for 0–3 yr; 12 (10·3–13·6) for 4–16 yr; combined = 12·5
Kasmini et al., 1993[b]	Malaysia	Upper-middle	Regional community, rural	ICD-9; RQC & FIC	Parents; best estimate	2	507	99·6	1–15	6·1
Benjet et al., 2009	Mexico	Upper middle	Regional community, urban	DSM-IV; WMH-CIDI	Adolescent	1	3005	71	12–17	39·4 (38–40·9)
Abiodun, 1993[a]	Nigeria	Lower middle	Regional community, rural	ICD-9; RQC & FIC	Parents	2	200	NA	5–15	15
Goodman et al., 2005	Russia	Upper middle	Regional school, urban and rural	ICD-10; SDQ & DAWBA	Parents, children (<11 yr) and teachers; best estimate	2	448	74	7–14	15·3 (10·4–20·1)
Wacharasindhu and Panyyayong, 2002	Thailand	Lower middle	Regional, school, urban	DSM-IV	Parent, teacher, child[d]	2	1480	83	8–11	37·58
Alyahri & Goodman, 2008	Yemen	Lower middle	Regional, school, urban and rural	DSM-IV; SDQ & DAWBA	Parents and teachers; best estimate	2	1210	91	7–10	15·7 (11·7–20·2)

[a]Although reported as a two stage study, the second stage was not adjusted for the performance of the screening test in the first stage. So, technically it is a one-stage study (second stage = random subsample of the first stage).

[b]Only screening positives assessed in the second stage.

[c]This was a convenience sample.

[d]Not clear how the information from different sources was combined.

RQC = Reporting questionnaire for children; FIC = Follow-up interview for children; NA = not assessed or not available; CPMS = Childhood Psychopathology Measurement Scale (Indian adaptation of the CBCL); SCL = Structured Interview Schedule; VSMS = Vineland social maturity scale; ISICMD = Investigation Screening Inventory for Child Mental Disorders; GHQ-12 = General Health Questionnaire—12 questions version; CDI = child depression inventory.

When the study reported on prevalence rates from different waves of assessment, we opted for including the prevalence rate of the first wave. When in addition to point prevalence/period prevalence (e.g., 12 month prevalence), lifetime prevalence was also presented, we included point prevalence/period prevalence to make findings comparable as the majority of studies report on this type of prevalence.

Source: Extracted from Kieling et al. (2011).

instruments was assessed in another recent study, in which data for 44 societies were presented, probably the most successful effort to compare studies across different cultures (Rescorla *et al.*, 2012). Age and gender patterns remained relatively stable across the international level, and a confirmatory factor analysis supported the proposed syndromes when tested separately in each context. However, although many societies showed comparable average scores, nine studies presented scores one standard deviation above and another seven studies one standard deviation below the overall mean. The authors proposed a categorization of societies according to low, medium, and high norms, thus allowing for specific set of norms to reflect regional variations. Despite the huge efforts that such studies represent, it is important to note that even for the most frequently used instrument (the CBCL) no data are currently available for more than 1.4 billion children and adolescents—those living outside the 44 societies investigated. Another factor to be taken into account is the fact that samples were mostly regional and not representative of entire countries, but heterogeneity within countries can be even greater than between nations (Kieling & Rohde, 2012a, b).

Challenges and opportunities

Despite the widespread recognition of the importance of mental health promotion and prevention in children and adolescents, there is an enormous gap between needs and resource availability (Belfer 2008). Building technical and scientific capacity in low resource settings has been recognized as a crucial step toward decreasing the global burden of disease. In many LMIC there is less than one psychiatrist per 100,000 people, and in most countries investment in mental health represents less than 1% of investments in health as a whole (Saxena *et al.*, 2006a, b). Despite the availability of cost-effective treatments for childhood and adolescence mental health problems, there is a huge gap between needs and implementation worldwide.

In order to reduce the gap, the World Health Organization (WHO) launched the Mental Health Gap Action Programme (mhGAP) to scale up services for people with mental disorders, especially in LMIC (WHO, 2008). One essential component of mhGAP is to develop management recommendations (guidelines) for mental disorders identified as conditions of high priority (Dua *et al.*, 2011). The priority conditions in children and adolescents include depression, psychosis, bipolar disorders, and developmental and behavioral disorders. The priority conditions were selected because they represent a large burden in terms of mortality, morbidity, or disability, have high economic costs, and are often associated with violations of human rights. WHO established a Guideline Development Group in 2008 to develop evidence-based recommendations that adhered to the Grading of Recommendations Assessment, Development and Evaluation (GRADE) principles for developing transparent, evidence-based WHO guidelines (Barbui *et al.*, 2010). The

guidelines recognize that in most LMIC settings, the interventions would be conducted by nonspecialist primary care personnel—feasibility was therefore a key consideration. The guidelines are summarized in Table 16.2. Further research, especially of the implementation type, is required to translate these guidelines into scaled-up services.

Research

It can be argued that evidence-based information is probably even more critical to the less developed settings, where resources are scarce. Research plays a crucial role in defining the local needs, assessing the required cultural adaptation strategies, evaluating already implemented actions, identifying potential barriers and monitoring results (Thornicroft *et al.*, 2012). In fact, general health professionals believe that research conducted in their own country is more likely to change clinical practice (Guindon *et al.*, 2010). Therefore, dissemination of scientific research plays a pivotal role in the development and implementation of evidence-based health policies and practices such as those proposed by the WHO mhGAP guidelines. Notwithstanding almost 90% of all children and adolescents in the world live in LMIC, only 10% of randomized controlled trials assessing treatments for mental health problems for this population come from LMIC (Figure 16.2). Of note, the vast majority of intervention research conducted in LMIC assessed psychopharmacological strategies, neglecting the need for culture-specific psychosocial interventions. Thus, WHO guidelines rely on evidence generated from HIC to produce their guidelines, and further research is required to culturally adapt these recommended interventions to their settings. Indeed, evidence from a recent meta-analysis suggested that psychosocial treatments for depression that underwent cultural adaptation exhibit larger effect sizes in terms of effectiveness (Chowdhary *et al.*, 2013).

A recent survey in the Web of Science database for items published in the 2002–2011 decade showed that, although the field of child and adolescent mental health grew from nearly 5000 items published in 2002 to more than 10,000 in 2011, marked discrepancies exist according to income classification of countries. While the immense majority of indexed items (90.69%) had at least one author from a HIC, authorship from LMIC was modest, concentrating predominantly among upper middle income countries (7.79%). Authors from lower middle and low income countries were present in 1.19% and 0.33% of the items, respectively. Confirming these results, GNI per capita was linearly correlated ($r = 0.65$; $p < 0.001$) to the number of items published in the period. Perhaps more striking, no single indexed publication could be identified for 42 nations—countries in which 76 million individuals under the age of 18 years currently live (Kieling & Rohde, 2012a, b).

Individual analyses per country revealed that almost half (48.19%) of the child and adolescent mental health literature in the last decade had at least one author from the United States. Other leading publishing nations were England (9.58%),

Table 16.2 Abridged recommendations for child and adolescent mental health conditions (CAMH 1–13).

Maternal mental health interventions	CAMH 1. For at-risk children, parenting interventions promoting mother-infant interactions, including psychosocial stimulation, should be offered to improve child development outcomes. To improve child development outcomes, mothers with depression or with any other mental, neurological or substance use condition should be treated using effective interventions (see recommendations for treatment of depression and other mental, neurological, or substance use conditions).
Parent skills training for behavioral disorders	CAMH 5. Parent skills training should be considered for the treatment of emotional and behavioral disorders in children age 0–7 years. The content should be culture sensitive but should not allow violation of children's basic human rights according to internationally endorsed principles.
Parent skills training for developmental disorders	CAMH 6. Parent skills training should be considered in the management of children with intellectual disabilities and pervasive developmental disorders (including autism). Such training should use culturally appropriate training material.
Child abuse	CAMH 2. Non-specialized health care facilities should consider home visiting and offer parent education to prevent child abuse, especially among at-risk individuals and families. They should also collaborate with school-based "sexual abuse prevention" programmes where available.
Intellectual disabilities	CAMH 3. Non-specialized health care provides should consider assessment and regular monitoring of children suspected of intellectual and other developmental delays by brief, locally validated questionnaires. Clinical assessment under the supervision of specialists to identify common causes of these conditions should be considered. CAMH 4. Non-specialized health care provides should consider supporting, collaborating with, and facilitating referral to and from community-based rehabilitation programmes.
Behavior disorders (attention deficit hyperactivity disorder [ADHD])	CAMH 7. Non-specialized health care providers at the secondary level should consider initiating parent education/training before starting medication for a child who has been diagnosed as suffering from ADHD. Initial interventions may include cognitive behavioral therapy (CBT) and social skills training if feasible. Methylphenidate may be considered, when available, after a careful assessment of the child, preferably in consultation with the relevant specialist and taking into consideration the preferences of parents and children.
Pharmacological interventions for children with disruptive behavior disorders or conduct disorder or oppositional defiant disorder	CAMH 8. Pharmacological interventions (such as methylphenidate, lithium, carbamazepine, and risperidone) should not be offered by nonspecialized health care providers to treat disruptive behavior disorders (DBD), conduct disorder (CD), oppositional defiant disorder (ODD), and comorbid ADHD. For these conditions, the patients should be referred to a specialist before prescribing any medicines.
Somatoform disorders	CAMH 9. Pharmacological interventions should not be considered by nonspecialized health care providers. Brief psychological interventions, including CBT, should be considered to treat somatoform disorders in children, if adequate training and supervision by specialists can be made available.
Antidepressants for children with depression	CAMH 10. Antidepressants should not be used for the treatment of children 6–12 years of age with depressive episode/disorder in nonspecialist setting.
Antidepressants for adolescents with depression	CAMH 11. Fluoxetine, but not tricyclic antidepressants (TCA) or other selective serotonin reuptake inhibitors (SSRI), may be considered as one possible treatment in nonspecialist settings of adolescents with depressive episodes. Adolescents on fluoxetine should be monitored closely for suicide ideas/behavior. Support and supervision from a mental health specialist should be obtained, if available.
Pharmacological interventions for anxiety disorders in children and adolescents	CAMH 12. Pharmacological interventions should not be considered in children and adolescents with anxiety disorders in nonspecialist settings.
Behavior change techniques for promoting mental health	CAMH 13. Non-specialized health care facilities should encourage and collaborate with school-based life skills education, if feasible, to promote mental health in children and adolescents.

Source: Reproduced with permission from Dua *et al.* (2011).

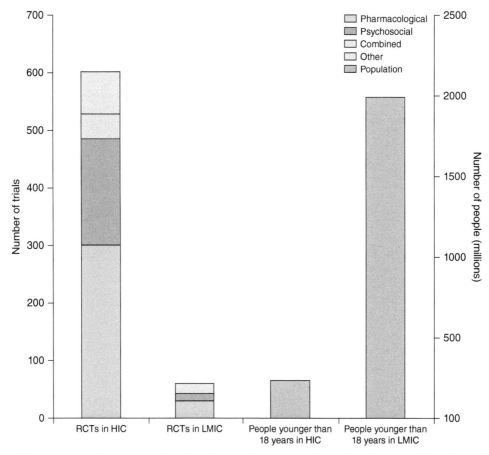

Figure 16.2 The 10/90 divide in research into treatment for childhood and adolescence mental health disorders (2001–2010). *Source:* Extracted from Kieling *et al.* (2011).

Canada (6.45%), Germany (6.29%), and Australia (5.08%). The LMIC with the highest representation were Turkey (1.64%; ranked 12th), China (1.53%; 14th), and Brazil (1.42%; 15th). Trend analyses suggest that this scenario might be changing: over the 2002–2011 period, the relative proportion of authorships from the United States decreased 26%, whereas leading LMIC exhibited a growing contribution: Turkey increased it share by 136%; China, 108%; and Brazil, 86% (Kieling & Rohde, 2012a, b). This scenario calls for a need to divert research resources and talent to LMIC.

Services

Integration of child mental health to systems of care imposes a set of challenges, such as cultural adaptation of strategies from one context to another; intersectoral collaboration; identification and inclusion of high risk groups (e.g., children who dropped out of school); cost-effectiveness determination (Jordans *et al.,* 2010). Collaboration with pediatric and primary care services might leverage benefits both to mental health and to general health outcomes.

Despite the burden imposed by mental health problems to children and adolescents, most countries do not provide satisfactory care to those in need (Belfer & Saxena, 2006). The Atlas

of Child and Adolescent Mental Health Resources included data for 66 countries, showing that less than a third of them had a specific entity responsible for child mental health promotion. Also, very few countries reported having an adequate and permanent budget for such programs. A more recent survey performed in 42 LMIC used a structured instrument developed by the WHO to assess key components of mental health systems. Unfortunately, findings confirmed the inadequacy of services to address mental health problems of children and adolescents, as well as the lack of professional training at multiple levels (Morris *et al.,* 2011).

Many factors are associated with the use of mental health services by children and adolescents, and their identification is crucial for planning. A systematic review of literature identified 57 studies investigating mental health services in community and school-based samples—however, with scarce data from LMIC (Graeff-Martins, 2010). Service utilization ranged from 2.2% to 63.0%, with lower rates associated with younger age and lack of impairment associated with symptomatology. Four reports also estimated the proportion of youth requiring but not receiving treatment (a measure of unmet need), with coverage rates varying between 17.1% and 87.1% (Flisher *et al.,* 1997; Goodman *et al.,* 1997; Kataoka *et al.,* 2002;

Sturm *et al.*, 2003). Notably, no quality or outcome assessment can be determined from these figures, as they only represent the proportion of children and adolescents having any contact with services.

Promising strategies to improve access to care include investments in gatekeepers such as parents, teachers, general practitioners or pediatricians, as even if children and adolescents do not reach specialized services, they are usually in contact with such professionals. Easy to read manuals and guides with culturally adapted strategies for management of childhood mental disorders in the nonspecialist primary care (Eapen *et al.*, 2012) and school settings (Patel *et al.*, 2013) have been recently published which can be a useful resource for practitioners intending to develop services in such settings.

Other innovative strategies to overcome obstacles in mental health promotion is the use of telemedicine or telepsychiatry, enhancing the interaction between multiple professionals in the community with specialists, allowing for discussion and supervision of complex clinical cases. One example of such initiative is currently being implemented in Brazil where specialists at the University of São Paulo supervise primary care physicians from the North and the Northeast, poorer and underserved regions of the country (Lowenthal, personal communication). The majority of these strategies, however, need to be rigorously tested (see Chapter 13). Also importantly, identification and intervention strategies should ideally be interconnected, in order to avoid a situation in which diagnosis is made but treatment is not available.

Training

In addition to concerted efforts to garner investments for the development of youth mental health services, innovative approaches will be needed to maximize the limited human resources in LMIC. The demand for training in global health today is a widespread phenomenon in HIC (Johnson *et al.*, 2012), and has also presented innovative initiatives from LMIC (Kerry *et al.*, 2011). A recent survey of the Consortium of Universities for Global Health, for example, found that the number of global health programs more than quadrupled in North America in recent years, going from eight to more than 40 between 2003 and 2009 (Merson & Page, 2008). In the UK, curriculum guidelines have been launched to define a set of basic skills that medical students should possess in relation to global health (Johnson *et al.*, 2012). Clinicians and researchers from LMIC can also benefit more on collaboration with their counterparts from other LMIC and not only from HIC. This is relevant, given the fact that many LMIC have similar problems and similar resources, together with a pressing need to improve local capacity.

Efforts need to be tailored to meet the specific needs of LMIC populations while considering local availability of resources. Although the role of child and adolescent psychiatrists and psychologists is essential, in many countries specialists may only be available in major urban centers. Nonspecialists, therefore,

may help fill this void, especially in the identification of mental health problems, making appropriate referrals and providing the support system that patients need. Increasingly, innovations in training and supervision models which involve redistribution of roles so that the more specialized personnel train and supervise large numbers of nonspecialists to deliver many of the interventions previously delivered by specialists (often referred to as Task-Shifting), are seen as key to meeting the human resource deficit in mental health (Murray *et al.*, 2011; Patel *et al.*, 2011a, b; Kazdin *et al.*, 2013).

Although key initiatives from global agents can offer research-based guidance on intervention strategies, the appropriate implementation of mental health services involves the recognition of local demands and, possibly, international collaboration among LMIC (Hamoda & Belfer (2010)). In addition to collaborations with the health sector, strategies such as school-based interventions represent encouraging approaches as education receives increasing investments in many LMIC; joint enterprise can also be developed with programs such as nutritional and antenatal care.

Coordinated efforts for training multidisciplinary providers for child and adolescent mental health are required to foster the development of the next generation of clinicians and researchers. Presence of local training capacity and the development of mechanisms to attract back LMIC professionals who underwent training in HIC may help limit the brain drain phenomenon. If professionals from LMIC who have immigrated to HIC cannot return, their expertise may still be valuable as consultants for program development in their home countries. Training programs in HIC planning to train professionals from LMIC should be sensitive to teaching skills that are applicable in LMIC (e.g., advanced psychopharmacology training might have limited relevance if basic drugs are not available in the country of origin). Other alternatives for LMIC collaboration include sharing training resources and expertise among countries in close proximity (Hamoda & Belfer (2010)).

The establishment of collaborative networks is also of extreme value, and can be achieved with or without the involvement of international professional organizations. An initiative that has shown encouraging results in the promotion of mental health worldwide is the Movement for Global Mental Health (MGMH) (Lancet, 2008). It is a coalition of individuals and institutions committed to collective actions to reduce the treatment gap for people with mental disorders. The MGMH promotes their actions based on two principles: evidence of effectiveness of treatment and human rights of people with mental disorders. The initiative seeks inspiration from successful experiences, such as the movement for the care of HIV-infected people in LMIC (Eaton & Patel, 2009; Patel *et al.*, 2011a, b).

The development of courses and mentorship programs can benefit further from longitudinal involvement between countries, allowing a better appreciation of the unique challenges that each country imposes and thus establishing more meaningful collaborations. In another promising initiative, multiple professional child and adolescent mental health organizations (including the International Association for Adolescent Psychiatry and Psychology, the International Association for Child and Adolescent Psychiatry and Allied Professions, the International Association for Child Mental Health in Schools, the World Association for Infant Mental Health, and the World Federation for Mental Health) have recently partnered in a global consortium to advance education and advocacy in the field of child mental health.

Future perspectives

Despite seemingly overwhelming challenges and limited resources, the field of global child mental health now faces a time of tremendous opportunities. While mental, neurologic, and substance-use disorders are among the most disabling conditions, global partnerships have sprouted, drawing attention to the unmet needs of child mental health worldwide. The greatest challenge ahead is to build on these partnerships to create sustainable, reliable, and cost-effective mental health services in resource-limited settings. Advancements in clinical, research, and training efforts in these underprivileged contexts are needed to answer critical questions through evidence-based research, reduce the treatment gap and the burden of mental health disorders.

Professionals in HIC can contribute to the developments in global child mental health. Research and capacity building of colleagues are two such arenas where the scope for collaboration is wide. Importantly, much can also be learnt from the experiences of professionals working in such settings—task-shifting strategies, innovative models of training and supervision, and the use of mobile phone and information technology to provide both service and training/supervision at a distance—are examples of developments which could apply to high income settings also.

References

Abiodun, O.A. (1993) Emotional illness in a pediatric population in Nigeria. *Journal of Tropical Pediatrics* **39**, 49–51.

Achenbach, T.M. *et al.* (2012) International epidemiology of child and adolescent psychopathology: 1. Diagnoses, dimensions, and conceptual issues. *Journal of the American Academy of Child and Adolescent Psychiatry* **51**, 1261–1272.

Alyahri, A. & Goodman, R. (2008) The prevalence of DSM-IV psychiatric disorders among 7-10 year old Yemeni school children. *Social Psychiatry and Psychiatric Epidemiology* **43**, 224–230.

Angelucci, M. & DiMaro, V. (2010) Program evaluation and spillover effects. In: *IDB Technical Note 136, Office of Strategic Planning and Development Effectiveness working papers.* Inter-American Development Bank, Washington.

Anselmi, L. *et al.* (2010) Prevalence of psychiatric disorders in a Brazilian birth cohort of 11-year-olds. *Social Psychiatry and Psychiatric Epidemiology* **45**: 135–142.

Barbui, C. *et al.* (2010) Challenges in developing evidence-based recommendations using the GRADE approach: the case of mental, neurological, and substance use disorders. *PLoS Medicine* **7**, e1000322.

Belfer, M.B. (2008) Child and adolescent mental disorders: the magnitude of the problem across the globe. *Journal of Child Psychology and Psychiatry* **49**, 226–236.

Belfer, M.L. & Saxena, S. (2006) WHO Child Atlas project. *Lancet* **367**, 551–552.

Benjet, C. *et al.* (2009) Youth mental health in a populous city of the developing world: results from the Mexican Adolescent Mental Health Survey. *Journal of Child Psychology and Psychiatry* **50**, 386–395.

Berlinguer, G. (1999) Globalização e saúde global. *Estudos Avançados* **13**, 21–38.

Betancourt, T.S. *et al.* (2009) Assessing local instrument reliability and validity: a field-based example from Northern Uganda. *Social Psychiatry and Psychiatric Epidemiology* **44**, 685–692.

Bradshaw, J.B. *et al.* (2013) Children's Subjective Well-being in Rich Countries, *Working Paper 2013–03.* UNICEF Office of Research, [Online]. Available: http://www.unicef-irc.org/publications/pdf/iwp_2013_3.pdf.

Brown, T.M. *et al.* (2006) The World Health Organization and the transition from "international" to "global" public health. *American Journal of Public Health* **96**, 62–72.

Canino, G. & Alegría, M. (2008) Psychiatric diagnosis - is it universal or relative to culture? *Journal of Child Psychology and Psychiatry* **49**, 237–250.

Chowdhary, N. *et al.* (2013) The methods and outcomes of cultural adaptations of psychological treatments for depressive disorders: a systematic review. *Psychological Medicine* **19**, 1–16.

Cluver, L. & Gardner, F. (2007) Excluded and Invisible. The mental health of children orphaned by AIDS: a review of international and southern African research. *Journal of Child and Adolescent Mental Health* **19**, 1–17.

Collins, P.Y. *et al.* (2011) Grand challenges in global mental health. *Nature* **475**, 27–30.

Demyttenaere, K. *et al.* (2004) Prevalence, severity, and unmet need for treatment of mental disorders in the World Health Organization World Mental Health Surveys. *JAMA* **291**, 2581–2590.

Dercon, S. & Krishnan, P. (2009) Poverty and the psychosocial competencies of children: evidence from the young lives sample in four developing countries. *Children, Youth and Environments* **19**, 138–163.

Dimitry, L. (2012) A systematic review on the mental health of children and adolescents in areas of armed conflict in the Middle East. *Child: Care, Health and Development* **38**, 153–161.

Dua, T. *et al.* (2011) Evidence-based guidelines for mental, neurological, and substance use disorders in low- and middle-income countries: summary of WHO recommendations. *PLoS Medicine* **8**, e1001122.

Eapen, V. *et al.* (2012) *Where There is No Child Psychiatrist. A Mental Health Care Manual.* Royal College of Psychiatrist, London.

Eaton, J. & Patel, V. (2009) A movement for global mental health. *African Journal of Psychiatry* **12**, 1–3.

Einfeld, S. & Emerson, E. (2008) Intellectual disability. In: *Rutter's Child and Adolescent Psychiatry.* (M. Rutter *et al.*), 5th edn, pp. 820–840. Blackwell, Oxford.

Einfeld, S.L. *et al.* (2011) Comorbidity of intellectual disability and mental disorder in children and adolescents: a systematic review. *Journal of Intellectual and Developmental Disability* **36**, 137–143.

Emerson, E. & Hatton, C. (2007) Mental health of children and adolescents with intellectual disabilities in Britain. *British Journal of Psychiatry* **191**, 493–499.

Engle, P.L. (2011) Strategies for reducing inequalities and improving developmental outcomes for young children in low-income and middle-income countries. *Lancet* **378**, 1339–1353.

Engle, P. & Black, M. (2010) The effect of poverty on child development and educational outcomes. *Annals of the New York Academy of Sciences* **1136**, 243–256.

Fekadu, D. *et al.* (2006) The prevalence of mental health problems in Ethiopian child laborers. *Journal of Child Psychology and Psychiatry* **47**, 954–959.

Fleitlich, B. & Goodman, R. (2001) Social factors associated with child mental health problems in Brazil: cross sectional survey. *BMJ* **323**, 599–600.

Fleitlich-Bilyk, B. & Goodman, R. (2004) Prevalence of child and adolescent psychiatric disorders in southeast Brazil. *Journal of American Academy of Child and Adolescent Psychiatry* **43**, 727–734.

Flisher, A.J. *et al.* (1997) Correlates of unmet need for mental health services by children and adolescents. *Psychological Medicine* **27**, 1145–1154.

Fremont, W.P. (2004) Childhood reactions to terrorism-induced trauma: a review of the past 10 years. *Journal of the American Academy of Child & Adolescent Psychiatry* **43**, 381–392.

Goodman, S.H. *et al.* (1997) Representativeness of clinical samples of youths with mental disorders: a preliminary population-based study. *Journal of Abnormal Psychology* **106**, 3–14.

Goodman, R. *et al.* The Ilha de Maré study: a survey of child mental health problems in a predominantly African-Brazilian rural community. *Social Psychiatry and Psychiatric Epidemiology* 2005a **40**, 11–17.

Goodman R, Slobodskaya H, Knyazev G. Russian child mental health--a cross-sectional study of prevalence and risk factors. *European Child & Adolescent Psychiatry* 2005b **14**, 28–33.

Gordon, D. *et al.* (2003) *Child Poverty in the Developing World*. The Policy Press, Bristol.

Gore, F.M. *et al.* (2011) Global burden of disease in young people aged 10–24 years: a systematic analysis. *Lancet* **377**, 2093–2102.

Graeff-Martins, A. (2010). *Serviços de saúde mental para crianças e adolescentes: recomendações para o planejamento de políticas de saúde mental* (PhD thesis), Universidade Federal de São Paulo, São Paulo.

Grantham-McGregor, S. (2007) Child Development in developing countries. Developmental potential in the first 5 years for children in developing countries. *Lancet* **369**, 60–70.

Guan, B.Q1. *et al.* (2010) Prevalence of psychiatric disorders in primary and middle school students in Hunan Province. *Zhongguo Dang Dai Er Ke Za Zhi* **12**, 123–127.

Guindon, G.E. *et al.* (2010) Bridging the gaps between research, policy and practice in low- and middle-income countries: a survey of health care providers. *Canadian Medical Association Journal* **182**, E362–E372.

Hackett, R. *et al.* (1999) The prevalence and associations of psychiatric disorder in children in Kerala, South India. *Journal of Child Psychology and Psychiatry* **40**, 801–807.

Hamoda, H. & Belfer, M. (2010) Challenges in international collaboration in child and adolescent psychiatry. *Journal of Child and Adolescent Mental Health* **22**, 83–89.

Heckman, J.J. & Krueger, A. (eds) (2003) *Inequality in America: What Role for Human Capital Policy?* MIT Press, Cambridge.

Hollifield, M. *et al.* (2002) Measuring trauma and health status in refugees: a critical review. *JAMA* **288**, 611–621.

Ickovics, J.R. *et al.* (2001) Mortality, CD4 cell count decline, and depressive symptoms among HIV-seropositive women: longitudinal analysis from the HIV Epidemiology Research Study. *JAMA* **285**, 1466–1474.

Institute of Medicine (1997) *America's Vital Interest in Global Health*. National Academy Press, Washington, DC.

Institute of Medicine (2001) *Neurological, Psychiatric, and Developmental Disorders: Meeting the Challenge in the Developing World*. National Academy Press, Washington, DC.

Johnson, O. *et al.* (2012) Global health learning outcomes for medical students in the UK. *Lancet* **379**, 2033–2035.

Jordans, M.J. *et al.* (2010) Development of a multi-layered psychosocial care system for children in areas of political violence. *International Journal of Mental Health Systems* **4**, 15.

Joshi, P.T. & O'Donnell, D.A. (2003) Consequences of child exposure to war and terrorism. *Clinical Child and Family Psychology Review* **6**, 275–292.

Kasmini, K. *et al.* (1993) A prevalence survey of mental disorders among children in a rural Malaysian village. *Acta Psychiatrica Scandinavica* **87**, 253–257.

Kataoka, S.H. *et al.* (2002) Unmet need for mental health care among U.S. children: variation by ethnicity and insurance status. *American Journal of Psychiatry* **159**, 1548–1555.

Kazdin, A.E. *et al.* (2013) Novel models for delivering mental health services and reducing the burdens of mental illness. *Clinical Psychological Science* **1**, 170–191.

Kerry, V.B. *et al.* (2011) Managing the demand for global health education. *PLoS Medicine* **8**, e1001118.

Kieling, C. & Rohde, L.A. (2012a) Child and adolescent mental health research across the globe. *Journal of the American Academy of Child and Adolescent Psychiatry* **51**, 945–947.

Kieling, C. & Rohde, L.A. (2012b) Going global: epidemiology of child and adolescent psychopathology. *Journal of the American Academy of Child and Adolescent Psychiatry* **51**, 1236–1237.

Kieling, C. *et al.* (2011) Child and adolescent mental health worldwide: evidence for action. *Lancet* **378**, 1515–1525.

Kleinman, A. (2009) Global mental health: a failure of humanity. *Lancet* **374**, 603–604.

Kletter, H. *et al.* (2013) Helping children exposed to war and violence: perspectives from an international work group on interventions for youth and families. *Child and Youth Care Forum* **42**, 1–18.

Koplan, J.P. *et al.* (2009) Towards a common definition of global health. *Lancet* **373**, 1993–1995.

Lancet [editorial] (2008) A movement for global mental health is launched. *Lancet* **372**, 1274.

Malhotra, S. *et al.* (2002) Prevalence of psychiatric disorders in school children in Chandigarh, India. *Indian Journal of Medical Research* **116**, 21–28.

Martorano, B. et al. (2013) *Child well-being in economically rich countries: changes in the first decade of the 21st century'*, Working Paper 2013-02, [Online], Available: http://www.unicef-irc.org/publications/pdf/iwp_2013_2.pdf

Matson, J.L. & Shoemaker, M. (2009) Intellectual disability and its relationship to autism spectrum disorders. *Research in Developmental Disabilities* **30**, 1107–1114.

Maulik, P.K. *et al.* (2011) Prevalence of intellectual disability: a meta-analysis of population-based studies. *Research in Developmental Disabilities* **32**, 419–436.

Merson, M. & Page, K. (2008) *The Dramatic Expansion of University Engagement in Global Health: Implications for US Policy.* Center for Strategic and International Studies, Washington, DC.

Morris, J. *et al.* (2011) Treated prevalence of and mental health services received by children and adolescents in 42 low-and-middle-income countries. *Journal of Child Psychology and Psychiatry* **52**, 1239–1246.

Mullick, M.S. & Goodman, R. (2005) The prevalence of psychiatric disorders among 5-10 year olds in rural, urban and slum areas in Bangladesh: an exploratory study. *Social Psychiatry and Psychiatric Epidemiology* **40**, 663–671.

Murray, L.K. *et al.* (2011) Building capacity in mental health interventions in low resource countries: an apprenticeship model for training local providers. *International Journal of Mental Health Systems* **5**, 30.

Murray, C.J. *et al.* (2012) Disability-adjusted life years (DALYs) for 291 diseases and injuries in 21 regions, 1990–2010: a systematic analysis for the Global Burden of Disease Study 2010. *Lancet* **380**, 2197–2223.

Nugent, R. & Jamison, D. (2011) What can a UN health summit do? *Science Translational Medicine* **3**, 1–3.

O'Connor, D.L. *et al.* (2000) Distribution of accidents, injuries, and illnesses by family type. *Pediatrics* **106**, e68.

Patel, V. & Prince, M. (2010) Global mental health: a new global health field comes of age. *JAMA* **303**, 1976–1977.

Patel, V. *et al.* (2011a) The movement for global mental health. *British Journal of Psychiatry* **198**, 88–90.

Patel, V. *et al.* (2011b) Improving access to psychological treatments: lessons from developing countries. *Behaviour Research and Therapy* **49**, 523–528.

Patel, V. *et al.* (2013) *A School Counsellor Casebook.* Byword Books, Delhi.

Pillai, A. *et al.* (2008) Non-traditional lifestyles and prevalence of mental disorders in adolescents in Goa. *India. British Journal of Psychiatry.* **192**, 45–51.

Prince, M. *et al.* (2007) No health without mental health. *Lancet* **370**, 859–877.

Rescorla, L. *et al.* (2012) International epidemiology of child and adolescent psychopathology: 2. Integration and applications of dimensional findings from 44 societies. *Journal of the American Academy of Child & Adolescent Psychiatry* **51**, 1273–1283.

Rohde, L.A. (2011) Commentary: do potential modifications in classificatory systems impact on child mental health in developing countries? Reflections on Rutter (2011). *Journal of Child Psychology and Psychiatry* **52**, 669–670.

Santa-Ana-Tellez, Y. *et al.* (2011) Costs of interventions for AIDS orphans and vulnerable children. *Tropical Medicine & International Health* **16**, 1417–1426.

Saxena, S. *et al.* (2006a) World Health Organization's mental health atlas 2005: implications for policy development. *World Psychiatry* **5**, 179–184.

Saxena, S. *et al.* (2006b) The 10/90 divide in mental health research: trends over a 10 year period. *British Journal of Psychiatry* **188**, 81–82.

Skotheim, B. *et al.* (2011) The World Health Organization and global health. *Tidsskrift for den Norske Lægeforening* **131**, 1793–1795.

Srinath, S. *et al.* (2005) Epidemiological study of child & adolescent psychiatric disorders in urban & rural areas of Bangalore. *India. Indian Journal of Medical Research* **122**, 67–79.

Sturm, R. *et al.* (2003) Geographic disparities in children's mental health care. *Pediatrics* **112**, e308.

Susser, E. (2012) Relation of childhood malnutrition to adult mental disorders. *American Journal of Psychiatry* **169**, 777–779.

Thornicroft, G. *et al.* (2012) Capacity building in global mental health research. *Harvard Review of Psychiatry* **20**, 13–24.

UNDP (United Nations Development Programme) (2013), [Online], Available: http://hdr.undp.org/en/statistics/hdi/

UNICEF (2006). *Progress for children: a report card on nutrition*, [Online] Available: http://www.unicef.org/progressforchildren/2006 n4/files/PFC4_EN_8X11.pdf

Wacharasindhu, A. & Panyyayong, B. (2002) Psychiatric disorders in Thai school-aged children: I Prevalence. *Journal of the Medical Association of Thailand* **85**, S125–S136.

Walker, S.P. *et al.* (2007) Child development: risk factors for adverse outcomes in developing countries. *Lancet* **369**, 145–157.

Walker, S.P. *et al.* (2011) Inequality in early childhood: risk and protective factors for early child development. *Lancet* **378**, 1325–1338.

Widenfelt, B.M. *et al.* (2005) Translation and cross-cultural adaptation of assessment instruments used in psychological research with children and families. *Clinical Child and Family Psychology Review* **8**, 135–147.

World Bank (2013a) *A short history*, [Online], Available: http://data.worldbank.org/about/country-classifications/a-short-history

World Bank (2013b) *How we classify countries*, [Online], Available: http://data.worldbank.org/about/country-classifications

World Health Organization (WHO) (2008) *Scaling up care for mental, neurological, and substance use disorders*, [Online], Available: http://www.who.int/mental_health/mhgap_final_english.pdf

Yeung, W.J. *et al.* (2002) How money matters for young children's development: parental investment and family processes. *Child Development* **73**, 1861–1879.

CHAPTER 17

Prevention of mental disorders and promotion of competence

Mark T. Greenberg[1] and Nathaniel R. Riggs[2]

[1] Prevention Research Center for the Promotion of Human Development, Pennsylvania State University, University Park, PA, USA
[2] Department of Human Development and Family Studies, Colorado State University, CO, USA

This chapter covers the broad area of prevention science, with a focus on universal and selective prevention. While space limitations prevent a comprehensive review of mental health prevention and promotion, we have selected issues and challenges that affect both researchers and practitioners. We include brief descriptions of a number of tested, effective prevention programs focused on childhood and adolescence and refer the reader to other sources for greater detail. The chapter is divided into sections on (1) epidemiology and rationale for preventive interventions, (2) the role of developmental theory in prevention and promotion, (3) defining prevention and its levels, (4) empirical advances of prevention research on mental health problems of children, (5) key issues in current and future prevention research, and (6) issues regarding dissemination, implementation, and sustainability. We conclude with recommendations to deal with the global challenges faced by research and practice in implementing effective preventive interventions.

Epidemiology and the rationale for preventive interventions

Prevention of mental, emotional, and behavioral disorders (MEBDs) in childhood and adolescence is a key avenue for improving public health and is also central to reducing morbidity from numerous related conditions. This is not only because childhood MEBD problems are predictive of adult mental health and substance use disorders but they also serve as risk factors for many other poor health outcomes in adolescence and adulthood. Mental health disorders account for 13% of the total disease burden worldwide (World Health Organization, 2009). By 2030, it is estimated that depression will be second, to HIV/AIDS, in global disease burden. In low- and middle-income (LAMI) countries, depression contributes

almost as much disease burden as malaria (World Health Organization, 2006). The rates of mental disorders increase across childhood and adolescence with one in five US adolescents reporting mental health problems (Knopf *et al.*, 2008). A striking 50% of adult mental disorders have an onset during or before adolescence (Belfer, 2008); thus, preventive models in childhood are key to reducing the burden of disorder.

The role of developmental theory in the prevention of MEBDs

One hallmark of prevention science is that it is steeped in developmental theory, which spans and integrates related fields including public health, epidemiology, neuroscience, behavioral genetics, and developmental psychopathology (Cicchetti & Cohen, 1995; Ialongo *et al.*, 2006; Bradshaw *et al.*, 2012). Developmental theory is conceived broadly to include multilevel social ecological and systems science perspectives, which incorporate layered contexts interacting in dynamic ways to influence risk and resilience (Bronfenbrenner, 1995; Green, 2006). This richness in theoretical breadth and depth provides a powerful framework for understanding the etiology of MEBDs and serves as the basis for conceptualizing, designing, and implementing preventive interventions that target their theoretically and empirically supported risk and protective factors. Risk factors increase the likelihood of MEBDs and can be characterized into one of six domains: child (e.g., self-regulation problems), family (e.g., the quality of parent–child attachment), peer (isolation), demographic (e.g., family income), school (school climate), and community/policy (e.g., neighborhood poverty and crime rates) (Coie *et al.*, 1993; Fagan *et al.*, 2007). It is clear that children living in poverty are at greatest risk for MEBDS (Yoshikawa *et al.*, 2012). Risk factors often co-occur and current theory

Rutter's Child and Adolescent Psychiatry, Sixth Edition.
Edited by Anita Thapar and Daniel S. Pine, James F. Leckman, Stephen Scott, Margaret J. Snowling, Eric Taylor.
© 2015 John Wiley & Sons Ltd. Published 2018 by John Wiley & Sons Ltd.

and research have resulted in several observations regarding the relation of risk factors to mental health problems. First, due to the complex nature of human development, it is likely that few mental health disorders are due to a single cause, or risk factor, residing in the child alone (Rutter, 1982). Rather, the development of mental health problems is often the result of multiple accumulated risks across time and contexts, potentially exhibiting nonlinear (i.e., exponential) relationship with psychopathology (Sameroff *et al.*, 1987). Second, not all children who experience any given risk factor, or set of risk factors, will develop adjustment problems, suggesting that children vary in their resilience in the face of adversity (see Chapter 27). Third, developmental epidemiology findings indicate multiple pathways to most psychological disorders; different combinations of risk factors may lead to the same disorder, and rarely are risk factors disorder-specific (Greenberg *et al.*, 1993). Thus, prevention efforts that focus on risk reduction of multiple interacting risk factors may have direct effects on diverse outcomes (Coie *et al.*, 1993).

The role of protective factors

Protective factors reduce the likelihood of maladaptive outcomes under conditions of risk and thus build resilience in particular contexts. Less is known about protective factors and their operation (Rutter 1979; Losel & Farrington, 2012), but they include domains operating at the level of the child (e.g., social-cognitive skills), family (e.g., parental warmth and monitoring), peer (peers with prosocial values), demographic (family structure), school (school quality), and community/policy (neighborhood social capital). By specifying links between protective factors, positive outcomes, and reduced problem behaviors, prevention researchers may more successfully identify relevant targets for intervention (Coie *et al.*, 1993; Fagan *et al.*, 2007) and nurture environments central to positive mental health and averting mental illness (Biglan *et al.*, 2012). It should be noted that although much of the theory regarding risk and protective factors occurs at the community level. There has been little investigation of the assumptions underlying this model (Feinberg, 2012) and much of the research on risk and protective factors has been correlational, not causal.

Developmental neuroscience and genetics

Advances in developmental neuroscience have recently advanced traditional theories of prevention science. Developmental neuroscience research has demonstrated the importance of the executive attention systems and executive function (EF) (Blair, 2002). There has been an enormous expansion of knowledge regarding both the development of EF skills and the growth and differentiation of the prefrontal area of the brain. Subsequently, there has been progress on the development of curricula and training programs to promote self-regulation, and a few programs have focused directly on developing EF skills (Davidson *et al.*, 2003; Riggs *et al.*, 2006; Diamond & Lee, 2011; Greenberg & Harris, 2011).

The growing field of developmental genetics has similarly altered models of developmental processes (Jaffee & Price, 2007). Recently, developmental models have focused on the issue of differential susceptibility to environments, with preventive interventions being a specific type of environment (Ellis *et al.*, 2011). This has heralded the initiation of research to examine Gene X Preventive Treatment interaction effects that might demonstrate that genetic endowment may lead to differential outcomes from interventions. Brody *et al.* (2014) provide one example showing that African American male teens with a *DRD4* gene variant with 7 or more repeats who received a family intervention model were more likely to show lower rates of substance use 2 years after intervention.

Promotion of competence

New and complementary models for the prevention of mental health problems also include strength-based models such as social-emotional learning (SEL) and positive youth development. For example, the Collaborative for Academic and Social-Emotional Learning (CASEL) approach to preventing mental health problems is to promote self-regulation, self-awareness, social awareness, positive peer relationships, and responsible decision-making as precursors to social-emotional competence (CASEL, 2003). Recent research shows that proficiency in each of these five domains of social competence is related to positive academic, behavioral, and mental health outcomes (Durlak *et al.*, 2011).

The specification of intervention goals is an important component of preventive intervention. Although these goals may include the prevention of difficulties (e.g., absence of psychopathology), they also involve the promotion of healthy outcomes and the enhancement of competency as mediators (e.g., effective social problem-solving mediating reduction in delinquency). This requires an understanding of how risk and protective factors contribute to outcomes, and the identification of competencies that mediate intervention outcomes.

Defining prevention

Levels of prevention

Prevention programs can take a number of forms depending upon factors such as community need and capacity. The Institute of Medicine placed preventive interventions within a broader mental health intervention framework that differentiates prevention from treatment (Institute of Medicine, 2009). Within prevention, programs can vary in terms of reach and focus.

Universal interventions target all children, are relatively low in cost, attempt to reduce a variety of risk factors, and promote a broad range of protective factors. Three common foci of school-based universal interventions are improvements to school structure (e.g., organizational features/rules), teacher's classroom management, and curricula that teach new social-emotional skills (CASEL, 2003). Common foci of universal family programs are parenting skills including communication, responsivity, management, and monitoring of child behavior. Advantages of universal programs are that they (a) contribute to adaptive coping/resilience across an array of experiences and settings; (b) are positive and provided independent of risk status, and therefore nonstigmatizing; and (c) reduce or prevent multiple behavior problems which share overlapping risk factors (Greenberg *et al.,* 2001).

Selective interventions are those that are delivered to a class of families or children because their characteristics place them at risk for later problems. There are two broad classes of selective interventions. The first group is based on risk characteristics of the child, family, or community (e.g., poverty, the children of parents who are depressed, and children with social skills difficulties). The second type of selective intervention is for children or families who have experienced a stress-triggered event that increases their risk for maladjustment (e.g., divorce, loss of a parent through death, other traumas, moving to a new school) (Wolchik *et al.,* 2007). In both instances, no child may yet have difficulties, but the circumstances in which children find themselves create risk. Selective interventions usually involve specialized services such as group interventions (Lochman *et al.,* 2012), that teach social emotional skills, social information processing, and decision-making. A major advantage of selective programs is that effort and resources will be spent on children and youth at greatest risk for developing mental health problems. Thus, selective interventions may provide greater conceptual precision, intensity, and focus for children at relatively high risk.

Indicated prevention is directed at children or families that are already showing substantial and sometimes even diagnostic levels of difficulty (see Chapters 36 and 42). These programs usually occur after a child has had substantial difficulties (e.g., have received psychiatric diagnoses or have been arrested). Such programs are intensive and expensive, but may be cost-effective given the high-cost and long-term effects of such experiences (Lee *et al.,* 2012). As this chapter is focused on universal and selective models, the reader is referred to other sources for further review (Vitaro & Tremblay, 2008; Greenberg & Lippold, 2013).

Universal and selective interventions may employ multiple components that target school, family, and community factors. Given their extra cost, multicomponent interventions are more often utilized with selective interventions, or with universal models in high-risk neighborhoods or schools. Universal programs are likely to be most effective when implemented as part of a comprehensive, potentially tiered, approach to prevention (Greenberg *et al.,* 2001), an example of which is the Seattle Social Development Project (Hawkins *et al.,* 2005).

A relative advantage of universal prevention is that selective and indicated approaches are not sensitive to a large percentage of MEBD that develops later in life. Durlak (1995) points out that if only 8% of well-adjusted children go on to have serious adjustment problems as adults (as opposed to 30% of clinically dysfunctional children), the well-adjusted children will represent 50% more of the population of maladjusted adults. This follows Rose's maxim that "a large number of people exposed to a small risk may generate many more cases than a small number exposed to a high risk." It may then be beneficial to provide universal preventive interventions regardless of the low prevalence rate of childhood psychopathology (Rose, 1985). Thus, when dealing with a common and costly disorder such as depression or conduct disorder, there may be justification for preventive efforts that are universal and provided at the population level (Merry & Spence, 2007; Shamblen & Derzon, 2009).

However, there are also "trade-offs" between universal and targeted (indicated or selective) approaches (Offord *et al.,* 1998). A potential disadvantage of universal programs is that if used in contexts with low prevalence of psychopathology, substantial effort will be spent on children who may not develop mental health problems. Further, because of relatively low dosage, universal intervention might not provide sufficient duration or intensity to alter pathways of children at most risk. Offord *et al.* (1998) also raises the question of whether universal programs have the greatest impact on lowest risk children, though some findings contradict this theory by demonstrating stronger effects for more at-risk subgroups (Kellam *et al.,* 2008; Spoth *et al.,* 2013a).

The implementation of universal interventions in schools also poses challenges (see Chapter 42). First, they require approval of schools that often appear overburdened with other priorities. They require multiple levels of approval from administrators, community partners, and local authorities. In general, universal interventions are likely to be most effective when they have sufficient duration and intensity, target the development of protective factors related to multiple disorders, or target problems with high prevalence (e.g., bullying, early alcohol use). Similarly, universal family-based programs face considerable challenges in effectively recruiting families to participate (Spoth *et al.,* 2013b).

Empirical advances in prevention research with children and families

The past two decades have brought clear progress and a stronger empirical base to the field of prevention (Institute of Medicine, 2009; Catalano *et al.,* 2012). Controlled trials over the past two decades have identified effective prevention programs that can reduce risk, increase protection, and reduce MEBDs. There are now a considerable number of broad reviews of evidence-based interventions (EBIs), classroom- and family-based curricula that have been shown to reduce mental health symptoms including anxiety, depression, antisocial behavior, and aggression (Greenberg *et al.,* 2001; Adi *et al.,* 2007; Hoagwood, *et al.,* 2007; Tenant *et al.,* 2007; Wilson & Lipsey, 2007; Durlak *et al.,* 2011; Sandler *et al.,* 2011; Henggeler & Sheidow, 2012; Furlong *et al.,* 2013). Program reviews are now widely available on a number of Internet sites; those with the most rigorous inclusion criteria are Blueprints for Healthy Youth Development (www.colorado.edu/cspv/blueprints), the Cochrane Collaboration (www.cochrane.org), and the Campbell Collaboration (www.campbellcollaboration.org). The following sections highlight successful programs included in many of these reviews. However, it should be noted that positive intervention effects are not universally found despite well-reasoned theory, fidelity of implementation, and rigorous evaluation design. Thus, the following successful programs should be viewed within the context of other prevention programs that have demonstrated effects limited to subsamples of participants or null effects on all or some MEBD outcomes (e.g., Scott *et al.*, 2010a, b).

Conduct problems and aggression

The prevention of conduct problems and aggression has dominated early prevention trials. A meta-analysis examining 249 experimental studies designed to prevent aggressive and disruptive behavior yielded significant effects (Wilson & Lipsey, 2007). When divided by type of intervention, the universal model effect size was 0.21; within these studies there were somewhat larger effects for younger children and those of lower SES. Effect size for selected and indicated interventions was 0.29; among the targeted students, those who showed greater problems showed greater improvements. In addition, behavioral strategies were more effective than cognitively oriented models. There was a significant impact of the quality of implementation on outcome with higher quality implementation related to greater effect size. The authors conclude that these effects are both statistically significant but also of practical significance and they forecast that such programs would lead to a 25–33% reduction in the base rate of aggressive problems in an average school.

A recent report from a Center for Disease Control taskforce also indicates the efficacy of universal school-based models for the prevention of violence (Hahn *et al.*, 2007). Fifty-three universal prevention studies were utilized in the meta-analysis and the median effect size was 0.15, with generally greater effect sizes with preschool and elementary school-aged children. Thus, there was substantial agreement between these two comprehensive studies that universal school-based violence prevention programs represent an important means of reducing violent and aggressive behavior in the United States as well as other countries (Adi *et al.*, 2007).

Incredible Years (IY) is an exemplary selective intervention designed to reduce child behavior problems through parent training, which focuses on improving parent competencies, parent involvement in school, and effective management of child behavior problems (see Chapter 37; Webster-Stratton & Reid, 2010). Although initially used with clinical populations, numerous studies in the United States and other countries (Brotman *et al.*, 2008; Scott *et al.*, 2010a, b; Baker-Henningham *et al.*, 2012) have shown its effectiveness in improving parenting and reducing child behavior problems with selective samples, including those at risk for maltreatment (Hurlburt *et al.*, 2013).

A second exemplary parenting model is the *Triple P Positive Parenting* program (Sanders, 2008), which employs a five-level comprehensive model using media, providing basic information, advice, and support from health workers, selective parenting groups, and treatment. One evaluation of this program employed a community level "workforce development strategy" to deliver the program across diverse family-helping agencies and showed county-wide reductions in child abuse and neglect (Prinz *et al.*, 2009). This model originated in Australia and has shown evidence of positive outcome in numerous countries (Sanders, 2008).

The *Coping Power Program* is a preventive intervention involving structured sessions for selected children and behavioral parent training groups delivered to their parenting adult(s). The program is delivered at schools in small groups with at-risk children in the late elementary school and early middle school years (Lochman, *et al.*, 2012). In most studies it has shown an impact on reducing conduct problems as well as reducing risk for substance use.

Depression

There has been a dramatic increase in the development and evaluation of both universal and targeted depression prevention models during the past decade. Although meta-analyses show inconsistency in findings, few follow-ups from universal models, and a need for further replication in school settings, in general the results show substantial effects of selective programs; however, effects vary by population and there is a need for further replication in school settings (Horowitz & Garber, 2006; Merry & Spence, 2007; Stice *et al.*, 2009; Calear & Christensen, 2010). Due to the absence of the need for screening, and the potential benefits of nondepressed peers as models, universal programs also show promise. One recent universal prevention study with US high school students illustrates that both cognitive models and interpersonal models show overall effectiveness compared to a control sample, and that students with higher pretest depression scores had the greatest reduction from intervention (Horowitz *et al.*, 2007). In contrast, a large-scale universal trial of *Beyond Blue* involving 25 secondary schools across Australia showed no effects and investigators note the difficulties in maintaining implementation quality across school settings (Sawyer *et al.*, 2010).

The *Penn Resiliency Program* (PRP; Gillham *et al.* 2008) has been one of the most widely researched depression prevention programs. A meta-analysis of 17 studies showed consistent small, but significant effects at 6- and 12-month follow-up in both universal and selective implementations (Brunwasser *et al.*, 2009). Arnarson and Craighead (2011) provide an exemplar universal study involving Icelandic children at risk for depression and showing significant reduction in the first depressive episode through one year of follow-up.

Anxiety

Anxiety disorders are the most frequent psychiatric disorders in adolescents, yet only recently have they been a focus for preventive interventions. Although there are relatively few studies that have examined preventive interventions for anxiety disorders, these programs appear quite promising (Neil & Christensen, 2009; Lau & Rapee, 2011). Both universal and indicated interventions have been conducted with populations from preschoolers through early teens and have shown significant reductions at post-test, with some effects maintained as long as two to three years after intervention. Initial studies have in some cases shown the largest impact on girls (although impact on boys is also reported) and on children around ages 11 and 12. Most of these studies have been conducted in Australia and require replication in other countries. Teubert and Pinquart (2011) conducted a recent meta-analysis of 65 trials. They reported small but significant effects on anxiety at posttest (effect size; symptoms = 0.22, diagnosis = 0.23) and follow-up (effect size; symptoms = 0.19, diagnosis = 0.32). Intervention effects at posttest varied by type of prevention. As expected, selective programs showed larger effect sizes than universal programs. As with depression prevention, there is a need for longer term follow-up of outcomes.

The *FRIENDS* program is an exemplar cognitive-behavioral universal anxiety prevention program used in school contexts (Barrett & Turner, 2011). The program involves 10 in-school sessions, 2 booster sessions, and information for parents. Across studies, the outcome from FRIENDS typically indicates a significant decrease in anxiety symptoms. Most studies in Australia have shown significant reduction in anxiety symptoms. However, there have been a few recent nonreplications in other countries (Lau & Rapee, 2011).

Early substance use

Spoth *et al.* (2008) reviewed 127 reports of prevention studies with alcohol-specific outcome measures. Most studies were in schools, taught social, cognitive, and peer resistance skills and fell into three age groups (below 10, 10–15, 16–20+). They classified interventions as "most promising evidence," "mixed or emerging evidence," and "insufficient or no evidence of impact." Twelve interventions met criteria for "most promising" and 28 met criteria for "mixed or emerging." The review indicated the need for greater emphasis on early teens, young adults not attending college, and non-majority populations, the need for longer longitudinal follow-up, replication studies, and dissemination research. Other reviews have shown that interventions in early adolescence can reduce the rates of alcohol, marijuana, other illegal drugs, and misuse of prescription drugs.

Life Skills Training is a 15-session school-based program with additional booster sessions that has been widely studied and implemented (Botvin *et al.*, 2006). When implemented with high quality it has been shown to reduce early use of alcohol, tobacco, and other drugs and has shown effects up to 5 years after intervention.

Unplugged is a universal prevention program tested in a European trial involving seven countries. Similar to LST, it is a 12 hour teacher-led program which includes interpersonal life skills through a social-cognition approach. Persisting beneficial program effects were found for past 30-day episodes of drunkenness and for frequent cannabis use (Faggiano *et al.*, 2010).

The *Strengthening Families Program: For Parents and Youth 10–14* (SFP 10–14) is a seven-session universal family-focused program that enhances parenting skills—specifically nurturance, limit setting, and communication, and youth substance refusal. SFP has shown effects on alcohol, tobacco, and illicit substance use up to 9 years after intervention (age 21) and its effects are mediated by improvements in the parent–youth relationship (Spoth *et al.*, 2012).

Promotion of social and emotional competence

Two recent meta-analyses have examined the effectiveness of universal school-based interventions (Durlak *et al.*, 2011; Sklad *et al.*, 2012). Durlak's analysis of US programs indicated that SEL (social and emotional learning) interventions have a substantial impact (effects sizes 0.15–0.35) on a variety of outcomes including aggression and disruption, social and emotional competence, school bonding, prosocial norms, disciplinary referrals, emotional distress, and academic achievement. Sklad's analysis included 25% of programs outside the United States and showed somewhat higher effect sizes at posttest and follow-up. It should be noted that few interventions that focus on promoting positive development or citizenship have been evaluated.

The *PATHS Curriculum* is a widely studied universal SEL program for preschool and elementary school-aged children. It is provided by classroom teachers and focuses on emotional awareness, self-control and social problem-solving. A series of RCTs have shown significant, modest improvements in prosocial behavior and reductions in aggressive/disruptive behaviors, and depressive symptoms as well as improvements in executive functions and classroom atmosphere (Kusché & Greenberg, 2012).

Event-triggered prevention: the prevention of trauma

A variety of selective prevention programs have been developed to support resilience in children who have experienced events that place them at risk (e.g., divorce, death of a parent, and trauma resulting from war or refugee status—see Chapter 59). Although these programs have different foci and techniques, results are quite promising. For example, studies have shown reduction in PTSD symptoms and depression in Israeli children subject to terrorist attacks (Gelkopf & Berger, 2009), Israeli students subject to ongoing rocket attacks (Wolmer *et al.*, 2011; Berger *et al.*, 2012), Russian children taken hostage in a school siege (Vetter *et al.*, 2010), and US children who experienced a potentially traumatic event (Berkowitz *et al.*, 2011). On the other hand, mixed results were found in a study of children experiencing war exposure in Sri Lanka (Tol *et al.*, 2012). Given the plight of refugee children in many countries, there is a need to develop further interventions to prevent and/or reduce the effects of PTSD (Pacione *et al.*, 2013; Schneider *et al.*, 2013).

The *New Beginnings Program* (NBP) (Wolchik *et al.*, 2007) is an 11-session program with the residential parent designed to improve children's coping with divorce by strengthening parenting. At six-year follow-up, youth in the NBP had lower rates of diagnosed mental disorder, less substance use and risky sexual behavior, and higher school grades.

Birth to five: early prevention

During the past three decades attention has focused on the effects of early prevention for children living in poverty or other at-risk circumstances (Manning *et al.*, 2010). Broadly, three types of programs have been effective in reducing early maltreatment and other early outcomes related to later mental disorders. First, high-quality home visiting programs beginning prenatally or after birth have demonstrated long-term impacts on both children and parents (MacMillan *et al.*, 2009; Olds, 2010). Second, preschool parenting interventions have reduced conduct problems both in group (Webster-Stratton & Reid, 2010) and individual contexts (Toth & Gravener, 2012) utilizing both attachment-focused and cognitive-behavioral orientations (Furlong *et al.*, 2013). Third, quality preschool experience has lowered risk for MEBDs and promoted healthy functioning into adulthood (Reynolds *et al.*, 2010). All three types of interventions have been found to have a high benefit-to-cost ratio (Conti & Heckman, 2012; Lee *et al.*, 2012).

The *Nurse Family Partnership* is a nurse-led home visiting intervention for first-time mothers at risk as a result of poverty and other risk factors (Olds, 2010). It has been tested in three RCTs in the United States. The intervention begins prenatally and ends at age 2 with a focus on both mother's life course and the mother–child relationship. This intensive intervention has resulted in lower rates of neglect and abuse, and lower rates of drug and alcohol use and arrests for the children in the transition to adulthood. In one trial, visited children showed higher school achievement at age 9.

Family Foundations is a universal eight-session intervention for expectant parents delivered through before and after birth by childbirth education departments (Feinberg *et al.*, 2010). The program prepares couples for parenthood by fostering attitudes and skills related to positive parenting teamwork (called "coparenting"). Through age 3, effects include reduced parental stress, depression, and harsh parenting, and improved child social competence. Significant effects were found for boys on child behavior problems and couple relationship quality.

Prevention in lower and lower-middle income countries

Mental health services for children in most lower and middle income countries (LAMIC) are scarce (see Chapters 16 and 44). An essential question is whether preventive interventions developed in Western technological societies will be transferable (albeit with modifications) to LAMI countries. During the past decade there has been a substantial rise in the number of preventive interventions focused on mental health in such countries

as Tanzania (Hermenau *et al.*, 2012), Iran (Oveisi *et al.*, 2010), Mauritius (Rivet-Duval *et al.*, 2011), and Romania (Stefan & Miclea, 2013). Mejia *et al.* (2012) provide a thoughtful discussion of the numerous issues in program modification and implementation. Future research should focus on the adaptation of existing programs and the development of indigenous, local programs.

Key issues in current prevention research

Researchers have paid increasing attention to improving methodology and most studies now use randomized designs that enhance the credibility of the outcomes. Nevertheless, the field has significant gaps that need to be addressed.

Limited longitudinal studies

One important issue is the collection of data over extended periods of time to track the longitudinal effects at different stages of development. This is especially important for universal studies as few children in a whole population have, or are at risk for, a disorder. Thus, the follow-up period should be sufficiently long in order to "allow" the control populations to develop symptoms/disorders. For example, if studies of the immunization of polio only provided a 6-month follow-up, it is likely that one would conclude that immunization was ineffective. One would need to follow the control (nonimmunized) population long enough for a substantial number of cases to manifest in order to document the vaccine effectiveness.

The need for independent replication studies

There has been substantial controversy regarding potential publication bias and the lack of independent replication of programs and policies (Holder, 2009; Axford & Morpeth, 2013). Surely, the concern regarding the potential bias introduced by studies that are not independent of the developer is a key issue (Eisner, 2009; Olds, 2009) and there is a need to verify findings in independent trials.

Limited long-term economic assessments have been conducted to date; however, existing cost–benefit analyses clearly indicate that EBIs (evidence-based intervention) can be cost effective (Lee *et al.*, 2012). This has yet to lead to a large-scale shift in policy to support widespread EBI dissemination and implementation. It is notable that few evaluations have assessed the costs and benefits of building the infrastructure necessary to successfully install and sustain large-scale prevention efforts (Crowley *et al.*, 2012). It is more likely that when research is conducted within actual service settings capable of sustainability, key factors relevant to economic outcomes will be included in evaluations. Given their relatively low cost, such analyses could be particularly important for universal and selective interventions.

Limited study of factors that moderate effects

It is essential to understand the factors that may moderate (i.e., increase or decrease) the magnitude of intervention effect.

This is especially important for universal interventions that target all members of a certain population. Is the intervention equally effective for all members of the population, regardless of their level of risk for mental health problems? Such analyses are necessary as it is unlikely that intervention effects are uniform for participants (Brown & Liao, 1999; Scott & O'Connor, 2012; Brody *et al.*, 2014).

Consistent standards for evidence and research reporting

Consistent standards for evaluating interventions, conducting replication trials, and reporting results are needed (Flay *et al.*, 2005). Although no single method fits all interventions, standards should include study design components such as randomization (where feasible); using multiple, unbiased reporters; examining follow-up effects; and fully reporting outcome data. Accordingly, an intervention could be considered efficacious if it produced consistent and statistically significant findings in high-quality, independent studies and the findings have public health significance. To be considered disseminable, an intervention also would provide manuals or training programs that allow it to be implemented by third parties and evaluated under real-world conditions (Flay *et al.*, 2005). To date, few intervention research programs meet these standards. The UN Office on Drug and Crime has recommended international standards for drug abuse prevention and similar standards are needed in mental health (UNODC, 2013).

Need for improved standards concerning intervention replications and cultural adaptations

When replication studies are conducted, standards are needed for judging when a study is truly a replication or when substantial program modifications would mean the study no longer qualifies as a replication (Valentine *et al.*, 2011). As preventive interventions are transported across cultures and contexts, there is a need to adapt and modify the interventions, at least in terms of their surface structure (Moore *et al.*, 2013). Conceptual and practical guidelines for the cultural adaptations are available and there are numerous examples of such adaptations (Castro *et al.*, 2004; Ferrer-Wreder *et al.*, 2012; Colby *et al.*, 2013). Studies are needed to examine the effects of systematic variations of the original intervention to understand the influence of culture and context and its generalizability.

Metrics for reporting and levels of prevention

Clear metrics are needed to report outcomes to the public and policy makers, and this may differ depending upon the level of prevention. Effect size may be the best metric for selective interventions, where participants begin with greater risk or symptoms and thus show greater change. However, it may be a poor metric for universal interventions where a large percentage of the population begins without symptoms and thus it is unlikely to show change. In most cases, it is only in the higher risk/symptom groups that larger effect sizes will be obtained (Wilson & Lipsey, 2007).

Thus, for universal interventions, other risk reduction metrics, potentially in combination with thoughtful use of effect sizes, are more appropriate (Davis *et al.*, 2003). For example, a universal depression program may reduce diagnoses from 10% to 5% of the population; thus, risk reduction would indicate a 50% reduction in prevalence. However, if 90% of the population shows no depression, the effect size for the entire population will surely be in the "small" range. Shamblen and Derzon (2009) use a population level adjustment model to illustrate the different interpretations that can be made from the same effect sizes. Thus, comparing effect sizes of selective versus universal programs to conclude which may be more effective is problematic (Horowitz & Garber, 2006).

Dissemination, implementation and sustainability; Type 2 questions

Much of the research covered is classified as Type 1 research: understanding basic developmental mechanisms and applying this research to the development, testing, and refinement of preventive interventions. As a growing number of programs have shown efficacy in controlled trials, the next stage in prevention research is studying program effectiveness under real-world conditions (Institute of Medicine, 2009) or with the use of new delivery models such as use of the Internet or telemedicine. There is also a significant gap between the availability of such preventive interventions and their widespread implementation across communities and nations (Glasgow *et al.*, 2003; Rhoades *et al.*, 2012).

Type 2 translation research investigates the complex processes and systems through which EBIs are adopted, implemented, and sustained on a large scale, as well as devising empirically driven strategies for increasing their population impact. Spoth *et al.* (2013a, b) have proposed a heuristic model, the Translation Science to Population Impact (TSci Impact) Framework, to conceptualize research and practice issues related to the four phases of pre-adoption, adoption, implementation, and sustainability.

In the preadoption phase, there are numerous issues including how information on EBIs is diffused by governments and NGOs, and understanding the communication channels used by prospective adopters. One strategy for assisting the diffusion process is to provide agencies, schools, and communities with guidelines and recommendations for choosing among EBIs. Numerous best-practice guidelines and reports have been published in the United States (e.g., Blueprints for Violence Prevention; National Registry of Evidence-based Programs and Practices (http://www.nrepp.samhsa.gov/), in Europe (Fundacion Marcelino Botin, 2008), and the United Kingdom (Allen, 2011). However, the lack of well-standardized criteria for selecting "model" or "effective" programs can be confusing to prospective adopters.

The selection of evidence-based prevention strategies is just the first step to achieving widespread, high-quality, and sustained prevention programming. Once selected, adopters require expert training and technical assistance to ensure high-fidelity implementation. Adopters must ensure that they are faithfully replicating the core intervention components and ongoing monitoring and technical assistance are necessary to ensure that implementation is congruent with the core principles associated with program success (Kelly & Perkins, 2012). Finally, to achieve population-level outcomes, communities must learn how to effectively recruit interventions participants via large-scale media or marketing campaigns. Implementation challenges will inevitably occur and communities will be more successful when they increase their capacity for effective implementation and are provided with proactive technical assistance to carefully monitor program needs. A key issue in implementation is the need to adapt EBIs to create a better fit with the nature of public mental health and social service systems (Little, 2010). This requires that public systems and program developers work together to understand issues of scaling as they design, test, and implement new interventions. To achieve long-term success, organizations need to enhance their internal capacity to support preventive interventions.

As effective programs become more widely adopted, the need for strategies to enhance their long-term sustainability becomes increasingly important. Program sustainability can be threatened by many causes, including implementation challenges, loss of funding, and changes in priorities among key players. Moving from funding based on discretionary, short-term grants to more stable funding streams is a substantial challenge. Research regarding the conditions which facilitate or undermine sustainability is only beginning to emerge. A study of 67 EBIs funded in Pennsylvania found that 5 years after state funding withdrawal, 45% of programs were operating at the same or a higher level, 22% at a reduced level, and 33% were no longer operating (Tibbits et al., 2010). Other research has indicated that long-term sustainability is associated with strong levels of staff and leaders support; widespread belief in the benefits of the innovation; and a strong integration between the new innovation and the agency's mission, schedule of services, and staffing profile (Scheirer & Dearing, 2011; Greenberg & Lippold, 2013). These factors also promote the adoption and quality implementation of new programs, indicating that efforts to increase organizational capacity for prevention can increase the likelihood of widespread, high-quality, and sustained prevention programming.

Adopting public health impact-oriented models

Methods for increasing the general and specific capacity of local communities to undertake successful prevention are only now beginning to emerge. Strong collaborations between researchers, practitioners, and governments are necessary to achieve this goal. One model is to develop an intermediary organization between government and local communities to support quality implementation and sustainability as conceptualized by Wandersman et al. (2008). Bumbarger and Campbell (2012) illustrate such a model from a decade-long partnership in Pennsylvania. In the United States and Europe, models have also been developed to create community-level infrastructure to facilitate prevention efforts including the Communities That Care (CTC) and The PROmoting School-community-university Partnerships to Enhance Resilience (PROSPER) models (Catalano et al., 2012). CTC includes structured training workshops and proactive technical assistance to assist communities in conducting needs assessments, selecting, and implementing EBIs that address these needs. The PROSPER model seeks to increase community capacity by explicitly linking community stakeholders with land-grant university faculty and researchers that undertake prevention activities in local schools (Spoth et al., 2013a). Both CTC and PROSPER have been moderately successful in enhancing community collaboration to undertake prevention activities, reducing rates of problem behaviors among youth, and sustaining prevention activities over time (Hawkins et al., 2012; Spoth et al., 2013a).

Conclusion

During the past two decades, prevention science has emerged as a new multidisciplinary science. Research primarily in high-income countries has demonstrated that major mental health problems can be moderately reduced through population-level preventive interventions as well as through programs that selectively intervene with children already at risk due to early behavioral risk and experience/context. However, few of these interventions have reached the status of "business as usual" in mental health or social service systems and only a small number of interventions have shown consistent outcomes. The expansion and broad use of these interventions will require changes in policy and practice, as well as further demonstrations of cost-effectiveness. New research is needed to understand for whom these interventions are most effective as well as how to modify interventions to fit cultural circumstances. Policy work is necessary to inform government officials regarding the importance of EBIs that have the potential to reduce health spending and other social costs. To create widespread adoption in LAMI countries, it is necessary to understand if there are unique risk and protective factors that might lead to new or modified interventions that better suit these contexts. Governments, agencies, schools, and local communities will vary in their capacity to incorporate EBIs into service systems and schools. A future goal of the field is to identify approaches that promote the readiness and capacity of prospective stakeholders to adopt effective interventions in a coordinated manner, implement them effectively, and sustain them over time. Such systematic process will be necessary to substantially reduce the public health burden and improve community-level well-being.

References

Adi, Y. *et al.* (2007). *A systematic review of interventions to promote mental wellbeing in children in primary education: Report 1: Universal approaches non-violence related outcomes.* University of Warwick, Report. Available: http://www.nice.org.uk/guidance/index.jsp?action=download&o=43911

Allen, G. (2011). *Early intervention: the next steps, An independent report to Her Majesty's Government.* HM Government. Available: https://www.gov.uk/government/news/graham-allen-launches-second-report-on-early-intervention

Arnarson, E.O. & Craighead, W.E. (2011) Prevention of depression among Icelandic adolescents: a 12-month follow-up. *Behaviour Research and Therapy* **49**, 170–174.

Axford, N. & Morpeth, L. (2013) Evidence-based programs in children's services: a critical appraisal. *Children and Youth Services Review* **35**, 268–277.

Baker-Henningham, H. *et al.* (2012) Reducing child conduct problems and promoting social skills a middle-income country: cluster randomised controlled trial. *British Journal of Psychiatry* **201**, 101–108.

Barrett, P. & Turner, C. (2011) Prevention of anxiety symptoms in primary school children: preliminary results from a universal school-based trial. *British Journal of Clinical Psychology* **40**, 399–410.

Belfer, M.L. (2008) Child and adolescent mental disorders: the magnitude of the problem across the globe. *Journal of Child Psychology and Psychiatry* **49**, 226–36.

Berger, R. *et al.* (2012) A teacher-delivered intervention for adolescents exposed to ongoing and intense traumatic war-related stress: a quasi-randomized controlled study. *Journal of Adolescent Health* **51**, 453–462.

Berkowitz, S.J. *et al.* (2011) The Child and Family Traumatic Stress Intervention: secondary prevention for youth at risk of developing PTSD. *Journal of Child Psychology and Psychiatry* **52**, 676–685.

Biglan, A. *et al.* (2012) The critical role of nurturing environments for promoting human well-being. *American Psychologist* **67**, 257–271.

Blair, C. (2002) School readiness: integrating cognition and emotion in a neurobiological conceptualization of children's functioning at school entry. *American Psychologist* **57**, 111–127.

Botvin, G.J. *et al.* (2006) Preventing youth violence and delinquency through a universal school-based prevention approach. *Prevention Science* **7**, 403–408.

Bradshaw, C.P. *et al.* (2012) Infusing developmental neuroscience into school-based preventive interventions: implications and future directions. *Journal of Adolescent Health* **51**, S41–S47.

Brody, G.H. *et al.* (2014) Differential sensitivity to prevention programming: a dopaminergic polymorphism-enhanced prevention effect on protective parenting and adolescent substance use. *Health Psychology* **33**, 182–191.

Bronfenbrenner, U. (1995) Developmental ecology through space and time: a future perspective. In: *Examining Lives in Context.* (eds P. Moen, G.H. Elder, Jr., & K. Luscher), pp. 619–647. American Psychological Association, Washington, DC.

Brotman, L.M. *et al.* (2008) Preventive intervention for preschoolers at high risk for antisocial behavior: long-term effects on child physical aggression and parenting practices. *Journal of Clinical Child Adolescent Psychology* **37**, 386–96.

Brown, C.H. & Liao, J. (1999) Principles for designing randomized preventive trials in mental health: an emerging developmental epidemiology paradigm. *American Journal of Community Psychology* **27**, 673–710.

Brunwasser, S.M. *et al.* (2009) A meta analytic review of the Penn Resiliency Program's effect on depressive symptoms. *Journal of Consulting and Clinical Psychology* **77**, 1042–1054.

Bumbarger, B.K. & Campbell, E.M. (2012) A state agency-university partnership for translational research and the dissemination of evidence-based prevention and intervention. *Administration and Policy in Mental Health and Mental Health Services Research* **39**, 268–277.

Calear, A.L. & Christensen, H. (2010) Systematic review of school-based prevention and early intervention programs for depression. *Journal of Adolescence* **33**, 429–438.

Castro, F.G. *et al.* (2004) The cultural adaptation of preventive interventions: resolving tensions between fidelity and fit. *Prevention Science* **5**, 41–45.

Catalano, R.F. *et al.* (2012) Adolescent health: global application of the prevention science research base. *Lancet* **379**, 1653–1664.

Cicchetti, D. & Cohen, D.J. (1995) *Developmental Psychopathology.* John Wiley & Sons, New York.

Coie, J.D. *et al.* (1993) The science of prevention: a conceptual framework and some directions for a national research program. *American Psychologist* **48**, 1013–1022.

Colby, M. *et al.* (2013) Adapting school based substance use prevention curriculum through cultural grounding. *American Journal of Community Psychology* **51**, 190–205.

Collaborative for Academic, Social, and Emotional Learning (CASEL) (2003). *Safe and sound: an educational leader's guide to evidence-based social and emotional learning programs.* Available: http://www.casel.org.

Conti, G. & Heckman, J.J. (2012). The economics of child well-being. National Bureau of Economic Research.

Crowley, D.M. *et al.* (2012) Resource consumption of a dissemination model for prevention programs: the PROSPER delivery system. *Journal of Adolescent Health* **50**, 256–263.

Davidson, R.J. *et al.* (2003) Alterations in brain and immune function produced by mindfulness meditation. *Psychosomatic Medicine* **65**, 564–570.

Davis, C.H. *et al.* (2003) Cumulative risk and population attributable fraction in prevention. *Journal of Clinical Child and Adolescent Psychology* **32**, 228–235.

Diamond, A. & Lee, K. (2011) Interventions shown to aid executive function development in children 4 to 12 years old. *Science* **333**, 959–964.

Durlak, J.A. (1995) *School-Based Prevention Programs for Children and Adolescents.* Sage, Thousand Oaks, CA.

Durlak, J.A. *et al.* (2011) The impact of enhancing students' social and emotional learning: a meta-analysis of school-based universal interventions. *Child Development* **82**, 405–432.

Eisner, M. (2009) No effects in independent prevention trials: can we reject the cynics' hypothesis? *Journal of Experimental Criminology* **5**, 163–183.

Ellis, B.J. *et al.* (2011) Differential susceptibility to the environment: an evolutionary–neurodevelopmental theory. *Development and Psychopathology* **23**, 7–28.

Fagan, A.A. *et al.* (2007) Using community and family risk and protective factors for community-based prevention planning. *Journal of Community Psychology* **35**, 535–555.

Faggiano, F. *et al.* (2010) The effectiveness of a school-based substance abuse prevention program: 18-month follow-up of the EU-Dap cluster randomized controlled trial. *Drug and Alcohol Dependence* **108**, 56–64.

Feinberg, M.E. (2012) Community epidemiology of risk and adolescent substance use: practical questions for enhancing prevention. *American Journal of Public Health* **102**, 457–468.

Feinberg, M.E. *et al.* (2010) Effects of a transition to parenthood program on parents, parenting, and children: 3.5 years after baseline. *Journal of Family Psychology* **24**, 532–542.

Ferrer-Wreder, L. *et al.* (2012) Tinkering with perfection: theory development in the intervention of cultural adaptation field. *Child Youth Care Forum* **41**, 149–171.

Flay, B.R. *et al.* (2005) Standards of evidence: criteria for efficacy, effectiveness and dissemination. *Prevention Science* **6**, 151–175.

Fundacion Marcelino Botin. (2008). *Social and emotional education: an international analysis.* Santander, Spain.

Furlong, M. *et al.* (2013) Cochrane review: behavioural and cognitive-behavioural group-based parenting programmes for early-onset conduct problems in children aged 3 to 12 years. *Evidence Based Child Health* **8**, 318–692.

Gelkopf, M. & Berger, R. (2009) A school-based, teacher-mediated prevention program (ERASE-Stress) for reducing terror-related traumatic reactions in Israeli youth: a quasi-randomized controlled trial. *Journal of Child Psychology and Psychiatry* **50**, 962–71.

Gillham, J.E. *et al.* (2008) Preventing depression in early adolescence: the Penn Resiliency Program. In: *Handbook of Depression in Children and Adolescents.* (eds J.R.Z. Abela & B.L. Hankin), pp. 309–322. Guilford Press, New York.

Glasgow, R.E. *et al.* (2003) Why don't we see more translation of health promotion research to practice? Rethinking the efficacy-to-effectiveness transition. *American Journal of Public Health* **93**, 1261–1267.

Green, L.W. (2006) Public health asks of systems science: to advance our evidence-based practice, can you help us get more practice-based evidence. *American Journal of Public Health* **96**, 406–413.

Greenberg, M.T. & Harris, A.R. (2011) Nurturing mindfulness in children and youth: current state of research. *Child Development Perspectives* **6**, 161–166.

Greenberg, M.T. & Lippold, M.A. (2013) Promoting healthy outcomes among youth with multiple risks: innovative approaches. *Annual Review of Public Health* **34**, 253–270.

Greenberg, M.T. *et al.* (1993) The role of attachment in the early development of disruptive behavior problems. *Development and Psychopathology* **5**, 191–213.

Greenberg, M.T. *et al.* (2001) The prevention of mental disorders in school-age children: current state of the field. *Prevention & Treatment* **4**, 1–62.

Hahn, R. *et al.* (2007) Effectiveness of universal school-based programs to prevent violent and aggressive behavior: a systematic review. *American Journal of Preventive Medicine* **33**, s114–s129.

Hawkins, J.D. *et al.* (2005) Promoting positive adult functioning through social development intervention in childhood: long-term effects from the Seattle Social Development Project. *Archives of Pediatrics & Adolescent Medicine* **159**, 25–31.

Hawkins, J.D. *et al.* (2012) Sustained decreases in risk exposure and youth problem behaviors after installation of the Communities That Care prevention system in a randomized trial. *Archives of Pediatrics and Adolescent Medicine* **166**, 141–148.

Henggeler, S.W. & Sheidow, A.J. (2012) Empirically supported family-based treatments for conduct disorder and delinquency in adolescents. *Journal of Marital and Family Therapy* **38**, 30–58.

Hermenau, K. *et al.* (2012) Childhood adversity, mental ill-health and aggressive behavior in an African orphanage: changes in response to trauma-focused therapy and the implementation of a new instructional system. *Child and Adolescent Psychiatry and Mental Health* **5**, 29–38.

Hoagwood, K.E. *et al.* (2007) Empirically based school interventions target at academic and mental health functioning. *Journal of Emotional and Behavioral Disorders* **15**, 66–94.

Holder, H. (2009) Prevention programs in the 21st century: what we do not discuss in public. *Addiction* **105**, 578–581.

Horowitz, J.L. & Garber, J. (2006) The prevention of depressive symptoms in children and adolescents: a meta-analytic review. *Journal of Consulting and Clinical Psychology* **74**, 401–415.

Horowitz, J.L. *et al.* (2007) Prevention of depressive symptoms in adolescents: a randomized trial of cognitive–behavioral and interpersonal prevention programs. *Journal of Consulting and Clinical Psychology* **75**, 693–706.

Hurlburt, M.S. *et al.* (2013). Efficacy of the Incredible Years group parent program with families in Head Start who self-reported a history of child maltreatment. *Child Abuse & Neglect* **37**, 531–543.

Ialongo, N.S. *et al.* (2006) A developmental psychopathology approach to the prevention of mental health disorders. In: *Developmental Psychopathology, Vol1: Theory and method.* (eds D. Cicchetti & J.D. Cohen), 2nd edn, pp. 968–1018. John Wiley & Sons, Hoboken, NJ.

Institute of Medicine (2009) *Preventing Mental, Emotional, and Behavioral Disorders Among Young People: progress and Possibilities.* (eds M.E. O'Connell, T. Boat & K.E. Warner). The National Academies Press, Washington, DC.

Jaffee, S.R. & Price, T.S. (2007) Gene-environment correlations: a review of the evidence and implications for prevention of mental illness. *Molecular Psychiatry* **12**, 1432–1442.

Kellam, S.G. *et al.* (2008) Effects of a universal classroom behavior management program in first and second grades on young adult behavioral, psychiatric, and social outcomes. *Drug and Alcohol Dependence* **95**, S5–S28.

Kelly, B. & Perkins, D.F. (2012) *Handbook of Implementation Science for Psychology in Education.* Cambridge University Press, New York.

Knopf, D. *et al.* (2008) *The Mental Health of Adolescents: A National Profile.* National Adolescent Health Information Center, San Francisco, CA.

Kusché, C. & Greenberg, M.T. (2012) The PATHS Curriculum: promoting emotional literacy, prosocial behavior, and caring classrooms. In: *The Handbook of School Violence and School Safety: International Research and Practice.* (eds S.R. Jimerson, *et al.*), pp. 435–446. Routledge, New York.

Lau, E.X. & Rapee, R.M. (2011) Prevention of anxiety disorders. *Current Psychiatric Report* **13**, 258–266.

Lee, S. *et al.* (2012) *Return on Investment: Evidence-Based Options to Improve Statewide Outcomes, April 2012 (Document No. 12-04-1201). Washington State Institute for Public Policy*, Olympia, WA.

Little, M. (2010) *Proof Positive*. Demos, London.

Lochman, J.E. *et al.* (2012) Cognitive-behavioral intervention for anger and aggression: the Coping Power Program. In: *Handbook of School Violence and School Safety: International Research and Practice*. (eds S.R. Jimerson, A.B. Nickerson, M.J. Mayer & M.J. Furlong), 2nd edn, pp. 579–591. Routledge, New York, NY.

Lösel, F. & Farrington, D.P. (2012) Direct protective and buffering protective factors in the development of youth violence. *American Journal of Preventive Medicine* **43**, S8–S23.

MacMillan, H.L. *et al.* (2009) Interventions to prevent child maltreatment and associated impairment. *Lancet* **373**, 251–266.

Manning, M. *et al.* (2010) A meta-analysis of the effects of early developmental prevention programs in at-risk populations on non-health outcomes in adolescence. *Children and Youth Services Review* **32**, 506–519.

Mejia, A. *et al.* (2012) A review of parenting programs in developing countries: opportunities and challenges for preventing emotional and behavioral difficulties in children. *Clinical Child & Family Psychology Review* **15**, 163–175.

Merry, S.N. & Spence, S.H. (2007) Attempting to prevent depression in youth: a systematic review of the evidence. *Early Intervention in Psychiatry* **1**, 128–137.

Moore, J.E. *et al.* (2013) Examining adaptations of evidence-based programs in natural contexts. *Journal of Primary Prevention* **34**, 147–161.

Neil, A.L. & Christensen, H. (2009) Efficacy and effectiveness of school-based prevention and early intervention programs for anxiety. *Clinical Psychology Review* **29**, 208–215.

Offord, D.R. *et al.* (1998) Lowering the burden of suffering from child psychiatric disorder: trade-offs among clinical, targeted, and universal interventions. *Journal of the American Academy of Child and Adolescent Psychiatry* **37**, 686–694.

Olds, D. (2009) In support of disciplined passion. *Journal of Experimental Criminology* **5**, 201–214.

Olds, D.L. (2010) The Nurse-Family Partnership: from trials to practice. In: *Childhood Programs and Practices in the First Decade of Life: A Human Capital Integration*, pp. 49–75. Cambridge University Press, New York.

Oveisi, S. *et al.* (2010) Primary prevention of parent–child conflict and abuse in Iranian mothers: a randomized-controlled trial. *Child Abuse and Neglect* **34**, 206–213.

Pacione, L. *et al.* (2013) Refugee children: mental health and effective interventions. *Current Psychiatric Report* **15**, 341–350.

Prinz, R.J. *et al.* (2009) Population-based prevention of child maltreatment: the U.S. Triple P system population trial. *Prevention Science* **10**, 1–12.

Reynolds, A. *et al.* (2010) Preschool-to-third grade programs and practices: a review of research. *Child and Youth Services Review* **32**, 1121–1131.

Rhoades, B.L. *et al.* (2012) The role of a state-level prevention support system in promoting high-quality implementation and sustainability of evidence-based programs. *American Journal of Community Psychology* **50**, 386–401.

Riggs, N.R. *et al.* (2006) The mediational role of neurocognition in the behavioral outcomes of a social–emotional prevention program in elementary school students: effects of the PATHS Curriculum. *Prevention Science* **7**, 91–102.

Rivet-Duval, E. *et al.* (2011) Preventing adolescent depression in Mauritius: a universal school-based program. *Child and Adolescent Mental Health* **16**, 86–91.

Rose, G. (1985) Sick individuals and sick populations. *International Journal of Epidemiology* **14**, 32–38.

Rutter, M. (1979) Protective factors in children's responses to stress and disadvantage. *Annals of Academy of Medicine, Singapore* **8**, 324–328.

Rutter, M. (1982) Prevention of children's psychosocial disorders: myth and substance. *Pediatrics* **70**, 883–894.

Sameroff, A.J. *et al.* (1987) Intelligence quotient scores of 4-year-old children: social-environmental risk factors. *Pediatrics* **79**, 343–350.

Sanders, M. (2008) Triple-P Positive Parenting Program as a public health approach to strengthening parenting. *Journal of Family Psychology* **22**, 506–517.

Sandler, I.N. *et al.* (2011) Long-term impact of prevention programs to promote effective parenting: lasting effects but uncertain processes. *Annual Review of Psychology* **62**, 299–329.

Sawyer, M.G. *et al.* (2010) School-based prevention of depression: a randomized controlled study of the beyond blueschools research initiative. *Journal of Child and Psychology and Psychiatry* **51**, 199–209.

Scheirer, M.A. & Dearing, J.W. (2011) An agenda for research on the sustainability of public health programs. *American Journal of Public Health* **101**, 2059–2067.

Schneider, S.J. *et al.* (2013) Evidence-based treatments for traumatized children and adolescents. *Current Psychiatric Report* **15**, 332–341.

Scott, S. & O'Connor, T.G. (2012) An experimental test of differential susceptibility to parenting among emotionally dysregulated children in a randomized controlled trial for oppositional behavior. *Journal of Child Psychology and Psychiatry* **53**, 1184–1193.

Scott, S. *et al.* (2010a) Impact of a parenting program in a high-risk, multi-ethnic community: the PALS trial. *Journal of Child Psychology and Psychiatry* **51**, 1331–1341.

Scott, S. *et al.* (2010b) Randomized controlled trial of parent groups for child antisocial behaviour targeting multiple risk factors: the SPOKES project. *Journal of Child Psychology and Psychiatry* **51**, 48–57.

Shamblen, S.R. & Derzon, J.H. (2009) A preliminary study of the population-adjusted effectiveness of substance abuse prevention programming: towards making IOM program types comparable. *Journal of Primary Prevention* **30**, 89–107.

Sklad, M. *et al.* (2012) Effectiveness of school-based social, emotional, and behavioural programs: do they enhance students' development in the area of skill, behavior, and adjustment? *Psychology in the Schools* **49**, 892–909.

Spoth, R.L. *et al.* (2008) Preventive interventions addressing underage drinking: state of the evidence and steps toward public health impact. *Pediatrics* **121**, S311–S336.

Spoth, R.L. *et al.* (2012) Benefits of universal intervention effects on a youth protective shield 10 years after baseline. *Journal of Adolescent Health* **50**, 414–417.

Spoth, R. *et al.* (2013a) Longitudinal effects of universal PROSPER community–university partnership delivery system effects on substance misuse through $6\frac{1}{2}$ years past baseline from a cluster randomized controlled intervention trial. *Preventive Medicine*, **56**, 190–196.

Spoth, R. *et al.* (2013b) Addressing challenges for the next generation of Type 2 translation research: the translation science to population impact framework. *Prevention Science* **14**, 319–351.

Stefan, C.A. & Miclea, M. (2013) Effects of a multifocused prevention program on preschool children's competencies and behavior problems. *Psychology in the School* **50**, 382–402.

Stice, E. *et al.* (2009) A meta-analytic review of depression prevention programs for children and adolescents: factors that predict magnitude of intervention effects. *Journal of Consulting and Clinical Psychology* **77**, 486–503.

Tenant, R. *et al.* (2007) A systematic review of interventions to promote mental health and prevent mental health problems in children and young people. *Journal of Public Mental Health* **6**, 25–34.

Teubert, D. & Pinquart, M. (2011) A meta-analytic review on the prevention of symptoms of anxiety in children and adolescents. *Journal of Anxiety Disorders* **25**, 1046–1059.

Tibbits, M.K. *et al.* (2010) Sustaining evidence-based interventions under real-world conditions: results from a large-scale diffusion project. *Prevention Science* **11**, 252–262.

Tol, W.A. *et al.* (2012) Outcomes and moderators of a preventive school-based mental health intervention for children affected by war in Sri Lanka: a cluster randomized trial. *World Psychiatry* **11**, 114–122.

Toth, S. & Gravener, J. (2012) Review: bridging research and practice: relational interventions for maltreated children. *Child and Adolescent Mental Health* **17**, 131–138.

United Nations Office of Drugs and Crime (2013). International standards on drug use prevention. Available: http://www.unodc.org/unodc/en/prevention/prevention-standards.html

Valentine, J.C. *et al.* (2011) Replication in prevention science. *Prevention Science* **12**, 103–117.

Vetter, S. *et al.* (2010) Impact of resilience enhancing programs on youth surviving the Beslan school siege. *Child and Adolescent Psychiatry and Mental Health* **4**, 1–11.

Vitaro, F. & Tremblay, R.E. (2008) Clarifying and maximizing the usefulness of targeted preventive interventions. In: *Rutter's Child and Adolescent Psychiatry.* (eds M. Rutter, *et al.*), 5th edn, pp. 989–1008. Wiley-Blackwell, London.

Wandersman, A. *et al.* (2008) Bridging the gap between prevention research and practice: the interactive systems framework for dissemination and implementation. *American Journal of Community Psychology* **41**, 171–181.

Webster-Stratton, C. & Reid, M.J. (2010) The incredible years parents, teachers and children training series: a multifaceted treatment approach for young children with conduct problems. In: *Evidence-Based Psychotherapies for Children and Adolescents.* (eds J. Weisz & A. Kazdin), 2nd edn, pp. 194–210. Guilford Press, New York.

Wilson, S.J. & Lipsey, M.J. (2007) Effectiveness of school-based intervention programs on aggressive behavior: update of a meta-analysis. *American Journal of Preventive Medicine* **33**, S130–S143.

Wolchik, S.A. *et al.* (2007) New beginnings: an empirically-based program to help divorced mothers promote resilience in their children. In: *Handbook of Parent Training: Helping Parents Prevent and Solve Problem Behaviors.* (eds J.M. Briesmeister & C.E. Schaefer), pp. 25–62. John Wiley & Sons, New York.

Wolmer, L. *et al.* (2011) Preventing children's posttraumatic stress after disaster with teacher-based intervention: a controlled study. *Journal of the American Academy of Child and Adolescent Psychiatry* **50**, 340–348.

World Health Organization. (2006). *Projections of Mortality and Burden of Disease to 2030, Projected Deaths for 2005, 2015 and 2030 by Country Income Group Under the Baseline Scenario.* Geneva, Switz. Available: http://www.who.int/entity/healthinfo/statistics/bod_deathbyincome.xls

World Health Organization. (2009) *Disease and Injury Regional Estimates for 2004.* Geneva, Switz. Available: http://www.who.int/healthinfo/global_burden_disease/estimates_regional/en/index.html

Yoshikawa, H. *et al.* (2012) The effects of poverty on the mental, emotional, and behavioral health of children and youth: implications for prevention. *American Psychologist* **67**, 272–284.

CHAPTER 18

Health economics

Martin Knapp[1] and Sara Evans-Lacko[2]

[1] Department of Social Policy, London School of Economics and Political Science, UK
[2] Institute of Psychiatry, Psychology and Neuroscience, King's College London, UK

Introduction

For better or for worse, money is a key consideration in policy and practice discussions, even if it sometimes lurks just below the surface. Although the professional delivering one-to-one therapy, or prescribing a course of medication or arranging a group activity might not have to be concerned about the associated costs, further along the management chain someone will be watching expenditure levels and trying to balance the books. And while the budget holder may be focused on avoiding a financial deficit at the end of the year, someone higher up in the health, education or social services system will need to consider wider strategic options and will be looking to achieve the best value for money in the use of available resources. If a new treatment (such as a new medicine, a new mode of family therapy, or a new arrangement for care and support) is introduced—and known to be effective—budget holders will want to know whether it is affordable and worth what it costs to provide. If needs and their consequences are enduring, governments will want to know the associated long-term expenditure implications and how to contain them.

The underlying challenge common to all of these wants or concerns is scarcity: there are never enough resources to meet all of society's needs. This is the most fundamental, pervasive, durable, and indeed important justification for a better understanding of the economics of child and adolescent mental health. Scarcity is an endemic, in fact permanent feature of all health and related systems, and is the reason why choices have to be made between alternative uses of a particular resource or service. As we shall see, those choices between alternative uses give meaning to costs. Economics—and, in particular, economic evaluation—aims to provide evidence to inform both professional practice and strategic decisions about how to allocate available resources so as to get more out of them (in terms of—for example—better outcomes for children and families, or

a fairer distribution of access to, or use of services), and about the incentives needed to help achieve those allocations.

Although the primary aim of any mental health system is to alleviate symptoms so as to improve personal functioning and promote quality of life, it is increasingly recognized that pursuit of such a laudable, fundamental objective cannot proceed without regard for the economic consequences of the therapies, support arrangements or broad policy strategies put into place. Awareness of this need to improve not only the effectiveness but also the cost-effectiveness of health care (and other) interventions and actions has produced various demands for economic evidence. There are requests for measures of the overall resource or cost impact of a particular health problem, (often called *cost-of-illness* studies). There are demands for *cost-effectiveness* and similar analyses of particular treatments or policies, carried out either alongside trials or independently: these are evaluations that compare not only the outcomes of two or more different interventions but also the relative costs of achieving them. There are searches for new service and system reconfigurations that can improve the efficiency of use of available resources. And there are searches for improved incentive structures that could positively alter the ways that resources are deployed.

Health economic methods provide a powerful way to help answer questions relevant to health professionals, budget holders, and governments and can aid in decision-making. Considerations around health care decisions are always relevant, however, as the global economic context changes, decisions, preferences, and social conditions may also change. For example, during the current economic "crisis" facing a number of countries, policymakers, and budget holders may seek austerity measures aimed at reducing costs (Wahlbeck & McDaid, 2012; Knapp, 2013); however, these choices need to be made carefully within the context of changes in population mental health and social conditions, and in cognizance of the preferences of children and families. Methods such

Rutter's Child and Adolescent Psychiatry, Sixth Edition.
Edited by Anita Thapar and Daniel S. Pine, James F. Leckman, Stephen Scott, Margaret J. Snowling, Eric Taylor.
© 2015 John Wiley & Sons Ltd. Published 2018 by John Wiley & Sons Ltd.

as cost, cost-offset analyses (comparing amounts expended with amounts saved), and cost-effectiveness analyses (comparing costs and the outcomes achieved) can support better, more informed decisions about the efficient ways of allocating resources during times of economic transition. It may be that increasing investment in interventions or services to alleviate the consequences of the recession could be associated with long-term savings. In addition, during times of economic growth, economic methods can help determine the most efficient ways of scaling up services. For instance, health economic methods could be especially relevant to countries such as Brazil, Russia, India, China, and South Africa, which are experiencing rapid economic and health transitions, generating a strong economic need for timely investment to address mental disorders. Recent estimation of the resources needed compared to the resources currently available in South Africa makes the case for further investment and scaling up of child and adolescent mental health services (Lund *et al.*, 2009).

Costs in childhood

Mental health problems—if they are recognized and responded to—have cost implications. The most obvious effect will be on health service utilization, but there may be contacts with special education, social work, public housing, criminal justice, and other service-delivering agencies. Indeed, the multiplicity of contacts and services is a marked and welcome characteristic of well-developed child and adolescent mental health systems (Glied & Cuellar, 2003). If needs or problems are not appropriately treated, then there could be adverse effects on functioning, with implications for educational engagement and attainment, employment and income (in later years), as well as effects on families. A number of studies have described these costs during childhood and adolescence.

Snell *et al.* (2013) demonstrate the substantial additional health care, social care, and education costs associated with childhood psychiatric disorders and the range of sectors impacted. National annual cost estimates associated with services used by young people aged 5–15 years were derived from the British Survey of Child and Adolescent Mental Health (Meltzer *et al.*, 2000) (see Figure 18.1). In addition to showing the large magnitude of costs associated with childhood psychiatric disorders, the study emphasized the substantial impact on the education sector. The cost of care delivered by frontline education services was more than twelve times greater than that delivered by specialty mental health services; the costs of special education services were also high. Cost also differed by type of child mental health problem with higher costs being associated with children with hyperkinetic and conduct disorders, compared to children with emotional disorders.

Romeo *et al.* (2006) looked at the impact across a range of sectors, but also estimated broad implications for families and the wider economy, in this case, for children referred for severe

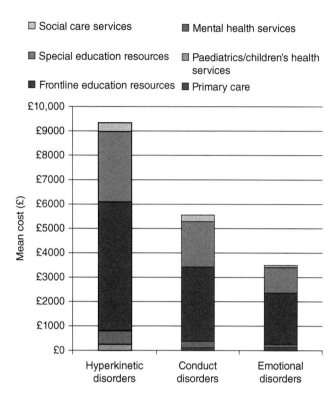

Figure 18.1 Health, social service and education resource use: mean cost over three-year follow-up for all children/young people with a disorder. *Note:* Costs can be converted from £ sterling to US$ by dividing the £ figures by 0.681. *Source:* Snell *et al.*, 2013. Reproduced with permission of John Wiley & Sons.

antisocial behavior. This study found considerable nonservice costs, with almost half of the total costs being borne by the family. Mean annual cost of care was £5960 (equivalent to US$8752 using the OECD purchasing power parity exchange rate (Organization for Economic Cooperation and Development, 2013) for which the same conversion rate is used throughout the chapter). Around this mean, costs varied by as much as a factor of more than 400, emphasizing the inherent heterogeneity in samples of children with mental health needs.

A third example points to the high and enduring costs of autistic spectrum disorder in both the United States and the UK. Integrating data from a number of studies on accommodation, medical services, nonmedical services, and out-of-pocket payments by families, combined with estimates of prevalence, Buescher *et al.* (2014) suggested that the discounted lifetime cost of someone with autism and intellectual disability were quite similar in the two countries. The study also found—similar to the evidence reported by Snell and colleagues discussed above—that high costs were borne by the education sector (specifically special education in this case), with parental productivity losses also found to be large.

What the Snell, Romeo and Buescher studies show very clearly is the breadth of economic impact across a variety of service sectors and on families, although they can only measure what is provided (in terms of service-related costs) or what impacts are recognized (in terms of indirect costs). We shall see in the next section that if behavioral problems in childhood or adolescence are inadequately addressed, then there are also likely to be substantial long-term costs stretching into adulthood.

The extent to which the resource (cost) consequences of childhood or adolescent mental health problems fall outside the health sector will obviously depend on how that and neighboring sectors are organized and configured: different boundaries between health, social services, education, housing, and other service sectors will mean redrawing the cost map. But it will not change the fact that many young people with mental health problems have needs in multiple life domains, each of them potentially with economic ramifications. Foster and Jones (2005), for example, describe the economic implications of conduct disorder among adolescents in four US communities over a seven-year period. The cost difference between youths with and without conduct disorder was nearly $70,000. The distribution of costs between budgets was different from that found in the UK partly because of differences in system structures.

These multiple impacts are obviously hard to measure, and much harder still to factor into decision-making. Not only does the decision-maker in, for example, the health sector need to find out the implications of their actions for other sectors, whether positive or negative, but they also have to think through the mechanisms needed to do something about them. A major problem in many systems is "silo budgeting": resources located in specific agencies or budgets cannot easily be shifted, indeed might be rigorously protected (Glied & Cuellar, 2003). Professional rivalry, myopic budget protection, performance assessment regimes or simply slowly churning bureaucratic processes could leave one agency unwilling or unable to devote more of its own resources in order for another agency or service to achieve savings, or for the broader system of treatment and support to achieve greater effectiveness or cost-effectiveness.

Costs continuing into adulthood

It is well known that mental health problems experienced in childhood or adolescence can have many and often serious adverse effects on psychosocial outcomes such as crime, relationships, substance misuse, and on quality of life. Many studies have traced these connections between behavioral and emotional problems in childhood and adverse experiences of various kinds in adulthood (see Chapter 1).

Mental health needs in childhood could also be associated with later physical health needs. Physical and mental comorbidities tend to cluster together and can thus lead to increased costs in childhood due particularly to increased service use (Guevara et al., 2001; Nelson et al., 2013). These comorbid health problems are likely to worsen in adulthood, with service costs being correspondingly higher (Naylor et al., 2012), plus there could be further costs associated with lower workforce participation and higher absenteeism (Molosankwe et al., 2012). Although

comorbidity seems to be the rule rather than the exception, there is a lack of research on how these comorbidities interact, the economic consequences of these disorders occurring together, and how best to evaluate the costs and outcomes of complex combinations of interventions aimed at addressing comorbid problems.

Many of the adulthood sequelae of child mental health problems and experiences will have measurable cost consequences, and while any computed monetary indicators cannot hope to represent or cover the full set of experiences of individual children and adults, they have the virtue of expressing some of these experiences in magnitudes that are readily understood by those key policy makers who hold the purse strings.

A few studies have explicitly explored the connections between childhood disorders and adulthood economic consequences. These studies demonstrate unusually high rates of utilization of health and other services (obviously with personal and societal costs), and impacts related to employment, such as not being economically active, or being active but unemployed, or being employed but frequently absent or unproductive, or working in a lower status occupation than would otherwise be expected. The employment effects will almost inevitably have impacts on earnings and could lead to individual and household poverty. Three examples can be offered.

Evidence from the Inner London Longitudinal Study

The Inner London Longitudinal Study collected data on 2281 10-year olds in 1970 and selected 228 of them for intensive study: a random 1 in 12 sample of the population and a 1 in 2 sample of children with emotional or behavioral problems (Maughan, 1989). This group was interviewed again at age 28. Neither interview set out to collect "economic" data as such, but it was possible to construct service-related costs from the information gathered (Scott et al. 2001). Nevertheless, the computed cost averages are undoubtedly underestimates of the full costs because the data collection did not cover all possible impacts and did not follow people continuously over time. Among the costs not measured were those associated with social work, voluntary sector service use, primary health care contacts, lost employment, divorce, undetected crime, the effects of crime on victims, the emotional impacts on other people, and other transmitted effects to other family members or children. Many of these omissions are known to be substantial (see below). Notwithstanding these missing elements, conduct disorder in childhood (which was found for the most antisocial 3% of the population studied) and conduct problems (which were found for the next 9%) led to greatly elevated costs in adulthood for a number of agencies, and especially for the criminal justice system (Figure 18.2).

The links between conduct problems and conduct disorder in childhood and service-related costs in early adulthood were further explored through multiple regression analysis, adjusting for gender, parental social class, reading age, number of primary

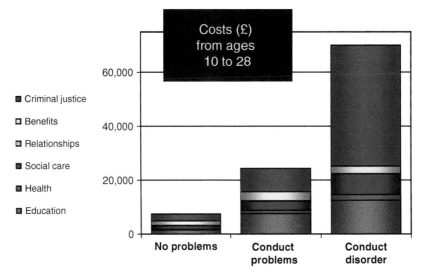

Figure 18.2 Costs in early adulthood from childhood conduct disorder. *Source:* Reproduced with permission of BMJ.

schools attended. A number of other factors were examined, but found not to be significant. Adjusting for those covariates, the estimated coefficient on the conduct disorder variable—the additional cost between the ages of 10 and 28 (aggregating across all 18 years) of having conduct disorder at age 10 compared to not having any antisocial behavior problems—was £40,784 (at 2004/05 prices; equivalent to US$59,888). The additional cost of having conduct problems (those who were less severely affected by antisocial behavior—the next 9% of the group) compared to having no such problems was £17,017 (US$24,988). Given the underdeveloped and underresourced nature of child and adolescent mental health services in the UK in the early 1970s, these cost differences might perhaps be interpreted as indicative of the economic consequences of not addressing (or only rather poorly addressing) antisocial behavior among 10-year olds.

Evidence from a British birth cohort study

The second example comes from the 1970 British birth cohort study (BCS70) and illustrates employment-related consequences of child and adolescent mental health problems. The BCS70 is a nationally representative birth cohort of 17,196 babies born in the UK during a particular week in 1970. Data were collected from young people and their families at ages 5, 10, 16, 26, 30, and 34. Knapp *et al.* (2011) looked at the links between childhood antisocial conduct, attention deficit, anxiety, and coordination problems at age 10 and employment experiences (economic inactivity, occupational status, and earnings) at age 30.

In general, mental health problems during childhood were associated with worse employment outcomes during adulthood; however, the consequences varied by gender and by type of mental health problem. Both women and men with childhood attention deficit problems had worse outcomes across all indicators (i.e., lower employment rates, worse jobs, lower earnings if employed, and lower expected earnings overall). Among individuals with anxiety problems, men had lower earnings if

employed and lower expected earnings overall. Women with childhood anxiety problems had lower expected overall earnings only. Individuals with childhood coordination problems had the fewest adverse consequences during adulthood: men with childhood coordination problems had lower expected earnings. Males with conduct problems at age 10 had an interesting pattern of mixed outcomes in adulthood. Males with childhood conduct problems were more likely to be unemployed at age 30. Unexpectedly, however, those who were employed had higher earnings and higher expected overall earnings (when taking economic inactivity into account). No such trend was evident for women with childhood conduct problems.

Other childhood social and psychosocial factors were also found to be important for later adult employment including: low cognitive attainment, living in a disadvantaged neighborhood, having a mother with higher educational qualifications, lower family income, and being looked after by a local authority (municipality).

Evidence from a 20-year follow-up of boys resident in the London Borough of Newham

D'Amico *et al.* (2014) describe the longitudinal trajectory of childhood behavior problems and their impact for a range of problems in adulthood. Eighty-three individuals were followed up from a population-based cohort of 6–7 year old boys resident in the London Borough of Newham who were attending mainstream schools (Taylor *et al.*, 1991) twenty years after baseline (participants were between the ages of 25 and 30 years at follow-up). For this study, participants were categorized into four groups based on their baseline responses: (a) hyperactivity problems only; (b) conduct problems only; (c) mixed conduct and hyperactivity problems and (d) no hyperactivity or conduct problems.

The study found that boys with baseline conduct problems had the highest costs in early adulthood, mostly because of the contacts with the criminal justice system. Childhood conduct problems were associated with a two- to three-fold increase in costs in early adulthood. The mixed group had the highest health and social care costs, but their overall costs were lower because they had the lowest criminal justice costs. After adjusting for socio-demographic factors, the average increased costs for individuals with conduct problems only were the highest £4033 (US$5922), while individuals with mixed conduct and hyperactivity problems had similar costs (£2208) to those with hyperactivity problems only (£2118). These figures are somewhat lower than those found by Scott *et al.* (2001).

Evidence of early prevention and intervention programs for young people

In 2004, Aos and colleagues (2004) were commissioned by the Washington State legislature to investigate the long-term costs and benefits of early prevention and intervention programs for young people. Specifically, they were asked to make recommendations about (a) whether prevention and early intervention programs were a good investment and (b) which programs would provide the best investment. To answer this question, they modeled the costs and benefits across seven key areas: education, crime, substance abuse, child abuse and neglect, teen pregnancy, and public assistance. Programs which performed a rigorous evaluation of at least one of the key outcomes were identified from the literature.

Importantly, the report concluded that some prevention and early intervention can provide a good return on investment to taxpayers. However, findings were mixed, with some interventions resulting in clear benefits while for others the benefits did not outweigh the costs. Thus, their findings emphasized the importance of rigorous evaluation and attention to fidelity and quality control when considering the implementation of a program.

Economic analysis showed that the highest net benefits were associated with programs for juvenile offenders, although outcomes varied widely even among effective programs (from $1900 to $31,200 per young person). Home visiting programs and early childhood education targeted at risk and/or low income families also provided good return on investment ($6000 to $17,200 for home visiting programs, and up to $9000 for early education programs). The net benefits associated with substance abuse programs were relatively low, but were still found to be cost-effective because most programs were inexpensive. A gap was identified among programs which were effective at reducing teen pregnancy.

Impact of child maltreatment

Another example—this time from the Netherlands—is the evaluation of the long-term impact of risk factors such as child maltreatment on health-related costs, specifically, costs that arise when people are confronted with mental disorders due to health care uptake and productivity losses when staying absent from work. Data for this analysis came from Netherlands Mental Health Survey and Incidence Study (NEMESIS) which included 5618 individuals in a large, population-based cohort. At the individual level, excess costs of child maltreatment at 1-year follow-up were between $2610 and $3666 when adjusting for socio-demographic factors in addition to parental anxiety and depression. At the population level, child maltreatment was associated with excess costs of between $203 million and $655 million per million people per year. Importantly, the study also found that certain protective factors, such as a high internal locus of control, ameliorated the onset of mental disorder and subsequently also reduced the associated economic consequences (Smit *et al.*, 2013).

Cost-offset considerations

A question that governments and other macrolevel decision-makers often want answering is whether investment in preventive measures or better treatments during (say) a child's early years will pay off in terms of reduced economic impacts in adolescence and in adulthood. This is what economists would call the *cost-offset* question: it asks about the balance between amounts expended and amounts saved.

There have been studies which have looked at the long-term cost-offsetting properties of such investments. An example comes from the United States where Foster and Connor (Foster & Connor, 2005) investigated the impact of improved community mental health services for young people on fiscal expenditures in other sectors. The study found that delivering child and adolescent mental health services as part of a system-of-care approach, while more expensive than standard services, reduced expenditure in other sectors (juvenile justice, child welfare, special education, inpatient services). Thus the reduced expenditures in other sectors partially offset the costs of improved community mental health services.

There have also been studies that have looked at the long-term cost-offsetting properties of such investments. Cohen (1998), for example, looked at "high-risk youth" in the United States and the *potential* economic advantages from "saving" each individual by estimating costs over the lifetime associated with crime, drug misuse and dropout from school. The estimated monetary value of "saving each high risk youth" was estimated to be between $1.7 million and $2.3 million. Another study by Bonin *et al.* (2011) looked at the effect of group parenting interventions for young people with conduct disorder using simulation modeling (see Box 18.1 for discussion of simulation modeling and other types of health economics study designs; and see Chapter 13). The study suggested that the parenting intervention resulted in long-term benefits to the public sector and to society by reducing the chance that conduct disorder persisted into adulthood. Long-term benefits of the program were greatest to the health and criminal justice sectors.

Cohen and Bonin's studies were based on hypothetical (simulated) valuations, whereas a second example—the High/Scope

Box 18.1 Examples of health economics study designs

Randomized controlled trial

The randomized controlled trial (RCT) is the gold standard experimental study design in which study participants are randomly assigned to two or more groups. Economic evaluations can be attached to an existing RCT, or an RCT might be designed specifically to evaluate, for example, the cost-effectiveness of a treatment. Although the design has high internal validity, it may not produce results that are widely generalizable.

Quasi-experimental study design

Quasi-experimental studies cover a range of designs and investigate the effect of an intervention without using random allocation. They tend to

have lower internal validity compared to RCTs. When performing economic evaluation, it is important to be confident about causality and that important confounding factors are taken into consideration.

Simulation modeling

Simulation modeling may use already published results from previous studies to estimate the impact of an intervention or changes in policy for a range of hypothetical scenarios. It may incorporate epidemiological or cost data from other sources to model costs and outcomes of intervention and control groups.

Perry Preschool Study—was based on direct observations. Although not focused on children with mental health problems, this well-known intervention has been quite influential because of its finding of substantial savings in relation to crime, education and welfare payments, as well as higher taxes paid by those people who went through the preschool program (see, e.g., the summary by Schweinhart, 2004; Heckman *et al.,* 2010). However, these findings relate to a very small sample of individuals, and generalization from this study has been far from straightforward.

Exploring cost-effectiveness

Knowing the costs in childhood associated with mental health problems helps decision-makers to gauge the component and overall societal impact of these conditions. Knowing what economic consequences these problems lead to in adulthood helps those same decision-makers focus their minds on the need for better preventive or treatment interventions in early years or subsequently. But neither of these bodies of evidence can tell a decision-maker how to make better use of available resources. For this purpose it is necessary to examine both the costs and the outcomes of different uses of those resources. This is what economists would recognize as the examination of *cost-effectiveness.*

Consider what happens following the development or introduction of a new treatment (say a new medication intended for treating childhood depression). Decision-makers face two central questions when considering whether to use or recommend this new drug as part of the treatment range. The first is the clinical question: is the medication effective in alleviating depressive symptoms and generally improving child health? Or, when considering two or more different drugs, which of them has the better outcome? If the answer to the clinical question is that the new medication is no better or perhaps actually worse than existing treatment options, then there is usually no need to consider its use any further, nor probably to look at relative costs. But if the new medication looks clinically effective, the decision-maker will then want an answer to a second question: is it cost-effective?

That is, does the treatment achieve the improved child outcomes at a cost that is worth paying?

These two questions (Is the treatment effective? Is it worth it?) are at the heart of cost-effectiveness analysis (CEA). It is important to emphasize that CEA does what it says on the label: it looks at *both* costs and effectiveness (outcomes). Comparing the costs of one intervention with the costs of another, without any evidence on outcomes, might be interesting but does not constitute an economic evaluation because it does not provide enough evidence to assist service professionals, managers or others to make informed choices between alternative uses of their scarce resources. Similarly, calculating and in some way comparing the costs and outcomes of a single intervention could be revealing, but again is not especially helpful (and not an economic evaluation) unless comparison is made with equivalent data for another service (or with the "do nothing" option), for otherwise the decision-maker will have no benchmark against which to judge whether the observed costs and outcomes are attractive enough to justify action.

Note that the second question in a CEA asks whether improved outcomes are "worth" the extra cost. Deciding what is or is not "worth" the cost is far from straightforward and not without controversy, as we discuss below.

There are different variants of cost-effectiveness that can be applied to decision-making in health and related contexts. They share a common approach to the conceptualization, definition, and measurement of costs, but they adopt different approaches when considering and measuring the outcome side of the evaluation, primarily because they seek to answer slightly different questions. There is, however, some potential for terminological confusion. The term "cost-effectiveness" is used to describe a specific variant of economic evaluation as well as to refer generically to the group of all such evaluations. In this chapter we are using the term in its generic sense, unless specifically stated to the contrary.

Question and perspective

The choice of evaluative approach therefore depends on the question to be addressed. If the question is essentially clinical—what is the most appropriate treatment for a child with particular needs in particular circumstances, and whether to opt for one therapeutic package or another—then information is needed on the comparative costs of the different therapies and the comparative outcomes measured in terms of symptom alleviation, improved functioning and so on. In these circumstances, a CEA (in the narrow sense of the term) would be appropriate and sufficient (see the section on "Effectiveness measurement").

If, to take a broader stance, the question is whether to invest available health system resources to treat either childhood depression or asthma, then decision-makers again need to know the relative costs of the two alternatives, but they now need a measure of effectiveness that uses a common metric across the fields of depression and asthma. The most common measure so employed is "utility," generated from health-related quality of life scales (see "Utility measurement" below). In these circumstances a cost-utility analysis (CUA) is needed (also see below).

To widen the perspective even further, if the question is whether to invest more money in the health system or more money in improving transport, launching a new environmental policy or bolstering a country's defense forces, then the research question becomes one of asking what are the comparative costs and merits of the different investment options, where "merit" will now need to be measured in a common unit across all of these broad areas of public policy. The usual choice of broad measure is monetary, leading to cost-benefit analysis (see "Benefit measurement").

The choice of question clearly influences the type of evaluation needed, but the choices are not mutually exclusive: a single study could support more than one type of analysis and address more than one policy or practice-related question. A body of evidence which is well located within the clinical domain will be exactly what the treating professional needs but may not be appropriate for a higher level decision-making body, such as a health ministry. The broader the research question, the more demanding are the data needs: brutally summarized, cost-benefit analyses are usually harder to do than cost-utility analyses, which in turn are usually more difficult than cost-effectiveness analyses.

Linked to the specification of the question to be addressed is the *perspective* to be adopted. Is the evaluative information needed to help resource allocation within a particular agency (such as a child and adolescent mental health service), or within a particular system (such as the health care system or education system), or within a particular sector (such as government), or within the whole society? The breadth of perspective will determine the breadth of both the measurement of costs and the choice of measures of effectiveness or outcomes.

Cost measurement

There are a number of ways to categorize the costs associated with mental health problems. There are *direct costs* associated with the treatment services and associated supports, some of them delivered by nonhealth agencies. There are also *indirect* costs, which may fall to families, or may be measured in terms of lost productivity because of future disruptions to employment patterns for children once they have reached adulthood, or current disruptions to employment for parents. There may also be some unmeasured costs, perhaps reflecting the burden carried by family members, or societal concerns about antisocial behavior. In evaluations, the usual approach is to try to measure these elements as long-run marginal opportunity costs (Knapp, 1993). This helps to ensure that a long-term perspective on resource implications is employed, that only those effects on resources attributable to the program or service user are counted, and that costs are reckoned as opportunities forgone, not just money expended. How broadly the costs are measured will depend upon the perspective taken for the evaluation, which in turn depends upon the purpose of the study.

In carrying out evaluations in practice, the economist would be looking for data on service use patterns from one or more source. The data might come from organizational "billing" systems, recording the amounts that are transferred between a payer and a provider for services used by individual children or families. This is a common approach in US research, for example (although usually only spanning one system—such as healthcare—at a time). In care systems without such payment mechanisms, there might nevertheless be routine information systems that record service contacts and referrals, which might provide the necessary data for an evaluation. However, in many countries there are no billing data, and organizational information systems are too rudimentary or inaccurate to provide the basis for cost calculation. In these circumstances, the usual approach is to collect information on patterns of service use through interviews with family members or service professionals (for which there are a number of tools, including the Client Service Receipt Inventory (Beecham & Knapp, 2001).

To the service use levels generated by information systems or from interviews the researcher would then attach unit cost estimates for each service. It is not always necessary to calculate these unit costs anew. In England, for example, there is an excellent annual compendium of such unit costs which is very widely used in applied research (Curtis, 2012). Nonservice costs are harder to measure than service costs, partly because of the difficulty of identifying the impacts (e.g., on parental employment patterns, or on a child's own future earning capacity) and partly because of the difficulty of then attaching a monetary value. (For further discussion of these issues see Johnston *et al.*, 1999; Brouwer *et al.*, 2001.)

Effectiveness measurement

Probably the most intuitive mode of economic evaluation is CEA: it measures costs as set out above, and measures outcomes using instruments, and scales familiar from clinical studies, because its focus is symptoms, behavior, functioning, peer-group integration, and so on. A CEA is employed to help decision-makers choose between alternative interventions available to or aimed at specific patient groups.

An analysis would look at a single outcome dimension—such as change in a behavioral measure, or symptom-free days or self-esteem—and would then compute and compare the ratio of the difference in costs between two treatments to the difference in (primary) outcome (the so-called incremental cost-effectiveness ratio). Certain areas of child mental health lack robust studies (see Box 18.2), however, there are good examples of cost-effectiveness analyses across many other areas. For example, an evaluation of a home-based social work intervention for children and adolescents who have deliberately poisoned themselves by Byford et al (Byford *et al.*, 1999) measured suicidal ideation, hopelessness and family functioning as the main outcomes, and health, education, social care, and voluntary sector services as the basis for cost measurement. Their randomized controlled trial, involving 162 children aged 16 years or under found no significant difference in the main outcomes for costs, although parental satisfaction with treatment was significantly greater in the group that received a new social work intervention compared to those who received routine care.

Another example of cost-effectiveness based on a randomized controlled trial comes from Domino et al (2009). The study looked at the relative cost-effectiveness of three treatments for major depression: (a) fluoxetine alone; (b) cognitive behavioral therapy alone, and (c) a combination of fluoxetine and cognitive behavioral therapy). Costs of service use of participants in this study were evaluated at 36 weeks follow-up in relation to the number of depression-free days and quality-adjusted life years. Although the combination treatment was the most costly, it was also found to be the most cost-effective treatment overall.

An obvious weakness with the strict cost-effectiveness methodology is the focus on a single outcome dimension (which is necessary to compute ratios) when children and adolescents with mental health problems often have multiple needs for support and when most clinicians would expect to achieve improvements in more than one area. For this reason,

cost-effectiveness ratios are sometimes computed for each of a *number* of outcome measures. This is sometimes called *cost-consequences analysis*. This approach has the advantage of breadth but poses a challenge if two or more ratios point to different interventions as the more cost-effective: in these circumstances, the decision-maker must weigh up the strength of evidence.

Making trade-offs

Many evaluations of new interventions find them to be both more effective (the outcome profiles are better than for old or current interventions) but simultaneously more expensive. For example, one study (Cunningham *et al.*, 1995) found that a group-training parenting program had better outcomes but slightly higher costs than an individual program. How is the trade-off to be made between the better outcomes and the higher expenditure necessary to achieve them?

The net benefit approach seeks to explicate the nature of the trade-off. It is most commonly seen today in the construction of *cost-effectiveness acceptability curves* (CEACs). These curves show the probability that a new intervention will be cost-effective for each of a number of prespecified or implicit valuations of an outcome improvement by the decision-maker. The advantage of the CEAC approach is that it makes transparent the trade-offs faced by decision-makers.

Two studies by Byford and colleagues illustrate this approach in the field of child and adolescent mental health. The first example examines the cost-effectiveness of treating adolescents with major depression using selective serotonin reuptake inhibitors (SSRI) and routine specialist care alone, or in conjunction with cognitive behavioral therapy (Byford *et al.*, 2007b). The latter intervention was both more costly and less effective: adding CBT to SSRI and usual treatment did not look economically attractive. The researchers plotted a CEAC as a way to address uncertainty in the data: this showed that, even at a value of £50,000 per one-point improvement in mental

Box 18.2 Cost and benefits of programs for learning disorders

Learning disorders represent one area for which there is little published evidence on the cost-effectiveness of programs. Some encouraging evidence using interventions data combined with various cohort data is available and described below; however, more robust study designs are still needed

Challen *et al.* identified indicators of learning difficulties from the 1970 British Cohort Survey (BCS70) and the Longitudinal Survey of Young People, and examined the association between the indicators and various social and economic outcomes later on (Challen *et al.*, 2008). Combining these data with intervention data from a phonological awareness intervention for kindergartners (Schneider *et al.*, 1997) allowed for estimates of potential cost-effectiveness of the program. The substantial effect size found in the evaluation (spelling improved by 0.57 and reading by 0.26 standard deviations) suggested that the intervention was potentially very cost-effective. This finding appears promising, but there are several caveats in that the evaluation of the intervention was too small

to look specifically at the effects for individuals with learning disorders and did not include a long term follow up.

Machin and McNally investigated the cost-effectiveness of a specific reading intervention called "the literacy hour" (Machin & McNally, 2008). The intervention was implemented in English primary schools and targeted young people aged 5–11 years. The program aimed to improve literacy through a teaching framework incorporating focused literacy instruction and effective classroom management. Evaluation of the program demonstrated significant impact on reading and on school achievement. Again the BCS70 data were combined with the intervention data to estimate the impact of the intervention (in terms of reading score improvement) on future earnings. As the cost of the intervention was quite low (£26 (US$38) per pupil per year), even with very conservative estimates of the impact, the economic benefits were between £1375 and £3581 (US$2019–US$5258).

health (measured by the Health of the Nation Outcome Scale for Children and Adolescents), the probability that adding CBT to SSRI treatment would be seen as cost-effective was only low (only 0.25). When the researchers used QALYs to measure outcomes, the probability that CBT added to SSRI would be cost-effective was considerably lower (no higher than 0.04).

The second study by Byford and colleagues compares three treatment options for adolescents with anorexia: inpatient psychiatric services, specialist outpatient psychiatric services, and general outpatient services (Byford et al., 2007a). The study showed that specialist outpatient treatment tended to cost less and be more effective as measured by the Morgan–Russell Average Outcome Scale (MRAOS) score, an indicator of severity of anorexia. The plotted CEAC showed that at two-year follow-up, if a decision-maker's willingness to pay for a unit increase in MRAOS score were zero, there was a 78% probability that the specialty outpatient services would be cost-effective. At higher levels of willingness to pay, the probability of being cost-effective actually decreased, but specialist outpatient services remained the most cost-effective of the three options.

Utility measurement

A mode of economic evaluation that seeks to reduce outcomes to a single dimension is CUA, which measures and then values the impact of an intervention in terms of improvements in preference-weighted, health-related quality of life. The value of the quality of life improvement is gauged in units of "utility," usually expressed by a combined index of the mortality and quality of life effects of an intervention. The best known and most robust such index is the Quality Adjusted Life Year (QALY).

CUA are being used increasingly in health economics evaluations. They have a number of advantages, including using a unidimensional measure of impact, a generic measure which allows comparisons to be made across diagnostic or clinical groups (e.g., comparing psychiatry with oncology or cardiology), and a fully explicit methodology for weighting preferences and valuing health states. But these same features have sometimes been seen as disadvantages: the utility measure may be seen as too reductionist; the generic quality of life indicator may be insufficiently sensitive to the kinds of change expected in schizophrenia treatment; and a transparent approach to scale construction paradoxically opens the approach to criticism from those who question the values thereby obtained. In particular, there are worries that the generic utility-generating instruments, such the EQ-5D (EuroQol Group, 1990), which is recommended by the National Institute for Health and Care Excellence (NICE), and the SF-6D (Brazier et al., 2002) and HUI3 (Petrou et al., 2010), are insufficiently sensitive to the kinds of symptoms and functioning change observed for people with mental health problems, and particularly for children and adolescents.

On the other hand, cost-utility analyses avoid the potential ambiguities with multi dimensional outcomes in cost-effectiveness studies. The transparency of approach should obviously also be welcomed. Such an approach to economic evaluation produces an estimate of the cost per QALY-gain from one therapy or intervention and another. Estimates of this kind can then inform health care resource allocation decisions or priority setting, such as in the work of the NICE which has responsibility in England and Wales for providing national guidance on promoting good health and preventing and treating ill health. NICE has a well-developed process for assessing economic evidence (NICE, 2008) and cost-effectiveness values certainly influence guideline development (NICE, 2008; Cerri et al., 2013).

There have been few published cost-utility analyses in the child and adolescent mental health area, the study by Byford et al. (2007a) summarized above being one of the few. Gilmore and Milne (2001) used the same evaluative approach to compare the costs and effects of methylphenidate and placebo for treating hyperactivity. Theirs was a modeling (simulation) exercise rather than a study that collected primary data. Another contribution to the literature on utility and cost measurement comes from Petrou et al. (2010). Although the study did not perform a full CUA, it did estimate the costs and utilities associated with a range of psychiatric disorders from participants of the EPICure cohort (Wood et al., 2000). EPICure is a population-based longitudinal study of infants born in the UK and Ireland. Utilities were based on parental responses to the Health Utilities Index (Torrance et al., 1995). Findings suggested a £2000 (US$2937) annual cost difference between children with and without psychiatric disorder.

There is a quandary facing researchers and decision-makers in the UK today, and in some other countries that have chosen a strategic evidence-based approach to health technology appraisal. A generic outcome measure such as the QALY, when combined with cost estimates, can point to ways of achieving improved value for money when decisions need to be taken across a broad area (such as across a number of diagnostic areas), but if that QALY measure is not sensitive enough to reflect all relevant differences in effectiveness, then it might not be a sound enough basis for such an important task.

Benefit measurement

Cost-benefit analysis asks whether the benefits of a treatment or policy exceed the costs. This would allow decision-makers to consider the merits not only of allocating resources within health care, but also to consider whether it would be more appropriate to invest in other sectors such as housing, education or defense. In this form of evaluation all costs and outcomes (benefits) are valued in the same (monetary) units. If benefits exceed costs, the evaluation would provide support for the treatment, and vice versa. With two or more alternatives, the treatment with the greatest net benefit would be deemed the most efficient. Cost-benefit analyses are thus intrinsically attractive, but conducting them is especially problematic because of the difficulty of valuing outcomes in monetary terms.

Comparing costs incurred (e.g., on treatments) with costs saved (e.g., on future health services no longer needed) is not a

Box 18.3 Determining the quality of economic evaluations

<table>
<tr>
<td>

1 Have all the relevant costs been taken into account? As we have seen, there are many and various inputs to a broadly defined mental health system—from health, social care, education, housing, social security and other agencies—plus economic consequences in terms of lost productivity, premature mortality and family impact. It might be necessary to measure all of these, depending on the policy or practice question that needs to be addressed and the perspective necessary for the evaluation.

</td>
<td>

2 Are all the dimensions of effectiveness taken into account? Good mental health care is obviously not just about tackling clinical symptoms, but about improving an individual's ability to function in ways that are valued by them (such as performing well at school and integrating with peers) and of course about promoting quality of life.

</td>
</tr>
</table>

cost-benefit analysis but a *cost-offset* comparison. This confusion is unfortunately still quite common. A cost-benefit analysis must measure outcomes (in terms of improved health or improved quality of life) and then convert them to monetary values. Consequently, studies such as that by Jacobson *et al.* (1998) of an early intensive behavioral program for children with pervasive development disorder or autism, which compared the costs of the intervention with cost savings into adulthood, are certainly interesting but not as helpful as studies that compare the costs and the outcomes of interventions.

The problem is that attaching values to the outcomes of child and adolescent mental health interventions is inherently complicated. Methodological advances in health economics may offer a way to obtain direct valuations of health outcomes by patients, relatives or the general public. These techniques ask individuals to state the amount they would be prepared to pay (hypothetically) to achieve a given health state or health gain, or they observe actual behavior and impute the implicit values (Olsen & Smith, 2001). They are likely to be quite difficult to apply in mental health contexts. Another approach that is beginning to be used more and more often to value health interventions is "conjoint analysis": individuals are asked to rank different real world scenarios, which may consist of several dimensions (including, for instance, health outcomes, quality of life, time inputs, discomfort, and stigma) and by including cost as one of these dimensions a monetary value can be elicited (provided that respondents can make the necessary trade-offs). While quite complex, the conjoint analysis approach has the advantage of not specifically asking individuals to put a monetary value on health states or health gain, which can make the technique easier to administer than traditional willingness-to-pay studies (Ryan, 1999). Bodies such as NICE provide useful recommendations for appropriate methods to be employed in economic evaluations. These resources may also be useful in judging the quality of economic analysis, which is an important consideration for any type of evaluation (see Box 18.3).

Conclusion

The starting point for an interest in the economics of child and adolescent mental health is clearly scarcity: it is the recognition

that there are not, and indeed there never will be, enough resources available to meet all mental health (or other) needs of all children and families. There is still a notion abroad in some parts of some health systems that incremental growth in budgets will gradually remove all need, but this is naively over-optimistic, indeed irrationally utopian. We cannot and we must not avoid facing up to the choices that have to be made in the face of scarcity. In making those choices we would want our decision-makers to be transparent about the criteria that they are employing. For instance, are they looking to maximize effectiveness in terms of symptom alleviation or aggregate quality of life, or to redistribute resources to poorer communities within society, or to ensure that access to skilled resources is equally available to every family?

Within this set of criteria, cost-effectiveness obviously has a role to play. As noted earlier, the cost-effectiveness criterion should probably be seen as secondary. If, for example, a therapeutic intervention has been shown to be effective in improving the well-being of children and families, and appears to be more effective than currently available therapies, then it would be natural to ask about the relative costs of the two options and to compare those costs with the outcome gains. Balancing outcome improvements with higher costs is, however, quite a challenge. A great many economic evaluations across the health spectrum today find that new therapies (whether pharmacological, psychological or organizational) offer better outcome profiles than currently prevalent interventions, but they do so at higher cost. The decision-maker, whether this is the individual care professional working with children and families, or their line manager and budget holder, or someone near the top of the health ministry, then faces a difficult trade-off: are the better outcomes from the new intervention worth the higher cost of introducing that intervention?

Heckman argues that we need a better understanding of the dynamics of the life course in order to identify the optimal time points for intervention (Heckman, 2012). A developmental approach which models early, intermediate and longer-term outcomes, and examines how interventions and consequences vary over time, would help those charged with the difficult tasks of allocating resources to consider the relative benefits of various approaches to prevention and treatment. In addition to considering life-course and timing, context is also important. Some cost-effective interventions could be prenatal, which could be important for global mental health: investing in sustainable prenatal interventions could make good sense in low and middle income countries (Panter-Brick & Leckman, 2013).

Requests for economic insights in the child and adolescent mental health field are of many kinds. In this chapter we have illustrated some of them, including requests to measure the overall cost impact of a particular disorder or diagnosis (so called cost-of-illness studies). Second, there are cost-offset studies that compare the amounts expended on interventions with the longer-term savings from introducing those interventions. Third, and the most powerful and useful, are cost-effectiveness studies (using the term generically also to include cost-benefit and cost-utility studies): these weigh up and compare costs *and* outcomes, and therefore give a more complete and rounded view as to the consequences of introducing different interventions.

There is a concern that most of the completed economic studies that can be found in the international literature today have been undertaken in North America, parts of Western Europe and Australia. Unfortunately, the results of economic evaluations often do not transfer well from one health or care system to another, and therefore not well between countries. This is primarily because of the differences in the structure of health systems, financing arrangements, incentive structures and relative price levels. There might also be differences in the appropriate choice of comparator: a new therapeutic approach might look attractive compared to current arrangements in one country but not in comparison to what is generally the norm elsewhere. It is infeasible and certainly unnecessary to carry out an evaluation every time a policy decision needs to be taken, but evidence-based decisions are generally thought to be better than evidence-free decisions. This could mean using the results from a study carried out in another country, or updating a previous study, or carrying out a modest adaptation to adjust for context.

The available economics evidence base in the child and adolescent mental health field is growing, but only slowly. It is disappointingly under-developed at present in high income countries and almost completely absent in low and middle income countries, but more is now being invested in the area, including a number of new studies that will—in time—offer valuable new insights into the resource consequences and cost-effectiveness properties of different interventions aimed at meeting the needs of children and families.

References

Aos, S. *et al.* (2004) *Benefits and Costs of Prevention and Early Intervention Programs for Youth*. Washington State Institute for Public Policy, Olympia, WA.

Beecham, J. & Knapp, M. (2001) Costing psychiatric interventions. In: *Measuring Mental Health Needs*. (ed G. Thornicroft), 2nd edn. Gaskell, London.

Bonin, E.M. *et al.* (2011) Costs and longer-term savings of parenting programmes for the prevention of persistent conduct disorder: a modelling study. *BMC Public Health* **11**, 803.

Brazier, J. *et al.* (2002) The estimation of a preference-based measure of health from the SF-36. *Journal of Health Economics* **21**, 271–292.

Brouwer, W. *et al.* (2001) Costing in economic evaluations. In: *Economic Evaluation in Health Care: Merging Theory with Practice*. Oxford University Press, New York.

Buescher, A. *et al.* (2014) Costs of autism spectrum disorders in the United Kingdom and the United States of America. *JAMA Pediatrics* **168**, 721–728.

Byford, S. *et al.* (1999) Cost-effectiveness analysis of a home-based social work intervention for children and adolescents who have deliberately poisoned themselves. Results of a randomised controlled trial. *British Journal of Psychiatry* **174**, 56–62.

Byford, S. *et al.* (2007a) Economic evaluation of a randomised controlled trial for anorexia nervosa in adolescents. *British Journal of Psychiatry* **191**, 436–440.

Byford, S. *et al.* (2007b) Cost-effectiveness of selective serotonin reuptake inhibitors and routine specialist care with and without cognitive behavioural therapy in adolescents with major depression. *British Journal of Psychiatry* **191**, 521–527.

Cerri, K.H. *et al.* (2013) Decision making by NICE: examining the influences of evidence, process and context. *Health Economics, Policy and Law* **9**, 119–141.

Challen, A., *et al.* 2008, *Economic Modeling for Foresight Project: Mental Capital and Wellbeing*, Working paper, Center for Economic Policy, LSE.

Cohen, M. (1998) The monetary value of saving a high-risk youth. *Journal of Quantitative Criminology* **14**, 5–33.

Cunningham, C.E. *et al.* (1995) Large group community-based parenting programs for families of preschoolers at risk for disruptive behaviour disorders: utilization, cost effectiveness, and outcome. *Journal of Child Psychology and Psychiatry* **36**, 1141–1159.

Curtis, L. (2012) *Unit Costs of Health and Social Care*. University of Kent, PSSRU.

D'Amico, F. *et al.* (2014) Use of services and associated costs for young adults with childhood hyperactivity/conduct problems: 20-year follow-up. *British Journal of Psychiatry* **204**, 441–447.

Domino, M.E. *et al.* (2009) Relative cost-effectiveness of treatments for adolescent depression: 36-week results from the TADS randomized trial. *Journal of the American Academy of Child and Adolescent Psychiatry* **48**, 711–720.

EuroQol Group (1990) EuroQol – a new facility for the measurement of health-related quality of life. *Health Policy* **16**, 199–208.

Foster, E.M. & Connor, T. (2005) Public costs of better mental health services for children and adolescents. *Psychiatric Services* **56**, 50–55.

Foster, E.M. & Jones, D.E. (2005) The high costs of aggression: public expenditures resulting from conduct disorder. *American Journal of Public Health* **95**, 1767–1772.

Gilmore, A. & Milne, R. (2001) Methylphenidate in children with hyperactivity: review and cost-utility analysis. *Pharmacoepidemiology and Drug Safety* **10**, 85–94.

Glied, S. & Cuellar, A.E. (2003) Trends and issues in child and adolescent mental health. *Health Affairs(Millwood)* **22**, 39–50.

Guevara, J. *et al.* (2001) Utilization and cost of health care services for children with attention-deficit/hyperactivity disorder. *Pediatrics* **108**, 71–78.

Heckman, J.J. (2012) The developmental origins of health. *Health Economics* **21**, 24–29.

Heckman, J.J. *et al.* (2010) The rate of return to the high/scope perry preschool program. *Journal of Public Economics* **94**, 114–128.

Jacobson, J. *et al.* (1998) Cost-benefit estimates for early intensive behavioral intervention for young children with autism – general model and single state case. *Behavioral Interventions* **13**, 201–226.

Johnston, K. *et al.* (1999) Assessing the costs of healthcare technologies in clinical trials. *Health Technology Assessment* **3**, 1–76.

Knapp, M. (1993) Principles of applied cost research. In: *Costing Community Care: Theory and Practice.* (eds A. Netten & J. Beecham). Ashgate, Aldershot.

Knapp, M. (2013) Mental health in an age of austerity. *Evidence-Based Mental Health* **15**, 54–55.

Knapp, M. *et al.* (2011) Economic outcomes in adulthood and their associations with antisocial conduct, attention deficit and anxiety problems in childhood. *Journal of Mental Health Policy and Economics* **14**, 137–147.

Lund, C. *et al.* (2009) Scaling up child and adolescent mental health services in South Africa: human resource requirements and costs. *Journal of Child Psychology and Psychiatry* **50**, 1121–1130.

Machin, S. & McNally, S. (2008) The literacy hour. *Journal of Public Economics* **92**, 1441–1462.

Maughan, B. (1989) Growing up in the inner city: findings from the inner London longitudinal study. *Paediatric and Perinatal Epidemiology* **3**, 195–215.

Meltzer, H. *et al.* (2000) *Mental Health of Children and Adolescents in Great Britain.* The Stationery Office, London.

Molosankwe, I. *et al.* (2012) Economic aspects of the association between diabetes and depression: a systematic review. *Journal of Affective Disorders* **142**, S42–S55.

National Institute for Health and Care Excellence (2008) *Guide to the Methods of Technology Appraisal.* National Institute for Health and Care Excellence, London.

Naylor, C. *et al.* (2012) *Long Term Conditions and Mental Health: The Cost of Comorbidities.* The King's Fund.

Nelson, T.D. *et al.* (2013) Psychopathology as a predictor of medical service utilization for youth in residential treatment. *Journal of Behavioral Health Services and Research* **40**, 36–45.

Olsen, J.A. & Smith, R.D. (2001) Theory versus practice: a review of 'willingness-to-pay' in health and health care. *Health Economics* **10**, 39–52.

Organization for Economic Cooperation and Development. (2013) PPPs and exchange rates. Available: http://stats.oecd.org/Index.aspx.

Panter-Brick, C. & Leckman, J.F. (2013) Editorial commentary: resilience in child development–interconnected pathways to wellbeing. *Journal of Child Psychology and Psychiatry* **54**, 333–336.

Petrou, S. *et al.* (2010) Economic costs and preference-based health-related quality of life outcomes associated with childhood psychiatric disorders. *British Journal of Psychiatry* **197**, 395–404.

Romeo, R. *et al.* (2006) Economic cost of severe antisocial behaviour in children–and who pays it. *British Journal of Psychiatry* **188**, 547–553.

Ryan, M. (1999) Using conjoint analysis to take account of patient preferences and go beyond health outcomes: an application to in vitro fertilisation. *Social Science and Medicine* **48**, 535–546.

Schneider, W. *et al.* (1997) Short- and long-term effects of training phonological awareness in kindergarten: evidence from two German studies. *Journal of Experimental Child Psychology* **66**, 311–340.

Schweinhart, L.J. (2004) *The High/Scope Perry Preschool Study through age 40: Summary, Conclusions and Frequently Asked Questions.* High\Scope Educational Research Foundation, Ypsilanti, MI.

Scott, S. *et al.* (2001) Financial cost of social exclusion: follow up study of antisocial children into adulthood. *BMJ* **323**, 191.

Smit, F., *et al.* 2013. Long-lasting economic consequences of childhood neglect and abuse: population-based. Unpublished Manuscript.

Snell, T. *et al.* (2013) Economic impact of childhood psychiatric disorder on public sector services in Britain: estimates from national survey data. *Journal of Child Psychology and Psychiatry* **54**, 977–985.

Taylor, E. *et al.* (1991) *The Epidemiology of Childhood Hyperactivity.* Oxford University Press, London.

Torrance, G.W. *et al.* (1995) Multi-attribute preference functions. Health Utilities Index. *Pharmacoeconomics* **7**, 503–520.

Wahlbeck, K. & McDaid, D. (2012) Actions to alleviate the mental health impact of the economic crisis. *World Psychiatry* **11**, 139–145.

Wood, N.S. *et al.* (2000) Neurologic and developmental disability after extremely preterm birth. EPICure Study Group. *New England Journal of Medicine* **343**, 378–384.

CHAPTER 19

Legal issues in the care and treatment of children with mental health problems

Brenda Hale[1] and Jane Fortin[2]

[1] The Supreme Court, UK
[2] Sussex Law School, University of Sussex, Brighton, UK

The universality of human rights

The issues are universal: how are mental health professionals to navigate their way between the responsibilities of the parents, the autonomy of the child, and their professional duties toward their patient or client? In this chapter we shall illustrate the relevant concepts by reference to the law of England and Wales.[1] But it is likely that the legal principles will be very similar in those western countries whose legal systems are derived from the common law of England and Wales, including Canada, Australia, New Zealand, and most of the United States.

Moreover, the issues engage with the human rights of both parents and child. The right to liberty and security of person, the right not to be subjected to torture or inhuman or degrading treatment or punishment, the right to physical and psychological integrity, the right to respect for family life, and the right to a fair trial have been recognized since the United Nations Universal Declaration of Human Rights in 1948, since translated into the binding International Covenants on Civil and Political Rights and Economic, Social and Cultural Rights in 1966, and supplemented by UN Conventions catering for specific groups, of which the Convention on the Rights of the Child (CRC) 1989 and the Convention on the Rights of Persons with Disabilities (CRPD) 2006 are the most relevant. In addition, members of the Council of Europe must become parties to the European Convention on Human Rights (ECHR) 1950.

In common law countries, such international treaties are binding in international law once ratified, but do not generally become part of the ordinary law of the land unless the national Parliament so provides. Under the United Kingdom's Human Rights Act 1998 (HRA), the rights guaranteed by the ECHR became rights enforceable in the UK law. The UK has not legislated to incorporate the whole of the CRC or the CRPD into its domestic law; but the European Court of Human Rights in Strasbourg interprets the ECHR rights in the light of other international human rights instruments; so the CRC is increasingly finding its way into both the Strasbourg and the UK courts' judgments on children's rights issues.[2] Under its influence there is further support for the general movement toward now giving young people greater rights concerning their own future while reducing the supervisory rights of their parents.[3] Something similar may eventually be said of the CRPD.

Most western style democracies have written constitutions which also protect fundamental rights. The oldest is the Constitution of the United States of America, with its Bill of Rights of 1791 and later Amendments. This does not explicitly protect many of the rights recognized in the Universal Declaration and other modern instruments, but a great deal has been achieved through interpretation, in particular of the "due process" and "equal protection" clauses in the 14th Amendment. The modern Constitutions of the independent Commonwealth countries protect enumerated fundamental rights which are largely based on those in the ECHR. In between are the "old" Commonwealth countries, which (apart from Australia) have their own Bill or Charter of Rights, such as the Canadian Charter of Rights and Freedoms 1982. National laws dealing with mental health issues have therefore to be judged against these constitutional standards.

---

[1] Scotland and Northern Ireland are separate jurisdictions with their own laws.

[2] E.g. *Neulinger and Shuruk v Switzerland* (2012) 54 EHRR 31; *R (Williamson and Others) v Secretary of State for Education* [2005] UKHL 15, [2005] 2 AC 246 [80].

[3] *R (Axon) v Secretary of State for Health and another* [2006] EWHC 37 (Admin), [2006] 2 FLR 206, [115].

Rutter's Child and Adolescent Psychiatry, Sixth Edition.
Edited by Anita Thapar and Daniel S. Pine, James F. Leckman, Stephen Scott, Margaret J. Snowling, Eric Taylor.
© 2015 John Wiley & Sons Ltd. Published 2018 by John Wiley & Sons Ltd.

The different roles of the mental health professional

Most commonly, of course, a mental health professional will encounter a child or young person as a patient. In the UK, health care is a universal service, free to all (apart from some "persons from abroad") at the point of need, regardless of ability to pay. Unlike both the education and social care services, however, the NHS can rarely be obliged to offer treatment or care which it does not wish to offer. However, mental health professionals, like all other professionals, owe a duty of care to their own patients. If they negligently fail to diagnose or to treat, and the patient suffers harm as a result, they may be held liable in damages: for example, a child psychologist who fails to diagnose dyslexia[4] or a child psychiatrist who negligently diagnoses child abuse.[5] The duty is owed only to their child patient and not to the child's parents. The courts here and elsewhere recognize that if professionals also owed a duty to the parents, they might hesitate to diagnose abuse and the child would go unprotected.[6]

If health professionals wish to provide treatment for a child with mental health problems and either the child or his family resist this, they have a range of options available. These include persuading an approved mental health professional (AMHP) to invoke the compulsory procedures under the Mental Health Act 1983, persuading the local children's services authority to bring care proceedings under the Children Act 1989 (CA), or themselves applying to a family court for an order authorising the treatment. The choice between these will depend on whether it is the parents or the child who are seen as the principal obstacle and what it is ultimately sought to achieve—treatment for the child or a different family environment. These are discussed in the next two sections. Any court proceedings are likely to require expert evidence from mental health professionals, discussed in the concluding section.

Mental health professionals may also be involved in providing advice to other statutory agencies. Thus, for example, psychological reports are part of the formal process of assessing and providing the child with a "statement" of his special educational needs, which the education authorities are then under a legal duty to meet.[7] Unlike the health and social care services, the education services can be ordered by a tribunal to provide an individual child with the education which the tribunal decides that he needs.[8] Occasionally, psychiatric reports are required in the criminal justice system, on those rare occasions when a specialist mental health disposal is made, such as a hospital or guardianship order under the Mental Health Act 1983, or a youth rehabilitation order with a mental health treatment requirement under the Criminal Justice and Immigration Act 2008.

Intervening against the parents

If health or social care professionals encounter opposition to what they believe to be in the best interests of an individual child, the first question is whether it is appropriate to take action against the parents or against the child. With older children, the obstacle may well be the child. With younger children, the obstacle is generally the authority of the parents, known in English law as "parental responsibility." The mother automatically has parental responsibility, sharing it with the father if they are married to one another, or if an unmarried father has acquired it by agreement, court order, or since 1 December 2003 by registration on the child's birth certificate (CA, ss 2(1), (2), and (4)). The great majority of unmarried fathers are now registered.

In western democratic legal systems it is parents and families, rather than the State, who have the primary right and the primary responsibility to bring up their children: to meet their claims for nurture, care, and upbringing and to decide for themselves how this will be done. It is the hallmark of a dictatorship to gain control of the children and distance them from the varied and subversive influences of their families (Hale, 2005: 5). Hence article 8 of the ECHR, drafted in 1950 in the twin shadows of the Nazi totalitarianism of the recent past and the Stalinist totalitarianism of the then present, guarantees to everyone, parents and children alike, the right to respect for their private and family life, their home and their correspondence. The CRC also requires States Parties to recognize that "parents or, as the case may be, legal guardians, have the primary responsibility for the upbringing and development of the child. The best interests of the child will be *their* basic concern" (article 18.1, emphasis added). States Parties must also recognize "the right of the child to the enjoyment of the highest attainable standard of health and to facilities for the treatment of illness and rehabilitation of health" (article 24.1) and "that a mentally or physically disabled child should enjoy a full and decent life, in conditions which ensure dignity, promote self-reliance and facilitate the child's active participation in the community" (article 23.1).

The rights of parents are not absolute, and there are various ways of overcoming their neglect of or opposition to treatment. The CA provides in section 3(5) that a person who does not have parental responsibility for a child but has care of the child may "do what is reasonable in all the circumstances of the case for the purpose of safeguarding or promoting the child's welfare." This provision would clearly authorize emergency treatment to save a child's life or prevent serious deterioration in the child's health whatever the parents said. It would also authorize routine measures where the parents' views were not known and could not be obtained within a reasonable time. But it would not

---

[4] *Phelps v Hillingdon London Borough Council* [2001] 2 AC 619 (none has succeeded).

[5] Cf *X and Others v Bedfordshire County Council* [1995] 2 AC 633.

[6] *D v East Berkshire Community Health NHS Trust and Others* [2005] UKHL 23; *B and Others v Attorney General of New Zealand* [2003] UKPC 61; [2003] 4 All ER 803.

[7] Education Act (EA) 1996, Part IV. But as from 1st Sept 2014, "statements" will be replaced by Education, Health and Care (EHC) plans; see Children and Families Act 2014, Part 3.

[8] EA 1996, s 326.

be reasonable to proceed with major non urgent interventions without consulting the parents.

Historically, the only means of putting pressure on the parents to agree to treatment was the threat of prosecution for child neglect or abuse.[9] Some legal systems are still reluctant to go beyond this threat to secure parental compliance, but this will not help the child unless it is effective. And it is least likely to be effective against inadequate parents who simply do not appreciate the risks.[10]

For one-off situations, where the child is being properly looked after in other respects, a hospital or health care professional can apply to a court for permission to override the parent's objections. In English law this can be done either by invoking the ancient *parens patriae* jurisdiction of the High Court or by a "specific issue" order (CA 1989, s 8) authorising the treatment: for example, a blood transfusion for the child of Jehovah's Witnesses. Where two or more people have parental responsibility, each of them may act alone and without the other in meeting it (CA, s 2(7)), so the consent of one parent will usually suffice. But where they disagree, the other parent can take steps to prohibit the treatment until the matter is resolved by the court, so in practice such disputes may have to be taken to court. The same procedures can also be invoked by a professional who wants to *prevent* treatment to which a parent had agreed: for example, the sterilization of an 11-year-old girl with Sotos' syndrome.[11]

Many children with mental health problems or learning difficulties are likely to present more long-term and complex problems. The family environment and dynamics may be an important part of the child's difficulties. If so, it may be necessary to bring proceedings to remove the child from the harmful environment. Indeed, in some cases, it may be thought necessary to remove the child at or soon after birth, in order to prevent his suffering harm to his mental or psychological health in the future. Responsibility for undertaking care proceedings lies, not with the health authorities, but with the local children's services authorities, which have the statutory responsibility to protect children from harm (CA, s 47 and Sched 2). This is because the eventual outcome of most care proceedings is that the authority will have to take parental responsibility for the child. Care by a local authority may not be ideal, but at least the authority should have, or have access to, the full range of facilities needed to take care of the child, including the health and education services. Neither the health nor the education services are equipped to cater for everything which parents should provide for their children, nor can they find alternative homes for children who need them.

It is not enough that such intervention is in the child's best interests. While some legal systems have a list of specific grounds for taking children into care, section 31(2) of the Children Act 1989 focusses on actual or likely harm to the child. First, it must be shown that the child is suffering or likely to suffer significant harm. "Harm" means ill-treatment or the impairment of health or development (see Chapters 29 and 30). "Health" means physical or mental health. "Development" means physical, intellectual, emotional, social or behavioral development. "Ill-treatment" includes sexual abuse and forms of ill-treatment which are not physical. Hence it is very likely that a child with mental health problems whose health or educational needs are not being met will be suffering or likely to suffer significant harm. But it is not the object of the Act to supply children with ideal parents to replace the less than ideal parents which we all are. It is not enough that the children might do better with different parents. As Hedley J said in *Re L (Care: Threshold Criteria)*,[12] which was a case about children of parents with quite serious learning difficulties, ". . . society must be able to tolerate very diverse standards of parenting, including the eccentric, the barely adequate, and the inconsistent. It follows too that children will inevitably have both very different experiences of parenting and very unequal consequences flowing from it." So one problem is to distinguish "significant harm" from the ordinary consequences of growing up with parents who are learning disabled, mentally ill, substance abusers, criminals or whatever.

"Likely" does not mean "probable," but simply "a real possibility, a possibility which cannot sensibly be ignored having regard to the nature and gravity of the feared harm in the particular case."[13] So quite a low risk of really serious harm might justify preventive action, whereas if the feared harm is less serious, a greater risk may be required. Section 31(2) also requires that the harm, or likelihood of harm, is attributable to a lack of reasonable parental care, because the child's carers have not provided or will not provide it, and not because the services themselves are failing to deliver what the child needs.

Once the harm threshold is crossed, the court can decide what order will be best for the child. It may be better for the child to make no order at all; but unless there is someone else (such as another family member) who is willing and able to take parental responsibility for the child, the only other choices are a supervision order and a care order. A supervision order places the child under the local authority's supervision, but without affecting the parents' own parental responsibility. Conditions for medical or psychiatric examination and treatment of the child can be imposed, if there is medical evidence to support it (CA, s 35 and Sched 3, paras 4 and 5). But supervision is rarely thought sufficient to protect the child from significant harm. A care order gives the designated local authority parental responsibility for the child, which can limit the parents' exercise of their responsibility. The court has no power to impose conditions or to insist that the local authority discharge their parental responsibilities in a particular way. This puts the court

---

[9] Children and Young Persons Act 1933, s 1(1). A parent is presumed to have neglected a child in a manner likely to cause unnecessary suffering or injury to health if he has failed to provide the child with adequate medical treatment: s 1(2)(a).

[10] *R v Sheppard* [1981] AC 394.

[11] *Re D (A Minor)(Wardship: Sterilisation)* [1976] Fam 185.

---

[12] [2007] 1 FLR 2050, 2063.

[13] *Re H (Minors) (Sexual Abuse: Standard of Proof)* [1996] AC 563, 585F.

in a quandary. How can it know whether the order will be in the best interests of the child unless it knows how the authority plan to look after him and has some confidence that the plan will be carried out? This can be a source of frustration both for courts and for health care professionals whose recommendations for treatment are not always adopted by the local authority (Thorpe & Clarke, 1998), but courts have neither the resources nor the expertise to act as substitute parents for children.

In most cases, the real choice is between planning to reunite the child with his family and planning to place him with a permanent alternative family. This raises an even greater dilemma. If the authorities intervene early, before a child suffers permanent harm, the more likely it is that he can be successfully placed for adoption with a new family. The later things are left, the more harm is done, and the more difficult it will be successfully to repair the damage. The dilemma is particularly acute with emotional neglect or abuse which may take many years to result in significant harm to the child, if indeed they ever do. But can such early intervention be justified in human rights terms?

Article 8(2) of the ECHR permits interference by a public authority with the right to respect for family life only if three conditions are fulfilled. First, the intervention must be "in accordance with the law"; this means that it must comply with a national law which is sufficiently clear and certain for people to be able to conduct themselves accordingly. Second, the interference must be for one of the legitimate aims laid down; in this case, for the protection of the "health or morals" or the "rights and freedoms" of the child. Third, and most important, the interference must be "necessary in a democratic society"; this means that the steps taken must be proportionate to the legitimate aim pursued and the reasons given must be relevant and sufficient. The Strasbourg court generally allows a wide "margin of appreciation" to the national authorities in deciding whether to take a child into public care.[14] But the aim when doing so must generally be to reunite the family; so steps which cut children off from their families of birth will be scrutinized with much more care. Permanent removal requires exceptional justification in the interests of the child.

If the court considers that the local authority should take steps to make possible the reunification of parent and child and the local authority fails to do this, a parent might complain that the authority was acting in breach of either her own or the child's convention rights. If the court considers that the child needs a permanent family elsewhere but the local authority fails to take timely steps to find one, the child might have a claim that his family life should not have been taken away from him without providing him with an alternative family.

Separate court authorisation is needed under the Adoption and Children Act 2002 if the child is to be placed for adoption without the parents' consent (see Chapter 22). This can be done at the same time as a care order is made or later. Parental consent can only be dispensed with if the court is satisfied that the welfare of the child requires this (s 52). This is a test of necessity, not desirability.[15] Compulsory adoption is clearly the most drastic possible interference in the family life of a child, his parents, and their wider family and the UK is unusual in allowing this. But in *R and H v United Kingdom*,[16] the Strasbourg court held that it was justifiable to free a child for adoption without parental consent when it was clear that the child could not go back to parents who had a long history of alcohol abuse. This was despite the expert evidence that the child needed to retain contact with her parents, so that every effort should be made to find adopters who would support that contact, and the proceedings should be adjourned to enable that to be done. But the Strasbourg court reiterated that "measures which deprive biological parents of the parental responsibilities and authorize adoption should only be applied in exceptional circumstances and can only be justified if they are motivated by overriding requirements pertaining to the child's welfare" (para 81).

The particular dilemmas arising where it is feared that a parent's mental health problems may cause psychological harm to a child in the future are well illustrated in the Supreme Court case of *Re B*.[17] The mother had a history of sexual abuse in childhood and had begun a long and abusive relationship with her controlling and violent stepfather when she was still under 16. She also had a history of presenting herself to many different hospitals and doctors with a variety of symptoms, some of which had a physical explanation, but the history satisfied the diagnostic criteria for somatisation disorder. There were also indications of factitious illness disorder, though not of the so-called Munchausen syndrome by proxy. Eventually she succeeded in extricating herself from the relationship with her stepfather (leaving behind their daughter, then aged 10) and formed a relationship with the father of her new baby. When the baby was born, there was such a confusion of accusation and counter-accusation from the mother and her stepfather, in which the dreaded word "Munchausen's' featured, that the child was removed on an interim care order shortly after birth. But the parents showed during regular contact that they were devoted to her and well able to cater for her immediate needs and she became strongly attached to them. The trial judge found that there was a risk that she would suffer psychological harm from her mother's somatisation disorder, and quite extraordinary propensity for lying and deceptive behavior, and some risk of her being exposed to unnecessary medical examinations and treatment. The judge also found that the parents would not be able to cooperate with social services in a programme of monitoring and support to avoid these risks, so there was no alternative but to agree to the local authority's plan for adoption.

Was this "significant harm" or was it just the ordinary risk that a child might pick up bad behaviors from her parents? Was the unquantified risk of the child doing so a sufficiently "real possibility" to justify compulsory preventive action? Above all, was

---

[14] E.g. *KA v Finland* (2001) 2 FLR 696.

[15] *S v L* [2012] UKSC 30, 2012 SLT 961.
[16] [2011] 2 FLR 1236.
[17] [2013] UKSC 33, [2013] 1 WLR 1911.

an unquantified risk of this sort of psychological or emotional harm at some time in the distant future sufficient to justify the most drastic step of all, the separation of the child from her parents at birth and placement in a closed adoption? The Supreme Court upheld the judge's decision, but one of the Justices dissented on the ground that this was not a proportionate response to the risk presented.

Intervening against the child

When health or social care professionals encounter opposition to what they believe to be in the best interests of an individual child, the source of the problem may be the child's own resistance. Traditionally the assumption was that the right to decide the medical treatment of a child rested with his parents. Today, this approach is being reassessed, particularly in relation to adolescents, many of whom have an intellectual development on a par with many adults. Although most countries have a relatively high age of legal majority (18 is the most common in countries in the EU), there has been a growing realization worldwide that long before this, many adolescents acquire a strong personal interest in taking responsibility for decisions affecting their future.

The child's right to consent to treatment

In England and Wales where the age of majority is 18, legislation enables 16 and 17 year-olds to consent to surgical, medical, or dental treatment themselves with no need to seek parental consent.[18] But what of those under the age of 16?

In the late 1980s, the groundbreaking decision of the House of Lords in *Gillick v West Norfolk and Wisbech Area Health Authority* (*Gillick*)[19] established that even a child under 16 who had sufficient understanding was able to give a valid consent to medical treatment and advice. It was a question of fact, to be decided on a case by case basis, whether the child had "sufficient understanding of what is involved to give a valid consent in law." If the child was competent to consent, the parents need not be involved. The notion of "*Gillick*-competence" (or the "mature minor" doctrine) became widely used in common law countries by doctors dealing with young patients. [20]

Although doctors were provided with more specific guidance when providing contraceptive advice and treatment without involving parents,[21] in a more general medical context the

"*Gillick*-competence" test has been criticized for its ambiguities (NSW, 2008: 4.10); for leaving doctors to assess competence, with the possibility of judges second-guessing them in the event of a parental challenge (Parkinson, 1986: 14); for ignoring the realities of every day medical practice (Cretney, 1985: 173); and for failing to provide doctors with clear guidelines (Brazier & Bridge, 1996: 91–92). In particular, it contains no guidance as to the extent to which an adjustment should be made for factors affecting adolescents' understanding, such as peer pressure, drug and substance abuse, family stress, emotional disturbance, risk taking, physical and mental illness—all matters which might radically influence their ability to attain *Gillick* competence (Fortin, 2009: 82–86).

Doctors may therefore be in some doubt over their precise legal standing regarding treatment without parental consent. In the UK, legal developments in relation to determining the capacity of adults with mental disorders or disabilities may prove useful. This topic was much explored through case law and by official bodies (e.g., Law Commission 1995), culminating in the test of capacity laid down in section 3 of the Mental Capacity Act 2005 (MCA). An adult is presumed to have capacity and is only unable to make a decision for himself if he is "unable (a) to understand the information relevant to the decision; (b) to retain that information; and (c) to use or weigh that information as part of the process of making the decision; or (d) to communicate his decision (whether by talking, using sign language or by any other means)." Although the Act only applies to adults, doctors may find that the same concepts are helpful when deciding whether a child is *Gillick*-competent.

It is not entirely clear how the concept of *Gillick* competence fits with the principles of human rights law. The CRC and the CRPD deliver a rather different message from the one sent out by *Gillick*. Article 12(1) of the CRC requires States to give all children who are capable of forming their own views, the right to express these freely in all matters affecting them and the right to have their views given "due weight in accordance with the age and maturity of the child." Article 7(3) of the CRPD requires children with disabilities to be given that right on an equal basis with other children, and to be provided with disability and age appropriate assistance to realize that right. This gives every child, not merely a *Gillick*-competent child, the right to *participate* in decision-making about himself, and (in the CRPD) to be helped to be able to do so. But, unlike *Gillick*, this right to be consulted is not about autonomy: it does not give children the right to decide matters for themselves.

Turning to the ECHR, one might assume that article 8 of the ECHR reinforces the concept of *Gillick* competence and autonomy. In case law concerning adults, the Strasbourg court has emphasized that it protects the right to respect for physical and psychological integrity, and includes the right to

---

[18] Family Law Reform Act 1969, section 8 (2). See also Age of Legal Capacity (Scotland) Act 1991, section 2(4).

[19] [1986] AC 112.

[20] E.g. *Secretary, Department of Health and Community Services v JWB* (*Marion's case*) (1992) 175 CLR 218 (Australia); *JSC v Wren* (1986), 76 AR 115 (CA) (Canada).

[21] Lord Fraser in *Gillick* stated that the doctor should be satisfied: (1) that the girl (although under 16) will understand his advice; (2) that he cannot persuade her to inform her parents or allow him to inform the parents that she is seeking contraceptive advice; (3) that she is very likely to begin or to continue having sexual intercourse with or without contraceptive treatment;

(4) that unless she receives contraceptive advice or treatment her physical or mental health or both are likely to suffer; and (5) that her best interests require him to give her contraceptive advice, treatment or both without the parental consent. And see Department of Health (2004).

self-determination or the "notion of autonomy"[22]; it protects against compulsory medical intervention even if that intervention is of minor importance.[23] In theory these rights are available to everyone, irrespective of age and certainly irrespective of opposition from third parties, such as parents. But in a rare (and controversial) early decision about the psychiatric care of a child, the European court adopted a conservative approach to the notion of children having rights against their parents.[24] Nevertheless, the High Court has since held that the concept of *Gillick* competence is unaffected by a mother's (article 8) right to bring up her daughters free from state interference—that her rights are not so extensive that they override her daughters' own (article 8) right to medical privacy.[25]

Overriding the child's refusal to consent to treatment

But where does this leave the "*Gillick*-competent" teenager who wishes to refuse consent to what is proposed? *Gillick* appeared to give mature minors the right to decide for themselves what medical treatment they should *or should not* receive. How then should a doctor respond to a desperately ill adolescent patient who rejects even lifesaving treatment (Ferguson, 2004; NSW, 2008; Irish Law Reform Commission, 2011)? Crucially, did Lord Scarman's words that the "parental right yields to the child's right to make his own decisions when he reaches a sufficient understanding and intelligence to be capable of making up his own mind on the matter requiring decision" (*Gillick*, p. 186) preserve the right of the parents to give an alternative consent (Fortin, 2011: 202–208; Herring *et al.* 2012: 62–68)?

While most doctors sympathize with the need to adopt more liberal attitudes toward adolescents' own powers of consent, they are also aware that some adolescents are particularly ill-equipped to reach decisions which affect their long-term well-being. An adolescent's capacity to make wise health care decisions may be greatly hampered by emotional and social immaturity, risk-taking behavior and a concern only for the short-term consequences of decisions (NSW, 2008: 2.29–2.34).

Given these factors, it is arguable that young people's capacity to make health care decisions should require not only the competence to understand information relating to the proposed health care and to consider multiple options, but also to choose voluntarily, free from outside influence, and to appreciate the nature of the decision—in terms of its gravity, immediacy, and the permanence of the choice. "Decision-making competence should be linked not just with developing cognition, but also to life experience and experience in making decisions" (NSW, 2008: 2.31). Arguably, the MCA definition (see above), with its emphasis on the ability to use the information understood in order to arrive at a free choice, would meet this concern.

On the other hand, in developmental terms, an adolescent's brain is more like that of an adult than that of a young child—and an adolescent patient may be just as intelligent as many adult patients. The fact that serious risks or consequences may result from an *adult's* refusal of medical treatment does not undermine his or her right to self-determination— a choice not to allow treatment must be respected, whether or not the professionals agree with the patient's decision.[26] Why should an adolescent patient be treated any differently, particularly now that society perceives young people as individuals with rights and points of view of their own?

In two English cases decided in the 1990s, doctors faced with adolescents refusing lifesaving treatment made their patients wards of court in order to side step that refusal. Both applications involved adolescents with serious psychological problems.[27] The Court of Appeal held that under its inherent jurisdiction it could override a young patient's wishes and authorize lifesaving treatment in his or her best interests. Although not necessary for the decision, it went further and said that *anyone* with parental responsibility for a minor patient could authorize doctors to carry out much needed treatment despite the patient's own clear opposition. This authority could be granted whatever the patient's age (over or under the age of 16) and whether or not he or she was *Gillick* competent. Such a judicial response is not surprising and has been followed in later cases. Given the courts' protective responsibility for all minors, they may find it impossible to conclude that it is in the child's best interests to be allowed to die.[28] The Court of Appeal was also concerned to provide doctors with a legal "flak jacket" protecting them against litigation where the minor has refused treatment.[29]

Although convenient for doctors, this principle makes substantial inroads into the principle of adolescent responsibility established in *Gillick* (Douglas, 1992). It has also produced a situation that appears illogical and confusing. The law allows a *Gillick* competent adolescent to consent to medical treatment, which the parents have no right to veto. But it allows those same parents to override that same adolescent's refusal to accept such treatment. Most of all, it is one thing to allow a *court* to override the child's decision after a fair hearing in which all sides of the argument have been properly ventilated. It is another thing to allow a parent—or worse still a local authority with parental

---

[22] *Pretty v United Kingdom* [2002] 2 FLR 45, [61].

[23] *YF v Turkey* (2004) 39 EHRR 34, para [33]: 'A person's body concerns the most intimate aspect of one's private life.'

[24] *Nielsen v Denmark* (1988) 11 EHRR 175.

[25] *R (Axon) v Secretary of State for Health and the Family Planning Association* [2006] EWCA 37 (Admin), [2006] 2 FLR 206.

[26] *Re B (Adult: Refusal of Medical Treatment)* [2002] EWHC 429 (Fam) [2002] 2 All ER 449, [94].

[27] *Re R (A Minor) (Wardship: Consent to Treatment)* [1992] Fam 11, authorizing the compulsory use of anti-psychotic drugs to treat a 15-year-old suffering from increasingly paranoid and disturbed behaviour; *Re W (A Minor) (Medical Treatment: Court's Jurisdiction)* [1993] Fam 64, authorizing the compulsory treatment of a 16-year-old in a dangerously anorexic state.

[28] See *Re E (A Minor) (Wardship: Medical Treatment)* [1993] 1 FLR 386, 394: a court 'should be very slow to allow an infant to martyr himself'.

[29] *Re W (A Minor) (Medical Treatment: Court's Jurisdiction)* [1993] Fam 64, 78.

responsibility—the right to force unwanted treatment on a competent child.

When considering this issue, the New South Wales law reformers considered that the parental right of veto should be jettisoned but that the *courts'* right to override their refusal should be retained where a young person's decision is considered to damage his or her best interests (NSW, 2008: paras 5.44–5.45). In their view it was important for the courts to retain this power; a paternalistic approach was justified because "young people, even as they reach the intellectual or cognitive capacities of adults, still as a group tend to lack a certain level of maturity and world experience because of their youth" (para 2.64). Furthermore, it was important for the courts to have the power to save adolescents from making medical decisions which they might later regret and which might hinder their longer life chances (para 2.73).

Cases of this kind may be complicated by the existence of a religious element. An adolescent growing up in a deeply religious home with parents opposed to certain kinds of medical treatment may have a limited opportunity for independent thought (Brazier & Bridge, 1996: 104); but overriding firmly held religious convictions will undoubtedly reinforce distress over enforced treatment. Courts here and abroad have shown little appetite for allowing the wishes of adolescents with strong religious views to dictate a fatal outcome.[30] English courts have sometimes found a way round this dilemma by adopting a stringent approach to the assessment of young patients' competence. Young Jehovah's Witnesses have been held to lack competence because they do not understand the manner of their impending death, together with the pain and distress accompanying it.[31] Critics point out that although few adults can comprehend the process of dying, the pain they would suffer, the fear they would undergo and relatives' distress in watching them die, neither doctors nor the courts are entitled to overrule their refusal to undergo treatment for similar reasons (McCafferty, 1999).

This issue has not so far reached the UK Supreme Court. But in *AC v Manitoba (Director of Child and Family Services)*,[32] the Supreme Court of Canada dealt with a challenge from AC, a 14-year-old Jehovah's Witness, forced to undergo blood transfusion treatment for a life-threatening condition. Its survey of international approaches to this problem, including that of the English Court of Appeal, showed that other jurisdictions were finding it equally difficult to allow adolescents to reject lifesaving treatment: " … courts … have generally not seen the 'mature minor' doctrine as dictating guaranteed outcomes, particularly where the consequences for the young person are catastrophic" (para 69). The majority considered that the provincial legislation giving the courts a discretionary power to authorize medical treatment for adolescents under the age of 16, even against their wishes, did not unduly infringe AC's constitutional right to freedom from forced medical treatment. The state had a legitimate

concern to protect younger adolescents as a vulnerable group from making decisions before attaining capacity for truly mature and independent thought.

While this judicial approach is comprehensible, it is also controversial.[33] Some have argued that enforced survival to adulthood might not be in every child's best interests (Lewis, 2001: 159; Harmon, 2010: 95). There is also a concern that the courts sometimes find themselves on a slope too slippery to resist and do not restrict their interventions to circumstances where paternalism can be justified on lifesaving grounds. While it may be morally justifiable to override the wishes of a competent adolescent patient to prevent "death or severe permanent injury," it is questionable where failure to treat will not produce such dire consequences—especially in mental health settings involving compulsory detention.[34] Furthermore, granting such authority may entail the use of physical force. As Gostin says, "Nothing degrades a human being more than to have intrusive treatment thrust on him despite his full understanding of its nature and purpose and his clear will to say 'no'" (Gostin, 1992: 76).

Does human rights law hold the key to this problem? It provides child patients, like adults, with a right to freedom from arbitrary deprivation of liberty,[35] an absolute right to protection from inhuman and degrading treatment, and a qualified right to respect for their physical and psychological integrity.[36] On the other hand, like adults, they also have a right to life, which in certain circumstances includes the right of a vulnerable patient or prisoner to be prevented from harming himself.[37] Perhaps Strasbourg would regard an adolescent refusing lifesaving treatment in the same light. Furthermore, it takes the view that, in principle, treatment which is a "medical necessity" infringes neither article 3 nor article 8.[38] But that is in the context of detained psychiatric patients. It remains to be seen what view both the UK and the Strasbourg courts would take of a human rights challenge to the power of either the parents or the courts to impose treatment on a competent child who refuses it. Strasbourg's decision in *Storck v Germany*,[39] holding that an 18 year old's right to liberty was infringed when she was detained in a psychiatric hospital on her father's authority suggests that they might be willing to reconsider their early and controversial stand favoring parents' rights against children's rights in the context of medical decision making.[40] It has been suggested that *Storck* sent out

---

[30] E.g. *Minister for Health v AS* [2004] WASC 286, 33 Fam LR 223.
[31] E.g. *Re E (A Minor)(Wardship: Medical Treatment)* [1993] 1 FLR 386.
[32] 2009 SCC 30, [2009] 2 SCR 181.

[33] Binnie J gave a strong dissenting judgment.
[34] E.g. *Re K, W and H (Minors)(Medical Treatment)* [1993] 1 FLR 854: psychiatric treatment unit authorized to use 'emergency medication' when treating mentally disturbed teenagers.
[35] ECHR, article 5; also CRC, article 37(b).
[36] ECHR, articles 3 and 8; also CRC article 19(a).
[37] *Savage v South Essex Partnership NHS Foundation Trust* [2008] UKHL 74, [2009] 1 AC 681; *Rabone v Pennine Care NHS Trust* [2012] UKSC 2, [2012] 2 AC 72.
[38] *Herczegfalvy v Austria* (1993) 15 EHRR 437.
[39] (2006) 43 EHRR 96.
[40] *Nielsen v Denmark* (1988) 11 EHRR 175.

"a clear message indicating a different approach to the personal autonomy of young people."[41]

Using mental health law

Sometimes children, more commonly adolescents, require specialized treatment for mental health problems and, rarely, their doctors need compulsory powers to ensure that this occurs. The Mental Health Act 1983 (MHA) applies to all patients requiring treatment for mental disorder, irrespective of their age (for a full account, see Hale, 2010). Where hospital treatment is needed, most patients are admitted informally under section 131(1), thereby avoiding the compulsory procedures.

In the past, the informal admission of mentally ill or behaviorally disturbed young people might be far from voluntary. Doctors were frequently reluctant to use the MHA to enforce their young patients' detention and treatment (BMA, 2001: 140), the most common objection being the perceived stigma for the child, when adult, attached to the use of compulsory powers. It was tempting, therefore, for doctors to utilize the 1990s case law discussed above, and thereby rely on parental authority to admit patients under 18 informally, even against their will, with none of the safeguards available for those compulsorily detained under the MHA. Alternatively doctors could ask the court to authorize admission.

The Mental Health Amendment Act 2007 introduced important new legal safeguards for older adolescents regarding their informal admission. This responded to critics arguing that children, whether competent or not, had liberty interests which should be protected against the well-meaning but possibly arbitrary decisions of their parents. Parents should not be able to "volunteer" their children for informal admission for psychiatric treatment without some additional safeguard, such as an automatic tribunal review (Gostin, 1975). Now, where a patient aged 16 or 17 has capacity to consent to informal admission to hospital for treatment for mental disorder, and does consent, the arrangements may be made on his or her authority, even though there are one or more persons who have parental responsibility for him (s 131 (2), (3)); and where such a patient does *not* consent, the arrangements may *not* be made, even though a person with parental responsibility does consent (s 131(2, (4)). So doctors can no longer bypass the refusal of a patient aged 16 or 17 who has capacity, by obtaining parental consent. They will have to choose between using compulsion under the MHA and going to court (Code of Practice, 2008: 36.27–36.33). The young patient's capacity to consent should be judged, not by the broad test of *Gillick* competence, but by the more explicit criteria of the Mental Capacity Act 2005 (s 3; discussed above).

The MHA does not deal with the position where a child under the age of 16 also has that capacity. Presumably, therefore, the *Gillick* principle will apply where the child does consent

to admission. Where a competent child refuses to agree to admission, the Code of Practice advises that "the trend in recent cases is to reflect greater autonomy for competent under 18s, so it may be unwise to rely on the consent of a person with parental responsibility" (para 36.43). If so, as with the older age group, the professionals will have to choose between the compulsory procedures in the MHA or asking the court to authorize admission and treatment.

Where a child of any age is not competent, or expresses no view about his admission, it will generally be possible to rely on parental consent to his or her informal admission. The Code points out that the child may have the intellectual capacity to make a decision but in fact be so overwhelmed by the situation that he is unable to do so (paras 36.28 and 36.37). But before doctors turn to parents for legal authority, they should perhaps reflect on the wisdom of doing so, given how difficult parents will find it to be objective over their children's mental health needs.

Admission and treatment are different matters legally. Informal patients may not be treated without valid consent or some other lawful justification, so the same legal principles as those discussed earlier will apply. In other words, for those aged between 16 and 17, their competence to consent to treatment will be assessed by the criteria set out by the MCA; competence to consent for those under 16 is assessed by the *Gillick* competence criterion.

Where informal admission or treatment is not possible, the same compulsory powers to admit for up to 28 days assessment (under section 2,), or for up to 72 hours in an emergency (under section 4), or longer term for treatment (under section 3) are available for patients of any age. Although, as noted below, these procedures have features designed to protect the human rights of mental patients, they must obviously be effective to overcome the objections of the patient and, when relevant, the objections of a parent. A patient's nearest relative (usually his parent, if the patient is a minor) has no right to prevent an approved mental health professional (AMHP) making an application for short-term admission under section 2 or section 4, although "before or within a reasonable time," the AMHP must "take such steps as are practicable" to inform that person that the application is to be or has been made (s 11(3)). An AMHP cannot make an application for long-term admission for treatment under section 3 without first consulting the nearest relative, unless this is not reasonably practicable or would involve unreasonable delay (s 11(4)(b)); active consent of the nearest relative is not required, but the application cannot be made if he objects (s 11(4)(a)). But there is a process for applying to a court to replace a nearest relative who unreasonably objects to the admission or is otherwise unsuitable (s 29).

The Act recognizes that removing a person's liberty in order to compel him to accept treatment is a drastic step and so the criteria, the procedures and the consequences are clearly defined. Most forms of treatment for mental disorder may be given without the patient's consent (s 63); this includes

---

[41] *Austin v Metropolitan Police Commissioner* [2009] UKHL 5, [2009] 1 AC 564, [45], Lord Walker.

force-feeding for anorexia nervosa.[42] There are special safeguards for neurosurgery, long-term medication and ECT (ss 57, 58, 58A). Neurosurgery cannot be performed on any patient, whether or not he is detained, unless the patient is capable of consenting to it, does so consent and an independent multidisciplinary team certify that it should be given (s 57). Patients under 18, whether or not they are detained, cannot be given ECT without the benefit of an independent second opinion (ss 56(5) and 58A). Patients also have the right to apply to a tribunal for their discharge.[43]

It appears that attitudes to the use of the MHA for minors are gradually changing and that, particularly when treating eating disorders in older adolescents, doctors are now more prepared to envisage its use. As discussed above, the law now acknowledges the autonomy rights of mentally ill or behaviorally disturbed 16- and 17-year-olds so far as informal admission is concerned. But in other respects, because of the law's complexity and uncertainty, young patients' rights can be overlooked. There is a difficult balance to be struck between the protection given by legal formalities and the stigma they are sometimes thought to bring. But doctors specializing in child and adolescent psychiatry are more used to negotiating these dilemmas than any lawyer could ever be.

Expert witnesses

Compulsory procedures under the MHA require the prescribed medical recommendations explaining that the statutory criteria are made out (MHA, s 12). The patient's responsible clinician will usually be called up to give evidence if the detention is challenged in a tribunal and the patient may have the benefit of an independent psychiatric report. Mental health professionals are also frequently called up to give expert evidence in court proceedings about a child's future, assessing either the parents' mental health or parenting capacities, or the child's mental health and development, or both. Experts differ from other witnesses in that they are permitted to give evidence, not only as to the facts, but also as to their opinions. In children's proceedings they are allowed to base those opinions on hearsay.[44] But they should be willing to acknowledge that medical records are not always perfectly accurate or complete and may from time to time repeat or rely on unverified hearsay.

Expert witnesses fall into two broad categories, although the distinction between them is not always clear cut. Professionals who are already working with the child or his family may be asked to report on the history, diagnosis and treatment to date, together with their assessment and recommendations

for the future. Independent experts may be commissioned to investigate, sometimes only on paper and sometimes also by seeing the parties, and to make a report and recommendations to the court.[45] Such reports may be commissioned by any of the parties to the case, but the court is in charge of whether and how many experts may be instructed and in which disciplines.[46] One original aim is to prevent the child being subjected to multiple examinations and assessments (Butler-Sloss, 1988). Another is to prevent the proceedings becoming unnecessarily prolonged and expensive.

The court has power to require an assessment of the child but not the treatment of the parents.[47] This does not always reflect the realities of psychiatric practice. In some of the most complex and difficult cases, it is not possible to separate the assessment of the child from the assessment of the parents.[48] What requires assessment is the relationship between them all and the capacities of the parents to meet the needs of the child. What begins as assessment may move into assessment with therapy and move again into therapy with continuing assessment. It has been forcefully argued that doctors are assessing their patients all the time (Kennedy, 2001). Our nice legal distinctions mean nothing to them. This would not matter were it not for the problems of funding the very specialist resources which some of these deeply damaged families require. The court can only require the parties to pay for an assessment which is necessary to enable the court to perform its own function of deciding what order to make.

There is another problem in child protection proceedings (Norgrove, 2011: para 33): the quality of evidence presented by local authorities to the courts is "not consistently good"; "this fuels distrust and lack of confidence in local authority social work"; and the reluctance of courts to rely on local authority social workers rather than other experts "encourages authorities to think there is little point in carrying out their own expert assessment before a case begins." Hence the courts became disinclined to rely on evidence provided by local authorities and turned to independent experts instead (Pearce *et al.*, 2011).

The court may require the parties to agree on a single, jointly instructed expert. Even then, some cases require expertise in more than one discipline.[49] And while the battle between separately instructed experts can be unedifying, especially if one or other is seen as a "hired gun" for the instructing party, a single joint expert brings problems for a party who wishes to challenge his conclusions. Parents or children's guardians who have serious concerns about the accuracy or rigor of an expert's report face formidable difficulties if they try to challenge it without expert evidence of their own. It is not easy to reconcile the need of the child to be spared multiple and intrusive investigations, and to

---

[42] *Riverside Mental Health NHS Trust v Fox* [1994] 1 FLR 614.

[43] Now the Health, Education and Social Care (HESC) Chamber within the First-tier Tribunal.

[44] Children Act 1989, s 96(3) to (7) and Children (Admissibility of Hearsay Evidence) Order 1993. But hearsay evidence is now generally admissible in civil proceedings in England and Wales: Civil Evidence Act 1995.

[45] *Re B (Sexual Abuse: Expert's Report)* [2000] 1 FLR 871.

[46] Family Proceedings Rules 2010, rule 25.1; Civil Procedure Rules 1998, rule 35.4.

[47] Children Act 1989, s 38(6); *Re G (A Child) (Interim Care Order: Residential Assessment)* [2005] UKHL 68; [2006] 1 AC 576.

[48] *Re C (A Minor) (Interim Care Order: Residential Assessment)* [1997] AC 489.

[49] E.g. *Re B*, above.

have the issues about his future resolved without delay, with the right (guaranteed by article 6 of the ECHR as well as the common law) of both the child and his family to a fair trial of the issues. Added to this was the reluctance of courts to make a final order which would hand over complete responsibility to the local authority (Norgrove, 2011).

The result was that by 2011 the more complicated care cases were taking more than a year to resolve. Experts were used in around 92% of care order applications, with a staggering average of 3.9 reports per case (Cassidy & Davey, 2011). The bulk of these were from adult or child psychiatrists or psychologists (Chief Medical Officer, 2006: para 2.13). They were prepared on a fee-paid basis, funded by the Legal Services Commission at levels which deterred the more experienced and better qualified practitioners from taking it on, leaving the task to more junior or retired practitioners. Hence there was also criticism of the quality of much of the psychological evidence given in care cases (Ireland, 2012).

In 2006, the Chief Medical Officer proposed that the NHS should recognize that its duty under the Children Act 2004 to safeguard and promote the welfare of children should extend beyond caring for the sick and injured and into providing expert medical evidence for the family courts as a public service. NHS Trusts should set up specialty and multidisciplinary teams for that purpose. But that proposal has still not been taken up, except in pilot projects. Instead, expert evidence can now only be commissioned where it is *necessary* to resolve the case and the information is not already available from other sources.[50] The court, rather than the parties, should decide what questions the expert should address. The expert's overriding duty is to the court and takes precedence over any duty to the party who instructs him. An expert witness enjoys immunity from suit in respect of his evidence but not the investigations leading up to it[51]; but this does not protect him from professional discipline if, for example, he goes beyond the limits of his expertise[52]; and he may be held liable in negligence to the party who instructs him.[53] In family proceedings, a lack of contradiction or opposition will place a heightened duty of independent professionalism on the expert witness and of vigilance on the court.

Conclusion

Children with mental health problems present more legal issues than do adults: there is the parents' responsibility for and authority over the child, as well as the more problematic question of the child's own autonomy. Mental health professionals are now much more aware of such questions than once they

were. Fortunately, most of the time they are able to treat their patients without disputes or challenge. It is always better to try and reach agreement rather than to resort to the blunt instrument of legal proceedings which may polarize positions and make future cooperation for the sake of the patient more difficult.

References

BMA (2001) *Consent, Rights and Choices in Health Care for Children and Young People.* BMJ Books, London.

Brazier, M. & Bridge, C. (1996) Coercion or caring: analysing adolescent autonomy. *Legal Studies* **16**, 84–109.

Butler-Sloss, L.J. (1988) *Report of the Inquiry into Child Abuse in Cleveland 1987* Cm 412. HMSO, London.

Cassidy, D and Davey, S (2011). *Family Justice Children's Proceedings – Review of Public and Private Case Files in England and Wales,* Research Summary *5/11.* London: Ministry of Justice.

Chief Medical Officer (2006) *Bearing Good Witness, Proposals for Reforming the Delivery of Medical Expert Evidence in Family Law Cases.* Department of Health, London.

Cretney, C. (1985) Family law. In *All ER Annual Review,* pp. 171–186.

Department of Health (2008) *Code of Practice: Mental Health Act 1983.* TSO, London.

Douglas, G. (1992) The retreat from Gillick. *Modern Law Review* **55**, 569–576.

Ferguson, L. (2004) *The End of an Age: Beyond Age Restrictions for Minors' Medical Treatment Decisions.* Law Commission of Canada, Ottawa.

Fortin, J. (2009) *Children's Rights and the Developing Law.* Cambridge University Press, Cambridge.

Fortin, J. (2011) The *Gillick* decision – not just a high water mark. In: *Landmark Cases in Family Law.* (eds S. Gilmore, J. Herring & R. Probert). Hart Publishing, Oxford.

Gostin, L. (1975) *A Human Condition: The Mental health Act from 1959 to 1975: Observations, Analysis and Proposals for Reform* 1. MIND, London.

Gostin, L. (1992) Consent to treatment: the incapable person. In: *Doctors, Patients and the Law.* (ed C. Dyer). Blackwell Scientific Publications, Oxford.

Hale, B. (2005) Understanding children's rights: theory and practice. *Childright* **216**, 3–8.

Hale, B. (2010) *Mental Health Law.* Sweet and Maxwell, London.

Harmon, S. (2010) Body blow: mature minors and the Supreme Court of Canada's Decision in *AC v Manitoba. McGill Journal of Law and Health* **4**, 83–96.

Herring, J. *et al.* (2012) *Great Debates: Family Law.* Palgrave Macmillan, Basingstoke.

Ireland, J (2012). *Evaluating Expert Witness Psychological Reports: Exploring Quality. Summary Report.* University of Central Lancashire, Preston.

Irish Law Reform Commission (2011). *Children and the Law: Medical Treatment,* Law Reform Commission, Dublin.

Kennedy, R. (2001) Assessment and treatment in family law – a valid distinction? *Family Law* **31**, 676–681.

Law Commission (1995) *Mental Incapacity,* Law Com No 231. HMSO, London.

---

[50] Family Procedure Rules 2010, Part 25, also PD25B and PD25C.
[51] *D v East Berkshire Community NHS Trust* [2003] EWCA Civ 1151, [2004] QB 358.
[52] *Meadow v General Medical Council* [2006] EWCA Civ 1390, [2007] QB 462.
[53] *Jones v Kaney* [2011] UKSC 13, [2011] 2 AC 398.

Lewis, P. (2001) The medical treatment of children. In: *Legal Concepts of Childhood*. (ed J. Fionda). Hart Publishing, Oxford.

McCafferty, C. (1999) Won't consent? Can't consent! Refusal of medical treatment. *Family Law* **29**, 335–336.

Norgrove, D. (2011) *Family Justice Review, Final Report*. Ministry of Justice, Department for Education and Welsh Government, London.

NSW Law Reform Commission (2008) *Report 119, Young People and Consent to Health Care*. New South Wales Law Reform Commission, Sydney.

Parkinson, P. (1986). The *Gillick* case – just what has it decided? *Family Law* 11–21.

Pearce, J. *et al.* (2011) *Just Following Instructions? The Representation of Parents in Care Proceedings*. School of Law, University of Bristol, Bristol.

Thorpe, M. & Clarke, E. (eds) (1998) *Divided Duties: Care Planning for Children Within the Family Justice System*. Family Law, Bristol.

CHAPTER 20

Children's testimony: a scientific framework for evaluating the reliability of children's statements

Maggie Bruck[1] and Stephen J. Ceci[2]

[1] School of Medicine, Johns Hopkins University, MD, USA
[2] Department of Human Development, Cornell University, NY, USA

In the past 30 years, there has been an outpouring of research on the accuracy and distortion of children's autobiographical memory. The major issues concern how much children can remember of their near and far past, and the degree to which such factors as age of the child, salience of the event, delay, stress level, and an array of psychological factors (e.g., intelligence, personality) influence their recall. A second major issue concerns the degree to which a variety of external factors, mainly viewed in the interviewing process (e.g., leading questions, false suggestions, rewards), can distort children's testimony to the point that children will falsely report unexperienced events. In this chapter we focus on the latter issue—one that has been termed "children's suggestibility."

In the 1990s and into the first decade of the 21st century, much of the research focused on preschool-aged children, and was framed to address issues concerned with sexual abuse. This was primarily due to significant numbers of criminal cases in the 1980s and early 1990s in which young children claimed that their parents or other adults, often in daycare settings, had sexually abused them. The claims were often fantastic and bizarre, involving reports of ritualistic abuse, animal sacrifice, pornography, witchcraft, multiple perpetrators, and multiple victims (Nathan & Snedeker, 1995; Bottoms & Davis, 1997; De Young, 2004). When these types of cases first came to trial in the 1980s, the major issue before the jury was whether to believe the children. Prosecutors argued that children do not lie about sexual abuse, that their reports were authentic, and that their bizarre and chilling accounts of events, which were beyond the realm of most preschoolers' knowledge and experience, confirmed the fact that the children had actually participated in them, otherwise how could they graphically describe events beyond the ken of the typical child. The defense in these cases argued that the children's reports were the product of repeated suggestive interviews by parents, law enforcement officials, social

workers, and therapists. Although the defense identified an array of potentially "suggestive" interview techniques that were associated with the evolution of children's allegations, at the time there was no direct scientific evidence to support the view that such techniques lead children to make incorrect disclosures of a sexual nature. Consequently, in many of these cases the defendants were found guilty and sentenced to long prison terms (Ceci & Bruck, 1995; Nathan & Snedeker, 1995). As a result of such cases, social scientists pioneered the path to providing a social-psychological explanation for the conditions that promulgated such accusations. In doing so, we acquired valuable knowledge about the normal development of the preschool child—a field that was relatively underresearched at that time. As a consequence of new research, many, but not all, of the alleged perpetrators successfully appealed and were pardoned.

Although the daycare cases have all but disappeared from the forensic arena, research on children's autobiographical memory has continued to flourish and to be used in the forensic arena where there is concern about the accuracy of the testimony of children who were alleged victims, participants, or witnesses to a variety of events (e.g., sexual abuse, physical abuse, eyewitness to a crime). This area of research also is important for professionals and caretakers who question children or try to get them to talk about less traumatic issues. In this chapter we highlight the most prominent scientific findings in this field and demonstrate how these findings provide an objective framework for evaluating the reliability of young children's false claims, focusing on allegations of sexual abuse that arose in the course of a divorce/custody case.

Before proceeding, it is important to emphasize that most cases that involve child allegations of sexual abuse do not raise issues about suggestion and about false reports (see Chapter 30). Many children readily disclose their abuse either spontaneously or when asked in a neutral setting (see review by London

Rutter's Child and Adolescent Psychiatry, Sixth Edition.
Edited by Anita Thapar and Daniel S. Pine, James F. Leckman, Stephen Scott, Margaret J. Snowling, Eric Taylor.
© 2015 John Wiley & Sons Ltd. Published 2018 by John Wiley & Sons Ltd.

et al., 2008). There are also many children who do not disclose abuse because they are afraid, ashamed, and embarrassed; these numbers are unknown. Nonetheless, the smaller proportion of children who make false allegations is an important area of study because the results indicate a number of measures that can be taken by experts and clinicians to avoid such outcomes in a variety of cases going beyond sex abuse allegations, and also because these studies are crucial for our understanding of the development of the child's autobiographical memory system.

We begin this chapter by defining a variety of concepts and experimental paradigms that characterize this scientific area.

Defining suggestibility. One's recall of past experiences is rarely error-free. Errors can occur for a variety of reasons such as forgetting, lapses of attention in experiencing the event or in recalling its details, blocking of the memory by other experiences, or blending of two or more different memories (e.g., see Schacter, 2001). Recall of one's past can also be distorted by one's beliefs or expectations about what should have happened. And finally, recall can be distorted by suggestions—interactions with others that result in incorporation of their beliefs and statements into one's own report.

Suggestions become incorporated into reports for a variety of social and cognitive reasons. Cognitive theories suggest that the original memory trace can be damaged, replaced or overshadowed by suggestions—both internally generated such as ruminations and scripted expectancies, and externally generated such as interviewer-provided misleading information (Brainerd & Reyna, 2005; Otgaar et al., 2012a, 2012b). In contrast, social theories posit that false reports reflect compliance with the interviewer or the group (Gudjonsson, 1989; Billings et al., 2007). Compliance reflects trust in the knowledge of the interviewer (e.g., Lampinen & Smith, 1995; Waterman et al., 2004; Mills, 2013), or at the other end of the continuum wanting to go along with the peer group (Pynoos & Nader, 1989). Compliance can occur when there is no memory or a gap in the memory and the suggestion is used to fill that gap. Both social and cognitive mechanisms may jointly lead to suggestibility effects: a child may initially acquiesce due to social factors (e.g., to please their interviewer) but over time the child comes to falsely believe that the suggestion actually occurred (e.g., Bruck & Ceci, 1999; Stolzenberg & Pezdek, 2013).

Reliability, competence, credibility. These three terms are often used interchangeably but inaccurately in the context of the legal arena. In the legal context, reliability refers to the "trustworthiness" of the evidence, not to the honesty or credibility of a witness. Statements or reports can be unreliable due to normal processes of forgetting, of distortion, and of reconstruction. Statements can also be rendered unreliable if they are elicited in certain suggestive contexts. Thus, the existing literature on reliability focuses on factors that enhance or degrade the quality of witness reports. Although an assessment of the credibility (believability) of the witness and of the guilt of the alleged perpetrator are issues within the province of the jury, not the expert witness, the provision of information on the reliability

of the evidence is crucial to allow jurors or judges to draw conclusions about the credibility of children's allegations and ultimately about the guilt of the defendant. For several reasons, the scientific literature on reliability is rarely used to evaluate the "competence" of a witness. There are several reasons for this. First, there appears to be little, if any, relationship between the accuracy of children's recall and their performance on competence-type interviews (e.g., knowing the difference between a truth and a lie) that are often used in the courtroom (e.g., London & Nunez, 2002; Talwar et al., 2004). Second, because the competence standard is quite undemanding (witnesses are deemed competent if they are sufficiently intelligent to observe, recollect, and recount an event, and have a moral sense of obligation to speak the truth), most witnesses are deemed competent by the court.

Experimental measures of suggestibility. There are two basic paradigms that have been used to examine the direct influence of various types of suggestions on the accuracy of reports. In the first paradigm, children are exposed to an event or activity about which the researcher has full knowledge of all the details, such as a staged robbery. After the event, children are asked to recall these experiences through the use of techniques that falsely suggest details that were not present during the event, or through neutral interviewing techniques that do not involve suggestion. Subsequently, children are asked to recall the original event. A comparison of the errors made in the suggestive and neutral conditions allows a determination of how much suggestions taint the child's reports. In the second major paradigm, children are given suggestions about whole events that (according to parent reports) their child had never experienced, such as going on a hot air balloon ride or having their finger caught in a mousetrap. The degree to which children assent to and provide details about nonexperienced events are measures of their suggestibility.

Outline of present case involving allegations of sexual abuse[1]

The father of two preschool-aged daughters was charged with abusing his children. The statements emerged at the beginning of a long, contentious divorce and custody battle in which the mother sought sole custody based on the children's allegations. The following provides the basic details of the case.

Mr. and Mrs. Smith were married in 1998. They had two daughters, Sophia (born in 2000) and Sally (born in 2002). Around 2001, the couple began marital counseling and at the same time the mother sought legal advice about divorce. In 2005, Mr. Smith left the home with a shared agreement of having three overnight visits per week with his children.

On September 25, 2005, after the father brought the children home, the parents had an argument. The father grabbed his

---

[1] We have changed all names and some descriptive details to protect the identities of family members and experts in this case.

wife's face and kissed her just before leaving, telling her the marriage was "done." The mother promptly obtained a temporary restraining order that prohibited the father from contacting her or the children. There was no mention of child abuse in the complaint.

On September 26, the mother brought the children to a crisis mental health evaluator (Ms. Kelly), recommended by her attorney. Sophia's (now 5 years 10 months) statements focused on her upset of her parents' yelling at each other. She said, "Mommy says Daddy is mean"; and that she would be sad if she couldn't see her father, but if she had to, she would choose her mother. Sally provided no information except that her father stopped the family credit card. (Sophia also made a similar statement.) Thus, 24 hours after they had just seen their father, the children did not allege sexual abuse nor did they exhibit any behaviors that caused the evaluator to suspect abuse.

The next day the mother called the school to inform them of the restraining order. At that time, she first expressed her concerns about sexual abuse. It was recommended that the school's crisis counselor (SG) interview Sophia.

On September 28, during a 45-min unrecorded interview, Sophia allegedly told SG in detail how her father had tried to abuse her sexually and how he had abused her sister. She also claimed he put feces in her face. Later in the presence of a school nurse, SG, and a teddy bear,[2] Sophia claimed that her father digitally penetrated both herself and Sally.

A third interview with Department of Youth and Family Services (DYFS) occurred later that day. Sophia described "bad things" such as yelling, fighting, and hitting. Importantly, she did not report sexually abusive acts.

In the fourth interview on that same day, Sophia was questioned by a detective at the prosecutor's office. During this interview (the only videotaped interview in the case), Sophia's claims were inconsistent and at times fantastic. She denied questions about sexual abuse while at other times making vague claims.

On that same day, the mother asked Sally if anyone touched her "peepee," Sally replied, "it's a secret." Later that day, Sally said that it was a friend. The next day, Sally made no allegations of abuse when interviewed by the detective.

Six weeks later, when the DYFS investigation continued, Sophia claimed that she kissed her father's private parts, that he digitally penetrated her, and all this also happened to her sister. Sally told the DYFS investigator that her father also put feces in front of her face and that her mother hit her with a belt.

December 2005, the father filed for divorce asking for liberal visitation. The mother counterclaimed, alleging the father had sexually abused his daughters. On June 20, 2006, the prosecutors' office decided the case was unsubstantiated and refused to intervene.

July 2006, the mother's attorney phoned psychologist, Dr. Sy, requesting an urgent evaluation of the children who, despite

allegations of sexual abuse, were to begin visitation with their father. Dr. Sy met with the mother for a few minutes and then interviewed Sophia for about 1 hour. At this point, Sophia had no contact with her father for almost 10 months. On the basis of this interview, and on the results of two checklists filled out by the mother, Dr. Sy concluded that Sophia had been abused.

From February 15, 2007 to April 16, 2009, a trial occurred over approximately 50 noncontinuous days concerning the issues of custody and sexual abuse. One of us (MB) was asked by the father to provide an expert opinion on the reliability of these children's allegations of sexual abuse as well as the particular factors that may have affected the reliability of their statements.

Research findings/major principles

The following research findings provide a scientific basis for interpreting the children's allegations in this case.

Preschoolers' reports are often very accurate.

Although preschoolers can remember events and details of experienced events over long periods of time, the age of their earliest memories changes as a function of their age of recall. Thus, according to the most recent review of this literature (Peterson, 2012), on average 6-year-olds can recall information from more than 2 years previously. However, these same memories are not available if the child is asked to retrieve them a few years later. Peterson also summarizes the research on the effects of stress on early recall: children can accurately recall stressful events several years after their occurrence. This characterization of children's memory pertains when they are interviewed by neutral interviewers who question them in a nonsuggestive manner, who test alternative hypotheses, and who have no motive to influence the child's testimony (e.g., Bruck *et al.*, 2006).

Biased interviewers can taint the child's report, rendering it unreliable

The concept of "interviewer bias" characterizes interviewers who hold *a priori* beliefs about the occurrence of events and, as a result, conduct their interviews to obtain confirmatory evidence. In so doing, biased interviewers do not test plausible alternative hypotheses. When children provide such interviewers with inconsistent or bizarre evidence, it is either ignored or interpreted within the framework of the biased interviewer's initial hypothesis.

Biased interviewers' beliefs are transmitted to the child through a range of suggestive techniques that are associated with the elicitation of false reports. Consequently, the child may come to inaccurately report the belief of the interviewer rather than the child's own experience. Finally, the concept of a biased interviewer is not limited to forensic interviewers but may also includes therapists, teachers, and parents (see Bruck *et al.*, 2006 for a review).

A study by Bruck *et al.* (1999) showed how interviewer bias can quickly develop in natural interviewing situations

---

[2] Although SG initially claimed that it was a doll, the nurse and police notes indicate that it was a bear. Thus allegations of insertion could not be physically demonstrated.

and how children will adopt the belief of the interviewer and wrongly report that they experienced an event. Importantly, interviewer bias also affects the memories and reports of the interviewers. Thus, even if a child correctly denied engaging in an experience which the interviewer believed had occurred, the interviewer will later report that the child, in fact, had engaged in that experience.

Biased interviewers use suggestive interviewing techniques

Interviewer bias influences the entire architecture of interviews as revealed through a variety of suggestive interviewing techniques. In the present case, we identified the undue presence of six techniques that also occurred in suggestive interviews in a range of cases involving child witnesses and consequently have been the subject of scientific study.

Specific questions

Asking the child "yes"/"no" questions (Did he do that?) or choice questions (Did he do A or B or C), or "loaded"/leading questions, (Her mom told me that happened to her, did it happen to you?) are particularly problematic when interviewing young children. These not only force the child to provide an answer but also indirectly give the child information about the suspected event or the interviewers' beliefs—thus, they are termed suggestive. One of the major problems with such questions is that young children rarely reply "I don't know" when questions are nonsensical or very misleading (e.g., Fritzley et al., 2013; Waterman & Blades, 2013). This is true even when they have been enjoined to say they do not know if they are not sure about something.

It is because of their poor performance on such questions that general guidelines for interviewing children emphasize the importance of asking open-ended questions (e.g., Tell me what you did today) to allow children to describe their experiences in their own words (e.g., Lamb et al., 2008).

Repeated specific questions within interviews

When children first deny the occurrence of an event, they will often change their answers if these same types of questions are repeated (Poole & White, 1991; Krähenbühl et al., 2009). Of particular concern is the finding that this pattern is more likely when children are asked misleading questions (about events they have not experienced). Thus, repetition of questions not only provides the child additional misinformation but can also result in shifting their initial accurate answers to inaccurate answers.

Repeated suggestive interviews

There are also adverse effects of repeating suggestive information (through the use of a variety of suggestive techniques, including asking specific questions) across multiple interviews (e.g., Bruck et al., 2002; Erdmann et al., 2004). Specifically, with each repeated suggestive interview, children are more likely to assent to previously denied nonexperienced events and these reports persist when children are later questioned by a neutral interviewer.

It is also the case that if children provide new information with repeated suggestive interviews, there is a high probability that it will be false (Pipe et al., 1999; Salmon & Pipe, 2000), even if children are suggestively interviewed about true events (Bruck et al., 2002; Scullin et al., 2002). When interviewers urge children to tell them more, these requests sometimes result in false reports by the children to comply with their perception of the interviewer's wishes. Often these false reports are highly detailed, even more so than true reports (see Bruck et al., 2002). Thus, in a suggestive interviewing context, the presence of many details is unrelated to accuracy.

It is also important to keep in mind that in some contexts repeated interviews can have positive effects on children's recall of an experienced event by providing them with additional opportunities and time to recall additional details; this is especially true if the interviews are nonsuggestive and occur close to the experienced event (La Rooy et al., 2010).

Stereotype induction

Suggestions do not always take the form of explicit (mis)leading questions, such as "Your Dad was mad, right?" A more subtle strategy of conveying the same information is to insert (often negative) characteristics about a person into the conversations, that is, vilification. A variety of studies have shown that when children are provided with information that a person does "bad things," they will creatively incorporate this into their own reports of wrongdoing (e.g., Lepore & Sesco, 1994). For example, when children were told that a man who visited their preschool was clumsy, they often later claimed to have observed him doing clumsy things like breaking toys (Leichtman & Ceci, 1995).

Peer contamination (cowitness contamination)

Although adults are usually the suggestive source, children (peers, siblings) can also contaminate each other's reports through natural conversations. Principe and Schindewolf (2012) have shown that young children will pick up information about an event from peers and even though they have never experienced this event, will elaborate it and later claim it also happened to them. Their false claims are indistinguishable in many ways from true claims made by other children.

Nonverbal props

Because of young children's limited language skills, nonverbal props (dolls, toys) have been used as a tool to question children who witnessed crimes, including those suspected of having been abused. Although the use of props seems intuitively useful, the scientific literature indicates they can be suggestive, particularly for younger children; they result in increased false reports about touching (see Poole & Bruck, 2012). A major reason for this is that children use the props as toys to play with and to explore, rather than to demonstrate experienced actions.

Although each suggestive technique is associated with error, the risk for false statements is greatly augmented when interviews contain a combination of different suggestive techniques (e.g., leading questions, peer pressure, vilification through stereotype induction), which increase the salience of the interviewer's bias (see Ceci & Bruck, 1995; Bruck *et al.*, 2006 for details and examples).

The first interview with a child provides the most reliable testimony

When children are interviewed over time, the general rule is that the statements in the first interview are the most reliable. This is because, compared to later interviews, there is less chance for forgetting, and less opportunity for suggestive and other influences to taint children's reports. However, if there is suggestion in the first interview or in conversations prior to it, the child's initial statements may be tainted and therefore unreliable.

Thus, in documenting the evolution of children's allegations, it is important to determine if (a) the child's first statement is spontaneous, unprompted, and made in the absence of previous suggestive elements, or (b) the first statement is associated with previous or concurrent suggestive interviewing techniques.

Suggestive interviewing techniques can result in false beliefs that are longlasting

Children may come to believe that they actually experienced false suggested events. Thus, asking them to tell the truth, to tell only what actually happened, or to say "don't know" when they are unsure, can be fruitless (Poole & Lindsay, 2001; Principe & Schindewolf, 2012) and will not detaint their reports.

A corollary of this principle is that once a child's statement has been tainted, it may be impossible to untaint it in subsequent interviews, regardless of the skill of the interviewer. In subsequent nonsuggestive neutral interviews, children will make spontaneous disclosures sometimes with many details about events that are thematically related to prior suggestions. They will do this even when a subsequent interviewer attempts to talk them out of their false statements or warn them that what they heard was untrue (Leichtman & Ceci, 1995; Erdmann *et al.*, 2004). No amount of probing and deprogramming can unearth the original, untainted memory because it may have been irrevocably modified by the prior suggestive questions and become a false belief, that is, part of the child's autobiographical memory. Recent evidence also shows that even after mildly suggestive interviewing has ceased for many months, children will still continue to make false reports (Akehurst *et al.*, 2009; London *et al.*, 2009; Price & Connolly, 2013).

Children's false reports can seem credible

Some professionals state that they can detect the effects of suggestive questioning because the children parrot the words of adults who interviewed them. However, evidence from the past decade provides no support for this assertion. First, children's false reports are not simply repetitions or monosyllabic responses to leading questions. Under some conditions, their answers go well beyond the suggestion and incorporate additional nonsuggested details and emotions (e.g., Bruck *et al.*, 1995, 2002). In fact, in some studies, children's narratives of false events contain more embellishments (including descriptive and emotional terms) and details than their narratives of true events (Bruck *et al.*, 2002). False narratives often contain more spontaneous statements than true narratives. Although for the most part the details in false stories are realistic, they often contain more bizarre details than true narratives (Bruck *et al.*, 2002; Powell *et al.*, 2003).

Relatedly, subjective ratings of children's reports after suggestive interviewing reveal that they appear highly credible to prospective jurors or trained professionals in the fields of child development, mental health, and forensics (e.g., Leichtman & Ceci, 1995; Laimon & Poole, 2008); these professionals cannot reliably discriminate children's accurate reports from suggestively induced inaccurate reports. In many of these studies, the children who provided the false reports spoke sincerely and provided accounts laden with emotion and perceptual details and used body language consistent with their reports. In summary, there are no scientifically acceptable markers for judging the child's truthfulness in interviews that have been preceded by suggestive interviews.

Electronic recordings of the full interview must be obtained in order to determine the degree of bias and suggestiveness of the interview

It is important to have an accurate verbatim record of everything that the child and the interviewer said. Although it may be impossible to electronically record all interviews and conversations (including ones with parents and peers), at the very least all forensic interviews should be recorded (see Bruck *et al.*, 1999).

The reason for electronic recording is because interviewers/observers cannot accurately write down all of the interactions and exact words of an interview. Notes of interviews omit many details and utterances that the recorder simply misses or deems unimportant. For example, the note may omit all instances where the child provided no information in response to questions, and may only contain information about details that the interviewer considers important to the investigation. (Cauchi *et al.*, 2010). Recorders also make mistakes in describing how statements are elicited; a common error is to claim the statement was spontaneous when, in fact, it was a monosyllabic response to a set of repeated leading questions (Bruck *et al.*, 1999; Warren & Woodall, 1999). When asked how specific information was obtained from a child, most interviewers erroneously reply that they never use leading questions when in reality they rely on them heavily (see Lamb *et al.*, 2000). Recorders, especially those with specific biases, also misinterpret or misperceive children's statements: even though a child may fail to confirm an interviewer's belief, the interviewer may nonetheless later inaccurately report that the child made a statement that was consistent with the belief (Bruck *et al.*, 2006).

Scientific analysis of the facts of the case

Sources of information about the children's reports

The only interviews that were videorecorded were those conducted with Sophia (September 28) and Sally (September 29) at the prosecutor's office. There was no electronic recording of SG's interview that elicited Sophia's first allegations of abuse (on September 28) and SG could not take notes due to a broken thumb. There is an audiotape of Sophia's interview with Dr. Sy but it is of such poor quality that Dr. Sy had to use her notes to produce a transcript. Thus, the following analysis of these interviews is made without reliable information on their structure or content. It is unknown how many of the children's statements were omitted or misinterpreted or if suggestive techniques were used to elicit them. Finally, the court ruled that the mother's diary notes were often manufactured or edited in anticipation of the upcoming trial.

Here we provide examples from the case materials of the children's allegations. We have edited these greatly to reduce the salacious language used by the children. We however do provide some examples because the statements in this case are similar in terms of their shock value to those in many cases that we have assessed. Also, it is important for the reader to appreciate the types of statements that are elicited in the context of interviewer bias and suggestive interviewing techniques.

The role of bias in the evolution of children's initial disclosures
Mother

Biased interviewers may have a conscious or unconscious motive to tilt children's testimony. This seems to have been the case for Mrs. Smith who had been actively seeking advice about divorce for several years before Sophia's disclosures. Months before Sophia's allegations of CSA, Mrs. Smith expressed concern (according to her diary entries) that the children may have been be abused or were at risk for abuse. Further she was concerned that her husband might gain custody. Mrs. Smith relayed these concerns to her children and their interviewers in a variety of ways. For example,

- She repeatedly told the girls that nobody should touch their private parts and that if this happened they should tell her.
- She estimated that she had discussed sexually abusive activities with both of her children approximately 90 times between September 25, 2005 and August 2006. These talks also included the "bad things that daddy did."
- Prior to the children's first interview with the crisis counselor, on September 26, she discussed the prior day's incidents involving their father with the children and corrected Sophia's recollections.

SG (The school's crisis counselor)

Before interviewing Sophia on September 28, SG had a phone conversation with Mrs. Smith who provided details about her husband's sexual violence, about her concerns about Sophia, particularly in light of what she felt were highly inappropriate and sexualized behaviors on the part of both Sophia and her husband. (Sophia probably heard the mother's side of the conversation.) Armed with this background, SG began her interview with Sophia.

Suggestive techniques on September 28

Although the SG interview was not recorded, there are a number of hints that throw some light on the atmosphere and interactions during this interview:

At the beginning of the interview, Sophia needed to go to the bathroom where the interview continued. As Sophia was on the toilet moving her bowels, she said that she had a really big secret that only her mother knew about. Instead of waiting to question her until they returned to the interview room, SG coaxed Sophia to tell about the secret. As Sophia exited the toilet stall, she took paper towels from SG's hands, crumbled them up and reported that Daddy puts feces (poop) in her face. Thus, the claim about feces being put in her face arose in this toileting scenario, not in a neutral forensic context.

Next, Sophia made a number of unusual allegations, for example, the father made her touch his private parts with a towel and then with a broom stick and he was wearing a business suit when he scooped the poop out of the toilet. The lack of follow-up questioning about these allegations reveals SG's belief that Sophia was telling the truth. Finally, although Sophia said she had run away when her father tried to touch her, she said she had seen him poke Sally's genitals with his fingers (in response to a leading question), and that she saved Sally. She was not asked how she did this nor was she challenged to explain seemingly implausible allegations.

Later, in the nurse's office with SG present, Sophia was given a bear and asked if she had been hurt and to show on the bear how. Sophia proceeded to hit the bear repeatedly. When asked if her father hurt her anywhere else, she demonstrated by poking the bear between the legs and said that her father did that to Sally, too.

A number of factors compromised the reliability of these reports. First, they were based on SG's memory, which changed as she reported this incident over time (e.g., SG claimed that a doll was used and not a bear). As discussed, adults are unable to accurately reconstruct verbatim accounts of what children told them even minutes following an interview, often misremembering the number of times a question was asked, its content, and the nature of the child's answers. The reliability of Sophia's allegations was also compromised by (i) the inappropriateness of questioning her during a toilet break; (ii) the possibility that the towels, along with the activity of having a bowel movement, prompted this child to make a report based on them; (iii) the possibility that these reports were not spontaneous but emerged as a result of constant questioning about the "secret." (Sophia later told another interviewer that there were hundreds of questions.) It is often found that when children are repeatedly questioned and feel pressured to answer, they will alight on something that captures their attention (as seen in transcripts of laboratory studies, e.g., Bruck *et al.*, 2002). Perhaps if Sophia had been interviewed in a cafeteria she would have seized upon a bowl or utensil and woven this into her narrative. (iv) the lack of follow-up questioning about Sophia's bizarre allegations revealing SG's firm belief (as reflected by her statement that she was certain that Sophia was telling the truth); (v) the first report of sexual touching was enacted on a prop (a bear) in response to repeated suggestive questions. These factors, along with SG's prior information about the mother's concerns that were also overheard by Sophia, render Sophia's statements unreliable.

In the early evening of September 28, 2005, Sophia was interviewed for the fourth time that day.[3] At the beginning of the interview, she reported that she had fun with daddy at his house but she was also aware that her mother was watching out for wrongdoing on his part. She did not make any derogatory statements about her father during this part of the interview.

When asked what she had talked to SG about, Sophia reported the incident of yelling and grabbing from Sunday, September 25. She claimed that Daddy was mean and he hit her. She said that her father tried to touch her private parts, but he never touched her or her sister. When prompted to tell more about what she had told SG, Sophia said, "I can't … because there was 100 questions." Sophia was very distracted and asked for the questioning to stop.

Still, the detective pursued her with repeated and pressurized request for more information about what she had told SG: "What did you tell her?", "What did you show her?", "Did you talk to SG and the nurse about daddy touching your peepee?" This is highly problematic because the task for Sophia became one of remembering what she told SG and the nurse rather than remembering what, if anything, really happened.

As now shown, it was the use of repeated questions that provoked an ambiguous response from Sophia that she was touched. She initially denied that her father had touched her private parts. To many repeated questions about what she showed on the bear, she either was silent or else replied that she showed how Daddy had hit her. Finally, Sophia was asked, "Poked you where?" at which point, she pointed to her stomach and her crotch. This interaction is significant because Sophia's nonverbal gesture was made in response to a leading question and to the directive to tell what she showed SG and the nurse. The response was also made after she was asked a number of similar questions where she denied touching or did not respond. When she was directly asked about the "poopy," Sophia didn't want to tell, repeating that it was a secret with her mother. During this period she was bombarded with questions and told that she could not see her mother, despite her many requests to leave the room. Thus, any of Sophia's statements could be a consequence of trying to please the interviewer (rather than report what actually happened) and to escape this aversive situation.

---

[3] Recall, that in the third interview with DYFS, Sophia made no sexual allegations.

November 2005 interviews

Six weeks after their last contact with their father, the two children were interviewed by DYFS. Their statements differed considerably from those made in September. First, Sally reported that her father had put poop in her face and that her mother had hit her with a belt.

Sophia now claimed that she did kiss her father's private parts, that he digitally penetrated her, and that these things happened to her sister, too. She claimed that the poop incident had happened at both parents' houses. Sophia stated her father should go to jail, evidence of a growing negative stereotype.

Although the children's new reports of sexual abuse may reflect a growing comfort and support in disclosing actual events, they are equally likely to reflect the repeated suggestive conversations with their mother and interviewers. This hypothesis was also raised by one of the November interviewers who expressed concern about the effects of the prior interviewing on the accuracy of Sophia's statements.

Evidence of peer contamination

Although Sally had yet to make any reports of sexual abuse to professional interviewers, her mother's diary included many such allegations. These were remarkably similar to those made by her sister and raise the concern that the children contaminated each others' reports. For example, one child reported a nightmare and the other child stated that she also had that one. In November, Sally's allegations of "poop" and being hit also mirror those of her sister.

Reports of hitting and of scatological behavior

Sophia's (and Sally's) first allegations involved hitting and also touching poop. We have observed this pattern in many cases in which young children are suggestively interviewed; often these reports precede more explicit reports of sexual abuse (e.g., New Jersey v. Michaels, 1994 and others). One interpretation often given by clinicians is that children begin to disclose abuse by describing the least abusive incident, which allows them to gauge the reactions of their interviewers. Some experts have claimed that scatological reports are consistent with the behavior of sexually addicted perpetrators, although there is no empirical evidence for this claim. Another interpretation that is consistent with research on stereotype induction (e.g., Ceci & Bruck, 1995) is that when young children are relentlessly asked to tell "bad" things about a suspect, in order to please their interviewers they think of the worst things within their realm of knowledge or fantasy—namely, physical abuse and scatological subjects. For example, Mrs. Smith recounted that Sophia's fear that her father would do "badder" things to her such as pushing her down the stairs.

This also leads to the conjecture that Sophia may have made allegations of sexual abuse without truly understanding the content of her statements, as further illustrated when Sophia said that she hadn't told her earlier of her father's bad acts because she didn't know they were bad. Then she asked her mother, "Why is it so bad?"

In summary, by definition, all reports provided by Sophia and Sally after September 26, 2005 were unreliable and tainted. Sophia's statements on September 28 were responses to "hundreds of questions" in both the school and police interviews. The idea of digital penetration seemed to emanate from being asked to show on a bear where she and her sister were touched. Furthermore, given the turmoil between parents that sometimes involved the children, including witnessing her father grab her mother and knowing that the police were called to protect her mother, it is not surprising that Sophia's major reports involved hitting, yelling, and descriptions of a mean father.

Thus, 6 weeks after the first allegations, Sally had yet to make an allegation of sexual abuse and Sophia's allegations were inconsistent with what she had previously reported (some details were added and others were omitted). New reports or changed reports that emerge in the context of suggestive interviewing have a high probability of being false (as reviewed). Consistent with this reasoning, the prosecutor's office decided that the case was unsubstantiated. Thus, based on legal, scientific, and clinical grounds, there was no reasonable foundation to interview the children about abuse again. Nonetheless, the interviewing did continue.

Dr. Sy Interviews Sophia on July 19, 2006, 10 months after her last contact with her father

Sophia readily engaged in conversation with Dr. Sy and without too much prompting revealed that she had to touch her father's feces and lick his private parts and Sally poked her with her finger. She also stated that Sally lied and she only saw her father hit Sally on her buttocks. Dr. Sy's diagnosis of child abuse was based on Sophia's spontaneity, credibility, and physiological reactivity while relating some of the events.

In general, experts in this case discounted the potential effects of any previous suggestion because Sophia's later disclosures were so credible and so consistent with previous reports. They also stated that her lack of contact with the perpetrator minimized false recantations and increased the probability of true disclosures. The experts also agreed that because Dr. Sy's interviewing techniques were impeccable, she could not only extract true disclosures but also evaluate the degree to which they were a product of coaching. All agreed that her interview with the child was neutral and nonsuggestive. In the remainder of this chapter, we discuss these and other claims in light of the scientific research literature.

Dr. Sy's recording and reporting techniques

Dr. Sy used a voice-activated audio recorder that kept shutting off during the interview and needed to be turned back on. She claimed that she was also taking contemporaneous verbatim notes, and used these to fill in gaps in the transcript of the interview.

Having to monitor the functioning of a machine, scrupulously observing nonverbal actions, and at times using props (such as dolls), would likely make it impossible to write virtually everything asked and answered. Furthermore, the claims that she could verify the child's trauma through body language such as "gag reflex" and holding her crotch (a sign that the child was in pain) are nonverifiable without a video record of this important interview.

Dr. Sy violated important interview guidelines

Dr. Sy portrayed her style as one of neutrality and nonsuggestiveness. She bolstered her neutrality by stating that she went into the interview "cold"; meaning that she did not review the previous records or speak to any of the previous professionals.

However, reviewing all records and sources is a cornerstone of good interviewing practices. Without this, she could not test hypotheses about the source of or influences on the child's statements. Thus, one is left with the paradigmatic model of an interviewer who has one major hypothesis and does not rule out competing ones. It turns out, however, that Dr. Sy did not go into the interview "cold"; she had spoken with the mother's attorney and with the mother who related the details of her sexual history with the father, among other things. Furthermore, it is clear in part of the interview that Dr. Sy knew some of the prior allegations because she asked questions about some of the content before the child had said anything. (In fact, Dr. Sy later did admit that she did know the content of the child's allegations.)

Despite her statements that she conducted a "state-of-the art" interview that would allow her to elicit the truth from the child and to avoid suggestions, this was not what occurred.

She used dolls to elicit a new allegation of penetration. Many of the current protocols discourage the use of dolls for young children and all warn of their potential suggestive powers. Because this interview was not recorded, it is unknown if the dolls were anatomically detailed; even if they were not, as we explain here, the use of dolls to elicit sexual information from children is very suggestive and can taint children's reports (Poole & Bruck, 2012). The following interaction in which Dr. Sy tried to get Sophie to elaborate shows how dolls can interfere with the reliability of a child's statements.

Sy:	If this were him and this were you, show me how he did that? (*she gives her a doll*). This is him and he is sitting just like this and this is you. Show me how he put you. I don't get it. He is sitting and you are standing and then what?
Sophia:	And then he pushed me down
Sy:	And then what?
Sophia:	He was on the couch.
Sy:	I don't see any pee pee's touching. I don't see pee pee's touching. Show me how the pee pee's started to touch. But I want you to just show me with the dolls. You are laying there and how does he get his pee pee to touch your pee pee, I still can't figure it out.
Sophia:	Standing up, standing up, standing up (*demonstrates with two dolls*).

…

Dr. Sy: Now how did that feel when that was touching that? How did that feel?

Sophia: It was actually poking inside it.

Here we see why dolls/props are suggestive Dr. Sy repeatedly demanded that Sophia show sexual touching on the dolls—a strategy that was associated with Sophia changing her initial response from "laying on the floor," "to sitting on the floor," "to standing." The latter is physically impossible for a man and a young child, but is nevertheless accepted by Dr. Sy. This is the first time, 10 months after the initial allegations, penile penetration is reported.

In other sections of the interview, Dr. Sy also used a number of leading questions and Sophia conceded to these rather than sticking with her original stories.

The experts vouched for the truth of Sophia's reports

Contrary to the scientific evidence, experts in this case remarked on the credibility and truth of the Sophia's statements. Dr. Sy's conclusion that Sophia was abused was based in part on the consistency of her reports. One expert claimed that most of Sophia's reports were consistent over 10 months. To the contrary, except for the consistency of her reports touching feces and hitting, her reports were not consistent but changed remarkably over time. Initially she told SG that her father tried to touch her and she saw him poke Sally. It was not until the November interview that she disclosed the sexual experiences. Much later she told Dr. Sy further details such as genital insertion, and she only saw her father hit her sister's butt. Given the amount of suggestion and discussion with the mother and her sister that has occurred over a period of 21 months, a major hypothesis is that these reports were suggestively induced.

The experts claimed that Sophia's reports were accurate because they were spontaneous and thus could not have been coached. The scientific literature supports the view that spontaneous reports in response to open questions are a good marker of children's accuracy. However, this is only if reports are free from previous or concurrent suggestive techniques. In much of the literature reviewed in this chapter, as a consequence of suggestive interviewing, children's subsequent reports become spontaneous, consistent, and detailed—albeit inaccurate. Sophia's narratives with Dr. Sy conform to the expected pattern of children whose reports emerge as a consequence of suggestion. This is not to imply that they are demonstrably inaccurate, only that their accuracy cannot be assumed.

The experts also dismissed the hypothesis of suggestion by claiming that there was no evidence of coercive interviewing or that the interviewers provided them with sexual information. Although there is reason to believe that the children were exposed to a highly suggestive environment where their father was vilified and where they were constantly engaged in conversations of abuse, taint could also occur in situations that were less toxic. The literature has shown that even after one or two suggestive interviews children can develop false memories about salient but nonexperienced events.

Also inherent in the experts' denial of the role of suggestibility was the view that it would be impossible to suggest sexual abuse to children who can only be led to make false reports about unemotional, unimportant events. Both views are incorrect. For example, in a series of studies, Otgaar and colleagues have implanted false memories in children by telling them their mother or teacher described an event that happened to the child in the past. Sometimes extra details were provided (showing the child a photograph or giving them more knowledge about the event). Using these rather mild short-lasting procedures, these researchers found significant rates of false memories for viewing a UFO (Otgaar et al., 2009), receiving an enema (Otgaar et al., 2010), and being caught by their teacher for cheating (Otgaar et al., 2008).

In addition, there have been a number of studies in which children have been led to make false allegations about bodily events which, were they to occur in the real world, could result in criminal investigation. For example, children have made false claims about "silly events" that involved body contact (e.g., "Did she blow in your ear?"), which persisted in subsequent interviews over a 3-month period (Ornstein et al., 1992). Children falsely reported that a man put something "yuckie" in their mouth (Poole & Lindsay, 2001), that their pediatrician inserted a finger or a stick into their genitals (Bruck et al., 1995), and that a man touched their friends, kissed them on the lips, and removed some of their clothes (Lepore & Sesco, 1994). A significant number of children falsely reported that someone touched their private parts, kissed them, and hugged them (Goodman et al., 1991; Bruck et al., 2000). Children assented to suggestions that a doctor cut a bone in the center of their nose to stop the bleeding (Quas et al., 1999). Finnila et al. (2003) reported a significant number of 4- to 8-year-olds falsely assented to misleading questions about keeping a secret, being touched, and having their picture taken. Children have also elaborated their false narratives with emotional terms (e.g., "It hurt"; "I cried"; "I was happy", see Bruck et al., 1995, 2002). Finally, some research has found that it is easier to create a false memory for a negative event than for a neutral event (Otgaar et al., 2008). Thus, the suggestibility literature is a valid basis for evaluating the possibility that suggestive interviewing can result in false allegations about emotionally evocative events, including, but not limited to, bodily harm.

In order to examine the reliability of the children's disclosures, one must follow the general principles described in this article. Specifically, the first interview with the crisis counselor, Ms. Kelly, on September 26, 2005 is the most reliable. Although the first interview did not focus on sexual abuse (the interviewer did not see any signs of abuse), it is important to note that this interview occurred closest to a very unpleasant event (parental fighting) when the children's memories were freshest. Sophia described that event clearly, but did not report any other significant negative events concerning her father. At this point, the mother had not communicated suspected sexual abuse that she supplied in the following days. Her relative lack of interference at this point may have produced the most neutral interview and the most reliable statements from the children.

Epilog

The judge barred Dr. Sy's testimony and report from the court proceedings. "Dr. Sy's methodology was not based on generally accepted science. Among other deficiencies, Dr. Sy also failed to test alternative hypotheses, record the interview, and generally failed to consider the totality of the circumstances leading to (Sophia's) interview." The judge also ruled that for all the reasons stated in this report that Sophia would not be allowed to testify, namely, because her testimony was potentially tainted. The judge issued a final judgment of divorce, awarding the father sole custody of his two daughters.

Beyond issues of sexual abuse

In this chapter we have focused on a case of alleged sexual abuse; however, the very same issues, guidelines, and scientific frameworks apply across a wide variety of situations when children are interviewed by adults. These include legal contexts in which the child is a potential observer or participant, such as claims of physical abuse or being an eyewitness to a crime. These issues are particularly important in the psychiatric milieu where the child is often the primary provider of information. Professionals must be aware of their own biases and attempt to question children in as neutral fashion as possible and above all to test alternative hypotheses.

References

Akehurst, L. *et al.* (2009) Effect of socially encountered misinformation and delay on children's eyewitness testimony. *Psychiatry, Psychology and Law* **16**, 125–136.

Billings, F.J. *et al.* (2007) Can reinforcement induce children to falsely incriminate themselves? *Law & Human Behavior* **31**, 125–139.

Bottoms, B. & Davis, S. (1997) The creation of satanic ritualistic abuse. *Journal of Social and Clinical Psychology* **16**, 112–132.

Brainerd, C. & Reyna, V. (2005) *The Science of False Memory*. Oxford University Press, New York.

Bruck, M. & Ceci, S. (1999) The suggestibility of children's memory. *Annual Review of Psychology* **50**, 419–439.

Bruck, M. *et al.* (1995) "I hardly cried when I got my shot!": influencing children's reports about a visit to their pediatrician. *Child Development* **66**, 193–208.

Bruck, M., *et al.* (1999) The effect of interviewer bias on the accuracy of children's reports and interviewer's reports. Paper presented at the Biennial Meeting of SRCD. Albuquerque, NM. 2–4 April.

Bruck, M. *et al.* (2000) A comparison of three- and four-year-old children's use of anatomically detailed dolls to report genital touching in a medical examination. *Journal of Experimental Psychology: Applied* **6**, 74–83.

Bruck, M. *et al.* (2002) The nature of children's true and false narratives. *Developmental Review* **22**, 520–554.

Bruck, M. *et al.* (2006) The child and the law. In: *Handbook of Child Psychology. Child Psychology in Practice.* (eds A.K. Renninger, *et al.*), 6th Vol. 4 edn, pp. 776–816. John Wiley & Sons, Hoboken, NJ.

Cauchi, R. *et al.* (2010) A controlled analysis of professionals' contemporaneous notes of interviews about alleged child abuse. *Child Abuse & Neglect* **34**, 318–323.

Ceci, S. & Bruck, M. (1995) *Jeopardy in the Courtroom: A Scientific Analysis of Children's Testimony*. American Psychological Association, Washington, DC.

De Young, M. (2004) *The Day Care Ritual Abuse Moral Panic*. McFarland & Co., Jefferson, North Carolina.

Erdmann, K. *et al.* (2004) Children report suggested events even when interviewed in a non-suggestive manner: implications for credibility assessment. *Applied Cognitive Psychology* **18**, 589–611.

Finnila, K. *et al.* (2003) Validity of a test of children's suggestibility for predicting responses to two interview situations differing in their degree of suggestiveness. *Journal of Experimental Child Psychology* **85**, 32–49.

Fritzley, H. *et al.* (2013) Young children's response tendencies toward yes-no questions concerning actions. *Child Development* **84**, 711–725.

Goodman, G. *et al.* (1991) Children's testimony about a stressful event: improving children's reports. *Journal of Narrative and Life History* **1**, 69–99.

Gudjonsson, G. (1989) Compliance in an interrogative situation: a new scale. *Personality and Individual Differences* **10**, 535–540.

Krähenbühl, S. *et al.* (2009) The effect of repeated questioning on children's accuracy and consistency in eyewitness testimony. *Legal and Criminological Psychology* **14**, 263–278.

La Rooy, D. *et al.* (2010) Do we need to rethink guidance on repeated interviews? *Psychology, Public Policy and Law* **16**, 373–392.

Laimon, R. & Poole, D. (2008) Adults usually believe young children: the influence of eliciting questions and suggestibility presentations on perceptions of children's disclosures. *Law and Human Behavior* **32**, 489–501.

Lamb, M. *et al.* (2000) Accuracy of investigators' verbatim notes of their forensic interviews with alleged child abuse victims. *Law and Human Behavior* **24**, 707.

Lamb, M. *et al.* (2008) *Tell Me What Happened: Structured Investigative Interviews of Child Victims and Witnesses*. John Wiley & Sons, Hoboken, NJ.

Lampinen, J.M. & Smith, V.L. (1995) The incredible (and sometimes incredulous) child witness: child eyewitnesses' sensitivity to source of credibility cues. *Journal of Applied Psychology* **80**, 621–627.

Leichtman, M. & Ceci, S. (1995) The effects of stereotypes and suggestions on preschoolers' reports. *Developmental Psychology* **31**, 568–578.

Lepore, S. & Sesco, B. (1994) Distorting children's reports and interpretations of events through suggestion. *Applied Psychology* **79**, 108–120.

London, K. & Nunez, N. (2002) Examining the efficacy of truth/lie discussions in predicting and increasing the veracity of children's reports. *Journal of Experimental Child Psychology* **83**, 131–147.

London, L. *et al.* (2008) A review of the contemporary literature on how children report sexual abuse. *Memory* **16**, 29–47.

London, K. *et al.* (2009) Post-event information affects children's autobiographical memory after one year. *Law and Human Behavior* **33**, 344–355.

Mills, C.M. (2013) Knowing when to doubt: developing a critical stance when learning from others. *Developmental Psychology* **49**, 404–418.

Nathan, D. & Snedeker, M. (1995) *Satan's Silence: Ritual Abuse and the Making of a Modern American Witch Hunt*. Basic Books, New York.

New Jersey v. Michaels (1994) 625 A.2d 579 aff'd 642 A.2d 1372.

Ornstein, P. *et al.* (1992) Children's memory for a personally experienced event: implications for testimony. *Applied Cognitive Psychology* **6**, 49–60.

Otgaar, H. *et al.* (2008) Children's false memories: easier to elicit for a negative than for a neutral event. *Acta Psychologica* **128**, 350–354.

Otgaar, H. *et al.* (2009) Abducted by a UFO: prevalence information affects young children's false memories for an implausible event. *Applied Cognitive Psychology* **23**, 115–125.

Otgaar, H. *et al.* (2010) Script knowledge enhances the development of children's false memories. *Acta Psychologica* **133**, 57–63.

Otgaar, H. *et al.* (2012a) Children's implanted false memories and additional script knowledge. *Applied Cognitive Psychology* **26**, 709–715.

Otgaar, H. *et al.* (2012b) The origin of children's implanted false memories: memory traces or compliance? *Acta Psychologica* **139**, 397–403.

Peterson, C. (2012) Children's autobiographical memories across the years: forensic implications of childhood amnesia and eyewitness memory for stressful events. *Developmental Review* **32**, 287–306.

Pipe, M.E. *et al.* (1999) Children's recall 1 or 2 years after an event. *Developmental Psychology* **35**, 781–789.

Poole, D. & Bruck, M. (2012) Divining testimony? The impact of interviewing props on children's reports of touching. *Developmental Review* **32**, 165–180.

Poole, D. & Lindsay, D. (2001) Children's eyewitness reports after exposure to misinformation from parents. *Journal of Experimental Psychology: Applied* **7**, 27–50.

Poole, D. & White, L. (1991) Effects of question repetition on the eyewitness testimony of children and adults. *Developmental Psychology* **27**, 975–986.

Powell, M. *et al.* (2003) A comparison of preschoolers' recall of experienced versus non-experienced events across multiple interviews. *Applied Cognitive Psychology* **17**, 935–952.

Price, H. & Connolly, D. (2013) Suggestibility effects persist after one year in children who experienced a single or repeated event. *Journal of Applied Research in Memory and Cognition* **2**, 89–94.

Principe, G. & Schindewolf, E. (2012) Natural conversations as a source of false memories in children. *Developmental Review* **32**, 205–223.

Pynoos, R. & Nader, K. (1989) Children's memory and proximity to violence. *Journal of the American Academy of Child and Adolescent Psychiatry* **28**, 236–241.

Quas, J. *et al.* (1999) Emotion and memory: children's long-term remembering, forgetting, and suggestibility. *Journal of Experimental Child Psychology* **72**, 235–270.

Salmon, K. & Pipe, M.E. (2000) Recalling an event one year later: the impact of props, drawing and a prior interview. *Applied Cognitive Psychology* **14**, 9–120.

Schacter, D. (2001) *The Seven Sins of Memory*. Houghton Mifflin, Boston, MA.

Scullin, M. *et al.* (2002) Measurement of individual differences in children's suggestibility across situations. *Journal of Experimental Psychology: Applied* **8**, 233–246.

Stolzenberg, S. & Pezdek, K. (2013) Interviewing child witnesses: the effect of forced confabulation on event memory. *Journal of Experimental Child Psychology* **114**, 77–88.

Talwar, V. *et al.* (2004) Children's lie-telling to conceal a parent's transgression. *Law and Human Behavior* **28**, 411–435.

Warren, A. & Woodall, C. (1999) The reliability of hearsay testimony: how well do interviewers recall their interviews with children? *Psychology, Public Policy and Law* **5**, 355–371.

Waterman, A. & Blades, M. (2013) The effect of delay and individual differences on children's tendency to guess. *Developmental Psychology* **49**, 215–226.

Waterman, A. *et al.* (2004) Indicating when you do not know the answer: the effect of question format and interviewer knowledge on children's 'don't know' responses. *British Journal of Developmental Psychology* **22**, 335–348.

CHAPTER 21

Residential and foster care

Marinus H. van IJzendoorn[1], Marian J. Bakermans-Kranenburg[1] and Stephen Scott[2,3]

[1] Centre for Child and Family Studies, Leiden University, The Netherlands
[2] Institute of Psychiatry, Psychology and Neuroscience, Kings's College London, UK
[3] National Conduct Problems and National Adoption and Fostering Services, Maudsley Hospital, London, UK

Introduction

Some children cannot be cared for by their biological parents or other relatives, so unless private arrangements are made, the state has to find a way to care for them. The reasons for coming into public care vary across individuals, societies, and time. Some parents are unable to look after their children through illness, death or disposition; others, especially historically, could not due to poverty or due to the stigma in case of children born out of wedlock; the majority in developed countries now come into care due to neglect or abuse. The proportion of children in public care varies by country; for example, in England it is around 0.5% of the child population, about 60,000 children, (Department for Education, 2013), whereas in the United States it is around 1% of the child population, about 500,000; about a fifth of these are in residential care, but with considerable variability by area/state (Children's Bureau, 2013). Many stays in public care are brief; in any year, about half of the children seen in the care system will have entered or left it. We define foster care as living with unrelated parent figures who provide care and take responsibility in a similar way that a birth parent would, but without full and final legal responsibility. As with parents who do have such responsibility, there may be a mother figure, a father figure, both, or other combinations, and there may be other children in the family. In contrast, in residential care, there is usually no one taking on the more committed, intense, and exclusive role that a parent does. Instead, there are usually a number of care staff, none of whom typically has primacy or an especially close relationship; usually they leave as time goes by and are replaced by new workers.

There are several types of residential care. In many countries, babies who cannot be looked after by their parents or immediate family are put into orphanages, and much of the section on residential care refers to this context, which is now less common in high-income Westernized countries, but is not uncommon in some eastern and southern European countries and other parts of the world. In countries where the prevalence of AIDS is high, particularly in sub-Saharan Africa, the number of children being orphaned is going up rapidly, and many are being taken into institutional care (see Chapter 46); it has been estimated that there are 143 million orphans worldwide (Whetten *et al.*, 2009), with an estimated 8 million children in residential care. A second, different kind of residential care that we discuss occurs where children cannot be looked after by their parents and prove too difficult to be looked after by foster carers. Such children often have relatively severe behavioral problems, and are more often adolescents. This form of residential care is common in high-income Westernized countries, and in the United States may be called group-care homes. A third type of residential care is that given to young offenders (see Chapter 49), a fourth is inpatient child and adolescent psychiatric units (see Chapter 50); also, there are residential schools for children with emotional and behavioral disorders.

Residential care

The nature of residential care

Residential care of children whom biological parents are unable to care for is widely used across the world, and its nature varies both between and within countries. Gunnar (2001) defined three levels, based on quality: (1) institutions characterized by global deprivation of the child's health, nutrition, stimulation, and relationship needs; (2) institutions with adequate health and nutrition support, but deprivation of the child's stimulation and relationship needs; and (3) institutions that meet all needs except for stable, long-term relationships with consistent caregivers. Logically, it is possible to add a fourth level, namely, an institutional environment that provides for stable and consistent

Rutter's Child and Adolescent Psychiatry, Sixth Edition.
Edited by Anita Thapar and Daniel S. Pine, James F. Leckman, Stephen Scott, Margaret J. Snowling, Eric Taylor.
© 2015 John Wiley & Sons Ltd. Published 2018 by John Wiley & Sons Ltd.

caregiving (Van IJzendoorn *et al.*, 2011). Some organizations try to provide this (The St. Petersburg-USA Orphanage Research Team, 2008; SOS Children's Villages, 2013).

However, in typical residential care, group sizes tend to be large, typically 9–16 children per unit, and the number of children per caregiver can be very large, from 8:1 to 31:1 (Van IJzendoorn *et al.*, 2011). Groups tend to be similar with respect to child age and to psychological or physical disability status. Children are periodically "graduated" from one group to another, with separation from potentially trusted group workers and peers. Continuity of carers is often compromised as professional group workers tend to change frequently because of high staff turnover; workers may work long shifts and then be off for some days; they may not be always assigned to the same group; and they are of course entitled to vacations. The result is that a child may see anywhere between 50 and 100 different caregivers in the first 19 months of life (McCall *et al.*, 2011) and older youth in residential care may not fare better.

An example of an institutional rearing setting that is characterized by many of the features described above—at least up until 10 years ago—is the *Metera Babies Center* (MBC), in Athens, Greece. Most MBC infants come from settings in which they are at high risk for neglect or abuse, relinquished shortly after birth by parents who are unable to provide for them (Vorria *et al.*, 2003). After a few months, infants are moved to pavilions housing children ranging in age from 5 months to 5 years. MBC provides adequate nutrition and health care but lacks stability in child–caregiver relationships and does not provide a playful and cognitively stimulating environment. In the unit for newborns, social contacts and interactions are very restricted. Each newborn is placed alone in a separate small room. One caregiver is responsible for as many as seven infants; caregivers limit their attention to feeding and cleaning the babies. Subsequently, when the babies move to the pavilions, they are housed in groups of 12 children who are looked after by 12 caregivers in total. Thus, in theory the infant/caregiver ratio is 1:1, but in practice, due to the 24 hour shifts, the actual ratio is 6:1, as each caregiver has to look after 4–6 infants at the same time. On a regular day, infants spend a total of 3 1/2 hours playing and 17 1/2 hours in their beds. During weekends and holidays, fewer caregivers are available. Although books and toys are available, the caregivers do not have enough time to interact with the infants using these materials in a stimulating way (Vorria *et al.*, 2003; Van IJzendoorn *et al.*, 2011). Many of the caregivers are not adequately trained for their jobs and their interactions with the infants were less sensitive than those of biological mothers in a comparison group of family-reared infants (Vorria *et al.*, 2003).

The "prototypical" institution described inevitably deprives children of sensitive reciprocal interactions with stable caregivers. In this respect, many institutions are characterized by *structural neglect*, which may include minimum but sufficient physical resources, unfavorable staffing patterns, and inadequate caregiver–child interactions (Van IJzendoorn *et al.*, 2011). Structural neglect should be located at the extreme end of the cumulative risk continuum, and as such it may be considered a special case of child maltreatment (Cyr *et al.*, 2010).

Development of children raised in institutional care

Children raised in residential care settings often suffer from marked developmental delays and may follow deviant developmental pathways. However, the various causes of these delays are difficult to disentangle. First, in some instances, it is difficult to know whether the institutional experience actually causes the deficits or simply maintains preexisting deficits. Second, the forms of deprivation experienced by institutionalized children rarely occur in isolation (Van IJzendoorn *et al.*, 2011). Here we present the (often severe) commoner developmental deficiencies that most institution-reared children display; others are described by Nelson *et al.* (2011).

Physical growth

Children who spend the first few years of their lives in institutional care often show retarded physical growth on parameters such as weight, height, and head circumference. In a meta-analysis of eight studies ($N = 893$), institutional stays prior to adoption were strongly and linearly associated with reduced height ($d = 1.71$), a dose–response relationship, illustrating the potentially causal, negative effect of institutional care on physical growth (Van IJzendoorn & Juffer, 2007), which persists through adolescence (Sonuga-Barke *et al.*, 2010).

Hormonal (HPA axis) development

Atypical patterns of diurnal cortisol activity for children living in institutions were first reported by Carlson and Earls (1997). None of the children exhibited a normal pattern of cortisol variation (high morning and low evening values). Instead, they showed low morning values and slightly elevated evening levels, a pattern replicated in postinstitutionalized children adopted from Russia and China (Gunnar, 2001). In all these studies showing impaired physical growth and HPA axis development, physical nutrition was judged to be adequate; the cause appears to be related to lack of cognitive and social/emotional stimulation (see also Dobrova-Krol *et al.*, 2008).

Cognitive development

Orphanages can be considered "natural experiments" on the necessary conditions for intellectual growth (MacLean, 2003; Rutter *et al.*, 2012). Recent research continues to show the delayed cognitive performance of children in residential care (Rutter & Sonuga-Barke, 2010; Fox *et al.*, 2011). Van IJzendoorn *et al.* (2008) covered 75 studies on more than 3800 children in 19 different countries in a meta-analysis and found a combined effect size of more than a standard deviation. The children reared in institutions showed on average an IQ/DQ 20 points lower than comparison children. Favorable caregiver–child ratios were associated with smaller cognitive delays, whereas early entry into residential care (before 12 months) was associated with larger delays. One or more years of family life prior to institutionalization may provide a basis for further intellectual development even when children grow up in a poor intellectual environment later on.

Attachment security

Institution-reared children experience separation from or loss of their birth parents and other caregivers. Institutionalized children show high rates of insecure and disorganized attachment, for example, rates of security were 17% versus 62% in family-reared children, with most extra insecurity in the form of disorganization: 5% versus 15% avoidant, 5% versus 9% resistant, and 73% versus 15% disorganized (Van IJzendoorn *et al.*, 1999; see Chapter 6).

The rate of disorganized attachment in a residential setting of structural neglect is larger than among maltreated children living in their families, 73% versus 51%, (Cyr *et al.*, 2010). What disorganized attachment means in the context of being raised in an institution remains to be determined (Rutter *et al.*, 2009; Bakermans-Kranenburg *et al.*, 2011a), since there is often a lack of any specific attachment figure; where there is more sensitive caregiving, attachment patterns are more clear-cut (Zeanah *et al.*, 2005; see Chapter 58). Among adolescents admitted to residential treatment settings in West European countries (often due to abuse), most have been found to be insecure and this seems difficult to change in these residential settings (Schleiffer & Muller, 2002; Zegers *et al.*, 2008).

Resilience of attachment security in the face of structural neglect

In spite of insufficient sensitive care in residential settings, in some studies, a proportion of children appear resilient. For example, one in five of the Greek institutionalized infants was securely attached with their caregiver. The securely attached infants were found to be "happier," more social, and to initiate interactions with their caregivers more often (Vorria *et al.*, 2006). It may be that the "happier" infants were more rewarding to interact with, eliciting more sensitive responding from their caregivers, thereby enabling the formation of secure attachment relationships. In contrast, in the English Romanian Adoptee (ERA) study, none of the institutionalized children was found to be securely attached. It is likely that the quality of care in the Romanian institutions was markedly more neglectful and impoverished than in the MBC in Athens. More similar to the Greek rate is the rate in a Chinese institution where 20% of children were rated secure in a study with decreased numbers of children per caregiver to enhance the quality of care (Steele *et al.*, 2009).

The role of genetic factors in resilience under structural neglect is unclear. It would seem likely that infant characteristics would elicit specific caregiving responses which, in turn, could influence the type of attachment security. However, a number of twin studies using the SSP found that the development of attachment security is mostly environmentally

shaped (Bokhorst *et al.*, 2003). A small study of Ukrainian preschoolers reared in institutional settings or in their biological families showed a moderating role of the serotonin transporter gene polymorphism (5HTTLPR). Institutionalized children with the long alleles showed lower levels of attachment disorganization than their institutionalized peers with short alleles (Bakermans-Kranenburg, *et al.*, 2011a). Similar protective effects of the long allele with respect to emotional problems after institutionalization were found elsewhere (Kumsta *et al.*, 2010). Thus, children may differ in their vulnerability to extremely adverse rearing experiences, depending on their genetic characteristics.

Indiscriminate friendliness

One of the most disturbing and confusing behaviors that seems to be typical of institutionalized children is disinhibited or indiscriminately social behavior, characterized as affectionate and friendly behavior toward all adults, including strangers, without the fear or caution that is characteristic of typically developing children. A normative period of indiscriminate behavior is present early in the first year of life. Beginning about 2–3 months of age, infants are quite interested in engaging in social interaction with almost anyone. At 7–9 months, this changes and infants begin to exhibit wariness with strangers. This suggests inhibition of the affiliative motivational system. In children who experience serious neglect, however, the sensitive period for inhibition may close without the development of a selective or specific attachment in the context of a more or less continuous relationship, so that indiscriminate friendliness might persist (Bakermans-Kranenburg *et al.*, 2011b).

In Tizard's study of young children placed in residential nurseries in London in the 1960s (Tizard & Hodges, 1978), all infants experienced residential nursery care for the first 2 years of life, involving a high turnover of caregivers. Subsequently, some went home or were adopted, whereas others remained in institutions. Nearly 38% of the institutionalized children were indiscriminate at age 4 years. A high level of indiscriminately friendly behavior has been confirmed in subsequent studies of institutions (Zeanah *et al.*, 2005; Rutter and Sonuga-Barke, 2010). Interestingly, levels of indiscriminate social behavior appear unrelated to length of stay in the institution and to having a preferred attachment figure or not. Indiscriminate behavior seems more persistent after adoption when institutionalized rearing extends beyond the age of 6 months (Rutter & Sonuga-Barke, 2010; Bakermans-Kranenburg *et al.*, 2011b).

This persistence of indiscriminate friendliness led Rutter *et al.* (2007) to suggest that some form of biological programming may be responsible, whereby the early neglectful environment affects the capacity for focused attention and effortful control. They and others (Bakermans-Kranenburg *et al.*, 2011b) suggest that the core difficulty is a lack of self-control, manifest in social contexts and perhaps also in nonsocial contexts; indiscriminate friendliness was related to inattention/overactivity. This thinking has influenced the change from reactive attachment disorder in DSM-IV to the DSM-5 condition "disinhibited social engagement disorder" that is related to insufficient care but can be present in children who show no signs of disordered attachment or current neglect (American Psychiatric Association, 2013; see Chapter 58).

Psychopathology

In the Tizard study, those who remained in institutions had higher levels of behavior problems at age 4 (Tizard & Rees, 1975). In adolescence, the ex-institution sample showed high levels of social difficulties (Hodges & Tizard, 1989). Quinton and Rutter (1988) studied outcomes of children who had disrupted early years, were taken into public care and then spent prolonged periods in group homes in the 1960s. Again, the living conditions were satisfactory physically, but there were multiple changes of staff.

In the representative survey of children in residential and foster care who were looked after by local authorities in England by the Office of National Statistics (ONS; Meltzer et al., 2003), nearly three-quarters of children living in residential care had a mental health disorder, compared to 10% in the general population. Children in residential care were twice as likely as those in foster care to have anxiety disorders (16% vs 8%), and four times as likely to have depression (8% vs 2%). Conduct disorders were commoner too, 56% versus 33%, as were autistic spectrum disorders, 11% versus 2%. However, the children had either been placed in residential care because they were too difficult to handle in foster care, or because the units they were in specialized in managing and treating the problem in question, for example, autistic spectrum disorders. Therefore, it would be wrong to conclude that it was the residential care that caused the difficulties.

Benefits and harms of residential care
Can institutional care be as good as family care?

The findings described are universally clear that orphanages that deprive children of a reasonably stimulating environment with opportunities for attachment are harmful, when compared to family or family-like care. However, not all institutions are configured like this, and the Positive Outcomes For Orphans (POFO) project argued that the alternative family care is not always so beneficial. They took orphans or abandoned children aged 6–12 in five low- and middle-income countries and compared institutional care with community care (Whetten et al., 2009). Physical growth and health, as well as emotional and cognitive functioning, were no worse for institution-living than community-living children looked after by families in the wider social network. Indeed, in some domains, institution-living children seemed to fare better. The authors concluded that "institutional care," per se, should not be categorically described as damaging or inappropriate for all children.

However, the POFO study was not a study of foster care, and the majority of community carers were the child's mother—usually the father had died (Bakermans-Kranenburg & Van IJzendoorn, 2009). Allocation was not random, and pre placement differences might have existed. It makes no sense to compare home-reared children with institutionalized children to answer the central question of where abandoned and orphaned children should be placed for whom their biological parent is no option. The quality of community care may have been suboptimal due to the death in the family and the emotional and financial consequences; the countries chosen all had a low human development index. Secondly, 75% of the children came into the institutions over 5 years old, so may have had comparatively normal upbringing in the most sensitive developmental stages. Thirdly, the characteristics of the institutions in the POFO study were very different from those in the studies cited. Many were small and locally organized in response to the need to care for new orphans, rather than large state-run institutions. Last, measurements did not address crucial issues such as attachment and neurobiological development.

Based on the solid set of studies reviewed (and in McCall et al., 2011), it is hard not to conclude that residential settings with structural neglect are pathogenic and should be seen as a type of child maltreatment.

Harmful effects of deviant groups

The notion of peer contagion or deviancy training refers to the idea that if antisocial youth are spending much time together in groups, they may reinforce each other to behave more antisocially (Dishion & Tipsord, 2011). In treatment contexts, however, the validity of deviancy training inevitably being harmful has been questioned; thus, in a meta-analysis by Weiss et al. (2005), on 17 out of 18 indices outcomes were no different between individual and group treatments. Nonetheless, there is some evidence for peer contagion in longer term residential care (Lee & Thompson, 2009). Certainly, the survey of residential care described subsequently found a high rate of victimization by other young residents.

Abuse and violence in residential care

Children and adolescents who are vulnerable because of their past experiences with poor parenting and child maltreatment deserve, like all children, to be protected from any sexual or physical abuse. The prevalence of child maltreatment in foster and residential care in the previous year was examined in a representative nation-wide sample of adolescents in the Netherlands in 2010. Based on professional worker reports, the prevalence rates of sexual abuse for foster care and residential care in 2010 were 2 per 1000 and 5 per 1000, respectively, but children in foster care were younger and allowing for this, the rates were similar. Compared to children in the general population, children in residential care had a ninefold increase in sexual abuse, whereas the prevalence in foster care was similar to the general population. The estimates based on youth self-report were 50–100 times higher: 168 per 1000 children in foster care, similar to the general population, and 280 per 1000 children in residential care, significantly higher (Euser et al., 2013b). Higher rates in residential care may be due to more antisocial behavior at entry, a peer group culture of reinforcing negativity and emotional and physical bullying, and less emotional commitment from residential workers, who typically receive low pay, little training, and turn over quickly. Likewise, the peer group often turns over quickly, making it hard for the children to develop trusting bonds with other residents. For children who have to be in care, better trained and supervised staff could reduce abuse.

Violence against residential group care workers

In the study cited, 81% of the group workers experienced some type of violence from the children in their care, about half of the participants experienced serious physical violence (Alink *et al.*, 2014). The high levels of violence in residential youth care indicate that residential care may neither be the best workplace for professionals nor the best therapeutic setting for youth. (Euser *et al.*, 2013a, b).

Effects of removal from orphanages to adoptive or foster care

The ERA study (Rutter & Sonuga-Barke, 2010; Rutter *et al.*, 2012) compared adopted children who had lived in severely depriving orphanages until at least age 6 months with a composite comparison group. Of particular interest were four strictly defined deprivation-specific patterns (DSPs): Quasi-autism, disinhibited attachment, inattention/overactivity, and cognitive impairment. Quasi-autism referred to a pattern that showed autistic-like features (particularly, intense circumscribed interests) but which differed from "ordinary" autism in greater social interest and flexibility. Disinhibited attachment involved a disregard of social boundaries and undue familiarity with strangers. Inattention/overactivity had to be persistent and accompanied by one of the first two patterns, as did cognitive impairment (IQ below 80).

Those adopted away from the institution before the age of 6 months showed no deficits at follow up, whereas those who remained in the institution from 6 to 12 months of age showed a large stepwise increase in deficits and no dose–response association with duration of deprivation thereafter. At age 15, 46% of children adopted after 6 months of age had DSPs, versus 1% of controls; DSPs were not mediated by cognitive deficits. The follow-up findings to the late teens indicated that some with quasi-autism showed a fading of autistic-like features but a persistence of disinhibited attachment-like features. Institutional deprivation was not associated with an increase in other forms of psychopathology that were not accompanied or preceded by one of the DSPs. Disturbed peer relations were strongly associated with all DSPs, whereas disruptive behavior was only associated with inattention/overactivity. Emotional disturbances were not increased at age 6, but started to emerge increasingly to age 15; they were largely accounted for by DSPs.

Cognitively, at age 4 years, the children adopted after 6 months had a severely delayed developmental quotient (43 vs 89). Theory of mind, executive planning, and scholastic achievement all showed comparable differences. There was substantial catch up by the age of 6 (cognitive index 84 vs 106), with further catch up from 11 to 15 years. Those who had definitely not suffered from malnutrition still had very substantial DSPs, suggesting that most of the developmental impact of the orphanages was through psychosocial deprivation (Rutter *et al.*, 2012).

Other studies of internationally adopted children yield similar results, showing massive catch up, but some deficits in those adopted after 1 year of age (Van der Vegt *et al.*, 2009; Audet & Le Mare, 2011). An exception was the British Chinese Adoption study (Rushton *et al.*, 2013). The study group consisted of refugees from China who put their children into institutional care in Hong Kong at the mean age of 3 months and were then adopted into British families at 23 months on average; they were followed up in midlife, in their 40s. On measures of mental health and well-being, there were no significant differences compared to control groups. Possible explanations are that the Hong Kong orphanages were not severely depriving (although the study team give examples of very poor social and emotional care), that the impact of negative institutional experiences may attenuate over decades, and that the quality of adoptive care was better than the care in the control groups. Clearly, more studies that examine these issues and, in particular, that measure the quality of early emotional care, and the effect of several decades of later normal experiences are needed.

In the unique Bucharest Early Intervention Project (BEIP, Fox *et al.*, 2011) children were randomized to stay in institutions or to receive foster care. Their cognitive development was tracked until early adolescence. The three main findings for the first 5 years of the children's life confirm the meta-analytic findings of Van IJzendoorn *et al.* (2008): first, children reared in institutions showed greatly diminished intellectual performance (borderline mental retardation). Second, children randomly assigned to foster care experienced significant gains in cognitive function. Lastly, the younger a child was when placed in foster care, the better the cognitive outcome. Indeed, there was a continuing "cost" to children who remained in the institution for longer. Overall then, adoption or foster care greatly enhance developmental prospects of most institutionalized children and lead to substantial catch-up growth in most domains (Juffer & van IJzendoorn, 2005; Van IJzendoorn & Juffer, 2006).

Summary of the effects of residential care

In summary, most children raised in institutional care show delays and maladaptation in various domains, including physical, cognitive, socio-emotional, and psychopathological. Not every child is affected in the same way by institutional care, and a small but significant proportion of children show remarkable resilience. Sadly, the majority of institutions worldwide even in modern times create a childrearing environment typified by structural neglect. Residential care for older children who cannot be fostered also does not seem to serve children well; often the climate is violent. Except for cases that cannot be contained despite intensive fostering interventions, residential care would seem to be an undesirable option.

Foster care

Prevalence and nature of foster care

In the United States, there were 410,000 children in foster care in 2012 (Children's Bureau, 2013); in England there were 55,000 children in foster care in 2012, with quite a lot of turnover, nearly half had come into care during the year with a similar number being returned home (Glenndenning, 2012). Foster children are usually placed because of caretaker incapacity or absence, child protection reasons, or parental incarceration. Nowadays, many foster placements include visits with the biological parent (Leathers, 2003; Joseph *et al.*, 2014). Ideally, if conditions at home improve, foster care is not long-lasting and children can be reunited permanently with their biological parent(s). However, in practice there are often frequent changes of placement. In one (not atypical) UK authority in 2012, two-thirds of children taken into foster care were returned within a few months to their birth families, suggesting social workers judged there was an improvement at home, but unfortunately two-thirds of these returners home were subsequently taken back into foster care, adding more separations and turmoil to their lives (Minnis *et al.*, 2010). These figures also show how difficult it can be to assess what is "good enough" parenting.

Development of children in foster care
Hormonal (HPA axis) development
Like other abused children (see Chapter 29), fostered children as a group show blunted early morning cortisol and a dysregulated diurnal pattern (Fisher *et al.*, 2006). Fortunately, good quality foster care can reduce the abnormal secretion patterns so that they become normal (Fisher *et al.*, 2006).

Attachment patterns
A meta-analysis of fostered infants and later placed foster children has shown that they are as securely attached to their foster carers as children living in their birth families (Van den Dries *et al.*, 2009). However, within the fostered children, rates of disorganization were higher than in controls (36% vs 15%). Both early- and late-placed children showed more disorganized attachments, probably reflecting their experiences of neglect and maltreatment early in life. Nonetheless, these rates show impressive improvements in comparison with institutionalized children, who in the same meta-analysis had rates of disorganized attachment between 66% and 93%.

Among adolescents, Joseph *et al.* (2014) directly compared attachment patterns to biological parents and foster carers within the same individuals using the Child Attachment Interview. While attachment insecurity to biological parents was almost the rule (90% to birth mothers and 100% to birth fathers), there was a high rate of recovery seen in foster care, with nearly half achieving security (46% to foster mothers and 49% to foster fathers)—rates similar to comparison children living in birth families. Factors associated with higher rates of security were longer duration in placement and warmer observed parenting style from foster carers.

Oosterman *et al.* (2010) found that foster children who were securely attached to their carers showed better physiological regulation of emotions during stress; in contrast, disorganized children did worst. In the Joseph *et al.* (2014) study, attachment security was associated with lower levels of emotional and behavioral problems, fewer psychiatric diagnoses, and less self-reported delinquency in both fostered and nonfostered adolescents.

These findings and the meta-analysis comparing separate fostered and nonfostered groups both counter the notion that because of their abusive past experiences lasting several years, late-placed foster children would have developed generalized internal working models that prevented them from forming trusting relationships with adults who care for them. On the contrary, many children who are placed after several years of abuse nonetheless show ability to recover in this aspect of their development.

Psychopathology
The ONS survey found that almost half of children in foster care had a mental health disorder, 45%, compared to 10% of the general population; all disorders were more frequent. Of course, these high rates are probably not only due to the children having experienced neglect and maltreatment; the genetic background of children taken into care will also predispose to high rates of psychopathology and the disruption from their parents and changes of carer may further increase rates of disorder.

Factors influencing successful foster placement
Sinclair *et al.* (2004) followed nearly 600 fostered children longitudinally and used two measures of placement success or failure, the judgments of carers and social workers, and placement breakdown. Five groups of factors were significant. First, within the child, success was more likely if the child wanted to be in the placement, if the child had attractive characteristics, and had few emotional and behavioral problems. Second, in the carers, success was more likely in those who were rated highly by the social workers for their parenting qualities, were "child oriented" on a questionnaire, and had experienced few allegations of abusive practices and few previous disruptions of children in their care. These factors remained important after taking into account child characteristics. Third, it was important how well the carers and the children "clicked," how well each felt they fitted together. Fourth, placements were more likely to be successful where children were happy at school and where their carers said they had been able to encourage them over school; contact with an educational psychologist was strongly associated with an absence of breakdown (again after taking other factors into account). Finally, where there was strong evidence of prior abuse and no birth family member was forbidden contact, breakdown was three times more likely than if it was forbidden.

These detailed findings have been largely confirmed in a meta-analyses and systematic reviews, which find placement breakdown is predominantly related to child behavior problems, but also is increased by older age at placement, a history of residential care, and more previous placements (Oosterman *et al.*, 2007; Day *et al.* 2013). Investigating the role of externalizing behavior in placement disruption, Fisher *et al.* (2011) used the parent daily report (PDR) telephone interview of antisocial child behaviors to monitor foster placements prospectively for a year. Children displaying fewer than five behaviors a day were at low risk of disruption, but after that each additional behavior increased the probability of disruption by 10%. Using a measure such as the PDR could help detect likely disruptions early on and hopefully lead to interventions to make them less likely.

Kinship care is not protective against placement breakdown, perhaps because of a lack of training and information on the part of kinship caregivers, and perhaps because some of the same factors that led to the biological parents being unable to cope with their children are present in the relatives who take over their care (Terling-Watt, 2001).

Assessment

Introduction

While children in residential or foster care may have had social work assessments, many will not have had a thorough mental health evaluation. It is helpful for the clinician to keep in mind the kind of information set out; thus, for example, as well as suffering abuse at the hands of their birth parents, children may have suffered further bullying or abuse while in care; intellectual levels may be low, rates of psychopathology are likely to be high. It is helpful to have a social worker who knows the child well attend the assessment, along with the foster carers. Although referrers may attribute many of the child's difficulties to insecure attachment or attachment disorders, the clinician should not overlook the presence of conventionally understood disorders.

Taking the history

It is important to ascertain as much detail as possible about the birth parents. Criminality, alcoholism, drug dependence, and other mental health disorders have a heritable component which may help understand the child presentation. Alcohol and substance misuse during pregnancy may have impaired the child's brain development. The intellectual level of the birth parents will also be important; enquiry should be made of the highest level of attainment and whether they appeared to have suffered from intellectual disability.

A careful chronology should be built up of the salient events in the child's life, obviously paying particular attention to the nature of neglect or maltreatment. What factors led the parents to be unable to care properly for the child? Were a series of stepparents involved, what changes of parent figure took place including the number of times the child has come into foster care? What medical conditions does the child have, have they been adequately treated? How is the child doing at school, do they need much extra help firstly for academic matters and secondly for their behavior? What are their grades, what are the prospects for getting any examination qualifications? Are they being bullied or racially harassed? What is the quality of their friendships, are their friends well adjusted or antisocial?

Turning to the current care arrangements, what is the reaction of the foster carers or residential care staff to the child, why did any previous placements break down? What is the current quality of care? What strategies do the foster carers or residential staff deploy when faced by challenging behavior from the child? What are their feelings toward the child, is there any warmth, what strengths do they see in the child? Will the child come to them to talk about emotional difficulties; will the child give and receive affection? How well can the carers support the child's education, and do they enforce homework?

With respect to the birth family, what kind of contact is occurring; for example, none, letter only, regular visits? Are there any legal orders prohibiting contact, does the child find a way round these through, for example, the Internet or Facebook? What happens during visits; is the child disturbed and upset afterwards? How often do they see their siblings, are they in different placements? How are the birth parents explaining to the child why they are now living at home; for example, are they making unrealistic promises about the child's return? Are the birth parents receiving support and training to improve the quality of their parenting, what are the criteria that would enable the child to return to the birth family? If this is impossible, is the long-term plan for adoption or long-term foster care? If the latter, the clinician will need to judge whether the current foster carers are up to the task of looking after the child, often not an easy task if the child is challenging. Is specialist foster care necessary, and if no such facilities are available, is residential care planned?

Systematic enquiry should ask about all the usual forms of psychopathology. Various forms of neurodevelopmental disorder and symptom clusters that do not quite fit textbook descriptions are quite often seen (Rutter & Sonuga-Barke, 2010), as is poor emotional regulation, with some children taking a long time (sometimes hours) to calm down from angry episodes. Some children will show indiscriminate friendliness. Among teenagers, drug misuse and sexual promiscuity are not uncommon, especially in residential homes that cannot prevent the young people going out at night; sexual abuse of girls by organized rings of men (sometimes in the institution) is not unknown.

Examination and investigations

Observation of the interaction between the foster carers and the child should assess the quality of care given. Is there good sensitivity to the children's needs and interest in their activity and point of view, is there to-and-fro mutuality, are the children acknowledged and praised for good behavior? Or are they dismissed and only talked about in negative terms?

Physical examination should include the nervous system and the presence of any dysmorphic features, for example, those seen in fetal alcohol syndrome. Height, weight, and head circumference should all be plotted as impaired growth is common; after a period of foster care, there may be catch up and this needs to be documented both for the child's benefit and sometimes to provide evidence for court. If the mental health professional does not have the skills to do the physical examination, they must ensure that a pediatrician carries it out.

Mental health state examination, as well as covering difficulties, should enquire about what the children enjoy doing and their aspirations. Their views and feelings toward their birth parents and foster parents should be ascertained. The former may be realistic, but may be either over-idealized or sometimes birth parents are demonized. Traumatic symptomatology in relation to abuse should be asked about; as with symptoms of depression and anxiety, it may be the first time they have been properly explored. Asking the child for their three wishes is often revealing.

A psychometric evaluation of intellectual ability is usually illuminating, and is mandatory if school performance is below average. Short forms of standardized tests of intelligence and reading can be completed in under an hour (see Chapter 34). If the history and mental state examination had revealed symptoms suggestive of a disorder, domain-specific questionnaires are helpful diagnostically and for monitoring progress.

Formulation and treatment planning

Formulation should follow the structure of any mental health assessment (see Chapter 32). The allure of rare disorders in maltreated children should be avoided; the American Professional Society on the Abuse of Children (APSAC) specifically advises "Although more common diagnoses, such as ADHD, conduct disorder, PTSD, or adjustment disorder, may be less exciting, they should be considered as *first line diagnoses* before contemplating any rare condition, such as Reactive Attachment Disorder or an unspecified attachment disorder" (Chaffin et al., 2006). These cautions are advised since many children in care have had treatable conditions missed but often have had years of counselling therapies not indicated for their disorders. This is not to say that insecure attachment patterns should not be recognized, nor on the rare occasions when present (see Chapter 58), attachment disorders should not be diagnosed. However, the best treatment for these is not an attachment therapy like holding (Chaffin et al., 2006) but prolonged sensitive care from a parent-like caregiver (see Chapter 6) supported by intervention.

In practical terms, it is important to explain the diagnosis and treatment to the social worker who is taking legal responsibility on behalf of the relevant authority; if changes of placement occur, the information should travel with the child. A meeting with the child's school is often fruitful; advice can be given on behavioral management in the school setting as well as the findings from psychometric testing and recommended intervention.

If the foster care quality is insufficient to meet the needs of the child, it is helpful to apply similar evaluation procedures as

in birth families: (1) carrying out an assessment of the carers' current functioning; (2) specifying operationally defined targets for change; (3) implementing an evidence-based intervention; and (4) objectively measuring progress over time, including evaluation of the carers' willingness to engage and cooperate with the intervention and the extent to which targets were achieved.

Intervention

Individual-level work

General principles

For children in residential and foster care, individual clinical work should be carried out using the same principles as for any child with mental health problems. Treatment should consist of the usual evidence-based psychological and pharmacological interventions. Likewise, in the educational domain, a specific educational plan should be drawn up in conjunction with the school authorities and educational psychologists and monitored for its effectiveness. Individual counseling should be offered to help the children make sense of their predicament and, where possible, come to terms with the possible doubt about with whom they will live in future; however, counseling and psychodynamic or creative art therapies are not evidence-based treatments for substantive mental health disorders or attachment problems. Helping residential workers and foster carers learn good management techniques should reduce the rate of prescription of antipsychotic medication for aggressive behavior, which should not be used routinely for severe behavior problems; a wide survey in the United States found that 12% of fostered children were being prescribed antipsychotics, half of whom were receiving two different medications (Rubin, 2012).

Managing contact with birth parents

The degree of contact with the birth parents will need to be managed; in high-risk cases, it will need to be supervised. Contrary to some received notions that contact with birth parents necessarily impedes children making secure attachments to their foster carers, the study of Joseph et al. (2014) found it had no effect. Indeed, a large study by McWey et al. (2010) found lower levels of conduct problems and depression in children who had frequent contact with their birth parents compared with none, but allowing contact is likely to have been confounded with fewer problems in the first place. Common problems reported by carers include unreliability of birth parents, the impact on children of rejecting parental behavior, and the propensity of parents to try to undermine the carers' discipline (Farmer et al., 2004; Sinclair et al., 2004). During episodes of foster care where there is the prospect of reunion, work with the birth parents should be happening to improve their capacity to care and increase the probability that the child may safely be returned home; unfortunately, this often does not occur.

Interventions to improve residential care
Improving cognitive development

Intervention efforts in institutions have been quite successful; in a meta-analysis, the effect size was large, $d = 0.84$ (Bakermans-Kranenburg et al., 2008). This may point to the extremely disadvantageous rearing environment of institutional settings, and to children's plasticity to overcome their cognitive delays. The timing of the intervention made a difference: those starting before the child's first birthday were significantly more effective ($d = 1.03$) than interventions starting later ($d = 0.58$). Similar effects have been found for children's physical growth (Van IJzendoorn & Juffer, 2007), school achievement, and attachment security (Van IJzendoorn & Juffer, 2006; Van den Dries, et al., 2009). The findings suggest a linear effect, with decreasing effects with children's increasing age at the start of the intervention, and again underline the detrimental effects of structural neglect in the first year of life.

Improving social development

The St-Petersburg-USA Orphanage Research Team (2008) initiated an intervention program to improve the social-emotional relationship experience of Russian children from birth to 4 years. It consisted of staff training (emphasizing sensitive, responsive, and developmentally appropriate interactions) and structural changes (assigning two primary caregivers to lower age and disability groups, terminating transitions of children to new wards, establishing a "Family Hour" for primary caregivers to be with their children). These interventions led to a significant change in the social and emotional behavior of children without and with disabilities, although the latter group needed longer exposure. Specifically, the intervention improved the caregiver–child relationship during free-play with better quality of play, more positive affect, and more positive reciprocal engagement. The rate of attachment disorganization was lower after the intervention (62%) compared to a training-only and no-treatment control orphanages (86% and 85%, respectively).

Interventions to improve foster care
Interventions for infants and young children

Interventions in foster families should support carers' sensitivity and enhance children's attachment security (Juffer et al., 2008a, b), and reduce their antisocial behavior (Leve et al., 2012). A meta-analysis of interventions including foster/adoptive families showed that increasing parental sensitivity led to enhanced attachment security (Bakermans-Kranenburg et al., 2003). The most successful used video interaction feedback, whereby the carer watches videotapes of themselves with the child and is taught to notice the child's reaction to their sensitive overtures and to increase these. The Video-feedback to Promote Positive Parenting-Sensitive Discipline program (VIPP-SD, Juffer et al., 2008a, b) is based on attachment and social learning theory and has been successfully tested with RCTs in maltreating families, adoptive families, and families with externalizing children. There are a number of interventions developed specifically for

foster carers, for example, the Attachment and Biobehavioral Catch-up program (Dozier et al., 2008; see Chapter 6). An RCT showed that as well as enhancing child attachment security, the intervention improved diurnal cortisol production, executive functioning, and emotional regulation (see Chapter 6). The New Orleans intervention is specifically for maltreated children in foster care and works on similar principles.

Starting from a social learning standpoint, Multidimensional Treatment Foster Care (MTFC), originally developed with adolescents, was adapted for younger children. An RCT showed that compared to usual foster care, there were fewer placement disruptions (Fisher et al., 2005), less caregiver stress (Fisher & Stoolmiller, 2008), more securely attached infants (Fisher & Kim, 2007), and more normal cortisol secretion (Fisher & Stoolmiller, 2008) but no evidence has been published that it improves child mental health or behavior. A further trial failed to find any reduction in placement disruptions compared to usual foster care (Fisher et al., 2011).

Interventions for older children

The RCT by Briskman et al. (2013) of the Fostering Changes group-based program showed it improved both disruptive behavior and attachment security as rated by carers. This program has now been disseminated to all 152 local authorities in England. A less intensive form of MTFC proved effective in reducing behavior problems by a smaller effect size ($d = 0.26$; Chamberlain et al., 2008). There have also been some less successful trials in middle childhood; thus, the adaptation of the Incredible Years parenting program for foster carers led to no improvement in externalizing behaviors but an improvement in parenting practices (Linares et al., 2006; Bywater et al., 2011). In summary, choosing programs that are specifically designed for foster children and that promote sensitive caregiving, an understanding of the child's predicament and firm limits seem to be most effective.

In adolescence, the best known foster program is MTFC. However, the original trial compared MTFC to incarceration, when it proved effective (Chamberlain & Reid, 1998). A small Swedish replication study showed positive effects in comparison to foster or residential care (Westermark et al., 2010), but a second Swedish trial comparing MTFC with mainly residential care got no effects on child symptoms, but reduced placement disruption (Hansson & Olsson, 2012). However, a trial in England comparing MTFC with a mixture of foster care and residential care failed to show any effects (Green et al., 2014). In summary, there are encouraging new programs to support foster carers that are often effective in improving attachment security, neurophysiological adaptation, and behavioral adjustment.

Conclusions

Much has been learned in recent years about the development of infants raised in institutions and of older children in residential care. For infants, the evidence clearly points to a very harmful effect of psychosocial deprivation in the first 6 months of life, with fewer effects after that. On the positive side, institutions can be made less depriving, but in most comparisons young children raised in an adoptive or foster care fare better on a wide range of outcomes. Likewise, residential care for older children may bring a different set of harms, including greater risk of sexual and physical abuse and violence than in foster care. While close relationships with people who care for children are the "golden thread" in their lives, the mental health professional must recognize symptoms and disorders when they are present and instigate appropriate treatment, also promoting the children's strengths.

Acknowledgments

MJBK and MHvIJ were supported by awards from the Netherlands Organization for Scientific Research (MJBK: VICI grant no. 453-09-003; MHvIJ: SPINOZA prize). The authors declare that there are no conflicts of interest.

References

Alink, L.R.A. *et al.* (2014) A challenging job: physical and sexual violence towards group workers in youth residential care. *Child and Youth Care Forum* **43**, 243–250.

American Psychiatric Association (2013) *Diagnostic and Statistical Manual*, 5th edn. American Psychiatric Association, Washington, DC.

Audet, K. & Le Mare, L. (2011) Inattention and overactivity in Canadian Romanian adoptees. *International Journal Behavioral Development* **35**, 107–115.

Bakermans-Kranenburg, M.J. & Van IJzendoorn, M.H. (2009) No evidence for orphanages being 'not so bad'. *PLoS ONE* **4**, e8169.

Bakermans-Kranenburg, M.J. *et al.* (2003) Less is more: meta-analyses of sensitivity and attachment interventions in early childhood. *Psychological Bulletin* **129**, 195–215.

Bakermans-Kranenburg, M.J. *et al.* (2008) Earlier is better: a meta-analysis of 70 years of intervention improving cognitive development in institutionalized children. *Monographs Society Research Child Development.* **73**, 279–293.

Bakermans-Kranenburg, M.J. *et al.* (2011a) Impact of institutional care on attachment disorganization and insecurity of Ukrainian preschoolers: protective effect of the long variant of the serotonin transporter gene (5HTT). *International Journal Behavioral Development* **36**, 11–18.

Bakermans-Kranenburg, M.J. *et al.* (2011b) Attachment and emotional development in institutional care: characteristics and catch-up. *Monographs Society Research Child Development* **76**, 62–91.

Bokhorst, C.L. *et al.* (2003) The importance of shared environment in mother-infant attachment security. *Child Development* **74**, 1769–1782.

Briskman, J. *et al.* (2013) Randomized controlled trial of the fostering changes programme. Department for Education Research Report RR237, London.

Bywater, T. *et al.* (2011) Incredible years parent training support for foster carers in Wales. *Child: Care, Health, Development* **37**, 233–243.

Carlson, M. & Earls, F. (1997) Psychological and neuro-endocrinological sequelae of early social deprivation in institutionalized children in Romania. *Annals New York Academy Sciences* **807**, 419–428.

Chaffin, M. *et al.* (2006) Report of the APSAC task force on attachment therapy. *Child Maltreatment* **11**, 76–89.

Chamberlain, P. & Reid, J. (1998) Comparison of two community alternatives to incarceration for chronic juvenile offenders. *Journal Consulting Clinical Psychology* **6**, 624–633.

Chamberlain, P. *et al.* (2008) Prevention of behavior problems for children in foster care: outcomes and mediation effects. *Prevention Science* **9**, 17–27.

Children's Bureau (2013) Child Welfare Outcomes 2008–2011: Report to Congress. US Department of Health and Human Services, Washington, Available: http://www.acf.hhs.gov/programs/cb/resource/cwo-08-11.

Cyr, C. *et al.* (2010) Attachment security and disorganization in maltreating and high-risk families: a series of meta-analyses. *Development Psychopathology* **22**, 87–108.

Dishion, T.J. & Tipsord, J.M. (2011) Peer contagion in child and adolescent social and emotional development. *Annual Review of Psychology* **62**, 189–214.

Department for Education (2013) *Children looked after in England (including adoption and care leavers) year ending 31 March 2013.* Department for Education Publications, London number SFR 36/2013.

Dobrova-Krol, N. *et al.* (2008) Physical growth delays and stress dysregulation in stunted and non-stunted Ukrainian institution-reared children. *Infant Behavior Development* **31**, 539–553.

Dozier, M. *et al.* (2008) Effects of an attachment-based intervention on the cortisol production of infants and toddlers in foster care. *Development and Psychopathology* **20**, 845–859.

Euser, S. *et al.* (2013a) The prevalence of child maltreatment in the Netherlands across a 5-year period. *Child Abuse & Neglect* **37**, 841–851.

Euser, S. *et al.* (2013b) The prevalence of child sexual abuse in out-of-home care: a comparison between abuse in residential and in foster care. *Child Maltreatment* **18**, 221–231.

Farmer, E. *et al.* (2004) *Fostering Adolescents*. Jessica Kingsley, London.

Fisher, P. & Kim, H. (2007) Intervention effects on foster preschoolers' attachment-related behaviors from a randomized trial. *Prevention Science* **8**, 161–170.

Fisher, P.A. & Stoolmiller, M. (2008) Intervention effects on foster parent stress: associations with children's cortisol levels. *Development and Psychopathology* **20**, 1003–1021.

Fisher, P. *et al.* (2005) The early intervention foster care program: permanent placement outcomes from a randomized trial. *Child Maltreatment* **10**, 61–71.

Fisher, P. *et al.* (2006) Effects of Therapeutic Interventions for foster children on behavioral problems, caregiver attachment, and stress regulatory neural systems. *Annals New York Academy Sciences* **1094**, 215–225.

Fisher, P.A. *et al.* (2011) Foster placement disruptions associated with problem behavior: mitigating a threshold effect. *Journal Consulting Clinical Psychology* **79**, 481–487.

Fox, N.A. *et al.* (2011) The effects of severe psychosocial deprivation and foster care intervention on cognitive development at 8 years of age:

findings from the Bucharest Early Intervention Project. *Journal Child Psychology Psychiatry* **52**, 919–928.

Glenndenning, J. (2012) *Children Looked After by Local Authorities in England in 2012*. Department for Education, London.

Green, J. et al. (2014) Multidimensional treatment foster care for adolescents in English care: randomised trial and observational cohort evaluation. *British Journal of Psychiatry* **204**, 214–221.

Gunnar, M. (2001) Effects of early deprivation. In: *Handbook of Developmental Cognitive Neuroscience*. (eds C.A. Nelson & M. Luciana), pp. 617–629. MIT Press, Cambridge.

Hansson, K. & Olsson, M. (2012) Effects of multidimensional treatment foster care (MTFC) in Sweden. *Children Youth Services Review* **34**, 1929–1936.

Hodges, J. & Tizard, B. (1989) Social and family relationships of ex-institutional adolescents. *Journal Child Psychology and Psychiatry* **30**, 77–97.

Joseph, M. et al. (2014) The formation of secure new attachments by children who were maltreated: an observational study of adolescents in foster care. *Development and Psychopathology* **26**, 67–80.

Juffer, F. & Van IJzendoorn, M.H. (2005) Behavior problems and mental health referrals of international adoptees: a meta-analytic approach. *Journal American Medical Association* **293**, 2501–2515.

Juffer, F. et al. (2008a) Attachment-based interventions in early childhood: an overview. In: *Promoting Positive Parenting: An Attachment-Based Intervention*. (eds F. Juffer, M. Bakermans-Kranenburg & M. van IJzendoorn), pp. 37–57. Erlbaum, NY.

Juffer, F. M.J. Bakermans-Kranenburg & M.H. van IJzendoorn, (eds) (2008b) *Promoting Positive Parenting: An Attachment-Based Intervention*. Erlbaum, New York.

Kumsta, R. et al. (2010) 5HTT genotype moderates the influence of early institutional deprivation on emotional problems in adolescence. *Journal Child Psychology Psychiatry* **51**, 755–762.

Leathers, S. (2003) Parental visiting, conflicting allegiances, and emotional and behavioral problems among foster children. *Family Relations* **52**, 53–63.

Lee, B.R. & Thompson, R. (2009) Examining externalizing behavior trajectories of youth in group homes: is there evidence for peer contagion? *Journal Abnormal Child Psychology* **37**, 31–44.

Leve, L. et al. (2012) Children in foster care—vulnerabilities and evidence-based interventions that promote resilience processes. *Journal Child Psychology Psychiatry* **53**, 1197–1211.

Linares, L. et al. (2006) A promising parenting intervention in foster care. *Journal Consulting Clinical Psychology* **74**, 32–41.

MacLean, K. (2003) The impact of institutionalization on child development. *Development and Psychopathology* **4**, 853–884.

McCall, R. et al. (2011) Children without permanent parents: research, practice, and policy: IX. *Monographs Society Research Child Development*. **76**, 223–272.

McWey, L.M. et al. (2010) The impact of continued contact with biological parents upon the mental health of children in foster care. *Children Youth Services Review* **32**, 1338–1345.

Meltzer, H. et al. (2003) *Mental Health of Children Living in England*. ONS, London.

Minnis, H. et al. (2010) Translating a model of intervention with maltreated children and their families for the Glasgow context. *Clinical Child Psychology and Psychiatry* **15**, 497–509.

Nelson, C. et al. (2011) The neurobiological toll of early human deprivation. *Monographs Society Research Child Development* **76**, 127–146.

Oosterman, M. et al. (2007) Disruptions in foster care: a review and meta-analysis. *Children and Youth Services Review* **29**, 53–76.

Oosterman, M. et al. (2010) Autonomic reactivity in relation to attachment and early adversity among foster children. *Development Psychopathology* **22**, 109–118.

Quinton, D. & Rutter, M. (1988) *Parenting Breakdown: The Making and Breaking of Inter- Generational Links Surrey*. Gower, UK.

Rock, S. et al. (2013) Understanding foster placement instability for looked after children. A systematic review and narrative synthesis of quantitative and qualitative evidence. *British Journal Social Work* **43**, 1–27.

Rubin, D. (2012) Interstate variation in trends of psychotropic medication use among Medicaid-enrolled children in foster care. *Children and Youth Services Review* **34**, 1492–1499.

Rushton, A. et al. (2013) the British Chinese adoption study. *Journal of Child Psychology and Psychiatry* **54**, 1215–1222.

Rutter, M. & Sonuga-Barke, E. (2010) Overview of findings from the ERA Study, inferences, and research implications. *Monographs of the Society for Research in Child Development* **76**, 212–229.

Rutter, M. et al. (2007) Early adolescent outcomes for institutionally-deprived and non-deprived adoptees. I: disinhibited attachment. *Journal of Child Psychology and Psychiatry*. **48**, 17–30.

Rutter, M. et al. (2009) Attachment insecurity, disinhibited attachment, and attachment disorders: where do research findings leave the concepts? *Journal of Child Psychology and Psychiatry*. **50**, 529–543.

Rutter, M. et al. (2012) Longitudinal studies using a "natural experiment" design: the case of adoptees from Romanian institutions. *Journal of the American Academy of Child and Adolescent Psychiatry* **51**, 762–770.

Schleiffer, R. & Muller, S. (2002) Attachment representations of adolescents in residential care. *Praxis Kinderpsychologie Kinderpsychiatrie* **51**, 747–765.

Sinclair, I. et al. (2004) *Foster Placements: Why They succeed and Why They Fail*. Jessica Kingsley, London.

Sonuga-Barke, E.J. et al. (2010) Differentiating developmental trajectories for conduct, emotion, and peer problems following early deprivation. *Monographs of the Society for Research in Child Development* **75**, 102–124.

SOS Children's villages (2013) Available: http://www.sos-childrens villages.org/what-we-do/research/approaching-capabilities-with -children-in-care

St. Petersburg-USA Orphanage Research Team (2008) The effects of early social-emotional and relationship experience on young orphanage children. *Monographs of the Society for Research in Child Development* **73**, 1–262.

Steele, M. et al. (2009) Attachment representations and adoption outcome. In: *International Advances in Adoption Research for Practice*. (eds G. Wrobel & E. Neil), pp. 193–215. John Wiley & Sons, NY.

Terling-Watt, T. (2001) Permanency in kinship care: an exploration of factors associated with placement disruption. *Children Youth Services Review* **23**, 111–126.

Tizard, B. & Hodges, J. (1978) The effect of early institutional rearing on the development of eight year old children. *Journal of Child Psychology and Psychiatry* **19**, 99–118.

Tizard, B. & Rees, J. (1975) The effect of early institutional rearing on four-year-old children. *Journal of Child Psychology and Psychiatry* **16**, 61–73.

Van den Dries, L. *et al.* (2009) Fostering security? A meta-analysis of attachment in adopted children. *Children and Youth Services Review* **31**, 410–421.

Van der Vegt, E.J. *et al.* (2009) Impact of early childhood adversities on adult psychiatric disorders: a study of international adoptees. *Social Psychiatry Psychiatric Epidemiology* **44**, 724–731.

Van IJzendoorn, M.H. & Juffer, F. (2006) Adoption as intervention. Meta-analytic evidence for massive catch-up and plasticity in physical, socio-emotional, and cognitive development. *Journal of Child Psychology and Psychiatry* **47**, 1228–1245.

Van IJzendoorn, M.H. & Juffer, F. (2007) Plasticity of growth in height, weight and head circumference: meta-analytic evidence of massive catch-up after international adoption. *Journal of Developmental and Behavioral Pediatrics* **28**, 334–343.

Van IJzendoorn, M.H. *et al.* (1999) Disorganized attachment in early childhood: meta-analysis of precursors, concomitants, and sequelae. *Development Psychopathology* **11**, 225–249.

Van IJzendoorn, M.H. *et al.* (2008) IQ of children growing up in children's homes: a meta-analysis on IQ delays in orphanages. *Merrill-Palmer Quarterly.* **54**, 341–366.

Van IJzendoorn, M.H. *et al.* (2011) Children without permanent parents: research, practice, and policy. *Monographs of the Society for Research in Child Development* **76**, 1–91.

Vorria, P. *et al.* (2003) Early experiences and attachment relationships of Greek infants raised in residential group care. *Journal of Child Psychology and Psychiatry* **44**, 1208–1220.

Vorria, P. *et al.* (2006) The development of adopted children after institutional care: a follow-up study. *Journal of Child Psychology and Psychiatry* **47**, 1246–1253.

Weiss, B. *et al.* (2005) Iatrogenic effects of group treatment for antisocial youth. *Journal of Consulting and Clinical Psychology* **73**, 1036–1044.

Westermark, P. *et al.* (2010) Multidimensional treatment foster care: results from an independent replication. *Journal Family Therapy* **33**, 20–41.

Whetten, K. *et al.* (2009) A comparison of the wellbeing of orphans and abandoned children ages 6–12 in institutional and community-based care settings in 5 less wealthy nations. *PLoS ONE* **4**, e8169.

Zeanah, C. *et al.* (2005) Attachment in institutionalized and community children in Romania. *Child Development* **76**, 1015–1028.

Zegers, M.A.M. *et al.* (2008) Attachment and problem behavior of adolescents during residential treatment. *Attachment Human Development* **10**, 91–103.

CHAPTER 22

Adoption

Nancy J. Cohen[1,2] and Fataneh Farnia[1,2]

[1] Department of Psychiatry, University of Toronto, Ontario, Canada
[2] Hincks-Dellcrest Centre, Gail Appel Institute, Toronto, Ontario, Canada

This chapter provides a review of contemporary trends in adoption, including diverse alternatives for those who want to adopt. The chapter proceeds to discuss outcomes of both domestic and intercountry adoptions and to consider issues related to selection, assessment, preparation, and support of families who adopt.

Contemporary trends in adoptive family formation

Decreases in domestic and intercountry adoption

Adoption statistics indicate a decrease in both domestic and intercountry adoptions worldwide. This trend in domestic adoption in developed countries is related to a decrease in available infants, preference for children without special needs and an increase in kinship adoption, adoption by a step-parent, and the accessibility of *in vitro* fertilization and other assisted reproductive technologies (United Nations, 2009). Other factors include politicized issues such as struggling to find an ethnic match and delays due to legal complications (Barn & Kirton, 2012). The decline also may be explained by the decrease in unplanned pregnancies and changing practices surrounding single parenthood.

Since 2007, intercountry adoption from major sending countries declined, while efforts were made to increase domestic adoption. For instance, Guatemala, Vietnam, and Cambodia have suspended their international adoption programs. In China, Russia, and Korea, the number of children available for intercountry adoption has dropped significantly. In 2011, Ethiopia reduced intercountry adoption by 90% (Selman, 2009). Some of the sending countries periodically place a moratorium on intercountry adoption because of concerns regarding unethical practices such as corruption, adoption fraud, bribery, child abduction and trafficking, and irregularities in the adoption process that are inconsistent with the Hague Convention for Protection of Children and Cooperating in Respect of Intercountry Adoption (2006).

In other countries, political and economic conditions precluded establishment of an adequate social welfare structure and provision of quality foster care and adoption. There is now increasing awareness of the detrimental effects of institutionalization on children and how caregivers' skills and, in turn, children's lives, can be improved (McCall, 2011; see Chapter 58). There has also been a push toward deinstitutionalization, improved social service delivery systems, and emphasis on reunification with birth families, placement in foster care, and adoption (Nedelcu & Groza, 2012).

Further, whereas in the past, children were adopted following natural disasters, local authorities have shifted from sending these children abroad in favor of local solutions. In this way, children are not doubly traumatized by the disaster that made them orphans and a rapid transition to an unfamiliar environment.

A variety of approaches have increased domestic adoptions. Korea provides monthly allowances and health benefits for children adopted domestically, and removed restrictions on prospective parents' qualifications such as age and single parenthood (Lee, 2007; Ministry of Health & Welfare, 2011). Russia removed stringent requirements for housing and income level (Moe, 2007). Immediately following Russia's ban on adoptions from the United States, the government facilitated domestic adoption (The Moscow Times, 2013). Ethiopia provides similar social (Buckner International, 2013) and legal (Ethiopian, 2013) support for domestic adoption.

In China, the number of orphans has increased 24% since 2005 (Shang, 2011). More than 80% of these orphans do not live in government institutions, are not legally adopted and have limited access to resources (Shang, 2008). Nevertheless, the government has maintained restrictions on domestic adoption and added hurdles for international prospective parents' qualifications (i.e., heterosexual married couples, willingness to adopt

Rutter's Child and Adolescent Psychiatry, Sixth Edition.
Edited by Anita Thapar and Daniel S. Pine, James F. Leckman, Stephen Scott, Margaret J. Snowling, Eric Taylor.
© 2015 John Wiley & Sons Ltd. Published 2018 by John Wiley & Sons Ltd.

children with special needs). Moreover, wait times are longer and procedures more costly.

In major receiving countries (e.g., the United States, United Kingdom, Canada, Australia), there has been a movement to increase domestic adoption. With fewer infants available for domestic adoption, prospective parents must consider adopting "hard to place" or "special needs" children, such as older children, sibling groups, and children with developmental, educational, social-emotional, or medical needs (Henry & Pollack, 2009; Denby et al., 2010). Factors contributing to acceptance of children with a disability include access to health insurance, a positive experience with an individual with a specific syndrome, and religious beliefs (Lindh et al., 2007).

In the United States, foster care special needs children can be adopted through subsidized public programs (Dalberth et al., 2005, National Council for Adoption, 2012). The Adoption Council of Canada (2013) expanded the federal adoption tax to support families who adopt domestically from the foster care system. Research has shown that children who are subsidy eligible are more likely to be adopted (Buckles, 2013).

Alternatives for individuals and families who want to adopt

Open adoption

A few decades ago, information on birth parents was kept sealed. A shift toward openness has now become the norm. A child's adoptive status cannot be kept secret from older children adopted from institutions or foster care, or from children adopted through international/interracial adoption. In domestic adoptions, children usually are aware of their adoptive status and often have some contact with their birth parents. Openness became more possible once birth mothers could choose conditions for adoption. A continuum of openness ranges from keeping identifying information secret to ongoing contact among members of the adoption triad.

Open adoption leads to greater satisfaction (Siegel & Smith, 2012). Birth parents' uncertainty about their child's well-being is reduced, and adoptive parents can obtain important historical information. Further, open adoption helps children to develop a sense of belonging (Grotevant et al., 2011; Child Welfare Information Gateway, 2013). Nevertheless, openness requires commitment and mutual respect from adoptive and birth parents. The best outcomes ensue when adoptive parents demonstrate sensitivity toward the child and birth parent(s) and help the child integrate past and present experiences (Neil, 2003). Openness agreements can vary among families. Because the agreement is not legally enforceable, adoptive families can use discretion to maintain children's interests. A higher level of satisfaction with contact predicts adoptees' social-emotional adjustment, especially a lower rate of externalizing behaviors (Von Korff et al., 2006; Grotevant et al., 2011). When disagreements among members of the triad arise, it is essential that they obtain help from trusted adoption workers or family therapists.

Foster care to adoption

Many children are placed in foster care due to maltreatment and neglect (Winokur et al., 2009; Munro & Manful, 2012). Once in foster care, children are unlikely to be reunited with their birth families (Farmer et al., 2011; Wade et al., 2011). In the United States, 54% of children are adopted by foster parents (US Department of Health and Human Services, 2012). This reduces time to permanency, ends uncertainty (Howard & Smith, 2003), and creates connectedness to permanent caregivers (Triseliotis, 2003) while helping children and youth to sustain contact with their birth families (Vandivere et al., 2009). Contact improves a sense of hereditary belonging and identity with the biological family (Grotevant et al., 2011).

Kinship care

Kinship care is another arrangement for children who are victims of maltreatment or whose parent(s) are incarcerated or deceased (Denby, 2012). This is a more stable placement than foster care, residential centers, or group homes (Hunt et al., 2008). It minimizes trauma from parental separation and provides a sense of belonging (Rubin et al., 2008; Winokur et al., 2009). Kinship care also poses challenges. Children in kinship care are often placed with grandparents, who may experience feelings of loss, guilt, and anger over what they believe is their contribution to the birth parent(s)' abuse or neglect (Kelley et al., 2011). Grandparents are likely to be less educated, unemployed, ill (Cuddeback, 2004; Hairston, 2007), and minimally aware of support services (Fechter-Leggett & O'Brien, 2010). Supporting kinship caregivers reduces stressors that affect permanency of the care (Denby, 2011).

Transracial adoption

The longstanding controversy over transracial adoption remains salient (Blackstock, 2003; Griffith & Bergeron, 2006). In certain jurisdictions, it is highly politicized when it comes to the domestic adoption of Black or Indigenous children by White parents. While child welfare policy identifies within-race adoption as optimal, it may take longer to find a matching family (Brooks et al., 1999; Adamec & Miller, 2007; Barn & Kirton, 2012). Some adoption experts believe that children available for adoption should be matched with families with at least one parent of the same race or ethnicity as the child. Prospective parents who intend to adopt interracially need training on a child's cultural, racial, religious, ethnic and linguistic background. To achieve positive outcomes, at a minimum, some of the child's heritage and culture must be integrated into family life (Simon, 1996).

Ethnic identity development also varies according to children's age and development (Lee, 2003). Because transracially adopted preadolescents tend to identify with their birth culture, it is important to place them in families sensitive to their cultural heritage (Evan B. Donaldson Institute, 2008).

In general, transracial adoption does not result in psychological problems or social adjustment issues in children. Seventy to eighty percent of transracial adoptees have few serious behavioral and emotional problems, similar to same-race adopted and nonadopted children (Lindblad *et al.*, 2003). However, transracially adopted children and their families face challenges including social discrimination. For example, parents who adopted children from Asia and Latin America reported more discrimination than those who adopted from Europe. Discrimination was associated with greater family stress and more child behavior problems (Lee *et al.*, 2010). Adoptive parents need to be aware of the social and emotional issues that they and their children may face. When parents facilitate their children's comfort with their ethnic identities, the children will have better psychological adjustment, higher self-esteem, greater ethnic pride, and less distress (Mohanty *et al.*, 2007; Johnston *et al.*, 2007).

Assistive reproductive technologies (ART): *in vitro* fertilization, intracytoplasmic sperm injection, donor insemination

ARTs have resulted in the birth of more than 4.3 million children worldwide (ESHRE, 2010) through intracytoplasmic sperm injection (ICSI), *in vitro* fertilization (IVF), and frozen embryo implantation. Where IVF is used, couples have to make ethical decisions, including the options of having their unused embryos cryopreserved and stored or destroyed, donating them for medical research, or putting them up for adoption by others.

The use of ARTs has been the subject of medical, legal, and ethical controversies. Some medical concerns are linked to the risk of pregnancy problems for mothers (Wen *et al.*, 2004) and their babies (Jauniaux, 2012) due to multiple gestations resulting from fertility-enhancing drugs taken before IVF or alternative insemination. Prospective mothers and women donating oocytes who undergo an IVF procedure must be informed of the medical risks associated with this procedure and provide informed consent (Brezina & Zhao, 2012).

Another ethical issue arises around the preimplantation genetic diagnosis (PGD) or screening (PGS) tests, used mainly to diagnose or screen specific genetic conditions or chromosomal anomalies. Since these procedures have become more affordable, an ethical concern is that parents not experiencing infertility may use the tests to create so-called "designer babies" by choosing nontherapeutic physical attributes such as eye color, skin tone, and sex of the baby (Calpern, 2007).

A further ethical issue arises for parents who adopt an embryo or receive a donor gamete. The adoptive parents often grieve losses with regard to infertility and the ability to pass on their genes to create a child genetically related to both. A donor's loss of a potential genetic child may also lead to grief. Frozen embryo donors must make a stressful decision over the future of their frozen embryos, their virtual child (DeLacey, 2005). Almost half of those who considered donating embryos for adoption felt an ongoing sense of responsibility for the well-being of their offspring, and concerns about the quality of adoptive parent caregiving (McMahon & Saunders, 2009).

While adoption openness benefits members of the adoption triad, the practice in ART has been donor anonymity. A review of studies on donor insemination concluded that only 1–30% of parents intended to tell their children about their genetic origins (Brewaeys, 2001). The reasons for this include social preference for biological parenthood, lack of awareness about the importance of openness, and fear of rejection by the child. However, parents are advised to disclose early on since lack of information about one's origin and genetic ties may negatively affect a person's health and well-being (Paul & Berger, 2007; Cushing, 2010).

In adolescence and young adulthood, the impact of donor anonymity and secrecy about genetic origin is described as a sense of isolation, disconnection, grief and loss, confusion, struggle with identity formation, and anger (Shanner, 2003; Marquardt *et al.*, 2010). These feelings may damage family relationships and place these individuals at risk for adjustment difficulties (Marquardt *et al.*, 2010; Golombok *et al.*, 2013). Therefore, as with adoptive families, it is important for parents to find age-appropriate means to include the truth about their child's genetic origins as early as possible. In some cases it also may be possible to encourage a relationship with the child's biological parent(s).

A higher rate of disclosure is reported among single mothers and lesbian couples (Jadva *et al.*, 2009; Beeson *et al.*, 2011). The situation is changing, however, and increasingly more parents of donor offspring are willing to disclose to their children their donor conceived status. Moreover, the policy of donor anonymity is being rethought, systems of open-identity donation are in place in some countries and the donor offspring are entitled to identifying information about their donors when they turn 18 (HFEA, 2009).

Another concern about donor anonymity is the number and identity of children conceived using the same donor. Laws regulating sperm donation address this issue. However, there is great variability in the number of children allowed to be born from each donor in different jurisdictions. The numbers range from 3 offspring in Hong Kong to 25 in Canada and the Netherlands. The Donor-Sibling Registry is a worldwide organization that helps individuals conceived by any ART practice and parents of donor offspring to find donors and genetic half siblings (Freeman *et al.*, 2009).

Gay and lesbian adoption

Single women have been able to adopt a child for some time, but adoption has not been so readily accepted for gay, lesbian, bisexual, and transgendered (GLBT) individuals or couples. While gay and lesbian parenting has become more common, little is known about parenting by bisexual and transgendered individuals and couples.

Gay and lesbian parenting began with consideration of the rights of parents coming out of a heterosexual marriage (Goldberg & Gianino, 2011). A new generation of gay and lesbian individuals assumes that parenting is a right and plan to become parents (Lev & Sennott, 2013). Some individuals have an agreement with a known partner to conceive a child. Others use ART or a surrogate or adopt a child (Berkowitz, 2013). Both legal and emotional issues inform the choice of the means for having a child. When one individual gives birth or adopts, the partner can adopt as coparent. This places the coparent at a disadvantage regarding legal status that can create difficulties if the couple separate. Where gay and lesbian marriage has become legal, the parental rights of both parents are respected, thus alleviating both legal and emotional concerns. Also, physiological changes in the parent giving birth, and the child's possible preferential reaction, can disturb the sense of equality. Some lesbian couples resolve this issue by taking turns going through a pregnancy and birth. Longitudinal studies of adolescents and adults indicate that it is not parents' sexual orientation but family process variables, important in all families, that are critical (Mellish et al., 2013). This includes low parenting stress and qualities of the couple's relationship with one another and with their children (Averett et al., 2009). Contextual factors, including acceptance of extended family, neighbors, schools, and religious institutions are related to children's outcomes. Children's overall adjustment, including gender role behavior, is not adversely affected (Goldberg et al., 2011; Patterson & Wainright, 2011). Moreover, children of gay and lesbian parents do not differ in their cognitive ability, school performance, or social-emotional health. Some individuals had problems with trust in adulthood primarily related to their parents' coming out unexpectedly and experiences of being teased and bullied (Goldberg, 2007).

In fact, gay and lesbian households may have low levels of parenting stress as adopting parents tend to be well educated and professionally and financially secure (Farr et al., 2010). Longitudinal studies also suggest that youth of lesbian and gay parents are more tolerant and have more flexible ideas about gender and sexuality (Goldberg, 2007). Moreover, being raised without a father from infancy does not seem to have negative consequences for social and emotional development for children (MacCallum & Golombok, 2004). Similar findings about motherless children are not yet available. Although there is little systematic study of lesbian and gay couples in open adoption arrangements, these couples may be more accepting of open adoption because they appreciate the concept of openness generally and more likely to view nonfamily related individuals as kin (Goldberg et al., 2010).

Lesbian and gay couples are more open to transracial and special needs adoptions (Goldberg & Gianino, 2011) and have been solicited for adoption of these children (Downing et al., 2009). This greater openness may result from their own experiences of being unaccepted or marginalized or having to wait longer than heterosexual couples for private domestic adoptions where a birth mother chooses the adoptive parents (Farr & Patterson, 2009; Ausbrooks & Russell, 2011).

Acceptance of gay and lesbian adoption is greater among private secular adoption agencies, and some faith-affiliated agencies (Matthews & Cramer, 2006; Brodzinsky, 2011). Training of adoption workers to facilitate such adoptions and to provide ongoing support is often limited as is having GLBT staff workers (Goldberg & Gianino, 2011; Mallon, 2011). Taken together, research concludes that decisions about children's and adolescents' placement into adoptive homes should not focus on parental sexual orientation.

It is important to discuss implications of the prospective parents' sexuality for their children within the extended family, at school, and in the community. The parents also will need to explore children's views of their parents' sexual orientation and their responses to potential reactions from teachers and peers. Clinicians can play an important role in understanding and supporting life course events and transitions for lesbian and gay individuals and couples and their adopted children.

Opening the birth records: search for birth parents (including ART donors)

Sealing birth and adoption records was meant to provide stability to adoptive families and a chance for a new start to birth parents. While adopted children have the highest stake, their rights to biological information, cultural heritage, and medical history were not considered. Research has shown that mothers who relinquish a child may experience persisting mental health issues (Novac et al., 2006). Legislative changes now allow more openness in adoption and take into account the constitutional rights of both adoptees and birth parents by facilitating search and contact between these parties.

Pursuit of birth parents or gamete donors often becomes important once adopted children reach adolescence or adulthood when unresolved psychological and identity issues come to the fore (Curtis & Pearson, 2010) or at a life cycle transition (Campbell et al., 1991). Gender, self-esteem, degree of openness in adoption, age at adoption, and quality of the adoption experience distinguish searchers from nonsearchers (Howe & Feast, 2000). The search tends to be stimulated by the desire to know the birth parent's history and motivation for placing a child for adoption or donating and to seek health information. For birth mothers/parents, the search and reunion is motivated by assuring their children's well-being, how they are being parented, letting them know that they were loved, and explaining the reasons they were given up (Petta & Steed, 2005).

Adoptees' search and hope for reunification often focuses on the birth mother (Trinder et al., 2004) although increasing numbers seek contact with their birth fathers (Clapton, 2003; Passmore & Chipuer, 2009). While some adoptive parents believe that this is their children's choice and right to know about their genetic origin, others are reluctant to have their child form an attachment relationship with a birth parent or gamete donor (Wallbank, 2004). Parents are more open to the possibility of their children developing attachment relationship with their donor siblings (Freeman et al., 2009).

Reunions have positive outcomes for adopted children and birth parents (Lifton, 1994; Cavoukian, 2005). However, unfulfilled hopes and unrealistic expectations of the reunion may negatively impact the emotional stability and security of both parties (Howe & Feast, 2001; Kelly, 2005; Feeney *et al.,* 2007).

While the majority of adoptive parents reported satisfaction with contact (Siegel & Smith, 2012), children's search for their birth parents may be the most emotionally loaded moment in adoptive parents' lives. They may feel that the unexpected, unplanned contact will harm their relationship with their children and their role and identity as parents (MacDonald & McSherry, 2013). Adoptive families who support their children's search and are involved in their reunion decision making are less stressed than those who disapprove of reunions (Silverman *et al.,* 1994). They are likely to remain active members of the adoption triad and establish friendly relationships with the birth family (Howe & Feast, 2000).

Outcomes of adoption

Outcomes of domestic adoption

The positive outcomes for domestically adopted infants have been well documented with respect to aspects of development and attachment security (van IJzendoorn & Juffer, 2006). Because there is a shortage of healthy infants available for adoption, older children and those with other special needs continue to be available for adoption in large numbers. Children who are older at adoption, or have other special needs, initially show more emotional and behavior problems that can make parenting more challenging. With respect to school performance, when compared to nonadopted siblings, adopted children performed better at school but lagged behind current nonadopted peers (van IJzendoorn, & Juffer, 2005). Nevertheless, once adopted, the outcomes for these children are generally positive (Rushton & Dance, 2006; Child Welfare Information Gateway, 2012).

Child, parent, and agency factors contribute to adjustment of children with special needs. Child factors include presence of emotional and behavioral problems, strong attachment to the birth mother, and being a victim of preadoption sexual abuse. Parent factors include being a new parent rather than the child's foster parent, receiving less support from relatives, being more highly educated and having unrealistic expectations of the child (Hussey, 2011). Agency factors include placement through a public rather than private agency and having a less experienced caseworker (Child Welfare Information Gateway, 2012). Accurate information about the child and the child's history, along with support through the preparation and placement process, help parents gain a realistic understanding of their child and the comfort to make a gradual transition to adoptive family life. It is important to keep in mind, however, that these families often move through stages of adjustment in the postadoption period, especially with children with special needs (Pinderhughes, 1996). In this process, families often have to relinquish fantasies of the adjustment process and make accommodations to a child

who tests limits. In doing so, parents' expectations are unmet, creating ambivalence about the adoption. Clinicians can help parents both to discuss and alter their expectations such that expectations and reality become more closely matched.

Outcomes of intercountry adoption

Intercountry adoptees typically lived in institutions prior to adoption and infrequently experienced foster care. Institutional living poses risks for infectious diseases and neurological problems and is associated with lack of adequate cognitive and social stimulation and individualized attention (van IJzendoorn & Juffer, 2006; Miller, 2012). These children tend to be short, weigh less, and have a small head circumference. Catch-up growth and improved health follow adoption, especially for children adopted by or before their first birthday and from relatively less depriving circumstances (van IJzendoorn *et al.,* 2007; Cohen *et al.,* 2008; Bakermans-Kranenburg *et al.,* 2011) compared to those raised in extremely depriving environments over an extended period (Sonuga-Barke *et al.,* 2008). Moreover, children adopted internationally are at risk for early puberty, often accompanied by shortened final height and more social-emotional problems (Teilmann *et al.,* 2006).

Research has shown that postadoption outcomes depend not only on age but also on the quality of institutional care. Children adopted by 1 year of age typically fare best in terms of language, cognitive and social-emotional development (van IJzendoorn & Juffer, 2006; van Londen *et al.,* 2007; Cohen *et al.,* 2008). However, children adopted from extremely depriving institutions after 6 months of age (e.g., in Romania) exhibited problems in language and cognition at 6, 11, and 15 years of age compared to Romanian children adopted younger than 6 months and children adopted within the United Kingdom (Rutter *et al.,* 2010).

Regarding attachment, infants adopted at a relatively early age (i.e., at or before 1 year) (Stams *et al.,* 2002; Pugliese *et al.,* 2010; Cohen & Farnia, 2011a) or raised in institutions that created conditions for forming a secure attachment (Vorria *et al.,* 2006) do not exhibit attachment difficulties. However, children adopted later, who did not experience sensitive and responsive individualized caregiving, often show signs of insecure or disorganized attachment and sometimes indiscriminate approach to strangers (Rutter *et al.,* 2007).

Intercountry adoptees are consistently overrepresented in mental health services, but the sources of emotional and behavioral disturbance may be different from those shown by domestic adoptees (Juffer & van IJzendoorn 2005), possibly as a consequence of preadoption conditions. A parent survey of internationally adopted children aged 4–18 years showed that early institutional rearing was associated with increased rates of attention and social problems, but not internalizing or externalizing problems (Gunnar *et al.,* 2007). Children adopted from Romania into the United Kingdom after the age of 6 months exhibited a unique constellation of symptoms that persisted into adolescence marked by inattentiveness/overactivity, quasi-autism, and disinhibited attachment, which were qualitatively different from such disorders observed in clinical settings (Kumsta *et al.*, 2011). Parenting stress is one factor related to behavior problems in school-aged internationally adopted children (Gagnon-Oosterwaal *et al.*, 2012).

More subtle behavior traits have been observed in some children adopted relatively early from a less depriving environment. Mothers of infants adopted from China, on average at 1 year of age, consistently rated their daughters as more emotionally reactive than nonadoptive mothers over four time points in their first 2 years postadoption (Cohen & Farnia, 2011b). In older children, Tan (2011) reported that internalizing problems in Chinese adoptees increased from preschool to school years.

Relatively little is known about intercountry adoptees in adulthood. Teilmann *et al.* (2006) found that adult male adoptees were less likely to have intimate relationships, to live with a partner, and to be married but did not differ in educational or professional attainment. In another study, girls adopted from Hong Kong by British parents at approximately 2 years of age were followed into midlife (Feast *et al.*, 2013). These women reported positive outcomes in health, education, occupation, close relationships, and social-emotional functioning.

Selection, preparation, and assessment

Prospective parent(s)' suitability for adoption is based on individual and joint interviews and documentation regarding health and finances and home and neighborhood environment. A history of secure attachment relationships, relationships with one another (for couples) and with extended family, parenting capacity and communicative openness are important parts of the equation. Personal references, including a criminal background check, are also required. In addition, adopting parents are asked about their reasons for pursuing adoption, characteristics of a child they are interested in adopting, and their readiness to adopt (Crea *et al.,* 2007). For families adopting children of a different race or with special needs, attention is paid to flexibility of parent expectations about children who may require additional attention. The adoption process can be especially complex and lengthy for older children who have a history of abuse, parent drug and alcohol use, or rejection by foster parents. Optimally, the process continues after these children join their adoptive family, with periodic visits by an adoption social worker to evaluate and facilitate the progress of family formation (Hanna, 2007). Comprehensive preparation has been related to less frequent use of both general and clinical postadoption services (Wind *et al.* 2007).

Assessment of adopting parents is done by a qualified individual through a publicly funded child welfare system, an international adoption agency, or an independent facilitator such as a lawyer. It is essential to ensure that children will be safe and supports appropriate to their needs provided. Prospective parents also need to know what to expect of the children's behavior and learning abilities (Rushton & Monck, 2009). When available,

adoptive parents need to be informed about genetic or biological factors that may influence children's health and adjustment.

The home study is often accompanied by group meetings with other potential adopters and parents whose adoptions are completed and can provide a realistic view of what to expect. In the case of intercountry adoptions, considerable time is spent talking about the conditions in which children lived, cultural practices that parents may want to continue, and what can be expected of children's health, development, and attachment. In a study of preparedness for intercountry adoption, many families felt minimally prepared for the adoption process and the emotional challenges they might face. Preparation was found to be positively associated with satisfaction with the adoption (Paulsen & Merighi, 2009).

Children also need to be prepared for adoption and encouraged to feel entitled to have permanent parents. Older children are given an age-appropriate explanation of why they will not be living with their birth or foster parents. Creating a life book helps children remember and put the various people and events in their lives into sequence and perspective and understand why their birth parents and/or foster parents could not continue to care for them. It also helps children reframe prior experiences in a realistic, yet positive light. Making children part of this process helps them to explore feelings of loss, anger, and confusion as well as remember positive experiences. For children who do not have such information, as is the case with intercountry adoptees, records of the events on children's birthday and photos of the institution or surrounding environment can be helpful. Adopting parents must understand the importance of this process without prematurely negating children's pasts in order to "move on." Having a life book also may prepare children to engage in classroom activities such as drawing a family tree. Unfortunately, life books are not consistently available (Hanna, 2007).

Postadoption services

Being adopted approximately doubles the chance of having contact with a mental health professional (Keyes *et al.*, 2008; Hussey *et al.*, 2012). This is likely determined by both longstanding effects of preadoption stressors and the tendency of adoptive parents to seek services. Moreover, the need for postadoption clinical services increases over time with changes in children's physical, behavioral, and emotional needs. It is also necessary to keep in mind that parents, particularly mothers who are less emotionally stable prior to adoption, are at risk for postadoption depression in the first year after a child joins the family (Payne *et al.*, 2010; Foli *et al.*, 2012). When this happens, it is important to provide clinical services as quickly as possible.

The increase in children adopted from foster care places expanding demands on postadoption preservation and clinical services for both parents and children. Parents often feel particularly unprepared to manage their child's emotional and behavioral problems (Rushton & Monck, 2009). Issues identified by families as areas of need include stress reduction, forming realistic expectations, attachment, separation, loss and grief, and child and youth identity formation. Moreover, medical and developmental conditions that require referral to specialized clinics may be present.

Given the varying experiences of adopted children, a one-size-fits-all model of intervention is insufficient. Postadoption services include ongoing meetings with the caseworker, participation in adoption support groups, clinical interventions, and crisis intervention (Howe, 2006; Wind et al., 2007; Vostanis, 2010). From a survey of families that adopted children with special needs, financial, medical, and dental supports and subsidies also emerged as postadoption service needs (Reilly & Platz, 2004). There are further needs for in-home supports such as respite care. Receiving financial and social work assistance and involvement in informal support groups are associated with higher parenting satisfaction. There is a particular need for support groups for families adopting transracially to address struggles around racial identity (Evan B. Donaldson Adoption Institute 2010; Adkison-Bradley et al., 2012).

Although many families seek clinical services, they often complain that mental health professionals are not "adoption competent" (Riley, 2009). An ongoing theme is the importance of educators and clinicians receiving specialized training related to the adoption family life cycle and mental health issues associated with adoption including loss and grief, identity, the birth family search process, and attachment (Evan B. Donaldson Adoption Institute 2010; Palacios 2012). In addition, families need information regarding the adoption kinship network, and genetic and other biological risks that contribute to adjustment (Palacios, 2009).

A specific concern is that clinicians view difficulties through a lens of family pathology rather than family development. This is especially important because children's understanding of adoption changes with age. Developmental turning points are most marked in the early school years when children truly understand the meaning of adoption and in adolescence when issues of identity and their reproductive future may cause emotional upset (Brodzinsky, 2011). Thus, it is essential for clinicians not to pathologize what might be part of an expectable adjustment process that includes adoptees' grief and anger, sensitivity to rejection, and fears about being unlovable, especially if they act out in some way. The importance of parents openly discussing adoption-related issues with their children as they emerge and supporting their child who may grieve is critical (Brodzinsky, 2011). In fact, adolescents who perceived greater communication openness reported more trust in their parents, fewer feelings of alienation, and better family functioning (Kohler et al., 2002).

Promoting a positive attachment relationship is an important step in the adoption process. For instance, a book and video-feedback program directed at increasing maternal sensitive responsiveness was found to improve both maternal sensitive responsiveness and infant competence and attachment

(Juffer et al., 1997). When seen again at 7 years of age, these children showed fewer internalizing behavior problems and more resilience than children who had not received the intervention (Stams et al., 2001). Attachment-based interventions used to help children form a relationship with foster parents might also be applied to adoptive families (see Chapters 6 and 58). Unfortunately, some parents use remedies that lack supporting evidence described on Internet sites for treating children with attachment problems.

In a study of older children, Rushton and Dance (2009) compared two manualized 10-week home-based parenting programs with families whose adopted children showed problems in the first 18 months postplacement. One program took a cognitive behavioral approach and the other an educational approach. Adoptive parents reported a significant reduction in negative parenting techniques (e.g., threats, telling off), but no significant differences in child behavior. Similarly, a survey of adoptive parents showed that postadoption services improved understanding of adoption and the adopted child but had less impact on behavior problems or peer and sibling relations (Dhami et al., 2007). These programs are time limited; in reality, there needs to be longer term programming or options for parents to return for service as their needs change over time. Clearly, more controlled studies of postadoption services are required and their outcomes followed longitudinally. Despite the challenges associated with adopting children with special needs, it is important to emphasize that the majority of adoptive parents report good adoption outcomes.

Adoptive families also pursue nonclinical service options. They seek or organize workshops around specialized topics, establish Internet chat groups, and search for websites to provide support and answers to their concerns. For parents who have adopted internationally, supports often are provided by organizations related to adoptions from a particular country (e.g., Families with Children from China). There also are group initiatives for the children themselves. It would be worthwhile to know the outcomes of participation in these various support groups.

Conclusions and future directions

Adoption continues to play a prominent role in the fabric of family life worldwide. Yet the nature of adoption has changed, and so too the topics for research. For instance, there is still a need to follow intercountry adoptees into adolescence and adulthood. Thus, it is important to understand the outcomes of a wide spectrum of early experiences. More research is also needed on the rights and needs of gay and lesbian individuals and couples and to understand the outcomes for transgendered and bisexual individuals who choose to be parents.

There is greater acceptance of openness in adoption. In the past, this applied primarily to adopted children but now is being considered for both younger and older children born from use of ARTs. There is a growing trend for intercountry adoptees to seek their birth families or siblings through the Internet and/or visits to their birth country. These continuing shifts in openness invite future research.

Historically, relinquishing a child for adoption was in the hands of the birth mother. More recently, an ethical dilemma has arisen for some infant adoptions when a birth father's agreement for adoption is not sought. In some jurisdictions, a putative father registry has been established to claim paternal rights. While such cases periodically appear in newspapers, empirical findings are sorely lacking.

Finally, it is essential to continue specialized training and evaluation of efforts to ensure the adoption competence of mental health professionals, teachers, social service workers, physicians, and lawyers. Moreover, there is increasing need for therapists who can work with gay, lesbian, bisexual, and transgendered parents and kinship adoptions. An important future goal is to provide a stronger evidence base for all postadoption services.

References

Adamec, C.A. & Miller, L.C. (2007) *The Encyclopedia of Adoption*. Facts On File, New York.

Adkison-Bradley, C. *et al.* (2012) Postadoption services utilization among African American transracial and White American parents; Counseling and legal implications. *The Family Journal: Counseling and Therapy for Couples and Families* **20**, 392–398.

Adoption Council of Canada (2013) *Government of Canada announces enhanced adoption tax credit*. Available: http://adoption.ca/adoption-news?news_id=130 [5 Apr 2013].

Ausbrooks, A.R. & Russell, A. (2011) Gay and lesbian family building: a strengths perspective of transracial adoption. *Journal of GLBT Family Studies* **7**, 201–216.

Averett, P. *et al.* (2009) An evaluation of gay/lesbian and heterosexual adoption. *Adoption Quarterly* **12**, 129–51.

Bakermans-Kranenburg, M.J. *et al.* (2011) Attachment and emotional development in institutional care: characteristics and catch-up. *Monographs of the Society for Research of Child Development* **76**, 62–91.

Barn, R. & Kirton, D. (2012) Transracial adoption in Britain: politics, ideology and reality. *Adoption and Fostering* **36**, 25–37.

Beeson, D.R. *et al.* (2011) Offspring searching for their sperm donors: how family type shapes the process. *Human Reproduction* **26**, 2415–2424.

Berkowitz, D. (2013) Gay men and surrogacy. In: (eds A.E. Goldberg & K.R. Allen) *LGBT-Parent Families: Innovations in Research And Implications For Practice*, pp. 71–86. Springer, New York, NY.

Blackstock, C. (2003) First Nations child and family services: restoring peace and harmony in First Nations communities. In: *Child Welfare: Connecting Research Policy and Practice*. (eds K. Kufeldt & B. McKenzie), pp. 331–342. Wilfred Laurier University Press, Waterloo, ON.

Brewaeys, A. (2001) Review: parent–child relationships and child development in donor insemination families. *Human Reproduction Update* **7**, 38–46.

Brezina, P.R. & Zhao, Y. (2012) The ethical, legal, and social issues impacted by modern assisted reproductive technologies. *Obstetrics and Gynecology International* **2012**, 686253.

Brodzinsky, D.M. (2011) Children's understanding of adoption: developmental and clinical implications. *Professional Psychology: Research and Practice* **42**, 200–207.

Brooks, D. *et al.* (1999) Adoption and race: implementing the multiethnic placement act and the interethnic adoption provisions. *Social Work* **44**, 167–179.

Buckles, K.S. (2013) Adoption subsidies and placement outcomes for children in foster care. *Journal of Human Resources* **48**, 596–627.

Buckner International (2013) *Ethiopia* [Online]. Available: http://www.buckner.org/locations/africa-ethiopia.shtml [5 Apr 2013].

Calpern, E. (2007) *Assisted reproductive technologies: overview and perspective using a reproductive justice framework. Information and Privacy Commissioner of Ontario* [Online]. Available: http://geneticsandsociety.org/downloads/ART.pdf [5 Apr 2013].

Campbell, L.H. *et al.* (1991) Reunions between adoptees and birth parents: the adoptees' experience. *Social Work* **36**, 329–335.

Cavoukian, A. (2005) *A review of the literature on adoption-related research: the implications for proposed legislation* [Online]. Available: http://www.ipc.on.ca/images/Resources/adoption.pdf [5 Apr 2013].

Child Welfare Information Gateway (2012) *Adoption disruption and dissolution* [Online]. Available: http://www.childwelfare.gov [5 Mar 2013].

Child Welfare Information Gateway (2013) *Openness in adoption building relationships between adoptive and birth families* [Online]. Available: http://adoption.ca/adoption-news? news_id=130 [5 Mar 2013].

Clapton, G. (2003) *Birth Fathers and their Adoption Experiences*. Jessica Kingsley, London.

Cohen, N.J. & Farnia, F. (2011a) Children adopted from China: attachment security two years later. *Child and Youth Services Review* **33**, 2342–2346.

Cohen, N.J. & Farina, F. (2011b) Social-emotional adjustment and attachment in children adopted from China: processes and predictors of change. *International Journal of Behavioral Development* **35**, 67–77.

Cohen, N.J. *et al.* (2008) Children adopted from China: a prospective study of their growth and development. *Journal of Child Psychology and Psychiatry* **49**, 458–468.

Crea, T. *et al.* (2007) Home study methods for evaluating prospective resource families: history and promising approaches. *Child Welfare* **86**, 141–159.

Cuddeback, G.S. (2004) Kinship family foster care: a methodological and substantive synthesis of research. *Children and Youth Services Review* **26**, 623–639.

Curtis, R. & Pearson, F. (2010) Contact with birth parents: differential psychological adjustment for adults adopted as infants. *Journal of Social Work* **10**, 347–367.

Cushing, A.L. (2010) 'I just want more information about who I am': the search experience of sperm-donor offspring, searching for information about their donors and genetic heritage. *Information Research – An International Electronic Journal* **15**, article number 428.

Dalberth, B., Gibbs, D., Berkman, N. (2005). *Understanding Adoption Subsidies: an Analysis of AFCARS Data*. Washington, DC: US Department of Health and Human Services. Office of the Assistant Secretary for Planning and Evaluation.

DeLacey, S. (2005) Parent identity and "virtual" children: why patients discard rather than donate unused embryos. *Human Reproduction* **20**, 1661–1669.

Denby, R.W. (2011) Kinship liaisons: a peer-to-peer approach to supporting kinship caregivers. *Children & Youth Services Review* **33**, 217–225.

Denby, R.W. (2012) Parental incarceration and kinship care: caregiver experiences, child well-being, and permanency intentions. *Social Work in Public Health* **27**, 104–128.

Denby, R.W. *et al.* (2010) The journey to adopt a child who has special needs: parents' perspectives. *Children and Youth Services Review* **33**, 1543–1554.

Dhami, M.K. *et al.* (2007) An evaluation of post-adoption services. *Children and Youth Services Review* **29**, 162–179.

Downing, J. *et al.* (2009) Making the decision: factors influencing gay men's choice of an adoption path. *Adoption Quarterly* **12**, 247–271.

ESHRE (2010) *Focus on Reproduction*. Grimbergen, Belgium: ESHRE.

Ethiopian Herald (2013) Encouraging *local adoption: positive stride for vulnerable children's rights* [Online]. Available: http://www.ethpress .gov.et/herald/index.php/herald/society/290-encouraging-local -adoption-positive-stride-for-vulnerable-children-rights [10 Apr 2013].

Evan B. Donaldson Adoption Institute (2008*) Finding Families for African American Children: the Role of Race and Law in Adoption from Foster Care*. Evan B. Donaldson, NY.

Evan B. Donaldson Adoption Institute (2010) *Keeping the Promise: the Critical Need for Post-adoption Services to Enable Children and Families to Succeed*. Evan B. Donaldson, NY.

Farmer, E. *et al.* (2011) *Achieving Successful Returns From Care: What Makes Reunification Work?* British Association for Adoption and Fostering, London.

Farr, R.H. & Patterson, C.J. (2009) Transracial adoption by lesbian, gay, and heterosexual couples: who completed transracial adoptions, and with what results? *Adoption Quarterly* **12**, 187–204.

Farr, R.H. *et al.* (2010) Parenting and child development in adoptive families: does parental sexual orientation matter? *Developmental Science* **14**, 164–178.

Feast, J. *et al.* (2013) *Adversity, Adoption and Afterwards: A Mid-Life Follow-Up Study of Women Adopted From Hong Kong*. British Association for Adoption and Fostering, London.

Fechter-Leggett, M.O. & O'Brien, K. (2010) The effects of kinship care on adult mental health outcomes of alumni of foster care. *Children and Youth Services Review* **32**, 206–213.

Feeney, J.A. *et al.* (2007) Adoption, attachment, and relationship concerns: a study of adult adoptees. *Personal Relationships* **14**, 129–147.

Foli, K.J. *et al.* (2012) Maternal postadoption depression, unmet expectations, and personality traits. *Journal of the American Psychiatric Nurses Association* **18**, 267–277.

Freeman, T. *et al.* (2009) Gamete donation: parents' experiences of searching for their child's donor siblings and donor. *Human Reproduction* **24**, 505–516.

Gagnon-Oosterwaal, N. *et al.* (2012) Preadoption adversity, maternal stress, and behaviour problems at school-age in international adoptees. *Journal of Applied Developmental Psychology* **33**, 236–242.

Goldberg, A.E. (2007) How does it make a difference? Perspectives of adults with lesbian, gay, and bisexual parents. *American Journal of Orthopsychiatry* **77**, 550–562.

Goldberg, A.E. & Gianino, M. (2011) Lesbian and gay adoptive families: assessment, clinical issues and intervention. In: *Adoption by Lesbians and Gay Men: A New Dimension in Family Diversity*. (eds D. Brodzinsky & A. Pertman), pp. 204–232. Oxford University Press, New York.

Goldberg, A.E. *et al.* (2010) Pre-adoptive factors predicting lesbian, gay, and heterosexual couples relationship quality across the transition to adoptive parenthood. *Journal of Family Psychology* **24**, 221–232.

Goldberg, A.E. *et al.* (2011) Perception and internalization of adoption stigma among gay, lesbian, and heterosexual adoptive parents. *Journal of GLBT Family Studies* **7**, 132–154.

Golombok, S. *et al.* (2013) Children born through reproductive donation: a longitudinal study of child adjustment. *Journal of Child Psychology and Psychiatry* **54**, 653–660.

Griffith, E.E.H. & Bergeron, R.L. (2006) Cultural stereotypes die hard: the case of transracial adoption. *Journal of the American Academy of Psychiatry and the Law* **34**, 303–314. Available: https://www.adoptioncouncil.org/images/stories/documents/439-452_PM0000_CH39.pdf [5 April 2013].

Grotevant, H.D. *et al.* (2011) Post-adoption contact, adoption communicative openness, and satisfaction with contact as predictors of externalizing behavior in adolescence and emerging adulthood. *Journal of Child Psychology and Psychiatry* **52**, 529–536.

Gunnar, M.R. *et al.* (2007) Behavior problems in postinstitutionalized internationally adopted children. *Development and Psychopathology* **19**, 129–148.

Hairston, C.F. (2007) *Focus on Children with Incarcerated Parents: An Overview of Research Literature*. Annie E. Casey Foundation, Baltimore, MD.

Hanna, M.D. (2007) Preparing school age children for adoption: perspectives of successful adoptive parents and caseworkers. *Adoption Quarterly* **10**, 1–32.

Henry, M.J. & Pollack, D. (2009) *Adoption in the United States: A Reference for Families, Professionals, and Students*. Lyceum Books, Chicago.

Howard, J. & Smith, S.L. (2003) *After Adoption: The Needs of Adopted Youth*. Child Welfare League of America, Washington, DC.

Howe, D. (2006) Developmental attachment psychotherapy with fostered and adopted children. *Child and Adolescent Mental Health* **11**, 128–134.

Howe, D. & Feast, J. (2000) *Adoption, Search & Reunion*. The Children's Society, London.

Howe, D. & Feast, J. (2001) The long term outcome of reunions between adult adopted people and their birth mothers. *British Journal of Social Work* **31**, 351–368.

Human Fertilisation and Embryology Authority (2009) *Code of Practice*, 8th edn. Available: http://www.hfea.gov.uk/docs/Code_of_Practice_8_-_October_2013.PDF.

Hunt, J. *et al.* (2008) *Keeping Them in the Family: Outcomes for Children Placed in Kinship Care Through Care Proceedings*. British Association for Adoption and Fostering, London.

Hussey, D.L. (2011) An in-depth analysis of domestically adopted children with special needs and their biological mothers. *Journal of Social Work* **12**, 528–544.

Hussey, D. *et al.* (2012) Risk factors for mental health diagnoses among children adopted from the public child welfare system. *Children and Youth Services Review* **34**, 2072–2080.

Jadva, V. *et al.* (2009) The experiences of adolescents and adults conceived by sperm donation: comparisons by age of disclosure and family type. *Human Reproduction* **24**, 1909–1919.

Jauniaux, E.R.M. (2012) Multiple gestation pregnancy after assisted reproductive technology. In: *Pregnancy After Assisted Reproductive Technology*. (eds Eric R.M. Jauniaux & Botros R.M.B. Rizk). Cambridge University Press.

Johnston, K.E. *et al.* (2007) Mothers' racial, ethnic, and cultural socialization of transracially adopted Asian children. *Family Relations* **56**, 390–402.

Juffer, F. & van IJzendoorn, M.H. (2005) Behavior problems and mental health referrals of international adoptees: a meta-analysis. *JAMA* **293**, 2501–2515.

Juffer, F. *et al.* (1997) Early intervention in adoptive families: supporting maternal sensitive responsiveness, infant-mother attachment and infant competence. *Journal of Child Psychology and Psychiatry* **38**, 1039–1050.

Kelley, S. *et al.* (2011) Behavior problems in children raised by grandmothers: the role of caregiver distress, family resources, and the home environment. *Children & Youth Services Review* **33**, 2138–2145.

Kelly, R. (2005) Reflection on adoption reunion-factors which contribute to satisfactory or unsatisfactory outcomes in post reunion relationships for natural mothers. In: *Motherhood Silenced – The Experiences of Natural Mothers on Adoption Reunion.* Liffey Press, Dublin.

Keyes, M.A. *et al.* (2008) The mental health of US adolescents adopted in infancy. *Archives of Pediatric and Adolescent Medicine* **162**, 419–425.

Kohler, J.K. *et al.* (2002) Adopted adolescents' preoccupation with adoption: the impact on adoptive family relationships. *Journal of Marriage and Family* **64**, 93–104.

von Korff, L. *et al.* (2006) Openness arrangements and psychological adjustment in adolescent adoptees. *Journal of Family Psychology* **20**, 531–534.

Kumsta, R. *et al.* (2011) Deprivation-specific psychological patterns: effects of institutional deprivation. *Monographs of the Society for Research in Child Development* **75**, 48–78.

Lee, R.M. (2003) The transracial adoption paradox: history, research, and counseling implications of cultural socialization. *Counseling Psychologist* **31**, 711–744.

Lee, B.J. (2007) Recent trends in child welfare and adoption in Korea: challenges and future directions. In: *International Korean Adoption: A Fifty-year History of Policy and Practice.* (eds K.J.S. Bergquist, *et al.*), pp. 189–206. The Haworth Press, New York.

Lee, R.M. & the Minnesota International Adoption Project Team (2010) Parental perceived discrimination as a post adoption risk factor for internationally adopted children and adolescents. *Cultural Diversity and Ethnic Minority Psychology* **16**, 493–500.

Lev, A.I. & Sennott, S. (2013) Clinical work with LGBT parents and prospective parents. In: *LGBT-Parent Families: Possibilities for New Research and Implications for Practice.* (eds A.E. Goldberg & K.R. Allen). Springer Press, NY.

Lifton, B.J. (1994) *Journal of the Adopted Self: A Quest for Wholeness.* Basic, New York.

Lindblad, F. *et al.* (2003) Intercountry adopted children as young adults: a Swedish cohort study. *American Journal of Orthopsychiatry* **73**, 190–202.

Lindh, H.L. *et al.* (2007) Characteristics and perspectives of families waiting to adopt a child with Down syndrome. *Genetics in Medicine* **9**, 235–240.

van Londen, M. *et al.* (2007) Attachment, cognitive and motor development in adopted children: short-term outcomes after international adoption. *Journal of Pediatric Psychology* **32**, 1249–1258.

MacCallum, F. & Golombok, S. (2004) Children raised in fatherless families from infancy: a follow-up of children of lesbian and single heterosexual mothers at early adolescence. *Journal of Child Psychology and Psychiatry* **45**, 1407–1419.

MacDonald, M. & McSherry, D. (2013) Constrained adoptive parenthood and family transition: adopters' experience of unplanned birth family contact in adolescence. *Child & Family Social Work* **18**, 87–96.

Mallon, G.P. (2011) Lesbian and gay prospective foster and adoptive families. In: *Adoption by Lesbians and Gay Men: A New Dimension in Family Diversity.* (eds D.B. Brodzinsky & A. Pertman), pp. 130–149. Oxford University Press, New York.

Marquardt, E. *et al.* (2010) *My Daddy's Name is Donor: A New Study of Young Adults Conceived Through Sperm Donation*, pp. 1–135. Institute for American Values, New York.

Matthews, J.D. & Cramer, E.P. (2006) Envisaging the adoption process to strengthen gay- and lesbian-headed families' recommendations for adoption professionals. *Child Welfare* **85**, 317–330.

McCall, R.B. (2011) Research, practice, and policy perspectives on issues of children without permanent parental care. In: *Children Without Permanent Parents: Research, Practice, and Policy* vol. **76**. (eds R.B. McCall, *et al.*), pp. 223–272. *Monographs of the Society for Research in Child Development.*

McMahon, C.A. & Saunders, D.M. (2009) Attitudes of couples with stored frozen embryos toward conditional embryo donation. *Fertility and Sterility* **91**, 140–147.

Mellish, L. *et al.* (2013) *Gay, Lesbian and Heterosexual Adoptive Families: Family Relationships, Child Adjustment and Adopters' Experiences.* British Association for Adoption and Fostering, London, UK.

Miller, L. (2012) Medical status of internationally adopted children. In: *Intercountry Adoption: Policies, Practices, and Outcomes.* (eds J.L. Gibbons & K.S. Rotabi), pp. 187–198. Ashgate Publishing Ltd, Farnham, UK.

Ministry of Health & Welfare (2008, 2011) *Yearly Statistical Report.* Seoul, Korea: Ministry of Health & Welfare.

Moe, B.A. (2007) *Adoption: A Reference Handbook*, 2nd edn. ABC-CLIO, Santa Barbara, CA.

Mohanty, J. *et al.* (2007) Family cultural socialization, ethnic identity, and self-esteem: web-based survey of international adult adoptees. *Journal of Ethnic & Cultural Diversity in Social Work* **15**, 153–172.

Munro, E.R. & Manful, E. (2012) *Safeguarding Children: A Comparison of England's Data with that of Australia, Norway and the United States.* (Research Report DFE-RR198). London: DFE [Online]. Available: https://www.education.gov.uk/publications/eOrderingDownload /DFE-RR198.pdf [5 Apr 2013].

National Council for Adoption (2012) *Adoption tax credit advocacy kit* [Online]. Available: www.adoptioncouncil.org [15 Apr 2013].

Nedelcu, C. & Groza, V. (2012) Child welfare in Romania. In: *Intercountry Adoption: Policies, Practices, and Outcomes.* (eds J. Gibbons & K. Rotabi). Ashgate Press, Surrey, UK.

Neil, E. (2003) Understanding other people's perspectives: tasks for adopters in open adoptions. *Adoption Quarterly* **6**, 3–30.

Novac S. *et al.* (2006*) A Visceral Grief: Young Homeless Mothers and Loss of Child Custody.* Centre for Urban and Community Studies, Research Bulletin, 34 [Online]. Available: http://www.urbancentre.utoronto .ca/pdfs/researchbulletins/CUCSRB34Novacetal.pdf [12 Apr 2013].

Palacios, J. (2009) The ecology of adoption. In: *International Advances in Adoption Research for Practice.* (eds G.M. Wrobel & E. Neil), pp. 71–94. Wiley-Blackwell, Chichester.

Palacios, J. (2012) Understanding and preventing intercountry adoption breakdown. In: *Intercountry Adoption: Policies, Practices, and Outcomes.* (eds J. Gibbons & K. Rotabi), pp. 273–282. Ashgate Publishing, Farnham, Surrey.

Passmore, N.L. & Chipuer, H.M. (2009) Female adoptees' perceptions of reunions with their birth fathers: factors that facilitate and hinder a successful reunion. *American Journal of Orthopsychiatry* **79**, 93–102.

Patterson, C.L. & Wainright, L. (2011) *Adolescents with same sex parents.* Findings from the National Longitudinal Study of Adolescent Health.

Paul, S. & Berger, R. (2007) Topic avoidance and family functioning in families conceived with donor insemination. *Human Reproduction* **22**, 2566–2571.

Paulsen, C. & Merighi, J.R. (2009) Adoption preparedness, cultural engagement and parental satisfaction in intercountry adoption. *Adoption Quarterly* **12**, 1–18.

Payne, J.L. *et al.* (2010) Post adoption depression. *Archives of Women's Mental Health* **13**, 147–151.

Petta, G.A. & Steed, L.G. (2005) The experience of adoptive parents in adoption reunion relationships: a qualitative study. *American Journal of Orthopsychiatry* **75**, 230–241.

Pinderhughes, E.E. (1996) Toward understanding family readjustment following older child adoption: the interplay between theory generation and empirical research. *Child and Youth Services Review* **18**, 115–138.

Pugliese, M. *et al.* (2010) The emerging attachment relationship between adopted Chinese infants and their mothers. *Child and Youth Services Review* **32**, 1719–1728.

Reilly, T. & Platz, L. (2004) Post-adoption service need of families with special needs children: use, helpfulness, and unmet needs. *Journal of Social Service Research* **30**, 51–67.

Riley, D. (2009) Training mental health professionals to be adoption competent. *Policy & Practice* **67**, 33.

Rubin, D.M. *et al.* (2008) The impact of kinship care on behavioral well-being for children in out-of-home care. *Archives of Pediatric and Adolescent Medicine* **162**, 550–556.

Rushton, A. & Dance, C. (2006) The adoption of children from public care: a prospective study of outcome in adolescence. *Journal of the American Academy of Child and Adolescent Psychiatry* **45**, 877–883.

Rushton, A. & Dance, C. (2009) *Adoption Support Services for Families in Difficulty.* British Association for Adoption and Fostering, London.

Rushton, A. & Monck, E. (2009) *Enhancing Positive Parenting.* British Association for Adoption and Fostering, London.

Rutter, M. *et al.* (2007) Early adolescent outcomes for institutionally deprived and non-deprived adoptees. I. Disinhibited attachment. *Journal of Child Psychology and Psychiatry* **48**, 17–30.

Rutter, M. *et al.* (2010) Deprivation-specific psychological patterns: effects of institutional deprivation. *Monographs of the Society for Research in Child Development* **75**, 212–229.

Selman, P. (2009) The rise and fall of intercountry adoption in the 21st century. *International Social Work* **52**, 575–594.

Shang, X. (2008) *A Study of the Condition of Orphans in China.* Shehui Kexue Wenxian Chubanshe, Beijing, China.

Shang, X. (2011) *Child Welfare in China: Stocking taking Report 2011,* (No. ARC—2011001—CW) [Online]. Available: http://www.bnu1.org/uploads/soft/1_11601085027.pdf [4 April 2013], p. 65. Beijing, China.

Shanner, L. (2003) Legal challenges to donor anonymity. *Health Law Review* **11**, 25–28.

Siegel, D.H. & Smith, S.L. (2012) *Openness in Adoption: From Secrecy and Stigma to Knowledge and Connections.* Evan B. Donaldson Adoption Institute, NY. Available: http://adoptioninstitute.org/research/2012_03_openness.php [4 Apr 2013].

Silverman, P.R. *et al.* (1994) Reunions between adoptees and birth parents: the adoptive parents' view. *Clinical Social Work Journal* **39**, 542–549.

Simon, R. (1996) Transracial adoptions: experiences of twenty-year study. *American Sociologist* **27**, 79–89.

Sonuga-Barke, E. *et al.* (2008) Is subnutrition necessary for a poor outcome following early institutional deprivation? *Developmental Medicine and Child Neurology* **50**, 664–671.

Stams, G.J. *et al.* (2001) Attachment based intervention in adoptive families in infancy and children's development at age 7: two follow-up studies. *British Journal of Developmental Psychology* **19**, 159–180.

Stams, G.-J.M. *et al.* (2002) Maternal sensitivity, infant attachment, and temperament in early childhood predict adjustment in middle childhood: the case of adopted children and their biologically unrelated parents. *Developmental Psychology* **38**, 806–821.

Tan, T.X. (2011) Two-year follow-up of girls adopted from China: continuity and change in behavioural adjustment. *Child and Adolescent Mental Health* **16**, 14–21.

Teilmann, G. *et al.* (2006) Increased risk of precocious puberty in internationally adopted children in Denmark. *Pediatrics* **118**, 391–399.

The Hague Convention for Protection of Children and Cooperating in Respect of Intercountry Adoption (2006) *Report of the Special Commission to Review the Practical Operation of the 1993 Hague Convention.* HDDH, The Hague. Available: http://www.hcch.net/upload/wop/adop2005_rep-e.pdf [3 Mar 2013].

The Moscow Times (2013) *Russians not lining up to adopt Americans* [Online]. Available: http://www.themoscowtimes.com/news/article/russians-not-lining-up-to-adopt-americans/474821.html [2 Mar 2013].

Tieman, W. *et al.* (2008) Young adult international adoptees' search for birth parents. *Journal of Family Psychology* **22**, 678–687.

Trinder, L. *et al.* (2004) *The Adoption Reunion Handbook.* John Wiley & Sons, Chichester.

Triseliotis, J. (2003) Long-term foster care or adoption? In: *Studies in the Assessment of Parenting.* (eds P. Reder, S. Duncan, & C. Lucey). Brunner-Routledge, New York.

United Nations Publications (2009). *Child Adoption: Trends and Policies.* United Nations, New York.

US Department of Health and Human Services (2011) *The AFCARS report: Preliminary FY 2011 estimates as of July 2012 (19).* Available: http://www.acf.hhs.gov/sites/default/files/main/afcarsreport19.pdf [24 Apr 2013].

van IJzendoorn, M.H. & Juffer, F. (2005) Adoption is a successful natural intervention enhancing adopted children's school performance. *Current Directions in Psychological Science* **14**, 326–330.

van IJzendoorn, M.H. & Juffer, F. (2006) The Emanuel Miller Memorial Lecture 2006: adoption as intervention. Meta-analytic evidence for massive catch-up and plasticity in physical, socio-emotional and cognitive development. *Journal of Child Psychology and Psychiatry* **47**, 1228–1245.

van IJzendoorn, M.H. *et al.* (2007) Plasticity of growth in height, weight, and head circumference: meta-analytic evidence of massive catch-up after international adoption. *Journal of Developmental and Behavioral Pediatrics* **28**, 334–343.

Vandivere, S. *et al.* (2009) *Adoption USA: a chartbook based on the 2007 National Survey of Adoptive Parents* [Online]. Available: http://aspe.hhs.gov/hsp/09/NSAP/ [3 Apr 2013].

Vorria, P. *et al.* (2006) The development of adopted children after institutional care: a follow-up study. *Journal of Child Psychology and Psychiatry* **47**, 1246–1253.

Vostanis, P. (2010) Mental health services for children in public care and other vulnerable groups: implications for international collaboration. *Clinical Child Psychology and Psychiatry* **15**, 555–571.

Wade, J. *et al.* (2011) *Caring for Abused and Neglected Children: Making the Right Decisions for Reunification or Long-Term Care.* Jessica Kingsley Publishers, London.

Wallbank, J. (2004) *The* role of rights and utility in instituting a child's right to know her genetic history. *Social and Legal Studies* **13**, 245–264.

Wen, S.W. *et al.* (2004) Maternal morbidity and obstetric complications in triplet pregnancies and quadruplet and higher-order multiple pregnancies. *American Journal of Obstetrics and Gynecology* **191**, 254–258.

Wind, L.H. *et al.* (2007) Influences of risk history and adoption preparation on post-adoption services use in US adoptions. *Family Relations* **56**, 378–389.

Winokur, M. *et al.* (2009) Kinship care for the safety, permanency, and well-being of children removed from the home for maltreatment. *Campbell Systematic Reviews* **1**, CD006546.

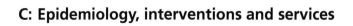

C: Epidemiology, interventions and services

PART I

Conceptual issues and research approaches

CHAPTER 23

Biology of environmental effects

Michael Rutter and Camilla Azis-Clauson

Institute of Psychiatry, Psychology and Neuroscience, King's College London, UK

Introduction

Throughout the previous five editions of this book, there was much discussion about the importance of experiences in the liability to different forms of psychopathology. However, this edition marks a substantial change in the way that the issues are considered. There is a chapter on the effects of psychosocial stressors and chronic adversities (see Chapter 26) and a separate chapter on resilience (see Chapter 27) in relation to those adversities. Here, however, the focus is exclusively on the biology of environmental effects. This has meant that the range of experiences being considered has widened considerably. Thus, experiences include the effects of treatment and the role of physical hazards of various kinds, as well as psychosocial influences. There is also an extension in the time periods covered, particularly the inclusion of the prenatal developmental period (see Chapter 9), and an extension into adult life. Finally, there is a focus on seeking to provide an understanding of causal pathways and mediating mechanisms. These include the role of epigenetics (concerning the processes involved in gene expression; see Chapter 25) on the hypothalamic-pituitary-adrenal (HPA) axis, and on inflammation, as well as attention to the effects of the dose and timing of experiences. There has been a substantial increase in the knowledge base on all of these, although we emphasize that much remains to be learned. Tottenham and Sheridan (2010) have argued for the importance of considering developmental timing when studying the biology of environmental effects. They noted the value of animal models (see Chapter 12) but also emphasized the need for prospective human studies with multiple data points. Nevertheless, what has been learned has enabled a considerable sharpening of the questions that have to be considered in relation to environmental effects on biology (Rutter, 2012a). We start the chapter by considering prenatal effects and then move on to a range of postnatal experiences.

Prenatal experiences

Maternal drinking of alcohol during pregnancy

In 1973, Jones *et al.* (1973) reported an unusual syndrome of malformations in the offspring of chronic alcoholic mothers. A distinctive set of facial features was evident and it was argued that these reflected damage to the developing brain brought about by exposure of a fetus to high alcohol levels in early pregnancy. Numerous reports in humans confirmed the observation and indicated that this was accompanied by abnormalities in behavioral development (Gray & Henderson, 2006). The causal inference was made more likely by the specific link with the first trimester of pregnancy (Day *et al.,* 1989). It was supported by studies in mice showing that the embryos developed craniofacial malformations closely resembling those seen in the human fetal alcohol syndrome (Sulik *et al.,* 1981). Later mouse studies went on to show strain differences in vulnerability to alcohol (Becker *et al.,* 1996) and reprogramming of genetic networks (Green *et al.,* 2007).

Studies of children exposed *in utero* to alcohol, but adopted or fostered in early infancy, have helped indicate the reality of the prenatal effects—because, despite rearing away, they still showed sequelae (Moe, 2002; Singer *et al.,* 2004). Human studies (Gray & Henderson, 2006) have shown that alcohol exposure in early pregnancy can lead to adverse developmental or psychopathological effects even when the characteristic congenital stigmata were absent. But uncertainty on how to diagnose these more subtle fetal alcohol effects remained. In addition, it was not clear whether the damage mainly reflected very high, but episodic, alcohol exposure (such as brought about through binge drinking), or whether it reflected an overall total "dosage" of alcohol exposure during the key time period. Uncertainty similarly remained on the extent to which the effects extended throughout later periods of the pregnancy and on whether even

Rutter's Child and Adolescent Psychiatry, Sixth Edition.
Edited by Anita Thapar and Daniel S. Pine, James F. Leckman, Stephen Scott, Margaret J. Snowling, Eric Taylor.
© 2015 John Wiley & Sons Ltd. Published 2018 by John Wiley & Sons Ltd.

low levels of alcohol exposure in early pregnancy can bring about adverse effects of brain development.

Two recent findings are potentially informative regarding fetal alcohol effects on brain development. First, there is the tentative evidence on neural associations. Yang *et al.* (2012) reported that abnormal cortical thickness was associated with disrupted brain development in a clinical study, with the suggestion that cortical thickness might serve as a biomarker for an abnormality in brain development. Somewhat similarly, Lebel *et al.* (2012), in a two-year follow-up study of alcohol-exposed and nonexposed individuals (the former being recruited from a teratology clinic and the latter being volunteers), found that the cortical volume trajectories differed between the two groups. However, as the authors noted, whether this difference reflected very heavy alcohol exposure or other more prolonged dysfunctional experiences during childhood and adolescence was uncertain.

The second finding reported by Lewis *et al.* (2012) was based on using a Mendelian randomization design with the Avon Longitudinal Study (ALSPAC) sample, finding that low to moderate amounts of alcohol exposure during the pregnancy had effects on IQ. It is unknown whether these were a function of effects on the brain. As indicated, there are still important questions to be considered in relation to alcohol exposure in the pregnancy, but what is clear is that there are teratogenic effects from alcohol exposure during the first trimester, with queries as to whether there are any effects later in pregnancy.

Exposure to mother's smoking during pregnancy

Smoking exposure during pregnancy has been shown by animal models to have effects on birth weight (Office of the US Surgeon General, 2006). Human studies, too, are informative on whether the effects are specific to a particular trimester of pregnancy. Lieberman *et al.* (1994) in a study of a cohort of some 11,000 women found that exposure to smoking during the second and third trimesters only, was associated with a doubling of the frequency of small by gestational age births. By contrast, smoking in the first trimester only, or first and second trimester only, gave rise to a frequency that did not differ from that found with nonsmokers. Bernstein *et al.* (2005) confirmed the substantial effect of smoking in the third trimester in leading to a reduction in birth weight but there was no comparison with earlier trimesters. Ordinarily, the effects of stopping smoking during the pregnancy ought to be helpful in inferring causation but interpretation is complicated by the substantial differences between mothers who give up smoking and those who do not (Nordström & Cnattingius, 1994; England *et al.*, 2001).

What is striking in the comparison between the effects of exposure to maternal drinking and exposure to maternal smoking is that, although there are effects on the fetus in both cases, the pattern is quite different. Smoking is not associated with the congenital anomalies found with fetal alcohol exposure and the timing is quite different. Alcohol effects are greatest in the first

trimester and smoking effects are greatest in the last trimester. Suter *et al.* (2013) discussed whether the reduced fetal growth following smoking exposure was a consequence of the genetic changes, but this is a possibility that has still to be systematically investigated.

One of the very few studies to examine the effects of maternal smoking on fetal growth during the pregnancy was undertaken by Jaddoe *et al.* (2007) using the prospective Generation R Study in the Netherlands, with a sample size of some 7000. Fetal ultrasound examinations were undertaken in early, mid, and late pregnancy. The findings showed that the babies of mothers who smoked until they discovered they were pregnant, but then gave up smoking, showed no difference in head circumference growth from the babies of nonsmokers. By contrast, mothers who continued smoking after the pregnancy was known had babies that showed a significant impairment in head growth, as well as impairment in other growth indices, such as abdominal circumference and femur length. These differences still held after adjusting for a range of confounders.

Although findings from natural experiments indicate that exposure to maternal smoking during the pregnancy does not show a significant association with behavioral outcomes, the same evidence also indicates that there is a robust effect in lowering the birth weight (a finding confirmed from animal models). Recent work suggests that the mechanism may lie in epigenetic mechanisms (Knopik *et al.*, 2012; see Chapter 25).

Haghighi *et al.* (2013) used magnetic resonance imaging (MRI) of the brain to compare adolescents who had and who had not been exposed prenatally to their mother's smoking. Those exposed had a slightly smaller amygdala volume. The findings were interpreted as broadly in line with studies in adolescent rats (Kane *et al.*, 2004; Slotkin 2004; Chen *et al.*, 2005).

Prenatal exposure to cocaine

The consequences on the fetal brain of gestational cocaine exposure are much less well documented and understood. One of the practical problems has been the fact that most use of drugs of abuse involves several drugs and isolating the effects of just one (in this case cocaine) is tricky. Nevertheless, such limited evidence as there is suggests that, in some cases, there can be effects on brain structures (Derauf *et al.*, 2009). Their review concluded that clinical evidence suggested that cocaine independently contributed to impairment in brain growth that was prenatal in origin and exhibited an inverse dose–response relationship. Nevertheless, this selective impairment of brain growth occurred in only a subset of infants. Part of this was mediated through an indirect effect of poor maternal nutrition as well as a direct effect of cocaine. Zuckerman *et al.* (1989) concluded that the resulting deficits from cocaine were more subtle than those with alcohol. Their prospective study of infants followed from pregnancy onward concluded that the use of marijuana or cocaine during pregnancy is associated with impaired fetal growth and that measuring a biological marker of such use is important to demonstrate the association (Zuckerman *et al.*, 1989).

Dow-Edwards (2011) has provided a useful review of how to evaluate animal models studying the effects of prenatal cocaine when applied to the human situation. It is noted that translation from preclinical studies is influenced by the dose of the drug administered, the timing of events in brain development in the animal compared to the human, and the pharmacokinetics of the drug in animals and humans. The review concluded that there is ample evidence for the biological effects of cocaine on cortical and mesolimbic dopamine system development, but the manipulation of the rearing environment can dramatically alter the manifestations of these effects, including function of the mesolimbic dopamine reward system.

Prenatal exposure to depression/anxiety and antidepressant medication

Rather little is known about the facts of prenatal exposure to antidepressants taken by the mother but such evidence as there is suggests that the risks are low. From a practical point of view, clinicians have to balance such risks as there may be from the medication against the risks associated with maternal anxiety or depression. Peña *et al.* (2012) summarized the literature showing that, in humans, the experience of stress during pregnancy is associated with an increase in preterm birth, reduced birth weight, and smaller head circumference. The long-term consequences for offspring have been demonstrated in laboratory studies using rodents. Stress-induced elevations in maternal glucocorticoids have emerged as a primary mechanism of prenatal stress effects, supported by studies in rats in which the effects have been prevented among adrenalectomized females. Peña *et al.* (2012) conducted a study in rats in which restraint stress was brought about by placement in a small cage that prevented vertical and horizontal movement for 1 hour per day from gestational days 14 to 20. The findings showed significant effects on the placenta and the details suggested epigenetic regulation as a likely mediator of effects on the offspring. Lupien *et al.* (2007) in their systematic review, noted that glucocorticoids could cross the blood–brain barrier and that this was likely to be a key feature in effects on the brain of the offspring.

Maternal depression and antidepressants compared

The question of whether maternal antidepressant treatment during pregnancy is better or worse for the offspring than untreated maternal depression constitutes a key question for clinical practice (Steiner, 2012). However, the question should not assume that there is a prenatal effect of either, because depression during pregnancy is a significant risk factor for post-partum depression (Nulman *et al.*, 2012). Nevertheless, animal models suggest that there may well be neurodevelopmental

effects of prenatal antidepressant exposure (Ansorge *et al.*, 2004; Oberlander *et al.*, 2009).

Animal studies have shown the fetal programming of the hypothalamic/pituitary adrenal (HPA) axis function and behavior by synthetic glucocorticoids. It appears that the changes in HPA axis function persist throughout life, indicating some kind of programming effect (Davis *et al.*, 2011). Because the findings go across multiple animal species, and because they derive from randomized experiments, there is every reason to infer a causal effect. In humans, maternal cortisol, as measured through gestation, is associated with a larger right amygdala volume in girls but not in boys. It remains unclear why there is such a definite sex difference but sex differences have been found in many functions (Buss *et al.*, 2012). The findings indicate that there are neural effects of maternal stress hormone levels and not just programming effects on the HPA axis (Sandman *et al.*, 2012).

There are now a number of studies making systematic comparisons between prenatal exposure to maternal stress or depression and prenatal exposure to antidepressants (Nulman *et al.*, 2002; Pedersen *et al.*, 2013). An important study by Weikum *et al.* (2012) similarly focused on the comparison between antidepressants and depression that had not been treated by medication, but differed in using infant speech perception as the outcome measure. The findings suggested that serotonin reuptake inhibitors (SRIs) were associated with an accelerated timing of perceptual attunement. By contrast, maternal depression had the opposite effect in delaying speech perception differences. The findings are important in their reminder that it is not sufficient to compare the same effects of maternal depression and maternal use of antidepressant medication but also to consider that the two may differ in their pattern of effects.

In their useful review, Hanley and Oberlander (2012) summarized three main themes. First, prenatal antidepressant exposure alters central 5HTT levels but the developmental outcomes do not necessarily reflect a main effect due to one causal factor, such as maternal mood, genetics or the drug. Rather, outcomes represent an interplay among psychological, pharmacological, genetic, and social factors relating to the mother and her child. Second, although medication is prescribed during pregnancy with the expectation of optimizing infant health outcomes following associated improved maternal mood, children may continue to be at risk because the treatment may not buffer or protect them from postnatal maternal mood disturbances. Third, there is a context of developmental vulnerability as well as plasticity.

Two further studies complicate the picture. First, Simpson *et al.* (2011) in a study of drug-exposed rat pups found that perinatal drug exposure seemed to affect males more than females and that drug exposure was accompanied by a reduction in callosal connectivity. Both the sex difference and the effects on neural function are different from what is found in humans but the reasons for this remain unclear. Second, Croen *et al.* (2011) reported a human study based on healthcare records, with a finding that prenatal exposure to antidepressant medication was associated with an approximate doubling of the risk of an autism spectrum disorder in the offspring. The authors point out that the causal inference could have been due to uncontrolled confounding by variables that were not measured and that it was also the case that the fraction of cases of autism spectrum disorder attributable to antidepressants was very low—less than 3%. Further research is obviously indicated but findings do not, as yet, warrant public health action.

Lastly, it is important to note that the rate of maternal depression tends to be increased in the context of poverty and disadvantage. The effects must be considered bearing that in mind.

We conclude that, on the evidence available so far, the risks to the fetus associated with maternal depression outweigh possible risks associated with antidepressant medication. Inevitably, in view of the limited direct evidence, that must be a provisional conclusion but we agree with the various commentators who have all argued that it remains important to treat maternal depression without undue concern for the unknown risks of antidepressant medication. On the other hand, this may be a circumstance in which the use of psychological treatments has much to recommend it.

Prenatal effects of subnutrition/famine

The problem of studying the effect of subnutrition/famine is that, in ordinary circumstances, it is very difficult to separate the effects of the famine from the effects of the characteristics that led to the particular individuals being subnourished. The way around this problem has been to study the effects of famine that applied to the total population. The Dutch famine during the winter of 1944–1945 provided the natural experiment (Stein *et al.*, 1975). Unlike other famines, the Dutch hunger winter struck at a precisely circumscribed time and place and in a society able to document the timing and severity of the nutritional deprivation as well as its effects on fertility and health (Susser *et al.*, 1998). A follow-up of military inductees showed an increased rate of congenital anomalies of the nervous system. This provided a possible neurodevelopmental basis for the finding that prenatal famine was associated with a doubling of the risk for schizophrenia (Susser *et al.*, 1996). More recent work carried the science further forward through a comparison of epigenetic findings for individuals prenatally exposed to famine and their unexposed same-sex siblings (Heijmans *et al.*, 2008; Tobi *et al.*, 2009; Tobi *et al.*, 2012). The findings showed a lower level of methylation (a chemical change associated with epigenetics) of the locus for the insulin-like growth factor II. This effect was seen only in those exposed to famine early in pregnancy and was not found for those exposed later in the pregnancy. Interestingly, the differences were found only in males. Animal models using mice have shown broadly comparable effects (Bale *et al.*, 2010; Monk *et al.*, 2013). Monk *et al.* (2013) have pointed out that the effects of maternal prenatal distress and poor nutrition have much in common and there is a lack of studies making a systematic comparison of these two risks.

Prenatal exposure to testosterone

The effects of testosterone on neurobehavioral development were first systematically studied by Phoenix *et al.* (1959) in an experimental study of the administration of testosterone to pregnant guinea pigs. Since then there have been a host of studies in a range of animal species (Hines 2004; Arnold 2009). The findings have shown an effect on the sexually dimorphic nucleus of the pre optic area and the inference has been that the hormone has an organizational effect on the brain, with consequent implications for behavior. There have been far fewer human studies of the effects of testosterone on the brain, although there are a number that deal with effects on gender-typical behavior. The main lack in the human research is a systematic examination of the link between neural sex differences and behavior sex differences. Hines (2011) concluded that the prenatal hormone environment contributed to both neural changes and behavioral changes but the effects were smaller than those found in the animal models. There are few demonstrated effects of female sex hormones on either the brain or behavior. A novel study of prenatal testosterone levels was provided by Vuoksimaa *et al.* (2010) through a comparison of left-handedness among females with male co-twins. The results do not deal directly with effects on the brain but they were suggestive of the effects of prenatal testosterone transfer.

Lombardo *et al.* (2012) studied the effects of fetal testosterone measured from amniotic fluid samples collected between 13 and 20 weeks of gestation in relation to MRI findings at the age of about 10 years. Higher levels of fetal testosterone were associated with local gray matter volume differences in brain regions congruent with sexual dimorphism. The findings were interpreted as suggestive of programming effect in humans but it should be noted that the study was done only in males and also other research (Moore, 2012) has shown weak associations between maternal testosterone and testosterone in the amniotic fluid.

Biological effects of prenatal stress

One study of infants exposed to higher levels of maternal plasma cortisol in the second and third trimesters had themselves a larger cortisol response to a heel-stick procedure (Davis *et al.*, 2011). Buss *et al.* (2010), in a prospective study, found that children exposed to maternal prenatal anxiety in the second trimester had a reduced gray matter volume in several areas involved with learning and memory. In another study, Buss *et al.* (2012) found that higher maternal cortisol levels in early pregnancy were associated with a larger right amygdala volume in girls but not in boys. Furthermore, higher maternal cortisol levels in early pregnancy were associated with more affective problems in girls that was partially mediated by amygdala volume. However, as Monk *et al.* (2012) pointed out, none of the available studies examined prenatal effects in the context of assessment of postnatal environment. In view of the continuities over time, that is a rather crucial omission. The effects of exposure to maternal distress during fetal development is highly correlated with continued exposure during postnatal development and that raises the question as to how far changes in mother–child interaction postpartum play a role in the apparent effects of prenatal stress. Monk *et al.* (2012) suggested that, in keeping with animal models, the genetic effects may have important consequences.

In a rather different approach, Stevens *et al.* (2013) used a well-established animal model of prenatal stress (plexiglass restraint), and found that prenatal stress led to early disruption in GABAergic progenitor migration. Mychasiuk *et al.* (2011) studied the effects of prenatal stress in rats in order to examine possible variation in effects according to the severity of the stress. Mild prenatal stress increased global DNA methylation levels in the cortex and hippocampus, whereas high prenatal stress was associated with a dramatic decrease. This difference is in keeping with human studies, as well as other animal models, dealing with resilience (see Chapter 27).

Valentino *et al.* (2012) discussed stress and arousal in relation to sex differences in emotional disorders in humans. They pointed to the evidence that there were sex differences in the locus coeruleus (LC)-norepinephrine arousal system. Sex differences in LC dendritic structure have been found and these are of a kind that suggest that there may be increased receipt and processing of limbic information in females.

Entringer *et al.*'s (2011) study of the effects of prenatal stress exposure on telomere length (see subsequent text) in the offspring found that it was a significant predictor of a shortened telomere length in adulthood. The study is limited by the fact that it was a retrospective assessment.

In summary, there is evidence suggesting effects of prenatal stress on the brain, on epigenetics, and on HPA functioning. The evidence on epigenetics needs to take into account the cell-specific features of much in the way of epigenetic processes and all the prenatal effects have to be considered in relation to postnatal continuities from the prenatal period. Nevertheless, although we lack understanding of the details, clearly there are biological effects of prenatal stress.

Postnatal maltreatment

One of the methodological problems that dogs the whole of the literature on maltreatment effects derives from the fact that there is a massive co-occurrence between maltreatment and psychopathology. That makes it an important topic to study with respect to mental disorders but the difficulty arises from the fact that the physiological effects of adversity are very similar to those found with depression and anxiety (Heim *et al.,* 2008b; Frodl & O'Keane, 2013; Heim and Binder, 2012). Heim *et al.* (2008a) showed the importance of using subgroups without child abuse but with current depression, a group with depression but no history of abuse, and those with both. Regrettably, few studies have done this. However, studying inflammation effects, Danese and McEwen (2012, 2008) did do so (see subsequent text).

A further issue concerns the question as to whether all forms of maltreatment should be combined or whether a separation should be made between physical abuse, sexual abuse, physical neglect, and supervisory neglect (Pears *et al.,* 2008; Petrenko *et al.,* 2012). There may well be biological differences in the effects of these different forms of maltreatment but there are far too few studies to draw any valid conclusions on this. However, the biology of the effects of child abuse has been usefully brought together by McCrory *et al.* (2010, 2012). The findings suggest that child abuse is associated with atypical HPA axis functioning in a substantial minority of abused children and that this, in turn, tends to be associated with difficulties in emotional and behavioral regulation. The ongoing exposure to early adversity tends to be associated with stress habituation over time, leading to reduced cortisol levels rather than the elevated levels associated with acute stress.

Sapolsky *et al.* (1986) put forward a glucocorticoid-cascade hypothesis. This led on to McEwen's (2012) concept of allostatic overload concerning the toxic effect of prolonged HPA overactivity. Allostasis refers to the body's physiological response to adversity and threat. In practice, the allostatic load is indexed by features such as systolic blood pressure, urinary cortisol, catecholamines, waist/hip ratio, and high-density lipoprotein (HDL). In short, allostatic load/overload refers to an imbalance in systems that promote adaptation. However, the situation is complicated by the evidence of differences between children and adults (Lupien *et al.,* 2011). The evidence suggests that exposure to maltreatment is associated with reduced hippocampal volume in adults but not in children. Children exposed to postnatal maternal depression show significantly larger amygdala volumes. This has also been shown in studies of children reared in orphanages (see subsequent text). A study of rats has shown that environmental enrichment can mitigate chronic stress effects on hippocampal neuronal architecture (Hutchinson *et al.,* 2012). Although stress effects on the hippocampus differ between childhood and adult life, in both age groups there seems to be a smaller volume of the prefrontal cortex as a result of allostatic overload (Danese and McEwen, 2012). It is evident that the biological effects of stress experiences are quite complicated. Heim and Binder (2012) have argued that in addition to the features discussed, gene–environment interactions may also be influential.

Animal research has shown that the hippocampus plays a central role in learning and memory and these functions are impaired when animals are exposed to chronic stress (McCrory *et al.,* 2010, 2012). Thus, one might expect that, as with studies of adults with post traumatic stress disorder (PTSD) or with a history of maltreatment, the hippocampus should be smaller but this is not what is found in children. By contrast, the amygdala, which plays a central role in processing emotions, tends to show an increased volume. Moreover, these effects on the brain are not only found soon after the adversity has been experienced but they also tend to persist over time, in line with animal models. The findings on the effects on the prefrontal cortex are somewhat inconsistent and it seems likely that there may be differences that relate to the age at which the abuse has occurred. A decreased volume of the cerebellum following maltreatment has been a consistent finding. Functional MRI (fMRI) studies have shown increased activation in the anterior cingulate cortex in young people who have experienced maltreatment, as compared with controls.

School-age children who have been exposed to physical abuse show increases in evoked response potential (ERP) brain activity specific to angry faces; see, for example, Pollak and Tolley-Schell (2003). One study (Andersen et al., 2008) looking at MRI scans from 26 women with repeated episodes of childhood sexual abuse and 17 healthy controls found that the brain changes varied according to the age at which the abuse occurred. The findings require replication but it is likely that there will be age-related differences in neural effects. However, the Andersen et al. study was based on a relatively small number of subjects experiencing abuse at each stage and the sample excluded subjects with other forms of abuse such as witnessing domestic violence.

We have chosen to separate the effects of institutional deprivation from those of abuse despite the fact that there are important similarities between them. Early studies showed that whereas acute stress led to an increase in HPA activation, repeated stresses or chronic adversity usually led to a flattening in response (Gunnar & Vazquez, 2006). However, it is now evident that the situation is somewhat more complicated because there are differences between rodents and humans with respect to sensitivity to stress, and because in humans there are age-related and sex-related variations (Lupien et al., 2009).

Telomere length

Telomeres are the repetitive TTAGGG sequence at the end of linear chromosomes. They are thought to function by capping and protecting the ends of chromosomes from DNA damage due to responses to stress and to aging. It is generally accepted that telomeres become shorter with each cell division and they have become established as a molecular clock for cellular replicative aging (Shalev et al., 2013). Because telomeres have been thought to be adversely affected by stress, it has been suggested that they constitute a key part of the etiological pathways linking early life stress with inflammatory disease and aging (see Price et al., 2013 for an overview). An important recent study by Shalev et al. (2013) used the British, nationally representative environmental risk (E-Risk) longitudinal twin study as a data source for examining the effects of exposure to violence during childhood. Telomere length was assessed at an age 5 baseline and age 10 follow-up. Four earlier studies had found an association between childhood adversity and shorter telomere length (TL) but there was one negative finding (Glass et al., 2010). The Shalev et al. report has two important advantages over the earlier research. First, violence was assessed prospectively rather than retrospectively and, secondly, the changes in TL from baseline were examined as well as the overall association with TL. The results showed significantly more telomere erosion between baseline and follow-up in children who experienced two or more kinds of violence exposure, the finding holding up after adjustment for sex, socioeconomic status, and body mass index. As Shalev (2012) pointed out, there are several different ways of measuring telomere length with continuing uncertainty as to which is the best. In addition, there may be differences according to whether TL is assessed in buccal cells (as obtained during a cheek swab) or blood products. The findings from Shalev et al. (2013) provide an important indication that TL may constitute a vital part of the pathways linking early life adversity and later disease but it should be noted that the study also showed that some children showed an increase in TL and it remains unclear whether that was simply a methodological artifact or reflected a meaningful change and, if it did, what influenced it.

Inflammation

Danese et al. (2008) used the Dunedin Multidisciplinary Health and Development Study (with a sample size of about 1000) where the follow-up was up to age 32 years in order to study inflammatory levels in individuals who had experienced maltreatment in childhood. Inflammation (referring to the body's response to trauma or infection) was assessed using high-sensitivity C-reactive protein and a dimensional inflammation factor indexing the shared variance of continuance measures of high-sensitivity C-reactive protein, fibrinogen, and white blood cells. The two measures of inflammation gave much the same picture. The key finding was that those who had experienced both maltreatment and depression showed a much increased level of inflammation as compared with either controls or a depressed only group (these two not differing significantly). Those with maltreatment only showed intermediate findings, leaving an uncertainty as to exactly what the combination of maltreatment and depression meant. The issue was further explored in a more recent study using the E-Risk Study that had the advantage of the prospective measure of maltreatment but the limitation of a follow-up only to age 12 years (Danese et al., 2011). Like the earlier Dunedin study findings, the largest effect on inflammation was found in the depressed plus maltreated group. In this case, the maltreated-only and the depressed-only groups did not differ from controls. As Danese and McEwen (2012) pointed out, maltreatment leads to changes in the HPA axis and changes in the brain, as well as in the immune system. Quite how these different features relate to one another remains uncertain.

One of the queries regarding the lasting effects on inflammation concern the mechanisms that might be involved in its persistence over many years. A recent study by Cole et al. (2012) comparing peer-reared and maternal-reared rhesus macaque monkeys was informative in showing that peer-rearing was associated with enhanced expression of genes involved in inflammation, cytokine signaling, and T-lymphocyte activation; as well as suppression of genes involved in several innate antimicrobial defenses. The study was limited by the lack of any direct measure of immune system functional activity but other analyses have shown that macaques exposed to the same adverse conditions in early life do show, as shown here, significantly elevated physical and behavioral sequelae (Conti *et al.*, 2012).

Institutional deprivation

Institutional deprivation has been dealt with here as a separate kind of experience because it involved a far greater and far wider level of deprivation than anything ordinarily experienced in family settings (Rutter & Sonuga-Barke, 2010). In addition, it did not necessarily involve individualized abuse. Rather, the key feature of the experience was neglect that involved both human interaction and conversation and global experiences. In the English and Romanian Study (Rutter & Sonuga-Barke, 2010), many of the children experienced marked subnutrition as well as psychosocial deprivation but it was possible to make comparisons between those who did and those who did not have subnutrition (Sonuga-Barke *et al.*, 2010; Rutter *et al.*, 2012). In the children without subnutrition, there was no impairment of head growth in children who left the institution before the age of 6 months but there was huge impairment of head growth in those whose institutional deprivation continued beyond the age of 6 months. It is known that head growth provides a good index of brain growth and therefore the strong inference is that the "pure" psychosocial deprivation led to major overall impairment in brain growth.

Sheridan *et al.* (2012), using data from the Bucharest Early Intervention project, compared children exposed to institutional rearing and children previously exposed to institutional rearing but then randomized to high-quality foster care intervention. There was also a comparison with typically developing children in Romania who were not in institutions. The findings showed that a history of institutional rearing was associated with a significantly smaller cortical gray matter volume. The effects on gray matter applied to those who had a history of institutionalization irrespective of whether they were later placed in foster care. On the other hand, cortical white matter did not differ between never-institutionalized children and children placed in foster care as part of the randomized design. The same study also looked at alpha frequencies in the overall electroencephalogram (EEG) signal. Children exposed to institutional rearing exhibited decreased alpha power, implying developmental delay in neural functioning. The association between institutional rearing and EEG alpha power was partially mediated by cortical matter volume for children not randomized to foster care. The alpha power finding (Marshall *et al.*, 2004) significantly moderated the associations between attachment security and social skills (Almas *et al.*, 2012). A separate study (Eluvathingal *et al.*, 2006) used diffusion tensor imaging in a study of children in North America adopted from Romania, showed a generally compromised white matter tract integrity. Yet another study

(Tottenham *et al.*, 2010) showed that prolonged institutional rearing was associated with an atypically large amygdala volume and difficulties in emotion regulation.

Bauer *et al.* (2009) compared post-institutionalized children from the Wisconsin International Adoption Project registry (meaning that these were volunteers) and controls acquired through community advertisements and flyers. The children were raised in orphanages in Romania, Russia, China and other countries—making it a somewhat heterogeneous group. The main finding was that the institutionally deprived group had smaller superior-posterior cerebellar lobe volumes than control subjects and that these two brain regions were related to two aspects of cognition. A smaller subgroup of the same sample was studied by Fries *et al.*, (2008) with the finding that the post-institutionalized children showed prolonged elevations in cortisol levels following a standardized interaction between the child and the mother, and not the interaction with a stranger. Results suggested that early institutional deprivation may contribute to long-term regulatory problems of the stress-responsive system, but these were evident only in the context of ongoing close interpersonal relationships. One limitation of the study was that it did not include a cortisol measurement immediately following the experimental session and hence it remains uncertain whether there was a hyperreactive response following the interaction, a prolonged response to the event, or both.

Studies from Carlson and Earls (1997) onward have shown that institution-reared children tend to show a low morning cortisol and a flat pattern of diurnal variation during the rest of the day. What has been somewhat uncertain is whether this dysregulation of the HPA axis persists after adoption. Kroupina *et al.* (2012) showed that it did persist, at least over the first 6 months (but with an increase in morning cortisol). The dysfunctional pattern was most evident in those who were stunted in their physical growth and the abnormal cortisol pattern was associated with externalizing behavior problems in adolescence and adults. Another study showed institutional rearing was associated with reduced telomere length (Drury *et al.*, 2011).

Conti *et al.* (2012) analyzed health records of rhesus monkeys across mother rearing, peer rearing, and surrogate peer rearing conditions, the latter being the closest to institutional rearing, and found that adverse rearing conditions had long-term detrimental effects on health that were not improved by subsequently improved rearing conditions (analogous to adoption).

Putting the available evidence together, it appears that the biological findings associated with profound institutional deprivation are broadly similar to those found with child abuse, but that what is different with institutional deprivation is the major effect on overall brain growth.

Social disadvantage

There is abundant evidence from cohort studies that social disadvantage in early life is associated with poor health in adult life, even after adjusting for social status in adult life (Kuh *et al.*, 2002; Power *et al.*, 2005). The question that arises, therefore, is what biological mechanism underlies this persistence. The conceptual and methodological issues were well reviewed by Adler *et al.* (2012). The first problem is the need to check that the causal inference is justified and the second is that social disadvantage is an ill-defined concept that incorporates a wide range of circumstances—spanning low social status, poverty, neighborhood, and stresses of many varieties and behaviors (such as smoking, heavy drinking, and lack of exercise) that carry health risks. As such, the biological effects are likely to reflect those associated with each of these various features (many discussed in other sections of this chapter; see also Adler and Rehkopf, 2008).

Hertzman (2012) discussed the biology in terms of geographical variations in social vulnerability—noting differences in HPA axis functioning and event-related potentials assessing focused attention and epigenetic processes. Essex *et al.* (2011) reported epigenetic differences in adolescence associated with early adversity; and Lam *et al.* (2012) found some significant methylation differences in relation to social background—albeit with weaker effects than reported by Borghol *et al.* (2012) and by Miller *et al.* (2009). Numerous experimental animal models confirm the causal effects of social status on epigenetics (see Fernald & Maruska 2012; Mashoodh *et al.*, 2012). The study of epigenetics in humans is problematic in that effects tend to be cell-specific (not just tissue-specific) and developmental phase-specific. Nevertheless, it may be concluded that social disadvantage does have epigenetic effects in humans as well as other animals (Rutter, 2012a). However, the findings do not carry much clinical meaning unless it can be shown that the patterns of epigenetic findings can, at an individual level, differentiate between the different patterns of disadvantage, and between stress resistance and stress sensitivity to mention just two out of a much larger list of alternatives. That has yet to be determined.

Two small-scale imaging studies have examined neural correlates—one using structural imaging (Noble *et al.*, 2012) and one fMRI (Noble *et al.*, 2006). It is of considerable interest that individual differences in social status were associated with regional brain volume variations in the hippocampus and amygdala, and that reading levels were associated with responsivity in the left perisylvian and left occipitotemporal regions. However, as the authors note, the findings derived from a cross-sectional analysis with a small sample and that the direction of causality could not be assumed.

Enrichment and deprivation studies

Prompted by Donald Hebb's now classic book proposing the concept of use-dependent plasticity of the nervous system, Rosenzweig and his colleagues (1962) reported studies comparing rats reared under three different conditions. First, there was the standard colony situation with three animals in a standard laboratory cage provided with food and water. Second, there was an impoverished condition in which the cages housed single animals only; and thirdly, animals housed in a large cage containing a group of 10–12 animals with a variety of stimulus objects, changed daily. Findings showed that differential experiences caused changes in cortical chemistry and in the weight of different regions of the neocortex. The findings were replicated by Greenough and Volkmar (1973). The early studies of enrichment and deprivation were undertaken with juvenile rats, with the expectation that plasticity might be confined to early life. However, later studies showed that closely comparable (although lesser) effects were found with adult rats (Rosenzweig & Bennett, 1996). Although the capacity for plastic changes to the nervous system remained in older animals, the effects of differential experience developed more rapidly in younger animals, with the effects being larger in the young.

These findings on enrichment and deprivation derived from animal models were later studied in humans. The human studies involved several different developments. First, there were comparisons of the relative efficacy of environmental enrichment, physical exercise, or formal training (see, e.g., van Praag *et al.*, 2000; Will *et al.*, 2004). Overall, the evidence suggested that specific training was more effective than physical exercise and that enriched experience was more effective than either of the other two. The other development involved the extrapolation of the findings to what might be done to enhance recovery after neurological damage (Taub *et al.*, 2002). While it was clear that the general principles applied as much to recovery from brain injury as to effects in normals, it remains uncertain how far the benefits come from neuronal regrowth following intervention. One recent study using an animal model (involving partial transsection of the spinal cord) suggested that there could be neuronal regrowth (van den Brand *et al.*, 2012), but the finding requires replication and human studies have yet to be undertaken. It also remains to be seen whether the evidence that environmental enrichment enhances neurogenesis (growth of nerve cells) in the adult hippocampus (Kempermann, 2008) is relevant for the concept of brain and cognitive reserve in relation to brain disorders (Nithianantharajah & Hannan, 2009). Further research is also needed to identify the molecular mechanisms involved in plasticity at different ages (Bavelier *et al.*, 2010).

Human studies of the effects of learning on the brain in adult life hit the headlines with Maguire *et al.*'s (2000, 2006) study of structural differences in the hippocampi of London taxi drivers as compared with bus drivers and controls. London taxi drivers are distinctive in being required to undergo extensive training followed by a test of "The Knowledge" involving the learning of the layout of some 25,000 streets and many thousands of places of interest. Compared with controls, the taxi drivers had a larger gray matter volume in the posterior hippocampus and a smaller volume in the anterior hippocampus. Because this was not an experimental study, it was not possible to rule out the possibility that taxi drivers who passed "The Knowledge" had a hippocampus that was different before the training started. However, the taxi drivers and their controls generally had average IQs (Woollett *et al.*, 2010). Later research went on to show that retired taxi drivers had a hippocampus pattern similar to practising taxi drivers but the pattern became closer to controls. In other words, although the effects of the intense prolonged training were lasting, they were not permanent.

Somewhat similar findings are evident in studies of musical training, except that the changes were in the motor and auditory areas critical for music training rather than the hippocampus (Elbert *et al.*, 1995). In this case, longitudinal data were used to test the hypothesis that the cerebral differences truly reflected the effects of training rather than preexisting brain differences. Hyde *et al.*, (2009) showed that there were no differences in the brain between young children who received 15 months of instrumental musical training compared with a group of children who did not. However, there were significant differences in the brain after training and, moreover, these were correlated with behavioral improvements. What this study did not do, because it was concerned with children, is test whether the same would apply to training in adult life.

A study of jugglers undertaken by Draganski *et al.*, (2004; Draganski & May, 2008) did show training-induced structural brain changes in adults. The music and the juggling studies are also crucial in their demonstration that the brain changes applied to areas of the brain other than the hippocampus.

Experience-expectant effects

Vision

As indicated, the biological effects of most experiences are not dependent on a narrowly defined sensitive period. However, there are exceptions. The Hubel and Weisel studies during the 1960s, (summarized in Hubel & Wiesel, 2005) were crucially important in showing that visual input was essential for the normal development of the visual cortex. These findings with cats have sometimes been considered to deal with a mechanism that applies more generally to brain development. The evidence clearly indicates that it does not, although it is likely that effects are not only confined to the visual system.

Hubel and Wiesel (2005) showed clearly, in a series of experiments with kittens, that profound sensory deprivation had a major effect on the development of the visual cortex. Kittens underwent monocular deprivation (i.e., one eye was sewn shut) during a critical period of visual development. Ordinarily, this period (4 weeks–3 months) corresponds to a period of preprogrammed ocular dominance but, with monocular deprivation, profound visual impairment was seen after the deprived eye was opened. Crucially, these effects were not seen if the deprivation occurred later (e.g., at 3–4 months). It seemed that the cortical areas functioned in relation to a competitive interaction between environmental inputs received during critical periods, rather than preprogrammed representation only. These findings, which resulted in a Nobel Prize, demonstrated the remarkable plasticity (modifiability) of the brain for the first time (Bryck & Fisher, 2012).

Pollutants

A study by Herr *et al.* (2010) showed that maternal exposure to pollution had an effect on the balance between T lymphocytes and B lymphocytes, which was interpreted as meaning an effect on immunity. This was seen only in early gestation. Evidence reviewed by Perera and Herbstman (2011) suggests that the prenatal effects may be concerned with regulating the fetal epigenome but, although plausible, the suggestion so far lacks empirical support. Also, implications for later consequences of these prenatal effects from pollutants remain quite uncertain.

One of the main groups of pollutants concerns endocrine disrupting compounds (EDCs) (DiVall, 2013). The findings on biological effects well illustrate the problems in assessing any pollutant. The National Toxicology Program (NTP) panel noted the uncertainties regarding both the epidemiological evidence and the animal studies. The NTP expressed negligible or minimal concern regarding most claimed ill effects (including those on birth weight and growth). However, it was noted that prenatal phthalate *might* predispose to congenital disorders of much reproductive tract development.

The Mexican studies (Calderón-Garcidueñas *et al.*, 2013) suggested that air pollution in Mexico City involved particulate matter metal neurotoxicity leading to a neuroinflammatory response and neural effects. However, the sample size was small and this is best considered as only a possibility warranting further study.

Lead

Rutter (1983) reviewed extensive evidence on low level lead exposure—with a major focus on the behavioral sequelae but also with attention to the biological findings. He noted that it had long been known that lead is a neurotoxin and that lead poisoning can cause encephalopathy and death. He concluded that there was no clear threshold below which there were no neural effects. Human evidence showed that blood/lead levels greater than 50 μg/dL, and probably at levels below that, led to impaired nerve conduction velocities. Similarly, children with raised lead levels had significantly increased amounts of low frequency delta activity on the EEG. One investigation also showed that slow wave voltage varies as a linear function of blood lead level. Animal studies are important in terms of the evidence that lead inhibits the heme biosynthetic pathway with effects measureable at lead levels below 30 μg/dL. In addition, lead has effects on several neurotransmitters and has been found to delay brain development in rat pups exposed to quite modest levels of lead in the neonatal period. It was concluded that increased levels of blood/body lead can and do cause impairment of biological functioning at levels well below those associated with recognizable signs and symptoms attributable to lead toxicity.

During the 1990s, a meta-analysis showed that there was a decline of 2–3 points for every 10 µg/dL increase in blood level (Schwartz, 1994). This was, however, based on studies in which most children had blood-lead levels in the range of 10–30 µg/dL. The situation since the 1980s and 1990s has changed greatly so that in most general populations the mean blood-lead level is now well below 10 µg/dL and sometimes it is as low as 1–2 µg/dL. Accordingly, the issue is whether lead has important adverse biological effects in this low range (Bellinger, 2008). The recent population-based brain imaging study by Cecil *et al.* (2008) found dose-dependent decreases in the volume of gray matter in the ventrolateral prefrontal cortex, the anterior cingulate cortex, the postcentral gyri, the inferior parietal lobule and the cerebellum, the reduction being particularly striking in males. Because this was an observational study, firm conclusions on causality were not possible. However, they attempted to get a handle on this by determining whether the brain changes were associated with neuropsychological functioning—with the finding of a lack of clear structure–function correlates, except in the case of motor skills. The conclusion now, unfortunately, has to be much the same as it was in the early 1980s. That is, there is no clear point below which there are no risks from lead toxicity but, equally, the effects are slight within a range of lower lead levels.

Traumatic brain injury

The first controlled, prospective psychiatric interview study of traumatic brain injury in children was undertaken by Rutter and colleagues in the late 1970s (Brown *et al.,* 1981). At that time brain imaging was not available and there had to be reliance only on duration of post traumatic amnesia as an index of the severity of the injury. There was good evidence that severe head injury played a crucial causal role in the development of psychiatric disorders arising during the 27 months subsequent to the accident but the risk was significantly influenced by the children's pre-accident behavior, their cognitive level, and their psychosocial circumstances. The only disorder specifically associated with the injury was a disinhibited state—a pattern that did not fit in with the usual psychiatric classifications at that time. A recent study by Max *et al.* (2012) took an understanding of the biology further through its use of diffusion tensor imaging (DTI)-derived fractional anisotropy (FA) and other brain imaging measures. The findings showed that new psychiatric disorders were not significantly related to volumetric measures of white or gray matter structures, volumetric measures of lesions or cortical thickness measures, but they were related to FA. It was concluded that lowered white matter integrity may be important in the pathophysiology of new psychiatric disorders following traumatic brain injury. It was notable that almost all the novel psychiatric disorders involved personality change—a finding in good keeping with the earlier study by Brown *et al.* (1981) showing disinhibited behavior.

Biological effects of different therapeutic interventions

There has long been an interest in the biology of depression (Mayberg, 2003; Nestler & Carlezon, 2006). The hope has been that treatments may alleviate symptoms through correction of dysregulated neural circuit activity (Ressler & Mayberg, 2007). Goldapple *et al.* (2004) reported a small study using functional brain imaging in which the findings suggested that cognitive behavior therapy (CBT) had a different neural effect than paroxetine, an antidepressant medication. Mayberg *et al.* (2000) noted changes in brain glucose metabolism measured using positron emission tomography (PET) in patients treated with fluoxetine that paralleled the clinical response. On the other hand, research also showed that imaging findings indicated that common regions of brain activation were targeted with pharmacological and somatic treatments as well as with emotional learning in psychotherapy (Ressler & Mayberg, 2007). Nemeroff *et al.* (2003) found that the effects of CBT and antidepressants were broadly similar but that responsivity did seem to be influenced by a history of childhood maltreatment. Tremblay *et al.* (2005) showed that individuals with a major depressive disorder had a hypersensitive response to the rewarding effects of dextroamphetamine, with altered brain activation in the ventrolateral PFC and the orbitofrontal cortex and the caudate and putamen.

We conclude that cognitive therapy and antidepressant medication of various sorts probably engage somewhat similar neural mechanisms although there may well be some mechanisms that are distinctive to each (DeRubeis *et al.,* 2008). It is necessary to be mindful, however, of the substantial conceptual, methodological, and statistical problems using brain imaging of all kinds in order to infer causal effects (Peterson, 2003), especially in relation to interventions (Bishop, 2013). There is little doubt that treatment is associated with a change in the neural features associated with depression and anxiety but some of these changes are also seen in people given placebos. In short, are the supposed treatment effects cause or consequence? In seeking to answer that question, it is necessary also to bear in mind that depression is associated with a somewhat heterogeneous range of biological differences (Ressler & Nemeroff, 2000).

Gene–environment interaction (G × E)

There is a wealth of data showing the reality of G × E based on research conducted with multiple species and from research using both observational and experimental methods (Rutter, 2006; Caspi *et al.,* 2010; Rutter, 2012b; Rutter, 2014). This is well summarized in State and Thapar (see Chapter 24). The focus in this chapter, however, is exclusively on the biology of the G × E effects.

These have been shown most clearly in the human experimental studies undertaken by Weinberger, Meyer-Lindenberg, Hariri and Pezawas (Hariri *et al.,* 2002; Hariri *et al.,* 2005; Pezawas *et al.,* 2005; Meyer-Lindenberg *et al.,* 2006;

Meyer-Lindenberg & Weinberger 2006; Buckholtz & Meyer-Lindenberg 2008). All of these studies were undertaken with normal volunteers who had been screened to be free of psychopathology. This had the important consequence that the findings applied, not just to patients with particular mental disorders but to the population as a whole. The findings apply to both the MAOA genotype and to the serotonin transporter-linked polymorphic region (5-HTTLPR) with the former concerned predominantly with impulsive violence and the latter with anxiety and depression. It is striking, however, that the impact on the structure and function of the amygdala (with increased reactivity) and the perigenual cingulate cortex, which implies a shared mechanism of emotional regulation under serotonergic control applied to both. Nevertheless, the MAOA genotype showed much more extensive effects on both structure and activation notably affecting more caudal regions of the cingulate associated with cognitive control, as well as the orbitofrontal cortex and hippocampus. All of these findings were derived from structural and functional magnetic resonance imaging (sMRI and fMRI respectively) and DNA findings on the genotype. The increase in bilateral orbitofrontal cortex was evident only in men. The 5-HTTLPR findings were associated with reduced gray matter volume in short allele carriers in limbic regions critical for the processing of negative emotion—particularly the perigenual cingulate and amygdala. Functional analysis during perceptual processing of fearful stimuli demonstrated tight coupling as the feedback circuit, the short allele carriers having a relative uncoupling of this circuit.

Nonhuman primate studies have shown that the G × E is associated with an increased HPA axis response to stress in infant macaques (Barr *et al.*, 2004). Rodent studies have been informative, through the study of genetically engineered 5HTT mutations. They have shown that the neural consequences extended well beyond the regulation of 5HTT availability. There were alterations throughout the system, in which the 5HTT knock-out mice exhibited an abnormally high density of excitatory dendritic spines on amygdala neurons and an increase in dendritic arborization of the prefrontal cortex neurons. This implication was confirmed in a rhesus macaque model (Jedema *et al.*, 2010). The last point to make is that many people have assumed that the G × E applies to responsivity to adverse experiences. However, it has been argued—particularly by Boyce and by Belsky—that evolutionary considerations suggest that it is more likely that it involves an increased sensitivity to the environment both good and bad (Ellis *et al.*, 2011). The evidence in support of this suggestion is growing, although it is still a bit too early to regard this as established. Nevertheless, it seems increasingly likely that it may prove to be valid.

Overall conclusions

Four key issues apply to all the biological effects discussed in this chapter. First there is the question as to whether the associations with experiences truly represent a causal influence of experiences on the biology. Second, there are questions on the specificity of the biological effects. Third, there is a lack of knowledge on the connections among the different biological features. Fourth, there is the question as to whether the biological features are responsible for the consequent effects on psychopathological functioning.

The causal inference has been considered in several different ways. To begin with, it has often been possible to use animal models and, where they have been available and relevant, we have briefly summarized the findings. In addition, we have paid attention to specificity of timing. Thus, this applied to the effects of exposure to maternal alcohol, to smoking and to testosterone. Also, in the few instances where such data were available, we noted the use of prospective data to look at changes in the biology as found following experiences. That applies, for example, to the telomere length research. There are not many instances where natural experiments have been available but they were informative with respect to the separation of prenatal from postnatal effects using adoptee data. Lastly, we have made use, whenever available, of the additional leverage provided by bringing together different measures. For example, this was useful with respect to the neural effects of institutional deprivation—as shown by the combination of MRI findings and alpha strength on the EEG. We conclude that the causal inference has had reasonable, albeit modest, support for most of the biological findings we have considered.

The second major issue concerns the specificity of the biological effects. What is immediately striking is that all clinically significant experiences have been shown to have biological effects. In some cases, questions remain on whether very mild experiences have measurable effects, but it is evident that if there is a threshold on dosage it must be a very low threshold. What is also very striking is that there is a huge diversity of biological consequences—including epigenetic effects, HPA axis effects, impact on telomere length, effects on the hippocampus, the amygdala and the cerebral cortex, on overall brain growth, on inflammation, and on birth weight. In addition, there appears to be variation according to sex, to the individual's age at the time of the experience, and to the specifics of the nature of the experience. There is likely to be an understandable meaning to the causes of this heterogeneity but, although good ideas have been put forward, there is no consensus so far on the mechanisms. Furthermore, the research undertaken so far has not provided a clear differentiation between the biologically negative consequences of adverse experiences and the biological changes that represent positive adaptational changes underpinning resilience.

Third, there is still a lack of understanding of the relationship among the various biological features. How, for example, do the epigenetic changes relate to the HPA effects and how do both of these relate to inflammation and telomere findings? The precise neural effects (such as between the hippocampus and the amygdala) seem to vary between children and adults. Is this because of structural and functional changes in the development of the brain, or do these reflect age-related variations in experiential effects? Clearly, much remains to be learned. Finally, major questions remain on the functional implications of the biological findings—particularly with respect to their role in the psychological and psychopathological outcomes of the experiences—as discussed by Rutter (2012a).

References

Adler, N.E. & Rehkopf, D.H. (2008) US disparities in health: descriptions, causes, and mechanisms. *Annual Review of Public Health* **29**, 235–252.

Adler, N. *et al.* (2012) Rigor, vigor, and the study of health disparities. *Proceedings of the National Academy of Sciences* **109**, 17154–17159.

Almas, A.N. *et al.* (2012) Effects of early intervention and the moderating effects of brain activity on institutionalized children's social skills at age 8. *Proceedings of the National Academy of Sciences* **109**, 17228–17231.

Andersen, S. *et al.* (2008) Preliminary evidence for sensitive periods in the effect of childhood sexual abuse on regional brain development. *Journal of Neuropsychiatry and Clinical Neurosciences* **20**, 292–301.

Ansorge, M.S. *et al.* (2004) Early-life blockade of the 5-HT transporter alters emotional behavior in adult mice. *Science* **306**, 879–881.

Arnold, A.P. (2009) The organizational–activational hypothesis as the foundation for a unified theory of sexual differentiation of all mammalian tissues. *Hormones and Behavior* **55**, 570–578.

Bale, T.L. *et al.* (2010) Early life programming and neurodevelopmental disorders. *Biological Psychiatry* **68**, 314–319.

Barr, C.S. *et al.* (2004) Rearing condition and rh5-HTTLPR interact to influence limbic-hypothalamic-pituitary-adrenal axis response to stress in infant macaques. *Biological Psychiatry* **55**, 733–738.

Bauer, P.M. *et al.* (2009) Cerebellar volume and cognitive functioning in children who experienced early deprivation. *Biological Psychiatry* **66**, 1100–1106.

Bavelier, D. *et al.* (2010) Removing brakes on adult brain plasticity: from molecular to behavioral interventions. *Journal of Neuroscience* **30**, 14964–14971.

Becker, H.C. *et al.* (1996) Teratogenic actions of ethanol in the mouse: a minireview. *Pharmacology Biochemistry and Behavior* **55**, 501–513.

Bellinger, D.C. (2008) Neurological and behavioral consequences of childhood lead exposure. *PLoS Medicine* **5**, e115.

Bernstein, I.M. *et al.* (2005) Maternal smoking and its association with birth weight. *Obstetrics & Gynecology* **106**, 986–991.

Bishop, D. (2013) Research Review: Emanuel Miller Memorial Lecture 2012—neuroscientific studies of intervention for language impairment in children: interpretive and methodological problems. *Journal of Child Psychology and Psychiatry* **54**, 247–259.

Borghol, N. *et al.* (2012) Associations with early-life socio-economic position in adult DNA methylation. *International Journal of Epidemiology* **41**, 62–74.

van den Brand, R. *et al.* (2012) Restoring voluntary control of locomotion after paralyzing spinal cord injury. *Science* **336**, 1182–1185.

Brown, G. *et al.* (1981) A prospective study of children with head injuries: III. Psychiatric sequelae. *Psychological Medicine* **11**, 63–78.

Bryck, R.L. & Fisher, P.A. (2012) Training the brain: practical applications of neural plasticity from the intersection of cognitive neuroscience, developmental psychology, and prevention science. *American Psychologist* **67**, 87–100.

Buckholtz, J.W. & Meyer-Lindenberg, A. (2008) MAOA and the neurogenetic architecture of human aggression. *Trends in Neurosciences* **31**, 120–129.

Buss, C. *et al.* (2010) High pregnancy anxiety during mid-gestation is associated with decreased gray matter density in 6–9-year-old children. *Psychoneuroendocrinology* **35**, 141–153.

Buss, C. *et al.* (2012) Maternal cortisol over the course of pregnancy and subsequent child amygdala and hippocampus volumes and affective problems. *Proceedings of the National Academy of Sciences* **109**, E1312–E1319.

Calderón-Garcidueñas, L. *et al.* (2013) The impact of environmental metals in young urbanites' brains. *Experimental and Toxicologic Pathology* **65**, 503–511.

Carlson, M. & Earls, F. (1997) Psychological and neuroendocrinological sequelae of early social deprivation in institutionalized children in Romania. *Annals of the New York Academy of Sciences* **807**, 419–428.

Caspi, A. *et al.* (2010) Genetic sensitivity to the environment: the case of the serotonin transporter gene and its implications for studying complex diseases and traits. *American Journal of Psychiatry* **167**, 509–527.

Cecil, K.M. *et al.* (2008) Decreased brain volume in adults with childhood lead exposure. *PLoS Medicine* **5**, e112.

Chen, H. *et al.* (2005) Gestational nicotine exposure reduces nicotinic cholinergic receptor (nAChR) expression in dopaminergic brain regions of adolescent rats. *European Journal of Neuroscience* **22**, 380–388.

Cole, S.W. *et al.* (2012) Transcriptional modulation of the developing immune system by early life social adversity. *Proceedings of the National Academy of Sciences* **109**, 20578–20583.

Conti, G. *et al.* (2012) Primate evidence on the late health effects of early-life adversity. *Proceedings of the National Academy of Sciences* **109**, 8866–8871.

Croen, L.A. *et al.* (2011) Antidepressant use during pregnancy and childhood autism spectrum disorders. *Archives of General Psychiatry* **68**, 1104–1112.

Danese, A. & McEwen, B.S. (2012) Adverse childhood experiences, allostasis, allostatic load, and age-related disease. *Physiology & Behavior* **106**, 29–39.

Danese, A. *et al.* (2008) Elevated inflammation levels in depressed adults with a history of childhood maltreatment. *Archives of General Psychiatry* **65**, 409–415.

Danese, A. *et al.* (2011) Biological embedding of stress through inflammation processes in childhood. *Molecular Psychiatry* **16**, 244–246.

Davis, E.P. *et al.* (2011) Prenatal maternal stress programs infant stress regulation. *Journal of Child Psychology and Psychiatry* **52**, 119–129.

Day, N.L. *et al.* (1989) Prenatal exposure to alcohol: effect on infant growth and morphologic characteristics. *Pediatrics* **84**, 536–541.

Derauf, C. *et al.* (2009) Neuroimaging of children following prenatal drug exposure. *Seminars in Cell & Developmental Biology* **20**, 441–454.

DeRubeis, R.J. *et al.* (2008) Cognitive therapy versus medication for depression: treatment outcomes and neural mechanisms. *Nature Reviews Neuroscience* **9**, 788–796.

DiVall, S.A. (2013) The influence of endocrine disruptors on growth and development of children. *Current Opinion in Endocrinology, Diabetes and Obesity* **20**, 50–55.

Dow-Edwards, D. (2011) Translational issues for prenatal cocaine studies and the role of environment. *Neurotoxicology and Teratology* **33**, 9–16.

Draganski, B. & May, A. (2008) Training-induced structural changes in the adult human brain. *Behavioural Brain Research* **192**, 137–142.

Draganski, B. *et al.* (2004) Neuroplasticity: changes in grey matter induced by training. *Nature* **427**, 311–312.

Drury, S. *et al.* (2011) Telomere length and early severe social deprivation: linking early adversity and cellular aging. *Molecular Psychiatry* **17**, 719–727.

Elbert, T. *et al.* (1995) Increased cortical representation of the fingers of the left hand in string players. *Science* **270**, 305–307.

Ellis, B.J. *et al.* (2011) Differential susceptibility to the environment: an evolutionary-neurodevelopmental theory. *Development and Psychopathology* **23**, 7–28.

Eluvathingal, T.J. *et al.* (2006) Abnormal brain connectivity in children after early severe socioemotional deprivation: a diffusion tensor imaging study. *Pediatrics* **117**, 2093–2100.

England, L.J. *et al.* (2001) Effects of smoking reduction during pregnancy on the birth weight of term infants. *American Journal of Epidemiology* **154**, 694–701.

Entringer, S. *et al.* (2011) Stress exposure in intrauterine life is associated with shorter telomere length in young adulthood. *Proceedings of the National Academy of Sciences* **108**, E513–E518.

Essex, M.J. *et al.* (2011) Epigenetic vestiges of early developmental adversity: childhood stress exposure and DNA methylation in adolescence. *Child Development* **84**, 58–75.

Fernald, R.D. & Maruska, K.P. (2012) Social information changes the brain. *Proceedings of the National Academy of Sciences* **109**, 17194–17199.

Fries, A.B.W. *et al.* (2008) Neuroendocrine dysregulation following early social deprivation in children. *Developmental Psychobiology* **50**, 588–599.

Frodl, T. & O'Keane, V. (2013) How does the brain deal with cumulative stress? A review with focus on developmental stress, HPA axis function and hippocampal structure in humans. *Neurobiology of Disease* **52**, 24–37.

Glass, D. *et al.* (2010) No correlation between childhood maltreatment and telomere length. *Biological Psychiatry* **68**, e21–e22.

Goldapple, K. *et al.* (2004) Modulation of cortical-limbic pathways in major depression: treatment-specific effects of cognitive behavior therapy. *Archives of General Psychiatry* **61**, 34–41.

Gray, R. & Henderson, J. (2006) *Review of the Fetal Effects of Prenatal Alcohol Exposure: Report to the Department of Health*. National Perinatal Epidemiology Unit, Oxford.

Green, M.L. *et al.* (2007) Reprogramming of genetic networks during initiation of the fetal alcohol syndrome. *Developmental Dynamics* **236**, 613–631.

Greenough, W.T. & Volkmar, F.R. (1973) Pattern of dendritic branching in occipital cortex of rats reared in complex environments. *Experimental Neurology* **40**, 491–504.

Gunnar, M.R. & Vazquez, D.M. (2006) Stress, neurobiology and developmental psychopathology. In: *Developmental Psychopathology*. (eds D. Cicchetti & D. Cohen), pp. 533–577. John Wiley & Sons, New York.

Haghighi, A. *et al.* (2013) Prenatal exposure to maternal cigarette smoking, amygdala volume, and fat intake in adolescence. *Archives of General Psychiatry* **70**, 98–105.

Hanley, G.E. & Oberlander, T.F. (2012) Neurodevelopmental outcomes following prenatal exposure to serotonin reuptake inhibitor antidepressants: a "social teratogen" or moderator of developmental risk? *Birth Defects Research Part A: Clinical and Molecular Teratology* **94**, 651–659.

Hariri, A.R. *et al.* (2002) Serotonin transporter genetic variation and the response of the human amygdala. *Science* **297**, 400–403.

Hariri, A.R. *et al.* (2005) A susceptibility gene for affective disorders and the response of the human amygdala. *Archives of General Psychiatry* **62**, 146–152.

Heijmans, B.T. *et al.* (2008) Persistent epigenetic differences associated with prenatal exposure to famine in humans. *Proceedings of the National Academy of Sciences* **105**, 17046–17049.

Heim, C. & Binder, E.B. (2012) Current research trends in early life stress and depression: review of human studies on sensitive periods, gene-environment interactions, and epigenetics. *Experimental Neurology* **233**, 102–111.

Heim, C. *et al.* (2008a) The dexamethasone/corticotropin-releasing factor test in men with major depression: role of childhood trauma. *Biological Psychiatry* **63**, 398–405.

Heim, C. *et al.* (2008b) The link between childhood trauma and depression: insights from HPA axis studies in humans. *Psychoneuroendocrinology* **33**, 693–710.

Herr, C.E. *et al.* (2010) Air pollution exposure during critical time periods in gestation and alterations in cord blood lymphocyte distribution: a cohort of live births. *Environmental Health* **9**, 46–58.

Hertzman, C. (2012) Putting the concept of biological embedding in historical perspective. *Proceedings of the National Academy of Sciences* **109**, 17160–17167.

Hines, M. (2004) *Brain Gender*. Oxford University Press, New York.

Hines, M. (2011) Gender development and the human brain. *Annual Review of Neuroscience* **34**, 69–88.

Hubel, D.H. & Wiesel, T.N. (2005) *Brain and Visual Perception: The Story of a 25-year Collaboration*. Oxford University Press, New York & Oxford.

Hutchinson, K.M. *et al.* (2012) Environmental enrichment protects against the effects of chronic stress on cognitive and morphological measures of hippocampal integrity. *Neurobiology of Learning and Memory* **97**, 250–260.

Hyde, L.W. *et al.* (2009) The effects of musical training on structural brain development. *Annals of New York Academy of Sciences* **1169**, 182–186.

Jaddoe, V.W.V. *et al.* (2007) Maternal smoking and fetal growth characteristics in different periods of pregnancy: the Generation R Study. *American Journal of Epidemiology* **165**, 1207–1215.

Jedema, H.P. *et al.* (2010) Cognitive impact of genetic variation of the serotonin transporter in primates is associated with differences in brain morphology rather than serotonin neurotransmission. *Molecular Psychiatry* **15**, 512–522.

Jones, K.L. *et al.* (1973) Pattern of malformation in offspring of chronic alcoholic mothers. *Lancet* **301**, 1267–1271.

Kane, V.B. *et al.* (2004) Gestational nicotine exposure attenuates nicotine-stimulated dopamine release in the nucleus accumbens shell of adolescent Lewis rats. *Journal of Pharmacology and Experimental Therapeutics* **308**, 521–528.

Kempermann, G. (2008) The neurogenic reserve hypothesis: what is adult hippocampal neurogenesis good for? *Trends in Neurosciences* **31**, 163–169.

Knopik, V.S. *et al.* (2012) The epigenetics of maternal cigarette smoking during pregnancy and effects on child development. *Development and Pychopathology* **24**, 1377–1390.

Kroupina, M.G. *et al.* (2012) Adoption as an intervention for institutionally reared children: HPA functioning and developmental status. *Infant Behavior and Development* **35**, 829–837.

Kuh, D. *et al.* (2002) Mortality in adults aged 26–54 years related to socioeconomic conditions in childhood and adulthood: post war birth cohort study. *British Medical Journal* **325**, 1076–1080.

Lam, L.L. *et al.* (2012) Factors underlying variable DNA methylation in a human community cohort. *Proceedings of the National Academy of Sciences* **109**, 17253–17260.

Lebel, C. *et al.* (2012) A longitudinal study of the long-term consequences of drinking during pregnancy: heavy in utero alcohol exposure disrupts the normal processes of brain development. *Journal of Neuroscience* **32**, 15243–15251.

Lewis, S.J. *et al.* (2012) Fetal alcohol exposure and IQ at age 8: evidence from a population-based birth-cohort study. *PLoS One* **7**, e49407.

Lieberman, E. *et al.* (1994) Low birthweight at term and the timing of fetal exposure to maternal smoking. *American Journal of Public Health* **84**, 1127–1131.

Lombardo, M.V. *et al.* (2012) Fetal testosterone influences sexually dimorphic gray matter in the human brain. *Journal of Neuroscience* **32**, 674–680.

Lupien, S. *et al.* (2007) The effects of stress and stress hormones on human cognition: implications for the field of brain and cognition. *Brain and Cognition* **65**, 209–237.

Lupien, S.J. *et al.* (2009) Effects of stress throughout the lifespan on the brain, behaviour and cognition. *Nature Reviews Neuroscience* **10**, 434–445.

Lupien, S.J. *et al.* (2011) Larger amygdala but no change in hippocampal volume in 10-year-old children exposed to maternal depressive symptomatology since birth. *Proceedings of the National Academy of Sciences* **108**, 14324–14329.

Maguire, E.A. *et al.* (2000) Navigation-related structural change in the hippocampi of taxi drivers. *Proceedings of the National Academy of Sciences* **97**, 4398–4403.

Maguire, E.A. *et al.* (2006) London taxi drivers and bus drivers: a structural MRI and neuropsychological analysis. *Hippocampus* **16**, 1091–1101.

Marshall, P.J. *et al.* (2004) A comparison of the electroencephalogram between institutionalized and community children in Romania. *Journal of Cognitive Neuroscience* **16**, 1327–1338.

Mashoodh, R. *et al.* (2012) Paternal social enrichment effects on maternal behavior and offspring growth. *Proceedings of the National Academy of Sciences* **109**, 17232–17238.

Max, J.E. *et al.* (2012) Neuroimaging correlates of novel psychiatric disorders after pediatric traumatic brain injury. *Journal of the American Academy of Child and Adolescent Psychiatry* **51**, 1208–1217.

Mayberg, H.S. (2003) Modulating dysfunctional limbic-cortical circuits in depression: towards development of brain-based algorithms for diagnosis and optimised treatment. *British Medical Bulletin* **65**, 193–207.

Mayberg, H.S. *et al.* (2000) Regional metabolic effects of fluoxetine in major depression: serial changes and relationship to clinical response. *Biological Psychiatry* **48**, 830–843.

McCrory, E. *et al.* (2010) Research review: the neurobiology and genetics of maltreatment and adversity. *Journal of Child Psychology and Psychiatry* **51**, 1079–1095.

McCrory, E. *et al.* (2012) The link between child abuse and psychopathology: a review of neurobiological and genetic research. *Journal of the Royal Society of Medicine* **105**, 151–156.

McEwen, B.S. (2012) Brain on stress: how the social environment gets under the skin. *Proceedings of the National Academy of Sciences* **109**, 17180–17185.

Meyer-Lindenberg, A. & Weinberger, D.R. (2006) Intermediate phenotypes and genetic mechanisms of psychiatric disorders. *Nature Reviews Neuroscience* **7**, 818–827.

Meyer-Lindenberg, A. *et al.* (2006) Neural mechanisms of genetic risk for impulsivity and violence in humans. *Proceedings of the National Academy of Sciences* **103**, 6269–6274.

Miller, G.E. *et al.* (2009) Low early-life social class leaves a biological residue manifested by decreased glucocorticoid and increased proinflammatory signaling. *Proceedings of the National Academy of Sciences* **106**, 14716–14721.

Moe, V. (2002) Foster-placed and adopted children exposed in utero to opiates and other substances: prediction and outcome at four and a half years. *Journal of Developmental & Behavioral Pediatrics* **23**, 330–339.

Monk, C. *et al.* (2012) Linking prenatal maternal adversity to developmental outcomes in infants: the role of epigenetic pathways. *Development and Psychopathology* **24**, 1361–1376.

Monk, C. *et al.* (2013) Research review: maternal prenatal distress and poor nutrition–mutually influencing risk factors affecting infant neurocognitive development. *Journal of Child Psychology and Psychiatry* **54**, 115–130.

Moore, D.S. (2012) Sex differences in normal fetuses and infants: a commentary. *Child Development Perspectives* **6**, 414–416.

Mychasiuk, R. *et al.* (2011) Intensity matters: brain, behavior and the epigenome of prenatally stressed rats. *Neuroscience* **180**, 105–110.

Nemeroff, C.B. *et al.* (2003) Differential responses to psychotherapy versus pharmacotherapy in patients with chronic forms of major depression and childhood trauma. *Proceedings of the National Academy of Sciences* **100**, 14293–14296.

Nestler, E.J. & Carlezon, W.A. (2006) The mesolimbic dopamine reward circuit in depression. *Biological Psychiatry* **59**, 1151–1159.

Nithianantharajah, J. & Hannan, A.J. (2009) The neurobiology of brain and cognitive reserve: mental and physical activity as modulators of brain disorders. *Progress in Neurobiology* **89**, 369–382.

Noble, K.G. *et al.* (2006) Brain–behavior relationships in reading acquisition are modulated by socioeconomic factors. *Developmental Science* **9**, 642–654.

Noble, K.G. *et al.* (2012) Neural correlates of socioeconomic status in the developing human brain. *Developmental Science* **15**, 516–527.

Nordström, M.L. & Cnattingius, S. (1994) Smoking habits and birthweights in two successive births in Sweden. *Early Human Development* **37**, 195–204.

Nulman, I. *et al.* (2002) Child development following exposure to tricyclic antidepressants or fluoxetine throughout fetal life: a prospective, controlled study. *American Journal of Psychiatry* **159**, 1889–1895.

Nulman, I. *et al.* (2012) Neurodevelopment of children following prenatal exposure to venlafaxine, selective serotonin reuptake inhibitors, or untreated maternal depression. *American Journal of Psychiatry* **169**, 1165–1174.

Oberlander, T. *et al.* (2009) Sustained neurobehavioral effects of exposure to SSRI antidepressants during development: molecular to clinical evidence. *Clinical Pharmacology & Therapeutics* **86**, 672–677.

Office of the US Surgeon General (2006) *Surgeon General's Report: The Health Consequences of Involuntary Exposure to Tobacco Smoke.* US Department of Health and Human Services, Atlanta.

Pears, K.C. *et al.* (2008) Psychosocial and cognitive functioning of children with specific profiles of maltreatment. *Child Abuse & Neglect* **32**, 958–971.

Pedersen, L.H. *et al.* (2013) Prenatal antidepressant exposure and behavioral problems in early childhood—a cohort study. *Acta Psychiatrica Scandinavica* **127**, 126–135.

Peña, C.J. *et al.* (2012) Epigenetic effects of prenatal stress on 11β-hydroxysteroid dehydrogenase-2 in the placenta and fetal brain. *PLoS One* **7**, e39791.

Perera, F. & Herbstman, J. (2011) Prenatal environmental exposures, epigenetics, and disease. *Reproductive Toxicology* **31**, 363–373.

Peterson, B.S. (2003) Conceptual, methodological, and statistical challenges in brain imaging studies of developmentally based psychopathologies. *Development and Psychopathology* **15**, 811–832.

Petrenko, C.L.M. *et al.* (2012) Does subtype matter? Assessing the effects of maltreatment on functioning in preadolescent youth in out-of-home care. *Child Abuse & Neglect* **36**, 633–644.

Pezawas, L. *et al.* (2005) 5-HTTLPR polymorphism impacts human cingulate-amygdala interactions: a genetic susceptibility mechanism for depression. *Nature Neuroscience* **8**, 828–834.

Phoenix, C.H. *et al.* (1959) Organizing action of prenatally administered testosterone propionate on the tissues mediating mating behavior in the female guinea pig. *Endocrinology* **65**, 369–382.

Pollak, S.D. & Tolley-Schell, S.A. (2003) Selective attention to facial emotion in physically abused children. *Journal of Abnormal Psychology* **112**, 323–338.

Power, C. *et al.* (2005) Socioeconomic position in childhood and early adult life and risk of mortality: a prospective study of the mothers of the 1958 British birth cohort. *American Journal of Public Health* **95**, 1396–1402.

van Praag, H. *et al.* (2000) Neural consequences of environmental enrichment. *Nature Reviews Neuroscience* **1**, 191–198.

Price, L.H. *et al.* (2013) Telomeres and early-life stress: an overview. *Biological Psychiatry* **73**, 15–23.

Ressler, K.J. & Mayberg, H.S. (2007) Targeting abnormal neural circuits in mood and anxiety disorders: from the laboratory to the clinic. *Nature Neuroscience* **10**, 1116–1124.

Ressler, K.J. & Nemeroff, C.B. (2000) Role of serotonergic and noradrenergic systems in the pathophysiology of depression and anxiety disorders. *Depression and Anxiety* **12**, 2–19.

Rosenzweig, M.R. & Bennett, E.L. (1996) Psychobiology of plasticity: effects of training and experience on brain and behavior. *Behavioural Brain Research* **78**, 57–65.

Rosenzweig, M.R. *et al.* (1962) Effects of environmental complexity and training on brain chemistry and anatomy: a replication and extension. *Journal of Comparative and Physiological Psychology* **55**, 429–437.

Rutter, M. (1983) Low level lead exposure: sources, effects and implications. In: *Lead Versus Health: Sources and Effects of Low Level Lead Exposure.* (eds M. Rutter & R. Jones), pp. 333–370. John Wiley & Sons, Chichester.

Rutter, M. (2006) *Genes and Behavior: Nature-Nurture Interplay Explained.* Blackwell Scientific, Oxford.

Rutter, M. (2012a) Achievements and challenges in the biology of environmental effects. *Proceedings of the National Academy of Sciences* **109**, 17149–17153.

Rutter, M. (2012b) Gene-environment interdependence. *European Journal of Developmental Psychology* **9**, 391–412.

Rutter, M. (2014) Nature-nurture integration. In: *Handbook of Developmental Psychopathology.* (eds M. Lewis & K. Rudolph), 3rd edn, pp. 45–66. Springer Science.

Rutter, M. & Sonuga-Barke, E.J. (2010) X. Conclusions: overview of findings from the E.R.A. study, inferences, and research implications. In: *Deprivation-Specific Psychological Patterns: Effects of Institutional Deprivation*, vol. **75**, pp. 212–229. Monographs of the Society for Research in Child Development, Oxford.

Rutter, M. *et al.* (2012) Longitudinal studies using a "natural experiment" design: the case of adoptees from Romanian institutions. *Journal of the American Academy of Child & Adolescent Psychiatry* **51**, 762–770.

Sandman, C.A. *et al.* (2012) Exposure to prenatal psychobiological stress exerts programming influences on the mother and her fetus. *Neuroendocrinology* **95**, 8–21.

Sapolsky, R.M. *et al.* (1986) The neuroendocrinology of stress and aging: the glucocorticoid cascade hypothesis. *Endocrine Reviews* **7**, 284–301.

Schwartz, J. (1994) Low-level lead exposure and children's IQ: a meta-analysis and search for a threshold. *Environmental Research* **65**, 42–55.

Shalev, I. (2012) Early life stress and telomere length: investigating the connection and possible mechanisms. *BioEssays* **34**, 943–952.

Shalev, I. *et al.* (2013) Exposure to violence during childhood is associated with telomere erosion from 5 to 10 years of age: a longitudinal study. *Molecular Psychiatry* **18**, 576–581.

Sheridan, M.A. *et al.* (2012) Variation in neural development as a result of exposure to institutionalization early in childhood. *Proceedings of the National Academy of Sciences* **109**, 12927–12932.

Simpson, K.L. *et al.* (2011) Perinatal antidepressant exposure alters cortical network function in rodents. *Proceedings of the National Academy of Sciences* **108**, 18465–18470.

Singer, L.T. *et al.* (2004) Cognitive outcomes of preschool children with prenatal cocaine exposure. *JAMA* **291**, 2448–2456.

Slotkin, T.A. (2004) Cholinergic systems in brain development and disruption by neurotoxicants: nicotine, environmental tobacco smoke, organophosphates. *Toxicology and Applied Pharmacology* **198**, 132–151.

Sonuga-Barke, E.J. *et al.* (2010) vii. Physical growth and maturation following early severe institutional deprivation: do they mediate specific psychopathological effects?. In: *Deprivation-Specific Psychological Patterns: Effects of Institutional Deprivation*, pp. 143–166. Monographs of the Society for Research in Child Development, Oxford.

Stein, Z.A. *et al.* (1975) *Famine and Human Development: The Dutch Hunger Winter of 1944–1945.* Oxford University Press, New York.

Steiner, M. (2012) Prenatal exposure to antidepressants: how safe are they? *American Journal of Psychiatry* **169**, 1130–1132.

Stevens, H.E. *et al.* (2013) Prenatal stress delays inhibitory neuron progenitor migration in the developing neocortex. *Psychoneuroendocrinology* **38**, 509–521.

Sulik, K.K. *et al.* (1981) Fetal alcohol syndrome: embryogenesis in a mouse model. *Science* **214**, 936–938.

Susser, E. *et al.* (1996) Schizophrenia after prenatal famine: further evidence. *Archives of General Psychiatry* **53**, 25–31.

Susser, E. *et al.* (1998) Neurodevelopmental disorders after prenatal famine: the story of the Dutch famine study. *American Journal of Epidemiology* **147**, 213–216.

Suter, M.A. *et al.* (2013) Maternal smoking as a model for environmental epigenetic changes affecting birthweight and fetal programming. *Molecular Human Reproduction* **19**, 1–6.

Taub, E. *et al.* (2002) New treatments in neurorehabilitation founded on basic research. *Nature Reviews Neuroscience* **3**, 228–236.

Tobi, E.W. *et al.* (2009) DNA methylation differences after exposure to prenatal famine are common and timing-and sex-specific. *Human Molecular Genetics* **18**, 4046–4053.

Tobi, E.W. *et al.* (2012) Prenatal famine and genetic variation are independently and additively associated with DNA methylation at regulatory loci within IGF2/H19. *PLoS One* **7**, e37933.

Tottenham, N. & Sheridan, M.A. (2010) A review of adversity, the amygdala and the hippocampus: a consideration of developmental timing. *Frontiers in Human Neuroscience* **3**, 1–18.

Tottenham, N. *et al.* (2010) Prolonged institutional rearing is associated with atypically large amygdala volume and difficulties in emotion regulation. *Developmental Science* **13**, 46–61.

Tremblay, L.K. *et al.* (2005) Functional neuroanatomical substrates of altered reward processing in major depressive disorder revealed by a dopaminergic probe. *Archives of General Psychiatry* **62**, 1228–1236.

Valentino, R.J. *et al.* (2012) Molecular and cellular sex differences at the intersection of stress and arousal. *Neuropharmacology* **62**, 13–20.

Vuoksimaa, E. *et al.* (2010) Decreased prevalence of left-handedness among females with male co-twins: evidence suggesting prenatal testosterone transfer in humans? *Psychoneuroendocrinology* **35**, 1462–1472.

Weikum, W.M. *et al.* (2012) Prenatal exposure to antidepressants and depressed maternal mood alter trajectory of infant speech perception. *Proceedings of the National Academy of Sciences* **109**, 17221–17227.

Will, B. *et al.* (2004) Recovery from brain injury in animals: relative efficacy of environmental enrichment, physical exercise or formal training (1990–2002). *Progress in Neurobiology* **72**, 167–182.

Woollett, K. *et al.* (2010) Talent in the taxi: a model system for exploring expertise. In: *Autism and Talent.* (eds F. Happé & U. Frith), pp. 89–104. Oxford University Press, Oxford & New York.

Yang, Y. *et al.* (2012) Abnormal cortical thickness alterations in fetal alcohol spectrum disorders and their relationships with facial dysmorphology. *Cerebral Cortex* **22**, 1170–1179.

Zuckerman, B. *et al.* (1989) Effects of maternal marijuana and cocaine use on fetal growth. *New England Journal of Medicine* **320**, 762–768.

CHAPTER 24

Genetics

Matthew W. State[1] and Anita Thapar[2]

[1] Department of Psychiatry, Langley Porter Psychiatric Institute, University of California, San Francisco, CA, USA
[2] Child and Adolescent Psychiatry Section, Institute of Psychological Medicine and Clinical Neurosciences, Cardiff University School of Medicine, Cardiff University, UK

Introduction

The past few years have heralded a new era in psychiatric genetics. After several decades of halting progress, a phase of steady and rapid advance is leading to consensus on a range of issues, including the identification of specific risk genes. These discoveries are paving the way for a deeper understanding of population risks, molecular, cellular and circuit-level mechanisms underpinning psychiatric pathophysiology and identification of novel treatment targets.

It is clear that identified genetic factors typically operate in a probabilistic fashion, increasing the risk for, rather than determining symptoms. Moreover, identical genetic mutations may lead to a range of psychiatric outcomes, defying the current psychiatric diagnostic nosology. These complexities, coupled with the rapid pace of gene discovery, mean that practicing clinicians will need to remain up to date on the basics of genetics and recent progress.

DNA, genes and chromosomes

DNA

The human genome is composed of DNA, deoxyribonucleic acid, which is in turn comprised of a sugar phosphate backbone and four nitrogenous bases: adenine (A), thymine (T), guanine (G), and cytosine (C). The structure of DNA is the well-known double helix: at each base position in the DNA code, there is both a base and a specific complementary base forming a "base-pair" (Figure 24.1). In human cells, the majority of hereditary material is carried in the nucleus and is referred to as the nuclear genome. It is ~3 billion bases long when counted end to end and contains about 21,000 genes. Human cells also contain a much smaller mitochondrial genome (~17,000 bases) in a single double stranded circular DNA molecule that is inherited through the maternal line.

Genes

The definition of a gene continues to be refined. In the late 1950s, a gene was conceptualized as a DNA sequence that was transcribed into a messenger ribonucleic acid (mRNA) and then translated into a protein (Figure 24.1). However, as the understanding of genomics has advanced, numerous exceptions to this definition have been identified. For example, DNA sequences may lead to transcribed RNA that is not translated into protein but has important biological functions nonetheless. Thus, a more contemporary notion of a gene is a code contained within the nucleic acid that gives rise to a functional product.

The characterization of all DNA elements and their function, including what was previously thought to be "junk DNA" between genes, is the goal of the international collaboration ENCODE (http://genome.ucsc.edu/encode/). However, for the sake of the current discussion, we focus largely on genes that code for proteins. These comprise only about 1% of the genome (~30,000,000 bases) and are collectively referred to as the "exome." Individual genes include multiple component parts (Figure 24.1). In addition, upstream of protein-coding genes are classical "promoter" elements that regulate gene expression. There are also regulatory regions widely distributed throughout the genome that can result in increased gene expression (enhancers), decreased gene expression (silencers), or provide boundaries between these two types of elements (insulators). In addition, DNA sequences, often in the 3′ untranslated region (UTR; Figure 24.1), that bind to small RNA molecules, called microRNAs, can regulate gene expression.

Chromosomes

The human genome is organized into 23 pairs of chromosomes. Each nuclear chromosome pair consists of one from the paternal lineage and the other from the maternal line. Pairs 1–22 are referred to as "autosomes," numbered from largest to smallest based on the length of the DNA strand. There is also one pair

Rutter's Child and Adolescent Psychiatry, Sixth Edition.
Edited by Anita Thapar and Daniel S. Pine, James F. Leckman, Stephen Scott, Margaret J. Snowling, Eric Taylor.
© 2015 John Wiley & Sons Ltd. Published 2018 by John Wiley & Sons Ltd.

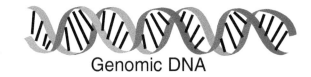

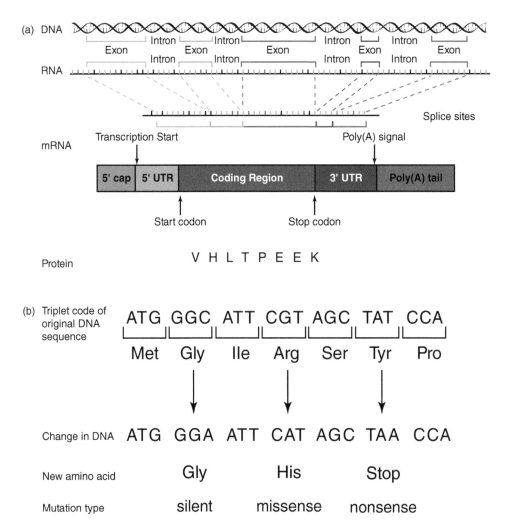

Figure 24.1 *DNA, Transcription, and Translation*

(a) The double helix structure of DNA is shown at the top. The translation of DNA to RNA to protein is diagrammed moving from top to bottom. The majority of human genes consist of multiple "exons"; segments of DNA that contain a series of three-letter nucleotide codes (codons) that specify individual amino acids. These are interspersed among "introns," which do not specify amino acids. The central dogma is that DNA (a) is transcribed into RNA and then translated into protein. In transcription, introns are spliced out of the gene, leading to the specification of a full-length mRNA that encodes a specific protein. In addition to the "coding portion" of the gene, additional sequence motifs are present in the DNA and remain in the mRNA including a region immediately upstream of a translation start site, known as the 5′ untranslated region (UTR) and a region just beyond the "stop codon" specifying the termination of translation. These regions are known to be involved in the regulation of gene expression. (b) Variations in the genetic code may lead to several classes of amino acid "substitutions." As the genetic code contains redundancies, some changes in the code of the DNA will not result in an amino acid change (GLY to GLY in the diagram). This is referred to as a "silent" mutation. When a nucleotide change alters one amino acid to a different amino acid, this is known as a "missense" mutation (ARG to HIS in the diagram). When a change in sequence results in the code for an amino acid changing to a termination (or stop) codon, the mutation is referred to as a nonsense mutation. Amino acid abbreviations: V = valine; H/his = histidine; L = leucine; T/tyr = tryrosine; P/pro = proline; E = glutamic acid; K = lysine; Met = methionine; gly = glycine; Ile = isoleucine; arg = arginine; ser = serine.

of sex chromosomes (X and Y). Mitochondrial chromosome is transmitted via the maternal line.

Chromosomes also contain proteins called histones around which the DNA is coiled. This combination of DNA and protein is referred to as chromatin. The compactness of the chromatin varies throughout the cell cycle. Chromosomes are particularly tightly condensed during metaphase, which renders them visible under the light microscope, as is seen in the typical karyotype. The degree of coiling or condensation of chromatin may be regulated, via a number of processes, including (but not limited to) chemical modification of the DNA through methylation, as well as histone protein modification, via acetylation, methylation, and phosphorylation. These processes regulate gene expression in part by regulating the "access" of the transcriptional and regulatory machinery to the DNA, and play a key role in epigenetics (see Chapter 25). These epigenetic mechanisms also contribute to genomic imprinting whereby the expression of a given gene or genes is silenced depending on the parent of origin; defects in this process can result in a range of important disorders such as Prader Willi syndrome (see Chapter 54).

Genetic variation and its detection

Genetic variation

Any two individuals are identical across ~99% of their genetic material. It is the 1% of the genome that varies that is a main preoccupation of those interested in disease risk, with the key question being how the DNA among affected individuals varies from those who are not at risk.

There are several important categories of variation. It has long been known that the sequence of the DNA varies between individuals. However, the fine structure of chromosomes also commonly varies between individuals. Indeed, genomes contain many regions, consisting of a thousand to several million bases of DNA, that are either missing or increased in the number of copies relative to a reference genome (Figure 24.2). When these changes remain below the level of detection afforded by the light microscope, they are referred to as copy number variants (CNVs).

A second important characteristic of DNA variation, whether sequence or structural, is its frequency in the population: variation is considered common when it exceeds an arbitrary threshold (typically 1% of individuals). Conversely, variation that does not reach this frequency is termed rare. These categories turn out to be relevant biologically. As a rule of thumb, variation that is common in the genome tends to carry smaller biological effects relative to variation that is rare in the genome (Figure 24.3).

It is also useful to review the nomenclature describing the frequency of variation: Single base changes in DNA present in more than 1% of a reference population are typically referred to as single nucleotide polymorphisms (SNPs). Rare single base changes are often referred to as single nucleotide

variants (SNVs). Changes in copy number variation common in the population are sometimes referred to as copy number polymorphisms (CNPs) as opposed to CNVs, which is a term most often used to refer to rare structural variation.

A third important distinction revolves around the temporal origin of the genetic variation. A variation present in a prior generation and passed from that generation to the next is termed "transmitted" variation. In contrast, in the generation in which a mutation first occurs, it is referred to as a "*de novo.*" If a spontaneous mutation occurs in a germ cell (egg or sperm) prior to conception and that egg or sperm is fertilized, then the mutation would lead to "germ line" *de novo* variation in the offspring. It will be present in every offspring cell but will not be detectable in their parents. Alternatively, if the mutation arises post conception, this somatic mutation is not present in every cell of the individual. Finally, when a somatic mutation occurs in the parent germ line and is not detectable more generally in the parent, it is referred to as a germ line mosaicism. This may lead to more than one child in a family with what appears to be a germ line *de novo* mutation.

Detecting variation

Currently, three broad types of DNA assays are in wide use. These include genotyping, sequencing, and copy number variation detection.

Genotyping evaluates for the presence or absence of a known genetic (typically sequence) variation. Initially, due to technological hurdles, genotyping assays involved one or a small number of SNPs, placing practical limits on the number of variations that could reasonably be assayed in a given experiment. However, the development of microarray technology resulted in the dramatic expansion of genotyping capacity, allowing currently, the simultaneous testing of millions of SNPs rapidly and at low cost.

DNA sequencing, in contrast to genotyping, involves the elaboration of the genetic code at each position in the genome, without the requirement of knowing, in advance, the identity of the base in the reference genome or the range of possible variations. The details of "next generation sequencing" are beyond the scope of this chapter. In 2013, it is now routine to sequence all 30,000,000 bases in the human exome for less than $1000 per person, a price point that is considered an approximate upper limit for feasible large-scale studies supported by traditional funding mechanisms. The cost of sequencing the entire 3 billion bases in the human genome is rapidly approaching this threshold.

Chromosomal copy number is currently typically evaluated either by comparative genomic hybridization (CGH) or genotyping microarrays (Figure 24.2). Importantly, both approaches infer copy number states from fluorescence signal in a way that, particularly for detection of *de novo* variation, often requires confirmation via an alternative method.

Next generation sequencing technology can also be used to assay copy number. These sequencing methods involve oversampling of DNA data to ensure that a complete picture

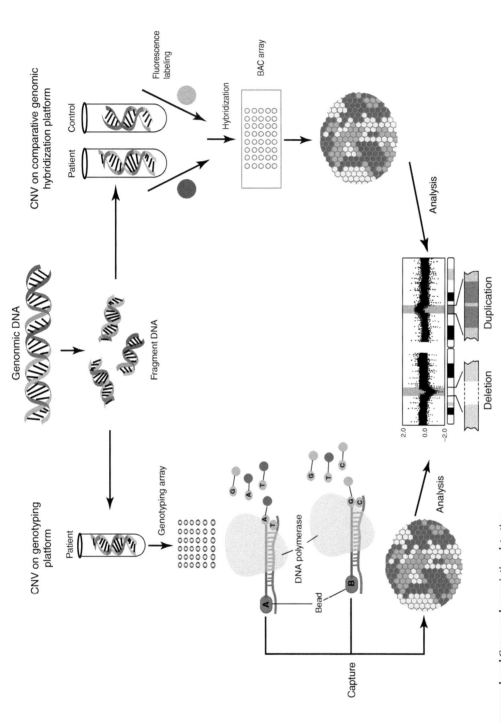

Figure 24.2 Microarray-based Copy number variation detection

Two commonly used methods for the detection of copy number variation are diagrammed. On the left, the use of a genotyping approach is shown. In this method, DNA only from a patient is used. Sheared DNA is prepared and hybridized to synthetic oligonucleotides maintained on a solid substrate (a microarray of beads in this figure). These synthetic nucleotides are specific sequences that bind to cognate sequences in the patient DNA. A single base reaction then takes place in the presence of fluorescently labeled nucleotides. The incorporation of a given nucleotide base leads to the incorporation of a distinct fluor depending on the sequence of the patient DNA at that position. Consequently, this platform provides genotyping data. In addition, there are many copies of each synthetic oligonucleotide on the array. The amount of input DNA from the patient can be inferred by the strength of the fluorescence signal that results. The signal is compared to a large group of controls that have been genotyped on the array. This signal strength for the subject is displayed relative to that from the group control (shown at the very bottom of the diagram). The right side of the figure shows a comparative genomic hybridization array. In this method, sheared patient and control DNA (either an individual or a group of controls) is prepared and hybridized to an array containing segments of the human genome (currently, typically carried in bacterial artificial chromosomes (BACs)). Patient and control are tagged with different fluorescence probes. The relative amounts of the patient signal and the control signal are then determined. An increase in patient signal is predicted to be a duplication or further amplification of the DNA copy number, and a relative paucity of patient DNA is inferred to be a deletion. For both types of assays, the inferences from the relative fluorescences signal may be subject to some confirmatory process either through a repeat or alternative assay.

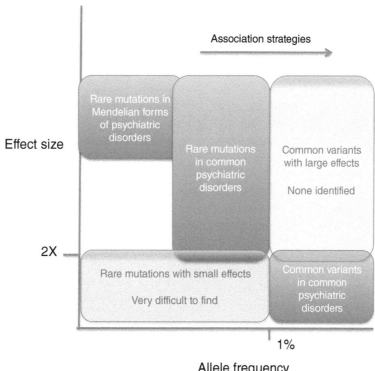

Figure 24.3 *Allele Frequency and Effect Size*

The figure provides an overview of the relationship between allele frequency and effect size in human disease, in this case psychiatric illness. Examples of Mendelian forms of psychiatric phenotypes have been identified in which a single gene is very strongly related to a specific definable phenotype. These involve very rare mutations generally carrying large effects. Their contribution to population risk for psychiatric disorders is limited. However, gene identification in these circumstances may provide avenues to identify molecular mechanisms relevant for more common forms of a disorder. Rare mutations have also been identified increasingly in common forms of psychiatric conditions. These have generally been found to confer intermediate risks and to do so in a probabilistic fashion (as shown in the diagram). Finally, specific common variations have been found to carry risk for several common psychiatric conditions, including schizophrenia and bipolar disorder and are highly suspect, but not yet confirmed, in others including autism, ADHD, and depression. These alleles are, by definition, common in the population and so far have been found to confer very small risks. Given the theoretical ease of finding common variants carrying large risks, the absence of such findings suggests that few, if any, of these types of variations will be found contributing to common psychiatric disorder. In a similar vein, rare variants carrying small risks may be relevant for psychiatric illness, but are likely to be impossible to find given limits on sample size.

of genetic variation is captured for every base. The number of "reads" produced for each interval is proportional to the amount of starting material in the reaction. Consequently, both read "depth" as well as an analysis of changes in the sequence output relative to a reference genome, can provide information regarding copy number changes as well as chromosomal rearrangements (e.g., inversions and translocations)—something that most common array-based CNV methods cannot detect.

Relating Genes to Behaviors

Genetic epidemiology

In traditional genetic epidemiological designs, the contribution of genetic factors is inferred rather than directly measured. This is achieved by assessing phenotype similarity between individuals who differ in genetic relatedness. A significant genetic contribution for a given trait or disorder is inferred when there is greater similarity between those who are more

closely genetically related versus those who are less closely related or unrelated. These traditional designs were initially important in demonstrating the contribution of familial and genetic influences to different psychiatric disorders. Subsequently they have proven useful for assessing a broader set of questions, for example, to test causal environmental risks (see Chapter 12), and gene–environment interplay (Rutter, 2012). More recently, traditional designs are being used to investigate biological questions (van Dongen *et al.*, 2012); for example, the contributions of DNA and epigenetic variation.

Family studies

These involve investigating whether the relatives of those with a given disorder show an increased rate of that disorder when compared with relatives of controls. These early studies demonstrated that psychiatric disorders show familial clustering although the magnitude varies for different disorders. For example, relative risks of a first-degree relative (e.g., parent, child, sibling) having the same disorder as the proband are around 2–4 for child and adolescent depression (Rice *et al.*, 2002), around 2–8 for ADHD (Attention Deficit Hyperactivity Disorder; Thapar *et al.*, 2012) and rates of recurrence in siblings of those with autism are around 25 times higher than in the general population (Devlin & Scherer, 2012).

Challenges with regard to developing precise estimates of familial risk include changing estimates of population prevalence over time, difficulties in establishing precise diagnostic boundaries, and taking into account phenotypes that may either emerge or change in character across development. The patterns of familial transmission observed in early family studies paved the way for modern molecular genetic studies and showed that psychiatric disorders, like other common diseases, were complex and multifactorial in origin.

Relatives share environments as well as genes. Consequently, family studies are unable to distinguish whether any observed aggregation is a consequence of shared environmental exposures or shared genetic risks. Twin and adoption study designs are thus a critical complement to help distinguish genetic and environmental influences.

Twin designs

The twin design is based on the premise that monozygotic (MZ) twins are genetically identical, whereas dizygotic (DZ) twins share on average 50% of their genes. A genetic contribution to a trait or disorder (phenotype) is inferred where MZ twins show greater similarity than DZ twin pairs for the phenotype in question. This similarity is indicated by higher MZ than DZ correlation coefficients for trait measures, and significant MZ–DZ differences in proband-wise concordance rates for categorical measures.

Data from such studies can be used to disaggregate phenotype variation (Falconer, 1989) in a given population into variance that is attributable to genetic influences (G) that will include additive (A) and nonadditive (D) contributions, shared or common environment (C) and nonshared environmental (E) factors. The nonshared environment component will also include measurement error and contributions from stochastic events. Traditionally, twin studies cannot simultaneously test C and D and are much better powered to detect G than C. Twin studies can be extended to include other types of relatives; for example, biological siblings, half siblings, and step siblings.

The proportion of total phenotypic variation explained by genetic factors is known as heritability (h^2), a quantity about which there is a good deal of misunderstanding (Tenesa & Haley, 2013). Heritability is a population attribute; it refers to differences *between* people from a given population. For example, the high heritability estimates (80–90% in some studies) for autism and ADHD do not mean that 80–90% of an individual's ADHD or autism is explained by genes. For example, if a population was universally exposed to the critical environmental risks, then there would be very little environmental variance and heritability estimates would accordingly be high.

The disparity between high h^2 estimates for many common psychiatric conditions and the amount of variance captured via genome-wide association studies has been the subject of much discussion (Lee *et al.*, 2011). There are many potential explanations for this so-called "missing heritability." Potential factors include the contribution of rare variation, which may not be detected in current studies of common variation; the likely importance of nonadditive genetic influences including epistasis (gene–gene interaction); the contribution of environmental risks (gene–environment correlation and interaction) (discussed later), and an overestimation of heritability from twin studies.

The strength of the twin design is that it can be used for multiple purposes beyond simply testing whether a disorder or trait is heritable. For example, many forms of psychopathology can be usefully viewed as dimensions as well as categorical disorders. Twin findings further suggested that genetic risks for many psychiatric disorders influence variation in trait measures of these phenotypes in the general population and that these operate across the spectrum of severity (Rutter, 2011; Thapar *et al.*, 2013).

Twin studies have also consistently shown that genetic risks operate beyond diagnostic boundaries and across diagnostic categories. In this case, recent molecular genetic findings are in keeping with this observation. The same common and rare genetic risk variants or sets of variants cross diagnostic boundaries (Cross-Disorder Group of the Psychiatric Genomics *et al.*, 2013). For example, twin studies have found that shared genetic contributions explain most of the comorbidity between different psychiatric disorders, while nonshared environmental influences appear to be more disorder specific (Lahey *et al.*, 2011).

A final major strength of twin study and other genetically informative designs is that by providing an indirect measure of genetic contributions, it becomes possible to test the effects of environment independent of associations that arise through genes. The uses of genetically informative designs in testing causal hypotheses in relation to environmental risks are described in Chapter 12.

It is nonetheless important to understand some of the limitations of twin designs. These include a reliance on MZ twins being genetically identical when there are differences between them, including post zygotic mutations and epigenetic variation. As a result, discordant MZ twin pairs are now being utilized not only to identify if measured aspects of environment contribute to psychopathology (see Chapter 12) but also to test whether biological markers such as epigenetic signatures distinguish affected and unaffected twins (van Dongen *et al.*, 2012). Another key assumption is that MZ and DZ twins share environment to the same extent. MZ twins likely have greater sharing of intrauterine influences and many later environmental risks will be shaped by genetically influenced dispositions, thereby also serving to inflate heritability estimates. For example, MZ twin similarity would be inflated through greater sharing of prenatal influences.

Adoption studies

In adoption study designs, the contribution of genetic factors is inferred when individuals show greater phenotypic similarity to their biological relatives than with their unrelated adoptive relatives. There have been three main variants of this design. First, there are the studies of adopted away offspring of parents with a psychiatric disorder. Early studies of this type showed a strong genetic contribution to schizophrenia that extended to risks for a broader "schizophrenia spectrum" (Tienari *et al.*, 2003). The second design focuses on individuals who have been adopted away and examining the rates of disorder in adoptive and biological relatives. These types of design have, for example, highlighted an important genetic contribution to ADHD (Thapar *et al.*, 2013) and shown that exposure to adoptive maternal depression contributes to adolescent depression (Tully *et al.*, 2008). Finally, cross-fostering designs are based on comparing rates of psychopathology in high genetic risk individuals who have been adopted away into low environmental risk families against the rates observed in (1) adoptees at low genetic risk, low adoptive environmental risk and (2) those at high genetic risk and who are exposed to high environmental adversity. Such studies are rare but have highlighted, for example, that while genetic liability is needed to manifest petty criminality, the risk effects are greatly magnified in those placed in adoptive homes with low social status (Cloninger *et al.*, 1982). Adoption studies provide a useful means of demonstrating gene-environment interaction that we discuss later.

Adoption studies also have their own set of assumptions and limitations (see Chapter 12). For example, the design is based on adoptive placements being nonselective. Adopted away children at genetic risk will likely also have been exposed to prenatal adversities influenced by biological maternal genetic dispositions and unless adoption takes place at birth, early environmental adversity provided by biological parents will also inflate phenotype similarities between biological relatives. Adoptive families tend to come from more advantaged backgrounds, thereby restricting the range of environmental exposures (Stoolmiller, 1999) and potentially reducing power to detect environmental contributions.

Approaches to gene discovery

Parametric linkage analysis

For many decades, parametric linkage has been the gold standard approach to gene discovery in disorders reflecting Mendelian inheritance, that is, an essentially one-to-one relationship between a particular mutation and a given disease or syndrome. Linkage is based on the idea that the position within the genome of an unknown disease mutation may be found by examining the transmission of known genetic variations (or markers) in an affected family or group of families. If the unknown disease-causing variant is sufficiently close to a known marker, these variants will very frequently be inherited together despite homologous recombination and are thus termed "linked."

Parametric linkage involves *a priori* hypotheses about the mode of inheritance (e.g., dominant, recessive, X-linked), the frequency of the disease mutation in the population (typically, very rare), the penetrance of mutation (i.e., what proportion of those with the mutation show the disease), and the frequency of phenocopies (i.e., what proportion of affected individuals show the disease who do not carry the sought after mutation). The genome is then examined for the inheritance of known markers within selected families and the probability of seeing the observed pattern of inheritance for each of these known markers under the model of linkage is compared to the probability of seeing the observed pattern under the null hypothesis. If a marker or markers that show a high probability of being linked are identified, this region or these regions of the genome are examined in more detail—using more markers to fine map the "linkage interval" or, more recently, via exome or genome sequencing—with the ultimate aim of identifying the rare disease-causing mutation.

Many mental disorders were originally thought likely to reflect Mendelian inheritance of one or a small number of disease genes. However, for the most part, psychiatric syndromes have subsequently been found to be the result of complex inheritance, involving many genes—both within the individual, as well as within the population—the contribution of nongenetic factors, and demonstrating a probabilistic relationship between having a mutation and any given phenotypic outcome. These characteristics have limited the usefulness of parametric linkage in psychiatric genetics.

However, a so-called "outlier" approach to gene discovery is based on the hypothesis that even within a genetically complex disorder or syndrome, there will be examples of simpler inheritance. Several of the earliest successes in psychiatric genetics involved taking just such an approach, including the identification of mutations in the gene Neuroligin 4X in autism spectrum disorder (ASD)(Jamain *et al.*, 2003). More recent applications of this approach have identified recessive mutations contributing to neurodevelopmental disorders (Morrow *et al.*, 2008).

Common variant / candidate gene studies

The combination of the failure of broader efforts at applying Mendelian approaches to psychiatric illness; a reconceptualization of psychiatric disorders as complex and likely involving common polymorphisms; and the relatively low cost of genotyping assays all led to a dramatic rise in candidate gene approaches. Initially, this involved identifying one or a small number of common variations or SNPs present in one or a small number of specific genes of interest. These variations were most often selected on the basis of biological plausibility and then assessed in some version of a case–control design to determine if the frequency of a specific variant (allele) was greater in affected individuals.

Such approaches were initially very attractive. From a conceptual standpoint, there is an understandable draw toward hypothesis-driven experiments. Moreover, the logistics of mounting a candidate gene association study were comparatively straightforward. Investigators were able to recruit tens to hundreds of affected individuals at one or a small number of sites. Genotyping assays were relatively inexpensive, and less computationally intensive than doing whole genome linkage analyses. Finally, there were a large number of biologically attractive candidates to evaluate, including multiple genes encoding components of neurotransmitter systems.

These investigations came to occupy a very large proportion of the psychiatric genetics literature. However, they suffered from a general lack of reproducibility (Hirschhorn *et al.*, 2002). The causes for these inconsistencies initially led to considerable debate. However, with the emergence of high-throughput parallel genotyping assays and the rise of so-called genome-wide association studies (GWAS), many of the sources for these early difficulties became readily apparent (Altshuler *et al.*, 2008).

Genome-wide association studies

GWAS focus on the contribution of common variation to common psychiatric disorders but take a hypothesis-free approach to gene discovery (Risch & Merikangas, 1996). The ability to do so was conditioned on the development of microarrays that allowed for the inexpensive and rapid detection of common polymorphisms at every gene in the genome. It became apparent that it would be necessary to evaluate multiple variations at any gene of interest to determine with confidence whether it played a role in a given phenotype. Consequently, the development of arrays capable to testing initially tens of thousands and now millions of SNPs simultaneously resulted in the ability to conduct a genome-wide, as opposed to a candidate gene, association study.

As this technology was employed, it became clear that the approach was capable of yielding highly reproducible results (Edwards *et al.*, 2005; Haines *et al.*, 2005; Klein *et al.*, 2005). Accordingly, in retrospect, the difficulties with prior candidate gene approaches became clear: first, the effect sizes hypothesized for most candidate gene studies were an order of magnitude or more higher than what eventually has been found to obtain for common variants; second, the likelihood of selecting, *a priori*, the correct variant(s) in the correct gene(s) turned out to be very low. Finally, any case and control cohort in GWAS or candidate gene association studies need to be matched for ancestral origin, a key confound in genetic association studies. It took the sequencing of the human genome and the development of high-throughput tools to reveal how sensitive case–control studies could be to occult differences in ancestry, and to provide the means to correct for this confound (Altshuler *et al.*, 2008).

The use of the GWAS approach, coupled with rigorous statistical thresholds that take into account the hundreds of thousands of comparisons being conducted simultaneously, has led to a spate of reliable and reproducible findings in psychiatric conditions, including schizophrenia and bipolar disorder. At the time of writing, for schizophrenia, 108 loci have been identified through GWAS but this has required around 40,000 cases and 40,000 controls (Schizophrenia Working Group of the Psychiatric Genomics Consortium, 2014). Several general observations from GWAS are notable: first, a substantial portion of the variation that has been found to be associated with disease risk maps to intergenic regions. This observation may be explained, at least in part, by a relative overrepresentation of noncoding common alleles on genotyping assays. However, the findings also raise the prospect of a prominent role for gene regulation in disease risk. Second, as noted earlier, the effect sizes for common alleles have been much smaller than anticipated. Associated loci rarely exceed a twofold increase in risk, and typically fall below a 50% increase.

These findings provide important data with regard to interpreting genetic association studies. As noted, the small effects, in retrospect, suggest that the majority of early candidate gene and candidate gene–environment interaction studies (see later) were dramatically under powered. In addition, the absence of statistically significant and reproducible GWAS results for some common complex psychiatric disorders, such as autism or Tourette's disorder, may still say less about the types of variation that contribute to disease risk and instead highlight the need to develop larger cohorts for these conditions; ones that rival those studied in schizophrenia.

Cytogenetics

The earliest efforts at rare variant discovery rested on either parametric linkage analysis, as described previously, or traditional cytogenetics. The study of chromosomal abnormalities has had considerable impact on psychiatric genetics. For example, the cloning of the fragile X gene, now appreciated to be associated with both autism as well as intellectual disability, was made possible by the observation of a chromosomal fragile site (Sutherland, 1977). Similarly Neuroligin 4X, a gene associated with autism risk, was discovered initially through the investigation of genomic intervals disrupted by chromosomal rearrangements (Jamain *et al.*, 2003).

Such investigations initially involved the light microscope and subsequently made use of fluorescent probes to increase resolution, an approach known broadly as molecular cytogenetics. However, these methods were largely restricted to fine mapping either one or a very small number of targeted chromosomal regions.

Copy number variation analysis

This limitation was eliminated, however, by the development of microarray technology and the identification of CNVs as part of typical human genetic variation. CNVs are now known to contribute risk of autism, schizophrenia, ADHD, and a range of other neurodevelopmental syndromes (Malhotra *et al.*, 2011).

It also became clear that copy number changes were not distributed randomly across the genome, but instead accumulated at particular regions in affected individuals, providing an avenue to identify specific chromosomal intervals, and in some cases specific genes, associated with disease (Kumar *et al.*, 2008; Marshall *et al.*, 2008; Weiss *et al.*, 2008).

Some early CNV studies focused on *de novo* copy number variation and so-called simplex families with only one clearly affected proband. These were based on the hypothesis that the apparently "spontaneous" emergence of a neurodevelopmental or neuropsychiatric phenotype in a family could be accounted for in some cases by a new mutation. This hypothesis was further supported by the reasoning that mutations carrying large effects, particularly for early-onset disorders, would be subject to "purifying" natural selection and would tend to be removed from the genome over generations (Figure 24.3). Indeed, for disorders in which CNVs have been found to play a role, the identification of *de novo* mutation has proved to be a particularly powerful means to identify associated loci, and overall these new mutations have been found to carry larger effects than either common or rare transmitted variation contributing to common psychiatric disorders (Malhotra & Sebat, 2012).

Next-generation sequencing

The rapid evolution of DNA sequencing over the past few years has now made possible the identification of rare and *de novo* mutations at single base resolution, across substantial portions of the genome. Two study designs have so far predominated, both focusing on rare mutations in exomes, either in traditional case–control cohorts or via the study of simplex families looking for *de novo* mutation. Both types of studies have evaluated the overall burden of mutations in comparison groups as well as the distribution of these mutations, looking for "recurrence." This refers to the identification of a *de novo* mutation in the same gene, as opposed to observing the precisely identical mutation.

Early applications have been quite productive. For example, in autism, the identification of recurrent *de novo* mutations that result in a loss of protein function has led to the identification of multiple associated genes (O'Roak *et al.*, 2011; Iossifov *et al.*, 2012; Neale *et al.*, 2012; O'Roak *et al.*, 2012; Sanders *et al.*, 2012).

An additional interesting observation (Iossifov *et al.* 2012; Neale *et al.*, 2012; O'Roak *et al.*, 2012; Sanders *et al.*, 2012; Kong *et al.*, 2012) has been that the rate of *de novo* single base mutations is strongly correlated with paternal age. This finding represents an important example, at the molecular level, of gene–environment interplay. In addition, it suggests that there are likely to be other environmental inputs that contribute to or protect against *de novo* mutation and consequently could influence the prevalence and population distribution of autism and other neurodevelopmental and psychiatric disorders.

Gene × environment interplay

Findings generated by traditional genetic epidemiological studies of psychopathology highlight that the effects of genes and environment are interdependent (see Chapter 23; Rutter, 2012). Environmental risks that are of the type most relevant to psychiatric disorder are not randomly allocated; they are shaped by genetically influenced dispositions and behaviors.

This is known as gene–environment correlation. The phenotypic manifestations of genetic liability captured indirectly through traditional studies or assessed at a molecular level depend on exposure to particular environmental conditions. Gene–environment interaction (G × E) is a well-established phenomenon in animal and plant genetics but has created more controversy in psychiatry. Whilst G × E has been more difficult to consistently detect at a molecular level in human studies, its importance is well established and undisputed for less complex organisms (Lehner, 2013).

Gene–environment correlation

Most types of environmental risks that have been considered important in relation to psychopathology, for example, adverse life events and quality of family relationships, have been found to be familial and heritable. This is unsurprising given that exposure to and perception of environmental risks are affected by genetically influenced attributes of parent and/or child (see Chapter 12). The correlation between parental genotype and environmental risks is known as passive gene–environment correlation. For example, a parent who has a genetic disposition toward being socially anxious, not only transmits risk genes to offspring but might, for example, also avoid situations that reduce socialization experiences for their children and magnify similar traits in their offspring. Passive gene–environment correlation effects (when postnatal in origin) are removed in adoption study designs. Genetically influenced attributes of children are also important as they shape environmental exposures, not only by seeking out experiences but also by evoking responses in others. These situations are considered as active and evocative gene–environment correlation. Adoption studies, for example, have found that this is important in relation to harsh discipline and negative parenting in adoptive parents of children who are genetically predisposed to being antisocial (as indexed by an antisocial biological parent). These environmental risks appear to be evoked by the children's behavior (Ge *et al.*, 1996).

There is now a wealth of literature highlighting that risk genes and environments often co-occur and show interdependence in this way.

Gene–environment interaction

In this chapter we consider G × E conceptually rather than as a statistical term. This phenomenon is where genetic predisposition, or a particular mutation or gene, only has risk effects or has much stronger risk effects in the presence of an environmental factor. Such a situation is much more easily assessed in experimental studies of organisms where the genetic background and environmental exposures are controlled by the researcher.

The situation is complicated in humans because we have to focus on phenotypes that are difficult to measure and complex in origin. Multiple genes and environmental risks are involved. Another issue is that whilst gene–environment interaction is a conceptual term, in observational studies, we rely on assessing statistical interaction that is not the same as biological interaction but does provide a start point (Rutter *et al.*, 2009). Also, it is impossible to exactly reproduce the same types of sample and control for multiple environmental exposures and genetic backgrounds.

Nevertheless, traditional genetic epidemiological studies have consistently highlighted that environmental risks do not have the same effects on all and that genetic and environmental risks work together. While family and twin studies have tested for gene–environment interaction (G×E), adoption studies have afforded an especially powerful means of investigating G×E. Such studies have found not only are those at higher genetic risk more likely to be exposed to environmental risks but the effects of environmental adversity appear to be stronger in genetically predisposed individuals. For example, family and twin studies of adults and adolescents have shown that the risk effects of life events are increased in those at increased genetic and familial risk of depression (Kendler *et al.*, 1995; Silberg *et al.*, 2001). As we have already discussed, adoption studies find that those at genetic risk of antisocial behavior appear to be much more sensitive to adverse rearing adoptive environments. Similar findings have been shown in adoption studies of schizophrenia.

As already mentioned, gene–environment interactions have been widely observed in organisms that are less complex than humans and other primates (Lehner, 2013). Thus, it is well recognized that the effect of a genetic mutation on a phenotype is influenced by exposure to a specific environmental condition or a specific environmental trigger (e.g., diet, exposure to pathogen). The environment can also influence interactions between genes and alter the phenotypic effect of mutations by changing other biological processes, for example, by altering proteins (Lehner, 2013).

However, while the rationale for studying G×E interactions is well established, human molecular genetic studies of gene–environment interaction have attracted controversy, largely due to concerns about the reliance on candidate gene strategies and the attendant confounds and limitations already noted. In addition, the challenge with regard to the identification and utilization of good measures of environment has also been highlighted (Rutter *et al.*, 2009; Caspi *et al.*, 2010).

A prime example of this controversy is a very highly cited finding regarding the risk for a depression based on the cross product of earlier experience and genotype (Caspi *et al.*, 2002). Specifically, a functional variant in the promoter region of the serotonin transporter gene was found to be associated with depression in the presence of life events. The findings have since been replicated in multiple studies, partly replicated and also nonreplicated by many. An initial meta-analysis found no evidence for association across studies (Risch *et al.*, 2009; Rutter *et al.*, 2009). However, a subsequent meta-analysis found significant evidence of gene–environment interaction and suggested that the key risk stemmed from exposure to early maltreatment (Karg *et al.*, 2011). Other studies have investigated alternative stress-related and behavioral phenotypes (Caspi *et al.*, 2010).

The back and forth regarding this study underscores the difficulties that have emerged as scepticism regarding candidate gene methodology has mounted. Indeed, the key issue is not whether this or other prior findings from candidate gene studies are "correct," but rather what types of evidence would be required at this point to confirm or refute these associations. Different investigators are likely to provide divergent answers. However, in general, it is reasonable to suspect that, just as GWAS has become the gold standard for identifying common variants contributing to common disorders, the rigorous application of genome-wide approaches will be an essential contributor to reaching a consensus on the interaction between common variation and environmental factors. The same issues are likely to apply to investigations of "differential susceptibility," whereby some individuals are more susceptible not only to environmental risks but also to potentially beneficial environmental conditions including those provided through intervention (Pluess & Belsky, 2013).

Pharmacogenetic/pharmacogenomics

All clinicians are familiar with the observation that individuals show considerable variation in their responses to pharmacological agents with respect to efficacy and side effects. Pharmacogenetic investigations aim to identify the genetic contributions to this variation in drug response that are a form of gene–environment interaction. There has been enormous interest in the idea of personalized medicine across the whole of medicine, whereby drug treatments are tailored to an individual according to biological and clinical profiles.

To date, most pharmacogenetic studies in psychiatry have involved candidate genes in neurotransmitter systems thought to be targeted by the pharmacological agent and involved in generating side effects (e.g., weight gain with atypical antipsychotic medication) or therapeutic responses. No strong, consistent findings have emerged. Other studies have dealt with genetic variation in pharmacokinetics that deals with drug metabolism; for example "slow" and "ultra-rapid" metabolizers of drugs metabolized by the enzyme CYP2D6. Consistent findings have so far been limited in psychiatry and one relevant issue here is that the efficacy of most psychotropic medications is not closely related to circulating plasma levels (Malhotra *et al.*, 2012).

For pharmacogenetics and other genetic studies of interventions to have clinical impact, genetic risks must have strong predictive value and replicate well across different populations. While it is theoretically possible that the genetic variants involved in responses to treatment and side effects have larger effect sizes than those that contribute to psychiatric phenotypes, there is little evidence so far to support this view.

Intermediate phenotypes

Investigating how genetic factors associated with psychiatric disorder might exert their risk effects can be conducted at many different levels. These span from the cellular and biological to encompass investigations of brain structure and function. Intermediate phenotypes such as cognitive and imaging measures have been viewed by some to represent biological substrates that might lie closer to genes than psychiatric diagnoses. For example in general medicine, cholesterol levels can be considered as an intermediate phenotype that lies along a causal risk pathway to ischemic heart disease. It is however difficult in psychiatry to determine if a hypothesized intermediate phenotype truly lies along a causal pathway. Such measures could, for example, simply reflect another aspect of the psychiatric disorder in question. Also, genetic variants have multiple pleiotropic risk effects on different brain/behavioral phenotypes. Genetic imaging and cognitive studies can nevertheless potentially provide some valuable insights into potential mechanisms and neural substrates that are influenced by genetic risks but that cross diagnostic boundaries. Intermediate phenotypes most commonly studied in psychiatry have involved cognitive and structural and functional imaging measures. Traditional genetic epidemiological studies have shown that most of these measures are heritable and for many, shared genetic influences contribute to their covariation or correlation with specific psychiatric disorders. Nevertheless, like psychiatric disorders, these sorts of phenotypes are still genetically complex and so far, there is little to suggest that their genetic architectures are simpler than those underlying psychiatric disorders. For example, recent very large-scale genetic studies of brain structure highlight that multiple genetic variants of very small effect size appear to contribute to phenotypic variation, appearing nearly identical to the types of findings seen in GWAS studies of categorical diagnoses.

Findings on how single genetic risk variants that have been found to be associated with a psychiatric phenotype relate to different neural measures are still at an early stage in terms of robust replications. While earlier studies utilized candidate genes that were not robustly associated with psychiatric disorder, more recent investigations are focusing on more strongly replicated genetic findings. For example, imaging has suggested that *ZNF804A*, a gene now known to be associated with schizophrenia, might be implicated in disrupting brain connectivity (Esslinger *et al.*, 2009).

Other studies are beginning to test the impact of common and rare risk variants on neural circuitry not only in humans but also using animal models. It is likely that the emergence of new techniques that enable improved characterization of neural circuitry and architecture (e.g., Chung & Deisseroth, 2013) (see Chapters 10 and 11) will be used in the future to further investigate mechanisms that mediate genetic risk effects.

Genetic testing

We conclude this chapter by considering clinical implications with regard to genetic testing and counseling. In most instances, the estimated recurrence rate of any psychiatric disorder has had to be estimated from family studies. This of course does not provide a risk estimate that is individually tailored. Molecular testing of individual and composite common genetic risk variants has so far been of limited predictive utility.

In contrast, it has long been accepted that when a rare chromosomal anomaly or syndrome is clinically suspected, the effects are more predictable and cytogenetic testing and/or targeted molecular investigation of that syndrome (e.g., tuberous sclerosis) is indicated. In the past few years, genome-wide chromosomal microarray clinical investigations have become routinely available in many countries. Potential benefits of testing individuals and their relatives for such mutations include an enhanced understanding of how the disorder has arisen, access to information and support groups for those with certain types of CNVs (e.g., 22q11 microdeletion), early recognition and treatment of medical conditions when known to be a feature of the mutation, and more individually tailored risk prediction estimates for those who wish. However, there are complexities with regard to accurately interpreting risks because CNVs are so highly pleiotropic and probabilistic in their effects. Moreover, there are multiple ethical issues that arise from identifying a mutation including potential stigma, discrimination, and family conflict; these require careful consideration and expert counseling (Gershon & Alliey-Rodriguez, 2013).

So, what does the child and adolescent mental health clinician need to do? We recommend that clinicians consult their local clinical genetics service and be familiar with national and local guidelines as there is considerable variation currently in recommendations for testing as well as the investigations and counseling resources available. Also, rapid changes in technology, its cost, and emergent findings mean that guidelines will inevitably change. For example, the American College of Medical Genetics and Genomics guideline revisions in 2013 (Schaefer *et al.*, 2013) highlight that for ASD, the diagnostic yield has risen from 6–10% a few years ago, to 30–40% because of advances in testing technology. They recommend that genetic testing should be discussed with all patients and families with ASDs. The current UK National Institute for Health and Care Excellence (NICE) guidelines on autism (see Chapter 51) suggest that genetic testing should only be routinely performed on those with dysmorphic features and/or intellectual disability but acknowledge technology is rapidly changing.

Overall, referral to clinical genetics services for investigation and counseling would likely be most appropriate for children with ID and for complex presentations of ASD, ADHD, or schizophrenia (i.e., accompanied by ID (intellectual disability), dysmorphic features, or a medical condition). Additional selection criteria will depend not only on genetic discoveries but also on consideration of how well placed local clinical genetics services are in interpreting risks and providing appropriate counseling. Moreover, these processes require a deeper understanding of the ethical implications, sensible use of limited resources, and consideration of clinical utility.

Summary: recent findings and changing conceptions

There is now the appreciation that a wide range of genetic variation can contribute to the same psychiatric phenotype (Figure 24.3). Moreover, it seems likely that the distribution of these classes of genetic variation is not uniform across all common psychiatric conditions. These observations suggest that the future success of gene discovery efforts will reflect a cross product of methodology, sufficient sample size, and the nature and distribution of the genetic risk for that phenotype.

A recent, conceptually challenging observation from both common and rare variant studies has been the wide range of phenotypic outcomes that have been related to the identical variation. Indeed, the means by which the identical variation may result in outcomes with very different natural histories and treatment responses is emerging as a major preoccupation. Perhaps the most important question emerging from these studies is why a genetic variation with such widely divergent outcomes will sometimes lead to no psychiatric phenotype at all.

Another notable observation is the extraordinary degree of genetic heterogeneity of psychiatric disorders. Estimates for genes contributing to ASD range from hundreds to as high as a thousand (Levy *et al.*, 2011; Sanders *et al.*, 2011; Iossifov *et al.*, 2012; Sanders *et al.*, 2012). So far, more than 100 common variant loci have been found to be associated with schizophrenia, with evidence of considerably more to be discovered (Lee *et al.*, 2012). These findings, along with the observations already noted, in which a single mutation may lead to a wide range of phenotypic outcomes, suggest that the study of individual mutations, one at a time, may not be sufficient to identify molecular mechanisms specifically relevant to a given disorder. Indeed, it is likely that it will be important to understand how, when, and where during brain development, multiple distinct mutations contributing to a given disorder converge (State & Sestan, 2012). Consequently, the application of systems biological approaches is likely to be increasingly relevant to making the transition for gene identification to the illumination of mechanisms of disease.

Fortunately, the tools necessary to make sense of findings are evolving as rapidly as the genomic tools that have made these discoveries possible. Traditional model systems, such as rodents, will continue to play a central role in linking genes to brain and behavior and the ability to manipulate these animal models is expanding dramatically (see Chapter 12). There are now a wide array of methods that allow for modeling temporally and spatially defined genetic alterations, ranging from conditional knock-outs to viral vectors to optogenetics. These advances have led to an unprecedented ability to manipulate and study specific neuronal cells and circuits. Moreover, the ability in model systems to recapitulate or correct specific mutations found in humans is being accelerated by the development of technologies that allow for the rapid introduction of highly specific mutations into the genome (Gaj *et al.*, 2013).

An equally exciting recent development facilitating the translation of genomic findings in psychiatry into an understanding of molecular mechanisms has been the evolution of induced pluripotent stem cells (IPSCs). IPSCs allow for the creation of specific neuronal cell types from a range of accessible human cells including skin fibroblasts, blood lymphocytes, and hair follicles. The attendant possibilities are numerous, from creating a neuronal cell from a patient with a given mutation and then correcting that mutation, to generating a series of disease-related mutations in a well-characterized so-called isogenic IPSC line, to implanting human neuronal IPSC lines into other model organisms to detect and study non-cell-autonomous effects.

Reliable and systematic methods to detect genetic risk factors for common psychiatric disorders are establishing a critically important foundation for the next generation of studies. Along with parallel advances in neurobiology, systems biology, computational sciences, and genetic epidemiology, the field is now poised to begin to elaborate the molecular-, cellular-, and circuit-level mechanisms of complex psychiatric illness and to clarify the complex interplay of environmental and genetic risk factors.

References

Altshuler, D. *et al.* (2008) Genetic mapping in human disease. *Science* **322** (5903), 881–888.

Caspi, A. *et al.* (2002) Role of genotype in the cycle of violence in maltreated children. *Science* **297** (5582), 851–854.

Caspi, A. *et al.* (2010) Genetic sensitivity to the environment: the case of the serotonin transporter gene and its implications for studying complex diseases and traits. *American Journal of Psychiatry* **167** (5), 509–527.

Chung, K. & Deisseroth, K. (2013) CLARITY for mapping the nervous system. *Nature Methods* **10** (6), 508–513.

Cloninger, C.R. *et al.* (1982) Predisposition to petty criminality in Swedish adoptees. II. Cross-fostering analysis of gene-environment interaction. *Archives of General Psychiatry* **39** (11), 1242–1247.

Cross-Disorder Group of the Psychiatric Genomics Consortium (2013) Identification of risk loci with shared effects on five major psychiatric disorders: a genome-wide analysis. *Lancet* **381** (9875), 1371–1379.

Devlin, B. & Scherer, S.W. (2012) Genetic architecture in autism spectrum disorder. *Current Opinion in Genetics and Development* **22** (3), 229–237.

van Dongen, J. *et al.* (2012) The continuing value of twin studies in the omics era. *Nature Reviews Genetics* **13** (9), 640–653.

Edwards, A.O. *et al.* (2005) Complement factor H polymorphism and age-related macular degeneration. *Science* **308** (5720), 421–424.

Esslinger, C. *et al.* (2009) Neural mechanisms of a genome-wide supported psychosis variant. *Science* **324** (5927), 605.

Falconer, D.S. (1989) *Introduction to quantitative genetics*, 3rd edn. John Wiley & Sons, New York.

Gaj, T. *et al.* (2013) ZFN, TALEN, and CRISPR/Cas-based methods for genome engineering. *Trends in Biotechnology* **31** (7), 397–405.

Ge, X.J. *et al.* (1996) The developmental interface between nature and nurture: a mutual influence model of child antisocial behavior and parent behaviors. *Developmental Psychology* **32** (4), 574–589.

Gershon, E.S. & Alliey-Rodriguez, N. (2013) New ethical issues for genetic counseling in common mental disorders. *Am J Psychiatry* **170** (9), 968–976.

Haines, J.L. *et al.* (2005) Complement factor H variant increases the risk of age-related macular degeneration. *Science* **308** (5720), 419–421.

Hirschhorn, J.N. *et al.* (2002) A comprehensive review of genetic association studies. *Genetics in Medicine* **4** (2), 45–61.

Iossifov, I. *et al.* (2012) De novo gene disruptions in children on the autistic spectrum. *Neuron* **74** (2), 285–299.

Jamain, S. *et al.* (2003) Mutations of the X-linked genes encoding neuroligins NLGN3 and NLGN4 are associated with autism. *Nature Genetics* **34** (1), 27–29.

Karg, K. *et al.* (2011) The serotonin transporter promoter variant (5-HTTLPR), stress, and depression meta-analysis revisited: evidence of genetic moderation. *Archives of General Psychiatry* **68** (5), 444–454.

Kendler, K.S. *et al.* (1995) Stressful life events, genetic liability, and onset of an episode of major depression in women. *American Journal of Psychiatry* **152** (6), 833–842.

Klein, R.J. *et al.* (2005) Complement factor H polymorphism in age-related macular degeneration. *Science* **308** (5720), 385–389.

Kong, A. *et al.* (2012) Rate of de novo mutations and the importance of father's age to disease risk. *Nature* **488** (7412), 471–475.

Kumar, R.A. *et al.* (2008) Recurrent 16p11.2 microdeletions in autism. *Human Molecular Genetics* **17** (4), 628–638.

Lahey, B.B. *et al.* (2011) Higher-order genetic and environmental structure of prevalent forms of child and adolescent psychopathology. *Archives of General Psychiatry* **68** (2), 181–189.

Lee, S.H. *et al.* (2011) Estimating missing heritability for disease from genome-wide association studies. *American Journal of Human Genetics* **88** (3), 294–305.

Lee, S.H. *et al.* (2012) Estimating the proportion of variation in susceptibility to schizophrenia captured by common SNPs. *Nature Genetics* **44** (3), 247–250.

Lehner, B. (2013) Genotype to phenotype: lessons from model organisms for human genetics. *Nature Reviews Genetics* **14** (3), 168–178.

Levy, D. *et al.* (2011) Rare de novo and transmitted copy-number variation in autistic spectrum disorders. *Neuron* **70** (5), 886–897.

Malhotra, D. & Sebat, J. (2012) CNVs: harbingers of a rare variant revolution in psychiatric genetics. *Cell* **148** (6), 1223–1241.

Malhotra, D. *et al.* (2011) High frequencies of de novo CNVs in bipolar disorder and schizophrenia. *Neuron* **72** (6), 951–963.

Malhotra, A.K. *et al.* (2012) Pharmacogenetics in psychiatry: translating research into clinical practice. *Mol Psychiatry* **17** (8), 760–9.

Marshall, C.R. *et al.* (2008) Structural variation of chromosomes in autism spectrum disorder. *American Journal of Human Genetics* **82** (2), 477–488.

Morrow, E.M. *et al.* (2008) Identifying autism loci and genes by tracing recent shared ancestry. *Science* **321** (5886), 218–223.

Neale, B.M. *et al.* (2012) Patterns and rates of exonic de novo mutations in autism spectrum disorders. *Nature* **485** (7397), 242–245.

O'Roak, B.J. *et al.* (2011) Exome sequencing in sporadic autism spectrum disorders identifies severe de novo mutations. *Nature Genetics* **43** (6), 585–589.

O'Roak, B.J. *et al.* (2012) Sporadic autism exomes reveal a highly interconnected protein network of de novo mutations. *Nature* **485** (7397), 246–250.

Pluess, M. & Belsky, J. (2013) Vantage sensitivity: individual differences in response to positive experiences. *Psychological Bulletin* **139** (4), 901–916.

Rice, F. *et al.* (2002) The genetic aetiology of childhood depression: a review. *Journal of Child Psychology and Psychiatry, and Allied Disciplines* **43** (1), 65–79.

Risch, N. & Merikangas, K. (1996) The future of genetic studies of complex human diseases. *Science* **273** (5281), 1516–1517.

Risch, N. *et al.* (2009) Interaction between the serotonin transporter gene (5-HTTLPR), stressful life events, and risk of depression a meta-analysis. *JAMA* **301** (23), 2462–2471.

Roffman, J.L. *et al.* (2008) MTHFR 677C -- > T genotype disrupts prefrontal function in schizophrenia through an interaction with COMT 158Val -- > Met. *Proceedings of the National Academy of Sciences of the United States of America* **105** (45), 17573–17578.

Rutter, M.L. (2011) Progress in understanding autism: 2007-2010. *Journal of Autism and Developmental Disorders* **41** (4), 395–404.

Rutter, M. (2012) Achievements and challenges in the biology of environmental effects. *Proceedings of the National Academy of Sciences of the United States of America* **109** (Suppl 2), 17149–17153.

Rutter, M. *et al.* (2009) Gene-environment interactions biologically valid pathway or artifact? *Archives of General Psychiatry* **66** (12), 1287–1289.

Sanders, S.J. *et al.* (2011) Multiple recurrent de novo CNVs, including duplications of the 7q11.23 Williams syndrome region, are strongly associated with autism. *Neuron* **70** (5), 863–885.

Sanders, S.J. *et al.* (2012) De novo mutations revealed by whole-exome sequencing are strongly associated with autism. *Nature* **485** (7397), 237–241.

Schaefer, G.B. & Mendelsohn, N.J. (2013) Professional practice and guidelines committee. Clinical genetics evaluation in identifying the etiology of autism spectrum disorders: 2013 guideline revisions. *Genet Med* **15** (5), 399–407.

Schizophrenia Working Group of the Psychiatric Genomics Consortium (2014) Biological insights from 108 schizophrenia-associated genetic loci. *Nature.* **511** (7510), 421–427.

Silberg, J. *et al.* (2001) Genetic moderation of environmental risk for depression and anxiety in adolescent girls. *British Journal of Psychiatry* **179**, 116–121.

State, M.W. & Sestan, N. (2012) Neuroscience. The emerging biology of autism spectrum disorders. *Science* **337** (6100), 1301–1303.

Stoolmiller, M. (1999) Implications of the restricted range of family environments for estimates of heritability and nonshared environment in behavior-genetic adoption studies. *Psychological Bulletin* **125** (4), 392–409.

Sutherland, G.R. (1977) Marker X chromosomes and mental retardation. *New England Journal of Medicine* **296** (24), 1415.

Tenesa, A. & Haley, C.S. (2013) The heritability of human disease: estimation, uses and abuses. *Nature Reviews Genetics* **14** (2), 139–149.

Thapar, A. *et al.* (2012) Depression in adolescence. *Lancet* **379** (9820), 1056–1067.

Thapar, A. *et al.* (2013) What have we learnt about the causes of ADHD? *Journal of Child Psychology and Psychiatry* **54** (1), 3–16.

Tienari, P. *et al.* (2003) Genetic boundaries of the schizophrenia spectrum: evidence from the Finnish Adoptive Family Study of Schizophrenia. *American Journal of Psychiatry* **160** (9), 1587–1594.

Tully, E.C. *et al.* (2008) An adoption study of parental depression as an environmental liability for adolescent depression and childhood disruptive disorders. *American Journal of Psychiatry* **165** (9), 1148–1154.

Weiss, L.A. *et al.* (2008) Association between microdeletion and microduplication at 16p11.2 and autism. *New England Journal of Medicine* **358** (7), 667–675.

CHAPTER 25

Epigenetics and the developmental origins of vulnerability for mental disorders

Michael J. Meaney[1,2] and Kieran J. O'Donnell[1]

[1] Ludmer Centre for Neuroinformatics and Mental Health, Douglas Mental Health University Institute, McGill University, Montreal, Canada
[2] Singapore Institute of Clinical Sciences, A*STAR, Brenner Centre for Molecular Medicine, Singapore

There are profound developmental origins for individual differences in mental health that extend over the lifespan. Maternal perinatal anxiety/depression, low socioeconomic status (SES) and child maltreatment, including emotional and physical neglect and abuse, all predict poor child and adolescent mental health. Importantly, child maltreatment not only predicts the risk for multiple mental disorders, but at least in the case of depression, also the severity and treatment response (Nanni et al., 2012).

An obvious question concerns the mechanism by which the effects of the early environment, including variations in parent–offspring interactions, are embedded in the molecular machinery that regulates genomic transcription (see Chapter 24). In this chapter we examine the evidence for the environmental epigenetics hypothesis, which proposes that the sustained effects of environmental conditions on gene expression are mediated by effects on the epigenetic mechanisms that regulate the transcriptional machinery. We also discuss the current status of translational research that examines the role of epigenetics in the context of the developmental origins of vulnerability for mental disorders in humans.

Parental influences

Studies with a remarkable range of species reveal profound parental influences on the phenotype of the offspring. Within evolutionary biology and ecology such parental effects are defined as instances in which the phenotype of the offspring is affected by that of the parent, independent of genetic inheritance. Such effects are considered as a primary mechanism for phenotypic plasticity (i.e., variation in genotype–phenotype relations). There are also examples of parental mediation where environment effects on the phenotype of the developing animals are directly regulated by parental signals. Such parentally induced variation in phenotype is considered to be adaptive (i.e., when the resulting phenotype enhances survival and reproduction). In the meadow vole, offspring growth, fur thickness and sexual maturation are influenced by the length of daylight experienced by the mother during the perinatal period, preparing her offspring for the approaching winter (Lee & Zucker, 1988; Lee, 1993). In the red squirrel, increased population density associates with greater offspring weight gain in the early postnatal period, which may enhance survival beyond the first year of life (Dantzer et al., 2013). Similarly, in the desert locust, maternal lifetime exposure to increased population density also has profound effects on the phenotype of her offspring. In areas of low population density, desert locusts produce cryptic, solitary offspring. In contrast, progeny from females exposed to high population density are more gregarious and demonstrate migratory behaviors, easing competition for resources in the local environment (Saiful Islam et al., 1994). Collectively, these examples serve to demonstrate the importance of environment-dependent parental signaling for offspring development, fitness and survival. The question arises as to the extent and mode of transmission of parental effects in humans, and their relevance for child development and vulnerability for later mental disorder.

Studies of children born to Holocaust survivors illustrate how early environmental adversity confers vulnerability for later mental health disorder. Yehuda and colleagues (2008) show an increased risk of posttraumatic stress disorder (PTSD) in children born to Holocaust survivors as a function of maternal, rather than paternal, PTSD. This group has also shown altered neuroendocrine function in children of Holocaust survivors, again more strongly associated with maternal PTSD, and most pronounced in children born soon after the Holocaust, suggesting some specificity for maternally mediated effects. Similar effects of maternal, rather than paternal, prenatal anxiety

Rutter's Child and Adolescent Psychiatry, Sixth Edition.
Edited by Anita Thapar and Daniel S. Pine, James F. Leckman, Stephen Scott, Margaret J. Snowling, Eric Taylor.
© 2015 John Wiley & Sons Ltd. Published 2018 by John Wiley & Sons Ltd.

and depression on child emotional/ behavioral development (O'Donnell *et al.*, 2013) and neuroendocrine function have also been reported (O'Donnell *et al.*, 2013) (see Chapter 5). Thus, the challenge includes not only that of understanding the immediate effects of the environment on parent–offspring interactions but also the persistence of such environmental influences on offspring development.

The critical assumptions for this parental signaling hypothesis are that (1) there is a systematic relation between the quality of the environment and the nature of the parental signal, (2) that the offspring have evolved the necessary mechanisms to respond to the parental signal, and (3) that the parental signal initiates the intracellular systems that reliably produce and maintain the specific phenotypic variation. Likewise, natural selection should favor offspring that are better able to decode accurately parental signals as a "forecast" of the conditions that lie ahead (see Hinde, 1986). Psychologists would suggest that the same argument extends to parental sensitivity (i.e., the ability to decode the signals from the offspring). We argue that the parental signaling implicit in the study of parental effects is widely apparent in studies of child development and that epigenetic mechanisms contribute to the biological embedding of parental signals. Here we introduce the topic of epigenetics and use examples from our studies in rodents to illustrate how epigenetic modifications to DNA can have lasting effects on gene transcription/expression and the phenotype of the organism. This is followed by a review of clinical epigenetic studies of relevance to child development and vulnerability to mental disorders. While this chapter focuses predominately on maternal care, and more broadly, the effects of early adversity, on epigenetic processes, it should be noted that there are other factors that may influence the epigenome across the lifespan. Examples include, but are not limited to, smoking and environmental toxins, psychotropic drugs, UV exposure and radiation, as well as several disease processes including cancer.

Epigenetics

Epigenetics, stemming from the Greek "*epi*" meaning "upon" and "*genetics*," refers to a series of chemical modifications to chromatin that regulate genomic transcription. Indeed, epigenetics has become largely synonymous with the study of transcriptional regulation, that is, the degree to which a gene is expressed or repressed.

For reasons of graphic simplicity, we often describe the organization of a gene as if the DNA were a linear molecule to which transcription factors (the proteins that read the DNA sequence and initiate gene expression) gain unimpeded access. The reality of protein–DNA interactions is very different. Figure 25.1 presents the classic crystallographic analysis of the organization of DNA (Luger *et al.*, 1997). DNA is commonly organized in a form that resembles beads lying along a string (Figure 25.2). The beads are nucleosomes comprised of ~146 base pairs wrapped around a core of histone proteins (Turner, 2001). The histones

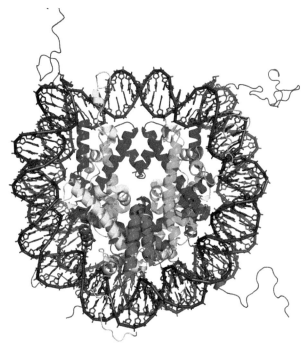

Figure 25.1 Nucleosome core particle.
Ribbon traces for the 146-bp DNA (grey double helix) wrapped around a single nucleosome consisting of eight histone proteins, with two copies of H2A (yellow), H2B (red), H3 (blue) and H4 (green). Histone tails, the sites of functional post-translational modifications, can be seen extending from the nucleosome core. (Source: www.commons.wikimedia.org/wiki/File: Nucleosome_1KX5_colour_coded.png).

and DNA together are referred to as chromatin; the nucleosome is the organization of chromatin.

Under normal conditions there is a tight physical relationship between the histone proteins and the accompanying DNA, resulting in a closed nucleosome configuration. This restrictive configuration is maintained, in part, by electrostatic bonds between the positively charged histones and the negatively charged DNA. The closed configuration impedes transcription factor binding and is associated with a reduced level of gene expression (Figure 25.2). Epigenetic modifications essentially favor a closed or open state of chromatin that either increases or decreases the ability of transcription factors to access regulatory sites on the DNA, which control gene transcription.

Chromatin modifications

The dynamic alteration of chromatin structure is achieved in part through covalent modifications to the histone proteins at the amino acids that form the histone protein tails extending out from the nucleosome (Figures 25.1 and 25.2). There are several examples of such modifications including, but not limited to, acetylation, phosphorylation, methylation and ubiquitylation (see Maze *et al.*, 2013). These modifications are achieved through a series of enzymes that bind to the histone tails and modify the local chemical properties of specific amino acids (Grunstein, 1997; Jenuwein & Allis, 2001). For example, the enzyme histone

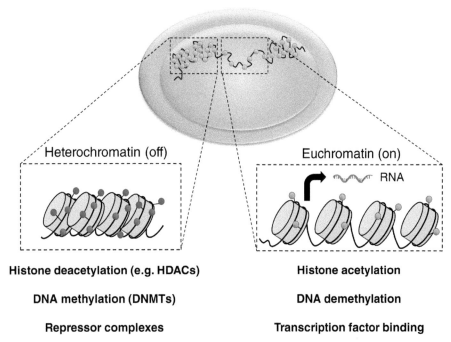

Figure 25.2 Chromatin dynamics and gene transcription.
DNA within a cell's nucleus coiled around histone proteins resembling beads on a string (upper panel: black lines/light blue circles). Increased repressive modifications to histone tails (red circles) and DNA methylation (dark blue circles) promote a closed conformation associated with gene inactivation (heterochromatin; lower left panel). Histone acetylation (green circles) and DNA demethylation associate with an open chromatin configuration, increased transcription factor binding and active gene transcription (euchromatin; lower right panel). DNMTs = DNA methytransferases, HDACs = histone deacetylases.

acetyltransferase "transfers" an acetyl group onto specific lysine amino acids on the histone tails. The addition of the acetyl group diminishes the positive charge, loosening the relation between the histones and DNA, opening the chromatin and improving the ability of transcription factors to access DNA sites. Thus, histone acetylation at specific lysine sites is commonly associated with active gene transcription. Nucleosomes in this open, permissive state are termed *euchromatin* (Figure 25.2).

The functional antagonists of the histone acetyltransferases are a class of enzymes known as histone deacetylases (HDACs). These enzymes remove acetyl groups and prevent further acetylation, thus maintaining a closed chromatin structure, decreasing transcription factor and gene expression. Both the acetylation and deacetylation of histones is a dynamic process that is regulated by environmental signals. Additional histone modifications, notably histone methylation, act less directly. Methylation can occur at multiple amino acid sites in the histone tails and then attracts protein complexes that mediate either the closure or opening of chromatin. Methylation or demethylation at individual sites is catalyzed by specific enzymes. Stability is an important feature of histone methylation; unlike acetylation, methylation marks can persist and have been shown to directly mediate the stable influence of environmental signals on gene transcription (Sun *et al.*, 2013).

DNA methylation

Another level of regulation occurs directly on the DNA. Indeed, the classic epigenetic alteration is that of DNA methylation, which involves the addition of a methyl group (CH_3) onto cytosines predominately bound to guanines (CpGs) in the DNA (Razin & Riggs, 1980; Bird, 1986). More recently non-CG methylation, occurring on cytosines usually followed by an adenine base, has been identified. Both CpG and non-CG methylation show dynamic change across human brain development and are relevant for the specification of neurons and glia (Lister *et al.*, 2013). As very little is currently known about non-CG methylation and mental health outcomes, this chapter focuses on CpG DNA methylation.

DNA methylation in the gene promoter, the regulatory region associated with the initiation of transcription, is typically associated with transcriptional repression. The repressive effect of DNA methylation on gene transcription appears to be mediated in one of two ways. First, wide swaths of densely methylated DNA preclude transcription factor binding to DNA sites, thus silencing transcription. The second manner is subtler, and probably far more prevalent in regions with more dynamic variations in gene transcription, such as the brain. In this case, the presence of the methyl group attracts a class of proteins known as methylated-DNA binding proteins (see Deaton & Bird, 2011). These proteins, in turn, attract an entire cluster of proteins that form a repressor complex, which includes active mediators of gene silencing. The HDACs (see preceding text) are a critical component of the repressor complex. HDACs prevent histone acetylation and favor a heterochromatin (closed) state that constrains transcription factor binding and gene expression (Figure 25.2 and see preceding text). DNA demethylation associates with a return to an open chromatin state that occurs subsequent to specific histone modifications (Weaver *et al.*, 2007).

Collectively, these modifications alter the structure and chemical properties of the DNA, and thus gene expression. As such, modifications to the DNA and its chromatin environment can be considered phenotypes which provide an additional layer of information on genomic function. Furthermore, unlike the underlying DNA sequence, which remains static across development, epigenetic modifications are dynamically regulated and responsive to changes in the environment. This is illustrated using the example of DNA methylation; however, it should be noted that other chromatin modifications also show dynamic change across development.

DNA methylation in development

DNA methylation patterns were once thought to be overlaid upon the genome only during early periods in embryonic development. Indeed, DNA methylation is considered a fundamental feature of cell differentiation. It is important to consider a simple feature of cell biology: all of the 300 or more cell types in the human body share the same DNA. Thus, the processes of cell specialization, whereby liver cells specialize in functions related to energy metabolism and brain cells establish the capacity for learning and memory, involve silencing certain regions of the genome in a manner that is specific for each cell type. Such processes define the function of the cell type. DNA methylation is considered a mechanism for the genomic silencing that underlies the cell specialization. Similarly, DNA methylation and other epigenetic mechanisms play a critical role in gene silencing during X chromosome inactivation (in females) and genomic imprinting. X inactivation is a mechanism to compensate for the greater number of genes found on the X sex chromosome relative to the Y sex chromosome. This results in the random silencing of one of the two X chromosomes in females (XX). X inactivation is implicated in childhood developmental disorders such as fragile X and Rett syndromes, which arise from the dysregulated expression of genes located on the X chromosome. Conversely genomic imprinting describes the silencing of one copy of a gene in a parent-of-origin fashion. Alleles which are "maternally imprinted" are silenced and thus "paternally expressed" and vice versa. Examples of imprinting-related disorders include Angelman and Prader–Willi syndromes arising from a cluster of imprinted genes on chromosome 15 (see Lee & Bartolomei, 2013; Keverne, 2014; and Chapter 54 for more information).

Such events, such as cell specialization and imprinting, occur early in development and are considered to be highly stable, such that de differentiation (whereby a cell loses its specialization) is rare, and often associated with organ dysfunction and pathology.

These developmental processes left the impression that under normal conditions DNA methylation occurs early in embryonic life and is irreversible. This perspective was further reinforced by findings showing that an alteration of DNA methylation at critical genomic targets (i.e., tumor suppressors) is associated with cancer (Hansen *et al.*, 2011).

At this point, dynamic changes in DNA methylation were of considerable interest for developmental biologists, but somewhat less so for mental health practitioners, who study the aftermath of more subtle variations in neuronal differentiation that occur in later periods of development or even in the fully mature brain. The studies reviewed here provide an important revision to this perspective.

There is now considerable evidence from neuroscience and other fields, including immunology and endocrinology, that the state of DNA methylation at specific genomic sites is indeed dynamic even in adult animals. Moreover, alterations in DNA methylation are emerging as the candidate mechanism for the effects of early experience in individual differences in neural function as well as in learning and memory. Thus, while the assumptions concerning DNA methylation appear valid for the examples cited, recent studies reveal that DNA methylation patterns are actively modified in mature (i.e., fully differentiated) cells, including, and perhaps especially, neurons, and that such modifications can occur in animals in response to cellular signals driven by environmental events. For example, variations in the diet of mice during gestation or later in development, such as the early post weaning period, can stably alter the methylation status of the DNA (Cooney *et al.*, 2002; Waterland & Jirtle, 2003). Likewise, both mature lymphocytes (Murayama *et al.*, 2006) and neural tissue (Martinowich *et al.*, 2003; Champagne *et al.*, 2006; Guo *et al.*, 2011; Herb *et al.*, 2012) show changes in the DNA methylation patterns at critical genomic regions in response to environmental stimuli that stably alter cellular function. The ability of environmental signals to actively remodel epigenetic marks that regulate gene expression is a rather radical change in our understanding of the environmental regulation of gene expression. Such epigenetic modifications are thus a candidate mechanism for the environmental "programming" of gene expression and, potentially, vulnerability to mental illness.

Studies of development are replete with examples of the environmental programming of gene expression. Such studies commonly report that a variation in the early environment associates with changes in gene expression and biological function that persists into adulthood and thus well beyond the duration of the relevant environmental event. In the rat, for example, prenatal nutrient deprivation or enhanced exposure to hormonal signals associated with stress stably alter, or program, the activity of genes in the liver and other sites that are associated with glucose and fat metabolism, including the gene for the glucocorticoid receptor (GR) (Gluckman & Hanson, 2007; Jirtle & Skinner, 2007; Meaney, 2007; Seckl & Holmes, 2007). These findings are assumed to represent instances in which the operation of a genomic region in adulthood varies as a function of early environmental influences. The results of recent studies suggest that such programming effects can derive from gene–environment interactions in early life that lead to a structural alteration of the DNA, which in turn mediates the effects on gene expression as well as more complex levels of phenotype. These studies were performed in rodents, but were inspired by the vast literature reporting the pervasive effects of family environment on health outcomes in humans (Repetti *et al.*, 2002).

Maternal regulation of stress reactivity in the offspring

Naturally occurring variations of maternal care in the rat are studied with simple, albeit time-consuming observations of animals in their home cages (Champagne *et al.*, 2003). One behavior, pup licking/grooming (LG), is highly variable across mothers. Dams for which the frequency of pup LG over the first week after delivery is 1 standard deviation (SD) > than the mean for the breeding cohort are designated as high LG mothers. Those for which the frequency of pup LG lies 1 SD < the mean are considered as low LG mothers. Such variations in the frequency of pup LG are highly stable over days and even across litters.

Pup LG is a major source of tactile stimulation for the neonatal rat that regulates endocrine and cardiovascular function in the pup (Hofer, 1984; Schanberg *et al.*, 1984; Levine, 1994).

The tactile stimulation derived from pup LG increases levels of growth hormone and decreases that of adrenal glucocorticoids. Together, these effects would be expected to promote somatic growth. The question then was whether such variations in pup LG might stably alter the development of individual differences in behavior and physiology.

Our findings revealed considerable evidence for the effect of maternal care on the behavioral and endocrine responses to stress in the offspring, as well as a range of associated phenotypes (Table 25.1). The male or female adult offspring of high LG mothers show more modest behavioral and endocrine responses to stress compared to animals reared by low LG mothers. Specifically, the offspring of high LG mothers show reduced fearfulness and more modest hypothalamic-pituitary-adrenal (HPA) responses to acute stress. Cross-fostering studies, where pups born to high LG mothers are fostered at birth to low LG mothers (and vice versa), or neonatal handling studies, which significantly increase maternal LG, reveal a direct relationship between maternal care and the postnatal development of individual differences in behavioral and HPA responses to stress (Francis *et al.*, 1999; Caldji *et al.*, 2000; Caldji *et al.*, 2003; Weaver *et al.*, 2004). In the cross-fostering studies, the rearing mother determined the phenotype of the offspring. Handling-induced increases in maternal LG also reverse the phenotypes associated

Table 25.1 Maternal postnatal licking and grooming (LG), offspring phenotype and reversal of maternal effects through cross-fostering or neonatal handling.

Measure/offspring phenotype	Maternal LG	Is it possible to reverse the maternal effect through cross fostering/neonatal handling?[a]
HPA-axis function/regulation		
ACTH response to acute stress	High < Low	–
CORT response to acute stress	High < Low	Yes, handling reduces the CORT response to stress
Hippocampal GR		
mRNA expression	High > Low	Yes, handling increases GR expression in offspring from low LG dams
Protein expression	High > Low	–
GC negative feedback sensitivity	High > Low	–
PVNh CRF mRNA expression	High < Low	Yes, handling decreases CRF in offspring from low LG dams
Fearfulness/Anxiety-like behavior		
Fear reactivity	High < Low	–
Novelty-suppression of feeding	High < Low	–
Contextual fear conditioning	High < Low	–
Open-field exploration	High > Low	Yes, reversed by cross-fostering
Learning and memory		
Morris water maze learning latency	High < Low	Yes, in part: low LG offspring raised by high LG dams show reduced latency. No cross-fostering effect in high LG offspring raised by low LG dams
Sexual maturation/behavior		
Vaginal opening	High > Low	–
Sexual receptivity (lordosis rating)	High < Low	Yes, in part: low LG offspring raised by high LG dams show improved decreased receptivity, no cross-fostering effect in high LG offspring raised by low LG dams

ACTH = adrenocorticotropic hormone; CRF = corticotropin releasing factor; CORT = corticosterone; GC = glucocorticoid; PVNh = hypothalamic paraventricular nucleus; HPA = hypothalamic pituitary adrenal; – = data not available.
[a] Neonatal handling significantly increases maternal LG to levels comparable with high LG dams.

with decreased maternal licking (Francis *et al.*, 1999). Thus, variations within a normal range of parental care can dramatically alter phenotypic development in the rat. It is nevertheless interesting to note that some of the phenotypic differences associated with variations in pup LG are only partly reversed with postnatal cross-fostering or neonatal handling (Table 25.1). These findings suggest possible *in utero* influences that have been confirmed at least with respect to the development of individual differences in hypothalamic-pituitary-ovarian function and sexual behavior in the female offspring (Cameron *et al.*, 2008; Borrow *et al.*, 2013) and metabolic function (Kappeler *et al.*, unpublished).

The differences in the HPA response to stress in the offspring of high and low LG mothers is mediated by a maternal effect on the expression of the GR gene (*Nr3c1*) in the hippocampus (Weaver *et al.*, 2004, Weaver *et al.*, 2007). The GR is a ligand-gated nuclear receptor, which, when bound by glucocorticoids (corticosterone in most rodents and cortisol in humans), is activated and translocated to the cell nucleus where it functions as a transcription factor that regulates gene expression. GR activation in the hippocampus associates with the activation of a negative-feedback signal that regulates corticotropin-releasing factor (CRF) expression in the hypothalamus. Since CRF serves to activate the pituitary-adrenal stress response, negative-feedback regulation serves to moderate the magnitude of the stress response. The offspring of high, compared with low LG mothers, show increased hippocampal GR expression, more efficient negative-feedback regulation of CRF, reduced hypothalamic CRF expression and more modest HPA responses to stress (Table 25.1).

Persistence is a critical feature of the maternal effects described. The differences in the frequency of pup LG between high and low LG mothers are limited to the first week of postnatal life. And yet the differences in gene expression and neural function are apparent well into adulthood. We hypothesized that maternal licking might activate intracellular signals that would lead to a stable epigenetic state on the region of the genome that regulates GR expression, thus serving to sustain the "maternal effect" on GR expression.

The focus of the epigenetic studies is the nerve growth factor-induced protein A (NGFI-A) binding site in exon 1_7, a specific coding region, of the GR gene promoter. Importantly, NGFI-A is a transcription factor that activates GR expression in hippocampal neurons. Pups reared by high LG mothers show increased NGFI-A expression in hippocampal neurons as well as an increased binding of NGFI-A to the exon 1_7 promoter sequence (Weaver *et al.*, 2007; Hellstrom *et al.*, 2012). Moreover, the binding of NGFI-A to the exon 1_7 promoter sequence is actively regulated by mother–pup interactions, such that there is increased NGFI-A bound to the exon 1_7 promoter immediately following a nursing bout, but not at a period that follows 25 min without mother–pup contact (Hellstrom *et al.*, 2012). This effect is mediated in part through the increased circulating levels of thyroid hormone (T3) in pups from high LG dams, which drives hippocampal serotonin (5-HT) activity and downstream effects

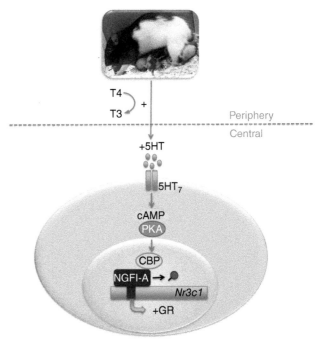

Figure 25.3 Maternal licking and grooming and demethylation of the glucocorticoid receptor gene in the hippocampus of her offspring. The tactile stimulation associated with pup licking and grooming leads to increased thyroid hormone (T3) conversion in the plasma of offspring from high LG dams. This increases levels of serotonin (5-HT, blue circles) within the hippocampus. Serotonin acts via 5-HT$_7$ receptors to activate an intracellular signaling cascade involving cyclic AMP (cAMP, light blue oval) and protein kinase A (PKA, dark blue oval). This culminates in increased binding of a CREB binding protein (CBP, light oval with navy border) and nerve growth factor inducible-A (NGFI-A, dark blue rectangle) complex with the NGFI-A binding site (dark blue square) in the promoter of the glucocorticoid receptor gene (*Nr3c1*). Binding of NGFI-A to its consensus binding site leads to the demethylation of a nearby methylated CpG (red circle) and increased expression of the glucocorticoid receptor (GR).

on NGFI-A signaling (see Figure 25.3). Binding of NGFI-A actively redesigns the methylation pattern at this region of the genome (Weaver *et al.*, 2004; Weaver *et al.*, 2007). Thus, as adults, the offspring reared by high LG mothers show very modest levels of methylation at the CpG close to the NGFI-A consensus sequence.

The demethylation of this CpG site occurs as a function of the same 5-HT-activated signals that regulate GR gene expression in cultured hippocampal neurons (Weaver *et al.*, 2007). Thus, when hippocampal neurons of embryonic origin are placed in culture and treated with 5-HT, which mimics the extracellular signal associated with maternal LG, this CpG site is demethylated; the binding of NGFI-A to the exon 1_7 site is critical. Hippocampal neurons that are rendered incapable of increasing NGFI-A show neither the demethylation of this CpG site nor the increase in GR expression (Weaver *et al.*, 2007). Likewise, a mutation of the NGFI-A site that completely abolishes the binding of NGFI-A to the exon 1_7 promoter also prevents the demethylation of this CpG. Finally, the infection of hippocampal neurons with a virus engineered to express high levels of

NGFI-A produces demethylation of this CpG in the exon 1_7 promoter sequence and increases GR expression. These findings provide evidence for transcription-factor-binding-dependent demethylation; however, the precise mechanism whereby the methylated cytosine is removed or modified to a demethylated state is still unknown.

In summary, the maternally induced changes in specific intracellular signals in hippocampal neurons can physically remodel the epigenome. The events described to date represent a model by which the biological pathways activated by a social event may become imprinted onto the genome. This imprint is then physically apparent in the adult genome, resulting in stable alterations (or programming) of gene expression. Importantly, our findings at the molecular level co-vary with marked and persistent differences in anxiety- and depressive-like behavior in these adult offspring, underscoring the influence of maternal care in early life on phenotypes of clinical relevance. Similar findings have been reported for other models of early life stress in rodents (Mueller & Bale, 2008; Murgatroyd et al., 2009) and non human primates (Provençal et al., 2012), demonstrating lasting maternal effects on the epigenome and the associated neurobehavioral phenotype of her offspring. The Murgatroyd study in particular parallels findings from our laboratory as it elegantly shows an influence of maternal separation on the expression of the hypothalamic vasopressin gene, which in turn regulates HPA responses to stress.

The human early environment and DNA methylation

The persisting effects of the early environment on DNA methylation were first documented in clinical studies of maternal undernutrition in the context of the Dutch Hunger Winter (see Chapter 12). Maternal periconceptual famine exposure was associated with decreased methylation of *IGF2*, an important regulator of metabolism, in prenatally exposed individuals (Heijmans et al., 2008). The results of these analyses are in line with rodent studies described earlier, which show a marked effect of maternal nutrition on epigenetic processes in her offspring. A critical question is whether familial influences operating during early development in humans are linked to the stable epigenetic regulation of gene expression in a manner comparable to that revealed in rodent studies, despite the multitude of environmental influences experienced during human development. Human studies using brain tissue collected from suicide victims have helped address this question.

Approximately a third of suicide victims have histories of childhood adversity, including childhood sexual and physical abuse, as well as parental neglect. At least two studies have shown decreased hippocampal GR expression in samples from suicide completers with histories of childhood maltreatment compared with controls (sudden, involuntary fatalities) (McGowan et al., 2009; Labonte et al., 2012). Forensic interviews that establish developmental history and mental health status of these suicide victims (Dumais et al., 2005; Zouk et al., 2006) showed that there was no significant correlation between major depressive disorder or substance disorders with hippocampal GR expression. Rather, the decreased hippocampal GR expression was associated with a history of childhood maltreatment. There were no differences in hippocampal GR expression in samples from suicides negative for a history of childhood maltreatment. Instead, the differences in hippocampal GR expression were unique to suicide completers with a history of childhood maltreatment. These expression differences correlated with differential DNA methylation patterns between groups in the corresponding exon 1 variant promoters. The exon 1_F sequence, of particular interest as it is the homologue of the rat exon 1_7, is highly expressed in the brain and contains an NGFI-A response element (Turner & Muller, 2005; McGowan et al., 2009). Moreover, the exon 1_F sequence shows increased DNA methylation and decreased NGFI-A binding in samples from suicide victims with a history of maltreatment. These findings bear considerable similarity to the maternal effect in the rat and are suggestive of early environmental regulation of the neural epigenome in humans. Recent studies in independent human samples investigating the effects of early environmental adversity on exon 1_F methylation reported consistent results (Radtke et al., 2011; Tyrka et al., 2012; and see later). In parallel, several studies have carried out genome-wide analyses characterising the widespread epigenetic changes observed following early adversity.

The English and Romanian Adoptee study (see Rutter et al., 2012) and the Bucharest Early Intervention Project highlight the profound influence of the early care environment on child neurodevelopment and vulnerability for mental disorder (O'Connor et al., 2000; Nelson et al., 2007; Rutter et al., 2012). Such cohorts are fertile ground for epigenetic studies. Recent findings indicate that children deprived of parental care show distinct epigenetic changes at least into adolescence (Naumova et al., 2012). Naumova and colleagues (2012) assessed the methylation status of approximately 27,000 CpGs (~0.1% of CpGs in the human genome) in 14 children raised in federal institutions and 14 controls, ranging in age between 7 and 10 years of age. The authors state that a shift toward hypermethylation of a small subset of target genes associated with immune response and cellular signaling was observed in the institutionalized group. While the functional effects of these epigenetic changes on vulnerability for psychopathology remain to be clarified, this study provides proof of principle that the absence of parental care influences DNA methylation in humans. Additional genome-wide analyses of DNA methylation reveal the persisting effect of early adversity on the methylome (Labonte et al., 2012; Essex et al., 2013; Mehta et al., 2013; Yang et al., 2013). Similarly, maternal stress, especially early in infancy, is predictive of DNA methylation profiles assessed in cheek swab DNA samples at age 15 years (Essex et al., 2013). More recently, Mehta and colleagues (2013) show that childhood adversity associates with coordinated epigenetic and transcriptional changes in peripheral blood cells from adults with PTSD (Mehta *et al.*, 2013). Interestingly, despite a similar clinical presentation for both groups (i.e., PTSD), early life adversity was associated with an almost unique transcriptional profile, relative to PTSD patients without early life exposure, suggesting differential regulation of gene transcription in this group. Collectively, these studies suggest that the early social environment influences epigenetic mechanisms both in neural tissue and peripheral sources. More specifically, the work of Essex and colleagues demonstrates a distinct maternal stress effect on DNA methylation in adolescent children. This effect was most pronounced when maternal stress was experienced early in life and associated with a greater number of CpGs than paternal stress. Similarly, Provençal *et al.* (2012) show a profound influence of maternal rearing on DNA methylation across blood and brain using samples from non human primates. A question remains about the functional importance of these changes, which will need to be addressed with appropriate *in vitro* models examining individual sites. Moreover, the statistical models used to detect affected CpGs remains an issue of some debate and existing reports of the actual number of differentially methylated CpG sites should be considered as estimates. Perhaps a greater concern is the degree to which DNA methylation profiles established in peripheral sources of DNA are informative about epigenetic mechanisms within the brain.

Tissue specificity: DNA methylation in blood and brain

As discussed, DNA methylation is, in part, responsible for cell-fate specification. As such DNA methylation is tissue and indeed cell-type specific (Deaton *et al.*, 2011). This poses a challenge to researchers studying DNA methylation in the context of child mental health where access to neural tissue is not possible. A number of recent studies have addressed this issue by comparing DNA methylation profiles in both blood and brain.

Ursini and colleagues (2011) report findings from a sample of healthy young adults in which an interaction between stressful life events and catechol-o-methyltransferase (*COMT*) genotype predicts *COMT* methylation in peripheral blood and working memory performance during an fMRI task. The authors use paired adult rat prefrontal cortex and blood samples to demonstrate a moderate correlation between *COMT* methylation across tissues ($r = 0.50$); however, the degree of association in human samples is unknown. This study uses a very appropriate approach. The correspondence between methylation states in brain and peripheral tissues is likely to vary as a function of genomic region. Focusing on candidate genes is a valuable complement to studies using genome-wide assessments.

Provençal *et al.* (2012) used a genome-wide approach to describe the long-term effects of the early rearing environment on DNA methylation in the blood and brain of adult rhesus macaques. Maternal versus peer rearing, a manipulation

which leads to persistent and marked changes in behavior and stress reactivity, associates with differential methylation of 1981 methylation sites in the prefrontal cortex, but only 227 sites in a selected peripheral T-cell population. A weak correlation was observed between differentially methylated sites between the two tissues ($r = 0.07$). It should be noted that this study focused exclusively on gene promoter methylation. In humans, Davies *et al.* (2012) provide a comprehensive description of DNA methylation in six cortical regions, the cerebellum and matched peripheral whole blood samples. DNA methylation within each brain region clusters together and is clearly distinct from blood. Remarkably, between-individual differences in DNA methylation identified in blood were correlated with between-individual differences in brain samples ($r = 0.66 - 0.76$). This study contrasts with the findings of Provencal *et al.*, which examined direct correlations of absolute methylation levels across tissues rather than between-individual differences across tissues. Collectively, these studies suggest that peripheral sources of DNA may be somewhat informative for identifying individual differences in DNA methylation of relevance to neural processes. However, an important caveat to the Davies *et al.* study, and to genome-wide analyses in general, is that large regions of the genome (e.g., retrotransposons) should be highly methylated regardless of cell type. The inclusion of such regions into analyses is likely to inflate the degree of correspondence across cell types. Indeed, it is highly likely that correspondence across tissues will depend upon the genomic region under study. Moreover, the effects of certain environmental conditions, such as those that activate steroid hormones or cytokines that act widely across a range of tissues, might reveal greater correspondence. In addition to questions regarding tissue specificity, an increasing number of studies assess the stability of methylation over time. This issue is critical for studies examining the potential of DNA methylation marks to serve as a peripheral biomarker for vulnerability to psychopathology.

The role of DNA methylation in developmental processes such as X-inactivation, genomic imprinting and tissue differentiation suggests that DNA methylation is a highly stable epigenetic modification. Nevertheless, at certain sites DNA methylation can be dynamic. Cross-sectional, longitudinal and twin studies now describe variation in DNA methylation across development. A study in newborns and centenarians reports more widespread hypomethylation and greater variability in DNA methylation between CpG sites in the elderly relative to the more uniformly methylated newborn DNA (Heyn *et al.*, 2012). Similarly, Fraga and colleagues (2005) show increasing epigenetic discordance in monozygotic twins across ages. Indeed, discordance in DNA methylation between monozygotic twins is evident at birth, suggestive of intrauterine and/or stochastic effects on DNA methylation early in life (Kaminsky *et al.*, 2009; Gordon *et al.*, 2012). Rates of change in DNA methylation may not be linear across the lifespan, with studies suggesting more dynamic change between 3 and 17 years, a period encompassing puberty (Alisch *et al.*, 2012). Two longitudinal studies examine the stability of DNA methylation in infancy. Wang and colleagues (2012) examine DNA methylation in umbilical cord and venous blood samples at birth and the first 24 months of life (average follow-up was 12 months of age). The authors report remarkable stability over time with significant changes occurring at <1% of methylation sites assessed. In contrast, Martino and colleagues (2011) show more dynamic change in mononuclear cell DNA methylation in their study of 0- to 5-year-olds. In DNA methylation profiles from female newborns, 1- and 5-year-olds tended to form distinct clusters, while the 2.5-year-old group clustered with both 1- and 5-year-olds. Such individual differences in DNA methylation in the postnatal period may point to differential susceptibility of certain individuals to environmental factors such as parenting behaviors, which can influence DNA methylation. Moreover, there is likely to be variation in the stability of DNA methylation as a function of cell type, with perhaps the more phenotypically variable cells associated with immune function showing greater variation than those in other cell types.

Collectively, these studies provide important information on the dynamics of DNA methylation over time and across tissues. The methylation data from twin and multigenerational studies are particularly noteworthy as they suggest a strong genetic influence on epigenetic modifications such as DNA methylation (see later). Indeed, an exciting area of current research in epigenetics is the characterization of gene × environment (G × E) interactions at the molecular level.

The molecular definition of gene × environment interaction

Genetic polymorphisms and epigenetic modifications both influence gene transcription. It is important to emphasize that these are coordinated and often interdependent processes. For example, a methylated cytosine is more readily mutated to thymine leading to mismatched guanine–thymine pairs, which are further modified to create an adenine–thymine (A–T) bond. This process may, in part, explain the reduced frequency of CpGs across the human genome (see Deaton & Bird, 2011). Similarly, genotype is an important determinant of the epigenetic landscape (Lienert *et al.*, 2011). An analysis of DNA methylation in six individuals from a three-generation family illustrates that DNA methylation reflects genetic relatedness (Gertz *et al.*, 2011). This study demonstrates that many of the genetic effects identified in related individuals are also seen in unrelated individuals with similar genotypes. There are widespread effects of genotype on DNA methylation in the human brain (Zhang *et al.*, 2010) with some evidence that genotype-methylation associations are conserved across peripheral and neural tissues (Docherty *et al.*, 2012; Klengel *et al.*, 2013).

Genotype may influence DNA methylation in a number of ways. Genetic polymorphisms (see Chapter 24) such as single nucleotide polymorphisms (SNPs), variable number tandem repeats and copy number variants may introduce or remove CpGs, thereby adding (or removing) potential sites for methylation. Genetic polymorphisms that modulate transcription factor binding may also influence DNA methylation events. Increased transcription factor binding can protect CpG islands from DNA methylation and vice versa (Lienert *et al.*, 2011; Stadler *et al.*, 2011). Both gene promoter and more distal regulatory regions appear to be influenced by transcription factor binding in this way. Collectively, these findings point to a strong association between genotype and DNA methylation. Furthermore, there is emerging evidence that such genotype-methylation interdependency may be influenced by the early environment (Ursini *et al.*, 2011; Vijayendran *et al.*, 2012; Klengel *et al.*, 2013). These allele-specific effects may provide a biological mechanism to explain statistical G × E associations.

The concept of G × E effects on vulnerability for mental disorder has been a major paradigm shift in child psychiatry (Caspi & Moffitt, 2006; Meaney, 2010). Environmental factors such as childhood maltreatment (Caspi *et al.*, 2002), stressful life events (Caspi *et al.*, 2003) and cannabis use (Caspi *et al.*, 2005) interact with genetic risk factors to predict risk of later mental disorder. These reports have been supported and extended by clinical and basic research over the past 15 years (however, see Risch *et al.*, 2009; but also Rutter *et al.*, 2009; Meaney, 2010). More recently, G × E effects have been reported, which provide preliminary support for the parental signaling hypothesis and vulnerability for mental disorder. For example, children carrying the dopamine receptor D4 (DRD4) 7-repeat polymorphism show both the *highest* and *lowest* risk of adverse neurodevelopmental outcomes as a function of maternal sensitivity or an enriched early care environment (Berry *et al.*, 2013; Belsky & Pluess, 2013). Replication of these findings is required, but such studies are beginning to provide some clues as to why some children may be more, or less, sensitive to the quality of the early care environment.

Despite an increased appreciation for the importance and biological plausibility of G × E effects, the molecular basis for these associations remains poorly defined. Epigenetic modifications, such as DNA methylation, provide a mechanism to link genetic and environmental risk to phenotype (Meaney, 2010; Klengel *et al.*, 2013). In addition to our work in rats, two recent human studies provide evidence for a molecular definition of G × E effects. The first, drawn from the Iowa adoption study, demonstrates that exposure to childhood sexual abuse and carriers of the short version of the serotonin transporter (*SLC6A4*) repeat polymorphism interact to predict decreased methylation of a CpG within *SLC6A4*. More recently, Klengel and colleagues (2013) provide a comprehensive description of allele-specific demethylation of the GR co-regulator FK506 Binding Protein 5 (FKBP5) in adults exposed to childhood trauma. This study demonstrated that polymorphisms in *FKBP5* influence the position of the nucleosome, which, when combined with childhood trauma (postulated to increase circulating cortisol), results in an increased risk of PTSD. At the molecular level, this interaction is associated with stable DNA demethylation, which in turn predicted symptoms of glucocorticoid resistance and hippocampal volume. In line with what is known about the capacity for transcription factors to modulate local DNA methylation levels, a large emphasis is placed on the presence of a glucocorticoid-binding site within the DNA, which may be an important factor for such demethylation events. Ursini and colleagues (2011) also provide evidence that environmental stress associates with allele-specific changes in *COMT* methylation, which associate with cognitive performance. In summary, these studies build on epidemiological analyses of G × E effects by providing a functional mechanism to link genetic risk factors and adverse environmental exposures to sustained physiological changes of relevance to mental health. Undoubtedly, both candidate gene and genome-wide analyses will uncover additional genomic regions which show epigenetic sensitivity to early adversity and the early care environment.

Methodological considerations in studies of epigenetics

The recent wave of epigenome-wide association studies reflects the growing interest in epigenetics in the field of child mental health. These analyses are beginning to uncover disease risk markers (in peripheral tissue) in conditions often associated with exposure to various adverse experiences early in life; examples include major depression (Sabunciyan *et al.*, 2012; Byrne *et al.*, 2013), PTSD (Smith *et al.*, 2011; Mehta *et al.*, 2013), schizophrenia and bipolar disorder (Dempster *et al.*, 2011). However, the application of conventional genome-wide association study (GWAS) designs may prove problematic for the field of epigenetic epidemiology. Chromatin modifications, such as DNA methylation, are dynamic and respond not only to environmental influences but also to disease processes. Therefore, it remains a challenge to identify epigenetic modifications that are causal, and not a consequence of disease processes (Mill & Heijmans, 2013). In addition, unlike conventional GWASs in which the predictor (presence or absence of genetic risk factor) is invariant over time and tissue, epigenetic phenotypes are considerably more variable. Prospective birth cohorts in which biological samples are collected longitudinally, across developmental periods and risk exposures, twin studies and *in vitro* functional analyses will all help to identify specific epigenetic phenotypes that are causally related to the risk of mental disorder (see Chapter 12).

Additional considerations for epigenome-wide analyses are the issues of statistical power and stringency. Many of the studies described employed microarray-based platforms for analysis of genome-wide DNA methylation. Currently, the Illumina human methylation 450 Beadchip (450 k) array provides the most comprehensive genome-wide coverage (~485,000 sites) at a cost that permits its use in larger scale, epidemiological-like studies. It should be noted that despite improved genome-wide coverage, this array provides quantitative data on less than 2% of the 28 million CpGs contained in the human genome. The ever-decreasing cost of sequencing technologies will undoubtedly increase the use of next-generation sequencing for whole genome methylation analyses. While such approaches may reveal novel genomic regions of relevance to child vulnerability for mental disorder, increasing genome-wide coverage poses analytical challenges. For example, in the field of mental health, few studies to date have identified between-group differences in DNA methylation that exceed 10%. These relatively small changes in DNA methylation, combined with the large number of comparisons (~485,000 for the Illumina 450 k array) require adequately powered sample sizes to detect subtle differences in DNA methylation (Michels *et al.*, 2013). In the absence of large sample sizes, replication in independent samples is important to increase confidence in novel findings. Somewhat similar to early candidate gene association studies, the emerging field of epigenetic epidemiology is likely to identify several false positives if studies are not adequately powered and controlled.

Finally, as noted, epigenetic modifications do not occur in isolation nor are they independent of the underlying DNA sequence. Genome-wide surveys of multiple epigenetic modifications, including different forms of DNA methylation, genotype and gene expression may prove useful in clinical studies of early adversity, and will help identify novel functional loci of relevance to child mental health.

Summary and concluding remarks

We have described how maternal effects operating early in life drive phenotypic diversity across species and summarized studies in the rat that systematically examined the influence of maternal care. The offspring of mothers differing in the frequency of LG have distinct developmental trajectories and behavioral profiles, mediated in part by epigenetic regulation of gene expression. Somewhat similar data has emerged from clinical studies of early adversity, highlighting epigenetic modifications such as DNA methylation as a potential mediator of maternal effects on vulnerability for mental disorder. A challenge as we move forward with a wider application of the environmental epigenetic hypothesis to the field of child mental health is to determine to what extent epigenetic modifications can be used to identify at-risk children and treatment responses. It is also unknown if the effects of early adversity on epigenetic processes can be reversed by therapeutic interventions or if such an outcome would be desirable, given the potential adaptive value of certain modifications. Thus, while epigenetics is an exciting and rapidly growing field, translating basic scientific findings to improve clinical care and child outcomes will require continued and cautious research efforts.

References

Alisch, R.S. *et al.* (2012) Age-associated DNA methylation in pediatric populations. *Genome Research* **22**, 623–632.

Belsky, J. & Pluess, M. (2013) Genetic moderation of early child-care effects on social functioning across childhood: a developmental analysis. *Child Development* **84**, 1209–1225.

Berry, D. *et al.* (2013) Gene-environment interaction between dopamine receptor d4 7-repeat polymorphism and early maternal sensitivity predicts inattention trajectories across middle childhood. *Development and Psychopathology* **25**, 291–306.

Bird, A.P. (1986) CpG-rich islands and the function of DNA methylation. *Nature* **321**, 209–213.

Borrow, A.P. *et al.* (2013) Perinatal testosterone exposure and maternal care effects on the female rat's development and sexual behaviour. *Journal of Neuroendocrinology* **25**, 528–536.

Byrne, E.M. *et al.* (2013) Monozygotic twins affected with major depressive disorder have greater variance in methylation than their unaffected co-twin. *Translational Psychiatry* **3**, e269.

Caldji, C. *et al.* (2000) The effects of early rearing environment on the development of GABAA and central benzodiazepine receptor levels and novelty-induced fearfulness in the rat. *Neuropsychopharmacology* **22**, 219–229.

Caldji, C. *et al.* (2003) Variations in maternal care alter GABAA receptor subunit expression in brain regions associated with fear. *Neuropsychopharmacology* **28**, 1950–1959.

Cameron, N. *et al.* (2008) Maternal programming of sexual behavior and hypothalamic-pituitary-gonadal function in the female rat. *PLoS One* **3**, e2210.

Caspi, A. & Moffitt, T.E. (2006) Gene-environment interactions in psychiatry: joining forces with neuroscience. *Nature Reviews Neuroscience* **7**, 583–590.

Caspi, A. *et al.* (2002) Role of genotype in the cycle of violence in maltreated children. *Science* **297**, 851–854.

Caspi, A. *et al.* (2003) Influence of life stress on depression: moderation by a polymorphism in the 5-HTT gene. *Science* **301**, 386–389.

Caspi, A. *et al.* (2005) Moderation of the effect of adolescent-onset cannabis use on adult psychosis by a functional polymorphism in the catechol-o-methyltransferase gene: longitudinal evidence of a gene x environment interaction. *Biological Psychiatry* **57**, 1117–1127.

Champagne, F.A. *et al.* (2003) Variations in maternal care in the rat as a mediating influence for the effects of environment on development. *Physiology and Behavior* **79**, 359–371.

Champagne, F.A. *et al.* (2006) Maternal care associated with methylation of the estrogen receptor-alpha1b promoter and estrogen receptor-alpha expression in the medial preoptic area of female offspring. *Endocrinology* **147**, 2909–2915.

Cooney, C.A. *et al.* (2002) Maternal methyl supplements in mice affect epigenetic variation and DNA methylation of offspring. *Journal of Nutrition* **132**, 2393S–2400S.

Dantzer, B. *et al.* (2013) Density triggers maternal hormones that increase adaptive offspring growth in a wild mammal. *Science* **340**, 1215–1217.

Davies, M.N. *et al.* (2012) Functional annotation of the human brain methylome identifies tissue-specific epigenetic variation across brain and blood. *Genome Biology* **13**, R43.

Deaton, A.M. & Bird, A. (2011) CpG islands and the regulation of transcription. *Genes and Development* **25**, 1010–1022.

Deaton, A.M. *et al.* (2011) Cell type–specific DNA methylation at intragenic CpG islands in the immune system. *Genome Research* **21**, 1074–1086.

Dempster, E.L. *et al.* (2011) Disease-associated epigenetic changes in monozygotic twins discordant for schizophrenia and bipolar disorder. *Human Molecular Genetics* **20**, 4786–4796.

Docherty, S. *et al.* (2012) A genetic association study of DNA methylation levels in the drd4 gene region finds associations with nearby SNPs. *Behavioral and Brain Functions* **8**, 31.

Dumais, A. *et al.* (2005) Is violent method of suicide a behavioral marker of lifetime aggression? *American Journal of Psychiatry* **162**, 1375–1378.

Essex, M.J. *et al.* (2013) Epigenetic vestiges of early developmental adversity: childhood stress exposure and DNA methylation in adolescence. *Child Development* **84**, 58–75.

Fraga, M.F. *et al.* (2005) Epigenetic differences arise during the lifetime of monozygotic twins. *Proceedings of the National Academy of Sciences of the United States of America* **102**, 10604–10609.

Francis, D. *et al.* (1999) Nongenomic transmission across generations of maternal behavior and stress responses in the rat. *Science* **286**, 1155–1158.

Gertz, J. *et al.* (2011) Analysis of DNA methylation in a three-generation family reveals widespread genetic influence on epigenetic regulation. *PLoS Genetics* **7**, e1002228.

Gluckman, P.D. & Hanson, M.A. (2007) Developmental plasticity and human disease: research directions. *Journal of Internal Medicine* **261**, 461–471.

Gordon, L. *et al.* (2012) Neonatal DNA methylation profile in human twins is specified by a complex interplay between intrauterine environmental and genetic factors, subject to tissue-specific influence. *Genome Research* **22**, 1395–1406.

Grunstein, M. (1997) Histone acetylation in chromatin structure and transcription. *Nature* **389**, 349–352.

Guo, J.U. *et al.* (2011) Neuronal activity modifies the DNA methylation landscape in the adult brain. *Nature Neuroscience* **14**, 1345–1351.

Hansen, K.D. *et al.* (2011) Increased methylation variation in epigenetic domains across cancer types. *Nature Genetics* **43**, 768–775.

Heijmans, B.T. *et al.* (2008) Persistent epigenetic differences associated with prenatal exposure to famine in humans. *Proceedings of the National Academy of Sciences* **105**, 17046–17049.

Hellstrom, I.C. *et al.* (2012) Maternal licking regulates hippocampal glucocorticoid receptor transcription through a thyroid hormone-serotonin-ngfi-a signalling cascade. *Philosophical Transactions of the Royal Society, B: Biological Sciences* **367**, 2495–2510.

Herb, B.R. *et al.* (2012) Reversible switching between epigenetic states in honeybee behavioral subcastes. *Nature Neuroscience* **15**, 1371–1373.

Heyn, H. *et al.* (2012) Distinct DNA methylomes of newborns and centenarians. *Proceedings of the National Academy of Sciences* **109**, 10522–10527.

Hinde, R.A. (ed) (1986) *Some Implications of Evolutionary Theory and Comparative Data for the Study of Human Prosocial and Aggressive Behavior.* Academic Press, Orlando, FL.

Hofer, M.A. (1984) Early stages in the organization of cardiovascular control. *Proceedings of the Society for Experimental Biology and Medicine* **175**, 147–157.

Jenuwein, T. & Allis, C.D. (2001) Translating the histone code. *Science* **293**, 1074–1080.

Jirtle, R.L. & Skinner, M.K. (2007) Environmental epigenomics and disease susceptibility. *Nature Reviews Genetics* **8**, 253–262.

Kaminsky, Z.A. *et al.* (2009) DNA methylation profiles in monozygotic and dizygotic twins. *Nature Genetics* **41**, 240–245.

Keverne, E.B. (2014) Significance of epigenetics for understanding brain development, brain evolution and behaviour. *Neuroscience* **264**, 207–217.

Klengel, T. *et al.* (2013) Allele-specific fkbp5 DNA demethylation mediates gene-childhood trauma interactions. *Nature Neuroscience* **16**, 33–41.

Labonte, B. *et al.* (2012) Genome-wide epigenetic regulation by early-life trauma. *Archives of General Psychiatry* **69**, 722–731.

Lee, T.M. (1993) Development of meadow voles is influenced postnatally by maternal photoperiodic history. *American Journal of Physiology - Regulatory, Integrative and Comparative Physiology* **265**, R749–R755.

Lee, J.T. & Bartolomei, M.S. (2013) X-inactivation, imprinting, and long noncoding RNAs in health and disease. *Cell* **152**, 1308–1323.

Lee, T.M. & Zucker, I. (1988) Vole infant development is influenced perinatally by maternal photoperiodic history. *American Journal of Physiology - Regulatory, Integrative and Comparative Physiology* **255**, R831–R838.

Levine, S. (1994) The ontogeny of the hypothalamic-pituitary-adrenal axis. The influence of maternal factors. *Annals of the New York Academy of Sciences* **746**, 275–288.

Lienert, F. *et al.* (2011) Identification of genetic elements that autonomously determine DNA methylation states. *Nature Genetics* **43**, 1091–1097.

Lister, R. *et al.* (2013) Global epigenomic reconfiguration during mammalian brain development. *Science* **341**, 1237905.

Luger, K. *et al.* (1997) Crystal structure of the nucleosome core particle at 2.8 a resolution. *Nature* **389**, 251–260.

Martino, D.J. *et al.* (2011) Evidence for age-related and individual-specific changes in DNA methylation profile of mononuclear cells during early immune development in humans. *Epigenetics* **6**, 1085–1094.

Martinowich, K. *et al.* (2003) DNA methylation-related chromatin remodeling in activity-dependent BDNF gene regulation. *Science* **302**, 890–893.

Maze, I. *et al.* (2013) Histone regulation in the CNS: basic principles of epigenetic plasticity. *Neuropsychopharmacology* **38**, 3–22.

McGowan, P.O. *et al.* (2009) Epigenetic regulation of the glucocorticoid receptor in human brain associates with childhood abuse. *Nature Neuroscience* **12**, 342–348.

Meaney, M.J. (2007) Environmental programming of phenotypic diversity in female reproductive strategies. In: *Advances in Genetics.* (ed Y. Daisuke). Academic Press, New York.

Meaney, M.J. (2010) Epigenetics and the biological definition of gene x environment interactions. *Child Development* **81**, 41–79.

Mehta, D. *et al.* (2013) Childhood maltreatment is associated with distinct genomic and epigenetic profiles in posttraumatic stress disorder. *Proceedings of the National Academy of Sciences of the United States of America* **110**, 8302–8307.

Michels, K.B. *et al.* (2013) Recommendations for the design and analysis of epigenome-wide association studies. *Nature Methods* **10**, 949–955.

Mill, J. & Heijmans, B.T. (2013) From promises to practical strategies in epigenetic epidemiology. *Nature Reviews Genetics* **14**, 585–594.

Mueller, B.R. & Bale, T.L. (2008) Sex-specific programming of offspring emotionality after stress early in pregnancy. *Journal of Neuroscience* **28**, 9055–9065.

Murayama, A. *et al.* (2006) A specific CpG site demethylation in the human interleukin 2 gene promoter is an epigenetic memory. *EMBO Journal* **25**, 1081–1092.

Murgatroyd, C. *et al.* (2009) Dynamic DNA methylation programs persistent adverse effects of early-life stress. *Nature Neuroscience* **12**, 1559–1566.

Nanni, V. *et al.* (2012) Childhood maltreatment predicts unfavorable course of illness and treatment outcome in depression: a meta-analysis. *American Journal of Psychiatry* **169**, 141–151.

Naumova, O.Y. *et al.* (2012) Differential patterns of whole-genome DNA methylation in institutionalized children and children raised by their biological parents. *Development and Psychopathology* **24**, 143–155.

Nelson, C.A. *et al.* (2007) Cognitive recovery in socially deprived young children: the Bucharest early intervention project. *Science* **318**, 1937–1940.

O'Connor, T.G. *et al.* (2000) The effects of global severe privation on cognitive competence: extension and longitudinal follow-up. *Child Development* **71**, 376–390.

O'Donnell, K.J. *et al.* (2013) Prenatal maternal mood is associated with altered diurnal cortisol in adolescence. *Psychoneuroendocrinology* **38**, 1630–1638.

Provençal, N. *et al.* (2012) The signature of maternal rearing in the methylome in rhesus macaque prefrontal cortex and t cells. *Journal of Neuroscience* **32**, 15626–15642.

Radtke, K.M. *et al.* (2011) Transgenerational impact of intimate partner violence on methylation in the promoter of the glucocorticoid receptor. *Translational Psychiatry* **1**, e21.

Razin, A. & Riggs, A.D. (1980) DNA methylation and gene function. *Science* **210**, 604–610.

Repetti, R.L. *et al.* (2002) Risky families: family social environments and the mental and physical health of offspring. *Psychological Bulletin* **128**, 330–366.

Risch, N. *et al.* (2009) Interaction between the serotonin transporter gene (5-httlpr), stressful life events, and risk of depression: a meta-analysis. *JAMA* **301**, 2462–2471.

Rutter, M. *et al.* (2009) Gene-environment interactions: biologically valid pathway or artifact? *Archives of General Psychiatry* **66**, 1287–1289.

Rutter, M. *et al.* (2012) Longitudinal studies using a "natural experiment" design: the case of adoptees from Romanian institutions. *Journal of the American Academy of Child & Adolescent Psychiatry* **51**, 762–770.

Sabunciyan, S. *et al.* (2012) Genome-wide DNA methylation scan in major depressive disorder. *PLoS One* **7**, e34451.

Saiful Islam, M. *et al.* (1994) Parental effects on the behaviour and colouration of nymphs of the desert locust schistocerca gregaria. *Journal of Insect Physiology* **40**, 173–181.

Schanberg, S.M. *et al.* (1984) Tactile and nutritional aspects of maternal care: specific regulators of neuroendocrine function and cellular development. *Proceedings of the Society for Experimental Biology and Medicine* **175**, 135–146.

Seckl, J.R. & Holmes, M.C. (2007) Mechanisms of disease: gluco-corticoids, their placental metabolism and fetal' programming' of adult pathophysiology. *Nature Clinical Practice Endocrinology and Metabolism* **3**, 479–488.

Smith, A.K. *et al.* (2011) Differential immune system DNA methylation and cytokine regulation in post-traumatic stress disorder. *American Journal of Medical Genetics Part B: Neuropsychiatric Genetics* **156**, 700–708.

Stadler, M.B. *et al.* (2011) DNA-binding factors shape the mouse methylome at distal regulatory regions. *Nature* **480**, 490–495.

Sun, H. *et al.* (2013) Epigenetics of the depressed brain: role of histone acetylation and methylation. *Neuropsychopharmacology* **38**, 124–137.

Turner, B.M. (2001) *Chromatin and Gene Regulation: Mechanisms in Epigenetics.* Blackwell Science, Cambridge, MA.

Turner, J.D. & Muller, C.P. (2005) Structure of the glucocorticoid receptor (nr3c1) gene 5′ untranslated region: identification, and tissue distribution of multiple new human exon 1. *Journal of Molecular Endocrinology* **35**, 283–292.

Tyrka, A.R. *et al.* (2012) Childhood adversity and epigenetic modulation of the leukocyte glucocorticoid receptor: preliminary findings in healthy adults. *PLoS One* **7**, e30148.

Ursini, G. *et al.* (2011) Stress-related methylation of the catechol-o-methyltransferase val158 allele predicts human prefrontal cognition and activity. *Journal of Neuroscience* **31**, 6692–6698.

Vijayendran, M. *et al.* (2012) Effects of genotype and child abuse on DNA methylation and gene expression at the serotonin transporter. *Frontiers in Psychiatry* **3**, 55.

Wang, D. *et al.* (2012) Individual variation and longitudinal pattern of genome-wide DNA methylation from birth to the first two years of life. *Epigenetics* **7**, 594–605.

Waterland, R.A. & Jirtle, R.L. (2003) Transposable elements: targets for early nutritional effects on epigenetic gene regulation. *Molecular and Cellular Biology* **23**, 5293–5300.

Weaver, I.C.G. *et al.* (2004) Epigenetic programming by maternal behavior. *Nature Neuroscience* **7**, 847–854.

Weaver, I.C.G. *et al.* (2007) The transcription factor nerve growth factor-inducible protein a mediates epigenetic programming: altering epigenetic marks by immediate-early genes. *Journal of Neuroscience* **27**, 1756–1768.

Yang, B.-Z. *et al.* (2013) Child abuse and epigenetic mechanisms of disease risk. *American Journal of Preventive Medicine* **44**, 101–107.

Yehuda, R. *et al.* (2008) Maternal, not paternal, PTSD is related to increased risk for PTSD in offspring of holocaust survivors. *Journal of Psychiatric Research* **42**, 1104–1111.

Zhang, D. *et al.* (2010) Genetic control of individual differences in gene-specific methylation in human brain. *American Journal of Human Genetics* **86**, 411–419.

Zouk, H. *et al.* (2006) Characterization of impulsivity in suicide completers: clinical, behavioral and psychosocial dimensions. *Journal of Affective Disorders* **92**, 195–204.

CHAPTER 26

Psychosocial adversity

Jennifer Jenkins[1], Sheri Madigan[1] and Louise Arseneault[2]

[1] Applied Psychology and Human Development, University of Toronto, Ontario, Canada
[2] Institute of Psychiatry, Psychology and Neuroscience, King's College London, UK

Introduction

Human development is the process of individual adaptation to a complex and ever-changing environment. At times the adaptation is smooth; the environment provides support to the individual and the individual is able to use his/her own skills in a successful adaptation to the circumstance. At other times, however, the adaptation of the individual fails. This may be because the challenges in the environment are too great or the individual's abilities in adapting to the environment are insufficient. It may also be that failure to adapt is explained by the combination of individual characteristics and a challenging environment (Rutter, 2012). Most of our knowledge about psychosocial adversities and their effect on children's mental health comes from correlational studies and specific designs are needed to help us identify the mechanisms that explain why adversity and mental health are correlated. These designs are discussed in Chapter 12.

Conceptual issues in the effects of psychosocial adversity on children

Transactional processes between individuals and their environments

Although we know that risky environments increase mental health problems in children, characteristics of children can also influence exposure to environmental adversities. Several types of mechanism operate. First, characteristics of children elicit environmental experiences. Children who are hyperactive, impulsive, and negative in their mood elicit more negativity from parents (Shaw *et al.*, 2001); certain children within families provoke marital conflict more than others (Jenkins *et al.*, 2005); infants who have less capacity for synchrony alter their mothers' attachment-related caregiving (Beebe *et al.*, 2010).

Second, individuals choose relationships/friends that have a negative effect on them subsequently: for example, individuals with behavioral problems befriend like individuals, who in turn increase the child's behavioral problems (Dishion & Owen, 2002). Thus, bidirectional influences are evident between people and their environment. Bidirectional effects are most often measured using cross-lagged designs (Steele *et al.*, 2013). In these designs, two processes that co-vary (e.g., parental harshness and difficult child behavior) are examined over time and the goal is to examine which of the two processes predicts change in the other more strongly. There is evidence for effects from children to parents and parents to children (Burt *et al.*, 2006).

Moderation processes in the effects of environmental adversity

Probably the most important principle in understanding the impact of psychosocial adversity is that children vary markedly in their susceptibility to environmental influences. Some are much more vulnerable to the adverse effects of psychosocial adversity. This means that although, on average, there is a raised risk to all children through exposure to risky environments, the effects come about because a subsample of children show marked responses to adversity, while others remain relatively unaffected. Individual vulnerability has been found to be explained by individual characteristics of children (El-Sheikh, 2005), but also by the presence of good relationships in children's lives (Gass *et al.*, 2007), issues discussed in Chapter 27.

Mediation: from distal to proximal risks

Bronfenbrenner (1977) proposed a model for understanding context effects on children. He suggested that development occurred within embedded "layers" of context to children, from macro systems (country and community influences) to micro systems (children's experiences in families, schools, peer groups, and childcare centers). Ecological models stress these

Rutter's Child and Adolescent Psychiatry, Sixth Edition.
Edited by Anita Thapar and Daniel S. Pine, James F. Leckman, Stephen Scott, Margaret J. Snowling, Eric Taylor.
© 2015 John Wiley & Sons Ltd. Published 2018 by John Wiley & Sons Ltd.

layered influences (Ungar *et al.*, 2013). Within these models, both "macro" and "distal" refer to more distant stressors and "micro" and "proximal" to stressors that are closer to the child. These terms are generally utilized within mediation models. A mediation model requires a significant pathway from the distal process to the child outcome, through the proximal process; for example, cumulative environmental risk leads to greater differential parenting, which in turn explains child behavior (Meunier *et al.*, 2013). Mediation models are considered to be "causal" models: the mediator is conceptualized as the active agent that is causally responsible for the relationship between two other variables. It is important to note, however, that theories of causation are very discipline based and influenced by our current scientific knowledge. For example, although "parenting" offers a causal mechanism for behavioral scientists, for neuroscientists mediation is about brain mechanism (Hanson *et al.*, 2013) and for cognitive psychologists it is about cognitions (White *et al.*, 2011). Further, our mediation models only represent short sequences of process when in reality long chains of sequenced influences, across many cognitive and neural systems, are likely to be operating.

Developmental timing

The effect of psychosocial adversity on mental health could vary depending on the developmental period during which it occurs. Such an impact, via the embedding of stress in biological and cognitive systems (see Chapter 23), could be greater in childhood when the brain is developing rapidly and cognition is still consolidating. Alternatively, adolescence, which brings pubertal changes, could also be a time of increased sensitivity to the effect of adversity. Questions relating to the timing of psychosocial adversity and stress on the development of mental health difficulties are hardly testable with human samples. Individual changes are examined in longitudinal observational studies but causality can only be implied by this study design, and not tested properly. Natural experiments, embedded in a longitudinal design, offer the strongest research opportunities to test questions of developmental timing. A useful example is the English and Romanian Adoptee Study, which follows the developmental milestones of children who were placed in institutional care at an early age (see Rutter *et al.*, 2012). The timing of institutional deprivation and its impact on children's development was extensively documented through the years. Findings indicate that when institutional deprivation ceased within children's first 12 months of life, poor outcomes are not as severe as when deprivation persists beyond the first year of life. Similar conclusions were reached by another study of adoptees, the Bucharest Early Intervention Project (Nelson *et al.*, 2007).

Studies examining the effect of developmental timing should consider the possibility that psychosocial adversity in infancy/early childhood may represent a longer duration or persistence of stress, and should control for this confounding effect. Controls should also be considered for factors that may predispose some children to experience psychosocial adversity

in the first place. Animal research allows a stricter control over the concept of adversity and stronger conclusions with regard to developmental timing. However, findings so far are still inconclusive (Tottenham & Sheridan, 2009).

Empirical findings on distal risk factors

Neighborhood influences

Deprived neighborhoods are characterized by high unemployment rates, predominantly minority populations, dense public housing, crime and violence, as well as social isolation. Research on the influence of neighborhoods on children's mental health has the challenge of differentiating between the impact of families' socioeconomic status (SES) and the neighborhood in which they live, given that SES constrains families' choice of neighborhood. One review estimated that effects of deprived neighborhoods accounted for between 5% and 10% of variance observed in children's developmental outcomes (Leventhal & Brooks-Gunn, 2000); however, because of the design of these studies, it remains possible that uncontrolled effects at the individual and family levels are misattributed to neighborhoods.

Results from an experimental study, the Move to Opportunity (MTO) program, provide more compelling causal data. Families recruited from high-poverty neighborhoods in the United States were randomly assigned to the experimental or control condition. Members of the experimental group were given vouchers to move to a low-poverty area. Approximately 40% of families in the experimental condition took up the option of moving and effects were calculated for all families. Although initially beneficial effects on school achievement were notable for both girls and boys, later follow-ups suggested that only girls benefited from the intervention (Ludwig *et al.*, 2012) and lasting effects were only seen for specific outcomes in girls (psychological distress and obesity).

One component of the neighborhood effect is likely to be exposure to violence. Gorman-Smith and Tolan (1998) interviewed African-American and Latino adolescents in public high schools in deprived neighborhoods in the Chicago area, with the majority of the sample living in poverty. They found that 16.5% reported that a family member had been robbed or attacked and 15.6% had seen someone shot or killed in the previous year. A meta-analysis of community violence and children's mental health showed that violence in neighborhoods was moderately to strongly associated with children's symptoms with the strongest effects seen for PTSD ($d = 0.79$) and behavior problems ($d = 0.63$). It should be noted, though, that these effect sizes are not independent of family SES (Fowler *et al.*, 2009).

Exposure to war

Children in war zones can be exposed to a wide range of traumatic events including famine and thirst, loss of family members and homes, seeing dead and injured people, rape, physical injury, threats to life and being taken prisoner (Drury & Williams, 2012). In a population of children who experienced the Rwandan genocide, 78% experienced a death in the family, while 70% saw someone being killed or injured, and 15% reported hiding under a dead body to escape detection during the massacre (Dyregrov *et al.*, 2000). A meta-analysis of mental disorders among children exposed to war showed that rates of PTSD were 47%, with rates of depression and anxiety also elevated (Attanayake *et al.*, 2009).

Socioeconomic status

Societies are hierarchically organized along an economic dimension. Both absolute levels of income and the extent of the difference between rich and poor members of the society have been found to be a consistent correlate of mental and physical health. With respect to absolute deprivation, Slopen *et al.* (2010) showed that children who had experienced persistent food insecurity were twice as likely to suffer from externalizing problems compared to children without such insecurity. Macmillan *et al.* (2004) found that the number of years of living in poverty was strongly associated with initial levels of antisocial behavior. Further, children exposed to persistent poverty, those who only moved out of poverty for a short time, and those who moved into poverty, showed faster *rates of change* on antisocial behavior than children who had never lived in poverty. Two direct effects to account for this relationship have been hypothesized: inequitable allocation of resources like nutrition, healthcare, housing, and education and the development of negative health behaviors such as low exercise and tobacco use (Bradley & Corwyn, 2002). SES effects on children's developing brains have been noted to be strongest for brain areas related to language, executive function, and attention (Hackman & Farah, 2009). Stevens *et al.* (2009) assessed children between 3 and 8 years using event-related potential and found that children in low SES homes, compared to their middle SES counterparts, showed a brain pattern indicative of trouble suppressing distracting information.

Relative income also plays a role in health outcomes. Wilkinson and Pickett (2009) developed an inequality metric by examining the ratio of incomes for the top and bottom 20% of a society across countries. This metric explained variation across countries in many health and learning outcomes for children. Absolute levels of income have been found to explain more variance in health outcomes than relative income (Kondo *et al.*, 2009; Olson *et al.*, 2010). A clever brain-imaging experiment (Dohman *et al.*, 2011) shows that a region of the brain that registers reward (the ventral striatum) becomes activated by relative income. This activation was evident the more discrepant the advantaged persons were from their partner with respect to financial rewards given for task performance. This finding provides evidence for one neurobiological system that may be implicated in the effects of relative income on health outcomes.

Effects of poverty on children mediated by parenting

Parenting has been found to play a mediating role in the relationship between socioeconomic adversity and children's well-being (Grant *et al.*, 2003). Low SES makes it more likely that parents show high levels of hostile inconsistent parenting, less sensitivity, and parental investment, and expose children to lower levels of cognitive stimulation. Several studies have tested mediation models in which the indirect effect of SES on children's mental health through exposure to adverse parenting has been supported (Grant *et al.*, 2003; Gershoff *et al.*, 2007).

Cumulative risk

Risk factors for children's development rarely operate in isolation. For example, living in poverty is associated with single parenthood, parental psychiatric disorders, and greater marital conflict. This means that by looking at the impact of single risks we fail to capture the degree of risk exposure that children experience. Cumulative risk indices are simply a count of the number of risks to which children are exposed and this has been found to explain more variance in child outcomes than single risks and both linear and nonlinear effects of cumulative risk are seen (Evans *et al.*, 2013). Nonlinear effects show that risks combine multiplicatively to influence child disorders. Effects of cumulative risk persist into adulthood and influence physical as well as mental health. For instance, adults who experienced four or more adverse childhood experiences were 3.9 times more likely to suffer from emphysema and chronic bronchitis and 2.2 times more likely to have ischemic heart disease than individuals with no adverse childhood experiences (Felitti *et al.*, 1998).

Cumulative social disadvantage and parenting

At higher levels of cumulative risk, the ability of parents to be attentive and sensitive to their children is compromised (Burchinal *et al.*, 2008). They also show more differential parenting across the sibship (Meunier *et al.*, 2013). Other mediators of cumulative risk include allostatic load (i.e., the physiological consequences of adapting to repeated stress) (Evans, 2003), sequences of risks in all periods of childhood (Appleyard *et al.*, 2005), and brain function. For instance, Hanson *et al.* (2013) show that prefrontal volume of adolescents is a mediator between cumulative life stress and spatial working memory.

Distal risks in low- and middle-income countries

The development of children growing up in developing countries and areas where conflicts prevail is precarious. Risk factors are numerous and resources scarce. The development of over 200 million children under the age of 5 years is compromised by factors such as poverty and stunting, which are common in countries in South Asia and sub-Saharan Africa (Grantham-McGregor *et al.*, 2007). These factors are associated with lower levels of achievement and poor cognitive outcomes, which in turn result in the perpetuation of poverty given the ill-preparedness of these children for the workforce in adulthood. Other factors that contribute to poor cognitive and mental health outcomes include inadequate cognitive stimulation, iodine and iron deficiencies, malaria, intrauterine growth restriction, maternal depression, and exposure to violence (Walker *et al.*, 2007).

Empirical findings on proximal risk factors: development in the context of close relationships

Parental responsivity

Parenting in early infancy centers on attachment processes. Bowlby (1971) proposed that the attachment system is a bio-behavioral system developed for the protection of the young. Human infants elicit caregiving through signals such as crying, and clinging, which are designed to maintain close proximity to a parent and, subsequently, safety and protection (Goldberg *et al.*, 1999). This biobehavioral system motivates the child to use the parent as a secure base from which to explore the world, and as a haven of safety in times of perceived threat or distress. The core parental mechanism of this theory is parental sensitive responding to child distress, that is, their ability to perceive and respond promptly, accurately, and sensitively to child signals and cues. Sensitive responding is associated with secure attachment relationships (van IJzendoorn, 1995). It is enduring and convincingly impacts child development across multiple domains of functioning (e.g., Fraley *et al.*, 2013). Recent theories of sensitivity suggest that synchronous responses between parents and children build the hardwiring that is essential for the social brain (Feldman, 2007).

More recently, researchers have called for a more multi-dimensional approach to parental responsivity to enhance our understanding of the transactional nature of the parent–child relationship, and child outcomes (Kobak & Madsen, 2008). One aspect of responsivity is maternal autonomy support, defined as the degree to which parents promote, encourage, and monitor the child's independent problem-solving and decision-making skills. The effective use of parental autonomy support predicts secure parent–child attachment and executive function (Whipple *et al.*, 2010) as well as academic success and peer relations (Joussemet *et al.*, 2005).

Recent research has focused on the parents' accurate understanding and interpretation of the child's behavior and the cognitive capacity to see things from the child's point of view, globally labeled as mind-mindedness (Meins *et al.*, 2001) and partially operationalized as mental state talk. Mental state talk is related to ratings of maternal sensitivity (Laranjo *et al.*, 2008), secure attachment (Meins *et al.*, 2001), children's later mentalistic vocabulary (Jenkins *et al.*, 2003), and harmonious peer interactions (McElwain *et al.*, 2011) (see also Chapter 37).

Parenting dimensions

The parenting dimensions described here have emerged as correlates of psychopathology in children. Associations tend to be nonspecific, with many types of parenting found to be associated with both emotional and behavioral psychopathology (Wang & Kenny, 2014; Wood *et al.*, 2003).

Harshness

The domain of parenting most consistently linked to psychopathology is parental harshness, with the most consistent links to children's externalizing behavior (Hoeve *et al.*, 2009). Harsh parenting can be viewed dimensionally with physical abuse at the extreme end of the continuum. Overt physical abuse is associated with an increased risk of both emotional and behavioral psychopathology in children (Kim & Cicchetti, 2010), as well as a myriad of physical and mental health problems in adulthood (Norman *et al.*, 2012). Effects, however, are evident all along the continuum and long before physical abuse is at issue. Harsh parenting involves verbal aggression, hostility, and criticism toward children. Even from an early age, children who are recipients of harsh and controlling interchanges with parents are more likely to show noncompliance, aggressive behavior with peers, and other behavioral problems (Smith *et al.*, 2004). Harsh parenting has been shown to predict *change* in child behavior using a longitudinal design that controls for previous behavior, lending support to the idea that harsh parenting plays a causal role in childhood disorders (Burt *et al.*, 2006) (see also Chapter 65).

Warmth

A complementary body of developmental research exists to demonstrate the importance of dyadic parent–child exchanges that are high in parental warmth. Parental warmth includes positive affect, affection, and admiration toward the child (Davidov & Grusec, 2006). Exposure to warm and responsive parenting has shown to buffer children from adverse outcomes, and, conversely, an absence of warmth has been linked to poor emotion regulation, and emotional and behavioral maladjustment (Keller *et al.*, 2008). Parental warmth moderates the association between harsh parenting and child behavioral problems, with the association being modest in high-warmth mothers and robust in low-warmth mothers (Deater-Deckard *et al.*, 2006).

Monitoring

Another dimension of parenting that is associated with psychopathology, particularly conduct problems and substance use, and particularly in adolescence, is lack of parental monitoring. Common indicators of parental monitoring include parental knowledge about where children are, who they are with and what they are doing, parental control of the child's activities and associations, and finally, the child's voluntary disclosure of information. Meta-analytic evidence suggests that all indicators of parental monitoring have a relatively similar impact on outcomes (Hoeve *et al.*, 2009). Research into parenting factors that predict a child's willingness to self-disclose suggest that a warm and responsive family climate is likely to influence the child's proclivity to disclose information (Soenens *et al.*, 2006) and this proclivity was found by Kerr and Stattin (2000) to be the best predictor of adolescent normbreaking behavior. Thus, both the child and the parent play an active role in protecting the child from maladaptive outcomes. Intervention efforts to enhance parental monitoring practices have been effective in reducing antisocial behavior and early adolescent substance use (Dishion *et al.*, 2003).

Parenting for cognitive development

A critical developmental milestone in early childhood is the acquisition of language. Individual differences in language skills show remarkable predictive power, with early oral language predicting later academic achievement and reading comprehension (Storch & Whitehurst, 2002; NICHD Early Child Care Research Network, 2005). Parental behaviors, including sensitivity, cognitive stimulation, and parental warmth, have been consistently implicated in child language development and its sequalae. Theoretically, it is postulated that the availability of warm and responsive parent–child exchanges provide opportunities for scaffolding the child's emergent language via focused and attuned parental behaviors that are attuned to the child's interests and needs. Rich and interactive learning environments also promote stimulating and rewarding reciprocal verbal and nonverbal exchanges between dyads (Pungello *et al.*, 2009). Accordingly, positive parenting has been shown to mediate associations between maternal and child language skills (Taylor *et al.*, 2009). The predictive role of parenting appears enduring as positive parenting in toddlerhood predicts academic skills through to fifth grade (Cook *et al.*, 2011). Intervention research has demonstrated that enhancing parental contingent responsiveness can significantly impact the child's language and cognitive development, supporting a causal role for responsiveness on child outcomes (Landry *et al.*, 2008).

Differential parenting

Parents have been found to be differentially positive and negative with siblings in the family. To some extent such differential treatment of children is explained by child characteristics, including age and temperament. Differential parenting predicts increased levels of disturbance in the child who receives less positivity or more negativity over time even after controlling for genetic influences (Caspi *et al.*, 2004). For a long time, differential parenting was thought of as something that was problematic for the health of the "disadvantaged" child. Recent research suggests that the dynamic is negative for the whole family. Thus, Meunier *et al.* (2013) showed that the within-family standard deviation on parenting is associated with the family average for children's behavior problems. This suggests that it may create a dynamic in the family of divisiveness, which is problematic for everyone involved. It is interesting to note that higher levels of differential parenting predict more negative sibling relationships and the negativity of these relationships can last a lifetime (Suitor *et al.*, 2008).

The childhoods of parents

An intergenerational transmission of parenting exists: parents who experienced poor parenting in their own childhoods are more likely to engage in poor parenting with their own children,

and individuals experiencing positivity and warmth in their childhoods grow up to be more responsive parents (Belsky *et al.*, 2005; Kovan *et al.*, 2009). The same intergenerational effects have been shown for hostile parenting behavior (Neppl *et al.*, 2009). Interestingly, these intergenerational continuities are also affected by an individual's partner choice. Conger and colleagues (Conger *et al.*, 2012) initially assessed the parenting that children received when they were young and then followed them up after they had their own children. Children who had been parented harshly were more likely, once they became adults, to choose partners who were harsh. Adults who had experienced harsh parenting in their childhoods were also more likely to parent harshly if their partner parented harshly. The impact of mental and physical illness in a parent on the children is described in Chapter 28.

Loss of a parent

The bereavement process involves demonstrations of sadness and distress that sometimes develop into more severe psychopathology. A proportion of children suffering from grief will demonstrate clinically relevant symptoms that require the attention of health professionals. For example, children who lost their parents had a higher rate of major depressive episode 2 months after their loss (24%) compared to children who did not experience such a loss (1%) (Gray *et al.*, 2011). Worryingly, 35% of bereaved children reported suicidal ideation compared to 10% of their nongrieving counterparts. Further, bereaved children had more depressive symptoms 2 years after the death of their parents than controls, but significantly less than clinically depressed children in the community (Cerel *et al.*, 2006). High family socioeconomic status and few depressive symptoms reported by the surviving parent were associated with better outcomes.

Siblings

Siblings have been shown to influence one another's mental health both positively and negatively. On the positive side, when children are in stressful circumstances but have a sibling with whom they are close, they are less likely to show emotional and behavioral problems as a result of life events (Gass *et al.*, 2007). On the negative side, there is some evidence that older aggressive or delinquent siblings may train younger siblings in these behaviors, particularly when the relationship is a close one (Slomkowski *et al.*, 2001). These designs, however, did not take into account clustering on aggressive and delinquent behavior, which may have come about through genetic similarity of siblings. When such clustering is taken into account, this "training" effect of a sibling is not evident (Steele *et al.* 2013).

The family environment

The earlier discussion is centered on dyadic family relationships. The "whole" family environment may also be important to children's well-being: the processes and atmosphere that operate beyond individuals and dyads. There are very few research designs that can effectively capture the influence of the whole family, because in order to do this we must first isolate the influence of individuals and specific dyads in the family. The family-based social relations model achieves this. Every family member interacts with all other family members. Through this the following components of family life can be isolated: (a) the consistency of behavior that an individual directs to, and elicits from, others; (b) interactional behavior that is specific to each dyad in the family; and (c) the similarity of dyads within the family to one another. By taking account of the components "further down" the family system (i.e., individuals and dyads), we can achieve a real estimate of the whole family system. These studies show us that there are whole family influences. About 16% of observed negativity occurs at the family level (Rasbash et al., 2011). Furthermore, when we examine change over time in sibling relationship quality based on child report and across multiple sibling dyads in the family, we find 32% of the variance for positive sibling relationships and 37% of the variance for negative sibling relationships is attributable to the family environment (Jenkins et al., 2012). This shows us that we must go beyond dyadic interactions when we consider the ways in which families influence child well-being.

Peers

A similar risk mechanism to that described for siblings is likely to operate for peers. Several studies, including one involving an experimental design, have shown that peers may train one another to increased levels of deviant behavior. The most convincing demonstration of the negative impact of deviant peers comes from a group treatment study (Dishion et al., 1999). The experimental group was offered treatment for their delinquency in a group setting. The treatment for the comparison group was individually administered. Boys were randomly assigned to treatments and the two groups were indistinguishable at the start of treatment. The investigators were surprised to find on follow-up that adolescents who were treated in group settings showed a major rise in delinquency over time. Through group treatment the investigators had inadvertently facilitated introductions to other delinquent youth. The boys formed groups outside of the sessions. They reinforced one another, exchanged techniques, and encouraged further delinquent activities.

Exposure to deviant peers is not only a problem in adolescence. Howes (2000) assessed levels of aggression in preschool classes in childcare settings. When the proportion of aggressive children was higher in the preschool daycare, this resulted in children being more aggressive themselves when they entered Grade 2, after taking account of children's own aggression in preschool.

A common form of peer abuse is bullying, which involves repeated hurtful actions between peers where an imbalance of power exists. Accumulating evidence demonstrates that bullying is harmful to children's well-being and increases the risk of psychopathology: victims are more at risk for anxiety, depression, self-harm, violent behavior, and psychotic symptoms than

nonvictims and these problems can last until late adolescence (Arseneault et al., 2010). The effects of victimization on mental health have been shown to be over and above other hardships and genetic confounds (Arseneault et al., 2008).

Being the victim of bullying is not a random event (Ball et al., 2008) and is related to child characteristics such as emotional and behavioral problems (Barker et al., 2008; Bowes et al., 2009). The family environment also plays a role in placing some children at risk of being the victims of bullying via factors like physical maltreatment (Bowes et al., 2009), parental depression (Beran & Violato, 2004), and low socioeconomic status (Wolke et al., 2001). Genetic and environmental factors such as physical maltreatment contribute to the continuity of bullying victimization over time (Bowes et al., 2013). Children who are victims of abuse often enter a cycle of victimization that perpetuates itself over time and across situations. Being a victim of violence places the child at increased risk of various forms of further violence (revictimization), including emotional abuse, physical abuse, sexual abuse, and Internet harassment (polyvictimization). Child victims of physical assaults were twice as likely to experience another assault a year later, and victims of sexual abuse were seven times more likely to experience the same form of abuse in that same period of time (Finkelhor et al., 2007a). Further, in a national survey in the United States, out of the 71% of children who reported experiencing violence in a year, one-third reported more than one type of victimization including bullying, assaults, sexual abuse, and maltreatment (Finkelhor et al., 2007b). Furthermore, children who experienced polyvictimization suffer from increased symptoms of mental health problems, irrespective of more recent victimization experiences. Factors such as having older siblings and friends were associated with desistence of victimization from one year to another while moving to a bad neighborhood was associated with persistence. Altogether, this body of evidence suggests that efforts aimed at reducing bullying victimization in childhood and adolescence should be strongly supported.

Bully-victims are children who are involved in bullying both as bullies and as victims (about 6% of bullies, Nansel et al., 2004). Bully-victims have the highest level of adjustment problems among all children involved in bullying (Nansel et al., 2001).

Marital conflict

Marital conflict has been found to be associated with a wide range of emotional and behavioral problems in children, with the association between the latter and marital conflict being particularly robust. A number of studies provide convincing longitudinal evidence that marital conflict influences child behavior (Davies et al., 2002; Jenkins et al., 2005).

The aspect of marital conflict found to be most harmful for children is openly expressed hostility or aggression. Silence, ignoring, or other unexpressed modes of unhappiness in marriage do not have the same negative impact on children, at least in the short term (Jenkins & Smith, 1991). Children rate themselves as feeling more upset by conflict that remains unresolved between parents than conflict that is resolved (Cummings & Davies, 1994). Conflict that is about children has been found to be more distressing than conflict that is about non-child-related issues (Grych & Fincham, 1993). There is enormous variability in the extent to which children are negatively affected by marital conflict. Children's attributional processes concerning the conflict explain some of this variability. Those who perceive the conflict as threatening to family well-being (Davies *et al.*, 2002) or who blame themselves for it are more adversely affected (Grych *et al.*, 2003). The quality of the parent–child relationship has been found to be a partial mediator of the relationship between marital conflict and children's well-being (Buehler & Gerard, 2002). It should also be noted that difficult children increase the conflict between parents (Jenkins *et al.*, 2005), showing that although parental conflict has an influence on children, difficult children generate more parental conflict.

Separation and divorce

The rate of divorce has been steadily climbing. Thus, the proportion of children living apart from a biological parent is on the rise. Compared to children of intact families, children of divorced parents experience a range of negative outcomes, including behavioral problems, academic failures, as well as problems with peer relations and self-concept (Amato, 2001), which continue into adulthood (Amato, 2001). Divorce is not a discrete event: the marital conflict that usually precedes it is more problematic for children than the separation event itself (Morrison & Coiro, 1999). Consequences of divorce include economic hardship, decline in effective parental control, and diminution of noncustodial parent–child contact (Amato, 2010).

Several factors have been examined as potential moderators of divorce on child adjustment. Marital quality prior to divorce can influence how divorce is experienced: children react more adversely when there has been low parental conflict prior to divorce. When conflict is high, little change or mild improvements in child adjustment are noted when the marriage dissolves, suggesting that divorce may be more welcome in high-conflict situations (Strohschein, 2005). An emerging body of research underscores the importance of father involvement following separation and suggests that fathers' higher level of involvement promotes favorable outcomes for children but only when the father is not antisocial (Coley & Medeiros, 2007). Race has also been identified as a moderator, with European-American children experiencing a more detrimental impact of divorce compared to African-American children (Amato & Keith, 1991). It has been proposed that the nominal change in household income, as well as the more accepted norm of single parent status in the African-American community may attenuate the impact of divorce and separation for this racial group (Lansford, 2009).

Childcare influences

Childcare is a core element of most industrial societies as the majority of children attend childcare prior to school entry.

Quality and number of hours in care appear to be particularly important predictors of outcomes. Some studies have reported that longer hours predict more behavioral problems in children, although effect sizes tend to be small (NICHD, 2004). The effect of longer hours was still present on impulsivity and risk taking at age 15 (Vandell *et al.*, 2010). A meta-analysis of 20 independent samples revealed that across all ages, children in higher quality childcare had better academic, language, and social skills outcomes (Burchinal *et al.*, 2011). Peisner-Feinberg *et al.* (2001) demonstrated that, after adjusting for child and family characteristics, children's cognitive, language, and social skill gains were evident into early elementary school in children who attended high-quality childcare centers and the NICHD follow-up to 15 years has shown the same. Positive effects of childcare have been found to be strongest among socially disadvantaged children (Coté *et al.*, 2008). Both the gains associated with high-quality childcare, as well as the adverse consequences of long hours in care are enduring, but it is important to note that parenting quality appears to be a far stronger and more consistent predictor of child developmental outcomes than childcare experience (Belsky *et al.*, 2007).

Chronic versus acute psychosocial adversity

Many of the adversities described are chronic in nature. High levels of stability have been seen in risks such as marital conflict (Birditt *et al.*, 2010) and the parent–child relationship (Burt *et al.*, 2006). Within chronic exposures there are acute elements (parents are highly conflicted and then separate) which make it hard to separate the effect of chronic and acute stressors. The study of the effect of natural disasters on child well-being provides, on the surface, a more precise test of the acute hypothesis. Here too, however, chronic and acute effects are obfuscated because acute disasters often precipitate long-term problems in living. In general, findings related to natural disasters mirror conclusions from the chronic adversity studies. First, there is a dosage effect: the closer and more intense the exposure, the more negative the outcome (Masten & Osofsky, 2010). Second, when the acute event is associated with an increase in chronic adversities in the home such as family tensions and violence, then the effects on children are worse (Fernando *et al.*, 2010). Third, there is marked heterogeneity in reactions to disaster with predisaster symptomatology explaining some of this heterogeneity (Pine *et al.*, 2005).

Summary of findings related to psychosocial adversity causing child psychopathology

The evidence suggests that exposure to a range of environmental adversities increases the risk of disorder in children through the biological embedding of environmental risk. Environmental influences are best conceptualized as embedded layers of context with macro environments influencing micro environments, which in turn have effects on children's development.

Poverty and social position in society, war, and exposure to violence in neighborhoods have all been shown to have influences on the development of child psychopathology. Some of this influence operates indirectly through the proximal environment (children's relationships), while some of the effect is direct to the child. Children's relationships with parents, peers, and siblings as well as their exposure to marital conflict are more negative and problematic, the more negative and problematic the macro-context. When these relationships are problematic, children show higher levels of disorder. Understanding the mechanism in this association is complex, however, as child characteristics influence children's experiences in family relationships and who they befriend. Finally, it is very important to recognize that the vulnerability of children to environmental stressors varies enormously, an issue discussed in Chapter 27.

Directions for future research

One of the most significant issues in this area is the extent to which proximal adversities such as parenting, peer, and sibling influences are independent of the individual. Designs that examine behavior over time or across interactional partners are helpful for improving our understanding of this issue. Second, issues related to the timing and sequence of risk exposure, as well as the vulnerability of individuals to timing and sequence, will become increasingly important as we gain a better understanding of biological embedding. Third, there have been successful randomized control trials related to reducing children's exposure to environmental adversities and thus improving behavioral outcomes. It would be valuable to combine these with measurement of brain structures and neuroendocrine and immune function in order to examine the extent to which these biological processes mediate the relationship between exposure to adversity and child behavior (see Chapter 25).

References

Amato, P.R. (2001) Children of divorce in the 1990s: an update of the Amato and Keith (1991) meta-analysis. *Journal of Family Psychology* **15**, 355–370.

Amato, P.R. (2010) Research on divorce: continuing trends and new developments. *Journal of Marriage and Family* **72**, 650–666.

Amato, P.R. & Keith, B. (1991) Parental divorce and the well-being of children: a meta-analysis. *Psychological Bulletin* **110**, 26–46.

Appleyard, K. *et al.* (2005) When more is not better: the role of cumulative risk in child behavior outcomes. *Journal of Child Psychology and Psychiatry* **46**, 235–245.

Arseneault, L. *et al.* (2008) Being bullied as an environmentally mediated contributing factor to children's internalizing problems: a study of twins discordant for victimization. *Archives of Pediatrics & Adolescent Medicine* **162**, 145–150.

Arseneault, L. *et al.* (2010) Bullying victimization in youths and mental health problems: 'much ado about nothing'. *Psychological Medicine* **40**, 717–729.

Attanayake, V. *et al.* (2009) Prevalence of mental disorders among children exposed to war: a systematic review of 7920 children. *Medicine Conflict and Survival* **25**, 4–19.

Ball, H. *et al.* (2008) Genetic and environmental influences on victims, bullies and bully-victims in childhood. *Journal of Child Psychology and Psychiatry* **49**, 104–112.

Barker, E.D. *et al.* (2008) The predictive validity and early predictors of peer victimization trajectories in preschool. *Archives of General Psychiatry* **65**, 1185–1192.

Beebe, B. *et al.* (2010) The origins of 12-month attachment: a micro-analysis of 4-month mother-infant interaction. *Attachment & Human Development* **12**, 6–141.

Belsky, J. *et al.* (2005) Intergenerational transmission of warm-sensitive-stimulating parenting: a prospective study of mothers and fathers of 3-year-olds. *Child Development* **76**, 384–396.

Belsky, J. *et al.* (2007) Are there long-term effects of early child care? *Child Development* **78**, 681–701.

Beran, T.N. & Violato, C. (2004) A model of childhood perceived peer harassment : analyses of the Canadian National Longitudinal Survey of Children and Youth Data. *Journal of Psychology* **138**, 129–147.

Birditt, K.S. *et al.* (2010) Marital conflict behaviors and implications for divorce over 16 years. *Journal of Marriage and the Family* **72**, 1188–1204.

Bowes, L. *et al.* (2009) School, neighborhood and family factors are associated with children's bullying involvement: a nationally-representative longitudinal study. *Journal of the American Academy of Child and Adolescent Psychiatry* **48**, 545–553.

Bowes, L. *et al.* (2013) Chronic bullying victimization across school transitions: the role of genetic and environmental influences. *Development and Psychopathology* **25**, 333–346.

Bowlby, J. (1971) *Attachment and Loss, Volume 1. Attachment*. Hogarth Press, London.

Bradley, R.H. & Corwyn, R.F. (2002) Socioeconomic status and child development. *Annual Review of Psychology* **53**, 371–399.

Bronfenbrenner, U. (1977) Toward an experimental ecology of human development. *American Psychologist* **32**, 513–531.

Buehler, C. & Gerard, J.M. (2002) Marital conflict, ineffective parenting, and children's and adolescents' maladjustment. *Journal of Marriage and Family* **64**, 78–92.

Burchinal, M.R. *et al.* (2008) Social risk and protective factors for African American children's academic achievement and adjustment during the transition to middle school. *Developmental Psychology* **44**, 286–292.

Burchinal, M. *et al.* (2011) How well do our measures of quality predict child outcomes? A meta-analysis and coordinated analysis of data from large-scale studies of early childhood settings. In I. Martinez-Beck, K. Tout, & T. Halle (Eds.), *Quality Measurement in Early Childhood Settings* (pp. 11–32). Paul H. Brookes Publishing Company, Baltimore.

Burt, S.A. *et al.* (2006) Differential parent–child relationships and adolescent externalizing symptoms: cross-lagged analyses within a monozygotic twin differences design. *Developmental Psychology* **42**, 1289–1298.

Caspi, A. *et al.* (2004) Maternal expressed emotion predicts children's antisocial behavior problems: using monozygotic-twin differences to identify environmental effects on behavioral development. *Developmental Psychology* **40**, 149–161.

Cerel, J. *et al.* (2006) Childhood bereavement: psychopathology in the 2 years postparental death. *Journal of the American Academy of Child & Adolescent Psychiatry* **45**, 681–690.

Coley, R.L. & Medeiros, B.L. (2007) Reciprocal longitudinal relations between nonresident father involvement and adolescent delinquency. *Child Development* **78**, 132–147.

Conger, R.D. *et al.* (2012) Intergenerational continuity and discontinuity in harsh parenting. *Parenting* **12**, 222–231.

Cook, G.A. *et al.* (2011) Fathers' and mothers' cognitive stimulation in early play with toddlers: predictors of 5th grade reading and math. *Family Science* **2**, 131–145.

Coté, S.M. *et al.* (2008) Nonmaternal care in infancy and emotional/behavioral difficulties at 4 years old: moderation by family risk characteristics. *Developmental Psychology* **44**, 155–168.

Cummings, E.M. & Davies, P. (1994) *Children and Marital Conflict: The Impact of Family Dispute and Resolution*. Guilford Press, New York.

Davidov, M. & Grusec, J.E. (2006) Untangling the links of parental responsiveness to distress and warmth to child outcomes. *Child Development* **77**, 44–58.

Davies, P.T. *et al.* (2002) Child emotional security and interparental conflict. *Monographs of the Society for Research in Child Development* **67**, 1–131.

Deater-Deckard, K. *et al.* (2006) Maternal warmth moderates the link between physical punishment and child externalizing problems: a parent-offspring behavior genetic analysis. *Parenting: Science and Practice* **6**, 59–78.

Dishion, T.J. & Owen, L.D. (2002) A longitudinal analysis of friendships and substance use: bidirectional influence from adolescence to adulthood. *Developmental Psychology* **38**, 480–491.

Dishion, T.J. *et al.* (1999) When interventions harm: peer groups and problem behavior. *American Psychologist* **54**, 755–764.

Dishion, T.J. *et al.* (2003) The family check-up with high-risk young adolescents: preventing early-onset substance use by parent monitoring. *Behavior Therapy* **34**, 553–571.

Dohman *et al.* (2011) Relative versus absolute income, joy of winning and gender: brain imaging evidence. *Journal of Public Economics* **95**, 279–285.

Drury, J. & Williams, R. (2012) Children and young people who are refugees, internally displaced persons or survivors or perpetrators of war, mass violence and terrorism. *Current Opinion in Psychiatry* **25**, 277–284.

Dyregrov, A. *et al.* (2000) Trauma exposure and psychological reactions to genocide among Rwandan children. *Journal of Traumatic Stress* **13**, 3–21.

El-Sheikh, M. (2005) Does vagal tone exacerbate child maladjustment in the context of parental problem drinking? A longitudinal examination. *Journal of Abnormal Psychology* **114**, 735–741.

Evans, G.W. (2003) A multimethodological analysis of cumulative risk and allostatic load among rural children. *Developmental Psychology* **39**, 924–933.

Evans, G.W. *et al.* (2013) Cumulative risk and child development. *Psychological Bulletin* **139**, 1342–1396.

Feldman, R. (2007) Parent-infant synchrony and the construction of shared timing: physiological precursors, developmental outcomes and risk conditions. *Journal of Child Psychology and Psychiatry* **48**, 329–354.

Felitti, V.J. *et al.* (1998) Relationship of childhood abuse and household dysfunction to many of the leading causes of death in adults. *American Journal of Preventive Medicine* **14**, 245–258.

Fernando, G.A. *et al.* (2010) Growing pains: the impact of disaster-related and daily stressors on the psychological functioning of youth in Sri Lanka. *Child Development* **81**, 1192–1210.

Finkelhor, D. *et al.* (2007a) Poly-victimization and trauma in a national longitudinal cohort. *Development and Psychopathology* **19**, 149–166.

Finkelhor, D. *et al.* (2007b) Poly-victimization: a neglected component in child victimization trauma. *Child Abuse & Neglect* **31**, 7–26.

Fowler, P.J. *et al.* (2009) Community violence: a meta-analysis on the effect of exposure and mental health outcomes of children and adolescents. *Development and Psychopathology* **21**, 227–259.

Fraley, R.C. *et al.* (2013) The legacy of early experiences in development: formalizing alternative models of how early experiences are carried forward over time. *Developmental Psychology* **49**, 109–126.

Gass, K.R. *et al.* (2007) Are sibling relationships protective? A longitudinal study. *Journal of Child Psychology and Psychiatry* **48**, 167–175.

Gershoff, E.T. *et al.* (2007) Income is not enough: incorporating material hardship into models of income associations with parenting and child development. *Child Development* **78**, 70–95.

Goldberg, S. *et al.* (1999) Confidence in protection: arguments for a narrow definition of attachment. *Journal of Family Psychology* **13**, 475–483.

Gorman-Smith, D. & Tolan, P. (1998) The role of exposure to community violence and developmental problems among inner-city youth. *Development and Psychopathology* **10**, 101–116.

Grant, K.E. *et al.* (2003) Stressors and Child and Adolescent Psychopathology: moving from markers to mechanisms of risk. *Psychological Bulletin* **129**, 447–466.

Grantham-McGregor, S. *et al.* (2007) Developmental potential in the first 5 years for children in developing countries. *Lancet* **369**, 60–70.

Gray, L.B. *et al.* (2011) Depression in children and adolescents two months after the death of a parent. *Journal of Affective Disorders* **135**, 277–283.

Grych, J.H. & Fincham, F.D. (1993) Children's appraisals of marital conflict: initial investigations of the cognitive-contextual framework. *Child Development* **64**, 215–230.

Grych, J.H. *et al.* (2003) A prospective investigation of appraisals as mediators of the link between interparental conflict and child adjustment. *Child Development* **74**, 1176–1193.

Hackman, D.A. & Farah, M.J. (2009) Socioeconomic status and the developing brain. *Trends in Cognitive Science* **13**, 65–73.

Hanson, J.L. *et al.* (2013) Structural variations in prefrontal cortex mediate the relationship between early childhood stress and spatial working memory. *Journal of Neuroscience* **32**, 7917–7925.

Hoeve, M. *et al.* (2009) The relationship between parenting and delinquency: a meta-analysis. *Journal of Abnormal Child Psychology* **37**, 749–775.

Howes, C. (2000) Social-emotional classroom climate in child care, child-teacher relationships and children's second grade peer relations. *Social Development* **9**, 191–204.

Jenkins, J.M. & Smith, M.A. (1991) Marital disharmony and children's behaviour problems: aspects of a poor marriage that affect children adversely. *Journal of Child Psychology and Psychiatry* **32**, 793–810.

Jenkins, J.M. *et al.* (2003) A longitudinal investigation of the dynamics of mental state talk in families. *Child Development* **74**, 905–920.

Jenkins, J. *et al.* (2005) Mutual influence of marital conflict and children's behavior problems: shared and nonshared family risks. *Child Development* **76**, 24–39.

Jenkins, J. *et al.* (2012) The role of maternal affect in sibling relationship quality: a multilevel study of multiple dyads per family. *Journal of Child Psychology and Psychiatry* **53**, 619–722.

Joussemet, M. *et al.* (2005) A longitudinal study of the relationship of maternal autonomy support to children's adjustment and achievement in school. *Journal of Personality* **73**, 1215–1236.

Keller, P.S. *et al.* (2008) Longitudinal relations between parental drinking problems, family functioning, and child adjustment. *Development and Psychopathology* **20**, 195–212.

Kerr, M. & Stattin, H. (2000) What parents know, how they know it, and several forms of adolescent adjustment: further support for a reinterpretation of monitoring. *Developmental Psychology* **36**, 366–380.

Kim, J. & Cicchetti, D. (2010) Longitudinal pathways linking child maltreatment, emotion regulation, peer relations, and psychopathology. *Journal of Child Psychology and Psychiatry* **51**, 706–716.

Kobak, R. & Madsen, S. (2008) Disruptions in attachment bonds: implications for theory, research, and clinical intervention. In: *Handbook of Attachment: Theory, Research, and Clinical.* (eds J. Cassidy & P. Shaver), 2nd edn. Guilford, New York.

Kondo, N. *et al.* (2009) Income inequality, mortality, and self rated health: meta-analysis of multilevel studies. *British Medical Journal* **339**, 1178–1181.

Kovan, N.M. *et al.* (2009) The intergenerational continuity of observed early parenting: a prospective, longitudinal study. *Developmental Psychology* **45**, 1205–1213.

Landry, S.H. *et al.* (2008) A responsive parenting intervention: the optimal timing across early childhood for impacting maternal behaviors and child outcomes. *Developmental Psychology* **44**, 1335–1353.

Lansford, J.E. (2009) Parental divorce and children's adjustment. *Perspectives on Psychological Science* **4**, 140–152.

Laranjo, J. *et al.* (2008) Associations between maternal mind-mindedness and infant attachment security: investigating the mediating role of maternal sensitivity. *Infant Behavior and Development* **31**, 688–695.

Leventhal, T. & Brooks-Gunn, J. (2000) The neighborhoods they live in: the effects of neighborhood residence on child and adolescent outcomes. *Psychological Bulletin* **126**, 309–337.

Ludwig, J. *et al.* (2012) Neighborhood effects on the long-term well-being of low-income adults. *Science*, **337**, 1505–1510.

Macmillan, R. *et al.* (2004) Linked lives: stability and change in maternal circumstances and trajectories of antisocial behavior in children. *Child Development* **75**, 205–220.

Masten, A.S. & Osofsky, J.D. (2010) Disasters and their impact on child development: introduction to the special section. *Child Development* **81**, 1029–1039.

McElwain, N.L. *et al.* (2011) Infant–mother attachment and children's friendship quality: maternal mental-state talk as an intervening mechanism. *Developmental Psychology* **47**, 1295–1311.

Meins, E. *et al.* (2001) Rethinking maternal sensitivity: mothers' comments on infants' mental processes predict security of attachment at 12 months. *Journal of Child Psychology and Psychiatry* **42**, 638–648.

Meunier, J.C. *et al.* (2013) Multilevel mediation: cumulative contextual risk, maternal differential treatment, and children's behavior within families. *Child Development* **84**, 1594–1615.

Morrison, D.R. & Coiro, M.J. (1999) Parental conflict and marital disruption: do children benefit when high-conflict marriages are dissolved? *Journal of Marriage and Family* **61**, 626–637.

Nansel, T.R. *et al.* (2001) Bullying behaviors among US youth: prevalence and association with psychosocial adjustment. *JAMA* **285**, 2094–2100.

Nansel, T.R. *et al.* (2004) Health behaviour in school-aged children bullying analyses working group. Cross-national consistency in the relationship between bullying behaviors and psychosocial adjustment. *Archives of Pediatric and Adolescent Medicine* **158**, 730–736.

Nelson, C.A. *et al.* (2007) Cognitive recovery in socially deprived young children: the Bucharest Early Intervention Project. *Science* **318**, 1937–1940.

Neppl, T.K. *et al.* (2009) Intergenerational continuity in parenting behavior: mediating pathways and child effects. *Developmental Psychology* **45**, 1241–1256.

NICHD Early Child Care Research Network (2004) Type of child care and children's development at 54 months. *Early Childhood Research Quarterly* **19**, 203–230.

NICHD Early Child Care Research Network (2005) Duration and developmental timing of poverty on children's cognitive and social development from birth to third grade. *Child Development* **76**, 795–810.

Norman, R.E. *et al.* (2012) The long-term health consequences of child physical abuse, emotional abuse, and neglect: a systematic review and meta-analysis. *PLoS Medicine* **9**, e1001349.

Olson, M. *et al.* (2010) Impact of income and income inequality on infant health outcomes in the United States. *Pediatrics* **126**, 1165–1173.

Peisner-Feinberg *et al.* (2001) The relation of preschool child-care quality to children's cognitive and social developmental trajectories through second grade. *Child Development* **72**, 1534–1553.

Pine, D.S. *et al.* (2005) Trauma, proximity, and developmental psychopathology: the effects of war and terrorism on children. *Neuropsychopharmacology* **30**, 1781–1792.

Pungello, E.P. *et al.* (2009) The effects of socioeconomic status, race, and parenting on language development in early childhood. *Developmental Psychology* **45**, 544–559.

Rasbash, J. *et al.* (2011) Social relations model of family negativity and positivity using a genetically-informative sample. *Journal of Personality and Social Psychology* **100**, 474–491.

Rutter, M. (2012) Resilience as a dynamic concept. *Development and Psychopathology* **24**, 335–344.

Rutter, M. *et al.* (2012) Longitudinal studies using a "natural experiment" design: the case of adoptees from Romanian institutions. *Journal of the American Academy of Child & Adolescent Psychiatry* **51**, 762–770.

Shaw, D.S. *et al.* (2001) Infant and toddler pathways leading to early externalizing disorders. *Journal of the American Academy of Child & Adolescent Psychiatry* **40**, 36–43.

Slomkowski, C. *et al.* (2001) Brothers, sisters, and delinquency: evaluating social influence from early to middle adolescence. *Child Development* **72**, 271–283.

Slopen, N. *et al.* (2010) Poverty, food insecurity, and the behavior for childhood internalizing and externalizing disorders. *Journal of the American Academy of Child & Adolescent Psychiatry* **49**, 444–452.

Smith, C.L. *et al.* (2004) Predicting stability and change in toddler behavior problems: contributions of maternal behavior and child gender. *Developmental Psychology* **40**, 29–42.

Soenens, B. *et al.* (2006) Parenting and adolescent problem behavior: an integrated model with adolescent self-disclosure and perceived parental knowledge as intervening variables. *Developmental Psychology* **42**, 305–318.

Steele, F. *et al.* (2013) A multilevel simultaneous equations model for within-cluster dynamic effects, with an application to reciprocal parent–child and sibling effects. *Psychological Methods* **18**, 87–100.

Stevens, C. *et al.* (2009) Differences in the neural mechanisms of selective attention in children from different socioeconomic backgrounds: an event-related brain potential study. *Developmental Science.* **12**, 634–646.

Storch, S.A. & Whitehurst, G.J. (2002) Oral language and code-related precursors to reading: evidence from a longitudinal structural model. *Developmental Psychology* **38**, 934–947.

Strohschein, L. (2005) Parental divorce and child mental health trajectories. *Journal of Marriage and Family* **67**, 1286–1300.

Suitor *et al.* (2008) Within-family differences in parent–child relations across the life course. *Current Directions in Psychological Science* **17**, 334–338.

Taylor, N. *et al.* (2009) Maternal control strategies, maternal language usage and children's language usage at two years. *Journal of Child Language* **36**, 381–404.

Tottenham, N. & Sheridan, M.A. (2009) A review of adversity, the amygdala and the hippocampus: a consideration of developmental timing. *Frontiers in Human Neuroscience* **3**, 68.

Ungar, M. *et al.* (2013) What is resilience within the social ecology of human development? *Journal of Child Psychology and Psychiatry* **54**, 348–366.

van IJzendoorn, M.H. (1995) Adult attachment representations, parental responsiveness, and infant attachment: a meta-analysis on the predictive validity of the adult attachment interview. *Psychological Bulletin* **117**, 387–403.

Vandell, D.L. *et al.* (2010) Do effects of early child care extend to age 15 years? Results from the NICHD study of early child care and youth development. *Child Development* **81**, 737–756.

Walker, S.P. *et al.* (2007) Child development: risk factors for adverse outcomes in developing countries. *Lancet* **369**, 145–157.

Wang, M.T. & Kenny, S. (2014) Longitudinal links between fathers' and mothers' harsh verbal discipline and adolescents' conduct problems and depressive symptoms. *Child Development* **85**, 908–923.

Whipple, N. *et al.* (2010) Broadening the study of infant security of attachment: maternal autonomy-support in the context of infant exploration. *Social Development* **20**, 17–32.

White, L. *et al.* (2011) Cascading effects: the influence of attention bias to threat on the interpretation of ambiguous information. *Behavior Research and Therapy* **49**, 244–251.

Wilkinson, R. & Pickett, K. (2009) *The Spirit Level: Why More Equal Societies Almost Always Do Better*. Allen Lane, London.

Wolke, D. *et al.* (2001) Bullying and victimization of primary school children in England and Germany: prevalence and school factors. *British Journal of Psychology* **92**, 673–696.

Wood, J.J. *et al.* (2003) Parenting and childhood anxiety: theory, empirical findings, and future directions. *Journal of Child Psychology and Psychiatry* **44**, 134–151.

CHAPTER 27

Resilience: concepts, findings, and clinical implications*

Michael Rutter

Institute of Psychiatry, Psychology & Neuroscience, King's College London, UK

Resilience, as used in this chapter, is a concept that brings together three essential features (Garmezy *et al.*, 1984; Garmezy & Tellegen, 1984; Rutter, 1987; Luthar, 2003). First, it can only be studied in individuals who have experienced significant adversity. Second, there is heterogeneity in outcome, with a resilience pattern being present when the individual is functioning much better than others who have experienced the same degree and type of adversity. Third, the resilience pattern is inferred from evidence of the relatively better outcome; that is, it is not a trait that can be measured directly. Also, a resilience pattern rarely operates in a categorical pattern. That means that it is seriously misleading to use the term "invulnerability" (as put forward by Anthony, 1974; Anthony & Cohler, 1987). A resilience pattern may be evident with respect to some types of adversity but not others. Thus, it should not be expected that resilience in relation to psychosocial hazards will also apply to infections or carcinogenesis. Similarly, it may be present at one developmental period but not others. Although resilience patterns are likely to show significant temporal stability, they can change markedly if social circumstances alter. For all these reasons, Luthar and Zelazo (2003) urged that it is best to avoid terms such as "resiliency" that imply a personality trait, that resilience should apply to patterns and not individuals, and that the concept should refer to a *process*.

Nevertheless, it has to be accepted that not everyone agrees. For some, the roots of resilience as a concept lie in the emergence of positive psychology (Seligman & Csikszentmihalyi, 2000) and the wish to emphasize the positive rather than the maladaptive (Mohaupt, 2009). A helpful aspect of this movement was the wish to urge that socioemotional well-being (including a sense of purpose) was as important as economic

success (Keyes, 2007). An unhelpful aspect was a downgrading of the seriousness of mental disorder in order to concentrate on variations in the degrees of happiness in the general population (Layard, 2005), as well as an ignoring of the methodological problems inherent in the concept of "positive mental health" (Jahoda, 1959) and the difficulties in differentiating between hedonic pleasure and excitement and the quiet satisfaction of a job well done (Rutter, 2011).

An alternative starting point is provided by the concept of psychosocial competence (Masten *et al.*, 1999). It has all the advantages of using a desirable quantifiable outcome, but it suffers from four important limitations. First, it implies that the causal influences will be much the same in nonstressed groups as in those suffering extreme adversity, with nonlinear effects (meaning those that vary across the span of outcomes) identifiable only through mathematical modeling (see, e.g., Maier *et al.*, 2012) with uncertainties involved in the assumptions required (Parker & Maestripieri, 2011, Seery, 2011). Second, it implies that outcome will ordinarily be identifiable on the balance between risk and protective factors, with both identifiable on the basis of their *nature* rather than their effects. Third, it assumes that most individuals will respond to stress and adversity in much the same way and to the same degree. Fourth, it assumes that competence can and should be measured in an absolute way rather than in terms of functioning that is unusually positive in relation to the adversities experienced.

The starting point for the concept of resilience is quite different. Rather than make untested assumptions, it begins with the extensive empirical evidence that there is enormous heterogeneity in people's responses to all manner of stresses and adversities (Rutter, 2006). Because of the evidence that resilience needs to incorporate recovery (partial or total) from earlier adversity and not just to good outcome despite current adversity, a life-course perspective is required. This indicates the

---

* This chapter is largely based on two papers by the author: Rutter (2012b, 2013a).

Rutter's Child and Adolescent Psychiatry, Sixth Edition.
Edited by Anita Thapar and Daniel S. Pine, James F. Leckman, Stephen Scott, Margaret J. Snowling, Eric Taylor.
© 2015 John Wiley & Sons Ltd. Published 2018 by John Wiley & Sons Ltd.

likelihood of a dynamic process rather than some "chemistry of the moment" effect operating at just one moment in time.

For all these reasons, resilience is quite different from positive psychology and from psychosocial competence. Both gave rise to findings that indicate beneficial effects of features that operate similarly across the population. They are most important both scientifically and clinically but to avoid the misleading implication that they are protecting against some risk, the term "promotive" factors should be used (Sameroff *et al.*, 2003; Luthar & Zelazo, 2003). But, how is resilience research different from traditional risk and protective factors research? To begin with, it is the same with respect to the essential need to determine risk and protective effects in order to go on to investigate individual differences in outcome. That is, to a considerable extent, variations in outcome *are* a function of individual differences in exposure to risk and protective influences (Sameroff *et al.*, 2003). Resilience is concerned only with the differences (albeit large differences) that remain *after* risk and protective factor variations have been taken into account. In short, resilience research has to begin with a careful study of risk and protective influences.

There are 10 main features that serve to characterize resilience research as different from the overall field of risk and protective factors research (Rutter, 2012b). First, there is a *direct* analysis of the features associated with heterogeneity rather than a reliance on statistical analyses to detect nonlinear interactive effects. Gene–environment interactions (G × E) research starts with the explicit expectation that environmental hazards will *not* have the same effect in everyone, and that genetic features may account for the individual differences.

Second, there is a requirement to test for environmental mediation of risk effects (Rutter, 2007, 2012a). It might be supposed that should apply equally to risk research, and indeed it should, but in fact most psychosocial researchers have ignored this need (Rutter, 2012a).

Third, there is an interest in variables that are without effects in the general population of low-risk individuals, but which have substantial effects in the presence of adversity. Adoption is the obvious example of this kind (Rutter & Sonuga-Barke, 2010; Rutter *et al.*, 2012). Adoption is not a particularly beneficial experience in the general population but it may be *very* protective for individuals experiencing abuse or neglect in their biological family.

Fourth, resilience requires an interest in the possible "steeling" or strengthening effects of coping successfully with stress or challenge. That is, it involves an interest in and focus on negative experiences that may nevertheless provide a protection against later stressors. That requires a focused hypothesis-testing approach—a feature of resilience research but not of risk research to the same extent.

Fifth, a specific example of hypothesis-driven research is that undertaken to study gene–environment interaction (G × E) (Rutter *et al.*, 2009; Rutter, 2014). A further key characteristic is the explicit acceptance that epidemiological approaches have

to be put to the test through experimental studies, and basic science (see Rutter, 2014).

Sixth, in resilience research, animal models constitute a key element in the research strategy (see later). The study of stress inoculation in squirrel monkeys provides a good example, in that it focused specifically on possible steeling effects and used an experimental approach (Parker *et al.*, 2004). There is absolutely no reason why this should not be done with risk research but it has rarely been done.

Seventh, resilience includes a study of possible turning point effects, such as evident in the beneficial effects of marriage (Sampson *et al.*, 2006) and of early service in the Armed Forces for individuals from a disadvantaged background (Sampson & Laub, 1996).

Eighth, a key feature of resilience research has been the use of qualitative data to determine the *meaning* of experiences—a crucial detail in understanding *how* resilience might come about. This is evident in the study of positive outcomes in young people hospitalized for mental disorders in adolescence (Hauser *et al.*, 2006), and Laub *et al.*'s (1998) study of the protective effects of marriage. Note that in both cases, qualitative and quantitative data were considered together. It is a major error to consider qualitative and quantitative research as competing opposites (Rutter, 2013b).

Ninth, there are the basic findings on brain plasticity (Hensch, 2005; Bavelier *et al.*, 2010; Rutter, 2012a) which underline the dynamic concept of brain changes in terms of their temporal limits and the openness to external influences (see Chapter 23).

Finally, resilience is defined in terms of a better outcome than that usually seen in other individuals from a similarly adverse background. That is, there is no requirement of functioning that is superior to the nondeprived population as a whole. The study of Romanian adoptees (Rutter & Sonuga-Barke, 2010; Rutter *et al.*, 2012) illustrates the point. A minority of individuals had superior outcomes in relation to the general population, but a large proportion did remarkably well in relation to the other adoptees who experienced profound institutional deprivation, although they were not generally superior in functioning to nondeprived individuals. Resilience is an interactive concept and hence what matters is the variation in response among individuals experiencing the same level and type of adversity.

Testing for environmental mediation of risks

Before considering the "natural experiment" strategies designed to test environmental risk mediation, it is necessary to consider the several reasons why a statistical association might not reflect causation (see Chapter 12 for a more detailed critique). First, the relevant aspect of an overall environmental risk situation may have been misidentified. For example, for many years, family breakup was viewed as a causal risk factor for antisocial behavior in the children. Fergusson *et al.* (1992), by statistically contrasting breakup with family discord/conflict, showed that the main risk stemmed from the latter. The implication was that resilience would have to be investigated in relation to discord/conflict rather than family breakup.

Second, the causal influence might be genetically mediated in part. Most risk effects stem from people's behavior rather than acts of fate. Thus, this would apply to physical abuse. In this case, twin analyses showed that abuse was largely environmentally mediated, whereas physical punishment was more often reactive to the child's behavior (Jaffee *et al.*, 2004). Resilience could reasonably be studied in relation to abuse but it would be problematic in the case of physical punishment because it carried such a minor environmentally mediated risk.

Third, the exposure to the risk situation might be a consequence of choice or social selection. For example, it has long been observed that members of delinquent gangs commit a large number of crimes. But, is this because of the characteristics of the individuals who join such gangs, or is it the result of an influence from the gang? Thornberry's longitudinal study (Thornberry *et al.*, 1993) showed that both applied but there was a significant tendency for more crimes to be committed while people were gang members. One of the ways in which social selection effects may be bypassed is by focusing on circumstances when *whole* populations were subject to some experience without the opportunity to exercise choice. The World War II Dutch famine (Stein *et al.*, 1975) and the somewhat comparable Chinese famine (St Clair *et al.*, 2005) provide examples in relation to the risks of schizophrenia associated with prenatal famine—because the famine affected the total population. The Casino study by Costello *et al.* (Costello *et al.*, 2003) did the same with respect to the effects of relieving poverty, and the Japanese cessation of using the MMR (measles, mumps and rubella) vaccine (Honda *et al.*, 2005) showed that MMR was not responsible for an "epidemic" of autism. Atladóttir *et al.* (2007) had the same negative findings with respect to the hypothesis that Thimerosal supposedly also had given rise to an epidemic of autism. The opportunity arose because Scandinavia ceased using this mercury preservative at a time when widespread usage was continuing in the rest of the world.

Types of features associated with resilience

A wide range of features have been described as ones fostering resilience (Luthar, 2003; Ungar, 2012) but an understanding of resilience may be more usefully aided by focusing on the key *types* of features associated with resilience, starting with those that do not fit easily into a standard risk model.

Features that are neutral or risky in the absence of a risk experience

The search for such features is predicated on the basis that risk and protection must be measured with respect to their *effects*, rather than appearing inherently negative or positive in nature. The best known medical example is heterozygote sickle cell status, which provides a substantial protective effect

against malaria, despite the fact that homozygote status leads to the very serious sickle cell disease (Aidoo *et al.*, 2002). A possible psychological equivalent may be adoption or long-term fostering, although this provides protection through an entirely different mechanism (namely, the provision of a new rearing environment that replaces, and is superior to, the abusive or neglectful environment that constituted the initial risk). It is not that adoption is always preferable to being reared by biological parents. Indeed, because adoption constitutes an atypical experience, it may involve a very slight psychopathological risk. On the other hand, the adoption of a child who has been reared in a profoundly depriving institutional environment (see Nelson *et al.*, 2007; Rutter & Sonuga-Barke, 2010; Rutter *et al.*, 2012), or who has been removed from parental care because of serious abuse or neglect (Duyme *et al.*, 1999), will lead to improved psychological functioning. This has been shown by group comparisons (as part of a randomized controlled trial) of children left in an institution versus those provided with good quality long-term fostering (see Nelson *et al.*, 2007; Fox *et al.*, 2011). It has also been demonstrated by the within-individual change over time of children who leave institutional care to move to an adoptive home (Vorria *et al.*, 2006; Rutter & Sonuga-Barke, 2010; Rutter *et al.*, 2012).

Nonmaternal care constitutes a different, but somewhat comparable, example. There is no reason to suppose that being cared for by someone other than the biological mother constitutes a generally beneficial experience if the care provided by the biological mother is good. Nevertheless, two Canadian studies have shown that nonmaternal care is associated with worthwhile benefits for children from disadvantaged families (Geoffroy *et al.*, 2007; Côté *et al.*, 2008). In short, the key question in each case is not whether some supposedly atypical rearing environment constitutes an unusual health-promoting experience, but rather whether it improves upon what the child would have had in the risky environment. When it does, it will foster better functioning than the child would have had being reared by the biological mother.

Mental features

Both quantitative and qualitative research have pointed to the role of mental features in resilience. Thus, Clausen (1993, 1991) referred to the importance of planfulness in overcoming adversity and disadvantage, and Quinton and Rutter (1988), in their study of institution-reared girls found that planning was important in key life decisions (Quinton *et al.*, 1993). It was not any particular planning skill that was crucial but, rather, the self-concept that they could have some control over their lives and hence could, and would, take active decisions instead of just assuming that they were at the mercy of other people's actions.

Two points are fundamental in thinking about these findings in relation to resilience. First, the empirical findings showed that neither planning with respect to choice of marriage partner nor choice of employment were influential in girls being reared in a low-risk environment. That is because their peer group was largely neither disadvantaged nor deviant. If they selected a marriage partner by random allocation, they were likely to choose one who was relatively well-functioning. Clearly, that was not at all the case with the institution-reared girls whose peers were mainly similar to themselves. Thus, there was an interaction effect. Second, it appeared that the main influence on planning derived from successes in some activity at school (the one other operative environment they experienced). Scarcely any girls had gained any kind of scholastic achievements but some had successes in music or sport on in gaining some position of responsibility. It seemed that the ability to exert control in one area of their life made it more likely that they would develop a positive self-concept and, most crucially, a cognitive set that they could and would deal successfully with life experiences. Also, Bandura (1995) has shown that what he called "self-efficacy" was more important than simply feeling good about yourself.

Hauser et al. (2006) undertook qualitative interviewing comparing young people who fared unusually well (as shown by quantitative analyses) despite a period of psychiatric institutional care in adolescence, as against those with an average outcome. Three main features were identified: (1) a style of self-reflection to assess what had worked or not worked for them; (2) a sense of agency or determination to deal with challenges (meaning *actions* to deal with the issues) and a self-confidence in being able to do so successfully (equivalent to Bandura's self-efficacy), and (3) a commitment to social relationships.

Moffitt et al. (2011), in the Dunedin longitudinal study, found that good self-control in childhood was associated with better health and social psychological outcomes. The effects were independent of IQ and social class and operated dimensionally across the population. The research included no intervention but the finding that improvements over time in self-control were associated with better outcomes suggested a probable causal effect. While this cannot be definitely considered as a resilience feature in the absence of a demonstrated interaction, it seems possible that this is also one component of mental features associated with resilience.

Turning points in life after childhood

Much of the literature on resilience focuses on the childhood years, but the evidence of positive turning points in adult life argues for the need for a life-course perspective. Two well-studied naturalistic examples from Sampson and Laub's long-term follow-up of the Gluecks' sample of incarcerated male delinquents serve to illustrate the point (Sampson & Laub, 1993; Laub et al., 1998; Laub & Sampson, 2003). First, it was found that men who married had a better outcome; the difference remaining after controlling for a range of possibly relevant confounding variables. They went on to test this further through examination of within-individual change across periods of being and not being married, capitalizing on the natural experiment provided by the rather high rate of marriage breakdown and remarriage in American society. They created a propensity score based on the 20 variables that best predicted whether individuals would get married. This was then used, in effect, to create groups matched on their propensity scores. The overall changes in crime rate according to age were then put into the model before examining crime variation according to whether the individual was or was not married. The findings showed an overall reduction of 36–43% in crime rate during periods of marriage—confirming the protective effect of marriage.

For this finding to be clinically useful, it was essential to determine what it was about marriage that brought about this effect. John Laub tackled this question by means of systematic qualitative interviews of a purposive sample of 52 of the men. The findings indicated that marriage had many facets. These included, as one might expect, a loving supportive relationship but it also included the regulating function of wives with respect to both employment and family activities, in turn associated with the acquisition of a new kinship group and new peer group. The crucial features seem to be the "knifing off" of the past, and the opening up of fresh opportunities for the future (Maruna & Roy, 2007). Of course, people varied in the extent to which they made good use of the opportunities that were available—the mental features already discussed probably playing a key role in this connection. There is a parallel in Costello et al.'s (2003) finding on the relief of poverty brought about by the distribution on an Indian reservation of casino proceeds—as required by US federal law. Not surprisingly, families varied in the extent (and way) to which use was made of the increase in income. Interviews suggested that the mediation might lie in an increased amount of parenting time with the children, accompanied by greater supervision.

The second example is provided by early service in the Armed Forces for individuals from a severely socially disadvantaged background at the time of the 1930s Great Economic Depression (Elder, 1986). Sampson and Laub (1996) showed that such Armed Services experiences were associated with significantly better outcomes as compared with individuals from a similar background who did not serve in the Armed Forces. This was a resilience effect, as evidenced by the finding that the benefits did not apply to individuals from a nondisadvantaged background. The key question was why and how the potentially stressful experience of Army service served to provide protection. It should be appreciated that serving in the Army at that time did not involve the very high risk of death and mutilation associated with recent experiences in Iraq and Afghanistan.

As with marriage, it turned out that Army service was multifaceted. Probably, two key features mattered most. First, most of the young men had dropped out of school and lacked scholastic qualifications. Education in the more "adult" arena of the Armed Forces re-engaged many with the consequent benefits of both enjoyable learning and the acquisition of qualifications. The Government Issue (GI) bill also provided funding for a later college education. Postponement of marriage constituted the second advantageous feature. Not only did it mean that marriage could take place after, rather than before, a career was established but also it opened up the pool of potential marriage partners beyond the group of similarly disadvantaged, and often delinquent, young people that constituted their peer group prior to Army service. The data did not allow determination of just which elements in the experiences were crucial but they did point to a likely chain of events and experiences that involved both a "knifing off" of the past and the provision of new opportunities. It is highly probable that mental features influenced the extent to which such opportunities were actually taken up and made good use of. However, although the quantitative findings provide strong evidence of a resilience effect from both marriage and Army service, the precise operative elements in resilience remain speculative (but they could, and should, be tested).

Enhancement of successful coping with stress/challenge

It might be assumed that the avoidance of all environmental hazards is always desirable but, in fact, this is not the case. This is evident from the medical example of the need to be *exposed* to infectious agents in order to acquire immunity from the infectious diseases that they bring about. The problems that arise from *lack* of exposure is well illustrated by the way in which the individuals evacuated to the United Kingdom from Tristan de Cunha following a volcanic eruption there, succumbed to measles, influenza, and the like to which they had not developed immunity (Tyrrell *et al.*, 1967). Immunization represents the protection provided by the induced exposure to a modified version of the pathogen. Incidentally, the development of immunization against smallpox arose from Edward Jenner's astute observation that people exposed to cowpox (an infectious agent similar to smallpox but much milder in the effects) were much less likely to develop smallpox.

In addition, there is evidence that exposure to microbacterial agents is protective against some forms of atopic disease—particularly asthma. Children reared on farms are less likely to get asthma because of the endotoxins to which they are exposed; marked hygiene seems to increase the risk (Strachan, 1989; von Mutius, 2007; Martinez, 2008; Obihara & Bardin, 2008).

A psychopathological parallel is possibly provided by the treatment of specific phobias (Marks, 1987; Rachman, 1990). It appears that *avoidance* of the feared object makes it particularly likely that the phobia will persist. Various forms of behavioral treatment have been shown to be effective but all involve some type of controlled exposure that leads to successful coping with encounters with the feared object.

Another possible example is evident in the naturalistic, non-experimental, observations by Stacey *et al.* (1970) that children who experienced happy separations from their parents (such as by sleepovers or staying with relatives) were better able to cope with the more complicated multiple stresses associated with hospital admission.

Glen Elder (1974) found that adolescents who had to take on additional family responsibilities during the Great Economic Depression of the 1940s, and who coped successfully with those responsibilities, often seemed strengthened by what they had to do. By contrast, this was not evident with younger children who appeared less able to cope with what was demanded of them. Of course, taking on unusual responsibilities should not be viewed as a psychological "pathogen," but it does seem that coping successfully with either stresses or challenges may be strengthening or "steeling."

The most convincing evidence of "steeling" effects of controlled exposure is provided by the squirrel monkey studies undertaken by David Lyons and his colleagues (Parker *et al.*, 2004; Lyons & Parker, 2007; Lyons *et al.*, 2009; Lyons *et al.*, 2010)—building on the early studies by Levine in the early 1960s and continued up to the time of his death (Levine & Mody, 2003).

In brief, they used a strategy that mimicked the normal tendency in nature for the occurrence of brief mother–infant separations brought about by the mothers going off to forage for food when the newly weaned infants reached 3–6 months of age. Socially housed squirrel monkeys were randomized at 17 weeks of age to either brief intermittent separations for a one-hour period once each week for a total of 10 weeks or a nonseparated control condition. After 27 weeks of age, both groups were reared in identical conditions. Behavioral, hormonal, and brain imaging data were obtained at specified ages up to adulthood.

At 9 months in a novel environment test, the two groups were initially similar but they became more different over repeated sessions. Cognitive control was assessed at $2\frac{1}{2}$ years. On all these measures, the separated group performed better and cortisol measures showed a decreased reactivity to stress. Neuroimaging showed that the separated monkeys had a larger ventromedial prefrontal cortex volume. Other experiments showed that the changes in arousal more closely corresponded to stress exposure than to separation-induced changes in maternal care.

Similar beneficial effects of *brief* exposure were found in rats but prolonged separation led to increased *sensitization* to later stress experiences, rather than steeling. The overall body of evidence from animal models suggests the reality of steeling effects from brief stress experiences that are not accompanied by overall adversity or deprivation. Rather than focus on the precise level of stress that can provide protection, it is probably preferable to focus on whether or not stress or challenge leads to effective physiological and psychological coping. Of course, that dodges the difficulties in defining and measuring coping but, nevertheless, that does seem the most appropriate focus.

Gene–environment interactions (G × E)

From the outset, studies of maternal deprivation, and other forms of family adversity, indicated the huge variation in children's responses to apparently comparable experiences. Rutter (1972) suggested that one element influencing this heterogeneity might lie in genetic influences on environment susceptibility. This would mean some form of gene–environment interaction (G × E).

Quantitative behavioral genetic studies provided many pointers to the likely occurrence of G × E—especially with respect to the outcomes of depression and antisocial behavior (Rutter & Silberg, 2002). However, this early evidence was severely limited by the necessity of having to deal with "anonymous" genes. The situation became transformed by the availability of molecular genetic methods to identify individual genes and by the greater availability of measures of specific environments with a tested environmental mediation of risk (Moffitt, 2005; Rutter, 2014).

The leadership in the field of epidemiological/longitudinal studies of G × E was undoubtedly provided by the Dunedin studies undertaken by Caspi, Moffitt, and their colleagues, using the Dunedin longitudinal study. They started with reports using polymorphic variants of the MAOA gene (Caspi *et al.*, 2002) and the serotonin transporter (5HTT) promoter genevariant (Caspi *et al.*, 2003). The environmental hazards studied included both maltreatment in early childhood and stressful life events in adolescence. The focus of the mistaken critique of G × E had been solely on stress (Risch *et al.*, 2009) but, not only is maltreatment the greater hazard but also a large-scale meta-analysis of a range of adverse experiences (Karg *et al.*, 2011) showed that there was only marginal statistical significance for G × E dealing with stressful life events but a much larger, highly significant G × E with respect to maltreatment.

Figure 27.1 uses the 5HTT interaction with maltreatment to illustrate what is meant by an interaction. The upper green line shows a strong effect of maltreatment in those who have two copies of the short allele, whereas the bottom line shows no effect of maltreatment in those with two copies of the long allele. The Risch *et al.* (2009) paper created a stir in its challenge to the validity of G × E. However, it was based on a biased sample and it paid no attention to measurement issues (Uher & McGuffin, 2010). Also, it failed to pay attention to nonepidemiological research strategies (Caspi *et al.*, 2010).

With respect to maltreatment, the findings were striking in showing that the psychopathological sequelae of depression and antisocial behavior were minimal in the case of one particular genotype and much greater in the case of other genotypes. In other words, one genetic variant was associated with a resilience pattern following an experience known to carry a major mental health risk. Four findings are particularly important with respect to resilience. First, the G × E effects are largely specific to a narrow range of outcomes. Thus, the MAOA genotype showed a resilience effect in relation to antisocial behavior but no such effect in relation to depression. Similarly, the 5HTT genotype showed a resilience effect with respect to depression but not at all in relation to antisocial behavior. The findings underline the implausibility of there being a generalized resilience trait. Second, the Karg *et al.* (2011) meta-analysis findings pointed to the likelihood of a biological process that extended over a long time period extending from early childhood into early adult

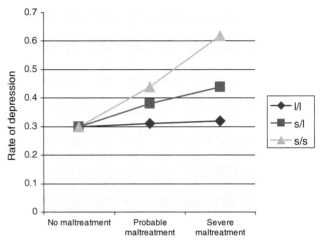

(l = long variant: s = short variant)

Figure 27.1 Effects of maltreatment on liability to depression moderated by the 5HTT gene (based on Caspi *et al.*, 2003). *Source:* Reprinted with permission of American Association for the Advancement of Science.

life—rather than one concerned with an immediate effect that involved a protection against the provoking of an onset of some mental disorder. Third, the human experimental studies of Weinberger, Hariri, and Meyer-Lindenberg (Meyer-Lindenberg & Weinberger, 2006; Hyde *et al.*, 2011) examining the neural effects of G × E as studied by brain imaging, showed that the G × E applied to individuals *without* psychopathology. In other words, although the G × E is relevant to disorder, it concerns processes that apply to all of us. Fourth, there is extensive evidence from animal models confirming the operation of G × E in relation to comparable genes to those operative in humans (Rutter, 2014).

The evidence available to date does not identify the precise mediating mechanisms for these resilience effects but the implication is that the existence of G × E is likely to mean that either the genetic and environmental influences operate on the same biological pathway or that the two pathways are close together. That possibility requires systematic testing because of the potential of determining how both G and E operate. From a practical point of view, it will also matter whether the genes affect susceptibility to adverse environments only or susceptibility to all environments. Evolutionary considerations and a growing amount of empirical evidence suggest that the latter is probably the case (Ellis *et al.*, 2011), although there may be some domain specificity (Obradović *et al.*, 2011; Essex *et al.*, 2013). The clinical implication is that the genetic polymorphisms associated with vulnerability to adverse environments may also be associated with greater responsivity to positive environments brought about through therapeutic interventions.

Supportive family warmth and cohesion

Humans are social beings and it might therefore be expected that the presence of supportive family relationships might aid resilience. Bowes *et al.* (2010) investigated this possibility using the UK Environmental Risk (E-Risk) prospective longitudinal study—focusing on the possible protective role of family warmth and positive family atmosphere in buffering the damaging effects of bullying victimization (shown through the twin design to be environmentally mediated). These positive family features assessed when the children were aged 5 and 10 years were significantly protective against the effects of bullying on emotional and behavioral disturbance at 10 and 12 years. The benefits were also evident in nonbullied children (indicating a promotive rather than a resilience effect) but a significant interaction with bullying indicated that they were greater in the bullied (indicating a resilience as well as a promotive effect). A discordant MZ twin strategy was used to test whether the beneficial effect of maternal warmth was environmentally mediated—finding that it was in the case of behavioral problems.

Overview of resilience features

By focusing on features that account for variations in the response to adversity, rather than risk/protective factors in the total population, resilience research has identified several different sorts of features that would have been less easily identified in traditional risk/protective factor analyses. The features identified included (1) features (such as adoption) that were neutral or risky in the absence of a risk experience; (2) mental features such as planfulness and self-efficacy; (3) beneficial turning point experiences in adult life such as marriage or service in the Armed Forces; (4) successful coping with stress/challenge (as brought about by exposure to the environmental hazard or challenge) and (5) gene–environment interaction. In addition, warm family support was found to have both promotive and resilience effects.

Clinical implications

There are six key conceptual considerations that need to guide all clinical implications of resilience findings. First, when resources are limited it makes sense to focus on those in greater need—those experiencing the chronic adversities considered in resilience patterns. Second, resilience findings have identified key causal influences that had not emerged from research into risk and protective factors (see later). Third, because some variable describes an environmental feature (such as poverty or social disadvantage), that does not mean that the psychopathological risks are environmentally mediated. At least some part of the effects may be genetically mediated, or represent reverse causation or bidirectional effects (see Chapter 12). Fourth, many influences are relatively context-specific (see Rutter, 1999), making it mandatory to consider the likely impact in each individual case. The findings on family breakup, marriage, and nonmaternal care well illustrate the point (see British Academy Working Group Report, 2010; Rutter, 2013a). Fifth, resilience operates as

a dynamic process across the lifespan, with restorative as well as protective effects. Sixth, the mediating mechanisms involved in resilience patterns may involve the biology (as shown, e.g., by $G \times E$), as well as mental operations (see Chapter 23).

Prevention

Although there have been programs designed to teach resilience (Ungar, 2012), these have a dubious validity because resilience is not a characteristic that can be taught or measured; it is an interactive concept that can only be identified in terms of the response to some adversity. On the other hand, it is appropriate to consider what can be done to provide individuals with the competencies that might make them better prepared to deal with adversity when it occurs.

First, in prevention, attention should be paid to the role of mental features such as planning, self-reflection, and active personal agency. Under the rubric of self-efficacy, Bandura (1995) has shown how this may be taught through experiential teaching (rather than didactic instruction), with demonstrated efficacy.

Second, there should be a focus in schools on the value of children taking responsibility, exercising a degree of autonomy, and having the opportunity of learning from their mistakes. Schools that do this well have been shown to have better pupil outcomes (Rutter *et al.*, 1979; Rutter & Maughan, 2002). More specifically, some schools have schemes to teach children how to deal with peer conflict in the classroom or playground by becoming peer mediators (Johnson & Johnson, 1996). The prime goal of such schemes is not the teaching of resilience in relation to children's own experiences but that is likely to be a worthwhile by-product.

Third, it should be worthwhile to take actions on the basis of the evidence of the protective effects of being exposed to and coping successfully with challenges and stresses. This means that children should be expected to be exposed to manageable risks, challenges, and responsibilities rather than being protected from the need to cope with them.

Fourth, attention should be paid to the value of adoption or long-term fostering when child abuse or neglect or serious parental problems have led to the child being removed from the care of the biological parents. A series of short-term foster care placements without any decision or action on long-term plans is not in the child's interest. On the other hand, adoption without the approval of the biological parents would not be ethically acceptable unless strenuous, well-focused efforts have been taken to determine whether the parents could be helped to cope effectively with their problems. This dilemma is particularly acute in the case of newborn babies being removed at birth on the basis of the severe risks associated with the mother's drug or alcohol problems. A novel initiative was set up, with the support of the Coram Foundation, in which remedial intervention was provided for a 6-month period after which a decision had to be taken on whether sufficient progress had been made to justify leaving the child in the care of the biological parents (with whatever further intervention seemed required) or, recognizing that adequate care was unlikely to be attainable, adoption should be made available without further procrastination (Harwin *et al.*, 2011). A further follow-up has been undertaken with the support of the Nuffield Foundation.

Fifth, possible turning point experiences after childhood need to be considered in terms of when they may make possible the "knifing off" of the adversities of the past and the provision of new opportunities for success and good relationships. Clearly, it is not practicable to prescribe good marriages (or other experiences) but it would be feasible to consider how such experiences may be guided or shaped to enable them to be most likely to provide a positive turning point.

Sixth, the findings on the resilience, as well as promotive, benefits of good warm family relationships indicate that therapeutic interventions designed to reduce family conflict and hostility and intervention to improve parenting, although not targeted on resilience, are likely to have resilience benefits (Bowes *et al.*, 2010).

Finally, the evidence on G × E draws attention to the potential value of paying attention to the biological pathways involved. At the moment, because the mechanism remains poorly understood there are no specific treatment pointers but they are likely to become available in the future. Although certainly not indicated at the moment, the treatment pointer might indicate a possible pharmacological intervention.

Treatment

Resilience concepts and findings do not point to a specific type of treatment but, nevertheless, they do have major implications for what is needed in any clinical assessment. Thus, the substantial evidence that there is huge heterogeneity in people's responses to all manner of environmental hazards means that, in addition to diagnosis, assessment must include an analysis of possible causal influences in that individual and a consideration of the mechanisms by which they might have operated. The focus must be on the present at least as much as on the past. Thus, there should be an appraisal of features in the child, or in the family and social circumstances, that provide either continuing risk or possible protection. This appraisal has to take account of social context because the context may alter the meaning of experiences (Rutter, 1999). There are four basic messages in considering positive or negative causal influences. First, attention needs to be focused on those for which there is good evidence of environmental mediation of effects. Second, some influences may have begun in early childhood but nevertheless have effects that persist even into adult life (Rutter & Sonuga-Barke, 2010; Karg *et al.*, 2011). Third, although acute negative life events may provoke the onset of a disorder, the long-term effects of chronic adversity tend to be much greater than those of acute events. Fourth, when considering the sequelae of early adversity, there needs to be attention to possible turning point experiences. Could there be a possibility of changing circumstances so that there might be some experience that both "knifed off" the past and provided new opportunities for success and good relationships. For example, are there youth

groups that could build on the individual's strengths? Could the school provide appropriate opportunities? Would it be helpful to seek the involvement of other family members? Does the individual's history provide clues on escape from, or successful coping with, past adversities or difficulties? How did the child (and family) deal with past crises or challenges, as success then may be relevant for the present situation? Sibling comparisons may also be informative in providing clues to possible coping strategies.

Resilience findings, both quantitative and qualitative, emphasize the importance of mental phenomena—ideas, attributes, self-reflection, and planning. Any adequate clinical assessment should assess these with an interest in those that might have the potential for overcoming adversity. In that connection, whatever treatment is implemented—whether psychological or pharmacological—it will be crucial to ensure that it is provided in a manner that encourages patients to consider that they can "act" to improve their situation, rather than feel that all benefits derive from what the clinician does. The goal of all treatments must be to pass the initiative back to the patient and so avoid a dependent reliance on the therapist. Attention also needs to be paid to the child's ongoing relationships; successful coping encompasses the social, as well as the psychological, dimension.

Conclusions

Resilience concepts and findings should be making an impact on clinical practice. It is a dynamic concept concerned with process rather than traits and it focuses attention on experiences that can foster improved coping. Such experiences are not necessarily unambiguously positive in appearance because the benefits may come from coping successfully with challenges and manageable stressors; from experiences that are neutral, or even slightly risky, in the absence of adversity; from experiences that provide fresh opportunities and a distancing from past troubles, from mental phenomena such as planning, self-reflection, and self-efficacy; and from biological pathways that bring together genes and environment in a biological pathway that extends over a long time period. Resilience is not an individual characteristic that can be taught but it should be possible through experiential influences to enable young people to be able to develop a style of functioning that will make resilience more likely.

References

Aidoo, M. *et al.* (2002) Protective effects of the sickle cell gene against malaria morbidity and mortality. *Lancet* **359**, 1311–1312.

Anthony, E.J. (1974) The syndrome of the psychologically invulnerable child. In: *The Child in his Family: Children at Psychiatric Risk.* (eds E.J. Anthony & C. Koupernik), pp. 529–545. John Wiley & Sons, New York.

Anthony, E.J. & Cohler, B.J. (1987) *The Invulnerable Child.* Guilford Press, New York.

Atladóttir, H. *et al.* (2007) Time trends in reported diagnoses of childhood neuropsychiatric disorders: a Danish cohort study. *Archives of Pediatric and Adolescent Medicine* **161**, 193–198.

Bandura, A. (1995) *Self-Efficacy in Changing Societies.* Cambridge University Press, Cambridge.

Bavelier, D. *et al.* (2010) Removing brakes on adult brain plasticity: from molecular to behavioral interventions. *Journal of Neuroscience* **30**, 14964–14971.

Bowes, L. *et al.* (2010) Families promote emotional and behavioural resilience to bullying: evidence of an environmental effect. *Journal of Child Psychology and Psychiatry* **51**, 809–817.

British Academy Working Group Report (2010) *Social Science and Family Policies.* British Academy Policy Centre, London.

Caspi, A. *et al.* (2002) Role of genotype in the cycle of violence in maltreated children. *Science* **297**, 851–854.

Caspi, A. *et al.* (2003) Influence of life stress on depression: moderation by a polymorphism in the 5-HTT gene. *Science* **301**, 386–389.

Caspi, A. *et al.* (2010) Genetic sensitivity to the environment: the case of the serotonin transporter gene and its implications for studying complex diseases and traits. *American Journal of Psychiatry* **167**, 509–527.

Clausen, J.S. (1991) Adolescent competence and the shaping of the life course. *American Journal of Sociology* **96**, 805–842.

Clausen, J.S. (1993) *American Lives: Looking Back at the Children of the Great Depression.* Free Press, New York.

Costello, E.J. *et al.* (2003) Relationships between poverty and psychopathology: a natural experiment. *JAMA* **290**, 2023–2029.

Côté, S.M. *et al.* (2008) Nonmaternal care in infancy and emotional/behavioral difficulties at 4 years old: moderation by family risk characteristics. *Developmental Psychology* **44**, 155–168.

Duyme, M. *et al.* (1999) How can we boost IQs of "dull children"? A late adoption study. *Proceedings of the National Academy of Sciences* **96**, 8790–8794.

Elder, G.H. (1974) *Children of the Great Depression.* University of Chicago Press, Chicago.

Elder, G.H. (1986) Military times and turning points in men's lives. *Developmental Psychology* **22**, 233–245.

Ellis, B.J. *et al.* (2011) Differential susceptibility to the environment: an evolutionary-neurodevelopmental theory. *Development and Psychopathology* **23**, 7–28.

Essex, M.J. *et al.* (2013) Epigenetic vestiges of early developmental adversity: childhood stress exposure and DNA methylation in adolescence. *Child Development* **84**, 58–75.

Fergusson, D.M. *et al.* (1992) Family change, parental discord and early offending. *Journal of Child Psychology and Psychiatry* **33**, 1059–1075.

Fox, N.A. *et al.* (2011) The effects of severe psychosocial deprivation and foster care intervention on cognitive development at 8 years of age: findings from the Bucharest Early Intervention Project. *Journal of Child Psychology and Psychiatry* **52**, 919–928.

Garmezy, N. & Tellegen, A. (1984) Studies of stress-resistant children: methods, variables, and preliminary findings. *Advances in Applied Developmental Psychology* **1**, 231–287.

Garmezy, N. *et al.* (1984) The study of stress and competence in children: a building block for developmental psychopathology. *Child Development* **55**, 97–111.

Geoffroy, M.C. *et al.* (2007) Association between nonmaternal care in the first year of life and children's receptive language skills prior to school entry: the moderating role of socioeconomic status. *Journal of Child Psychology and Psychiatry* **48**, 490–497.

Harwin, J. *et al.* (2011) *The Family Drug & Alcohol Court (FDAC) Evaluation Project.* Brunel University, London.

Hauser, S. *et al.* (2006) *Out of the Woods: Tales of Resilient Teens.* Harvard University Press, Cambridge, MA.

Hensch, T.K. (2005) Critical period plasticity in local cortical circuits. *Nature Reviews Neuroscience* **6**, 877–888.

Honda, H. *et al.* (2005) No effect of MMR withdrawal on the incidence of autism: a total population study. *Journal of Child Psychology and Psychiatry* **46**, 572–579.

Hyde, L.W. *et al.* (2011) Understanding risk for psychopathology through imaging gene-environment interactions. *Trends in Cognitive Sciences* **15**, 417–427.

Jaffee, S.R. *et al.* (2004) The limits of child effects: evidence for genetically mediated child effects on corporal punishment but not on physical maltreatment. *Developmental Psychology* **40**, 1047–1058.

Jahoda, M. (1959) *Current Concepts of Positive Mental Health.* Basic Books, New York.

Johnson, D.W. & Johnson, R.T. (1996) Conflict resolution and peer mediation programs in elementary and secondary schools: a review of the research. *Review of Educational Research* **66**, 459–506.

Karg, K. *et al.* (2011) The serotonin transporter promoter variant (5-HTTLPR), stress, and depression meta-analysis revisited: evidence of genetic moderation. *Archives of General Psychiatry* **68**, 444–454.

Keyes, C.L.M. (2007) Promoting and protecting mental health as flourishing: a complementary strategy for improving national mental health. *American Psychologist* **62**, 95–108.

Laub, J.H. & Sampson, R.J. (2003) *Shared Beginnings, Divergent Lives: Delinquent Boys to Age 70.* Harvard University Press, Cambridge, Massachusetts & London.

Laub, J.H. *et al.* (1998) Trajectories of change in criminal offending: good marriages and the desistance process. *American Sociological Review* **63**, 225–238.

Layard, R. (2005) *Happiness: Lessons From a New Science.* Allen Lane, London.

Levine, S. & Mody, T. (2003) The long-term psychobiological consequences of intermittent postnatal separation in the squirrel monkey. *Neuroscience & Biobehavioral Reviews* **27**, 83–89.

Luthar, S.S. (2003) *Resilience and Vulnerability: Adaptation in the Context of Childhood Adversities.* Cambridge University Press, Cambridge, UK.

Luthar, S.S. & Zelazo, L.B. (2003) Research on resilience: an integrative review. In: *Resilience and Vulnerability: Adaptation in the Context of Childhood Adversities.* (ed S.S. Luthar), pp. 510–549. Cambridge University Press, Cambridge.

Lyons, D.M. & Parker, K.J. (2007) Stress inoculation-induced indications of resilience in monkeys. *Journal of Traumatic stress* **20**, 423–433.

Lyons, D.M. *et al.* (2009) Developmental cascades linking stress inoculation, arousal regulation, and resilience. *Frontiers in Behavioral Neuroscience* **3**, 1–6. Article 32.

Lyons, D.M. *et al.* (2010) Stress coping stimulates hippocampal neurogenesis in adult monkeys. *Proceedings of the National Academy of Sciences* **107**, 14823–14827.

Maier, M.F. *et al.* (2012) A multilevel model of child-and classroom-level psychosocial factors that support language and literacy resilience of children in Head Start. *Early Childhood Research Quarterly* **27**, 104–114.

Marks, I. (1987) *Fears, Phobias and Rituals: Panic, Anxiety, and their Disorders*. Oxford University Press, New York.

Martinez, F.D. (2008) Gene–environment interaction in complex diseases: asthma as an illustrative case. In: *Genetic Effects on Environmental Vulnerability to Disease*. (ed M. Rutter), pp. 184–197. John Wiley & Sons, Chichester.

Maruna, S. & Roy, K. (2007) Amputation or reconstruction? Notes on the concept of "knifing off" and desistance from crime. *Journal of Contemporary Criminal Justice* **23**, 104–124.

Masten, A.S. *et al.* (1999) Competence in the context of adversity: pathways to resilience and maladaptation from childhood to late adolescence. *Development and Psychopathology* **11**, 143–169.

Meyer-Lindenberg, A. & Weinberger, D.R. (2006) Intermediate phenotypes and genetic mechanisms of psychiatric disorders. *Nature Reviews Neuroscience* **7**, 818–827.

Moffitt, T. *et al.* (2011) A gradient of childhood self-control predicts health, wealth, and public safety. *Proceedings of the National Academy of Sciences* **108**, 2693–2698.

Moffitt, T.E. (2005) Genetic and environmental influences on antisocial behaviors: evidence from behavioral–genetic research. *Advances in Genetics* **55**, 41–104.

Mohaupt, S. (2009) Review article: resilience and social exclusion. *Social Policy and Society* **8**, 63–71.

von Mutius, E. (2007) Allergies, infections and the hygiene hypothesis - the epidemiological evidence. *Immunobiology* **212**, 433–439.

Nelson, C.A. *et al.* (2007) Cognitive recovery in socially deprived young children: the Bucharest Early Intervention Project. *Science* **318**, 1937–1940.

Obihara, C.C. & Bardin, P.G. (2008) Hygiene hypothesis, allergy and BCG: a dirty mix? *Clinical & Experimental Allergy* **38**, 388–392.

Obradović, J. *et al.* (2011) The interactive effect of marital conflict and stress reactivity on externalizing and internalizing symptoms: the role of laboratory stressors. *Development and Psychopathology* **23**, 101–114.

Parker, K.J. & Maestripieri, D. (2011) Identifying key features of early stressful experiences that produce stress vulnerability and resilience in primates. *Neuroscience & Biobehavioral Reviews* **35**, 1466–1483.

Parker, K.J. *et al.* (2004) Prospective investigation of stress inoculation in young monkeys. *Archives of General Psychiatry* **61**, 933–941.

Quinton, D. & Rutter, M. (1988) *Parenting Breakdown: The Making and Breaking of Inter-Generational Links*. Avebury, Aldershot, UK.

Quinton, D. *et al.* (1993) Partners, peers, and pathways: assortative pairing and continuities in conduct disorder. *Development and Psychopathology* **5**, 763–763.

Rachman, S.J. (1990) *Fear and Courage*. WH Freeman/Times Books/Henry Holt & Co., New York.

Risch, N. *et al.* (2009) Interaction between the serotonin transporter gene (5-HTTLPR), stressful life events, and risk of depression. *JAMA* **301**, 2462–2471.

Rutter, M. (1972) Maternal deprivation reconsidered. *Journal of Psychosomatic Research* **16**, 241–250.

Rutter, M. (1987) Psychosocial resilience and protective mechanisms. *American Journal of Orthopsychiatry* **57**, 316–331.

Rutter, M. (1999) Psychosocial adversity and child psychopathology. *British Journal of Psychiatry* **174**, 480–493.

Rutter, M. (2006) Implications of resilience concepts for scientific understanding. *Annals of N Y Academy of Sciences* **1094**, 1–12.

Rutter, M. (2007) Proceeding from observed correlation to causal inference: the use of natural experiments. *Perspectives on Psychological Science* **2**, 377–395.

Rutter, M. (2011) Biological and experiential influences on psychological development. In: *Nature and Nurture in Early Child Development*. (ed D. Keating), pp. 7–44. Cambridge University Press, New York.

Rutter, M. (2012a) Achievements and challenges in the biology of environmental effects. *Proceedings of the National Academy of Sciences* **109**, 17149–17153.

Rutter, M. (2012b) Resilience as a dynamic concept. *Development and Psychopathology* **24**, 335–344.

Rutter, M. (2013a) Resilience: clinical implications. *Journal of Child Psychology and Psychiatry* **54**, 474–487.

Rutter, M. (2013b) The role of science in understanding family troubles. In: *Family Troubles? Exploring Changes and Challenges in the Family Lives of Children and Young People*. (eds J.R. McCarthy, C.-A. Hooper & V. Gillies), pp. 45–58. The Policy Press, Bristol.

Rutter, M. (2014) Nature-nurture integration. In: *Handbook of Developmental Psychopathology*. (eds M. Lewis & K. Rudolph), 3rd edn, pp. 45–66. Springer Science.

Rutter, M. & Maughan, B. (2002) School effectiveness findings 1979-2002. *Journal of School Psychology* **40**, 451–475.

Rutter, M. & Silberg, J. (2002) Gene-environment interplay in relation to emotional and behavioral disturbance. *Annual Review of Psychology* **53**, 463–490.

Rutter, M. & Sonuga-Barke, E.J. (2010) X. Conclusions: overview of findings from the E.R.A. study, inferences, and research implications. In: *Deprivation-Specific Psychological Patterns: Effects of Institutional Deprivation*, vol. 75, pp. 212–229. Monographs of the Society for Research in Child Development, Oxford.

Rutter, M. *et al.* (1979) *Fifteen Thousand Hours: Secondary Schools and their Effects on Children*. Harvard University Press, Cambridge, MA.

Rutter, M. *et al.* (2009) Gene-environment interactions: biologically valid pathway or artifact? *Archives of General Psychiatry* **66**, 1287–1289.

Rutter, M. *et al.* (2012) Longitudinal studies using a "natural experiment" design: the case of adoptees from Romanian institutions. *Journal of the American Academy of Child & Adolescent Psychiatry* **51**, 762–770.

Sameroff, A. *et al.* (2003) Adaptation among youth facing multiple risks: prospective research findings. In: *Resilience and Vulnerability: Adaptation in the Context of Childhood Adversities*. (ed S.S. Luthar), pp. 364–391. Cambridge University Press, Cambridge.

Sampson, R.J. & Laub, J.H. (1993) *Crime in the Making: Pathways and Turning Points Through Life*. Harvard University Press, Cambridge MA.

Sampson, R.J. & Laub, J.H. (1996) Socioeconomic achievement in the life course of disadvantaged men: military service as a turning point, circa 1940-1965. *American Sociological Review* **61**, 347–367.

Sampson *et al.* (2006) Does marriage reduce crime? A counterfactual approach to within-individual causal effects. *Criminology* **44**, 465–508.

Seery, M.D. (2011) Resilience a silver lining to experiencing adverse life events? *Current Directions in Psychological Science* **20**, 390–394.

Seligman, M.E.P. & Csikszentmihalyi, M. (2000) Positive psychology: an introduction. *American Psychologist* **55**, 5–14.

St Clair, D. *et al.* (2005) Rates of adult schizophrenia following prenatal exposure to the Chinese famine of 1959-1961. *Journal of the American Medical Association* **294**, 557–562.

Stacey, M. *et al.* (1970) *Hospitals, Children and their Families. The Report of a Pilot Study.* Routledge & Kegan Paul, London.

Stein, Z.A. *et al.* (1975) *Famine and Human Development: The Dutch Hunger Winter of 1944–1945.* Oxford University Press, New York.

Strachan, D.P. (1989) Hay fever, hygiene, and household size. *British Medical Journal* **299**, 1259–1260.

Thornberry, T.P. *et al.* (1993) The role of juvenile gangs in facilitating delinquent behavior. *Journal of Research in Crime & Delinquency* **30**, 55–87.

Tyrrell, D. *et al.* (1967) Serological studies on infections by respiratory viruses of the inhabitants of Tristan da Cunha. *Journal of Hygiene* **65**, 327–341.

Uher, R. & McGuffin, P. (2010) The moderation by the serotonin transporter gene of environmental adversity in the etiology of depression: 2009 update. *Molecular Psychiatry* **15**, 18–22.

Ungar, M.E. (2012) *The Social Ecology of Resilience: A Handbook of Theory and Practice.* Springer, New York.

Vorria, P. *et al.* (2006) The development of adopted children after institutional care: a follow-up study. *Journal of Child Psychology and Psychiatry* **47**, 1246–1253.

CHAPTER 28

Impact of parental psychiatric disorder and physical illness

Alan Stein[1] and Gordon Harold[2]

[1] Department of Psychiatry, Child and Adolescent Psychiatry, Warneford Hospital, University of Oxford, UK
[2] Rudd Centre for Adoption Research and Practice, School of Psychology, University of Sussex, Brighton, UK

There is a substantial body of evidence that psychiatric and physical disorders in parents are associated with an increased rate of psychological disturbances in children. However, contemporary research evidence is illuminating the mechanisms through which some children experience elevated psychological disturbances in response to parental psychiatric disorder, while other children show resilience to such intergenerational transmission. The elucidation of the mechanisms involved in the intergenerational transmission of disorder is scientifically important in helping to understand the pathways to both healthy and disturbed development, and informative in developing interventions aimed at reducing the intergenerational transmission of psychopathology to children.

Intergenerational transmission of psychiatric disorder: a conceptual and theoretical overview

One of the most consistent correlates of psychiatric dysfunction is having a parent with a history of psychiatric disorder. Offspring of depressed parents, for example, are at least three times more likely to develop a mood disorder as well as other psychiatric problems and impairment compared to children of nondepressed parents (Weissman *et al.*, 1997). The intergenerational transmission of psychiatric disorders is a complex and multifaceted process (Serbin *et al.*, 2004).

Specifically relating to depression, for example, Goodman and Gotlib (1999) proposed four general explanations for the transmission of depression from mothers to children: heritability; innate neuroregulatory dysfunction; exposure to maternal negative affect, cognitions, and behaviors; and increased stress in the family (see Garber *et al.*, 2010). We offer an integrated

theoretical model that conveys the complex and multifaceted processes through which early exposure to parental psychiatric disorder may confer developmental risk to children (see Figure 28.1). In this figure, parental psychiatric disorder is presented as an early risk factor that sets the stage for a cascade of processes through which elevated risk for offspring psychopathology is conveyed.

Contemporary research models have moved beyond examining simple bivariate associations between specific risks and related risk outcomes, to examining the pathways and processes through which early parental risk may confer elevated risk outcomes for children. Specifically, factors that mediate and moderate initial associations are examined as mechanisms through which risk effects are conveyed, and thus offer sites through which intervention targets may be directed in order to reduce or ameliorate the intergenerational transmission of risk outcomes. For example, parental depression has been linked to disruptions in children's neurobiological functioning (e.g., HPA axis dysregulation), cognitive-emotional-social processing (e.g., negative attributions, emotional regulation, social skills), as well as disrupted patterns of family functioning (e.g., heightened interparental conflict, negative parent–child relationships). These, in turn, could link to elevated symptoms of depression in children. While each of these theoretical domains offers a mediating process through which associations between parental depression and child depression may be explained (see Figure 28.1, e.g., Paths E + I; Paths F + J; Paths M + N), each intervening domain may also offer further mediation (e.g., G + K; L + H). One possible explanatory sequence underlying the intergenerational transmission of psychopathology may emanate from early psychiatric risk leading to dysregulated neurobiological functioning, which in turn disrupts cognitive, emotional and social processing, offering the propensity to

Rutter's Child and Adolescent Psychiatry, Sixth Edition.
Edited by Anita Thapar and Daniel S. Pine, James F. Leckman, Stephen Scott, Margaret J. Snowling, Eric Taylor.

Parental influences Neurobiological, cognitive, social Child outcomes
Mechanisms

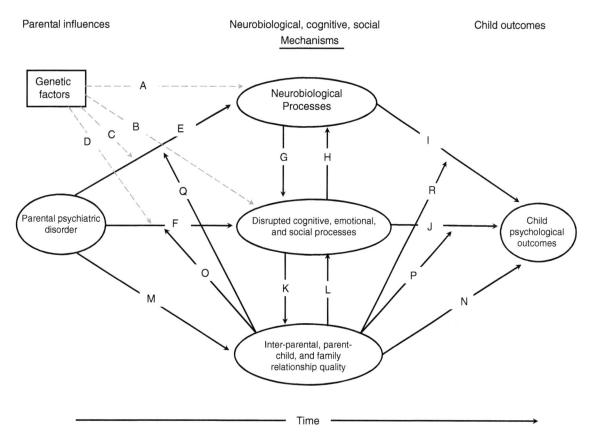

Figure 28.1 Theoretical model of the intergenerational transmission of psychopathology.

disrupt patterns of functional family relationships (e.g., parenting practices), which then leads to elevated psychopathology in children (see Figure 28.1, i.e., Paths E + G + K + N).

Other theoretical possibilities also exist (e.g., Paths E + G + H + I; F + K + L + J), capturing not only unidirectional processes, but bidirectional and transactional patterns. While these respective configurations of intergenerational transmission of psychopathology represent plausible mediating processes, the model also incorporates the propensity for possible moderating influences. For example, genetic factors are recognized as relevant to the transmission of psychopathology from parent to offspring (see Chapters 12 and 24). Children born to mothers who are depressed might inherit DNA that places them at elevated risk for depression (Goodman & Gotlib, 1991). These susceptibility factors may also disrupt neurobiological and cognitive-emotional-social processing (Paths A and B). Specifically relating to the role of genetic transmission in studies that examine the etiology of psychopathology in childhood, recent molecular genetic studies have reported allele (G) × environment (E; specifically child maltreatment) interactions (genetic moderation) predicting children's antisocial behavior and conduct problems (Caspi et al., 2002; Kim-Cohen et al., 2006; Rutter et al., 2009). Building on this body of evidence, it is increasingly recognized that rather than serve as a

direct cause of disrupted individual psychological functioning, genetic factors may interact with adverse environmental conditions (gene–environment interplay), promoting more negative developmental outcomes (e.g., Paths C and D).

As a further example of a process-orientated approach to understanding the intergenerational transmission of psychopathology, each of the proposed mediators presented in Figure 28.1 may also serve to moderate specific pathways linking parental psychiatric disorder to offspring outcomes. For example, negative family interaction patterns may accentuate the association between parental psychiatric disorder and disruptions in children's neurobiological processing (Path Q), or between levels of cognitive-emotional-social processing and children's symptoms of psychopathology (Path P). The model presented in Figure 28.1 offers a conceptual framework through which understanding of intergenerational transmission processes may be represented schematically, offering testable hypotheses that may be extended and amended relative to the specific index of parental psychiatric disorder that is being examined. We review primary areas of psychiatric disorder and associated outcomes for children in the following sections. First, however, we provide (1) a very brief synopsis of research findings that illuminate the heterogeneous nature of psychopathology as conveyed through intergenerational risk and the mediating and moderating mechanisms through which this heterogeneity may be explained, and (2) we provide a brief primer for the clinical reader of the specifics of mediating and moderating variables as they are conceptually and statistically examined, with features of mediation and moderation also addressed in other relevant chapters (see Chapters 12 and 24).

Intergenerational transmission of psychopathology: one size does not fit all

Despite evidence that increased risk for psychopathology is conferred to children of parents with psychiatric disorder, emerging evidence suggests that a given psychiatric risk in a parent (e.g., depression) may convey one or more risk outcomes in children (e.g., depression and/or conduct problems); intergenerational transmission of psychopathology is not necessarily phenotype specific (e.g., parent depression to child depression; parent antisocial behavior to child conduct problems). Further, the transmission mechanisms (e.g., parenting behavior) that underlie any such association may vary depending on the particular index of psychopathology considered. As outlined above, past research has suggested that genetic factors passed on from parents to children (G) may explain the pattern of association between specific indices of parent psychopathology and associated outcomes for children, other studies suggest that the environmental conditions (E) experienced by children in the context of parent psychopathology explain transmission effects, with recent studies suggesting that the combination of genetic susceptibility factors and adverse environments (G × E) explain intergenerational transmission associations (see Chapters 12 and 24). Recent studies employing novel research designs that allow disaggregation of genetic and environmental factors underlying associations between parent and child psychopathology find differential results for the relative role of G versus E. For example, Silberg *et al.* (2010), using a Children of Twins (COT) design, noted that associations between parent antisocial behavior and child depression were entirely mediated by environmental factors, with genetic and environmental factors mediating association with child antisocial behavior, and genetic factors mediating association with child ADHD. Specifically relating to the role of parenting as an environmental mediator of associations between parent and child psychopathology, Silberg *et al.* (2010) noted the role of parenting as a mediator in the case of parent antisocial behavior and both child conduct problems and depression. Harold and colleagues echo this pattern of results using a sample of differentially related parents and children conceived through *in vitro* fertilization (IVF) (Harold *et al.*, 2013). Findings from studies using this design, suggest that genetically unconfounded associations between parent and child antisocial behavior are mediated by hostile parenting, while parenting does not mediate the association between parent and child depression (Harold *et al.*, 2011). Findings from these studies illuminate the complexity of genetic and/or environmental processes that underlie associations between parent and child psychopathology.

The mechanics of mechanism: mediators versus moderators in clinical research

Any question that engages the hypothesized role of a third variable, such that the initial association or link between an independent variable (X, cause) and a dependent variable (Y, criterion) is explained by a mid-level variable may be described as a *mediating variable*. According to MacKinnon (2011), there are two overlapping ways in which mediating variables have been used in prior research, with particular relevance to clinical applications. First, mediation for design where interventions are employed to change a mechanism (mediator) through which a factor exerts influence over an outcome or criterion. Second, mediation for explanation where mediators are selected after an effect of X to Y has been demonstrated to explain the mediating process by which X affects Y. The use of mediating variables for design is central to interventions designed to affect or influence behavior (e.g., hostile parenting practices in the context of parental antisocial behavior). A *moderating variable* is a variable that modifies the form or strength of the relationship between an independent and a dependent variable. Moderated effects are also more commonly known as interaction effects. Unlike a mediating variable, a moderating variable is not part of a causal sequence or chain; rather, the moderator qualifies the relationship between X and Y (e.g., sex, group allocation, genetic predisposition, IQ, temperament).

Moderating and mediating variables may also work together in explaining psychiatric risk effects on psychological outcomes in children. There are two major types of effects that combine moderation and mediation as described in the literature (see Preacher *et al.*, 2007) (1) moderation of a mediated effect, where the mediated effect is different at different levels of a moderator variable (e.g., hostile parenting practices (Med) in the context of parent antisocial behavior (X) and child conduct problems (Y) affects behavioral outcomes for boys but not girls, the role of the mediator is therefore moderated by child gender, (2) mediation of a moderated effect, where the effect of an interaction (moderated effect) on a dependent variable is mediated (e.g., a parenting-focused intervention targeting adult antisocial behavior on child depression may be explained by parent gender, such that the interaction between the intervention and adult antisocial behavior is due to differential time spent with child between mothers versus fathers, the role of the moderator is therefore mediated by parental gender as measured through time spent with child). Despite the conceptual appeal of moderated-mediation and mediated-moderation, particularly from a clinical standpoint, few research studies simultaneously include both mediating and moderating variables, at least in part because of the difficulty of specifying and interpreting these models, relative to clinical applications.

Parental psychiatric disorders

The issue of the effects of parental disorder on children applies both to mothers and fathers, although the majority of research has been conducted with mothers (Ramchandani et al., 2009). Some disorders are especially common in the child-bearing years, such as depression, anxiety, eating disorders, and alcoholism. In the following section, we primarily focus on the psychiatric or psychosocial outcomes for children. Alongside these, other difficulties, such as the impact on family functioning, need to be considered.

Depression

Depression is the most common psychiatric condition among women of childbearing age and has a point prevalence of over 8% (Weissman et al., 1988). Depression affecting parents of older children has revealed consistent associations with difficulties in their children. A recent meta-analysis of the impact of maternal depression on four domains of offspring psychopathology: emotional disorders, behavioral disorders, general psychopathology, and negative/positive affect or behavior found that the risks were increased in all four domains (Goodman et al., 2011). The effect sizes, however, were relatively small. Children from low-income families, children of single mothers, and girls seem to be most affected. More severe and chronic parental depression is associated with a higher risk for offspring disorder (Goodman et al., 2011), more specifically, an increased risk of behavioral problems, such as conduct disorder in school-aged children, and an increased risk of psychiatric disorder in adolescents, particularly depression and anxiety disorders (Tully et al., 2008; Harold et al., 2011). This risk persists into adulthood; a 20-year longitudinal study found that offspring of depressed parents had a threefold increase in depressive and anxiety disorders and substance dependence, as well as an increased risk of physical health problems and greater social impairment (Weissman et al., 2006). Other research has found an increased risk of insecure attachment to the depressed parent (Martins et al., 2000). Compared to controls, young children of mothers with depression score lower on measures of language and general cognitive development, but again effect sizes were relatively small (Stein et al., 2008; Murray et al., 2010). In low- and middle-income countries (LMICs), there is also substantial evidence that child growth is associated with maternal depression, with an increased risk of child stunting and children being underweight (Surkan et al., 2011).

The postnatal period has been a particular focus of research and clinical work in recent years. This is partly because the infant is entirely dependent on carers for his/her health and development at this time, and because of the emphasis on the benefits of early intervention and prevention (Doyle et al., 2009). Estimates of depression occurring specifically in the postnatal period are approximately 13% (O'Hara et al., 1996). A recent review from high-income countries (HICs) indicates that the prevalence of "major depression" using diagnostic interviews is lower (4.7% in the 3 months postpartum) (Gavin et al., 2005). Recent studies of LMICs have shown rates to be substantially higher than in HICs, although with considerable variability in rates (Parsons et al., 2012). Those at particular risk of developing postnatal depression (PND) include women with a past history of depression and those who lack social support. Other factors include socioeconomic deprivation and social isolation (Boyce, 2003).

An increasing number of longitudinal studies have identified associations between maternal PND and adverse child outcomes (Murray et al., 2010, Stein et al., 2014.). PND can affect a mother's ability to cope with the care of her infant and limits her capacity to engage positively with the infant in social interactions. PND is also associated with poorer functioning in a number of developmental domains, including child behavior, attachment, and social and cognitive development. The children at most risk are those whose parents are socioeconomically disadvantaged or those where the mother's depression persists (Goodman et al., 2011). The few studies which have followed up children into adolescence, suggest that at 18 years they are at an increased risk for depression themselves (Pearson et al., 2013). Experimental evidence indicates that maternal cognitions associated with depression (rumination) and anxiety (worry) make it difficult for the mother to attend to the child's signals, which in turn impact negatively on mother–child interactions (Stein et al., 2012).

Evidence suggests that parenting is an important mediator of the effects of depression on young children (Leve et al., 2009). However, the effects are not inevitable and are moderated by socioeconomic status, social adversity, education (Lovejoy et al., 2000), and the health status of the non-ill parent (Engle et al., 2013). Thus, in more adverse circumstances or where parents have low levels of education, depression is more likely to impact on the quality of parenting and thereby child development (Stein et al., 2008), but wider healthy family relationships may ameliorate (moderate) this relationship.

Antenatal psychiatric disorders are also associated with disturbances in child development (Van den Bergh et al., 2005; Talge et al., 2007). Whether the associations observed arise directly through effects on the fetus, genetic confounds or because depression continues into the postnatal period, are difficult to determine (Batenburg-Eddes et al., 2012). There is now some evidence of association with increased rates of ADHD (Galéra et al., 2011), and depression in late adolescence for those whose mothers had antenatal psychiatric disorders (Pearson et al., 2013). However, the causal underpinnings underlying these associations remain unclear.

There has been some research on the effects of depression in fathers in the postnatal period. One large longitudinal study showed that paternal depression was associated with increased risk of behavioral problems at 3 years, largely in boys. There was also an increased risk of both conduct and emotional problems for both sexes at 8 years (Ramchandani et al., 2009).

Anxiety

Anxiety disorders in parents are also common. Social phobia is the most prevalent of the anxiety disorders and it has a lifetime rate of 13% (Kessler *et al.*, 1994). Children of parents with anxiety disorders have been shown to have a markedly increased rate of anxiety disorder themselves (up to 7 times) (Turner *et al.*, 1987) and an increased rate even compared with offspring of substance-abusing parents (Merikangas *et al.*, 1998; Biederman *et al.*, 2006). Social phobia has been reported in almost a quarter of the children of patients with social phobia (Mancini *et al.*, 1996). Antenatal anxiety has also been associated with a range of offspring problems, including both emotional and behavioral problems (Glover, 2011). Postnatal anxiety also shows negative effects on both psychological and somatic outcomes (Murray *et al.*, 2009; Glasheen *et al.*, 2010).

Two aspects of parenting as modes of transmission of anxiety have been of particular interest. The first is through modeling of anxious behavior, for example, where parents respond to strangers in an anxious/wary way, young children may show avoidant behavior (Murray *et al.*, 2009). The second is via the transfer of information through parental cognitions, for example, in conversations with children, anxious parents express fear, particularly of threat about the future, or the consequences of actions. These in turn impact on the child's behavior and cognitions (Murray *et al.*, 2009). When cognitions of mothers with postnatal anxiety disorders were primed, adverse effects on their responsiveness to their infants were evident, which in turn was associated with infant withdrawal and negative mood (Stein *et al.*, 2012).

Eating disorders

Eating disorders are common among women of child-bearing age (Fairburn *et al.*, 2003), and the prevalence may be rising. The majority of such women suffer from bulimia nervosa or eating disorder not otherwise specified (EDNOS), which are significantly impairing but do not fulfill all the criteria for anorexia or bulimia nervosa. Only a small minority suffer from anorexia nervosa as low weight affects their fertility. Maternal anorexia nervosa (active or past) is associated with low birth weight, increased rates of prematurity, and even an increased risk of miscarriage. This is likely to be mediated by both low maternal BMI prepregnancy and smoking (see Micali *et al.*, 2009 for a review).

Children of mothers with eating disorders are particularly vulnerable during infancy and adolescence (Patel *et al.*, 2002). Such children are more likely to grow more slowly and some even fail to thrive (Patel *et al.*, 2002). Two longitudinal studies have shown that children of mothers with eating psychopathology are more likely to experience conflict during mealtimes when 5 years of age. They are also more likely to have concerns about their body shape and weight and to use dietary restraint; this is possibly more common in girls (Stice *et al.*, 1999; Jacobi *et al.*, 2001; Stein *et al.*, 2006a, also see Chapter 71). Data from the Avon Longitudinal Study of Parents and Children (ALSPAC) study showed that children whose mothers had a history of anorexia nervosa or bulimia nervosa were at increased risk in the preschool period of a range of difficulties such as emotional, conduct, and hyperactivity disorders for girls and emotional problems for boys for children of women with anorexia nervosa (Micali *et al.*, 2014). Girls of mothers with bulimia nervosa were more likely to show hyperactivity and boys had more emotional and conduct disorders.

Alcohol and substance misuse

Alcoholism and substance misuse are conditions that are easily overlooked. They are not uncommon among adults of child-bearing age, and are associated with higher risks among the children (Lieberman, 2000). Heavy alcohol consumption during pregnancy has been recognized as potentially harmful to the fetus (Stratton *et al.*, 1996). In particular, it may result in fetal alcohol syndrome, which is characterized by minor facial anomalies, impaired growth, and developmental delay (Jones *et al.*, 1973).

The worldwide prevalence of this condition varies with estimated rates of 2–7 per thousand children in the United States contrasting with rates of around 50 per thousand in the Western Cape of South Africa (May *et al.*, 2009). It is a condition associated with poverty and disadvantage (Abel, 1995). In addition to this well-described syndrome, it seems plausible that prenatal alcohol exposure could exert neurotoxic effects in the absence of facial or other abnormalities. Such a condition has been termed alcohol-related neurodevelopmental disorder (Stratton *et al.*, 1996). Although this condition is purported to be more common than fetal alcohol syndrome, making a causal link in an individual case is very difficult and more research is warranted (Gray *et al.*, 2009). Alcohol and drug problems can exist alone, but often coexist with depressive disorder. With regard to problems in older children, a large longitudinal study found that adult children of alcoholics had an increased lifetime prevalence of mood, anxiety, and abuse/dependence disorders and possibly also schizophrenia when compared to offspring of nonalcoholic parents (Cuijpers *et al.*, 1999). Rates were especially high for the children of fathers with drinking problems.

Of particular relevance to the early postpartum period is the problem of withdrawal syndrome. Newborn babies of mothers who are drug-dependent are already at higher risk than nonexposed infants for perinatal complications such as prematurity and low birth weight. A withdrawal syndrome can develop in cases where the mother has been using opiates, but this can also occur with other drugs such as benzodiazepines. The symptoms and signs seen in the infant depend on the drug used, and the risk and severity of these symptoms diminish significantly if the mother has been abstinent for more than a few days (Hudak *et al.*, 2012). In circumstances where a child exhibits a withdrawal reaction, the issue of child protection will also require careful consideration and, where parents have a continuing substance addiction, child protection will be a continuing concern for the professionals involved (Gray *et al.*, 2009).

Schizophrenia and other psychoses

Some severe psychiatric disorders, such as schizophrenia, are associated with reduced fertility. Compared with the general population, parents with schizophrenia have a greatly increased risk of having a child who later develops schizophrenia (Gottesman *et al.*, 1991; Bergman *et al.*, 1995). In addition, although most of the study samples have historically been relatively small, they do suggest that children of affected parents have a raised risk of a range of other psychiatric diagnoses; including ADHD, autism, anxiety disorders, and depressive disorder. More recent, larger scale population studies affirm this pattern of results (see Sullivan *et al.*, 2012). Children of parents with such disorders may have to cope with enormous variations in parental mood and behavior as well as sometimes having to provide substantial care for their parents.

With respect to bipolar disorder there is a high risk of offspring developing affective disorders with a smaller specific risk of bipolar disorder. For example, in a 12-year prospective study of the adolescent children of parents with bipolar disorder, lifetime prevalence was found to be 13% for bipolar spectrum disorders and 45% for mood disorders (Mesman *et al.*, 2013). Other studies report even higher rates for both bipolar disorder (morbidity risk 33.0 vs 2.8) and earlier onset depression (by age 12 years, morbidity risk 34.2 vs 7.5) in children of parents with bipolar disorder (Henin *et al.*, 2005).

Postpartum psychosis is less common, affecting between 1 and 2 women per 1000. Episodes are usually affective in type and the most notable risk factor is a past or family history of affective psychosis. These disorders can have a devastating effect on the family. The impact on an infant can manifest both in terms of a mother's ability to care for herself and her infant (poorer quality caregiving), and by the infant becoming the focus of a mother's delusional beliefs. Fortunately, this latter problem is a relatively rare occurrence; nevertheless, when it does occur, provision of a high level of treatment, supervision, and support becomes necessary. Longer term studies, have generally been very small in size and some suggest a relative absence of ill effects. However, one study which followed-up offspring for an average of 23 years following an episode of severe puerperal disorder, found an increase in adult psychiatric illness amongst offspring whose mothers had a puerperal episode compared to siblings not exposed to a postnatal episode (Abbott *et al.*, 2004). These were mainly anxiety and depression. One of the most important issues concerns further pregnancies. The risks for subsequent psychotic episodes rise markedly with each additional episode and it is important that parents are counseled about future pregnancies and that if they decide to go ahead, appropriate measures are put in place to support the family and to promptly deal with any problems that arise.

Overall patterns of association suggest a degree of specificity in some of the links between the disorders in parents and offspring, but more recent studies highlight more nonspecific intergenerational associations.

Psychiatric disorders in fathers

Where relevant the effects of paternal disorders have been mentioned. Overall, most psychiatric disorders that affect fathers are associated with an increased risk of behavioral and emotional difficulties in their children, similar in magnitude to that due to maternal psychiatric disorders (see Ramchandani *et al.*, 2009). Findings indicate that boys are at greater risk than girls, and that paternal compared with maternal disorders might be associated with an increased risk of behavioral rather than emotional problems and be independent from maternal psychiatric disorders.

Parental physical disorders

The association between physical illnesses and child disturbance and development has received less attention than parental psychiatric disorder. Nonetheless, some physical illnesses are relatively common in adults of parenting age, and a number of chronic conditions have been shown to affect women of childbearing age; almost 10% of women aged 18–44 report some restriction of activity caused by chronic disease (Misra *et al.*, 2000).

In this relatively limited research field, much of the research has focused on cancers that affect parents. Approximately 21% of newly diagnosed cancer patients are between the ages of 25 and 54; a time when people are likely to have dependent children (Krattenmacher *et al.*, 2012). Breast cancer alone affects 1 in 9 women in the Western world. Over a quarter of those affected have children living with them and consequently this has tended to be the most frequently studied condition. Reviews of the effects of parental cancer on children's development reveal a relatively complex story. A significant minority of children become distressed or develop psychological problems. There is a relatively consistent increase in emotional problems seen in adolescent offspring of parents with cancer (Krattenmacher *et al.*, 2012). However, there is less evidence regarding emotional problems in younger children. This lack of research does not mean that they are unaffected, as qualitative interview studies have highlighted common feelings of guilt and distress, but these may not always translate to changes in measured scores on psychological questionnaires. The effects on children appear to be moderated by a number of similar factors that amplify or ameliorate the effects of parental psychiatric illness on children. A recent systematic review highlighted that the most important factors influencing children's adjustment were family-related factors, with better family functioning, including marital adjustment, being associated with better child adjustment (Krattenmacher *et al.*, 2012). Parental depressive mood was associated with more problems in children's psychosocial functioning as was the severity of disease.

HIV/AIDS has become the largest ever pandemic and in sub-Saharan Africa it has reached catastrophic proportions. Young people of child-bearing age, particularly women, are most affected, with, for example, 10 million people in sub-Saharan Africa aged 15–24 being infected—the next generation of parents. There is now substantial evidence that the offspring of mothers with HIV are at increased risk of poor development, psychological problems, compromised growth, and even survival (Sherr *et al.*, 2013; Clark *et al.*, 2013). Furthermore, these risks also apply to uninfected children of mothers with HIV (Sherr *et al.*, 2013). One of the most important mechanisms is likely to be through compromised maternal care, especially in the context of maternal depression. Maternal depression has been shown to be relatively common among women attending antenatal clinics and being tested for HIV/AIDS (Rochat *et al.*, 2006), which is when most women in Africa receive their diagnosis.

A recent review (Chi *et al.*, 2013) found that AIDS orphans and vulnerable children had poorer psychological well-being compared to children from HIV-free families or children orphaned by other diseases. In terms of mechanisms, Cluver *et al.* (2013) found that neither AIDS orphanhood nor parental AIDS illness were directly associated with psychological distress, educational access, or sexual health. Rather, the influences on the child are derived from indirect effects such as parental disability, poverty, community violence, stigma, and child abuse, which together interact through chain effects (see Chapter 46).

Studies of parents with other illnesses have included diverse groups of physical health problems, such as diabetes and multiple sclerosis (Korneluk *et al.*, 1998). Some studies have compared children of these parents with children from "healthy" families, and some with families where a parent has a psychiatric disorder. Overall, children in families where a parent has a physical illness have higher rates of anxiety and depression than children in "healthy" families. It should be stressed that most of the studies were relatively small, and had limited scope to investigate the mechanisms by which any increased risk may occur. Similar moderating influences, such as those apparent in the literature on parental cancer outlined earlier, are likely to operate (Pederson *et al.*, 2005), although there is a lack of research addressing this at present. Given the high prevalence of chronic physical illnesses in adults of parenting age, further research to understand the way in which increased risk to the child occurs is important, particularly as it may lead to the development of effective interventions. Anxiety and depression are clearly only two areas of child functioning that may be affected by parental ill-health. They are the most studied, but some studies of functional disorders, such as irritable bowel syndrome, have also examined responses to illness in the children themselves (Crane *et al.*, 2004). These studies suggest that a lower parental threshold for seeking help may potentially affect children's interpretations of symptoms as they grow up to take increasing responsibility for their own health.

Clinical implications

Parental psychiatric disorders

It is important to be aware when seeing parents with psychiatric problems that their children may be at risk, and that a careful assessment needs to be made. A helpful overall framework for assessing the potential risks to children where a parent has a psychiatric disorder is provided by Rutter (1989). Careful assessment should include the areas which are most likely to be affected by the parental disorder. These have been outlined, but include specific difficulties in parental interaction with their children, the quality and type of care the parent is able to provide, the presence of extended family, and the quality of the parental relationship. Review of these factors in the past history, as well as at the present time, can give useful insight into any potential areas of difficulty that may exist. A thorough and individualized assessment of this kind will be the best guide to the areas where intervention (if required) is most likely to be of benefit. Clinicians can also play a practical, positive role in providing support, information, and treatment to parents affected by psychiatric disorder. There is sufficient evidence to suggest that treating parental psychiatric difficulties will, in many cases, contribute to better outcomes for the child and family (Cobham *et al.*, 1998; Weissman *et al.*, 2006).

When children are referred for psychiatric problems, clinicians should again be aware that their parents may have a disorder and that assessing the parent's mental health and treating any disorders found, may be an important part of the overall treatment package. This is now being recognized in treatment guidelines; for example, the UK NICE (National Institute for Health and Care Excellence) guidelines for the treatment of depression in children and young people specifically identify the assessment of parental mood as part of the clinical assessment. It can be helpful to involve adult mental health services, although this is not always possible. Clearly, assessments need to be conducted cautiously and sensitively as parents can easily feel blamed. When children are referred for problems and the family is being seen, parents can sometimes appear relatively lively at initial appointments, belying underlying difficulties. It is important, with parental consent, to obtain information from people outside the immediate family about the situation at home. For example, parents may be reluctant to acknowledge that they spend long periods of time in bed and are unable to provide necessary support for their children. The establishment of close collaborative links with adult psychiatric services is likely to lead to the most positive outcomes for families where a parent has chronic, severe psychiatric difficulties. However, this is not always possible either because such services are not readily available, or because of differences in thresholds for accepting referrals. The decision about treatment can sometimes be a difficult clinical judgment. When the ideal circumstance of close joint management with adult services is not available, a clinician might be able to liaise with the parent's general practitioner, but in some circumstances provision of treatment directly to the parent within the child and adolescent mental health setting may be most appropriate, such as systemic family therapy.

Occasionally, in very serious cases, there is a concern about neglect and maltreatment in which case social services may need to be involved (see Chapter 29). The critical point is to assess, recognize, and arrange appropriate management of parental difficulties, as well as the child's presenting problem. In addition, it is important to monitor treatment progress. Face-to-face follow-up appointments are ideal, but with the widespread use of mobile phones, a great deal can be achieved through telephone calls and text messages (Miklowitz et al., 2012).

Common psychiatric disorders in parents

There is substantial research literature on the treatment of children who are diagnosed with a psychiatric disorder. However, there is less research on interventions to help families where a parent has such a disorder; to either prevent or manage problems in the children if they manifest themselves. Studies that have addressed this question have mainly concerned parental depression, and it has become clear that it is essential to treat the parental disorder to improve child outcome. One large treatment trial of 7- to 17-year-old children whose mothers were treated with antidepressant medication found that maternal remission within three months (occurring in approximately one-third of women) was associated with a significant decrease in child and adolescent disorders and symptoms (Weissman et al., 2006). A recent meta-analysis of preventative interventions for children of mentally ill parents found a range of benefits (Siegenthaler et al., 2012). The risk of developing the same illness as the parent was decreased by 40% and emotional symptoms (depression, anxiety) specifically were decreased. Some trials found benefits for behavioral symptoms but overall this was not significant. The trials comprised interventions directed at the parent, the couple, and the family but there were no differences across these groups. The authors suggest that the positive effects may have been due to more nonspecific factors such as attention and empathy, which are common to most treatment. However, it should be noted that all treatments in their meta-analysis were structured with a clear focus and therefore may not generalize to treatments with less structure and a more general focus. A number of studies have specifically been aimed at preventing depression among adolescents of depressed parents. One trial of a group cognitive intervention for adolescents of depressed parents found that the treatment reduced the risk of depression up to 15 months posttreatment. At the two year follow-up, a significant preventative effect persisted but at a diminished level (Clarke et al., 2001). A recent large trial, using a group cognitive behavior prevention program targeting a similar group, added six-monthly continuation sessions with the aim of prolonging the effects. This trial showed significant sustained benefits in terms of preventing onset of depressive disorders at the 3-year follow-up (Beardslee et al., 2013). A cautionary note should be applied in interpreting this body of evidence, in that recommendations highlighting the benefits of treating parent symptoms in relation to offsetting expression of symptoms in the child (offspring) do not preclude recommendations to continue to treat/focus on child symptoms.

With respect to parental depression occurring in the early years, treating the depression alone does not generally improve parent–child interaction and specific efforts need to be targeted at improving mother–child interaction in order to improve child outcome (Forman et al., 2007). There is now emerging evidence for the benefit of therapies such as video-feedback, which aim to focus parents' attention on infant cues and communication, leading to improvements in both child attachment security and child competence (Van Doesum et al., 2008). A similar study using video-feedback, in the context of maternal postnatal eating disorders, compared to control treatment, showed benefits in terms of reduced rates of mother–child conflict, enhanced maternal facilitation of infant behavior, and increased infant autonomy. Both groups maintained good infant weight with no differences between them (Stein et al., 2006b).

Emerging evidence suggests that disturbed parental cognitions may be a feature of the transmission mechanism from parental depression to child outcomes. These cognitive disturbances comprise a narrowed state of attention, where the parent is overwhelmed by recurrent intrusive thoughts known as rumination in depression and worry in anxiety (Watkins, 2008). This narrowed focus of attention can have adverse effects on an individual's capacity to attend and respond to the outside world. This may affect appropriate responsiveness and attention to a child. It is critical to help a parent to attend to a child's communication, especially facial cues, speech, and mood, and to respond appropriately in order to move the parent's focus of attention from internal thoughts to those of communication patterns with children (Juffer et al., 2008; Stein et al., 2009, 2012).

In LMICs where trained healthcare professionals may not be available, local community health workers can play an invaluable role in supporting families and can be trained to provide interventions for parents and young children (Rahman et al., 2008; Cooper et al., 2009). In particular, a small number of randomized trials in LMICs have demonstrated that psychological interventions delivered by local health workers may be helpful in reducing maternal depression and may have a positive impact on some aspects of child development. In Pakistan, a perinatal intervention program using cognitive behavioral principles delivered by primary care health workers, compared with enhanced usual care, reduced rates of maternal depression, although infant growth was not affected (the principal outcome) (Rahman et al., 2008). Parents reported that they played more with their children, although the quality of parent–child interaction was not measured. A second study was conducted in a socioeconomically disadvantaged South African community, although not specifically in the context of depression (Cooper et al., 2009). The home-based intervention focused specifically on helping mothers to attend to the details of the infant's communication and to respond sensitively. It led to improvements in the quality of mother–child interaction and increased rates of secure attachment. There is some evidence that community "participatory learning and action" groups (focused on education and maternal and newborn health practices) which are principally aimed at reducing neonatal mortality rates, may also reduce maternal depression (Tripathy et al., 2010).

Psychotic disorder

Children of parents with psychotic disorders often experience substantial unpredictability and lack of consistency in the household as well as occasional absences due to hospital admissions. Parents often display major fluctuations in mood and behavior. Children need support not only to cope with these but also to realize that such behavior is part of their parent's illness. They need time and care from "healthy adults" as well as opportunities to have positive experiences with their ill parent. Children often want to know whether they are also likely to develop the disorder and thus supportive and open discussions at age appropriate times are necessary. Mothers with puerperal psychosis will often require in-patient care, ideally in a specialist mother and baby unit, where the baby can remain with her mother in all but the most extreme of presentations, and where experienced, skilled staff can provide the level of care and supervision necessary. It is in these circumstances that clinicians have to be particularly aware of the potential danger to the child's well-being, either through direct risk from a mother with delusional beliefs and/or hallucinations, or through neglect of the child. The need to balance the risk (to mother and child) with the desire to keep families together to promote the development of a positive relationship and facilitate the mother's recovery requires experienced clinical judgment.

Substance misuse

There have been a number of studies which have investigated the effectiveness of comprehensive programs for mothers with substance misuse in relation to child outcomes (Niccols et al., 2012). Such programs deal not only with substance misuse but also with maternal and child well-being through prenatal services, parenting programs and child-care, or other child-centered services (Niccols et al., 2012). They found that such interventions had positive impacts on birth outcomes and on children's behavior, growth, and development. This emphasizes the importance of dealing with the associated family environment and parenting factors when attempting to mitigate effects on children. This is especially important given the evidence that there is higher risk for child maltreatment and poorer outcomes for such children (Dunn et al., 2002; Niccols et al., 2012).

Parental physical disorders

There has been little research examining how to mitigate the potential impact of a serious parental physical disorder on children's development. However, a number of studies have focused on the nature of the communication between parents and children in the context of maternal breast cancer and provide guidance to intervention (Forrest et al., 2006). Individual

differences, as well as age, developmental stage, and previous experience need to be taken into account. Many children will have already become aware that something is seriously wrong from changes in their parents' mood or behavior. From as young as 7, children may associate the diagnosis of cancer with the threat of dying. Not talking about this connection does not protect children from anxiety. Children's behavioral reactions to bad news may belie their feelings. Thus, withdrawal and lack of upset or angry challenging behavior does not necessarily indicate indifference or lack of sympathy or empathy. Parents diagnosed with cancer or other serious illnesses should be offered help to think about whether, what, and how to tell their children about their illness, and about what the children can understand, especially as the parents may be struggling themselves to come to terms with their illness. In the first instance, this is most appropriately led by the clinicians involved with the illness, but guidance or even direct involvement of mental health professionals may be of particular benefit. Involving the healthy parent (or another carer) in the discussions is important (Forrest et al., 2006, 2009).

Young carers and parental psychiatric and physical illness

It is estimated that large numbers of children provide informal (and unpaid) care for parents with either physical or psychiatric disorders. This is a common and underrecognized concern, and is especially important in chronic illnesses where children often take on a range of physical and medical caring roles as well as providing emotional support for their parents (Becker, 2007). In sub-Saharan Africa, a much higher proportion of young children with parents who have physical or psychiatric illnesses are involved in care, largely because of the lack of social or health care support (Becker, 2007). Very large numbers of children are looking after sick and dying relatives and at a much younger age, often with older siblings going out to work. Children's roles can include, for example, accompanying for medical appointments, collecting and administering medication, bathing and toileting their unwell parent (Cluver et al., 2012), as well as high levels of housework and, in low-resource settings, earning money to support the family (Bauman et al., 2006). A number of reports (e.g., Aldridge et al., 2003) rightly stress that each family and presentation is different, and that the carer role is not always detrimental to the child's well-being. Nonetheless, there are important potential difficulties and risks for a child required to take on a caring role. These include missing out on school and developing peer relationships, absent or inconsistent parental support and discipline, as well as having anxiety about their parent's health and fearing separations for either hospital admission or because their parent is terminally unwell. It has been argued that when children have to play these roles in the context of parental depression, they are at particular risk of psychological disturbance (Radke-Yarrow et al., 1994). The involvement of the healthier parent or carer can be vital for children. Strengthening families to care for such vulnerable children and strengthening community responses is critical (Richter *et al.*, 2009; Betancourt *et al.*, 2011).

Concluding comments in relation to both parental physical and psychiatric disorders

Health care professionals should always enquire about whether patients have children, their well-being, and the extent to which they are involved in care of the parent. Hospitals and other clinical facilities should provide space and facilities to allow children to visit and spend time with their parents. Emotional support for such children is critical. Advice on how and where they can obtain help and liaison with social services to provide practical support in the home is invaluable. Where "young carer" groups exist, these can provide emotional support and respite.

Summary

In summary, there is evidence that parental psychiatric and physical disorders are associated with a range of psychological and physical sequelae in children. However, it is crucial to be aware that children are not invariably adversely affected, and the outcomes emanating from and mechanisms through which parental psychiatric disorder may affect outcomes for children are heterogeneous. Recent research has moved from assuming traditional causal models to process-orientated models, whereby the aim is to understand why an association exists between parent risk and child outcome (mediation) and under what conditions the risk may be accentuated or ameliorated (moderation). A number of high-quality intervention studies have informed both clinical practice and policy; however, much remains to be done to improve child outcomes and support families. Furthermore, much can be learnt from children who thrive despite adversity, and a focus on resilience is critical for the future (see Chapter 27).

Finally, it is important to note that much of the burden of the impact of parental psychiatric disorder falls in LMICs. However, most of the research on parental psychiatric disorder has been conducted in high-income settings, with uncertainty about the applicability of these findings across different LMIC settings. Much less research, especially treatment trials, has been conducted in LMICs, and this omission needs to be rectified (Patel *et al.*, 2011).

References

Abbott, R. *et al.* (2004) Long-term outcome of offspring after maternal severe puerperal disorder. *Acta Psychiatrica Scandinavica* **110**, 365–373.

Abel, E.L. (1995) An update on incidence of FAS: FAS is not an equal opportunity birth defect. *Neurotoxicology and Teratology* **17**, 437–443.

Aldridge, J. *et al.* (2003) *Children Caring for Parents with Mental Illness: Perspectives of Young Carers, Parents and Professionals*, Policy Press. Bristol.

Van Batenburg-Eddes, T. *et al.* (2012) Parental depressive and anxiety symptoms during pregnancy and attention problems in children: a cross-cohort consistency study. *Journal of Child Psychology and Psychiatry* **54**, 591–600.

Bauman, L. *et al.* (2006) Children caring for their ill parents with HIV/AIDS. *Vulnerable Children and Youth Studies* **1**, 56–70.

Beardslee, W.R. *et al.* (2013) Prevention of depression in at-risk adolescents: longer-term effects. *JAMA Psychiatry* **70**, 1161–1170.

Becker, S. (2007) Global perspectives on children's unpaid caregiving in the family: research and policy on 'young carers' in the UK, Australia, the USA and Sub-Saharan Africa. *Global Social Policy* **7**, 23–50.

Bergman, A.J. *et al.* (1995) The relationship between cognitive functions and behavioral deviance in children at risk for psychopathology. *Journal of Child Psychology and Psychiatry* **36**, 265–278.

Betancourt, T.S. *et al.* (2011) Nothing can defeat combined hands (Abashize hamwe ntakibananira): protective processes and resilience in Rwandan children and families affected by HIV/AIDS. *Social Science & Medicine* **73**, 693–701.

Biederman, J. *et al.* (2006) Effects of parental anxiety disorders in children at high risk for panic disorder: a controlled study. *Journal of Affective Disorders* **94**, 191–197.

Boyce, P. (2003) Risk factors for postnatal depression: a review and risk factors in Australian populations. *Archives of Women's Mental Health* **6**, s43–s50.

Caspi, A. *et al.* (2002) Role of genotype in the cycle of violence in maltreated children. *Science* **297**, 851–854.

Chi, P. *et al.* (2013) Impact of parental HIV/AIDS on children's psychological well-being: a systematic review of global literature. *AIDS and Behavior* **17**, 2554–2574.

Clark, S.J. *et al.* (2013) Young children's probability of dying before and after their mother's death: a rural South African population-based surveillance study. *PLoS Medicine* **10**, e1001409.

Clarke, G.N. *et al.* (2001) A randomized trial of a group cognitive intervention for preventing depression in adolescent offspring of depressed parents. *Archives of General Psychiatry* **58**, 1127–1134.

Cluver, L. *et al.* (2012) 'I can't go to school and leave her in so much pain' Educational shortfalls among adolescent young carers in the South African AIDS epidemic. *Journal of Adolescent Research* **27**, 581–605.

Cluver, L. *et al.* (2013) Pathways from parental AIDS to child psychological, educational and sexual risk: developing an empirically-based interactive theoretical model, *Social Science & Medicine*. **87**, 185–193.

Cobham, V.E. *et al.* (1998) The role of parental anxiety in the treatment of childhood anxiety. *Journal of Consulting and Clinical Psychology* **66**, 893.

Cooper, P.J. *et al.* (2009) Improving quality of mother-infant relationship and infant attachment in socioeconomically deprived community in South Africa: randomised controlled trial. *British Medical Journal* **338**, b974.

Crane, C. *et al.* (2004) Illness-related parenting in mothers with functional gastrointestinal symptoms. *American Journal of Gastroenterology* **99**, 694–702.

Cuijpers, P. *et al.* (1999) Psychiatric disorders in adult children of problem drinkers: prevalence, first onset and comparison with other risk factors. *Addiction* **94**, 1489–1498.

Doyle, O. *et al.* (2009) Investing in early human development: timing and economic efficiency. *Economics & Human Biology* **7**, 1–6.

Dunn, M.G. *et al.* (2002) Origins and consequences of child neglect in substance abuse families. *Clinical Psychology Review* **22**, 1063–1090.

Engle, J.M. *et al.* (2013) Parental depressive symptoms and marital intimacy at 4.5 years: joint contributions to mother–child and father–child interaction at 6.5 years. *Developmental Psychology* **49**, 2225–2235.

Fairburn, C.G. *et al.* (2003) Eating disorders. *Lancet* **361**, 407–416.

Forman, D.R. *et al.* (2007) Effective treatment for postpartum depression is not sufficient to improve the developing mother-child relationship. *Development and Psychopathology* **19**, 585–602.

Forrest, G. *et al.* (2006) Breast cancer in the family—children's perceptions of their mother's cancer and its initial treatment: qualitative study. *BMJ* **332**, 998–1003.

Forrest, G. *et al.* (2009) Breast cancer in young families: a qualitative interview study of fathers and their role and communication with their children following the diagnosis of maternal breast cancer. *Psycho-Oncology* **18**, 96–103.

Galéra, C. *et al.* (2011) Early risk factors for hyperactivity-impulsivity and inattention trajectories from age 17 months to 8 years. *Archives of General Psychiatry* **68**, 1267–1275.

Garber, J. *et al.* (2010) Intergenerational transmission of depression: a launch and grow model of change across adolescence. *Development and Psychopathology* **22**, 819–830.

Gavin, N.I. *et al.* (2005) Perinatal depression: a systematic review of prevalence and incidence. *Obstetrics & Gynecology* **106**, 1071–1083.

Glasheen, C. *et al.* (2010) A systematic review of the effects of postnatal maternal anxiety on children. *Archives of Women's Mental Health* **13**, 61–74.

Glover, V. (2011) Annual research review: prenatal stress and the origins of psychopathology: an evolutionary perspective. *Journal of Child Psychology and Psychiatry* **52**, 356–367.

Goodman, S.H. & Gotlib, I.H. (1991) Risk for psychopathology in the children of depressed mothers: a developmental model for understanding mechanisms of transmission. *Psychological Review* **106**, 458–490.

Goodman, S.H. *et al.* (2011) Maternal depression and child psychopathology: a meta-analytic review. *Clinical Child and Family Psychology Review* **14**, 1–27.

Gottesman, I.I. *et al.* (1991) *Schizophrenia Genesis: The Origins of Madness*. WH Freeman, New York.

Gray, R. *et al.* (2009) Alcohol consumption during pregnancy and its effects on neurodevelopment: what is known and what remains uncertain. *Addiction* **104**, 1270–1273.

Harold, G.T. *et al.* (2011) Familial transmission of depression and antisocial behavior symptoms: disentangling the contribution of inherited and environmental factors and testing the mediating role of parenting. *Psychological Medicine* **41**, 1175–1185.

Harold, G.T. *et al.* (2013) Integrating family socialization and intergenerational transmission hypotheses underlying childhood antisocial behavior: the role of inter-parental conflict and passive-genotype environment correlation. *Development and Psychopathology* **25**, 37–50.

Henin, A. *et al.* (2005) Psychopathology in the offspring of parents with bipolar disorder: a controlled study. *Biological Psychiatry* **58**, 554–561.

Hudak, M.L. *et al.* (2012) Neonatal drug withdrawal. *Pediatrics* **129**, e540–e560.

Jacobi, C. *et al.* (2001) Predicting children's reported eating disturbances at 8 years of age. *Journal of the American Academy of Child and Adolescent Psychiatry* **40**, 364–372.

Jones, K. *et al.* (1973) Recognition of the fetal alcohol syndrome in early infancy. *Lancet* **302**, 999–1001.

Juffer, F. *et al.* (2008) *Promoting Positive Parenting: An Attachment-Based Intervention*. Lawrence Erlbaum, New York.

Kessler, R.C. *et al.* (1994) Lifetime and 12-month prevalence of DSM-III-R psychiatric disorders in the United States: results from the National Comorbidity Survey. *Archives of General Psychiatry* **51**, 8–19.

Kim-Cohen, J. *et al.* (2006) MAOA, maltreatment, and gene–environment interaction predicting children's mental health: new evidence and a meta-analysis. *Molecular Psychiatry* **11**, 903–913.

Korneluk, Y.G. *et al.* (1998) Children's adjustment to parental physical illness. *Clinical Child and Family Psychology Review* **1**, 179–193.

Krattenmacher, T. *et al.* (2012) Parental cancer: factors associated with children's psychosocial adjustment—a systematic review. *Journal of Psychosomatic Research* **72**, 344–356.

Leve, L.D. *et al.* (2009) Structured parenting of toddlers at high versus low genetic risk: two pathways to child problems. *Journal of the American Academy of Child and Adolescent Psychiatry* **48**, 1102–1109.

Lieberman, D. (2000) Children of alcoholics: an update. *Current Opinion in Pediatrics* **12**, 336–340.

Lovejoy, M.C. *et al.* (2000) Maternal depression and parenting behavior: a meta-analytic review. *Clinical Psychology Review* **20**, 561–592.

MacKinnon, D.P. (2011) Integrating mediators and moderators in research design. *Research on Social Work Practice* **21**, 675–681.

Mancini, C. *et al.* (1996) A high-risk pilot study of the children of adults with social phobia. *Journal of the American Academy of Child and Adolescent Psychiatry* **35**, 1511–1517.

Martins, C. *et al.* (2000) Effects of early maternal depression on patterns of infant-mother attachment: a meta-analytic investigation. *Journal of Child Psychology and Psychiatry* **41**, 737–746.

May, P.A. *et al.* (2009) Prevalence and epidemiologic characteristics of FASD from various research methods with an emphasis on recent in-school studies. *Developmental Disabilities Research Reviews* **15**, 176–192.

Merikangas, K.R. *et al.* (1998) Psychopathology among offspring of parents with substance abuse and/or anxiety disorders: a high-risk study. *Journal of Child Psychology and Psychiatry, and Allied Disciplines* **39**, 711–720.

Mesman, E. *et al.* (2013) The dutch bipolar offspring study: 12-year follow-up. *American Journal of Psychiatry* **170**, 542–549.

Micali, N. *et al.* (2009) Biological effects of a maternal ED on pregnancy and foetal development: a review. *European Eating Disorders Review* **17**, 448–454.

Micali, N. *et al.* (2014) Childhood psychopathology in children of women with eating disorders: understanding risk mechanisms. *Journal of Child Psychology and Psychiatry* **55**, 124–134.

Miklowitz, D.J. *et al.* (2012) Facilitated integrated mood management for adults with bipolar disorder. *Bipolar Disorders* **14**, 185–197.

Misra, D.P. *et al.* (2000) An intersection of women's and perinatal health: the role of chronic conditions. *Women's Health Issues* **10**, 256–267.

Murray, L. *et al.* (2009) The development of anxiety disorders in childhood: an integrative review. *Psychological Medicine* **39**, 1413–1423.

Murray, L. *et al.* (2010) Effects of postnatal depression on mother–infant interactions and child development. In: *Handbook of Infant Development*, (eds J. Bremner & T. Wachs), 2nd edn Vol. 2, pp. 192–220. Wiley-Blackwell, Oxford.

Niccols, A. *et al.* (2012) Integrated programs for mothers with substance abuse issues and their children: a systematic review of studies reporting on child outcomes. *Child Abuse & Neglect* **36**, 308–322.

O'Hara, M. *et al.* (1996) Rates and risk of postpartum depression: a meta-analysis. *International Review of Psychiatry* **8**, 37–54.

Parsons, C.E. *et al.* (2012) Postnatal depression and its effects on child development: a review of evidence from low-and middle-income countries. *British Medical Bulletin* **101**, 57–79.

Patel, P. *et al.* (2002) The children of mothers with eating disorders. *Clinical Child and Family Psychology Review* **5**, 1–19.

Patel, V. *et al.* (2011) A renewed agenda for global mental health. *Lancet* **378**, 1441–1442.

Pearson, R.M. *et al.* (2013) Maternal depression during pregnancy and the postnatal period: risks and possible mechanisms for offspring depression at age 18 years. *JAMA Psychiatry* **70**, 1312–1319.

Pederson, S. *et al.* (2005) Parental illness, family functioning, and adolescent well-being: a family ecology framework to guide research. *Journal of Family Psychology* **19**, 404–419.

Preacher, K.J. *et al.* (2007) Addressing moderated mediation hypotheses: theory, methods, and prescriptions. *Multivariate Behavioral Research* **42**, 185–227.

Radke-Yarrow, M. *et al.* (1994) Caring behavior in children of clinically depressed and well mothers. *Child Development* **65**, 1405–1414.

Rahman, A. *et al.* (2008) Cognitive behaviour therapy-based intervention by community health workers for mothers with depression and their infants in rural Pakistan: a cluster-randomised controlled trial. *Lancet* **372**, 902–909.

Ramchandani, P. *et al.* (2009) Paternal psychiatric disorders and children's psychosocial development. *Lancet* **374**, 646–653.

Richter, L.M. *et al.* (2009) Strengthening families to support children affected by HIV and AIDS. *AIDS Care* **21**, 3–12.

Rochat, T. *et al.* (2006) Depression among pregnant rural South African women undergoing HIV testing. *JAMA* **295**, 1376–1378.

Rutter, M. (1989) Pathways from childhood to adult life. *Journal of Child Psychology and Psychiatry* **30**, 23–51.

Rutter, M. *et al.* (2009) Gene-environment interactions: biologically valid pathway or artifact? *Archives of General Psychiatry* **66**, 1287–1289.

Serbin, L.A. *et al.* (2004) The intergenerational transfer of psychosocial risk: mediators of vulnerability and resilience. *Annual Review of Psychology* **55**, 333–363.

Sherr, L. *et al.* (2013) *Pathways to Psychological Impacts and Responses of HIV and AIDS on Children*. USAID.

Siegenthaler, E. *et al.* (2012) Effect of preventive interventions in mentally ill parents on the mental health of the offspring: systematic review and meta-analysis. *Journal of the American Academy of Child & Adolescent Psychiatry* **51**, 8–17.

Silberg, J.L. *et al.* (2010) Genetic and environmental influences on the transmission of parental depression to children's depression and conduct disturbance: an extended Children of Twins study. *Journal of Child Psychology and Psychiatry* **51**, 734–744.

Stein, A. *et al.* (2006a) Treating disturbances in the relationship between mothers with bulimic eating disorders and their infants: a randomized, controlled trial of video feedback. *American Journal of Psychiatry* **163**, 899–906.

Stein, A. *et al.* (2006b) Eating habits and attitudes among 10-year-old children of mothers with eating disorders. A longitudinal study. *British Journal of Psychiatry* **189**, 324–329.

Stein, A. *et al.* (2008) The influence of maternal depression, caregiving, and socioeconomic status in the post-natal year on children's language development. *Child: Care, Health and Development* **34**, 603–612.

Stein, A. *et al.* (2009) The influence of postnatal psychiatric disorder on child development: is maternal preoccupation one of the key underlying processes? *Psychopathology* **42**, 11–21.

Stein, A. *et al.* (2012) Maternal cognitions and mother-infant interaction in postnatal depression and generalized anxiety disorder. *Journal of Abnormal Psychology* **121**, 795–809.

Stein, A. *et al.* (2014) Effects of perinatal mental disorders on the fetus and child. *Lancet* **384**, 1800–1819.

Stice, E. *et al.* (1999) Risk factors for the emergence of childhood eating disturbances: a five-year prospective study. *International Journal of Eating Disorders* **25**, 375–387.

Stratton, K.R. *et al.* (1996) *Fetal Alcohol Syndrome: Diagnosis, Epidemiology, Prevention, and Treatment*. National Academy Press, Washington.

Sullivan, P.F. *et al.* (2012) Family history of schizophrenia and bipolar disorder as risk factors for autism. *Archives of General Psychiatry* **69**, 1099–1103.

Surkan, P.J. *et al.* (2011) Maternal depression and early childhood growth in developing countries: systematic review and meta-analysis. *Bulletin of the World Health Organization* **89**, 607–615.

Talge, N. *et al.* (2007) Antenatal maternal stress and long-term effects on child neurodevelopment: how and why? *Journal of Child Psychology and Psychiatry* **48**, 245–261.

Tripathy, P. *et al.* (2010) Effect of a participatory intervention with women's groups on birth outcomes and maternal depression in Jharkhand and Orissa, India: a cluster-randomised controlled trial. *Lancet* **375**, 1182–1192.

Tully, E.C. *et al.* (2008) An adoption study of parental depression as an environmental liability for adolescent depression and childhood disruptive disorders. *American Journal of Psychiatry* **165**, 1148–1154.

Turner, S.M. *et al.* (1987) Psychopathology in the offspring of anxiety disorders patients. *Journal of Consulting and Clinical Psychology* **55**, 229–235.

Van Den Bergh, B.R.H. *et al.* (2005) Antenatal maternal anxiety and stress and the neurobehavioural development of the fetus and child: links and possible mechanisms. A review. *Neuroscience & Biobehavioral Reviews* **29**, 237–258.

Van Doesum, K. *et al.* (2008) A randomized controlled trial of a home-visiting intervention aimed at preventing relationship problems in depressed mothers and their infants. *Child Development* **79**, 547–561.

Watkins, E.R. (2008) Constructive and unconstructive repetitive thought. *Psychological Bulletin* **134**, 163–206.

Weissman, M.M. *et al.* (1988) Affective disorders in five United States communities. *Psychological Medicine* **18**, 141–53.

Weissman, M.M. *et al.* (1997) Offspring of depressed parents: 10 years later. *Archives of General Psychiatry* **54**, 932–940.

Weissman, M. *et al.* (2006) Remissions in maternal depression and child psychopathology. A STAR*D-Child Report. *JAMA* **295**, 1389–1398.

CHAPTER 29

Child maltreatment

Andrea Danese[1,2] and Eamon McCrory[3,4]

[1] Institute of Psychiatry, Psychology and Neuroscience, King's College London, UK
[2] National and Specialist Clinic for Child Traumatic Stress and Anxiety Disorders, South London and Maudsley NHS Foundation Trust, London, UK
[3] Division of Psychology and Language Sciences, University College London, UK
[4] Anna Freud Centre, London, UK

Safeguarding children: a pressing global challenge

Child maltreatment is a prevalent risk factor associated with later illness, socio-economic disadvantage, and crime (Gilbert *et al.*, 2009b). Worldwide, many children are exposed to abusive or neglectful experiences that violate their rights (Pinheiro, 2006). Some of these children die as a result of maltreatment, while many more develop psychiatric and medical disorders, at significantly higher rates than non-maltreated children. The detrimental health consequences of child maltreatment are not limited to the childhood years. Rather, they can endure well into adult life (Danese *et al.*, 2009). Maltreated children are not only at high risk of adult psychiatric and medical disorders but may also respond more poorly to traditional treatment (Nanni *et al.*, 2012). Even when they do not develop diagnosable disorders, they often suffer significant distress and impairment in cognitive, social, and emotional development and functioning. In addition, individuals with a history of childhood maltreatment often have poorer educational achievements, lower earnings, and higher risk of engaging in criminal activities compared to non-maltreated individuals (Currie & Widom, 2010). Because child maltreatment is associated with significant personal and societal costs, prevention, identification, and treatment of child maltreatment cases should be conceptualized not only as a moral responsibility but also as an urgent economic target.

However, protecting children remains a challenging task for several reasons. First, simply trying to define maltreatment can be difficult given the variations in boundaries around parenting practices and the variation in norms and attitudes about violence across cultures and across generations. Clarity of definitions is important to ensure recognition of maltreatment cases. Second, professionals may be challenged by the diversity of the theoretical frameworks used to understand acts of abuse and neglect of children. Child protection work necessarily involves the close collaboration of professionals with backgrounds in medicine, psychology, education, social work, law, law enforcement, and policy. Harmonization of knowledge from these diverse fields is crucial, in order to promote interdisciplinary work. Finally, professionals may find it difficult to make sense of the complex and diverse nature of the consequences associated with maltreatment. Better understanding of how child maltreatment relates to these various outcomes is important to promote effective interventions for maltreated children (Shonkoff *et al.*, 2009).

Child protection also represents a significant challenge for governments worldwide. Maltreatment of children continues to occur in all societies and possibly more frequently in low- and middle-income countries (Pinheiro, 2006). To affirm universal children's rights, the 1989 United Nations (UN) Convention on the Rights of the Child sets a legal framework for implementing policy, accountability, and social justice. This UN Convention emphasizes that the best interest of the child is paramount. Rights across three main areas were established. First, children have rights of protection, including the right to be protected from any form of maltreatment or exploitation resulting in threats to their survival, development, or well-being. This implies that effective prevention should be a primary focus. Second, children have rights of participation, including the right to be actively involved in decisions and actions affecting them. Finally, children have rights of provision, including the right to education and the obligations of the state to support families. Although nearly every government worldwide has ratified the UN Convention on the Rights of the Child, its practical implementation remains incomplete in several countries. Furthermore, resources dedicated to child protection are insufficient in most countries.

Definitions: maltreatment types

The World Health Organization (WHO) has defined child maltreatment as: "…all forms of physical and/or emotional ill treatment, sexual abuse, neglect or negligent treatment or commercial or other exploitation, resulting in actual or potential harm to the child's health, survival, development or dignity in the context of a relationship of responsibility, trust or power" (Krug *et al.*, 2002). However, it is widely acknowledged that such a concise definition belies a complex issue that can vary in relation to the victim's age and identity, the motivation and actions of the perpetrator and the cultural context. Four primary types of child maltreatment will be reviewed here (Butchart *et al.*, 2006); other forms of child maltreatment (e.g., child trafficking, children exposed to combat, etc.) are beyond the scope of this chapter.

Sexual abuse has been defined as "…forcing or enticing a child or young person to take part in sexual activities, not necessarily involving a high level of violence, whether or not the child is aware of what is happening" (UK DoE, 2013). Sexual abuse can include activities that involve physical contact (e.g., touching, kissing, and penetration), non-contact activities (e.g., involving children in looking at, or in the production of, sexual images), child sexual exploitation (e.g., prostitution), and grooming (in England).

Physical abuse of a child has been defined as the intentional use of physical force (often to inflict punishment) against a child "…that results in—or has a high likelihood of resulting in—harm for the child's health, survival, development, or dignity" (Butchart *et al.*, 2006). This includes a variety of acts, such as hitting, beating, kicking, shaking, biting, strangling, scalding, burning, poisoning, and suffocating. The definition includes fabricated or induced illness in the United Kingdom (UK DoE, 2013), while the US definition requires threat of harm (U.S. DHHS, 2010). Domestic corporal punishment is classified as unlawful and regarded as physical abuse in twenty-nine countries but remains lawful (albeit controversial) in several countries, including England, Australia, and the United States of America.

Emotional and psychological abuse has been defined as: "the persistent emotional maltreatment of a child such as to cause severe and persistent adverse effects on the child's emotional development" (UK DoE, 2013). It may involve conveying to a child that they are worthless, unloved, or inadequate, not giving the child opportunities to express their views, or imposing developmentally-inappropriate expectations on children. England, the United States of America and Canada include exposure to domestic violence within their definitions of emotional abuse (Munro *et al.*, 2011); in addition, the United States of America and Canada have a separate category on witnessing violence (U.S. DHHS, 2010). In England, serious bullying and cyber-bulling are included in the definition of emotional abuse (UK DoE, 2013).

Neglect has been defined as "The persistent failure to meet a child's basic physical and/or psychological needs, likely to result in the serious impairment of the child's health or development" (UK DoE, 2013). Neglect may relate to a failure to provide adequate nutrition, shelter, protection from harm or access to medical care or treatment. In England and Canada, reference is also made to failure to adequately supervise a child, which has the potential to lead to harm (Munro *et al.*, 2011).

Epidemiology

The exact prevalence of child maltreatment varies depending not only on the definition used but also on the method of assessment, namely self-reports of victims who are old enough to participate in surveys; parent-reports on child abuse or neglect and patterns of care; or official statistics from statutory agencies (e.g., child protection services and police).

Several community studies based on self- and parent-reports have been undertaken to study the prevalence of various maltreatment types in high-income countries (Gilbert *et al.*, 2009b). The cumulative prevalence of any *sexual abuse* in community studies ranges between 15% and 30% in girls and between 5% and 15% in boys, while the cumulative prevalence of penetrative sexual abuse ranges between 5% and 10% in girls and between 1% and 5% in boys. The cumulative prevalence of *physical abuse* ranges between 5% and 35%. The cumulative prevalence of *emotional abuse* ranges between 4% and 9%. In addition, 10–20% of children and adolescents witness intimate-partner violence in their homes. The cumulative prevalence of *neglect* ranges between 6% and 12% in the United Kingdom and United States of America. In contrast to these high prevalence figures from community studies, official reports showed that only 5% of children are referred to social welfare in the United Kingdom and in the United States of America, and that 0.3–1% of children were substantiated as cases of maltreatment. Among the substantiated cases, neglect is by far the most common form of maltreatment (44–60%), followed by emotional abuse (11–23%), physical abuse (10–15%), and sexual abuse (7%).

A community study by the UK National Society for the Prevention of Cruelty to Children (NSPCC) found that nearly 1 in 5 children (18.6%) experience some forms of maltreatment (Radford *et al.*, 2011). Consistent with previous studies, the NSPCC survey showed that children who experienced one form of maltreatment were 2–3 times more likely to also experience other forms of maltreatment and to be victimized by other perpetrators over time. The evidence of such poly-victimization, namely the recurrent and cumulative nature of different types of maltreatment, emphasizes the importance of secondary prevention strategies in child protection (Finkelhor et al., 2007a, b).

Despite these high prevalence estimates, evidence suggests that some forms of maltreatment may have decreased over the past two decades, although this topic remains hotly debated (Gilbert *et al.*, 2012; Radford *et al.*, 2012; Finkelhor & Jones, 2012). It should be noted that the prevalence of child abuse codes from hospitalized children has not declined in the same period. In contrast to the downward trends for sexual and physical abuse (62% and 56% decline, respectively), data indicated a relatively stable prevalence of neglect (10% decline) over the past two decades (Olson & Stroud, 2012).

Factors associated with occurrence of maltreatment

Although several risk factors show a statistical association with maltreatment, it is often unclear whether such factors have a causal role in its occurrence. Making inferences about causality is complicated by a number of issues. To begin with, several factors associated with maltreatment (e.g., a child's behavior problems, parents' mental illness, and poverty) are correlated, that is, they tend to co-occur, and it may be difficult to isolate causal elements within a complex mixture of correlated factors in observational studies. Advances in this area have been aided by the development of multilevel, ecological models encompassing individual, family, and community risk factors (Belsky, 1993), and by the recognition of the bidirectional interaction between individual factors in children and their parents/carers (Bell, 1968). A peculiar form of bidirectional interaction is the genetic predisposition to environmental exposure, or gene–environment correlation (Jaffee & Price, 2007). For example, children may inherit from their parents a predisposition to exhibit problem behaviors, which in turn may increase the odds of evoking harsh parenting. An additional challenge to causal inference is that risk factors for maltreatment are non-deterministic, that is, no single risk factor is either necessary or sufficient for maltreatment to occur. For example, although parental mental illness is a risk factor for child maltreatment, most parents with mental illness do not abuse their children and most maltreated children do not have parents with mental illness (Kaufman & Zigler, 1987; Dixon et al., 2005). Different risk factors could be conceptualized as component causes that interact with each other and with protective factors in linear or non-linear fashion. Therefore, risk of maltreatment is likely to be more accurately predicted by examining a comprehensive set of risk and protective factors. The available evidence provides a framework for the informed clinician to make judgments about children most likely to be at risk and target resources appropriately. The following risk factors may help identify children at risk of maltreatment and maltreatment recurrence (Goldman et al., 2003).

Child's individual risk factors for victimization

A number of child-specific factors have been associated with increased risk of being maltreated. The presence of such factors does not imply that the child holds any responsibility for their maltreatment; rather, such factors can be understood as potentially aggravating other parental, family, and community risk factors for perpetration. Some of these risk factors could be targeted by interventions to reduce the risk of maltreatment or its recurrence. Young children (age 5 and younger) are disproportionally represented among reported cases of maltreatment and cases of death due to maltreatment (U.S. Child Welfare, 2013), presumably because of their physical vulnerability, developmental immaturity, and more dependent relationship with carers. However, teenagers are at greater risk for sexual abuse both from family members and from strangers. Other characteristics of the child that increase strain for the parents or carers have also been associated with greater maltreatment risk, including broadly defined disability (Jones et al., 2012), and difficult temperament or problem behaviors.

Parents' or carers' individual risk factors for perpetration

Maltreatment may be more likely when parents or carers struggle to understand the needs of the developing child or to modulate their own behavior accordingly. For example, young age of parent, low education, inaccurate knowledge of child development, unrealistic expectations of their children and impaired capacity for empathy have all been linked to elevated risk of maltreatment (Zeanah & Zeanah, 1989; Dixon et al., 2005). Furthermore, elevated risk of maltreatment has been associated with impaired emotion regulation in parents, as manifested through both emotional symptoms (e.g., low self-esteem, neurotic personality, and depression) and behavior problems (e.g., impulsive behavior and substance abuse). As child maltreatment predicts several of these risk factors in adult life (see below), it is not surprising that parents' own history of maltreatment is, in turn, associated with elevated risk of maltreatment perpetration.

Family risk factors

Heightened maltreatment risk has been linked to a constellation of inter-related factors that increase strain on the family, including large family size, single parenthood, non biological transient carers in the home and intimate-partner violence (Finkelhor et al., 2007b). Furthermore, maltreatment risk is greater in families that cannot access support because of social isolation (Crouch et al., 2001), socio economic disadvantage, or lower levels of education (Brown et al., 1998).

Community risk factors

In addition to individual and family factors, maltreatment risk is also influenced by the broader context in which children and their families live. Child maltreatment cases are concentrated in more impoverished neighborhoods and research suggests that poverty and unemployment are particularly associated with risk of neglect and physical abuse, with mixed evidence in relation to sexual abuse (Coulton et al., 1995). Community violence and collective efficacy (i.e., mutual trust among neighbors and willingness to intervene on behalf of the common good) may also contribute to maltreatment rates (Sampson *et al.*, 1997). These distal factors may be associated with more proximal risk factors, such as unstable housing, childcare burden, greater strain on families, and attitudes toward violence.

Consequences of maltreatment

The most tragic and widely publicized consequence of maltreatment is death due to deliberate acts of physical or sexual abuse or severe neglect. Despite the likely under-reporting owing to insufficient investigation of child deaths in most countries, WHO estimated that 155,000 deaths in children younger than 15 years occur worldwide every year as a result of abuse or neglect, which is 0.6% of all deaths and 12.7% of deaths due to any injury (Pinheiro, 2006). Homicide occurs most frequently during infancy but also peaks in adolescence, largely at the hands of biological or step-parents (UNICEF, 2003).

Child maltreatment has also been associated with a variety of consequences for health, wealth, and crime. However, establishing the causal mechanisms linking maltreatment with these outcomes remains challenging. On the one hand, because maltreatment is not randomly distributed in the population but rather clusters with other risk factors, maltreated individuals differ from non-maltreated individuals in relation to several other characteristics in addition to maltreatment. These differences may represent confounds that, in turn, bias the interpretation of the effects of maltreatment. On the other hand, several studies have investigated the association of retrospective reports of childhood maltreatment with various outcomes, introducing the possibility that outcome status could influence the recall of maltreatment (recall bias) and that an apparent outcome may have actually preceded maltreatment exposure (selection bias). When weighing the strength of the available evidence, it is therefore important to consider whether studies have adequately considered the presence of co-occurring risk factors, report findings consistent with those observed in animals randomly exposed to early life stress and report results consistent with longitudinal-prospective investigations (Danese & Tan, 2014).

Figure 29.1 lists the range of phenomena associated with child maltreatment. First, child maltreatment has been associated with a variety of physical health problems. The most consistent effects observed in longitudinal-prospective studies are arguably in relation to obesity (Gilbert *et al.*, 2009b; Danese & Tan, 2014). In addition, cross-sectional and case–control studies also showed elevated risk for several chronic medical conditions in maltreated compared to non-maltreated adults. Second, child maltreatment has been associated with a variety of mental

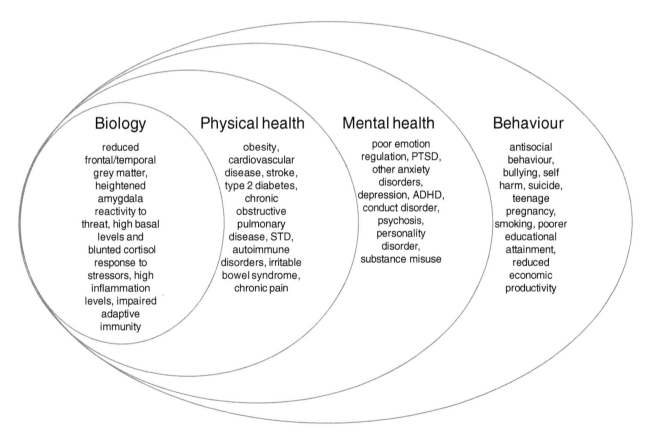

Figure 29.1 Biological/psychological/medical consequences of maltreatment in children and adults exposed to maltreatment in childhood.

health problems, both in childhood and adult years. Because of its enduring effects, it is possible that maltreatment could affect not only the risk of psychiatric disorders but also their longitudinal course (Nanni *et al.*, 2012). Third, child maltreatment has been associated with poor educational achievement and economic productivity (Currie & Widom, 2010). Finally, child maltreatment has been associated with violence, antisocial behavior, and criminal offenses. It is important to stress that such outcomes are associated with only a minority of children who experience abuse, but they are important in understanding the risk of inter-generational cycles of violence that characterize some families (Dodge *et al.*, 1990).

The experience of being maltreated often co-occurs with a range of familial disadvantages and can impact development at a number of levels. Psychologically, children commonly experience feelings of powerlessness and shame and internalize their experiences to signify that they are neither valued nor loved. Over time, such feelings can contribute to patterns of low self-esteem and negative self-schemata, reducing a sense of self-efficacy and increasing vulnerability to psychopathology. Exposure to poor or erratic physical and emotional boundaries and a failure of adults to help the child reflect on their own emotions and social behavior can lead to poor socialization and manifest as disorganized or insecure attachment patterns. This absence of normative "emotional scaffolding" by carers, paired with a sense that adults are a source of danger rather than protection, can create an experience of chronic stress that also impacts at the biological level (McCrory *et al.*, 2010; Danese & McEwen, 2012). Studies of the biological mechanisms through which maltreatment affects clinical outcome (or "biological embedding") have the potential to identify latent neurobiological risk factors that may shed light on the ways in which clinical symptoms emerge. For example, at the structural level, maltreated children compared to typically developing peers show reduced gray matter volume in a number of brain regions, including frontal and temporal regions. The reduced volume of the orbitofrontal cortex in particular may represent a neural basis for possible deficits in social and cognitive functioning (Hanson *et al.*, 2010; De Brito *et al.*, 2013). At the functional level, maltreated children show heightened reactivity to threat cues in the amygdala (McCrory *et al.*, 2011), even when these are presented subliminally (McCrory *et al.*, 2013), suggesting increased vigilance to social threat in their environment. Consistent with this, it has been shown that maltreated children generally show higher basal (unstimulated) levels of the stress-hormone cortisol and blunted cortisol response to psychosocial stress tasks or pharmacological challenges (Danese & McEwen, 2012). They also have been reported to show higher circulating levels of inflammation proteins and impaired adaptive immune response to pathogens (Shirtcliff *et al.*, 2009; Danese *et al.*, 2011). Although such biological adaptations may confer short-term benefits, for example, in increasing vigilance in the face of threat, they are likely to incur longer-term costs, ultimately increasing vulnerability to psychiatric and medical disorder (McCrory & Viding, in press;

Danese & McEwen, 2012). Indeed, compared to non-maltreated adults, adults with a history of maltreatment continue to show alterations in brain structure and function (McCrory *et al.*, 2010; Danese & McEwen, 2012) and persistent abnormalities in endocrine and immune functioning (Heim *et al.*, 2000; Danese *et al.*, 2007). Such biological changes may be brought about by the molecular effects of stress on the biochemical composition of a child's DNA, or epigenetic changes (Chapter 25), which may affect expression of key regulatory genes (Meaney, 2010).

Further research is required to establish if the association between child maltreatment and biological abnormalities or clinical outcomes is sensitive to the type of maltreatment considered or to the timing of maltreatment, although preliminary evidence suggests that earlier timing might lead to more detrimental effects (Andersen & Teicher, 2008; Tottenham *et al.*, 2010; McCrory *et al.*, 2011; McCrory *et al.*, 2013). Consistent with the cumulative effects of other life stressors (McEwen, 1998), different types of maltreatment at different ages may exert cumulative effects on biology and health (Felitti *et al.*, 1998; Danese *et al.*, 2007). Clinically, maltreated children are commonly exposed to multiple types of maltreatment with repeated experiences over time and such chronicity is a strong predictor of poor outcomes (Finkelhor *et al.*, 2007a, b; Radford *et al.*, 2011; Jonson-Reid *et al.*, 2012). Therefore, identification of independent effects of specific forms of maltreatment is difficult in epidemiological and clinical studies, and distinctions may be artificial.

Finally, it is important to emphasize that the aforementioned studies largely looked at differences between groups of maltreated and non-maltreated children. However, there are broad individual differences within groups of maltreated children, many of whom do not develop some or indeed any of these outcomes. Child-level, family-level, and community-level factors may act to increase or reduce resilience in the face of adversity (Cicchetti, 2013). For example, there is ample evidence that genetic influences may affect an individual's sensitivity to environmental stressors, such as maltreatment, and their likelihood of developing depression (Caspi *et al.*, 2010). Furthermore, a more flexible personality style, a warm and loving relationship with parents and more secure attachments, positive peer relationships in adolescence, and positive romantic relationships in adulthood could reduce the risk of developing adult psychopathology after child maltreatment (Jaffee *et al.*, 2007; Collishaw *et al.*, 2007).

Recognizing child maltreatment

The discrepancies in maltreatment prevalence estimates based on official statistics and on self-/parent-reports suggest that child protection referrals account for only a fraction of maltreatment cases. Training in child protection may address these discrepancies by increasing recognition and reporting (Jones *et al.*, 2008). Recognition and reporting may also be increased by reducing structural barriers and empowering young people to make self-referrals through voluntary organizations, such as ChildLine in the United Kingdom and the Italian Telefono Azzurro.

Data from Europe and the United States of America has shown that schools contribute a large proportion of the child protection cases referred to professionals, followed by law enforcement agencies, social services, and health professionals (Gilbert *et al.*, 2009a). Although referrals by health professionals constitute only a minority of the overall number, these often relate to the children who have experienced the most severe forms of abuse and present with injuries and symptoms.

Mental health professionals should be vigilant of the possibility of maltreatment while working with children and families who present with some of the risk characteristics outlined in the section "Factors associated with occurrence of maltreatment." For example, increased risk of maltreatment has been associated with parental substance/alcohol misuse, mental health problems, history of violent offending, own history of maltreatment, cruelty to animals, young age, low education, poor understanding of child development, unrealistic expectations, and lack of empathy. Equally, a child's disability, difficult temperament, and problem behaviors may also increase risk of being a victim of maltreatment.

Recognizing maltreatment often requires health professionals to piece together information from different sources and agencies and from their own assessment (NICE, 2009). During their assessment, professionals should observe a child's appearance and behavior, their interaction with parents and signs and symptoms. They should also listen carefully to the history reported and particularly to any reports or disclosures of maltreatment. Systematic reviews of the literature on the validity and discriminatory ability of various possible signs of maltreatment (Kempe *et al.*, 1962) have informed guidelines to improve recognition of child maltreatment by health professionals. For example, in the United Kingdom, the National Institute for Health and Care Excellence (NICE) has produced a list of features that should prompt professionals to consider or to suspect maltreatment (see Table 29.1) (NICE, 2009). Similar guidelines have also been developed in the United States of America by the American Professional Society on the Abuse of Children (APSAC) and the US Child Welfare/US Department of Health & Human Services (U.S. Child Welfare, 2007; Myers & APSAC, 2010). Professionals should seek an explanation for observed injuries or presentations, speaking to carers and to the child and any siblings (if appropriate), as well as collecting collateral information. Because recognition of maltreatment is generally more difficult in children with disability, professionals should seek support from colleagues with relevant expertise in these circumstances. Professionals should then consider if they have been provided with a suitable explanation for the alerting features they identified. For example, explanations may be unsuitable when they are implausible or inadequate. Explanations may also be unsuitable when they are inconsistent with a child's developmental stage, normal activities, or medical condition, or when they are inconsistent between different people or over time. Professionals should discuss their conclusions with experienced colleagues, such as pediatricians, child and adolescent mental health professionals, and designated members of staff with experience in child protection. Based on the information gathered, professionals may decide to exclude the occurrence of maltreatment, or to suspect it and, thus, to act to address their concerns (see section "Responding to child maltreatment").

It is common for mental health professionals to find themselves in a delicate position where they not only work with children and their families but also contribute to multi-agency child protection work. Clinical dilemmas related to confidentiality, divided loyalty and professional responsibility are common in everyday practice. First, professionals should make clear from the beginning that they cannot necessarily keep information about risk of significant harm to young patients, their siblings or other people as confidential (UK DoE, 2008). Rather, they have a duty to take action, including, where necessary, disclosing relevant confidential information to statutory agencies. Second, professionals working with both children and their parents may have a sense of divided loyalty as they may have professional responsibilities to both parties. However, all professionals should be mindful that the child's interest is always paramount, as they are more vulnerable. Finally, professionals may believe that the person or agency with whom they shared their concerns have not acted on them appropriately. In this case, they should follow up their concerns and take them to the next level of authority.

Table 29.1 NICE guidelines on recognition of child maltreatment.

Emotional abuse
Age-inappropriate behavior, aggression, body rocking, change in emotional or behavioral state, cutting, dissociation, drug taking, eating and feeding behavior, encopresis, fearful, runaway behavior, self-esteem, self-harm, sexual behavior, smearing (feces) and wetting

Physical abuse
Abrasions, bites (human), bruises, burns, cold injuries, cuts, eye injuries, fractures, hypothermia, intra-abdominal injuries, intracranial injuries, intrathoracic injuries, lacerations, ligature marks, oral injuries, petechiae, retinal hemorrhage, scalds, scars, spinal injuries, strangulation, subdural hemorrhage and teeth marks

Sexual abuse
Anal symptoms and signs, anogenital injuries, dysuria, foreign bodies, genital symptoms and signs, pregnancy, sexual exploitation, sexualized behavior (also see Emotional, behavioral, interpersonal and social functioning), sexually transmitted infections (STIs) and vaginal discharge

Neglect
Abandonment, bites (animal), clothing, dirty child, failure to thrive, faltering growth, footwear, head lice, health promotion, health reviews, home conditions, immunization, lack of provision, lack of supervision, medication adherence, parental interaction with medical services, persistent infestations, poor hygiene, scabies, screening, smelly child, sunburn and tooth decay

Source: Adapted from http://www.nice.org.uk/nicemedia/live/12183/44872/44872.pdf.

To document actions and improve clarity of communication, it is important that professionals keep clear, accurate, comprehensive and contemporaneous notes, reporting what they have observed and heard from whom and when, what is of concern in their opinion, and what action they have taken. They should also follow up oral communications with other professionals in writing.

Responding to child maltreatment

Decisions about how best to respond to maltreatment concerns involve a degree of risk, particularly when signs of abuse or neglect are not clear-cut and the evidence is ambiguous. At one extreme, there is a risk of leaving the child in a harmful environment. At the other extreme, there is a risk of removing the child unnecessarily from the family. In general, it is important that mental health professionals do not ignore warning signs because risk to children may only become apparent when several professionals express even minor concerns on the same child or family.

When professionals recognize signs of abuse or neglect or consider maltreatment as a possible explanation for a child's clinical presentation or unmet needs, they should initially discuss their concerns with their manager and with a designated member of staff with experience in child protection. If concerns persist, it is also possible to discuss them with senior colleagues from other agencies, including social services, without disclosing the identity of the child or family.

If concerns about child maltreatment persist after discussion, professionals must refer the case to statutory agencies, such as the local authority social services (other statutory agencies are the police and, in the United Kingdom, the National Society for the Prevention of Cruelty to Children, or NSPCC), and follow up in writing. If the child is already known to the agency, the allocated social worker should be informed of the concerns.

Referrals to social services should be discussed with the children and their parents in order to seek their agreement. Children should be involved in this process as appropriate for their competence and understanding, and through open discussion without leading questions that may jeopardize later police investigation. These discussions with parents and children help ensure that children's rights to protection and participation and parents' right to family life are respected. Moreover, they are an important means to build trust and collaboration. If children or parents refuse to give consent, professionals should assess whether the possible benefits of sharing information outweigh those of keeping the information confidential. Furthermore, professionals may decide not to seek consent if they believe that this would place the child at significant risk of increased harm.

Referral to social services prompts responses that may differ based on the legal and administrative frameworks set in different countries but overall adhere to common principles. They are discussed here with reference to the UK child protection procedures (UK DoE, 2013).

Following a referral, social services (or other statutory agencies) make a rapid assessment of the child's needs and risks to plan initial actions. At one extreme, where risk is deemed to be low, social services may decide that the child's needs could be addressed through universal and targeted services supporting parents (e.g., parenting programs, assistance with mental health

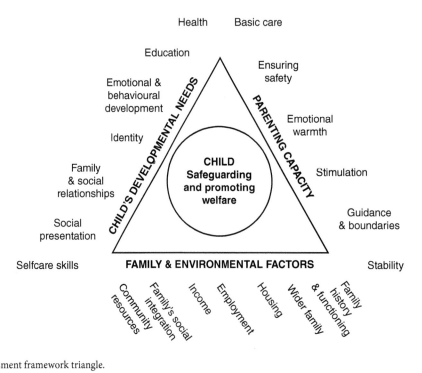

Figure 29.2 Family assessment framework triangle.

problems). At the other extreme, where risk is deemed to be immediate and life-threatening, social services may decide that it is in the child's best interest to be removed from the family and placed elsewhere (e.g., under section 20 or section 31 of the UK Children Act 1989). However, most cases are not clear-cut and require further investigation.

Many cases involve children found in the initial assessment to be "in need," that is (according to the UK Children Act 1989), children who are unlikely to achieve or maintain a satisfactory level of health or development, who are disabled or asylum seeker, or whose parents are in prison. In these cases, social services are mandated to undertake a multidisciplinary, holistic assessment of the child's needs in the context of their family and wider community ("core" assessment, under section 17 of the UK Children Act 1989). The Common Assessment Framework (CAF, Figure 29.2) (UK DoE, 2012) remains a helpful tool for this assessment, guiding the comprehensive evaluation of the child's developmental needs (including whether they are suffering or likely to suffer significant harm), parenting capacity, and family environment. Tools used to further evaluate these areas include the Strengths and Difficulties Questionnaire (Goodman, 1997), the Family Assessment (Bentovim & Bingley, 2001), and the HOME inventory (Cox & Walker, 2002), respectively. The assessment typically considers the needs of the child in relation to the capacity and motivation of the parents or carers to meet those needs, in order to evaluate potential for remediation and set objectives for subsequent interventions.

During initial or "core" assessment, evidence may emerge leading the social worker to suspect that the child is suffering or likely to suffer significant harm. There are no absolute criteria by which significant harm can be judged, but decisions in this area involve a consideration of the effect of any ill treatment on the child's overall physical and psychological health and development. In these circumstances, social services are mandated to investigate further by convening a multi-agency discussion (strategy meeting) and, if significant risk is identified, by undertaking further enquiries (under section 47 of the UK Children Act 1989), along with law enforcement investigation by the police. The findings from these investigations are discussed in multi-agency meetings (child protection conference) and, if future risk to a child is likely, a tailored child protection plan is put in place and reviewed periodically to monitor progress.

Interventions

As discussed earlier, child maltreatment is not a disorder but rather an exposure to an adverse experience or set of experiences during development. Therefore, safeguarding interventions are best conceptualized not as treatment of child maltreatment but rather as prevention of recurrence (i.e., re-exposure to maltreatment) or impairment (i.e., clinical symptoms) linked to maltreatment (MacMillan *et al.*, 2009).

Prevention of recurrence of child maltreatment

Interventions in this category are generally carried out under the auspices of child protection services in collaboration with different professionals and agencies. The first aim of any intervention is to ensure safety for the maltreated child (and the non-abusing parent in cases of domestic violence), working with the family whenever possible or removing the child (and siblings) from severely abusive or neglectful families. In order to identify the most effective elements for intervention in a particular case of maltreatment, it is important to recognize the particular strengths and vulnerabilities of the individual child and the family during the assessment phase. Although exposure to a single type of maltreatment is unusual, interventions nevertheless commonly focus on one prevailing type of maltreatment. Parent–child interaction therapy (PCIT) has been shown to reduce the recurrence of physical abuse but not neglect, according to child protection services reports (Chaffin *et al.*, 2004). Limited evidence supports the use of parent-training programs to prevent recurrence of physical and emotional abuse (Barlow *et al.*, 2006). For example, parenting programs such as 'The Incredible Years' have been shown to be effective in reducing abusive parenting in maltreating families (Letarte *et al.*, 2010). A large cluster randomized trial showed that a structured, home-based behavioral-skill training program (SafeCare) was associated with reduction in neglect recurrence over the 6 years of follow-up (Chaffin *et al.*, 2012). Limited evidence from small studies suggests that resilient-peer training, imaginative play, therapeutic day training, and multisystemic therapy might reduce recurrence of neglect. One program of intensive nurse visitation failed to prevent recurrence of physical abuse or neglect (MacMillan *et al.*, 2005). A number of studies addressed prevention of maltreatment recurrence by investigating the effect of foster care (MacMillan *et al.*, 2009). Compared to children who remained at home, fostered children often showed better behavioral and educational outcomes. Furthermore, a remarkable randomized trial of postinstitutionalized children showed that foster care placement could remediate the detrimental effects of early deprivation on cognition in institutionalized children (Nelson *et al.*, 2007).

Prevention and treatment of impairment

Interventions targeting mental health needs are generally carried out by child and adolescent mental health services. Because not all children exposed to maltreatment develop psychiatric disorders and maltreatment may lead to different psychiatric disorders (see Figure 29.1), it is important to identify psychopathology and levels of clinical symptoms and everyday functioning during the assessment phase. Systematic review (Ramchandani & Jones, 2003) and meta-analysis (Macdonald *et al.*, 2006) of this literature suggested that Trauma-Focused Cognitive-Behavioral Therapy is effective in treating sexually abused young people with post-traumatic stress disorder, anxiety, and depressive symptoms, but is not effective in treating externalizing disorders symptoms or sexualized behavior.

Effective components of Trauma-Focused Cognitive-Behavioral Therapy after child sexual abuse include psycho-education, relaxation, affect modulation, cognitive restructuring, trauma narrative and in vivo exposure modules for young people, and also seek active involvement of parents (Cohen *et al.*, 2006). In addition, there is preliminary evidence supporting the efficacy of short-term community-based interventions for mothers and children exposed to interpersonal violence, in relation to both behavior problems and emotional symptoms (Graham-Bermann *et al.*, 2007).

Prevention of maltreatment occurrence

Over the last two decades, there has been an increasing focus on evaluating the effectiveness of universal and targeted approaches to prevent the occurrence of childhood maltreatment (MacMillan *et al.*, 2009). Universal approaches include public awareness and education campaigns as well as more practically focused programs that aim to improve parenting practices. While universal approaches are applied to whole communities, targeted approaches are delivered specifically to high-risk groups such as low-income first time mothers.

Universal interventions

Evidence supporting the effectiveness of universal approaches has generally been limited. However, there is preliminary but strong evidence from one randomized controlled trial (RCT) of the Positive Parenting Program (or Triple P) professional training alongside a media and communication strategy (Prinz *et al.*, 2009). The RCT found that compared to the services-as-usual control condition, areas where Triple P was delivered showed significant reductions in rates of substantiated cases of child maltreatment, child out-of-home placements, and child maltreatment injuries after two years of dissemination.

Education programs delivered in school represent another universal approach—typically targeting the prevention of sexual abuse by covering themes such as identifying potential abuse situations, differentiating "good touch" from "bad touch" and how and whom to tell if abuse has occurred. One recent systematic review summarized the evidence from 15 RCTs or quasi RCTs that tested programs aiming to teach children about sexual abuse and how to protect themselves from it (Zwi *et al.*, 2007). Although these programs were found to be generally effective in improving knowledge and protective behaviors, studies have been characterized by a number of methodological weaknesses, such as lack of blinding and short follow-up periods. In addition, some studies have reported negative outcomes, including increased anxiety. Most crucially, however, there is as yet no evidence that increased knowledge translates into actual reduction in risk of sexual abuse (Zwi *et al.*, 2007).

Targeted interventions

Targeted home-visitation programs, such as the Nurse Family Partnership and Early Start, have been shown to be effective in preventing child maltreatment in several studies (Dodge & Coleman, 2011). Visitation programs vary in their models of delivery, focus and practitioner training.

The Nurse Family Partnership (NFP) is probably the most rigorously evaluated example, having undergone three RCTs with high retention rates in different samples in the United States, both in urban and semi-rural areas. Nurses visit low-income first-time mothers during pregnancy and into infancy in order to develop a trusting relationship with the mother and other family members and to promote sensitive parenting. The program aims to ensure prenatal and postnatal health of the child and to improve the mother's economic self-sufficiency (MacMillan *et al.*, 2009). Three published trials have reported reductions in emergency department visits, fewer cases of child abuse and neglect in the whole sample after a 15-year follow-up (Olds *et al.*, 1997), fewer health-care encounters (Kitzman *et al.*, 1997), and preliminary evidence of an overall reduction in the likelihood of child death by age 9 years. However, the positive effects of the NFP intervention were not observed in families where moderate-to-high levels of intimate partner violence were reported (Eckenrode *et al.*, 2000).

The Early Start program is an intensive home-visiting program targeted at families experiencing stress that includes an assessment of the family's needs and resources, a collaborative problem solving approach and provision of support and advice. The intervention aims to improve child health, reduce risk of abuse, and improve parenting, relationship stability, and material well-being. There is preliminary support that this program is associated with lower hospital attendance for childhood injuries and lower parent-rated physical abuse (Fergusson *et al.*, 2005). RCTs evaluating home visiting programs employing paraprofessionals have overall been less effective (Geeraert *et al.*, 2004).

Future directions

Although there is an increasing appreciation of the negative impact of maltreatment on children across a range of outcomes, there remain significant gaps in our understanding of the underlying causal mechanisms and of best practice in this context.

Prevention of child maltreatment remains the priority for all professionals involved in safeguarding. The need for effective preventive interventions is emphasized, for example, by the continuing high prevalence of different types of maltreatment, by the severity of its immediate potential consequences, by the lack of knowledge about the ability of treatment to remediate biological abnormalities before the onset of clinical conditions, and by the poor outcomes of clinical conditions in maltreated individuals. Future preventive interventions will need to explore the value of new conceptual approaches. For example, the idea of "blending" universal and targeted approaches aims to improve matching the intensity of interventions with the severity of a family's risk profile (Prinz *et al.*, 2009). Furthermore, the idea of "common elements" aims to identify the components shared by different effective interventions and to improve matching these components with the family's risk profile (Chorpita *et al.*, 2007, Bentovim & Elliot, 2014). Finally, the "New Orleans Model" aims to improve the initial phase of assessment and intervention for families with children in foster care, in order to more clearly establish the potential for remediation in parents, to promptly achieve a permanent plan of reunion or adoption, and to minimize risk of maltreatment recurrence (Zeanah *et al.*, 2001). While prevention of child maltreatment is a pressing priority, it will be crucial to rigorously evaluate promising preliminary findings before dissemination.

Despite the efforts promoting prevention, it is naïve to assume that child maltreatment can be easily or entirely eradicated from society. Therefore, it is equally important to ensure that as clinicians we are effective in recognizing, responding to, and alleviating the consequences of maltreatment. Research emphasizes two important directions that have the potential to significantly impact on future clinical care.

Research suggests that focus should be placed not only on clinical conditions but also on preclinical vulnerabilities that are evident at the biological level in community samples of maltreated children (Danese *et al.*, 2011; McCrory & Viding, in press). However, the current configuration of health services is centered on the identification and treatment of clinical conditions, with few tools or resources deployed to identify and help those children at elevated risk for future problems. Even in the absence of clinical conditions, it appears that maltreated children show stress-related biological changes that confer what has been conceptualized as 'Latent Vulnerability' for future disorders (McCrory & Viding, in press). To the extent that they predict disease risk and could be remediated, preclinical biomarkers represent missed opportunities for the design of effective therapeutic and secondary-preventative interventions. Longitudinal research is required to isolate and identify risk markers that could be incorporated into routine clinical practice. Furthermore, clinical trials are needed to test whether currently available interventions are effective in modifying clinically relevant biological abnormalities (Fisher *et al.*, 2007; Dozier *et al.*, 2008; Pace *et al.*, 2013).

Finally, research on the mechanisms of biological embedding of early life stress suggests that the potential consequences of maltreatment may go far beyond the traditionally recognized psychological symptoms and also impact physical health in children and adults (Danese *et al.*, 2009; Danese & McEwen, 2012). Stress-related endocrine and immune abnormalities in maltreated children could increase risk of medical conditions, such as obesity (Danese & Tan, 2014) and inflammatory/immune disorders (Dube *et al.*, 2009), as well as cardiovascular disease and other age-related disorders in later life (Dong *et al.*, 2004; Danese *et al.*, 2009). However, children's liability to non-acute medical conditions is often overlooked in clinical practice. To the extent that alleviation of trauma-related psychological symptoms could remediate the biological liability to medical conditions, an integrative brain/body approach to assessment and treatment may significantly improve outcomes of maltreated children.

References

Andersen, S.L. & Teicher, M.H. (2008) Stress, sensitive periods and maturational events in adolescent depression. *Trends in Neurosciences* **31**, 183–191.

Barlow, J., *et al.* 2006. Individual and group-based parenting programmes for the treatment of physical child abuse and neglect. *Cochrane Database of Systematic Reviews*, CD005463, http://online library.wiley.com/doi/10.1002/14651858.CD005463.pub2/abstract; jsessionid=1FE24020443BDDA37F9145A1FF088C3F.f03t03.

Bell, R.Q. (1968) A reinterpretation of the direction of effects in studies of socialization. *Psychological Review* **75**, 81–95.

Belsky, J. (1993) Etiology of child maltreatment: a developmental-ecological analysis. *Psychological Bulletin* **114**, 413–434.

Bentovim, A. & Bingley, M.L. (2001) *The Family Assessment of Family Competence, Strengths, and Difficulties*. Brighton Publishing, Brighton.

Bentovim, A. & Elliott, I. (2014) Hope for children and families: targeting abusive parenting and the associated impairment of children. *Journal of Clinical Child & Adolescent Psychology* **43**, 270–285

Brown, J. *et al.* (1998) A longitudinal analysis of risk factors for child maltreatment: findings of a 17-year prospective study of officially recorded and self-reported child abuse and neglect. *Child Abuse & Neglect* **22**, 1065–1078.

Butchart, A. *et al.* (2006) *Preventing Child Maltreatment: A Guide to Taking Action and Generating Evidence*. World Health Organization and International Society for Prevention of Child Abuse and Neglect.

Caspi, A. *et al.* (2010) Genetic sensitivity to the environment: the case of the serotonin transporter gene and its implications for studying complex diseases and traits. *American Journal of Psychiatry* **167**, 509–527.

Chaffin, M. *et al.* (2004) Parent–child interaction therapy with physically abusive parents: efficacy for reducing future abuse reports. *Journal of Consulting and Clinical Psychology* **72**, 500–510.

Chaffin, M. *et al.* (2012) A statewide trial of the SafeCare home-based services model with parents in Child Protective Services. *Pediatrics* **129**, 509–515.

Chorpita, B.F. *et al.* (2007) Understanding the common elements of evidence-based practice: misconceptions and clinical examples. *Journal American Academy Child and Adolescent Psychiatry* **46**, 647–652.

Cicchetti, D. (2013) Annual research review: resilient functioning in maltreated children—past, present, and future perspectives. *Journal of Child Psychology and Psychiatry, and Allied Disciplines* **54**, 402–422.

Cohen, J.A. *et al.* (2006) *Treating Trauma and Traumatic Grief in Children and Adolescents*. Guilford Press, New York.

Collishaw, S. *et al.* (2007) Resilience to adult psychopathology following childhood maltreatment: evidence from a community sample. *Child Abuse & Neglect* **31**, 211–229.

Coulton, C.J. *et al.* (1995) Community level factors and child maltreatment rates. *Child Development* **66**, 1262–1276.

Cox, A. & Walker, S. (2002) *The HOME Inventory—Home Observation and Measurement of the Environment*. Brighton Publishing, Brighton.

Crouch, J. *et al.* (2001) Childhood physical abuse, early social support, and risk for maltreatment: current social support as a mediator of risk for child physical abuse. *Child Abuse & Neglect* **25**, 93–107.

Currie, J. & Widom, C.S. (2010) Long-term consequences of child abuse and neglect on adult economic well-being. *Child Maltreatment* **15**, 111–120.

Danese, A. & McEwen, B.S. (2012) Adverse childhood experiences, allostasis, allostatic load, and age-related disease. *Physiology & Behavior* **106**, 29–39.

Danese, A. & Tan, M. (2014) Childhood maltreatment and obesity: systematic review and meta-analysis. *Molecular Psychiatry* **19**, 544–554.

Danese, A. *et al.* (2007) Childhood maltreatment predicts adult inflammation in a life-course study. *Proceedings of the National Academy of Sciences of the United States of America* **104**, 1319–1324.

Danese, A. *et al.* (2009) Adverse childhood experiences and adult risk factors for age-related disease: depression, inflammation, and clustering of metabolic risk markers. *Archives of Pediatrics & Adolescent Medicine* **163**, 1135–1143.

Danese, A. *et al.* (2011) Biological embedding of stress through inflammation processes in childhood. *Molecular Psychiatry* **16**, 244–246.

De Brito, S.A. *et al.* (2013) Reduced orbitofrontal and temporal grey matter in a community sample of maltreated children. *Journal of Child Psychology and Psychiatry, and Allied Disciplines* **54**, 105–112.

Dixon, L. *et al.* (2005) Risk factors of parents abused as children: a mediational analysis of the intergenerational continuity of child maltreatment (Part I). *Journal of Child Psychology and Psychiatry* **46**, 47–57.

Dodge, K.A. & Coleman, D. (2011) *Preventing Child Maltreatment: Community Approaches.* Guilford Press, London.

Dodge, K.A. *et al.* (1990) Mechanisms in the cycle of violence. *Science* **250**, 1678–1683.

Dong, M. *et al.* (2004) Insights into causal pathways for ischemic heart disease: adverse childhood experiences study. *Circulation* **110**, 1761–1766.

Dozier, M. *et al.* (2008) Effects of an attachment-based intervention on the cortisol production of infants and toddlers in foster care. *Development and Psychopathology* **20**, 845–859.

Dube, S.R. *et al.* (2009) Cumulative childhood stress and autoimmune diseases in adults. *Psychosomatic Medicine* **71**, 243–250.

Eckenrode, J. *et al.* (2000) Preventing child abuse and neglect with a program of nurse home visitation. *JAMA* **284**, 1385–1391.

Felitti, V.J. *et al.* (1998) Relationship of childhood abuse and household dysfunction to many of the leading causes of death in adults. The Adverse Childhood Experiences (ACE) Study. *American Journal of Preventive Medicine* **14**, 245–258.

Fergusson, D.M. *et al.* (2005) Randomized trial of the Early Start program of home visitation. *Pediatrics* **116**, e803–e809.

Finkelhor, D. & Jones, L. (2012) Trends in child maltreatment. *Lancet* **379**, 2048–2049.

Finkelhor, D. *et al.* (2007a) Poly-victimization: a neglected component in child victimization. *Child Abuse & Neglect* **31**, 7–26.

Finkelhor, D. *et al.* (2007b) Re-victimization patterns in a national longitudinal sample of children and youth. *Child Abuse & Neglect* **31**, 479–502.

Fisher, P.A. *et al.* (2007) Effects of a therapeutic intervention for foster preschoolers on diurnal cortisol activity. *Psychoneuroendocrinology* **32**, 892–905.

Geeraert, L. *et al.* (2004) The effects of early prevention programs for families with young children at risk for physical child abuse and neglect: a meta-analysis. *Child Maltreatment* **9**, 277–291.

Gilbert, R. *et al.* (2009a) Recognising and responding to child maltreatment. *Lancet* **373**, 167–180.

Gilbert, R. *et al.* (2009b) Burden and consequences of child maltreatment in high-income countries. *Lancet* **373**, 68–81.

Gilbert, R. *et al.* (2012) Child maltreatment: variation in trends and policies in six developed countries. *Lancet* **379**, 758–772.

Goldman, J., *et al.* 2003. *What Factors Contribute to Child Abuse and Neglect?* U.S. Department of Health and Human Services [Online]. Available: http://www.childwelfare.gov/pubs/usermanuals/foundation/foundatione.cfm

Goodman, R. (1997) The strengths and difficulties questionnaire: a research note. *Journal of Child Psychology and Psychiatry, and Allied Disciplines* **38**, 581–586.

Graham-Bermann, S.A. *et al.* (2007) Community-based intervention for children exposed to intimate partner violence: an efficacy trial. *Journal of Consulting and Clinical Psychology* **75**, 199–209.

Hanson, J.L. *et al.* (2010) Early stress is associated with alterations in the orbitofrontal cortex: a tensor-based morphometry investigation of brain structure and behavioral risk. *Journal of Neuroscience* **30**, 7466–7472.

Heim, C. *et al.* (2000) Pituitary-adrenal and autonomic responses to stress in women after sexual and physical abuse in childhood. *JAMA* **284**, 592–597.

Jaffee, S.R. & Price, T.S. (2007) Gene-environment correlations: a review of the evidence and implications for prevention of mental illness. *Molecular Psychiatry* **12**, 432–442.

Jaffee, S.R. *et al.* (2007) Individual, family, and neighborhood factors distinguish resilient from non-resilient maltreated children: a cumulative stressors model. *Child Abuse & Neglect* **31**, 231–253.

Jones, R. *et al.* (2008) Clinicians' description of factors influencing their reporting of suspected child abuse: report of the Child Abuse Reporting Experience Study Research Group. *Pediatrics* **122**, 259–266.

Jones, L. *et al.* (2012) Prevalence and risk of violence against children with disabilities: a systematic review and meta-analysis of observational studies. *Lancet* **380**, 899–907.

Jonson-Reid, M. *et al.* (2012) Child and adult outcomes of chronic child maltreatment. *Pediatrics* **129**, 839–845.

Kaufman, J. & Zigler, E. (1987) Do abused children become abusive parents? *American Journal of Orthopsychiatry* **57**, 186–192.

Kempe, C.H. *et al.* (1962) The battered-child syndrome. *JAMA* **181**, 17–24.

Kitzman, H. *et al.* (1997) Effect of prenatal and infancy home visitation by nurses on pregnancy outcomes, childhood injuries, and repeated childbearing. *JAMA* **278**, 644–652.

Krug, E.G. *et al.* (2002) The world report on violence and health. *Lancet* **360**, 1083–1088.

Letarte, M.-J. *et al.* (2010) Effectiveness of a parent training program "Incredible Years" in a child protection service. *Child Abuse & Neglect* **34**, 253–261.

Macdonald, G.M., *et al.* 2006. Cognitive-behavioural interventions for children who have been sexually abused *Cochrane Database of Systematic Reviews*, CD001930, http://onlinelibrary.wiley.com/doi/10.1002/14651858.CD001930.pub3/abstract

MacMillan, H.L. *et al.* (2005) Effectiveness of home visitation by public-health nurses in prevention of the recurrence of child physical abuse and neglect: a randomised controlled trial. *Lancet* **365**, 1786–1793.

MacMillan, H.L. *et al.* (2009) Interventions to prevent child maltreatment and associated impairment. *Lancet* **373**, 250–266.

McCrory, E. *et al.* (2010) Research review: the neurobiology and genetics of maltreatment and adversity. *Journal of Child Psychology and Psychiatry, and Allied Disciplines* **51**, 1079–1095.

McCrory, E.J. *et al.* (2011) Heightened neural reactivity to threat in child victims of family violence. *Current Biology* **21**, R947–R948.

McCrory, E.J. *et al.* (2013) Amygdala activation in maltreated children during pre-attentive emotional processing. *British Journal of Psychiatry : The Journal of Mental Science* **202**, 269–276.

McCrory, E.J. & Viding, E. (in press) The theory of latent vulnerability: reconceptualizing the link between childhood maltreatment and psychiatric disorder. *Development and Psychopathology*.

McEwen, B.S. (1998) Protective and damaging effects of stress mediators. *New England Journal of Medicine* **338**, 171–179.

Meaney, M.J. (2010) Epigenetics and the biological definition of gene x environment interactions. *Child Development* **81**, 41–79.

Munro, E.R., *et al.* 2011. Scoping review to draw together data on child injury and safeguarding and to compare the position of England with that in other countries. Department for Education.

Myers, J.E.B. & APSAC (2010) *The APSAC Handbook on Child Maltreatment*. SAGE Publications.

Nanni, V. *et al.* (2012) Childhood maltreatment predicts unfavorable course of illness and treatment outcome in depression: a meta-analysis. *American journal of psychiatry* **169**, 141–151.

Nelson, C.A. *et al.* (2007) Cognitive recovery in socially deprived young children: the Bucharest Early Intervention Project. *Science* **318**, 1937–1940.

National Institute for Health and Care Excellence. 2009. When to suspect child maltreatment [Online]. Available: http://guidance.nice.org.uk/CG89

Olds, D.L. *et al.* (1997) Long-term effects of home visitation on maternal life course and child abuse and neglect. *JAMA* **278**, 637–643.

Olson, S. & Stroud, C. 2012. *Child Maltreatment Research, Policy, and Practice for the Next Decade: Workshop Summary*. US National Academy of Sciences [Online]. Available: http://www.nap.edu/catalog.php?record_id=13368

Pace, T.W. *et al.* (2013) Engagement with cognitively-based compassion training is associated with reduced salivary C-reactive protein from before to after training in foster care program adolescents. *Psychoneuroendocrinology* **38**, 294–299.

Pinheiro, P.S. 2006. *World Report on Violence against Children*. New York: United Nations [Online]. Available: http://www.unicef.org/lac/full_tex(3).pdf

Prinz, R.J. *et al.* (2009) Population-based prevention of child maltreatment: the US Triple P system population trial. *Prevention Science* **10**, 1–12.

Radford, L. *et al.* (2011) *Child Abuse and Neglect in UK Today*. NSPCC, London.

Radford, L. *et al.* (2012) Trends in child maltreatment. *Lancet* **379**, 2048–2049.

Ramchandani, P. & Jones, D.P. (2003) Treating psychological symptoms in sexually abused children: from research findings to service provision. *British Journal of Psychiatry: The Journal of Mental Science* **183**, 484–490.

Sampson, R.J. *et al.* (1997) Neighborhoods and violent crime: a multilevel study of collective efficacy. *Science* **277**, 918–924.

Shirtcliff, E.A. *et al.* (2009) Early childhood stress is associated with elevated antibody levels to herpes simplex virus type 1. *Proceedings of the National Academy of Sciences of the United States of America* **106**, 2963–2967.

Shonkoff, J.P. *et al.* (2009) Neuroscience, molecular biology, and the childhood roots of health disparities: building a new framework for health promotion and disease prevention. *JAMA* **301**, 2252–2259.

Tottenham, N. *et al.* (2010) Prolonged institutional rearing is associated with atypically large amygdala volume and difficulties in emotion regulation. *Developmental Science* **13**, 46–61.

U.S. Child Welfare 2007. *Recognising Child Abuse and Neglect: Signs and Symptoms* [Online]. Available: http://www.childwelfare.gov/pubs/factsheets/signs.cfm

U.S. Child Welfare 2013. *Child Abuse and Neglect Fatalities 2011: Statistics and Interventions* [Online]. Available: http://www.childwelfare.gov/pubs/factsheets/fatality.cfm

U.S. DHHS 2010. *Child Maltreatment 2008* [Online]. Available: http://www.acf.hhs.gov/programs/cb/resource/child-maltreatment-2008

UK DoE 2008. *Information Sharing: Guidance for Practitioners and Managers* [Online]. Available: http://www.education.gov.uk/publications/standard/publicationdetail/page1/DCSF-00807-2008

UK DoE 2012. *Common Assessment Framework (CAF)* [Online]. Available: http://www.education.gov.uk/childrenandyoungpeople/strategy/integratedworking/caf

UK DoE 2013. *Working Together to Safeguard Children: A Guide to Inter-Agency Working to Safeguard and Promote the Welfare of Children*, London [Online]. Available: http://www.education.gov.uk/publications/standard/publicationDetail/Page1/DFE-00030-2013

UNICEF. 2003. *Child Maltreatment Deaths in Rich Nations*, Florence [Online]. Available: http://www.unicef-irc.org/publications/pdf/repcard5e.pdf

Zeanah, C.H. & Zeanah, P.D. (1989) Intergenerational transmission of maltreatment: insights from attachment theory and research. *Psychiatry: Interpersonal and Biological Processes* **52**, 177–196.

Zeanah, C.H. *et al.* (2001) Evaluation of a preventive intervention for maltreated infants and toddlers in foster care. *Journal of the American Academy of Child and Adolescent Psychiatry* **40**, 214–221.

Zwi, K.J., et al. 2007. School-based education programmes for the prevention of child sexual abuse *Cochrane Database of Systematic Reviews*, CD004380, http://onlinelibrary.wiley.com/doi/10.1002/14651858.CD004380.pub2/abstract

CHAPTER 30

Child sexual abuse

Danya Glaser

Department of Child and Adolescent Psychiatrist, Great Ormond Street Hospital for Children, London, UK

Introduction

While child sexual abuse (CSA) involves the child in a physical act, its deleterious consequences are primarily psychological. It is a significant risk factor for the development of psychopathology in childhood, adolescence and adulthood.

CSA may be the explicit reason for referral to CAMHS (child and adolescent mental health services), but may also be discovered incidentally during assessment or treatment, especially when common sequelae are encountered. At times, an unsolicited disclosure is made by a child during therapeutic work. Child psychologists, psychiatrists, and psychotherapists may contribute to investigations of CSA, particularly in assessment interviews of young or very traumatized children, or in children with communication difficulties. Consultation to social services in case management and to caregivers of children who have been sexually abused is often requested. Risk assessments of adolescent abusers may also be required. It is therefore of importance to CAMHS.

The hallmarks of CSA are its secret nature and the very frequent denial of alleged abuse by the abuser. Sexual abuse extends beyond incest, occurring both within and outside the family but the abuser is frequently already known to the child. Indeed this acquaintance may follow a deliberate befriending or "grooming" of the child by the abuser.

CSA is not a new phenomenon. General Booth, founder of the Salvation Army, wrote in 1890: "I understand that the Society for the Protection of Children prosecuted last year a fabulous number of fathers for unnatural sins with their children" (Booth, 1890). However, CSA only began to be noted as a significant form of child maltreatment in the 1970s. Increasing recognition came with the development of the women's movement, reports by women survivors of their childhood abuse and a greater openness regarding sexuality. There have been successive reports from many countries in the scientific press, in particular in *Child Abuse and Neglect, the International Journal*.

In the United Kingdom and many other jurisdictions, disapproval of CSA is expressed by the legal prohibition of incest and sexual contact between an adult and a child. However, some of the harmful effects of child sexual abuse are largely consequent on societal disapproval. Despite the high frequency of CSA reports (see later), most suspicions of sexual abuse continue to be met with caution, and disclosures are often regarded with suspicion. This is probably explained by the social taboo surrounding adult sexual contact with children, the absence of noninvolved witnesses to this (secret) activity and the potentially serious consequences for the alleged abuser if found guilty. Thus the rates of criminal prosecution and conviction are low (Hagborg *et al.*, 2012) and lower in comparison with other crimes (Cross *et al.*, 2003).

Controversy has surrounded disputed memories of childhood sexual abuse recovered in adulthood, (Davies & Dalgleish, 2001). Some memories have returned spontaneously whereas others have been triggered by reminders or recalled in response to enquiry that include leading questions and other forms of suggestion (Loftus *et al.*, 1994; see also Chapter 20). A few have been induced by over-zealous therapists. While this debate has (inappropriately) rekindled doubts about the general truth of allegations made by children, there has now been recognition of considerable magnitude of CSA outside the family by clergy and media persons who have gained access to children.

Definitions

A myriad of definitions for legal, research and other purposes continue to be used. A recent definition guiding child protection work in England states: "Sexual abuse involves forcing or enticing a child or young person to take part in sexual activities, not necessarily involving a high level of violence, whether or not the

Rutter's Child and Adolescent Psychiatry, Sixth Edition.
Edited by Anita Thapar and Daniel S. Pine, James F. Leckman, Stephen Scott, Margaret J. Snowling, Eric Taylor.
© 2015 John Wiley & Sons Ltd. Published 2018 by John Wiley & Sons Ltd.

child is aware of what is happening. The activities may involve physical contact, including assault by penetration (for example, rape or oral sex) or non-penetrative acts such as masturbation, kissing, rubbing and touching outside of clothing. They may also include noncontact activities, such as involving children in looking at, or in the production of, sexual images, watching sexual activities, encouraging children to behave in sexually inappropriate ways, or grooming a child in preparation for abuse (including via the internet). Sexual abuse is not solely perpetrated by adult males. Women can also commit acts of sexual abuse, as can other children" (Department for Education, 2013). The United Nations Committee on the Rights of the Child (UNCRC, 2011) in its General Comment 13 (a detailed guidance on Article 19 which deals with violence against children) has the following definition: "Sexual abuse and exploitation includes: (a) The inducement or coercion of a child to engage in any unlawful or psychologically harmful sexual activity. Sexual abuse comprises any sexual activities imposed by an adult on a child against which the child is entitled to protection by criminal law. Sexual activities are also considered as abuse when committed against a child by another child, if the child offender is significantly older than the child victim or uses power, threat or other means of pressure. Sexual activities between children are not considered as sexual abuse if the children are older than the age limit defined by the State party for consensual sexual activities; (b) The use of children in commercial sexual exploitation; and (c) The use of children in audio or visual images of CSA; (d) Child prostitution, sexual slavery, sexual exploitation in travel and tourism, trafficking (within and between countries) and sale of children for sexual purposes and forced marriage. Many children experience sexual victimization which is not accompanied by physical force or restraint but which is nonetheless psychologically intrusive, exploitive and traumatic." It is important to note that the abuser's intentions or motivations are not considered necessary to be included in definitions.

The term pedophilia applies to a sexual attraction to, and arousal by prepubertal children, of either gender. It is clear that many sexual abusers are therefore not pedophiles.

Cultural aspects

Culturally sanctioned and normative practices may be harmful (McKee, 1984) and "cultural practice … should not justify hurting a child or young person" (National Institute for Health and Care Excellence (NICE), 2009). A particular example of harmful cultural practice is female genital mutilation (Powell *et al.*, 2004), which is regarded as a clear form of child abuse in many jurisdictions.

Legal considerations

The differences between the civil – family and child protection law and criminal law are pertinent to CSA. The threshold for a criminal prosecution, which is solely concerned with the innocence or guilt of the alleged abuser, is higher than that required for the civil legal protection of the child.

In some jurisdictions, such as in England and the United Stated of America, civil and criminal proceedings can continue in parallel and independently of each other. Thus, a child may be protected from an abuser by being moved from his care under civil law, when there has been no criminal trial, or a failed prosecution. In other jurisdictions, child protective procedures will only follow a criminal conviction of the abuser; the CRC definition (see earlier) refers to the criminal law. This confers considerably less protection for children, especially as the rate of convictions worldwide is low relative to the number of allegations.

Demographics

The victims

Age of victims
Children may be abused from infancy onwards but frequency and severity increase with age (Finkelhor *et al.*, 2009; Radford *et al.*, 2011).

Gender of victims
Girls are more commonly victims of sexual abuse than boys. There is a tendency for sexual abuse of boys to be under-reported (Holmes & Slap, 1998), in part because of shame and the fear of homosexuality. Extrafamilial abuse more commonly involves boys although there is no agreement about whether boys are more commonly abused by strangers (Watkins & Bentovim, 1992).

Disability
The rate of sexual abuse of children with disabilities is 2 or 3 times greater than in "normal" children (Sullivan & Knutson, 2000), the reasons for this including: the children's difficulties in communicating about abuse (Morris, 1999); their dependency on intimate physical care; social isolation in institutional care (Utting *et al.*, 1997); and care by staff rather than parents (Westcott & Jones, 1999).

Abusers
Adults
Sexual abusers constitute a heterogeneous group in terms of personal, social, and demographic factors. The majority of abusers (85–95%) are male. Men in old age may well continue to abuse children. Pedophiles, who abuse prepubertal children, may target both boys and girls (Strassberg *et al.*, 2012). A small proportion of CSA is carried out by female abusers (Saradjian, 1996), often in conjunction with a man. Women abusers on their own are more likely to abuse boys (Faller, 1989). There is no unitary psychological profile of abusers. Moreover, whereas many will have experienced disruption and physical abuse in their formative years, sexual abuse in childhood is only one

predisposing factor (summarized in Watkins & Bentovim, 1992) and is not a prerequisite to sexual abuse.

Children and adolescents

Sexual abuse by both children and adolescents, mostly boys, has become widely recognized and is no longer considered an acceptable variant of childhood or adolescent sexual development. A significant proportion of adolescent abusers are of low intellectual ability and show heterogeneous maladaptive mental schemata regarding social interaction and abuse (Richardson, 2005). Most children and adolescents who sexually abuse other children have experienced psychosocial adversity. They include material neglect, lack of supervision, sexual abuse by a female person and witnessing intrafamilial violence (Salter *et al.*, 2003), discontinuity of care, and experience of physical violence and emotional abuse (Skuse *et al.*, 1998). Sixty six per cent of contact sexual abuse reported by children and young people in the United Kingdom was perpetrated by other children and young people under the age of 18 (Radford *et al.*, 2011).

Many adult abusers report the onset of their abusive activities in adolescence and abuse by an adolescent cannot necessarily be considered safely to "burn out" in adulthood (Vizard *et al.*, 1995). However, there is evidence of good response to treatment of adolescent abusers (see later).

Abuser–child relationship

The majority of children know their abuser and abuse by strangers is rare. However, the abuser may befriend the child as part of the grooming process, or the abuser and child may be part of the same family, or social network. In community studies, the commonest relationship is step-father – step-daughter (Finkelhor, 1984). The same abuser may abuse children both within and outside the family and include biological as well as step-children. Intrafamilial abuse continues for longer than sexual abuse outside the family, and some forms, such as parent-child abuse, have more serious and lasting consequences (Finkelhor, 1994.)

The nature and circumstances of the abuse

Frequency and duration of abuse for an individual child

Whereas some population studies include a majority with a single episode of abuse, for many children and in clinical samples there has been repeated abuse by the same abuser, often continuing for several years.

Contact abuse

Broadly, any physical contact between the breasts and genitalia of a child or adult and a part of the other's body, with the exception of isolated accidental touch or for developmentally- and age-appropriate cleaning or for applying medication or ointment, is considered to be sexual abuse. It includes fondling, masturbation, oral-genital contact or penetration, attempted or actual digital and penal penetration of, and the insertion of objects into, the vagina or anus. There is, typically, a gradual progression from touching to more penetrative abuse (Berliner & Conte, 1990), so as to avoid causing initial pain or injury which would be more likely to lead the child to complain about or report the abuse. Anal abuse is understandably commoner in boys, although younger girls are not infrequently anally abused (Hobbs & Wynne, 1989). In a small proportion of cases, actual physical violence is used, either as a way of intimidating or coercing the child, or as an integral aspect of the abuse.

Noncontact abuse

This includes deliberate exposure of children to adult genitalia or sexual activity, either live or depicted in photographs or film. It also includes intrusive looking at the young person's body, inducing children to interact sexually with each other and taking photographs for pornographic purposes. Although the most serious effects of sexual abuse are associated with contact, and especially penetrative, abuse, many young persons report the experience of being intrusively observed as humiliating and intimidating, with greater coercion increasing the harm.

The use of the internet and mobile phone technology

The internet and mobile phone technology have become sources of sexual abuse of children by a number of different ways (Taylor & Quayle, 2003). Children may view pornographic images inadvertently or by deliberately searching for them. This exposure is increasing (Wolak *et al.*, 2006) and is reported by children as very disturbing (Finkelhor *et al.*, 2000). The internet is also increasingly used by adults in a variety of ways (CEOP, 2013) including requests for children's pictures of themselves or for grooming with the intention of luring children into sexual activity (O'Connell, 2003). In addition, children are being made the subjects of abuse images (Palmer, 2005). Lastly, child pornography may act as a motivator or reinforcer of sexually abusive activity by adolescents (Quayle & Taylor, 2006). Children are also distributing images of themselves and of other children captured on mobile phones. As with other forms of sexual abuse, children and adolescents are often reluctant to talk about this activity, which may be discovered in the course of criminal investigations regarding material found on computers, rather than disclosed by the child.

Organized abuse

Most abusers abuse in isolation. However, there are also organized forms of abuse involving more than one abuser and multiple children, some of whom are recruited in sex rings (Wild & Wynne, 1986). Some adolescents are being targeted on the basis of their vulnerability, for example, living in care and institutions. Organized abuse also includes the use of children and young persons for the production of child pornography. Questions remain about the reliability, verifiability, and credibility (Young *et al.*, 1991) of the reports of formalized rituals (Frude, 1996).

Commercial sexual exploitation of children

Commercial sexual exploitation or "transactional sex" (Williams *et al.*, 2012), involving both boys and girls, takes the inter-related forms of prostitution and trafficking – usually across borders (Chase & Statham 2005). While an accurate scale of the problem is difficult to determine (Dottridge, 2008), it is likely to be global and increasing with economic hardship (ECPAT International, 2009). Sexual exploitation can provide a source of money to support drug dependency and introduces the young person to addictive drugs as a means of gaining control over them for subsequent sexual exploitation.

Abuse by clergy, media personnel, and in institutions

Sexual abuse by clergy and media personnel has come to light in a number of countries including the United Kingdom, Ireland, the United States of America and Australia. It includes abuse of both single and multiple victims, across the age-range and of both genders (Haywood *et al.*, 1996), although boys were over-represented (Parkinson *et al.*, 2012). Finkelhor (2003) mentions negative as well as some positive consequences including increased public belief in the existence of CSA; enabling more children and adolescents to talk of their own abuse; lessening the stigma of sexual abuse for boys; and recognition of corporate or organizational responsibility for employees' behavior.

Children in residential settings are particularly vulnerable, being dependent on staff and often isolated from confiding contact with adults outside the residential setting (Utting *et al.*, 1997).

Epidemiology

Published figures for incidence and prevalence of CSA vary considerably according to the definition used, the source of data, and the population studied. Whereas broad definitions point to the extent of the problem, they are less helpful in indicating severity and the kind of therapeutic services required.

Prevalence

The most accurate prevalence figures are from population studies (Finkelhor *et al.*, 1990). Even here, responses to interviews or questionnaires may be underestimates, due to reluctance to report, or a lack of recall of previous abuse, even when this had been documented at the time (Williams, 1994).

In population, as opposed to victim samples, nonpenetrative contact abuse is more commonly described than in clinical samples. A meta-analysis of self-report studies across a number of countries (Andrews *et al.*, 2004) found the following prevalence rates (see Table 30.1).

Table 30.1 Prevalence rates of sexual abuse.

	Girls (%)	Boys (%)
Any sexual abuse	25.3	8.7
Contact abuse	13.2	3.7
Penetrative abuse	5.3	1.9

In a retrospective study using a questionnaire with a random probability sample of 18–24 years olds in the United Kingdom (May-Chahal & Cawson, 2005) 10% reported experiencing contact sexual abuse while under 16 years of age (15% girls and 6% boys). A retrospective study from the United States, using a mailed questionnaire to a national geographically stratified, random sample of 1442 subjects with mean age 46 years (range of 18–90) yielded a response by 64.8% and 32.3% female and 14.2% male respondents reported childhood sexual abuse. Rates of abuse within the immediate or extended family (46.8%) and penetrative abuse (52.8%) did not differ according to gender of subject (Briere & Elliott, 2003). Prevalence rates of maltreatment including CSA were reported in a recent large random probability sample from the United Kingdom, in which there were interviews with parents of children under the age of 11 years, children aged 11–17 and their caregivers, and young adults aged 18–24, respectively (Radford *et al.*, 2011). Percentage of contact and overall, including noncontact, sexual abuse in the samples was reported as follows (see Tables 30.2 and 30.3).

Considerable co-occurrence of different forms of maltreatment is reported in many of these studies.

Fluctuations in rates of reported cases

Rates of reporting increased over the 20 years after 1970, both in the United Kingdom (Markowe, 1988) and in the United States of America (Finkelhor, 1991) probably due to increased awareness with little evidence that the actual incidence had been changing significantly (Feldman *et al.*, 1991). However, the number of substantiated cases of CSA in the United States

Table 30.2 Percentage contact child sexual abuse experienced by age.

AGE (years)	<11	11–17	18–24
Girls (%)	0.8	7	17.8
Boys (%)	0.2	2.6	5.1
Total (%)	0.5	4.8	11.3

Table 30.3 Percentage overall child sexual abuse experienced by age.

AGE (years)	<11	11–17	18–24
Total (%)	1.2	16.5	24.1

of America has decreased by an estimated 49% between 1990 and 2004 with fewer disclosures, confessions by abusers and a reduction in emotional and behavioral problems associated with CSA (Finkelhor & Jones, 2006). A similar finding, of declining rates of sexual abuse of males over some decades and of females more recently, has been reported from Australia (Dunne *et al.*, 2003) and a possible decline in substantiated cases in Canada (Collin-Vézina *et al.*, 2010) and the United Kingdom (see Radford *et al.*, 2011 above). There could be several reasons for these findings: (a) an actual decline (Finkelhor & Jones, 2004) possibly signaling a positive effect of interventions for reported CSA; growing awareness of children's rights or greater vigilance and child-focused parenting; (b) a decline in reporting due, for instance, to fear of legal repercussions or (c) changes in agency responses to reported abuse, such as increased cautiousness and a raised threshold for an active professional response. It is likely that this decline in substantiated cases of sexual abuse reflects some actual reduction in incidence.

Country, ethnicity, culture, socioeconomic, and family status

CSA is now reported from most, including developing countries (e.g., Luo *et al.*, 2008) with some 5% of children in sub-Saharan Africa reportedly experienced penetrative sexual abuse in childhood (Lalor, 2004).

Within the United Kingdom and the United States of America, population-based studies have shown no ethnic differences in the rates of CSA (Fontes, 1995). However, data on CSA incidence in minority and different ethnic communities are lacking, partly due to decisions on data collection criteria, which do not classify racial/ethnic background sufficiently finely, and partly because shame and denial about sexual abuse within some minority cultures conspire against reporting. Incidence within a particular ethnic group may reflect effects of that group's recent traumatic and migration experiences, rather than aspects of the particular culture. Lastly, some societies continue to find difficulty in facilitating open acknowledgment of the existence of child maltreatment in general and sexual abuse in particular.

Socioeconomic status is unrelated to the incidence of CSA in population studies (Berliner & Elliott, 1996) but there is an overrepresentation of lower socioeconomic groups in clinic samples (Bentovim *et al.*, 1987). This may be because these groups are more likely to come to the attention of child protective agencies than middle class families who may find ways of hiding the abuse or avoiding its reporting (Gomes-Schwartz *et al.*, 1990). Different forms of child abuse and neglect are not infrequently found in the same family and the same child (Mullen *et al.*, 1994), especially among the socially disadvantaged. CSA is associated with troubled family life including family disruption (Russel, 1986), reconstituted families, intrafamilial violence (Bifulco *et al.*, 1991), and parents who are perceived as emotionally distant and uncaring (Alexander & Lupfer, 1987).

Risk and maintaining factors for child sexual abuse

There is no unitary theory of causation to explain CSA. Although, by definition, it is an interaction between the abuser/perpetrator and child/victim, intention and responsibility rest with the abuser. The abuser's wish for sexual gratification and for power are the two main motivators. Pedophilia is based on sexual arousal to prepubertal children. An explanatory theory needs to include biological, psychological, cultural, and situational factors (Ward & Siegert, 2002).

Finkelhor's (1984) systemic model of four preconditions continues to provide a basis for understanding CSA. They are:

1 **Motivation to sexually abuse children**
   Motivations include pedophilia, fear/avoidance of peer intimate and sexual relationships, sadism; interpersonal motivators such as a need to overpower or gain mastery over more vulnerable persons, often as a result of one's own past abuse and low self-esteem. Sexual interest in children and a consequent predisposition to sexual abuse is far commoner than the action, requiring other factors to exist before abuse will actually occur. Mothers who sexually abuse have been described as simultaneously attacking and emotionally engulfing or possessing their children (Welldon, 1988).

2 **Absence of internal inhibitors**
   Absence of internal inhibitors includes the effects of alcohol and emotional dysregulation. Abusers also use cognitive distortions or rationalizations including minimization of the harm to the child; conceptualizing the abuse as "love" or "education"; and placing responsibility on the child or adolescent who is described as inviting or requesting the abuse.

3 **Absence of external inhibitors**
   External inhibitors of sexual abuse include cultural, social, and family protective structures and relationships surrounding the child, in particular a secure attachment to primary caregiver(s), good monitoring of the child's whereabouts and the existence of confiding relationships for the child. Their absence renders the child or adolescent vulnerable to sexual abuse.

4 **Child's vulnerability**
   The particular child's vulnerability by virtue of age, disability, neglect, being orphaned and homeless, social isolation, and previous sexual abuse all increase the likelihood of sexual abuse, all of which abusers recognize.

This explanatory schema does not remove the abuser's responsibility for the abuse, whatever the nature of contributory risk factors.

Maintaining factors

Despite a growing recognition of CSA worldwide, the censure surrounding it leads to secrecy, denial, and disbelief of children about its occurrence. About 1 in 3 young people show no outward indicators (Kendall-Tackett *et al.*, 1993), allowing abuse to be undetected over prolonged periods. This is particularly likely with children as compared with adolescents (McLeer *et al.*, 1998). By the time sexual abuse is discovered in childhood, it has often occurred repeatedly. In the Radford *et al.* (2011) study, in 34% of cases of sexual assault by an adult and 82.7% of cases of sexual assault by a peer nobody else knew about it at the time of the interview. Children's own coping through a psychological accommodation process may help to maintain the secret.

Effects of child sexual abuse

Charting the "natural history" of sexual abuse-related symptomatology is difficult for a number of reasons. Most studies have been retrospective and have variously included clinical, convenience, and population samples. While there is no post CSA syndrome (Kendall-Tackett *et al.*, 1993; Paolucci *et al.*, 2001), CSA is a significant risk factor for mental health disorders both in childhood and adulthood (Cutajar *et al.*, 2010) as well as having effects on physical health. There has been little systematic study of the effects of CSA on people with learning disability. Findings suggest that the effects are similar to those in the general population (Sequeira & Hollins, 2003).

Effects in childhood and adolescence

Not all children who have been sexually abused will develop difficulties and some will develop them only later (Saywitz *et al.*, 2000). However, a wide range of difficulties, which may not appear immediately, has been found with considerable effect sizes: depression, anxiety, PTSD, self-harm, low self-esteem, conduct disorder, drug misuse, age-inappropriate sexual activity (Friedrich, 1993) and promiscuity, sexual victimization of other children, and academic underachievement (Kendall-Tackett *et al.*, 1993; Paolucci *et al.*, 2001; Cutajar *et al.*, 2010). Some symptoms – post-traumatic phenomena and sexualized behavior, attenuate only slowly (Beitchman *et al.*, 1991) even with treatment (Lanktree & Briere, 1995). Bulimia has also been found following CSA (Carter *et al.*, 2006). Sexual abuse may lead to unwanted pregnancy or sexually transmitted disease including HIV. Rarely, it may cause genital injuries. However, the search for conclusive evidence of CSA on the basis of physical signs is now deemed of limited value (Adams, 2010).

Useful instruments to assess effects include Children's Impact of Traumatic Events Scale – Revised (CITES-R) (Wolfe *et al.*, 1991) and the Trauma Symptom Checklist for Children (Briere *et al.*, 2001).

Factors and postulated explanations for variability

Paolucci *et al.* (2001) found that gender, socioeconomic status, type of abuse, age when abused, relationship to perpetrator, and number of incidents of abuse did not moderate the effects of CSA on depression, PTSD, self-harm, inappropriate sexual activity, and academic achievement. Cutajar *et al.* (2010) found that affective, anxiety, conduct, and other childhood Axis I disorders and drug abuse, but not PTSD, were significantly

associated with sexual abuse at a younger age. Penetrative abuse and abuse by more than one perpetrator were associated with mental health disorders.

The variability of post-sexual abuse difficulties, and the search for possible protective or ameliorating factors, has led to much research on moderating factors, with conflicting results, summarized in Yancey *et al.* 2013. They have grouped potential factors into (i) child's personal factors (age at abuse, gender, and attributions about the abuse); (ii) family factors (parental own sexual abuse and mental health and family stress); and (iii) abuse-specific factors (victim-perpetrator relationship and abuse duration and severity). Using a cluster analysis, they established four distinct subtypes of clinical presentation following CSA: (a) a highly distressed group with clinical levels of child-reported depression, anxiety and PTSD symptoms, and parent-reported internalizing, externalizing, and sexualized behaviors; (b) a problem behavior group with parent-reported difficulties as in (a); (c) a self-reported distress group of children reporting difficulties as in (a); (d) a subclinical group with low level child and parent reports, respectively. They found that (i) a child's negative attributions about the abuse such as self-blame and shame correlated significantly with being in the highly distressed and problem behaviors groups; (ii) children in the highly distressed group had parents with depression; (iii) children whose sexual abuse included penetration were more often in the highly distressed group.

Other influences on outcomes have been found. Maternal coping through avoidance strategies correlates with deterioration in behavior (Oates *et al.*, 1994). Onset of sexual abuse before the age of 7, appears to be a risk factor for later inappropriate sexualized behavior (McClellan *et al.*, 1996; Mian *et al.*, 1996). Boys experience anxiety about their own latent homosexuality or having been rendered homosexual by the abuse (Watkins & Bentovim, 1992). Distress following CSA is greater in girls with higher cognitive functioning (Shapiro *et al.*, 1992). Interestingly, the child's coping strategies and cognitive evaluation of the abusive experiences have been shown to contribute less to the child's later functioning than severity of the abuse and the support of the non-abusing caregiver (Spaccarelli & Kim, 1995). Bal *et al.* (2003) suggest that for adolescents, avoidant coping strategies following sexual abuse are associated with more distress.

Protective factors

The non-abusing parent(s)' belief, support, and active protection of the child are significant determinants of a better outcome for the child regardless of the nature of the sexual abuse (e.g., Everson *et al.*, 1989). Conversely, the closer the relationship between the abuser and the non-abusing caregiver(s), the less the child will be supported by her caregiver(s) (Berliner & Elliott, 1996).

Effects in adulthood
Mental health
CSA is followed by significant adult mental health problems (Fergusson *et al.*, 1996) and has been estimated to contribute

independently to 13.1% of adult psychopathology (Fergusson *et al.*, 2008). Findings from many retrospective studies have been confirmed by a large, controlled prospective study from Australia (Cutajar *et al.*, 2010), which found that 23.3% (22.5% female, 26.5% male) of adult survivors of substantiated CSA required lifetime (childhood or adulthood) mental health services, in comparison with 7.7% of a comparison population sample. Effects are summarized in the Table 30.4.

Stigma and self-blame, but not betrayal and powerlessness, have been found to mediate the effects of sexual abuse on adult psychological functioning (Coffey *et al.*, 1996). Contrary to common belief, a systematic review of the impact of CSA on health (Maniglio, 2009) did not find that a number of variables concerning aspects of the abuse experience, such as age when abused, incestuous abuse, level of contact, use of force, frequency, and duration of abuse, influence the outcomes of CSA.

Only a minority of homosexual men have been sexually abused in childhood, and they have no greater sexual interest in children than heterosexual men.

Physical health

CSA, among other forms of maltreatment and other adverse childhood experiences, is significantly associated with adult physical illnesses and earlier death (Felitti *et al.*, 1998).

Neurobiological effects

There has been a burgeoning of empirical findings regarding neurobiological effects of childhood stressors and maltreatment, including CSA. These findings describe, and to some extent, explain the observed and reported effects following CSA (for details, see Chapter 29).

Suspicion, recognition, investigation, validation, and protection

Principles

Whenever sexual abuse is suspected or presented explicitly to a professional, including child mental health practitioners, a multi-agency professional involvement will follow. Its broad aims are to ascertain what, if anything, has happened to the child and to gain an understanding of the child's current functioning, family context, and needs. If the child has been abused, the child's needs will include:

(a) immediate and long-term protection
(b) amelioration of the effects of the abuse including
   (i) reduction of distress and the resolution of internal conflicts and mental health disorders
   (ii) resolution of interpersonal conflicts surrounding the child
   (iii) treating physical consequences of the abuse
(c) ensuring optimal development for the child following cessation of abuse.

The achievement of these aims is, in practice, fraught with difficulties. Suspicions need to be verified and a child's account tested, because protection comes at a cost and therapy can only follow protection. As there are rarely witnesses to the abuse, establishing whether it has occurred will rest heavily on the child's verbal description, which may be retracted even if it was true. Discovery of abuse is often accompanied by denial by the alleged abuser, and some doubt or disbelief, and usually constitutes a crisis for the family and a challenge to the professional system. The child's ultimate well-being will, to a significant extent, be determined by the support given by the family. The nature of the early intervention by professionals, and their consideration of the position and needs of the mother or non-abusing caregivers, will have long-lasting effects on the child's and the family's subsequent expectations and attitudes toward professionals with whom they may need to continue to work.

In most countries, the responsibility for protecting the child rests with social services or the courts to whom suspicions of, or actual abuse are reported. The subsequent multidisciplinary and multi-agency process involves, in addition, the police, health, education, and the courts. A number of well established, coordinated steps in the process have been identified, each step depending on the outcome of the previous one, and involving a number of agencies:

1 Suspicion or recognition leading to referral to (child protection) social services
2 Establishing whether there is a need for immediate protection
3 Planning the investigation including
   ° interagency discussion
   ° interviewing the child
   ° medical examination of the child
   ° initial assessment of the family
4 Validation and initial child protection meeting (conference) leading to a protection plan and a more comprehensive assessment
5 Implementation of plans and review
6 Possible criminal prosecution
7 Therapy.

Suspicion, recognition, and disclosure

CSA either comes to light when a child talks about it to a friend, relative, or a teacher or is suspected on the basis of one or more indicators which are more or less specific. Spontaneous and intentional disclosures are likely to be credible. Specific indicators include: age-inappropriate sexualized behavior, and rarer genital physical signs, sexually transmitted diseases, and pregnancy in a young girl or when the identity of the father is unclear (NICE, 2009). Nonspecific indicators include sudden onset of unexplained difficulties in a previously untroubled child such as distractibility, educational deterioration, social isolation, aggressiveness, low self-esteem, marked unhappiness, disturbed sleep and nightmares, fearfulness, and separation

Table 30.4 Adulthood effects of CSA.

Studies	Gender effects	Effect	Precursors and explanations
Cutajar et al. (2010)	Women = men	Anxiety, Drug misuse	
	Men > women	Antisocial personality disorder	
Cutajar et al. (2010), Morgan and Fisher (2007), and Read et al. (2005)	Women > men	PTSD, depression, alcohol misuse, borderline personality disorder, schizophrenia	CSA in adolescence, penetrative abuse, >1 perpetrator
Mullen et al. (1994)	Women	Suicidal behavior, difficulties in sexual functioning & intimate interpersonal relationships, low self-esteem, unskilled or semi-skilled work	
Kendler et al. (2000)		Major depression, anxiety, drug & alcohol misuse	Not confounded by genetic factors or mediated by common environmental factors

anxiety. Depression, running away, deliberate self-harm, and drug and alcohol misuse may arise later.

CSA of other children in the family and known contact with a sexual abuser should also raise the possibility of abuse of a particular child.

Source and explanations for indicators of CSA need to be explored in a non-leading way. This is important as children (especially younger ones) will not usually describe sexual abuse during a formal interview, unless they have previously spoken about it (Keary & Fitzpatrick, 1994). (The converse is not, however, true). As a result of such enquiries, sexual abuse may come to light.

Disclosure of sexual abuse needs to be reported to social services or police who will inform each other; confidentiality will need to be overridden. A child may not wish for their disclosure to be passed on. As this cannot be honored, the child's misgivings need to be explored, and the child requires an explanation for the need to report the abuse. Referral is usually made with the knowledge of the family, unless there are indicators that this will place the child at increased risk which includes placing pressure on the child to retract an allegation.

The investigation, protection, and formal interview

The need for immediate protection is a decision of social services or the court in consultation with other professionals and agencies. There are helpful guidelines in most developed countries, including those by the American Academy of Child and Adolescent Psychiatry on evaluation and treatment of trauma abuse (AACAP, 1997).

Children will be interviewed formally if there are clear suspicions of abuse or if the child has already disclosed the abuse informally. The formal interview should be carried out by trained professionals, usually police and social workers, and video-recorded evidence can be used both for criminal prosecution and/or civil legal child protection proceedings. It is therefore carried out according to strictly specified guidelines

(Lamb et al., 2007). Rarely, when children are too distressed or traumatized or have significant difficulties in communication, a child mental health professional may be required to interview the child. Facilitated Communication with autistic children who are suspected of having been abused is not recommended (Howlin & Jones, 1996). Anatomically-correct dolls should not be used as a screening tool or cue despite little evidence that young, non-abused children proceed beyond exploration of the dolls' genitalia (Glaser & Collins, 1989).

Validation

Validation of CSA requires assessment of the evolution of suspicions and the circumstances as well as the crucially important content of the child's first description or disclosure of abuse; the outcome of a formal interview; findings in a medical examination; family circumstances; the child's relationship with the alleged abuser; and the responses to the allegation by the mother or the non-abusing caregivers and by the alleged abuser. In a retrospective review of 551 case notes of reported concerns about possible CSA, 43% were substantiated, 21% were inconclusive, and 34% were not considered to be abuse cases. Only 2.5% were erroneous concerns emanating from children, and included only 8 (1.5%) of false allegations originating from the child, and 3 made in collusion with a parent (Oates et al., 2000). In other studies, false allegations are found to be most commonly made by a parent in the context of contact or residence disputes between warring parents, or rarely under the influence of a parent in the context of inter-parental disputes (Faller, 2005).

The nature of protection

A child can only be protected from further harm when all contact with the alleged abuser is either fully supervised or stopped and when the child is believed and not blamed for the abuse or the disclosure. Children abused by persons outside the family tend to be excluded from child protective services on the, sometimes erroneous (Tebbutt et al., 1997), assumption that they will be protected by their families. If protection is achieved, and if no legal proceedings ensue, there may never be a formal record of the validated fact of the abuse.

Legal proceedings

In cases of alleged CSA, both civil family and criminal proceedings may be involved in parallel and often independently. Civil proceedings concern the future safety of the child within which the child's welfare is usually paramount and hearsay and expert evidence are allowed. Civil proceedings determine whether the child has been harmed and how the child's well-being is to be ensured in future. Criminal proceedings are concerned with determining the guilt or innocence of the alleged abuser and the child is a mere accessory or witness whose testimony will be heavily scrutinized. In some jurisdictions, the child's account, previously video-recorded in the formal interview, can be produced but the child will still be cross-examined, preferably through a video link. Expert opinion regarding the child's credibility is not permitted in English criminal courts, that being an issue for the jury and the judge to decide.

In some jurisdictions, protection of the child by social services, on the basis of civil law, relies on the outcome of a prior criminal trial. If there is no prosecution or no conviction, the child will remain unprotected.

Therapeutic work, which can only meaningfully commence after protection, may need to be postponed until the child's evidence has been heard in a criminal trial.

Therapeutic work

Therapeutic work follows closely on protection. A systemic treatment approach to the effects of CSA attends to the child's needs both individually and in the context of the family. Relationships between the three participants in the "abuse triangle" – the abuser, the child, and the non-abusive caregiver(s) (Glaser, 1991) are important. Some of the child's acute difficulties may be related more to their family's response to the abuse or to moves and separation from the family than to the sexual abuse. Work with the child needs to be linked with work with the parent(s) or caregivers and family, separately and together.

Fulfilment of children's therapeutic needs

Not all children who have been sexually abused require therapy. However, a minimum requirement is for the child to have an appropriate narrative about their abuse and to have access to an identified person who believes the child and is able to listen to the child supportively and uncritically. Coping by avoidance, which includes not being able to talk about the abuse when appropriate, is a predisposing factor for the development of PTSD (Kaplow et al., 2005). Children who have been sexually abused also require age-appropriate education about sexuality and the nature and risks of sexual abuse.

Although some symptoms such as sexualized behavior are readily apparent, others such as PTSD or depression may need

to be actively sought within a full assessment of the child's functioning. It is important to include children who have been abused by strangers or by someone outside the family (Grosz et al., 2000), as their therapeutic needs may be overlooked when protection from re-abuse is not required.

There are several ways in which treatment approaches for children can be categorized. Children may be treated individually or in groups; treatment may be offered to a sexually abused child or directed at specific symptoms; there is a range of different treatments including psycho-education about sexual abuse, sexuality and self-protection, comprehensive brief trauma-focused work with the child and parents, and intensive and more prolonged therapeutic work. Finkelhor & Berliner (1995) found that overall, therapy facilitated recovery independently of time elapsed from the abuse and other external factors and particularly when directed at specific difficulties. Others have found no effects of treatment (Oates et al., 1994; Tebbutt et al., 1997) or some deterioration during therapy for a minority of children (Jones & Ramchandani, 1999). It is not clear what contribution intercurrent developments in the child's life or therapy made to the reported deterioration. Despite this, treatment should be offered to symptomatic children.

Several meta-analyses have found large to moderate effect sizes for psychotherapy, group treatment, and CBT combined with supportive, psychodynamic, or play therapy. King et al. (2000) found that, compared with wait-list controls, children with PTSD who received CBT either individually or as a family intervention improved equally in both treatment conditions.

Group therapy

Overall good outcomes have been reported for group therapy in terms of general psychological distress, internalizing and externalizing symptoms, sexual behaviors, self-esteem, and knowledge of sexual abuse/prevention (Reeker et al., 1997). Several reviews have shown individual and group treatments to be equally effective (Trask et al., 2011).

Parallel groups for caregivers support the process (Rushton & Miles, 2000).

Individual therapy

Several meta-analyses (Hetzel-Riggin et al., 2007; Sánchez-Meca et al., 2011; Trask et al., 2011) have found an overall improvement in the many difficulties studied. Longer duration of treatment was associated with larger effect sizes and treatment effects tended to be maintained. There were conflicting results regarding the inclusion of the caregiver. Boys did well.

Specifically, several studies of trauma-focused cognitive behavioral therapy (TF-CBT) (Cohen et al., 2006) were included in the meta-analyses. This programmatic, trauma-focused work involves the child and parent. It includes psycho-education, parenting skills, and relaxation for the child; recognition of feelings and learning to master and modulate affect are followed by cognitive coping. A narrative account is followed by beginning of reprocessing of the traumatic experience, correcting inaccurate recollections and unhelpful cognitions and mastering traumatic reminders. Despite some uncertainty regarding the outcomes (Macdonald *et al.*, 2012), it is likely that TF-CBT is helpful for PTSD, anxiety, and depressive symptoms but may be less effective in treating externalizing behaviors. Nondirective supportive therapy does not appear to be of much benefit. Adolescent depression following sexual abuse appears to respond less well to CBT (Barbe *et al.*, 2004).

Therapeutic work with caregivers and family
Non-abusing caregivers
The outcome for the abused child is, in part, determined by the mental health of the non-abusing caregivers, who are often faced with a conflict of loyalties between the abuser and the child, as well as guilt for not protecting the child and possibly memories of their own past abuse. Lack of belief in and support of the child may lead to removal of the child. Individual or group work is therefore important.

Siblings and the family
Siblings are sometimes the silent witnesses of abuse and may be overlooked. Whole family meetings are important in enabling the family to talk openly about the fact of the abuse but would not include an abuser unless he has taken responsibility for the abuse and is receiving treatment. Other dysfunctional aspects of family interactions that are associated with CSA include, in particular, inappropriate intergenerational boundaries, and parental neglect and unavailability which also need to be addressed (Elton, 1988).

Work with abusers
Child and adolescent abusers
The treatment of child and adolescent abusers requires coordinated support by child protective and youth justice systems as well as support by the young person's parents or primary caregivers. Cognitive behavioral therapy (Kolko et al., 2004) which may be offered individually or in groups, includes:

- challenging denial and minimization of the abuse and responsibility for it
- sex education
- development of social skills
- victim awareness
- recognition of cognitive distortions concerning the abuse
- mapping the abuse cycle (Hawkes, 1999) and learning to halt its progression.

Structured group work for children and young adolescents who had sexually abused has been shown to be effective with a long follow-up showing little recurrence (Carpentier *et al.*, 2006).

A small number of children and adolescents may show features of lack of empathy and cruelty, which will indicate a more serious problem and call for careful monitoring of the child and very skilled therapy, sometimes requiring residential care (Vizard *et al.*, 1995).

Adult abusers
Treatment for adult abuser is important for those children who wish to resume a meaningful relationship with him and for society in general. Therapy addresses denial of the extent of the abuse, responsibility for the abuse, and the harm caused to the child. CBT has shown significant reduction in recidivism in sex offenders (Hanson *et al.*, 2002).

Conclusions

CSA is a definable and often repeated event that is embedded in a complex web of contextual factors, both historical and relational. Its antecedents and consequences are manifold and not necessarily specific. For these reasons, specific prevention is particularly difficult and alertness to the possibility and early recognition offer the best hope for damage limitation. Children cannot be relied upon to protect themselves. Secrecy, denial, and disbelief are integrally related to sexual abuse and exert a very significant influence on the professional response and outcome for the children and their families.

References

AACAP (1997) Practice parameters for evaluation and treatment of trauma abuse. *Journal of the American Academy of Child and Adolescent Psychiatry* **36**, 423–442.

Adams, J. (2010) Medical evaluation of suspected child sexual abuse: 2009 update. *APSAC Advisor* **22**, 2–7.

Alexander, P. & Lupfer, S. (1987) Family characteristics and long-term consequences associated with sexual abuse. *Archives of Sexual Behavior* **16**, 235–245.

Andrews, G. *et al.* (2004) Child sexual abuse. In: *Comparative Quantification of Health Risks: Global and Regional Burden of Disease Attributable to Selected Major Risk Factors.* (eds M. Ezzati, *et al.*), vol. **2**, pp. 1851–1940. WHO, Geneva.

Bal, S. *et al.* (2003) Avoidant coping as a mediator between self-reported sexual abuse and stress-related symptoms in adolescents. *Child Abuse & Neglect* **27**, 883–897.

Barbe, R. *et al.* (2004) Lifetime history of sexual abuse, clinical presentation, and outcome in a clinical trial for adolescent depression. *Journal of Clinical Psychiatry* **65**, 77–83.

Beitchman, J. *et al.* (1991) A review of the short-term effects of child sexual abuse. *Child Abuse & Neglect* **15**, 537–556.

Bentovim, A. *et al.* (1987) Child sexual abuse – children and families referred to a treatment project and the effects of intervention. *British Medical Journal* **295**, 1453–1457.

Berliner, L. & Conte, J. (1990) The process of victimization: the victim's perspective. *Child Abuse & Neglect* **14**, 29–40.

Berliner, L. & Elliott, D. (1996) Sexual abuse of children. In: *The APSAC Handbook on Child Maltreatment.* (eds J. Briere, *et al.*), pp. 51–71. Sage, London.

Bifulco, A. *et al.* (1991) Early sexual abuse and clinical depression in adult life. *British Journal of Psychiatry* **159**, 115–122.

Booth, W. (1890) A preventive home for unfallen girls when in danger. In: *Darkest England and the Way Out*, pp. 192–193. International Headquarters of the Salvation Army, London.

Briere, J. & Elliott, D. (2003) Prevalence and psychological sequelae of self-reported childhood physical and sexual abuse in a general population sample of men and women. *Child Abuse & Neglect* **27**, 1205–1222.

Briere, J. *et al.* (2001) The Trauma Symptom Checklist for Young Children (TSCYC): reliability and association with abuse exposure in a multi-site study. *Child Abuse & Neglect* **25**, 1001–1014.

Carpentier, M. *et al.* (2006) Randomized trial of treatment for children with sexual behavior problems: ten-year follow-up. *Journal of Consulting and Clinical Psychology* **74**, 482–488.

Carter, J. *et al.* (2006) The impact of childhood sexual abuse in anorexia nervosa. *Child Abuse & Neglect* **30**, 257–269.

CEOP (2013) Threat Assessment of Child Sexual Exploitation and Abuse.

Chase, E. & Statham, J. (2005) Commercial and sexual exploitation of children and young people in the UK – a review. *Child Abuse Review* **14**, 4–25.

Coffey, P. *et al.* (1996) Mediators of the long-term impact of child sexual abuse: perceived stigma, betrayal, powerlessness, and self-blame. *Child Abuse & Neglect* **20**, 447–455.

Cohen, J. *et al.* (2006) *Treating Trauma and Traumatic Grief in Children Adolescents.* Guilford, London.

Collin-Vézina, d. *et al.* (2010) Is child sexual abuse declining in Canada? An analysis of child welfare data. *Child Abuse & Neglect* **34**, 807–812.

Committee on the Rights of the Child (2011) *General Comment No. 13: The Right of the Child to Freedom from all Forms of Violence.* United Nations, Geneva.

Cross, T. *et al.* (2003) Prosecution of child abuse : a meta-analysis of rates of criminal justice decisions. *Trauma Violence Abuse* **4**, 323–340.

Cutajar, M. *et al.* (2010) Psychopathology in a large cohort of sexually abused children followed up to 43 years. *Child Abuse & Neglect* **34**, 813–822.

Davies, G. & Dalgleish, T. (2001) *Recovered Memories: Seeking the Middle Ground.* Chichester.

Department for Education (2013) *Working Together to Safeguard Children: A Guide to Inter-Agency Working to Safeguard and Promote the Welfare of Children.* HM Government, London.

Dottridge, M. (2008) *Child Trafficking for Sexual Purposes.* ECPAT International, Bangkok.

Dunne, M. *et al.* (2003) Is child sexual abuse declining? Evidence from a population-based survey of men and women in Australia. *Child Abuse & Neglect* **27**, 141–152.

ECPAT International (2009) *Their Protection Is in Our Hands: The State of Global Child Trafficking for Sexual Purposes.* ECPAT International, Bangkok.

Elton, A. (1988) Working with substitute carers. In: *Child Sexual Abuse Within the Family: Assessment and Treatment.* (eds A. Bentovim, *et al.*), pp. 238–251. John Wright, London.

Everson, M. *et al.* (1989) Maternal support following disclosure of incest. *American Journal of Orthopsychiatry* **59**, 198–207.

Faller, K. (1989) Characteristics of a clinical sample of sexually abused children: how boy and girl victims differ. *Child Abuse & Neglect* **13**, 281–291.

Faller, K. (2005) False accusations of child maltreatment: a contested issue. *Child Abuse & Neglect* **29**, 1327–1331.

Feldman, W. *et al.* (1991) Is child sexual abuse really increasing in prevalence? Analysis of the evidence. *Pediatrics* **88**, 29–33.

Felitti, V. *et al.* (1998) Relationship of childhood abuse and household dysfunction to many of the leading causes of death in adults: the Adverse Childhood Experiences (ACE) Study. *American Journal of Preventive Medicine* **14**, 245–258.

Fergusson, D. *et al.* (1996) Childhood sexual abuse and psychiatric disorder in young adulthood: II. Psychiatric outcomes of childhood sexual abuse. *Journal of the American Academy of Child and Adolescent Psychiatry* **35**, 1365–1374.

Fergusson, D. *et al.* (2008) Exposure to childhood sexual and physical abuse and adjustment in early adulthood. *Child Abuse & Neglect* **32**, 607–619.

Finkelhor, D. (1984) *Child Sexual Abuse.* Free Press, New York.

Finkelhor, D. (1991) The scope of the problem. In: *Intervening in Child Sexual Abuse.* (eds K. Murray & D. Gough), pp. 9–17. Scottish Academic Press, Glasgow.

Finkelhor, D. (1994) Child sexual abuse. *The Future of Children* **4**, 31–53.

Finkelhor, D. (2003) The legacy of the clergy abuse scandal. *Child Abuse & Neglect* **27**, 1225–1229.

Finkelhor, D. & Berliner, L. (1995) Research on the treatment of sexually abused children: a review and recommendations. *Journal of the American Academy of Child and Adolescent Psychiatry* **34**, 1408–1423.

Finkelhor, D. & Jones, L. (2004) *Explanations for the Decline in Child Sexual Abuse Cases.* Juvenile Justice Bulletin No. NC199298. Office of Juvenile Justice and Delinquency Prevention, Washington, DC.

Finkelhor, D. & Jones, L. (2006) Why have child maltreatment and child victimization declined? *Journal of Social Issues* **62**, 685–716.

Finkelhor, D. *et al.* (1990) Sexual abuse in a national survey of adult men and women: prevalence, characteristics and risk factors. *Child Abuse & Neglect* **14**, 19–28.

Finkelhor, D. *et al.* (2000) *Online Victimization: A Report on the Nation's Youth.* National Center for Missing and Exploited Children, Alexandria, VA.

Finkelhor, D. *et al.* (2009) Violence, abuse, and crime exposure in a national sample of children and youth. *Pediatrics* **124**, 1411–1423.

Fontes, L. (ed) (1995) *Sexual Abuse in Nine North American Cultures.* Sage, California.

Friedrich, W. (1993) Sexual victimization and sexual behavior in children: a review of recent literature. *Child Abuse & Neglect* **17**, 59–66.

Frude, N. (1996) Ritual abuse: conceptions and reality. *Clinical Child Psychology and Psychiatry* **1**, 59–77.

Glaser, D. (1991) Treatment issues in child sexual abuse. *British Journal of Psychiatry* **159**, 769–782.

Glaser, D. & Collins, C. (1989) The response of young non-sexually abused children to anatomically correct dolls. *Journal of Child Psychology and Psychiatry* **30**, 547–560.

Gomes-Schwartz, B. *et al.* (1990) *Child Sexual Abuse: The Initial Effects.* Sage, California.

Grosz, C. *et al.* (2000) Extrafamilial sexual abuse: treatment for child victims and their families. *Child Abuse & Neglect* **24**, 9–23.

Hagborg, J. *et al.* (2012) Prosecution rate and quality of the investigative interview in child sexual abuse cases. *Journal of Investigative Psychology and Offender Profiling* **9**, 161–173.

Hanson, R. *et al.* (2002) First report of the collaborative outcome data project on the effectiveness of psychological treatment for sex offenders. *Sexual Abuse* **14**, 169–194.

Hawkes, C. (1999) Linking thoughts to actions: using the integrated abuse cycle. In: *Good Practice in Working with Violence.* (eds H. Kemshall & J. Pritchard), pp. 149–167. Jessica Kingsley, London.

Haywood, T. *et al.* (1996) Psychological aspects of sexual functioning among cleric and noncleric alleged sex offenders. *Child Abuse & Neglect* **20**, 527–536.

Hetzel-Riggin, M. *et al.* (2007) A meta-analytic investigation of therapy modality outcomes for sexually abused children and adolescents: an exploratory study. *Child Abuse & Neglect* **31**, 125–141.

Hobbs, C. & Wynne, J. (1989) Sexual abuse of English boys and girls: the importance of anal examination. *Child Abuse & Neglect* **13**, 195–210.

Holmes, W. & Slap, G. (1998) Sexual abuse of boys: definition, prevalence, correlates, sequelae and management. *JAMA* **280**, 1855–1862.

Howlin, P. & Jones, D.P.H. (1996) An assessment approach to abuse allegations made through facilitated communication. *Child Abuse and Neglect* **20**, 103–110.

Jones, D.P.H. & Ramchandani, P. (1999) *Child Sexual Abuse: Informing Practice from Research.* Radcliffe Medical Press, Abingdon.

Kaplow, J. *et al.* (2005) Pathways to PTSD, part II: sexually abused children. *American Journal of Psychiatry* **162**, 1305–1310.

Keary, K. & Fitzpatrick, C. (1994) Children's disclosure of sexual abuse during formal investigations. *Child Abuse & Neglect* **18**, 543–548.

Kendall-Tackett, K. *et al.* (1993) Impact of sexual abuse on children: a review and synthesis of recent empirical studies. *Psychological Bulletin* **113**, 164–180.

Kendler, K. *et al.* (2000) Childhood sexual abuse and adult psychiatric and substance use disorders in women. *Archives of General Psychiatry* **57**, 953–959.

King, N. *et al.* (2000) Treating sexually abused children with posttraumatic stress symptoms: a randomized clinical trial. *Journal of the American Academy of Child & Adolescent Psychiatry* **39**, 1347–1355.

Kolko, D. *et al.* (2004) Cognitive-behavioral treatment for adolescents who sexually offend and their families: individual and family applications in a collaborative outpatient program. *Journal of Child Sexual Abuse* **13**, 157–192.

Lalor, K. (2004) Child sexual abuse in sub-Saharan Africa: a literature review. *Child Abuse & Neglect* **28**, 439–460.

Lamb, M. *et al.* (2007) A structured forensic interview protocol improves the quality and informativeness of investigative interviews with children. *Child Abuse & Neglect* **31**, 1201–1231.

Lanktree, C. & Briere, J. (1995) Outcome of therapy for sexually abused children: a repeated measures study. *Child Abuse & Neglect* **19**, 1145–1156.

Loftus, E.F. *et al.* (1994) Forgetting sexual trauma – what does it mean when 38-percent forget. *Journal of Consulting and Clinical Psychology* **62**, 1177–1181.

Luo, Y. *et al.* (2008) A population-based study of childhood sexual contact in China: prevalence and long-term consequences. *Child Abuse & Neglect* **32**, 721–731.

Macdonald, G. *et al.* (2012) Cognitive-behavioural interventions for children who have been sexually abused. *Cochrane Database of Systematic Reviews* **5**, CD001930.

Maniglio, R. (2009) The impact of child sexual abuse on health: a systematic review of reviews. *Clinical Psychology Review* **29**, 647–657.

Markowe, H. (1988) The frequency of child sexual abuse in the UK. *Health Trends* **20**, 2–6.

May-Chahal, C. & Cawson, P. (2005) Measuring child maltreatment in the United Kingdom: a study of the prevalence of child abuse and neglect. *Child Abuse & Neglect* **29**, 969–984.

McClellan, J. *et al.* (1996) Age of onset of sexual abuse: relationship to sexually inappropriate behaviours. *Journal of the American Academy of Child and Adolescent Psychiatry* **35**, 1375–1383.

McKee, L. (1984) Sex differentials in survivorship and customary treatment of infants and children. *Medical Anthropology* **8**, 91–108.

McLeer, S. *et al.* (1998) Psychopathology in non-clinically referred sexually abused children. *Journal of the American Academy of Child and Adolescent Psychiatry* **37**, 1326–1333.

Mian, M. *et al.* (1996) The effects of sexual abuse on 3-to-5-year old girls. *Child Abuse & Neglect* **20**, 731–745.

Morgan, C. & Fisher, H. (2007) Environmental factors in schizophrenia: childhood trauma. *Schizophrenia Bulletin* **33**, 3–10.

Morris, J. (1999) Disabled children, child protection systems and the Children Act 1989. *Child Abuse Review* **8**, 91–108.

Mullen, P. *et al.* (1994) The effect of child sexual abuse on social, interpersonal and sexual function in adult life. *British Journal of Psychiatry* **165**, 35–47.

National Institute for Health and Care Excellence (2009) *When to Suspect Child Maltreatment.* National Institute for Health and Care Excellence, London.

O'Connell, R. (2003). *A Typology of Cybersexploitation and On-Line Grooming Practices.* Cyberspace Research Unit, University of Central Lancashire.

Oates, R. *et al.* (1994) Stability and change in outcomes for sexually abused children. *Journal of the American Academy of Child and Adolescent Psychiatry* **33**, 945–953.

Oates, R. *et al.* (2000) Erroneous concerns about child sexual abuse. *Child Abuse & Neglect* **24**, 149–157.

Palmer, T. (2005) Behind the screen: children who are the subjects of abuse images. In: *Viewing Child Pornography on the Internet.* (eds E. Quayle & M. Taylor), pp. 61–74. Russell House, Lyme Regis.

Paolucci, E. *et al.* (2001) A meta-analysis of the published research on the effects of child sexual abuse. *Journal of Psychology* **135**, 17–36.

Parkinson, P. *et al.* (2012) Child sexual abuse in the Anglican Church of Australia. *Journal of Child Sexual Abuse* **21**, 553–570.

Powell, R. *et al.* (2004) Female genital mutilation, asylum seekers and refugees: the need for an integrated European Union agenda. *Health Policy* **70**, 151–162.

Quayle, E. & Taylor, M. (2006) Young people who sexually abuse: the role of the new technologies. In: *People Who Sexually Abuse Others.* (eds M. Erooga & H. Masson), pp. 115–128. Routledge, London.

Radford, L. *et al.* (2011) *Child Abuse and Neglect in the UK Today.* NSPCC, London.

Read, J. *et al.* (2005) Childhood trauma, psychosis and schizophrenia: a literature review with theoretical and clinical implications. *Acta Psychiatrica Scandinavica* **112**, 330–350.

Reeker, J. *et al.* (1997) A meta-analytical investigation of group treatment outcomes for sexually abused children. *Child Abuse & Neglect* **21**, 669–680.

Richardson, G. (2005) Early maladaptive schemas in a sample of British adolescent sexual abusers: implications for therapy. *Journal of Sexual Aggression* **11**, 259–276.

Rushton, A. & Miles, G. (2000) A study of a support service for the current carers of sexually abused girls. *Clinical Child Psychology and Psychiatry* **5**, 411–426.

Russel, D. (1986) *The Secret Trauma: Incest in the Lives of Girls and Women*. Basic Books, New York.

Salter, D. *et al.* (2003) Development of sexually abusive behaviour in sexually victimized males: a longitudinal study. *Lancet* **361**, 471–476.

Sánchez-Meca, J. *et al.* (2011) The psychological treatment of sexual abuse in children and adolescents: a meta-analysis. *International Journal of Clinical and Health Psychology* **11**, 67–93.

Saradjian, J. (1996) *Women Who Sexually Abuse Children*. John Wiley & Sons, Chichester.

Saywitz, K.J. *et al.* (2000) Treatment for sexually abused children and adolescents. *American Psychologist* **55**, 1040–1049.

Sequeira, H. & Hollins, S. (2003) Clinical effects of sexual abuse on people with learning disability. *British Journal of Psychiatry* **182**, 13–19.

Shapiro, J. *et al.* (1992) Cognitive functioning and social competence as predictors of maladjustment in sexually abused girls. *Journal of Interpersonal Violence* **7**, 156–164.

Skuse, D. *et al.* (1998) Risk factors for the development of sexually abusive behaviour in sexually victimised adolescent males: cross sectional study. *British Medical Journal* **317**, 175–179.

Spaccarelli, S. & Kim, S. (1995) Resilience criteria and factors associated with resilience in sexually abused girls. *Child Abuse & Neglect* **19**, 1171–1182.

Strassberg, D. *et al.* (2012) Psychopathy among pedophilic and nonpedophilic child molesters. *Child Abuse & Neglect* **36**, 379–382.

Sullivan, P. & Knutson, J. (2000) Maltreatment and disabilities: a population-based epidemiological study. *Child Abuse & Neglect* **10**, 1257–1273.

Taylor, M. & Quayle, E. (2003) *Child Pornography. An Internet Crime.* Bruner Routledge, London.

Tebbutt, J. *et al.* (1997) Five years after child sexual abuse: persisting dysfunction and problems of prediction. *Journal of the American Academy of Child and Adolescent Psychiatry* **36**, 330–339.

Trask, E.V. *et al.* (2011) Treatment effects for common outcomes of child sexual abuse: a current meta-analysis. *Aggression & Violent Behavior* **16**, 6–19.

Utting, W. *et al.* (1997) *People Like Us. The Report of the Review of the Safeguards for Children Living Away from Home.* The Stationery Office, London.

Vizard, E. *et al.* (1995) Child and adolescent sex abuse perpetrators: a review. *Journal of Child Psychology and Psychiatry* **36**, 731–756.

Ward, T. & Siegert, R. (2002) Toward a comprehensive theory of child sexual abuse: a theory knitting perspective. *Psychology, Crime & Law* **8**, 319–351.

Watkins, B. & Bentovim, A. (1992) The sexual abuse of male children and adolescents: a review of current research. *Journal of Child Psychology and Psychiatry* **33**, 197–248.

Welldon, E. (1988) *Mother, Madonna, Whore*. Free Association Books, London.

Westcott, H. & Jones, D.P.H. (1999) The abuse of disabled children. *Journal of Child Psychology and Psychiatry* **40**, 497–506.

Wild, N. & Wynne, J. (1986) Child sex rings. *British Medical Journal* **293**, 183–185.

Williams, L. (1994) Recall of childhood trauma: a prospective study of women's memories of child sexual abuse. *Journal of Consulting and Clinical Psychology* **62**, 1167–1176.

Williams, T. *et al.* (2012) Transactional sex as a form of child sexual exploitation and abuse in Rwanda: implications for child security and protection. *Child Abuse & Neglect* **36**, 354–361.

Wolak, J. *et al.* (2006) *Online Victimization of Youth: Five Years Later.* National Center for Missing and Exploited Children, Alexandria, VA.

Wolfe, V. *et al.* (1991) The children's impact of traumatic events scale: a measure of post-sexual abuse PTSD symptoms. *Behavioral Assessment* **13**, 359–383.

Yancey, C. *et al.* (2013) The relationship of personal, family, and abuse-specific factors to children's clinical presentation following childhood sexual abuse. *Journal of Family Violence* **28**, 31–42.

Young, W. *et al.* (1991) Patients reporting ritual abuse in childhood: a clinical syndrome. *Child Abuse & Neglect* **15**, 181–189.

PART II

Influences on psychopathology

CHAPTER 31

Brain disorders and psychopathology

Isobel Heyman[1,2], David Skuse[2] and Robert Goodman[3]

[1] Psychological Medicine, Great Ormond Street Hospital for Children, London, UK
[2] Institute of Child Health, UCL School of Life and Medical Sciences, University College London, UK
[3] Institute of Psychiatry, Psychology and Neuroscience, King's College London, UK

This chapter focuses on the psychiatric features of childhood brain disorders, including epilepsy. This topic has variously been called "organic child psychiatry," "pediatric behavioral neurology," and "developmental neuropsychiatry." The terms "functional" and "organic" have previously been used to differentiate between idiopathic mental illness, where no neurological basis for the disorder could be found, and conditions in which there was clear evidence of neural dysfunction. The terms used to make the distinction are now rarely employed. A wide range of evidence shows that there is often a neural substrate for neurodevelopmental disorders that were at one time regarded as being "functional" in origin, including autism (see Chapter 51), schizophrenia (see Chapter 57) and ADHD (see Chapter 55) (Steen *et al.*, 2006; Amaral *et al.*, 2008; Rapoport *et al.*, 2012; Arnsten & Rubia, 2012; Lai *et al.*, 2013). For many clinicians and researchers in child mental health, the claim that persistent abnormalities in behavior and emotion often have an underlying neural basis is neither surprising nor controversial. Therefore, to make a distinction between disorders of "brain" and "mind" could be regarded as misleading or even meaningless. Cognizant as we are of this potential criticism, we are discussing in this chapter conditions where there is a relatively direct link between neurological disorder and psychopathology, with a focus on epilepsy and cerebral palsy.

In trying to understand the relationships between disorders of brain and their impact upon specific psychopathologies, we need to draw on knowledge from both child psychiatry and child neurology. Unfortunately, relatively little is known about how best to classify such conditions based on their etiology, course and management, from the perspective of psychiatry or neurology. For that reason, making firm statements about the relationship to be anticipated between disorders of brain and behavioral problems in childhood is unwise. The task is made all the more difficult because of changing classification rules for both psychiatric disorders and neurological

conditions such as epilepsy. These difficulties are not mentioned to discourage readers, but to put them on their guard against expecting a summary that draws simplistic conclusions from inadequate data.

Brain damage?

This chapter is deliberately entitled "Brain Disorders and Psychopathology" rather than "Brain Damage and Psychopathology." The term "damage" suggests that the brain was developing normally until something happened to damage it. While this description accurately portrays a pathological process in a few conditions, such as athetoid cerebral palsy (which can follow rhesus hemolytic disease), hydrocephalus that may arise from the consequences of tuberculous meningitis and epilepsy following a penetrating head injury, it is more usual for neural development to have been following an abnormal developmental path from embryonic life. The neural anomalies that are associated with child psychopathology usually have a genetic substrate, although their developmental trajectories are shaped in part by environmental conditions encountered both in utero and beyond. Such anomalies include novel genetic mutations as well as structural chromosomal aberrations (Cooper *et al.*, 2011). As far as the common brain disorders in childhood are concerned, we do not know if acquired or intrinsic etiologies are more important. Sometimes, children with cerebral palsy or (intellectual disability) ID (formerly called "mental retardation") are labeled as "brain damaged"; parents and researchers therefore tend to assume that the cause must be some insult, such as a difficult birth. In such cases, the role of genetically or chromosomally determined malformations tends to be overlooked. The term "brain damage" is, however, capable of wide interpretation, and some have used it to include the impact of persistent inflammation or even epigenetic changes (Fleiss & Gressens, 2012).

Rutter's Child and Adolescent Psychiatry, Sixth Edition.
Edited by Anita Thapar and Daniel S. Pine, James F. Leckman, Stephen Scott, Margaret J. Snowling, Eric Taylor.
© 2015 John Wiley & Sons Ltd. Published 2018 by John Wiley & Sons Ltd.

A disadvantage of the term "brain damage" is that it suggests permanence to anyone who has been taught that the brain cannot regenerate lost or damaged parts. This connotation of irreversibility is potentially misleading. Take the example of epilepsy. Children do commonly "grow out of" epilepsy. Reversible "organic" brain disorders of this type may arise not from fixed abnormalities of neuronal organization but from delayed or precocious neuronal maturation. It is plausible (although currently unproven) that transient childhood epilepsy reflects temporarily delayed development of inhibitory neurotransmitter systems (or prematurely accelerated development of excitatory systems). We are also learning more about the structure of the brain in normal and abnormal development and the relationship between structure and psychopathology (Giedd & Rapoport, 2010; Shaw *et al.*, 2010). On the other hand, although there are, in broad terms, different developmental brain trajectories in disorders such as autism, schizophrenia and ADHD, the science is still not at a level where we can interpret an individual scan and find it informs us about the psychopathology of an individual child. Some authors believe that evidence that brain imaging can guide diagnosis or treatment in conditions such as developmental language disorders has not been forthcoming, and also that imaging has not significantly advanced our understanding of brain and behavior relationships (Bishop, 2013).

Birth damage

The best-known "brain damage" theories are those that propose that trauma at birth is a frequent cause of later developmental disorders with neurological correlates. Generations of medical students have been taught that cerebral palsy, epilepsy, and severe intellectual disabilities are commonly caused by brain abnormalities arising from perinatal complications. This view is almost certainly false.

Obstetric and neonatal complications are common but are generally innocuous. Even severe perinatal complications are usually harmless. Most children who experience birth asphyxia do not develop cerebral palsy. Conversely, even the approximately 20% of children with cerebral palsy who do have a history of birth asphyxia, have been subject to other risk factors that antedated birth. They are found to possess, for example, congenital malformations or microcephaly at birth; the fetuses were already abnormal before labor began (Bilder *et al.*, 2013), therefore the birth process could be regarded as a "harmless marker."

The fetus is an active participant in the delivery process, not simply a passive passenger who is expelled when his or her time is up. Accordingly, it is not surprising that a genetically abnormal fetus has an enhanced liability to an abnormal birth (Bilder *et al.*, 2013), although it is possible that perinatal complications compound anomalies that have already occurred prenatally. The "harmless marker" hypothesis is supported by findings

that cerebral palsy rates in children born at term have been fairly steady in recent years, despite major advances in perinatal management and a dramatic fall in perinatal mortality (Paneth *et al.*, 2006). If perinatal complications commonly converted normal or vulnerable fetuses into cerebral palsied children, improvements in obstetrics and neonatal pediatrics should have resulted in a clear fall in the rate of cerebral palsy, but this does not appear to have occurred. More recent work has suggested that some single-gene disorders can lead to cerebral palsy, although this is controversial (O'Callaghan *et al.*, 2012) and it is likely that, as in other neurodevelopmental conditions, many cases are caused by multiple gene effects (Moreno-De-Luca *et al.*, 2013).

Although this account has focused on the extent to which birth complications are largely irrelevant to cerebral palsy (probably accounting for fewer than 10% of cases), similar considerations may apply to severe intellectual disabilities. There is a higher rate of perinatal complications in children whose severe ID is genetic or chromosomal in origin. Intellectual disabilities can be caused by environmental and/or genetic factors, although in 60% of cases no identifiable cause can be found (Rauch *et al.*, 2012). Increasing evidence indicates that genetic influences are causal in a substantial minority of cases, and the proportion is rising (Kaufman *et al.*, 2010). For epilepsy too, prenatal risk factors appear far more important than perinatal risk factors (Wallace, 2004).

In some circumstances, complications arising from birth can cause brain damage that results in behavioral and cognitive problems in later life, even in the absence of neurological signs (Moore *et al.*, 2012). Substantial research has shown that children born very prematurely, especially those born before 30 weeks gestation, are at high risk. Follow-up studies of children born weighing less than 1500 g show that, even when those with overt neurological disorders are excluded, there is a consistently higher rate of attention-deficit hyperactivity disorder (ADHD). Rather less evidence has been adduced for an increase in the rate of conduct or emotional disorders (Johnson, 2007). Studies using neonatal ultrasound scans have shown that the periventricular white matter damage that commonly occurs in children born before 28 weeks gestation (see Figure 31.1 Brain scan PVL) is strongly associated with subsequent cognitive and psychiatric problems, even when the children do not develop overt neurological disorders (Woodward *et al.*, 2012). White matter damage in very prematurely born children results in cerebral palsy and is associated with an especially high risk of comorbid psychiatric problems (Elgen *et al.*, 2012).

Brain dysfunction increases the risk of child psychiatric disorders

The neuropsychiatric component of the classical Isle of Wight epidemiological study showed that brain disorders were powerful risk factors for psychiatric disorders. Among children with

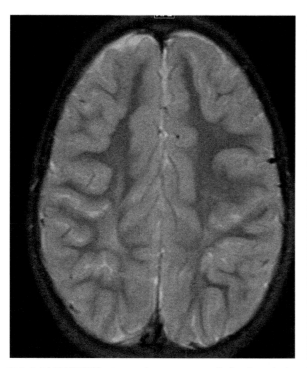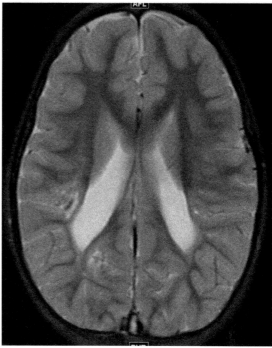

Figure 31.1 Axial T2W MRI brain scan demonstrates marked periventricular white matter injury in an ex-premature baby. There is lateral ventricular dilatation secondary to white matter volume loss in keeping with Periventricular Leukomalacia (PVL).

structural brain anomalies (evidenced by neurological signs rather than by neuroimaging), the rates of psychiatric disorders were 44% compared with 29% among children with idiopathic epilepsy and just 12% among children with non-cerebral physical disorders (such as diabetes). The equivalent figure was 7% among children free from physical disorders (Rutter *et al.*, 1970). Almost 30 years later, the British Child and Adolescent Mental Health Survey reported strikingly similar results (Davies *et al.*, 2003). The finding that cerebral disorders conferred a much higher psychiatric risk than non-cerebral disorders strongly suggested the existence of direct brain-behavior links. Many other studies have since confirmed that psychiatric problems are more likely to result from brain disorders than from physical disorders that do not involve the brain (e.g., Howe *et al.*, 1993; Baca *et al.*, 2011).

At risk for which psychiatric disorders?

There is a long running controversy about the extent to which brain disorders are risk factors for particular sorts of psychiatric problems, as opposed to non-specific risk factors for all types of psychiatric problems. The truth lies between these two extremes: brain disorders increase the risk of most psychiatric problems, but not to the same extent. For example, ADHD (then known as Hyperkinetic Disorder) was exceptionally over-represented among children with cerebral palsy or epilepsy on the Isle of Wight (Rutter *et al.*, 1970). A more recent UK epidemiological study showed that autism is relatively common among children with epilepsy (Davies *et al.*, 2003). There is specificity

between certain neurological disorders and the type of psychiatric disorder associated with them. The risk of autism is increased in cases of tuberous sclerosis (Tsai & Sahin, 2011); Pediatric Autoimmune Neuropsychiatric Disorders (PANDAS) are associated with streptococcal infections, and include tic-like conditions as well as obsessive-compulsive disorder (Snider & Swedo, 2004). When the neurological disorder has a genetic basis, as in the case of tuberous sclerosis (Figure 31.2 Brain scan TS), the associated psychiatric problems comprise a "behavioral phenotype" of the underlying genetic disorder. Behavioral phenotypes are not specific to a disorder; there is a considerable overlap between symptoms associated with a wide range of genetic risks, but statistically significant associations do exist (see www.ssbp.org.uk which provides information sheets on many genetic syndromes).

How do neurological and non neurological risk factors interact?

As described in the rest of this volume, a multitude of psychosocial and genetic factors influence a child's liability to psychiatric disorders. How do these "ordinary" risk factors interact with neurological risk factors? First, children with brain disorders are also subject to common environmental risk factors and these may interact with the underlying biological vulnerability. In the Isle of Wight study, children with evidence of structural brain anomalies were exceptionally likely to have a psychiatric problem if they also came from a "broken home" or had an emotionally disturbed mother (Rutter *et al.*, 1970). A plausible

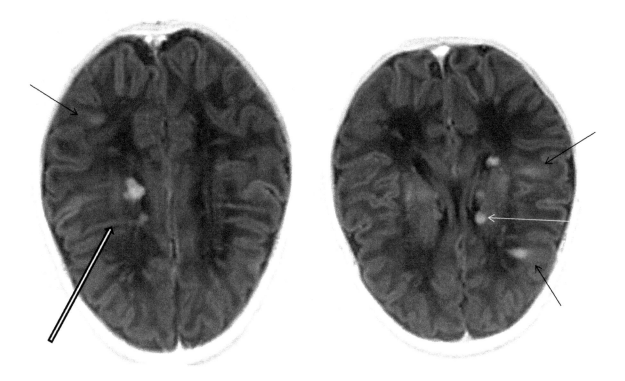

Figure 31.2 Axial FLAIR MRI in a two year old demonstrate typical findings of tuberous sclerosis: Several cortical/subcortical tubers (black arrows), "white matter radial migration lines" (open arrow) associated with "subependymal nodules" (white arrow) are demonstrated.

explanation is that neurologically determined behavioral problems had been responsible for an adverse impact on the parents' marriage and on the parents' mental state. Cross-sectional studies cannot determine the direction of causation. In a longitudinal study that is designed to disentangle causal pathways, evidence may be found for a causal process. Consider the prospective study of childhood head injury carried out by Rutter *et al.* (1984). Although the severity of head injury was the most powerful single predictor of whether a child would develop a psychiatric problem, ordinary risk factors for disorders (such as psychosocial adversity) were also influential. Among children with severe head injuries, new psychiatric disorders developed in 60% of those who prior to the injury had experienced high levels, but in just 14% of the children who had experienced low levels of psychosocial adversity.

Occasionally, the impact of neurological impairment may confer such substantially greater risk for child psychiatric problems that prosaic factors normally associated with risk no longer impact. For example, among prepubertal children without neurological problems, boys are at considerably greater psychiatric risk than girls, especially of behavioral or externalizing conditions (e.g., Rutter *et al.*, 1975). By contrast, several studies of children with neurological brain disorders have reported that psychiatric risk is not differentiated by sex. This lack of sexual dimorphism was reported in the Isle of Wight sample of children with brain disorders (Rutter *et al.*, 1970), and (Rutter

et al.'s 1984) study of children followed prospectively after a severe head injury.

Our current understanding of the interaction between neurological and environmental risk factors suggests two lessons for clinicians. First, children with brain disorders are as vulnerable as any other children to social and other environmental risk factors. Accordingly, the severity and frequency of psychiatric problems in this high-risk group could be reduced by non specific interventions, such as improving the quality of the care provided by parents. Interventions that are designed to reduce discord between parents and/or siblings, to provide consistency of supervision, and to increase the child's confidence through praise and shaping of prosocial behavior would all be beneficial. Secondly, for some children the "behavioral phenotype" may be exceptionally strongly influenced by the underlying neurological dysfunction. Vulnerability in these children to psychopathology is therefore relatively unaffected by psychosocial adversity. In cases with "strong" behavioral phenotypes, psychiatric problems will be found even in the most favorable of environments. Examples include the hyperphagia associated with Prader-Willi syndrome (McAllister *et al.*, 2011). Clinicians who bear this in mind should reassure parents, and teachers, who sometimes blame themselves for not having done enough to prevent the emergence of psychiatric problems. Families and schools who are doing a good-enough job with an extremely challenging group of children should feel admired rather than blamed.

What are the mediating links?

Why do children with "organic" brain disorders have relatively high rates of psychiatric problems? This question should be posed at the beginning rather than at the end of neuropsychiatric investigations. Uncovering the mechanisms that link brain disorder to behavioral dysfunction will shed light on the biological determinants of normal psychological development, as well as on prevention and treatment. Thus, practical implications of clarifying brain-behavior relationships are substantial. For example, in our clinical practice, we often encounter children with disorders of neural development in which there are severe, but unrecognized specific learning difficulties (see Chapter 52). Because the nature of the cognitive deficits are not obvious (and may be uncovered only by specialist testing) they go unrecognized. The child cannot keep up with his or her lessons and that engenders marked frustration with schooling, leading on to defiant and disruptive behavior in class. In other circumstances, the presence of an overt neurological problem might lead to psychiatric problems as a consequence of parental overprotectiveness, or from inconsistent discipline provided by a parent who is suffering guilt because they regard themselves to blame for the child's neurological disorder. The capacity of even highly educated and intelligent parents to inflict blame on themselves (or on their child's medical care), based on the most tenuous of presumed causal events, is remarkable and must be addressed by clinicians.

Unfortunately, because there is a dearth of relevant empirical studies, current accounts of mediating processes are based largely on clinical plausibility. It is worth reiterating that just because a child has both neurological and psychiatric symptoms, it does not necessarily follow that the former caused the latter: a child with cerebral palsy who is disrupting the class may be doing so because of school stresses that are unrelated to the child's brain disorder. Alternatively, the two sets of problems may reflect a common origin. A child's head injury and an associated conduct disorder may both be due to inadequate parental supervision. Alternatively, in some cases the psychiatric problem could have caused the neurological disorder. Children with ADHD may run impulsively into the road, get hit by a car, and suffer brain damage as a consequence. With these reservations, it is now appropriate to consider instances in which the child's brain disorder will have played some direct or indirect part in the origin of the concomitant psychiatric problems. For the sake of clarity, it is helpful to distinguish between the organic and psychosocial consequences of a brain disorder (see Figure 31.3), acknowledging that these are often intimately interrelated.

An "organic" brain disorder may lead to developmental problems in physical, educational and neurobehavioral domains. If there are associated physical disabilities (ranging, for example, from easy fatigability to lack of independent mobility) these may have an indirect impact on psychological well-being. The child who is exhausted by everyday playground activities could suffer reduced self-esteem, compounded by their limited

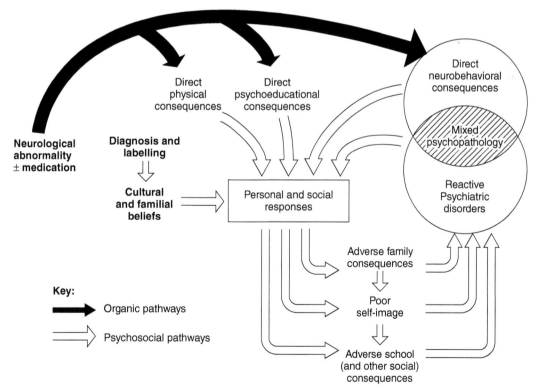

Figure 31.3 A simplified representation of organic and psychosocial pathways from brain to behavioral abnormalities.

opportunities to develop peer relationships. Treatment regimes for physical problems can be disruptive to the child's life. For instance, many hours each week could be spent in physiotherapy, during which the child is sacrificing time when they would prefer to have been playing. Reluctance to engage with treatment occasions "I don't want to do it" battles. In more serious cases of neurological impairment, children experience repeated hospital admissions, with attendant separations and an impact on family integrity.

Specific learning problems and below-average intelligence are common psycho-educational correlates of structural brain abnormalities (e.g., Rutter *et al.*, 1970; Reilly & Neville, 2011). There is often a direct link between the impact of the underlying brain disorder on neural functioning and impaired cognitive processing. On the other hand, risk is sometimes aggravated by restricted educational opportunities, lower expectations, and lengthy absences from school for therapy or operations. For children with epilepsy, their cognitive and scholastic skills can be disrupted not only by clinical and subclinical seizures, but also by the effects of antiepileptic medication.

The evidence that brain disorders arising from genetic risk lead directly to specific childhood psychopathology is largely circumstantial. Recent research with animal models for genetic risk is beginning to illuminate causal mechanisms (see Nestler & Hyman, 2010). Medical treatments, provided for neurological dysfunction, can also have an adverse impact on children's behavior. These include steroids, which affect activity and mood (Stuart *et al.*, 2005), and antiepileptic drugs (Bath & Scharfman, 2013). Thirdly, biologically mediated mechanisms can provide an adequate explanation for some specific neuropsychiatric associations in childhood, such as the association between Prader–Willi syndrome and characteristic sleep and appetite problems, or the association between Lesch–Nyhan syndrome and severe self-injury (see Chapter 24). In summary, brain disorders can have a multitude of psychosocial consequences. Physical disabilities can result in teasing, poor self-image and reduced opportunities for peer interaction. Repeated hospitalizations may disrupt friendships and predispose to behavioral disorders, perhaps as a result of repeated separations from family. Specific learning problems and low intelligence are also associated with a much higher rate of psychiatric problems in children with brain disorders, just as they are in ordinary children (Rutter *et al.*, 1970; Ryland *et al.*, 2010). Many organic brain disorders also have neurobehavioral consequences, especially poor attention, hyperactivity and an impaired ability to decipher social and emotional cues. While these consequences are relatively non-specific, they may, in turn, have adverse effects on family relationships as well as the ability to make and sustain friendships at school and elsewhere outside the home.

The beliefs and attitudes of the family and the wider social world also have a major impact on emotions and behavior in the child. Parents, teachers and peers respond to a neurologically impaired child in the light of their beliefs and prejudices about "brain damaged" children. These beliefs influence the likelihood of overprotection, peer rejection and unrealistic expectations. Unhelpful attitudes about the nature of their child's condition can interfere with parents' abilities to set limits to unacceptable behaviors. Some parents assume that all bad behavior is driven by the neurological abnormality and that it is therefore beyond the child's control. Others fear that any reproof will trigger an epileptic seizure and further damage the child's brain. Family relationships can be disrupted for other reasons as well. Sibling rivalry, for example, can be fuelled by the resentment of disabled children who see themselves being overtaken by younger siblings, or by the resentment of non-disabled siblings who feel they are missing out on parental attention. These are only a few of the many possible psychosocial pathways from brain disorders to child psychiatric problems. In a recent study of children with epilepsy, factors that most compromised quality of life included impaired cognitive ability and disrupted family functioning (Speechley *et al.*, 2012).

Longitudinal studies provide a valuable research strategy for investigating the causal mechanisms underlying cross-sectional associations. A longitudinal study of children with hemiplegic cerebral palsy found that adverse family factors, including low parental warmth or marital discord, were more likely to be consequences than causes of the child's psychiatric problems (Goodman, 1998). Thus adverse family circumstances at baseline did not independently predict whether the hemiplegic child improved or deteriorated by the time of follow-up. Intervention studies could also be powerful research strategies for investigating the causal mechanisms underlying brain-behavior links—this potential has hardly been tapped to date.

The psychiatric consequences of specific brain disorders

Turning from the general to the particular, the following sections review a range of childhood brain disorders from a psychiatric perspective. Because we cannot cover the whole of pediatric neurology and neurosurgery in a few pages, disorders have been selected on the basis of frequency, severity or particular relevance to child psychiatry. The main clinical features of each disorder are reviewed along with the psychiatric consequences. For readers who want to learn more about specific aspects of pediatric neurology, we recommend Aicardi *et al.* (2009) or Piña-Garza (2013) for good accounts.

Epilepsy

Convulsions are the commonest problem encountered in pediatric neurology. At least one child in 200 experiences repeated epileptic seizures without a detectable extracerebral cause. This constitutes the usual definition of epilepsy. By "extracerebral" causes, we refer to conditions such as hypoglycaemic seizures (in context of diabetes) or anoxic seizures (associated with faints or breath-holding attacks). The definition also excludes the 3% of preschool children who have one or more convulsions provoked by febrile illnesses. Febrile convulsions are usually benign; about 98% of affected individuals do not go on to develop persistent epilepsy. In practice, distinguishing epilepsy from other sorts of paroxysmal disorders (such as faints and parasomnias) can be surprisingly difficult. Misdiagnoses are all too common in both directions (Crompton & Berkovic, 2009).

Psychiatrists may be asked to help distinguish between "true" seizures and non-epileptic seizures. This is not an easy task. Most children with non-epileptic seizures also suffer from true seizures. Emotional stresses can precipitate true seizures; many children with true epilepsy have psychiatric problems too. Clinically, we seek to make the distinction on the grounds of behavioral observations. Pointers indicating that a child is having non-epileptic seizures include: occurrence when the child is being observed but not when the child is alone; a gradual rather than sudden onset; a paroxysm that involves quivering or uncontrolled flailing rather than true clonus; theatrical semipurposive movements accompanied by loud screaming or shouting; the fact that painful stimuli are actively avoided during an attack and serious injury does not occur; the offset is sudden with an immediate return to an alert and responsive state. Finally, to determine with reasonable validity the nature of the convulsion, it will be necessary to establish whether or not the EEG shows any paroxysmal discharge during an episode. All these observations are easier to make when the child is assessed with combined EEG and video monitoring. None of the pointers is infallible; however, and some sorts of true seizures (most notably frontal lobe seizures) are easily mistaken for non-epileptic seizures (Cuthill & Espie, 2005; Caplan *et al.*, 2011).

For the purpose of deciding how to manage non-epileptic seizures, there are few treatment studies in children. The most promising treatments emerging from the adult literature include cognitive behavioral treatments that have been used successfully in other medically unexplained symptoms (see, for example, Goldstein *et al.*, 2010). Clinical consensus suggests incorporating a careful behavioral analysis of antecedents and underlying stressors, and remediation of these as far as possible. This should be followed by a focus on a consistent, calm and optimistic management approach. In general terms, everyone should deal with the child in such a way that they pay as little attention as possible to the attacks and avoid medical interventions.

The classification of epileptic seizures and syndromes has changed repeatedly over recent decades. In the current classification of the International League Against Epilepsy (ILAE), the most basic distinction in seizure type is between generalized and focal seizures (Berg *et al.*, 2010; see Figure 31.4). Generalized seizures are bilaterally generated and the first clinical symptoms do *not* suggest a focal onset. Examples of generalized seizures include generalized tonic-clonic seizures, absence seizures, atypical absences, tonic seizures, atonic seizures, and myoclonic seizures. In the recent reclassification of the epilepsies, it has been concluded somewhat controversially that no natural classification for focal seizures exists, therefore focal

Table I. Classification of seizures[a]
Generalized seizures
Tonic—clonic (in any combination)
Absence
Typical
Atypical
Absence with special features
Myoclonic absence
Eyelid myoclonic
Myoclonic
Myoclonic
Myoclonic atonic
Myoclonic tonic
Clonic
Tonic
Atonic
Focal seizures
Unknown
Epileptic spasms
[a]Seizure that cannot be clearly diagnosed in one of the preceding categories should be considered unclassified until further information allows their accurate diagnosis. This is not considered a classification category, however.

Figure 31.4 Revised terminology and concepts for organization of seizures and epilepsies: report of the ILAE Commission on Classification and Terminology, 2005–2009. (From Berg *et al.*, 2010.)

seizures should be described according to their manifestations (e.g., dyscognitive, focal motor). Focal seizures arise in a single hemisphere and can generalize. The previous terms, "simple" and "complex" partial seizures, have been abandoned.

The link between epilepsy and cognitive impairment is complex (Reilly & Neville, 2011). Rates of intellectual disability (ID) (IQ < 70) in children with epilepsy range from 18% to 30%. We do not know for sure why the average IQ of children with seizures is reduced. Although it is often assumed that the seizures themselves cause neural disruption, there is an alternative viewpoint that proposes that seizures can be markers for adversity. That adversity is, according to this theory, the proximal cause of ID and can arise from family factors (social or genetic) or from other non-epilepsy related neurological abnormalities. Children whose epilepsy is associated with additional neurological abnormalities have a significantly lower mean IQ than children with idiopathic epilepsy. Lower IQ is also associated with early onset seizures, more frequent seizures, and with a longer duration of epilepsy (Kernan *et al.*, 2012). Permanent intellectual deterioration as a direct result of the seizures themselves is probably rare. Rasmussen's syndrome (Figure 31.5) is an example of a rare, progressive (usually unihemispheric) epilepsy syndrome in which the impact of persistent seizures on the unaffected hemisphere is thought to contribute to the characteristically associated cognitive deterioration (Bien *et al.*, 2005).

Clinical studies suggest that cognitive impairment over the short term is associated with the frequency of seizures, with the presence of multiple seizure types, an early onset, and chronicity. On the other hand, the development of psychiatric disorders and behavioral problems over the longer term does not appear to be linked so closely to seizure burden (Jones *et al.*, 2010).

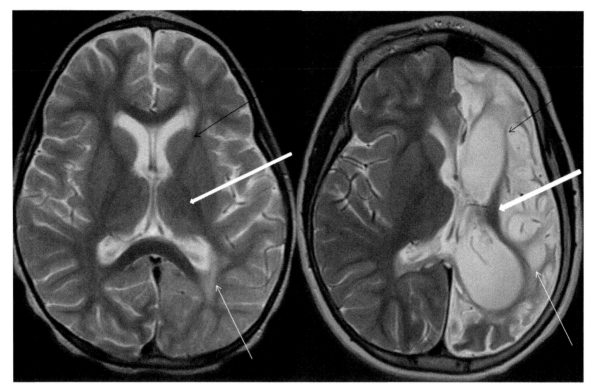

Figure 31.5 *Rasmussen's encephalitis:* Axial T2 MRI demonstrates atrophy of the left cerebral hemisphere. There is severe loss of white matter (white arrow) associated with damage of the left basal ganglia (black arrow) and thalamus (white arrow). Note significant progression of the disease over 4 years.

Two other factors are potentially relevant to cognitive impairments in children with epilepsy. Firstly, subclinical seizure discharges (as measured by EEG) are associated with significant impairments in cognitive processing in about 50% of individuals in whom they are recorded (Binnie, 2003). Secondly, antiepileptic medication may impair cognition too. Older drugs, such as phenobarbitone and phenytoin, are the worst offenders. Carbamazepine and sodium valproate are probably less harmful, particularly when given singly rather than in combination. Determining whether antiepileptic medications have an independent adverse impact on cognition is complicated by the fact that children with recent onset epilepsy, previously unmedicated, also have impaired cognitive functioning. Although most studies of cognition and epilepsy have focused on IQ, there is good evidence that children with seizures also have a high rate of specific learning problems *after allowing for their IQ*. These specific learning difficulties include language and reading problems (Rutter *et al.*, 1970; Kernan *et al.*, 2012).

Epilepsy in childhood is a powerful risk factor for emotional and behavioral disorders. In the Isle of Wight study (Rutter *et al.*, 1970), 29% of 63 children with idiopathic epilepsy had a psychiatric disorder. This was four times the rate in children without physical disorders and over twice the rate in children with physical disorders not affecting the brain. Davies *et al.* (2003) reported that 37% of an epidemiological sample of schoolchildren with epilepsy had at least one psychiatric diagnosis, compared with 10% of community controls. Although

children with epilepsy have a high rate of psychiatric problems, the nature of these problems is not particularly distinctive (with a few rare exceptions). Despite many attempts to establish whether particular types of epilepsy are associated with specific psychiatric problems, the presence or absence of associated neurological abnormalities provides a better predictor. In the Isle of Wight study, for example, psychiatric disorders were twice as common among children with epilepsy in the presence of additional neurological problems (Rutter *et al.*, 1970). Accordingly, some predictors of psychopathology, such as the frequency of seizures or the presence of generalized cognitive impairment, are probably just markers for the extensiveness of underlying brain abnormalities (Kanner *et al.*, 2012). Cognitive predictors of psychopathology therefore include impaired neuropsychological functioning and specific reading difficulties, the effects of which may be directly or indirectly related to mental health problems.

There is rather weak evidence that antiepileptic medication influences the risk and type of psychopathology, at least in adults (Piedad *et al.*, 2012). Few properly controlled trials have been performed, almost none in children. Antiepileptic drugs can have beneficial as well as adverse psychotropic influences. The impact of medication upon the risk of a psychiatric disorder such as depression is hard to distinguish in practice from reporting bias. Adults who are coincidentally depressed may report undesirable side effects of antiepileptic medication. If they reduce their medication as a consequence, their seizure frequency may increase. If they are suffering from increased seizure frequency and severity they may be prescribed higher doses of antiepileptic medication. Higher doses may influence the risk and reporting of side effects. Directions of effect are therefore difficult to establish in the absence of properly controlled trials. The wise clinician will take seriously parental reports of behavioral or emotional side effects that could be due to medication and will monitor them carefully (Caplan, 2012).

Social pressures can also influence psychiatric adjustment in cases of epilepsy. One potential social predictor is the extent to which the child is rejected or stigmatized as a result of community prejudices about epilepsy. Peer rejection is, however, more often a consequence than a cause of psychiatric problems in children with epilepsy. Interrelationships between risk of psychiatric disorder, social, family and other risk factors are complex. There is increasing evidence that behavioral problems are present very early in the course of epilepsy (or even before its onset). In such cases, underlying cerebral pathology is probably a risk factor for both epilepsy and the associated psychiatric disorder (see Lin *et al.*, 2012 for a review).

The interested reader is advised to seek more detailed accounts of the epilepsies than we have been able to provide here. Wallace (2004) provides a good introductory text, and there is a three-volume textbook by Engel and colleagues (2007) for a more detailed and densely referenced account. References are only provided in this section for topics that are not well covered in the main texts. There are also several good charity websites that give valuable information (e.g., www.epilepsyaction.org.uk).

Cerebral palsy

Cerebral palsy (CP) is the single greatest cause of severe physical disability in childhood. The label refers to a heterogeneous group of congenital and early-acquired brain disorders that meet three criteria. First, the disorders are chronic rather than transient. Secondly, the underlying brain lesions are static, although the clinical manifestations may change as the child grows up (thereby ruling out progressive neurodegenerative conditions or brain tumors). Thirdly, the clinical manifestations include abnormalities of motor function. These motor defects are often accompanied by other clinical manifestations of brain abnormalities, including epilepsy, learning problems and sensory impairments. More recently it has become apparent that children with CP have up to five times the probability of neurologically intact children in the general population of developing emotional and behavioral problems of clinical significance (Parkes *et al.*, 2008).

In the Isle of Wight study (Rutter *et al.*, 1970), psychiatric problems were evident in almost half of the children with CP and related disorders. The likelihood of psychiatric problems was significantly increased by low intelligence and specific reading difficulties, both of which commonly accompanied the condition. If the child with CP also had epileptic seizures, the rate of psychiatric disorder was even higher (58% vs 38%). No specific type of psychiatric disorder was associated with CP, though there was a hint that attention deficit/hyperactivity disorder was disproportionately common.

Hemiplegic CP has been the focus of many psychiatric studies (Goodman & Yude, 2000), making it the best-characterized type of CP from a psychiatric perspective. Hemiplegia is a relatively mild physical disability and most children with hemiplegia are of normal intelligence and attend mainstream schools. Even so, about half of all children with hemiplegia have at least one psychiatric disorder. A recent study of 270 children with hemiplegia found that over 70% had difficulties with emotional regulation, concentration, behavior and getting on with other people (Parkes *et al.*, 2009).

Childhood dementias and other conditions involving the loss of skills

Childhood dementias usually present with an insidious loss of skills. They are often accompanied by non-specific psychiatric symptoms. Child psychiatrists must learn to recognize these disorders at an early stage, so that the child can be referred to a pediatric neurologist. Some conditions, such as Wilson's Disease, are now capable of being treated effectively. Any delay in diagnosis and treatment can result in unnecessary and irreversible brain damage. We do not have firm data on the prevalence of childhood dementia, but estimates of 20/100,000 population have been made, of which at least one third are of uncertain etiology (Nunn *et al.*, 2002).

In cases of cognitive deterioration, until the organic basis is recognized, the child's problems may be blamed on his or her laziness, or on parental mishandling, causing unnecessary anguish and subsequent guilt or anger. If the disease were inherited, genetic counseling might avert the birth of a second affected child. Finally, once the diagnosis has been made, a child psychiatrist may be able to offer useful help to the child, the parents, and the siblings—and this help is much more likely to be accepted if the child psychiatrist referred the case on to a pediatrician for appropriate physical investigations at an early stage.

Although desirable, prompt recognition of a dementing disorder is undoubtedly difficult. Normal development often involves some degree of "two steps forward, one step back"; many children revert to more babyish ways when physically ill or under stress. It is often claimed that a high proportion of children with autistic disorders suffer early regression, within the first 2 years or so of life (see Chapter 51). While true loss of skills, particularly of language, is indeed occasionally verified, it appears likely that "regression" is in truth more often a plateauing of skill acquisition especially of language (Baird *et al.*, 2008).

Many psychiatric disorders can interfere with concentration or application at school, leading to a falling off in classroom performance. A marked loss of skills in several areas is more likely to be caused by psychosocial rather than organic factors. In some rare conditions, psychosocial and biological risk factors interact. The children of prostitutes or drug addicts are clearly at psychiatric risk for psychosocial reasons. On the other hand, they are also at risk of HIV infection and its associated dementia (see Chapter 46). Children of a parent with Huntington disease have a 50% chance of carrying the gene themselves. Although the onset of typical symptoms is in adulthood, psychiatric problems are often prominent in those with a juvenile onset (about 10% of all cases). While movement disorders are a frequent comorbid symptom, the diagnosis may be missed in circumstances where there is abuse, neglect and disorganization—commonly encountered in affected families (Julien *et al.*, 2007).

In practice, an organic cause for cognitive deterioration needs to be considered (and appropriate referrals or investigations initiated) when the child meets one or more of the following three criteria:

(a) Progressive loss of well-established linguistic, academic or self-help skills—with performance being well below previous levels even when the child appears content, motivated and not preoccupied. Psychometric testing is sometimes helpful, particularly if repeated measures are available.

(b) Emergence of other features suggestive of a brain disorder, such as seizures, evidence of visual impairment, tremor or postural disturbance.

(c) Risk factors for relevant genetic or infectious diseases, such as a parent with Huntington disease, or who is known to have HIV/AIDS. Clinicians who make a practice of reviewing their initial diagnostic formulation at regular intervals will be less likely to miss insidiously progressive disorders that initially present with apparently straightforward psychiatric symptoms.

The dementing disorders that are most likely to present to child psychiatrists are:

Batten's Disease (also known as Neuronal Ceroid Lipofuscinosis). The diagnosis refers to a group of inherited neurodegenerative disorders, most of which are autosomal recessive (www.bdsra.org). Child psychiatrists are most likely to encounter the juvenile form. It is the most common neurodegenerative disorder of childhood, affecting up to one in 25,000 births, and onset is between 5 and 7 years of age. The presentation is usually visual failure; the disease progresses to obvious dementia after a few years. Because the presentation is with an unusual symptom, if no obvious cause is initially found for the visual failure, the child may be referred for psychiatric assessment of "hysterical" blindness. Alternatively, the initial pediatric assessment may attribute the visual impairment to a non-progressive cause. Because cognitive decline is delayed, psychiatric referral may occur several years later when deteriorating schoolwork and non-specific behavioral problems (such as disruptive and aggressive behavior) are mistakenly attributed to the psychological consequences of blindness or family stresses. Seizures may occur fairly early in the disorder, but the emergence of hard neurological signs is usually a late feature. Causal genes have now been identified (containing several hundred mutations). Accordingly, genetic tests can be helpful in diagnosing the disorder and permitting the identification of carrier status in the parents (Kousi *et al.*, 2012).

Wilson's Disease is an autosomal recessive disorder of copper metabolism. It occurs in about 1/30,000 live births (www.wilsonsdisease.org). The presentation in children at elementary school age is usually with progressive liver failure. Overt symptoms presenting after the age of 10 include neurological features, insidious dementia, or non-specific emotional or behavioral problems. Early neurological features include extrapyramidal and cerebellar signs. Dystonic movements and postures can be bizarre, unilateral and exacerbated by stress. Misdiagnosis of the condition as conversion disorder is all too easy. The key investigation is to ascertain whether urinary copper is high, while plasma copper and caeruloplasmin are both low. Ophthalmological examination with a slit lamp may reveal the pathognomonic Kayser–Fleischer ring on the iris. A liver biopsy is necessary in doubtful cases. The disorder can be treated successfully by copper chelation, and earlier treatment results in a better outcome. Genetic testing to assist in diagnosis and screen relatives is now available (Ala *et al.*, 2007).

Huntington Disease is very rare, although recent research has suggested that the prevalence in the UK population could be as high as 12.3/100,000 (Evans *et al.*, 2013). It is an autosomal dominant disorder that typically presents with chorea and dementia in mid-adult life (Ha & Fung, 2012; hda.org.uk). The juvenile form occurs in 5–10% of cases, with onset under 21 years. The early onset form is characterized by psychiatric symptoms accompanied by a motor disorder. Chorea may occur but a rigid Parkinsonian picture is more common. Epilepsy is an early feature in a substantial minority. The first presentation may be with disturbed or withdrawn behavior, including loss of interest in games and lessons. These psychiatric features are particularly difficult to interpret in the context of the marked psychosocial disturbance that is common in families where one parent has Huntington disease. The child's fear of developing the same disease may also be important. Just as a positive family history should not lead to the assumption of a positive diagnosis, a negative family history does not rule out the diagnosis as the presence of affected relatives may be concealed, may be masked by misdiagnosis or may not be apparent due to "non paternity."

The substantial increase in identified cases in the United Kingdom over the past few years confirms that 'hidden' pathology does exist in the general population. Identification of the disorder in younger people with early or prodromal symptoms is important now, but will become more so if there are developments in disease modifying treatments that need to be started before the cerebral degeneration becomes advanced. Brain imaging may reveal atrophy; striatal atrophy and white matter changes predominate in the prodromal stages. Huntington's disease is caused by a CAG triplet repeat expansion in the Huntington's disease gene, huntingtin (*HTT*). Longer CAG repeats predict earlier onset, (Ross & Tabrizi, 2011). A simple genetic test can confirm the presence of the expanded repeat, although the timing and impact of testing needs careful specialist consideration with the family, particularly regarding predictive testing of children (for a discussion of ethics, see Hawkins *et al.*, 2011).

Adrenoleucodystrophy is an X-linked recessive disorder, thus affects males primarily, although female carriers may have a partial phenotype. It is characterized by a combination of adrenal insufficiency, progressive dementia and neurological features (Moser *et al.*, 2007). Even within the same family, however, the presentation can be very variable. Adrenal failure predominates in some affected boys; dementia and neurological features predominate in others. The earliest manifestations include non specific symptoms such as restlessness, poor coordination, disruptiveness and deteriorating progress at school. Occasionally, the condition may initially be confused with ADHD, if the associated adrenal failure is not recognized. Unequivocal neurological abnormalities usually begin between 5 and 9 years of age. There are both pyramidal and extrapyramidal signs, together with convulsions, deafness or visual failure (sometimes due to cortical blindness). In cases where the child has adrenal failure, there will be diarrhea, vomiting, hypotension and pigmentation. Mild adrenocortical insufficiency may only be evident from the results of an ACTH challenge. A leucodystrophy with occipital predominance is often evident on brain scan. The combination of leucodystrophy and adrenal failure is pathognomonic. The diagnosis can be confirmed by high levels of saturated very long chain fatty acids in tissues and body fluids, and by molecular genetic tests for mutations in the ABCD1 gene. This rare, but devastating, condition is one where gene therapies hold promise in terms of modifying disease progression (Cartier *et al.*, 2009).

Treatment of psychiatric problems in children with brain disorders

The psychiatric problems of children with brain disorders can be treated in just the same ways as the psychiatric problems of neurologically intact children and biological treatments are neither more nor less useful. There is no empirical basis, for example, for expecting greater success in treating a child's disruptive behavior disorder with carbamazepine rather than with parent training simply because the child also has a brain disorder. Individual, family and school-based treatment approaches can all be helpful. Children with brain illness such as epilepsy are almost always excluded from randomized controlled trials of therapeutic interventions so there is little systematic information on response to psychological, or psychotropic drug, treatment. However, clinical experience suggested that children with epilepsy and an additional mental health problem such as oppositional defiant disorder, respond just as well, if not better, to the current best evidence-based interventions (parent training programs—see Chapter 37). Similarly, although there are very few studies, children with depression and epilepsy appear to respond well to antidepressants (Thomé-Souza *et al.*, 2007), and children with anxiety and epilepsy to cognitive behavior therapy (Blocher *et al.*, 2013). In each of these examples, the

treatment is an evidence-based intervention for these conditions in children *without* epilepsy, so should be the treatment of choice for children with epilepsy, until there is evidence to the contrary.

As far as drug treatment is concerned, four points are worth emphasizing. First, the indications for, and choice of, psychotropic medication differs little from standard practice (see Chapter 43). Secondly, epilepsy is not a strong contraindication to using antipsychotics or antidepressants even though these drugs may increase seizure frequency. In practice, an increase in seizure frequency is rarely a major problem and can often be countered by adjusting the dose of antiepileptic medication. Most of the second generation antipsychotic drugs such as risperidone are probably less likely than chlorpromazine to exacerbate seizures, while olanzapine and clozapine are better avoided if possible because they are associated with a particularly high risk of seizures. Thirdly, stimulant medication can be very helpful for children with ADHD who also have a neurological problem such as epilepsy. A recent trial has confirmed that methylphenidate appears to be safe and effective for children with epilepsy (Santos *et al.*, 2013). Finally, when children with epilepsy develop behavioral problems, changing the type or dosage of antiepileptic medication can sometimes help, although there are few systematic or consistent findings. Changes in antiepileptic medication should obviously be discussed with the child's pediatrician.

In summary, there is substantial evidence that children with a brain illness are likely also to have a psychiatric disorder. Above all, this association demands good collaboration between professionals to ensure effective detection and treatment of mental health problems. Some of the most common and impairing disorders of childhood such as anxiety can be treated successfully with methods that achieve 80% good outcomes. Such success is associated with some of the largest effect-sizes in medicine (see e.g., Walkup *et al.*, 2008). Parents and children, if asked, often rate the psychiatric disorder as having a larger negative impact on quality of life, than the physical condition, yet the mental health problem may be quicker and easier to treat. For example, one study which looked at a 5 year follow-up of children with epilepsy, and their quality of life, showed that presence or absence of seizures did not affect quality of life ratings. However, the presence of a psychiatric disorder was associated with significantly reduced quality of life, as rated by both parents and children (Baca *et al.*, 2011). Pediatricians may lack the time or skills to diagnose an associated psychiatric disorder, and even if they did detect such a disorder they are often unaware of its significant functional impact.

Mental health professionals are often alarmed by a clinical encounter with a child who has active epilepsy, or severe cerebral palsy. Their discomfiture distracts them from recognizing and treating coexisting mental health problems, because their initial response is to feel the child's problems lie outside their area of expertise. However, the most effective and acceptable services for children with brain illnesses are likely to have physical and mental health professionals working closely together. Joint clinical discussions, in which each expert's professional skills are recognized and valued, should ensure that these children do not suffer the double-disadvantage of having both a neurological illness and an untreated, yet usually treatable, mental illness too.

References

Aicardi, J. et al. (2009) Diseases of the nervous system in children. In: *Clinics in Developmental Medicine*, 3rd edn. Mac Keith Press, London.

Ala, A. et al. (2007) Wilson's disease. *Lancet* **369**, 397–408.

Amaral, D.G. et al. (2008) Neuroanatomy of autism. *Trends in Neurosciences* **31**, 137–145.

Arnsten, A.F. & Rubia, K. (2012) Neurobiological circuits regulating attention, cognitive control, motivation, and emotion: disruptions in neurodevelopmental psychiatric disorders. *Journal of the American Academy of Child and Adolescent Psychiatry* **51**, 356–367.

Baca, C.B. et al. (2011) Psychiatric and medical comorbidity and quality of life outcomes in childhood-onset epilepsy. *Pediatrics* **128**, 532–1543.

Baird, G. et al. (2008) Regression, developmental trajectory and associated problems in disorders in the autism spectrum: the SNAP study. *Journal of Autism and Developmental Disorders* **38**, 1827–1836.

Bath, K.G.J. & Scharfman, H.E. (2013) Impact of early life exposure to antiepileptic drugs on neurobehavioral outcomes based on laboratory animal and clinical research. *Epilepsy and Behavior* **26**, 427–439.

Berg, A.T. et al. (2010) Revised terminology and concepts for organization of seizures and epilepsies: report of the ILAE Commission on Classification and Terminology, 2005–2009. *Epilepsia* **51**, 676–685.

Bien, C.G. et al. (2005) Pathogenesis, diagnosis and treatment of Rasmussen encephalitis: a European consensus statement. *Brain* **128**, 454–471.

Bilder, D.A. et al. (2013) Prenatal and perinatal factors associated with intellectual disability. *American Journal on Intellectual and Developmental Disabilities* **118**, 156–176.

Binnie, C.D. (2003) Cognitive impairment during epileptiform discharges: is it ever justifiable to treat the EEG? *Lancet Neurology* **2**, 725–730.

Bishop, D.V. (2013) Research Review: Emanuel Miller Memorial Lecture 2012 – neuroscientific studies of intervention for language impairment in children: interpretive and methodological problems. *Journal of Child Psychology & Psychiatry* **54**, 247–259.

Blocher, J.B. et al. (2013) Computer-assisted cognitive behavioral therapy for children with epilepsy and anxiety: a pilot study. *Epilepsy and Behavior* **27**, 70–76.

Caplan, R. (2012) Psychopathology in pediatric epilepsy: role of antiepileptic drugs. *Frontiers in Neurology* **3**, 163.

Caplan, J.P. et al. (2011) Pseudopseudoseizures: conditions that may mimic psychogenic non-epileptic seizures. *Psychosomatics* **52**, 501–506.

Cartier, N. et al. (2009) Hematopoietic stem cell gene therapy with a lentiviral vector in X-linked adrenoleukodystrophy. *Science* **326**, 818–823.

Cooper, G. M. et al. (2011). A copy number variation morbidity map of developmental delay. *Nature Genetics* **43**, 838–846.

Crompton, D.E. & Berkovic, S.F. (2009) The borderland of epilepsy: clinical and molecular features of phenomena that mimic epileptic seizures. *Lancet Neurology* **8**, 370–381.

Cuthill, F.M. & Espie, C.A. (2005) Sensitivity and specificity of procedures for the differential diagnosis of epileptic and non-epileptic seizures: a systematic review. *Seizure* **14**, 293–303.

Davies, S. et al. (2003) A population survey of mental health problems in children with epilepsy. *Developmental Medicine and Child Neurology* **45**, 292–295.

Elgen, S.K. et al. (2012) Mental health at 5 years among children born extremely preterm: a national population-based study. *European Child & Adolescent Psychiatry* **21**, 583–589.

Engel, J. et al. (2007) *Epilepsy: A Comprehensive Textbook*. Lippincott, Williams & Wilkins, Philadelphia.

Evans, S.J.W. et al. (2013) Prevalence of adult Huntington's disease in the UK based on diagnoses recorded in general practice records. *Journal of Neurology, Neurosurgery and Psychiatry* **84**, 1156–1160.

Fleiss, B. & Gressens, P. (2012) Tertiary mechanisms of brain damage: a new hope for treatment of cerebral palsy? *Lancet Neurology* **11**, 556–566.

Giedd, J.N. & Rapoport, J.L. (2010) Structural MRI of pediatric brain development: what have we learned and where are we going? *Neuron* **67**, 728–734.

Goldstein, L.H. et al. (2010) Cognitive-behavioral therapy for psychogenic nonepileptic seizures: a pilot RCT. *Neurology* **74**, 1986–1994.

Goodman, R. (1998) The longitudinal stability of psychiatric problems in children with hemiplegia. *Journal of Child Psychology and Psychiatry* **39**, 347–354.

Goodman, R. & Yude, C. (2000) Emotional, behavioural and social consequences. In: *Congenital Hemiplegia, Clinics in Developmental Medicine No. 150.* (eds B. Neville & R. Goodman), pp. 166–178. Mac Keith Press, London.

Ha, A.D. & Fung, V.S. (2012) Huntington's disease. *Current Opinion in Neurology* **25**, 491–498.

Hawkins, A.K. et al. (2011) Lessons from predictive testing for Huntington disease: 25 years on. *Journal of Medical Genetics* **48**, 649–650.

Howe, G.W. et al. (1993) Adolescent adjustment to chronic physical disorders – I. Comparing neurological and non-neurological conditions. *Journal of Child Psychology and Psychiatry* **34**, 1153–1171.

Johnson, S. (2007) Cognitive and behavioural outcomes following very preterm birth. *Seminars in Fetal and Neonatal Medicine* **12**, 363–373.

Jones, J.E. et al. (2010) Cognition, academic achievement, language, and psychopathology in pediatric chronic epilepsy: short-term outcomes. *Epilepsy and Behavior* **18**, 211–217.

Julien, C.L. et al. (2007) Psychiatric disorders in preclinical Huntington's disease. *Journal of Neurology, Neurosurgery and Psychiatry* **78**, 939–943.

Kanner, A.M. et al. (2012) Depression and epilepsy, pain and psychogenic non-epileptic seizures: clinical and therapeutic perspectives. *Epilepsy and Behavior* **24**, 169–181.

Kaufman, L. et al. (2010) The genetic basis of non-syndromic intellectual disability: a review. *Journal of Neurodevelopmental Disorders* **2**, 182–209.

Kernan, C.L. et al. (2012) Neurocognitive profiles in children with epilepsy. *Epilepsia* **53**, 2156–2163.

Kousi, M. *et al.* (2012) Update of the mutation spectrum and clinical correlations of over 360 mutations in eight genes that underlie the neuronal ceroid lipofuscinoses. *Human Mutation* **33**, 42–63.

Lai, M.C. *et al.* (2013) Biological sex affects the neurobiology of autism. *Brain* **136**, 2799–2815.

Lin, J.J. *et al.* (2012) Uncovering the neurobehavioural comorbidities of epilepsy over the lifespan. *Lancet* **380**, 1180–1192.

McAllister, C.J. *et al.* (2011) Development of the eating behaviour in Prader-Willi Syndrome: advances in our understanding. *International Journal of Obesity* **35**, 188–197.

Moore, T. *et al.* (2012) Neurological and developmental outcome in extremely preterm children born in England in 1995 and 2006: the EPICure studies. *BMJ* **345**, 7961.

Moreno-De-Luca, A. *et al.* (2013) Developmental brain dysfunction: revival and expansion of old concepts based on new genetic evidence. *Lancet Neurology* **12**, 406–414.

Moser, H.W. *et al.* (2007) X-linked adrenoleukodystrophy. *Nature Clinical Practice Neurology* **3**, 140–151.

Nestler, E.J. & Hyman, S.E. (2010) Animal models of neuropsychiatric disorders. *Nature Neuroscience* **13**, 1161–1169.

Nunn, K. *et al.* (2002) The Australian Childhood Dementia Study. *European Child and Adolescent Psychiatry* **11**, 63–70.

O'Callaghan, M.E. *et al.* (2012) Fetal and maternal candidate single nucleotide polymorphism associations with cerebral palsy: a case–control study. *Pediatrics* **129**, e414–e423.

Paneth, N. *et al.* (2006) The descriptive epidemiology of cerebral palsy. *Clinics in Perinatology* **33**, 251–267.

Parkes, J. *et al.* (2008) Psychological problems in children with cerebral palsy: a cross-sectional European Study. *Journal of Child Psychology & Psychiatry* **49**, 405–413.

Parkes, J. *et al.* (2009) Psychological problems in children with hemiplegia: a European multicentre survey. *Archives of Disease in Childhood* **94**, 429–433.

Piedad, J. *et al.* (2012) Beneficial and adverse psychotropic effects of antiepileptic drugs in patients with epilepsy: a summary of prevalence, underlying mechanisms and data limitations. *CNS Drugs* **26**, 319–335.

Piña-Garza, J.E. (2013) *Fenichel's Clinical Pediatric Neurology: A Signs and Symptoms Approach 7e Saunders.* Elsevier.

Rapoport, J.L. *et al.* (2012) Neurodevelopmental model of schizophrenia: update 2012. *Molecular Psychiatry* **17**, 1228–1238.

Rauch A, *et al.* (2012) Range of genetic mutations associated with severe non-syndromic sporadic intellectual disability: an exome sequencing study. *Lancet* **380**, 1674–1682.

Reilly, C. & Neville, B.G. (2011) Academic achievement in children with epilepsy: a review. *Epilepsy Research* **97**, 112–123.

Ross, C.A. & Tabrizi, S.J. (2011) Huntington's disease: from molecular pathogenesis to clinical treatment. *Lancet Neurology* **10**, 83–98.

Rutter, M. *et al.* (1970) *A Neuropsychiatric Study in Childhood. Clinics in Developmental Medicine Nos. 35/36.* S.I.M.P./Heinemann, London.

Rutter, M. *et al.* (1975) Attainment and adjustment in two geographical areas - I. The prevalence of psychiatric disorder. *British Journal of Psychiatry* **126**, 493–509.

Rutter, M. *et al.* (1984) Head injury. In: *Developmental Neuropsychiatry.* (ed M. Rutter), pp. 83–111. Churchill Livingstone, Edinburgh.

Ryland, H.K. *et al.* (2010) Is there a protective effect of normal to high intellectual function on mental health in children with chronic illness? *Child and Adolescent Psychiatry and Mental Health* **4**, 3.

Santos, K. *et al.* (2013) The impact of methylphenidate on seizure frequency and severity in children with attention-deficit-hyperactivity disorder and difficult-to-treat epilepsies. *Developmental Medicine and Child Neurology* **55**, 654–660.

Shaw, P. *et al.* (2010) Childhood psychiatric disorders as anomalies in neurodevelopmental trajectories. *Human Brain Mapping* **31**, 917–925.

Snider, L.A. & Swedo, S.E. (2004) PANDAS: current status and directions for research. *Molecular Psychiatry* **9**, 900–907.

Speechley, K.N. *et al.* (2012) Quality of life in children with new-onset epilepsy: a 2-year prospective cohort study. *Neurology* **79**, 1548–1555.

Steen, R.G. *et al.* (2006) Brain volume in first-episode schizophrenia: systematic review and meta-analysis of magnetic resonance imaging studies. *British Journal of Psychiatry* **188**, 510–518.

Stuart, F.A. *et al.* (2005) Adverse psychological effects of corticosteroids in children and adolescents. *Archives of Disease in Childhood* **90**, 500–506.

Thomé-Souza, M.S. *et al.* (2007) Sertraline and fluoxetine: safe treatments for children and adolescents with epilepsy and depression. *Epilepsy and Behavior* **10**, 417–425.

Tsai, P. & Sahin, M. (2011) Mechanisms of neurocognitive dysfunction and therapeutic considerations in tuberous sclerosis complex. *Current Opinion in Neurology* **24**, 106–113.

Walkup, J.T. *et al.* (2008) Cognitive behavioral therapy, sertraline, or a combination in childhood anxiety. *New England Journal of Medicine* **359**, 2753–2766.

Wallace, S. (2004) *Epilepsy in Children.* Arnold, London.

Woodward, L.J. *et al.* (2012) Neonatal white matter abnormalities an important predictor of neurocognitive outcome for very preterm children. *PLoS One* **7**, e51879.

CHAPTER 32

Clinical assessment and diagnostic formulation

James F. Leckman[1] and Eric Taylor[2]

[1] Child Study Center and the Departments of Psychiatry, Pediatrics and Psychology, Yale University, New Haven, CT, USA
[2] Department of Child and Adolescent Psychiatry, Institute of Psychiatry, Psychology and Neuroscience, King's College London, UK

Introduction

The goal of clinical assessments is to identify the presence of psychopathology and, if indicated, to make a diagnosis and to develop a plan to initiate treatment in partnership with the parents and/or other providers often within a larger system of care. This is a multistep process that involves complex and conscientious decision-making based upon the available evidence from multiple sources (Bostic & King, 2007; Rutter & Taylor, 2008). Beyond the nature and progression of the child's symptoms (past and present) within and across multiple contexts (somatic, family, peers, school, and cultural background), it is important to consider the child's developmental and medical histories, exposure to adversity (acute or chronic) as well as the child's strengths and abilities and the presence of protective and resilience factors that may impact treatment outcomes. Another important goal is the formation of a therapeutic alliance with family. An alliance is more than just being liked by the patient and the family, but involves negotiating to identify shared goals (Green, 2006). Consequently, the formulation and prioritization of treatment goals with the family should involve a collaborative, problem-solving, hypothesis-generating, and hypothesis-testing approach that is based both on the available scientific evidence concerning potential risks and benefits of specific interventions, and on the child's and the family's knowledge-base and their attitudes concerning various treatment options and opportunities. Consequently, clinical assessments often need to include a psychoeducational component. Less frequently, clinical assessments of children and adolescents are conducted in a more focused and circumscribed fashion to address immediate safety, forensic, or research issues. Regardless of the scope, clinical assessments of children and adolescents are complex in nature and vary a good deal across the globe.

This chapter addresses each of these assessment components (Table 32.1) before moving on to consider the diagnostic process and initial treatment planning. We begin by addressing the reasons for the referral and the need to understand the intentions of the person or agency requesting the clinical assessment.

Initial questions regarding referral

Children are usually referred to practitioners by someone with a focused question in mind. Clarity about why the referral was initiated (and by whom) is an essential ingredient for the evaluation to be a success. Children rarely initiate the referral and often their presenting symptoms are a greater source of concern for the parents or others in their environment than they are for the child. Many clinicians, based on their training and a traditional medical model of care, may choose to focus on whether or not the child meets criteria for a particular disorder; but this question may not be foremost in the mind of the person making the referral. For example, parents are often proactive in seeking the assessment based upon their worry that the child's current symptoms may portend the emergence of a more serious mental disorder that is thought to run in the family. The child's behavior at school may be much more problematic than it is judged to be at home. Not infrequently, the parties involved may not view the situation in the same way. Parents may be seeking special services or be in need of an evaluation for the child to return to school. In other instances, the referral source may be asking for an opinion concerning the legal status of the child—whether the child should be removed from the family or what the custody arrangements should be (see Chapters 19 and 49). Because of this broad range of possibilities, procedures need to be in place to clarify questions about the referral (Kanner, 1957; Rutter, 1975). Who made the referral? What prompted the referral? Are there differing points of view concerning the need for a clinical assessment? What are the key questions to be addressed? Are there clear administrative issues that need

---

Rutter's Child and Adolescent Psychiatry, Sixth Edition.
Edited by Anita Thapar and Daniel S. Pine, James F. Leckman, Stephen Scott, Margaret J. Snowling, Eric Taylor.
© 2015 John Wiley & Sons Ltd. Published 2018 by John Wiley & Sons Ltd.

Table 32.1 Basic elements in child and adolescent psychiatric assessments.

Content	Informant	Resources	Goals
Reason for referral; *Why this child? Why now?*	Parent, guardian, school personnel, and health-care provider(s)	Referral letters and conversations from school personnel and other health-care providers	Clarity concerning reasons for the assessment; Potentially different perspectives; Opportunity to build therapeutic alliance; Initial opinions concerning potential treatment options
Child's strengths, talents and interests and environmental supports How the family members interact with one another *Who is this child?*	Parents, child, other family members, peers, teachers, coaches	Parent- and self-reports about areas of interest and excellence Nature of the observed interactions between and among family members	Clarity concerning how the child is viewed within the family Opportunity to build trust and establish a therapeutic alliance and promote resiliency
History of present illness Comorbid conditions; Past psychiatric history and treatment response *What is the nature of the problem?*	Parents, child, other family members Past psychiatric evaluations and mental health records	Review of parent-, teacher- and self-reports; questionnaires; diagnostic interviews; videotapes Previous evaluations, therapies, treatments, medications (including dietary supplements); hospitalizations	Clarity concerning the course and function of the symptoms, accommodation, intervening stressors or associated changes in life circumstances Success of prior interventions Initial impressions concerning treatment priorities
Developmental, educational, and medical history	Parent, guardian, school personnel, and health-care provider(s)	Review of birth and pediatric records; education evaluations (see Chapters 35 and 42)	Presence of developmental or medical disorders as well as traumatic events that may have an impact on the child
Family history	Parent, guardian, school personnel, and health-care provider(s)	Review of structured and unstructured questionnaires; Genogram (see Chapters 24 and 28)	Presence of familial vulnerabilities relevant to prognosis
Home, school, and community environment	Parents, child, other family members	Parental self-esteem and psychopathology, parental strain, partial discord, sibling conflicts, level of hubbub, computer/video games, access to the internet; family resources including pets and neighbors (see Chapters 26 and 28)	To inform intervention strategies and identify challenges that will be faced by the treatment team; potential targets for adjunctive interventions
Mental Status examination	Child	Structured assessments of appearance, mood, orientation, adaptive functioning, attention, memory, fund of knowledge, judgment, insight, thought (coherence, speed, and content)	Assess the child's interaction with the clinician; screen for overt psychiatric symptoms that impact the child's behavior, adjustment and cognitive functioning
Neuropsychological evaluation	Child	Optional standardized assessments of intelligence, memory, receptive and expressive language, reading, executive function, visuo-spatial skills and motor coordination (see Chapter 34)	Clarify nature of the child's interaction with the psychologist; characterize the child's pattern of cognitive, linguistic strengths and weaknesses relative to same aged peers
Physical and neurological examination, laboratory testing, electrophysiological assessment and brain imaging	Child	Optional examinations to identify body dysmorphic features and evaluate the child's somatic, metabolic, and neurological status as well as brain structure and function (see Chapters 11, 24, and 35)	Identify any genetic, medical, metabolic, endocrine, or neurological disorders that may impact the child's course of illness and treatment

to be considered? Based on the answers to these questions, one should also consider whether the assessment team that has been approached is the one best suited to undertake the assessment. For example, depending on the clarity of the issues and the health-care system, it may make sense to refer the family on to another provider with greater expertise who is better positioned to intervene with the appropriate services.

Many of these questions can be clarified by direct contact with the referral source and by review of any relevant documents. If privacy and confidentiality can be assured, direct contact by telephone or via the internet may be of great benefit and lead to requests for additional information. Many clinicians and health-care systems have found the use of structured and semi-structured questionnaires and well-validated parent, teacher, and self-reports to be invaluable in preparing for clinical assessments. Some of the widely used parent-report instruments with excellent psychometric properties provide a preliminary assessment of the child's mood and anxiety level, attentional and disruptive behavioral problems, and the child's perceived level of psychosocial stress as well as the parents' well-being, the home environment and the level of caregiver strain (see Chapter 33). At times this information may point to other important problems that had not been previously identified and that need to be considered during the course of the evaluation. It is also often helpful to ask families for prior authorization to contact other relevant parties (school personnel and primary care providers).

At the beginning of the in-person assessment, practitioners often use open-ended questions such as, "Because we want to be sure to address your primary concerns, please briefly tell us how we can best be of service to you." Typically, the parents are asked this question with and without the child present and the child is asked as well. Questions of this sort, as well as other efforts to gain greater clarity concerning the motivation to seek a clinical assessment can also be very useful in setting the stage for the development of a positive therapeutic alliance, which has been shown to be associated with improved outcomes for both children with disruptive behaviors and those with severe anxiety (Kazdin & Durbin, 2012; Marker et al., 2013).

Observations of the family

Attitudes to referral, disorder and treatment

From the initial contact with the family, it is important to be attentive to the nature of the parents' attitudes to their child and to each other as well as to the professionals involved in the case. For example, did the mother or father take the lead in making the referral and deciding on the timing of the assessment? How did they describe their child and were there any hints as to the nature of the communication between the parents? What are their fears and expectations? How important is the family's cultural background as they consider their child's difficulties? Clinicians should be attentive to these attitudes throughout the assessment and initial treatment planning. Often they shift to

some degree as the assessment process takes place and as the family recognizes the inherently collaborative nature of the process. When clinicians show respect and a positive attitude during the assessment, it can make a difference.

Patterns of interaction

Among the sources of information that the clinician has available during the assessment, one of the most important is the nature of the interactions within the family. Patterns of dyadic reciprocity, sensitivity, and intrusiveness are often remarkably stable over the course of development (Feldman, 2010). Opportunities to observe these interactions abound beginning with how the family members position themselves in the waiting room and where they choose during the interview assessment.

Regardless of how the later stages of the assessment are organized, it is often beneficial to have a brief meeting with the family all together to explain what will be taking place and to sort out who will be seeing whom for what purpose. This is another time to closely monitor the nature of the verbal and nonverbal communication among the family members. After welcoming the family, making any further introductions, and thanking them for coming in and filling out the questionnaires and parent-reports, some clinicians have found that asking the parents to "brag" about their child is a useful starting point. "What talents and favorite activities does your child have?" This can usefully engage the family and set the stage for a successful encounter as well as providing clues as to how one might foster resilience in the child and the family (see Chapter 27). Each of the family members should be asked to share their perspective (Brown & Rutter, 1966). The clinician may ask, "What questions do you have for us? We will do our best to answer each of them before you leave today." Other open-ended questions such as, "I wonder how much you have talked together about why you are here to see us?" or "Have you had a family discussion about your reasons for coming in today?" or "How did you feel about the referral?" are often more informative than making more specific inquiries. This approach also provides opportunities for the clinician to observe interactions among family members as well as to identify any conflicting viewpoints that will need to be reconciled if the recommended interventions will be adhered to and successfully implemented. Depending on the age of the child, some of these questions should be repeated when the child is no longer in the room.

Naturally, during this initial portion of the interview when the family is together, care needs to be taken to make the child feel as comfortable as possible. For younger children, the availability of toys, paper and crayons ,and other play materials, for example, Lego, makes good sense. Access to videogames on the parents' cell phone may be more problematic and distracting. Whatever the circumstance, observing what the child decides to do and how they interact with their parents and the clinician at the very beginning of the assessment can be informative. Likewise, if the child becomes distressed or starts to display disruptive behavior, this provides another opportunity to monitor the parent's response as well as to intervene in a sensitive fashion by encouraging the parents to respond in a way that they find the most appropriate.

Basic elements in the diagnostic clinical assessment

Other key elements in the assessment include interviewing the child and interviewing the parents. The sequence and organization of these interviews depend on the child's age and developmental level as well as the clinician's best judgment about how best to proceed.

Interview with the child

The cardinal aim of the interview is to help the child relax with the interviewer and to lay a foundation of trust (Nurcombe, 2008). Without trust little can be achieved. If a modicum of trust does develop, the clinician will be able to ascertain how the child perceives problems in his or her life, evaluate the child's affect and capacity to relate to the interviewer, and catch a glimpse of his or her family life. The age, developmental level, personality, and expectations of the child matter and will shape the course and content of the interview.

The clinical assessment of young children differs fundamentally from that of adults and adolescents. While it is useful to monitor the child's behavior and social interactions in various contexts including when the parents are present, it is also crucial to interview the child separately. Care needs to be taken to minimize the child's distress when being separated from their parents. This can be performed by reassuring the child that they can be reunited with their parents as needed. The child also needs to see exactly where their parents will be located during their interview. If the assessment is being completed by a team of clinicians, often the parental interview will occur simultaneously with the child's interview. Under such circumstances, having the parents accompany the child to the room set aside for his/her assessment makes sense and can be a source of comfort for the child.

For younger children, the opportunity to play and interact in a less structured fashion with the clinician can help put the child at ease. For example, asking the child talk about what they enjoy doing and to elaborate on the areas identified as strengths and interests is a good place to start. Having an on-going activity, for example, drawing a picture or building something with Lego, permits the child to respond more spontaneously and openly to the clinician's queries. Intermittently praising the child's work and positioning oneself at the child's eye-level, that is, sitting on the floor, can facilitate the dyadic interaction between child and clinician. Some clinicians find it helpful to ask the child questions such as, "If I were a magician and could give you three wishes, what would those be?"

Eventually the clinician will need to address the behaviors and emotional issues that prompted the referral. People of all ages are open to the influence of suggestions, but none more

so than young children. Open-ended questions will work the best and be the least prone to distortion and suggestion: "What did your parents say about why you were coming in to see me today?" "What is most upsetting to you?" "What do you wish might be different?" "Is there anything you worry about every day?" Moreover, when assessing any symptom, to ask the child to give it a rating out of 10, where zero is "not a problem" and 10 is "awful, couldn't be worse" can provide a baseline for future assessments. Once the child provides some insight into their difficulties, it will be important for the clinician to contextualize the problem in terms of where and when and in relation to whom these problems occur. "How does your mom respond when that happens?" "Do you remember what was going on just before that happened yesterday?"

The issues for older children and adolescents vary and may reflect their reluctance to be open with an "adult" who is likely to try to impose their will. While it is almost always possible to establish rapport and collect information from adolescents, it can be a challenge. Being respectful and curious about the adolescent's perspective is important. While it is important for the assessments of children of all ages to have an appropriate degree of structure and standardization, the clinician also needs to be open to the unexpected. Otherwise, important information and insights may be missed (Cox *et al.*, 1981; Rutter *et al.*, 1981; Cox & Rutter, 1985). Variations in the style and content of the interview may differ considerably depending on the child's symptoms, and on cognitive and sensory impairments, if any (see Chapters 47 and 51–72). The interview with the child will also include many elements of the mental status examination (see later). At the end of the interview, the clinician should review with the child what they have both learned about the child's reasons for being seen and how he or she feels about it.

Parental interview

The parental interview is focused on the child's presenting problems, medical and family history, early development, school progress, and peer relations as well as on gathering information concerning the home and family environment including the parents' child rearing techniques and the methods of discipline used (Table 32.1). The best place to start is to address the **reason for referral** and determine what it is about the child's behavior, feelings, or social interactions that are of the greatest concern to the parents and what prompted the assessment. How do the parents understand their child's problems?

Context is critically important. How predictable are the symptoms in a given set of circumstances? How much do they vary depending upon which parent is there or which class the child is in? Are there other contextual features that appear to make the situation better or worse? Identifying specific antecedents and precipitants can provide valuable clues to what *function* the symptoms have. What has been the parents' response? Anxiety in children will often trigger behaviors in their parents. At times the parent's efforts to comfort and reassure the child can have unforeseen negative consequences by providing a form of reinforcement that may lead the symptoms to persist and intensify. Although accommodation of this sort has been studied extensively in Obsessive-compulsive disorder, it is commonplace among other pediatric onset anxiety disorders (Lebowitz et al., 2013). How have others in the family or at school responded? What has worked in the past and what has not? Is there any hint of secondary gain? Here it is important to move beyond general answers (such as mentioning efforts to comfort, admonish, or punish the child) and to obtain a more detailed sequential account of how this has been performed and how the child responded. Often asking the parents to recall specific recent episodes can be useful. This can provide some clarity about how things have progressed from the onset and if there were any precipitating events or predisposing factors. It is important to ask for detailed examples of the child's symptoms from the last week, and then determine if these were typical of the past month as well.

Do these symptoms reflect an underlying disorder or do they reveal problems within the child's environment? It is also important to be vigilant about the parents' state of mind and their possible embarrassment, ambivalence, or shame in seeking professional advice. "What did we do wrong?" "Is it my fault?"—are common unspoken questions. Echoes of the parents' memories of their own experiences while growing up are often part of the unspoken dialogue.

Beyond the immediate reason for referral, the assessment team also needs to consider the presence of any co-occurring symptoms as well as any significant past psychiatric and neurodevelopmental problems. Many services now ask parents to complete questionnaires to screen for possible co-occurring conditions, but clinicians still need to be alert in the course of the parental interview to the presence of co-occurring symptoms and past disorders.

Next, asking the parents to review their child's developmental history will allow the clinician to gain a clear perspective on the child's somatic, psychomotor, neurocognitive, linguistic, social, temperamental, and emotional development. Parents can vary a great deal in terms of their ability to recall specific developmental milestones. Often it is useful to ask the parents to complete a structured questionnaire and for the clinician to review this information prior to the time of the in-person assessment. This will allow the clinician to be knowledgeable and relatively expeditious.

It is also important to review the child's educational history, starting with nursery and kindergarten. Then in later schooling, what did the parents hear from the teachers? What were their peer interactions like? How easy was it for them to make good friends? What pastimes did they enjoy most and excel at?

Another important component of the parental interview concerns the child's medical history. Major influences on neural development occur during embryonic and fetal development (see Chapter 9). Consequently, this history needs to proceed from conception and include any difficulties the mother had in becoming pregnant and the use of any interventions (such as

in vitro fertilization), any pregnancy and birth complications including the mother's emotional state and level of psychosocial stress during the pregnancy. The parents' smoking habits, alcohol consumption, and use of illicit drugs should also be included in the medical history. Chapter 35 describes the detection of physical illness and injury, past and present. Allergies should be carefully documented and results of previous medications noted.

The mental status examination is another essential part of the initial clinical assessment. It includes a description of the child's appearance; patterns of interaction; current affect and reactivity; orientation to person, place and time; attention and apparent intelligence; fluency of speech; and the speed, coherence and content of the child's cognitive processes. The mental status examination also serves as a useful opportunity to screen for organic or neurological conditions and serves as a prelude to conducting further psychological, medical, and/or neurological examinations (see Chapters 34 and 35). Although the mental status examination is conceptualized as being distinct from other portions of the assessment, it serves to summarize the clinician's impressions from the interviews with the family and with the child. Some components, however, do require specific inquiries (such as the child's orientation to person, place and time, and their fund of knowledge and memory).

Finally, while some clinicians prefer to conduct the entire diagnostic assessment in a conjoint family setting, in our view this approach has some inherent disadvantages. Context matters and individuals do not behave the same when everyone in the family is present. Indeed, there are circumstances when spending time with each parent individually can be important: as in the case of parental divorce and joint custody arrangements. Some time spent with each parent may be useful even if there is no obvious discord between them. However, being open to the parents' preferences in this matter also makes good sense especially as the team continues to build a therapeutic alliance collaboratively with the parents and child and attends to the treatment priorities (Cox et al., 1995).

School reports and direct contact with teachers

After securing parental agreement and in advance of the initial interview, it is useful for the clinician to review school reports. This is particularly true of reports related to academic performance and any special education services that the child may currently be receiving or received in the past. Children may behave differently in the classroom or in other school settings than they do at home. Educational difficulties are frequently associated with psychopathology, and parents and teachers may only partially agree on the presence of particular symptoms such as inattentiveness, hyperactivity-impulsivity, and oppositionality (Bussing et al., 2008). While there are advantages to using standardized teacher-report questionnaires (see Chapter 33), it also is useful to have teachers express their own concerns and report on the child's behavior and response to directives. If special services have been provided, it is important to review their impact on the child's behavior and academic performance over the course of time. Being attentive to cultural differences in the educational context is also important especially if the child has recently relocated from their home country. Even with the teacher and school reports in hand, it is often the case that specific queries will arise that will prompt a member of the assessment team to contact the school personnel directly. In some instances, if there are persistent differences of opinion concerning the child's behavior at home and at school, visits to observe the child in both settings may be useful. Efforts to build a collaborative alliance with the teachers and other professionals at the school will bode well for the child's outcome. This is particularly true as the initial treatment plan is developed and implemented due to the fact that some treatment components may focus on the school environment in terms of advocacy, services, accommodations, opportunities for resilience, or simply monitoring changes in the child's behavior over the course of treatment.

Psychological testing and medical assessment

These important aspects of assessment are reviewed in Chapters 34 and 35. The initial assessment needs to be informed by knowledge of previous assessments and screening (e.g., for hearing) and there must be enough expertise to appreciate when there is a need for further referral.

Standardization of clinical assessment

Standardized approaches and the use of structured interviews, rating scales, and observational methods constitute an important part of a clinical assessment (see Chapter 33), but there is also a clear need to look beyond the diagnostic formulation to consider factors that might be important in the causation of the disorder and its course and prognosis and that inform therapeutic planning.

Viewed from a global perspective, the availability of standardized interviews is a step forward. This is particularly true in many parts of the world where child and adolescent mental health professionals and other clinicians are forced to make decisions about diagnosis and treatment in imperfect situations within a limited time period and with incomplete information. For example, the Development and Well-Being Assessment (DAWBA) is a package of interviews, questionnaires, and rating techniques designed to generate ICD-10 and DSM-IV psychiatric diagnoses on 5–17-year-olds based on information provided from multiple informants (parents, youth over 11-year-old and teachers) and is now available, free and with computer algorithms, in more than 20 languages (Goodman *et al.*, 2000) (http://www.dawba.info/a0.html).

However, there are clear downsides to being overly reliant on diagnostic instruments. One reason for caution is the high frequency of idiosyncratic but clinically significant information that may be missed. Despite recent efforts to revise and validate the DSM and ICD diagnostic categories, they remain imperfect (see Chapter 2). Additionally, the much debated and carefully chosen wording of these criteria rarely matches the complex presentations of the children referred for assessment.

As it formulates a narrative concerning the nature of the child's problems, the assessment team needs to consider how a given child's symptoms resemble those observed in other children as well as what aspects of the presentation are unique to this child and this family. These considerations will allow them to frame an initial set of hypotheses concerning what factors will influence response to treatment while building a strong therapeutic alliance. This is a key step in the problem-solving, hypothesis-generating, and hypothesis-testing approach needed to formulate and prioritize treatment goals with the child and the family.

Presence/absence of clinically significant psychopathology

Formulation in child and adolescent psychiatry is a complex and iterative process that distills the information from multiple sources into a meaningful narrative and establishes a set of hypotheses about the child and his or her presentation that then helps to shape the initial treatment priorities. One basic question underlying this process is whether or not the child's problems are clinically significant. One of the hallmarks of many psychiatric symptoms is their dimensional character and continuity with normal emotional and behavioral states. Care needs to be taken not to "pathologise the normal." This raises the important issue of how to establish thresholds that distinguish developmental normal traits and emotional states from those that are indicative of pathology. Relevant questions include: Does their intensity go beyond the range of normal variation given the child's age and temperamental predisposition? Do these symptoms reflect a clear substantial change from the child's usual emotional state? Are they pervasive across interpersonal and social contexts? How much time do they consume in a typical day? To what extent can the child control these symptoms by means of distraction or engagement in pleasurable activities? Many of these questions are embedded in symptom-specific rating scales. These scales allow clinicians to better characterize each child relative to other children with similar problems across a range of symptom dimensions including anxiety, obsessive-compulsive, manic and depressive symptoms as well as symptoms of post traumatic stress disorder, motor and vocal tics, and attentional and behavioral symptoms, among others (see Chapter 33). Repeat assessments with these instruments can provide an important tool to clinicians so that they can regularly monitor the child's progress. Despite the potential benefits associated with the use of these scales, they are no substitute for the practitioner's clinical judgment concerning whether or not the presenting symptoms are clinically significant. In addition, the usefulness of these scales may be limited depending on the child's age, the need for specific informants (parent, teacher, self, and expert clinician), the variable time periods that are assessed (current, past week, past 6 months, etc.), idiosyncratic scoring paradigms, their potential cost, and, in some cases, the need for formal training to establish the rater's reliability.

In other instances, clinical interventions may not be indicated even if the level of distress is high. For example, a serious grief reaction following the death of a loved one is quite common and a source of distress. In some cases, the emotional distress of the parents and family members contributes to the intensity of the child's reaction. The passage of time and supportive counseling may be sufficient (see Chapter 36).

Finally, the assessment team may determine that although the severity of the presenting problem is not great enough to warrant an immediate intervention, it is clinically significant. This is true of many medical disorders as they herald recurrent difficulties and an increased likelihood of a range of negative health outcomes, for example, high blood pressure. Many neurodevelopmental disorders are chronic conditions which require long-term monitoring and interventions across a number of contexts (home, school, and social). The waxing and waning course of tic disorders is a good example. Often parents or the primary care provider will request a consultation when the tics are severe, but by the time the child is observed in evaluation they have all but disappeared (Leckman, 2002). Here psychoeducational interventions with the child, the parents, school personnel, and peers, concerning the nature and course of tic disorders may be indicated (see Chapter 56).

Assessment of psychosocial impairment and safety

Efforts to determine the degree of impairment in psychosocial functioning are another key consideration in establishing the clinical significance of a child's presenting symptoms. From the time of the Isle of Wight studies onward, the assessment of impairment has been a standard part of the assessment of children and adolescents (Rutter *et al.*, 1970). The need to establish the level of psychosocial impairment associated with various forms of psychopathology was given further impetus by subsequent epidemiological surveys that reported remarkably high prevalence rates of psychiatric disorders (Kessler *et al.*, 1994). This in turn directly led the developers of DSM-IV (American Psychiatric Association, 2000) to incorporate a clinical significance criterion in more than 70% of all diagnostic criteria. The precise wording varied but generally followed: "The disturbance causes clinically significant distress or impairment in social, academic, occupational, or other important areas of functioning." Not surprisingly, the inclusion of this criterion dramatically reduced the prevalence rates for many disorders and increased the proportion of cases likely needing mental health services. The debate continues and the clinical significance criterion has been removed from many of the DSM-5 diagnostic criteria (American Psychiatric Association, 2013). It is therefore all the more important that the presence and degree of impairment are noted separately and consistently. Are the features of the disorder(s) distressing the child? Is their school

work suffering? Are they held back from social activities, or victimized, or unable to make friends?

The assessment of safety is another important topic. In the case of younger children, this may focus on the child's risk of injury as a result of abuse or neglect (see Chapters 29 and 30). For older children and adolescents, the assessment concerns the risk of violence to self or others (see Chapters 49 and 64–68). In some instances, the referral itself may have been prompted by these concerns. If so, the person making the referral will often be directed immediately to seek emergency services which in turn may lead to psychiatric hospitalization or to the involvement of government agencies charged with protecting the safety of the child and of specialized forensic assessment services. In any case, the clinical assessment team, in nonemergency settings, needs to be alert to issues of safety. Based on the information provided by the child and the parents, the clinician may need to determine whether the child or others is in immediate danger. Relevant information includes the presence of current or past ideation or acts that indicate a significant risk to self or others as well as a range of risk factors (explicit plans, cognitive distortions, mood state, impulsivity, personality, and a range of environmental stress factors involving family psychopathology and conflict) (see Chapter 64). In addition to self-harm with clear suicidal intent, acts of intentional self-harm (cutting, burning, etc.) to provide temporary relief from intense dysphoria have become more common over the past two decades among adolescents and young adults (Zetterqvist *et al.*, 2013). Acts of nonsuicidal self-injury need to be carefully documented and understood and, if present, need to be considered in the formulation of the initial treatment plan. Other serious risks during adolescence include unplanned pregnancies due to reckless and hypersexual behaviors associated with bipolar disorder (see Chapter 62).

Duration and timing of disorder

The duration and timing of psychopathological states are two other features that contribute to an understanding of their clinical significance. Many diagnostic classification systems specify a duration criterion—the minimal time period the symptoms need to be present in order for a diagnosis to be made. In the case of DSM-IV and DSM-5, the panels of experts came up with a very broad range of required periods, currently: 2 weeks for major depressive disorder; 3 months for bulimia nervosa; 6 months for generalized anxiety disorder, 12 months for conduct disorder; and 2 years for persistent depressive disorder (American Psychiatric Association, 2000, 2013). While these time periods are based on the consensus of experts, they remain opinions and are somewhat arbitrary. For other diagnoses, such as ADHD, the DSM criteria specify that the symptoms being considered must have been present prior to a certain age. In many instances, establishing a clear onset or estimating the duration can be problematic given the retrospective nature of the information provided by multiple informants and concerning multiple potentially interrelated psychiatric symptoms. Apart from possible reporting biases, it may well be that many psychiatric disorders do not, in fact, have a clear-cut onset. Frequently, symptomatology gradually builds up over time when new symptoms become evident or when psychosocial impairment is manifested (Sandberg *et al.*, 2001). By contrast, other disorders are defined in part by their sudden, overnight onset, for example, the recently proposed pediatric acute-onset neuropsychiatric syndrome (PANS) (Swedo *et al.*, 2012). While clinicians need to take the necessary time to clarify as much as possible the onset, course and timing of the presenting symptoms as well as the points of remission and exacerbation, this is usually an imperfect science. As a consequence, a slavish adherence to diagnostic criteria that specify symptom duration makes little sense.

In sum, the process of determining whether or not the child's problems are clinically significant requires the assessment team to distill information from multiple sources into a meaningful narrative and to establish a set of hypotheses about the nature, origin (onset), course (exacerbations and duration), and current severity (impairment) of the child's presenting neurodevelopmental, emotional, and behavioral symptoms.

Diagnostic formulation: integration and synthesis

As noted earlier, formulation in child and adolescent psychiatry is a complex and iterative process that distills information from multiple sources into a meaningful narrative and establishes a set of hypotheses about the child and his or her presentation that then shape the initial treatment priorities. What symptoms are causing the greatest degree of difficulty for the child and for others in his or her immediate environments? When and why did these problems arise and how long have they been present? What can be done to ameliorate them? Are there any proximal risk mechanisms that, if addressed, might have a positive impact? What else is going on in the environment (acute or chronic stressors, etc) that is having an impact on these symptoms? What new knowledge could we provide that would be useful for the family and others directly involved in the case (peers, teachers, etc.) to be aware of, for example, evidence-based knowledge concerning the natural history, treatment, and prognosis? Can everyone agree regarding the nature of these difficulties and what the best course of action would be to address them?

Diagnoses are one element in this formulation and they provide a succinct summary of some aspects of what has been learned over the course of the evaluation. Ultimately, the clinician's judgment in integrating all the available information into a "best estimate" diagnosis is key (Leckman *et al.*, 1982). However, care needs to be taken not to "reify" the diagnosis. When a specific disorder is reified by the clinicians, there is a risk that the child is no longer viewed as a unique human entity but is instead viewed as "a case of X disorder." We need to focus on "the whole child" including his/her strengths, interests and abilities, not just his/her "diagnosis."

Diagnoses allow for "informed" communication between professionals and researchers, for example, what interventions have the strongest evidence base for a specific disorder, or as record keeping, for example, health-care systems that need to monitor the prevalence of disorders as well as track service delivery. In putting the clinical information together to establish a set of hypotheses about the child, the clinician needs to consider the source of the information and the context within which it was obtained. In cases of divorce and parental discord, the parents may not agree even with regard to the presence of specific symptoms or their importance. Parents, teachers, and other informants may also disagree on the importance of specific symptoms. It is also important to consider the knowledge-base of the informants. Are there other family members with a similar condition and how did this condition impact that individual over the course of his/her life? How much information has the family gleaned from various sources including the internet and how accurate is their understanding of the condition and its course and treatment? Given the iterative nature of assessments and treatment planning, the clinician always needs to ask—what information am I lacking and what would be the best source(s) to gain a more complete view of the child and a deeper understanding of their psychopathology?

Psychoeducation

Psychoeducation can be a key ingredient leading to a successful intervention. Given the incremental advances in our understanding of the etiology, course and treatment of childhood-onset psychiatric disorders, providing families with accessible, user-friendly sources of information can be enormously helpful (Lucksted *et al.*, 2012). Most involved family members of children and adolescents with mental illnesses need information, assistance, and support to best assist their ill family member and to cope with the challenges posed to their family system. Ideally, this information will include content about the nature of the disorder (etiology, course, and outcome), as well as expanding social support networks. For example, in the case of Tourette's disorder, familiarizing the family (and in some instances teachers and peers) with the existence of premonitory sensory urges and the momentary "sense of relief" experienced by many individuals suffering from this condition is truly enlightening and sets the stage for a greater level of interest and acceptance of recommendations to initiate cognitive-behavioral therapy (CBT) such as Habit Reversal Training (see Chapter 56; Martino & Leckman, 2013). Advocacy organizations are often an excellent source of such information. Indeed, providing the parents with the web links to such organizations can be very helpful and may initiate an interconnection that will be useful to everyone involved.

Another dimension of psychoeducation, for both the clinician and the family, is the need to be acquainted with the available evidence concerning the efficacy of various therapeutic interventions. *Evidence-based medicine* (*EBM*) is the conscientious, explicit, and judicious use of current best evidence in making decisions about the care of individual patients. This evidence includes meta-analyses of the relevant clinical trials in an effort to guide clinical practice. EBM has driven a transformation of clinical practice in medicine and has been adopted by major organizations including the center for Evidence Based Medicine (http://www.cebm.net/) and the Cochrane Collaboration (http://www.cochrane.org/). EBM seeks to assess the strength of the evidence regarding the risks and benefits of treatments (including lack of treatment) and diagnostic tests. Evidence quality can be gauged based on the source type (from meta-analyses and systematic reviews), as well as other factors including statistical validity, clinical relevance, currency, and peer-review acceptance. EBM recognizes that many aspects of health care depend on individual factors such as quality- and value-of-life judgments, which are only partially subject to quantitative scientific methods. In addition to EBM resources, clinical practice guidelines are also available from professional organizations including the National Institute for Health and Care Excellence in the United Kingdom and the American Academy of Child and Adolescent Psychiatry, and the European Society for Child and Adolescent Psychiatry, among others. The decision on which course of action to follow remains subject to input from personal, political, philosophical, ethical, economic, and esthetic values as well as the imperative to minimize the potential for doing harm to the child.

Treatment planning

Once the assessment nears completion and a meaningful narrative has been formulated that summarizes the information from multiple sources, the next step is to build a consensus and to propose a set of hypotheses that can be tested. Following a range of psychoeducation interventions, the clinician and the family are ready to embark on treatment planning. Although setting forth a "diagnosis" is important, relying solely on the "diagnosis" to guide a treatment plan can be problematic (Rutter, 2011). Seldom does our current state of knowledge allow for "the diagnosis" by itself to dictate the intervention. For example, if Johnny's (an 8-year-old boy) increasing separation anxiety at home and his increasing social isolation and, at times, his disruptive behavior at school are based, in part, on his parents' hostile estrangement from one another and on his need to transition back and forth between two residences, then it may make sense to engage the family in a therapeutic intervention that seeks to help the parents recognize the negative consequences of their hostile interactions on their child and to provide a neutral therapist to explore with the child his or her understanding of the situation (see Chapters 26, 39, and 40). This in turn may help the estranged parents refocus on their child and find ways to support and celebrate jointly the child's interests and abilities. By contrast, if the child's anxiety is long-standing and a reflection of a shy or inhibited temperament manifested by being socially awkward, withdrawn, and avoidant, a course of CBT or pharmacotherapy or both may be indicated depending on the family's willingness to pursue one of these interventions (see Chapter 60). Other principles that are key to treatment planning include: safety (to do no harm); building on the child's strengths (as a way to foster resilience and keep the child's development "on track") (see Chapter 27); and work as a collaborative team with the patients, the family, the school, and other providers to ensure coordination and continuity of culturally appropriate care.

Safety

Just as safety is a key issue to consider during the course of an assessment, it has no less a role in the initial phase of treatment planning. This is always a balance. In situations with the potential for child abuse or neglect, care needs to be taken to ensure the protection of the child as well as the rights of the child's care takers in accordance the legal and ethical guidelines that are in place (see Chapters 19–22, 29, 30, and 49). The initiation of pharmacological treatment also requires that the family and the patient have a clear grasp of the risks and benefits. Often it is useful to delay the initiation of medications. The experience of going through an evaluation, learning about the disorder through psychoeducation, and giving voice to the child's and family's concerns can have a positive impact on the clinical picture. Simply having someone who understands the situation and is committed to working with the family and other practitioners can make a real difference. Likewise, given the increasing number of CBT interventions with proven efficacy, pharmacotherapy may not be the first agreed upon intervention (Leckman, 2013). Often the major problem is finding a clinician with the necessary skills and experience to provide the CBT with fidelity. However, once the joint decision is made to initiate medication, it is important for the child and family to "commit" to completing an adequate trial unless untoward side effects are clinically significant even after making any necessary adjustments in dosage or the timing of drug administration.

Build on strengths, foster resilience, and keep development "on track"

In our experience, supporting the positive elements of the child's life is always an important part of the initial treatment planning. This is especially true if there are opportunities to build on the child's talents and interests (music, sports activities, etc.). The child's continued engagement in such activities provides something for him/her to be "proud of" and is a source of positive reenforcement. Physical exercise can also have a positive impact on the brain and there is some evidence to support its use across a range of conditions from ADHD to depressive mood (Petty *et al.*, 2009; Berwid & Halperin, 2012). It is also very important to emphasize with the patient and the parents the need to keep the child's development "on track." Almost invariably this means finding ways to continue the child's life with others outside the home. Withdrawal and isolation is a prescription for on-going self-doubt, low self-esteem, as well as problematic interactions in the home. For example, children with ADHD often have major difficulties with social acceptance and this can create a vicious cycle that involves a degree of social isolation, peer rejection, and an increased risk of being bullied (Murray-Close *et al.*, 2010; McQuade *et al.*, 2014). Depending on the child's developmental level, efforts to keep development on track may involve identifying opportunities for the child in question to interact with younger or older children rather than with their same-aged peers, for example, in religious groups or scouting or outdoor activities. In these contexts, the child with impaired social skills can interact with younger (as a mentor) or older peers (as a mentee). These new settings provide an opportunity for the child to be resilient in the face of continuing adversity (peer rejection, bullying, etc.) (see Chapter 27 and Panter-Brick & Leckman, 2013).

Team building with the child and the parents

Optional treatment planning and the willingness of the family to engage in treatment interventions depend on consensus building within the therapeutic alliance. This step can be problematic if the parents are in conflict and can easily provoke each other. In such instances, separate interactions with each parent may be of value in reenforcing the merits of a specific intervention as viewed from that parent's unique perspective. Encouraging acceptance of the realities of their lives and circumstances may permit a lessening of the anger and distress that continue to distract them from the needs of their child.

Interface with school personnel, pediatricians, and other practitioners

Often, the therapeutic team needs to involve other practitioners and professionals. Multiple examples come to mind. For example, autism spectrum disorders, and speech and language and other learning disorders, including ADHD, will often involve working with school personnel and other professionals and medical disciplines (see Chapters 51–55). In these complex situations, someone, besides a parent, needs to serve as the coordinator and convener as the child matures.

Cultural appropriateness

It is also important that clinicians do not lose sight of the unique cultural and religious background of the family during the treatment planning process. Attrition is a long-standing problem in mental health centers serving youth (Warnick *et al.*, 2012). Ethnicity is a consistent predictor of attrition particularly when the treatment provider is not from the same ethnic or religious background. Likewise, a family's ethnic and cultural background may influence their choice of various treatment alternatives. Although enduring therapeutic alliances are possible across ethnic and cultural backgrounds, a careful appraisal of the match between the mental health service providers and the family in question is encouraged.

Standards for Practice

Clinical practice must be performed under a variety of administrative, financial, and legal constraints. This chapter outlines what is needed to complete a psychiatric assessment. However, health services may not provide adequate time or resources and may require burdensome administrative tasks all of which compromise one's ability to complete a meaningful psychiatric assessment. In some instances, a short period of time may be sufficient, if the presenting problems are straight forward and not particularly worrisome, for example, uncomplicated bedwetting or parental "over-concern" about a preschool child's age-appropriate behavior toward siblings. However, when the presenting problems are substantial and context dependent, it is critical for the clinician to address each of the areas mentioned earlier in order to formulate a coherent narrative concerning the child's condition. Almost invariably this will require multiple sources of information and a degree of professional judgment. Clinicians must also act in accordance with the legal and ethical guidelines that are in place to ensure the safety of the child (see Chapters 19–22, 29, 30, and 49).

Approaches to assessment and treatment planning across the globe

Health-care systems vary widely across the world. Wonderfully, even in some Low and Middle Income countries, such as Brazil, health care is considered as a right not a privilege. On the other hand, in some of the wealthier countries, for example, the United States, marked disparities are still in place. In addition to access, the question of the quality of the services that are available is significant especially given the stigma associated with mental disorders and the shortage of well-trained practitioners (see Chapter 16). Often, the issues of access to and the availability of well-trained professionals means that the task of assessment falls to primary care clinicians, pediatricians, and to professionals in settings outside of medical centers, for example, school-based programs (see Chapters 42 and 48). In these contexts, the availability of expert consultants and the existence of sustainable programs to train professionals in school settings are an important focus for health care planning. Innovative approaches are needed to address these barriers and to improve access to care. Options to consider include the use of screening measures for detection of children at high risk coupled with a more complete second-stage diagnostic assessment and the use of nonspecialist workers in community and school settings for the delivery of psychosocial interventions (Patel *et al.*, 2013). One of the most promising emerging strategies is through the empowerment of existing human resources, for example, parents and other members of the extended families, through innovative technologies, such as mobile health, with the necessary skills for the detection and treatment of child mental disorders (see Chapter 16). The increasing use of electronic medical records, e-mail, and the social media is also transforming aspects of referral and clinical assessments as well as treatment planning. For example, some interventions are now available online (Spence *et al.*, 2011). The internet is also an expanding source of information and misinformation increasingly used by parents as a guide to decision-making. Additionally, telemedicine is being increasingly used to provide mental health assessments and services at a distance (Grady & Nelson, 2011).

Conclusions

This chapter has sought to stress the importance of forming an alliance with the child and family, keeping in mind their cultural background and family milieu, their developmental status, and their perspective (as well as that of those around them) on their child's symptoms. The approach outlined requires multiple sources of information and clinical judgment; and sharing the information with the child and the family along with an honest appraisal of the child's prognosis. Treatment planning can then build on the child's strengths as a way to foster resilience and keep the child's development "on track." The child's response to treatment will indicate whether or not the therapeutic hypothesis was correct and what modifications are needed to ensure a path to recovery.

References

American Psychiatric Association (2000) *Diagnostic and Statistical Manual of Mental Disorders*, 4th edn. American Psychiatric Association, Washington, DC.

American Psychiatric Association (2013) *Diagnostic and Statistical Manual of Mental Disorders*, 5th edn. American Psychiatric Association, Washington, DC.

Berwid, O.G. & Halperin, J.M. (2012) Emerging support for a role of exercise in attention-deficit/hyperactivity disorder intervention planning. *Current Psychiatry Reports* **14**, 543–551.

Bostic, J.F. & King, R.A. (2007) Clinical assessment in children and adolescents: content and structure. In: *Lewis's Child and Adolescent Psychiatry: A Comprehensive Textbook*. (eds A. Martin & F.R. Volkmar), 4th edn, pp. 323–344. Lippincott, Williams & Wilkins, Philadelphia.

Brown, G. & Rutter, M. (1966) The measurement of family activities and relationships: a methodological study. *Human Relations* **19**, 241–263.

Bussing, R. *et al.* (2008) Parent and teacher SNAP-IV ratings of attention deficit hyperactivity disorder symptoms: psychometric properties and normative ratings from a school district sample. *Assessment* **15**, 317–328.

Cox, A. & Rutter, M. (1985) Diagnostic appraisal and interviewing. In: *Child and Adolescent Psychiatry Modern Approaches*. (eds M. Rutter & L. Hersov), 2nd edn, pp. 233–248. Blackwell Scientific Publications, Oxford.

Cox, A. *et al.* (1981) Psychiatric interviewing techniques. *British Journal of Psychiatry* **139**, 29–37.

Cox, A. *et al.* (1995) A comparison of individual and family approaches to initial assessment. *European Child and Adolescent Psychiatry* **4**, 94–101.

Feldman, R. (2010) The relational basis of adolescent adjustment: trajectories of mother-child interactive behaviors from infancy to adolescence shape adolescents' adaptation. *Attachment and Human Development* **12**, 173–192.

Goodman, R. *et al.* (2000) The development and well-being assessment: description and initial validation of an integrated assessment of child and adolescent psychopathology. *Journal of Child Psychology and Psychiatry* **41**, 645–655.

Grady, B.J. & Nelson, E.L. (eds) (2011) Telepsychiatry and telemental health. *Child and Adolescent Psychiatric Clinics of North America* **20**, 1–178.

Green, J. (2006) The therapeutic alliance--a significant but neglected variable in child mental health treatment studies. *Journal of Child Psychology and Psychiatry* **47**, 425–435.

Kanner, L. (1957) *Child Psychiatry*, 3rd edn. Charles. C. Thomas, Springfield, IL.

Kazdin, A.E. & Durbin, K.A. (2012) Predictors of child-therapist alliance in cognitive-behavioral treatment of children referred for oppositional and antisocial behavior. *Psychotherapy (Chicago)* **49**, 202–217.

Kessler, R.C. *et al.* (1994) Lifetime and 12-month prevalence of DSM-III-R psychiatric disorders in the United States. Results from the National Comorbidity Survey. *Archives of General Psychiatry* **51**, 8–19.

Lebowitz, E.R. *et al.* (2013) Family accommodation in pediatric anxiety disorders. *Depression and Anxiety* **30**, 47–54.

Leckman, J.F. (2002) Tourette's syndrome. *Lancet* **360**, 1577–1586.

Leckman, J.F. (2013) What's next for developmental psychiatry? *World Psychiatry* **12**, 125–126.

Leckman, J.F. *et al.* (1982) Best estimate of lifetime psychiatric diagnosis: a methodologic study. *Archives of General Psychiatry* **39**, 879–883.

Lucksted, A. *et al.* (2012) Recent developments in family psychoeducation as an evidence-based practice. *Journal of Marital and Family Therapy* **38**, 101–121.

Marker, C.D. *et al.* (2013) The reciprocal relationship between alliance and symptom improvement across the treatment of childhood anxiety. *Journal of Clinical Child and Adolescent Psychology* **42**, 22–33.

Martino, D. & Leckman, J.F. (eds) (2013) *Tourette's Syndrome*. Oxford University Press, Oxford.

McQuade, J.D. *et al.* (2014) Perceived social acceptance and peer status differentially predict adjustment in youth with and without ADHD. *Journal of Attention Disorders* **18**, 31–43.

Murray-Close, D. *et al.* (2010) Developmental processes in peer problems of children with attention-deficit/hyperactivity disorder in the Multimodal Treatment Study of Children with ADHD. *Developmental Psychopathology* **22**, 785–802.

Nurcombe, B. 2008. Diagnostic encounter for children and adolescents. In: Ebert, M. H., Loosen, P. T., Nurcombe, B., & Leckman, J. F. *Current Diagnosis & Treatment in Psychiatry*, 2nd edn, New York: McGraw-Hill.

Panter-Brick, C. & Leckman, J.F. (2013) Resilience in child development—interconnected pathways to wellbeing. *Journal of Child Psychology and Psychiatry* **54**, 333–336.

Patel, V. *et al.* (2013) Improving access to care for children with mental disorders: a global perspective. *Archives of Diseases of Childhood* **98**, 323–327.

Petty, K.H. *et al.* (2009) Exercise effects on depressive symptoms and self-worth in overweight children: a randomized controlled trial. *Journal of Pediatric Psychology* **34**, 929–939.

Rutter, M. (1975) *Helping Troubled Children*. Penguin Books, Harmondsworth, Middlesex.

Rutter, M. (2011) Child psychiatric diagnosis and classification: concepts, findings, challenges and potential. *Journal of Child Psychology and Psychiatry* **52**, 647–660.

Rutter, M. & Taylor, E. (2008) Clinical assessment and diagnostic formulation. In: *Rutter's Child and Adolescent Psychiatry*. (eds M. Rutter, D. Bishop, E. Pine, S. Scott, J. Stevenson, E. Taylor & A. Thapar), 5th edn, pp. 42–57. Blackwell Publishing, London.

Rutter, M. *et al.* (1970) *Education, Health and Behaviour*. Lonhmans, London. Melbourne: F.A, Reprint 1981.

Rutter, M. *et al.* (1981) Psychiatric interviewing techniques. IV. Experimental study. *British Journal of Psychiatry* **138**, 456–465.

Sandberg, S. *et al.* (2001) Do high-threat life events really provoke the onset of psychiatric disorder in children? *Journal of Child Psychology and Psychiatry* **42**, 523–532.

Spence, S.H. *et al.* (2011) A randomized controlled trial of online versus clinic-based CBT for adolescent anxiety. *Journal of Consulting and Clinical Psychology* **79**, 629–642.

Swedo, S.E. *et al.* (2012) From research subgroup to clinical syndrome: modifying the PANDAS criteria to describe PANS (Pediatric Acute-onset Neuropsychiatric Syndrome). *Pediatrics and Therapeutics* **2**, 113.

Warnick, E. *et al.* (2012) Defining dropout from youth psychotherapy: how definitions shape the prevalence and predictors of attrition. *Child and Adolescent Mental Health* **17**, 76–85.

Zetterqvist, M. *et al.* (2013) Prevalence and function of non-suicidal self-injury (NSSI) in a community sample of adolescents. *Journal of Abnormal Child Psychology* **41**, 759–773.

CHAPTER 33

Use of structured interviews, rating scales, and observational methods in clinical settings

Prudence W. Fisher[1], Erica M. Chin[2] and Hilary B. Vidair[3]

[1] Division of Child and Adolescent Psychiatry, New York State Psychiatric Institute, Columbia University, New York, USA
[2] Division of Child and Adolescent Psychiatry, New York Presbyterian Hospital, Columbia University Medical Center, New York, USA
[3] Clinical Psychology Doctoral Program, Department of Psychology, Long Island University, Post Campus, Brookville, NY, USA

Assessment procedures lie at the heart of healing professions. In this chapter we review procedures for selecting measures, summarize available measures, and discuss the importance of measurement in providing high quality clinical care.

Introduction

Systematic assessment is an essential part of any mental health evaluation. Assessment of youth differs fundamentally from that of adults. Unlike adults, children rarely initiate mental health contact. Typically, a parent, but sometimes a teacher or primary care doctor, has found the child's behavior problematic or noticed the child's distress. Hence, children are more likely to be referred for disruptive behavior than for anxiety, although anxiety is more prevalent. Most children coming for treatment have multiple disorders. Often, the most important or impairing problem is not the reason for seeking help. Moreover, youth assessment is complex. Younger children have limited insight and are poor informants about the timing, duration, and severity of their problems. Thus, assessment typically includes information from adults who know the child *and* from the child. These sources often disagree, sometimes because informants see youth in different settings or because informant characteristics influence their view of the child, but it is generally accepted that all information is diagnostically useful. Finally, youth are often reluctant reporters about embarrassing, distressing, or socially undesirable behaviors, even when directly questioned, a problem that might be addressed by automated measures (Bachman, 2003).

Treatment decisions should follow from a thorough initial assessment, ideally completed by a skilled clinician who interviews the child/adolescent and his/her parent(s), obtains a detailed history, collects information about social development, and gathers information from third parties, such as teachers (see Chapter 32). The clinician also may review records and administer questionnaires. This initial assessment should include a "psychiatric review of systems" to identify possible diagnoses to be evaluated more thoroughly and ensure consideration of alternative diagnoses, as many symptoms (e.g., irritability, concentration problems) are shared across disorders. This ideal situation does not always occur. Instead, clinicians often make diagnostic decisions based on insufficient information ("premature closure") before considering information that might contradict initial hypotheses ("confirmation bias"). Clinicians also often neglect "rare" conditions and are influenced in diagnostic decision making by cases recently seen in clinics or discussed at meetings (the "availability heuristic"), and by the context in which the evaluation occurs (see discussion in Galanter & Patel, 2005). After the initial evaluation, it is important to undertake systematic (re)evaluations to identify conditions either missed or that arise during treatment.

Currently available assessment tools emerged after DSM-III (American Psychiatric Association, 1980) and expansion in child psychiatric research. By clearly delimited diagnostic criteria, DSM-III represented a radical new approach for diagnosis, which enhanced diagnostic reliability, improved communication, and facilitated the development of assessment instruments. Later revisions, culminating with DSM-5 in 2013 (American Psychiatric Association, 2013), extended this approach, with synergy between the DSM and ICD systems. Although the ICD classification code remains the standard for official morbidity and mortality reports, the DSM is often used to determine psychiatric diagnoses and create a medical record. Both systems include explicit criteria, which can be assessed with standardized instruments useful in both research and clinical settings.

Rutter's Child and Adolescent Psychiatry, Sixth Edition.
Edited by Anita Thapar and Daniel S. Pine, James F. Leckman, Stephen Scott, Margaret J. Snowling, Eric Taylor.
© 2015 John Wiley & Sons Ltd. Published 2018 by John Wiley & Sons Ltd.

During this period, rapid expansion in mental health research created a growing need for standardized assessments. Systematic errors plague routine clinical assessment, and research tools can aid clinical care. Historically, as clinicians faced increasing pressure to justify interventions, track progress, and report to third parties, clinical use of standard measures grew and yielded benefits. These included more comprehensive descriptions of patient populations, better monitoring of diagnostic changes over time, better tracking of treatment responses, and possible identification of homogeneous patient subgroups. Finally, educational value was shown; standard measures increase efficiency and help clinicians consider diagnoses they previously may have ignored.

Selecting measures

Purpose

The purpose of an assessment determines selection of measures, in terms of targeted symptoms and level of detail. For initial evaluations, broadband measures facilitate triage and identification of problems to be more intensively probed. Typically, an initial evaluation will assess material covered in comprehensive diagnostic interviews described later, supplemented by family factors and other social relationships. If the purpose of the assessment is to screen for a particular condition, one might choose a measure designed to identify that condition. For measuring severity or monitoring treatment, one would choose a measure that rates the severity of symptoms or the disorder.

Psychometrics

Reliability and validity should inform measurement selection. These properties are constrained by sampling and procedural factors. Measures tested in inpatient settings often work differently in outpatient settings. Measures which perform well in highly educated samples may perform less well in other samples.

Reliability refers to "repeatability" or "reproducibility," the degree to which repeated administration yields the same results/answers. This can be quantified in several ways. "Internal reliability" or "internal consistency" quantifies the degree to which individual scale items measure one underlying construct (i.e., "repeat" each other). "Inter-rater reliability" quantifies the degree to which different raters generate the same result with the measure, which benefits from focused training. Thirty years ago, poor parent–child agreement was viewed as a "problem," but this is now expected, and different informants' perspectives are valued. A third type of reliability is test-retest, the degree to which repeated administration generates similar results in the absence of a change in the patient's status. Good test-retest can only be documented by the readministration of measures, typically after a week to 10 days. It is necessary if an instrument is going to be used to measure change. Assessment of reliability of diagnostic interviews involves many challenges (see Shaffer *et al.*, 1999).

Validity refers to the degree to which an instrument actually measures the targeted construct. It is difficult to assess since most mental health constructs lack accepted "gold standards" against which to compare the measure. As with reliability, there are many types of validity. "Face validity" involves mere inspection (or on the "face" of it), to evaluate if the measure seems to assess the relevant construct. "Concurrent validity" involves comparisons with other measures of the construct; "discriminate validity" involves determining if the measure differentiates cases with the targeted problem, relative to other, possibly similar problems. For screening, ability to identify cases with (sensitivity) or without (specificity) problems is of particular importance.

Practical considerations

In selecting measures, one set of practical issues includes the patient's developmental level, sociocultural background, family literacy levels, and spoken language. The availability of private space, forms tested in the patient's culture, and the length of time available are additional practical factors. For example, acquiring information before a face-to-face assessment can save time. Some measures require trained clinicians; others require even more specialized training; and still others can be administered on a computer. Other factors relate to ease of use, scoring, and interpretability, as well as history of use in similar settings. Diagnostic measures should reliably assess relevant disorder criteria at an appropriate level of specification. A final consideration is cost. Some instruments only can be used on a pay-per-administration cost; some require expensive training, others are "free" but may have hidden costs, related to staff time or questionable measurement properties.

Interviews

There are several interviews, which generate useful diagnostic information and differ in their structure. "Highly structured," or "respondent-based," interviews (RBI) require questions to be read *exactly as written* with few, predefined response options. The *respondent* must interpret questions. The Diagnostic Interview Schedule for Children (DISC, Shaffer *et al.*, 2000) is one widely used RBI. "Semistructured" or "interviewer-based" interviews (IBI) give the interviewer a pivotal role: she/he decides how to elicit and interpret information. Although IBIs may contain questions, these are "suggested"; the interviewer (re)words questions as appropriate and continues to ask questions until she/he decides the ratings. The Child and Adolescent Psychiatric Assessment (CAPA, Angold *et al.*, 1995) and versions of the Schedule for Affective Disorders and Schizophrenia for School Age Children (K-SADS, Kaufman *et al.*, 1997; Geller *et al.*, 2001) are examples of IBIs.

There are advantages and disadvantages to each approach. RBIs may be more standardized, are less expensive, and require far less training. However, they cannot address invalid responses and may miss atypical presentations. IBIs give interviewers the leeway to clarify discrepancies and use redundant questioning, but these require highly paid clinicians and extensive, ongoing training to minimize interviewer variability and rater "drift." The Development and Well-Being Assessment (DAWBA, Goodman *et al.*, 2000) combines these approaches. It includes an RBI comprising closed- and open-ended questions (responses are typed in) that is administered either by computer or interviewer with responses/results sent to an experienced clinical rater to make final diagnostic decisions.

Table 33.1 summarizes properties of commonly used interviews. Each yields DSM-IV (and for some ICD-10) diagnoses and will likely be revised for DSM-5. All are administered to parents and, depending on age of the youth, children separately, and information is combined using different procedures. Many have alternative versions for younger and older persons. For youth with multiple diagnoses, all can require hours to use. Each is used widely in research; few are routinely used in clinical services. The Anxiety Disorders Interview Schedule for Children (A-DIS-C, Silverman & Albano, 1996) has found use in specialized anxiety treatment centers, and the KSADS is used in some specialized mood clinics. The DAWBA and the DISC are both useful in settings where trained clinicians are not readily available. Although they cannot substitute for comprehensive clinical evaluation, they can greatly aid in screening and triage.

Scales

This section reviews data on various rating scales. This includes comprehensive scales and scales that assess more focused domains.

Comprehensive and broad-based scales

These scales are designed to efficiently assess diverse behavioral and emotional problems. Frequently utilized as screening instruments, broad-based scales present an efficient first assessment step. They may also be useful for public health and clinic administration review. We describe three widely used comprehensive and broad-based measures.

The Achenbach System of Empirically Based Assessment (ASEBA, Achenbach, 2009; www.aseba.org), which must be purchased, is the most widely used family of measures. This includes a Child Behavior Checklist for Ages 6–18 (CBCL/6–18), Teacher Report Form (TRF/6–18), Youth Self Report (YSR/11–18), Child Behavior Checklist for Ages 11/2–5 (CBCL/11/2–5) and Caretaker–Teacher Report Form (C–TRF), as well as forms for assessing adults. The ASEBA forms average 99–120 items to generate several syndrome scales with a strong research base in many languages and cultures (see Rescorla *et al.*, 2013).

The Behavioral Assessment System for Children (BASC-2, Reynolds & Kamphaus, 2004, www.pearsonclinical.com), another widely used cross-informant system that must be purchased, was designed to assess youth ages 4–18. BASC-2 forms contain 139–160 items. Inclusion of positive and adaptive adjustment is a distinctive feature of the BASC-2. Like the ASEBA, the BASC has broad- and narrowband scales,

with norms for general and clinical samples; it also has strong research support and validity scales to assess possible informant bias. The BASC-2 is available in Spanish, and psychometrics are good. For an in-depth comparison of ASEBA and BASC systems, see Rescorla (2009).

The Strength and Difficulties Questionnaire (SDQ, Goodman, 1997, 2001; Goodman & Scott, 1999), which is freely available (www.sdqinfo.org), was designed to be used as a brief behavioral screening tool for youth 2–17 years old that can be completed in 5 min. It contains just 25 items, has cross-informant forms, and yields five subscales. The SDQ has been translated into over 75 languages, possesses strong psychometrics (Hysing *et al.*, 2007), and correlates with CBCL scores (Goodman & Scott, 1999).

We limited our review to measures that are most widely used. Other measures include the Pediatric Symptom Checklist (PSC, Murphy & Jellinek, 1985), the Vanderbilt ADHD Rating Scales (discussed below) and the Child Symptom Inventories-4 (Gadow & Sprafkin, 1994). In addition, locally created checklists are often implemented in clinical settings as part of the intake to identify patient symptoms and probable diagnoses.

Anxiety and depression (also see Chapters 60 and 63)

Many measures are clinically useful. Because youth are considered the best source of information regarding their internal states, some measures began as "youth-only" measures. Informant agreement is typically low to moderate. Table 33.2 summarizes the properties of widely used measures with adequate psychometrics; many other measures are also available.

Anxiety

The Revised Children's Manifest Anxiety Scale (RCMAS, Reynolds & Richmond, 1985), a downward extension of the adult Manifest Anxiety Scale (Taylor, 1953), must be purchased; it uses simple language to assess chronic, "manifest" anxiety as opposed to specific diagnoses in school-aged children, although it can also be used with older youth. The revised version, RCMAS-2 (Reynolds & Richmond, 2008), has a slightly different factor structure. While the psychometric properties are reasonable, the scale has been criticized for insufficient discriminant validity and lack of data on treatment-related change.

The State-Trait Anxiety Inventory for Children (STAIC; Spielberger *et al.*, 1973), another downward extension of an adult instrument, also must be purchased. It contains two 20-item self-rated scales to quantify "state" and "trait" anxiety and has no corresponding parent-informant version. The STAIC also has reasonable psychometrics and mixed discriminant validity with somewhat better specificity than sensitivity. The STAIC has been shown to be sensitive to change in transient and more general anxiety levels, making the state scale useful in assessing response to stress.

The Multidimensional Anxiety Scale for Children (MASC, March, 1997, March *et al.*, 1997; MASC-2, MASC-2-P, March, 2012) is another self-rated scale that must be purchased. It was

Table 33.1 Structured diagnostic interviews.

Instrument (Author)	Recommended age range	Time period assessed	Items/response format	Structure/ organization	Interviews and training	Scoring/reports	Other information
Diagnostic Interview Schedule for Children, Version IV (DISC-IV) Shaffer et al. (2000)	6–17 years (6–8 parent only); young child and young adult versions available	Past year Past 4 weeks "Whole life" Voice & Present State version: past 4 weeks	All questions asked are coded usually "yes" or "no"; few open-ended questions; Responses entered into computer	RBI; questions read exactly as written; self-contained modules, can choose which diagnoses to assess; Few symptom skips within modules	Lay interviewer (2–3 days training CAPI) A-CASI: self-administered (half day training for administrator) Same or different interviewer for parent & youth	Scored by computer algorithm based on parent alone, youth alone, and combined parent and youth using "or rule"; symptom and criterion scales available	CAPI and A-CASI formats used Obtain information and interview from DISCGroup@nyspi.columbia.edu
The Development and Well-Being Assessment (DAWBA) Goodman et al. (2000)	5–17 years (5–10 parent only); teacher questionnaire	Current (but varies by diagnosis)	Most close-ended questions rated on a 3-point scale; for open-ended questions, responses typed verbatim with suggested follow-up probes if sparse answers	RBI; questions read as written, open-ended questions asked at end of each section or at end of interview; Clinician rater makes ratings based on information from all sources; Many symptom skips	Lay interviewer (1–3 days and "online" training available); Experienced clinician for final ratings; training varies by experience; Same or different interviewer for parent & youth	Preliminary scoring; "semi-automated" ("likelihood" and provisional diagnoses) by computer; Clinician assigns formal diagnoses based on clinical judgment	CAPI and CASI available ; Obtain information and interview from http://www.dawba.com/
Missouri Assessment for Genetics Interview for Children (MAGIC) Reich and Todd (1997)	7–17 years; different child and adolescent versions	MAGIC: Lifetime (and also past month for mood)	All questions asked are rated using categorical responses	MAGIC: RBI; with suggested follow up/clarifying probes; Some symptom skips	Lay interviewer (2–4 weeks of training); Same or different interviewer for parent & youth	Scored by computer algorithm for parent and youth separately	MAGIC: CAPI or CASI format; revision of a previous DICA version; Obtain information and MAGIC from author, Wendy4912@aol.com
Diagnostic Interview for Children and Adolescents-IV (DICA-IV) Reich (2000)		DICA: lifetime (not specified); current and past symp-tomatology	All questions asked are rated using categorical responses	DICA: RBI; usually CAPI or CASI; on paper some suggested follow-up probes (older versions); Some symptom skips	Lay interviewer (2–3 days); computerized (self) version; Same or different interviewer for parent & youth	Scored by computer algorithm for parent and youth separately	DICA: CAPI or CASI format; Obtain information and DICA from www.mhs.com
Child and Adolescent Psychiatric Assessment, Version 5.0 (CAPA) Angold et al. (1995)	8–17 years; young child and young adult versions available	Past 3 months	For most symptoms, separate scaled ratings of aspects of severity (intensity, frequency, duration, onset, resultant impairment)	IBI; extensive glossary defining symptoms and ratings; Few symptom skips	Lay interviewer (2–4 weeks training); Same or different interviewer for parent & youth	Scored by computer algorithm using "or rule"; utilizing "supervisor" ratings	Obtain information and interview from http://devepi.duhs.duke.edu/capa.html

Measure	Age	Time frame	Rating	Interview structure	Administration	Scoring/DSM criteria	Availability
Schedule for Affective Disorders and Schizophrenia for School-Age Children: Present and Lifetime (K-SADS-PL) Kaufman et al. (1997)	6–18 years	Current Past year without 2-month remission Lifetime: most severe	Most criteria/symptoms rated on 3-point scale, not present, subthreshold, threshold (definitions provided); some rated "yes" or "no"	IBI, interview starts with open-ended psychiatric/medical history; "Screen interview" determines which diagnoses to assess in "supplemental" modules; suggested questions; Many symptom skips	Clinician (3–4 days training); Same interviewer for parent & youth	DSM criteria rated by clinician based on all informants (including records); using clinician consensus ratings	DSM-5 version available; Obtain information and interview from joan.kaufman@yale.edu
Washington University Schedule for Affective Disorders and Schizophrenia for School-Age Children (WASH U K-SADS) Geller et al. (2001)	6–18 years	Current and lifetime onset, offset, and duration for most symptoms	Most criteria/symptoms rated on 7-point severity scale (from none to extremely profound); some on 4- or 5-point scale	IBI; interviewer starts with open-ended psychiatric/medical history suggested questions; Some symptom skips	Clinician (3–4 days training); Same or different interviewers for parent and youth	All symptoms occurring in same time period "count" towards diagnosis; DSM criteria rated by clinician based on all informants using "or" rule	Obtain information and interview from gellerb@wustl.edu
Anxiety Disorders Interview Schedule for Children (A-DIS-C) Silverman and Albano (1996)	6-17 years	Current and lifetime	Many questions rated "yes" or "no", "Thermometers" used to obtain severity, fear/avoidance, distress, interference information; Interviewer makes clinician severity rating from 0 to 8 for each diagnosis	IBI; probes provided adapted by interviewer as appropriate; Some symptom skips	Clinician (1–3 days training; length depends on experience with child anxiety disorders); Same or different interviewers for parent and youth	Scored by clinician; Composite diagnoses from child & parent interviews derived by comparing responses. When symptom is endorsed on one version but not another both severity ratings and level of interference with functioning are considered.	Obtain information and interview from Oxford University Press

RBI = respondent-based interview.

IBI = interviewer-based interview.

A-CASI = audio-computer-assisted self-interview.

CAPI = Computer-assisted personal interview.

CASI = Computer-assisted self interview.

"or rule" = criterion/symptom counted as positive if endorsed by parent or youth.

Table 33.2 Measures focusing on anxiety and depression.

Anxiety: Questionnaires

Instrument (Author)	Construct(s) assessed	Recommended age range	Time period assessed	Time to complete	Version: items (long/short)	Response format	Scoring/reports	Computerized?	Any cost?
Revised Children's Manifest Anxiety Scale: Second Edition (RCMAS-2) Reynolds and Richmond (2008)	Total anxiety; 3 subscales: physiological anxiety, worry, social anxiety; also assesses "defensiveness" (lie scale) and has "inconsistent reporting index"	6–19 years	Not specified; current; "true of you" trait	10–15 min	Youth: 49/10	Each item rated true or not true	Sum of items; total scores with cutoff points	Audio CD available for poor readers	Yes; WPS
State-Trait Anxiety Inventory for Children (STAIC, Spielberger et al. 1973)	State anxiety Trait anxiety	8–14 years	Current; "Right now" state and "Usually feel" trait	<20 min	Youth: 40	Each item rated on 3-point frequency scale: "hardly ever," "sometimes," "often"	Sum of items on each scale (norms available)	Computer software available for scoring	Yes; PAR
Multidimensional Anxiety Scale for Children (MASC) March et al. (1997)	Anxiety symptoms; 4 factors: physical symptoms, social anxiety, harm avoidance, separation anxiety (many DSM symptoms)	8–19 years	"Recently"	<15 min	Youth: 50/10 Parent: 50	Each item rated on 4-point scale ranging from "never true about me" to "often true about me"	Sum of items; T-score cutoffs for different severity levels and for "caseness"	Yes	Yes; MHS
Screen for Child Anxiety Related Emotional Disorders (SCARED) Birmaher et al. (1999)	DSM-IV anxiety disorder, including school avoidance	9–19 years	Last 3 months	10–15 min	Youth and Parent: 41/5	Each item rated on 3-point scale, "not true," "sometimes true," "very true"	Total scores with recommended cutoff points by age/gender	No	No; available at www.psychiatry.pitt.edu/research/tools-research/assessment-instruments
Spence Children's Anxiety Scale (SCAS) Spence (1998)	DSM-IV anxiety disorder	7–17 years	Not specified; current (items written in present tense)	10 min	Youth and Parent: 38	Each item rated on 4-point scale ranging from "never" to "always"; some items reverse scored	Sum of items; subscale scores for specific anxiety d/o given	Computer scoring	No; available at www.scaswebsite.com
Revised Child Anxiety and Depression Scales (RCADS) Chorpita et al. (2000)	DSM-IV anxiety disorder; depression	Grades 3–12	Not specified; current (items written in present tense)	10 min	Youth and Parent: 47	Each item comprises 4 statements of increasing intensity/severity (never to always)	Sum of items; T-score from appropriate grade level	Automated scoring online	No; available from authors, www.childfirst.ucla.edu

	Construct(s) assessed	Recommend age range	Time period assessed	Time to complete	Versions: items (long/short)	Response format	Scoring/reports	Computerized?	Any cost?
Hamilton Anxiety Rating Scale (HAM-A) Hamilton (1959)	Psychic anxiety (mental agitation and psychological distress) and somatic anxiety (physical complaints related to anxiety)	Children, adolescents, adults	Current (not specified)	10–15 min	Youth only: 14 items	Each item has 4 statements of increasing intensity/severity (none to severe)	Sum of items; suggested cutoffs for different severity levels and for "caseness"	No	No; public domain
Pediatric Anxiety Rating Scale (PARS) RUPP Anxiety Study Group (2002)	DSM-IV criteria and impairment for social phobia, separation anxiety, generalized anxiety disorder	6–17 years	Last week	<20 min	Youth and Parent: 50 symptom items; 7 global items	Each symptom item scored as present or absent (yes/no); global ratings rated by clinician on 7 dimensions of severity using a 6-point scale of increasing severity	Total score is sum of 7 global severity items	No	No; obtain information and scale from Mark Riddle, MD, mriddle1@jhmi.edu

Depression: Questionnaires

Instrument (Author)	Construct(s) assessed	Recommend age range	Time period assessed	Time to complete	Versions: items (long/short)	Response format	Scoring/reports	Computerized?	Any cost?
Beck Depression Inventory–II (BDI-II) Beck et al. (1996)	All DSM-IV MDD[a] symptoms	13–80 years	Last 2 weeks	5–10 min	Youth: 21	Each item comprises 4 statements of increasing intensity/severity	Sum of items; suggested cutoffs for different severity levels and for "caseness"	Yes	Yes; PsychCorp
Children's Depression Inventory 2 (CDI 2) Kovacs (2010)	Most DSM-IV MDD[a] symptoms Other associated symptoms	7–17 years	Last 2 weeks	5–15 min	Youth: 28/12 Teacher: 12 Parent: 17/12	Each item comprises 3 statements of increasing severity/intensity; (some items reverse scored)	Sum of items; corresponding T-score, suggested cutoffs for different severity levels and for "caseness"	Yes	Yes; MHS
Center for Epidemiological Studies-Depression Scale (CES-D) Radloff (1977) Center for Epidemiological Studies-Depression Scale for Children (CES-DC) Weissman et al. (1980)	Some DSM-IV MDD[a] symptoms	CES-D: 12–96 years CES-DC: 6–17 years	Last week	5–10 min	Youth: 20	Each item rated on 4 point scale of frequency, "rarely or none of the time" to "most or all of the time"; (some items reverse scored)	Sum of items; suggested cutoffs for different severity levels and for "caseness"	Yes	No; available online on various websites

(continued overleaf)

Table 33.2 (*continued*)

Anxiety: Questionnaires

Instrument (Author)	Construct(s) assessed	Recommended age range	Time period assessed	Time to complete	Version: items (long/short)	Response format	Scoring/reports	Computerized?	Any cost?
Mood and Feelings Questionnaire (MFQ) Costello et al. (1991)	Long: All DSM-IV MDD symptoms; other associated symptoms Short: Some DSM-IV symptoms	8–18 years; modified for 6–12 years	Last 2 weeks	5–10 min	Youth: 33/13 (6–12 years): 14 Parent: 34/13	Each item rated on 3 point scale, "true," "sometimes true," "not true"	Sum of items; no prescribed cutoffs (up to user)	No	No; obtain information and scale from: http://devepi.duhs.duke.edu/MFQ.html
Quick Inventory of Depressive Symptomatology (QIDS) Rush et al. (2003) Quick Inventory of Depressive Symptomatology—Adolescent (QIDS-A) Moore et al. (2007)	All DSM-IV MDD symptoms	QIDS: 18–75 years QIDS-A: 12–17 years	Last week	5–8 min	QIDS: Youth and Clinician: 16 QIDS-A: Youth, Parent, and Clinician: 17	Each item comprises 4 statements of increasing severity/intensity	Sum of highest score items; suggested cutoffs for different severity levels and for "caseness"	No	No; QIDS:<www.ids-qids.org>/ QIDS-A: <graham.emslie@utsouthwestern.edu>
Reynolds Adolescent Depression Scale, Second Edition (RADS-2) Reynolds (2002) Reynolds Child Depression Scale, Second Edition (RCDS-2) Reynolds (2010)	Long/Short: Most DSM-IV MDD symptoms; Other associated symptoms	RADS: 11–20 years RCDS: 7–13 years	RADS: current; not specified RCDS: Last 2 weeks	RADS: 5–10 min RCDS: 10–15 min	RADS: Youth: 30/11 RCDS: Youth: 30/10	Each item rated on 4-point scale of frequency from "almost never" to "all the time"; (some items reverse scored); RCDS-2 includes additional global item	Sum of items; corresponding T-score, suggested cutoffs for different severity levels and for "caseness"	No	Yes; PAR

Depression: clinician-administered measures

Instrument (Author)	Construct(s) assessed	Age range	Time period assessed	Time to complete	Informant: items (long/short)	Response format	Scoring/reports	Computerized?	Any cost?
Hamilton Rating Scale for Depression (HAM-D) Hamilton (1960), Warren (1997)	Most DSM-IV MDD symptoms	13+ years	Current (not specified)	5–10 min	Youth only: 17, 19, 21 (different versions)	Each item rated on 5-point or 3-point scale with increasing symptom severity	Sum of first 17 items; cutoffs for different severity levels and for "caseness"	Yes	No; public domain
Children's Depression Rating Scale-Revised (CDRS-R) Poznanski and Mokros (1996)	All DSM-IV MDD symptoms	6–12 years (often used with adolescents)	Current (not specified)	20–30 min	Youth and Parent and Other: 17 items	Each item rated on 5 point or 7-point scale with increasing symptom severity	Sum of items; T-scores, cutoffs for probable diagnosis	No	Yes; WPS

aMDD = Major depressive disorder.

developed on the basis of research to improve upon earlier anxiety scales, such as the RCMAS and STAIC. The MASC has been translated into over 15 languages. The psychometrics properties of this scale are good, and the measure is sensitive to treatment. The current version, MASC-2, contains 50 items assessing features of DSM diagnoses and includes a parent form. Less is known about the MASC-2 and the parent version, but initial results are promising.

The Screen for Child Anxiety Related Emotional States (SCARED, Birmaher *et al.*, 1999) is a freely-available self-rated scale also developed to improve upon earlier scales. Like the MASC, it assesses features of DSM diagnoses, has self- and parent-rated versions, and has been translated into multiple languages. It has both long, 41-item, and short, 5-item versions. The psychometrics are good, and the measure is sensitive to treatment effects.

The Spence Children's Anxiety Scale (SCAS, Spence, 1998) is a freely available youth-completed instrument with corresponding parent (Nauta *et al.*, 2004) and preschool versions (Spence *et al.*, 2001). The psychometrics are good, the scale has been translated into several languages, and it is sensitive to treatment effects. The Revised Children's Anxiety and Depression Scale (RCADS, Chorpita *et al.*, 2000), another freely available scale, closely resembles the SCAS, and also assesses depression, which is useful in many settings. The scale's psychometric properties are good, and the scale has been translated into several languages.

The Hamilton Anxiety Rating Scale (HAM-A, HARS, Hamilton, 1959) is a freely available clinician-rated measure that quantifies the severity of global anxiety by requiring clinicians to make five-point ratings of multiple physiologic and psychic-anxiety symptoms. No guidelines inform clinicians on procedures for generating scores. The HAM-A has been used with adolescents in addition to adults, with whom it is a widely used outcome measure. The measure requires extensive training and tends to focus heavily on somatic symptoms.

The Pediatric Anxiety Rating Scale (PARS, RUPP Anxiety Study Group, 2002) is another freely available clinician-rated measure. It targets symptoms not covered adequately by the HAM-A or HARS, and it is modeled on the Children's Yale-Brown Obsessive Compulsive Scale (CY-BOCS, Scahill *et al.*, 1997) (see subsequent text). After a review of symptoms, clinicians rate severity on seven dimensions using a six-point scale. The psychometrics are good, and the scale is sensitive to treatment effects. However, administration is lengthy, and it requires extensive training.

Depression

The Beck Depression Inventory (BDI-II, Beck *et al.*, 1996) is a widely used self-report scale that must be purchased and maps onto DSM criteria. This easy-to-use scale has good psychometrics, is sensitive to treatment effects (at least among adults), and it includes an item about suicidality. Modeled after the BDI, the Children's Depression Inventory (CDI-2, Kovacs, 2010) is widely used in 6-to-17 year-olds. While the psychometrics generally are good and the scale is sensitive to treatment effects, results are mixed in terms of distinguishing depression from other disorders. Although the scale is widely used for screening, sensitivity may be poor. The CDI has been translated into several languages. It also includes an item about suicidality.

The Center for Epidemiological Studies Depression Scale (CES-D, Radloff, 1977) is a freely available self-report depression scale developed for use in adult epidemiological studies. However, it does not cover suicidality and many DSM criteria. The Center for Epidemiological Studies Depression Scale for Children (CES-DC) is a version for youth, without a "parent-informant" version. Both are available in several languages. Criticisms of these scales focus on the incomplete coverage of depression items and nonspecificity for depression.

The Mood and Feelings Questionnaire (MFQ, Costello *et al.*, 1991) is a freely available self-report depression scale that allows rapid evaluation. A parallel parent report exists, as do short forms. The psychometrics are strong, and discriminability for depression appears better than for other self-report measures.

The Quick Inventory of Depressive Symptomatology (QIDS Rush *et al.*, 2003) and QIDS-A (adapted for adolescents, Moore *et al.*, 2007) are short forms of the Inventory of Depressive Symptomatology (IDS, Rush *et al.*, 1996). These freely available forms assess symptom criteria of Major Depressive Episode and are well suited for tracking treatment response. Both self- and clinician-rated versions exist, as well as a structured interview guide. The QIDS is widely translated, has strong psychometrics and has been adapted specifically for use with children and adolescents.

The Reynolds Adolescent Depression Scale, Second Edition (RADS-2) ("About Myself") (Reynolds, 2002) and the corresponding Reynolds Child Depression Scale, Second Edition (RCDS-2)" ("About Me") (Reynolds, 2010) are two scales that must be purchased and can be used for screening, research, and monitoring treatment. There are no corresponding parent forms. The psychometrics are strong, norms are available, and the scales are easy to use.

The Hamilton Rating Scale for Depression (HDRS or HAM-D, Hamilton, 1960) is a freely available, clinician-rated measure that has been widely used in treatment studies of adult depression. Several versions exist, with the HAM-D used most widely (Guy, 1976). The measure does not cover all depressive items, since it was developed long before DSM-III, and it has been criticized for its psychometrics (Bagby *et al.*, 2004). Nevertheless, it has played an important role in evaluating many treatments for depression over the past three decades.

Modeled after the HAM-D, the Children's Depression Rating Scale—Revised (CDRS-R, Poznanski & Mokros, 1996) is a clinician-rated measure that must be purchased. The scale is completed after the clinician interviews the patient and a parental informant. For youth, the CDRS-R is the measure of choice for most treatment outcome studies. The CDRS has been translated into several languages. The psychometrics are generally strong, provided that clinicians are properly trained and monitored, and the scale assesses suicidality. Norms are available, but are not typically used. Like the HAM-D, in typical clinical settings the CDRS-R might best be used as a measure with children who have been determined to or suspected of having a depressive illness to quantify severity and track change.

Disorders of attention, impulsivity, hyperactivity and disruptive behavior (also see Chapters 55 and 65)

There are many scales to assess disruptive behaviors. In contrast to mood and anxiety symptoms, disruptive behaviors are more readily observable, leading parents and teachers to provide highly valued information (Loeber et al., 1990). Both should be used to generate a comprehensive assessment, supplemented by children's reports, particularly for covert behaviors, such as lying or stealing, although children may conceal such behaviors from the clinician. Table 33.3 summarizes properties of the broadest, most widely used measures with adequate psychometric properties, while chapter text highlights key features.

There are several widely used scales developed by C. Keith Conners and colleagues to assess attention deficit hyperactivity disorder (ADHD) and disruptive disorders. The current version, which must be purchased, is the Conner 3 (third edition). It has parent, teacher, and self-rated forms with good psychometrics, especially for ADHD and disruptive behaviors. It has been used to track treatment and screen for ADHD.

The Swanson, Nolan, and Pelham Rating Scale, Fourth Edition (SNAP-IV, Swanson et al., 2001) assesses DSM ADHD, oppositional-defiant disorder (ODD) and related criteria via parent and teacher reports. There is no self-report. This freely available widely-used scale has strong psychometrics, especially for ADHD, and is sensitive to treatment effects. The Strengths and Weaknesses of ADHD Symptoms and Normal Behavior (SWAN, Swanson et al., 2006) is another freely available scale developed to address concerns about the SNAP-IV's exclusive focus on pathological behaviors. Unlike those for the SNAP-IV, SWAN items are rated using a scale ranging from "far below average" to "far above average" to reflect both weaknesses and strengths. The SWAN is easy to use and is available in several languages, but few treatment studies have used the SWAN.

The Vanderbilt ADHD Rating Scales (VARS, Wolraich et al., 1998, 2003) are more recent DSM-IV focused parent and teacher reports that assess for ADHD, ODD, and conduct disorder, though they also have features similar to comprehensive measures. The scales have good psychometrics and have been translated into several languages. English versions can be found on various Internet sites (e.g., www.childrenshospital.vanderbilt.org/services.php?mid=5734). One advantage of the VARS is the ability to assess comorbid externalizing and internalizing symptoms.

The Eyberg Child Behavior Inventory (ECBI, Eyberg & Pincus, 1999) is a parent report scale, widely used in both treatment studies and clinical settings, for assessing symptoms of disruptive behavior disorders. This easy-to-use scale must be purchased, is available in many languages, and has a corresponding teacher scale, the Sutter-Eyberg Student Behavior Inventory. The scales have been normed.

The Overt Aggression Scale (OAS, Yudofsky et al., 1986) and Modified Overt Aggression Scale (Sorgi et al., 1991) are both freely available (for OAS see, www.bcm.edu/departments/psychiatry-and-behavioral-sciences/index.cfm?pmid=3896; for MOAS see www.thereachinstitute.org/files/documents/moas.pdf). These scales track severity in real time, with the OAS focusing on behavior present "in the moment," and the MOAS including ratings for the past week. An observer rates the presence of various aggressive events during a specific time interval. While the scale has novel features, limited psychometric data are available.

The Children's Aggression Scale (CAS, Halperin et al., 2002, 2003), which must be purchased, was developed to focus specifically on aggression. It has parent and teacher scales that weight items to account for severity. The scale has strong psychometrics and is normed.

The Buss-Durkee Hostility Inventory (BDHI, Buss et al., 2003) is a self-report scale that is unique for its focus on hostility. Developed for college students, the scale was modified for youth. The original version has reasonable psychometrics. However, many versions exist and the psychometrics have not been examined for all of them. The scale is available in several languages.

Scales for other specific disorders

Part IV of this volume comprises chapters on specific syndromes, with discussions of assessment measures. Here, we review some commonly used measures.

For autism spectrum disorders (see Chapter 51), there are several good screening measures, including the Social Communication Questionnaire (SCQ, Rutter et al., 2003a, b), the Autism Spectrum Screening Questionnaire (ASSQ, Ehlers et al., 1999), the Childhood Autism Rating Scale, Second Edition (CARS 2, Schopler et al., 2010) and, for very young children, the Modified Checklist for Autism in Toddlers (M-CHAT, Robins et al., 1999). The Autism Diagnostic Interview—Revised (ADI-R, Rutter et al., 2003a, b) and the Autism Diagnostic Observation Schedule (ADOS-2) discussed subsequently are state-of-the art diagnostic measures.

For tic disorders (see Chapter 56), the clinician-rated Yale Global Tic Severity Scale (YGTSS, Leckman et al., 1989) quantifies overall tic severity in the week preceding evaluation. This is the measure of choice for treatment outcome studies, is a useful aid for clinicians, and is freely available. The Premonitory Urge for Tics Scale (PUTS; Woods et al., 2005) is a brief self-report measure, which can be useful when using behavioral interventions to treat these disorders.

For obsessive compulsive disorder (see Chapter 61), the Leyton Obsessional Inventory-Child Version (LOI-CV; Berg et al., 1986) has utility as a screen and good psychometric

Table 33.3 Measures focusing on behavioral and disruptive symptoms.

Instrument (Author)	Construct(s) assessed	Age range	Time period assessed	Time to complete	Version: items (long/short)	Items/response format	Scoring/ reports	Compu- terized?	Any cost?
Conners Third Edition (Conners 3) Conners (2008)	DSM-IV criteria, assesses ADHD, CD, ODD, learning problems, executive functioning, aggression, peer/family relations in home, social, school settings.	6–18 years 8–18 years (self-report)	Last month	10–20 min	Youth: 99/41 Parent: 110/45 Teacher: 115/41	Each item rated on increasing frequency on a 4-point scale from "not true at all/never" to "very much true/very often"	Sum of items with suggested cutoffs and percentages with T score for different severity levels	Yes	Yes; MHS
Swanson, Nolan, and Pelham Rating Scale, Fourth Edition (SNAP-IV) Swanson et al. (2001)	DSM-IV ADHD, ODD, other related diagnoses	6–18 years	User choice	10 min	Parent and Teacher: 26/90	Each item rated on 4-point scale of frequency from "not at all" to "very much"	Sum of items; cutoffs percentages for caseness	No	No; www.ADHD.net
Strengths and Weaknesses of ADHD symptoms and Normal behavior scale (SWAN) Swanson (2006)	DSM-IV ADHD; adaptive and impaired ends of ADHD symptom dimensions	6–18 years	Last 6 months	5 min	Parent and Teacher: 18	Each item rated on a 7-point scale with "average behavior" scored in the middle and "far below average" and "far above average" at the extremes	Sum of items; cutoffs percentages for caseness	No	No; www.ADHD.net
Vanderbilt ADHD Rating Scales (VARS) Wolraich (1998, 2003)	DSM-IV; inattention, hyper-activity/impulsivity, oppositional-defiant/conduct disorder, anxiety/depression, academic and classroom behavioral performance	Kindergarten to fifth grade	Current	10 min	Parent: 55 Teacher: 43	Each item rated on a 4-point scale of increasing frequency from "never" to "very often"; performance section rated on a 5-point scale of increasing performance from "problematic" to "above average"	Suggested score of select items required for "caseness"	No	No; www.childrenshospital.vanderbilt.org/services.php?mid=5734

(continued overleaf)

Table 33.3 (*continued*)

Instrument (Author)	Construct(s) assessed	Age range	Time period assessed	Time to complete	Version: items (long/short)	Items/response format	Scoring/reports	Computerized?	Any cost?
Eyberg Child Behavior Inventory (ECBI) Eyberg and Pincus (1999)	Conduct problems; intensity scale; problem scale	2–16 years	Current	5 min	Parent: 36	Each item on the intensity scale is rated on a 7-point scale of increasing frequency from "never" to "always"; problem scale asks parents to indicate "yes" or "no" to whether behavior is a problem	Sum of items, weighted depending on severity; suggested cutoffs with T-score for clinical range of problems	No	Yes; PAR, Inc.
Overt Aggression Scale (OAS) Yudofsky et al. (1986)	Verbal aggression, physical aggression against objects, physical aggression against self, physical aggression against other people, staff intervention	6–17 years, adults	Last 24 hours	5 min	Clinician: 7	Each behavior item has 4 levels of severity; type of staff intervention and severity of intervention are also ranked	Sum of items, weighted depending on severity; suggested cutoffs with T-score for clinical range of problems	No	No; https://www.bcm.edu/departments/psychiatry-and-behavioral-sciences/index.cfm?pmid=3896
Children's Aggression Scale (CAS) Halperin et al. (2002)	Frequency/severity of aggressive acts, distinct from oppositional and defiant behaviors, within and outside of home setting	5–18 years	Last year	10–15 min	Parent: 33 Teacher: 23	Each item is scored on a 5-point scale with increasing frequency/severity of symptom from "never" to "most days"	Sum of items, weighted depending on severity; suggested cutoffs and percentages with T-score for different severity levels	Yes	Yes; PAR
Buss-Durkee Hostility Inventory (BDHI) Aggression Questionnaire (AQ) Buss and Warren (2000)	Physical aggression, hostility, verbal aggression, anger, indirect aggression	9–88 years	Not specified	10 min	Youth: 34	Each item rated on 5-point scale from "not at all like me" to "completely like me"	Sum of items; corresponding T-score, suggested cutoffs for different severity levels and for "caseness"	Yes	Yes; WPS

properties. The Children's Yale-Brown Obsessive-Compulsive Scale (CY-BOCS, Scahill et al., 1997), a clinician-rated measure, is the measure of choice for tracking treatment outcome.

Two frequently used self-completed measures to screen for symptoms of traumatic stress (see Chapter 59) are the Children's Revised Impact of Event Scale (CRIES, Smith et al., 2003; Yule, 1997) and UCLA Post Traumatic Stress Disorder (PTSD) Reaction Index (USLA-PTSD-RI) Steinberg & Brymer, 2008; Steinberg et al., 2013). The Children's PTSD Inventory (CPTSDI, Saigh et al., 2000) is a clinician-rated measure. The Child PTSD Symptom Scale (CPSS, Foa et al., 2001) can be used as an interview measure by a clinician or can be self-completed. Except for the CRIES, all can be used to assess PTSD as defined by DSM-IV. For eating disorders (see Chapter 71) both the Eating Attitudes Test (EAT-26, Garner et al., 1982) and the Eating Disorder Exam Questionnaire (EDE-Q, Fairburn & Beglin, 1994) may be used for screening.

For bipolar disorder (see Chapter 62), a problematic diagnosis for youth, there is no consensus on a good screening instrument (see Youngstrom et al., 2001; Gracious et al., 2002; Pavuluri et al., 2006; Wagner et al., 2006). Potentially useful clinician-rated measures include the Young Mania Rating Scale (Young et al., 1978) and the K-SADS Mania Rating Scale (Axelson et al., 2003).

Finally, there are many freely available, psychometrically strong screens for substance use (see Chapter 66). These include the CRAFFT Screen tool (Knight et al., 2002), the Adolescent Alcohol and Drug Involvement Scale (AADIS, Moberg, 2000); the CAGE (for alcohol problems) (Ewing, 1984), the Drug Abuse Screening Test for Adolescents (DAST-A, Skinner, 1982; Martino et al., 2000) and the Michigan Alcoholism Screening Test (MAST, Selzer, 1971).

Impairment and functioning

This section focuses on well-known measures with adequate psychometrics. Measures not reviewed include those used primarily in service delivery systems, such as the Child and Adolescent Functional Assessment Scale (CAFAS, Hodges, 2000a, b) and the Child and Adolescent Needs and Strengths-Mental Health (CANS-MH, Lyons et al., 1999), or that are less widely used outside a pure research setting, for example, the Social Adjustment Inventory for Children (John, et al., 1987). In addition, the diagnostic interviews and the omnibus measures reviewed earlier, each include some assessment of impairment.

The Children's Global Assessment Scale (CGAS, Shaffer et al., 1983) is a global, one-item rating scale that asks clinicians to rate the child's most impaired level of functioning from 1 (needs constant supervision) to 100 (superior functioning) within the time period the user selects (typically 1 month) based on all available information. This easy and widely used measure has good psychometrics, though the scale has been criticized for subjective descriptions. A parent-rated version (Bird, 1999) is also available. The scales are available in many languages. Both scales are available at no charge from the authors (DISCGroup@nyspi.columbia.edu).

The Columbia Impairment Scale (CIS, Bird et al., 1993; Bird, 1999) is a global scale completed by parents of children ages 6–17 or to children themselves ages 9 and older. The Brief Impairment Scale (BIS, Bird et al., 2005) contains 10 additional items and evaluates three domains of functioning. These scales have an advantage over the CGAS in that they are respondent based. Both are psychometrically sound; however, neither has been normed or used as often as the CGAS. Both are free from the authors (DISCGroup@nyspi.columbia.edu)

The Vineland Adaptive Behavior Scales, Second Edition (Vineland-II, Sparrow et al., 1984) must be purchased (see www.pearsonclinical.com) and have been widely used in both clinical and research settings, particularly for children with developmental delays, ADHD, or on the "autism spectrum." The Vineland-II covers most of the lifespan, has multiple versions, is useful in various settings, with norms and good psychometrics, and effectively tracks children's developmental progress.

Observations

Observational measures record behaviors at the time they occur. Observations assess children with limited communication and may be less affected by respondent biases than teacher or parent scales. Validity may be affected by both type (e.g., naturalistic versus structured) and setting (e.g., home, school, or clinic) (Gardner, 2000). Because cognitive and internal states must be inferred by physical manifestations, observational methodologies complement but do not replace other assessments (Gardner, 2000).

Some measures directly assess environmental triggers, reinforcers, and factors that maintain behavior, as may occur during social interactions. Some schemes are explicitly designed to "press" for behaviors that may not occur without a trigger, like asking a child to clean up after play or separate from a caregiver. Concrete environmental factors can also be assessed. The Dyadic Parent Child Interaction Coding System (DPICS), the observational assessment in Parent Child Interaction Therapy (PCIT), has proved useful in treating disruptive behaviors.

Observational measures require significant time investments to master coding. Observational assessments can be made in naturalistic, behavioral analog, and standardized settings, usually attempting to capture settings where problematic behaviors typically occur (Skinner et al., 2000). Naturalistic observations have the advantage of ecological validity but may fail to capture relevant, infrequently occurring behavior. Analog observation methods mimic real-life conditions in a clinic setting, sometimes through enactments. For example, a parent and child may be asked to engage in a play activity, where the parent is asked to direct the child to clean up toys. Analog methods facilitate controlled opportunities to elicit low-frequency behaviors (Mash & Foster, 2001). With standardized diagnostic observations, the examiner directly participates as an observer and as a confederate in a systematic protocol that elicits behaviors relevant to a specific diagnosis. The examiner follows a protocol that provides contextual "presses" for specific behaviors.

Below we highlight features of common observational systems.

The Autism Diagnostic Observation Schedule (ADOS-2) involves standardized interactive activities introduced by the clinician in an effort to elicit social interactions and other settings where autism symptoms manifest (Lord *et al.*, 2000, 2001). The ADOS-2 has considerable empirical support and is recommended as a best-practice guideline (National Research Council, 2001). The psychometrics of the ADOS-2 are adequate, provided the user has been properly trained. The ADOS-2 is utilized in conjunction with a parent interview (e.g., the Autism Diagnostic Interview, Revised) and developmental history report. The ADOS-2 is standardized in terms of materials and activities, requiring hierarchical sequences of presses or prompts. It takes 40–60 min to administer, during which time the observer continuously takes qualitative notes. Afterward, the behaviors are coded and entered into an algorithm to rate features of an autism spectrum disorder.

The Disruptive Behavior Diagnostic Observation Schedule (DB-DOS) is a 50-min structured observation method that utilizes behavioral presses. It combines both examiner and parent behavioral observation with parallel sets of presses. Two core domains are assessed: problems in behavioral regulation and problems in anger modulation. The DB-DOS coding system attempts to distinguish normative from clinically concerning misbehavior through clinician judgment. Like the ADOS, the psychometrics are adequate with appropriate training.

The Direct Observation Form (DOF, Achenbach, 1986; Achenbach & Rescorla, 2001), like other components of the ASEBA system, must be purchased. The DOF obtains ratings of problem behaviors and on-task behavior through direct observations of a child over 10 min periods in the classroom and during group activities (such as recess). Because children's behavior may vary across occasions, three to six separate observations are recommended. The DOF is normed and has adequate psychometrics. Clinical utility is a notable strength.

The Student Observation System (SOS) is part of the BASC-2 system, so must be purchased. SOS is designed to assess both adaptive and maladaptive classroom behaviors during a 30-min observation session, typically repeated across 3 or 4 days in different classrooms. The system utilizes a time-sampling method, which has observers recoding student and teacher behavior in 30-s intervals. Student adaptive and maladaptive behaviors are recorded in the last 3 s of the observation. The BASC-2 system also offers a Portable Observation Program (POP), which allows the observer to utilize the SOS template or design their own template for classroom observations on their laptop. The BASC-2 SOS has limited published data regarding psychometric properties.

The Coding Interactive Behavior (CIB, Feldman, 1998) system is a measure that assesses the quality of dyadic interaction with versions for newborns, infants, children, adolescents, and adults.

The CIB has good psychometrics, has been validated, and is sensitive to important sociocultural parameters (Feldman 2003; Feldman & Eidelman, 2007). Training is offered by authors of the measure and qualified trainers with annual monitoring to address rater drift.

Implementing standardized assessments in clinical settings

Clinical use of standardized measures presents several challenges. Many clinicians trust their own clinical judgment and impressions and see little need to change their usual practice; some may already feel overwhelmed by paperwork and record keeping and see little value in adding to that load; and some may worry that their performance will come into question should they not agree with the findings of standard tools. Clinicians may think that using questionnaires may be off-putting to patients and families and will interfere with the clinical process—although research suggests that this is not usually a problem—and that introducing standard diagnostic interviews will constrain their inquiry. Thus, it is important to recognize potential biases, understand the uses of standardized measures, and educate clinical staff about advantages and disadvantages of each measure. For example, if introducing a diagnostic interview, one can point out that structure mimics a typical clinical evaluation; if using the DISC, DAWBA, ASEBA, or BASC systems, efficiency might be emphasized. When using all such measures, it is important to systematically consider procedures for generating the most useful information from each measure. Standardized measures provide efficient assessment structures that are best viewed as aids in the assessment process, which increase consistency. They do not substitute for a comprehensive clinical evaluation, described in Chapter 32.

Conclusion

Standardized measures can be used to assist the clinical process. They include a range of diagnostic interviews, comprehensive questionnaires, more targeted scales, and structured clinical observation schedules. Evidence-based assessments require both effective measurement and sound clinical judgment, with standardized measures aiding, but not replacing clinical skills in assessment.

References

Achenbach, T.M. (1986) *The Direct Observation Form of the Child Behavior Checklist (rev ed).* University of Vermont, Department of Psychiatry, Burlington, VT.

Achenbach, T.M. (2009) *The Achenbach System of Empirically Based Assessment (ASEBA): Development, Findings, Theory, and Applications.* University of Vermont Research Center for Children, Youth and Families, Burlington, VT.

Achenbach, T.M. & Rescorla, L.A. (2001) *Manual for the ASEBA School-Age Forms & Profiles* . Research Center for Children, Youth, and Families, Burlington, VT.

American Psychiatric Association (1980) *Diagnostic and Statistical Manual of Mental Disorders*, 3rd edn. American Psychiatric Association, Washington, DC.

American Psychiatric Association (2013) *Diagnostic and Statistical Manual of Mental Disorders*, 5th edn. American Psychiatric Association, Washington, DC.

Angold, A. *et al.* (1995) The child and adolescent psychiatric assessment (CAPA). *Psychological Medicine* **25**, 739–753.

Axelson, D. *et al.* (2003) A preliminary study of the Kiddie Schedule for Affective Disorders and Schizophrenia for School-Age Children mania rating scale for children and adolescents. *Journal of Child and Adolescent Psychopharmacology* **13**, 463–470.

Bachman, J.W. (2003) The patient-computer interview: a neglected tool that can aid the clinician. *Mayo Clinic Proceedings* **78**, 67–78.

Bagby, R.M. *et al.* (2004) The Hamilton depression rating scale: has the gold standard become a lead weight? *American Journal of Psychiatry* **161**, 2163–2177.

Beck, A.T. *et al.* (1996) *Manual for the Beck Depression Inventory-II*. Psychological Corporation, San Antonio, TX.

Berg, C.J. *et al.* (1986) The Leyton obsessional inventory-child version. *Journal of the American Academy of Child Psychiatry* **25**, 84–91.

Bird, H.R. (1999) The assessment of functional impairment. In: *Diagnostic Assessment in Child and Adolescent Psychopathology*. (eds D. Shaffer, J. Richters & C.P. Lucas), pp. 209–229. Guilford, New York.

Bird, H.R. *et al.* (1993) The Columbia Impairment Scale (CIS): pilot findings on a measure of global impairment for children and adolescents. *International Journal of Methods in Psychiatric Research* **3**, 167–176.

Bird, H.R. *et al.* (2005) The brief impairment scale (BIS): a multidimensional scale of functional impairment for children and adolescents. *Journal of the American Academy of Child & Adolescent Psychiatry* **44**, 699–707.

Birmaher, B. *et al.* (1999) Psychometric properties of the Screen for Child Anxiety Related Emotional Disorders (SCARED): a replication study. *Journal of the American Academy of Child & Adolescent Psychiatry* **38**, 1230–1236.

Buss, A.H. *et al.* (2003) *Rating Scales in Mental Health*, 2nd edn. Lexi-Comp, Hudson, OH.

Buss, A.H. & Warren, W.L. (2000) *Aggression Questionnaire: Manual*. Western Psychological Services. Los Angeles, CA.

Chorpita, B.F. *et al.* (2000) Assessment of symptoms of DSM-IV anxiety and depression in children: a revised child anxiety and depression scale. *Behaviour Research and Therapy* **38**, 835–855.

Conners, K.C. (2008) *Conners*, 3rd edn. Multi-Health Systems, Toronto, Ontario, Canada.

Costello, E.J. *et al.* (1991) Mood variability in adolescents: a study of depressed, nondepressed and comorbid patients. *Journal of Affective Disorders* **23**, 199–212.

Ehlers, S. *et al.* (1999) A screening questionnaire for Asperger syndrome and other high-functioning autism spectrum disorders in school age children. *Journal of Autism and Developmental Disorders* **29**, 129–141.

Ewing, J.A. (1984) Detecting alcoholism. The CAGE questionnaire. *JAMA* **252**, 1905–1907.

Eyberg, S.M. & Pincus, D. (1999) *Eyberg Child Behavior Inventory and Sutter-Eyberg Student Behavior Inventory-Revised: Professional Manual*. Psychological Assessment Resources, Odessa, FL.

Fairburn, C.G. & Beglin, S.J. (1994) Assessment of eating disorder psychopathology: interview for self-report questionnaire? *International Journal of Eating Disorders* **16**, 363–370.

Feldman, R. (1998) *Coding Interactive Behavior Manual*. Unpublished manual. Bar-Ilan University, Israel.

Feldman, R. (2003) Testing a family intervention hypothesis: the contribution of mother-infant skin to skin contact (kangaroo care) to family interaction, proximity, and touch. *Journal of Family Psychology* **17**, 94–107.

Feldman, R. & Eidelman, A.I. (2007) Maternal postpartum behavior and the emergence of infant-mother and infant-father synchrony in preterm and full-term infants: the role of neonatal vagal tone. *Developmental Psychobiology* **49**, 290–302.

Foa, E.B. *et al.* (2001) The child PTSD Symptom Scale: a preliminary examination of its psychometric properties. *Journal of Clinical Child Psychology* **30**, 376–384.

Gadow, K.D. & Sprafkin, J. (1994) *Child Symptom Inventories Manual*. Checkmate Plus, Stony Brook, NY.

Galanter, C.A. & Patel, V.L. (2005) Medical decision making: a selective review for child psychiatrists and psychologists. *Journal of Child Psychology and Psychiatry* **46**, 675–689.

Garner, D.M. *et al.* (1982) The eating attitudes test: psychometric features and clinical correlates. *Psychological Medicine* **12**, 871–878.

Gardner, F. (2000) Methodological issues in the direct observation of parent–child interactions: do observational findings reflect the natural behavior of participants? *Clinical Child and Family Psychology Review* **3**, 185–198.

Geller, B. *et al.* (2001) Reliability of the Washington University in St. Louis Kiddie Schedule for Affective Disorders and Schizophrenia (WASH-UKSADS) mania and rapid cycling sections. *Journal of the American Academy of Child and Adolescent Psychiatry* **40**, 450–455.

Goodman, R. (1997) The strengths and difficulties questionnaire: a research note. *Journal of Child Psychology and Psychiatry* **38**, 581–586.

Goodman, R. (2001) Psychometric properties of the strengths and difficulties questionnaire. *Journal of the American Academy of Child & Adolescent Psychiatry* **40**, 1337–1345.

Goodman, R. & Scott, S. (1999) Comparing the strengths and difficulties questionnaire and the child behavior checklist: is small beautiful? *Journal of Abnormal Child Psychology* **27**, 17–24.

Goodman, R. *et al.* (2000) The development and well-being assessment: description and initial validation of an integrated assessment of child and adolescent psychopathology. *Journal of Child Psychology and Psychiatry* **41**, 645–655.

Gracious, B.L. *et al.* (2002) Discriminative validity of a parent version of the Young Mania Rating Scale. *Journal of the American Academy of Child & Adolescent Psychiatry* **41**, 1350–1359.

Guy, W. (1976) *ECDEU Assessment Manual for Psychopharmacology*, pp. 218–222. U.S. Department of Health, Education, and Welfare, Public Health Service, Alcohol, Drug Abuse, and Mental Health Administration, NIMH Psychopharmacology Research Branch, Division of Extramural Research Programs, Rockville, MD.

Halperin, J.M. *et al.* (2002) Development, reliability, and validity of the children's aggression scale-parent version. *Journal of the American Academy of Child & Adolescent Psychiatry* **41**, 245–252.

Halperin, J.M. *et al.* (2003) Reliability, validity, and preliminary normative data for the Children's Aggression Scale-Teacher Version. *Journal of the American Academy of Child & Adolescent Psychiatry* **42**, 965–971.

Hamilton, M. (1959) The assessment of anxiety states by rating. *British Journal of Medical Psychology* **32**, 50–55.

Hamilton, M. (1960) A rating scale for depression. *Journal of Neurology, Neurosurgery, and Psychiatry* **23**, 56–62.

Hodges, K. (2000a) *Child and Adolescent Functional Assessment Scale.* Eastern Michigan University, Ypsilanti, MI.

Hodges, K. (2000b) *Child and Adolescent Functional Assessment Scale Self-Training Manual.* Eastern Michigan University, Ypsilanti, MI.

Hysing, M. *et al.* (2007) Chronic physical illness and mental health in children. Results from a large-scale population study. *Journal of Child Psychology and Psychiatry* **48**, 785–792.

John, K. *et al.* (1987) The Social Adjustment Inventory for Children and Adolescents (SAICA): testing of a new semi-structured interview. *Journal of the American Academy of Child & Adolescent Psychiatry* **26**, 898–911.

Kaufman, J. *et al.* (1997) Schedule for Affective Disorders and Schizophrenia for school-age children present and lifetime version (K-SADS-PL): initial reliability and validity data. *Journal of the American Academy of Child & Adolescent Psychiatry* **36**, 980–988.

Knight, J.R. *et al.* (2002) Validity of the CRAFFT substance abuse screening test among adolescent clinic patients. *Archives of Pediatrics & Adolescent Medicine* **156**, 607–614.

Kovacs, M. (2010) *Children's Depression Inventory Manual.* Multi-Health Systems Inc, Toronto, ON.

Leckman, J.F. *et al.* (1989) The Yale Global Tic Severity Scale: initial testing of a clinician-rated scale of tic severity. *Journal of the American Academy of Child and Adolescent Psychiatry* **28**, 566–573.

Loeber, R. *et al.* (1990) Mental health professionals' perception of the utility of children, mothers, and teachers as informants on childhood psychopathology. *Journal of Clinical Child Psychology* **19**, 136–143.

Lord, C. *et al.* (2000) The Autism Diagnostic Observation Schedule-generic: a standard measure of social and communication deficits associated with the spectrum of autism. *Journal of Autism and Developmental Disorders* **30**, 205–223.

Lord, C. *et al.* (2001) *Autism Diagnostic Observation Schedule.* Western Psychological Services, Los Angeles, CA.

Lyons, J.S. *et al.* (1999) *Child and Adolescent Needs and Strengths: An Information Integration Tool for Children and Adolescents With Mental Health Challenges (CANS-MH), Manual.* Buddin Praed Foundation, Chicago.

March, J.S. (1997) *Manual for the Multidimensional Anxiety Scale for Children (MASC).* Multi-Health Systems Inc, Toronto, ON.

March, J.S. (2012) *Manual for the Multidimensional Anxiety Scale for Children (MASC).* Multi-Health Systems Inc, Toronto, ON.

March, J.S. *et al.* (1997) The Multidimensional Anxiety Scale for Children (MASC): factor structure, reliability, and validity. *Journal of American Academy of Child & Adolescent Psychiatry* **36**, 554–65.

Martino, S. *et al.* (2000) Development of the drug abuse screening test for adolescents (DAST-A). *Addictive Behaviors* **25**, 57–70.

Mash, E.J. & Foster, S.L. (2001) Exporting analogue behavioral observation from research to clinical practice: useful or cost-defective? *Psychological Assessment* **13**, 86–98.

Moberg, D.P. (2000) *The Adolescent Alcohol and Drug Involvement Scale.* University of Wisconsin, Center for Health Policy and Program Evaluation, Madison, WI.

Moore, H.K. *et al.* (2007) A pilot study of an electronic, adolescent, version of the quick inventory of depressive symptomatology. *Journal of Clinical Psychiatry* **68**, 1436–1440.

Murphy, J.M. & Jellinek, M.S. (1985) *Development of a Brief Psycho-Social Screening Instrument for Pediatric Practice: Final Report. NIMH Contract No: 84 M0213612.* National Institute of Mental Health, Rockville, MD.

National Research Council (2001) *Educating Children with Autism.* National Academy Press, Washington, DC.

Nauta, M.H. *et al.* (2004) A parent-report measure of children's anxiety: psychometric properties and comparison with child-report in a clinic and normal sample. *Behaviour Research and Therapy* **42**, 813–839.

Pavuluri, M.N. *et al.* (2006) Child mania rating scale: development, reliability, and validity. *Journal of the American Academy of Child & Adolescent Psychiatry* **45**, 550–560.

Poznanski, E. & Mokros, H. (1996) *Children's Depression Rating Scale–Revised (CDRS-R).* Western Psychological Services, Los Angeles, CA.

Radloff, L.S. (1977) The CES-D scale: a self-report depression scale for research in the general population. *Applied Psychological Measurement* **1**, 385–401.

Reich, W. (2000) Diagnostic interview for children and adolescents (DICA). *Journal of American Academy of Child & Adolescent Psychiatry* **39**, 59–66.

Reich, W. & Todd, R.D. (1997) Missouri Assessment of Genetics Interview for Children (MAGIC). [Copyright authors].

Rescorla, L. (2009) Rating scale systems for assessing psychopathology: the Achenbach System of Empirically Based Assessment (ASEBA) and the Behavioral Assessment System for Children-2 (BASC-2). In: *Assessing Childhood Psychopathology and Developmental Disabilities.* (eds J.L. Matson *et al.*), pp. 117–149. Springer, New York.

Rescorla, L.A. *et al.* (2013) Cross-informant agreement between parent-reported and adolescent self-reported problems in 25 societies. *Journal of Clinical Child and Adolescent Psychology* **42**, 262–273.

Reynolds, C.R. & Kamphaus, R.W. (2004) *The BASC-2: Behavior Assessment System for Children*, 2nd edn. Pearson, Bloomington, Minnesota.

Reynolds, C.R. & Richmond, B.O. (1985) *Revised Children's Manifest Anxiety Scale. RCMAS Manual.* Western Psychological Services, Los Angeles, CA.

Reynolds, W.M. (2002) *Reynolds Adolescent Depression Scale: Professional Manual*, 2nd edn. Psychological Assessment Resources, Lutz, FL.

Reynolds, W.M. (2010) *Reynolds Child Depression Scale-2.* Psychological Assessment Resources, Lutz, FL.

Reynolds, C.R. & Richmond, B.O. (2008) *The Revised Children's Manifest Anxiety Scale*, 2nd edn. Western Psychological Services, Los Angeles, CA.

Robins, D.L. *et al.* (1999) *The Modified Checklist for Autism in Toddlers. (M-CHAT).* Self-published, Storrs, CT.

RUPP Anxiety Study Group (2002) The Pediatric Anxiety Rating Scale (PARS): development and psychometric properties. *Journal of the American Academy of Child & Adolescent Psychiatry* **41**, 1061–1069.

Rush, A.J. *et al.* (1996) The Inventory of Depressive Symptomatology (IDS) psychometric properties. *Psychological Medicine* **26**, 477–486.

Rush, A.J. *et al.* (2003) The 16-Item Quick Inventory of Depressive Symptomatology (QIDS), clinician rating (QIDS-C), and self-report (QIDS-SR): a psychometric evaluation in patients with chronic major depression. *Biological Psychiatry* **54**, 573–583.

Rutter, M. *et al.* (2003a) *The Social Communication Questionnaire manual.* Western Psychological Services, Los Angeles, CA.

Rutter, M. *et al.* (2003b) *Autism Diagnostic Interview-Revised.* Western Psychological Services, Los Angeles, CA.

Saigh, P. *et al.* (2000) The children's PTSD inventory: development and reliability. *Journal of Traumatic Stress* **13**, 369–380.

Scahill, L. *et al.* (1997) Children's Yale-Brown obsessive compulsive scale: reliability and validity. *Journal of the American Academy of Child and Adolescent Psychiatry* **36**, 844–852.

Schopler, E. *et al.* (2010) *Childhood Autism Rating Scale*, 2nd edn. Western Psychological Services, Los Angeles, CA.

Selzer, M.L. (1971) The Michigan Alcoholism Screening test (MAST): the quest for a new diagnostic instrument. *American Journal of Psychiatry* **127**, 1653–1658.

Shaffer, D. *et al.* (1983) A children's global assessment scale (CGAS). *Archives of General Psychiatry* **40**, 1228–1231.

Shaffer, D. *et al.* (1999) Respondent-based interviews. In: *Diagnostic Assessment in Child and Adolescent Psychopathology.* (eds D. Shaffer & C.P. Lucas), 1st edn, pp. 3–33. The Guilford Press, New York.

Shaffer, D. *et al.* (2000) NIMH diagnostic interview schedule for children, version IV (NIMH DISC-IV): description, differences from previous versions, and reliability of some common diagnoses. *Journal of the American Academy of Child & Adolescent Psychiatry* **39**, 28–38.

Silverman, W.K. & Albano, A.M. (1996) *The Anxiety Disorders Interview Schedule for DSM-IV-Child and Parent Versions.* Oxford University Press, London.

Skinner, H.A. (1982) The drug abuse screening test. *Addictive Behaviors* **7**, 363–371.

Skinner, C. *et al.* (2000) Increasing tootling: the effects of a peer-monitored group contingency program on students' reports of peers' prosocial behaviors. *Psychology in the Schools* **37**, 263–269.

Smith, P. *et al.* (2003) Principal components analysis of the Impact of Event Scale with children in war. *Personality and Individual Differences* **34**, 315–22.

Sorgi, P. *et al.* (1991) Rating aggression in the clinical setting. A retrospective adaptation of the overt aggression scale: preliminary results. *Journal of Neuropsychiatry* **3**, S52–S56.

Sparrow, S.S. *et al.* (1984) *Vineland Adaptive Behavior Scales.* Pearson Assessments, Bloomington, MN.

Spence, S.H. (1998) A measure of anxiety symptoms among children. *Behavior Research and Therapy* **36**, 545–566.

Spence, S.H. *et al.* (2001) The structure of anxiety symptoms among preschoolers. *Behaviour Research and Therapy* **39**, 1293–1316.

Spielberger, C.D. *et al.* (1973) *Preliminary Manual for the State-Trait Anxiety Inventory for Children.* Consulting Psychologists Press, Palo Alto, CA.

Steinberg, A.M. & Brymer, M.J. (2008) The UCLA PTSD reaction index. In: *Encyclopedia of Psychological Trauma.* (eds G. Reyes, J. Elhai & J. Ford), pp. 673–674. John Wiley & Sons, Hoboken, NJ.

Steinberg, A.M. *et al.* (2013) Psychometric properties of the UCLA PTSD reaction index: part I. *Journal of Traumatic Stress* **26**, 1–9.

Swanson, J.M. *et al.* (2001) Clinical relevance of the primary findings of the MTA: success rates based on severity of ADHD and ODD symptoms at the end of treatment. *Journal of the American Academy of Child and Adolescent Psychiatry* **40**, 168–179.

Swanson, J. *et al.* (2006) *Categorical and Dimensional Definitions and Evaluations of Symptoms of ADHD: The SNAP and SWAN Rating Scales.* University of California, Irvine, CA.

Taylor, J. (1953) A personality scale of manifest anxiety. *Journal of Abnormal and Social Psychology* **48**, 285–90.

Wagner, K.D. *et al.* (2006) Validation of the Mood Disorder Questionnaire for bipolar disorders in adolescents. *Journal of Clinical Psychiatry* **67**, 827–830.

Warren, W.L. (1997) *Revised Hamilton Rating Scale for Depression (HRSD): Manual.* Western Psychological Services, Los Angeles, CA.

Weissman, M.M. *et al.* (1980) Children's symptom and social functioning self-report scales: comparison of mothers' and children's reports. *Journal of Nervous Mental Disorders* **168**, 736–740.

Wolraich, M.L. *et al.* (1998) Obtaining systematic teacher reports of disruptive behavior disorders utilizing DSM-IV. *Journal of Abnormal Child Psychology* **26**, 141–152.

Wolraich, M.L. *et al.* (2003) Psychometric properties of the Vanderbilt ADHD diagnostic parent rating scale in a referred population. *Journal of Pediatric Psychology* **28**, 559–567.

Woods, D.W. *et al.* (2005) Premonitory Urge for Tics Scale (PUTS): initial psychometric results and examination of the premonitory urge phenomenon in youths with tic disorders. *Journal of Developmental and Behavioral Pediatrics* **26**, 397–403.

Young, R.C. *et al.* (1978) A rating scale for mania: reliability, validity and sensitivity. *British Journal of Psychiatry* **33**, 429–435.

Youngstrom, E.A. *et al.* (2001) Discriminative validity of parent report of hypomanic and depressive symptoms on the General Behavior Inventory. *Psychological Assessment* **13**, 267.

Yudofsky, S.C. *et al.* (1986) The Overt Aggression Scale for the objective rating of verbal and physical aggression. *American Journal of Psychiatry* **143**, 35–39.

Yule, W. (1997) Anxiety, depression and post-traumatic stress in childhood. In: *Child Psychology Portfolio.* (ed I. Sclare). Windsor, NFER-Nelson. Berkshire, UK.

CHAPTER 34

Psychological assessment in the clinical context

Tony Charman[1], Jane Hood[2] and Patricia Howlin[1]
[1] Department of Psychology, Institute of Psychiatry, Psychology and Neuroscience, King's College London, UK
[2] Centre for Developmental Neuropsychology, Oxon, UK

Introduction

Psychological assessment of young people may be needed for many reasons. Usually, the assessment will be a response to concerns that an adult has about the young person. The assessment domains that need to be considered are wide and, given the well-established link between developmental, cognitive or learning difficulties and emotional and behavioral difficulties, most assessments should consider both development and behavior, alongside the child's emotional well-being. The family, home, and school environment should also be considered. Psychological assessment will often include some direct assessment of the child's functioning, observations of the child, interviews with parents and, where appropriate, relevant information from school. Depending on the setting, both formal and informal measurement and testing may be required. Psychological assessment should adopt a "scientist-practitioner" model whereby a theory-driven assessment generates and tests hypotheses. Thus, the assessment provides a framework for difficulties to be targeted for remediation (see Figure 34.1).

Many professionals will use aspects of psychological assessments. In communities with well-developed professional structures these will typically include clinical (health service) and educational (school) psychologists as well as other professionals. In such communities, the most common service settings in which psychological assessments take place are child psychiatric services, child development/pediatric services, education settings and child health settings, as well as some specialist medical settings (e.g., neurology, genetic counseling services). Other practitioners will also benefit from material covered in this chapter, which also apply to many non-psychological practitioners in low- and middle-income countries where professional training in psychology is less well established.

This chapter first describes broad principles underpinning assessments. We then summarize information on commonly-used norm-referenced measures. We conclude by discussing how psychological assessment informs interventions.

Psychological assessment within the broader context

Later in the chapter, we describe tests of intelligence. However, psychological assessment is much more than intelligence testing! Although psychometric tests serve important functions, children rarely are referred solely to measure their intelligence quotient (IQ). Psychological assessment is more often requested because of wider concerns—Why has a child suddenly become withdrawn and sullen? Why is she/he having so many problems within the classroom? Why is she/he falling behind the rest of the class, or is unable to relate to peers? The primary purpose of psychological assessment is to gain insight into a young person's behavioral, mental-health, educational, or learning difficulties, by developing and testing formulations about underlying influences and thus guiding interventions. It involves many methods, informal as well as formal, based in the context of the younger person's family and other key environments (e.g., school, peer group, and wider society). In other words, psychological assessment is not merely the administration of tests but involves the identification of key clinical issues pertaining to each *individual* case; the formulation of clinical issues into testable hypotheses; and the recurrent implementation and evaluation of hypothesis-driven interventions (see Chapter 32).

Informal and semi-formal clinical assessments

Pre-assessment assessments

Individual clinical assessments are costly in terms of both time and personnel, but appropriate use of pre-existing information

---

Rutter's Child and Adolescent Psychiatry, Sixth Edition.
Edited by Anita Thapar and Daniel S. Pine, James F. Leckman, Stephen Scott, Margaret J. Snowling, Eric Taylor.
© 2015 John Wiley & Sons Ltd. Published 2018 by John Wiley & Sons Ltd.

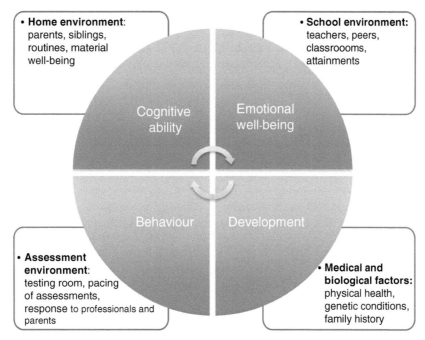

Figure 34.1 Child and environmental factors relevant to psychological assessment.

can greatly improve assessment efficiency and effectiveness. Detailed referral information can provide extremely helpful history, which can ensure availability of necessary clinical expertise and relevant individuals to inform the assessment. Information from parents, schools, and other services also can focus the assessment on the most pressing needs of the child and family. School reports should always be obtained prior to the assessment. Parent or teacher-based questionnaires (e.g., Strengths and Difficulties Questionnaire (SDQ; Goodman, 1997), Developmental Behaviour Checklist (DBC; Einfeld & Tonge, 2002) can identify general difficulties, while longer informant-based instruments such as the Development and Well Being Assessment (DAWBA; Goodman et al., 2000) can provide information about diagnosis. For specialist clinics (e.g., for children with autism), which frequently have long waiting lists, diagnosis-based questionnaires such as the Social Communication Questionnaire (SCQ; Rutter et al., 2003) can help to avoid costly assessments of children who clearly do not meet diagnostic criteria. However, the value of such pre-assessment information relies heavily on the quality of the information provided, and should not constrain either the range of areas covered by the assessment or the potential formulations explored as part of the assessment.

Clinic-based assessments

Careful child observation in the clinic, with parents and with unfamiliar adults, provides important information. Thus, even before testing begins, much can be learned from observing the young person in the waiting room (see Chapter 33). Clinical observations can also inform which formal assessments to undertake, how best to conduct them and how results should

be interpreted. In addition, clinic-based assessments enable the clinician to control environmental variables in order to obtain the best standardized sample of behavior. They also make it possible systematically to vary environmental "presses" and the structure in which the child is observed to assess impact on behavior. Structured observational schedules exist for some specific disorders (e.g., Autism Diagnostic Observation Schedule (ADOS-2; Lord et al., 2012); Disruptive Behavior Diagnostic Observation Schedule (DB-DOS; Wakschlag et al., 2008)). However, some measures are expensive and require extensive training.

Interviewing children and young people and parents

Structured interviews are a crucial part of any clinical assessment, and many different instruments are available (see Chapter 33). These include those designed to assess a range of possible psychopathologies (e.g., Kiddie-SADS-Present and Lifetime Version (K-SADS-PL; Kaufman et al., 1997) and measures that focus on specific disorders (e.g., the Autism Diagnostic Interview-Revised (ADI-R; Lord et al., 1994)). It is also important to obtain the child's own views of his or her difficulties and for school-aged children of average intellectual and language ability a range of well-standardized and -validated instruments, of varying lengths and complexity is available (see Chapter 33). However, informal conversation (e.g., about home life, school, friends, hobbies, likes, and dislikes, why they think they have come to the clinic, how they are feeling generally, etc.) can provide invaluable additional information. Tone of voice, facial expression, general attitude can also reveal a great deal about the young person's mood and emotional state. Many young people will be understandably reluctant to disclose information about personal issues or worries in front of their parents and will need to be interviewed alone, and this is clearly essential if child abuse or maltreatment is suspected. However, if appropriate, some time spent with both the young person and their parents together can provide important information about family relationships.

Interviewing very young or developmentally impaired children presents more difficulties, as standardized interviews tend to be inappropriate for their cognitive and/or linguistic level. Engaging them in play or viewing age-appropriate media may be informative (Beresford *et al.*, 2004). Because such children are distressed if separated from their parents it will usually be necessary to see them in the presence of a parent, which can provide additional valuable information.

Non-clinic-based assessment

A good-quality clinical assessment is time-consuming and requires expertise, but a few-hour assessment provides only a limited snap-shot of the child's functioning. Moreover, children's behavior in the clinic may not be representative of their behavior elsewhere. For example, a child who is polite, quiet and compliant may be highly disruptive in familiar settings. Parental reports may misrepresent the child's difficulties because of biases related to parents' background or problems. The father of a child with autism, for example, may underplay the difficulties, noting "I was just like that at his age and I don't have any problems now." School reports, too, can be biased. A well-behaved child with severe learning problems may be described as having no discernible difficulties, while a disruptive child of average IQ may be reported as failing academically as well as socially. Despite standardization in questionnaires, these, too, are not bias-free, and if respondents have intellectual or language problems they may not necessarily interpret questions correctly. In such circumstances, the only way to obtain more reliable information on the child and the factors that contribute to his or her difficulties is to supplement the clinical assessment with direct observations.

The need for non-clinic-based assessment is especially important when there is a discrepancy between the various accounts of behavior, for example, disagreements between parents and teachers concerning the nature or severity of the presenting difficulties, or when the behavior observed in the clinic does not tally with other reports. For example, a child referred for learning or behavioral difficulties at school may, on testing, show no obvious intellectual impairment. If more detailed assessment also fails to identify any specific cognitive/learning impairments then further investigation will be needed to explore possible home- or school-based factors (family disruption, parent–child relationship problems, bullying or emotional or mental health problems) that are affecting progress.

Difficulties in social relationships are a common reason for referrals to child and mental health services and informal observations can provide valuable information on the child's interaction with others across a range of different settings—for example, with teachers and assistants within the classroom or with peers in the playground at school. Although difficulties in social interactions and social behavior (ranging from peer interactions to attachment relationships with parents/carers) are often the primary focus of such observations they can also provide information about many other aspects of the child or young person's functioning, including emotional responses (e.g., shyness, anxiety), activity levels, and motor skills.

Unstandardized assessments are particularly important for children who cannot complete other measures due to profound learning difficulties. Informal observations of the child interacting with a familiar adult can provide valuable information. The adults involved can also provide information about their interpretation of the child's responses or what is triggering a specific behavior. However, behaviors may be misinterpreted. For example, aggressive behavior may be a severely impaired child's main way of indicating distress, which adults can misinterpret as deliberate attempts to harm others. Alternatively, a classroom assistant may insist that the child "understands every word you say" although the child is, in fact, able to follow only a few simple commands in specific contexts (e.g., will respond to "Get your coat" because all the other children are going outside).

Psychological assessments conducted outside the clinic may also produce unpredicted findings. For example, in group settings (the home, classroom or a residential unit) reports of difficulties often focus on one particular individual. However, systematic observations sometimes indicate that the problem is not restricted to the referral case. For example, a teacher in a school for children with moderate learning difficulties had asked for help with a particular student who was described as being constantly off task and disrupting other pupils. Classroom assessments included counts of on task behaviors using very simple time sampling techniques (child not/sitting at desk at 15 min intervals). These indicated that the child concerned was off task no more than other pupils. However, when out of his desk he had a habit of dribbling and smearing saliva and it was this specific undesirable behavior that needed to be the focus of intervention.

In families, too, although one child is the focus of parental concerns, there may also be difficulties with regard to other siblings. A broad psychological assessment can be crucial in identifying these and in refocusing intervention on the wider family dynamics (see Chapter 39).

Formal psychometric assessment

Intelligence testing

Since the emergence of "intelligence testing" (Galton, 1883; Cattell, 1890), there has been much debate about what "intelligence" is and how to measure it. One approach defines intelligence as "what intelligence tests measure" (Sparrow & Davis, 2000). Spearman (1904) proposed his concept of a "g" or general factor, empirically derived from factor analysis. While the subsequent century-long debate about the existence and nature of "g" has failed to reach consensus, most contemporary theories admit the presence of a general factor, with recent indications that this may have an identifiable brain basis (Duncan, 2010). There is strong evidence that intelligence tests measure something meaningful about development, cognitive abilities, and adaptive behavior. Thus, IQ scores show moderate (0.6) to high (0.8) stability (Watkins & Smith, 2013) and correlate highly with real-life outcomes, such as academic achievements and income (Fergusson *et al.*, 2005).

Standardized assessments

Understanding of psychometric theory and the statistical methods used to derive standardized scores is essential for evaluation of intelligence tests. Statistical methods, primarily factor analysis, have been used to derive global metrics of psychological constructs from individual test items. Many standardized tests have scaled scores with means of 100 and standard deviations of 15 although others use T-scores with means of 50 and standard deviations of 10. Standard scores are then used to define average, below average or superior ability depending on how many standard deviations above or below the general population mean a child's performance lies (see Kaplan & Saccuzzo, 2013; for a comprehensive review). Figure 34.2 shows a model standardization/normal curve with the percentages of a population who would fall above/below the various standard deviation scores and the standard and T-scores derived in many IQ and developmental tests.

Findings from standardized tests then have to be related to the educational or clinical classification systems that operate in any country. These may differ from those used in the ICD-10 (WHO, 1993) and DSM-5 (American Psychiatric Association, 2013) classification systems—sometimes creating a tension between medical-led clinical teams and education-led school services. Thus, within the UK education system, an IQ between 70 and 50/55 is described as "moderate learning difficulty,"

whereas ICD-10/DSM-5 criteria define an IQ in this range as being indicative of "mild" intellectual impairment. Furthermore, terms such as "learning difficulty," "learning disability" and "intellectual disability" tend to be used interchangeably, and confusingly. It is important in clinical practice for a technical summary of psychometric assessment results to be clear about the definition and use of terms employed to minimize misunderstanding.

What makes a "good" test?

In determining the applicability of any test, consideration should be given to the size, composition and diversity of the standardization sample in relation to the individual, group or setting for which it is to be used. Characteristics such as age, sex, educational, social, racial, economic, and geographical backgrounds of the normative sample are all important. For example, individuals with low IQ are often omitted from school-based standardization samples (Simonoff *et al.*, 2006)—leading to problems in the use of many IQ tests with children with more severe intellectual disabilities. *When* the test was normed is also crucial as there is likely to be an increase in scores in successive cohorts of children from any one country (the so-called "Flynn effect"), generally due to a combination of improvements in diet and education (Nijenhuis & van der Flier, 2013). Clinical reports should state the nature of the normative sample when this differs from the testing situation (e.g., test was normed in a different country).

Other critical test parameters are *reliability* and *validity*. The different types of reliability that are most relevant are split-half and test-retest reliability—the latter is particularly important for indicating the minimum test-retest time period that is vulnerable to practice and other learning effects. Some tests provide parallel forms to enable such difficulties to be minimized. Construct validity is usually documented by comparing test scores from the normative sample to scores on another established IQ test or to a previous version of the same test.

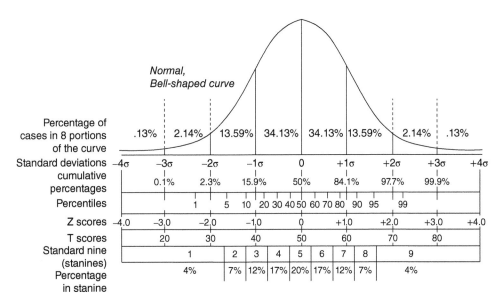

Figure 34.2 A model standardization/normal curve with percentages, *Z*-score and *T*-scores.

The final "test of a good test" is the *accessibility* and *relevance* of the test items to the population on whom the test is to be used. Particular considerations (e.g., on timed items) apply for children with sensory or physical limitations such as those with cerebral palsy or sight or hearing-impairments. Some tests of general intelligence, such as the Wechsler tests, rely heavily on understanding verbal instructions; others specifically eliminate the need for verbal comprehension (see later). Another consideration is how attractive and engaging the materials are and more recent editions of many of the most widely used intelligence tests now use colorful and modern test stimuli.

Tests of general intelligence

Among the best-established tests are the Stanford-Binet—fifth edition (SB-5; Roid, 2003); the Differential Abilities Scale (DAS-II; Elliot, 2007) and its UK counterpart the British Abilities Scale (BAS-3; Elliot & Smith, 2011) and the suite of Wechsler tests (Wechsler Preschool and Primary Scale of Intelligence—fourth edition (WPPSI-IV; Wechsler, 2012); Wechsler Intelligence Scale for Children—fourth edition (WISC-IV; Wechsler, 2003); Wechsler Adult Intelligence Scale—fourth edition (WAIS-IV; Wechsler, 2008)). The age ranges and derived standardized scores of these widely used tests are summarized in Table 34.1. There is less emphasis than in previous versions on the Performance (PIQ) and Verbal (VIQ) Intelligence Scale scores, with a more neuropsychological approach to grouping different abilities, supported by results of factor analysis. These index scores are more closely tied to empirically based theories of intelligence and have greater potential remedial value in identifying individual profiles of cognitive strengths and weaknesses.

Other tests are modeled on different theories of intelligence and are also more explicitly linked to strategies for remediation. For example, the Kaufman Assessment Battery for Children-II (KABC-II; Kaufman & Kaufman, 2004) is derived from Luria's (1966) neuropsychological model of information processing (simultaneous vs sequential) as opposed to information content (verbal vs visual-spatial). A valuable component of the Kaufman tests is the reduced reliance on verbal understanding/responding, so that non-verbal subtests can be both administered and responded to without speech. Many other tests of general intelligence are also available, as reviewed in Flanagan and Harrison (2012).

A general approach for supporting children's progress and learning is to help them (and their parents and teachers) to use areas of relative strength to compensate for areas of relative weakness, for example, by using additional visual materials and structure for a child or young person with weaker verbal comprehension skills.

There are many brief IQ assessments available, such as the Wechsler Abbreviated Scale of Intelligence (WASI-II; Wechsler, 2011) and the Kaufman Brief Intelligence Test—second edition (K-BIT-2; Kaufman & Kaufman, 2006) and others that can be administered across whole school populations, such as the Cognitive Abilities Test—third edition (CAT3; Lohman *et al.*, 2001). Such measures can usefully index general functioning for research purposes and can guide the clinician when a child with prior testing requires updated assessments to monitor progress. However, results can be misleading if wrongly applied in clinical settings. For example, achieving an average range IQ on a brief assessment does not rule out the presence of significant specific learning difficulties, which is more likely (but not always) to be picked up by a comprehensive omnibus test. Similarly, a low score alone does not provide detailed information about the nature of the child's difficulties.

Assessments for infants and toddlers

Psychological assessment of infants and toddlers requires particular expertise with this age group (see Chapters 6 and 7).

Until the 1990s, the use of intelligence tests with preschool children and toddlers was controversial, both because of unease about the appropriateness of such testing and concerns regarding stability (Flanagan & Alfonso, 1995). However, in the past two decades, there has been considerable development of preschool tests. Several of the instruments reviewed earlier have extended the age range downwards to 2–3 years (e.g., SB-5; DAS-II/BAS-3; WPPSI IV). There has also been more cross-fertilization between the approach that psychologists have traditionally taken and that taken by developmental pediatricians in which there was a decades-old tradition of pediatric developmental assessments.

Stemming from the work of Ruth Griffiths (1935) and Mary Sheridan (1945), but also influenced by Piaget's stages of infant and child development, several developmental assessments for infants and preschoolers have been developed. These include the Griffiths Mental Development Scales (Griffiths, 2006), Bayley Scales of Infant and Toddler Development (Bayley-III, 2005), and Mullen Scales of Early Learning (Mullen, 1995) (see Snow & Van Hemel, 2008 for comprehensive reviews of preschool assessments and Table 1). These tests involve direct assessments of young children's abilities using play-based materials as well as observations of the child in the clinic and, in some cases, parental reports of the child's functioning. They provide age-equivalent scores in domains of behavior such as fine and gross motor skills, expressive and receptive language ability, and early non-verbal conceptual reasoning and also allow an overall developmental quotient (akin to an IQ score for older children) to be calculated.

Caution needs to be employed in interpreting findings from assessments with infants under 2 years of age, particularly in terms of making judgements about likely outcome and prognosis. Even in cohorts of typically developing children, correlations between scores obtained in infancy and scores on tests completed later in childhood are only moderate, particularly when subdomains of functioning are considered (Aylward, 2004). In clinical samples including preterm infants (Hack *et al.*, 2005) and infants with autism (Charman *et al.*, 2005), the association between very early IQ/DQ scores and scores in mid-childhood

Table 34.1 Age ranges and derived standarization scores of widely used IQ and developmental assessments.

Test	Age range (years: months)	Key Standardized scores/subscales
General Intelligence tests		
British Abilities Scale—third edition (BAS-3; Elliot & Smith, 2011)	3:00 to 17:11	General conceptual ability Verbal ability Non-verbal reasoning ability Spatial ability Special non-verbal composite
Differential Abilities Scale—second edition (DAS-II; Elliot, 2007)	2:6 to 17:11	General conceptual ability score Verbal ability Non-verbal reasoning ability Spatial ability Special non-verbal composite
Stanford-Binet—fifth edition (SB-5; Roid, 2003)	2:00 to 85+	Full scale IQ Verbal IQ Non-verbal IQ Brief IQ 5 Factors scores: fluid, knowledge, quantitative, visual-spatial, and working memory
Wechsler Preschool and Primary Scale of Intelligence—fourth edition (WPPSI-IV; Wechsler, 2012)	2:6 to 7:7	Full scale IQ Verbal comprehension index Visual spatial index Working memory index Fluid reasoning index Processing speed index
Wechsler Intelligence Scale for Children—fourth edition (WISC-IV; Wechsler, 2003)	6:00 to 16:11	Full scale IQ Verbal comprehension index Perceptual reasoning Working memory index Processing speed index
Wechsler Adult Intelligence Scale—fourth edition (WAIS-IV; Wechsler, 2008)	16:00 to 90:11	Full Scale IQ Verbal comprehension index Perceptual reasoning Working memory index Processing speed index
Kaufman Assessment Battery for Children-II (KABC-II; Kaufman & Kaufman, 2004)	3:00 to 18:11	Mental processing composite Fluid-crystallized index Non-verbal composite Simultaneous processing Sequential processing

Test *Developmental tests*	*Age range (months)*	*Key Standardized scores/subscales*
Bayley Scales of Infant and Toddler Development—third edition (Bayley-III, 2005)	1–42	Adaptive behavior Cognitive Language Motor Social–emotional
Griffiths Mental Development Scales (Griffiths, 2006)	1–96	General quotient Locomotor Personal–social Language Eye and hand co-ordination Performance
Mullen Scales of Early Learning (Mullen, 1995)	1–68	Early learning composite Gross motor Fine motor Visual reception Expressive language Receptive language

is modest to poor. This partly reflects difficulties inherent in infant testing due to the different nature of infant vs. childhood developmental accomplishments and hence the skills tested at different ages, as well as the fact that environmental influences become more evident after 2 years of age. After the age of 2 years, the stability of test scores significantly increases (Aylward, 2009).

Tests of other abilities

Although the types of tests described earlier will provide an indication of the child's overall level in verbal and visuo-spatial skills, developmental difficulties in other domains also have a significant impact on functioning. Thus, a comprehensive assessment of a child's skills should also include an evaluation of his/her functional language and communication (see Chapter 52), psychomotor and sensory difficulties (see Chapter 47), executive functioning (including working memory and attention) and semantic and episodic memory.

Assessment of executive functioning, attention, and memory

Assessments of attention and executive functioning include the Delis-Kaplan Executive Functions System (Delis *et al.*, 2001), the Test of Everyday Attention for Children (TEA-Ch; Manly *et al.*, 1998), the Conners' Continuous Performance Test (Conners, 2004), the Developmental NEuroPSYchological Assessment (NEPSY; Korkman *et al.*, 2007), and the Behavioral Assessment of the Dysexecutive Syndrome in Children (BADS-C; Emslie *et al.*, 2003). It has also been observed that clinic-based assessments of executive functioning often do not reflect how children behave in other settings, for example, in class (Barney *et al.*, 2011). Clinic-based assessments using structured tests should perhaps be considered to indicate children's *optimum* or potential level of skill, whereas observations of their skills in their everyday environment (as elicited by observation and the use of structured questionnaires such as the Behavior Rating Inventory of Executive Functioning (BRIEF; Gioia *et al.*, 2000)) show the impact of their difficulties on their lives.

Assessments of memory include measures of verbal and visual memory for immediate and delayed recall. It is useful to assess both retrieval and recognition abilities, as the child's performance under different conditions will inform intervention methods. Batteries of tests such as the Children's Memory Scale (Cohen, 1997), the Rivermead Behavioral Memory Test for Children (Wilson *et al.*, 1991), the Test of Memory and Learning (Reynolds & Bigler, 2007), and the Wide Range Assessment of Memory and Learning (Sheslow & Adams, 1990) cover these various facets of memory. Additionally, working memory can be assessed in more detail (e.g., the Working Memory Test Battery for Children, Gathercole & Pickering, 2001). Children's everyday (episodic) memory should be considered and their rate of forgetting should be determined. Parents and teachers often observe that children appear to learn something one day and have forgotten it the next. Memory tests generally

only test 20–30 min later in the delayed condition and the rate of forgetting over longer periods of time may need to be considered.

Some psychologists, usually those with training in neuropsychology, are able to assess skills within all these domains. The benefit of a single assessment, covering a broad range of areas, is that the assessor can provide an overview of how areas of specific strength and weakness inter-relate and contribute toward the child's behavioral presentation. More typically, however, a multi-professional assessment is required to ensure that skills in all areas are adequately assessed.

Achievement tests

Assessments of school-based attainments, including reading, spelling, and maths are important because these skills are so critical to children's progress through school. It is useful to use batteries that are co-normed with measures of intellectual ability so that clinical discrepancies between skills can be measured. Batteries such as the Wide Range Achievement Test (Wilkinson & Robertson, 2006) and the Wechsler Individual Achievement Test (Wechsler, 2009) are designed to be used alongside the Wechsler IQ tests. Assessments that measure literacy usually focus on word reading, reading fluency, reading comprehension, and spelling. An area that can be hard to assess formally is children's ability to express their ideas on paper, an observed difficulty often commented on by teachers and parents.

When schools assess children's early academic progress, measures to determine their reading level and mathematical skills are usually administered, that is, skills that have been explicitly taught and possibly over-learned. Such assessments do not take into account the development of children's learning and thinking skills more broadly and do not consider how other cognitive difficulties can have a longer-term impact on the ability to succeed beyond school. Rather than focussing only on specific difficulties a broader-based assessment that incorporates academic attainments as well as screening for difficulties in the dynamic application of learned skills (e.g., tasks requiring a degree of working memory and problem-solving) would perhaps highlight where individuals needed a more wide-reaching learning intervention (see Chapter 53).

Special considerations

When undertaking any psychological assessment, it is important to consider diverse issues, highlighted earlier, particularly when testing children with special needs. Specialists have informed much of our knowledge about these issues.

Low IQ

The most likely reasons for very young children to be referred to clinical services are delays in motor, cognitive or language development. Pediatric assessments based on semi-structured observations of the child, reviewed earlier, can identify children with severe and global delays, but they may fail to detect more subtle developmental problems. If direct testing is not possible, or the results are considered unreliable because the child is too distressed or anxious, it will be necessary to rely on parental information.

Several informant-based measures are available that provide information on the child's progress across a range of different domains. Some, such as the Assessment of Basic Language and Learning Skills—Revised (ABLLS-R; Partington, 2006) are designed to identify specific areas of deficit in order to guide skill remediation programmes. Others (e.g., the Vineland Adaptive Behavior Scales (VABS-II; Sparrow *et al.*, 2005) or the Adaptive Behavior Assessment System (ABAS; Harrison & Oakland, 2003)) allow assessment of the child's level in comparison to other children of the same age. Because these measures are based on parental report they lack the objectivity of standardized, child-based assessments. Thus, some parents may overestimate the child's level of ability in certain areas, or, if the environment is very restrictive, the child may not have had the opportunity to demonstrate skills in some domains. However, these issues can often be resolved by careful questioning. It is also important to be aware that adaptive behavior scores are not equivalent to IQ scores and in some conditions, such as autism, a child's Vineland score, for example, may be much lower than his or her score on a standard IQ test (Charman *et al.*, 2011). Nevertheless, these types of assessment can be particularly helpful in providing a picture of a young person's developmental profile and everyday functioning. For very young or severely developmentally delayed children the information they provide can be more useful for planning educational and intervention programmes than a standard IQ score.

Testing hearing and/or language impaired children

Among tests that have been specifically developed for children with hearing or language difficulties are the Leiter International Performance Scale—Revised (Leiter-R; Roid & Miller, 1997) and the Snijders-Oomen Nonverbal Intelligence Scale—Revised (SON-R; Snijders *et al.*, 1989). These can be administered without spoken instructions, using demonstrations of correct responses. Ideally, a comprehensive clinical assessment should include measures of language understanding and expression (in the child's own language, if possible; if not, in the language in which he/she is being educated), as communicative function (note this is not the same as spoken language nor the same as Verbal IQ) is key to adaptive learning, behavior and development (see Chapter 52).

Rare disorders

Psychologists occasionally will be asked to assess children with specific and/or rare genetic syndromes, many involving particular cognitive profiles (Simons, 2007). For example, children with Williams syndrome tend to have mild—to moderate global intellectual disabilities and specific learning difficulties (e.g., in mathematics) but expressive language and social skills

are relatively well preserved; children with Fragile X show weaknesses in quantitative skills and in short-term memory for abstract stimuli, whereas short-term memory for visually presented, meaningful stimuli is a relative strength. Although, within all genetic disorders, there is considerable individual variation, it is important that the psychologist is aware of the cognitive profiles typically related to the condition; the assessment should also focus on highlighting the child's particular pattern of strengths and weaknesses.

Different cultures and communities

There are significant limitations and challenges in adapting and/or using tests outside the culture and community in which they have been developed and normed. Carter *et al.* (2005) identified five broad categories relevant to cross-cultural assessment: the influence of culture on performance, familiarity with the testing situation, the effect of formal education, language issues, and picture recognition. Even when translation of tests has been undertaken, there is a need to be cautious in interpreting and reporting standardized scores. Sánchez-Escobedo *et al.* (2011) compared performance across English-speaking children in American schools, Spanish-speaking children in American schools and Spanish-speaking children in Mexican schools on parallel versions of the WISC-IV. Subtest standard scores derived from the same raw score differed by as much as 1 standard deviation. Differences in the nature of the standardization samples, including hard-to-measure factors such as differential exposure to formal testing in schools and familiarity even with adapted test materials, most likely underlie the differences found. Encouraged by the test publishing houses, there are an increasing number of translations of some of the most widely available psychometric tests that are to be welcomed. However, the difficulties inherent in adapting a test developed in one culture and community to another need to be borne in mind. In communities where no culturally appropriate formal tests are available, greater reliance on information from parents and from schools will be required although, when possible, this should be augmented by direct observation both during structured and unstructured activities.

Interpreting and reporting test scores in "atypical" children

Standardized, clinic-based assessments are designed to provide information about a child's progress compared to that of a typically developing, same age, peer group. However, particularly in the case of children with developmental or other disabilities, it is possible for children to achieve a score that is within the normal range for their age while completing the test in an unusual way. For example, a child with autism tested on the WISC might obtain scores at ceiling on the subtests of Vocabulary and Information because of his or her extensive knowledge of facts and ability to define words. Although scores on other verbal subtests (e.g., Similarities or Comprehension) may be very low, the overall verbal ability score can, nevertheless, be well within the average range. Moreover, informal interactions with that same child may indicate that his social–communication skills are highly impaired. Another child might obtain very low scores on non-verbal tests not because of poor psychomotor or processing skills, but because he or she is highly anxious or suffering from Obsessive Compulsive Disorder (OCD). Thus, although the score on any psychometric assessment is important, careful observations of the child's performance provide some of the most clinically useful information. Test scores alone should never be considered in the absence of a description of test behavior.

Unstandardized assessments

With children with intellectual or learning disabilities who are functioning at a level well below their age, clinicians will often use assessments standardized for younger children because they are more appealing and accessible. Using tests in such a way can elicit useful information about a child's ability to respond to novel stimuli and co-operate with the formal assessment process. However, in such circumstances, it is important to be aware of the problems inherent in using and interpreting out-of-age tests results or relying on age equivalents to provide an indication of a child's ability. When using out-of-norm tests, the clinician uses the raw score to determine at what age such a raw score would be typical. In such cases, it is important to be aware of the statistical basis upon which such scores are calculated and the extent to which the skill being assessed develops in a linear or step-wise fashion. The clinician should also be explicit about exactly what is being measured and how the presentation of that skill would compare with a typically developing child with the same age equivalent (Bracken, 1988). For example, if a typically developing 3 year old child obtains an age equivalent score of 3 years (standard score = 100) on a measure of expressive language that involves naming single pictures, it is reasonable to assume that other aspects of his or her language competence are at a similar level. If a 12-year-old child with autism is able to name enough pictures to achieve the same raw score this may have been acquired via a very different process, for example, by learning to repeat large numbers of common words. Other aspects of his or her language development may be at a very different level. Thus, although the children's raw scores on the test are identical, there may be little else that is similar about their language abilities or communication skills.

Considerations in the testing environment

Psychologists need to be aware of factors that influence test performance, such as having observers during the assessment (e.g., parents or trainees), testing the child in a familiar versus unfamiliar environment and testing the child at the end of the school day. Occasionally, too, particularly when testing children with significant comprehension problems, it may be necessary to modify test instructions somewhat, perhaps giving additional verbal or non-verbal cues on early test items, or starting at a lower level than the testing manual indicates, to ensure that the child understands what is expected. Although these modifications can help to increase co-operation and test compliance, it is always important to record any deviations from standard administration procedures.

At all times, psychologists need to ensure the validity of their assessment and, where appropriate, assess the child's effort during testing (Blaskewitz *et al.*, 2008; Kirkwood *et al.*, 2012). Children need to be encouraged to do their best before the session commences. If there are suspicions that the child is not co-operating, for whatever reason, there are tests that can be used to determine whether or not she/he is performing optimally (e.g., Test of Memory and Malingering; Tombaugh, 1996; Reliable Digit Span test; Kirkwood *et al.*, 2011).

It is also important to ensure that poor performance is only interpreted as lack of effort when this is clearly the case. Children with specific learning difficulties may fail some assessments because of the extra effort involved, and it is normal for children's attention to vary during the assessment process. Children may also be tired after a long journey, anxious about the unfamiliar assessment situation or not feeling well. The clinician needs to take these variables into account before concluding a poor performance is down to lack of effort.

Finally, there may be times when testing is not appropriate at all, for example, where there have been previous recent administrations of the same or similar batteries. This might be the case, for example, if parents are determined to enroll their child in a programme for gifted children and have previously sent him or her for several other assessments. While the time needed between repeat assessments is not usually explicitly stated in test instructions, the utility and reliability of repeat testing needs to be considered by the practitioner to avoid scores being inflated by practice effects (or possibly deflated because the child sees no reason to repeat the same activities over again) (Calamia *et al.*, 2012).

What to report and how

Once the assessment is complete, the next step is to pass on this information to those involved in the most accessible and informative way. Some teams provide immediate feedback even if this is sometimes preliminary. Others ask the family to return when all the information has been fully collated. Whichever option is taken, it is essential that the child and family are aware what will happen at the end of the assessment, when oral feedback will be given, and when they will receive written reports. Decisions also need to be taken as to whether feedback will be given to the child and family together or individually. This will depend on the age and developmental level of the child as well as the quality of family relationships. The child and family must also be given time to raise their own questions and concerns, either on the day of the assessment or at a pre-arranged time thereafter.

Written reports must be provided within a set period and be appropriate for the recipients. Many families (and indeed many professionals) are unable to interpret technical details such as t-scores, confidence intervals, percentiles or algorithm scores. Even IQ scores can give rise to confusion, with some families being very upset that their child has an "IQ of 99" when they had been told previously he was of "average ability"! Instead, it is usually better to report IQ results in terms of ranges, rather than a single score.

In general, the findings from the assessment should be reported in as concise and straightforward a way, as appropriate for each family. Detailed scores of IQ or other assessments can be included as a separate appendix that can be supplied to the family or other services as needed. When summarizing the outcome of the assessment to the child, the style of the report letter should be carefully adapted to suit his or her developmental, linguistic, and emotional needs. Following a psychological assessment, especially when undertaken as part of a multi-disciplinary team assessment, the results should be discussed not only with other team members but also with education professionals working with the child or young person so that a jointly agreed approach can be developed to support the child's learning and/or behavior management. It is important that a consistent approach to support and intervention is adopted at home and school.

Reports to schools should provide all relevant educational information but it is important that any confidential personal information provided by the family is not inadvertently included. In reporting to court or social services, impressions of the relationship between the child and parents, or information on the young person's behavior and social history may be more important than a focus on details of IQ scores

Professional issues for psychologists

Psychologists are normally regulated by a professional body (e.g., the Health and Care Professions Council in the United Kingdom; the American Psychological Association in the United Stated of America) and have a responsibility to maintain their Continuing Professional Development (CPD). This usually means ensuring that they have spent a certain amount of time each year up-dating their knowledge through attendance at conferences and reading current research material and having regular professional supervision. Accessing supervision and current literature can be more challenging for psychologists working independently but is no less critical.

Psychologists are bound by a code of practice that is designed to ensure the safety of their clients, both through regulating their behavior toward the people with whom they work and to ensure a certain standard of practice. Having a regulated profession means that psychologists should work in a reasonably uniform way. They have a responsibility to maintain test security, to share test results with other psychologists where appropriate to avoid skewing later test results (e.g., through a practice effect or test fatigue), to report any unusual administration methods, such as testing the limits, which may affect later administration of the same test.

Using psychological assessments to inform intervention

Assessing behavioral functions

One of the most common reasons why children are referred to specialist clinical services is the presence of behaviors that are disturbing or distressing for themselves, their families, peers, teachers or society more generally. Such behaviors may result from many different, and often multiple, causes. They may be a reaction to environmental factors (e.g., neglect, abuse, bullying, excessive demands from school or family) or, for example, in the case of children with developmental disorders, they may be the individual's most effective means of escaping from undesired situations or of gaining attention. Emotional or psychiatric disorders may also present initially as behavioral disturbance. Successful intervention necessitates a clear understanding of the factors that may be causing or maintaining problem behaviors or interfering with learning but very often it is not possible to determine these from the initial referral. In such cases, the psychological assessment will also require a detailed analysis of the problem(s) (see Chapter 38). Anxiety, for example, is frequently associated with high levels of arousal (see Chapter 60); irritability is a common symptom of depression (see Chapter 63); attention deficit hyperactivity disorder (ADHD) is typically related to poor impulse control (see Chapter 55) and these secondary symptoms can often lead to apparently unprovoked explosions of anger, disruption, or aggression.

One critical aspect of psychological assessments used within the context of an intervention is the extent to which they are sensitive to change. Some aspects of the development of standardized psychometric tests have been influenced by the notion of a stable constitutional factor such as IQ. Non-standardized assessments can be of value to evaluate interventions, though they need to be systematic and reliable. The combination of formal and informal psychological assessments may also indicate that a child has more fundamental learning or behavior problems than were initially recognized, as well as revealing inadequacies or inconsistencies in the ways these are dealt with at home or at school. In such cases, these assessments can be essential in establishing the basis for more systematic cognitive, behavioral, or pharmacological interventions and for monitoring the effects of the intervention over time (see Chapter 14).

Although there are many different and widely used interventions for children with learning and behavioral difficulties few have a sound evidence base, particularly when applied in non-experimental settings. For example, the Response to Intervention model has become a standard model of intervention for children with learning difficulties across the United States. Response to Intervention was intended to provide a means of delivering early intervention to all children presenting with learning difficulties in school, with interventions of greater intensity and specificity being delivered to those who failed to respond to the earlier, broader intervention input. The tiered approach to intervention has some similarity to Dynamic Assessment, which is intended to provide a specific analysis of individual children's approaches to problems to enable the generation of a process-oriented model of intervention, for example, through providing graduated prompts to enable a child to achieve successful task completion (Tzuriel, 2000). However, providing this intervention in a group format, as is needed in the Response to Intervention model, rather diminishes the potential strengths of the model because children with severe difficulties are not identified at the early stages and potential intervention time is lost (Reynolds & Shaywitz, 2009). Information gleaned from observing individual children's response to interventions, if rigidly measured, could provide valuable information about intervention efficacy (initially on a single-case basis). A wide range of literacy and educational interventions are available; some but not all of which have a sound evidence base (see Chapters 41, 52, and 53).

There are a few intervention strategies available to tackle difficulties arising from specific neuropsychological impairments. These include computer-based working memory systems, such as Cogmed Working Memory Training for children with clearly assessed specific working memory weaknesses, although it is not clear the extent to which gains made during training have a functional impact (Shipstead *et al.*, 2012). Memory support strategies, such as errorless learning, for children with episodic memory and executive functioning weaknesses, are increasingly being developed because of evidence from neuropsychological investigations of children's learning abilities. By using psychological assessments to provide detailed information about the individual's strengths and weaknesses, targeted interventions of this kind can be evaluated through single-case designs. These allow the broader impact of an intervention, such as working memory training on academic attainments and behavior, to be accurately monitored.

The value of single case research

All interventions are likely to be based, at least initially, on information from single-case data and, although evidence from randomized control trials is considered the gold-standard on which to base therapy, many aspects of behavioral interventions have a strong evidence base from multiple case series data (Kratochwill *et al.*, 2013). Single case design methodology, employing strategies such as multiple baseline and reversal techniques is also important in demonstrating the potential effectiveness of novel or individualized treatments. Note that it is important not to overlook information on interventions that have been effective for individual children or young people and robust methods for evaluating the efficacy of single-case interventions can be applied (Perdices & Tate, 2009).

For all children, even when well-established intervention methods are used, these need to be assessed in terms of the benefit for that individual. For example, in schools, children who are making slow progress in the acquisition of early literacy skills may automatically be assigned to a phonics intervention group without any formal assessment to determine whether phonological difficulties are indeed the root of their literacy difficulties. Assessment of the child's skills and difficulties prior to and during the intervention is essential in order to determine if the child is learning the skill being taught and whether it is generalizing to improve access to the curriculum more broadly.

Single case-study design is particularly useful for assessing the best learning environment for a child. For example, when children have specific difficulties, such as specific language impairment, a split placement may be used, with the child dividing their time between a language unit and the mainstream class. Individual assessment over a period of time can determine their level of learning and social engagement in both settings to aid in future placement decisions. The data collected should include time on task, work completed independently and learning targets achieved as well as progress with language targets.

Detailed monitoring of individual children's progress is needed to ensure that strategies, assumed to be beneficial, are not inadvertently harming children's learning. Although children with special needs are often provided with additional support in mainstream classes using teaching assistants, this input can potentially limit the child's contact time with the teacher and has been shown to slow, rather than accelerate progress (Blatchford *et al.*, 2009). All too often classroom assistants for children with special needs have little or no training or support to ensure that they are actively facilitating learning. However, with adequate training and supervision non-professional staff are able to implement evidence-based intervention programmes effectively (see Chapter 41).

Conclusions

Psychological assessment of children and young people may be undertaken for a variety of reasons. Usually, the assessment will be a response to concerns that a parent, other health-care professional or teacher has about the child or young person's development or behavior. The domains that need to be considered in any assessment are wide and most assessments should consider both development and behavior, alongside the child's emotional well-being (Murray & Farrington, 2010). The family, home and school environment—its impact on the child and the child's impact on those with whom they come into contact—should also usually be considered as part of any psychological assessment.

Cognitive assessment can be a vital part of the assessment process, and requires a rigorous and methodological approach to testing together with an understanding of psychological and statistical theory. However, psychometric assessment is neither the psychologist's only nor indeed primary role. Thus, we have emphasized the crucial importance that far broader, wide-ranging and theory-driven assessment plays in formulating and systematically testing hypotheses about a child's difficulties. The results of a hypothesis-led assessment will provide a psychological framework for conceptualizing the child or young person's difficulties that, in turn, should guide and underpin approaches to intervention and remediation within the same hypothesis-testing framework.

References

American Psychiatric Association (2013) *Diagnostic and Statistical Manual of Mental Disorders—Text Revision (DSM-5)*, 5th edn. American Psychiatric Association, Washington, DC.

Aylward, G.P. (2004) Predictions of function from infancy to early childhood: implications for pediatric psychology. *Journal of Pediatric Psychology* **29**, 555–564.

Aylward, G.P. (2009) Developmental screening and assessment: what are we thinking? *Journal of Developmental & Behavioral Pediatrics* **30**, 169–173.

Barney, S.J. *et al.* (2011) Neuropsychological and behavioural measures of attention assess different constructs in children with traumatic brain injury. *Clinical Neuropsychologist* **25**, 1145–1157.

Bayley, N. (2005) *Bayley Scales of Infant Development*, 3rd edn. Harcourt Assessment, San Antonio, TX.

Beresford, B. *et al.* (2004) Developing an approach to involving children with autistic spectrum disorders in a social care research project. *British Journal of Learning Disabilities* **32**, 180–185.

Blaskewitz, N. *et al.* (2008) Performance of children on symptom validity tests: TOMM, MSVT and FIT. *Archives of Clinical Neuropsychology* **23**, 379–391.

Blatchford, P. *et al.* (2009) The effect of support staff on pupil engagement and individual attention. *British Journal of Educational Psychology* **35**, 661–686.

Bracken, B.A. (1988) Ten psychometric reasons why similar tests produce dissimilar results. *Journal of School Psychology* **26**, 155–166.

Calamia, M. *et al.* (2012) Scoring higher the second time around: meta-analyses of practice effects in neuropsychological assessment. *Clinical Neuropsychologist* **26**, 543–570.

Carter, J.A. *et al.* (2005) Issues in the development of cross-cultural assessments of speech and language for children. *International Journal of Language and Communication Disorders* **40**, 385–401.

Cattell, J.M.K. (1890) Mental tests and measurements. *Mind* **15**, 373–380.

Charman, T. *et al.* (2005) Outcome at 7 years of children diagnosed with autism at age 2: predictive validity of assessments conducted at 2 and 3 years of age and pattern of symptom change over time. *Journal of Child Psychology and Psychiatry* **46**, 500–513.

Charman, T. *et al.* (2011) IQ in children with autism spectrum disorders: population data from the SNAP Project. *Psychological Medicine* **41**, 619–627.

Cohen, M. (1997) *Children's Memory Scale*. Harcourt, San Antonio, TX.

Conners, C.K. (2004) *Continuous Performance Test II (CPT-II)*. Multi-Health Systems Inc., New York.

Delis, D.C. *et al.* (2001) *Delis-Kaplan Executive Function System (D-KEFS)*. Harcourt, San Antonio, TX.

Duncan, J. (2010) The multiple demand (MD) system of the primate brain: multiple programs for intelligent behaviour. *Trends in Cognitive Science* **14**, 172–179.

Einfeld, S.L. & Tonge, B.J. (2002) *Developmental Behaviour Checklist*. Monash University, Australia.

Elliot, C.D. (2007) *Differential Abilities Scale-II (DAS-II)*. Psychological Corporation, San Antonio, TX.

Elliot, C.D. & Smith, P. (2011) *British Abilities Scale-3 (BAS-3)*. NFER-Nelson, Windsor, Berks, England.

Emslie, H. *et al.* (2003) *Behavioural Assessment of the Dysexecutive Syndrome for Children (BADS-C)*. Psychological Assessment Resources, Lutz.

Fergusson, D.M. *et al.* (2005) Show me the child at seven II: childhood intelligence and later outcomes in adolescence and young adulthood. *Journal of Child Psychology and Psychiatry* **46**, 850–858.

Flanagan, D.P. & Alfonso, V.C. (1995) A critical review of the technical characteristics of new and recently revised intelligence tests for preschool children. *Journal of Psychoeducational Assessment* **13**, 66–90.

Flanagan, D.P. & Harrison, P.L. (eds) (2012) *Contemporary Intellectual Assessment: Theories, Tests and Issues*, 3rd edn. New York, Guilford.

Galton, F. (1883) *Inquiries Into Human Faculty and Its Development*. AMS Press, New York.

Gathercole, S. & Pickering, S. (2001) *Working Memory Test Battery for Children*. Pearson Education, Oxford.

Gioia, G.A. *et al.* (2000) *Behaviour Rating Inventory of Executive Function*. Harcourt, San Antonio, TX.

Goodman, R. (1997) The Strengths and Difficulties Questionnaire: a research note. *Journal of Child Psychology and Psychiatry* **38**, 581–586.

Goodman, R. *et al.* (2000) The Development and Well-Being Assessment: description and initial validation of an integrated assessment of child and adolescent psychopathology. *Journal of Child Psychology and Psychiatry* **41**, 645–55.

Griffiths, R.F. (1935) *Imagination in Early Childhood*. Routledge, London.

Hack, M. *et al.* (2005) Poor predictive validity of the Bayley Scales of Infant Development for cognitive function of extremely low birth weight children at school age. *Pediatrics* **116**, 333–341.

Harrison, P. & Oakland, T. (2003) *Adaptive Behavior Assessment System, 2nd edn* edn. Harcourt, San Antonio, TX.

Kaplan, R.M. & Saccuzzo, D.P. (2013) *Psychological Testing: Principles, Applications, and Issues*, 8th edn. Cengage Learning, Independence, KY.

Kaufman, A.S. & Kaufman, N.J. (2004) *Kaufman Assessment Battery for Children*, 2nd edn. American Guidance Services, Circle Pines, MN.

Kaufman, A.S. & Kaufman, N.J. (2006) *Kaufman Brief Intelligence Test*, 2nd edn. Pearson Assessment, Bloomington, MN.

Kaufman, J. *et al.* (1997) Schedule for Affective Disorders and Schizophrenia for School-Age Children-Present and Lifetime Version (K-SADS-PL): initial reliability and validity data. *Journal of the American Academy of Child and Adolescent Psychiatry* **36**, 980–988.

Kirkwood, M.W. *et al.* (2011) The value of the WISC-IV Digit Span test in detecting non-credible performance during paediatric neuropsychological examinations. *Archives of Clinical Neuropsychology* **26**, 377–384.

Kirkwood, M.W. *et al.* (2012) The implications of symptom validity test failure for ability-based test performance in a pediatric sample. *Psychological Assessment* **24**, 36–45.

Korkman, M. *et al.* (2007) *NEPSY-II*. Pearson Education, Oxford.

Kratochwill, T.R. *et al.* (2013) Single-case intervention research design standards. *Remedial and Special Education* **34**, 26–38.

Lohman, D.F. *et al.* (2001) *Cognitive Abilities Test*, 3rd edn. NFER Nelson, London.

Lord, C. *et al.* (1994) Autism Diagnostic Interview—Revised: a revised version of a diagnostic interview for caregivers of individuals with possible pervasive developmental disorders. *Journal of Autism and Developmental Disorders* **24**, 659–685.

Lord, C. *et al.* (2012) *The Autism Diagnostic Observation Schedule*, 2nd edn. Western Psychological Services, Los Angeles, CA.

Luiz, D. *et al.* (2006) *Griffiths Mental Developmental Scales—Extended Revised*. Hogrefe, Oxford.

Luria, A.R. (1966) *Higher Cortical Functions in Man*. Tavistock Publication, Andover, Hants.

Manly, T. *et al.* (1998) *Test of Everyday Attention for Children (TEA-Ch)*. Harcourt, London.

Mullen, E.M. (1995) *Mullen Scales of Early Learning*. American Guidance Services, Circle Pines, MN.

Murray, J. & Farrington, D.P. (2010) Risk factors for conduct disorder and delinquency: key findings from longitudinal studies. *Canadian Journal of Psychiatry* **55**, 633–642.

Nijenhuis, J.T. & van der Flier, H. (2013) Is the Flynn effect on g? A meta-analysis. *Intelligence* **41**, 802–807.

Partington, J.W. (2006) *Assessment of Basic Language and Learning Skills-Revised (ABLLS-R)*. Western Psychological Services, Torrance, CA.

Perdices, M. & Tate, R.L. (2009) Single-subject designs as a tool for evidence-based clinical practice: are they unrecognized and undervalued. *Neuropsychological Rehabilitation* **19**, 904–927.

Reynolds, C.R. & Bigler, E.D. (2007) *Test of Memory and Learning*, 2nd edn. Pearson Education, Oxford.

Reynolds, C.R. & Shaywitz, S.E. (2009) Response to intervention: ready or not? Or, from wait-to-fail to watch-them-fail. *School Psychology Quarterly* **32**, e130.

Roid, G.H. (2003) *Stanford-Binet Test—Fifth Edition (SB-5)*. Riverside, Itasca, IL.

Roid, G.H. & Miller, L.J. (1997) *Leiter International Performance Scale—Revised (Leiter-R)*. Stoelting, Wood Dale, IL.

Rutter, M. *et al.* (2003) *Social Communication Questionnaire (SCQ)*. Western Psychological Services, Los Angeles, CA.

Sánchez-Escobedo, P. *et al.* (2011) A cross-cultural, comparative study of the American, Spanish, and Mexican versions of the WISC-IV. *TESOL Quarterly* **45**, 781–792.

Sheridan, M.D. (1945) The child's acquisition of speech. *British Medical Journal* **4402**, 707–709.

Sheslow, D. & Adams, W. (1990) *Wide Range Assessment of Memory and Learning WRAML*. Jastak Associates, Wilmington, DE.

Shipstead, Z. *et al.* (2012) Cogmed Working Memory Training: does the evidence support the claims. *Journal of Applied Research in Memory and Cognition.* **1**, 185–193.

Simonoff, E. *et al.* (2006) The Croydon assessment of learning study: prevalence and educational identification of mild mental retardation. *Journal of Child Psychology and Psychiatry* **47**, 828–839.

Simons, T.J. (2007) Cognitive characteristics of children with genetic syndromes. *Child and Adolescent Psychiatric Clinics of North America* **16**, 599–616.

Snijders, J.T. *et al.* (1989) *Snijders-Oomen Non-Verbal Intelligence Test (SON-R 5.5-17)*. Wolters-Noordhoff, Groningen.

Snow, C.E. & Van Hemel, S.B. (2008) *Early Childhood Assessment: Why, What and How?* National Academies Press, Atlanta, GA.

Sparrow, S.S. & Davis, S.M. (2000) Recent advances in the assessment of intelligence and cognition. *Journal of Child Psychology and Psychiatry* **41**, 117–131.

Sparrow, S.S. *et al.* (2005) *Vineland Adaptive Behavior Scales, Survey Edition*, 2nd edn. American Guidance Service, Circle Pines, MN.

Spearman, C. (1904) "General intelligence" objectively determined and measured. *American Journal of Psychology* **15**, 201–293.

Tombaugh, T.N. (1996) *Test of Memory and Malingering (TOMM)*. Multi-Health Systems, New York.

Tzuriel, D. (2000) Dynamic assessment of young children: educational and intervention perspectives. *Educational Psychology Review* **12**, 385–434.

Wakschlag, L.S. *et al.* (2008) Observational assessment of preschool disruptive behavior, part I: reliability of the Disruptive Behavior Diagnostic Observation Schedule (DB-DOS). *Journal of the American Academy of Child & Adolescent Psychiatry* **47**, 622–631.

Watkins, M.W. & Smith, L.G. (2013) Long-term stability of the Wechsler Intelligence Scale for children—4th edn. *Psychological Assessment* **25**, 477–483.

Wechsler, D. (2003) *Wechsler Intelligence Scale for Children*, 4th edn. Psychological Corporation, San Antonio, TX.

Wechsler, D. (2008) *Wechsler Adult Intelligence Scale*, 4th edn. Psychological Corporation, San Antonio, TX.

Wechsler, D. (2009) *Wechsler Individual Achievement Test*, 3rd edn. Harcourt, San Antonio, TX.

Wechsler, D. (2011) *Wechsler Abbreviated Scale of Intelligence*, 2nd edn. Psychological Corporation, San Antonio, TX.

Wechsler, D. (2012) *Wechsler Preschool and Primary Scale of Intelligence*, 4th edn. Psychological Corporation, San Antonio, TX.

Wilkinson, G.S. & Robertson, G.J. (2006) *Wide Range Achievement Test 4 (WRAT4)*. Psychological Corporation, San Antonio, TX.

Wilson, B.A. *et al.* (1991) *Rivermead Behavioural Memory Test for Children*. Pearson Education, Oxford.

World Health Organisation (1993) *Mental Disorders: 10th Revision of the International Classification of Diseases: Research Diagnostic Criteria (ICD-10)*. WHO, Geneva.

A: The clinical assessment

CHAPTER 35

Physical examination and medical investigation

Kenneth E. Towbin

Emotion and Development Branch, National Institute of Mental Health, Intramural Research Program, Bethesda, MD, USA
Department of Psychiatry and Behavioral Health, The George Washington University School of Medicine, Washington, DC, USA

Introduction

Child psychiatry is a medical subspecialty that is closely related to child neurology and general pediatrics. While the primary focus of child psychiatry is mental disorders, practitioners must be ever mindful of the inextricable links among "mental," "neurological," and other "medical" symptoms. Furthermore, a basic principle of the field is that mental disorders are brain disorders that affect perception, thinking, learning, behavior, social interaction, and mood. Therefore, when making a diagnosis and during treatment, the child psychiatrist and all child mental health professionals must be alert to medical and neurological disorders that produce psychiatric symptoms, influence treatment interventions, and affect the outcome. Modern child psychiatry sees conditions as rooted in both biology and the mind, and it acknowledges the continuous interplay between these domains. Child mental health professionals recognize that a child's body is affected by the child's environment and by the way that child thinks and acts. Clearly, psychiatric disorders (e.g., eating disorders, depression, psychosis, psychosomatic fatigue, conversion symptoms), as well as the somatic treatments that are often prescribed, can affect pediatric growth and general medical health. However, child mental health professionals also know that various medical problems influence the child's development and mental well-being. For these reasons, the physical examination and evaluation of the patient—drawing information from what is reported and an examination of the patient's body—are fundamental to a comprehensive understanding of that individual.

There are other influences to be considered along with biomedical processes. It is equally fundamental to our field to appreciate the power of experiences, relationships, and the context of a child's life. These have a formidable effect on how that child develops and thinks; one must account for them in formulating the child's problems and treatment. The

sophisticated, modern view is that the course of development and disorders (e.g., onset, severity) are a function of biological and nonbiological forces acting through a complex interaction of risk and protective factors (Rutter *et al.*, 2006; Kendler & Baker, 2007; Meaney, 2010; Rutter, 2012).

The purpose of this chapter is to provide guidelines for clinicians to follow as part of a standard medical assessment of the child. The need to perform such an assessment follows from the fundamental principle that it is essential to discover biologically manifest features or observable risks (constitutional or acquired) that contribute to symptoms associated with a mental disorder. However, the astute clinician knows that physical and medical investigations are not sufficient to have a full grasp of the determinants of a patient's condition.

The physical examination in child psychiatry is a part of the doctor's relationship with the patient, the patient's family, and in many cases, other healthcare providers in the patient's life. Physicians are mindful of this as they approach their patients and their patients' families. The manner with which the examination is conducted will communicate a great deal, much of it non-verbally, to the patient; the psychiatrist's way of conducting the examination plainly conveys how the patient's identity, thoughts, emotions, and physical feelings are regarded. Similarly, most parents are keenly aware that physical contact with their child has profound significance; it arouses concern and invites protective instincts.

The medical examination reflects a scientific approach. Physicians begin with gathering data, such as the primary complaint and the history of its onset and course. As the data are being gathered, they consider hypotheses about the differential diagnosis, potential contributions to the expression of those symptoms, and prognosis. Medical and laboratory assessments are not "fishing expeditions"; they test specific hypotheses that arise from listening carefully to the chief complaint(s) and history. Laboratory and medical evaluations are tools that facilitate the

Rutter's Child and Adolescent Psychiatry, Sixth Edition.
Edited by Anita Thapar and Daniel S. Pine, James F. Leckman, Stephen Scott, Margaret J. Snowling, Eric Taylor.
© 2015 John Wiley & Sons Ltd. Published 2018 by John Wiley & Sons Ltd.

process of narrowing the differential diagnosis and hypotheses into a workable treatment plan and approach to the child's care. The process is a "two-way street" in which laboratory and medical data can raise new hypotheses, support existing ones, and refute others (see Chapter 32).

All child mental health professionals consider the context of their patients' healthcare because this will guide what role and which parts of the examination they must perform in detail. Thus, the medical evaluation entails more than the basic history and course of illness. Child mental health professionals consider the scope of their involvement and their place in their patients' overall medical care. Child mental health professionals should be mindful of what is feasible, what part of their patients' care falls to them alone, who has the most expertise to pursue the workup, and what should be performed by (or in collaboration) with others. It is common sense that a child without basic healthcare or access to care will face insurmountable barriers to fulfilling recommendations for various forms of ancillary medical tests, such as MRI scans or extensive metabolic assessments. Conversely, when a child has ready access to routine pediatric care, the approach should take this into account when planning the workup and ordering tests. Child mental health professionals consider their patients' general health, history of prior assessments, and current healthcare relationships. When a child's care includes other healthcare providers, child mental health professionals think about the basic data others will need in order to pursue more focused, additional studies. Child mental health professionals consider these collaborations carefully and frame specific questions or hypotheses for their collaborators. For example, if a psychiatrist believes a child might have anemia, it is logical to confirm this by obtaining a complete blood count, serum hemoglobin, and hematocrit prior to referring the child for a more comprehensive workup.

The medical history

The medical history is a cornerstone of the medical evaluation and should not be omitted. It encompasses the child's current general health, health history, developmental health history, and family medical history.

The current health history is generally understood to include all current illnesses, recurrent conditions, allergies, and current and past medications. In the context of psychiatric care, it also should include the child's living conditions, socioeconomic circumstances, and access to healthcare. In more developed countries clinicians may make the tacit assumption that children have primary care providers, satisfactory nutrition, and everything they need for basic hygiene. However, one should not assume this to be the case for all children. For example, some children reside in homes or communities where they face deprivation and/or neglect, in low- and middle-income countries (LAMIC), or in poverty (in developed or LAMIC countries)

where principal foundations of health are lacking. Thus, inquiring about these components is necessary. As a part of a routine medical history, it is important to ask about the child's diet, activity/exercise level, and whether either parent or child has concerns about how the child is growing or feeling physically. These questions are particularly salient when evaluating children for the possibility of an eating disorder or depression.

The developmental history can also inform the clinician about a broad range of risks in the child's life. This can also influence the clinician's evaluation of any concurrent mental health problem. When exploring the prenatal history one can listen for significant risks prior to the child's birth, such as family medical/psychiatric history, sources of stress for the family, how the family coped with those stressors, and the barriers to healthcare. The course of the pregnancy can convey information about constitutional and environmental influences and perinatal events. These deserve further exploration because they may continue to affect the child. As in general pediatrics the developmental history includes the review of developmental milestones and includes the feeding history, development of gross and fine motor skills, coordination, language, social abilities (including peer relationships), school/academic functioning, and overall adaptive functioning in communication, daily living skills, socialization, and motor domains (Gerber *et al.*, 2010; Wilks *et al.*, 2010; Gerber *et al.*, 2011). There are established norms for many of these milestones and screening instruments (Sparrow *et al.*, 1984; Frankenburg *et al.*, 1992; Sparrow *et al.*, 2005; Drotar *et al.*, 2008; CDC (Centers for Disease Control and Prevention), 2011) that are helpful when acquiring information about delays or deficits in the past or present. A history of developmental delays and deviances should alert the clinician to the possibility of a neurodevelopmental disorder (see Chapter 32). For older children, it is important to gather a history of work activities. Also, it is now standard practice to inquire about past or recent exposure to traumatic events (interpersonal or natural), abuse, being victimized or bullied, and any exposure to violence at home, in the community, or at school.

The past medical history typically includes the patient's past and current medical illnesses, surgical history, any hospitalizations, and a review of any complications from common childhood illnesses or from medications. As suggested, learning the history may raise questions that go beyond mere medical data. The past medical history relays important information about the context of the child's past and present. Medical illness can impair the child's psychological health and the family's relationship with the child. Juvenile onset conditions (e.g., diabetes, cancer, epilepsy, or rheumatoid arthritis) or congenital disorders (e.g., heart, blood, or immune diseases) will have profound effects on psychological, social, and physical development. Even seemingly ordinary childhood events can cue the child mental health professional to potentially relevant psychiatric concerns. For example, a history of repeated accidents, fractures, or injuries (particularly concussions) could lead to questions about safety, supervision of the patient, impulsivity, thrill-seeking, mood disorder, or risk-taking. Some psychiatric conditions, such as attention deficit hyperactivity disorder (ADHD) or a depressive disorder could also contribute to such events. Similarly, relatively common chronic or recurrent childhood maladies can shape the child's perspective on the world. Asking about asthma, bowel and bladder function, headaches, ear infections, and tics (and other repetitive movements) is important because these conditions may associate with psychiatric symptoms, influence psychological development, have profound effects on a child's day-to-day life, and/or involve treatments that affect mood and behavior. Also, a child psychiatrist will need to know whether psychotropic medications will interact with drugs that are already being taken for other conditions. In addition, asking about unusual reactions to any drugs may inform the psychiatrist about adverse effects that could arise with future psychotropic medications.

The family medical history is a major part of the patient's medical history. The family's medical history informs the child mental health professional about the patient's risk for developing medical and psychiatric disorders and suggests possible medical disorders that produce psychiatric symptoms. Furthermore, should a parent, guardian, or sibling have a serious medical or psychiatric disorder it is likely to have an impact on the family's life and the child. Learning the family medical history can inform the mental health professional about past and current events and circumstances in the patient's life that are troubling and have an influence on the patient's psychological development. While a single chapter could never catalog all the ways a medical disorder can influence a child or family, some conditions are mentioned here because they are relatively more heritable, particularly likely to produce psychiatric symptoms, or convey an elevated risk of adverse reactions to somatic treatments.

A family history of cardiac illness is an exemplar. While family history for cardiac disease in elderly relatives is common, such a history assumes compelling relevance for the child's medical and psychiatric care when there is a family history of childhood onset cardiac disorders (e.g., malformations, arrhythmias), or sudden death in young family members. A family history for myocardial infarction or sudden death in young family members indicates an elevated risk of cardiac conduction or myocardial diseases in the patient (Tan & Judge, 2012). Moreover, some psychiatric medications can increase the risk of a cardiac event in a vulnerable patient (Beach et al., 2013). There has been a particular increase in concerns about cardiovascular effects of psychostimulant medications, and these concerns should require more extensive evaluations in children with a family history of heart conditions, particular sudden death or arrhythmias. In this instance, learning this history would prompt a more thorough characterization of the patient's current cardiac function (e.g., a baseline electrocardiogram (ECG), exercise stress testing) and close monitoring for ECG changes during initiation and subsequent to dose increments with some medications. Consultations with the child's usual pediatric care provider also would likely be indicated. Some aspects of the relationship between cardiac history and symptomatic presentation of

mental health problems remain contentious. For example, focus on a relationship between mitral valve prolapse (in the child or family) and anxiety was popular in the 1980s and 1990s. However, more recent evidence suggests that the relationship is weak if it exists at all (Weisse, 2007; Filho et al., 2011).

A family history of endocrine disorders is another example. A family history of diabetes or hypothyroidism can increase the likelihood that the patient will have a similar disorder contributing to the psychiatric symptoms. A family history of diabetes type 2 (DM2) is a risk factor for developing DM2 (Wareham et al., 2002; Rodríguez-Moran et al., 2010). An overweight child who presents with depression and a strong family history for DM2 warrants consideration of hyperglycemia contributing to depression (Hannon et al., 2013). A family history of diabetes also increases the risk for additional weight gain and developing diabetes while on psychotropic medication (Amed et al., 2011). Similarly, there are major genetic contributions to development of both hyperthyroidism and Hashimoto's thyroiditis, which produces hypothyroidism (Ban & Tomer, 2005; Cooper et al., 2012). When a patient is being evaluated for depression and gives a family history of thyroid disease, this suggests a greater risk for a contribution from thyroid dysfunction compared with someone without such a family history.

A family history of neurological disorders should be reviewed. Although the most common severe inherited neurological disorders have a very early onset, often in infancy (e.g., gangliosidoses), or typically begin in adulthood (e.g., Huntington chorea, dementia), a few begin in childhood and adolescence (e.g., Wilson's disease). Family and personal history is often the first clue to the presence of such problems. In addition, less severe, more common inherited neurological conditions that produce psychiatric symptoms, such as chronic tic disorders, have their peak incidence during childhood. The family history may be important for treatment as well. For example, a family history of glaucoma increases the risk of developing it with some pharmacological treatments such as selective serotonin reuptake inhibitors (SSRIs) and atypical antipsychotic drugs (Richa & Yazbek, 2010).

Summary key points of the medical history

- It is essential to maintain a continuous awareness of medical disorders that can produce or result from psychiatric disorders.
- Recognizing the context of psychiatric care within the patient's overall healthcare guides the role and what parts of the examination the psychiatrist will perform.
- The medical history is a cornerstone of the medical evaluation.
- The medical examination reflects a scientific approach. The history should suggest a number of possible disorders that might explain the symptoms and course of illness (see Chapter 32).
- The history includes the child's current general health, medical health history, developmental history, and family medical history.
- Attention to a family history of cardiac, endocrine, psychiatric, or neurological illness is pivotal.

The physical examination

All physicians must be aware that a physical examination can affect the patient and family in many ways. Those who see children should be particularly attuned to how pediatric patients may perceive the examination. Most children and adolescents think that psychiatric care, which focuses on mood, "feelings," and behavior, is fundamentally different from pediatric healthcare, which focuses on general heath (well child care), infections (e.g., colds, flu, otitis), or injury. Patients may be surprised that the psychiatrist will be examining them. In addition, for many children, the mind and the body are such separate entities that if the child is not in physical pain, the logic of performing a physical examination will be obscure. They may not understand intuitively how a problem affecting their thinking, mood, or behavior would have any connection with their body.

The physician must also be aware of and protect the patient's modesty and anxiety. Thoughtfulness about modesty makes it imperative that a parent (or guardian) and/or another healthcare provider be with the physician at all times during the physical examination. Physicians should refrain from physical contact whenever they are alone with their patients. The rationale for keeping this boundary includes therapeutic, psychological, ethical, and legal principles.

This awareness should also lead the physician to help the patient understand what will be done and why. One cannot assume that all children will understand and interpret the physician's intentions correctly. Explaining what will be done before doing it allows anxious or confused children to anticipate the procedures of the examination and to see the point of the doctor's requests. Furthermore, compared to healthy children, children with severe psychiatric disorders have a greater risk of misunderstanding physical interactions. There also may be cultural beliefs about physical contact to consider when examining a child and these should be raised and discussed with the parent(s) in advance.

The physician must also be aware of how developmental features come into play when examining a child. Creating an environment in which a child can ask questions and exercise some choice over the examination is important. The space used for the examination should be well lit, large enough to move around comfortably, and protect privacy. Part of the art of examining developmentally younger children is gathering neurological information from observations while the child is engaged in ordinary actions or playing simple games. For a child with a psychiatric disorder, the examination will be less invasive and distressing when one uses techniques that include toys, observations, and games, rather than simply running through a series of requests to perform movements or actions.

As generally described in the introduction, the decision about who should examine the child will depend on the circumstances and the context of that child's general health care. When a child has an established pediatric care provider, the onus falls on the doctors to reach a mutual decision about who will perform the examination. In some cases, it is desirable for each doctor to perform some segments of the examination. For children who are being seen for psychiatric care, the mental status/neurological examination is the principal focus and attention is given to other sections of the physical as dictated by additional signs and symptoms (e.g., sign of encephalopathy, dysmorphic features, intellectual disability). In other circumstances, such as when a child is admitted to an inpatient or intensive psychiatric care facility or there are no other medical care providers available, a psychiatrist may do the entire physical examination.

There are excellent texts available for methods and techniques of the physical examination (e.g., LeBlond *et al.*, 2008; Bickley, 2012). A complete review of techniques and methods exceeds the scope of a single chapter of guidelines. Generally, practitioners have a standard, systematic, highly practiced routine for performing the examination. Nevertheless, some areas encompass findings that deserve comment because of their relevance for child psychiatric assessment. While few symptoms are pathognomonic of any disorder, the presence of a physical sign will raise hypotheses about possible underlying disorders, any one of which can be confirmed or refuted by the pattern of additional findings.

By convention, the examination typically begins with obtaining vital signs. The patient's height, weight, blood pressure, and pulse are important baseline measures. It is quite important for physicians to plot height, weight and head circumference on a growth chart so that this can be tracked over time. Vital signs assume even more salience when one is considering pharmacological interventions that might affect weight or cardiovascular function. When vital signs fall significantly above or below the normal range, this may signal the presence of a variety of medical and/or psychiatric conditions. For example, acquired low weight could reflect the presence of protein-calorie malnutrition, an eating disorder, depression with loss of appetite, hyperthyroidism, celiac disease, anemia, cancer, or another primary medical condition. As part of obtaining such data, careful attention also is needed regarding the child's growth. Signs of alteration in height or weight can provide clues to various changes in the child's medical well-being. In addition, some medications, such as SSRIs or psychostimulants, can alter the child's growth. As a result, it is important to be aware of the child's current growth trajectory when initiating treatment.

Plotting the patient's weight using standard growth charts will also assist physicians in recognizing excessive weight or obesity. When obesity is found, the risks to psychological and physiological health should be reflected in the history, physical examination, and any laboratory/medical tests that the physician considers and monitors. Obesity carries risks for psychopathology (Swallen *et al.*, 2005) and may generate sleep apnea, which, in turn, may produce or exacerbate psychiatric symptoms (Sateia, 2009).

The examination of the skin, which includes lesions, skin texture, and color variations, can reveal systemic illness or signal the presence of noteworthy behaviors. Common skin lesions, such as scars may also be informative and reflect intentional self-injury, repeated accidents, or past physical trauma (e.g., abuse). Acne, while very common, may be a notable source of distress, particularly among socially anxious adolescents. Skin hygiene could suggest loss of self-care or parental neglect, particularly when accompanied by parasitic infections such as lice and scabies. The skin also may show active lesions resulting from picking (dermatotillomania), pinching (tics), abrasions (from compulsive behaviors), petechia (especially around the eyes suggestive of self-induced choking), abuse (welts, bruising, petechia in specific patterns such as grip marks or ligatures, burns, wounds) or self-inflicted wounds. Examination of hair distribution and texture may reflect systemic illness or trichotillomania. The skin examination may also show dramatic hair styles, skin piercings, and tattoos that while not pathological, open avenues to learn about the patient's life, interests, and relationships.

Abnormalities in skin and hair texture could point to thyroid disease as a contribution to depression or cognitive changes.

Areas of hyperpigmentation may suggest neurocutaneous disorders that correlate with central nervous system disease such as neurofibromatosis. Examination of facial skin may reveal other neurocutaneous disorders such as Sturge Weber syndrome or tuberous sclerosis that carry risks for disruptive/mood disorders (Chapieski et al., 2000) and autism spectrum disorders (Numis et al., 2011), respectively.

The head, eyes, ears, nose, and throat examination bundle a number of signs that can be psychiatrically important. Head shape can reflect environmental risks from neglect or genetic risks from craniosynostosis (Speltz et al., 2004), particularly in intellectually disabled children. Head circumference, like other physical measures, may be excessively large or small and suggest genetic and neurological disorders with behavioral features. Similarly, highly characteristic dysmorphic facial features may suggest specific genetic disorders such as trisomy 21, Fragile X, Prader-Willi, Angelman, Klinefelter, Velo-cardio-facial (VCF), Williams, or Turner syndrome. There is a wide range of facial abnormalities in VCFS but cleft palate, particularly involving the soft palate, and elongated face, wide nose, and small ears are frequently seen with this disorder. Characteristic facial features are also seen with repeated fetal exposure to alcohol. Deprivation or neglect may lead to poor dental hygiene and severely damaged teeth and gums that are observed on examination of the mouth and throat. Inspection of the mouth can also reveal signs of self-induced vomiting, such as erosion of teeth and lesions in the mouth. Lesions from sexually transmitted diseases may be visible. Examination of the appearance of the eyes may uncover disorders affecting genetic/metabolic (e.g., Wilson's disease, neurofibromatosis) or endocrine (thyroid) function. Systemic and infectious diseases can influence eye function such as pupillary responses to light and accommodation.

A quick examination of vision may be conducted by having the patient view a hand-held pocket vision screener (or an E-chart) card at 14 in. or 36 cm, or copy drawings of familiar geometric shapes. Disorders that produce dysmorphic facial features like those mentioned could affect the shape, size, and placement of the ears. Limited or loss of hearing affects language acquisition in young children. Any concerns about hearing should be assessed by an audiologist, but a screening assessment can be performed in a quiet room by asking if the child can hear the sound of the clinician rubbing a forefinger and thumb together at a distance of about 13–14 in. (or 35–36 cm) from the ear.

Pediatric psychiatric disorders have many fewer specific associations with examination of the neck, heart, lungs, and abdomen. One major exception is the size of the thyroid gland, and, in asthmatic children, the presence of wheezing. Genetic disorders like the ones noted, may affect cardiac hemodynamics and auscultation.

The circumstances that require a psychiatrist to perform a genital examination are rare. It is generally recognized that psychiatric care providers should refrain from genital examinations. When other features of the physical examination suggest a pattern that requires inspection of the genitals in order to winnow the differential diagnosis (such as Fragile X, Klinefelter, or Prader–Willi syndrome, or disorders of sexual development), arrangements for another provider to perform a genital examination should be made. If it is necessary, such an examination demands the utmost of attention to the patient's comfort and modesty. Unless there are extraordinary circumstances, one should never examine a patient's genitals without a parent/guardian being present. If a genital examination is essential, the psychiatrist must explain and give a clear rationale for it in advance.

The examination of the extremities may reveal picking, bruising, scarring or recent evidence of self-injury. Much less commonly, one may see signs of dysmorphology in the extremities or back that suggest genetic disorders with psychiatric manifestations such as Smith-Magenis Syndrome (Gropman et al., 2006). Also, disorders such as Prader–Willi Syndrome (Kroonen et al., 2006; Cassidy et al., 2012) or XXX syndrome (Otter et al., 2010) may produce scoliosis and are associated with psychiatric symptoms.

The neurological examination is highly relevant to child psychiatric care and to resolving hypotheses about the diagnosis (see Chapter 32). Many pediatric neurological conditions produce psychiatric symptoms; discussing each of them exceeds the scope of this chapter. However, physicians should be mindful of behavioral and emotional changes that may be the first sign of a progressive neurological condition. The neurological examination should assess the cranial nerves, motor system (strength and tone), sensory system, balance and coordination, reflexes and mental status. Particular attention should be paid to sudden changes in cognitive and emotional functions since these may signal progressive and acute conditions (Wilne *et al.*, 2006; Reulecke *et al.*, 2008). A great deal can be learned by carefully observing the patient during an ordinary interview or, with younger children, while playing age appropriate games such as throwing or kicking a ball. Fine motor coordination skills can be observed from playing a game of copying geometric figures or simply asking the child to make a drawing. How the child walks, gets up from the floor, or moves during conversation can provide leads for a more focused examination. Observing repetitive movements, mannerisms, voice quality, articulation, gait, gaze, and coordination can be accomplished during a typical interview.

The mental status examination is central to the child psychiatric examination. The basic elements of the mental status examination focus on the patient's capacities and current function in the context of their developmental level. As with the examination of adults, the mental status examination begins with the patient's appearance, mood, and affect. The clinician notes the variations and range of mood and affect during the interview. Inquiring about current or past suicidal ideation or thoughts/plans to harm others should be a routine part of the examination. Observations are made of the patient's speech and language. Behaviors are noted including stereotyped motor movements, capacity to sit calmly, and use of nonverbal communication such as gestures, facial expressions, and eye gaze. Changes in behavior during the interview are important, too. Cognitive capacity can be estimated from the patient's vocabulary, the coherence of the patient's ideas, and complexity of the patient's language construction. The child's narrative provides information on major themes and contents of the patient's thoughts. Spontaneous comments convey information about the flow of the child's thoughts and whether there is perseveration, developmentally immature thinking, frankly odd or bizarre ideas, or reason to have concerns about delusional beliefs, hallucinations, or perceptual distortions. When considering the presence of hallucinations, it is important to inquire whether they arise exclusively in a pattern of falling off to sleep (hypnagogic) or upon awakening from sleep (hypnopompic). It is also useful to learn whether they are vivid, frightening to the child, can be summoned or dismissed easily, and if the child is convinced they are caused by an outside source rather than his or her mind (Pilowsky & Chambers, 1986). A great deal about the patient's mental status can be learned from ordinary conversation. Features of orientation, mood, affect, intelligence, fund of knowledge, judgment, memory, attention, and abstracting abilities can be readily noted. When a child performs well academically without accommodations at school, this usually reflects at least average general intelligence. The mental status examination traditionally includes comments on the manner of the child's relating to the examiner over the course of the interview(s) and on any changes in that manner of relating with time and topics.

> ### Summary key points of the physical examination
>
> - Performing a physical examination is basic to a comprehensive understanding of the patient.
> - Sensitivity to the patient's past experiences, current state, culture, and developmental and cognitive levels should be foremost.
> - Protecting the patient's modesty and providing reassurance by explaining what will be done before doing it are key.
> - Components of the physical examination that require touching the patient should be performed while the parent/guardian is present.
> - The physical examination includes vital signs and follows with a systematic approach for each segment of the body.
> - It is generally recognized that psychiatric care providers should refrain from genital examinations.
> - The neurological and mental status examinations are pivotal for a child psychiatry physical examination.

Laboratory investigation

The laboratory investigation flows from the same rubric as the physical examination. The physical examination is guided by thoughtfully listening to the chief complaint, being alert to any patterns that emerge as one hears about additional symptoms, narrowing the range of possible conditions to a differential diagnosis, using observation and examination to further narrow the possibilities, and ultimately gauging the likelihood that a condition is contributing to the child's impairment. The laboratory investigation provides additional data to support or refute the diagnostic possibilities that are raised by the history and physical examination. The decision about which additional studies to pursue should grow out of consideration of the context of the child's usual healthcare, the hypotheses about the most likely conditions, and clinical judgment about whether there may be an acute problem that poses immediate risk. Figure 35.1 offers an example of this kind of deductive process. There are risks and problems that arise from obtaining laboratory data using a scattershot approach that ignores the foundations of a considered differential diagnosis.

Under the optimal circumstances a child will have regular healthcare and will have been followed by a pediatric or family medical doctor. If so, the physicians should confer, discuss possible medical contributions to the patient's symptoms, and come to a consensus about the need and direction for any laboratory workup. Typically the laboratory evaluation will be the purview of the care provider who oversees the child's general medical health. As with the physical examination, the decision about who should order and follow the laboratory investigation and tests will depend on the circumstances and the context of that child's general health care. However, there may be suboptimal circumstances or extenuating situations that

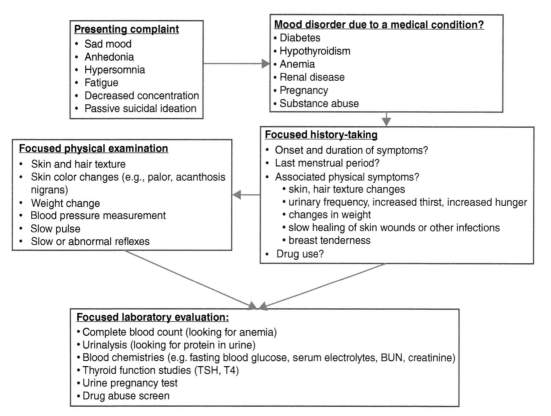

Presenting complaint
- Sad mood
- Anhedonia
- Hypersomnia
- Fatigue
- Decreased concentration
- Passive suicidal ideation

Mood disorder due to a medical condition?
- Diabetes
- Hypothyroidism
- Anemia
- Renal disease
- Pregnancy
- Substance abuse

Focused physical examination
- Skin and hair texture
- Skin color changes (e.g., palor, acanthosis nigrans)
- Weight change
- Blood pressure measurement
- Slow pulse
- Slow or abnormal reflexes

Focused history-taking
- Onset and duration of symptoms?
- Last menstrual period?
- Associated physical symptoms?
  - skin, hair texture changes
  - urinary frequency, increased thirst, increased hunger
  - changes in weight
  - slow healing of skin wounds or other infections
  - breast tenderness
- Drug use?

Focused laboratory evaluation:
- Complete blood count (looking for anemia)
- Urinalysis (looking for protein in urine)
- Blood chemistries (e.g. fasting blood glucose, serum electrolytes, BUN, creatinine)
- Thyroid function studies (TSH, T4)
- Urine pregnancy test
- Drug abuse screen

Figure 35.1 Medical assessment of a 16-year-old female with "possible depression." BUN, blood urea nitrogen; TSH, thyroid-stimulating hormone.

shift the responsibility to the psychiatrist. If so, then one should think about the medical evaluation as composed of steps and consider what a subspecialist might need in order to proceed subsequently with a more focused and specific evaluation. For example, if following considerable weight gain there were concerns about fatigue, polyuria, persistent thirst, and increased appetite, then the psychiatrist might obtain a fasting blood sugar, glycosylated hemoglobin level (HbA_{1c}), and, if possible, an oral glucose tolerance test before referring the child to a diabetic subspecialist (Copeland *et al.*, 2013).

The attuned clinician will also consider the impact that laboratory procedures have on the patient. On casual consideration, phlebotomy, an ECG, or an electroencephalogram (EEG) might seem minor, but these procedures can make children highly anxious. Therefore, it is important to explain, in developmentally informed terms, what will happen and why.

The timing of these laboratory studies is relevant. The laboratory evaluation may unfold over time as initial findings raise questions that need additional studies for answers. Also, the impact on parents of requesting these studies should be considered. In some situations, laboratory results may be needed urgently, but others may be deferred. Thought should be given to who will need the results and efforts should be made to avoid unnecessary repetition of studies. For example, if a child

has abdominal pain that could be due to gastro-esophageal reflux or anxiety, one might defer a medical workup (when the patient has relatively easy access to healthcare providers) until a pediatrician or family medical doctor has seen and examined the patient.

There is no standard battery of laboratory tests for psychiatric disorders and laboratory studies should never be ordered simply to assess "general health." However, when one suspects the presence of a specific condition, a focused laboratory assessment should be performed. For example, if there are concerns about anemia or bleeding problems then obtaining a complete blood count with differential count, hemoglobin, hematocrit, and coagulation indices such as a prothrombin time and partial thromboplastin time are warranted. If one is starting medications that might worsen anemia or bleeding, it would be important to obtain premedication, baseline measures. For example, SSRIs may cause changes in coagulation and, rarely, anemia, and therefore a full blood count (or a complete blood count in the United States) with differential count could be a reasonable baseline study to obtain.

Where the history suggests recurrent infections, symptoms of neurological problems with weakness and/or coordination, and weight loss, the physician might pursue whether there has been exposure to human immunodeficiency virus (HIV). Under these circumstances, or in parts of the world where the virus is highly endemic, HIV testing is warranted. In some parts of the world, this is standard testing for anyone admitted to hospitals or residential care facilities.

There is no standard battery of laboratory tests that must be obtained for all psychotropic medication. The selection of the tests and recommendations for ongoing monitoring will depend on the agent and other risk factors that individual patients bring to treatment. Generally, the laboratory tests and monitoring follow from the "Warnings" or "Warnings and Precautions" sections of the package insert or drug information for each specific agent. These sections typically recommend screening procedures, risks of concomitant medications, as well as clinical signs and symptoms that should be monitored. They often include what tests should be obtained.

Fortunately, most children have healthy kidney function. But if there are concerns about kidney impairment, or if one is starting a drug that is primarily excreted through the kidneys such as lithium, then obtaining a serum creatinine level, blood urea nitrogen, and basic electrolytes (sodium, potassium, chloride, carbon dioxide) would be important. Also, basic urine analysis would allow one to know whether there is proteinuria, any evidence of infection, or presence of particular metabolic conditions.

Primary liver disease is rare in children. However, since many medications can affect liver function, obtaining liver function tests becomes important prior to starting some medications. Generally liver function tests include alanine aminotransferase (ALT), aspartate aminotransferase (AST), alkaline phosphatase (ALP), and measures of direct and indirect bilirubin. Since high rates of hepatitis are to be found among children in some locales, results of these indices might lead one to proceed with obtaining measures of serum hepatitis antibodies.

Similarly, when there are concerns about cognitive function along with attentional problems and disruptive behaviors in a child who resides where environmental conditions produce a high risk of exposure to lead, one might obtain a serum lead level. The need for this would be more compelling if the child was young and had not had a lead level measured at any earlier point, or at any point while residing at his or her current address.

The decision to obtain thyroid function studies should be based on the examination (e.g., thin hair, puffy face, dry skin, bradycardia, muscle weakness) and symptom profile (depression, constipation, fatigue, cold sensitivity, impaired memory). However, even if there are fewer suggestive symptoms, a child who resides in a region where iodine deficiency is endemic (such as mountainous regions, areas of the northern Ganges River (India), or in North Africa) gives one more impetus for obtaining thyroid-stimulating hormone (TSH) and thyroxine (T4) (Zimmerman, 2009).

When considering additional medical studies, such as an ECG or EEG, the indications should be clear. Some medications, such as atypical antipsychotic medications or noradrenergic antagonists, may change cardiac conduction. Therefore, it is prudent to obtain a baseline ECG prior to starting these agents and to observe for any changes as the dose is increased. This is particularly important in children who have a family history of sudden death in young relatives, have a family history of cardiac anomalies or conduction disorders such as Wolff–Parkinson–White syndrome, or have a personal history of symptoms such as syncope, severe shortness of breath during exercise, prolonged or very significant fatigue, or, on routine ECG, borderline cardiac indices. This also is important when considering use of stimulant medication. The increase in pulse, blood pressure and cardiac work that methylphenidate or dextro-amphetamine produce, or direct cardiac conduction effects that agents like atomoxetine might induce, could exacerbate occult underlying cardiac problems (Stiefel & Besag, 2010; Martinez-Raga et al., 2013). In addition, children with known cardiac anomalies may be more likely to have symptoms of inattention, restlessness, and impulsivity, making them at particularly high risk for developing side effects when treated with these agents.

The decision to obtain an EEG should follow from the history and any symptoms that have been observed. The yield of clinically meaningful information from routine EEGs in children with generic psychiatric disorders is low (Camfield & Camfield, 2000; Smith, 2005; Raybould et al., 2012) and does not offset the cost, inconvenience, and discomfort to the patient. Conversely, when there is a history of paroxysmal events, with motor and/or psychomotor events, a prior history of serious head injury, the presence of disorders with a high likelihood of comorbid epilepsy, such as intellectual disability, specific genetic disorders, or autism spectrum disorders, then there is a compelling case to be made for obtaining an EEG. It is useful to pursue a careful history for any stereotyped symptoms that precede the psychomotor events or any "post-ictal" symptoms such as fatigue, cognitive dulling, or confusion that typically follow the event. Similarly, any disorder that presents with a decline in, or loss of previously acquired skills warrants an evaluation that includes an EEG.

The likelihood of finding clinically useful information from routine neuroimaging of child psychiatric patients is low. This is discussed thoroughly in Chapter 11. At this point there is a limited role for neuroimaging in general child and adolescent psychiatry.

Similarly, there is a very limited role for routine genetic evaluations. There are circumstances when the physical examination or concerns about intellectual disabilities (see Chapter 54) may require obtaining chromosomal and/or genetic studies. In addition, in the future, there may be a role for obtaining genetic studies when the patient gives a personal or family history of adverse drug reactions that raise a possibility of hyper- or hypo-metabolism of specific agents (e.g., codeine) (Kuehn, 2013). However, obtaining genetic assessments as a routine part of an evaluation is premature now. This is a controversial

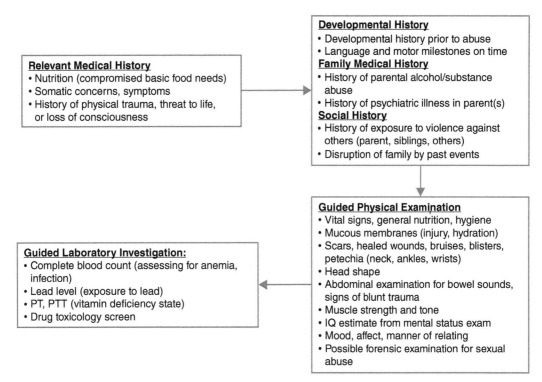

Relevant Medical History
• Nutrition (compromised basic food needs)
• Somatic concerns, symptoms
• History of physical trauma, threat to life, or loss of consciousness

Developmental History
• Developmental history prior to abuse
• Language and motor milestones on time
Family Medical History
• History of parental alcohol/substance abuse
• History of psychiatric illness in parent(s)
Social History
• History of exposure to violence against others (parent, siblings, others)
• Disruption of family by past events

Guided Physical Examination
• Vital signs, general nutrition, hygiene
• Mucous membranes (injury, hydration)
• Scars, healed wounds, bruises, blisters, petechia (neck, ankles, wrists)
• Head shape
• Abdominal examination for bowel sounds, signs of blunt trauma
• Muscle strength and tone
• IQ estimate from mental status exam
• Mood, affect, manner of relating
• Possible forensic examination for sexual abuse

Guided Laboratory Investigation:
• Complete blood count (assessing for anemia, infection)
• Lead level (exposure to lead)
• PT, PTT (vitamin deficiency state)
• Drug toxicology screen

Figure 35.2 Medical assessment of an 8-year-old female with "possible post traumatic stress disorder," recently removed from an abusive/neglectful home. PT, prothrombin time; PTT, partial thromboplastin time.

area with proponents who recommend genetic studies to guide selection of pharmacological agents (Wall *et al.*, 2012).

Assessment of cognitive functions should also flow from the history and physical examination. The history may point to consistent problems with learning and/or reaching social and cognitive milestones. This would prompt the clinician to consider obtaining a standard assessment of intellectual function (see Chapter 54). Similarly, specific patterns of impairment may emerge from the history, or arise from interviewing the child. A review of the child's academic history will provide essential data when considering the need for subsequent evaluations. Specific impairments in receptive language (e.g., problems with understanding instructions or explanations that use simple vocabulary), word finding, expressive language (e.g., problems in expressing thoughts, using appropriate length of utterances, using age- and culturally-appropriate vocabulary), or organization of language would prompt one to obtain a focused evaluation of language function from a speech pathologist (see Chapter 52).

Two examples of the flow of information and what the physician might consider during the examination are offered (Figures 35.1 and 35.2).

An example: the evaluation of psychosis

The differential diagnosis of psychotic conditions in children and adolescents is extensive (see Chapter 57; Yudofsky & Hales, 2007; Lishman's Organic Psychiatry (Anthony *et al.*, 2012).

The general grouping of etiologies parallels the many causes of delirium and mental status changes in adults (Table 35.1). In approaching the evaluation of the patient with new-onset psychosis, the psychiatrist must place particularly strong emphasis on the history, examination, and presentation of symptoms.

Despite the long list of disorders in Table 35.1, the probability that a child will have any one of these conditions is less than 1–2/10,000. For this reason, the preliminary laboratory examination should proceed from the presence of additional signs or symptoms. Laboratory assessments should also consider the most common etiologies first. For acute onset psychoses, it is reasonable to begin with a drug screen, complete blood count with differential (to consider infectious etiologies), serum electrolytes, urine analysis (for specific gravity, glucose, drugs of abuse, porphobilinogen, infection), thyroid function studies, and, if there are neurological symptoms or history that denote lead intoxication or seizures, a lead level, and an EEG.

> **Summary key points of the laboratory investigation**
>
> • The laboratory investigation provides additional data to narrow diagnostic possibilities raised by the history and physical examination.
>
> • The decision about which additional studies to pursue considers the context of the child's usual healthcare, the hypotheses about the most likely conditions, and clinical judgment about whether there may be an acute problem that poses immediate risk.

- There is no standard battery of laboratory tests for psychiatric disorders and laboratory studies should not simply assess "general health."
- When one suspects the presence of a specific condition, a focused laboratory assessment should be performed.
- Acquiring additional medical assessments such as ECG, EEG, genetics, cognitive testing, and language/communication evaluations follows from the history and physical examination.
- Routine use of neuroimaging in child psychiatry has a low yield of clinically useful information at this point.

Summary

Examination of the child psychiatric patient routinely includes all the basic elements of medical inquiry: the chief complaint, history of current illness, past medical and psychiatric history, family medical and psychiatric history, and a physical examination. Following the leads from these data, the psychiatrist may confer with a medical provider to plan for focused laboratory and other clinical evaluations that will reduce the differential diagnosis in a logical manner. Generally, that child's medical provider conducts the direct physical examination of the child, but there are occasions and situations when the psychiatrist may be required to examine his or her patient. If so, the sensitivity of the physician to the patient's past experiences, current state, culture, and developmental and cognitive levels should be foremost. The components of the examination that require touching the patient should occur in the presence of a parent or guardian. Perhaps one of the most vital skills in obtaining data from the history and physical examination is the mental health professional's capacity for observation. A great deal can be learned about cognitive and neurological functions from close observation of the patient during interviews, simple requests, and ordinary interactions.

Table 35.1 Differential diagnosis of delirium/psychosis.

I Toxic conditions (such as)
  (a) Substance abuse (amphetamines, bath salts, cocaine, 3,4-methylenedioxy-N-methylamphetamine (MDMA), hallucinogens)
  (b) Acute lead encephalopathy
  (c) Neuroleptic malignant syndrome
  (d) Drug-induced delirium
II Metabolic disorders (such as)
  (a) Adrenoleukodystrophy
  (b) GM2 gangliosidoses
  (c) Neimann–Pick disease
  (d) Beta-mannosidosis
  (e) Acute intermittent porphyria
  (f) Homocysteinuria
III Endocrinological disorders (such as)
  (a) Thyrotoxicosis
  (b) Hypothyroidism
  (c) Addison's disease
  (d) Cushing syndrome
  (e) Hyperparathyroidism
IV Infectious diseases (such as)
  (a) Viral encephalitis
  (b) Bacterial encephalitis
  (c) Post-infectious encephalitis
  (d) Fungal encephalitis (e.g., Cryptococcus)
  (e) Prion diseases
  (f) Spirochetal infections
V Structural neurological lesions (such as)
  (a) Temporal lobe glioma
VI Autoimmune disorders (such as)
  (a) Systemic lupus erythematosus
  (b) Sarcoidosis
VII Paroxysmal disorders (such as)
  (a) Temporal lobe epilepsy
  (b) Partial complex status epilepticus
  (c) Post-ictal psychosis
VIII Specific genetic disorders (such as)
  (a) Huntington's disease
  (b) Wilson's disease
  (c) Parkinson's disease
  (d) Fahr's disease

References

Amed, S. *et al.* (2011) Risk factors for medication-induced diabetes and type 2 diabetes. *Journal of Pediatrics* **159**, 291–296.

Anthony, D. *et al.* (2012) *Lishman's Organic Psychiatry: A Textbook of Neuropsychiatry*, 4th edn. Wiley-Blackwell, Hoboken, NJ.

Ban, Y. & Tomer, Y. (2005) Genetic susceptibility in thyroid autoimmunity. *Pediatric Endocrinology Reviews* **3**, 20–32.

Beach, S.R. *et al.* (2013) QTc prolongation, torsades de pointes, and psychotropic medications. *Psychosomatics* **54**, 1–13.

Bickley, L.S. (2012) *Bates' Guide to Physical Examination and History Taking*, 11th edn. Lippincott Williams & Wilkins Publisher, Philadelphia, PA.

Camfield, P. & Camfield, C. (2000) How often does routine pediatric EEG have an important unexpected result? *Canadian Journal of Neurological Sciences* **27**, 321–324.

Cassidy, S.B. *et al.* (2012) Prader-Willi syndrome. *Genetics in Medicine* **14**, 10–26.

CDC (Centers for Disease Control and Prevention) (2011) *Facts About Child Development*. Available: http://www.cdc.gov/ncbddd/childdevelopment/facts.html [13 May 2013]

Chapieski, L. *et al.* (2000) Psychological functioning in children and adolescents with Sturge-Weber syndrome. *Journal of Child Neurology* **15**, 660–665.

Cooper, J.D. *et al.* (2012) Seven newly identified loci for autoimmune thyroid disease. *Human Molecular Genetics* **21**, 5202–5208.

Copeland, K.C. *et al.* (2013) Management of newly diagnosed type 2 Diabetes Mellitus (T2DM) in children and adolescents. *Pediatrics* **131**, 364–382.

Drotar, D. *et al.* (2008) Selecting developmental surveillance and screening tools. *Pediatrics in Review* **29**, e52–e58.

Filho, A.S. *et al.* (2011) Mitral valve prolapse and anxiety disorders. *British Journal of Psychiatry* **199**, 247–248.

Frankenburg, W.K. *et al.* (1992) The DENVER II: a major revision and restandardization of the Denver Developmental Screening Test. *Pediatrics* **89**, 91–97.

Gerber, R.J. *et al.* (2010) Developmental milestones: motor development. *Pediatrics in Review* **31**, 267–276.

Gerber, R.J. *et al.* (2011) Developmental milestones 3: social-emotional development. *Pediatrics in Review* **32**, 533–536.

Gropman, A.L. *et al.* (2006) Neurologic and developmental features of the Smith-Magenis syndrome (del 17p11.2). *Pediatric Neurology* **34**, 337–350.

Hannon, T.S. *et al.* (2013) Depressive symptoms and metabolic markers of risk for type 2 diabetes in obese adolescents. *Pediatric Diabetes* **14**, 497–503.

Kendler, K.S. & Baker, J. (2007) Genetic influences on measures of the environment: a systematic review. *Psychological Medicine* **37**, 615–626.

Kroonen, L.T. *et al.* (2006) Prader-Willi Syndrome: clinical concerns for the orthopaedic surgeon. *Journal of Pediatric Orthopaedics* **26**, 673–679.

Kuehn, B.M. (2013) FDA: no codeine after tonsillectomy for children. *JAMA* **309**, 1100.

LeBlond, R.F. *et al.* (2008) *DeGowin's Diagnostic Examination*, 9th edn. McGraw Hill Professional Publishing, NY.

Martinez-Raga, J. *et al.* (2013) Risk of serious cardiovascular problems with medications for attention-deficit hyperactivity disorder. *CNS Drugs* **27**, 15–30.

Meaney, M.J. (2010) Epigenetics and the biological definition of gene x environment interactions. *Child Development* **81**, 47–79.

Numis, A.L. *et al.* (2011) Identification of risk factors for autism spectrum disorders in tuberous sclerosis complex. *Neurology* **76**, 981–987.

Otter, M. *et al.* (2010) Triple X syndrome: a review of the literature. *European Journal of Human Genetics* **18**, 265–271.

Pilowsky, D. & Chambers, W. (1986) *Hallucinations in children*. American Psychiatric Association, Washington, DC.

Raybould, J.E. *et al.* (2012) EEG screening for temporal lobe epilepsy in patients with acute psychosis. *Journal of Neuropsychiatry and Clinical Neurosciences* **24**, 452–457.

Reulecke, B.C. *et al.* (2008) Brain tumors in children: initial symptoms and their influence on the time span between symptom onset and diagnosis. *Journal of Child Neurology* **23**, 178–183.

Richa, S. & Yazbek, J.C. (2010) Ocular adverse effects of common psychotropic agents: a review. *CNS Drugs* **24**, 501–526.

Rodríguez-Moran, M. *et al.* (2010) Obesity and family history of diabetes as risk factors of impaired fasting glucose: implications for the early detection of prediabetes. *Pediatric Diabetes* **11**, 331–336.

Rutter, M. (2012) Resilience as a dynamic concept. *Development and Psychopathology* **24**, 335–344.

Rutter, M. *et al.* (2006) Gene-environment interplay and psychopathology: multiple varieties but real effects. *Journal of Child Psychology and Psychiatry* **47**, 226–261.

Sateia, M.J. (2009) Update on sleep and psychiatric disorders. *Chest* **135**, 1370–1379.

Smith, S.J. (2005) EEG in neurological conditions other than epilepsy: when does it help, what does it add? *Journal of Neurology, Neurosurgery, and Psychiatry* **76** (Suppl 2), ii8–ii12.

Sparrow, S.S. *et al.* (1984) *The Vineland Adaptive Behavior Scales*. America Guidance Service, Circle Pines, MN.

Sparrow, S.S. *et al.* (2005) *Vineland Adaptive Behavior Scales Second Edition Survey Forms Manual*. America Guidance Service AGS Publishing, Circle Pines, MN.

Speltz, M.L. *et al.* (2004) Single-suture craniosynostosis: a review of neurobehavioral research and theory. *J Pediatric Psychology* **29**, 651–668.

Stiefel, G. & Besag, F.M. (2010) Cardiovascular effects of methylphenidate, amphetamines and atomoxetine in the treatment of attention-deficit hyperactivity disorder. *Drug Safety* **33**, 821–842.

Swallen, K.C. *et al.* (2005) Overweight, obesity, and health-related quality of life among adolescents: the National Longitudinal Study of Adolescent Health. *Pediatrics* **115**, 340–347.

Tan, B.Y. & Judge, D.P. (2012) A clinical approach to a family history of sudden death. *Circulation Cardiovascular Genetics* **5**, 697–705.

Wall, C.A. *et al.* (2012) Psychiatric pharmacogenomics in pediatric psychopharmacology. *Child and Adolescent Psychiatric Clinics of North America* **21**, 773–788.

Wareham, N.J. *et al.* (2002) Establishing the role of gene-environment interactions in the etiology of type 2 diabetes. *Endocrinology and Metabolism Clinics of North America* **31**, 553–566.

Weisse, A.B. (2007) Mitral valve prolapse: now you see it; now you don't: recalling the discovery, rise and decline of a diagnosis. *American Journal of Cardiology* **99**, 129–133.

Wilks, T. *et al.* (2010) Developmental milestones: cognitive development. *Pediatrics in Review* **31**, 364–367.

Wilne, S.H. *et al.* (2006) The presenting features of brain tumours: a review of 200 cases. *Archives of Disease in Childhood* **91**, 502–506.

Yudofsky, S.C. & Hales, R.E. (2007) *The American Psychiatric Publishing Textbook of Neuropsychiatry and Behavioral Neurosciences*, 5th edn. American Psychiatric Association, Washington, DC.

Zimmerman, M.B. (2009) Iodine Deficiency. *Endocrine Reviews* **30**, 376–408.

CHAPTER 36

Psychological interventions: overview and critical issues for the field

John R. Weisz, Mei Yi Ng and Nancy Lau
Department of Psychology, Harvard University, Cambridge, MA, USA

Psychological intervention has deep historical roots. These extend at least as far back as ancient religious teachings about values for proper living, to Greek philosophers' use of discourse to alter perspectives and sharpen understanding, and to the long evolution of medical science and the healing traditions. Interventions for children and adolescents (henceforth "youths") share these ancient roots, but designation of youth psychotherapy as a distinctive specialty owes much to Sigmund Freud (1856–1939), notably his analysis of the "Little Hans" case of horse phobia and his psychoanalysis of his own daughter, Anna (1895–1982). Subsequent growth of youth psychotherapy was fueled by Freud's intellectual heirs, by the grand theories of personality and development, and by models and methods as different from psychoanalysis as behaviorism and cognitive psychology. By the end of the 20th century, Kazdin (2000) had identified 551 different named therapies used with youths. Of course, many more therapies are used in clinical practice, as hundreds of thousands of unique practitioners shape their own approaches.

While youth psychotherapy practice accelerated quickly over the past century, psychotherapy research developed slowly. In 1952, Eysenck's influential review of adult psychotherapy studies suggested that therapy might be ineffective. Levitt's (1957, 1963) reviews, which included youth treatment, reached a similar conclusion. Since the time of Eysenck and Levitt, youth treatment outcome research has grown more rigorous, and its volume has mushroomed (see Silverman & Hinshaw, 2008; Weisz & Kazdin, 2010).

Studying the effects of youth psychotherapy: methods and findings

Youth treatment effects are often assessed via randomized controlled trials (RCTs), and these RCTs can be pooled and synthesized within meta-analyses (discussed later). Multiple baseline designs, ABAB (sometimes called "reversal") designs, and other single-subject methods are also useful. These methods (see Barlow et al., 2009; Kazdin, 2011) have been used in diverse treatment situations—such as programs for ADHD (see, e.g., Pelham et al., 2010), studies of intervention for an entire classroom (see e.g., Wurtele & Drabman, 1984), or for only one or two youngsters with a rare condition (e.g., McGrath et al., 1987; Tarnowski et al., 1987). Studies using these designs have produced a rich body of outcome evidence and some meta-analyses—for example, on treatment for disruptive behavior (Chen & Ma, 2007), autism spectrum disorders (Campbell, 2003), and social skill deficits (Mathur et al., 1998). That said, youth psychotherapy meta-analyses have mainly focused on RCTs.

Meta-analytic findings

Among the meta-analyses of youth RCTs, four have synthesized findings from diverse treatments and treated conditions. Casey and Berman (1985) focused on studies with children aged 12 and younger. Weisz et al. (1987) included studies with 4- to 18-year-olds. Kazdin et al. (1990) included studies with 4- to 18-year-olds. Finally, Weisz et al. (1995) spanned ages 2–18. Mean effect sizes found in these four meta-analyses are shown in Figure 36.1, with a comparison to two widely cited meta-analyses of predominantly adult psychotherapy (Smith & Glass, 1977; Shapiro & Shapiro, 1982). The figure shows that youth treatment effect sizes fall mainly within the range found for adult therapy, and on average between Cohen's (1988) benchmarks for medium (i.e., 0.5) and large (0.8) effects.

Two other youth meta-analytic findings sharpen the picture in an encouraging way. First, findings (Weisz et al., 1987, 1995) showed that effects measured immediately after treatment were quite similar to effects measured at follow-up assessments, which

Rutter's Child and Adolescent Psychiatry, Sixth Edition.
Edited by Anita Thapar and Daniel S. Pine, James F. Leckman, Stephen Scott, Margaret J. Snowling, Eric Taylor.
© 2015 John Wiley & Sons Ltd. Published 2018 by John Wiley & Sons Ltd.

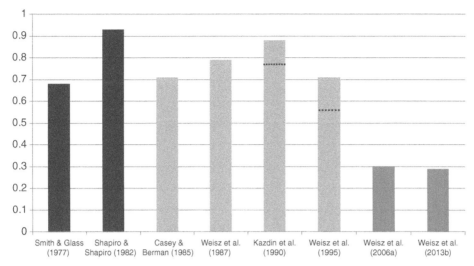

Figure 36.1 Mean effect sizes found in two broad-based meta-analyses of adult psychotherapy effects (the two bars at the left: Smith & Glass, 1977; Shapiro & Shapiro, 1982), four broad-based meta-analyses of youth psychotherapy effects (the four middle bars: Casey & Berman, 1985; Weisz *et al.*, 1987; Kazdin *et al.*, 1990; Weisz *et al.*, 1995), and two meta-analyses of RCTs comparing evidence-based youth psychotherapies to usual clinical care (the two bars at the right: Weisz *et al.*, 2006a, 2013b). The full bar for Kazdin *et al.* (1990) shows the mean effect size for treatment vs. inert control group comparisons; the dashed line shows the mean for treatment vs. active control group comparisons. The full bar for Weisz *et al.* (1995) shows the mean effect size when unweighted least squares analyses were conducted; the dashed line shows the mean for weighted least squares analyses. *Source:* Reprinted with permission from John R. Weisz.

averaged about 6 months after the end of treatment. This suggests reasonable holding power of treatment benefit over time. Second, findings indicated that effects are larger for the specific problems targeted in treatment than for problems that were not specifically addressed (Weisz *et al.*, 1995). This suggests that the tested therapies did not just create nonspecific good feelings but instead impacted rather precisely the kinds of dysfunction they were designed to treat.

These findings suggest certain strengths of youth psychotherapies, but meta-analysis can also highlight challenges, critical questions, and areas in which intervention needs to be strengthened. A meta-analysis of psychotherapy for youth depression, for example, showed beneficial effects that were statistically significant (mean effect size: 0.34) but also significantly smaller than effects of treatments for other youth problems and disorders; even the very popular cognitive approaches, including cognitive behavioral therapy (CBT), were no more successful than alternative treatments in alleviating depression (see Weisz *et al.*, 2006b). Such findings provide a reality check, potentially suggesting a need to strengthen or even reenvision youth depression treatment.

Identifying "evidence-based psychotherapies"

As treatment outcome evidence accumulated over the years, and documentation of the tested treatments grew more precise (typically in the form of detailed treatment manuals), efforts were launched to identify the specific therapies sufficiently well supported to be considered "evidence-based psychotherapies" (EBPs). Task forces and review teams were formed

(see e.g., Chambless *et al.*, 1998) to distill the research evidence and identify therapies that met standards for different levels of empirical support. Building on this work, experts in youth psychotherapy compiled their own reports in two journal special issues (Lonigan *et al.*, 1998; Silverman & Hinshaw, 2008). In the most recent report (Silverman & Hinshaw, 2008), reviewers identified therapies at four levels of empirical support: (1) *well-established* (i.e., two good group-design experiments by different research teams in two different settings, showing the treatment to be "superior to pill, psychological placebo, or another treatment"), (2) *probably efficacious* (i.e., " … at least two good experiments showing the treatment is superior … to a wait-list control group"), (3) *possibly efficacious* (i.e., " … at least one 'good' study showing the treatment to be efficacious in the absence of conflicting evidence"), or (4) *experimental* (i.e., " … not yet tested in trials meeting task force criteria").

This 2008 report identified dozens of youth psychotherapies as either *well-established* or *probably efficacious,* encompassing multiple disorders and problems. Table 36.1 shows the youth treatments classified at these two highest levels in the Silverman and Hinshaw (2008) special issue. Throughout this chapter, we refer to these interventions as EBPs.

The evidence-based psychotherapies: "well-established" and "probably efficacious"
Autism

In the autism review (Rogers & Vismara, 2008), only one treatment was designated well-established: Ivar Lovaas's Early Intensive Behavioral Intervention (EIBI; Smith, 2010); this is a form

Table 36.1 Evidence-based youth psychotherapies[a,b].

Problem/disorder category	Well-established (WE) or Probably efficacious (PE) psychotherapy
Early autism (Rogers & Vismara, 2008)	• Lovaas Model: Early Intensive Behavioral Intervention (WE) • Pivotal Response Treatment (PE)
Eating disorders in adolescence (Keel & Haedt, 2008)	• Family Therapy for Anorexia Nervosa (WE)
Depression (David-Ferdon & Kaslow, 2008)	• CBT for Children (WE) • CBT for Adolescents (WE) • Interpersonal Psychotherapy for Adolescents (WE) • Behavior Therapy for Children (PE)
Phobic & anxiety disorders (Silverman et al., 2008b)	• Group CBT (PE) • Group CBT for Social Phobia (PE) • Group CBT with Parents (PE) • Individual CBT (PE) • Social Effectiveness Training for Social Phobia (PE)
Obsessive-compulsive disorder (Barrett et al., 2008)	• Individual Exposure-Based CBT (PE)
Youths exposed to traumatic events (Silverman et al., 2008a)	• Trauma-Focused CBT (WE) • School-Based Group CBT (PE)
Attention-deficit/hyperactivity disorder (Pelham & Fabiano, 2008)	• Behavioral Classroom Management (WE) • Behavioral Parent Training (WE) • Intensive Peer-Focused Behavioral Interventions in Recreational Settings (WE)
Disruptive behavior (Eyberg et al., 2008)	• Parent Management Training Oregon Model (WE) • Anger Control Training (PE) • Group Assertive Training (PE) • Helping the Noncompliant Child (PE) • Incredible Years Parent Training (PE) • Incredible Years Child Training (PE) • Multidimensional Treatment Foster Care (PE) • Multisystemic Therapy (PE) • Parent–Child Interaction Therapy (PE) • Positive Parenting Program-Standard (PE) • Positive Parenting Program-Enhanced (PE) • Problem-Solving Skills Training (PSST) (PE) • PSST + Practice (PE) • PSST + Parent Management Training (PE) • Rational-Emotive Mental Health Program (PE)
Adolescent substance abuse (Waldron & Turner, 2008)	• Functional Family Therapy (WE) • Group CBT (WE) • Individual CBT (WE) • Multidimensional Family Therapy (WE) • Behavioral Family Therapy (PE) • Brief Strategic Family Therapy (PE) • Multisystemic Therapy (PE)

[a]*Data source:* Silverman, W.K. & Hinshaw, S.P. (eds) (2008) Evidence-based psychosocial treatments for children and adolescents: A ten year update [Special issue]. *Journal of Child and Adolescent Clinical Psychology* **37**, 1–301.
[b]This table shows classifications for broad forms of psychotherapy (e.g., Cognitive behavioral therapy; CBT); some reports in the special issue of the journal also classified specific treatment subtypes (e.g., group CBT for children, individual adolescent CBT plus parent/family component), which are not included in the table, given space limitations.

of applied behavior analysis that entails individual discreet trials training, often 30 hours per week or more, building specific core skills in language, social interaction, self-help, and other domains critical to children's development. Therapists treat the children and train parents to continue the intervention at home.

A related intervention, Pivotal Response Training (PRT; Koegel *et al.*, 2010) was rated probably efficacious; PRT uses core skills of the Lovaas model but with an expanded emphasis on treatment in the child's natural environment and on strategies for boosting the child's motivation to learn (e.g., relying on activities the child chooses, identifying natural reinforcers). PRT teaches communication, academic, self-help, social, and even recreational skills; like EIBI, PRT relies heavily on training parents to deliver the intervention.

Eating disorders

Only one treatment for eating disorders was identified as an EBP (see Keel & Haedt, 2008): family therapy for anorexia nervosa, and in particular the Maudsley model (Lock *et al.*, 2001). This model includes (a) relying on family members to return the client to more normal eating behavior—a process called "refeeding the client"; (b) negotiating restructured relationships in areas that influence eating behavior (e.g., if deceit is used by the family to avoid conflict *and* by the youth to conceal binging, therapy may focus on alternatives to deceit); and (c) termination, including planning ways to sustain healthy eating by sustaining healthy intrafamily relationships and youth autonomy. No EBP was identified for bulimia nervosa in adolescents, but the reviewers (Keel & Haedt, 2008) noted that CBT (e.g., addressing distorted cognitions about body shape and size, using behavioral procedures to structure healthy eating habits) is a well-established treatment for bulimia in young adults and older adolescents. A special challenge in the eating domain is that eating disorders can take multiple forms, and in fact the most prevalent diagnostic category is "not otherwise specified." Thus, even effective treatments for anorexia and bulimia will not necessarily fit most eating disordered youths (see Chapter 71).

Anxiety disorders

For phobic and anxiety disorders in youth (reviewed by Silverman *et al.*, 2008b), the most thoroughly tested psychotherapies are the CBTs; these most often blend graduated exposure to feared stimuli with efforts to identify and modify distorted cognitions that can spark and sustain fears. The treatments rated as EBPs included individual CBT, group CBT, group CBT with parents, and Social Effectiveness Therapy for Children (SET-C; Beidel *et al.*, 2000). SET-C, designed for social phobia, includes group sessions for youngsters, *in vivo* exposure sessions (e.g., practicing interacting with nonanxious peers), and teaching parents to notice and reward their children's steps toward less anxious behavior in social situations.

In their review of interventions for obsessive compulsive disorder, Barrett *et al.* (2008) identified only one treatment that met EBP criteria: individual exposure-based CBT. Youths are exposed to stimuli that lead to their obsessive fears but then told not to engage in the compulsive behavior those fears usually trigger. Ideally, across repeated exposures, the anxiety-obsession-compulsion cycle is weakened via autonomic habituation and altered cognition, as youths learn that bad things they fear do not actually happen when they say no to their compulsions.

Finally, reviewing treatments for youths exposed to traumatic events, Silverman *et al.* (2008a) identified trauma-focused CBT (Cohen *et al.*, 2010) as an EBP. This treatment, designed for young victims of sexual abuse and other forms of maltreatment, uses components of CBT for anxiety, plus additional elements designed to fit the situations in which trauma occurred. The components include, for example, safety planning (to reduce environmental risk) and "trauma narrative," in which young people write, then read, descriptions of their traumatic experiences. The draft narrative is repeatedly read to the therapist, as a form of exposure therapy. Distorted cognitions in the narrative (e.g., inappropriate self-blame) are modified through discussion between the youth and therapist. Caregivers participate, by joining the youth and therapist at later readings of the narrative and by supporting the youth's courage in sharing the story. Silverman *et al.* (2008a) also identified school-based group CBT (Kataoka *et al.*, 2003; Stein *et al.*, 2003) as an EBP. This treatment, designed for youths exposed to community violence, includes psychoeducation, cognitive work, coping skills training, social skills training, and graduated exposures carried out through writing and/or drawing.

Depression

David-Ferdon and Kaslow (2008), reviewing depression treatments, identified two broad approaches as EBPs: Interpersonal Psychotherapy for Adolescents (IPT-A; Mufson *et al.*, 1999) and CBT. IPT-A focuses on interpersonal issues that are common among adolescents, such as the ways roles shift in the parent–teen relationship as teens mature; the intervention focuses on helping adolescents build effective strategies for dealing with role transitions, disputes, grief, and interpersonal deficits. As for CBT, its content varies across programs, but it typically includes such components as identifying and scheduling mood-boosting activities, identifying and modifying unrealistic negative thoughts, self-calming and relaxation, and building problem-solving skills. An approach called "behavior therapy" was also identified as a probably efficacious EBP (e.g., Kahn *et al.*, 1990); its contents resembled CBT in most respects.

Attention deficit/hyperactivity disorder

Pelham and Fabiano (2008), reviewing treatments for ADHD, identified three as well-established. One was behavioral parent training, in which parents learn techniques for effective behavior management (e.g., clear instructions, differential attention for desired versus undesired behavior, use of praise and reward, time-out). The second was behavioral contingency management in classrooms, often carried out by school personnel. The third was intensive peer-focused behavioral interventions in recreational settings. A model program of this type is Pelham's Summer Treatment Program (Pelham *et al.*, 2010), in which youngsters are immersed in sports, academic, and social skill-building activities, all within the context of a highly structured environment with clear behavioral contingencies; caregivers also participate, learning effective behavior management strategies for use at home. Importantly, Pelham and Fabiano did not find convincing support for CBT or nonbehavioral treatments for ADHD youths.

Conduct-related problems and disorders

In the review of treatments for conduct-related problems and disorders, Eyberg *et al.* (2008) identified 16 EBPs. These included behavioral parent training programs, some involving parent management training (Forgatch & Patterson, 2010; Kazdin, 2010; Sanders & Murphy-Brennan, 2010) and some involving coaching during actual parent–child interactions (e.g., McMahon & Forehand, 2003; Zisser & Eyberg, 2010). The Incredible Years program (Webster-Stratton & Reid, 2010) includes a behaviorally oriented video-guided series involving group sessions for parents (who view and discuss video clips illustrating effective and ineffective parenting strategies), and social skills and problem-solving training groups for children (ages 3–8); the parent and child programs have been shown to be beneficial separately and in combination. Other EBPs for conduct problems include behavioral and cognitive training to enhance anger management (Lochman *et al.*, 2010), problem-solving skills (Kazdin, 2010), and socially appropriate assertiveness (Huey & Rank, 1984), as well as a school-based program designed to reduce misbehavior by training youths to make accurate appraisals of the self and social situations (Block, 1978).

Finally, two of the EBPs identified by Eyberg *et al.* (2008) blend behavioral training for caregivers with strategies for building support within the youth's social system. These include the extensively studied Multisystemic Therapy (MST; Henggeler & Schaeffer, 2010), developed originally for delinquent youths but later extended to other forms of dysfunction (e.g., sexual offending, suicidal behavior), and Multidimensional Treatment Foster Care (MTFC; Smith & Chamberlain, 2010), designed to support effective care for disruptive youths who have been placed in foster care. We later discuss MST and MTFC in greater detail.

Adolescent substance abuse

In their review of treatments for adolescent substance abuse, Waldron and Turner (2008) reported that interventions qualifying for EBP status have focused mainly on alcohol and marijuana use. The three EBPs they identified use a blend of behavioral methods, family systems work, and outreach to broader social systems. One of the EBPs, Functional Family Therapy (FFT; Alexander & Parsons, 1982), relies on core behavioral techniques and a family systems orientation to establish new patterns of family interaction, and therapists also work with extrafamilial systems such as schools and probation offices to help ensure that benefits will generalize to the community. In addition, both individual and group CBT approaches (see Waldron & Kaminer, 2004) were identified as EBPs. In general, the CBT approaches focus on identifying and modifying distorted cognitions, plus training and practice in the behavioral coping skills needed to avoid substance use (e.g., coping with cravings, resisting social pressure to get high, and avoiding situations where substance use might be likely).

Investigating the strength, causes, and conditions of effective treatment

Initially, researchers were most interested in identifying which psychotherapies work. Over time, however, interest has grown in *how* treatments work (i.e., through what processes), *with whom* they work, and *under what conditions*—questions to which we now turn.

Mediators and mechanisms of change

Understanding how a treatment works requires identifying mechanisms of change, the specific processes through which the treatment produces outcomes. A sound understanding of these mechanisms could help treatment developers strengthen the active ingredients of psychotherapy and minimize inactive components, thereby increasing treatment efficacy and cost-effectiveness (Kraemer *et al.*, 2002). A first step in identifying change mechanisms is testing whether a particular variable is a mediator of treatment outcome in an RCT, that is, an intermediate variable evident during treatment that statistically accounts for the treatment–outcome relationship (Kraemer *et al.*, 2002; Kazdin, 2007).

Moderators of treatment outcome

Understanding with whom treatments work and under what conditions requires identifying moderators of treatment outcome. In an RCT, a moderator is a variable present prior to randomization that interacts with treatment condition, such that treatment effects depend on the level of the moderator (Kraemer *et al.*, 2002). Identifying client characteristics that moderate treatment effects can reveal which client subgroups benefit most, and least, from various treatments. That information could help inform clinicians' efforts to identify the best-fit treatments for specific subgroups of patients (Kraemer *et al.*, 2002).

Mediators of evidence-based psychotherapies

To illustrate the search for mediators, we focus here on research testing two variables frequently studied in RCTs of youth EBPs—negative cognitions and parenting practices.

Negative cognitions

Negative cognitions have often been tested as candidate mediators of EBPs for internalizing disorders. This reflects the CBT theoretical model, which holds that symptoms can be reduced by changing cognitions that are unrealistically negative to cognitions that are more positive, realistic, or adaptive.

Mediation tests within RCTs of CBT for youth depression have yielded mixed findings. Shifts to less pessimistic or more optimistic explanatory styles have been found to mediate reductions in children's depressive symptoms (Jaycox *et al.*, 1994; Yu & Seligman, 2002). Decreases in negative automatic thoughts and in dysfunctional core beliefs were significant mediators in some RCTs of CBT for adolescent depression, but not in others (Ackerson *et al.*, 1998; Kaufman *et al.*, 2005; Stice *et al.*, 2010).

There have been fewer studies of mediation in CBT for youth anxiety. However, the studies have rather consistently found that decreases in anxious self-statements mediate reductions in anxiety symptoms in individual CBT (Treadwell & Kendall, 1996; Kendall & Treadwell, 2007) and group CBT (Lau *et al.*, 2010).

Parenting practices

Parenting practices have often been tested as mediators of EBPs for externalizing problems. Most such EBPs aim to reduce youth problems partly through changing their caregivers' behaviors. These EBPs include behavioral parent training for mild conduct problems, MTFC and MST for severe conduct problems, MDFT for adolescent substance abuse, and behavioral treatment for ADHD.

Effective, consistent parental discipline has been found to mediate treatment effects on child conduct problems in RCTs of Parent Management Training—Oregon model (PMTO; Amlund Hagen *et al.*, 2011) and anger control training (Lochman & Wells, 2002). For MTFC and MST—EBPs for adolescent offenders—mediators include not only caregivers' disciplinary practices, but also their ability to limit adolescents' association with deviant peers (Eddy & Chamberlain, 2000; Henggeler *et al.*, 2009). Both caregiver supervision and positive caregiver–youth relationship were also significant mediators of MTFC (Eddy & Chamberlain, 2000). In contrast, caregiver supervision and caregiver–youth communication were not mediators of MST (Henggeler *et al.*, 2009), and family cohesion was not a mediator of PMTO (Amlund Hagen *et al.*, 2011).

For substance use problems, parent monitoring of adolescents' activities and peers has mediated the effects of MDFT, relative to peer group intervention, on adolescents' 12-month abstinence from substance use (Henderson *et al.*, 2009). Intriguingly, mediation was found only when the outcome measured was the proportion of abstinent youths, but not when substance use frequency was the outcome; the authors concluded that parent monitoring may work when it prevents, but not when it merely reduces, substance use. Improved parent–adolescent relationship was not a mediator (Henderson *et al.*, 2009).

Research on ADHD intervention in the Multimodal Treatment Study of Children with ADHD (MTA; MTA Cooperative Group, 1999) has identified parents' discipline practices as a mediator. In the MTA, medication (methylphenidate, Ritalin) only and combined medication and behavioral treatment (i.e., behavioral parent training, summer treatment program, and behavioral classroom management) outperformed behavioral treatment only, as well as community care. Curiously, discipline practices mediated treatment effects on children's social skills at school only when combination treatment—but not behavioral treatment or medication only—was compared to community care; other parenting practices (i.e., positive involvement, deficient monitoring) were not mediators (Hinshaw *et al.*, 2000).

Discussion

The mediation research reviewed may shed some light on the EBPs' potential mechanisms of change. However, many questions remain. First, the small number of published mediation studies raises a concern that some of the mediators identified may represent chance findings, with many unpublished null findings languishing in file drawers. More replications are needed to confirm that even our best-supported candidate mediators, negative cognitions and parenting practices, are in fact robust mediators of EBP effects.

Second, findings were mixed; for example, negative cognitions did not consistently mediate CBT for depression, and parenting practices other than caregiver discipline did not consistently mediate EBPs for conduct problems. It is not clear whether these mixed findings reflect methodological artifacts, failure to differentiate related but distinct mediators, or true mediators that emerge only for certain conditions, age ranges, symptom severity, problem type, or protocol used; if so, this would represent what is called *moderated* mediation.

Third, we have not found clear evidence that change in any mediator preceded change in outcome; that temporal sequence is necessary for a mediator to be considered a true mechanism of change (Kazdin, 2007). Many studies measured the mediator and outcome at pre- and posttreatment only, precluding efforts to clarify the temporal sequence. For example, Hinshaw and colleagues (2000) could not determine whether combination treatment of methylphenidate plus behavioral therapy in the MTA (a) reduced parents' ineffective discipline, which in turn improved children's social skills; (b) improved children's social skills, which in turn led parents to reduce ineffective discipline; or (c) changed something else that caused improvement in both child social skills and parent discipline. Some (e.g., Henderson *et al.*, 2009) have demonstrated that an earlier measurement of change in the mediator predicted a later measurement of change in outcome, but a mediator change that was *measured* earlier does not equate to a mediator change that *occurred* earlier. Frequent measurement of *both* candidate mediators *and* outcomes throughout and after treatment will be needed to determine which changes occur in which order (Kazdin, 2007). When Stice and colleagues (2010) attempted such frequent measurement, they identified a paltry 8% of participants who met the temporal precedence criterion.

Fourth, a number of variables that have been conceptualized as change mechanisms have rarely been studied as mediators. Mediation studies of youth CBT have generally focused on cognitive variables, not behavioral variables such as engagement in pleasant activities or exposures, which are major components of CBT for depression and anxiety respectively (for exceptions, see Kaufman *et al.*, 2005; Stice *et al.*, 2010). In addition, mediation studies of EBPs for externalizing disorders have often neglected youth cognitive and behavioral variables such as hostile attributions, expectations of outcomes from aggressive behavior, locus of control, and school engagement, which have in fact been found to mediate treatment effects (Lochman & Wells, 2002; Leve & Chamberlain, 2007). Furthermore, few published studies have examined common factors (i.e., hypothesized change mechanisms shared by different psychotherapies, for different disorders, such as therapeutic alliance, hope, and readiness for change) as mediators in RCTs of youth EBPs. The therapeutic alliance, despite having been documented as a significant predictor of outcome in a meta-analysis of 38 studies of youth psychotherapy (McLeod, 2011), has, to our knowledge, been subjected to a mediation test in only a single study (Kaufman et al., 2005). Moreover, we are not aware of any published mediation studies for several EBPs (e.g., EIBI, IPT-A, FFT), which each have theoretical change models that could be empirically tested in mediation studies.

Fifth, at least two major multisite trials have found that combination treatment involving medication plus EBP was superior to medication alone and EBP alone—suggesting a need to study mediators and change mechanisms of combination treatments. As mentioned earlier, methylphenidate plus behavioral therapy was the most efficacious treatment in the MTA (MTA Cooperative Group, 1999); in addition fluoxetine (Prozac) plus CBT was the most efficacious treatment in the Treatment for Adolescents with Depression Study (TADS; TADS Team, 2004). Soberingly, in both these trials, combination treatment and medication alone, but not EBP alone, outperformed the control group (community care and pill placebo, respectively). In the MTA, both combination treatment and behavioral treatment alone improved parent discipline, but only for combination treatment was improved parent discipline related to improved child social skills and disruptive behavior (Hinshaw et al., 2000). In TADS, both combination treatment and CBT alone increased adolescents' readiness to change (specifically, their action orientation), and increases in readiness to change were associated with reductions in depressive symptoms (Lewis et al., 2009). However, pairwise contrasts of TADS treatment conditions were not conducted; thus, it is unclear if the mediation effect reported by Lewis and colleagues applies to both combination treatment and CBT. The bottom line is that we simply do not know exactly how medication and EBP combine synergistically to bring about superior effects; we need to uncover the mediators and change mechanisms targeted by combination treatments.

Moderators of evidence-based psychotherapies

Here, we review three categories of moderators—youth, caregiver, and methodological variables—found to be significant in meta-analyses of youth psychotherapies (encompassing multiple treatments, not exclusively EBPs) or in selected RCTs of youth EBPs.

Youth characteristics

Youth symptom severity, comorbidity, demographics, and other pretreatment characteristics are often tested as potential moderators of EBPs. The specific youth variables that emerge as significant moderators have varied across EBP and disorder. We exclude here a number of youth characteristics for which evidence is extremely mixed (e.g., age and gender), but we offer two examples of factors for which findings have been intriguing.

Pretreatment symptom severity was identified as a significant moderator in several meta-analyses and RCTs. Higher severity was associated with larger treatment effects in two meta-analyses—one of psychotherapy for youth depression (Watanabe et al., 2007), the other of behavioral parent training for youth disruptive behavior (Lundahl et al., 2006)—possibly because there is more room for improvement among severely symptomatic youths. However, higher severity has also been linked to *smaller* effects of combination treatment and medication alone in the MTA (Hinshaw, 2007). In addition, several RCTs have demonstrated that more symptomatic youths—unlike less symptomatic youths—derive greater benefit from more comprehensive, more intense, or family-focused therapies, compared to less comprehensive, less intense, or individual-focused therapies. For example, youths with more severe substance use and comorbidity at pretreatment benefited more from MDFT, which targets more risk factors including family interactions, than individual CBT or enhanced treatment as usual (Henderson et al., 2010). Moreover, among adolescents with anorexia nervosa, those with more severe overall symptoms or eating/weight-related obsessions and compulsions benefited more from a year-long course of family therapy compared to adolescent focused therapy of the same duration (Le Grange et al., 2012), and compared to a shorter 6-month course of family therapy (Lock et al., 2005).

Comorbid diagnoses have moderated treatment effects among children with ADHD; for example, the subgroup with comorbid anxiety but no CD/ODD (conduct disorder/oppositional defiant disorder) responded equally well to behavioral treatment alone and medication alone, pointing toward behavior treatment as a potential first-line treatment for this subgroup of youths (Jensen et al., 2001; Hinshaw, 2007).

Caregiver and family characteristics

Caregiver psychopathology, expressed emotion, and family demographics have been documented as significant moderators of EBPs. Here too, there is considerable variation across EBP and disorder in terms of which specific caregiver and family variables are treatment moderators, so again we offer just two examples of interesting findings.

Critical, hostile, and emotionally overinvolved attitudes toward the patient by close family members—termed expressed emotion (EE; Hooley & Parker, 2006)—moderated family therapy outcomes for adolescent anorexia nervosa in one RCT but not in another. High EE was associated with better response to separated family therapy than to conjoint family therapy (Eisler et al., 2007). However, EE did not moderate outcome in another RCT comparing family therapy to adolescent focused therapy (Le Grange et al., 2012). The authors surmised that separated family therapy may be especially suitable for adolescents from high EE families as it aims to reduce parent criticism while avoiding parent criticism during treatment sessions themselves. On the other hand, adolescent focused therapy aims to increase adolescent autonomy and does not thoroughly address the high levels of parent criticism in high EE families.

RCTs of several EBPs have documented family structure and socioeconomic status (SES) as moderators. Meta-analyses of behavioral parent training for disruptive behavior (Lundahl *et al.*, 2006) and of behavioral and cognitive-behavioral interventions for ADHD (Corcoran & Dattalo, 2006) documented smaller treatment gains for youths from nonintact families; the first meta-analysis also documented smaller gains for low SES families. A plausible explanation is that single and low SES parents have less time and energy to attend therapy sessions and practice the skills learned during therapy in order to implement them effectively at home. Fortunately, there is also evidence that nonintact or low SES families benefit more from some versions of EBPs. Lundahl and colleagues' meta-analysis found that low SES families gained more from individual than group parent training, perhaps because the individual format allows greater attention to fitting the treatment to individual families' needs. In addition, adolescents with anorexia nervosa from nonintact families responded better to a year-long course than a 6-month course of family therapy (Lock *et al.*, 2005), suggesting that adolescents from nonintact families may need longer treatment to derive meaningful benefit. These findings could potentially guide treatment decisions for youths based on their family demographics.

Method factors

The previous sections have focused on sample characteristics; we turn now to methodological factors that may moderate treatment outcome.

One of these involves the fact that different informants can differ markedly in their perspectives on the same youth's behavior, and on the outcome of treatment. Youth psychotherapy studies usually include outcome and process measures from multiple informants; these may include the youths themselves, caregivers, therapists, assessors not involved in providing treatment, siblings, peers, and teachers. Informant discrepancies are common and may be due to informant differences in both perspective and opportunities to observe the youth (De Los Reyes & Kazdin, 2005). Understandably, the presence, magnitude, and even *direction* of treatment effects can depend on the particular outcome measure used, and which informant completes that measure. Treatment effects were larger for youth-report than for parent-report measures in a meta-analysis of youth depression psychotherapy RCTs (Weisz *et al.*, 2006b). Perhaps depressive symptoms such as sad mood are most salient to the youths experiencing them, and less so for outside observers, such that youths would be more sensitive to changes in their depressive symptoms than their parents would be. In a multisite trial of treatments for social phobia among children, parent–youth disagreement on youth symptoms at pretreatment were significantly associated with disagreement at posttreatment only among nonresponders to treatment (De Los Reyes *et al.*, 2010).

Another aspect of informant report that may moderate treatment outcome is whether the informants are blind to treatment assignment. One relevant finding emerged from a recent meta-analysis of 52 RCTs comparing youth EBPs for an array of internalizing and externalizing disorders to usual clinical care (Weisz *et al.*, 2013b): the benefit of EBPs over usual care was significant only for youth-report and parent-report measures (i.e., reports by those who had sought treatment and knew what the treatment was). Another recent meta-analysis obtained significant effects of behavioral treatments for ADHD that did not hold up when analyses were limited to outcome measures for which informants were likely to be blind to treatment condition (Sonuga-Barke *et al.*, 2013; but note also that significant effects of *dietary* interventions for ADHD were evident with both blind and unblinded informants). Several explanations may account for better outcomes reported by unblinded informants: (a) informants who know about the treatment may be more invested in perceiving it as successful; (b) unblinded informants (e.g., youths and their caregivers) tend to also be those who have the most accurate and complete information about youth functioning; or (c) the measures most often taken via blinded informants are lacking in validity (e.g., observational ratings may not adequately sample the youth's behavior, or youths may behave in atypical ways when being observed).

A third method factor warranting attention is the setting in which treatment takes place and in which youth behavior and outcomes are assessed. Numerous reviews (e.g., Weisz, 2004) have noted that distinctive settings can carry distinctive constraints and can facilitate and inhibit very different behavior. The same youth may be very well regulated within a highly structured residential program but quite dysregulated at home or in school when the potent structure is no longer present. An effective behavioral parent training intervention may produce marked improvements in youth behavior at home that do not generalize to behavior in school. Prompted in part by such findings, the 2013 National Institute for Health and Care Excellence (NICE) guidelines for treatment of youth conduct problems in the UK recommend a multimodal approach (see Scott *et al.*, 2013, p. 33) in which treatment within the family is complemented by treatment focused on the school and other settings where youth behavior may be at issue. The challenge of cross-setting differences and the closely linked challenge of effect generalization warrant careful research attention in the days ahead.

Therapist adherence and competence

We end this section on a puzzling note: findings across multiple studies have been quite mixed in regard to whether higher levels of therapist adherence to treatment manuals, and higher levels of measured therapist competence in the component skills, are actually associated with better or worse treatment outcomes, or no difference (see, e.g., Hogue *et al.*, 2008; Webb *et al.*, 2010; Weisz *et al.*, 2012). Until there are more convergent findings (and perhaps refined measurement strategies will help), this important topic may remain shrouded in uncertainty, awaiting an empirical breakthrough.

Adapting and testing psychotherapies for diverse populations

In recent years, investigators have begun to examine the potency and reach of youth EBPs by evaluating their impact across a more and more diverse array of at-risk populations. We illustrate by focusing on four populations of special interest.

Ethnic minority populations
The massive movement of population groups across national boundaries—due to violent conflict, repression, and pursuit of educational and employment opportunity—has created ever-higher percentages of "minority youths" in countries around the world. In the United States, for example, 2008 statistics showed that 43% of youths belonged to ethnic minority groups, and that percentage has continued to increase (Mather & Pollard, 2009). About 13% of minority youths receive mental health services in the United States each year (Stagman & Cooper, 2010), but some reports on treatment process and outcome have not been encouraging. For example, a US Department of Health and Human Services report (DHHS, 2001) showed that only a small number of ethnic minorities had participated in psychotherapy RCTs, and these studies did not assess the efficacy of the treatment by ethnic status. In addition, some research found that ethnic minority youths were significantly more likely than European-Americans to drop out of treatment (Kazdin & Whitley, 2003), and less likely to show significant clinical improvement when treated for depression (Weersing & Weisz, 2002a).

The results of a selective review conducted by Huey and Polo (2008) of youth treatment outcome studies from 1960 to 2006 were more promising. At least 75% of participants in each study were ethnic minorities. Using the levels-of-support criteria described earlier (see Silverman & Hinshaw, 2008), Huey and Polo found no "well-established" treatments for ethnic minority youths, but they identified a number of "probably efficacious" and "possibly efficacious" treatments for a range of psychological disorders including anxiety, ADHD, depression, conduct problems, substance use, posttraumatic stress, and suicide risk, with CBT as the best-documented EBP for anxiety disorders, depression, and trauma-related disorders. Adding a meta-analysis of 25 studies, Huey and Polo found a mean pre–posttreatment effect size for ethnic minority youths averaging 0.44, just below a medium effect (Cohen, 1988).

Lower and middle-income countries and war-exposed youths
Limited research on mental health has been conducted in lower- and middle-income countries (LAMICs); this constitutes 3–6% of published mental health research (Saxena et al., 2006). This research gap is attributed to a range of factors, including limited mental health resources, a lack of trained mental health professionals, and child mortality concerns taking priority over morbidity (Patel et al., 2008).

Mental health efforts in LAMICs have primarily focused on the youths most in need of support: youths exposed to armed conflict in war-torn regions (see Chapters 16 and 44). These youths have experienced extreme psychosocial stressors such as military assault, sexual trauma, conscription as "child soldiers," and various consequences associated with involuntary displacement (e.g., refugee camps, a new and unfamiliar local language and culture, separation from family members). Thus, war-exposed youths are at heightened risk for substance use, depression, anxiety, conduct problems, posttraumatic stress, and suicidal ideation (Shaw, 2003; Lustig et al., 2004).

The modest research conducted to date on treatment for war-exposed youths is somewhat encouraging. Bolton et al. (2007) assessed a group interpersonal therapy (IPT) intervention for depression among adolescent Ugandan war refugees. Compared to a creative play program and wait-list control, IPT was significantly more effective in reducing depression symptoms (but not anxiety or conduct problems) for girls; symptom reductions occurred for boys but were nonsignificant. Dybdahl (2001) assessed a psychosocial treatment focused on parent trauma-processing and improving mother–youth interactions for mother–youth refugee dyads internally displaced within Bosnia. The treatment group showed significantly greater improvement in mothers' PTSD symptoms and youths' psychosocial functioning (youths' PSTD symptoms were not explicitly assessed), as compared to a control group.

Large-scale RCTs have also been conducted as school-based interventions. Trauma and grief component therapy (TGCT) has been widely disseminated in Bosnia as part of a UNICEF mental health program. Layne et al. (2008) assessed the effectiveness of school-based TGCT for Bosnian adolescents with PTSD, depression, or grief symptoms. Students participated in one of two treatment conditions consisting of components of TGCT: trauma- and grief-centered therapy with psychoeducation and social skills training (treatment condition), or psychoeducation with social skills training (active comparison group). Both TGCT groups showed a significant reduction in PTSD and depression symptoms, but only the treatment condition showed a significant reduction in grief symptoms. Jordans et al. (2010) assessed a classroom-based intervention in civil-war-affected Nepal designed to improve general well-being and psychosocial functioning among adolescents. The intervention consisted of CBT, narrative exposure techniques, and structured play. Compared to a wait-list control, the treatment group experienced significantly greater improvements in overall functioning, general psychological functioning, and greater reduction in depression and anxiety symptoms. PTSD symptoms decreased and feelings of hope increased to a similarly significant degree in both groups. Tol et al. (2008) tested a similar CBT intervention for PTSD symptoms among youths in

Indonesia exposed to political violence, and the treatment group showed a significantly greater reduction in PTSD symptoms (but not depression or anxiety symptoms) compared to a wait-list control. These studies show promising initial dissemination efforts of evidence-based treatments to war-exposed youths even in remote and limited-resource regions. Perhaps these early findings will be a springboard for work with other LAMIC populations greatly in need of support.

Youth offenders in the juvenile and criminal justice system

Previous studies have found a high prevalence of psychological disorders in incarcerated youth offenders. Teplin and colleagues (2006) found that the most common disorders included conduct-related, substance use, and affective disorders, with comorbidity quite substantial. The primary objective of the juvenile justice system is rehabilitation, and treatment for mental health problems is widely viewed as essential. However, there is little empirical support for many of the interventions used, and some may be ineffective or harmful. Lipsey and Wilson (1998) conducted a meta-analysis of 200 intervention studies for juvenile offenders and found a small effect for reduction in rate of reoffending (average effect size of 0.1).

The Blueprints for Violence Prevention project of the Center for the Study and Prevention of Violence, at the University of Colorado, has evaluated over 900 programs designed to rehabilitate juvenile delinquents (Mihalic et al., 2002). Evidence in support of most of these programs (e.g., boot camp, summer job programs) was found to be either disappointing or entirely lacking. Arguably the strongest evidence supports Multisystemic Therapy (MST; Glisson et al., 2010; Henggeler & Schaeffer, 2010; Schoenwald, 2010), an intensive intervention targeting multiple systems in youths' lives, including family support and relationships, neighborhood and peer networks, and their teachers and school. Across multiple trials, MST has been shown to significantly reduce rate of reoffending, improve parenting skills and family relations, enhance positive social networks and prosocial activities, and improve grades and vocational skills. MST has been shown to be more effective than common "usual care" alternatives, including probation services, child-welfare systems, and individual outpatient therapy (Weisz et al., 2013b). Unfortunately, practices found to be ineffective, or even harmful, continue to be widely used.

Youths cared for in child protection programs

Child protection and child welfare systems are typically designed to balance the value of family cohesion against the need to protect children from maltreatment. These systems may remove children from their home or assist parents in child rearing. The youths involved often have significant mental health needs, sometimes related to family stress or maltreatment they experienced, sometimes to the process of foster placement (often a series of placements), and sometimes to diverse factors not all of which can be identified. Unsurprisingly, admittance into the child protection system is a common precursor to mental health services (see Garland et al., 1996; Garland et al., 2001a, b).

Successful interventions for these youngsters often engage multiple systems in the youths' lives. One example, Multisystemic Therapy for Child Abuse and Neglect (MST-CAN), consists of the standard components of MST in addition to safety planning, parental anger management, and family problem-solving and communication training. In one RCT, MST-CAN was shown to be more effective than enhanced outpatient treatment in reducing youth psychopathology symptoms and placement changes, and improving parent functioning, including reduced maltreatment (Swenson et al., 2010).

Another successful approach is Multidimensional Treatment Foster Care (MTFC; Smith & Chamberlain, 2010). MTFC involves working with youths, biological parents, and foster parents using a multilevel intervention implemented in family, community, and school settings. Each youth is placed in a foster home for 6–9 months, where an intensive individualized behavior management program is implemented. Parents attend family therapy, and learn parenting strategies including limit-setting and positive reinforcement of prosocial behaviors. MTFC has been shown to be more effective in reducing youth delinquent behavior than standard group care (Chamberlain & Reid, 1998; Chamberlain et al., 2007). Other MTFC trials have found reductions in severe youth mental health problems (Chamberlain et al., 1992).

Youths in the child welfare system with histories of maltreatment who are at increased risk for PTSD may need trauma-focused mental health services. The most thoroughly tested of these is Trauma-Focused Cognitive Behavioral Therapy (TF-CBT; Cohen et al., 2010). TF-CBT integrates traditional CBT with trauma-specific methods, including narrative exposure therapy, safety planning, and graduated exposure to trauma-related cues. RCTs have shown TF-CBT to be more effective in reducing PTSD symptoms than wait-list control, "supportive therapy," and "child-centered therapy" (see review in Cohen et al., 2010).

Putting science into practice: EBPs and the clinical practice of youth mental health care

A central goal for so many who develop treatments and conduct treatment outcome research is to improve mental health care for the many girls and boys who struggle with problems and disorders in their everyday lives. Because most of these youngsters will never participate in a treatment trial, prospects for them to benefit from the research will depend on the extent to which that research informs and improves everyday clinical practice. This means that the interventions developed and tested will need to be appropriate for and adopted by clinical practice, and when used in practice will actually lead to improved outcomes. We now take stock of how well youth treatment research is doing in relation to these objectives.

Dissemination and implementation of evidence-based practices

The objectives are closely related to the subfield now known as dissemination and implementation science. Dissemination has been defined (National Institute of Mental Health [NIMH] 2009) as:

> ….the targeted distribution of information and intervention materials to a specific public health or clinical practice audience. The intent is to spread knowledge and the associated evidence-based interventions.

Implementation has been defined (NIMH, 2009) as:

> the use of strategies to adopt and integrate evidence-based health interventions and change practice patterns within specific settings.

What grade should we give youth psychotherapy research on the complementary tasks of dissemination and implementation? On the one hand, there is now extensive publicity for EBPs, within prominent journals and through government entities in many nations. On the other hand, despite all the publicity, most of the tested treatments are still used mainly in treatment trials; most have not made significant inroads into everyday clinical care. Studies in North America show very low levels of EBP use in everyday practice (see Weisz *et al.*, 2009; Brookman-Frazee *et al.*, 2010; Garland *et al.*, 2010; Southam-Gerow *et al.*, 2010). Complementing these reports, a UK survey published in 2006 by the Association for Child and Adolescent Mental Health (see http://www.acamh.org.uk/POOLED/articles/bf_eventart/view .asp?Q=bf_eventart_213513) found that CBT was the dominant approach of only 20% of practitioner respondents, despite very substantial government pressure favoring CBT (e.g., via the NICE guidelines). While the data from North America and the United Kingdom certainly do not cover all practice or training sites, they do suggest that EBPs are not making their way into training or practice very quickly. Why not? Why wouldn't professionals who chose careers to help young people be eager to adopt practices that have been tested and shown to work?

Goodness-of-fit issues in the design of evidence-based practices

One answer may relate to the design of the tested practices. Research in clinical care settings and with practitioner partners (e.g., Weisz, 2004; Weisz *et al.*, 2005b, 2013a) has raised significant design concerns. One is the fact that most of the EBPs (see Table 36.1) are designed for single problems or disorders (or homogeneous clusters—e.g., a few depressive disorders). For practitioners, whose caseloads tend to be broad and heterogeneous, with an array of disorders and significant comorbidity within cases, learning one or two single-disorder EBPs may not be seen as useful enough to warrant the time and cost. An additional concern is that EBPs tend to ask a lot of therapists—learning a detailed manual, much more advance preparation for each session than may seem feasible in everyday

practice, working from an agenda rather than letting the session flow freely, and devising ways to make the manualized content engaging and motivating for the youth. None of these challenges is insurmountable, but each may require attention in efforts to disseminate EBPs, and even in the very development and testing of EBPs, a topic to which we turn next.

Context of EBP development and testing versus conditions of everyday practice

The structure and content of EBPs, and the degree to which they fit the conditions of everyday practice, may have a lot to do with the conditions under which they are created and tested. In general, these conditions have differed markedly from the conditions of actual clinical practice (Weisz *et al.*, 2005a; Weisz & Gray, 2008). This difference may impose certain limits on prospects for extrapolating from research findings to treatment in youth clinical service settings. The difference may also have slowed the pace of dissemination and implementation, to some degree, in part by raising practitioner concern over whether these treatments that look promising in research are actually appropriate for their use in real-world clinical practice.

The research versus clinical practice differences surface in multiple areas, including therapy participants, treatment settings, and even the broader policy and fiscal context. Youths treated in clinical practice settings may differ from those recruited for RCTs in diverse ways, including severity and family adversity (Hammen *et al.*, 1999; Southam-Gerow *et al.*, 2003). Clinicians employed in clinics differ from research-employee therapists in background and training, daily working conditions, incentive structure, and professional goals (see Weisz & Addis, 2006; Palinkas *et al.*, 2008). In addition, clinical practice and research organizations differ in multiple ways relevant to implementation of EBPs; for example, in practice settings, time, productivity, financial, and other work pressures can make it hard to allocate time to the training and ongoing case consultation needed for successful implementation of EBPs (Weisz & Addis, 2006). Such differences—encompassing the patients, therapists, and settings of therapy—illustrate the stark gap between the world of clinical research and that of clinical practice.

(Un)Representativeness of most research on evidence-based youth psychotherapies

In principle, that gap might be addressed by conducting much of the research that leads to EBPs in representative clinical practice contexts. In fact, though, such research has been rare, to date. The problem is illustrated by Table 36.2, which summarizes relevant details of 461 youth psychotherapy RCTs from the 1960s to 2009. As shown in the table, the large majority of trials used (a) recruited (not clinically referred) samples, (b) therapists who were research employees (not practicing clinicians), and (c) university lab or other nonpractice settings. The table also shows that representativeness has increased somewhat in recent decades, but only 2.1% of all the studies, and only 4.5% of studies in the most recent decade, focused on clinically referred clients, treated by practitioners, in clinical practice settings (see also Weisz *et al.,* 2005a, for a similar analysis and similar conclusions). What seems clear is that most of the research that leads to the establishment of EBPs has been carried out in contexts quite different from the world of clinical practice for which the EBPs are ultimately intended. One result may be a collection of treatments that are a less than perfect fit to that clinical practice world.

Do EBPs actually produce better outcomes than usual clinical care?

Concerns about the fit between EBPs and usual clinical practice lead quite naturally to a critical question: Do EBPs produce better outcomes than the treatments youths would otherwise receive through usual clinical care? In some respects, this is the most basic question many in clinical practice might ask. Given the very substantial funding and time required to build competence in a typical manual-guided EBP, it is reasonable for practitioners, clinic directors, policy makers, and funders to ask whether shifting from usual treatment practices to EBPs will, in fact, lead to better youth outcomes than current practices do. Youth treatment research has not emphasized the kinds of studies that could answer that question—that is, RCTs in which youths with significant mental health problems or disorders are randomly assigned to a specific EBP or to usual clinical care. However, a limited pool of such studies does exist, and we turn to those studies next.

Our search for relevant studies has led to two meta-analyses focused on methodologically acceptable studies that have directly compared usual care to youth psychotherapies that have been formally classified as EBPs. In these two meta-analyses (32 studies in Weisz *et al.,* 2006b; 52 studies in Weisz *et al.,* 2013b) studies spanned the years 1973–2010, and youth ages ranged from 3 to 18 years. Most of the EBPs were specific behavioral or CBT interventions, and about a fourth were systems-oriented approaches such as MST. On average, the EBPs did outperform usual care. However, the mean posttreatment effect size was only 0.30 and 0.29, in the first and second meta-analysis, respectively, falling between conventional cutoffs for "small" and "medium," and markedly lower than mean effects found in prior meta-analyses (see Figure 36.1). To put the findings into context, a mean effect size of 0.29–0.30 translates into a probability of only 58% that a randomly selected youth receiving an EBP would be better off after treatment than a randomly selected youth receiving usual care. Also worrisome: in the 2013 meta-analysis, there was no significant advantage of the EBPs with two key subgroups: clinically referred samples and youths in samples severe enough to be clinically diagnosed. A more pessimistic picture was presented in Spielmans and colleagues' (2010) reanalysis of the Weisz *et al.* (2006b) meta-analysis. These authors controlled for factors they believed might bias study findings in favor of EBPs, and concluded that EBPs did not significantly outperform usual care. Readers might also find some support in both the Spielmans *et al.* and Weisz *et al.*

meta-analyses for the notion that effect sizes shrink when EBPs are tested by independent investigators with no involvement by the program developers (see Eisner, 2009). One conclusion on which all the meta-analysts would likely agree is that outcomes have been highly variable across studies, with a number of studies showing usual care outcomes to be similar or superior to EBPs outcomes. This variability is shown in Figure 36.2, for the Weisz *et al.* (2013b) meta-analysis study sample.

Strategies for strengthening youth psychotherapies and intervention science

The findings reviewed thus far point to a lively field with committed researchers actively searching for beneficial youth treatments. The findings also suggest strategies for building stronger treatments and improving the evidence base on youth psychotherapy.

Making intervention research look more like practice

A significant limitation of the evidence base, shown in Table 36.2, is that intervention research shows relatively low relevance to actual clinical practice. We have argued (e.g., Weisz, 2004; Weisz & Gray, 2008) for a *deployment-focused model* within which interventions are developed and tested, as soon as feasible, with the kinds of therapists and clients, and in the kinds of settings, for which the interventions are ultimately intended. If this model were adopted, the form of research known as efficacy testing (e.g., with recruited samples treated by research-employee therapists under experimenter-designed conditions) would be only a brief initial phase in intervention development, used to establish potential for benefit, and effectiveness testing under clinically representative conditions would be the dominant research approach. This in turn would provide a more direct path than now exists between research on youth psychotherapy and effective applications of the products of that research within everyday youth clinical care.

Tapping the heuristic potential of usual care

Speaking of usual care, our evidence suggests that it may have something to teach us. Figure 36.2 revealed that some forms of usual care produced outcomes comparable to or better than the outcomes of EBPs, suggesting that some treatments arising from everyday practice may deserve to be documented in written protocols and tested in their own right. For this to be feasible, however, investigators will need to stop treating usual care as a mere "control condition" and think of it instead as a source of ideas and methods. Weisz *et al.* (2006a) noted that the studies in their meta-analysis generally provided excellent documentation of EBP content but very poor documentation of the usual care conditions to which the EBPs were compared, leaving it unclear what "usual care" actually consisted of. This problem needs to be solved if we are to maximize the hypothesis-generating potential

Table 36.2 Percentage of groups in youth psychotherapy outcome studies that employed clinically representative youths, therapists, and treatment settings.

Decade	1960s	1970s	1980s	1990s	2000s	All decades
Number of studies	13	62	99	100	187	461
Number of groups	35	183	273	244	425	1160
How youths were enrolled in study						
Recruited, nontreatment-seeking	62.9	85.8	65.9	57.8	62.8	66.1
Clinic-referred, treatment-seeking	5.7	4.9	24.2	26.2	24.5	21.1
Required via court/justice system	17.1	8.2	8.8	11.5	7.8	9.1
Enrollment method not reported	14.3	1.1	1.1	4.5	4.9	3.6
Who provided the treatment						
≤50% therapists are practitioners	65.7	42.1	55.3	40.2	35.5	43.1
>50% therapists are practitioners	2.9	9.8	7.7	10.7	19.1	12.7
Therapist vocation not reported	14.3	27.9	23.4	32.0	25.4	26.4
No treatment/wait-list	17.1	20.2	13.6	17.2	20.0	17.8
Where treatment took place						
Research setting	11.4	6.6	9.9	18.4	19.5	14.7
Custodial, school, supervised setting	8.6	29.5	32.6	20.5	22.6	25.2
Clinical service setting	0	2.7	5.9	11.5	14.8	9.7
Correctional setting	14.3	1.1	5.1	4.1	2.1	3.4
Treatment setting not reported	48.6	39.9	33.0	28.3	20.9	29.1
No treatment/wait-list	17.1	20.2	13.6	17.2	20.0	17.8
Number of representativeness factors						
No factors reported	91.4	83.6	70.0	63.9	61.2	68.3
One factor reported	8.6	15.3	22.7	25.4	23.8	22.1
Two factors reported	0	1.1	7.0	9.0	10.6	7.6
Three factors reported	0	0	0.4	1.6	4.5	2.1

Note: Because treatment provider and setting are group-level variables, percentages of groups rather than percentages of studies are reported for all three variables. Three studies that employed a combination of nontreatment seeking and treatment seeking youths, and one study with a treatment condition that employed a combination of clinical and research settings, were excluded from analyses.
Source: Reprinted with permission from John R. Weisz.

of EBP versus usual care research. Methods are now available for documenting usual care contents through a standardized clinician checklist (Weersing *et al.* 2002) and through a system for observer coding of intervention sessions (McLeod & Weisz, 2005, 2010). The checklist has been used to describe usual care for a variety of youth problems and conditions (Weersing *et al.*, 2002), and the observational coding system has been used to document characteristics of usual care in treatment of youth disruptive disorders (Brookman-Frazee *et al.*, 2010; Garland *et al.*, 2010) and depressive and anxiety disorders (Weisz *et al.*, 2009; Southam-Gerow *et al.*, 2010). In the next generation of studies, these and related methods could be used to characterize those patterns of usual care that show evidence of benefit.

Taking risks and learning from both failure and harm

The need for more potent treatments argues for testing creative ideas and daring ventures—high-risk/high-gain efforts toward breakthrough innovations in treatment. However, taking risks with daring innovations virtually ensures some failures. Each

failure may add valuable information on treatments that *do not* work—an important complement to learning what *does* work; both form the empirical tapestry of our science. As any meta-analyst would note, reporting failures is critical to a balanced picture; woe be the science in which only positive results are published. Failure can also be a springboard for treatment refinement and improvement, as when group intervention with antisocial youths was found to produce iatrogenic "peer contagion" or "deviancy training" effects, suggesting the need for a different approach (Dishion & Dodge, 2005), or when the discovery that a particular implementation of parent training did not work suggested innovative enrichment strategies (Scott & Dadds, 2009). Evidence indicates that even evidence-based treatments can have harmful effects if poorly executed (Scott, 2013), thus highlighting the need for rigorous implementation. Treatment failure or weak effects can also prompt useful tests of dose-augmenting strategies, such as boosters and relapse prevention, in programs for both internalizing and externalizing problems (see e.g., Tolan *et al.*, 2009; Clarke & DeBar, 2010).

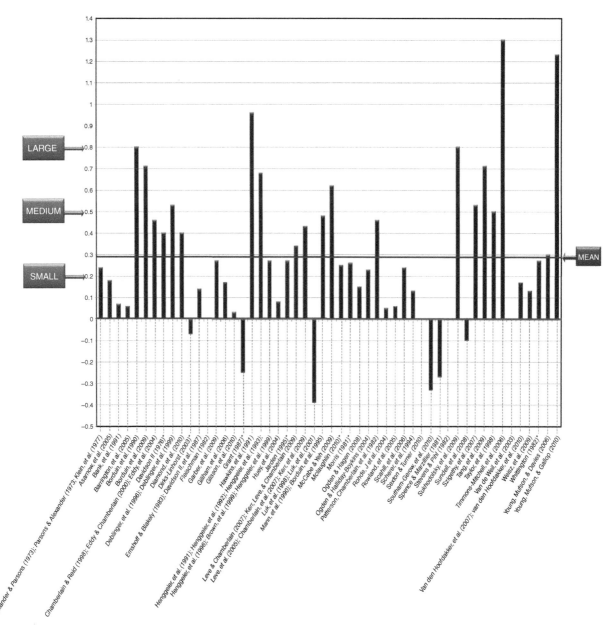

Figure 36.2 Effect sizes of individual studies comparing evidence-based youth psychotherapies (EBPs) to usual care. Horizontal bar at 0.29 shows mean effect size across the full study set. Bars below zero show studies in which usual care produced outcomes superior to those of EBPs. Note the number of studies for which usual care showed effects similar to or superior to EBPs. *Source:* Reprinted with permission from John R. Weisz.

Restructuring evidence-based psychotherapies to fit clinical practice needs

We suggested earlier that many EBPs are designed in ways that may not match up well with the clients, clinicians, and settings of everyday clinical care. For example, most EBPs are built for a single disorder or a small homogeneous cluster, whereas most clinicians carry diverse caseloads, such that one EBP for one disorder may fit only a tiny portion of their clientele. Single-disorder EBPs may also not mesh well with the fact that most referred clients have comorbid conditions, and that the most pressing problems that need attention can

shift during treatment, rendering the single focus with which treatment began to then be no longer so relevant. One approach to addressing the problems of diverse caseload, client comorbidity, and flux in treatment is to build integrative treatments that combine intervention components from multiple EBPs, encompassing multiple different problems and disorders. As an example, Chorpita and Weisz (2009) developed a *modular* protocol for child and adolescent disorders and problems involving anxiety, depression, and disruptive conduct. In a recent randomized effectiveness trial, this protocol produced significantly better clinical outcomes than (a) usual outpatient care and

(b) standard single-disorder protocols (Weisz *et al.*, 2012). Such integrative treatments may not only improve effectiveness but boost efficiency, reducing the need to do multiple trainings and to navigate multiple single-disorder protocols.

Improving care through monitoring and feedback

Another development that may improve clinical care and outcomes is the design and regular use of information systems that provide feedback on client response. Such a system was used with the modular protocol for youth, described in the previous paragraph (Chorpita & Weisz, 2009); the system provided weekly feedback on youth progress throughout treatment using two brief, psychometrically sound measures (Chorpita *et al.*, 2010; Weisz *et al.*, 2011), displayed on a "client dashboard" within an accessible web-based system. Recent research indicates that providing such client progress feedback to clinicians, even in the absence of EBPs, may improve therapy success and reduce deterioration among adults (Lambert *et al.*, 2002; Anker *et al.*, 2009) and improve therapeutic relationships and outcomes among youths (Stein *et al.*, 2010; Bickman *et al.*, 2011).

Enriching our understanding of what makes treatments work

Although we listed 40 youth EBPs at the beginning of this chapter, we have found very few replicated mediators of youth EBPs, and there is literally no evidence on whether any of these actually preceded changes in outcome. In fact, reviews (Weersing & Weisz, 2002b; Chu & Harrison, 2007) indicate that potential mediators of youth EBPs are often measured but not subjected to formal mediation testing. Consequently, we know a lot about *which* psychotherapies work for youth, but we know remarkably little about *how* these treatments work. This is unfortunate because understanding change mechanisms can help us build potent models of behavior change that can, in turn, inform development of powerful treatments (Kazdin & Nock, 2003). Identifying true mechanisms of change is resource-intensive, requiring frequent measurement of multiple candidate mediators and outcomes as well as experimental manipulation of mediators (Kazdin, 2007). But the effort may well be warranted, especially as we now have particularly promising statistical methods (e.g., bias-corrected bootstrapping, joint significance testing, and PRODCLIN asymmetric confidence-intervals testing; see Fritz & MacKinnon, 2007) for drawing strong inferences about the active ingredients that make treatments work.

Building efficient and accessible delivery methods and models

To increase accessibility and cost-effectiveness of treatment, some researchers have deviated from traditional in-person talk therapy. In fact, Kazdin and Blase (2011) have proposed a "portfolio" of treatment delivery methods to increase the public health impact of psychotherapies. These methods may include

(but certainly not be limited to) self-help books that impart EBP-related skills (e.g., Forehand & Long, 2010), treatments enlivened through video materials (e.g., Webster-Stratton & Reid, 2010), therapies delivered by paraprofessionals (e.g., Yu & Seligman, 2002), and therapies embedded within everyday settings such as summer camps (e.g., Pelham *et al.*, 2010). Such approaches may increase the uptake and spread of EBPs by reducing cost, travel time, logistical barriers, and even the stigma associated with traditional treatment methods, and by boosting engagement for many.

Another approach noted by Kazdin and Blase (2011) deserves special attention: the use of computer and internet technology (see Enock & McNally, 2013, for a review and relevant model). As one example, Kendall and Khanna (2008) developed a computer-assisted treatment for youth anxiety disorders, Camp Cope-A-Lot, based on the Coping Cat program. The youngster interacts with animated figures on the monitor to complete session activities, and the therapist coaches the patient through the program. Merry and colleagues (2012) developed SPARX, a computer-based treatment for youth depression. SPARX is a video game that conveys CBT skills such as problem solving, cognitive restructuring, and relaxation. Initial evidence suggests that both Camp Cope-A-Lot (Kendall *et al.*, 2011) and SPARX (Merry *et al.*, 2012) may be as effective as standard individual CBT.

Technology-assisted interventions for conduct problems also appear promising. As one example, Enebrink and colleagues (2012) developed an Internet-based version of parent management training that includes illustrations and video clips illustrating positive parenting strategies; this Internet PMT significantly outperformed a wait-list control condition in reducing youth conduct problems, increasing youth prosocial behavior, and enhancing positive parenting. Thus, early evidence suggests that some efficient, low-cost technology-assisted approaches to treatment may be no less effective than costly traditional methods. With further advances in technology, expansion of these alternatives seems quite likely and potentially promising.

Ideally, efforts to improve efficiency and cost-effectiveness would be guided by precise methods of calculating the cost of each approach. However, the calculations for, say, implementing a traditional manualized EBP may include the expense of initial training, ongoing expert supervision, therapist time preparing for sessions, therapist billing time foregone (during trainings and supervision), clinic administrative time, and other factors for many of which precise costs may be difficult to nail down. This may make it difficult to nail down the benchmark cost of standard approaches, and thus how much costs have been reduced by the use of technology and the other innovations noted in this section. Future collaboration with our health care economist colleagues could sharpen our ability to calculate costs precisely and thus assess whether, and if so how much, cost-effectiveness is boosted by these new approaches.

Summary and concluding comment

Research on youth psychotherapy has achieved remarkable gains in only five decades. There is now a rich treasury of tested treatments for an array of youth problems and disorders, an evolving process for evaluating the strength of the evidence for each of these, a vibrant intervention science focused on understanding how these treatments work and under what conditions, and a groundswell of interest and enterprise focused on strategies for making these treatments more and more accessible to more and more youths and families. There is a great deal of room for improvement in the interventions themselves and in the science that guides their development and refinement. Nonetheless, 50 years of research have produced a remarkable body of work and a remarkable launch for the scientific study of youth psychotherapy.

References

Ackerson, J. et al. (1998) Cognitive bibliotherapy for mild and moderate adolescent depressive symptomatology. *Journal of Consulting and Clinical Psychology* **66**, 685–690.

Alexander, J.F. & Parsons, B.V. (1982) *Functional Family Therapy: Principles and Procedures*. Brooks/Cole, Monterey, CA.

Amlund Hagen, K. et al. (2011) Treatment outcomes and mediators of parent management training: a one-year follow-up of children with conduct problems. *Journal of Clinical Child and Adolescent Psychology* **40**, 165–178.

Anker, M.G. et al. (2009) Using client feedback to improve couple therapy outcomes: a randomized clinical trial in a naturalistic setting. *Journal of Consulting and Clinical Psychology* **77**, 693–704.

Barlow, D.H. et al. (2009) *Single Case Experimental Designs: Strategies For Studying Behavior Change*. Allyn & Bacon, Boston, MA.

Barrett, P.M. et al. (2008) Evidence-based psychosocial treatments for child and adolescent obsessive-compulsive disorders. *Journal of Child and Adolescent Clinical Psychology* **37**, 131–155.

Beidel, D.C. et al. (2000) Behavioral treatment of childhood social phobia. *Journal of Consulting and Clinical Psychology* **68**, 1072–1080.

Bickman, L. et al. (2011) Effects of routine feedback to clinicians on mental health outcomes of youths: results of a randomized trial. *Psychiatric Services* **62**, 1423–1429.

Block, J. (1978) Effects of a rational-emotive mental health program on poorly achieving, disruptive high school students. *Journal of Counseling Psychology* **25**, 61–65.

Bolton, P. et al. (2007) Interventions for depression symptoms among adolescent survivors of war and displacement in Northern Uganda: a randomized controlled trial. *JAMA* **298**, 519–527.

Brookman-Frazee, L. et al. (2010) Factors associated with use of evidence-based practice strategies in usual care youth psychotherapy. *Administration & Policy in Mental Health & Mental Health Services Research* **37**, 254–269.

Campbell, J.M. (2003) Efficacy of behavioral interventions for reducing problem behavior in persons with autism: a quantitative synthesis of single-subject research. *Research in Developmental Disabilities* **24**, 120–138.

Casey, R.J. & Berman, J.S. (1985) The outcome of psychotherapy with children. *Psychological Bulletin* **98**, 388–400.

Chamberlain, P. & Reid, J.B. (1998) Comparison of two community alternatives to incarceration for chronic juvenile offenders. *Journal of Consulting and Clinical Psychology* **66**, 624–633.

Chamberlain, P. et al. (1992) Enhanced services and stipends for foster parents: effects on retention rates and outcomes for children. *Child Welfare* **5**, 387–401.

Chamberlain, P. et al. (2007) Multidimensional treatment foster care for girls in the juvenile justice system: a 2-year follow-up of a randomized clinical trial. *Journal of Consulting and Clinical Psychology* **75**, 187–193.

Chambless, D.L. et al. (1998) Update on empirically validated therapies II. *Clinical Psychologist* **51**, 3–16.

Chen, C. & Ma, H. (2007) Effects of treatment on disruptive behaviors: a quantitative synthesis of single-subject researches using the PEM approach. *Behavior Analyst Today* **8**, 380–397.

Chorpita, B.F. & Weisz, J.R. (2009) *Modular Approach to Therapy for Children with Anxiety, Depression, Trauma, or Conduct Problems (MATCH-ADC)*. PracticeWise, Satellite Beach, FL.

Chorpita, B.F. et al. (2010) Evaluation of the brief problem checklist: child and caregiver interviews to measure clinical progress. *Journal of Consulting and Clinical Psychology* **78**, 526–536.

Chu, B.C. & Harrison, T.L. (2007) Disorder-specific effects of CBT for anxious and depressed youth: a meta-analysis of candidate mediators of change. *Clinical Child and Family Psychology Review* **20**, 352–372.

Clarke, G.N. & DeBar, L. (2010) Group cognitive-behavioral treatment for adolescent depression. In: *Evidence-Based Psychotherapies for Children and Adolescents*. (eds J.R. Weisz & A.E. Kazdin), 2nd edn, pp. 110–125. Guilford Press, New York, NY.

Cohen, J. (1988) *Statistical Power Analysis for the Behavioral Sciences* Erlbaum. Hillsdale, NJ.

Cohen, J.A. et al. (2010) Trauma-focused cognitive-behavioral therapy for traumatized children. In: *Evidence-Based Psychotherapies for Children and Adolescents*. (eds J.R. Weisz & A.E. Kazdin), 2nd edn, pp. 295–311. Guilford Press, New York, NY.

Corcoran, J. & Dattalo, P. (2006) Parent involvement in treatment for ADHD: a meta-analysis of the published studies. *Research on Social Work Practice* **16**, 561–570.

David-Ferdon, C. & Kaslow, N.J. (2008) Evidence-based psychosocial treatments for child and adolescent depression. *Journal of Child and Adolescent Clinical Psychology* **37**, 62–104.

De Los Reyes, A. & Kazdin, A.E. (2005) Informant discrepancies in the assessment of childhood psychopathology: a critical review, theoretical framework, and recommendations for further study. *Psychological Bulletin* **131**, 483–509.

De Los Reyes, A. et al. (2010) The relations among measurements of informant discrepancies within a multisite trial of treatments for childhood social phobia. *Journal of Abnormal Child Psychology* **38**, 395–404.

Dishion, T.J. & Dodge, K.A. (2005) Peer contagion in interventions for children and adolescents: moving toward an understanding of the ecology and dynamics of change. *Journal of Abnormal Child Psychology* **33**, 395–400.

Dybdahl, R. (2001) Children and mothers in war: an outcome study of a psychosocial intervention program. *Child Development* **71**, 1214–1230.

Eddy, J.M. & Chamberlain, P. (2000) Family management and deviant peer association as mediators of the impact of treatment condition on youth antisocial behavior. *Journal of Consulting and Clinical Psychology* **68**, 857–863.

Eisler, I. *et al.* (2007) A randomized controlled treatment trial of two forms of family therapy in adolescent anorexia nervosa: a 5-year follow-up. *Journal of Child Psychology and Psychiatry* **48**, 552–560.

Eisner, M. (2009) No effects in independent prevention trials: can we reject the cynical view? *Journal of Experimental Criminology* **5**, 163–183.

Enebrink, P. *et al.* (2012) Internet-based parent management training: a randomized controlled study. *Behaviour Research and Therapy* **50**, 240–249.

Enock, P.M. & McNally, R.J. (2013) How mobile apps and other web-based interventions can transform psychological treatment and the treatment development cycle. *Behavior Therapist* **36**, 56–63.

Eyberg, S.M. *et al.* (2008) Evidence-based psychosocial treatments for children and adolescents with disruptive behavior. *Journal of Child and Adolescent Clinical Psychology* **37**, 215–237.

Eysenck, H.J. (1952) The effects of psychotherapy: an evaluation. *Journal of Consulting Psychology* **16**, 319–324.

Forehand, R. & Long, N. (2010) *Parenting the Strong-Willed Child*, 3rd edn. McGraw-Hill, New York, NY.

Forgatch, M.S. & Patterson, G.R. (2010) Parent management training—Oregon model: an intervention for antisocial behavior in children and adolescents. In: *Evidence-Based Psychotherapies for Children and Adolescents*. (eds J.R. Weisz & A.E. Kazdin), 2nd edn, pp. 159–177. Guilford Press, New York, NY.

Fritz, M.S. & MacKinnon, D.P. (2007) Required sample size to detect the mediated effect. *Psychological Science* **18**, 233–239.

Garland, A.F. *et al.* (1996) Type of maltreatment as a predictor of mental health service use for children in foster care. *Child Abuse and Neglect* **20**, 675–688.

Garland, A.F. *et al.* (2001a) Multi-sector complexity of systems of care for youth with mental health needs. *Children's Services: Social Policy, Research, and Practice* **4**, 123–140.

Garland, A.F. *et al.* (2001b) Prevalence of psychiatric disorders in youths across five sectors of care. *Journal of the American Academy of Child and Adolescent Psychiatry* **40**, 409–418.

Garland, A.F. *et al.* (2010) Mental health care for children with disruptive behavior problems: a view inside therapists' offices. *Psychiatric Services* **61**, 788–795.

Glisson, C. *et al.* (2010) Randomized trial of MST and ARC in a two-level evidence-based treatment implementation strategy. *Journal of Consulting Psychology* **78**, 537–550.

Hammen, C. *et al.* (1999) The context of depression in clinic-referred youth: neglected areas in treatment. *Journal of the American Academy of Child and Adolescent Psychiatry* **38**, 64–71.

Henderson, C.E. *et al.* (2009) Parenting practices as mediators of treatment effects in an early-intervention trial of multidimensional family therapy. *American Journal of Drug and Alcohol Abuse* **35**, 220–226.

Henderson, C.E. *et al.* (2010) Effectiveness of multidimensional family therapy with higher severity substance-abusing adolescents: report from two randomized controlled trials. *Journal of Consulting and Clinical Psychology* **78**, 885–897.

Henggeler, S.W. & Schaeffer, C. (2010) Treating serious antisocial behavior using Multisystemic Therapy. In: *Evidence-Based Psychotherapies for Children and Adolescents*. (eds J.R. Weisz & A.E. Kazdin), 2nd edn, pp. 259–276. Guilford Press, New York, NY.

Henggeler, S.W. *et al.* (2009) Mediators of change for multisystemic therapy with juvenile sexual offenders. *Journal of Consulting and Clinical Psychology* **77**, 451–462.

Hinshaw, S.P. (2007) Moderators and mediators of treatment outcome for youth outcome for youth with ADHD: understanding for whom and how interventions work. *Journal of Pediatric Psychology* **32**, 664–675.

Hinshaw, S.P. *et al.* (2000) Family processes and treatment outcome in the MTA: negative/ineffective parenting practices in relation to multimodal treatment. *Journal of Abnormal Child Psychology* **28**, 555–568.

Hogue, A. *et al.* (2008) Treatment adherence, competence, and outcome in individual and family therapy for adolescent behavior problems. *Journal of Consulting and Clinical Psychology* **76**, 544–555.

Hooley, J.M. & Parker, H.A. (2006) Measuring expressed emotion: an evaluation of the shortcuts. *Journal of Family Psychology* **20**, 386–396.

Huey, S.J. Jr. & Polo, A.J. (2008) Evidence-based psychosocial treatments for ethnic minority youth. *Journal of Clinical Child and Adolescent Psychology* **37**, 262–301.

Huey, W.C. & Rank, R.C. (1984) Effects of counselor and peer-led group assertive training on black-adolescent aggression. *Journal of Counseling Psychology* **31**, 95–98.

Jaycox, L. *et al.* (1994) Prevention of depressive symptoms in school children. *Behavioral Research and Therapy* **32**, 801–816.

Jensen, P.S. *et al.* (2001) Findings from the NIMH multimodal treatment study of ADHD (MTA): implications and applications for primary care providers. *Journal of Developmental and Behavioral Pediatrics* **22**, 60–73.

Jordans, M.J.D. *et al.* (2010) Evaluation of a classroom-based psychosocial intervention in conflict-afflicted Nepal: a cluster randomized controlled trial. *Journal of Child Psychology and Psychiatry* **51**, 818–826.

Kahn, J. *et al.* (1990) Comparison of cognitive-behavioral, relaxation, and self-modeling interventions for depression among middle-school students. *School Psychology Review* **19**, 196–211.

Kataoka, S.H. *et al.* (2003) A school-based mental health program for traumatized Latino immigrant children. *Journal of the American Academy of Child and Adolescent Psychiatry* **42**, 311–318.

Kaufman, N.K. *et al.* (2005) Potential mediators of cognitive-behavioral therapy for adolescents with co-morbid major depression and conduct disorder. *Journal of Consulting and Clinical Psychology* **73**, 38–46.

Kazdin, A.E. (2000) *Psychotherapy for Children and Adolescents: Directions for Research and Practice*. Oxford University Press, New York.

Kazdin, A.E. (2007) Mediators and mechanisms of change in psychotherapy research. *Annual Review of Clinical Psychology* **3**, 1–27.

Kazdin, A.E. (2010) Problem-solving skills training and parent management training for oppositional defiant disorder and conduct disorder. In: *Evidence-Based Psychotherapies for Children and Adolescents*. (eds J.R. Weisz & A.E. Kazdin), 2nd edn, pp. 211–226. Guilford Press, New York, NY.

Kazdin, A.E. (2011) *Single-Case Research Designs: Methods for Clinical and Applied Settings*. Oxford University Press, Oxford.

Kazdin, A.E. & Blase, S.L. (2011) Rebooting psychotherapy research and practice to reduce the burden of mental illness. *Perspectives on Psychological Science* **6**, 21–37.

Kazdin, A.E. & Nock, M.K. (2003) Delineating mechanisms of change in child and adolescent therapy: methodological issues and research recommendations. *Journal of Child Psychology and Psychiatry* **44**, 1116–1129.

Kazdin, A.E. & Whitley, M.K. (2003) Treatment of parental stress to enhance therapeutic change among children referred for aggressive and antisocial behavior. *Journal of Consulting & Clinical Psychology* **71**, 504–515.

Kazdin, A.E. *et al.* (1990) Empirical and clinical focus of child and adolescent psychotherapy research. *Journal of Consulting & Clinical Psychology* **58**, 729–740.

Keel, P.K. & Haedt, A. (2008) Evidence-based psychosocial treatments for eating problems and eating disorders. *Journal of Child and Adolescent Clinical Psychology* **37**, 39–61.

Kendall, P.C. & Khanna, M.S. (2008) *Camp Cope-A-Lot: The Coping Cat DVD*, [DVD], Workbook, Ardmore, PA. Available: http://workbookpublishing.com

Kendall, P.C. & Treadwell, K.H. (2007) The role of self-statements as a mediator in treatment for youth with anxiety disorders. *Journal of Consulting and Clinical Psychology* **75**, 380–389.

Kendall, P.C. *et al.* (2011) Computers and psychosocial treatment for child anxiety: recent advances and ongoing efforts. *Depression and Anxiety* **28**, 58–66.

Koegel, R.L. *et al.* (2010) Empirically supported pivotal response treatment for children with autism spectrum disorders. In: *Evidence-Based Psychotherapies for Children and Adolescents.* (eds J.R. Weisz & A.E. Kazdin), 2nd edn, pp. 327–344. Guilford Press, New York, NY.

Kraemer, H.C. *et al.* (2002) Mediators and moderators of treatment effects in randomized clinical trials. *Archives of General Psychiatry* **59**, 877–883.

Lambert, M.J. *et al.* (2002) Enhancing psychotherapy outcomes via providing feedback on client progress: a replication. *Clinical Psychology & Psychotherapy* **9**, 91–103.

Lau, W.Y. *et al.* (2010) Effectiveness of group cognitive-behavioral treatment for childhood anxiety in community clinics. *Behaviour Research and Therapy* **48**, 1067–1077.

Layne, C.M. *et al.* (2008) Effectiveness of a school-based group psychotherapy program for war-exposed adolescents: a randomized controlled trial. *Journal of the American Academy of Child and Adolescent Psychiatry* **47**, 1048–1062.

Le Grange, D. *et al.* (2012) Moderators and mediators of remission in family-based treatment and adolescent focused therapy for anorexia nervosa. *Behaviour Research and Therapy* **50**, 85–92.

Leve, L.D. & Chamberlain, P. (2007) A randomized evaluation of multidimensional treatment foster care: effects on school attendance and homework completion in juvenile justice girls. *Research on Social Work Practice* **17**, 657–663.

Levitt, E.E. (1957) The results of psychotherapy with children: an evaluation. *Journal of Consulting Psychology* **21**, 189–196.

Levitt, E.E. (1963) Psychotherapy with children: a further evaluation. *Behaviour Research and Therapy* **60**, 326–329.

Lewis, C.C. *et al.* (2009) The role of readiness to change in response to treatment of adolescent depression. *Journal of Consulting and Clinical Psychology* **77**, 422–428.

Lipsey, M.W. & Wilson, D.B. (1998) Effective intervention for serious juvenile offenders: a synthesis of research. In: *Serious & Violent Juvenile Offenders: Risk Factors and Successful Interventions.* (eds R. Loeber & D.P. Farrington), pp. 313–345. Sage Publications, Inc., Thousand Oaks, CA.

Lochman, J.E. & Wells, K.C. (2002) Contextual social-cognitive mediators and child outcome: a test of the theoretical model in the coping power program. *Development and Psychopathology* **14**, 971–993.

Lochman, J.E. *et al.* (2010) Anger control training for aggressive youth. In: *Evidence-Based Psychotherapies for Children and Adolescents.* (eds J.R. Weisz & A.E. Kazdin), 2nd edn, pp. 227–242. Guilford Press, New York.

Lock, J. *et al.* (2001) *A Treatment Manual for Anorexia Nervosa: A Family-Based Approach.* Guilford Press, New York.

Lock, J. *et al.* (2005) A comparison of short- and long-term family therapy for adolescent anorexia nervosa. *Journal of the American Academy of Child and Adolescent Psychiatry* **44**, 632–639.

Lonigan, C.J. *et al.* (1998) Empirically supported psychosocial interventions for children: an overview. *Journal of Clinical Child Psychology* **27**, 138–145.

Lundahl, B. *et al.* (2006) A meta-analysis of parent training: moderators and follow-up effects. *Clinical Psychology Review* **26**, 86–104.

Lustig, S.L. *et al.* (2004) Review of child and adolescent refugee mental health. *Journal of the American Academy of Child & Adolescent Psychiatry* **43**, 24–36.

Mather, M. & Pollard, K. (2009) *U.S. Hispanic and Asian Population Growth Levels Off* [Online]. Available: www.prb.org/Articles/2009/hispanicasian.aspx?p=1 [11 May 2009].

Mathur, S.R. *et al.* (1998) Social skills interventions with students with emotional and behavioral problems: a quantitative synthesis of single-subject research. *Behavioral Disorders* **23**, 193–201.

McGrath, M.L. *et al.* (1987) "Beat-the-buzzer": a method for decreasing parent–child morning conflicts. *Child and Family Behavior Therapy* **9**, 35–48.

McLeod, B.D. (2011) Relation of the alliance with outcomes in youth psychotherapy: a meta-analysis. *Clinical Psychology Review* **31**, 603–616.

McLeod, B.D. & Weisz, J.R. (2005) The therapy process observational coding system—alliance scale: measure characteristics and prediction of outcome in usual clinical practice. *Journal of Consulting and Clinical Psychology* **73**, 323–333.

McLeod, B.D. & Weisz, J.R. (2010) Therapy process observational coding system for child psychotherapy strategies scale. *Journal of Clinical Child and Adolescent Psychology* **39**, 436–443.

McMahon, R.J. & Forehand, R. (2003) *Helping the Noncompliant Child: Family Based Treatment for Oppositional Behavior.* Guilford Press, New York.

Merry, S.N. *et al.* (2012) The effectiveness of SPARX, a computerized self help intervention for adolescents seeking help for depression: randomized controlled non-inferiority trial. *British Medical Journal* **344**, 1–16.

Mihalic, S. *et al.* (2002) *Blueprints for Violence Prevention Replications: Factors for Implementation Success.* Center for the Study and Prevention of Violence, Boulder, CO.

MTA Cooperative Group (1999) A 14-month randomized clinical trial of treatment strategies for attention-deficit/hyperactivity disorder. *Archives of General Psychiatry* **56**, 1073–1086.

Mufson, L.H. *et al.* (1999) Efficacy of interpersonal therapy for depressed adolescents. *Archives of General Psychiatry* **56**, 573–579.

NIMH (2009) *Dissemination and Implementation Research in Health (R21)* [Online]. Available: http://grants.nih.gov/grants/guide/pa-files/par-10-040.html [14 Mar 2013].

Palinkas, L.A. *et al.* (2008) An ethnographic study of implementation of evidence-based practice in child mental health: first steps. *Psychiatric Services* **59**, 738–746.

Patel, V. *et al.* (2008) Promoting child and adolescent mental health in low and middle income countries. *Journal of Child Psychology and Psychiatry* **49**, 313–334.

Pelham, W.E. & Fabiano, G.A. (2008) Evidence-based psychosocial treatments for attention-deficit/hyperactivity disorder. *Journal of Clinical Child and Adolescent Psychology* **37**, 184–214.

Pelham, W.E. *et al.* (2010) Summer treatment programs for attention-deficit/hyperactivity disorder. In: *Evidence-Based Psychotherapies for Children and Adolescents.* (eds J.R. Weisz & A.E. Kazdin), 2nd edn, pp. 277–292. Guilford Press, New York.

Rogers, S.J. & Vismara, L.A. (2008) Evidence-based comprehensive treatments for early autism. *Journal of Child and Adolescent Clinical Psychology* **37**, 8–38.

Sanders, M.R. & Murphy-Brennan, M. (2010) The international dissemination of the triple P—Positive parenting program. In: *Evidence-Based Psychotherapies for Children and Adolescents.* (eds J.R. Weisz & A.E. Kazdin), 2nd edn, pp. 519–537. Guilford Press, New York.

Saxena, S. *et al.* (2006) The 10/90 divide in mental health research: trends over a 10-year period. *British Journal of Psychiatry* **188**, 81–82.

Schoenwald, S.K. (2010) From policy pinball to purposeful partnership: the policy contexts of Multisystemic Therapy transport and dissemination. In: *Evidence-Based Psychotherapies for Children and Adolescents.* (eds J.R. Weisz & A.E. Kazdin), 2nd edn, pp. 538–553. Guilford Press, New York.

Scott, S. (2013). Section leader presentation In *Translation of Evidence-Based Knowledge into Real-World Settings.* Marbach Castle Conference, Lake Constance, Germany.

Scott, S. & Guideline Development Group Members (2013) *Antisocial Behavior and Conduct Disorders in Children and Young People: Recognition, Intervention and Management.* National Institute for Health and Care Excellence, London, United Kingdom.

Scott, S. & Dadds, M.R. (2009) Practitioner review: when parent training doesn't work: theory-driven clinical strategies. *Journal of Child Psychology and Psychiatry* **50**, 1441–1450.

Shapiro, D.A. & Shapiro, D. (1982) Meta-analysis of comparative therapy outcome studies: a replication and refinement. *Psychological Bulletin* **92**, 581–604.

Shaw, J.A. (2003) Children exposed to war/terrorism. *Clinical Child and Family Psychology Review* **6**, 237–246.

Silverman, W.K. & Hinshaw, S.P. (2008) The second special issue on evidence-based psychosocial treatments for children and adolescents: a 10-year update. *Journal of Child and Adolescent Clinical Psychology* **37**, 1–7.

Silverman, W.K. *et al.* (2008a) Evidence-based psychosocial treatments for children and adolescents exposed to traumatic events. *Journal of Child and Adolescent Clinical Psychology* **37**, 156–183.

Silverman, W.K. *et al.* (2008b) Evidence-based psychosocial treatments for phobic and anxiety disorders in children and adolescents. *Journal of Child and Adolescent Clinical Psychology* **37**, 105–130.

Smith, T. (2010) Early and intensive behavioral intervention in autism. In: *Evidence-Based Psychotherapies for Children and Adolescents.* (eds J.R. Weisz & A.E. Kazdin), 2nd edn, pp. 312–326. Guilford Press, New York.

Smith, D.K. & Chamberlain, P. (2010) Multidimensional treatment foster care for adolescents: processes and outcomes. In: *Evidence-Based Psychotherapies for Children and Adolescents.* (eds J.R. Weisz & A.E. Kazdin), 2nd edn, pp. 243–258. Guilford Press, New York.

Smith, M.L. & Glass, G.V. (1977) Meta-analysis of psychotherapy outcome studies. *American Psychologist* **32**, 752–760.

Sonuga-Barke, E.J.S. *et al.* (2013) Nonpharmacological interventions for ADHD: systematic review and meta-analysis of randomized controlled trials of dietary and psychological treatment. *American Journal of Psychiatry* **170**, 275–289.

Southam-Gerow, M.A. *et al.* (2003) Youth with anxiety disorders in research and service clinics: examining client differences and similarities. *Journal of Clinical Child and Adolescent Psychology* **32**, 375–385.

Southam-Gerow, M.A. *et al.* (2010) Does CBT for youth anxiety outperform usual care in community clinics? An initial effectiveness test. *Journal of the American Academy of Child & Adolescent Psychiatry* **49**, 1043–1052.

Spielmans, G.I. *et al.* (2010) The efficacy of evidence-based psychotherapies versus usual care for youths: controlling confounds in a meta-reanalysis. *Psychotherapy Research* **20**, 234–246.

Stagman, S. & Cooper, J.L. (2010) *Children's Mental Health: What Every Policymaker Should Know.* National Center for Children in Poverty, Columbia University Mailman School of Public Health, New York, NY.

Stein, B.D. *et al.* (2003) A mental health intervention for schoolchildren exposed to violence. *Journal of the American Medical Association* **290**, 603–611.

Stein, B.D. *et al.* (2010) Use of outcomes information in child mental health treatment: results from a pilot study. *Psychiatric Services* **61**, 1211–1216.

Stice, E. *et al.* (2010) Testing mediators of intervention effects in randomized controlled trials: an evaluation of three depression prevention programs. *Journal of Consulting and Clinical Psychology* **78**, 273–280.

Swenson, C.C. *et al.* (2010) Multisystemic therapy for child abuse and neglect: a randomized effectiveness trial. *Journal of Family Psychology* **24**, 497–507.

Tarnowski, K.J. *et al.* (1987) A modified habit reversal procedure in a recalcitrant case of trichotillomania. *Journal of Behavior Therapy and Experimental Psychiatry* **18**, 157–163.

Teplin, L.A. *et al.* (2006) *Psychiatric Disorders of Youth in Detention.* U.S. Department of Justice, Washington, DC.

Tol, W.A. *et al.* (2008) School-based mental health intervention for children affected by political violence in Indonesia: a cluster randomized trial. *JAMA* **300**, 655–662.

Tolan, P.H. *et al.* (2009) The benefits of booster interventions: evidence from a family-focused prevention program. *Prevention Science* **10**, 287–297.

Treadwell, K.H. & Kendall, P.C. (1996) Self-talk in youth with anxiety disorders: states of mind, content specificity. *Journal of Consulting and Clinical Psychology* **64**, 941–950.

Treatment for Adolescents With Depression Study (TADS) Team (2004) Fluoxetine, cognitive behavioral therapy, and their combination for adolescents with depression: treatment for adolescents with depression study (TADS) randomized controlled trial. *JAMA* **292**, 807–820.

U.S. Department of Health and Human Services (2001) *Mental Health: Culture, Race, and Ethnicity–A Supplement to Mental Health: A Report of the Surgeon General.* U.S. Department of Health and Human Services, Public Health Service, Office of the Surgeon General, Rockville, MD.

Waldron, H.B. & Kaminer, Y. (2004) On the learning curve: the emerging evidence supporting cognitive-behavioral therapies for adolescent substance abuse. *Addiction* **99**, 93–105.

Waldron, H.B. & Turner, C.W. (2008) Evidence-based psychosocial treatments for adolescent substance abuse. *Journal of Child and Adolescent Clinical Psychology* **37**, 238–261.

Watanabe, N. *et al.* (2007) Psychotherapy for depression among children and adolescents: a systematic review. *Acta Psychiatrica Scandinavica* **116**, 84–95.

Webb, C. *et al.* (2010) Therapist adherence/competence and treatment outcome: a meta-analytic review. *Journal of Consulting and Clinical Psychology* **78**, 200–211.

Webster-Stratton, C. & Reid, M.J. (2010) The incredible years parents, teachers, and children's training series: a multifaceted treatment approach for young children with conduct problems. In: *Evidence-Based Psychotherapies for Children and Adolescents.* (eds J.R. Weisz & A.E. Kazdin), 2nd edn, pp. 194–210. Guilford Press, New York.

Weersing, V.R. & Weisz, J.R. (2002a) Community clinic treatment of depressed youth: benchmarking usual care against CBT clinical trials. *Journal of Consulting and Clinical Psychology* **70**, 299–310.

Weersing, V.R. & Weisz, J.R. (2002b) Mechanisms of action in youth psychotherapy. *Journal of Child Psychology and Psychiatry* **43**, 3–29.

Weersing, V.R. *et al.* (2002) Development of the therapy procedures checklist: a therapist-report measure of technique use in child and adolescent treatment. *Journal of Clinical Child and Adolescent Psychology* **31**, 168–180.

Weisz, J.R. (2004) *Psychotherapy for Children and Adolescents: Evidence-Based Treatments and Case Examples.* Cambridge University Press, Cambridge, UK.

Weisz, J.R. & Addis, M.E. (2006) The research–practice tango and other choreographic challenges: using and testing evidence-based psychotherapies in clinical care settings. In: *Evidence-Based Psychotherapy: Where Practice and Research Meet.* (eds C.D. Goodheart, A.E. Kazdin & R.J. Sternberg), pp. 179–206. American Psychological Association, Washington, DC.

Weisz, J.R. & Gray, J.S. (2008) Evidence-based psychotherapies for children and adolescents: data from the present and a model for the future. *Child and Adolescent Mental Health* **13**, 54–65.

Weisz, J.R. & Kazdin, A.E. (eds) (2010) *Evidence-Based Psychotherapies for Children and Adolescents*, 2nd edn. Guilford Press, New York.

Weisz, J.R. *et al.* (1987) Effectiveness of psychotherapy with children and adolescents: a meta-analysis for clinicians. *Journal of Consulting & Clinical Psychology* **55**, 542–549.

Weisz, J.R. *et al.* (1995) Effects of psychotherapy with children and adolescents revisited: a meta-analysis of treatment outcome studies. *Psychological Bulletin* **117**, 450–468.

Weisz, J.R. *et al.* (2005a) Youth psychotherapy outcome research: a review and critique of the evidence base. *Annual Review of Psychology* **56**, 337–363.

Weisz, J.R. *et al.* (2005b) Promoting and protecting youth mental health through evidence-based prevention and treatment. *American Psychologist* **60**, 628–648.

Weisz, J.R. *et al.* (2006a) Evidence-based youth psychotherapies versus usual clinical care: a meta-analysis of direct comparisons. *American Psychologist* **61**, 671–689.

Weisz, J.R. *et al.* (2006b) Effects of psychotherapy for depression in children and adolescents: a meta-analysis. *Psychological Bulletin* **132**, 132–149.

Weisz, J.R. *et al.* (2009) Cognitive-behavioral therapy versus usual clinical care for youth depression: an initial test of transportability to community clinics and clinicians. *Journal of Consulting and Clinical Psychology* **77**, 383–396.

Weisz, J.R. *et al.* (2011) Youth top problems: using idiographic, consumer-guided assessment to identify treatment needs and track change during psychotherapy. *Journal of Consulting and Clinical Psychology* **79**, 369–380.

Weisz, J.R. *et al.* (2012) Testing standard and modular designs for psychotherapy with youth depression, anxiety, and conduct problems: a randomized effectiveness trial. *Archives of General Psychiatry* **69**, 274–282.

Weisz, J.R. *et al.* (2013a) Evidence-based youth psychotherapy in the mental health ecosystem. *Journal of Clinical Child & Adolescent Psychology* **42**, 274–286.

Weisz, J.R. *et al.* (2013b) Performance of evidence-based youth psychotherapies compared with usual clinical care: a multilevel meta-analysis. *JAMA Psychiatry* **70**, 750–761.

Wurtele, S.K. & Drabman, R.S. (1984) "Beat the buzzer" for classroom dawdling: a one-year trial. *Behavior Therapy* **15**, 403–409.

Yu, D.L. & Seligman, M.E.P. (2002) Preventing depressive symptoms in Chinese children. *Prevention and Treatment* **5**. Article 9.

Zisser, A. & Eyberg, S.M. (2010) Parent–child interaction therapy and the treatment of disruptive behavior disorders. In: *Evidence-Based Psychotherapies for Children and Adolescents.* (eds J.R. Weisz & A.E. Kazdin), 2nd edn, pp. 179–193. Guilford Press, New York.

CHAPTER 37

Parenting programs

Stephen Scott[1,2] and Frances Gardner[3]

[1] Department of Child and Adolescent Psychiatry, Institute of Psychiatry, Psychology and Neuroscience, King's College London, UK
[2] National Conduct Problems and National Adoption and Fostering Services, Maudsley Hospital, London, UK
[3] Centre for Evidence-Based Intervention, Department of Social Policy and Intervention, University of Oxford, UK

Introduction

A parenting program is a specific intervention designed to improve the overall quality of parenting that a child receives. Parenting programs aim to help the way mothers and fathers relate to their child: primarily by changing their behavior in moment-to-moment interchanges throughout the day, although they also address parental beliefs and feelings. Change is achieved through the training of specific skills such as collaborative play, selective attention and praise to promote sociable behavior, and clear rules backed by consistently applied consequences to reduce misbehavior. There is a structured sequence of sessions that build up each of the competencies. This approach to intervention, in which the emphasis is usually on understanding the parents' views and giving them nondirective general support, but not coaching them, is distinct from counseling (see Chapter 40); it differs from psycho-education in which a parent is informed about the nature of the child's disorder and given advice on management but not trained. In family therapy, the therapist typically addresses the whole family system, often with a primary emphasis on a deeper understanding of interpersonal processes and meanings; it is the change in understanding, rather than skills, that should lead to changes in relationships (see Chapter 39).

Parenting programs often aim to improve child symptoms as well as improving the quality of the relationship, but this is not inevitable. Thus where neglectful or abusive parenting has been uncovered, the goal may be to improve positive parental engagement with the child and reduce harsh emotional and physical practices, whether or not the child is displaying problems (see Chapter 29). Moreover, where there are child-specific emotional or behavioral problems, parenting programs may help, whether or not suboptimal parenting has contributed to causing the problem. Thus programs can help parents to better manage children with problems that are mainly genetically influenced, such as autistic spectrum disorders (see Chapter 51) or children

with obsessive-compulsive disorder (see Chapter 61) although parenting quality is satisfactory at the outset.

Furthermore, where there are child symptoms and parenting is less than optimal, this does not necessarily mean that the parenting caused the child's problems. Parent–child relationships are bidirectional and more difficult child behavior can elicit harsher parenting. Several lines of evidence show this, from the classic experiment in which parents with relatively well-behaved children were asked to look after children with behavioral problems and became harsher and more critical (Anderson *et al.*, 1986), to experiments showing that where disruptive child behavior such as ADHD is reduced by medication, parenting quality improves (Schachar *et al.*, 1987). Two areas of child functioning where parenting has been strongly implicated as causing difficulties are conduct problems and insecure attachment; we concentrate on these domains in this chapter, but refer to others.

Styles of parenting addressed by parenting programs

As there are many different theories of what constitutes good parenting, there are many different approaches incorporated in intervention programs. We focus here on those dimensions that are well empirically supported and that have led to proven intervention programs.

Dimensions of parenting addressed in interventions derived from social learning theory

Social learning theory evolved from general learning theory and behaviorism (Bandura, 1977). The notion is that children's real-life experiences and exposures directly or indirectly shape behavior; processes underlying this learning can be diverse. In interventions, there has historically been a near-exclusive focus on externally observable behavior rather than children's inner mental states (Patterson, 1982). Operant behavioral principles of reinforcement and (noncoercive) consequences are applied immediately after the child has acted/responded; there is less

Rutter's Child and Adolescent Psychiatry, Sixth Edition.
Edited by Anita Thapar and Daniel S. Pine, James F. Leckman, Stephen Scott, Margaret J. Snowling, Eric Taylor.
© 2015 John Wiley & Sons Ltd. Published 2018 by John Wiley & Sons Ltd.

emphasis on classical, stimulus-controlled conditioning (Scott, 2008). Moment-to-moment exchanges are crucial: if a child receives an immediate reward for their behavior, such as getting parental attention or approval, then they are more likely to repeat the behavior, whereas if they are ignored or an unwelcome sanction is applied, then they are less likely to do it again.

Patterson (1982) showed how children's aggressive behaviors were learned from and reinforced by parallel negative behaviors by parents. A negative parenting style appears to have a causal role in leading to conduct problems, even after allowing for child effects. The association has been repeatedly found in (i) large-scale epidemiological investigations, such as those in New Zealand and UK (e.g., Isle of Wight); (ii) intensive clinical investigations such as Patterson's work mentioned earlier; and (iii) numerous naturalistic studies of diverse samples using a mixture of methods (e.g., Gardner *et al.*, 1999; Denham *et al.*, 2000). The parenting behaviors identified are high criticism and hostility, harsh punishment, inconsistent discipline, low warmth, involvement and encouragement, and poor supervision.

A further important dimension is supervision of child activity, and monitoring their whereabouts and activities outside the home. Careful monitoring has greater effects in neighborhoods where there are many risks such as drugs and violence (Pettit *et al.*, 1999). Monitoring is not just a matter of parents being good "policemen", as knowing the whereabouts of a child depends in part on the child having a good enough relationship to tell the parent what they are doing (Racz & McMahon, 2011). Therefore, enabling parents to impose effective discipline depends on their also developing a positive relationship, skills addressed in most modern programs. These elements promote child positive behavior and affect and provide a more positive relationship context for parental disciplinary interventions. They improve child behavior (Gardner, 1987) and attachment (Scott *et al.*, 2011).

More recently, social learning models have increasingly considered inner cognitive or "mindful" processes, such as attributions and expectations that underlie parents' behavior (Snarr *et al.*, 2009). More negative attributions about a child predict poorer child outcomes over and above observed parental behavior (Doolan, 2006), and addressing them in interventions leads to better child outcomes (Sanders *et al.*, 2004). Beliefs can vary considerably across cultures, with more traditional societies showing more authoritarian views, particularly among fathers. Parenting programs based on "Western" values need to address different cultural beliefs regarding how best to bring up a child, but if they do this, they can be equally effective in improving parenting in ethnic minority groups (Reid *et al.*, 2001; Scott *et al.*, 2010a).

Dimensions of parenting addressed in interventions derived from attachment theory

Attachment theory (Bowlby, 1969/1982; see Chapter 6) focuses on the extent to which the relationship provides the child with protection against harm and a sense of emotional security,

resulting in a "secure base" for exploration. The theory proposes that the quality of parental care, particularly sensitivity and responsiveness to the child's emotional needs ("sensitive responding"), promotes a relationship characterized by warm, expressive to-and-fro interchanges ("mutuality"), leading to secure attachment. Evidence shows that sensitive responding is important in promoting attachment security, but less than theorized (De Wolff & van IJzendoorn, 1997; see Chapter 6). Longitudinal studies confirm that attachment security does not shape subsequent development deterministically, but interacts with child and family factors to influence outcome (Sroufe *et al.*, 2010). A particularly harmful parenting style is frightening and abusive parenting, which is associated with "disorganised" attachment patterns—meta-analyses confirm a strong association with maltreatment (Cyr *et al.*, 2010). Disorganization is associated with many forms of child psychopathology, especially conduct problems (Fearon *et al.*, 2010), although it is important to note that it occurs in 15% or more of normal populations.

Over time, attachment relationships are internalized and carried forward to influence expectations for other important relationships, by an "internal working model." In the last decade, progress has been made in measuring internal working models, in childhood using doll-play story-stems (Green *et al.*, 2007) and in adolescence using semi-structured interviews (Shmueli-Goetz *et al.*, 2008). These measures have shown that attachment insecurity continues to be associated with higher levels of psychopathology in middle childhood (Green *et al.*, 2007; Futh *et al.*, 2008) and adolescence (Scott *et al.*, 2011), and with less sensitive parenting in both periods (Scott *et al.*, 2011; Matias *et al.*, 2013). Some aspects of parenting, however, are not emphasized in attachment accounts of parenting, such as cognitive stimulation or consistent discipline; yet studies of child (Matias *et al.*, 2013) and adolescent (Scott *et al.*, 2011) security found that consistent discipline independently predicted secure attachment, beyond sensitive responding. Intervention programs designed to increase attachment security could beneficially target limit-setting as well as sensitive responding (O'Connor *et al.*, 2013).

Biological effects of parenting

Besides affecting children's psychological processes, parenting influences a wide array of biological processes. Physiologically, harsh and abusive parenting often leads to altered stress hormone levels, with chronically elevated cortisol and much greater secretion in response to threat or stress, with slower rates of return to normal levels (see Chapters 23 and 29). Moreover, inflammatory responses are elevated in those who are abused and depressed (see Chapters 29 and 30), and harsh parenting is associated with structural brain changes (see Chapters 23 and 29). Finally, a series of elegant studies in rats led by Meaney and in chimpanzees by Suomi have shown that changes in parenting lead to epigenetic changes (notably acetylation and methylation) in sections of genes that control protein synthesis (see Chapter 25).

The implications of these biological findings for parenting interventions are not yet clear. The physiological changes may be partly reversible by intervention, thus children taken away from abusive parenting into foster care show improved cortisol secretion patterns (Fisher *et al.*, 2006). Whether improving the parenting environment leads to measurable epigenetic or brain changes is uncertain at present. Even if biological changes are alterable, they may contribute to behavioral traits that reduce susceptibility to improved parenting, a subject we now address.

Child characteristics that may affect susceptibility to the effects of parenting

Some child disorders and traits have high heritability, for example, ADHD, autism, and callous-unemotional traits, leading some to assume that they are less susceptible to intervention efforts. However, as we shall see, this is not always the case.

Inherited characteristics and behavioral phenotypes

The effects of parenting can differ according to the characteristics of children. Adoption studies are one way of investigating this (see Chapter 24). In a large follow-up study, Bohman (1996) divided early adopted infants into those whose birth parents had been criminal or alcoholic, representing higher congenital (genetic plus early environmental) risk, versus those who were not. Adopting parents were categorized the same way, to index more and less favorable child-rearing conditions. Police contact by age 17 was 3% versus 12% for children with low versus high congenital risk favorably reared, suggesting a substantial inherited component under good conditions. For those raised under unfavorable conditions, the rates were 7% and 40% respectively. This study, replicated since, shows that some children have a much greater liability to poorer outcomes under stressful rearing conditions, a so-called diathesis-stress model. An implication is that higher congenital risk does not necessarily condemn a child to poor outcomes, indeed improving parenting may have larger effects with such individuals. Moreover, better parenting can help mitigate congenital risk through attachment security. Bergman *et al.* (2010) showed that mothers who had higher amniotic fluid cortisol levels had infants with poorer cognitive development at 17 months, but this effect disappeared if the infant was securely attached.

Longitudinal observational studies suggest that children with different characteristics may need different parenting styles. Kochanska (1997) reported that, for temperamentally fearful children, gentle parental control was associated with optimal behavioral/emotional regulation whereas temperamentally more aggressive ("fearless") children required firmer control to achieve the same positive results, a finding that has been replicated for children with difficult/irritable temperament, who fare better under conditions of firmer control (Bates *et al.*, 1998).

More recently, the possibility has been explored that rather than just confer liability to poorer outcomes under stressful rearing, some child characteristics may also confer liability to better outcomes under benign conditions, the so-called differential susceptibility hypothesis (Ellis *et al.*, 2011), whereby some children are relatively impermeable to their surroundings while others are more sensitive. Experimentally, Scott and O'Connor (2012) found that antisocial children who were more emotionally dysregulated (tantrums and anger outbursts) showed a greater response to improved parenting than those who were disobedient in a more controlled way. However, while differential susceptibility is an exciting theory, more replication of findings is necessary to characterize the scope and size of its impact.

These findings have implications for parenting programs. Firstly, intervention effects are likely to vary according to child characteristics- for example, children with autistic traits may change less, whereas those with irritable temperaments may change more. Secondly, parenting programs should not follow a "one size fits all" rigid approach, but rather the content should be varied according to child characteristics.

Specific genotypes

In a classic paper, Caspi *et al.* (2002) found that a variant of a gene coding for an enzyme involved in the breakdown of CNS neurotransmitters Monoamine Oxidase A (MAOA) conferred worse antisocial outcomes in the presence of harsh parenting. The effect has been confirmed in meta-analyses, but it is small. Furthermore, emerging studies identify genotypes that confer differential susceptibility to interventions. However, the field is beset by failure to replicate findings and if found, we will need to know the specific mechanism of action through which such genes exert their effect.

Programs for children with conduct problems

These are almost exclusively based on social learning theory. Characteristics of some of the more widely used programs are given in Table 37.1, the basic content of a typical program in Table 37.2 and pros and cons of a group-based versus individual-based delivery in Table 37.3.

Effectiveness

Outcomes

Programs based on social learning theory have evolved over 50 years and there is a larger evidence base for this intervention than any other psychological intervention in child mental health. The National Institute for Health and Care Excellence (NICE) for England and Wales conducted a meta-analysis of 54 randomized controlled trials (RCTs) of parenting programs for prevention or treatment of conduct problems/disorders in 4150 children aged 3–10 years against any control (43 studies vs. waiting list or no treatment controls, 11 vs. management as usual) (NICE, 2013). The result was a moderate effect size of 0.54 SD on parent-rated outcomes, 0.40 SD by independent observation, and 0.69 SD by independent researcher evaluation. Follow-up 1 year later showed persistent effects but a halving of

Table 37.1 Characteristics of some widely used programs.

Name	Target population	Levels and delivery modes	Evidence	Comments, website, dissemination
Incredible Years	A series of parent group programs from babyhood to age 12	*Universal prevention*: 6 weeks *Indicated prevention*: 14 week *Treatment*: 18–24 weeks	50 RCTs, 10 by developer, 40 independent replications confirm effects	Developer Carolyn Webster-Stratton. One of the most intensive programs in clinical process and supervision www.incredibleyears.com
Triple P	A range of programs at all levels and ages	*Universal prevention*: On line; broadcast media *Selective prevention*: short one off sessions up to 4 weeks *Indicated* 6–8 weeks	Over 50 RCTs by developer; 3 independent replications, some failing to show effects	Developer: Matt Sanders. Comprehensive range of levels www1.triplep.net/
Parent–Child Interaction Therapy	Child disruptive and parenting difficulties including maltreatment	Parent/child dyad is live coached by therapist over 12–20 sessions.	Several RCTs by developer and independent evaluators show effects	Developed by Sheila Eyberg. www.pcit.org/
Parent Management Training Oregon	Behavioral problems age 4–12; parents with mental health problems or separating	Individual program: 19–30 sessions, Group: 14 sessions	RCTs by program developer and independents show effects	Developer: Marion Forgatch. http://evidencebasedprograms.org/1366–2/
Strengthening Families (10–14)	Universal preventive program for age 10-14	Seven 2 hour sessions which include whole family and separate parent and child groups.	Two RCTs by program developer show some effects	Developer Karol Kumpfer. Well developed across many countries www.strengtheningfamiliesprogram.org/
Nurse Family Partnership	Preventive for young, disadvantaged first time mothers	Trained nurses visit mother at home during pregnancy and first 24 months of child's life	Three RCTs have shown varied and long-lasting effects	Developer: David Olds. www.nursefamilypartnership.org

Table 37.2 Content of a typical social learning program.

Part 1: Promoting a child-centered approach
Play is covered in the first 2–3 sessions. Instead of giving directions, teaching, and asking questions during play, parents are instructed simply to give a running commentary on their child's actions. Parents are asked to practice these techniques for 10 minutes every day

Part 2: Increasing acceptable child behavior
Praise and Rewards. The parent is required to praise their child for lots of simple, desirable everyday behaviors such as playing quietly on their own, eating nicely, getting dressed the first time they are asked, and so on. Later sessions go through the use of reward charts.

Part 3: Setting clear expectations
Clear Commands. Parents are taught to reduce the number of commands, but to make them much more authoritative. The manner should be forceful (not sitting down, timidly requesting from the other end of the room; instead, standing over the child, fixing him in the eye, and in a clear firm voice giving the instruction). Commands should specify what the parent *does* want the child to do, not what he or she should *stop* doing ("please speak quietly" rather than "stop shouting").

Part 4: Reducing unacceptable child behavior
Consequences for unacceptable behavior should be applied as soon as possible. They must always be followed through and simple logical consequences are encouraged: if water is splashed out of the bath, the bath will end; if a child refuses to eat dinner, there will be no pudding; etc.
Ignoring This sounds easy but is a hard skill to teach parents. Whining, arguing, swearing, and tantrums are not dangerous and can usually safely be ignored. The technique is very effective.
Time Out from positive reinforcement remains the final "big one" as a sanction for unacceptable behavior. The child is put in some boring place for a previously agreed reason (hitting, breaking things, etc —not minor infringements) for a short time (say 5 min). However, the child must be quiet for the last minute.

their magnitude. Interestingly, there was no generalization to the school setting—overall, for all programs, teacher ratings showed no change. No adverse effects or harms were recorded. However, it may be that modest changes in teacher-rated behavior occur with some more intensive programs —for example, a recent meta-analysis (Menting *et al.*, 2013) of 50 trials of Incredible Years found a small but significant effect on classroom behavior (0.13 SD). Similar findings for parent-reported outcomes were reported in other meta-analyses, for example, by Cochrane Collaboration (Furlong *et al.*, 2012). The latter also analyzed

Table 37.3 Pros and cons of delivering parenting programs in individual versus group format.

Individual	Group
Case selection	
Can take on special cases unsuitable for groups: shy parents, failed group parenting programs, high risk/abusive parents	Can take on a variety of cases, can be hard to stop some parents falling behind.
Depth of work	
Therapist can go into greater depth of skills that need to be taught	Less detailed due to time constraints and exposure to other parents
Can observe parent interacting with child and pick up styles they are unaware of	Restricted to parents' accounts of what goes on with the child.
Can adapt the program for particular child needs for example, attachment problems, autistic tendencies, learning disabilities, ADHD etc	
Flexibility	
Flexible order of delivery of program, for example, time out can be given early	Fixed order—for example, Limit-setting and time-out have to wait till end
Flexible timing to attend to suit parent	Groups held at a fixed time when parent may be busy
Can easily be delivered in the home context,	Parents have to come to clinic or community venue
No need to set up a crèche for child	May need to set up a crèche
Support from other parents	
No support from other parents	Other parents can provide validation for their efforts; normalize having a child with problems; enable parents to learn from and support each other
Therapists skills and support	
Can work as a solo therapist	Requires a second group leader plus group management skills
Duration and cost-effectiveness	
Typical program takes around 8 sessions, more complex 10-12	Triple P level 4 has 4 group sessions plus 4 phone sessions; IY minimum 14 sessions, 18–22 recommended for clinical cases
Cost will vary, typically £2000/€2200/$2500	Costs typically lower per case, £1200/€1350/$1800

impacts on parental mental health and found it improved by 0.36 SD. Positive parenting and harsh practices improved, assessed by both parent report and independent observation. It is less clear how the effects are sustainable in the long term: many trials have used waiting list control groups that are offered the intervention 6 months later. As a result, no long-term randomized comparison can be made (e.g., Gardner *et al.*, 2006; Bywater *et al.*, 2009). A small number of trials based on selective prevention samples have retained their randomized control group and show good long-term outcomes (Forgatch *et al.*, 2009). In summary, there is convincing evidence that parenting programs substantially improve parenting practices, parental mental health, and child antisocial behavior, and importantly that behavior change is reported both by parent report and independent observations. The evidence for longer-term effects is less conclusive.

Comparison with nonbehavioral programs

There have been rather few head-to-head comparisons of social learning theory parenting programs with nonbehavioral, humanistic approaches. For children with severe conduct problems, the classic paper by Bank *et al.* (1991) found that behavioral parent management training was effective whereas usual family therapy was ineffective on objective measures, despite favorable reports from parents. Most other studies have found that the humanistic approach usually had no effect

whereas the more behavioral programs changed child outcomes (Scott, 2008). A trial of a universal parenting program based primarily on emotional communication (the Family Links Nurturing Programme) found no effects on parenting or child behaviour (Simkiss *et al.*, 2013). It would appear that for child behavior problems, programs with a practical slant and strong focus on parental behavior change are more effective.

Programs for infants

Most programs draw on attachment theory and in the last 20 years or so, several interventions have been developed and validated (see Chapter 6). The more effective interventions for infants typically last 8–20 sessions and videotape parent–infant interactions and then replay them to the parent. The great strength of this approach is that (i) it allows parents to get an accurate picture of what is actually happening (rather than just talking about their perception of their relationship with their infant, as in traditional parent–infant psychotherapies); (ii) it enables them to observe for themselves that when they change their behavior, this impacts on their infant (iii) it allows simultaneous exploration of the mother's mental state, so that mental blocks to more sensitive responding can be explored and often overcome. The Leiden group has tested video feedback programs in RCTs (Velderman *et al.*, 2006).

The Attachment and Biobehavioral Catch-up (ABC; Dozier *et al.*, 2012) is another well-proven intervention. It targets three issues known to affect children's attachment and self-regulation. First, parents are helped to behave in nurturing ways when children are distressed. Second, similarly to social learning approaches, parents are helped to follow children's lead, to enable children to better regulate their emotions. Third, parents are helped to reduce frightening behavior as it is associated with disorganized attachment. These issues are targeted through 10 sessions implemented in families' homes with parents and children present. Other attachment-based programs are discussed in Chapter 6.

Some interventions for infants do not use video-feedback. They include more lengthy and intensive psychodynamic ones, for example, Slade *et al.* (2005). Olds (2006), by contrast, developed a home visiting program delivered by nurses (Nurse Family Partnership), based not on attachment theory but on systematic evaluation of, and evidence-based interventions for, risk factors from pregnancy to age 2 years. Thus parents are encouraged to reduce smoking and alcohol in pregnancy through understanding the effects on their babies; once the baby is born, parent–child interaction is coached, including how to stimulate the baby appropriately, and wider issues such as partner violence and general education for the mother are addressed.

Effectiveness

A meta-analysis by Bakermans-Kranenburg *et al.* (2003) found 81 studies, with over 7000 parent–infant pairs. Overall, they improved parental sensitivity by 0.33 SD and attachment security by 0.20 SD. The most effective interventions were relatively short (under 26 sessions) and started later (after the infant was 6 months). Both of these findings go against cherished notions that early intervention must be better, and that more effort should lead to more change (mean effect size for long interventions was −0.03). Recently, an RCT of the Attachment and Biobehavioural catch up (ABC) intervention showed that as well as enhancing child attachment security, it improved diurnal cortisol production, executive functioning, and emotional regulation (see Chapter 6).

For programs that do not rely on attachment theory, those that focus on specified risk factors appear to fare better. Thus the Nurse–Family Partnership approach has been evaluated in three RCTs involving over 1000 mother–infant pairs. This has shown benefits for the child in terms of improved cognitive and emotional development and fewer accidents and injuries, and for the mothers in terms of less harmful health behaviors (e.g., smoking) and higher take-up of further education, less use of public handouts, and a longer interval until subsequent pregnancy (Olds, 2006). By contrast, programs that draw upon a more general notion that if the parents are supported, then they in turn will relate better to their infants appear less effective. For example, in a trial of a home visiting program with 97 hours of face-to-face contact with mothers, none of the many mother or child variables measured changed (Barnes *et al.*, 2006); a similar lack of effectiveness was found for the Oxfordshire Home Visiting project (Barlow *et al.*, 2007).

Father involvement in parenting programs

Most literature refers to "parenting" as if it made no difference whether fathers or mothers were involved. While in the great majority of cultures it is more often mothers who spend most time looking after younger children, fathers have a particular role, which often increases as children become older (Lamb, 2004). When it comes to parenting programs, it should not necessarily be assumed that evidence about effectiveness applies equally to mothers and fathers. In practice, however, it is mainly mothers who attend parenting programs and participate in research evaluations. The under-representation of fathers in these interventions is perhaps surprising, given that in many countries their role now reflects greater equality of gender roles and increased sharing of parenting (Maughan & Gardner, 2010). Furthermore, there is considerable research suggesting that amount and quality of father involvement in parenting is beneficial to children's mental health and development, over and above the level of the mother's involvement (Lamb, 2004; Ramchandani *et al.*, 2013). A systematic review by Lundahl *et al.* (2008) suggested that if intervention trials involve fathers, they produce stronger effects on child behavior. Some interventions have been designed to engage couples and fathers, with improved outcomes when couples attend (Cowan *et al.*, 2009). However, as it would be very difficult to randomize to one versus two parents attending a program (but see Besnard *et al.*, 2013), it is unclear if father attendance *per se* causes these changes, or whether outcomes are better in families with two parents (as found by Gardner *et al.*, 2009), and in families where the couple relationship is healthier (Cowan *et al.*, 2009), so fathers are more likely to attend. Irrespective of trial data, it is highly desirable that interventions should involve both parents. Studies of fathers' views (Stahlschmidt *et al.*, 2013) suggest a number of barriers (and potential solutions), including time of day of the intervention, and that many interventions are run by women, who may find it easier to communicate with mothers than fathers. This effect can be pronounced in group-based interventions where fathers may feel out of place if they are in a minority.

Application of programs to specific populations

Although designed for conduct problems, these programs can improve other clinical outcomes, even with minor or no adaptation; they can reduce children's anxiety disorders (Cartwright-Hatton *et al.*, 2011), ADHD (Jones *et al.*, 2008; Charach *et al.*, 2013); obesity (Brotman *et al.*, 2012), and parental depression (Hutchings *et al.* 2007; Barlow *et al.*, 2012).

However, adaptation and extension of these parenting programs is now increasingly occurring for a range of child psychiatric problems and parental contexts.

Programs for particular child issues and contexts
Depression, anxiety, and other emotional problems

Evidence supporting a link between quality of parent–child relationships and depression, anxiety, and other emotional problems (e.g., somatic complaints and social withdrawal) is clear, although smaller than that found for disruptive outcomes (Dadds *et al.*, 1996; Wood *et al.*, 2003). Low warmth and conflict are both linked with depression and anxiety; however, the influence of control strategies is generally much weaker. Additionally, emotional symptoms in children are linked with over-protectiveness (e.g., Dadds *et al.*, 1996). The elements of parenting programs aimed primarily at conduct problems are likely to be helpful for children showing emotional symptoms, but generally an individual-based intervention should probably be added, although Cartwright-Hatton *et al.* (2011) tested the effects of a group-based parenting program for diagnosed clinically anxious children (aged 3–9) and found strong effects on reducing anxiety disorders. The majority of sessions focused on components of traditional social learning theory-based parent management skills (e.g., child-centered play, rewards, and limit setting), with about one third of the sessions focusing on components specifically aimed at dealing with anxious children (e.g., anxiety education; fear hierarchies).

ADHD

A number of parenting programs designed for conduct problems have shown improvements in ADHD symptoms as well (Scott *et al.* 2001, 2010b; Webster-Stratton, 2011; Charach *et al.*, 2013). Additionally, parenting interventions have been developed specifically for children with ADHD, for example, the New Forest program in the UK, which showed good effects on ADHD symptoms in preschoolers in a clinic-based trial, but not in routine services (Sonuga-Barke *et al.*, 2001). Recent systematic reviews conclude that behavioral parenting interventions are effective for younger children with ADHD, more so than methylphenidate (Charach *et al.*, 2013), and are probably effective for older children (Zwi *et al.*, 2011). European and UK (NICE) guidelines, both recommend parenting programs as the first line treatment for ADHD. However, Sonuga-Barke *et al.* (2013) found that while effects were good on parent-report, they were negligible using direct observation.

Callous unemotional traits

Despite the common belief that children with conduct problems who also show callous unemotional traits are insensitive to parenting, and to parenting interventions, Waller *et al.* (2013) found little evidence to support this belief, either from longitudinal studies or from randomized trials. Nevertheless,

specific programs are being developed for them (Dadds *et al.*, 2013).

Programs for particular parent issues and contexts
Specific parental issues and contexts

There is some promising evidence that social learning theory based programs, with some adaptation and extension, can be effective for parents who maltreat their children (MacMillan *et al.*, 2009; Ch 30). For drug misusing parents, the program "Parents under Pressure" has shown promising results (Dawe & Harnett, 2007). For children in the foster care system, some trials suggest that parenting interventions aimed at foster-caregivers, can be effective in reducing problem behavior in this often very troubled group of young people (Briskman & Scott, 2013), although other trials have been more disappointing (MacDonald & Turner, 2005; Turner *et al.*, 2007), perhaps where the interventions have been less intensive.

Transportability of parenting programs to different cultures and countries

Parenting programs appear to transport well across cultures, despite different parenting norms and values. A systematic review of programs developed in the USA and Australia found comparable effect sizes in recipient countries, including Europe and Asia (Gardner *et al.*, 2015). Surprisingly perhaps, in many cases, "imported" programs were more effective in culturally very different settings (for example, Hong Kong). These findings are consistent with studies of effects in ethnic minority groups within one country. For example, Reid *et al.* (2001), in a large study of low income families in the USA found no ethnic differences in outcomes, engagement, or satisfaction across four ethnic groups, and Scott *et al.* (2010a) found a similar lack of ethnic differences in outcomes in London.

Given the high levels of international concern about youth crime and violence in developing countries (WHO, 2013), and the loss of children's developmental potential due to poverty and conflict, it is important to know if parenting programs work in low and middle-income countries (LAMICs). A recent systematic review (Knerr *et al.*, 2013) found promising evidence from randomized trials that parenting programs can be effective in LAMICs for improving harsh parenting, and potentially for reducing conduct problems. Broader parenting interventions that also target early cognitive stimulation can also be effective for improving parenting skills and children's developmental potential (Engle *et al.*, 2007; Rahman *et al.*, 2009). WHO (2013) have begun an important initiative to develop, adapt, and test through RCTs programs in LAMICs, where home-based parenting interventions have already shown good results for infants (Cooper *et al.*, 2009; Knerr *et al.*, 2013). There are many other examples of promising practice in developing countries, but very few have been tested in rigorous trials (Knerr *et al.*, 2013), as recommended by WHO, and sustainability will be challenging.

What makes parenting programs work?

Predictors and moderators of outcome

In a controlled trial, if a characteristic of the participants (e.g., child age or symptom severity) predicts outcome in both the intervention and control groups, then it is a predictor. If, however, there is an interaction with treatment, so that one subgroup (say younger children) does better than another (older children) in the intervention group only, then the characteristic is operating as a moderator. Until recently, analyses have mainly been at the level of predictors only, with one or two exceptions. It is crucial that treatment and policy decisions are based on evidence from moderator, rather than predictor analyses. Without these comparisons between intervention and control group, it is not possible to tell if a group that appears to benefit to a greater extent from treatment (e.g., girls or younger children), would not have done equally well untreated.

Child age and gender

Clinicians often gain the impression that boys and older children, especially adolescents, perform worse, and Bank *et al.* (1991) found a smaller effect size with adolescents than with younger children at the same institution. However, meta-analyses of interventions for antisocial behavior are mixed. For example, the Cochrane reviews of parenting interventions for antisocial behavior found an effect size of 0.56SD in teenagers (Woolfenden *et al.*, 2001), 0.53SD in middle childhood (Furlong *et al.*, 2012) and 0.25SD in early childhood (Barlow *et al.*, 2010), thus showing *smaller* effects in younger children. Within the middle childhood age range, Furlong *et al.* (2012) found no effect of age on outcome. Teenagers may appear less tractable for a number of reasons. Firstly, many studies on adolescents include the most severe cases (Lipsey, 2003; Leijten *et al.*, 2013). Often, when severity is controlled for, there is no age effect—across a wide age range (2–16 years), Ruma *et al.* (1996) found that the adolescent group did slightly less well, but the difference disappeared after taking into account initial severity. Within prepubertal children, there also do not appear to be age effects when using direct observation (Dishion & Patterson, 1992; Beauchaine *et al.*, 2005). By contrast, the meta-analysis by Serketich and Dumas (1996) found that across (not within) 36 studies ranging from 3 to 10 years, effectiveness was *greater* in older children. In summary, it appears that age is not a clear determinant of outcome. Likewise, boys are as likely to improve as girls (e.g., see Beauchaine *et al.*, 2005; Scott, 2005). Therefore, there is room for some optimism when treating adolescents.

Child psychopathology

The meta-analysis by Reyno and McGrath (2006) found that more severe initial antisocial behavior predicted (not

moderated) *less* change, but this was a bivariate association with no controlling for other factors. By contrast, taking other factors into account, Scott (2005) found the opposite, namely that higher initial levels of antisocial behavior predicted more change. Most recent reviews and meta-analyses tend to concur. Although Furlong *et al.*'s (2012) Cochrane review found no difference by conduct problem severity (coded at the trial level), Shelleby & Shaw's (2014) narrative review, and meta-analyses by Lundahl *et al.* (2006) and Leijten *et al.* (2013) found larger effect sizes with higher initial severity. Future studies need to address this issue using multivariate statistics and larger pooled samples. Child ADHD predicts a less good response in some studies (MTA, 1999; Scott, 2005) but not others (Beauchaine *et al.*, 2005; Ollendick *et al.*, 2008). In the MTA study, direct observations in the psychological treatment-only arm showed that parents had changed their behavior, whereas child ADHD symptoms had not (Wells *et al.*, 2006). This suggests that it is the characteristics of the children with ADHD that make them less sensitive to change, rather than parents not implementing more effective parenting practices. By contrast, when studied, comorbid anxiety appears to predict better treatment response for children with behavior problems (Beauchaine *et al.*, 2005). A broad review by Ollendick *et al.* (2008) concluded that for conduct problem interventions, comorbidity did not affect outcomes.

Family factors

Demographic predictors of outcome such as single parenthood, lower maternal education, poverty, and larger family size have traditionally been found in meta-analyses to have a small but negative effect on outcomes (Lundahl *et al.*, 2006; Reyno & McGrath, 2006). However, a recent systematic review (Leijten *et al.*, 2013) that controlled for confounders, especially initial child problem severity, found no diminished effects of parenting interventions in low socio-economic status families, consistent with moderator analyses in recent trials of more flexible interventions (Dishion *et al.*, 2008; Gardner *et al.*, 2009, 2010).

Similarly, reviews have traditionally found that parental psychopathology, especially maternal depression, predicts worse outcomes, as do life events and harsher initial parenting practices (Reyno & McGrath, 2006). However, Gardner *et al.* (2010) found *larger* child improvement with depressed parents. For mothers with the most negative beliefs about their children, Doolan (2006) found no change in child behavior at all. Overall, these conflicting subgroup findings from small trials suggest that the field would benefit from pooling individual patient-level data from multiple randomized trials (Brown *et al.*, 2013).

Mediators of change

In recent years, researchers have begun to investigate what mediates outcome, as recommended by Rutter (2005). To mediate treatment outcome, the treatment has to (i) change outcome (ii) change the mediator (iii) the mediator has to correlate with outcome, and (iv) the effect of treatment on outcome has to reduce or disappear after controlling for the mediator (Kraemer *et al.*, 2002). It would seem likely that for parenting programs to change child behavior, some aspect of parenting would first have to change. This is worth testing as it might not be the case—for example, the parenting program could make a couple realize that they should for example, stop arguing in front of their child, but still use the same disciplinary strategies.

Beauchaine *et al.* (2005) and Tein *et al.* (2004) found that changes in critical and ineffective parenting mediated child change in antisocial behavior, whereas several studies have found that positive parenting mediated change (Gardner *et al.*, 2006, 2010; Dishion *et al.*, 2008). Gardner *et al.* (2006) tested competing mediators, finding that it was change in positive parenting skill, rather than confidence in parenting, that predicted change in child problem behavior. In adolescents, Eddy and Chamberlain (2000) found for parenting, quality of supervision and discipline, and a positive adult–youth relationship all mediated change, as did time spent with deviant peers and the degree of their influence. Taken together, these four factors accounted for a substantial 32% of variance in subsequent antisocial behavior. Similarly, Huey *et al.* (2000) in a trial of MultiSystemic Therapy for delinquency showed that a positive relationship and firm discipline mediated outcome and good supervision mediated deviant peer association which in turn mediated subsequent antisocial behavior. These studies indicate which variables need to change for a good outcome and have led to changes in programs, for example, there is now a much stronger emphasis on preventing deviant peer association—the OSLC Treatment Fostercare program penalizes youth for every minute that they cannot verifiably account for their whereabouts.

Implementation and dissemination

Implementation

Most of the trials cited earlier were carried out using (i) specially recruited cases rather than clinical referrals, (ii) specially trained research therapists rather than regular clinicians (iii) university rather than clinical settings; indeed Weisz's studies show that fewer than 5% of psychosocial child mental health trials meet all three "real-life" criteria (see Chapter 36). There is therefore considerable concern whether the good effects seen in trials will be replicated in everyday life, where cases have a high degree of comorbid conditions and most therapists do not use evidence-based approaches and do not get skill-specific supervision. Trials that compared evidence-based approaches in real-life with usual services nonetheless get a clear advantage, by 0.3 SDs (see Chapter 36). The challenge is therefore to disseminate best practice more widely and to ensure that it is well implemented (Fixsen *et al.*, 2011).

Therapist effects

Therapist performance can be divided into three elements. (i) the *alliance*, which includes how well client and therapist get on together and agree shared goals. A meta-analysis of youth studies of the alliance found it contributed on average an effect size of 0.21 SD to outcome (Shirk & Karver, 2003). (ii) *fidelity* or adherence to specific components of a model that concerns the extent to which the therapist follows the actions prescribed in the manual. In a large real-life study of the implementation of a family program for antisocial youths, Sexton and Turner (2011) found that therapists who were highly adherent to the model obtained good results, with a larger effect size on more severe cases, whereas low adherent therapists actually obtained poorer results than the control group, implying that they might have perpetrated harm. (iii) the *skill* or competence with which the therapist carries out the tasks, that is, how well the therapist performs the actions. Skill can include aspects of the alliance and fidelity. Both Forgatch *et al.* (2005) and Eames *et al.* (2009) found that therapist skill significantly predicted change in independently observed parenting. In summary, there is good evidence that therapist variables make a crucial difference to parenting programs for antisocial behavior.

Dissemination

Although formal surveys are lacking in most countries, from the paucity of professionals trained in evidence-based programs, we can conclude that the vast majority of children with conduct problems or insecure attachment are not offered proven approaches. There are examples of initiatives to address this. Norway has set up a national training center to roll out and support a portfolio of parenting programs. In England, the National Academy for Parenting Practitioners was set up in 2007 and by 2010 had trained 4000 practitioners in a small number of carefully chosen evidence-based programs, estimated to have benefited 150,000 children (Scott, 2010). This was accompanied by a sizeable research program and a detailed evaluation of over 100 parenting programs, with the results posted on a searchable site for parents and commissioners (www.education.gov.uk/commissioning-toolkit). For clinically referred cases, the Children and Young People's Increasing Access to Psychological Therapies (CYP-IAPT) initiative is training up 5 staff from each local health authority in England in either parent training for conduct problems or cognitive behavioral therapy (CBT) for depression and anxiety. The training is intense, 3 days a week over a year, with close supervision of skills. A further element likely to lead to effectiveness is insistence on session-by-session outcome monitoring (http://www.iapt.nhs.uk/cyp-iapt). More is now known about how to achieve successful dissemination, including training managers as well as clinicians, educating both that regular supervision is necessary, and making the case for the cost-effectiveness of parenting programs.

Prevention

In an ideal public health preventive strategy, all parents would learn effective parenting skills, which would help to improve parent–child relationships and child well-being, and reduce the population rate of harsh and abusive parenting. There would be a tiered set of interventions available in primary and then in increasingly specialist levels of care, to help those with continuing difficulties. This vision has been well articulated by Sanders (1999) and appropriate programs developed by his group for each level. It is clear that we have good evidence for the effectiveness of parenting interventions for selective and indicated prevention and for treatment of conduct problems. However, it is less clear whether universal prevention parenting programs work: there have been many successful trials, but also many unsuccessful ones (Malti *et al.*, 2011; Simkiss *et al.*, 2013). Further studies need to understand under which conditions and using which delivery mechanisms, universal parenting programs can be helpful; if they are not, then the conclusion might be that targeted programs are more useful. Prevention is covered in more detail in Chapter 17.

Conclusions

Parenting programs have developed considerably in recent years. Findings from scores of randomized trials present a positive view of their effectiveness, with widespread implementation in many countries. Recent moderator analyses suggest that for many groups considered as hard-to-treat, for reasons of social disadvantage or psychopathology, parenting interventions can improve child behavior. For families with very complex needs, such as those in the child protection system, the evidence is promising. Future developments need to include evaluation of the long-term effects of programs and the mechanisms that mediate changes in parenting behavior. As parenting programs tend to have small effects on children's behavior in school, further evidence on school-based programs is warranted. Finally, future studies need to investigate which families can improve with minimal intervention such as computer-based self-instruction.

References

Anderson, K. *et al.* (1986) Mothers' interactions with normal and conduct disordered boys: who affects whom? *Developmental Psychology* **22**, 604–609.

Bakermans-Kranenburg, M. *et al.* (2003) Less is more: meta-analyses of sensitivity and attachment interventions in early childhood. *Psychological Bulletin* **129**, 195–215.

Bandura, A. (1977) *Social Learning Theory*. General Learning Corporation, NY.

Bank, L. *et al.* (1991) Comparative evaluation of parent-training interventions for families of chronic delinquents. *Journal of Abnormal Child Psychology* **19**, 15–33.

Barlow, J. *et al.* (2007) Role of home visiting in improving parenting and health in families at risk of abuse and neglect: results of a multicentre randomised trial and economic evaluation. *Archives of Disease in Childhood* **92**, 229–233.

Barlow, J. *et al.* (2010) Group-based parent-training programmes for improving emotional and behavioural adjustment in children from birth to three. *Cochrane Systematic Reviews* (3), CD003680.

Barlow, J. *et al.* (2012) Group-based parenting programmes for improving parental psychosocial health. *Cochrane Systematic Reviews* 6, CD002020.

Barnes, J. *et al.* (2006) The impact on parenting and the home environment of early support to mothers with new babies. *Journal of Children's Services* **1**, 4–20.

Bates, J. *et al.* (1998) Interaction of temperamental resistance-to-control and restrictive parenting in the development of externalizing behavior. *Developmental Psychology* **34**, 982–995.

Beauchaine, T. *et al.* (2005) Mediators, moderators and predictors of 1-year outcomes among children treated for early-onset problems. *Journal of Consulting and Clinical Psychology* **75**, 371–388.

Bergman, K. *et al.* (2010) Maternal prenatal cortisol and infant cognitive development: moderation by infant-mother attachment. *Biological Psychiatry* **67**, 1026–1032.

Besnard, T. *et al.* (2013) Moms and Dads count in a prevention program for kindergarten children with behavioural problems. *Canadian Journal of School Psychology* **28**, 219–238.

Bohman, M. (1996) Predisposition to criminality: Swedish adoption studies in retrospect. In: *Genetics of Criminal and Antisocial Behaviour*. (eds G. Bock & J. Goode), pp. 99–114. John Wiley & Sons, Chichester.

Bowlby, J. (1969/1982) *Attachment and Loss: Attachment*. Basic, New York.

Briskman, J. & Scott, S. (2013) *Randomised Controlled Trial of Fostering Changes Parenting Groups for Fostered Children*. DfE, London.

Brotman, L. *et al.* (2012) Early childhood family intervention and long-term obesity prevention. *Pediatrics* **129**, e621–e628.

Brown, C.H. *et al.* (2013) Methods for synthesizing findings on moderation effects across multiple randomized trials. *Prevention Science* **13**, 144–156.

Bywater, T. *et al.* (2009) Long-term effectiveness of the incredible years parenting programme. *British Journal of Psychiatry* **195**, 1–7.

Cartwright-Hatton, S. *et al.* (2011) A new parenting-based group intervention for young anxious children: RCT results. *Journal of the American Academy of Child and Adolescent Psychiatry* **50**, 242–251.

Caspi, A. *et al.* (2002) Evidence that the cycle of violence in maltreated children depends on genotype. *Science* **297**, 851–854.

Charach, A. *et al.* (2013) Interventions for preschool children at high risk for ADHD: comparative effectiveness review. *Pediatrics* **131**, e1584–e1604.

Cooper, P. *et al.* (2009) Improving quality of mother-infant relationship and infant attachment in South Africa: randomised trial. *British Medical Journal* **338**, b974.

Cowan, P. *et al.* (2009) Promoting fathers engagement with children: preventive interventions for low income families. *Journal of Marriage and Family* **71**, 663–679.

Cyr, C. *et al.* (2010) Attachment security and disorganization in maltreating and high-risk families: a series of meta-analyses. *Development and Psychopathology* **22**, 87–108.

Dadds, M. *et al.* (1996) Family process, child anxiety and aggression: observational analysis. *Journal of Abnormal Child Psychology* **24**, 715–734.

Dadds, M. *et al.* (2013) Callous-unemotional traits in children and mechanisms of impaired eye contact: a treatment target? *Journal of Child Psychology and Psychiatry* **55**, 771–780.

Dawe, S. & Harnett, P. (2007) Reducing potential for child abuse among methadone-maintained parents: results from a randomized trial. *Journal of Substance Abuse Treatment* **32**, 381–390.

De Wolff, M. & van IJzendoorn, M. (1997) Sensitivity and attachment: a meta-analysis. *Child Development* **68**, 571–591.

Denham, S. *et al.* (2000) Prediction of externalizing behavior problems from early to middle childhood: role of parental socialization and emotion expression. *Development and Psychopathology* **12**, 23–45.

Dishion, T. & Patterson, G. (1992) Age effects in parent training outcome. *Behavior Therapy* **23**, 719–229.

Dishion, T. *et al.* (2008) The family check-up: preventing problem behavior by increasing parents' positive behavior support. *Child Development* **79**, 1395–1414.

Doolan, M. (2006). *Mothers' emotional valence representations of children with antisocial behaviour and their role in treatment outcome.* PhD Thesis, King's College London.

Dozier, M. *et al.* (2012). *Attachment and biobehavioral catch-up*, University of Delaware, Newark.

Eames, C. *et al.* (2009) Treatment fidelity as a predictor of behaviour change in parents attending group-based parent-training. *Child: Care, Health and Development* **35**, 603–612.

Eddy, M. & Chamberlain, P. (2000) Family management and deviant peer association as mediators of the impact of treatment on youth antisocial behavior. *Journal of Consulting and Clinical Psychology* **68**, 857–863.

Ellis, B. *et al.* (2011) Differential susceptibility to the environment: an evolutionary-neurodevelopmental theory. *Development and Psychopathology* **23**, 7–28.

Engle, P. *et al.* (2007) Child development in developing countries: strategies to avoid the loss of developmental potential in over 200 million children in the developing world. *The Lancet* **369**, 229–242.

Fearon, P. *et al.* (2010) Insecure attachment and disorganization in children's externalizing behavior: a meta-analysis. *Child Development* **81**, 435–456.

Fisher, P. *et al.* (2006) Effects of therapeutic interventions for foster children on behavior, attachment, and stress regulatory systems. *Annals of the New York Academy of Sciences* **1094**, 215–225.

Fixsen, D. *et al.* (2011) Mobilizing communities for implementing evidence-based youth violence prevention. *American Journal of Community Psychology* **48**, 133–137.

Forgatch, M. *et al.* (2005) Evaluating fidelity: predictive validity for a measure of competent adherence to the Oregon model of parent training. *Behavior Therapy* **36**, 3–13.

Forgatch, M. *et al.* (2009) Testing the Oregon delinquency model: 9-year follow up of the Oregon divorce study. *Development and Psychopathology* **21**, 637–660.

Furlong, M. *et al.* (2012) Behavioural/cognitive-behavioural group-based parenting interventions for children age 3–12 with early onset conduct problems. *Cochrane Database of Systematic Reviews* **2**, CD008225.

Futh, A. *et al.* (2008) Attachment narratives and behavioural and emotional symptoms in an ethnically diverse, at-risk sample. *Journal of the American Academy of Child and Adolescent Psychiatry* **47**, 709–718.

Gardner, F. (1987) Positive interaction between mothers and conduct-problem children: is there training for harmony as well as fighting? *Journal of Abnormal Child Psychology* **15**, 283–293.

Gardner, F. *et al.* (1999) Parents anticipating misbehaviour: an observational study of strategies parents use to prevent conflict. *Journal of Child Psychology and Psychiatry* **40**, 1185–1196.

Gardner, F. *et al.* (2006) RCT of a parenting intervention in the voluntary sector for reducing child conduct problems. *Journal of Child Psychology and Psychiatry* **47**, 1123–1132.

Gardner, F. *et al.* (2009) Moderators of outcome in a brief family-centred intervention for preventing early problem behaviour. *Journal of Consulting and Clinical Psychology* **77**, 543–553.

Gardner, F. *et al.* (2010) Moderators and mediators of outcomes in a randomised trial of parenting interventions. *Journal of Clinical Child & Adolescent Psychology* **39**, 568–80.

Gardner, F., *et al.* (2015). Transporting evidence-based parenting programs for child problem behavior (age 3–10) between countries: systematic review and meta-analysis. Special Issue in press, *From Adoption to Adaptation, Journal of Clinical Child & Adolescent Psychology.*

Green, J. *et al.* (2007) Disorganized attachment representation and atypical parenting in young school age children with externalizing disorder. *Attachment & Human Development* **9**, 207–222.

Huey, S.J. *et al.* (2000) Mechanisms of change in MST: reducing delinquent behavior through therapist adherence and improved family and peer functioning. *Journal of Consulting and Clinical Psychology* **68**, 451–467.

Hutchings, J. *et al.* (2007) Parenting intervention in Sure Start services for children at risk of developing conduct disorder: pragmatic randomised trial. *British Medical Journal* **334**, 678–685.

Jones, K. *et al.* (2008) Efficacy of the Incredible Years basic parent training programme as an early intervention for children with conduct disorder and ADHD: long-term follow-up. *Child: Care, Health and Development* **34**, 380–390.

Knerr, W. *et al.* (2013) Improving positive parenting skills and reducing harsh and abusive parenting in low- and middle-income countries: a systematic review. *Prevention Science* **14**, 352–363.

Kochanska, G. (1997) Multiple pathways to conscience for children with different temperaments: from toddlerhood to age 5. *Developmental Psychology* **33**, 228–240.

Kraemer, H. *et al.* (2002) Mediators and moderators of treatment effects. *Archives of General Psychiatry* **59**, 877–883.

Lamb, M. (2004) *The Role of the Father in Child Development.* John Wiley & Sons, New York.

Leijten, P. *et al.* (2013) Does socioeconomic status matter? A meta-analysis on parent training effectiveness for disruptive child behavior. *Journal of Clinical Child & Adolescent Psychology* **42**, 384–392.

Lipsey, M. (2003) Those confounded moderators in meta-analysis: good, bad, and ugly. *Annals of the American Academy of Political and Social Science* **587**, 69–81.

Lundahl, B. *et al.* (2006) A meta-analysis of parent training: moderators and follow-up effects. *Clinical Psychology Review* **26**, 86–104.

Lundahl, B. *et al.* (2008) A meta-analysis of father involvement in parent training. *Research on Social Work Practice* **18**, 97–108.

MacDonald, G. & Turner, W. (2005) An experiment in helping foster-carers manage challenging behaviour. *British Journal of Social Work* **35**, 1265–1282.

MacMillan, H.L. *et al.* (2009) Interventions to prevent child maltreatment and associated impairment. *The Lancet* **373**, 250–266.

Malti, T. *et al.* (2011) Effectiveness of two universal preventive interventions in reducing children's externalizing behavior: cluster randomized trial. *Journal of Clinical Child & Adolescent Psychology* **40**, 677–692.

Matias, C. *et al.* (2013) Observational attachment theory-based parenting measures predict children's attachment narratives. *Attachment and Human Development* **16**, 77–92.

Maughan, B. & Gardner, F. (2010) Family and parenting influences on antisocial behaviour. In: *A New Response to Youth Crime.* (ed D. Smith). Devon: Willan, Cullompton.

Menting, A. *et al.* (2013) Effectiveness of Incredible Years parent training: meta-analysis. *Clinical Psychology Review* **33**, 913–901.

MTA Cooperative Group (1999) A 14-month RCT of treatment strategies for ADHD: multimodal treatment study of children with ADHD. *Archives of General Psychiatry* **56**, 1073–1086.

National Institute for Health and Care Excellence (2013) *Recognition, Intervention and Management of Antisocial Behaviour and Conduct Disorders in Children & Young People.* National Institute for Health and Care Excellence, London.

O'Connor, T. *et al.* (2013) Social learning theory-based parenting intervention promotes attachment-based caregiving: results from a randomized trial. *Journal of Clinical Child & Adolescent Psychology* **42**, 358–420.

Olds, D. (2006) The nurse-family partnership: an evidence-based preventive intervention. *Infant Mental Health Journal* **27**, 3–25.

Ollendick, T.H. *et al.* (2008) Comorbidity as a predictor and moderator of treatment outcome in youth with anxiety, affective, ADHD, and ODD/CD. *Clinical Psychology Review* **28**, 1447–1471.

Patterson, G. (1982) *Coercive Family Process.* Castalia, Eugene, Oregon.

Pettit, G. *et al.* (1999) The impact of peer contact on adolescent externalizing problems is moderated by parental monitoring, perceived neighborhood safety, and prior adjustment. *Child Development* **70**, 768–78.

Racz, S.J. & McMahon, R.J. (2011) The relationship between parental knowledge and monitoring and child conduct problems: 10 year update. *Clinical Child and Family Psychology Review* **14**, 377–398.

Rahman, A. *et al.* (2009) Cluster randomized trial of a parent-based intervention to support early development of children in a low-income country. *Child: Care, Health and Development* **35**, 56–62.

Ramchandani, P. *et al.* (2013) Do early father-infant interactions predict onset of externalising behaviours in young children? Findings from a longitudinal cohort study. *Journal of Child Psychology and Psychiatry* **54**, 56–64.

Reid, M. *et al.* (2001) Parent training in HeadStart: a comparison of response among African-American, Asian-American, Caucasian, and Hispanic mothers. *Prevention Science* **2**, 209–227.

Reyno, S.M. & McGrath, P.J. (2006) Predictors of parent training efficacy for child externalizing behavior problems – a meta-analytic review. *Journal of Child Psychology and Psychiatry* **47**, 99–111.

Ruma, P. *et al.* (1996) Group parent training: is it effective for children of all ages? *Behaviour Therapy* **27**, 159–169.

Rutter, M. (2005) Environmentally mediated risks for psychopathology: research strategies and findings. *Journal of the American Academy of Child and Adolescent Psychiatry* **44**, 3–18.

Sanders, M. (1999) Triple P-positive parenting program. *Clinical Child and Family Psychology Review* **2**, 71–90.

Sanders, M. *et al.* (2004) Does parental attributional retraining and anger management enhance the effects of the triple P-positive parenting program? *Behavior Therapy* **35**, 513–535.

Schachar, R. *et al.* (1987) Changes in family functioning and relationships in children who respond to methylphenidate. *Journal of the American Academy of Child and Adolescent Psychiatry* **26**, 728–732.

Scott, S. (2005) Do parenting programmes for severe child antisocial behaviour work over the longer term, and for whom? 1 year follow up of a multi-centre controlled trial. *Behavioural and Cognitive Psychotherapy* **33**, 403–421.

Scott, S. (2008) Parenting programs. In: *Rutter's Child and Adolescent Psychiatry.* (eds M. Rutter, *et al.*). Blackwell, Oxford.

Scott, S. (2010) National dissemination of effective parenting programmes to improve child outcomes. *British Journal of Psychiatry* **196**, 1–3.

Scott, S. & O'Connor, T. (2012) An experimental test of differential susceptibility to parenting among emotionally dysregulated children. *Journal of Child Psychology and Psychiatry* **53**, 1184–1193.

Scott, S. *et al.* (2001) Multicentre controlled trial of parenting groups for childhood antisocial behaviour in clinical practice. *BMJ* **323**, 194–201.

Scott, S. *et al.* (2010a) Impact of a parenting program in a high-risk, multi-ethnic community: the PALS trial. *Journal of Child Psychology and Psychiatry* **51**, 1331–1341.

Scott, S. *et al.* (2010b) Randomized controlled trial of parenting groups for child antisocial behavior targeting multiple risk factors: the SPOKES project. *Journal of Child Psychology and Psychiatry* **51**, 48–57.

Scott, S. *et al.* (2011) Attachment in adolescence: overlap with parenting and unique prediction of behavioural adjustment. *Journal of Child Psychology and Psychiatry* **52**, 1052–1062.

Serketich, W.J. & Dumas, J.E. (1996) The effectiveness of behavioral parent training to modify antisocial behavior in children: a meta-analysis. *Behavior Therapy* **27**, 171–186.

Sexton, T. & Turner, C. (2011) The effectiveness of functional family therapy for youth with behavioral problems. *Journal of Family Psychology* **24**, 339–348.

Shelleby, E.C. & Shaw, D.S. (2014) Outcomes of parenting interventions for child conduct problems: a review of differential effectiveness. *Child Psychiatry & Human Development*, **45**, 628–645.

Shirk, S.R. & Karver, M. (2003) Prediction of treatment outcome from relationship variables in child and adolescent therapy: a meta-analytic review. *Journal of Consulting and Clinical Psychology* **71**, 452–464.

Shmueli-Goetz, Y. *et al.* (2008) The child attachment interview. *Developmental Psychology* **44**, 939–956.

Simkiss, D. *et al.* (2013) Effectiveness and cost-effectiveness of a universal parenting skills programme in deprived communities: multicentre randomised controlled trial. *BMJ Open* **3**, e002851.

Slade, A. *et al.* (2005). In: *Enhancing Early Attachment: Theory, Research, Intervention and Policy.* (eds L. Berlin, *et al.*). Guilford Press, New York.

Snarr, J. *et al.* (2009) Validation of a new self-report measure of parental attributions. *Psychological Assessment* **21**, 390–401.

Sonuga-Barke, E.J. *et al.* (2001) Parent-based therapies for ADHD: RCT in a community sample. *Journal of the American Academy of Child and Adolescent Psychiatry* **40**, 402–408.

Sonuga-Barke, E.J. *et al.* (2013) Non-pharmacological interventions for ADHD: systematic review. *American Journal of Psychiatry* **170**, 275–289.

Sroufe, A. *et al.* (2010) Conceptualising the role of early experience: lessons from the Minnesota longitudinal study. *Developmental Review* **30**, 36–51.

Stahlschmidt, M. *et al.* (2013) Recruiting fathers to parenting programs: advice from dads and fatherhood program providers. *Children Youth Services Review* **35**, 1734–1741.

Tein, J.-Y. *et al.* (2004) Mediation in the context of a moderated prevention effect for children of divorce. *Journal of Consulting and Clinical Psychology* **72**, 617–624.

Turner, W. *et al.* (2007) Behavioural and cognitive behavioural training interventions for assisting foster carers in the management of difficult behaviour. *Cochrane Systematic Reviews* **1**, 1–63.

Velderman, M. *et al.* (2006) Preventing preschool externalizing behavior problems through video-feedback intervention in infancy. *Infant Mental Health Journal* **27**, 466–493.

Waller, R. *et al.* (2013) Parenting as predictor of callous unemotional traits in young people: systematic review. *Clinical Psychology Review* **33**, 593–608.

Webster-Stratton, C. (2011) Combining parent and child training for young children with ADHD. *Journal of Clinical Child & Adolescent Psychology* **40**, 191–203.

Wells, K. *et al.* (2006) Treatment related changes in objectively measured parent behaviors in the multimodal treatment study of ADHD children. *Journal of Consulting and Clinical Psychology* **74**, 649–657.

WHO (2013) *Preventing Violence: Evaluating Outcomes of Parenting Interventions.* WHO, Geneva.

Wood, J. *et al.* (2003) Parenting and childhood anxiety. *Journal of Child Psychology and Psychiatry* **44**, 134–151.

Woolfenden, S. *et al.* (2001) Family and parenting interventions in children and adolescents with conduct disorder and delinquency aged 10–17. *Cochrane Systematic Reviews* (2), CD003015.

Zwi, M. *et al.* (2011) Parent training interventions for ADHD in children aged 5 to 18 years. *Cochrane Systematic Reviews* (12), CD003018.

CHAPTER 38

Cognitive-behavioral therapy, behavioral therapy, and related treatments in children

Philip C. Kendall, Jeremy S. Peterman and Colleen M. Cummings
Department of Psychology, Temple University, Philadelphia, PA, USA

Understanding cognitive-behavioral therapy (CBT)

Cognitive-behavioral therapy (CBT) represents an integration of both cognitive and behavioral models of psychopathology. Given that CBT expanded from behavior therapy (BT), behavioral theories are a starting point in understanding CBT. In the 1930s, behaviorism emerged as a reaction to introspective psychology (e.g., examination of one's own conscious thoughts and feelings). Behavioral theories de-emphasize the "active mind" and consciousness as these phenomena cannot be readily observed or measured, and hold that environmental events shape behavior. For example, in respondent conditioning, youth learn behavior through associations. When a feared stimulus (unconditioned stimulus) is temporally paired with a neutral stimulus (conditioned stimulus), the initially neutral stimulus consequently provokes a fear response, even when presented in isolation. Therapeutic strategies born from respondent conditioning, such as extinction (presenting the conditioned stimulus without the unconditioned stimulus), and habituation (experiencing the conditioned stimulus over a prolonged period of time) have been integrated into treatment.

Operant conditioning (Skinner, 1969) marks a cornerstone in BT. Operant learning theories are based on learning due to consequences from a response (e.g., an increase or decrease a specific behavior via reinforcement and punishment, respectively). For example, an oppositional youth may act out to receive attention. When the parent attends to the behavior, by acquiescing to the youth's demands, the youth's behavior is reinforced and is likely to remerge in the future. On the other hand, when the parent provides reinforcement (e.g., praise)

for a counter-behavior, prosocial behaviors may increase over time. Thus, reinforcement (and punishment) can be both the problem and solution and is utilized within CBT. A common way that reinforcement is integrated is through shaping, in which a complex behavior is broken into several simpler steps and completion of each small step is rewarded.

CBT evolved from BT with the addition of cognitive theory. Cognitive theory emphasizes the importance of social information-processing (e.g., memory, attention, and flexible thinking) and cognitive distortions in psychopathology. Thus, cognitive theory brought "mind" back to psychology, positing that one's interpretation and processing of stimuli and events impact behavior. Specific theories regarding the latter have been pioneered by Aaron Beck and Albert Ellis. Though using different language, Beck and Ellis converge on the idea that cognition mediates the relationship between life stress and psychopathology. Rigid and distorted beliefs about oneself, the world, or the future are accordingly targeted in cognitive therapies. In other words, altering one's belief system can modify behavior. Additionally, the influence of information-processing theory has translated to therapies that target problem solving skills. CBT was also influenced by Bandura (1977) who described how learning can occur through observation. Observational learning has influenced specific CBT techniques, such as modeling and role-play.

Overall, CBT and BT are grounded in complementary theories that explain the psychology behind the emergence of psychopathology. Accordingly, CBT has developed a set of treatments, derived from behavioral and cognitive theory, to treat psychopathology. CBT has evidenced success across many diagnostic categories. In the following section, some of the supporting evidence will be considered.

Rutter's Child and Adolescent Psychiatry, Sixth Edition.
Edited by Anita Thapar and Daniel S. Pine, James F. Leckman, Stephen Scott, Margaret J. Snowling, Eric Taylor.
© 2015 John Wiley & Sons Ltd. Published 2018 by John Wiley & Sons Ltd.

Empirically-supported CBTs and BTs for youth

Several CBTs, BTs (and some other treatments) for youth psychopathology have emerged as having varying levels of empirical support (Kendall, 2012) according to guidelines by Chambless and Hollon (1998) and Chapter 36.

Treatment modalities

CBT and BT may be provided in individual, group, or family-based modalities. Individual treatment optimizes personalized treatment. Group treatment increases "reach" by working with multiple youth at a time, with opportunities for social skills practice and the ability to complete therapeutic activities (e.g., exposure tasks) with the support of peers. Treatment must still meet the individual needs of each group member and may not be indicated for children with multiple comorbidities (e.g., Farrell et al., 2012), environmental stressors, or other characteristics that decrease participation in group therapy (e.g., severe social anxiety or antisocial behaviors). Family-based treatment can target familial patterns and parenting practices that may serve to maintain youth psychopathology if not adequately addressed. Typically, youth CBTs and BTs include some form of parental involvement, which can vary from a few parent sessions to family-based treatment. Overall, the degree to which family members participate in youth treatment may depend on several factors (e.g., presence of a parental psychological disorder; maladaptive parenting behavior and family patterns; Creswell & Cartwright-Hatton, 2007).

Anxiety disorders

CBT for youth with anxiety is a well-established treatment (Hollon & Beck, 2013). Individual treatments are common for child anxiety. One is the *Coping Cat program* (Kendall & Hedtke, 2006a, b). It consists of 16 sessions, separated into two segments: skills training and skills practice (exposure tasks) and has been adapted for adolescents (i.e., *The C.A.T. Project*; Kendall et al., 2002). Several RCTs have supported its efficacy (Walkup et al., 2008). Additionally, gains have been found to be maintained at 1-year to 7.4-year follow-ups, and a meaningful percentage of successfully treated participants had reduced problems associated with substance use (Kendall et al., 2004; Puleo et al., 2011).

The largest randomized controlled trial (RCT), the Child/Adolescent Anxiety Multimodal Study (CAMS), evaluated the efficacy of CBT (the *Coping Cat/ C.A.T. Project*), medication (sertraline), a combination of the two (COMB), and a pill placebo (PBO) among 488 youth (ages 7–17). 80% of COMB (effect size = 0.86), 60% of CBT (effect size = 0.31), 55% of sertraline (effect size = 0.45), and 24% of placebo were considered treatment responders (rated by independent evaluators) at week 12 (Walkup et al., 2008). Rates of remission (i.e., identified as almost symptom-free) were lower but demonstrated the same pattern as rates of response (i.e., 68% of COMB, 36% of CBT, 46% of sertraline, and 27% of placebo; Ginsburg et al., 2011). The results were maintained at 36 week follow-up, with additional improvement to monotherapy conditions (i.e. 58% of CBT and 63% of sertraline; Piacentini et al., 2014). Data from RCTs suggest predictors: youth with a combination of more severity of symptoms at baseline, a primary diagnosis of social phobia, and comorbid internalizing disorders have a less favorable response to CBT (Crawley et al., 2008; Ginsburg et al., 2011).

Obsessive compulsive disorder

Exposure and response prevention (ERP) for obsessive compulsive disorder (OCD) in youth has been classified as probably efficacious (Weisz et al., 2013). The focus of ERP is to expose youth to stimuli that trigger obsessions, while encouraging the youth to refrain from engaging in compulsions that provide immediate, but transient, relief from anxiety (Foa & Kozak, 1986). The Pediatric OCD Treatment Study (POTS) was a multisite trial for 112 youth, aged 7 to 17, who were randomly assigned to CBT, sertraline, combined CBT and sertraline (COMB), or PBO for 12 weeks. All three active treatments outperformed PBO, and COMB was superior to CBT and sertraline. Furthermore, a greater number of CBT patients entered remission than sertraline patients.

In POTS predictors of attenuated response included higher OCD severity, higher levels of OCD-related functional impairment, higher levels of comorbid externalizing symptoms, and higher levels of family accommodation. Interestingly, family history of OCD moderated the effect of treatment condition: for participants with a positive family history of OCD, there were no differences in outcomes across the treatment groups, whereas for those with no family history, COMB outperformed PBO and SER and CBT outperformed PBO. Additionally, treatment effect sizes were smaller for those with a family history of OCD, and this reduction in effect sizes was particularly high for the CBT group (Garcia et al., 2010). The presence of a comorbid tic disorder moderated outcomes: among patients with a tic disorder, SER did not differ from PBO, whereas COMB remained superior to CBT and CBT remained superior to PBO (March et al., 2007).

Post traumatic stress disorder

For youth with PTSD, exposure-based CBT has been designated as well-established (Weisz et al., 2013). Exposures consist of confrontation with fearful memories of the trauma and can be imaginal or *in vivo*. The components of Trauma Focused-CBT (TF-CBT) are summarized by the acronym "PRACTICE," including psychoeducation/parenting component, relaxation, affect modulation, cognitive processing, trauma narrative, *in vivo* exposure and mastery of trauma reminders, conjoint child–parent session, and enhancing safety and future development (Cohen et al., 2007; see http://tfcbt.musc.edu). TF-CBT has demonstrated efficacy in RCTs. One study compared TF-CBT to child-centered therapy among 229 children (aged 8–14) who had been sexually abused. TF-CBT was superior on almost all measures, although 21% of children treated with TF-CBT still met diagnostic criteria for PTSD (Cohen *et al.*, 2004).

Depressive disorders

CBT is a well-established intervention, and BT is a probably efficacious intervention for youth depression (Weisz *et al.*, 2013). CBT for depression seeks to identify negative thoughts and encourages behaving in more positive and engaging ways. Core cognitive strategies include self-monitoring (i.e., using a CBT Thought Record), restructuring, and the identification of underlying assumptions. Core behavioral strategies include contingencies, self-reinforcement, activity scheduling, and relaxation training. CBTs that have received empirical support among youth include school-based approaches (Stark *et al.*, 2007) and Primary and Secondary Control Enhancement Training (PASCET; Weisz *et al.*, 1997). Among depressed adolescents, efficacy has been found for a CBT group treatment: the Adolescent Coping with Depression Course (CWD-A; Clarke *et al.*, 2001; Rohde *et al.*, 2001). TADS was a multicenter RCT that compared the effectiveness of fluoxetine alone, CBT alone, CBT plus fluoxetine, and placebo. Results supported the combination treatment (TADS Team, 2004): CBT plus fluoxetine led to the highest rates of response, followed by fluoxetine alone, CBT alone, and finally placebo, with response rates of 71%, 61%, 43%, and 35%, respectively. Adolescents with mild or moderate depression had better results with CBT plus fluoxetine than fluoxetine alone or CBT alone. Patients with severe depression responded equally well to CBT plus fluoxetine and fluoxetine alone (Curry *et al.*, 2006) with maintenance of gains for longer term TADS treatment (36 weeks) to 1-year follow-up (TADS Team, 2009). The Adolescent Depression Antidepressant and Psychotherapy Trial (ADAPT) randomized adolescents to SSRI (fluoxetine) + CBT or SSRI only conditions. ADAPT included participants with moderate to severe MDD and active self-harm. After the acute and maintenance treatment phases, response rates did not differ by condition, with 61% in the SSRI only condition and 53% in the SSRI + CBT rated to be much or very much improved (Goodyer *et al.*, 2007).

What about nonresponders? The Treatment of SSRI-Resistant Depression in Adolescents (TORDIA) randomized adolescents with MDD who did not respond to an 8-week trial of an SSRI to the following conditions: (i) switch to a different SSRI, (ii) switch to venlafaxine, (iii) switch to a second SSRI + CBT, (iv) switch to venlafaxine + CBT. Results indicated that treatment arms that included CBT outperformed medication-only (54.8% and 47% responders, respectively; Brent *et al.*, 2008).

Interventions are more efficacious for adolescents compared to children, albeit most effective for younger adolescents (e.g., Michael & Crowley, 2002). Ethnicity may moderate treatment, and Rohde and colleagues (2006) found that CBT outperformed control for only White youth, whereas non-White adolescents demonstrated no difference across conditions. In terms of gender, it has been suggested that female youth respond better to treatments with an interpersonal orientation (Garber,

2006). Findings suggest that more chronic depression, suicidality, melancholic features, poorer expectations for treatment success, and comorbidity (i.e., anxiety, attention deficit hyperactivity disorder (ADHD), disruptive behavior disorders, and substance abuse) may impede progress in depression treatment (Rohde *et al.*, 2001; Curry *et al.*, 2006).

Bipolar disorder

Treatment guidelines describe psychological treatment as an essential adjunct to pharmacological treatment for children with bipolar disorder. Psychosocial treatment targets psychoeducation, relapse prevention, individual therapy, social and family functioning, academic and occupational functioning, and community consultation (McClellan *et al.*, 2007). Adjunctive psychoeducation teaches families about the symptoms of bipolar disorder as well as its biopsychosocial management (e.g., improving family problem-solving and communication skills). Psychological therapy has demonstrated efficacy for bipolar disorder in youth (West *et al.*, 2007; Fristad *et al.*, 2009) and can be considered a probably efficacious treatment.

Psychosocial treatments that have been evaluated in youth with bipolar disorder include Fristad *et al.*'s work with multifamily psychoeducational psychotherapy groups (MF-PEP; Fristad *et al.*, 2011) and individual family psychoeducation (IFP), Miklowitz *et al.*'s family-focused treatment (FFT), and Pavuluri and colleagues' child- and family-focused CBT (CFF-CBT). These treatments showed improvements in their samples, including increases in parental knowledge of these treatments, lower ratings of symptom severity, improved family climate (Pavuluri *et al.*, 2004; Miklowitz *et al.*, 2008, 2013; Fristad *et al.*, 2009). At this juncture, the efficacy of FFT and MF-PEP is evidenced by RCTs, while empirical evidence of CFF-CBT includes only pilot studies.

Disruptive behavior disorders

A number of treatments for children and adolescents with disruptive behavior disorders (i.e., oppositional defiant disorder; conduct disorder) have garnered empirical support (Eyberg *et al.*, 2008). These are described in depth in Chapter 65 of this volume. Parenting programs alone (see Chapter 37) are well-supported, but individual programs are increasingly being shown to be effective. One CBT, the Coping Power Program (Lochman *et al.*, 2008), is based on a social-cognitive model of aggression (Lochman & Gresham, 2008), taking into account individual and environmental risk factors. Coping Power includes a 34-session child component (delivered either individually or in a group) and a 16-session group parent component. Children learn relaxation, emotion awareness, goal setting, and social skills such as how to manage peer pressure. Parents learn parent training techniques (e.g., positive reinforcement; ignoring), as well as strategies to manage their child's academic environment, family conflict, and their own stressors. RCTs have documented its efficacy (i.e., Lochman & Wells,

2004) and effectiveness (i.e., Lochman & Wells, 2003). Regarding predictors, (McMahon *et al.*, 2006), economic disadvantage and single parent household has been associated with poorer outcomes (Lundahl *et al.*, 2006).

Eating disorders

Adolescent eating disorders typically include anorexia nervosa (AN) and bulimia nervosa (BN) (see Chapter 71). CBT focuses on (i) addressing distorted cognition related to body shape and weight and (ii) working to directly alter maladaptive eating patterns, including restricting and purging. Although examined among samples including younger and older adolescents, CBT in general meets the criteria for an established treatment for BN (Keel & Haedt, 2008). The Maudsley model of family therapy for eating disorders includes the family in treatment (Lock *et al.*, 2001). Keel and Haedt (2008) determined that family therapy was a well-established treatment for adolescent AN (e.g., Robin *et al.*, 1999; Lock *et al.*, 2005) and a possibly efficacious treatment for adolescent BN (e.g., le Grange *et al.*, 2007).

Attention deficit/hyperactivity disorder

Stimulant medication has considerable evidence supporting its use for reduction of ADHD symptoms in youth (see Chapter 55). Nonetheless, BT is recommended as a first line intervention for youth with more mild levels of ADHD (see guidelines by the National Institute for Health and Care Excellence, 2008). For youth with more severe symptoms, BT has its place as a second line intervention or adjunctive intervention to medication that may add to long-term benefit (see guidelines by the American Academy of Child and Adolescent Psychiatry, 2007). BT, rather than CBT and nonbehavioral approaches, has empirical support for youth with ADHD (Pelham & Fabiano, 2008), although a recent meta-analysis suggested limited effect sizes (overall standard mean difference = 0.02) when blinded outcome assessments were used (Sonuga-Barke *et al.*, 2013). Established treatments for ADHD in youth include behavioral parent training, behavioral contingency management in classrooms, and intensive peer-focused interventions (e.g., summer camps).

In the Multimodal Treatment of Attention Deficit Hyperactivity Disorder (MTA) Study (MTA Cooperative Group, 1999a) Children were randomized to either 14 months of medication management (MedMgt), behavior therapy (Beh), their combination (Comb), or usual community care (CC). Findings post treatment (14 months) indicated that Comb and MedMgt showed greater improvements in ADHD and disruptive behavior disorder symptoms than Beh or CC (MTA Cooperative Group, 1999a). Comb outperformed Beh and CC in terms of internalizing symptoms, teacher-rated social skills, parent–child relationships, and reading achievement (MTA Cooperative Group, 1999a). Important to note, at 10-month, 3-year, and 8-year follow-ups, differences among the treatments were no longer apparent (MTA Cooperative Group, 2004a, b; Jensen *et al.*, 2007; Molina *et al.*, 2009).

Behavioral Classroom Management involves contingency management procedures in the classroom and teacher training in discipline procedures. RCTs of behavioral classroom management have demonstrated efficacy (e.g., Pelham & Fabiano, 2008). RCTs of summer treatment programs have also demonstrated efficacy (e.g., Pelham & Fabiano, 2008). Pelham and Fabiano (2008) concluded that due to its chronic nature, ADHD requires long-term, multisystemic, often multi component treatment to ensure long-term gains. There is evidence that low income and ethnic minority families may respond less well (Chronis *et al.*, 2004), but comorbidity and gender each have little association (Pelham & Fabiano, 2008).

Common treatment components

CBT and BTs are time-limited, typically manual-based, present-focused, and require active participation from youth and families. They address current problems rather than exploring early childhood conflicts. However, CBT and BT do take time to understand family interactions and previous traumas that may influence current disorder. Finally, CBT and BT require youth to actively contribute and participate in therapy, including activities between sessions (e.g., homework).

Psychoeducation

Typically an early feature of CBT interventions, psychoeducation involves information about possible explanations for the presenting problem, an overview of the treatment process, and affective education. First, the therapist provides a general framework for understanding the presenting problem. As part of this framework, there is, within reason, an effort to normalize certain emotional difficulties and reduce parent- and self-blame. For example, in the treatment of OCD the brain can be described as "short circuiting," or for younger youth, "having brain hiccups" (March & Mulle, 1998).

Another aspect of psychoeducation involves an overview of the treatment plan. From the onset, therapists note the subsequent sessions and the goals of therapy, while integrating feedback from the client to tailor the program. An overview of therapy also involves a discussion of each individual's part in the therapeutic process. The therapist may explain his/her own role using the metaphor of a "coach" (Kendall, 2012), in which the therapist provides support, encouragement, and training throughout treatment. Collaboration between the youth and the therapist, and with parents, is emphasized.

Finally, affective education promotes the youth's ability to become aware of, distinguish among, and appropriately express various emotions. Some youth do not have the vocabulary to properly express their feelings and the therapist can work to normalize some emotions and create a common emotional language. However, other youth may still struggle to distinguish between emotions. Thus, affective education focuses on emotional differentiation. For example, in the *Coping Cat program* for anxiety, the youth and therapist play *Feelings*

Detective in which the youth walks outside of the clinic and looks at other people ("spies") to label their likely emotions using facial and bodily cues (Kendall & Hedtke, 2006a). Other youth encounter problems when they interpret emotions (e.g., as an all-or-nothing phenomenon) and benefit from the presentation of a dimensional emotional model. For instance, some treatments introduce a "feelings thermometer" in which youth create a visual scale for the target emotional problem (e.g., anxiety, sadness). The scale may be numerical (e.g., 1 to 5), or use metaphors relevant to the child (e.g., least to most favorite color; characters from a comic book ranked least to most scary; the size of sports balls, from golf to basketball). The youth uses the scale to self-monitor mood, and consequently, as a signal to engage in emotion-regulating behavior when they reach a threshold. Finally, affective education involves a review of the three component model of feelings, thoughts, and behaviors (Figure 38.1). Youth gain experience in differentiating the components and in recognizing the interactions among them.

Relaxation

Although not always a part of CBT or BT with youth, relaxation training can be taught to youth to modulate their physiological arousal. Relaxation can be a useful first step in self-regulation. Decreased arousal from relaxation may permit the use of other coping strategies that necessitate higher ordered cognitive resources. Relaxation is part of the treatment for anxiety (Kendall & Hedtke, 2006a, b), depression (Reinecke & Ginsburg, 2008), and c) anger (Lochman *et al.*, 2008). Although some studies have shown beneficial outcomes of relaxation (Deffenbacher *et al.*, 1996; Norton, 2012), other data suggest that relaxation may not be a necessary component of CBT (Rapee, 2000; Hudson, 2005).

Youth are introduced to relaxation with a conversation that contrasts somatic tenseness to feelings of relaxation.

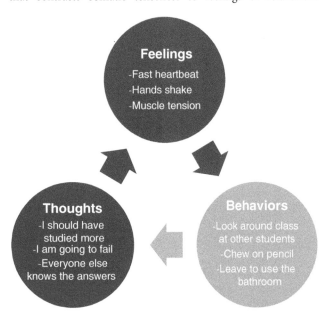

Figure 38.1 Three component model: test anxiety.

The metaphor of cooked versus uncooked spaghetti is one developmentally appropriate way to convey the somatic distinction. Scripts adapted from adults (e.g., Ollendick & Cerny, 1981) are used to teach relaxation techniques. A popular form of relaxation is diaphragmic breathing, involving deep inhalations into the nose and exhalations out the mouth. Progressive muscle relaxation (PMR) is another example in which youth alternate between tensing and relaxing specific muscles groups. Youth are encouraged to count when tensing (approximately 5 seconds), quickly release the muscle, and contrast the two feelings. Once again, metaphors assist in teaching youth relaxation. For example, in PMR, youth who tighten stomach muscles are encouraged to "fit through a tight fence," and when clenching their fists they may imagine "squeeze lemons to make lemonade" (Podell *et al.*, 2010). Therapists can make personalized relaxation recordings for youth to practice at home.

Problem-solving

Psychological disorders in youth are often associated with deficits in conceptualizing problems, generating feasible solutions, and putting solutions to action (Lochman & Dodge, 1994; Becker-Weidman *et al.*, 2010). Thus, problem-solving is commonly used in interventions (Shure, 2001; Kazdin, 2003; Kendall & Hedtke, 2006a, b). Problem-solving (D'Zurilla & Goldfried, 1971) teaches youth a systematic way to approach and reduce conflicts, and accordingly, provides a sense of control over the situation. Problem-solving differentiates itself from cognitive restructuring and relaxation: The latter are done to cope with an unavoidable situation, whereas the former is used when the youth has agency over their circumstances (Stark *et al.*, 2010).

Although CBT treatments often provide their own version of problem-solving, the core steps are universal and follow the same order. The steps of problem-solving include: (i) define the problem, (ii) generate as many solutions as possible, (iii) eliminate the unfeasible solutions, (iv) choose the best 1–2 solutions, and (v) implement the chosen solution, evaluate its outcome, and reevaluate as needed (Friedberg *et al.*, 2009). It is often helpful for the therapist to introduce problem solving by attempting to solve a low-threat problem (e.g., "it is time to leave for school but you cannot find your shoes"), and then move to problems related to the youth's presenting concern. Therapists encourage creative thinking and allow for any suggestion, no matter how outlandish, to be included in the solution generation step (e.g., "wear mommy's heels to school," "walk to school on my hands").

Homework

Homework is a central component of CBT with youth (as well as with adults). According to Hudson and Kendall (2002), homework allows the youth to practice and generalize therapeutic skills in a real-world setting, and provide feedback to the therapist regarding the youth's comprehension of session material. Although some studies have found that more positive outcomes are associated with homework compliance (Kazantzis *et al.*, 2010; Puleo & Kendall, 2011), some others have not (Clarke *et al.*, 1992; Hughes & Kendall, 2007). Research shows that homework compliance declines over time (Gaynor *et al.*, 2006).

Homework is used to bridge across sessions. Usually homework is assigned at the end of one session and reviewed at the beginning of the next one. Homework is collaborated with the family and negotiated with the youth. Homework compliance is often rewarded by the therapist (e.g., earning checks that can be exchanged for prizes). Compliance may be defined more in terms of *effort*, rather than *outcome*. Initial homework assignments may focus on monitoring symptoms, whereas later assignments require the youth to practice skills learned in therapy.

Work with parents

Parent's involvement in therapy will vary depending on the age of the youth, presenting problem, and stage in treatment. For example, with very young children therapy is usually centered upon parent management training (Van der Sluis *et al.*, 2012). However, even with older youth parents can participate by being consultants (presenting information about youth), collaborators (assisting in treatment components), or co-clients (using skills to manage their own symptomatology; Kendall, 2012). As therapy progresses, there is a gradual shift or "transfer of control" from therapist to parents in terms of helping the youth manage their stress (Ginsburg *et al.*, 1995).

The content of work with parents will vary by disorder. For example, in the treatment of anxiety disorders parents learn how to help with and even administer exposure tasks. They also are taught to reduce their accommodation of their child's anxious behaviors (e.g., assisting in compulsive rituals, permitting reassurance seeking; Freeman & Marrs Garcia, 2009). Parent management for oppositional youth will involve different skills, such as selective ignoring, praising for prosocial behavior, and learning to deliver effective commands (Barkley, 1997).

Social skills training

Social skills deficits are common across youth disorders. Social skill training is part of CBT when the objective is to "promote skill acquisition, enhance existing skills, and facilitate the generalization of skills across settings and persons" (Bellini & Peters, 2008, p. 858). Social skills training is often conducted in a group format where youth practice newly acquired skills with peers. Typically, a particular skill is introduced by the therapist, the behavior is role-played, the youth practices the skill with another peer or with the therapist, the youth is reinforced and receives corrective feedback, and the youth practices the skill for homework (Foster & Bussman, 2008).

The target social skills vary by presenting concern. For example, internalizing youth may require training that includes speaking up for themselves, giving and receiving compliments, and initiating conversations. On the other hand, externalizing youth may require empathy training (e.g., understanding other's perspective and interpretation of other's facial and bodily cues). Training for this population commonly focuses on conflict resolution skills, such as: walking away, ignoring, and acceptance and communication of feelings. Social skills programs are particularly popular for treating Autistic youth, and depending on severity, require more intensive training guided by shaping procedures. Basic social skills, including maintaining eye contact and asking the conversation partner questions, are taught. Despite the enthusiasm for social skills training, there is mixed data regarding the efficacy of these programs (Antshel & Barkley, 2008) and uncertainty to the extent that skills generalize to real world situations (Williams White *et al.*, 2007). Research suggests that conducting social skills training in the youth's natural setting may promote more generalizable and enduring effects (Bellini & Peters, 2008).

Contingency management

Contingency management strategies are used for encouragement and learning. Rewards are the cornerstone of contingency management and must be meaningful to the youth to have an effect on behavior (Gosch *et al.*, 2006). It is important to spend time speaking with the youth about potential rewards to be earned for homework completion, practicing therapy skills, and other desired behaviors. Parents of younger children are often instructed to create behavioral charts in which youth receive a point or sticker for a particular behavior. Earned points can be exchanged for various predetermined rewards. Rewards include both tangible (e.g., baseball cards, gift certificates) and nontangible options (e.g., choosing the family movie, cooking with dad). Praise is a key reinforcing agent and is given immediately following a desired behavior. It is important that praise be labeled and specific to the situation (e.g., "I like that you put your clothes in the closet" versus "good job;" Eyberg & Bussing, 2010). Ideally, throughout therapy, the youth moves from reinforcement from others to self-reinforcement.

Another side of contingency management is punishment. Punishment is often misunderstood by parents, and consequently overused or misused, potentially contributing to an exacerbation of the problem. Removal of a privilege (e.g., electronic devices and dessert) comes with the opportunity for the youth to earn it back with good behavior. Time-out, used for younger youth with externalizing issues, is considered to be "a temporary removal from reinforcement" and should be short-lasting (roughly 1 minute per 1 year of child).

Modeling and role play

CBT makes use of modeling, a strategy based on observational learning (Bandura, 1977). Stated simply, learning and behavioral change can result from the direct observation of others. Various behaviors, such as approaching a feared stimulus, refining a social skill, or practicing relaxation, can be modeled by the therapist. Therapists model *coping* with stressors (identifying distress, a way to address the distress, and then coping), rather than *mastery* (showing only a solution). Modeling often follows a sequence: The therapist models a desired behavior, the therapist and youth attempt the behavior together, and eventually the youth conducts the behavior independently. In addition to therapists, teachers, parents, and even other youth can serve as models. For example, in Social Effectiveness Therapy for social phobia, socially competent peers are invited to interact with phobic youth and model socially appropriate behaviors (Beidel *et al.*, 2000).

In "role plays," the therapist and youth "act out" various real-life situations and rehearse skills. For example, youth with an anger problem can role-play conflict resolution with the therapist who acts as a provocateur. The role play provides information to the therapist about the youth's proficiency of a skill and areas where it needs refinement. Likewise, role play affords an opportunity for the youth to literally practice the skill and receive feedback. For younger children, role play with puppets can be used. Following a role play, the youth is encouraged to practice their skills outside of session as homework.

Cognitive restructuring

Cognitive restructuring is a phrase often used to refer to changing the way that youth think about situations. It challenges distorted and negative thinking and encourages reasonable self-talk and "coping thoughts." A first step in cognitive restructuring is developing an awareness of distorted thoughts and their relationship to behavior. In group treatment for adolescent depression, youth are instructed to shout "negative thought" when someone in the group says one (Stark *et al.*, 2007). For homework, youth monitor and record their thoughts. In a next step, youth can become "thinking detectives" or "scientists" and challenge the validity of thoughts with a list of questions (e.g., "Am I sure that it is true," "Has it ever happened before," "What's the worst the can happen"). It is important that youth not merely ask these questions, but answer them. From their answers, they can derive coping thoughts (e.g., "I can do it," "No one is perfect"). As part of collaboration in CBT, therapists or the youth can write coping thoughts on index cards to create "coping cards" that the youth carry around outside of session.

Flexible adaptations of CBT

Although CBT and BT are typically manual-based, treatments are meant to be applied flexibly to meet the needs of each individual youth. This section reviews ways that CBT can be tailored to the individual.

"Flexibility within fidelity"

Manual-based treatments for childhood psychopathology have gained considerable research support. At the same time, critics have described them as "cookbooks" that dehumanize the therapeutic process, discourage flexibility, and interfere with the therapeutic relationship (discussed in Addis *et al.*, 2006). Advocates of manuals point out that they are to be applied by balancing judicious use with clinical judgment (Kendall & Beidas, 2007).

One suggestion is an emphasis on "empirically supported procedures," or the overarching principles within manuals

(Abramowitz, 2006). Similarly, Kendall and Beidas (2007) call for "flexibility within fidelity," an umbrella approach that applies important strategies/components of treatment, while individualizing each to the child. Research could inform the boundaries of flexibility (Kendall & Beidas, 2007), just as research has found that the program has been implemented in RCTs with flexibility (Chu & Kendall, 2009). When considering the boundaries to flexibility, consider: (i) the stated goals of the session, (ii) conceptualizations of the child's struggles within a CBT perspective, and (iii) action-oriented, rather than passive, treatment (Kendall *et al.*, 2012). As Shirk and colleagues (2012) argued, an increased understanding of core processes will likely increase both an acceptance of manuals by practicing clinicians and the flexible application of manual-based treatments to a variety of youth.

Modular treatments

Difficulties applying treatment manuals in clinical practice have arisen from suggestions that youth in clinical settings may be more complicated than those participating in research trials (Weisz & Gray, 2008). Modular treatment may address these concerns. Modular treatments are considered clinician-friendly and flexible, with the ability to tailor treatment toward each child's strengths and needs (Chorpita *et al.*, 2004).

One modular CBT for child anxiety disorders, the Building Confidence Program (Wood & McLeod, 2008), has demonstrated initial effectiveness in an individual format for 24 children (ages 5–12) with diagnoses of separation anxiety disorder, social phobia, or generalized anxiety disorder. Specifically, 72% of modular CBT participants were considered treatment responders, compared with 6% of the wait-list control (Chiu *et al.*, 2013). One year following treatment, 71% of children who received modular CBT continued to demonstrate a positive treatment response. Results are considered preliminary based on the sample size and high attrition at follow-up, but nonetheless demonstrate initial promise for the approach in the school setting (Galla *et al.*, 2012).

The Modular Approach to Therapy for Children with Anxiety, Depression, or Conduct Problems (MATCH; Chorpita & Weisz, 2005) has modules that contain elements of other empirically supported programs, the *Coping Cat*, Primary and Secondary Control Enhancement Training, and the Defiant Child therapies. With MATCH, the therapist focuses on the most salient presenting problem, and follows a flow chart that specifies a set of modules to apply. The therapist may then adapt strategies to target comorbidities. MATCH has been found to outperform usual care (Weisz *et al.*, 2012) and a modular treatment (based on prior treatments; Kazdin, 2005) for youth behavior disorders has been found to lead to comparable improvements in both an outpatient clinic and community settings such as the home or school (Kolko *et al.*, 2011). Although the studies suggest initial promise for modular treatments, given their reliance on clinical decision making, some suggest that modular approaches may be less appropriate for novice clinicians (Becker *et al.*, 2012).

Obstacles to treatment

A large disparity has been identified between children in need of mental health services and those who receive treatment (e.g., Collins *et al.*, 2004), such that many children with mental health problems are not receiving adequate treatment. Parents report barriers to children's mental health care, including structure constraints (e.g., cost, convenience, and uncertainty on where to seek care), perceptions of mental health problems (e.g., problems perceived as not serious enough), and perceptions of services (e.g., child refused to go, service was not recommended, and stigma from others). Additionally, parents with life stressors (e.g., unemployment, and divorce) were more likely to perceive barriers to seeking treatment for their child (Owens *et al.*, 2002). Barriers to treatment are key concerns, prompting dissemination and implementation research, discussed in the following sections.

Not all children respond to treatment. When treatment is less than effective, the therapist may wish to contemplate alternate treatment schedules, format, or delivery style. In some cases, an adjunctive treatment (e.g., family therapy) may be indicated. Consider also the possibility of misdiagnosis or poor case conceptualization. Moreover, the therapist may consider relevant process variables, such as giving more time to establish a collaborative relationship with the child. The therapist should be alert to increase child involvement by establishing shared goals. Therapist (e.g., a "preachy" therapist style) and patient characteristics (e.g., impairing behavioral problems) can also be considered.

Internet provided CBT

Given the disjunction between empirically supported treatments and those available in the community, computer-assisted treatments may help facilitate the dissemination of CBT while promoting fidelity to approaches that have empirical support. There are several potential advantages of computer-based CBT programs (Kendall *et al.*, 2011). First, computers reduce the cost of treatment (Olmstead *et al.*, 2010) and they can be available in a variety of settings (e.g., home and school). Computers can provide anonymity and privacy for those hesitant to seek treatment, thereby extending the reach of services. Computers may improve standardization and adherence to key treatment strategies while offering customization for individuals. Data can easily be collected and stored during the use of computer-assisted programs, an effective time and cost saver for clinicians (Khanna *et al.*, 2007).

Research findings have supported several computer-assisted programs for the treatment of child and adolescent psychopathologies; such as *Camp Cope-A-Lot* (CCAL; Kendall & Khanna, 2008) and *Cool Teens* (Cunningham *et al.*, 2007) for anxiety, and SPARX (Merry *et al.*, 2012) and Stressbusters (Abeles *et al.*, 2009) for depression. Ethnically diverse and low-income families have expressed particular interest in online parenting programs (Love *et al.*, 2013). The Triple P Positive Parenting Program (Sanders, 2012) was developed into an internet-delivered treatment (www.triplep.net) for young children with disruptive behavior disorders and was reported to be superior to an internet help as usual condition (Sanders *et al.*, 2012). Additionally, the Incredible Years parenting program demonstrated initial promise when administered online (Taylor *et al.*, 2008).

Developmental considerations

Although CBT with youth shares similarities with its adult counterpart, there are important differences that reflect developmentally sensitive adaptations. First, there is no such thing as pure "individual therapy" when working with youth. Therapists collaborate with individuals within the child's immediate environment, such as parents and teachers, to develop a therapy plan to assure skills are generalized. Likewise, the therapist negotiates the goals of all involved parties, particularly when working with adolescents.

Unlike adults, youth often do not enter therapy by their own volition. Accordingly, youth may not be motivated to participate in therapy tasks and the therapist may need to spend considerable time fostering incentive in the youth and forging an alliance. With children, rapport is often built by playing games, whereas adolescents may be more engaged by casual conversation regarding topics of their interest. To increase motivation in children, tangible and short-term rewards are used in behavioral contingency systems. Social rewards, such as autonomy to spend time with friends or drive a car, are more appropriate rewards for adolescents. It is also helpful to raise intrinsic motivation of adolescents by discussing how therapy may improve their quality of life and help them achieve their personal goals (e.g., friendship building; getting into college).

Given cognitive and emotional variations in youth, therapy materials are best presented in a way that promotes engagement and comprehension. For younger children the content is presented concretely, with visual aids, handouts (or metaphors) to promote understanding. Therapists are best when they avoid using jargon and over explaining CBT theories. Moreover, it is paramount that therapists provide material interactively and collaboratively. Material can be presented didactically to adolescents, more closely resembling therapy with adults. Likewise adolescents may be able to provide direct feedback when elicited, but children may be reticent because they feel intimidated or struggle to verbally express their thoughts. Using alternative means to receive feedback (e.g., drawings), or simplifying questions so they only require "yes/no" responses can aid the process. As always, it is worth noting that the therapist reassures the youth that their feedback will not get them into trouble.

CBT and BT for intellectual disabilities

As mentioned, cognitive distortions involve a belief about something that is maladaptive, rigid, and/or untrue. By contrast, a deficit reflects a youth underperforming in a particular domain with reference to their culture group and developmental age.

CBT is often used to address disorders that are characterized by distorted thinking (e.g., anxiety disorders and depression), whereas BT is implemented for disorders marked more by deficits (e.g., ADHD, autism, and elimination disorders). Young children, (age 6 and under) and youth with an intellectual disability may have difficulty grasping some CBT content (e.g., not yet ready for perspective taking, meta-cognition) and may be more responsive to BT. Deficits are on a continuum, so cases of high-functioning intellectual disability can respond to CBT with a behavioral emphasis (e.g., more regular reinforcement; Storch et al., 2013). Moreover, the auxiliary visual aids are used to adapt CBT for youth with intellectual deficits or mild to moderate language impairments.

Criticisms of CBT

CBT and BT interventions are not without criticism. Some have argued that the approaches are too narrowly focused on symptom reduction, rather than emphasizing personal growth or the functionality of the family system. Additionally, psychodynamic theorists believe that an emphasis on current symptomatology neglects deeper underlying issues. Finally, although CBT and BT have considerable empirical support, the findings do indicate that a percentage of individuals are treatment "nonresponders" or later relapse.

CBT related therapies

CBT and BT are recommended approaches, but they do not result in remission for all youth participants. Accordingly, alternate therapies, derived from behavioral and/or cognitive theories, have emerged. Mindfulness-Based Cognitive Therapy, Acceptance and Commitment Therapy (ACT) and Dialectical Behavioral Therapy (DBT) are three such therapies.

Mindfulness-based cognitive therapy (MBCT)

Mindfulness, defined as regulating attention toward the present moment while adapting an attitude of curiosity, openness, and acceptance (Bishop et al., 2004), has gained interest as an adjunct to CBT. Grounded in Buddhist traditions, mindfulness includes a variety of techniques that may be applied to youth, such as imagery, meditation, and even yoga. Mindfulness based therapies have yielded moderate effect sizes for adult internalizing disorders, with effects maintained at follow-up (Hofmann et al., 2010). Research with youth is in its nascent stages, but the literature suggests that mindfulness is acceptable and feasible with youth. Preliminary outcomes show some improvement in areas such as anxiety, attention, pain, and academic problems (Burke, 2010). Nonetheless, effect sizes are smaller than in adult samples, youth samples are heterogeneous, and mindfulness has yet to be tested for several types of psychopathology. Moreover, there is a need for more RCTs to determine if the addition of mindfulness adds a significant benefit to CBT or BT.

Acceptance and commitment therapy (ACT)

ACT strives to increase psychological flexibility, defined as being present in the moment and adapting one's behavior according to chosen values (Hayes et al., 2006). Psychological inflexibility is said to be caused by six interrelated problems: cognitive fusion (attachment to one's thoughts), experiential avoidance (attempts to deny or eradicate negative thoughts and feelings), detachment from the present moment (processing past or future events at the expense of present awareness), conceptualized self perspective (fusion with one's self-description), unclear or absent values, and unworkable action (engaging in behaviors incompatible with personal values and counter to desired goals). Each area is targeted in therapy. For example, defusion exercises illustrate that thoughts are transient, can be observed without needing to be controlled, and are nothing more than words. In one exercise, youth repeat a negative word (e.g., ugly) for a minute, after which they are asked to notice that the word sounds funny and has lost much of its meaning. As another example, the therapist may elicit the youth's values by inquiring how they would live their lives in a world without positive or negative consequences for actions. These and other processes are interconnected and clinical judgment determines the area that the therapist initially targets.

ACT is said to contrast with CBT in its philosophical foundations. First, there is a difference in the stated goals: Whereas CBT strives to reduce psychopathology (e.g., emotion regulation) ACT can be said to increase valued living. Although reduction in psychopathology is a concern, ACT theorists argue that it is secondary. Second, CBT questions "distorted" thoughts, seeking a more rational and "adaptive" thinking pattern. ACT rejects the idea of inherently good or bad thoughts and attempts to change one's relationship to one's thoughts. Others have argued that the differences between ACT and CBT are overstated and reflect more differences in philosophy rather than implementation (Arch & Craske, 2008). Both therapies are present-focused, use homework, require active client participation and use behavioral and cognitive strategies to facilitate change.

The literature on ACT with youth is mostly uncontrolled and case studies. Accordingly, conclusions about efficacy are premature (Murrell & Scherbarth, 2011). One study of youth with chronic pain found that ACT outperformed usual treatment at posttreatment and 6.5 month follow-up on pain intensity and interference (Wicksell et al., 2009). Systematic research is needed regarding ACT with youth.

Dialectical behavior therapy

Dialectical Behavior Therapy (DBT) is akin to CBT (e.g., problem solving, behavioral strategies, skills training, and practice), but differs a bit in its delivery and philosophy. DBT was developed for individuals with chronic suicidality (Linehan, 1993a, b) but has been applied to adolescents with severe behavioral and emotional dysregulation. DBT theory combines elements of Zen, behavioral science, and dialectical philosophy. In brief, DBT postulates a worldview through which opposing forces exist simultaneously and can lead to conflict. As a result, dialectical change occurs when opposing forces are resolved. The DBT therapist strives to help patients by reducing maladaptive behavior, promoting positive behavior, and helping to "build a life worth living" by providing a validating, supportive environment (MacPherson et al., 2013).

DBT consists of stages: (i) pretreatment, including orientation and commitment of the patient to goals, (ii) reduction of life-threatening behavior and behavior that interferes with therapy and quality of life, (iii) reduction of posttraumatic distress and increase of normative emotional experiences, (iv) working toward achieving typical levels of happiness through goal achievement and increasing self-respect, and (v) working toward achieving lasting contentment by resolving sense of incompleteness. Therapy includes individual sessions, group skills training and telephone coaching for the participant, and consultative/supportive sessions for the therapist (MacPherson et al., 2013) and is intended to be provided flexibly. A DBT manual for adolescents (Miller et al., 2007) was adapted from the adult version and research suggests that DBT has some support for the treatment of adolescent borderline personality disorder, bipolar disorder, suicidality, oppositional defiant disorder, and eating disorders (Macpherson et al., 2013).

Future directions

There is good news! Treatments for youth psychopathologies described here have been developed, evaluated, and often determined to be efficacious (Kendall, 2012). Given this status, the field needs to focus on transporting these treatments into use in everyday practice (Kendall & Beidas, 2007). Related to this, dissemination and implementation (DI) is rapidly growing. An American Psychiatric Association (APA) Task Force issued a policy statement calling for effective mental health care for youth across settings and clinicians that is "based on scientific knowledge and integrated with clinical experience in the context of patient characteristics, culture, and preferences" (APA Task Force on Evidence-Based Practice for Children and Adolescents, 2008, p. 6). Despite this recognition and related efforts, CBT remains underutilized in the community (Shafran et al., 2009). In a national survey, 47% of therapists reported never having used a treatment manual (Addis & Krasnow, 2000). ESTs can call for extensive training and ongoing consultation of clinicians (Edmunds et al., 2013), which can be costly. However, such efforts are likely warranted to ensure fidelity to the essential "ingredients" of ESTs particularly in the context of community clinics. With this in mind, emerging efforts to disseminate treatment for a variety of psychological disorders exhibit promise (Spence & Shortt, 2007; Loeb et al., 2007; Southam-Gerow et al., 2010).

Ethnic minorities have been under represented in ESTs (Silverman et al., 2008) and some studies suggest that minority status may be associated with poorer outcomes (Chronis et al., 2004), whereas others suggest comparable outcomes across ethnicities

(Pina et al., 2003). Future research should consider the development of culturally sensitive and culturally adaptive therapies. Will outcomes be superior if treatments are modified to integrate differing values (e.g., parenting practices and religious preferences)? How does a family's level of acculturation influence treatment compliance, completion, and outcome?

A next step toward personalizing treatment is to examine and better understand the mechanisms of change. In their review, Shirk and colleagues (2012) determined that although research on therapy process in CBT for youth has grown, unanswered questions remain. They argued that we need research to understand the essential mechanisms of change. The results of such work may in turn, increase the overall efficacy of treatments, inform the training of future therapists, and increase the cost-effectiveness of therapy by streamlining manuals to the essential elements (Chu & Harrison, 2007). The identification of treatment mediators represents a worthy effort to identify variables that account for therapeutic change. Research suggests potential treatment mediators, such as parenting practices within disruptive behavior disorders (Beauchaine et al., 2005) and cognitive processes in anxiety (Kendall & Treadwell, 2007) and depression (Chu & Harrison, 2007).

Finally, a relatively new area in the field of child and adolescent psychopathology is the development and testing of transdiagnostic treatments. Given that comorbidity in youth psychopathology is the rule, rather than the exception, transdiagnostic therapies can be tailored to address the complex needs of youth with comorbid diagnoses. Such therapies may be more efficient and cost-effective, reduce attrition, and promote dissemination (Rohde, 2012). Recent efforts to test transdiagnostic treatments for youth mood and anxiety disorders offer initial promise (e.g., Chu et al. 2009; Bilek & Ehrenreich-May, 2012).

Acknowledgment

Preparation of this chapter was facilitated by grants awarded to Philip C. Kendall (MH086438; MH063747) from NIMH.

References

Abeles, P. et al. (2009) Computerized CBT for adolescent depression ('stressbusters') and its initial evaluation through an extended case series. *Behavioural and Cognitive Psychotherapy* **37**, 151–165.

Abramowitz, J.S. (2006) 'Toward a functional analytic approach to psychologically complex patients. *Clinical Psychology: Science and Practice* **13**, 163–166.

Addis, M.E. et al. (2006) Does manualization improve therapy outcomes?. In: *Evidence-Based Practices in Mental Health: Debate and Dialogue on the Fundamental Questions*. (eds J.C. Norcross, et al.), pp. 131–160. American Psychological Association, Washington, DC.

Addis, M. & Krasnow, A. (2000) A national survey of practicing psychologists' attitudes toward psychotherapy treatment manuals. *Journal of Consulting and Clinical Psychology* **68**, 331–339.

American Academy Child and Adolescent Psychiatry (2007) Practice parameter for the assessment and treatment of children and adolescents with attention-deficit/hyperactivity disorder. *Journal of the American Academy Child & Adolescent Psychiatry* **46**, 894–921.

American Psychological Association Task Force on Evidence-Based Practice for Children and Adolescents (2008) *Disseminating Evidence-Based Practice for Children and Adolescents: A Systems Approach to Enhancing Care.* American Psychiatric Association, Washington, DC.

Antshel, K. & Barkley, R. (2008) Psychosocial interventions in attention deficit hyperactivity disorder. *Child and Adolescent Psychiatric Clinics of North America* **17**, 421–437.

Arch, J. & Craske, M. (2008) Acceptance and commitment therapy and cognitive behavioral therapy for anxiety disorders: different treatments, similar mechanisms? *Clinical Psychology: Science and Practice* **15**, 263–279.

Bandura, A. (1977) *Social Learning Theory.* Prentice-Hall, Oxford England.

Barkley, R.A. (1997) *Defiant Children: A Clinician's Manual for Assessment and Parent Training,* 2nd edn. Guilford Press, New York.

Beauchaine, T.P. *et al.* (2005) Mediators, moderators, and predictors of 1-year outcomes among children treated for early-onset conduct problems: a latent growth curve analysis. *Journal of Consulting and Clinical Psychology* **73**, 371–388.

Becker, E. *et al.* (2012) Modular cognitive behavioral therapy for youth with anxiety disorders: a closer look at the use of specific modules and their relation to treatment process and response. *School Mental Health* **4**, 243–253.

Becker-Weidman, E. *et al.* (2010) Social problem-solving among adolescents treated for depression. *Behaviour Research and Therapy* **48**, 11–18.

Beidas, R. *et al.* (2013) Brief cognitive-behavioral therapy for anxious youth: the inner workings. *Cognitive and Behavioral Practice* **20**, 134–146.

Beidel, D. *et al.* (2000) Behavioral treatment of childhood social phobia. *Journal of Consulting and Clinical Psychology* **68**, 1072–1080.

Bellini, S. & Peters, J. (2008) Social skills training for youth with autism spectrum disorders. *Child and Adolescent Psychiatric Clinics of North America* **17**, 857–873.

Bilek, E. & Ehrenreich-May, J. (2012) An open trial investigation of a transdiagnostic group treatment for children with anxiety and depressive symptoms. *Behavior Therapy* **43**, 887–897.

Bishop, S. *et al.* (2004) Mindfulness: a proposed operational definition. *Clinical Psychology: Science and Practice* **11**, 230–241.

Brent, D. *et al.* (2008) Switching to another SSRI or to venlafaxine with or without cognitive behavioral therapy for adolescents with SSRI-resistant depression: the TORDIA randomized controlled trial. *JAMA* **299**, 901–913.

Burke, C.A. (2010) Mindfulness-based approaches with children and adolescents: a preliminary review of current research in an emergent field. *Journal of Child and Family Studies* **19**, 133–144.

Chambless, D. & Hollon, S. (1998) Defining empirically supported therapies. *Journal of Consulting and Clinical Psychology* **66**, 7–18.

Chiu, A.W. *et al.* (2013) Effectiveness of modular CBT for child anxiety in elementary schools. *School Psychology Quarterly* **28**, 141–153.

Chorpita, B. *et al.* (2004) Efficacy of modular cognitive behavior therapy for childhood anxiety disorders. *Behavior Therapy* **35**, 263–287.

Chorpita, B.F. & Weisz, J.R. (2005) *Modular Approach to Therapy for Children with Anxiety, Depression, or Conduct Problems.* Judge Baker Children's Center, Harvard Medical School, Boston, MA.

Chronis, A. *et al.* (2004) Enhancements to the behavioral parent training paradigm for families of children with ADHD: review and future directions. *Clinical Child and Family Psychology Review* **7**, 1–27.

Chu, B. *et al.* (2009) An initial description and pilot of group behavioral activation therapy for anxious and depressed youth. *Cognitive and Behavioral Practice* **16**, 408–419.

Chu, B. & Harrison, T. (2007) Disorder-specific effects of CBT for anxious and depressed youth: a meta-analysis of candidate mediators of change. *Clinical Child and Family Psychology Review* **10**, 352–372.

Chu, B. & Kendall, P. (2009) Therapist responsiveness to child engagement: flexibility within manual-based CBT for anxious youth. *Journal of Clinical Psychology* **65**, 736–754.

Clarke, G. *et al.* (1992) Cognitive-behavioral group treatment of adolescent depression: prediction of outcome. *Behavior Therapy* **23**, 341–354.

Clarke, G. *et al.* (2001) A randomized trial of a group cognitive intervention for preventing depression in adolescent offspring of depressed parents. *Archives of General Psychiatry* **58**, 1127–1134.

Cohen, J. *et al.* (2004) A multisite, randomized controlled trial for children with sexual abuse-related PTSD symptoms. *Journal of the American Academy Child & Adolescent Psychiatry* **43**, 393–402.

Cohen, J. *et al.* (2007) A pilot randomized controlled trial of combined trauma-focused CBT and setraline for childhood PSTD symptoms. *Journal of the American Academy Child & Adolescent Psychiatry* **46**, 811–819.

Collins, K.A. *et al.* (2004) Gaps in accessing treatment for anxiety and depression: challenges for the delivery of care. *Clinical Psychology Review* **24**, 583–515.

Crawley, S. *et al.* (2008) Treating socially phobic youth with CBT: differential outcomes and treatment considerations. *Behavioural and Cognitive Psychotherapy* **36**, 379–389.

Creswell, C. & Cartwright-Hatton, S. (2007) Family treatment of child anxiety: outcomes, limitations and future directions. *Clinical Child and Family Psychology Review* **10**, 232–252.

Cunningham, M. *et al.* (2007) Overview of the cool teens CD-ROM for anxiety disorders in adolescents. *The Behavior Therapist* **30**, 15–19.

Curry, J. *et al.* (2006) Predictors and moderators of acute outcome in the treatment for adolescents with depression study (TADS). *Journal of the American Academy Child & Adolescent Psychiatry* **45**, 1427–1439.

Deffenbacher, J.L. *et al.* (1996) Anger reduction in early adolescents. *Journal of Counseling Psychology* **43**, 149–157.

D'Zurilla, T. & Goldfried, M. (1971) Problem solving and behavior modification. *Journal of Abnormal Psychology* **78**, 107–126.

Edmunds, J. *et al.* (2013) Dissemination and implementation of evidence–based practices: training and consultation as implementation strategies. *Clinical Psychology: Science and Practice* **20**, 152–165.

Eyberg, S. & Bussing, R. (2010) Parent-child interaction therapy for preschool children with conduct problems. In: *Clinical Handbook of Assessing and Treating Conduct Problems in Youth,* pp. 139–162. Springer, New York.

Eyberg, S. *et al.* (2008) Evidence-based psychosocial treatments for children and adolescents with disruptive behavior. *Journal of Clinical and Child Adolescent Psychology* **37**, 215–237.

Farrell, L. *et al.* (2012) Comorbidity and treatment response in pediatric obsessive-compulsive disorder: a pilot study of group cognitive-behavioral treatment. *Psychiatry Research* **199**, 115–123.

Foa, E. & Kozak, M. (1986) Emotional processing of fear: exposure to corrective information. *Psychological Bulletin* **99**, 20–35.

Foster, S. & Bussman, J. (2008) Evidence-based approaches to social skills training with children and adolescents. In: *Handbook of Evidence-Based Therapies for Children and Adolescents*, pp. 409–427. Springer, New York.

Freeman, J. & Marrs Garcia, A. (2009) *Family-Based Treatment for Young Children with OCD: Therapist Guide*. Oxford University Press, New York.

Friedberg, R.D. *et al.* (2009) *Cognitive Therapy Techniques for Children and Adolescents: Tools for Enhancing Practice*. Guilford Press, New York.

Fristad, M. *et al.* (2011) *Psychotherapy for Children with Bipolar and Depressive Disorders*. Guilford Press, New York.

Fristad, M. *et al.* (2009) Impact of multifamily psychoeducational psychotherapy in treating children aged 8 to 12 years with mood disorders. *Archives of General Psychiatry* **66**, 1013–1020.

Galla, B. *et al.* (2012) One year follow-up to modular cognitive behavioral therapy for the treatment of pediatric anxiety disorders in an elementary school setting. *Child Psychiatry & Human Development* **43**, 219–226.

Garber, J. (2006) Depression in children and adolescents: linking risk research and prevention. *American Journal of Preventive Medicine* **31**, S104–S125.

Garcia, A. *et al.* (2010) Predictors and moderators of treatment outcome in the pediatric obsessive compulsive treatment study (POTS I). *Journal of the American Academy of Child & Adolescent Psychiatry* **49**, 1024–1033.

Gaynor, S. *et al.* (2006) Measuring homework compliance in cognitive-behavioral therapy for adolescent depression. *Behavior Modification* **30**, 647–672.

Ginsburg, G. *et al.* (2011) Remission after acute treatment in children and adolescents with anxiety disorders: findings from the CAMS. *Journal of Consulting and Clinical Psychology* **79**, 806–813.

Ginsburg, G. *et al.* (1995) Family involvement in treating children with phobic and anxiety disorders: a look ahead. *Clinical Psychology Review* **15**, 457–473.

Goodyer, I. *et al.* (2007) Selective serotonin reuptake inhibitors (SSRIs) and routine specialist care with and without cognitive behaviour therapy in adolescents with major depression: randomised controlled trial. *British Medical Journal* **335**, 7611.

Gosch, E. *et al.* (2006) Principles of cognitive-behavioral therapy for anxiety disorders in children. *Journal of Cognitive Psychotherapy* **20**, 247–262.

Hayes, S. *et al.* (2006) Acceptance and commitment therapy: model, processes and outcomes. *Behaviour Research and Therapy* **44**, 1–25.

Hofmann, S. *et al.* (2010) The effect of mindfulness-based therapy on anxiety and depression: a meta-analytic review. *Journal of Consulting and Clinical Psychology* **78**, 169–183.

Hollon, S.D. & Beck, A.T. (2013) Cognitive and cognitive-behavioral therapies. In: *Handbook of Psychotherapy and Behavior Change*. (ed M.J. Lambert), pp. 393–442. John Wiley & Sons, Hoboken, New Jersey.

Hudson, J.L. (2005) Mechanisms of change in cognitive behavioral therapy for anxious youth. *Clinical Psychology: Science and Practice* **12**, 161–165.

Hudson, J. & Kendall, P. (2002) Showing you can do it: homework in therapy for children and adolescents with anxiety disorders. *Journal of Clinical Psychology* **58**, 525–534.

Hughes, A. & Kendall, P. (2007) Prediction of cognitive behavior treatment outcome for children with anxiety disorders: therapeutic relationship and homework compliance. *Behavioural and Cognitive Psychotherapy* **35**, 487–494.

Jensen, P. *et al.* (2007) 3-year follow-up of the NIMH MTA study. *Journal of the American Academy Child & Adolescent Psychiatry* **46**, 989–1002.

Kazantzis, N. *et al.* (2010) Meta-analysis of homework effects in cognitive and behavioral therapy: a replication and extension. *Clinical Psychology: Science and Practice* **17**, 144–156.

Kazdin, A.E. (2003) Problem-solving skills training and parent management training for conduct disorder. In: *Evidence-Based Psychotherapies for Children and Adolescents*, pp. 241–262. Guilford Press, New York.

Kazdin, A.E. (2005) Child, parent, and family-based treatment of aggressive and antisocial child behavior. In: *Psychological Treatments for Child and Adolescent Disorders: Empirically based Strategies for Clinical Practice*. (eds E.D. Hibbs & P.S. Jensen), 2nd edn, pp. 445–476. American Psychological Association, Washington, DC.

Keel, P. & Haedt, A. (2008) Evidence-based psychosocial treatments for eating problems and eating disorders. *Journal of Clinical Child and Adolescent Psychology* **37**, 39–61.

Kendall, P.C. (2012) Guiding theory for therapy with children and adolescents. In: *Child and Adolescent Therapy: Cognitive-Behavioral Procedures*. (ed P.C. Kendall), 4th edn, pp. 3–24. Guilford Press, New York.

Kendall, P.C. & Beidas, R. (2007) Smoothing the trail for dissemination of evidence-based practices for youth: flexibility within fidelity. *Professional Psychology: Research and Practice* **38**, 13–20.

Kendall, P.C. *et al.* (2002) *The C.A.T. Project Therapist Manual*. Workbook Publishing, Ardmore, PA.

Kendall, P.C. & Khanna, M.S. (2008) *Camp Cope-A-Lot* [DVD]. Workbook Publishing, Ardmore, PA.

Kendall, P.C. & Hedtke, K. (2006a) *Cognitive-Behavioral Therapy for Anxious Children: Therapist Manual*, 3rd edn. Workbook Publishing, Ardmore, PA.

Kendall, P.C. & Hedtke, K. (2006b) *Coping Cat Workbook*, 3rd edn. Workbook Publishing, Ardmore, PA.

Kendall, P.C. *et al.* (2011) Computers and psychosocial treatment for child anxiety: recent advances and ongoing efforts. *Depression and Anxiety* **28**, 58–66.

Kendall, P. *et al.* (2004) Child anxiety treatment: outcomes in adolescence and impact on substance use and depression at 7.4-year follow-up. *Journal of Consulting and Clinical Psychology* **72**, 276–287.

Kendall, P. *et al.* (2012) No need to worry: the promising future of child anxiety research. *Journal of Clinical Child and Adolescent Psychology* **41**, 103–115.

Kendall, P. & Treadwell, K. (2007) The role of self-statements as a mediator in treatment for youth with anxiety disorders. *Journal of Consulting and Clinical Psychology* **75**, 380–389.

Khanna, M. *et al.* (2007) New frontiers: computer technology in the treatment of anxious youth. *The Behavior Therapist* **30**, 22–25.

Kolko, D. *et al.* (2011) Moderators and predictors of clinical outcome in a randomized trial for behavior problems in pediatric primary care. *Journal of Pediatric Psychology* **36**, 753–765.

Le Grange, D. *et al.* (2007) A randomized controlled comparison of family-based treatment and supportive psychotherapy for adolescent bulimia nervosa. *Archives of General Psychiatry* **64**, 1049–1056.

Linehan, M.M. (1993a) *Cognitive-Behavioral Treatment of Borderline Personality Disorder*. Guilford Press, New York.

Linehan, M.M. (1993b) *Skills Training Manual for Treating Borderline Personality Disorder*. Guilford Press, New York.

Lochman, J. & Dodge, K. (1994) Social-cognitive processes of severely violent, moderately aggressive, and nonaggressive boys. *Journal of Consulting and Clinical Psychology* **62**, 366–374.

Lochman, J. & Gresham, F.M. (2008) Intervention development, assessment, planning and adaptation: importance of developmental models. In: *Cognitive Behavioral Interventions for Emotional and Behavioral Disorders: School-Based Practice*. (eds M.J. Mayer, R. Van Acker, J.E. Lochman & F.M. Gresham), pp. 29–57. Guilford, New York.

Lochman, J.E. & Wells, K.C. (2003) Effectiveness of the Coping Power Program and of classroom intervention with aggressive children: outcomes at a 1-year follow-up. *Behavior Therapy* **34**, 493–515.

Lochman, J.E. & Wells, K.C. (2004) The coping power program for preadolescent aggressive boys and their parents: outcome effects at the 1-year follow-up. *Journal of Consulting and Clinical Psychology* **72**, 571–578.

Lochman, J.W. *et al.* (2008) *Coping Power: Child Group Program, Facilitator Guide*. Oxford University Press, New York.

Lock, J. *et al.* (2005) A comparison of short- and long-term family therapy for adolescent anorexia nervosa. *Journal of the American Academy Child & Adolescent Psychiatry* **44**, 632–639.

Lock, J. *et al.* (2001) *Treatment Manual For Anorexia Nervosa: A Family-Based Approach*. Guilford Press, New York.

Loeb, K. *et al.* (2007) Open trial of family-based treatment for full and partial anorexia nervosa in adolescene: evidence of successful dissemination. *Journal of the American Academy Child & Adolescent Psychiatry* **46**, 792–800.

Love, S. *et al.* (2013) Enhancing accessibility and engagement in evidence-based parenting programs to reduce maltreatment: conversations with vulnerable parents. *Journal of Public Child Welfare* **7**, 20–38.

Lundahl, B. *et al.* (2006) A meta-analysis of parent training: moderators and follow-up effects. *Clinical Psychology Review* **26**, 86–104.

MacPherson, H. *et al.* (2013) Dialectical behavior therapy for adolescents: theory, treatment adaptations, and empirical outcomes. *Clinical Child and Family Psychology Review* **16**, 59–80.

March, J. *et al.* (2007) Tics moderate treatment outcome with sertraline but not cognitive-behavior therapy in pediatric obsessive-compulsive disorder. *Biological Psychiatry* **61**, 344–347.

March, J.S. & Mulle, K. (1998) *ODC in Children and Adolescents: A Cognitive-Behavioral Treatment Manual*. Guilford Press, New York.

McClellan, J. *et al.* (2007) Practice parameter for the assessment and treatment of children and adolescents with bipolar disorder. *Journal of the American Academy Child & Adolescent Psychiatry* **46**, 107–125.

McMahon, R. *et al.* (2006) Conduct problems. In: *Treatment of Childhood Disorders*. (eds E. Mash & R. Barkley), 3rd edn, pp. 137–268. Guilford Press, New York.

Merry, S. *et al.* (2012) The effectiveness of SPARX, a computerised self help intervention for adolescents seeking help for depression: randomised controlled non-inferiority trial. *British Medical Journal* **344**, 1–16.

Michael, K. & Crowley, S. (2002) How effective are treatments for child and adolescent depression? A meta-analytic review. *Clinical Psychology Review* **22**, 247–269.

Miklowitz, D. *et al.* (2008) Family-focused treatment for adolescents with bipolar disorder: results of a 2-year randomized trial. *Archives of General Psychiatry* **65**, 1053–1061.

Miklowitz, D. *et al.* (2013) Early intervention for symptomatic youth at risk for bipolar disorder: a randomized trial of family-focused therapy. *Journal of the American Academy Child & Adolescent Psychiatry* **52**, 121–131.

Miller, A. *et al.* (2007) *Dialectical Behavior Therapy with Suicidal Adolescents*. Guilford Press, New York.

MTA Cooperative Group (1999) A 14-month randomized clinical trial of treatment strategies for attention-deficit/hyperactivity disorder. *Archives of General Psychiatry* **56**, 1073–1086.

Molina, B. *et al.* (2009) The MTA at 8 years: prospective follow-up of children treated for combined-type ADHD in a multisite study. *Journal of the American Academy Child & Adolescent Psychiatry* **48**, 484–500.

MTA Cooperative Group (2004a) National Institute of Mental Health Multimodal Treatment Study of ADHD follow-up: changes in effectiveness and growth after the end of treatment. *Pediatrics* **113**, 754–761.

MTA Cooperative Group (2004b) National Institute of Mental Health Multimodal Treatment Study of ADHD follow-up: 24-month outcomes of treatment strategies for attention-deficit/hyperactivity disorder. *Pediatrics* **113**, 762–769.

Murrell, A. & Scherbarth, A. (2011) State of the research & literature address: ACT with children, adolescents and parents. *International Journal of Behavioral Consultation and Therapy* **7**, 15–22.

National Institute for Health and Care Excellence (2008) *Attention Deficit Hyperactivity Disorder: Diagnosis and Management of ADHD in Children, Young People, and Adults*. National Institute for Health and Care Excellence, Manchester, UK.

Norton, P.J. (2012) A randomized clinical trial of transdiagnostic cognitve-behavioral treatments for anxiety disorder by comparison to relaxation training. *Behavior Therapy* **43**, 506–517.

Ollendick, T.H. & Cerny, J.A. (1981) *Clinical Behavior Therapy with Children*. Plenum Press, New York.

Olmstead, T. *et al.* (2010) Cost-effectiveness of computer-assisted training in cognitive-behavioral therapy as an adjunct to standard care for addiction. *Drug and Alcohol Dependence* **110**, 200–207.

Owens, P.L. *et al.* (2002) Barriers to children's mental health services. *Journal of the American Academy of Child & Adolescent Psychiatry* **41**, 731–738.

Pavuluri, M. *et al.* (2004) Child- and family-focused cognitive-behavioral therapy for pediatric bipolar disorder. *Journal of the American Academy of Child & Adolescent Psychiatry* **43**, 528–537.

Pelham, W. & Fabiano, G. (2008) Evidence-based psychosocial treatments for attention-deficit/hyperactivity disorder. *Journal of Clinical and Child Adolescent Psychology* **37**, 184–214.

Piacentini, J. *et al.* (2014) 24- and 36-week outcomes for the child/adolescent anxiety multimodal study (CAMS). *Journal of the American Academy of Child & Adolescent Psychiatry* **53**, 297–310.

Pina, A. *et al.* (2003) Exposure-based cognitive-behavioral treatment for phobic and anxiety disorders: treatment effects and maintenance.

Journal of the American Academy of Child & Adolescent Psychiatry **42**, 1179–1187.

Podell, J. et al. (2010) The Coping Cat Program for anxious youth: the FEAR plan comes to life. *Cognitive and Behavioral Practice* **17**, 132–141.

Puleo, C. et al. (2011) CBT for childhood anxiety and substance use at 7.4-year follow-up: a reassessment controlling for known predictors. *Journal of Anxiety Disorders* **25**, 690–696.

Puleo, C. & Kendall, P. (2011) Anxiety disorders in typically developing youth: Autism spectrum symptoms as a predictor of cognitive-behavioral treatment. *Journal of Autism and Developmental Disorders* **41**, 275–286.

Rapee, R.M. (2000) Group treatment of children with anxiety disorders: outcomes and predictors of treatment response. *Australian Journal of Psychology* **52**, 125–130.

Reinecke, M. & Ginsburg, G. (2008) Cognitive-behavioral treatment of depression during childhood and adolescence. In: *Handbook of Depression in Children and Adolescents*, pp. 179–206. Guilford Press, New York.

Robin, A. et al. (1999) A controlled comparison of family versus individual therapy for adolescents with anorexia nervosa. *Journal of the American Academy Child & Adolescent Psychiatry* **38**, 1482–1489.

Rohde, P. (2012) Applying transdiagnostic approaches to treatments with children and adolescents: innovative models that are ready for more systematic evaluation. *Cognitive Behavioral Practice* **19**, 83–86.

Rohde, P. et al. (2001) Impact of comorbidity on a cognitive-behavioral group treatment for adolescent depression. *Journal of the American Academy Child & Adolescent Psychiatry* **40**, 795–802.

Rohde, P. et al. (2006) Predicting time to recovery among depressed adolescents treated in two psychosocial group interventions. *Journal of Consulting and Clinical Psychology* **74**, 80–88.

Sanders, M. et al. (2012) A randomized controlled trial evaluating the efficacy of Triple P online with parents of children with early-onset conduct problems. *Behaviour Research and Therapy* **50**, 675–684.

Sanders, M.R. (2012) Development, evaluation, and multinational dissemination of the triple P-positive parenting program. *Annual Review of Clinical Psychology* **8**, 345–379.

Shafran, R. et al. (2009) Mind the gap: improving the dissemination of CBT. *Behaviour Research and Therapy* **47**, 902–909.

Shirk, S. et al. (2012) Change processes and active components. In: *Child and Adolescent Therapy: Cognitive-Behavioral Procedures*, 4th edn, pp. 471–498. Guilford Press, New York.

Shure, M.B. (2001) I can problem solve (ICPS): an interpersonal cognitive problem solving program for children. *Residential Treatment for Children & Youth* **18**, 3–14.

Silverman, W.K. et al. (2008) Evidence-based psychosocial treatments for phobic and anxiety disorders in children and adolescents. *Journal of Clinical and Child Adolescent Psychology* **37**, 105–130.

Skinner, B.F. (1969) *Contingencies of Reinforcement: A Theoretical Analysis*. Appleton, New York.

Sonuga-Barke, E. et al. (2013) Nonpharmalogical interventions for ADHD: systematic review and meta analyses of randomized controlled trials of dietary and psychological treatments. *American Journal of Psychiatry* **170**, 275–289.

Southam-Gerow, M. et al. (2010) Does cognitive behavioral therapy for youth anxiety outperform usual care in community clinics? *Journal of the American Academy Child & Adolescent Psychiatry* **49**, 1043–1052.

Spence, S. & Shortt, A. (2007) Can we justify the widespread dissemination of universal, school-based interventions for the prevention of depression among children and adolescents? *Journal of Child Psychology and Psychiatry* **48**, 526–542.

Stark, K.D. et al. (2007) *Treating Depressed Youth: Therapist Manual for ACTION*. Workbook Publishing, Ardmore, PA.

Stark, K. et al. (2010) Cognitive-behavioral therapy for depression: the ACTION treatment program for girls. In: *Evidence-Based Psychotherapies for Children and Adolescents*, 2nd edn, pp. 93–109. Guilford Press, New York.

Storch, E. et al. (2013) The effect of cognitive-behavioral therapy versus treatment as usual for anxiety in children with autism spectrum disorders: a randomized, controlled trial. *Journal of the American Academy Child & Adolescent Psychiatry* **52**, 132–142.

TADS Team (2004) Fluoxetine, cognitive-behavioral therapy, and their combination for adolescents with depression: treatment for adolescents with depression study (TADS) randomized controlled trial' 2004. *JAMA* **292**, 807–820.

TADS Team (2009) The treatment for adolescents with depression study (TADS): long-term effectiveness and safety outcomes' 2007. *Archives of General Psychiatry* **64**, 1132–1144.

Taylor, T. et al. (2008) Computer-based intervention with coaching: an example using the incredible years program. *Cognitive Behaviour Therapy* **37**, 233–246.

Van der Sluis, C. et al. (2012) Parent-directed cognitive behavioral therapy for young anxious children: a pilot study. *Behavior Therapy* **43**, 583–592.

Walkup, J. et al. (2008) Cognitive behavioral therapy, sertraline, or a combination in childhood anxiety. *New England Journal of Medicine* **359**, 2753–2766.

Weisz, J. et al. (2012) Testing standard and modular designs for psychotherapy treating depression, anxiety, and conduct problems in youth: a randomized effectiveness trial. *Archives of General Psychiatry* **69**, 274–282.

Weisz, J.R. et al. (2013) Psychotherapy for children and adolescents. In: *Handbook of Psychotherapy and Behavior Change*. (eds A. Bergen & S. Garfield), pp. 541–586. John Wiley & Sons, New Jersey.

Weisz, J. & Gray, J. (2008) Evidence-based psychotherapy for children and adolescents: data from the present and a model for the future. *Child and Adolescent Mental Health* **13**, 54–65.

Weisz, J. et al. (1997) Brief treatment of mild-to-moderate child depression using primary and secondary control enhancement training. *Journal of Consulting and Clinical Psychology* **65**, 703–707.

West, A. et al. (2007) Maintenance model of integrated psychosocial treatment in pediatric bipolar disorder: a pilot feasibility study. *Journal of the American Academy Child & Adolescent Psychiatry* **46**, 205–212.

Wicksell, R.K. et al. (2009) Evaluating the effectiveness of exposure and acceptance strategies to improve functioning and quality of life in longstanding pediatric pain – A randomized controlled trial. *Pain* **141**, 1–10.

Williams White, S. et al. (2007) Social skills development in children with autism spectrum disorders: a review of the intervention research. *Journal of Autism and Developmental Disorders* **37**, 1858–1868.

Wood, J. & McLeod, B.D. (2008) *Child Anxiety Disorders: A Family-Based Treatment Manual for Practitioners*. Norton & Co, New York.

CHAPTER 39
Family interventions

Ivan Eisler[1] and Judith Lask[2]
[1] Institute of Psychiatry, Psychology and Neuroscience, King's College London, UK
[2] University of Exeter, Exeter, UK

There is a wide acceptance of the role of the family environment in contributing to the emotional and psychological well being of a child. When a child presents with mental health difficulties professionals need to form an effective working relationship with those who care for the child. Work with the family can take many forms and will be based to a considerable degree on our particular understanding of the role that family factors play in relation to the development, maintenance, and above all the resolution of presenting problems.

We will discuss why clinicians need to be cautious in attempting to translate research data on family factors into putative etiological explanations at the level of the individual child and the implications this has for how we engage families in treatment. The chapter will examine different approaches for working with families and the factors which may indicate whether this is an appropriate approach.

Family interventions in the broader context of other psychological treatments

Family therapy, like other psychotherapies, has evolved over several decades and today includes a broad range of ideas and techniques that are often described as representing discrete theoretical models (e.g., structural, strategic, Milan systemic, and narrative—see Carr, 2012 for an overview). In practice, the conceptual ideas and techniques associated with each of these tend to be adopted quite widely and most family therapists integrate ideas from different approaches in their work as single theoretical models often do not provide sufficient conceptual breadth or choice of interventions to address the wide range of difficulties presented to clinicians. The boundaries between systemic family therapy and other therapeutic approaches are also frequently blurred with many overlaps.

The role of the family therapist in the multidisciplinary team

Most clinicians working with children and adolescents will include families in their work. This is sometimes referred to as "family work" or "family interventions" to distinguish it from "family therapy," although the distinction is somewhat artificial and usually refers more to the level of training of the clinician rather than necessarily to a different approach. Family therapists by virtue of their training will have developed specialist skills in working with families, may take on more complex work and should be more able to adapt interventions to suit the needs of individual families. However, where there is an indication for family interventions, the same principles should apply whether the specialist family therapist or the nonspecialist carries out the work. The role of the family therapist within the multidisciplinary team is of course much wider than just seeing families. They will be able to identify when a family approach is likely to be helpful and the different styles of work that might be best suited for the specific problem or a particular family. Moreover, the family therapist can also provide support and supervision for other team members working with families.

There is a wide continuum of ways that the family may be involved in treatment. This includes taking part in assessments, providing a supportive role in relation to other, more child focused interventions such as cognitive behavioral therapy (CBT), through the family being the main vehicle of engagement for a reluctant child or adolescent, to family therapy being the main focus of treatment. It is helpful for all clinicians involved with children to have basic skills in engaging and communicating with families and for teams to have sufficient expertize to offer specific, family-focused interventions as well as clinicians trained to offer more flexible systemic family treatments for more complex problems or more difficult family situations.

Rutter's Child and Adolescent Psychiatry, Sixth Edition.
Edited by Anita Thapar and Daniel S. Pine, James F. Leckman, Stephen Scott, Margaret J. Snowling, Eric Taylor.
© 2015 John Wiley & Sons Ltd. Published 2018 by John Wiley & Sons Ltd.

Theoretical considerations informing work with families

The family context of individual problems and the broader social environment

Observing the child in the presence of his/her family will provide a rich source of information that contextualizes and often provides new meaning to the child's behaviors. It also provides insights about the strengths and resources of the family and the community in which they belong as well as constraints that may come from lack of time, relationship difficulties, other family stressors, and factors such as social deprivation or the threat of crime or racism. It is important to consider the wider contexts surrounding the family, including culture, the diversity of family life across cultures, and the considerable change that families have undergone in most societies, as these will affect basic values and beliefs around family relationships. The notion of what family life means in terms of the nature of family relationships, the expectations of the way in which families change over time or the roles of different family members varies hugely. Children may grow up in foster and adoptive families or a succession of different families or may be part of more than one family constellation following marriage break up. Single-parent families, same-sex parent partnerships, and friendship networks provide different forms of family life. While much of this may appear self-evident, it is crucial to be open to the different experiences and expectations that families bring with them. Moreover, we have to be aware that as professionals our own personal and cultural perspectives will inevitably color our observations and assessments.

Exploring the family's social and cultural contexts will also provide information on stresses (e.g., specific social expectations in the community) and resources such as sources of networking and support (Falicov, 1995). An evaluation of the role of professionals in the referral process and the history and relationship of the family with other helping systems is important, particularly where there has been multiagency involvement, which may itself have become disabling for the family (Asen, 2002).

The family as a system

Family Systems Theory, the conceptual framework for much of the thinking about working with families, has evolved considerably over the years. The original notion of the family as a system described a number of features such as the recursive nature of relationships, the multilevel nature of communication (Bateson, 1972), the development of recognizable patterns of interaction, the role of relationships and beliefs, and the allocation of family roles (Carr, 2012). Minuchin (1974) described aspects of family organization such as boundaries and hierarchy and placed a particular emphasis on promoting an effective parental alliance and maintaining boundaries in a way that fostered the development of a secure sense of identity with appropriate individuation. In the 1980s and early 1990s, a major theoretical shift in systems theory emphasized the interplay between being an observer of a system and being part of the same system (Hoffman, 1985).

This has had key implications for understanding the active role that individuals have in construing reality, the limitations to the objectivity of observations (Hoffman, 1990) and the role of language, culture, history, and other social discourses in influencing our perceptions of the world around us (Gergen, 1999). This has shaped the practice of family therapy, moving it away from the notion of "treating families" to "treatment in collaboration with families"; in other words seeing families first and foremost as a resource to help their child overcome problems rather than the origin or source of dysfunction.

The role of the family in the development and maintenance of psychopathology

The family environment is the main social context that shapes and modifies the individual, biologically determined predispositions of the child and is also the context where the main developmental psychological needs should be met. The family context provides meaning to behaviors and is where individuals learn and practice how to manage emotions and feelings and manage the idiosyncrasies of their temperament and personality. The research literature highlighting the role of the family is huge and cannot be reviewed here in detail but the factors that would need to be considered include a range of prenatal factors such as being an unwanted child (Kubička et al., 2002) or maternal stress (Huizink et al., 2002), the consequences of growing up in an environment characterized by negative emotion, harsh parenting, high levels of discord or hostility (Waller et al., 2012), or the impact of neglect (Rutter & O'Connor, 2004). Of course, as many have pointed out, such negative family factors have to be considered alongside those factors that may have a protective role or promote resilience (Rutter, 2006; Bowes et al., 2010).

When considering family factors in relation to the development of specific problems, however, considerable caution is needed. Explanatory family models of particular disorders have often been proposed with limited empirical support other than clinical observations. Where associations are found between family factors and a disorder, these may be risk factors (often nonspecific) or maintaining factors rather than causal etiological factors. Even where there is robust evidence for particular family factors increasing the risk of a disorder(s), their relative contribution is often small. A good example is the evidence concerning parenting styles. These have been consistently shown to be associated with a range of child and adolescent difficulties but they account for less than 10% of the variance (McLeod et al., 2007a, b; Buschgens et al., 2010).

The dynamic relationship between family, child, and problem is complex and clinicians should desist from drawing simplistic conclusions and in particular making causal etiological inferences based on here-and-now observations. What we observe when assessing a family is the outcome of a complex interaction over time between the effect of the family environment, personality, and temperamental characteristics of the child, the impact of the developing disorder on the family, and resilience factors as well as mediating genetic factors (Kraemer et al., 2001; Plomin &

Daniels, 2011; Rutter, 2013). There is also evidence that even the most adverse factors do not have uniform effects (O'Connor *et al.*, 2000) and what applies at a group level may not translate to the individual child.

It is important that clinicians hold the empirical evidence about the role of family factors as part of a broad background without making assumptions too readily about their direct relevance to the current family. This is partly to avoid the pitfall of drawing unwarranted causal inferences but also helps to engage families in positive ways instead of adding to their sense of failure and self-blame.

Impact of individual problems on family life

When one member of a family begins to develop a problem, it affects other members and the family as a whole. Some effects may be readily apparent such as aggression toward siblings from a young person with attention deficit hyperactivity disorder (ADHD), some may be less obvious, for example, "well" siblings receiving less attention from parents (Areemit *et al.*, 2010). The stress of dealing with difficulties may put a strain on the parents' relationship or the relationships with wider family. The way the family adapts to the impact of illness tends to be gradual and will often start through the activation of protective and supportive processes in the family but can in time become part of what reinforces or maintains the problem. For example, what may start as supportive reassurance of an anxious and perhaps somewhat perfectionist child may with hindsight turn out to be the start of a process of parents being drawn into the emerging rituals of a developing obsessive-compulsive disorder (OCD) (Amir *et al.*, 2000). Useful models for understanding the process through which the family accommodates to the child's problem can be found in the studies of the impact on the family of enduring physical illness and disability (Cole & Reiss, 2013) as well as psychiatric illness (Muhlbauer, 2002).

The way families respond to a developing illness depends both on family factors and the specific problems that the illness brings but there is a general tendency for the problem to magnify certain aspects of the family's dynamics and narrow the range of their adaptive behaviors (Eisler, 2005). As the illness increasingly takes a central role in family life, what may be normal variations in family functioning become more pronounced and take on new meanings. Concern may begin to feel like overprotection and intrusiveness, while attempts to promote independence may feel like lack of care. Much of what we observe in families we meet as clinicians can be understood, at least in part, as an outcome of the process of family adjustment to the problem and should not be too readily labeled as dysfunctional.

The family life cycle

The Family Life Cycle model (McGoldrick *et al.*, 2010) provides a "developmental lens" for understanding the way the family as a system evolves over time and how families adjust to different cultural and social expectations and pressures. Families need to provide stability but also have to be able to change in order to adapt to new circumstances and the developmental demands of family members. For instance, the child's need for dependence and attachment requires a degree of stability and constancy in the family but, as the child develops, the family must find ways of meeting his or her needs for independence and separation too. As the family evolves through the family life cycle stages, it needs to be able to adapt and change its habitual style of functioning. These stages can be complicated by unexpected events such as illness, death, family separation, unemployment, or migration, and the combined stress can contribute to the development of problems. There is evidence that at these transitional times there is an increased vulnerability and increased psychological morbidity (Hetherington, 1989; Lueck & Wilson, 2011). The way the family responds to an emerging problem is a crucial factor in determining the extent of individual vulnerability to such pressures (Walsh, 2006). It is useful to explore with families how they managed key transitions and significant life events, the impact these may have had on family life and family relationships and the resources and strengths that helped them to manage these in the past.

A conceptual framework for working with families

Creating a safe context for working together toward change

Part of the effectiveness of family therapy will be the skill of the therapist to develop and maintain the engagement and motivation of family members. In many ways, this is not different from engagement in any other kind of therapy and requires the development of an emotional connection with the family and an agreement on the tasks and goals of therapy (Bordin, 1979) but additional factors come into play when working with families with a key aspect of alliance being the development of a shared purpose of treatment by the whole family (Escudero *et al.*, 2008). It is important to overtly recognize that there may be multiple viewpoints and ensure that everyone is engaged and heard. Therapists have to balance their position as experts (often a key element of creating a sense of safety in the early stages of treatment) with the need to ensure as collaborative an atmosphere as possible (Mason, 2005) while also respecting individual, social, and cultural differences in expectations of professionals.

Even very young children can be effectively included in family interviews, provided this is carried out in an age-appropriate way. Engaging a child effectively is often reassuring for parents, who may be concerned whether bringing the child to a psychiatric setting is the right thing to do. The choice of language in talking to parents about their child's problems is also important as it may be difficult for the child to understand what is being said. Often it is better to ask the parents to explain things to the child, as this may be less threatening for the child, and reinforces the sense that the parents are the experts in their own child.

Young people may not be too keen to take part in discussions at first, particularly if they feel blamed for the problems. Making it clear that it is OK to sit and listen is often important to avoid making the child or adolescent feel that they are being put on the spot and can help avoid unhelpful battles. When the pressure on them to join in is removed, they will often join themselves. The advantage of a family interview is that even a reluctant or unwilling participant can be included in an interview through indirect means, for example, making nonverbal contact, making observations or comments that include the young person and so on. With young children, this may include joining with a child in creative play, talking about a drawing he or she has made or using puppets or story making (Wilson, 1998).

Frameworks for change

In recent years, there has been a growing move toward integrating different approaches, both from within the family therapy field and outside it (Norcross & Goldfried, 2005). As Fraenkel and Pinsof (2001) point out clinicians either include techniques or ideas from other approaches without modifying their own conceptual framework or they integrate them at a theoretical level making it possible for different conceptualizations of the therapy process to be used and applied depending on the nature of the problem, stage of treatment, or difficulties encountered in treatment.

In this section, we outline a set of conceptual frameworks that provide an integrative way of thinking about different interventions and the process of change. They draw on earlier models of family therapy and the specific processes that these focus on but recognize that change happens on a number of levels. These frameworks are, of course, not mutually exclusive and most interventions will include elements of each.

Maintenance framework

Much of the early theory informing family therapy was concerned with the idea of the family as a self-regulating social system, the way in which family interactions and family structures maintain problems and two influential strands of family therapy (Structural and Behavioral) have drawn heavily on these ideas. The notion of maintenance does not make any assumptions about the origin of difficulties but postulates that families become organized around problems in a way that may contribute to their maintenance either by directly reinforcing problems or by disrupting adaptive or change processes.

The here-and-now focus of structural and behavioral interventions is of particular relevance for the understanding and intervening in possible maintenance mechanisms. Enquiring about the usual way in which the family operates, family rules, family roles, and boundaries and how this has changed around the problem will give insight to family strengths as well as potential areas of difficulties. When discussing patterns that may be connected to a specific problem, the clinician has an important role to help frame or ask questions that evoke non-blaming descriptions. The aim here is partly to avoid reinforcing

disabling feelings of guilt and blame and partly to set a context which encourages family members to be self-reflective and consider their own part in the pattern and what they can do to bring about change.

From the perspective of a maintenance framework, change can take place through interventions that are aimed at directly changing patterns or sequences of behaviors including actively intervening in the process of discussion with encouraging language, highlighting success, interrupting repetitive or escalating patterns, or exploring opportunities for the therapist to help the family to "do it differently." Parents may be encouraged in the session to have more constructive conversations about parenting or to tell their child what they want him to do rather than just complain about what he does do. Similarly, the adolescent might be asked to reflect what he would do if he thought that the parents had started listening more. While generally these are interventions that require the therapist to take an active and often quite directive role, it is also important to invite self-reflection by the family on their patterns and to assess the impact of following a different pattern.

Influencing framework

All psychotherapies are concerned with bringing about change but what characterizes this framework and the approaches that have this as their key focus is the interest in how change is brought about and the purposeful role therapists have in bringing about change. The two groups of systemic therapies that are most clearly identified by this framework are Strategic therapies (Haley, 1963) and Brief therapies (Weakland et al., 1974) the latter eventually developing into what is now known as Solution-focused therapy (de Shazer, 1985). The focus was on the interactive process that interfered with change, rather than the processes that maintained problems and the role of the therapist was to intervene strategically to interrupt the processes that blocked change.

Many of the minutiae of the therapy process, such as the choice and sequencing of interventions, how and when therapists use their expert knowledge, or when on the other hand they emphasize the limits of their expertize and invite families to look for their own solutions, can be understood as part of this framework. While all interventions can be considered from the perspective of an influencing framework, clinicians should consider in particular how they use interventions that aim to change behaviors or perceptions in specific ways and the way they use, directly or indirectly, their authority as therapists to achieve this. In doing this, they need to consider the broader context, for example, the choice of whether to have a conversation with the adolescent or with one of the parents, how different family members might respond to different questions as opposed to being "participant listeners," the effect on the therapeutic relationship and so on. The importance of considering this framework is that it overtly acknowledges the power of the therapist (positive as well as potentially negative) and requires therapists to be aware of and reflect carefully on their own motivation, their position in the system, on the impact they are having and the effect of their interventions on their relationship with the family. For instance, there is evidence from both individual psychotherapy research (Castonguay *et al.*, 2010) and family therapy research (Escudero *et al.*, 2012; Lambert *et al.*, 2012) that when there is a disruption to the therapeutic alliance, continuing with interventions that are usually effective can be counterproductive and may undermine treatment and in some cases cause harm.

The framework is also useful when considering tasks outside of the direct "therapy setting." For instance when writing letters to referrers which will be copied to the family, clinicians should always reflect on how the letter will be perceived by family members (children as well as parents). Such letters are not just a means of conveying information about an assessment, they also provide an opportunity to frame such information in ways that can be helpful or less helpful for the family and influence shared understanding by the family.

Frameworks focusing on changes in belief and meaning

An important idea that underpins all family therapy approaches is that problems are embedded and shaped by their social context and to a lesser extent help to shape the context. If we try to understand the interpersonal nature of problems, it is almost inevitable that we become concerned with language, beliefs, cognitions, and narratives because these are central to understanding the process of social interaction and the shaping of behavior through the meaning attached to it.

Several influential therapy approaches have placed language and narratives center stage of treatment, most notably Narrative Therapy (White, 2005) and the Collaborative Language approaches (Anderson & Goolishian, 1988). These emphasize the role of language and narratives as the vehicle through which people acquire their definitions of self. Individual problems are understood to be, at least in part, the result of the filtering of experiences through narratives that people have about themselves. From the perspective of this framework, change occurs through the emergence of new narratives, which alter the understanding of self as well of relationships with others. The skill of the therapist is to focus attention on small aspects of neglected or unnoticed narratives, which then may acquire a greater salience for the individual or the family. A negative, constraining narrative may thus be replaced by a more positively supported alternative. Part of the work is to identify "dominant stories" and help to identify exceptions or unique outcomes to counter the power of the (usually unhelpful) story. For example, a mother may have a firm idea that she will not be able to stand up to her children and may therefore withdraw or become over-disciplinarian. Uncovering examples of her effectiveness and skill as a parent or times she has stood up for herself in everyday life may help her change her view of herself and enable her to take another approach.

Increasingly, therapeutic work with families also includes explorations of the role that emotions and feelings have as specific organizers of beliefs, behaviors, and relationships. This may include exploration of attachment relationships, which may have become important components in problem behaviors, arousing overwhelming emotions that can direct individuals toward self-protective behaviors rather than ones that take into account others in the situation (Vetere & Dallos, 2008).

Practical issues and techniques of family interventions

Whom to see and when

Although it is always useful to witness the whole family interacting together, conjoint interviews also have their limitations in both the assessment and treatment phases. During assessment, there may be indications that some individuals do not have an effective voice in the family group or the presence of the whole family may seriously inhibit some aspect of discussion. An adolescent may not want parents to know about drug use or there may be concern that a child has been abused and may be unwilling to talk about this in front of parents. Similarly, there may be issues that parents may not wish to discuss with the child present (e.g., when parents of a child with disability may not be able to share negative feelings in front of the child). For these reasons, it is generally useful to make at least some separate sessions a routine part of practice even when family therapy is indicated as the main mode of treatment.

There are several other considerations that should be taken into account when deciding on individual or conjoint sessions. For instance, the therapist might decide that it is age-appropriate to see an adolescent on their own, particularly if they express a wish for this. The therapist should consider (and enquire about) to what extent this is determined by a wish to avoid talking about a painful or upsetting issue, which may not necessarily be a helpful thing to do. Some topics may appear difficult to address in a conjoint meeting although the discomfort may at times be largely to do with the clinician's own uncertainty about how or whether to raise the issue. Asking questions about what is acceptable or usual in the particular family will tell the clinician what can or cannot be easily talked about and may open up the topic for discussion. Questions such as "If your parents thought you were smoking dope, what would they do?" or "Some teenagers are very up-front about what they get up to, others keep things closer to their chest—what is your son like?" may quickly lead to frank and open conversations. More importantly, this kind of discussion will clarify what the actual boundaries in the family are rather than being assumed by the therapist.

The family interview is an important component in a comprehensive assessment. It provides the clinician with an opportunity to observe the family in direct interaction, to assess patterns of relationships, the emotional climate of the family and a chance to consider how the family is organized around the child's problem. Interviewing the family for purposes of assessment is a good starting point for making an effective treatment alliance with the family. Hearing the concerns of family members and their hopes for the future is as important as gathering information and making an assessment of the problem and can determine the most effective ways of helping the family to promote change.

In families where there is much hostility, criticism or open conflict, conjoint meetings may not always be helpful, particularly if the hostility or conflict simply escalates in sessions. There is evidence that families with high parental scores on criticism are more likely to drop out of treatment (Szmukler *et al.*, 1985) and outcomes may be better if parents and the young person are seen separately (Eisler *et al.*, 2000, 2007).

The context of family sessions

The context in which family sessions take place will have significant impact. If it is in the clinic, it may appear strange and inhibiting especially to small children but on the other hand may appear "neutral and safe." In some settings, such as inpatient units, it may be necessary to more clearly delineate boundaries for other staff and ensure that there is a quiet space for interviews and that there are no other competing demands. Family therapy in an inpatient context is of necessity different in that the child or adolescent is not with the family between sessions, and day-to-day responsibility does not rest with parents. This limits the possibility of the family working on changing ways of dealing with the child's problems and can reinforce the sense that it is the hospital's responsibility to "fix the child." The hospital context, on the other hand, can provide a sense that the child is in a safe place and may allow addressing upsetting or painful issues that at other times would feel too risky and would be avoided. Home-based interviews can be very useful in learning more about the family and may make it easier to engage some families. However, it may be difficult to manage interruptions and it is easier for a family member to leave the room if they become upset. Moreover, it may be more difficult for a session to end and some of the feelings may remain for longer. If the whole treatment takes place in the family home, families may also feel that they have less control how long treatment continues for and how it should end. The setting is important and the therapist must consider how best to make the most of the advantages and guard as far as possible against the disadvantages.

Specific interview and intervention techniques

It is beyond the scope of this chapter to cover in depth the variety of techniques that have been developed for working with families (Dallos & Draper, 2005; Carr, 2012) but questioning techniques play a central role. They not only gather useful information about patterns of interaction, family differences, and the connections between relationships, behavior, beliefs, and emotions, they also invite family members to reflect and become observers of themselves. Questions can also be used to invite action or they may include embedded suggestions—for example, a mother may be asked "What would happen if you were able to hide your worry when your daughter got depressed?" to encourage her to think about protecting her

daughter. Tomm (1987a, b, 1988) provides a useful overview of different kinds of "circular questioning" which provide a basis for describing the problem in a more contextual way and also allow for alternative descriptions to be heard.

One way of organizing the use of circular questions is to connect them to a systemic hypothesis. The therapist links information about the family to form a hypothesis about the family and their relationship to the presenting problem. This hypothesis is tested through circular questions and revised in the light of feedback until an idea is arrived at that fits well enough with the family to provide useful new information for them. Relative influence questions are specifically linked with the technique of externalizing the problem and explore the influence the problem has had on the person(s) and, more importantly, the influence the person has had on the problem. Through the process (e.g., of exploring how the family has helped a young child with fears or anxiety), it may be possible to establish exceptions or unique outcomes when there has been some control over the problem and how these can be developed further.

There are numerous techniques for intervening in the process of family interaction (Minuchin & Fishman, 1981) including blocking repetitive patterns that reinforce unwanted behaviors, highlighting constructive behaviors such as positive parenting, or setting rules to prevent repetitive escalation of arguments. Interventions may be fairly unobtrusive nonverbal ones (fixing the gaze of the person who is speaking, making it more difficult for others to interrupt) or more overt, even dramatic gestures ("Why don't you go and sit next to your dad and try to work out a compromise, without getting mum to help?") and may include specific suggestions or homework tasks. Alternatively, the therapist may comment in a way that draws attention to what is happening.

Genograms, family drawings, and other techniques

Genograms have great value in family work and are used to map out the family and family relationships, to explore beliefs, traditions and identify strengths, resources, and areas of resilience (Gil *et al.*, 2008). It is useful to include family members over three generations (to gather information on transgenerational influences), their occupations, gender, and dates of events such as marriage, relational breakdown and death, and a pictorial representation of positive or negative relationships. While gathering information is an important part of a genogram, far more important is that it is an opportunity for the family to reflect on how they view themselves, their values and sense of identity and engendering a sense of shared history. It is also an opportunity to move beyond problem talk and to identify strengths, evidence of courage and resilience and family resources that can be used to overcome problems. Family members who have been less central can also be more actively involved in completing a genogram. As with all techniques, care must be taken to be aware when sad or upsetting things are revealed. It may be particularly difficult for those who have lost important family members or who are alone or whose families are not known. The culture of the family should be taken into account throughout all work with families but is of particular importance when doing genograms as it provides an opportunity to talk about family beliefs, family history and culture, and the way that these have shaped the way of dealing with different problems.

A range of other visual and drawing tasks can be used with families, particularly when engaging children. Some more common ones are maps of relationships, which place the child in the center and place people at different distances on the map. This will sometimes reveal important people outside of the family. Simple drawings of the family or a family activity can provide important information and a focus for discussion. Progress in overcoming difficulties can be set out in a visual way. One example is an image of a mountain with "success" at the top. The child's "team" can be listed and hopefully this will include family members and the way they can help.

Contraindications for family interventions and/or indications to proceed with special care

Criticism, family conflict, hostility, and violence

Many family sessions will include some negative comments and hostile attitudes, which will hopefully change as family members become more confident in the setting. However, if this persists, it is important to make a judgment about the level of harm it may do to the more vulnerable members. If the hostility is between parents, it may be important to have a separate session to discuss whether their relationship issues are getting in the way of their ability to work together as parents in dealing with the child's problem. If criticism is difficult to contain, parallel sessions with parents and the young person may be more helpful at least in early in treatment.

If there are indications that there is violence in the family (e.g., aggressive atmosphere in the session or allusions to violent behavior), it is important to consider the possibility of how this is best explored in a safe way to minimize the risk of violence escalating after the session (Goldner *et al.*, 1990). In such situations, family sessions may be problematic but the information gained from an initial family assessment can still be useful in deciding about future interventions. If parents share concerns about what is happening and want to make changes, work with the family alongside other safeguarding measures may be very useful. If therapy with the whole family does proceed, it can only be undertaken with an agreement to stop the violence and a clear safety plan for the person(s) at risk.

Abuse and neglect

Abuse or neglect may not always be directly evident in sessions (e.g., there may be no overt hostility) but there may be other indications of abuse and neglect. From the start, it is important to be clear that if concerns about safety arise it will be necessary

to act on those (usually with the knowledge of the parents). An assessment must be made about levels of concern and safeguarding steps taken if there is fear of ongoing physical, sexual, or emotional abuse. While work with the family can be helpful, work with the whole family requires an acknowledgement of the abuse and an acceptance of responsibility (Barratt, 2012). The safety and protection of children has to always take precedence over other therapeutic needs.

Disorganized and poorly functioning families

It is sometimes assumed that family dysfunction should be the main indication for family therapy. In fact, the opposite is the case. Several studies have shown (Hampson & Beavers, 1996a; Barrett *et al.*, 2004) that family factors moderate the effect of family therapy, with poorly functioning families gaining less benefit. This should not be taken to mean that more dysfunction simply leads to poor outcome, as there is evidence that these effects might be specific to particular types of family intervention. For instance, collaborative treatment approaches (often favored by therapists) are less effective with disorganized families (Hampson & Beavers, 1996b), who tend to respond better to more directive and less open styles whereas the opposite is true of more balanced type families. Evidence of disorganization or poor family functioning does not mean that family therapy is contraindicated, rather that we need to proceed cautiously and that a higher degree of expertize or team support is needed to ensure that family interventions are both safe and effective.

Research evidence informing family therapy practice

The evidence showing the efficacy of family interventions is increasingly strong with a growing number of well designed, appropriately powered multisite studies appearing in recent years. A number of reviews provide both a general overview of the empirical evidence for the field as a whole (Kaslow *et al.*, 2012; Sprenkle, 2012; Retzlaff *et al.*, 2013; Sydow *et al.*, 2013) as well as for problem specific areas such as alcohol and drug abuse (Waldron & Turner, 2008; Baldwin *et al.*, 2012; Rowe, 2012), conduct disorder and delinquency (Baldwin *et al.*, 2012; Henggeler & Sheidow, 2012), eating disorders (Downs & Blow, 2013; Couturier *et al.*, 2013), anxiety disorders (Breinholst *et al.*, 2012; Simpson *et al.*, 2012), or mood disorders (Carr, 2008; Cosgrove *et al.*, 2013).

General reviews show family therapy to be effective when compared to no treatment or wait list controls (with an average effect size of 0.65—Shadish & Baldwin, 2003). With most problems, the differences between family therapy and other active treatments are relatively small but with some there is consistent evidence of family therapy leading to better outcomes. This is particularly the case for behavior problems and youth offending (Henggeler & Sheidow, 2012; Sydow *et al.*, 2013) and substance misuse (Baldwin *et al.*, 2012; Tanner-Smith *et al.*, 2013) where the evidence from around 30 RCTs provides clear support for the use of family therapy both in terms of outcome (with small but consistent between-treatment effect sizes of around 0.26—Baldwin *et al.*, 2012; Tanner-Smith *et al.*, 2013) but also because family therapy appears to be more effective in engaging and maintaining young people in treatment than individual therapy (Stanton, 2004).

Similarly, there is now compelling evidence for family therapy in the treatment of eating disorders (Downs & Blow, 2013; Couturier *et al.*, 2013) with recent larger studies confirming its superiority in the treatment of anorexia nervosa in comparison with an adolescent-focused individual therapy (Lock *et al.*, 2010) as well as its role in the treatment of bulimia nervosa (Le Grange *et al.*, 2007; Schmidt *et al.*, 2007).

For other problems such as anxiety disorders (including OCD), depression, or bipolar disorder, there is evidence that family interventions are effective but the comparison with other treatments is less straightforward. In anxiety disorders, most of the family intervention research has compared different versions of individual or family-based CBT. Generally, individual and family-based CBT tend to have similar outcomes, but the overall picture is more complex. Some studies have shown that where the parents themselves are anxious, including a family component in treatment may increase effectiveness (Kendall *et al.*, 2008) but this is not the case in other studies (Bodden *et al.*, 2008). There are also data suggesting that even when there is no difference between changes in anxiety symptoms, the family intervention leads to greater changes in general functioning both at the individual and family level (Khanna & Kendall, 2009) and some studies also indicate a better longer term maintenance of posttreatment gains (Barrett *et al.*, 2001; Cobham *et al.*, 2010). In mood disorders, a wider range of family interventions have been evaluated. These have included CBT with a family component where the findings are similar to anxiety disorders, that is, they are effective in comparison with a control but are similar to individual CBT, although again there is some indication of greater change in family relationships (Stark *et al.*, 2012). Two groups have evaluated systemic family therapy for depression in children and adolescents and shown them to be effective in comparison with control (Diamond *et al.*, 2002, 2009) and comparable to psychodynamic psychotherapy (Trowell *et al.*, 2007). There is also evidence that improvements in family functioning mediates changes in mood (Garoff *et al.*, 2012)

Moreover, there have been several studies of multifamily interventions for both depression and bipolar disorder (Miklowitz *et al.*, 2008; Fristad *et al.*, 2009), which show considerable promise. There are a growing number of treatment programs that include a multifamily component in the therapy for a range of problems and there is evidence that bringing groups of families together may improve outcomes (McKay *et al.*, 2011; MacPherson *et al.*, 2013) and is also a powerful way of addressing feelings of isolation, stigmatization, and helplessness that families often experience (Asen & Scholz, 2010); in these contexts, the family work is usually added to disorder-specific treatment.

Implications for clinical practice

As many have pointed out (e.g., Sackett *et al.*, 1996; Kazdin, 2008), evidence-based practice should not be understood simply as the adoption of treatments supported by results from randomized trials. For instance, the treatment research studies in anxiety and mood disorders indicate that a largely individual CBT and family-based CBT lead to similar outcomes at least in terms of symptom improvement. Nevertheless, it would be a mistake to conclude that the family, therefore, need not be involved in treatment. The potential positive effects go beyond improvements for the referred child and hopefully strengthen the network around the child and may provide protection for other vulnerable family members. Even putting aside the potential of the broader benefits and possibly better longer-term outcomes, family-based interventions have a clearly important contribution. At the very least individual and family-oriented treatments provide alternatives, the choice of which can be guided by factors other than efficacy. Many parents feel that they are to blame for their child's problem and a supportive nonblaming role in treatment can help to make them feel that they are a solution rather than the cause of the problem.

Even where there is clear evidence that family therapy is efficacious, implementing the research findings in clinical practice is by no means straightforward (see Chapter 36). The first limitation is our lack of understanding of the mechanisms of treatments and the difficulty therefore of defining what constitutes a distinct treatment. For example, the best researched areas of family therapy (behavior problems and substance misuse) have been dominated by the evaluation of several brand named therapies developed in the US (Multi-Systemic Therapy, Multi-Dimensional Family Therapy, Functional Family Therapy, and Brief Strategic Family Therapy). Notwithstanding the claims by the developers of these treatments as to the uniqueness of each approach and the need to implement the treatments strictly adhering to the treatment manuals, the evidence for this is weak. As the clinical commentary in a study by Baldwin *et al.* (2012) points out, the vast majority of the research has been undertaken by the developers and there is a lack of any significant comparison between the treatments. Many of the treatments are disseminated under license, making comparisons more difficult to undertake. The argument in favor of this is that this ensures that the treatments are evaluated and disseminated in an adherent way making them more robust. This, however, comes up against the second dissemination problem, namely the extent to which, and under what conditions, adherence improves outcomes. There are a number of studies undertaken by the developers of these treatments suggesting that improved adherence improves outcomes (e.g., Hogue & Liddle, 2009; Sexton & Turner, 2010). However, the broader literature on adherence shows a much more complicated picture indicating that adherence does not have a strong linear relationship with outcome (Barber *et al.*, 2006; Webb *et al.*, 2010) and may be moderated by factors such as therapeutic alliance, competence, and therapist experience (Castonguay *et al.*, 2010). The third dissemination complexity concerns the role of service context in which treatments are delivered. This has been shown in a recent naturalistic study (House *et al.*, 2012) comparing specialist and nonspecialist outpatient services providing treatment for adolescent anorexia nervosa in different parts of London. Three fundamental difference characterized areas with access to specialist services: first, identification of those requiring treatment was 2–3 times higher than in areas with no specialist provisions, second, hospital admissions were 2–3 times lower in specialist areas and third, 80% of those referred to generic CAMHS (child and adolescent mental health services) were at some stage referred on to other services which was true of less than 20% of those referred straight to a specialist service. The impact of these differences far outweigh the differences between treatment outcomes found in randomized control trials (RCTs) and suggests that specialist expertize (which includes but is not limited to knowledge of evidence-based treatments), referrer and family expectation may play a greater role than the treatments themselves.

Conclusions

Family interventions have been established as an essential treatment within a multidisciplinary team when working with children and adolescents with increasingly strong evidence for its efficacy. We have emphasized that the role of the family in treatment needs to be considered broadly and not just as part of an evidence-based equation of treatment efficacy related to a specific problem although clearly with behavior problems, youth offending, substance misuse and also eating disorders family therapy should be considered a key intervention. A great deal more research is needed to gain a better understanding of how family interventions work to bring about change and the similarities and differences between the mechanisms of change of different treatments. Much of the current discussion about evidence-based practice is concerned with the relative contribution of model specific and common factors in psychotherapy (Sprenkle *et al.*, 2009; Duncan *et al.*, 2010) and the extent to which careful adherence to very precisely defined treatment models need to be balanced by flexibility and clinical judgment in tailoring treatments to the specific needs of individual families (Sexton *et al.*, 2008). Thus while our knowledge of what works is clearly increasing, our understanding of how treatments work and the way in which research evidence is best disseminated has still a long way to go.

References

Amir, N. *et al.* (2000) Family distress and involvement in relatives of obsessive-compulsive disorder patients. *Journal of Anxiety Disorders* **14**, 209–217.

Anderson, H. & Goolishian, H. (1988) Human systems as linguistic systems: evolving ideas for the implications in theory and practice. *Family Process* **27**, 371–393.

Areemit, R.S. *et al.* (2010) The experience of siblings of adolescents with eating disorders. *Journal of Adolescent Health* **46**, 569–576.

Asen, E. (2002) Multiple family therapy: an overview. *Journal of Family Therapy* **24**, 3–16.

Asen, E. & Scholz, M. (2010) *Multi-Family Therapy: Concepts and Techniques*. Routledge, London.

Baldwin, S.A. *et al.* (2012) The effects of family therapies for adolescent delinquency and substance abuse: a meta-analysis. *Journal of Marital and Family Therapy* **38**, 281–304.

Barber, J.P. *et al.* (2006) The role of therapist adherence, therapist competence and alliance in predicting outcome of individual drug counseling: results from the National Institute drug abuse collaborative cocaine treatment study. *Psychotherapy Research* **16**, 229–240.

Barratt, S. (2012) Incorporating multi-family days into parenting assessments: the Writtle Wick model. *Child & Family Social Work* **17**, 222–232.

Barrett, P.M. *et al.* (2001) Cognitive-behavioural treatment of anxiety disorders in children: long-term (6 year) follow up. *Journal of Consulting and Clinical Psychology* **69**, 135–141.

Barrett, P. *et al.* (2004) Cognitive behavioral family treatment of childhood OCD: a controlled trial. *Journal of the American Academy of Child and Adolescent Psychiatry* **34**, 46–62.

Bateson, G. (1972) *Steps to an Ecology of Mind*. Ballentine, New York.

Bodden, D.H. *et al.* (2008) Child versus family cognitive-behavioral therapy in clinically anxious youth: an efficacy and partial effectiveness study. *Journal of the American Academy of Child & Adolescent Psychiatry* **47**, 1384–1394.

Bordin, E.S. (1979) The generalizability of the psychoanalytic concept of the working alliance. *Psychotherapy* **16**, 252–260.

Bowes, L. *et al.* (2010) Families promote emotional and behavioural resilience to bullying: evidence of an environmental effect. *Journal of Child Psychology and Psychiatry* **51**, 809–817.

Breinholst, S. *et al.* (2012) CBT for the treatment of child anxiety disorders: a review of why parental involvement has not enhanced outcomes. *Journal of Anxiety Disorders* **26**, 416–424.

Buschgens, C.J. *et al.* (2010) Externalizing behaviors in preadolescents: familial risk to externalizing behaviors and perceived parenting styles. *European Child & Adolescent Psychiatry* **19**, 567–575.

Carr, A. (2008) Depression in young people: description, assessment and evidence-based treatment. *Developmental Neurorehabilitation* **11**, 3–15.

Carr, A. (2012) *Family Therapy: Concepts, Process and Practice*, 3rd edn. Wiley-Blackwell, Chichester.

Castonguay, L.G. *et al.* (2010) Training implications of harmful effects of psychological treatments. *American Psychologist* **65**, 34–49.

Cobham, V.E. *et al.* (2010) Parental anxiety in the treatment of childhood anxiety: a different story three years later. *Journal of Clinical Child & Adolescent Psychology* **39**, 410–420.

Cole, R. & Reiss, D. (2013) *How Do Families Cope With Chronic Illness?* Routledge, Abingdon, Oxon.

Cosgrove, V.E. *et al.* (2013) Bipolar depression in pediatric populations: epidemiology and management. *Paediatric Drugs* **2115**, 83–91.

Couturier, J. *et al.* (2013) Efficacy of family-based treatment for adolescents with eating disorders: a systematic review and meta-analysis. *International Journal of Eating Disorders* **46**, 3–11.

Dallos, R. & Draper, R. (2005) *An Introduction to Family Therapy and Systemic Practice*. Open University Press, Maidenhead.

De Shazer, S. (1985) *Keys to Solutions in Brief Therapy*. Norton, New York.

Diamond, G.S. *et al.* (2002) Attachment-based family therapy for depressed adolescents: a treatment development study. *Journal of the American Academy of Child and Adolescent Psychiatry* **41**, 1190–1196.

Diamond, G.S. *et al.* (2009) Attachment-based family therapy for depressed adolescents. In: *Treatments for Adolescent Depression: Theory and Practice*. (ed C.A. Essau), pp. 215–237. xii, 328. Oxford University Press, New York.

Downs, K.J. & Blow, A.J. (2013) A substantive and methodological review of family-based treatment for eating disorders: the last 25 years of research. *Journal of Family Therapy* **35**, 3–28.

Duncan, B.L. *et al.* (2010) *The Heart and Soul of Change: Delivering What Works in Therapy*, 2nd edn. American Psychological Association, Washington, DC.

Eisler, I. (2005) The empirical and theoretical base of family therapy and multiple family day therapy for adolescent anorexia nervosa. *Journal of Family Therapy* **27**, 104–131.

Eisler, I. *et al.* (2000) Family therapy for adolescent anorexia nervosa: the results of a controlled comparison of two family interventions. *Journal of Child Psychology and Psychiatry* **41**, 727–736.

Eisler, I. *et al.* (2007) Long-term follow up of outcome of two forms of family therapy for adolescent anorexia nervosa. *Journal of Child Psychology and Psychiatry* **48**, 552–560.

Escudero, V. *et al.* (2008) Observing the therapeutic alliance in family therapy: associations with participants' perceptions and therapeutic outcomes. *Journal of Family Therapy* **30**, 194–214.

Escudero, V. *et al.* (2012) Alliance rupture and repair in conjoint family therapy: an exploratory study. *Psychotherapy* **49**, 26–37.

Falicov, C. (1995) Training to think culturally: a multidimensional comparative framework. *Family Process* **34**, 373–388.

Fraenkel, P. & Pinsof, W. (2001) Teaching family therapy-centred integration: assimilation and beyond. *Journal of Psychotherapy Integration* **11**, 59–86.

Fristad, M.A. *et al.* (2009) Impact of multifamily psychoeducational psychotherapy in treating children aged 8 to 12 years with mood disorders. *Archives of General Psychiatry* **66**, 1013–1020.

Garoff, F.F. *et al.* (2012) Depressed youth: treatment outcome and changes in family functioning in individual and family therapy. *Journal of Family Therapy* **34**, 4–23.

Gergen, K.J. (1999) *An Invitation to Social Construction*. Sage, London.

Gil, E. *et al.* (2008) *Genograms: Assessment and Intervention*. Norton, New York.

Goldner, V. *et al.* (1990) Love and violence: gender paradoxes in volatile attachments. *Family Process* **29**, 343–364.

Haley, J. (1963) *Strategies of Psychotherapy*. Grune & Stratton, New York.

Hampson, R.B. & Beavers, R. (1996a) Family therapy and outcome: relationships between therapists and family styles. *Contemporary Family Therapy* **18**, 345–370.

Hampson, R.B. & Beavers, R. (1996b) Measuring family therapy outcome in a clinical setting. *Family Process* **35**, 347–360.

Henggeler, S.W. & Sheidow, A.J. (2012) Empirically supported family-based treatments for conduct disorder and delinquency in adolescents. *Journal of Marital and Family Therapy* **38**, 30–58.

Hetherington, M.E. (1989) Coping with family transitions: winners, losers and survivors. *Child Development* **60**, 1–14.

Hoffman, L. (1985) Beyond power and control: towards a second order' family systems therapy. *Family Systems Medicine* **3**, 381–396.

Hoffman, L. (1990) Constructing realities: an art of lenses. *Family Process* **29**, 1–12.

Hogue, A. & Liddle, H.A. (2009) Family-based treatment for adolescent substance abuse: controlled trials and new horizons in services research. *Journal of Family Therapy* **31**, 126–154.

House, J. *et al.* (2012) Comparison of specialist and non-specialist care pathways for adolescents with anorexia nervosa and related eating disorders. *International Journal of Eating Disorders* **45**, 949–956.

Huizink, A.C. *et al.* (2002) Psychological measures of prenatal stress as predictors of infant temperament. *Journal of the American Academy of Child and Adolescent Psychiatry* **41**, 1078–1085.

Kaslow, N.J. *et al.* (2012) Family-based interventions for child and adolescent disorders. *Journal of Marital and Family Therapy* **38**, 82–100.

Kazdin, A.E. (2008) Evidence-based treatment and practice: new opportunities to bridge clinical research and practice, enhance the knowledge base, and improve patient care. *American Psychologist* **63**, 146–159.

Kendall, P.C. *et al.* (2008) Cognitive-behavioral therapy for anxiety disordered youth: a randomized clinical trial evaluating child and family modalities. *Journal of Consulting and Clinical Psychology* **76**, 282.

Khanna, M.S. & Kendall, P.C. (2009) Exploring the role of parent training in the treatment of childhood anxiety. *Journal of Consulting and Clinical Psychology* **77**, 981.

Kraemer, H.C. *et al.* (2001) How do risk factors work together? Mediators, moderators & independent overlapping and proxy risk factors. *American Journal of Psychiatry* **158**, 848–856.

Kubička, L. *et al.* (2002) The mental health of adults born from unwanted pregnancies, their siblings, and matched controls: a 35-year follow-up study from Prague, Czech Republic. *Journal of Nervous and Mental Disease* **190**, 653–662.

Lambert, J.E. *et al.* (2012) Problematic within-family alliances in conjoint family therapy: a close look at five cases. *Journal of Marital and Family Therapy* **38**, 417–428.

Le Grange, D. *et al.* (2007) A randomized controlled comparison of family-based treatment and supportive psychotherapy for adolescent bulimia nervosa. *Archives of General Psychiatry* **64**, 1049.

Lock, J. *et al.* (2010) Randomized clinical trial comparing family-based treatment with adolescent-focused individual therapy for adolescents with anorexia nervosa. *Archives of General Psychiatry* **67**, 1025.

Lueck, K. & Wilson, M. (2011) Acculturative stress in Latino immigrants: the impact of social, socio-psychological and migration-related factors. *International Journal of Intercultural Relations* **35**, 186–195.

MacPherson, H.A. *et al.* (2013) Implementation of multi-family psychoeducational psychotherapy for childhood mood disorders in an outpatient community setting. *Journal of Marital and Family Therapy* **40**, 193–211.

Mason, B. (2005) Relational risk-taking and the training of supervisors. *Journal of Family Therapy* **27**, 298–301.

McGoldrick, M. *et al.* (2010) *The Expanded Family Life Cycle: Individual, Family, and Social Perspectives*. Prentice Hall, NJ.

McKay, M.M. *et al.* (2011) A collaboratively designed child mental health service model: multiple family groups for urban children with conduct difficulties. *Research on Social Work Practice* **21**, 664–674.

McLeod, B.D. *et al.* (2007a) Examining the association between parenting and childhood anxiety: a meta-analysis. *Clinical Psychology Review* **27**, 155–172.

McLeod, B.D. *et al.* (2007b) Examining the association between parenting and childhood depression: a meta-analysis. *Clinical Psychology Review* **27**, 986–1003.

Miklowitz, D.A. *et al.* (2008) Family-focused treatment for adolescents with bipolar disorder: results of a 2-year randomized trial. *Archives of General Psychiatry* **65**, 1053–1061.

Minuchin, S. (1974) *Families and Family Therapy*. Harvard University Press, Cambridge, MA.

Minuchin, S. & Fishman, H.C. (1981) *Family Therapy Techniques*. Harvard University Press, Cambridge, MA.

Muhlbauer, S.A. (2002) Navigating the storm of mental illness: phases in the family's journey. *Qualitative Health Research* **12**, 1076–1092.

Norcross, J. & Goldfried, M. (2005) *Handbook of Psychotherapy Integration*, 2nd edn. Oxford University Press, New York.

O'Connor, T.G. *et al.* (2000) The effects of global severe privation on cognitive competence: extension and longitudinal follow-up. *Child Development* **71**, 376–390.

Plomin, R. & Daniels, D. (2011) Why are children in the same family so different from one another? *International Journal of Epidemiology* **40**, 563–582.

Retzlaff, R. *et al.* (2013) The efficacy of systemic therapy for internalizing and other disorders of childhood and adolescence: a systematic review of 38 randomized trials. *Family Process* **52**, 619–652.

Rowe, C.L. (2012) Family therapy for drug abuse: review and updates 2003–2010. *Journal of Marital and Family Therapy* **38**, 59–81.

Rutter, M. (2006) The promotion of resilience in the face of adversity. In: *Families Count: Effects on Child and Adolescent Development*. (eds A. Clarke-Stewart & J. Dunn). Cambridge University Press, Cambridge.

Rutter, M. (2013) Annual research review: resilience – clinical implications. *Journal of Child Psychology and Psychiatry* **54**, 474–487.

Rutter, M. & O'Connor, T.G. (2004) Are there biological programming effects for psychological development? Findings from a study of Romanian adoptees. *Developmental Psychology* **40**, 81–94.

Sackett, D.L. *et al.* (1996) Evidence based medicine: what it is and what it isn't. *British Medical Journal* **312**, 71–72.

Schmidt, U. *et al.* (2007) A randomized controlled trial of family therapy and cognitive-behavioral guided self-care for adolescents with bulimia nervosa or related disorders. *American Journal of Psychiatry* **164**, 591–598.

Sexton, T. & Turner, C.W. (2010) The effectiveness of functional family therapy for youth with behavioral problems in a community practice setting. *Journal of Family Psychology* **24**, 339–348.

Sexton, T.L. *et al.* (2008) Beyond a single standard: levels of evidence approach for evaluating marriage and family therapy research and practice. *Journal of Family Therapy* **30**, 386–398.

Shadish, W.R. & Baldwin, S.A. (2003) Meta analysis of MFT interventions. *Journal of Marital and Family Therapy* **29**, 547–570.

Simpson, D. *et al.* (2012) Treatment and outcomes for anxiety disorders among children and adolescents: a review of coping strategies and parental behaviors. *Current Psychiatry Reports* **14**, 87–95.

Sprenkle, D.H. (2012) Intervention research in couple and family therapy: a methodological and substantive review and an introduction to the special issue. *Journal of Marital and Family Therapy* **38**, 3–29.

Sprenkle, D.H. *et al.* (2009) *Common Factors in Couple and Family Therapy: The Overlooked Foundation for Effective Practice*. Guilford Press, New York.

Stanton, M.D. (2004) Getting reluctant substance abusers to engage in treatment/self-help: a review of outcomes and clinical options. *Journal of Marital and Family Therapy* **30**, 165–182.

Stark, K.D. *et al.* (2012) Child and adolescent depression in the family. *Couple and Family Psychology: Research and Practice* **1**, 161–184.

Sydow, K. *et al.* (2013) The efficacy of systemic therapy for childhood and adolescent externalizing disorders: a systematic review of 48 RCTs. *Family Process* **52**, 576–618.

Szmukler, G.I. *et al.* (1985) Parental expressed emotion, anorexia nervosa and dropping out of treatment. *British Journal of Psychiatry* **147**, 265–271.

Tanner-Smith, E.E. *et al.* (2013) The comparative effectiveness of outpatient treatment for adolescent substance abuse: a meta-analysis. *Journal of Substance Abuse Treatment* **44**, 145–158.

Tomm, K. (1987a) Interventive interviewing. Part I. Strategising as a fourth guideline for the therapist. *Family Process* **25**, 4–13.

Tomm, K. (1987b) Interventive interviewing. Part II. Reflective questioning as a means to enable self healing. *Family Process* **26**, 167–183.

Tomm, K. (1988) Interventive interviewing. Part III. Intended to ask linear, circular, strategic or reflexive questions. *Family Process* **27**, 1–15.

Trowell, J. *et al.* (2007) Childhood depression: a place for psychotherapy; an outcome study comparing individual psychodynamic and psychotherapy and family therapy. *European Child & Adolescent Psychiatry* **6**, 157–167.

Vetere, A. & Dallos, R. (2008) Systemic therapy and attachment narratives. *Journal of Family Therapy* **30**, 374–385.

Waldron, H.B. & Turner, C.W. (2008) Evidence-based psychosocial treatments for adolescent substance abuse. *Journal of Clinical Child & Adolescent Psychology* **37**, 238–261.

Waller, R. *et al.* (2012) Do harsh and positive parenting predict parent reports of deceitful-callous behavior in early childhood? *Journal of Child Psychology and Psychiatry* **53**, 946–953.

Walsh, F. (2006) *Strengthening Family Resilience*, 2nd edn. Guilford Press, New York.

Weakland, J.H. *et al.* (1974) Brief therapy: focused problem resolution. *Family Process* **13**, 141–168.

Webb, C.A. *et al.* (2010) Therapist adherence/competence and treatment outcome: a meta-analytic review. *Journal of Consulting and Clinical Psychology* **78**, 200–211.

White, M. (2005) *Narrative Practice and Exotic Lives: Resurrecting Diversity in Everyday Life*. Dulwich Centre Publications, Adelaide.

Wilson, J. (1998) *Child-Focused Practice: A Collaborative Systemic Approach*. Karnac Books, London.

CHAPTER 40

Relationship-based treatments

Jonathan Green

Child and Adolescent Psychiatry, Institute of Brain, Behaviour and Mental Health, University of Manchester and the Royal Manchester Children's Hospital, Manchester, UK

Introduction

"Relationship-based treatments" are defined in this chapter as those that have, as their prime aim, either the improvement of a child or adolescent's key relationships or else use relationships as a core mechanism through which they are delivered and generate psychological and behavioral change. The quality of early relationships with caregivers and others has a recognized impact on later social development, social competency, mental health and well-being and a central role in developmental science and developmental psychopathology. Additionally, much learning and development takes place within the context of social relating and is in that sense truly "social" learning. Theories of how maturational and extrinsic influences interact together at behavioral, cognitive, emotional and neural system levels within developmental psychopathology are increasingly important to the design of interventions.

The chapter covers three main areas: (i) interventions that aim to improve the relatedness between children and significant caregivers in early childhood, both in the context of parental risk such as trauma or mood disorder and child risk such as individual difference or atypical development; (ii) the nature and impact of the relationship between therapist and patient in the process of treatment, referring to non-specific factors such as the therapeutic alliance that operate across different forms of therapy; (iii) interventions in later childhood and adolescence that either have a particular focus on improving social relationships or are defined by the use of the therapist–patient relationship as a major mechanism for effecting change. Treatments are included for discussion if they are informed by modern developmental science and/or have an evidence base for the treatment itself or its key components. General approaches considered include Secure Base Therapy, Motivational Interviewing (MI) and Mentalization-Based Therapy (MBT); along with a number of specific forms of psychotherapy such as Short Term Psychodynamic Psychotherapy (STPP), Interpersonal Therapy

(IPT) and Cognitive Analytic Therapy (CAT). Not covered here are treatments marked by a more cognitive or social learning focus that are specifically addressed in other chapters, such as cognitive behavior therapy (CBT) (see Chapter 38), parent training (see Chapter 37) and multimodal approaches such as multisystemic therapy (see Chapter 50).

Taking a crosscutting approach, material in the chapter will overlap with a number of other chapters in this book, to which reference will be made.

Treatments targeted at early relationships

A number of interventions aim to improve early dyadic caregiver-infant and caregiver-child relationships, particular early infant attachment. These have been implemented and studied in the context both of known *parental risks* for relationship difficulties, such unresolved trauma or mental illness; and *child risks* such as early maltreatment, temperamental vulnerability or other biological risk exposure.

Context of parental risk
Parent-mediated video-aided interventions
For interventions in infancy focused on attachment, a meta-analysis of 51 randomized trials (Bakermans-Kranenburg *et al.*, 2003) has suggested that developmentally based, carefully tailored, brief (<16 sessions) and individualized interventions often using video-aided techniques are most effective in optimizing attachment-related parental behaviors such as sensitive responding (overall $d = 0.45$); whereas general parental support or longer term therapy aimed at altering maternal mental state showed less effectiveness ($d = 0.27$). The subsequent impact of the treatment on infant development, however, is consistently less, with modest improvement found in infant insecure attachments ($d = 0.22$) and none on disorganized attachment ($d = 0.05$). In these interventions, caregivers typically review with the therapist videotapes of their naturalistic interactions

Rutter's Child and Adolescent Psychiatry, Sixth Edition.
Edited by Anita Thapar and Daniel S. Pine, James F. Leckman, Stephen Scott, Margaret J. Snowling, Eric Taylor.
© 2015 John Wiley & Sons Ltd. Published 2018 by John Wiley & Sons Ltd.

with their infant. The therapist uses the video material to help sensitize the caregiver to the signals of and meaning behind infant social communication. The focus on real time learning through videotape is a powerful way of increasing parental awareness, sensitivity, and enjoyment with their infant. An example of such intervention is the Video Intervention for Positive Parenting (VIPP; Juffer et al., 2008), which has shown effectiveness in early parental risk and for children with vulnerable temperaments (Velderman et al., 2006). Adaptation of the model shows positive impact on interaction and patterns of early feeding in mothers with eating disorder (Stein et al., 2006) and an extension for preschool children with early externalizing behaviors incorporates positive disciplining practices (VIPP-Sensitive Discipline). This latter has been tested in a relatively large efficacy randomized control trial (RCT) ($N = 237$, Van Zeijl et al., 2006), showing positive effect on parental disciplining behaviors although not parental sensitivity; there was no overall effect on child externalizing behavior, but an improvement in child overactivity symptoms in a subset of families with high marital and daily hassle stress. In parents at significant risk, or showing early signs of, maltreatment of their children, an 8 week parent-mediated video-aided attachment-focused intervention in the early years (Moss et al., 2011) showed success in improving observed parental sensitivity in the home, and this was associated with a shift in the child from insecure and disorganized child attachment behaviors toward more organized and secure attachments. There was, however, no robust change here in parent-rated child internalizing or externalizing behaviors. The "attachment and bio-behavioral catch up" (ABC) program developed by Dozier and colleagues has a similar focus on parental support, nurturing and video-aided intervention to improve responsiveness and sensitive responding to children in contexts of parents at risk of maltreating their child or whose child is in foster care (Dozier et al., 2008; see Chapter 6).

Psychotherapeutic interventions

In contrast to the focus on detailed parent–infant interaction, psychotherapeutic approaches address the emotional and mental state of caregivers, who often have complex personal histories impacting on their parenting ability and relationships. A psychotherapy approach with depressed mothers and their toddlers at mean age 20 months showed a positive effect on infant attachment security at 36 months (Cicchetti et al., 1999), but psychotherapy intervention (21 sessions over 1 year) in maltreating parents of children aged about 12 months showed no additional benefit over a psychoeducational intervention (25 sessions over 1 year), although both showed benefit compared with standard community services (Cicchetti et al., 2006). Similar interventions focused on changing parents' own underlying cognitions ("representations") in relation to attachment relationships have found positive effects on maternal mood (Cooper et al., 2003) and sensitivity (Murray et al., 2003) but not on child attachment status (see Chapter 26).

Group support and counselling

Psychosocial support and counseling for caregivers is probably the most widely used intervention over the prenatal period or first 2 years. Three RCTs have shown benefits of such programmes on general maternal functioning and sensitivity in high social adversity situations but no associated effect on infant attachment (Barnard et al., 1988; Beckwith, 1988; Murray et al., 2003). By contrast, two studies showed no effect on maternal sensitivity but some increase in infant security over controls (Jacobson & Frye, 1991). Attachment-focused group interventions for parents have not been tested in randomized trials; observational studies indicate an increase in secure child attachment (Cassidy et al., 2007) and reduction in attachment disorganization (Hoffman et al., 2006); but this evidence is preliminary.

Context of child developmental risk or disability

There is a recent shift away from an exclusive focus on parenting sensitivity irrespective of child characteristics toward more consideration of individual differences in children. Video-aided parenting approaches have been used successfully to improve attachment and relatedness in infants at risk due to extreme or difficult temperaments (Van den Boom, 1994; Cassidy et al., 2011); they have also been targeted at improving relationships between parents and children with developmental disability. Here, it is the child's atypical development that is the main influence on impaired interaction and interaction-dependent development and outcomes. In autism for instance, developmental evidence (Wan et al., 2013) suggests that infant atypicality is associated with disrupted parent–infant interaction. This disruption itself could then amplify the atypical trajectory and create poorer developmental outcomes through direct effect on the evolving social brain within environmentally expectant neural systems (Johnson, 2011), or at the level of relationship development, language, or general psychological development. Social communication interventions here work with parents (or for older children, teaching assistants, or peers), often using video-aided methods, to enhance awareness of the child's communication and to enhance dyadic communication designed to promote child social communication, attention, shared enjoyment, and language. Such interventions have been recommended for consideration by UK National Institute for Health and Care Excellence in treatment of core features of autism (Kendall et al., 2013). An RCT ($n = 152$) of a 12 month parent-mediated intervention of this kind for preschool children with autism (Green et al., 2010) showed strong effects on parental synchronous communication responses to the child (effect size 1.22) and child dyadic communication to parent (effect size 0.41), but an attenuation in relation to generalized autism symptoms (effect size 0.24, non significant on ADOS-G), despite parental reports of language, social communication, and family well-being being positive. An RCT of another parent-mediated social communication intervention programme that focused on joint engagement ($n = 38$) showed a similar pattern of positive short-range effects on the targeted interaction variables (Kasari *et al.*, 2010), while a related intervention with separate procedures to enhance joint attention and symbolic play in relation to language outcomes ($n = 58$) that worked more directly with the child reported additional downstream improvement on assessed language (Kasari *et al.*, 2008), although this has not been replicated (Kaale *et al.*, 2014). These kinds of intervention studies presuppose that children with atypical neurodevelopment have the same relational needs as children with neuro-typical development and that the difficulties in interaction and relational development consequent on their disability may act in turn to amplify adverse mental health and social outcomes. The evidence suggests that such interventions can positively shift atypical transactional developmental patterns in the short term; the challenge is how to generalize and sustain these child changes through time.

Differential susceptibility theory (Belsky *et al.*, 2007) suggests that children may differ in their sensitivity to both positive and negative aspects of the environment and predicts that some children with atypical development may respond particularly positively to the improved environment through social interventions of this kind. Partial support of this comes from the treatment arms of infancy RCTs (Velderman *et al.*, 2006; Cassidy *et al.*, 2011) showing that brief parent-mediated interventions improving sensitivity are differentially efficacious in infants with high temperamental reactivity.

Summary

Across a variety of risk contexts, including parental psychosocial adversity, maltreatment history, or mood disorder and childhood developmental disability or temperamental vulnerability, interventions can improve parental behaviors understood to promote positive developmental relationships. Associated gains in infant or child dyadic behaviors such as communication initiations or attachment behaviors toward the parent are found, but attenuated compared to the effect on parental behaviors. Aspects of childhood vulnerability may be associated with increased response to such interventions. The interventions themselves are flexibly adapted to specific child needs, and in this the intervention design mirrors the kind of adaptive responding in parents that leads to increased sensitivity. There is well-established short-term effectiveness and it is theoretically reasonable to hope that altering relationship dynamics in this way will have longer-term benefits on child development; however, evidence for this downstream impact is currently much weaker, and this is even true of the non blinded parent-rated outcomes which would be expected to be most sensitive to treatment effect. Most of these interventions take an individual approach within which specific attention can be given to the needs of the dyad and there has been little testing of group approaches. For the future, there are two challenges: firstly to show generalization of treatment effect beyond the context of the specific dyadic relationship, including adding additional intervention elements to promote such generalization; secondly, to demonstrate sustained impact through time, again including additional elements such as repeated intervention or booster sessions to maximize developmental gains.

Therapist–patient relationship as a mode of treatment

Focus on the therapist–patient relationship as a mechanism of therapeutic change is a central theoretical feature of various traditions in psychotherapy, including transference theory in psychoanalysis and notions of 'unconditional positive regard' in humanistic traditions. Construed as the 'therapeutic alliance', it has been increasingly understood and studied as a non-specific therapeutic factor operating across different kinds of psychotherapy and broader treatments.

Therapeutic alliance

The therapeutic alliance is a term encompassing a variety of relational variables between patient and therapist (Green, 2006; see Chapter 36). Its description and measurement has evolved in parallel with changing theory (Elvins *et al.*, 2008); an empirically based review (Hougaard, 1994) identified key dimensions of "Personal Alliance," the relationship of engagement and personal trust between therapist and client, and "Task Alliance," a more contractual relationship around agreement on the focus, goals, method and depth of the intervention. These two dimensions were generally inter-correlated. The impact of therapeutic alliance is observed across many different types of intervention, extending well beyond psychotherapy. In adult mental health, for instance, an important study (Krupnick *et al.*, 1996) independently measured alliance from sessional transcripts in a large RCT for depression, with intervention arms ranging from medication management to cognitive therapy. The quality of the measured alliance was independent of the type of treatment, identity of therapist, or baseline symptom severity. It was, however, highly correlated with treatment outcome across *all arms* of the trial (overall $r = 0.46$) and predicted remission of depression caseness (OR 17.2) more strongly than the individual treatments themselves. Subsequent broader meta-analysis across both adult (Martin *et al.*, 2000) and child and adolescent (Shirk & Karver, 2003) mental health studies found an overall robust albeit modest association between alliance quality and outcome; in the child studies, this was $r = 0.24$ across 23 studies of differing methodology, independent of child age and type of treatment. Alliance is, however, a complex phenomenon and there are methodological limitations on some of these reports (Kazdin & Nock, 2003; Green, 2006; Dunn & Bentall, 2007); for instance, 57% of 49 studies in a recent meta-analysis (Karver *et al.*, 2006) showed significant problems with common method and rater biases (for instance, the same person rating both alliance and outcome) that may inflate apparent alliance effects. Moreover, because alliance emerges *during treatment* it is by definition a post-baseline variable that is subject to confounds that cannot be controlled by initial randomization in trials. Newer analytic methods addressing these problems still confirm a modest but significant impact of alliance on treatment outcomes in adult schizophrenia (Dunn & Bentall, 2007) and evidence of similar effect in adolescent depression (Elvins, 2012).

Therapist qualities such as active listening, accurate empathy, and commitment, as well as "direct influence" from good communication, clear treatment rationale, and collaborative planning all showed a moderate to strong association with alliance quality in a meta-analysis of 49 studies (Karver *et al.*, 2006), but therapist self-disclosure showed no relationship. Patient characteristics are also important. The alliance is usually found to be independent of severity of baseline symptomatology, but it is theoretically likely that the patient's prior capacity to form general social relationships of collaboration and trust will influence their capacity to form a productive therapeutic alliance in the therapy setting. An effect of child pretreatment social competence and intellectual functioning on early alliance was found in an RCT for child behavior problems ($n = 97$; Kazdin & Durbin, 2012), and pretreatment personality disorder independently predicted alliance and outcome in an RCT of adolescents with repeated self-harm (Ayodeji *et al.*, 2015).

The evidence thus supports the modest but important impact of quality of therapist–patient alliance relationship on outcomes across many intervention types, but we still do not know exactly how the alliance impacts on outcome. Does it just work by promoting good engagement with an efficacious treatment or does it have its own independent therapeutic effect in parallel to the specific treatment technique? Do prior patient qualities associated with good alliance formation themselves predict a good outcome? These questions have important implications for clinical practice and training in relation to what actually are the important components of successful treatment; and in research design, where careful methodological thinking is necessary to test the complexities of alliance phenomena (Kraemer *et al.*, 2002). We await experimental trials of whether specific methods to enhance alliance *alone* would be as effective as specific intervention protocols (a key question). Notwithstanding this, there is enough evidence to suggest that promotion of the alliance should be a core feature of professional training and intervention development; understanding family and child variables predicting alliance will also help us better individualize treatment approaches.

Alliance, treatment fidelity, and adherence

The effect of non specific factors such as alliance suggests that fidelity to a specific model may not always be the most important influence on treatment outcome. However, some studies do suggest an association between better model fidelity and outcome (for instance in Multisystemic Therapy; Schoenwald *et al.*, 2000). Maximizing *both* the quality of alliance and model fidelity may naturally have additive value; however, their relative effect is an important empirical question for training and service planning and has been under-studied. Castonguay *et al.* (1996) for instance directly compared quality of therapeutic alliance, the relational focus of sessions and therapist fidelity to a cognitively-focused CBT protocol, as predictors of outcome in adult depression. Alliance and relationship focus were found to carry the bulk of the treatment effect, and a rigid adherence to the cognitive model in the face of patient resistance tended to produce a poor outcome. This study emphasizes the dangers of "cook book" therapy routines and the need for manualized models of any kind to be applied with flexibility and sensitivity to patient need; but the broader question of the relative value of different treatment types as against non specific factors remains understudied. This will be considered further below in relation to individual psychotherapies.

Relational aspects are also implicated in the important area of treatment adherence. A study of 344 children (7–18 years) attending community mental health clinics in the US (Garcia & Weisz, 2002) found that premature termination of treatment was more associated with problems in the "therapeutic relationship" than lack of family motivation, practical difficulties, time concerns, or perceived lack of symptom improvement. Breaking off treatment in this way might arguably be protective; in a study of adult schizophrenia, continuing with session attendance in the face of a poor alliance actually produced adverse outcomes compared to no treatment (Dunn *et al.*, 2007); a similar finding is suggested in adolescent depression (Elvins, 2012). More specialist techniques of engagement in "hard-to-reach" groups has had some success; discussed in the following sections on MI and Mentalization Based Therapy.

Attachment-based therapy

Shirk and Russell (1996) argued that the large literature on interpersonal processes in developmental psychology should be applied to the study of the therapeutic relationship. Therapist qualities promoting a positive personal alliance are similar to those described in the developmental attachment literature as promoting secure-base attachment. In John Bowlby's concept of "secure base" therapy (Bowlby, 1988), this idea is extended to form the core of the therapy process. Bowlby used a juxtaposition central to attachment theory; that proximity to a secure attachment figure assuages anxiety which then acts to facilitate an exploratory movement away from the attachment figure toward exploration, development, other-directedness, and new learning. In Bowlby's formulation, the initial therapy task is to provide an interpersonal context within which the patient can work through attachment difficulties to experience the equivalent of such a "secure base" with the therapist; once achieved the patient may then naturally enter an "exploratory" mode in which problem solving and new learning in relation to the realities of the patient's life would emerge. In this solution-focused phase of therapy, the therapist might well act to guide or facilitate but because the ideas came largely from the patient they would be most likely appropriate to circumstance and experienced as self-generated and empowering. Bowlby also maintained that this solution-focused phase of therapy should not be directed by prior theory, but left open to be influenced by knowledge from developmental science. He thus crafted a therapist stance that was responsive, in that the patient would provide themselves many of the ideas for change, and also in the therapist's openness to emerging scientific understanding. This stance marked a break from the theory-driven models underlying psychoanalytic transference and has had a formative legacy for subsequent developments. Bowlby's articulation of a more collaborative therapeutic stance with the patient has become the norm across most varieties of psychotherapeutic work. His opening up of the content of therapeutic discussion to the findings of developmental science allows the possibility of flexible therapeutic strategies in dialogue with research. The result can be seen in contemporary developments such as MBT (see below) and in the adaptations of therapeutic approaches to emerging understanding of developmental disorders considered earlier.

Bowlby's formulation, however, begs a number of questions of detail, which have been insufficiently explored (Eagle, 2006). For instance, what is the process of therapeutic change here? Is a "corrective emotional experience" with the therapist enough to alter the internal assumptions and working models of attachment within the therapeutic relationship, or is some further procedure necessary? Detailed technical and procedural aspects of helping change in this model are beyond the scope of this chapter; but will involve inevitably a range of elements at the therapist's disposal, including cognitive restructuring, emotional rehearsal, desensitization, management of anxiety, modeling and others. In contemporary practice, therapeutic procedures can be informed by developmental research as to moderators of change from longitudinal or epidemiological studies; for instance, when working with vulnerable female adolescents, planning or the choice of a partner might be critical elements to consider and in working with children with externalizing behaviors, aspects of attention deficit hyperactivity disorder (ADHD) or Callous and Unemotional Traits might be important. The point is the integration of psychological therapy practice with empirical information from emerging developmental studies. In Bowlby's formulation a common feature is the initial need to engage the patient into a secure alliance. This will be easier in some patients than others, depending on their prior attachment and interpersonal experience. Bowlby's procedures were predicated on his clients having underlying difficulties with insecure relationships; next we consider adaptations to more complex ambivalence and disorganized mental states.

Motivational interviewing

It is a subtle paradox—observed also in other kinds of reciprocal relationship such as childhood attachment or joint attention in infancy—that while clinicians will wish to enhance patient alliance and relatedness in treatment, they cannot impose or control this—indeed trying to do so is likely to be particularly counterproductive. Motivational Interviewing (MI) is an approach to this paradox that was first developed in the context of substance misuse in adults but whose principles have been generalized to child and adolescent work (Baer & Peterson, 2002; Naar-King & Suarez, 2011). The interpersonal therapeutic stance in MI pays great attention to the details of the therapists' communication, working to enhance alliance and to identify discrepancies between the client's current situation or behavior and their own values or wishes, thus eliciting and reinforcing the seeds of a motivation towards change. In keeping with a respect for patient autonomy, "resistance to change" is considered in interpersonal terms as a meaningful reaction to external pressure or demand; the therapist sidesteps this by not suggesting or imposing change themselves but rather with a pattern of reflective questioning to identify and reinforce "change talk" or elements of change behaviors emerging in the client (reminiscent of the emerging solution-focused talk identified by Bowlby). Similarly there are techniques to reduce "sustain" ideas, which serve to maintain the status quo. MI theorists stress that this is not just a set of "techniques"; rather a sustained interpersonal stance with the patient, which reflects, questions and affirms their control of the path toward change. MI thus builds on alliance theory through articulating a set of therapeutic skills particularly well adapted for situations where patients are ambivalent or resistant to change: maintaining collaboration while also undertaking structured assessment or other questioning. MI can be applied to conditions such as substance misuse or eating disorder but also to therapeutic regimes such as medication adherence or behavioral programs. The stance is well adapted to the sensitivities of childhood and adolescence in which young people have often not actively chosen to seek treatment and experience external family or social pressure.

There is limited empirical evidence on the effectiveness of MI in childhood and adolescence. A preliminary study has shown that the addition of MI as a precursor to CBT in adolescent OCD demonstrated faster treatment gains compared to psychoeducation plus CBT (Merlo et al., 2010). In anorexia nervosa, a large RCT comparing outpatient CBT plus MI with standard outpatient and inpatient care (Gowers et al., 2007), found motivation for the therapy improved after the initial MI session and the MI + CBT arm as more cost-effective than the comparators. A variation on MI, Motivational Enhancement Training (MET), improved the speed and cost effectiveness of family therapy in reducing bulimic symptoms (Schmidt et al., 2007).

Psychotherapeutic treatments for children and adolescents

Mentalization based treatment

A further elaboration of the therapeutic relationship in treatment, particularly in the context of more complex psychopathology such as borderline states, is found in MBT.

This is possibly the most important therapeutic extension to attachment-related therapy since Bowlby's secure-base treatment, adding to it a more developed theory of mentalization. It is particularly applicable in the context of patients whose mental state is highly unstable or showing borderline personality traits, where MBT takes evidence-based theory to illuminate the therapeutic relationship. The empirical basis of MBT arises from work following Bowlby on states of disorganized attachment, commonly related to intergenerational trauma. Disorganized attachment is associated with significant child psychopathology and in adults particularly with borderline mental states. One of the development consequences of disorganized attachment is a relative failure of reflective function or "mentalization"; and it is the particular focus of MBT to recover such reflective function in patients' lives as a condition for developing mental health (Fonagy et al., 2002). Like CBT, therapist and patient in MBT occupy a shared empirical stance—but whereas in CBT the object of common regard is the pattern of client cognition in relation to affect and behavior, in MBT an important focus is the therapeutic relationship itself and a capacity to reflect on the mental states (thoughts, feelings and beliefs) arising within it. The mechanism of treatment is also different. In CBT, techniques of probabilistic reasoning are used, whereas in MBT, the therapist models for the patient in real time within the therapy how action, reflection, and insight have to be worked for authentically. The patient experiences the therapist monitoring and correcting their own mentalizing failures, "not knowing" prior answers, accepting differences in therapist and patient perspectives, actively questioning ("what questions") rather than explaining ("why questions"), and clarifying unclear communication (Bateman & Fonagy, 2008).

MBT is not presented as a "new form" of psychotherapy—rather it offers series of technical approaches to promote reflective function, which can be applied in the context of diverse forms of therapy. In that sense (although the details of approach are different), it bears some comparison with MI and alliance theory, as well as having origins in Bowlby's therapeutic orientation. Each of these approaches is grounded in empirical research and takes a more "modular" approach to elements of therapeutic strategy in contrast to self-contained "named" or "labeled" therapies. The logical extension of this approach is an empirically based psychotherapy combining evidenced effective elements utilized according to individual patient need. This is not to advocate an arbitrary "pick-and-mix," because coherence is important; but instead for a reconceptualization of what promotes therapeutic change in specific conditions. Bateman has elaborated this idea in the context of Borderline Personality Disorder (Bateman, 2012).

MBT has been adapted in a number of different settings for work with children and families (Midgley & Vrouva, 2012). In an RCT with adolescents who self-harmed and had depression, MBT-A was compared with treatment as usual, which was predominantly CBT and counseling intervention ($n = 80$; Rossouw & Fonagy, 2012), MBT-A was delivered in weekly individual sessions with monthly family-based sessions focused on affect regulation and mentalization. A moderate effect size in favor of MBT-A was found in both self-reported and interview-based self-harm estimates after 1 year of treatment, most strikingly in numbers reporting no self harm over 3 months (chi^2 5, $p = 0.01$; NNT (number needed to treat) 3.66). Treatment effect was associated with relative reduction in self-reported attachment avoidance and borderline features, with evidence of mediation from both on the reduction in self harm. This study needs replication on larger samples (there was considerable treatment dropout in both arms) but is an important preliminary result given the lack of treatment effect found over many years in other interventions for the important problem of adolescent self harm (Ougrin et al., 2012). Related developments are an adaptation of MBT for mood disorders called Dynamic Interpersonal Therapy (DIT, Lemma et al., 2011), a version for working with families (MBT-F; Keaveny et al., 2012) and an adaptation of a mentalizing focus within systemic multidisciplinary work for "hard to reach" young people, called AMBIT (Bevington et al., 2013). Each of these approaches is in development and has yet to be evaluated using randomized clinical trials.

Short term psychodynamic psychotherapy (STPP)

Any evaluation of current psychodynamic psychotherapy depends on its definition. One influential account (Shedler, 2010) takes a process orientated generic approach, defining psychodynamic psychotherapy in terms of its focus on a client's emotions and attempts to avoid distressing thoughts and feelings, discussion of past experiences and interpersonal relationships, exploration of wishes and fantasies, and relevance of the current therapy relationship. Other contemporary practitioners (e.g., Delgado, 2008) emphasize a more traditional psychoanalytic theory-driven account, giving central importance to the unconscious in mental functioning, the existence of internalised unconscious conflicts, the symbolic meaning of behaviors and the analysis in therapy of transference-based thoughts and behaviors. The more generic process-orientated account underlies recent reviews of the adult literature (Shedler, 2010), arguing for the increasing evidence of effectiveness of psychotherapy intervention and asserting that psychodynamic principles are common relational factors, which carry the treatment effect in a number of other treatment methods (for instance CBT). This makes psychodynamic therapy theory convergent with common-factors theory and therapeutic alliance. A narrative review of child and adolescent STPP (Midgley & Kennedy, 2011) included any trial described by its authors as involving STPP, but because such studies rarely used manuals (a situation that is improving), it is difficult to know what really is being studied. The review identified eight randomized trials but most had significant methodological difficulties mainly related to small sample size. In a randomized equivalence trial of a manualized STPP versus family therapy for child depression, Trowell *et al.* (2007) found that both groups improved, with no between-group effects. A quasi-experimental non randomized trial of an 11 week manualized form of STPP for anxiety and depression in middle childhood was studied against usual care in Italy (Muratori *et al.*, 2003). The focus was on parent-mediated treatment but with the addition of child sessions. No treatment effect was observed at 6 months but at 2 year follow-up an effect in favor of experimental treatment was observed on parent-CBCL, particularly on anxiety-related symptoms and in clinician Childhood Global Assessment Scale (both outcomes were non-blinded assessments). A recent meta-analysis of short-term (under 40 sessions) STPP for children and adolescents (Abbass *et al.*, 2013) found 11 RCT or quasi-experimental studies (total $n = 655$) with mean child age of 11.3 years (SD 2.7). Studies varied greatly in size and quality, overall classed as moderate. The majority represented equivalence trials against a total of 13 comparator treatments such as CBT, long-term psychotherapy, IPT, FT; only three studies had an attention control or non treatment control group. Patient groups included emotional disorder, mixed disorders, anxiety disorders and personality problems. Overall, there were generally high within-group effects in both arms of studies but very few between-group differences separating STPP from comparators. Sensitivity analysis suggested that there might be the possibility of some sleeper effects with increasing gains at follow-up (echoing findings also in adulthood; Shedler, 2010) and a positive effect of therapist adherence to the model. The greatest between-group effect in favor of STPP was found in mixed disorders and emotional/behavioral disorders; CBT comparators were more effective than STPP in mood disorder. The findings from this meta-analysis suggest that short-term psychoanalytic psychotherapy may fare no worse than comparators or treatment as usual in some contexts. However, it is difficult to make robust inference on efficacy given the lack of between group differences and non equivalence controls. The body of trial evidence for psychotherapy is considerably smaller than that for CBT or even family therapy, with the best evidence in relation to mood disorder. The quality of intervention studies is showing some signs of improvement, for instance, the large IMPACT trial underway of STPP, CBT, and specialist clinical care for adolescent depression shows considerable increase in sophistication over previous psychotherapy studies, (Goodyer *et al.*, 2011).

Interpersonal psychotherapy

IPT is a manualized psychotherapy that focuses on the reciprocal relationship between mood-state and the client's current real-world social relationships; it is pragmatic rather than theory driven in its focus on disruption in interpersonal relationships as an antecedent for mood change and improvement of relationships as a route into improving mood (Weissman *et al.*, 2000). IPT is time-limited (12–16 weekly sessions) and particularly focused on and evidenced in adults for depressive

illness, although adaptations for other mood and eating disorders have been made. Developed from a root in counseling rather than dynamic psychotherapy, there is less emphasis than STPP or MBT on the interpersonal relationship between therapist and patient during treatment, although the establishment of therapeutic alliance is incorporated into the therapy process. In the assessment phase of IPT, the client undertakes a review of current relationships, identifies how their mood problems interact with these and the relationship features associated with the onset of mood disorder. This allows the selection of a focus for therapeutic work from a number of typical areas of difficulty in depression, such as grief after the loss of a loved one, conflict in significant relationships, difficulties adapting to changes in relationships or life circumstances; or difficulties stemming from social isolation. In the adaptation of IPT for adolescence (IPT-A) additional areas are included such as separation from parents, single parent families, development of romantic relationships and initial experience with death of a relative or friend. In the treatment phase, the client learns to link changes in mood to events occurring in his/her relationships within the problem areas, identifies communication and problem-solving techniques for that problem area and practises these in the therapy sessions prior to using them outside of the session in the context of significant relationships (Mufson, 2010). IPT-A thus aims to help the adolescent identify and develop more adaptive methods for dealing with the interpersonal issues associated with the onset or maintenance of their depression. Although the treatment involves primarily individual sessions with the teenager, parents are asked to participate in a few sessions to receive education about depression, to address any relationship difficulties that may be occurring between the adolescent and his/her parents and to help support the adolescent's treatment. The final sessions work with issues of termination of treatment and maintenance of change.

In adolescents, an initial RCT ($n = 48$; Mufson *et al.*, 1999) found that 18 (75%) of 24 patients who completed IPT-A met recovery criterion on the Hamilton Rating Scale for Depression at 12 week endpoint compared to 11 (46%) in the control condition ($p = 0.04$, no effect size (ES) quoted), but there was no group effect in suicidality or global functioning or self-rated Beck depression inventory. A different parallel adaptation of the adult IPT model was tested in Puerto Rico in an equivalence trial against CBT and wait-list (Rossello & Bernal, 1999). Both IPT ($n = 23$; ES 0.72) and CBT ($n = 25$; ES 0.43) showed improvement over wait-list ($n = 23$) but endpoint was self-report and baseline inclusion was not standardized. A slightly larger community-based effectiveness study (Mufson *et al.*, 2004) implemented IPT-A with community-based physicians in frontline school health clinics for 63 low-income depressed adolescents. IPT-A showed benefits over treatment as usual on clinician-rated depression scores (Hamilton Depression Inventory; ES 0.5, $p = 0.04$) and global functioning (Child Global Assessment Scale; ES 0.54, $p = 0.04$) in ITT (intention to treat) analysis. Post hoc analysis suggested that high level of conflict with mother and friends at baseline moderated greater treatment effect (Gunlicks-Stoessel *et al.*, 2010). There were limitations around internal validity and sample size indicating the need for further replication; a study in Taiwan (Tang *et al.*, 2009) has recruited adolescents screened in school and diagnosed with moderate to severe depression and suicidality, randomized to a modified shortened form of IPT-A ($n = 35$) against in-school counseling ($n = 38$). The IPT group showed significant improvement over TAU on self-rated Beck Depression, Anxiety and Hopelessness Inventories at the 6-week endpoint in this trial. IPT-A thus has a promising evidence base for adolescent depression and has been evaluated in community settings (see Chapter 63).

Cognitive analytic therapy

CAT is a structured short-term form of psychotherapy that integrates psychodynamic principles with a cognitive focus based on personal construct theory. It is probably the closest to CBT of the psychotherapies and takes a shared stance toward developing a formulation with the patient and tackling cognitive traps, dilemmas and snags in therapeutic progress. CAT differs from IPT in greater use of the therapist–patient relationship in the therapy process and a theoretical focus on the effects of early experience. In the early stages, there is development of a shared written formulation of the key problems for the patient, their origins in previous relationships and experiences and the priorities for therapeutic change. The treatment phase uses problem-orientated discussion and reflection on the therapeutic relationship to gain insight into the operation of learned patterns both in and out of the therapy room and how these relate to the problems in focus. There is relatively little systematic RCT study of CAT and little evidence in adolescence but one study on borderline personality disorder and self harm showed no group effect over general clinical care (Chanen *et al.*, 2008).

Summary

Relationship-based treatments range from a core of process research into common factors across different therapies; to incorporation within an attachment framework around secure base therapy; and then elaboration for difficult client groups, such as those with ambivalent or resistant motivation and complex borderline mental states. Quality of therapist–patient relationship within therapeutic alliance shows consistent modest effects on treatment outcome across a number of types of therapy, although methodology may have historically inflated some of these alliance-outcome correlations. Alliance is affected by prior patient social and psychological functioning as well as therapist behaviors. Bowlby's secure base therapy develops the idea of attachment-relatedness between patient and therapist into a core component of treatment, underpinned by research into insecure attachment-related psychopathology. MBT extends this idea to address the more complex psychopathology associated with disorganized attachment and unstable mental states and MI takes technical development of therapeutic communication in a different direction to address ambivalence and resistance to change. Each of these developments consist of theory-based generic techniques which are designed to be applied across the range of "named" treatment types—indeed there is evidence that it is these non-specific relational factors in therapy that often carry the positive effect of treatment. MBT and MI have particular added value for clients traditionally hard to reach by psychotherapy. Of specific "labeled" therapies: STPP shares some common therapeutic characteristics with the attachment-based therapies and a set of similar relationship-based therapeutic skills, but it is differentiated by therapy content and theory of change based on historical psychoanalytic theory, with little evidenced rationale and variably operationalized in different STPP models. Manualization and systematic testing of STPP approaches has only just begun and the evidence is preliminary. IPT in contrast has a simpler style originating more in humanistic counseling and is focused on approaches to optimize patient social functioning. It has a growing evidence base for depressive disorders in relatively uncomplicated client contexts. CAT is structured and cognitively based with influences from personal construct theory but its evidence base in adolescence is slim.

Implementation science

Each of these relationship-based techniques-building alliance, using secure base theory as a skill in generic therapy and the more complex differentiated skills in MBT and MI are robust core skill sets with an evidence base that should be incorporated into systematic training of child mental health professionals. Implementation science (Eccles *et al.*, 2009; Green, 2012) looks to identify the process and barriers to implementation at a practitioner, system and organizational level. At a practitioner level, training is available for these approaches, but the success of cognitively oriented manualized treatments in recent years may have led to less awareness of these relational techniques. On the other hand, they are at the core of traditional client centred therapeutic practice and are intuitively appealing to many professionals, who often prefer a relational approach (Castonguay *et al.*, 1996; Shenley, 2012) and consider the therapeutic relationship is a key component of practice and outcome (Kazdin *et al.*, 1990; Siegel *et al.*, 1990). At a systems level the introduction in England of the "increasing access to psychological treatment" (IAPT) initiative provides an opportunity to standardize implementation and training in approaches that have empirical support and will increase practice quality. Traditionally psychotherapies have been considered as intensive and expensive; however, the difficulty of helping the increasingly complex cases that access child mental health services and the success of some of these complex theory-based approaches in tackling such difficulties provide a counterbalancing argument. The kind of process-orientated approach advocated by alliance theory, MI and MBT lends itself to flexible usage and empirical testing, which needs to embrace process research and equivalence trials designed to establish the most appropriate treatment methods for different disorders.

Treatment selection

For relationship-based treatments taken as a whole, the theory and current evidence reviewed here suggests that treatment selection be informed by the quality of prior relationship experience and capacity for social functioning. This can be assessed from clinical and developmental history supplemented with measures such as Strengths and Difficulties Questionnaire (SDQ), and attachment-related questionnaires such as the relationships questionnaire (Bartholomew & Horowitz, 1991). A positive prior social functioning and relationship suggests that a positive therapeutic alliance is likely and then a variety of therapeutic modalities have a good chance of effectiveness, with little current evidence that one therapeutic modality has advantage over another except for patient or therapist preference. For cases with disrupted or vulnerable prior relationships or an insecure attachment organisation, therapeutic alliance will be harder and specific techniques of the kind outlined in Bowlby's secure base therapy are needed. Cases presenting with motivational conflict in relation to change will need more sophisticated techniques to establish a therapeutic alliance, such as MI. Finally, there are cases with evidence of a disorganized attachment history, inconsistent relationships, and unstable mental state, often with a history of unresolved trauma; such as young people with borderline personality development, severe relational disturbance, or self-harm. Here, much attention needs to be paid to the establishment of the therapeutic alliance and the best-evidenced approach currently is Mentalization-Based techniques, which can then be combined with an appropriate evidence-based modality of choice. Patients who have no progress in one modality should not be discharged without escalation to a higher risk pathway to attempt further engagement.

Global health

A disproportionate number of young people live in Low and Medium Income Countries (LMIC) and it is a priority for the global health agenda to address early developmental mental health in these countries (Collins *et al.*, 2011). Recent review (Kieling *et al.*, 2011; see Chapter 16) has identified some adaptation of early relationship-focused interventions to LMIC. These include early stimulation intervention for parents and children to improve parental responsiveness in Ethopia (Klein & Rye, 2004), Russia (St Petersberg Orphanage Team, 2008) and Turkey (Kagitcibasi *et al.*, 2009) and in relation to child disability in Vietnam (Shin *et al.*, 2009). No studies into the implementation of specific psychotherapies with older children or adults are reported. There should be no reason why therapeutic alliance and relationship-based work should not form as central a part of mental health provision in LMIC as in high-income countries and there is an urgent need to adapt, test, and deliver evidence-based interventions to LMIC. The core therapeutic modular skills described earlier are relatively accessible and intuitive, but would need systematizing and training for an adaptation to global health.

References

Abbass, A. *et al.* (2013) Psychodynamic psychotherapy for children and adolescents: a meta-analysis of short-term psychodynamic models. *Journal of the American Academy of Child and Adolescent Psychiatry* **52**, 863–75.

Baer, J.S. & Peterson, P.L. (2002) Motivational interviewing with adolescents and young adults. In: *Motivational Interviewing: Preparing People for Change.* (eds W.R. Miller & S. Rollnick), 2nd edn, pp. 217–250. Guilford Press, New York.

Bakermans-Kranenburg, M.J. *et al.* (2003) Less is more: meta-analyses of sensitivity and attachment interventions in early childhood. *Psychological Bulletin* **129**, 195–215.

Barnard, K.E. *et al.* (1988) Prevention of parenting alterations for women with low social support. *Psychiatry* **51**, 248–253.

Bartholomew, K. & Horowitz, L.M. (1991) Attachment styles among young adults: a test of a four-category model. *Journal of Personality and Social Psychology* **61**, 226–244.

Bateman, A.W. (2012) Editorial: treating borderline personality disorder in clinical practice. *American Journal of Psychiatry* **169**, 560–563.

Bateman, A. & Fonagy, P. (1999) Effectiveness of partial hospitalisation in the treatment of borderline personally personality disorder: a randomised controlled trial. *American Journal of Psychiatry* **156**, 1563–1569.

Bateman, A. & Fonagy, P. (2008) Eight year follow-up of patients treated for borderline personality disorder: mentalisation-based treatment versus treatment as usual. *American Journal of Psychiatry* **165**, 631–638.

Beckwith, L. (1988) Intervention with disadvantaged parents of sick preterm infants. *Psychiatry* **51**, 242–247.

Belsky, J. *et al.* (2007) For better and for worse: differential susceptibility to environmental influences. *Current Directions in Psychological Science* **16**, 300–304.

Bevington, D. *et al.* (2013) Innovations in practice: adolescent mentalization-based integrative therapy (AMBIT)—a new integrated approach to working with the most hard to reach adolescents with severe complex mental health needs. *Child and Adolescent Mental Health* **18**, 46–51.

Bowlby, J. (1988) *A Secure Base.* Basic Books, New York.

Cassidy, J. *et al.* (2011) Enhancing infant attachment security: an examination of treatment efficacy and differential susceptibility. *Development and Psychopathology* **23**, 131–148.

Castonguay, L.G. *et al.* (1996) Predicting the effect of cognitive therapy for depression: a study of unique and common factors. *Journal of Consulting and Clinical Psychology* **64**, 497–504.

Chanen, A.M. *et al.* (2008) Early intervention for adolescents with borderline personality disorder using cognitive analytic therapy: randomized controlled trial. *British Journal of Psychiatry* **193**, 477–484.

Cicchetti, D. *et al.* (1999) The efficacy of toddler-parent psychotherapy to increase attachment security in off-spring of depressed mothers. *Attachment and Human Development* **1**, 34–66.

Cicchetti, D. *et al.* (2006) Fostering secure attachment in infants in maltreating families through preventive interventions. *Development and Psychopathology* **18**, 623–649.

Collins, P.Y. *et al.* (2011) Grand challenges in global mental health. *Nature* **475**, 27–30.

Cooper, P.J. *et al.* (2003) Controlled trial of the short- and long-term effect of psychological treatment of post-partum depression. 1. Impact on maternal mood. *British Journal of Psychiatry* **182**, 412–419.

Delgado, S.V. (2008) Psychodynamic psychotherapy for children and adolescents: an old friend revisited. *Psychiatry (Edgmont).* **5**, 67–72.

Dozier, M. *et al.* (2008) Effects of an attachment based intervention on the cortisol production of infants and toddlers in foster care. *Development and Psychopathology* **20**, 845–859.

Dunn, G. & Bentall, R. (2007) Modelling treatment-effect heterogeneity in randomized controlled trials of complex interventions (psychological treatments). *Statistics in Medicine* **26**, 4719–4745.

Eagle, M.N. (2006) Attachment, psychotherapy, and assessment: a commentary. *Journal of Consulting and Clinical Psychology* **74**, 1086–1097.

Eccles, M. *et al.* (2009) An implementation research agenda. *Implementation Science* **4**, 18.

Elvins R (2012) *Therapeutic alliance in a treatment trial of depressed adolescents.* Unpublished MD Thesis, University of Manchester.

Elvins, R. & Green, J. (2008) The conceptualization and measurement of therapeutic alliance: an empirical review. *Clinical Psychology Review* **28**, 1167–1187.

Fonagy, P. *et al.* (eds) (2002) *Affect Regulation Mentalisation and the Development of the Self.* Other Press, New York.

Garcia, J.A. & Weisz, J.R. (2002) When youth mental health care stops: therapeutic relationship problems and other reasons for ending youth outpatient treatment. *Journal of Consulting and Clinical Psychology* **70**, 439–443.

Goodyer, I.M. *et al.* (2011) Improving mood with psychoanalytic and cognitive therapies (IMPACT): a pragmatic effectiveness superiority trial to investigate whether specialised psychological treatment reduces the risk for relapse in adolescents with moderate to severe unipolar depression: study protocol for a randomised controlled trial. *Trials* **12**, 175.

Gowers, S. & North, C. (1999) Difficulties in family functioning and adolescent anorexia nervosa. *British Journal of Psychiatry* **174**, 63–66.

Gowers, S.G. *et al.* (2007) Clinical effectiveness of treatments for anorexia nervosa in adolescents: randomised controlled trial. *The British Journal of Psychiatry* **191**, 427–435.

Green, J. (2006) The therapeutic alliance—a significant but neglected variable in child mental health treatment studies. *Journal of Child Psychology and Psychiatry* **47**, 425–435.

Green, J. (2012) Editorial: science, implementation, and implementation science. *Journal of Child Psychology and Psychiatry* **53**, 333–336.

Green, J. & Dunn, G. (2008) Using intervention trials in developmental psychiatry to illuminate basic science. *British Journal of Psychiatry* **192**, 323–325.

Green, J. *et al.* (2010) Parent-mediated communication-focused treatment for preschool children with autism (PACT): a randomised controlled trial. *The Lancet* **375**, 2152–2160.

Green, J. *et al.* (2011) Group therapy for adolescents with repeated self harm: randomised controlled trial with economic evaluation. *British Medical Journal* **342**, d682.

Gunlicks-Stoessel, M. *et al.* (2010) The impact of perceived interpersonal functioning on treatment for adolescent depression: IPT-A versus treatment as usual in school-based health clinics. *Journal of Consulting and Clinical Psychology* **78**, 260–267.

Heywood, S. *et al.* (2003) A brief consultation and advisory approach for use in child and adolescent mental services: a pilot study. *Journal of Clinical Child Psychology and Psychiatry* **8**, 1359–1045.

Hoffman, K.T. *et al.* (2006) Changing toddlers' and preschoolers' attachment classifications: the circle of security intervention. *Journal of Consulting and Clinical Psychology* **74**, 1017–1026.

Hougaard, E. (1994) The therapeutic alliance—a conceptual analysis. *Scandinavian Journal of Psychology* **35**, 67–85.

Jacobson, S.W. & Frye, K.F. (1991) Effects of maternal social support on attachment: experimental evidence. *Child Development* **62**, 572–582.

Johnson, M.H. (2011) Interactive specialization: a domain-general framework for human functional brain development? *Developmental Cognitive Neuroscience* **1**, 7–21.

Juffer, F. *et al.* (2008) *Promoting Positive Parenting: An Attachment-Based Intervention.* Taylor Francis Group, New York.

Kaale, A. *et al.* (2014) Preschool-based social communication treatment for children with autism: 12-month follow-up of a randomized trial. *Journal of the American Academy of Child and Adolescent Psychiatry* **53**, 188–198.

Kagitcibasi, C. *et al.* (2009) Continuing effects of early enrichment in adult life: the Turkish early enrichment project 22 years later. *Journal of Applied Developmental Psychology* **30**, 764–79.

Karver, M.S. *et al.* (2005) A theoretical model of common process factors in youth and family therapy. *Mental Health Services Research* **7**, 35–51.

Karver, M.S. *et al.* (2006) Meta-analysis of therapeutic relationship variables in youth and family therapy: the evidence for different relationship variables in the child and adolescent treatment outcome literature. *Clinical Psychology Review* **26**, 50–65.

Kasari, C. *et al.* (2008) Language outcome in autism: randomized comparison of joint attention and play interventions. *Journal of Consulting and Clinical Psychology* **76**, 125–37.

Kasari, C. *et al.* (2010) Randomized controlled caregiver mediated joint engagement intervention for toddlers with autism. *Journal of Autism and Developmental Disorders* **40**, 1045–1056.

Kazdin, A.E. & Durbin, K.A. (2012) Predictors of child-therapist alliance in cognitive-behavioural treatment of children referred for oppositional and antisocial behaviour. *Psychotherapy* **49**, 202–217.

Kazdin, A.E. & Nock, M.K. (2003) Delineating mechanisms of change in child and adolescent therapy: methodological issues and research recommendations. *Journal of Child Psychology and Psychiatry and Allied Disciplines* **44**, 1116–1129.

Kazdin, A.E. & Whitley, M. (2006) Pretreatment social relations, therapeutic alliance and improvements in parenting practices in parent management training. *Journal of Consulting and Clinical Psychology* **74**, 345–355.

Kazdin, A. *et al.* (1990) Drawing on clinical-practice to inform research on child and adolescent psychotherapy—survey of practitioners. *Professional Psychology-Research and Practice* **21**, 189–198.

Keaveny, E. *et al.* (2012) Minding the family mind: the development and initial evaluation of mentalization based treatment for families. In:

Minding the Child: Mentalization-Based Interventions with Children, Young People and Their Families. (eds N. Midgley & I. Vrouva). Routledge, London.

Kendall, T. *et al.* (2013) Guideline development group. *British Medical Journal* **347**, f4865.

Kieling, C. *et al.* (2011) Child and adolescent mental health worldwide: evidence for action. *The Lancet* **378**, 1515–1525.

Klein, P. & Rye, H. (2004) Interaction-oriented early intervention in Ethiopia. The MISC approach. *Infants Young Child* **17**, 340–354.

Kraemer, H.C. *et al.* (2002) Mediators and moderators of treatment effects in randomized clinical trials. *Archives of General Psychiatry* **59**, 877–883.

Krupnick, J.L. *et al.* (1996) The role of the therapeutic alliance in psychotherapy and pharmacotherapy outcome: findings in the national institute of mental health treatment of depression collaborative research program. *Journal of Consulting and Clinical Psychology* **64**, 532–539.

Lemma, A. *et al.* (2011) *Brief Dynamic Interpersonal Therapy: A Clinician's Guide.* Oxford University Press, Oxford.

Lieberman, A. *et al.* (1991) Preventive intervention and outcome with anxiously attached dyads. *Child Development* **62**, 199–209.

Lozoff, B. *et al.* (2010) Home intervention improves cognitive and social-emotional scores in iron-deficient anemic infants. *Pediatrics* **126**, e884–e894.

Martin, D.J. *et al.* (2000) Relation of the therapeutic alliance with outcome and other variables: a meta-analytic review. *Journal of Consulting and Clinical Psychology* **68**, 438–450.

Merlo, L.J. *et al.* (2010) Cognitive behavioral therapy plus motivational interviewing improves outcome for pediatric obsessive–compulsive disorder: a preliminary study. *Cognitive Behaviour Therapy* **39**, 24–27.

Midgley, N. & Kennedy, E. (2011) Psychodynamic psychotherapy for children and adolescents: a critical review of the evidence base. *Journal of Child Psychotherapy* **37**, 1–29.

Midgley, N. & Vrouva, I. (eds) (2012) *Minding the Child: Mentalization-Based Interventions with Children, Young People and Their Families.* Routledge, London.

Midgley, N. *et al.* (2006) The outcome of child psychoanalysis from the patient's point of view: a qualitative analysis of a long-term follow-up study. *Psychology and Psychotherapy: Theory, Practice, Research.* **79**, 257–269.

Moss, E. *et al.* (2011) Efficacy of a home-visiting intervention aimed at improving maternal sensitivity, child attachment, and behavioral outcomes for maltreated children: a randomized control trial. *Development and Psychopathology* **23**, 195–210.

Mufson, L. (2010) Interpersonal psychotherapy for depressed adolescents (IPT-A): extending the reach from academic to community settings. *Child and Adolescent Mental Health* **15**, 66–72.

Mufson, L. *et al.* (1999) Efficacy of interpersonal psychotherapy for depressed adolescents. *Archives of General Psychiatry* **56**, 573–579.

Mufson, L. *et al.* (2004) A randomized effectiveness trial of interpersonal psychotherapy for depressed adolescents. *Archives of General Psychiatry* **61**, 577–584.

Muratori, F. *et al.* (2003) A two year follow up of psychodynamic psychotherapy for internalizing disorders in children. *Journal of the American Academy of Child and Adolescent Psychiatry* **42**, 331–339.

Murray, L. *et al.* (2003) Controlled trial of the short- and long-term effect of psychological treatment of post-partum depression.

2. Impact on the mother-child relationship and child outcome. *British Journal of Psychiatry* **182**, 420–427.

Naar-King, S. & Suarez, M. (eds) (2011) *Motivational Interviewing with Adolescents and Young Adults.* Guilford Press, New York.

Ougrin, D. *et al.* (2012) Practitioner review: self harm in adolescence. *Journal of Child Psychology and Psychiatry* **53**, 337–350.

Rossello, J. & Bernal, G. (1999) The efficacy of cognitive-behavioural and interpersonal treatments for depression in Puerto Rican adolescents. *Journal of Consulting and Clinical Psychology* **6**, 734–745.

Rossouw, T. & Fonagy, P. (2012) Mentalisation-based treatment for self harm in adolescence: a randomised controlled trial. *Journal of the American Academy of Child and Adolescent Psychiatry* **51**, 1304–1313.

Schmidt, U. *et al.* (2007) A randomized controlled trial of family therapy and cognitive behavior therapy guided self-care for adolescents with bulimia nervosa and related disorders. *American Journal of Psychiatry* **164**, 591–598.

Schoenwald, S.K. *et al.* (2000) Multisystemic therapy: monitoring treatment fidelity. *Family Process* **39**, 83–103.

Shedler, J. (2010) The efficacy of psychodynamic psychotherapy. *American Psychologist* **65**, 98–109.

Shin, J.Y. *et al.* (2009) The effects of a home-based intervention for young children with intellectual disabilities in Vietnam. *Journal of Intellectual Disability Research* **53**, 339–352.

Shirk, S.R. & Karver, M. (2003) Prediction of treatment outcome from relationship variables in child and adolescent therapy: a meta-analytic review. *Journal of Consulting and Clinical Psychology* **71**, 452–464.

Shirk, S.R. & Russell, R.L. (1996) *Change Processes in Child Psychotherapy; Revitalising Treatment and Research.* The Guilford Press, New York.

Stein, A. *et al.* (2006) Treating disturbances in the relationship between mothers with bulimic eating disorders and their infants: a randomized, controlled trial of video feedback. *The American Journal of Psychiatry* **163**, 899–906.

Tang, T.C. *et al.* (2009) Randomized study of school-based intensive interpersonal psychotherapy for depressed adolescents with suicidal risk and parasuicide behaviors. *Psychiatry and Clinical Neurosciences* **63**, 463–70.

The St. Petersburg-USA Orphanage Research Team (2008) The effects of early social-emotional and relationship experience on the development of young orphanage children. *Monographs of the Society for Research in Child Development* **73**, 1–297.

Trowell, J. *et al.* (2002) Psychotherapy for sexually abused girls: psychopathological outcome findings and patterns of change. *British Journal of Psychiatry* **180**, 234–47.

Trowell, J. *et al.* (2007) Childhood depression: a place for psychotherapy. An outcome study comparing individual psychodynamic psychotherapy and family therapy. *European Child and Adolescent Psychiatry* **16**, 157–167.

Van den Boom, D.C. (1994) The influence of temperament and mothering on attachment and exploration—an experimental manipulation of sensitive responsiveness among lower-class mothers with irritable infants. *Child Development* **65**, 1457–1477.

Van Zeijl, J. *et al.* (2006) Attachment-based intervention for enhancing sensitive discipline in mothers of one—to three-year-old children at risk for externalizing behavior problems. A Randomized controlled trial. *Journal of Consulting and Clinical Psychology* **74**, 994–1005.

Velderman, K.M. *et al.* (2006) Effects of attachment –based interventions on maternal sensitivity and infant attachment: differential susceptibility of highly reactive infants. *Journal of Family Psychology* **20**, 266–274.

Walker, S.P. *et al.* (2010) The effect of psychosocial stimulation on cognition and behaviour at 6 years in a cohort of term, low-birthweight Jamaican children. *Developmental Medicine & Child Neurology* **52**, e148–e154.

Wan, M.W. *et al.* (2013) Quality of interaction between at-risk infants and caregiver at 12–15 months is associated with 3-year autism outcome. *Journal of Child Psychology and Psychiatry* **54**, 763–71.

Weissman, M.M. *et al.* (eds) (2000) *Comprehensive Guide to Interpersonal Psychotherapy*. Basic Books, Inc., New York.

CHAPTER 41

Educational interventions for children's learning difficulties

Charles Hulme[1] and Monica Melby-Lervåg[2]

[1] Division of Psychology and Language Sciences, University College London, UK
[2] Department of Special Needs Education, University of Oslo, Norway

Conceptual and methodological issues

Educational or psychological interventions, whatever they are for, should be based on sound principles. Preferably, interventions should be based on a theory of the nature and causes of a disorder that the intervention is designed to help. It is worth emphasizing that the fields of education and special education are plagued by interventions that lack a sound theoretical rationale. It is always possible that such interventions will have effects, but we should demand very high levels of evidence to convince us that interventions that are not based on a sound theoretical foundation really are effective.

We would emphasize that clinicians should evaluate claims for the effectiveness of new educational treatments with caution. For any proposed treatment, a clinician should ask two basic questions: (1) Is the proposed intervention theoretically plausible (i.e., does the intervention directly target a skill that is deficient in a given population, or target a process which has been identified as a likely cause of a disorder)? (2) If the answer to question (1) is positive, is there evidence from one or more randomized controlled trials (RCTs) to indicate that the intervention has beneficial effects (with reasonable effect sizes)?

In this chapter, we will concentrate on interventions for which there is good evidence for their effectiveness. We will not deal with interventions for which we believe evidence for their effectiveness is lacking or negative. Two examples of such interventions would be the Dore programme which focussed on training balance skills (Reynolds *et al.*, 2003) and the use of colored overlays or lenses, both of which appear to be ineffective as treatments for dyslexia (Snowling & Hulme, 2003; Henderson *et al.*, 2012). Our silence in this chapter on these interventions (and many others that lack a sound theoretical rationale) reflects our judgement that adequate evidence for their efficacy is simply lacking.

Although methodological issues have been dealt with elsewhere (see Chapter 14), we believe that it is important to emphasize the types of evidence that can establish that interventions "work." In practice, this means the use of RCTs, quasi-experiments, or regression discontinuity designs. In the sections that follow, we will summarize a great deal of evidence (mostly from RCTs). The studies we review show that a range of educational interventions have been developed that are effective when delivered to children selected for having difficulties in developing key educational skills (problems of reading accuracy and fluency, problems of reading comprehension and problems with arithmetic skills). The studies usually involve specialist teaching delivered either to individual children or children in small groups.

Dyslexia and decoding impairments

Nature and causes of dyslexia and decoding impairments

Dyslexia, a severe difficulty in learning to read (in the sense of recognizing printed words accurately and fluently), is a relatively common disorder. Historically, dyslexia was typically defined using a discrepancy definition whereby a child's reading attainment needed to be out of line with their age and IQ (e.g., Rutter & Yule, 1975). Such a definition though still widely used has fallen from favor and DSM-5 makes no explicit reference to this (see Chapter 53). For children within the normal range of intellectual ability (IQs above 70), IQ appears only weakly correlated with reading accuracy and there is little evidence that IQ is predictive of variations in children's response to specialist reading instruction to improve decoding skills (e.g., Hatcher & Hulme, 1999).

Dyslexia is typically diagnosed when a person has severe difficulties with reading accuracy as assessed by a well standardized test. Given that reading skills have a continuous distribution in the population, the cut-off point for defining "dyslexia" is inherently arbitrary. Epidemiological studies suggest that, depending on where the diagnostic cut off is set, dyslexia affects approximately 3–8% of children (Peterson & Pennington, 2012). Decoding problems will not only affect the ability to read accurately at a word level, but also impair reading fluency and reading comprehension (Hulme & Snowling, 2009).

The currently accepted view is that the most powerful causal risk factor for dyslexia lies in the phonological system of language (i.e., the system responsible for representing sound structure of spoken words, see Chapter 53). Although the precise nature of this phonological deficit has been much debated, it appears that phonemic skills (being able to identify and manipulate the constituent sounds in spoken words) measured in children at the earliest stages of learning to read are closely related to the growth in children's word reading skills (Melby-Lervåg, et al., 2012). On this basis, it has been argued that the core problem in dyslexia is a difficulty in creating well-specified phonemic representations of speech (Hulme & Snowling, 2009). These findings have important applied implications because they suggest that the early teaching of reading, and the remedial teaching given to children with dyslexia, should emphasize the direct teaching of phonemic skills.

However, another key problem for children with dyslexia is learning letter-sound correspondences and poor letter-sound knowledge is another longitudinal predictor of learning to read (Lervåg et al., 2009). Furthermore, analyses from an intervention designed to improve decoding skills in children at risk of reading difficulties showed that improvements in phoneme awareness (the ability to identify and manipulate the individual speech sounds in spoken words) and letter-sound knowledge at the end of the intervention were two key mediators of subsequent increases in word level reading skills (Hulme et al., 2012). This suggests that children with weak word reading skills require help targeting phonemic awareness and letter-sound knowledge. However, it is important to emphasize that to be maximally effective, such interventions also need to be coupled with direct instruction in word recognition and book reading practice (Hatcher et al., 1994).

Interventions targeting phonology
Meta-analyses of outcome studies
Several meta-analyses have been published summarizing the effectiveness of phonological interventions designed to improve reading skills in children with reading difficulties (Bus & van Ijzendoorn, 1999; Ehri et al., 2000; Lonigan et al., 2008a, b). The most recent meta-analysis (Lonigan et al., 2008a, b), includes 83 well-controlled intervention studies (RCTs or quasi experiments with a control group and a pre-test–post-test design). The studies reviewed aimed to develop phonological awareness, alphabet

knowledge, and early decoding skills in unselected children and children with learning disorders in kindergarten or preschool. Virtually all of the studies had interventions that included some form of phonological awareness training delivered either individually or in small groups. This training taught children to identify phonemes in words (i.e., to match words with the same initial sound) or to manipulate phonemes in words (i.e., combine sounds to form spoken words or segment or delete parts of spoken words) and was typically combined with phonic reading instruction (training letter knowledge and training children to relate the letters in printed words to the sounds they represent). The intervention programmes were typically given in addition to any instruction children were already receiving, and usually the control group was untreated (i.e., they received whatever was typical teaching in their preschool or kindergarten). The meta-analysis showed that these interventions produced large improvements in phonological awareness ($d = 0.82$, that is, children who received an intervention targeting phonology improved by 0.82 of a standard deviation more on measures of phonological awareness than the control children). Importantly, word reading also improved more in the intervention than the control children ($d = 0.42$) as did spelling ($d = 0.61$).

It should also be noted that a recent meta-analysis focusing exclusively on children and adults with reading difficulties showed that phonic reading instruction (teaching that focusses on getting children to understand letter-sound rules) with or without phonological awareness training had positive effects on word reading accuracy ($d = 0.47$) and word reading fluency ($d = 0.51$; McArthur et al., 2012). Similarly, another recent meta-analysis (Coleman et al., 2013) examining interventions targeting phonology and phonic reading instruction in children with language disorders produced moderate to large improvements ($d = 0.45$–2.91) on measures of word reading and spelling. In summary, we can conclude that interventions targeting phonology along with letter-sound training and phonic reading instruction have clear and positive effects on children's reading, spelling, and phonological skills. This conclusion is also consistent with earlier meta-analyses (Bus & van Ijzendoorn, 1999; Ehri et al., 2000).

Moderators of outcome
Lonigan et al. (2008a, b) examined a large range of moderators that may help to explain variations in the size of intervention effects across the studies included in their meta-analysis. There was no evidence that the size of the effect was dependent on age or developmental level of the children or how the study was designed, nor were there any significant differences in effects between the different interventions. However, there were large differences between the interventions used, making it difficult to detect systematic variations in their effectiveness. Nevertheless, the results suggest that the best intervention effects are likely to be achieved when phonological awareness training is combined with teaching related to letter knowledge or phonically based reading instruction. Moreover, notably, phonological awareness

training appeared to be more effective when focusing on smaller units in speech such as phonemes (say the sounds in the word CAT -> /k/ /ae/ /t/) rather than larger units such as rimes (a rime unit is the part of a spoken syllable that follows the initial consonant (if there is one); so the rime unit in CAT is /at/) or syllables (Melby-Lervag *et al.*, 2012).

Interventions targeting reading fluency
Meta-analyses of outcome studies

In older children with dyslexia, basic word-level decoding skills may be mastered, but reading often remains dysfluent (slow and labored). Poor reading fluency can be a significant impediment to success in formal education. In a meta-analysis, Samuels *et al.* (2000) summarized the effects of interventions designed to remediate problems with reading fluency. These interventions all involved some form of guided repeated oral reading, which involves pupils reading and re-reading a text repeatedly, until a pre-specified level of proficiency has been met. The meta-analysis included studies where a training group had received a repeated reading intervention, with an untreated control group. Studies had to have pre-test and post-test measures of reading that were not based on the material used for training. Sixteen studies were included with children ranging in age from Grades 2 to 9 (6 to 13 years) and with both normally achieving children and children with reading difficulties. The results showed moderate effects from repeated reading on the different reading outcomes (decoding fluency $d = 0.44$, word recognition $d = 0.55$ and reading comprehension $d = 0.35$). The small number of studies did not allow for a conventional moderator analysis. The results from Samuels *et al.* (2000) were supported by those from another meta-analysis by Therrien (2004) that found substantial effects of repeated reading practice on measures of reading fluency ($d = 0.83$) and comprehension ($d = 0.67$). However, there are very few well-designed studies of repeated reading practice and both these meta-analyses included studies that had poor designs. We badly need more evidence concerning the effectiveness of repeated reading practice and other possible interventions to help remediate problems of reading fluency.

Recent studies targeting phonology and decoding

A number of recent studies were not included in the meta-analyses summarized earlier. Wolff (2011) studied the effects of a phonics-based reading intervention programme in 9-year-old Swedish children. The children ($n = 112$) were randomly assigned to either an intervention or a control group and received one-to-one tutoring for 12 weeks for a total of 40 hours. About 60% of the intervention time was spent on phonemic awareness training (learning to segment and manipulate the constituent phonemes in spoken words) and decoding (practising reading words and non words aloud, by sequentially "sounding out" unfamiliar words if necessary), with the rest of the time being spent on comprehension strategies and fluency

training. The results showed immediate improvements after intervention in spelling ($d = 0.30$), reading comprehension ($d = 0.41$), reading speed ($d = 0.15$) and phoneme awareness ($d = 0.43$). At follow-up a year later, significant effects on spelling and reading comprehension remained. The follow-up effects were mediated by the effects on phoneme awareness immediately after the intervention (supporting the finding of Hulme *et al.*, 2012).

Bowyer-Crane *et al.* (2008) reported a randomized trial that compared the efficacy of a phonology with reading intervention and an oral language intervention in children selected for poor language skills ($n = 152$). The children were just under 5 years old at the beginning of the study. The phonology with reading intervention involved training in letter-sound knowledge, phonological awareness (including articulatory awareness) and reading books at the instructional level. Direct teaching in sight word recognition was also included in order to build up children's reading vocabulary. The oral language intervention programme included direct instruction to develop vocabulary, inferencing, expressive language, and listening skills. Both programmes were delivered by specially trained teaching assistants working in the children's schools. Teaching sessions alternated between individual and small group lessons on different days. After 20 weeks of intervention, children in the phonology with reading group showed an advantage over the oral language group on literacy and phonological measures ($d = 0.4$ for decoding accuracy; $d = 0.4$ for spelling accuracy and $d = 0.7$ for phoneme blending (the examiner says a sequence of sounds and the child has to produce the target word (/k/ /ae/ /t// -> "cat") and segmentation (the examiner says a word and the child has to break it into its constituent sounds CAT -> /k/ /ae/ /t/)). By contrast, children in the oral language group showed an advantage over the phonology with reading group on measures of vocabulary and grammatical skills. These gains were maintained over a 5-month period after the intervention had ceased.

Finally, Vadasy and Sanders (2010) reported a randomized trial evaluating the effects of phonics based instruction in a group of kindergarten children who performed in the bottom half of their class on measures of phonological awareness and letter knowledge. The intervention consisted of individual instruction in phonics, phonemic awareness, early decoding, and spelling skills for 30 min a day, 4 times per week for 18 weeks. The intervention produced improvements in phonological awareness ($d = 0.29$) and word decoding ($d = 1.27$) in the intervention group immediately after training.

Summary: interventions for decoding and reading fluency problems

Interventions for children who have decoding problems are well developed and there is now strong evidence from many randomized trials that teaching that targets phoneme awareness and letter-sound knowledge, in the context of structured phonic teaching, is highly effective in improving decoding skills.

There is less evidence concerning interventions for the reading fluency problems that often persist after basic decoding skills are mastered in children with dyslexia. Nevertheless, there is suggestive evidence that repeated oral reading programmes can help to improve reading fluency, although such interventions may be least effective for the children who need them most. Clinically, it is widely believed that maintaining an interest in reading and ensuring that children with dyslexia engage in frequent reading practice are important for helping to reduce the reading fluency problems that are a persistent problem in this group of children.

Reading comprehension impairment

Nature and causes of reading comprehension impairment

Children with reading comprehension impairment decode words accurately, but have problems understanding the meaning of texts that they can read (Hulme & Snowling, 2009, 2011). Such children may often go unnoticed in school because they read aloud normally. These children have been much less studied than children with dyslexia (see Chapter 53 for a detailed account).

Reading comprehension impairment is typically diagnosed if a child shows a large (at least 1 SD) discrepancy between reading accuracy and reading comprehension on a well standardized test, coupled with a reading comprehension standard score of 90 or below. In a recent standardization of a reading test involving a nationally representative sample of 1324 UK primary-school children, 3.3% of the sample met these diagnostic criteria (Hulme & Snowling, 2011).

A great deal of evidence points to the conclusion that the cause of reading comprehension problems is a broader language comprehension deficit (Hulme & Snowling, 2011). This theoretical position leads directly to the view that interventions targeting language comprehension skills are likely to ameliorate these children's reading comprehension difficulties.

Interventions targeting reading comprehension impairment

Meta-analyses of outcome studies

Several different meta-analyses have been published examining interventions to improve children's reading comprehension (Stahl & Fairbanks, 1986; Edmonds et al., 2009; Elleman et al., 2009; Swanson et al., 2011). The most recent by Elleman et al. (2009) examines effects from interventions that target language comprehension skills. Studies in this meta-analysis had to employ either a pre-test – post-test control group design, post-test control with randomization, or a pre-test – post-test within subjects design using counterbalanced conditions. The studies included both unselected groups of children as well as children with learning disorders from pre-kindergarten to grade 12 (ages roughly 4 to 16 years) with English as their first language. The interventions all involved instructional methods

that aimed to increase word knowledge or reading comprehension that could be implemented in a classroom setting. Results showed that on reading comprehension tests that contained the words that were trained the mean effect size was moderate ($d = 0.50$, $k = 23$ groups). However, when effects were measured on standardized reading comprehension tests, effects were small ($d = 0.10$, $k = 16$). Notably, this meta-analysis included studies with short training durations (number of treatment hours ranging from 1–37.5), and this perhaps reduces the likelihood of effects on standardized measures. Nevertheless, the benefits from the interventions summarized by Elleman et al. are small in magnitude and arguably unlikely to be of clinical or educational importance.

Moderators of outcome

The moderator analyses in the study by Elleman et al. (2009) showed that when considering only custom measures and controlling for method variables, students with reading disabilities benefited more than three times as much as students without reading problems from the interventions. There were no overall differences between different teaching methods.

Recent studies targeting reading comprehension impairments

In a randomized trial, Clarke et al. (2010) examined the effects from three interventions designed to enhance reading comprehension in 8–9 year old children with reading comprehension problems ($n = 160$); text comprehension training, oral language training and text comprehension and oral language training combined. The two basic interventions (text comprehension training and oral language training) had very different characteristics. Text comprehension training involved working with children's reading books and involved teaching a range of strategies such as visualizing what was being conveyed in a text or making inferences from a text. The oral language training on the other hand involved working exclusively with spoken language. Children were taught the meanings of words they did not know, practised listening to stories and answering questions about their meanings and also practised generating their own narratives (stories) from sets of pictures. Children in this intervention also received instruction in understanding the figurative (nonliteral) use of language, such as learning the meaning of riddles and jokes. The combined intervention programme involved the key elements from both the text comprehension and oral language training programmes, which were combined to form an integrated instructional package. The interventions lasted for 20 weeks, with three 30-min (individual and small group) sessions per week. Compared with an untreated control group, all groups made significant and moderate to large gains on standardized tests of reading comprehension at post-test (for WIAT II $d = 0.59$ for text comprehension training, $d = 0.69$ for oral language training and $d = 0.99$ for text comprehension and oral language combined). Thus, in contrast to the meta-analysis by Elleman et al. (2009), large effects were demonstrated on standardized measures. Although all groups maintained effects at follow-up 11 months later, gains were greater in the oral language group ($d = 1.24$ on WIAT II) than the other groups. Both the oral language and the combined groups demonstrated significant improvements in expressive vocabulary and this was a mediator of their improved reading comprehension.

Cantrell *et al.* (2010) examined the effects from a reading comprehension strategy programme in a randomized trial with 6th and 9th graders (approximate ages 10 and 13 years respectively). Students were taught strategies of word identification, visual imagery, self-questioning, paraphrasing and sentence writing. After a year of intervention (50–60 min a day), 6th graders ($n = 131$) receiving the intervention performed better than the control group ($n = 171$) on a standardized measure of reading comprehension, but the effect size was small (estimated effect size $d = 0.22$). For the 9th graders ($n = 353$), there was no significant improvement and the effect size was very small (estimated $d = 0.1$).

The difference in results between the Clarke *et al.* study and the Cantrell *et al.* study are difficult to explain. The participants in the Cantrell *et al.*, study were older and possibly had more severe reading problems. It also appears that the group reading test used for selecting children for the Cantrell trial (the Group Reading and Diagnostic Evaluation) places heavy emphasis on reading accuracy as well as comprehension skills, so there is no evidence that the children in the trial had specific problems in comprehension that were out of line with their decoding skills. Overall the results from the Cantrell et al. study are clearly disappointing especially in relation to the amount of intervention received (roughly 1 hour per day for 1 school year). The results from the Clarke *et al.*, study, which involved considerably less teaching time and produced larger effects on reading comprehension, suggests that targeting oral language skills in children with reading comprehension impairment may be particularly important.

Finally, it is worth noting that Fricke *et al.* (2013) reported a randomized trial examining the effects of an oral language intervention delivered to children who represented roughly the bottom 30% of children in nursery classes in terms of their oral language proficiency. The intervention started in the last term of nursery school and continued through the first two terms of reception class (a total of 30 weeks of intervention). Children in the intervention group showed significantly better reading comprehension scores ($d = 0.52$) at a 6-month delayed follow-up test. This effect was completely mediated by changes in language comprehension scores obtained at the end of the intervention. This study therefore replicates, with a younger sample, the effects found by Clarke *et al.* (2010) that oral language intervention can be a highly effective means of improving children's reading comprehension skills.

Summary: interventions for reading comprehension impairment

There are many fewer studies of interventions for reading comprehension impairment than for dyslexia. The assessment of reading comprehension skills is inherently much more complex than the assessment of reading accuracy, as are the teaching methods required for improving reading comprehension. Current evidence nevertheless suggests that this disorder reflects an underlying weakness in oral language comprehension abilities and that interventions targeting oral language comprehension skills can be highly effective for improving children's reading comprehension skills. The interventions with the largest effects here (Clarke *et al.*, 2010; Fricke *et al.*, 2013) have involved teaching individual children, or children in small groups, over roughly four sessions a week for between 20 and 30 weeks in school. It should be emphasized that the children in these trials could all be considered to have significant educational weaknesses but the majority would not be viewed as having clinically severe language problems. Moreover, it should be emphasized that many children with language and reading difficulties would be likely to benefit from longer lasting interventions than the 20 to 30 week interventions that were delivered in these research studies. Further work in this area is badly needed. We need large scale trials of adequate duration that seek to establish generalized effects to standardized tests of reading and language comprehension.

Specific language impairment

Nature and causes of specific language impairment

Specific language impairment (SLI) has traditionally been defined as oral language skills that are much poorer than expected from a child's non verbal abilities and where other known causes (such as deafness) have been excluded (Bishop & Snowling, 2004). As in the case of dyslexia, however, there has been much controversy about the use of a discrepancy definition for this disorder and DSM-5 has now abandoned the use of such a definition. SLI, or more simply language impairment (LI) is thought to arise from deficits in both phonological and broader oral language skills (Bishop & Snowling, 2004) whereas dyslexia, in contrast, reflects a circumscribed difficulty with the phonological aspects of language.

Specific language impairment appears to be a relatively common disorder. In a large epidemiological study, Tomblin *et al.* (1997) examined a stratified cluster kindergarten sample ($n = 7218$) with a language screening test. The children who failed the screening were given a further diagnostic battery of tests. The diagnosis of SLI required normal hearing and non verbal IQ and a score of 1.25 SD below the mean for the child's age on two out of five language tests. Results showed an overall prevalence for SLI of 7.4%, with 8% for boys and 6% for girls. However, it should be noted that there are high levels of comorbidity between SLI, dyslexia, speech disorders, motor coordination disorder, general learning disorders, and ADHD (Beitchman *et al.*, 1990; Botting, 2005; Pennington, 2009; see Chapter 3), which may lead some to question the use of the term "specific" in relation to this disorder.

The causes of SLI remain poorly understood. Descriptively, children with SLI appear to have pronounced problems in word learning (vocabulary knowledge), grammar learning and phonology. In practice, the major approaches to intervention target different aspects of these children's language learning weaknesses head on in a direct and highly structured way. The interventions evaluated in this section generally include children with significant language learning weaknesses without imposing any restrictive diagnostic criteria for including children who require intervention.

Interventions targeting specific language impairment
Meta-analyses of outcome studies

Given that word learning is a major area of difficulty for children with SLI, interventions focusing on direct vocabulary instruction are relevant to treating the disorder as are interventions involving joint book reading, which help to improve oral language skills (for interventions related to phonology refer the earlier section on dyslexia). Several meta-analyses of the effects from such interventions have been published.

Elleman *et al.* (2009) analyzed effects from interventions implemented in classroom settings that aimed to increase word knowledge or comprehension. The studies included had to employ either a pre-test–post-test control group design, post-test control with randomization or pre-test–post-test within subjects design using counterbalanced conditions. The samples were first language learners from pre-kindergarten (approximate age 3–4 years) to grade 12 (approximate age 16 years) both with and without learning disorders. Results showed that effects from interventions were small to moderate when vocabulary was measured with standardized measures ($d = 0.29$, $k = 14$) and large when vocabulary was measured with tests constructed to assess knowledge of words directly taught in the study ($d = 0.79$, $k = 18$). In this analysis, effect size was correlated with control group strength and effect sizes were smaller for randomized trials: both of these findings suggest that the overall effect sizes reported overestimate the "true" effects of the interventions evaluated. Higher levels of discussion were associated with larger effect sizes.

A second line of research relevant to enhancing language comprehension and word learning involves studies of joint book reading. In joint book reading, a child and an adult take turns to read aloud from the same book and the adult engages the child in discussion about the passage being read. Lonigan *et al.* (2008a, b) evaluated the effects from studies of shared book reading interventions (represented by change in frequency or in the style of shared reading activities), implemented either by parents or in school settings. Studies had to use a randomized experiment or a quasi-experiment that was not seriously confounded. The results showed a large effect of shared book reading on measures of oral language ($d = 0.73$, $d = 0.57$ with

outlier excluded, $k = 16$). In this study, there were no differences between older and younger children, no differences between at risk and not at risk children and no difference between parent or teacher delivered interventions. Moderate to large effects from joint book reading interventions were also found in a meta-analysis by Mol *et al.* (2009).

Recent studies targeting language comprehension

In a cluster randomized trial, Neuman *et al.* (2011) examined whether helping Headstart preschoolers ($n = 604$) to learn words through categorization could enhance new word learning. The intervention program was organized on topics that represented different taxonomies of constructs. The children received the intervention for 12–15 min each day in addition to their regular teaching. Overall, results showed a small effect from the intervention immediately after training ($d = 0.07$) on a standardized vocabulary test (W-J picture vocabulary test). There were, however, larger effects on a custom measure of word knowledge, based on words that were used in the study.

Tuckwiller *et al.* (2010) used a regression discontinuity design to examine the effect of vocabulary instruction on kindergarten children (children were selected to be given intervention based on low scores at pre-test on the PPVT IV). The vocabulary instruction was based on a storybook with just 4 target words taught to children in small groups over 2 days. At post-test measures of children's ability to give meanings for these four words showed small to moderate improvements ($d = 0.33$), and the effect lasted on a delayed post-test. The very limited amount of intervention delivered here, the small number of words taught, and the fact that these children were from a typically developing population, greatly limits any conclusions that can be drawn from this study for clinical practice.

Bowyer-Crane *et al.* (2008) identified children at school entry with poorly developed oral language skills and provided them with either an oral language intervention focusing on vocabulary and narrative skills, or a phonology with reading intervention focusing on letter-sound knowledge, phonological awareness, and book reading. Both interventions were delivered by specially trained and supported teaching assistants working in the children's schools, using two scripted interventions. The intervention sessions alternated between small group and individual teaching sessions, over a period of two school terms (20 weeks). The oral language intervention, in comparison to the phonology with reading intervention, produced improvements in specifically taught vocabulary ($d = 1.00$) and expressive grammatical skills ($d = 0.31$).

In a similar study, Fricke *et al.* (2013) reported a randomized trial examining the effects of an oral language intervention delivered to children starting in the last term of nursery school (age 4 years) and continuing through the first two terms of reception class. Children in the intervention group showed significantly better performance ($d = 0.8$) on a latent oral language factor (defined by measures of vocabulary, listening comprehension, and expressive language) as well as on a latent spoken narrative factor ($d = 0.38$). Both effects were maintained at a 6-month delayed follow-up test.

Summary: interventions for oral language impairments in children

Current evidence suggests that structured language intervention programs that involve teaching vocabulary, listening comprehension and narrative skills are effective in improving oral language skills in the early years of formal schooling. The effect sizes from such interventions are moderate to large. Most of these studies, however, have arguably involved children whose language difficulties are not particularly severe, and we have little evidence about the effectiveness of interventions for children with severe oral language difficulties. More studies with such populations are badly needed.

Mathematics disorder

Nature and causes of mathematics disorder (see Chapter 53)

There have been great advances in research on mathematical development and performance in the last two decades. However, compared with studies of reading and its disorders, where we now have extensive knowledge about their causes and treatment, much work is still to be carried out in the field of mathematical skills and mathematics disorder. The diagnostic criteria for mathematics disorder in DSM-IV (American Psychiatric Association, 1994), was based on a discrepancy definition in which mathematics abilities as measured by a standardized test, needs to be substantially below the expected given chronological age, measured intelligence, and age appropriate education. However, in DSM-5 mathematics disorder is conflated with other forms of difficulty under the rubric of specific learning disorders and a discrepancy definition is not adhered to (this appears unfortunate—see Chapter 53).

Mathematics disorder, like other disorders considered in this chapter, is also relatively common. Lewis *et al.* (1994) assessed reading, arithmetic and non verbal ability in all 9- and 10-year old children in a single school district in the UK. Using a cutoff of a mathematics standard score of 85 or less coupled with normal non verbal ability (at or above a standard score of 90), some 3.6% of children were classified as having mathematics disorder (of these children roughly two thirds also had a reading disorder diagnosed in an analogous way).

In relation to theories of the causes of mathematics disorder, the main discussion in the field has been whether the core deficit is in an abstract approximate number sense system (Dehaene,

1997; Butterworth *et al.*, 2011) or whether it is the result of a more general deficit in working memory or visuo spatial abilities (e.g., Geary, 2004) or perhaps a verbally based deficit that involves problems in learning counting skills (Hulme & Snowling, 2009; see Chapter 53). Arguably, to date there has been little linkage between debates about the causes of mathematics disorder and interventions for these children.

Interventions targeting mathematics abilities
Meta-analyses of treatment studies

There has been an increase in the number of intervention studies for mathematics disorder in the last 10 years. A meta-analysis by Gersten *et al.* (2009) examined interventions for mathematics targeted toward children with identified learning disorders. To be included studies had to evaluate the effectiveness of a well-defined method for improving mathematics proficiency and be randomized controlled trials or quasi experiments where participants were matched on pre-test data. Large effects were obtained for interventions that contained explicit instruction in specific mathematic skills ($d = 1.22$, $k = 11$), instruction in a general strategy for solving problems ($d = 1.56$, $k = 4$), teaching children verbalizations of reasoning (i.e., teaching children to give explicit verbal descriptions of the reasoning processes used to solve problems; $d = 1.04$, $k = 8$) and using a specific sequence and range of examples ($d = 0.82$, $k = 9$). Moderate effects were demonstrated in interventions that focused on using visual representations for teacher and student ($d = 0.47$, $k = 12$). Studies with treated controls generated smaller effect sizes than untreated controls and studies using norm referenced tests showed smaller effect sizes than studies using researcher developed tests, all of these factors suggest that the effect sizes reported here may overestimate the "true" effects of the studies reviewed.

Recent studies targeting mathematical abilities

Klein *et al.* (2008) examined effects from a pre-kindergarten mathematics intervention in a randomized trial ($n = 278$). The intervention consisted of small group mathematics activities with concrete materials based on early numeracy skills, numerical operations, and logical reasoning for use both in educational settings and at home. Total intervention duration was 58 small group sessions of 20 min. The intervention group achieved significantly greater gains on a broad test of arithmetic skills (Child Math Assessment) than the control group ($d = 0.50$).

Clements and Sarama (2008) reported a clustered randomized trial of their "Building Blocks" pre-school mathematics programme. Groups of children in 36 pre-school classrooms (276 children) were assigned to receive the Building Blocks curriculum, which involved small group as well as individual and whole class instruction designed to improve children's counting and early number skills, or to receive an alternative preschool mathematics curriculum or to an untreated control. All programmes were implemented over 26 weeks. The children who received the Building Blocks programme showed significant improvements in early mathematical skills (assessed by the Early Mathematics Assessment of children's mathematical knowledge) compared to the untreated control children ($d = 1.07$) or those given an alternative preschool mathematics curriculum ($d = 0.47$). A follow-up study of the Building Blocks programme (Clements *et al.*, 2011) used a cluster randomized trial ($n = 1375$ children in 106 classrooms) and showed a sizable benefit from the intervention at post-test on children's mathematical understanding ($d = 0.72$).

In the United Kingdom, Torgerson *et al.* (2010) reported the results of a randomized trial evaluating the efficacy of a school-based intervention for 6–7 year old children with poor mathematical skills. The intervention, Numbers Count, is a 12 week programme, consisting of daily 30 min one-to-one sessions, delivered by specially trained teachers. Teaching in the programme uses shape, space measures and handling data as contexts for the development and application of children's number skills. The programme is scripted, but individualized, with teachers identifying teaching points based on continuing assessments of a child's mathematical skills. In the trial, 144 children who received the Numbers Count intervention showed reliably higher scores immediately after the intervention had finished on a standardized test of mathematical ability ($d = 0.33$) compared with a waiting list control group ($N = 274$).

Finally, in a small scale experimental study Ramani and Siegler (2008) randomly assigned 124 young children (aged 5.4 years) from low income backgrounds to two experimental conditions. One group played a linear board game involving counting. Here consecutive squares on the board were labeled with the numerals 1–10 and to advance children turned a spinner that was labeled with the numerals 1 or 2 on its two sides. The other group played a similar game in which squares were simply colored and the spinner had two different colors on it. The children played the game for just four 15–20 min sessions over 2 weeks. The children in the experimental group showed advantages over the control group on measures of numerical magnitude comparison, number line estimation, counting and numeral identification, which remained 9 weeks after the intervention (effect sizes were moderate to large). This study suggests that practice in counting can have beneficial effects on early arithmetic development in children from disadvantaged backgrounds.

Summary of interventions for mathematical abilities

There are relatively few well controlled studies of interventions for mathematical abilities. However, two published programmes (Building Blocks (for pre-school children) and Numbers Count (for 6–7 year old children)) have reasonable evidence for their efficacy.

The effectiveness of educational interventions for children with general learning difficulties

So far in this chapter, we have concentrated on interventions for children with specific learning difficulties. There have been a number of experimental and quasi-experimental studies that have evaluated the effectiveness of interventions for children with general learning difficulties (intellectual disabilities in US terminology); all of these studies concentrate on reading (or reading and language) skills.

Allor *et al.* (2010a, b) evaluated the effectiveness of a phonic reading programme with 28 children with moderate intellectual disabilities (IQs 40–79). Children were randomly assigned to daily small group reading instruction or "typical special education" ($N = 16$ intervention, $N = 12$ control). The programme was delivered for between 1 and 1.5 years and produced medium to large effect sizes on a standardized measure, the Test Of Word Reading Efficiency (TOWRE $d = 0.72$) and non word reading efficiency (TOWRE $d = 1.00$); these tests simply assess how many words or non words a child can read aloud in 90 s.

In a similar study with a larger sample, Allor *et al.* (2010a, b) evaluated the effectiveness of a comprehensive reading programme that involved teaching phonological and phonemic awareness, oral language skills, letter knowledge, word reading, vocabulary, reading fluency and comprehension. Fifty-nine children with moderate intellectual disabilities (IQs 40–79) were randomly assigned to either the treatment or a business as usual control group. Teaching for the intervention children was delivered in daily small group sessions across 2 to 3 school years. The intervention group showed greater gains, with small to moderate effect sizes, on measures of phoneme awareness (d's = 0.53 to 0.66) non word reading (d's = 0.49 to 0.58) and word reading (d's = 0.26 to 0.51).

In another small-scale RCT Finnegan (2012) investigated methods of teaching reading to children with intellectual disabilities. Here 52 children (mean age 8.6 years; mean IQ where available 56) were randomly assigned to three groups: synthetic phonics, an analogy-based phonic reading programme, or an untreated control. The synthetic phonics programme involved teaching children to "sound out" unknown words on a letter by letter basis and blend the sounds together to form the word. The analogy-based phonics programme focussed on larger segments of spoken words when trying to decode them (for example, given the word HAT the child might be asked to think of other words that share the same ending (CAT, SAT) or the same initial letter (HIT, HIS) and work out from this the pronunciation of HAT). Teaching only involved 12 sessions. Both phonics programmes resulted in improvements compared to the control group for children's ability to read words taught in the programme ($d = 0.54$ and 0.52) and on a measure of transfer to untaught words there was also an advantage for the synthetic phonics group compared to the control group ($d = 0.33$). Clearly, this study has low power but suggests that phonic reading instruction can be beneficial for children with general intellectual disability.

Burgoyne *et al.* (2012) reported a randomized trial evaluating the effects of an integrated reading and language intervention programme for children with Down Syndrome. The intervention involved a highly structured phonic reading programme (comparable to that used by Bowyer-Crane *et al.*, 2008) coupled with vocabulary instruction and was delivered by teaching assistants in 40 min sessions on each school day over 20-weeks. After 20 weeks of teaching, the intervention group ($N = 28$) showed significantly greater progress than the waiting control group ($N = 26$) (with small to medium to small effect sizes) on measures of single word reading ($d = 0.23$), letter-sound knowledge ($d = 0.42$), phoneme blending ($d = 0.54$) and knowledge of words meanings taught in the programme ($d = 0.47$). However, there was no statistically reliable generalization to skills not directly taught (non word reading, spelling, standardized expressive and receptive vocabulary, expressive information, and grammar).

Summary

These studies of children with general learning difficulties are typically small scale, and hence suffer from limited statistical power, nevertheless the results are consistent in suggesting that reading accuracy problems in this population can be ameliorated by phonically based reading instruction coupled with phonological (phonemic) awareness training. In short, the same approach to teaching reading to children with dyslexia appears to be effective for children with general learning difficulties also.

The effectiveness of interventions targeting general cognitive functions

In recent years, strong claims have been made for interventions that aim to enhance language and reading skills by training more general cognitive capacities (e.g., Merzenich & Jenkins, 1998; Klingberg, 2010). One such category of interventions aims to train working memory capacity, a cognitive system that has been observed as providing an all-purpose "work-space" for diverse cognitive functions such as reading, language, maths, and general attentional abilities. It has been claimed that working memory impairment is a contributory cause to many different forms of learning difficulty including language impairment, dyslexia, reading comprehension impairment, mathematics disorder, and attention deficits (Melby-Lervåg & Hulme, 2012; Melby-Lervåg *et al.*, 2012). According to such a theory, if working memory capacity can be increased through training, this would have diverse effects on people's ability to perform cognitive tasks, such reading and language comprehension, arithmetic and reasoning.

In the last decade, a number of studies have examined the effects from working memory training. In a meta-analysis, Melby-Lervåg and Hulme (2012) summarized the effects from such training in studies that used a design with a pre-test and post-test and a control group (both randomized and non randomized studies, and studies with both trained and untrained control groups). Twenty-three studies with 30 group comparisons met the criteria for inclusion. The studies involved clinical samples and samples of typically developing children and adults. Meta-analyses showed that the working memory programmes produced reliable short-term improvements in working memory skills. However, there was no convincing evidence of generalization from working memory training to other skills (non verbal and verbal ability, inhibitory processes in attention, word decoding and arithmetic). These programs appear to produce short-term, specific training effects that do not generalize to skills that are important for children with learning difficulties. Moreover, this pattern been confirmed in a recent well controlled study with adults (Redick *et al.*, 2012) and for the Cogmed training program in a further meta-analysis (Hulme & Melby-Lervåg, 2012).

A second category of interventions based on an approach that seeks to train general cognitive skills derives from a theory that language and literacy learning difficulties in children arise from problems related to rapid auditory temporal processing (Tallal, 2004). According to this theory, a basic deficit in perceiving rapidly changing auditory signals results in problems in perceiving speech which in turn lead to language learning difficulties. It has been claimed that neuroplasticity means that training of auditory processing skills can lead to improvements in underlying neural systems and thereby ameliorate children's language and reading problems (Merzenich & Jenkins, 1998). One such training program is called Fast ForWord which is marketed by the Scientific Learning Corporation in the US. In this program, children are trained with computer modified speech in which critical cues in speech are slowed down in order to make them more discriminable to children with auditory temporal processing impairments. In a meta-analysis by Strong *et al.* (2011) the effects of the Fast ForWord training programmes were examined. Six studies that met the inclusion criteria of randomized controlled trials or matched group comparison studies with baseline equivalence published in refereed journals were found. The results showed that there was no significant effect of Fast ForWord on language and reading measures when the training groups were compared with active or untreated control groups. Thus, Fast ForWord cannot be recommended for treating language and reading problems.

Conclusions and future directions for clinical practice and research

We have considered evidence for the efficacy of educational interventions for reading disorders (dyslexia and reading comprehension impairment), language disorders and mathematics disorder. It is clear that research on dyslexia is most advanced and we have good evidence that phonics reading instruction coupled with oral phoneme awareness training works relatively well as a way of reducing the severity of these children's reading problems. However, problems with spelling and reading fluency appear to be more difficult to remediate in this population. There is encouraging evidence that interventions for young children with weak oral language skills can be effective and that such interventions have knock on effects to improve reading comprehension skills. Work on interventions for mathematical difficulties is perhaps least advanced, but there is evidence for moderate effects for two published intervention programs.

It may be worth emphasizing some limitations to the evidence considered. First, nearly all the studies considered have fairly liberal criteria for including children to be treated and we have rather little evidence about the effectiveness of the interventions reviewed for children with severe difficulties. Second, nearly all the studies considered involve interventions of quite short duration with only short-term follow-up. A third issue that needs more evidence is the cost effectiveness of the interventions considered. However, given that a number of the interventions considered can be delivered by trained teaching assistants with small groups of children, it is likely that they could be considered potentially highly cost effective. Finally, it is notable that most intervention studies focus on evaluating the direct effects that a given intervention has on a given area of educational attainment (reading, language, or maths skills). For interventions with demonstrated effectiveness on such measures, it would be useful to have longer-term studies that included broader outcome measures, since clinically it is often claimed that effective educational interventions can have quite broad effects on well-being and self-esteem.

References

Allor, J.H. et al. (2010a) Comprehensive reading instruction for students with intellectual disabilities: findings from the first three years of a longitudinal study. *Psychology in the Schools* **47**, 445–466.

Allor, J.H. et al. (2010b) Teaching students with moderate intellectual disabilities to read: an experimental examination of a comprehensive reading intervention reading instruction for students with intellectual disabilities. *Education and Training in Autism and Developmental Disabilities* **45**, 3–22.

American Psychiatric Association (1994) *DSM-IV Diagnostic and Statistical Manual of Mental Disorders*. American Psychiatric Association, Washington, DC.

Beitchman, J.H. et al. (1990) Psychiatric risk in children with speech and language disorders. *Journal of Abnormal Child Psychology* **18**, 283–296.

Bishop, D.V.M. & Snowling, M.J. (2004) Developmental dyslexia and specific language impairment: same or different? *Psychological Bulletin* **130**, 858–886.

Botting, N. (2005) Non-verbal cognitive development and language impairment. *Journal of Child Psychology and Psychiatry* **46**, 317–326.

Bowyer-Crane, C. et al. (2008) Improving early language and literacy skills: differential effects of an oral language versus a phonology with reading intervention. *Journal of Child Psychology and Psychiatry* **49**, 422–432.

Burgoyne, K. et al. (2012) Efficacy of a reading and language intervention for children with Down syndrome: a randomized controlled trial. *Journal of Child Psychology and Psychiatry* **53**, 1044.

Bus, A.G. & van IJzendoorn, M.H. (1999) Phonological awareness and early reading: a meta-analysis of experimental training studies. *Journal of Educational Psychology* **91**, 403–414.

Butterworth, B. et al. (2011) Dyscalculia: from brain to education. *Science* **332**, 1049.

Cantrell, S.C. et al. (2010) The impact of a strategy-based intervention on the comprehension and strategy use of struggling adolescent readers. *Journal of Educational Psychology* **102**, 257–280.

Clarke, P. et al. (2010) Ameliorating children's reading comprehension difficulties: a randomised controlled trial. *Psychological Science* **21**, 1106–1116.

Clements, D.H. & Sarama, J. (2008) Experimental evaluation of the effects of a research-based preschool mathematics curriculum. *American Educational Research Journal* **45**, 443–494.

Clements, D.H. et al. (2011) Mathematics learned by young children in an intervention based on learning trajectories: a large-scale cluster randomized trial. *Journal for Research in Mathematics Education* **42**, 127–166.

Coleman, J. et al. (2013) *Impact of literacy intervention on achievement outcomes of children with developmental language disorders: a systematic review*. ASHA's National Center for Evidence-Based Practice in Communication Disorders, July 2013.

Dehaene, S. (1997) *The Number Sense: How the Mind Creates Mathematics*. Oxford University Press, New York.

Edmonds, M.S. et al. (2009) A synthesis of reading interventions and effects on reading comprehension outcomes for older struggling readers. *Review of Educational Research* **79**, 262–300.

Ehri, L. et al. (2000) Alphabetics. In the National Institute of Child Health and Human Development, Report of the National Reading Panel. Teaching Children to Read. An Evidence-Based Assessment of the Scientific Literature and its Implication for Reading Instruction. Reports of the Subgroups (NIH publication No. 00-4754, pp. 2-1-2-176). US government printing office, Washington, DC.

Elleman, A. et al. (2009) The impact of vocabulary instruction on passage-level comprehension of school-age children: a meta-analysis. *Journal of Educational Effectiveness* **2**, 1–44.

Finnegan, E.G. (2012) Two approaches to phonics instruction: comparison of effects with children with significant cognitive disability. *Education and Training in Autism and Developmental Disabilities* **47**, 269–279.

Fricke, S. *et al.* (2013) Efficacy of language intervention in the early years. *Journal of Child Psychology & Psychiatry* **54**, 280–290.

Geary, D.C. (2004) Mathematics and learning disabilities. *Journal of Learning Disabilities* **37**, 4–15.

Gersten, R. *et al.* (2009) Mathematics instruction for students with learning disabilities: a meta-analysis of instructional components. *Review of Educational Research* **79**, 1202–1242.

Hatcher, P.J. & Hulme, C. (1999) Phonemes, rhymes, and intelligence as predictors of children's responsiveness to remedial reading instruction: evidence from a longitudinal intervention study. *Journal of Experimental Child Psychology* **72**, 130–153.

Hatcher, P.J. *et al.* (1994) Ameliorating early reading failure by integrating the teaching of reading and phonological skills: the phonological linkage hypothesis. *Child Development* **65**, 41–57.

Henderson, L.M. *et al.* (2012) Questioning the benefits that coloured overlays can have for reading in students with and without dyslexia. *Journal of Research in Special Educational Needs* **13**, 57–65.

Hulme, C. & Melby-Lervåg, M. (2012) Current evidence does not support the claims made for CogMed working memory training. *Journal of Applied Research in Memory and Cognition* **1**, 197–200.

Hulme, C. & Snowling, M. (2009) *Developmental Cognitive Disorders*. Wiley-Blackwell, Oxford.

Hulme, C. & Snowling, M. (2011) Children's reading comprehension difficulties: nature, causes, and treatments. *Psychological Science* **20**, 139–142.

Hulme, C. *et al.* (2012) The causal role of phoneme awareness and letter-sound knowledge in learning to read: combining intervention studies with mediation analyses. *Psychological Science* **23**, 572–577.

Klein, A. *et al.* (2008) Effects of a pre-kindergarten mathematics intervention: a randomized experiment. *Journal of Research on Educational Effectiveness* **1**, 155–178.

Klingberg, T. (2010) Training and plasticity of working memory. *Trends in Cognitive Sciences* **14**, 317–324.

Lervåg, A. *et al.* (2009) The cognitive and linguistic foundations of early reading development: a Norwegian latent variable longitudinal study. *Developmental Psychology* **45**, 764–781.

Lewis, C. *et al.* (1994) The prevalence of specific arithmetic difficulties and specific reading difficulties in 9 to 10-year-old boys and girls. *Journal of Child Psychology* **35**, 283–292.

Lonigan, C.J. *et al.* (2008a) Impact of code-focused interventions on young children's early literacy skills. In: *Developing Early Literacy: SREE Spring 2012 Conference Abstract Template A-1 Report of the National Early Literacy Panel*, pp. 107–151. National Institute for Literacy, Washington, DC.

Lonigan, C.J. *et al.* (2008b) Impact of shared-reading interventions on young children's early literacy skills. In: *Developing early literacy: Report of the National Early Literacy Panel*, pp. 153–171. National Institute for Literacy, Washington, DC.

McArthur, G. *et al.* (2012). *Phonics training for English-speaking poor readers* [Online]. Available: http://www.thecochranelibrary.com

Melby-Lervåg, M. & Hulme, C. (2012) Is working memory training effective? A meta-analytic review. *Developmental Psychology* **49**, 270–291.

Melby-Lervåg, M. *et al.* (2012) Phonological skills and their role in learning to read: a meta-analytic review. *Psychological Bulletin* **138**, 322–352.

Merzenich, M.M. & Jenkins, W.M. (1998) Cortical plasticity, learning, and learning dysfunction. In: *Maturational Windows and Adult Cortical Plasticity*. (eds B. Julesz & I. Kovacs), pp. 247–272. Addison-Wesley Publishing, New York.

Mol, S. *et al.* (2009) Interactive book reading in early education: a tool to stimulate print knowledge as well as oral language. *Review of Educational Research* **79**, 979–1007.

Neuman, S.B. *et al.* (2011) Educational effects of a vocabulary intervention on preschoolers' word knowledge and conceptual development: a cluster-randomized trial. *Reading Research Quarterly* **46**, 249–272.

Pennington, B.F. (2009) *Diagnosing Learning Disorders: A Neuropsychological Framework*, 2nd edn. Guilford, New York.

Peterson, R.L. & Pennington, B.F. (2012) Developmental dyslexia. *The Lancet* **379**, 1997–2007.

Ramani, G.B. & Siegler, R.S. (2008) Promoting broad and stable improvements in low-income children's numerical knowledge through playing number board games. *Child Development* **79**, 375–394.

Redick, T.S. *et al.* (2012) No evidence of intelligence improvement after working memory training: a randomized, placebo-controlled study. *Journal of Experimental Psychology: General* **142**, 359–379.

Reynolds, D. *et al.* (2003) Evaluation of an exercise-based treatment for children with reading difficulties. *Dyslexia* **9**, 48–71.

Rutter, M. & Yule, W. (1975) The concept of specific reading retardation. *Journal of Child Psychology and Psychiatry* **16**, 181–197.

Samuels, S.J. *et al.* (2000) Fluency. In: *National Reading Panel, Teaching Children to Read: An Evidence-Based Assessment of the Scientific Research Literature on Reading and its Implications for Reading Instruction, Reports of the Subgroups (sections 3.1–3.43)*. National Institutes of Health, Washington, D.C.

Snowling, M. & Hulme, C. (2003) A critique of claims from Reynolds, Nicolson & Hambly (2003) that DDAT is an effective treatment for reading problems: lies, damned lies and (inappropriate) statistics. *Dyslexia: An International Journal of Research & Practice* **9**, 1–7.

Stahl, S.A. & Fairbanks, M.M. (1986) The effects of vocabulary instruction: a model-based meta-analysis. *Review of Educational Research* **56**, 72–110.

Strong, G.K. *et al.* (2011) A systematic meta-analytic review of evidence for the effectiveness of the Fast ForWord' language intervention program. *Journal of Child Psychology and Psychiatry* **52**, 224–235.

Swanson, E. *et al.* (2011) A synthesis of read-aloud interventions on early reading outcomes among preschool through third graders at risk for reading difficulties. *Journal of Learning Disabilities* **44**, 258–275.

Tallal, P. (2004) Improving language and literacy is a matter of time. *Nature Reviews Neuroscience* **5**, 721–728.

Therrien, W. (2004) Fluency and comprehension gains as a result of repeated reading: a meta-analysis. *Remedial and Special Education* **25**, 252–61.

Tomblin, J.B. *et al.* (1997) Prevalence of specific language impairment in kindergarten children. *Journal of Speech, Language, and Hearing Research* **40**, 1245–1260.

Torgerson, C.J. *et al.* (2010). *Every child counts: the independent evaluation technical report UK*, Department for Education [Online]. Available: https://www.gov.uk/government/publications/every-child-counts-the-independent-evaluation-technical-report [11 Aug 2014].

Tuckwiller, E.D. *et al.* (2010) An investigation of at-risk kindergarten students' response to a two-tiered vocabulary intervention: a regression discontinuity design. *Learning Disabilities Research and Practice* **25**, 137–150.

Vadasy, P.F. & Sanders, E.A. (2010) Efficacy of supplemental phonics-based instruction for lowskilled kindergarteners in the context of language minority status and classroom phonics instruction. *Journal of Educational Psychology* **102**, 786–803.

Wollf, U. (2011) Effects of a randomised reading intervention study: an application of structural equation modelling. *Dyslexia* **17**, 295–311.

CHAPTER 42

School-based mental health interventions

Sally N. Merry[1] and Stephanie Moor[2]

[1] Department of Psychological Medicine, Auckland School of Medicine, University of Auckland, Auckland, New Zealand
[2] Department of Psychological Medicine, Christchurch School of Medicine, University of Otago, Christchurch, New Zealand

Introduction

Ensuring that children with mental health needs receive effective care is challenging, and many who need care do not receive help (Burns *et al.*, 1995; Mariu *et al.*, 2012). Schools potentially provide a setting in which interventions can be delivered in an environment designed to meet the developmental needs of children and adolescents. While the primary purpose of schools is to provide education, poor mental health impacts adversely on educational outcomes and learning difficulties and mental health problems frequently co-exist, so that addressing mental health needs within the school setting is likely to lead to educational gains.

Schools are complex institutions that have the potential to exert a positive influence on behavior and academic attainment of students, regardless of their background (Rutter *et al.*, 1979). They can also increase risk for later mental health problems; the negative impact of bullying is clear (Jimenez Barbero *et al.*, 2012) and problematic teacher–pupil relationships are related to higher levels of psychiatric disorder in pupils at 3 year follow-up (Lang *et al.*, 2013).

Global school mental health

Schools vary in the way they address mental health problems, with socioeconomic status, geography, political stability, religion and culture all having an impact. There have been some global school mental health initiatives. The World Health Organization (WHO) developed a school mental health model incorporating mental health promotion, prevention, treatment and psycho-education (Hendren *et al.*, 1994). This led to initiatives such as the Health Promoting Schools approach, now applied in over 40 countries (Wei and Kutcher, 2012). The Education for All movement developed by UNESCO has included initiatives to address mental health and emotional support and to ensure that the school environment is supportive by preventing bullying, violence and by promoting good interpersonal

relationships and teaching life skills. The International Alliance for Child and Adolescent Mental Health and Schools, a relatively new initiative involving over 35 countries, aims to promote the mental health and well-being of children and young people.

There have been a number of countrywide initiatives, such as the Social and Emotional Aspects of Learning initiative in the United Kingdom and the European Network of Health Promoting Schools, which has 40 different member nations.

These initiatives tend to be taken up by high income countries with middle and low income countries lagging well behind. To address this disparity, a Child Mental Health Awareness Task Force was set up by the World Psychiatric Association, the WHO and the International Association for Child and Adolescent Psychiatry and Allied Professions. A mental health education resource was developed and introduced in nine countries. The impact is not known but this initiative has provided valuable information about the feasibility of developing and implementing school mental health programs in diverse settings (Wei & Kutcher, 2012).

Addressing mental health problems at schools

School-based services should be considered in the wider context of the family, the health system and other community resources. In an ideal world, services should be delivered in collaboration with a coherent over-arching framework, but in practice services are often delivered in parallel, or not at all. Working toward a more organized system would be of value in most parts of the world (Weisz *et al.*, 2005).

The role of the school differs according to the prevalence of disorder, the extent and nature of the resultant disability and the impact on the functioning of the class or school. For disorders with *high prevalence* rates, such as disruptive behavior disorders, consideration should be given to management within the school

Rutter's Child and Adolescent Psychiatry, Sixth Edition.
Edited by Anita Thapar and Daniel S. Pine, James F. Leckman, Stephen Scott, Margaret J. Snowling, Eric Taylor.

setting, using whole school, whole class, or indicated programs. For *lower prevalence* disorders, which affect the ability of the individual student to function at school, such as autistic spectrum disorders (ASDs), individual interventions may be needed to support individual students. Individuals with mental health problems are often stigmatized, even by young school children. While there have been some school-based interventions to try and address this problem, evidence of their efficacy is insufficient to warrant their introduction (Schachter *et al.*, 2008).

Strengths and weaknesses of school-based interventions

In schools, preventive interventions can be provided to a large proportion of the target population and school clinics can potentially provide treatment conveniently and without the stigma inherent in attending a mental health service. Integration with specialist mental health services can be achieved by having a close liaison between staff in both settings. While this rationale is appealing, there are practical difficulties including competing demands on the time of teachers and their pupils and lack of attendance at school by some students with mental health difficulties. In some parts of the world, the provision of education is not universal, resources are limited and the provision of mental health care within schools a distant aim. Families play a vital role in the mental health of young people but involving them in school-based interventions can be challenging.

Identifying risk and disorder
Given the high rates of undetected and untreated mental health problems in children and adolescents, mental health screening at schools has been advocated (U.S. Department of Education Office of Special Education and Rehabilitative Services, 2002; US Preventive Services Task Force, 2009). There are advantages of broad access to young people and students may be more likely to attend interventions if they are in the school setting (Levitt *et al.*, 2007). However, there has been some opposition to school-based screening because of potential stigmatization, limitations of screening instruments, and potential difficulties around consent (National Research Council and Institute of Medicine, 2009). The evidence that screening can lead to improved outcomes is limited. For example, there is evidence to support screening for the identification of depressive disorder in adolescents (but not children) but no evidence to show that this has resulted in improved mental health outcomes, or in increased uptake of services (Williams *et al.*, 2009).

Given the complex nature of screening in schools, the cost and benefits of screening should be carefully weighed up after considering the following:

- Evidence that screening results in improved outcomes;
- The availability of validated screening tools of adequate sensitivity and specificity;
- The acceptability of screening to young people and school staff;

- The potential for stigmatization of identified youth;
- The provision of information about the purpose, risks and benefits of screening;
- Consent processes;
- The availability of the resources and skills to confirm screening results, assess risk and clarify the need for intervention;
- The development of pathways for prevention and intervention following screening; and
- The availability and cost of subsequent intervention.

Methods of delivering interventions at school

Mental health interventions may be delivered in schools in a number of ways. Generally health promotion interventions are delivered to the *whole school* to try to create a positive school climate, which promotes mental health and pro-social behavior. These may integrate interventions for parents and the community. *Universal preventive interventions* are typically delivered to *whole classes*, or sub-groups of these classes, while *targeted* interventions can be delivered to groups *selected* because of a risk factor or where there are signs or symptoms *indicating* an incipient problem.

Some preventive interventions incorporate a stepped care approach to provide an *integrated range* of interventions, delivered universally with embedded systems to identify and intervene with students at elevated risk. There is evidence that school-based programs may be cost effective, for example, social and emotional learning programs have been estimated to save £84 for each pound invested, while programs to reduce bullying result in savings of £14 per pound invested (Campion, 2013).

There are different options for providing *treatment* for mental health problems within schools. Schools may provide specific settings for young people with specific needs: (i) through the provision of *special classes*, typically with low numbers of students and a high staff student ratio; and (ii) through *special schools*. Some schools have resident *school clinics* that may provide interventions for mental health problems. A recent meta-analysis of counseling and psychotherapy in schools showed the broad range of interventions delivered, but overall there was a small effect size, although this analysis was limited by the quality of the included studies (Baskin *et al.*, 2010). Mental health clinicians from specialist services may provide *consultation and liaison* services to schools. School staff may help ensure administration of medication, provide adjunctive support and work with mental health clinicians and the family to ensure an integrated approach to the difficulties faced by the young person.

A national survey of a representative sample of the 83,000 schools in the USA was carried out to determine the types of mental health problems presenting, the interventions delivered and wider issues of funding and administration of the services. Findings indicated that there was a recognition of the need to respond to mental health problems in schools and that services were widely available, mostly comprising assessment, behavior management, crisis intervention, and counseling. Concerns over rising need and decreasing resources to address the need were raised. The authors identified a need for further research to explore the way in which these services are delivered, the adequacy of training of school personnel and the effectiveness of combinations of prevention and treatment in the services provided (Teich *et al.*, 2007).

In a large survey of 599 primary schools and 137 secondary schools carried out in the UK, two thirds of schools reported that they provided mental health interventions. These were mostly for those with symptoms and clear evidence of mental health problems and were aimed at treatment, not prevention. Of concern were reports that the interventions were mostly not based on evidence and training of teachers was limited (Vostanis *et al.*, 2013).

Staff delivering interventions

School-based guidance counselors deliver psychological support for large numbers of young people in schools and the ease of access and timeliness makes this a valuable resource (Pattison & Harris, 2006). The humanistic counseling model most often used, helps students resolve crises and improve mental health and emotional well-being (Cooper, 2013). In US schools, a review of 132 counseling and psychotherapy interventions found them to have a moderately beneficial effect (effect size [ES] = 0.44). Interventions for adolescents outperformed those for children, and although group and individual interventions were equally effective, single sex groups did better than mixed sex groups. Well-trained mental health professionals outperformed less well-trained staff (Baskin *et al.*, 2010).

There is evidence that *school-based social workers* have a positive impact on students' mental health with a small effect on conduct problems (ES = 0.23) and a moderate effect on anxiety and depression (ES = 0.4) (Franklin *et al.*, 2009).

Mental health work is a key part of the role of *school nurses* who also provide an important link between the school and outside agencies such as social services, special education and specialist child mental health services (Pryjmachuk *et al.*, 2012).

Teachers may provide interventions directly, for example, providing class-based behavioral management programs and individual students with specific needs may have support from *teacher aids*.

School psychologists, child psychiatrists, and other *child mental health professionals* may provide interventions to patients within school clinics and may support school staff to address the mental health needs of their students.

Types of intervention

Interventions provided at a school level to promote mental health may include educating staff about how to interact positively with young people, ensuring that teachers are trained to develop positive and supportive relationships with their pupils and teaching teachers to manage difficult student behaviors. Interventions may be psycho-educational, delivered to whole classes as part of the syllabus, often as part of health education. Group interventions may be provided in schools for young people with mental health needs. Individual counseling may be provided and teacher aids may provide within-class interventions, for example, providing support for children with disruptive behavior. Some interventions may involve families, who may be invited to attend group sessions that are run in parallel with groups for students, or are stand-alone for parents only.

More recently, the use of technology has been considered. Interventions delivered through computers potentially offer some advantages over traditional implementation methods as they require less staff training and preparation time, guarantee consistency, provide flexibility in delivery, and, if well designed, can engage and maintain student interest and involvement. Mobile phones and tablets are likely to be used increasingly to deliver mental health interventions, although to date, phones are generally adjunctive to other interventions, and there is no evidence as yet, that an intervention delivered solely on mobile phones can prevent or treat mental health problems.

Programs developed for delivery at school
Programs targeting overall mental well-being

In addition to the development of cognitive and academic skills, schools are viewed as important settings for the fostering and development of social and emotional skills and a multitude of programs, based on social learning theory and cognitive behavioral approaches have been introduced as life skills programs. Social and emotional competencies include self-awareness, self-management, social awareness, goal setting, relationship skills and responsible decision making. Many programs teach specific skills, such as how to refuse drugs, alcohol or premature sexual behavior. A recent meta-analysis of social and emotional learning programs across the age-range of 6–16 years demonstrated initial moderate beneficial effects on social skills, pro-social behavior, positive self-image and academic achievement and reductions in antisocial behavior with initial small effects on reducing substance abuse and mental health problems (depression, anxiety and self-harm) (Sklad *et al.*, 2012). At 6 months follow up, there was a drop to a small effect in all areas, but within a population, these may be of public health benefit (Knapp *et al.*, 2011; Campion, 2013).

Problem behaviors and conduct disorder

Early behavioral difficulties are often evident in classroom settings from a young age and can herald developing conduct disorder but even when identified early, there is limited evidence about the effectiveness of classroom-based interventions in the prevention of conduct disorder. For schools with a high proportion of children at known risk of developing conduct disorder, offering classroom-based emotional learning and problem-solving programs for children between 3 and 7 years of age has been recommended (NICE, 2013). Enhancing the skills of teachers using behavioural techniques shown to be effective for parents is a promising approach. Early evaluation of the Incredible Years Teacher Training Program has shown benefits for both teacher practices and child behavior but await replication (Baker-Henningham et al., 2012).

The Good Behavior Game (GBG), is a widely utilized universal behavioral management intervention delivered by elementary teachers to reduce aggressive and disruptive behavior in the classroom and its effectiveness is currently being evaluated in several countries in large-scale trials (National Research Council and Institute of Medicine, 2009).

For classroom conduct problems in older children and adolescents, contingency behavioral management programs have been developed from social learning principles. Teachers use techniques such as giving clear instructions, planned ignoring, time-out and token reinforcement in class with children with disruptive or aggressive behavior. These programs achieve a moderate reduction in aggression, sustained to at least 12 months, in both primary and secondary school students (Mytton et al., 2006; Matjasko et al., 2012).

Programs with the strongest evidence include: Programme for Academic Skills, Contingencies for Learning Academic and Social Skills and Reprogramming Environmental Contingencies for Effective Social Skills (Blissett et al., 2009).

In adolescence conduct problems often intensify with more severe and wide-ranging consequences. Thus multimodal treatment interventions targeting the school as well as home and the wider community have been developed. The Fast Track intervention targeted social cognitive skills, reading, and modification of the disruptive and rejecting classroom environment as well as home visiting, mentoring and parent behavior-management. Despite the intensity of this well-funded program, at long-term follow up a reduction in conduct disorder was only demonstrated for those at the highest risk and not for the intervention group as a whole (Conduct Problems Prevention Research Group, 2011).

Students whose behavior cannot be managed in a typical classroom may be placed in an alternate education setting. This is often the last attempt to intervene for students who are at increased risk of a range of negative outcomes over the life span. The most effective behavioral management strategies have been identified by clinical consensus (Tobin and Sprague, 2000) resulting in a comprehensive framework for preventing and responding to challenging behavior by building a predictable environment with structure and routine, and with reinforcement delivered contingent on the student displaying the desired behavior. However, a review of alternate education settings showed that while the recommended low student to teacher ratio in this framework was implemented, most did not use recommended behavioral strategies (Flower et al., 2011).

Attention hyperactivity disorder (ADHD)

For children with attention hyperactivity disorder (ADHD), a comprehensive management plan that includes psychological and behavioral management at school as well as home has been recommended (NICE, 2008).

As teachers have limited training about mental health, in-service training sessions to increase teachers' knowledge about ADHD and practical ways to manage children with ADHD in the classroom have been developed. These include how to adapt lessons and structure the classroom environment to reduce distraction and how to implement behavioral management plans (Merrell, 2009). The importance of giving clear concise instructions, ensuring that tasks are broken down into small manageable steps, reinforcing desired behavior, planned ignoring and effectively managing undesirable behaviors is emphasized and reinforced with practice.

Behavioral management interventions by teachers result in moderate beneficial effects on behavior of children with ADHD (Fabiano et al., 2009) with less robust evidence for effects on academic achievement or the core ADHD symptoms (DuPaul et al., 2012). The dose or intensity of treatment, or the setting required to effect a meaningful change is not yet established, although there is some evidence from open studies and case reports that equivalent effects may be witnessed in special classes and general settings (DuPaul et al., 2012). There are important gaps in the literature about the long-term effectiveness of classroom-based interventions, how best to sequence interventions and, as the current evidence comes mostly from primary schools, how these interventions might be implemented in the high school environment.

Computers have been used to assist the presentation of academic material (Rabiner et al., 2010). Immediate and frequent feedback is given along with reinforcement and the highlighting of important information. Computer attention training (CAT) has been used as a training tool to decrease inattention (Steiner et al., 2011) but the effectiveness of these technologies for children with ADHD requires further evaluation.

Although parents of adolescents with ADHD often report school difficulties as a primary concern, the evidence for strategies in this age group is inconclusive (Young and Amarasinghe, 2010). In practice, a pragmatic approach is usually taken to develop individualized interventions for students.

Substance use disorders

Early initiation into drug use is a risk factor for the development of substance abuse and the high cost of this disorder, both to the individual and to society, has led to the development of early intervention programs, delivered to increasingly younger students in schools. Many of these programs are generic for all substances and some target specific drugs.

Universal generic school-based preventive programs include education about the risks of drugs of abuse; skills training to address the social influence of peers and the media; and cognitive behavioral approaches to address the modeling and reinforcement of substance use that children may have been exposed to. Susceptibility is increased by social vulnerability such as poor personal and social skills and some programs also address these difficulties. In addition, multi-modal programs combine curricular approaches with wider initiatives that may include programs for parents and communities.

Universal interventions that target substance abuse using social skills programs have been shown to be effective in increasing knowledge about drugs, decision-making skills and resistance to peer pressure and decreasing illicit drug use, although most did not have long-term follow-up (Faggiano *et al.*, 2005; Jackson *et al.*, 2012; Karki *et al.*, 2012; Teesson *et al.*, 2012; Norberg *et al.*, 2013).

Universal preventive programs: alcohol

Until recently, several systematic reviews concluded that classroom-based preventive education was not effective in reducing alcohol-related harm and the importance of restricting access and reducing alcohol advertising were emphasized (Anderson *et al.*, 2009). However, evidence is now accumulating to support the value of some (15 of 39 reviewed) generic interventions and some (6 of 11 reviewed) alcohol-specific interventions for reduced drunkenness and binge drinking (Foxcroft & Tsertsvadze, 2011). Effective interventions include the Life Skills Training Program and the Unplugged program. There is also evidence accumulating that programs targeting children with disruptive behavior in elementary school, such as the GBG (Good Behavior Game) also reduce the risk of substance use in adolescence (Castellanos-Ryan *et al.*, 2013).

Universal preventive programs: nicotine

The probability of quitting smoking is directly proportional to the age of initiation so that delaying the age of smoking initiation is crucial.

In a well conducted meta-analysis, combined social competence and social influence programs showed, on average, a 12% reduction in smoking onset but these effects were only observed a year or more after follow up. There was no evidence that any programs changed smoking behavior (Table 42.1) (Thomas *et al.*, 2013)

An incentive-based program, the Smoke Free Competition, targeting 11–14 year olds, has been implemented widely (16,000 students in three European countries) although incentive programs have not been shown to prevent smoking initiation in youth (Isensee and Hanewinkel, 2012; Johnston *et al.*, 2012). However, approaches using peers show promise. The ASSIST study from the UK (Campbell *et al.*, 2008), used "trained" students aged 12–13 years to spread and sustain new norms of nonsmoking behavior through informal everyday conversations using social networks in schools over a 10 week intervention. Evaluation of 10,000 students 1 year after the intervention showed a 23% reduction in the likelihood of being a regular smoker and was estimated to be cost effective, even though the effects of the intervention attenuated by 2 years.

Targeted programs

Programs targeting children at high risk of substance abuse that involve both school and home show some promise (Carney and Myers, 2012; Bröning *et al.*, 2012). A recent systematic review of ten targeted prevention programs in school settings reported a mean effect size of 0.2 but effects between programs varied widely (Norberg *et al.*, 2013).

Mentoring programs used particularly in the US to deter alcohol and other drug initiation in high risk youth have yet to show effectiveness (Thomas *et al.*, 2011).

Use of computers

Computerized drug prevention programs in schools have been shown to delay smoking initiation and reduce alcohol and illicit drug use, albeit with small effect sizes (Champion *et al.*, 2013) but this is a rapidly growing field and technology may assist delivery and increase access to interventions in the future.

Depression and anxiety

Given the prevalence and cost of depression and anxiety in children and adolescents, (World Health Organization, 2008) a number of school-based programs have been developed to try and prevent the onset of disorder or to intervene early. Schools may also play an important role in supporting the recognition and treatment of anxiety and depressive disorders. While depressive and anxiety disorders have different presentations and trajectories over time, they are frequently comorbid and prevention and early intervention studies typically measure symptoms of both types of disorders, and, if effective, usually have a significant effect on both disorders.

Generally, school-based depression and anxiety prevention programs, both universal and targeted, are based around cognitive behavioral or, less commonly, interpersonal therapy strategies, typically delivered in groups lasting 8 to 12 sessions. While some targeted approaches have been selective (e.g., for students affected by bereavement), usually students at risk are identified using screening for elevated symptoms of anxiety or depression. Groups are run at school by teachers or trained facilitators from a variety of backgrounds. The interventions are usually manualized and some include booster sessions to enhance long-term effect. More recently the use of computers or mobile phones to deliver interventions has been investigated. Some of the better-known programs include the Penn Prevention Programme, the Coping with Stress Course and the Resourceful Adolescent, all targeting depression (Merry *et al.*, 2011) and FRIENDS; and Cool Little Kids targeting anxiety (Mychailyszyn *et al.*, 2012).

Although the rationale for prevention and early intervention for anxiety and depression using school-based programs is clear, it has been difficult to show that the programs are truly effective and studies have a number of weaknesses, most importantly

Table 42.1 Evidence of effectiveness of school-based interventions.

Review	Studies and participants	Intervention	Age range	Outcome	Effect size	Quality of studies	Comment
School wide mental health promotion							
Sklad et al. (2012)	MA 75 studies, 56% RCTs	Social, emotional, and/or behavioral programs. Delivered by teachers	Elementary and high school	Improved social, emotional and academic skills	Initial ES 0.39–0.46 Follow-up ES 0.07–0.26	Significant heterogeneity	Promising
Durlak et al. (2011)	MA 213 studies 270,034 students 47% RCTs	Social and emotional learning. Delivered by teachers	Kindergarten through high school	Improved social and emotional skills, behavior, and academic performance	ES 0.30 (95% CI = 0.26–0.33) SE skills ES 0.57 (95% CI 0.48 to 0.67)	Significant heterogeneity	Promising
Depression and anxiety							
Merry et al. (2011)	MA 68 RCTs (53 in meta-analysis) 14,406 participants	Targeted and universal depression prevention programs. Psychological and educational, mostly CBT-based groups in schools	5–19 years	Reduced risk of depressive disorder up to 12-month follow up	Postintervention risk difference (RD) −0.09; 95% CI −0.14 to −0.05 **Follow-up** 3 to 9 month RD −0.11; 95% CI −0.16 to −0.06; 12 months RD −0.06; 95% CI −0.11 to −0.01)	Positive findings but heterogeneity and methodological shortcomings in the studies	Promising but not suitable for implementation on current evidence
Mychailyszyn et al. (2012)	MA 63 studies, 44 RCTs 15,211 participants	Targeted and universal school-based CBT for anxious (and depressed) youth		Moderately effective Targeted > universal School staff = research staff	Anxiety: ES = 0.50 (95% CI [0.40–0.60] Depression: ES = 0.3 (95% CI [0.21, 0.40]	Review weakened by inclusion of nonRCTS. Heterogeneity in findings	Promising for anxiety > depression
Problem behaviors							
Mytton et al. (2006)	MA 56 studies 34 trials with data All RCTs	Secondary prevention of violence for children identified with aggression	Primary and secondary schools	Aggressive behaviour was significantly reduced to 12-month follow up	Aggressive behavior postintervention ES −0.41; (95% CI −0.56 to −0.26); 12-month follow up: ES −0.40, (95% CI −0.73 to −0.06)	Improving social skills better than teaching nonresponse to provocation	Interventions appear effective
Matjasko et al. (2012)	Meta-review including 11 MAs and 4 SRs	Youth violence prevention or intervention		Majority found moderate effects	Moderate effects on youth violence		Interventions appear effective

Truancy

Study	Type of review / studies	Intervention	Population	Results	Effect size / statistics	Findings	Conclusion
Maynard et al. (2012)	MA 28 studies 5 RCTs 11 QED	School-, court-, or community-based programs		Improved attendance by an average of 4.69 days	ES for RCTs = 0.57 (95% CI 0.17 to 0.96)	Heterogeneous findings. Different approaches had similar findings No difference in effect between RCTs and QEDs	Possibly effective

Alcohol or Drugs

Study	Type of review / studies	Intervention	Population	Results	Effect size / statistics	Findings	Conclusion
Faggiano et al. (2005)	MA 32 studies 46,539 participants 29 RCTs 3 CPS	Universal school-based prevention of use of illicit drug use	6th–7th grade students	Significantly improved drug knowledge, decision-making skills, self-esteem, peer pressure resistance compared with usual curricula Reduced drug use 2 years after intervention	Improves peer pressure resistance (Relative risk (RR) =2.05 Decreased drug use: RR = 0.81. 95% CI 0.64 to 1.02 marijuana use RR 0.82; 95% CI 0.73 to 0.92) and hard drug use RR 0.45; 95% CI 0.24 to 0.85)	Programs targeting social skills are the most effective No long-term follow-up	Very promising but need replication in rigorous long-term studies
Foxcroft and Tsertsvadze (2011)	SR 53 trials All RCTS	Universal school-based alcohol prevention programs	< 18 years	About half the interventions showed a reduction in alcohol misuse	Reduced drunkenness and binge drinking Alcohol specific interventions no better than generic interventions	Variable findings Most promising programs Life Skills Training Program, Unplugged program, Good Behaviour Game	Rigorous review, Meta-analysis not conducted because of poor quality of the studies
Norberg et al. (2013)	MA 25 RCTs	Cannabis prevention mostly in school settings	<=24 years	Some universal multi-modal programs associated with large effect sizes	Wide range in ES (0.07–5.26). Majority were small	Overall quality of studies poor	Findings inconclusive
Teesson et al. (2012)	SR 8 RCTs (7 interventions)	Universal school-based prevention programs for alcohol and other drugs. Mostly based on social learning principles	13–14 years of age	5/7 programs achieved reductions in substance use at follow-up	Modest ES	Australian studies only	Promising

(continued overleaf)

Table 42.1 (*continued*)

Review	Studies and participants	Intervention	Age range	Outcome	Effect size	Quality of studies	Comment
Thomas et al. (2013)	MA Smoking prevention 49 RCTS N = 142,447 Change in smoking 15 RCTS N = 45,555	Smoking prevention and intervention	10–14 years	Prevention programs effective OR 0.49, (95% CI 0.28 to 0.87); P = 0.01 Change in smoking programs ineffective	Effectiveness only 1 year after intervention	Mixed findings	Social competence and social influences approaches are promising prevention programs but follow-up for longer than a year needed to show effect
Bullying							
Jimenez Barbero et al. (2012)	SR 32 studies	School programs aimed at reducing violence	6–16 years	Some evidence of effectiveness where focus is on social and interpersonal skills			Promising
Ttofi and Farrington (2011)	MA 44 programs	School-based programs to reduce bullying and victimization		Reduced bullying by 20–23% and victimization by 17–20%	Bullying SMD = 0.17 Victimization: SMD = 0.14	High quality Some individual programs for example OBPP in Norway, KiVa in Finland, have yielded reductions of around 40–50% in some age groups	Evidence that some programs are effective

Only meta-analyses with clear aims, search strategies and inclusion criteria have been used.
SR, Systematic Review; MA, Meta-analysis; RCT, Randomized controlled trials; QED, Quasi-experimental design CCTs case controlled trials; CPS, controlled prospective studies.

the lack of attention control groups. It has been difficult to confirm initial positive results in large-scale implementation trials. Many rigorous systematic reviews and meta-analyses of programs focusing on depression have not found a convincing effect and have outlined these concerns (Merry & Spence, 2007; Gladstone & Beardslee, 2009). A more recent meta-analysis was more hopeful about effectiveness (Merry et al., 2011), although there were still a number of weaknesses in the studies. Disappointingly, a subsequent large-scale study in the UK, did not show effect despite rigorous design and the use of a program previously shown to have some efficacy (Stallard et al., 2012).

A recent meta-analysis of cognitive–behavioral school-based interventions focusing on anxiety, particularly those targeted to students at higher risk, were moderately effective for both anxiety and depression, with larger effect sizes for anxiety (Table 42.1) (Mychailyszyn et al., 2012). The quality of the studies included in this analysis was variable.

Over the last decade, a large number of programs targeting internalizing problems in schools have been developed and evaluated but results have been mixed, and attempts to roll-out interventions have not led to clear improved outcomes. The evidence may be more robust for anxiety disorders. Until robustly designed implementation studies show good effect, it would be premature to disseminate these programs widely.

Schools have an important role to play in providing or supporting *treatment* of anxiety and depression in students. The prevalence of the disorders is such that secondary mental health services will not be able to provide treatment for all those affected by these disorders. Furthermore, a large proportion of young people with these disorders are never treated. Screening for depressive disorder and providing treatment in school settings could help address this problem, although evidence supporting this approach is not yet available (Williams et al., 2009).

Posttraumatic stress disorder

Traumatic stress reactions may be displayed in the school setting as increased aggression, anxiety, behavioral problems, developmental regression, psychosomatic complaints and school avoidance. Universal school-based programs have been developed using psycho-education, cognitive-behavioral strategies and a variety of other approaches to address the impact of a variety of disasters. These are delivered by teachers and aim both to increase resilience by preventing PTSD and other symptoms, and by treating PTSD. Examples include the ERASE-STRESS program (Berger & Gelkopf, 2009) and the "Cognitive Behavioral Intervention for Trauma in Schools" (CBITS) (Stein et al., 2003). The evaluation of these programs is complicated by marked heterogeneity in the populations studied, noncomparability of trauma exposure, and the lack of replication studies. Systematic reviews of studies that use primarily CBT techniques have shown small to moderate effects on depression and anxiety symptoms and small beneficial effects on PTSD symptoms in some reviews (Rolfsnes and Idsoe, 2011), but not others (Tol et al., 2011).

Eating disorders

While preventing the onset of eating disorders is appealing and a number of programs have been developed, there is little evidence of efficacy (Pratt & Woolfenden, 2002).

Autistic spectrum disorders (ASD)

There is increasing interest in how the educational environment can support inclusion for the growing numbers of students with ASD in mainstream school (Crosland & Dunlap, 2012). A pragmatic approach has been taken by schools using strategies including; managing challenging behaviors using positive behavioral support techniques; teaching self-management and social skills and anticipating and mitigating the effects of the inevitable changes in routine that occur in schools. It has been postulated that the school setting will provide opportunities for more appropriate socialization by increasing the number of interactions with typically developing peers such as a specialist intervention targeting conversational language skills (Adams et al., 2012) and using trained teachers supporting small peer social skills groups in the classroom (Cappadocia & Weiss, 2011). While these approaches appear sensible, there is no evidence that they are effective.

Computer-based interventions programs have been developed to teach social, emotional and literacy skills to young children with ASD and may be useful for children who are less responsive to traditional teaching approaches (Ramdoss et al., 2012) but whether these therapies facilitate generalizability into real world social interactions is not known (Rao et al., 2008).

Suicide prevention and postvention

Youth suicide is of concern and school-based suicide prevention strategies that include approaches that encourage positive mental health, and improve the detection and management of underlying mental illness, particularly depression, are well accepted as sensible by many mental health professionals even though there is no clear evidence that they are effective. It is logistically difficult to carry out studies to prove effectiveness. There is no evidence that school-based programs that target awareness of suicide directly are effective, and some evidence that they may do harm (Collings & Beautrais, 2005; Beautrais & Mishara, 2007) and on current evidence, these should not be implemented.

Schools will also sometimes have to deal with the aftermath of the suicide of one of their pupils and in doing so should work with local child and adolescent mental health services. Recommended steps in "postvention" usually include strategies to reduce contagion. Because of the known phenomenon of cluster suicides, schools are encouraged not to sensationalize suicide, to restrict the amount of detail about the method of suicide and to avoid either glorifying or condemning the victim of suicide. Identification of vulnerable students known to have risk factors and for whom the suicide may act as a trigger is often advocated. Providing support for the school community and families are important components of the school response. There are some good web-based resources providing detailed information about postvention responses for example http://www.nasponline.org/resources/intonline/HCHS2_weekley.pdf and http://www.headspace.org.au.

School absenteeism

There are a number of different problems that may lead to absenteeism from school. These have been variously defined but include truancy (unexcused, illegal, and surreptitious absences) school refusal (difficulty attending school associated with emotional distress), and school phobia (difficulty attending school because of a specific phobia) (Maynard et al., 2012).

A large number of programs have been developed to reduce truancy with model programs listed on the OJJDP website (U.S. Department of Justice), although the criteria for choosing the model programs on this site are not clear. These programs most commonly include school interventions, with counseling, CBT, mentoring, behavioral interventions, and social work being common components.

School refusal and school phobia are usually treated with CBT and a coordinated approach between the clinician, the family, and the school is necessary for a good outcome (Chapter 38).

A review of the literature on programs for persistently truant students showed modest benefit from targeted interventions on attendance outcomes (Maynard et al., 2012). There were minimal differences in effects across program types and modalities with no one program type or modality standing out as being more effective than any other. There was insufficient evidence to support the current "best-practice" recommendations that collaborative and multimodal interventions are more effective than programs that are not collaborative and single modal interventions.

Evidence for managing the anxiety that underlies school refusal is reviewed in Chapter 60.

School absenteeism is of concern and requires active intervention. For truancy, mentoring and behavioral strategies are likely be most effective, while school refusal is best managed by addressing the underlying anxiety. In both cases, the involvement of school personnel and families will be key to successful management.

Bullying

Bullying is defined as physical, verbal or psychological abuse or intimidation intended to cause distress or harm to the victim. There is an imbalance in power so that the more powerful oppressor bullies the less powerful victim. Bullying is usually perpetrated over a prolonged period. Cyber bullying, where bullying is perpetrated through mobile phones or the internet with a potentially very large audience, has been of increasing concern particularly given the ease with which an anonymous person can attack (Pearce et al., 2011).

Although bullying in schools has probably always been present there is increasing public attention and concern over recent years. Prevalence rates are around 20–30%, with clear adverse effects on mental health (Jimenez Barbero et al., 2012).

Anti-bullying programs, from kindergartens to high schools, generally comprise developmentally appropriate components of both universal and targeted approaches. These include:

1 a global school policy that encourages and supports the value of all individuals;
2 classroom-based strategies targeting behaviors, student attitudes and beliefs to improve relationships both between students and between teachers and students; and
3 increased supervision in the playground.

The first national anti-bullying programs were developed and implemented in Norway in the 1980s (Olweus, 1996). Although early meta-analyses showed minimal effects, more recent analyses have produced more encouraging findings (Ttofi and Farrington, 2011) (Table 42.1).

There is ongoing debate about the optimal time to intervene (Smith, 2011) and about the effectiveness of various components of the programs, particularly the possible negative effect of peer support schemes such as peer mediation and peer mentoring for bullied students and the type of disciplinary practices used for bullies (Ttofi & Farrington, 2011). The current view is that the most effective approach is implementation of anti-bullying programs across the entire school age range with multi-disciplinary professional support and parental involvement to ensure that the social and cultural milieu of the school is considered.

Currently the KiVa anti-bullying program is being implemented and evaluated nationwide in Finland with impressive initial results (Salmivalli et al., 2011). There is mounting evidence of the public health importance of anti-bullying programs in schools (Knapp et al., 2011). There is a large overlap between cyber-bullying and other bullying (Lindfors et al., 2012) and while evidence on specific approaches to address cyber-bullying is accumulating, appropriate modification of known anti-bullying strategies should be used to tackle this problem (Pearce et al., 2011).

School-based mental health in practice

As discussed earlier implementation of school-based mental health services may take many different forms. It is important first to establish the priorities for the school and for local mental health services. Because of the different focus of schools and mental health services, liaison with school personnel to establish a shared model for intervention is essential. Tensions may arise when mental health professionals believe that services can be delivered effectively in schools, while school personnel are more focused on the delivery of education. Similarly, it is important to ensure that there is clear communication with all the relevant staff, both those managing the schools and those who would deliver the services.

Addressing mental health problems in the school context requires adequate staffing and adequate training. Both should be addressed in any plan to enhance the provision of mental health care in the school setting. Clinicians from child and adolescent

Box 42.1 Tips and traps for practitioners working in schools

Do make sure that you have talked to all the relevant people	Do understand that there is a different culture within the education sector around confidentiality, parental involvement and consent
Do establish relationships with key people: visiting schools in the area served by a clinical service	Do take into account the school year including the term structure, and the need to work around particularly busy times, like exams and major school activities.
Do use technology—skype, text etc	Do plan ahead. It is often easier to start things at the beginning of a school year, which requires planning well before the end of the previous year.
Do be active about communication—check up on progress, have a strategy so the school is in the loop about what is happening in the mental health service	
Do check you have a shared understanding about what happens	

mental health services may play a key role in providing training. It should be noted that the use of manuals may not appeal to school teachers, who are used to tailoring their teaching to the educational and developmental levels of their students.

Child mental health professionals may support school staff to help children and adolescents with mental health problems in a number of ways. Active liaison with school personnel over individual students with mental health problems is useful. Having a meeting with some of the key teachers involved with the student may allow the clinician to provide essential information about the disorder, what level of function could be expected, the symptoms experienced and the likely course of these, appropriate ways to respond, signs of relapse or need for specific care, side-effects of medications and the ongoing role of the child and adolescent mental health team. Schools may appreciate resources to support them as they implement interventions, but unless these are regularly updated and are appealing and practical they may sit unused on shelves.

In England, the nationwide program, targeting mental health in schools (TaMHS), was started in 2008 and provides a framework to guide schools in the development of services for students at risk of or experiencing mental health problems suitable for their particular community and context. The framework provides practical information to guide. Three studies evaluating the impact have been carried out:

1 A large RCT;
2 A 3-year longitudinal study; and
3 Qualitative interviews with TaMHS workers, school staff, parents and pupils.

Overall, the findings supported the use of this approach although findings were mixed. TaMHS led to reduced behavioral but not emotional problems in younger but not older students. Providing information and good inter-agency working correlated with better outcomes in secondary schools. Overall, the intervention was well received (Wolpert *et al.*, 2013). This is a recent and promising initiative and further refinement is likely to lead to improved outcomes in the future.

Conclusions

In summary, schools provide a good site for the detection and intervention of mental health difficulties in students, although young people who do not attend school generally have higher mental health needs than those who so.

A wide range of interventions for health promotion and universal and targeted prevention have been developed, with some encouraging results from studies, particularly those targeting behavior. Translating programs shown to be effective in research settings into effective programs in practice has been difficult, while a number of programs that have been implemented in practice do not have data supporting their effectiveness. Further work is needed in most areas to ensure that implementation is optimized and positive effects confirmed.

Developing school-based services requires a strategic approach, with collaboration with school personnel and attention to the wider context of the child or adolescent. Variable resources globally result in variable distribution of school-based mental health services across different nations, and those most in need of services often have very poor access. Global initiatives to address this disparity have been developed and enhancing and extending these will require support from mental health professionals in more advantaged countries.

The appeal of school-based services is undoubted, but given the gaps in evidence it is important that enthusiasm for this approach does not trump evidence and that rigorous implementation trials on promising programs are carried out in the coming years.

REFERENCES

Adams, C. *et al.* (2012) Implementation of a manualized communication intervention for school-aged children with pragmatic and social communication needs in a randomized controlled trial: the social communication intervention project. *International Journal of Language & Communication Disorders* **47**, 245–256.

Anderson, P. *et al.* (2009) Effectiveness and cost-effectiveness of policies and programmes to reduce the harm caused by alcohol. *Lancet* **373**, 2234–2246.

Baker-Henningham, H. *et al.* (2012) Reducing child conduct problems and promoting social skills in a middle-income country: cluster randomised controlled trial. *The British Journal of Psychiatry* **201**, 101–108.

Baskin, T.W. *et al.* (2010) Efficacy of counseling and psychotherapy in schools: a meta-analytic review of treatment outcome studies. *The Counseling Psychologist* **38**, 878–903.

Beautrais, A. & Mishara, B. (2007) World Suicide Prevention Day-September 10, 2007: "suicide prevention across the life span". *Crisis* **28**, 57–60.

Berger, R. & Gelkopf, M. (2009) School-based intervention for the treatment of tsunami-related distress in children: a quasi-randomized controlled trial. *Psychotherapy and Psychosomatics* **78**, 364–371.

Blissett, W. *et al.* (2009) *Conduct Problems Best Practice Report*. Ministry of Social Development, Wellington, New Zealand.

Bröning, S. *et al.* (2012) Selective prevention programs for children from substance-affected families: a comprehensive systematic review. *Substance Abuse Treatment, Prevention, and Policy* **7**, 23.

Burns, B.J. *et al.* (1995) Children's mental health service use across service sectors. *Health Affairs* **14**, 147–159.

Campbell, R. *et al.* (2008) An informal school-based peer-led intervention for smoking prevention in adolescence (ASSIST): a cluster randomised trial. *Lancet* **371**, 1595–1602.

Campion, J. (2013) Public mental health: the local tangibles. *The Psychiatrist* **37**, 238–243.

Cappadocia, M. & Weiss, J.A. (2011) Review of social skills training groups for youth with asperger syndrome and high functioning autism. *Research in Autism Spectrum Disorders* **5**, 70–78.

Carney, T. & Myers, B. (2012) Effectiveness of early interventions for substance-using adolescents: findings from a systematic review and meta-analysis. *Substance Abuse Treatment, Prevention, and Policy* **7**, 25.

Castellanos-Ryan, N. *et al.* (2013) Impact of a 2-year multimodal intervention for disruptive 6-year-olds on substance use in adolescence: randomised controlled trial. *British Journal of Psychiatry* **203**, 188–195.

Champion, K.E. *et al.* (2013) A systematic review of school-based alcohol and other drug prevention programs facilitated by computers or the internet. *Drug and Alcohol Review* **32**, 115–123.

Collings, S. & Beautrais, A. (2005) *Suicide Prevention in New Zealand: A Contemporary Perspective*. Ministry of Health, Wellington.

Conduct Problems Prevention Research Group (2011) The effects of the fast track preventive intervention on the development of conduct disorder across childhood. *Child Development* **82**, 331–345.

Cooper, M. (2013) *School-Based Counselling in UK Secondary Schools: A Review and Critical Evaluation*. University of Strathclyde, Glasgow.

Crosland, K. & Dunlap, G. (2012) Effective strategies for the inclusion of children with autism in general education classrooms. *Behavior Modification* **36**, 251–269.

DuPaul, G.J. *et al.* (2012) The effects of school-based interventions for attention deficit hyperactivity disorder: a meta-analysis 1996–2010. *School Psychology Review* **41**, 387–412.

Durlak, J.A. *et al.* (2011) The impact of enhancing students' social and emotional learning: a meta-analysis of school-based universal interventions. *Child Development* **82**, 405–432.

Fabiano, G.A. *et al.* (2009) A meta-analysis of behavioral treatments for attention-deficit/hyperactivity disorder. *Clinical Psychology Review* **29**, 129–140.

Faggiano, F. *et al.* (2005) School-based prevention for illicit drugs' use. *Cochrane Database of Systematic Reviews* (2, Art. No.: CD003020).

Flower, A. *et al.* (2011) A literature review of research quality and effective practices in alternative education settings. *Education & Treatment of Children* **34**, 489–510.

Foxcroft, D.R. & Tsertsvadze, A. (2011) Universal school-based prevention programs for alcohol misuse in young people. *Cochrane Database of Systematic Reviews* (5, Art. No.: CD009113).

Franklin, C. *et al.* (2009) A meta-analysis of published school social work practice studies: 1980–2007. *Research on Social Work Practice* **19**, 667–677.

Gladstone, T.R. & Beardslee, W.R. (2009) The prevention of depression in children and adolescents: a review. *The Canadian Journal of Psychiatry* **54**, 212–221.

Hendren, R. *et al.* (1994) *Mental Health Programmes in Schools*. Division of Mental Health World Health Organization, Geneva.

Isensee, B. & Hanewinkel, R. (2012) Meta-analysis on the effects of the smoke-free class competition on smoking prevention in adolescents. *European Addiction Research* **18**, 110–115.

Jackson, C. *et al.* (2012) Interventions to prevent substance use and risky sexual behaviour in young people: a systematic review. *Addiction* **107**, 733–747.

Jimenez Barbero, J.A. *et al.* (2012) Effectiveness of antibullying school programmes: a systematic review by evidence levels. *Children and Youth Services Review* **34**, 1646–1658.

Johnston, V. *et al.* (2012) Incentives for preventing smoking in children and adolescents. *Cochrane Database of Systematic Reviews* (10, Art. No.: CD008645).

Karki, S. *et al.* (2012) The effects of interventions to prevent substance use among adolescents: a systematic review. *Journal of Child & Adolescent Substance Abuse* **21**, 383–413.

Knapp, M. *et al.* (eds) (2011) *Mental Health Promotion and Prevention: The Economic Case*. Department of Health, London.

Lang, I.A. *et al.* (2013) Influence of problematic child-teacher relationships on future psychiatric disorder: population survey with 3-year follow-up. *The British Journal of Psychiatry* **202**, 336–341.

Levitt, J.M. *et al.* (2007) Early identification of mental health problems in schools: the status of instrumentation. *Journal of School Psychology* **45**, 163–191.

Lindfors, P.L. *et al.* (2012) Cyberbullying among Finnish adolescents – a population-based study. *BMC Public Health* **12**, 1027.

Mariu, K.R. *et al.* (2012) Seeking professional help for mental health problems, among New Zealand secondary school students. *Clinical Child Psychology and Psychiatry* **17**, 284–297.

Matjasko, J.L. *et al.* (2012) A systematic meta-review of evaluations of youth violence prevention programs: common and divergent findings from 25 years of meta-analyses and systematic reviews. *Aggression and Violent Behavior* **17**, 540–552.

Maynard, B.R. *et al.* (2012) Indicated truancy interventions: effects on school attendance among chronic truant students. *Campbell Systematic Reviews* **8** (10), 48–50.

Merrell, C. (2009) Interventions for Children with ADHD in Educational Settings. *Attention Deficit Hyperactivity Disorder: The NICE Guideline on Diagnosis and Management of ADHD in Children, Young People and Adults*. The British Psychological Society and The Royal College of Psychiatrists, Leicester (UK).

Merry, S.N. & Spence, S.H. (2007) Attempting to prevent depression in youth: a systematic review of the evidence. *Early Intervention in Psychiatry* **1**, 128–137.

Merry, S.N. *et al.* (2011) Psychological and educational interventions for preventing depression in children and adolescents. *Cochrane Database of Systematic Reviews* (12, Art. No.: CD003380).

Mychailyszyn, M.P. *et al.* (2012) Cognitive-behavioral school-based interventions for anxious and depressed youth: a meta-analysis of outcomes. *Clinical Psychology: Science and Practice* **19**, 129–153.

Mytton, J. *et al.* (2006) School-based secondary prevention programmes for preventing violence. *Cochrane Database of Systematic Reviews* (3, Art. No.: CD004606).

National Institute for Health and Care Excellence (2008) Attention deficit hyperactivity disorder: diagnosis and management of ADHD in children, young people and adults. *NICE Clinical Guideline 72*. National Institute for Health and Care Excellence, London.

National Institute for Health and Care Excellence (2013) Antisocial behaviour and conduct disorders in children and young people: Recognition, intervention and management. *NICE Clinical Guideline 158*. National Institute for Health and Care Excellence, London.

National Research Council and Institute of Medicine (2009) Preventing mental, emotional, and behavioral disorders among young people: progress and possibilities. In: *Committee on the Prevention of Mental Disorders and Substance Abuse Among Children, Youth, and Young Adults: Research Advances and Promising Interventions.* (eds M.E. O'Connell, *et al.*). The National Academies Press, Washington, DC.

Norberg, M.M. *et al.* (2013) Primary prevention of cannabis use: a systematic review of randomized controlled trials. *PloS One* **8**, e53187.

Olweus, D. (1996) Bullying at school: knowledge base and an effective intervention program. *Annals of the New York Academy of Sciences* **794**, 265–276.

Pattison, S. & Harris, B. (2006) Adding value to education through improved mental health: a review of the research evidence on the effectiveness of counselling for children and young people. *The Australian Educational Researcher* **33**, 97–121.

Pearce, N. *et al.* (2011) Current evidence of best practice in whole-school bullying intervention and its potential to inform cyberbullying interventions. *Australian Journal of Guidance and Counselling* **21**, 1–21.

Pratt, B.M. & Woolfenden, S.R. (2002) Interventions for preventing eating disorders in children and adolescents. *Cochrane Database of Systematic Reviews* (2, Art. No.: CD002891).

Pryjmachuk, S. *et al.* (2012) School nurses' perspectives on managing mental health problems in children and young people. *Journal of Clinical Nursing* **21**, 850–859.

Rabiner, D.L. *et al.* (2010) A randomized trial of two promising computer-based interventions for students with attention difficulties. *Journal of Abnormal Child Psychology* **38**, 131–142.

Ramdoss, S. *et al.* (2012) Computer-based interventions to improve social and emotional skills in individuals with autism spectrum disorders: a systematic review. *Developmental Neurorehabilitation* **15**, 119–135.

Rao, P.A. *et al.* (2008) Social skills interventions for children with asperger's syndrome or high-functioning autism: a review and recommendations. *Journal of Autism and Developmental Disorders* **38**, 353–361.

Rolfsnes, E.S. & Idsoe, T. (2011) School-based intervention programs for PTSD symptoms: a review and meta-analysis. *Journal of Traumatic Stress* **24**, 155–165.

Rutter, M. *et al.* (1979) *Fifteen Thousand Hours: Secondary Schools and Their Effects on Children.* Harvard University Press, Cambridge, MA.

Salmivalli, C. *et al.* (2011) Counteracting bullying in Finland: The KiVa program and its effects on different forms of being bullied. *International Journal of Behavioral Development* **35**, 405–411.

Schachter, H.M. *et al.* (2008) Effects of school-based interventions on mental health stigmatization: a systematic review. *Child and Adolescent Psychiatry and Mental Health* **2**, 18.

Sklad, M. *et al.* (2012) Effectiveness of school-based universal social, emotional, and behavioral programs: do they enhance students' development in the area of skill, behavior, and adjustment? *Psychology in the Schools* **49**, 892–909.

Smith, P.K. (2011) Why interventions to reduce bullying and violence in schools may (or may not) succeed: comments on this special section. *International Journal of Behavioral Development* **35**, 419–423.

Stallard, P. *et al.* (2012) Classroom based cognitive behavioural therapy in reducing symptoms of depression in high risk adolescents: pragmatic cluster randomised controlled trial. *British Medical Journal* **345**, e6058.

Stein, B.D. *et al.* (2003) A mental health intervention for school children exposed to violence: a randomized controlled trial. *JAMA* **290**, 603–611.

Steiner, N.J. *et al.* (2011) Computer-based attention training in the schools for children with attention deficit/hyperactivity disorder: a preliminary trial. *Clinical Pediatrics* **50**, 615–622.

Teesson, M. *et al.* (2012) Australian school-based prevention programs for alcohol and other drugs: a systematic review. *Drug and Alcohol Review* **31**, 731–736.

Teich, J.L. *et al.* (2007) What kinds of mental health services do public schools in the United States provide? *Advances in School Mental Health Promotion* **1**, 13–22.

Thomas, R.E. *et al.* (2011) Mentoring adolescents to prevent drug and alcohol use. *Cochrane Database of Systematic Reviews* (11, Art. No.: CD007381).

Thomas, R.E. *et al.* (2013) School-based programmes for preventing smoking. *Cochrane Database of Systematic Reviews* (5, Art. No.: CD001293).

Tobin, T. & Sprague, J. (2000) Alternative education strategies: reducing violence in school and the community. *Journal of Emotional and Behavioral Disorders* **8**, 177–186.

Tol, W.A. *et al.* (2011) Mental health and psychosocial support in humanitarian settings: linking practice and research. *Lancet* **378**, 1581–1591.

Ttofi, M.M. & Farrington, D.P. (2011) Effectiveness of school-based programs to reduce bullying: a systematic and meta-analytic review. *Journal of Experimental Criminology* **7**, 27–56.

U.S. Department of Education Office of Special Education and Rehabilitative Services (2002) *A New Era: Revitalizing Special Education for Children and Their Families.* ED Pubs, Education Publications Center, U.S. Department of Education, Washington, DC.

U.S. Department of Justice. *OJJDP model programs guide*, [Online], Available: http://www.ojjdp.gov/mpg/progTypesTruancy.aspx [15 Jul 2013].

US Preventive Services Task Force (2009) Screening and treatment for major depressive disorder in children and adolescents: US preventive services task force recommendation statement. *Pediatrics* **123**, 1223–1228.

Vostanis, P. *et al.* (2013) How do schools promote emotional well-being among their pupils? Findings from a national scoping survey of mental health provision in English schools. *Child and Adolescent Mental Health* **18**, 151–157.

Wei, Y. & Kutcher, S. (2012) International school mental health: global approaches, global challenges, and global opportunities. *Child and Adolescent Psychiatric Clinics of North America* **21**, 11–27.

Weisz, J.R. *et al.* (2005) Promoting and protecting youth mental health through evidence-based prevention and treatment. *American Psychologist* **60**, 628–648.

Williams, S.B. *et al.* (2009) Screening for child and adolescent depression in primary care settings: a systematic evidence review for the US preventive services task force. *Pediatrics*, [Online], 123, Available: www.pediatrics.org/cgi/doi/10.1542/peds.2008-2415 [18 Oct 2013].

Wolpert, M. *et al.* (2013) Embedding mental health support in schools: learning from the Targeted Mental Health in Schools (TaMHS) national evaluation. *Emotional and Behavioural Difficulties* **18**, 270–283.

World Health Organization (2008) *The Global Burden of Disease: 2004 Update*. World Health Organization, Geneva.

Young, S. & Amarasinghe, J.M. (2010) Practitioner review: non-pharmacological treatments for ADHD: a lifespan approach. *Journal of Child Psychology and Psychiatry* **51**, 116–133.

CHAPTER 43

Pharmacological, medically-led and related treatments

Eric Taylor

Department of Child and Adolescent Psychiatry, Institute of Psychiatry, Psychology and Neuroscience, King's College London, UK

Introduction and regulation of psychoactive drugs

Discovery

The initial discovery of psychotropic actions of drugs has usually relied on unplanned clinical observation. Drugs used for other purposes have been found to have beneficial actions on the mind. Historical examples include: the central nervous stimulants—benzedrine having been introduced for postlumbar puncture headache, isoniazid for tuberculosis, and neuroleptics for premedication, especially hypothermia. A current example includes a drug modifying glutamate (riluzole), whose main indication is for amyotrophic lateral sclerosis, but which appears to have potential for treating some forms of depression. It is likely that systematic analysis of large databases will eventually find psychiatric potential in medicines used for other illnesses.

More recently, ideas for new drugs have come to be derived from the understanding of neurochemical targets and the screening of many molecules for their actions on those targets in vitro and in animal studies. The full potential of this method is still to be realized, so serendipitous discovery will keep a place for some years to come. The small number emerging as having therapeutic potential then undergo a planned—and expensive—process of clinical trials. Figure 43.1 illustrates the phases of testing and development

Young people are seldom involved in the early phases, because of the unpredictability of a new drug and the need for safety.

Even at Phase 3, where trials are designed to persuade drug regulators that a market license should be given, children have often been excluded; with the result that pediatric use is inadequately researched and very often not licensed.

Judging clinical trials

Clinicians will therefore need to understand the trial literature as it develops and extends. The quality of a trial needs to be judged in order to understand how much weight can be given to its conclusions. Its power (and therefore number of subjects), clarity and appropriateness of aim, outcome measure and comparator group, randomization, "blindness," and correct analysis all enter the judgment, as described in Chapter 14. In practice, therefore, prescribers are strongly influenced by systematic reviews, guidelines, and the advice of expert "opinion formers."

Difficulties emerge when a new drug has a substantial evidence base in its favor, but has not yet gone through the official procedure of approval. In general, caution is advised, especially for the nonspecialist prescriber. Safety concerns sometimes appear only in the later stages of drug development. An experimental treatment should not be preferred to an established one unless the evidence is very clear; its place would be when the full range of standard therapies has failed.

Recommendations, guidelines, and protocols

The process of developing evidence-based practice usually starts with a systematic review of Phase 3 (and other) trials. All the published evidence needs to be collected—and often unpublished as well, to safeguard against bias from nonpublication of negative or inconclusive results. When the evidence allows, estimates of effect size are made, tested for whether there is a consistent story, and pooled for an overall conclusion about efficacy. This is not yet a recommendation, but only a description of the trial evidence; it requires experts on trials and analysis rather than clinicians. The draft then receives a critique from expert clinicians who can incorporate considerations of what is

Rutter's Child and Adolescent Psychiatry, Sixth Edition.
Edited by Anita Thapar and Daniel S. Pine, James F. Leckman, Stephen Scott, Margaret J. Snowling, Eric Taylor.
© 2015 John Wiley & Sons Ltd. Published 2018 by John Wiley & Sons Ltd.

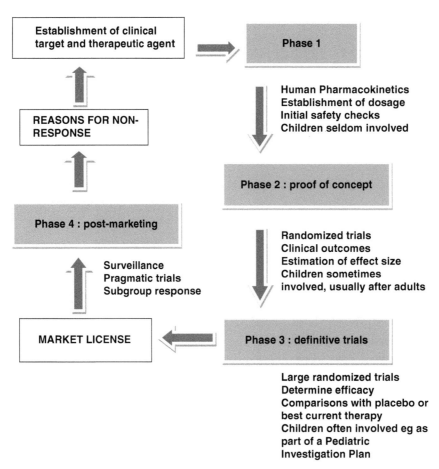

Figure 43.1 Establishing a new medication.

realistic and safe, the impact on quality of life, and the extent to which a new treatment compares favorably with existing practice. For instance, the literature review for attention deficit hyperactivity disorder (ADHD) undertaken by the (English and Welsh) National Institute for Health and Care Excellence (NICE, 2009) would on its own indicate that dexamfetamine (dextroamphetamine) should be the first choice of therapy because of high efficacy and low cost; but expert consensus did not adopt the recommendation because of uncertainty about its safety record and its popularity as a recreational drug.

The resulting recommendation can then be modulated into a guideline—typically, at a national level. The cost of the intervention and its acceptability to the public need to be brought in; they vary from country to country; and economists, users and clinicians from primary and secondary care need to be added to the review. Guidelines by their nature cannot apply to every individual. The prescriber, not the guideline, has the responsibility and must consider the individual circumstances. A particular service may want to draw up a detailed protocol of how treatment should be given—in which case it will need to consider whether it will be applicable to all groups in the community it serves. Guidelines do not have formal legal status. In many jurisdictions, however,

a demonstration that guidelines have been followed has been a successful defense against malpractice litigation.

Licensing, international differences, and off-label use

National and supranational regulators issue a license to a company to market a drug, not usually to individual professionals to prescribe it. (In a few instances, for example for controlled drugs [including stimulants], governments have restricted prescribing to specified centers). Countries vary in their requirements. The classical requirement in the USA has been for two trials, from different centers, showing superiority to placebo; in Europe, for demonstration of superiority to current standard therapy. In many countries there is consideration, not only of efficacy and safety, but of cost. For many drugs, a license has been issued only for adults. They may still be prescribed "off-label" for young people, but the absence of official dosages and safety surveillance can cause confusion. The problem is not only for psychotropic drugs, but occurs across the whole of medicine. In some countries, however, there is officially formulated advice, such as the pediatric version of the National Formulary in the UK (Pediatric Formulary Committee, 2012); or the market license holder will give its recommendations.

International differences and secular trends

There have been large, recent increases of drug prescription of certain drugs in many countries. The number of outpatient visits, by young people in the USA, at which antipsychotics were prescribed rose by some 600% during the decade from 1993 to 2002 (Olfson *et al.*, 2006). In the UK, stimulant drug prescriptions approximately doubled between 2003 and 2008 (McCarthy *et al.*, 2012); and the diagnosis of ADHD increased in tandem (see Chapter 55). Stimulant use in the Netherlands increased some eightfold between 1996 and 2006 (Trip *et al.*, 2009).

Different reasons apply for these increases in different places. In the UK and Netherlands, the increase in stimulants was from a very low base rate (4.8 per 1000 in UK, 2.6 in Netherlands) and followed the reintroduction of methylphenidate to the market and an increased willingness by the medical profession to recognize ADHD as a medical problem. In the USA, increased prescription for adults with ADHD and increased willingness to diagnose bipolar disorder in young children may well have contributed to rising rates. Nevertheless, Rapoport (2013) has argued that the USA now suffers overmedication and an excessive exposure of children to the dangers of antipsychotics (and indeed of other drugs). She attributes this to the economic contingencies applying to medical practice, such as an insistence by managed care that expensive physicians should be used for what they are uniquely qualified to do—prescribing—and so confining their work to medication clinics. Reimbursement policies may also favor the use of drugs over psychological approaches.

There are sometimes cultural reasons for very low drug use, as in France where (for instance) stimulants are used at a rate as low as 1.8 per 1000 (Knellwolf *et al.*, 2008). In many parts of the world, however, medicines are simply unavailable (Taylor, 2013). Medicines may be priced too high to be available (as in China) or there may be too few medical doctors to deliver them (as in most low- and middle-income countries). The World Health Organization advises on which drugs are economically affordable. Paramedical workers can be trained to deliver drugs effectively, provided that protocols are clear and there is access to specialist advice.

Place of medication in therapeutic planning

Targets for medication

Different medicines have different effects. Serotonin reuptake inhibitors (SSRIs) affect anxiety but not ADHD; the opposite is the case for stimulants; some tricyclic antidepressants affect obsessionality but not depression, while others affect ADHD but not depression.

Treatment planning, therefore, needs the physician to formulate a clear target. It should be clear enough to allow explicit monitoring, practical enough to be susceptible to change, simple enough to allow explanation to the child and family, and acceptable enough to be followed by them. There may of course be multiple targets (for instance, to reduce obsessionality, lift mood,

and improve social relating)—but it is best to keep clarity about the intended gains and review them separately.

Targets are very often symptomatic rather than diagnostic. They stem from the formulation of the whole case, not simply the diagnosis (see Chapter 32). They are frequently directed, not at the whole diagnosis but at one component of it (e.g., at reducing the hallucinations and delusions in schizophrenia, so that persistence of negative symptoms is not necessarily taken to show that the drug is failing). Furthermore, many child mental health problems act as dimensions that cut across formal diagnoses: stimulants, for instance, may reduce the component of impulsive hyperactivity even if it occurs in the presence of autism, or epilepsy, or conduct disorder. From this perspective, it was an error that DSM-IV did not allow the recognition of ADHD in the presence of autism, and DSM-5 has rightly changed the policy. Similarly, it may be valuable to recognize the presence of depression in a person whose major diagnosis is that of a reaction to trauma and to consider antidepressant treatment.

Targets can also refer to the course of a condition rather than immediate symptom reduction. Reducing the risk of future episodes in a person with recurrent depression is a valid target and can be measured. Each target can be observed as a hypothesis about the nature of the child's condition (see Chapter 32) and each treatment trial is testing a hypothesis.

Ultimately, people are treated, not symptoms. One should not lose sight of the wider picture in pursuit of a targeted symptom reduction. For many people with Tourette's disorder, for instance, the hazards of drugs used in assertive tic reduction will outweigh the benefits of partial suppression; and learning to be more accepting of their tic symptoms and resist the taunts of others can be a better long-term strategy than medication.

Pharmacological versus psychological interventions

Prescribers should know in detail about the benefits and hazards of the available interventions for the chosen target—or be able to find out. Furthermore, they should be able to advise their patients of the best treatment for them, even if they are not in a position personally to provide it. Behavior modification approaches, for example, are in general a safer approach than medication for aggressive behavior and can often be effective (see meta-analysis by NICE, 2013). The practitioner should, therefore, be guiding the family towards the appropriate provision rather than moving straight to medication.

On the other hand, it is often incorrectly thought that medication is a last resort, to be used only after all other methods have failed. The hazards of nonphysical treatments need also to be taken into consideration. In some families, for instance, a prolonged failure to identify improvement may lead to such lack of confidence in the treating service that effective medication is never started. (This can happen, for instance, in blindly following NICE recommendations for a 3-month period of psychotherapy before antidepressant medication). If, as suggested by the TADS research (March *et al.*, 2004), there is a lower rate of suicidal thinking in depressed young people treated with the combination of fluoxetine and CBT than in cases treated with either monotherapy, then including an antidepressant from the start could prove a safer policy. The judgments about the initial treatment should be based on the individual case, taking into account: The safety and efficacy as known from trials, any predictive factors that apply to the individual, the need for rapid action in urgent cases, the wishes of the child and the family and (other things being equal) the cost of the treatment. The family should be taken firmly into the decision-making process—especially when the balance of evidence is not tilted strongly towards one or the other treatment.

The choice of physical or psychological intervention does not usually depend upon judgments about cause. The physical changes in the brain after trauma (see Chapter 59) do not imply that medication is the best form of intervention for posttraumatic stress disorders. Similarly, the potential of psychological deprivation to give rise to ADHD features (see Chapter 55) does not imply that the treatment of such cases should be only psychological. The rationale for most drugs in current knowledge is based on symptom reduction rather than modification of initiating cause.

Pretreatment assessment

The specification of the target(s) for treatment will lead to a decision about how to measure them and track the impact of intervention. The rating scales used in research trials will be a good starting point and are usually used when the goal is a reduction in complex behavior patterns, such as ADHD. Sometimes, however, it will make better sense for effectiveness to be judged by its impact on a single symptom (such as an isolated phobia), or to include a symptom of particular importance to the child and/or family (e.g., insomnia). An individualized problem rating can then be employed. The overall impact on children's function should also be assessed and an evaluation made of the pretreatment status of any anticipated hazards of medication. A checklist of those hazards should also be set up and used in the monitoring of drug actions along with the selected outcome measures.

Explanation and advice

Families and children come with very different sets of knowledge and attitudes about medication. The internet has made detailed information very much more available to the public—sometimes so contradictory that the result has been more to confuse than to empower. For some, medication is welcome as an affirmation of the medical status of the child's problem and a relief from accusations of poor parenting. Others will have been led to very high expectation of what drugs can achieve. On the other hand, some parents will be strongly opposed to the use of drugs as unnatural and dangerous. Children may understand a "drug" as something that is dangerous, belittling or addictive. Most will bring a mixture of hope and fear. The assessment should include an appreciation of the mix in the individual case and of how the family's views interact with its community of friends, relatives, neighbors, teachers, and previous professionals.

Cultural and national differences and controversies help to inform the variety of beliefs. Public attitudes in many countries have been strongly influenced by perceptions of whether the treatments are natural or artificial. Some families, for instance, request the provision of St John's Wort (hypericum)—a chemical which carries greater hazards (e.g., of immunological and cardiovascular problems) than do the licensed drugs for depression and ADHD, but which brings the (false) reassurance of coming from a plant rather than a laboratory. The (UK) Academy of Medical Sciences (2008) made a public consultation about the use of drugs in people without formal psychiatric diagnoses: approval or disapproval was closely connected with whether the substance was natural and acceptable (e.g., caffeine) or synthetic (e.g., "Prozac"). Some spiritual leaders discourage their disciples from accepting drugs rather than relying on their faith.

Another strand in the debate in some countries has come from distrust of commercial practices. In many cultures, deference to physicians is being replaced by a view that medical psychiatrists have come to be untrustworthy and even venal. Medical opinion leaders have often been seen to accept money from pharmaceutical companies, which can be viewed as disqualifying their advice. Prescribers are advised to refrain from accepting gifts or other benefits that they would be unhappy to be known to their patients or revealed in the media.

A key task for the prescriber is therefore to understand, and responsively discuss, the understanding that children and their families bring to a recommendation for medication. Children will have a changing understanding as they develop and will need the opportunity to discuss their treatment in different ways as they grow older. Singh (2012) applied methods of qualitative interviewing for children and her findings emphasized that they frequently attain a sophistication of understanding, identifying positive and negative aspects of the treatment. Autonomy and authenticity become important ways in which adolescents come to think about themselves. Responsive discussion is needed and it is an influence on how the child and family make large decisions about whether to take the treatment at all, and smaller ones about dosing regimes. Families need to be willing partners in issues such as the generation of the clinical hypotheses and the need to test them with a trial that is long enough—depending on the drug—to test the hypothesis that the drug is effective.

Consent

Consent to medication means the uncoerced and informed agreement to treatment by a person who is competent to give it. Children may not be competent to make the decision, and their parents or guardians do it on their behalf; but their assent should be sought and their views respected even if they are over-ruled. The amount of information that needs to be given should be tailored to the person. The detailed information in the product package is legally specified and often useless to the reader by virtue of its length and lack of prioritization. The

Box 43.1 Information necessary for consent.

The condition to be treated	Physician's inability to predict results
Nature of proposed treatment	Irreversibility (if applicable)
Nature and probability of material risks	Likely results of no treatment
Benefits to be expected	Likely results/risks/benefits of alternatives

prescriber becomes the key source of information. He or she has the professional duty to brief with enough information to enable a rational choice, if the patient is fit to receive the information and wishes to receive it. One legal formulation of the information that should be given derives from the case of *Hamish v Children's Medical Center 1982* and is summarized in Box 43.1.

Compliance

A necessary step for a drug to be fully effective is that it should be swallowed. A lack of adherence to the prescriber's intentions is very common and the reasons for it need to be understood. There are many people in a child's network who can exercise an effective veto over medication, and some of them will not have had the benefit of full explanation. Estranged parents, grandparents, teachers who are new to the child, and professionals from disciplines hostile to medication are the commonest obstacles to the therapy. The remedy will probably be to explain the rationale to them. Sometimes, they will be able to observe the difference between medication and the lack of it with their own eyes (as with a temporary discontinuation of stimulants); but for many types of drugs (e.g., antidepressants) a premature discontinuation can have adverse effects. The responsible parent will then need to draw on the trust that has been built up with the prescriber and her (or his) own resolve.

Moreover, children's own attitudes play a strong part in adherence to expected regimes. There are several influences that can lead to their not taking the treatment, and they call for different types of action. Simple forgetfulness is common, especially when child or parent is afflicted with problems of memory or attention. Dispensing in calendar packs can help, as can charts in which medication is included with other daily chores. Taking tablets can be treated as a learned behavior and encouraged with star charts and the like. Simplicity of administration also helps—longer-acting drugs can be taken once a day and can therefore be more clearly under parental control. Children can often encounter considerable stigma if they are known to take psychotropic medication, especially from other children but sometimes from teachers. Extended-release preparations or long-acting drugs can then allow a single daily dose in the morning or evening and children often value the privacy and confidentiality that this brings.

Many children, especially those with autism spectrum disorders or intellectual disability, have an inability or a marked reluctance to swallow. Liquid preparations are often available; when they are not (e.g., for most controlled drugs) then granular preparations can often be swallowed much more readily, for instance by being sprinkled on food. (Surreptitious administration is not advocated, however, partly because of the breakdown of trust that can follow when the child discovers the truth). The taste of drugs can also be aversive; and some antidepressants (fluoxetine, escitalopram and bupropion) are particularly likely to cause a dysgeusia and need to be replaced with another antidepressant. Tart juices (such as lemonade), cold or iced drinks and food, and sugar-free chewing gum can all help to get rid of unpleasant taste sensations.

Adverse effects are also a reason for noncompliance and some of them may not be obvious because they are not volunteered or included in checklists of adverse effects. Sexual problems, for instance in ejaculation, are quite common with SSRIs and can be distressing to adolescents. A feeling that one has lost one's funny side can be expressed by children treated for ADHD: it is not always veridical, because it may be that children have stopped laughing *at* one rather than *with* one; but it may be a pointer to a lack of spontaneity and an overly high dosage. Some young people, who have rightly been warned against the dangerous effects of cannabis, may have understood or been told that it must never be combined with prescribed medicine and prefer to omit the medicine than forgo the cannabis. There is in fact no major interaction between stimulants and cannabis, and it is often better to permit the combination than to lose the benefit of the medicine. Other illegal drugs (see Chapter 66) are rightly regarded as contraindications outside very specialist settings.

In adolescents, development issues of autonomy become very important. If during childhood medication has been imposed coercively then a hostile reaction to it is only to be expected. In these circumstances, it is often possible to return responsibility to the teenager, to allow discontinuation, and to suggest the experiment of finding out how the absence of medicine affects ones progress—as seen by others (e.g., teachers and friends) as well as by subjective experience and family reaction. The goals of therapy may then be renegotiated to be more meaningful to the young person and most of those who need long-term treatment will indeed decide to return to it. The most ominous of the attitude changes is probably emotional: the nihilistic belief that nothing can be done to help one's predicament. This should be taken seriously and addressed vigorously with cognitive (or antidepressive) approaches.

A self-report scale has been developed by Ferrin *et al.* (2012) for young people to describe both positive and negative attitudes to drug therapy, and it may be helpful to track individuals' progress in this way. It is important to maintain positive attitudes. Good compliance was in one study associated with good outcome over a 5-year period (Charach *et al.*, 2004). This may not be wholly cause and effect. In a meta-analysis across a wide range of adult medical specialties, Simpson *et al.* (2006) found good compliance to be associated with good outcome—even when the treatment was a placebo. The healthy comply well. "Compliance" may be an oversimple goal, if it is taken to mean only accurate obedience to the wishes of doctors and parents. In the long run, perhaps, the model should be that of the intelligent consumer who has learned when and how to take medication in his or her best interest.

All the aforementioned obstacles to compliance can lead to multiple agents being tried but stopped prematurely, before they have had a chance to be effective. It may be necessary to return to such agents later; for instance to a reduced dosage of a drug that was discontinued because of an adverse effect that might well have subsided with time.

Involvement of multidisciplinary team: knowledge and attitudes, communication

Where prescribers have the advantage of working in a multidisciplinary team, care can readily be made comprehensive. Nurses, psychologists, and pharmacists can take on prescribing and monitoring. The initial decision to prescribe can be made after an assessment including several perspectives. The impact of physical treatment on ongoing psychological work can be explicitly considered. In neurodevelopmental disorders, it may be possible to apply therapies such as speech and language therapy for the first time when behavioral disturbance has been controlled medically. It may be possible for the management of anxiety to proceed when initial panics have restricted the opportunities for graded exposure. Conversely, therapists encouraging the exposure to anxiety-provoking situations may be able to request that anxiety-reducing drugs should be withheld.

Two possible problems need to be overcome. First, there needs to be an atmosphere of mutual respect for differing therapeutic approaches so that families are not confused. Second, there should be continuity for the children in their key worker, so that they can have extended conversations over time about their condition and its therapy.

Prescribing: evidence and practice

Developmental changes in pharmacokinetics

The body changes with age in the ways that it absorbs, distributes, and metabolizes drugs. The experience of adult psychiatry cannot be applied without careful revision. Adult doses cannot simply be scaled down on the basis of body weight.

Developmental differences are present at many stages of a drug's journey from mouth to brain. Ionized drugs (many are weak acids) may be less well absorbed from a child's less acid stomach. The great activity of the young liver may oxidize and conjugate drugs more swiftly than that of the adult. Distribution—which is often in the extracellular fluid—may

result in greater dilution for children, in whom there is a greater ratio of water to fat than applies after puberty. For most, the resultant is less bioavailability in children and therefore a need for a higher dose in mg/kg terms. On the other hand, the greater permeability of the blood–brain barrier in children may mean a greater than predicted effect. The complexity forbids accurate calculation and correspondingly Tables 43.1–43.3 show, for the most part, approximate dose ranges rather than mg/kg specifications. Titration according to the individual's clinical response is therefore required. "Start low and go slow" is not only the conventional wisdom, but good advice.

Prescribing errors and avoiding errors

Errors in prescribing and dispensing are responsible for many of the adverse effects reported. Prescribers are advised to have a restricted group of drugs that they know well (e.g., one from each major class) and to be particularly cautious when they go outside that range. They should have a prescribing manual at their side so that they do not have to rely on memory concerning doses at different ages and can check on interactions with other drugs or foodstuffs (e.g., Taylor *et al.*, 2012). They should keep a reference on specific problems about which to warn families in advance (e.g., suicidality with selective serotonin reuptake inhibitors and atomoxetine; and overeating in antipsychotic use). Monitoring should be carefully matched to the expectations of guidelines and protocols.

Stimulants and other antihyperkinetic agents

Methylphenidate, amphetamines, and atomoxetine comprise the approved range of therapies for ADHD (Attention Deficit/ Hyperactivity Disorder), in most countries. There is a sound evidence base for them, based on good quality trials and systematic reviews: Seixas *et al.* (2012) review national guidelines: there is a consensus that the licensed drugs all have large effects in reducing the features of ADHD. They are also used in the treatment of narcolepsy and in counteracting the obtunding effects of anticonvulsant drugs. Table 43.1 indicates their dosage ranges, duration of action, and legal status and Chapter 55 describes their application to the clinical problems of inattention, impulsivity, and inattention. The controlled status of the stimulants reflects their capacity for inducing euphoria and craving if they are taken by a rapidly acting route (such as intravenous injection or inhalation). Taken orally, however, and in therapeutic doses, there is little such risk, and its management is described in Chapter 55.

The pharmacology of efficacious drugs is rather diverse, but all have effects on catecholamine receptors (Heal *et al.*, 2012). Methylphenidate and the amphetamines inhibit the dopamine transporter; this and other actions create large increases in dopamine and norepinephrine in the prefrontal cortex and dopamine in the striatum. Atomoxetine inhibits the norepinephrine transporter; the functional effects include enhancing the brain levels not only of norepinephrine itself, but also of dopamine in many parts of the brain except the

Table 43.1 Considerations specific to individual antihyperkinetic drugs.

Drug	Preparations	Dose (per day)	Duration	Legal status
Methylphenidate	Immediate-release	5–60 mg in divided doses	2–4 hours	Licensed for children in many countries; controlled as a misusable drug
Extended release Methylphenidate (proprietary names given)	OROS (osmotic release) Concerta Equasym-XL (beaded) Medikinet-retard (beaded)	18–72 mg single dose 10–60 mg single dose 10–60 mg single dose	Up to 12 hours up to 8 hours up to 8 hours	Controlled drugs
Dexamfetamine	Immediate-release	2.5–40 mg	3–6 hours	Licensed in many countries for children. Controlled drug
	Lisdexamfetamine	20–70 mg	10–13 hours	Licensed in many countries. Controlled drug
Atomoxetine		0.5 mg/kg for first week, then 1.2 mg/kg; max. 1.8 mg/kg	Prolonged	Licensed in many countries for children and adults (in Europe, only if treatment started before 18). Not controlled
Alternative antihyperkinetics				
Bupropion		50–200 mg divided doses (or single dose of XL formulation)	c. 6 hours	Not licensed, even for depression, in UK Not controlled Caution re seizures
Clonidine		0.05–0.4 mg divided doses (or single dose of XL formulation)	c. 4 hours	Not licensed for children in most countries Not controlled
Guanfacine (extended-release formulation)		1–4 mg single dose	Prolonged	Licensed in USA, not Europe. Not controlled
Modafinil		200–425 mg single dose	Prolonged	Not licensed for children, due to concerns re skin problems Not controlled

Doses for children aged 6 years or more. They should be regarded as indicative only; individual titration against response is required and some children may need higher doses after appropriate review. Financial costs are not included as they vary greatly between countries. "Alternative antihyperkinetics" includes only those with evidence from randomized controlled trials. The table does not include drugs considered too hazardous for this purpose (e.g., pemoline and desipramine). Dexamfetamine is also known as dextroamphetamine.

striatum. Of the alternative antihyperkinetic agents that lack European approval, bupropion has several actions (including nicotinic) but its value as an antihyperkinetic is probably related to the inhibition of norepinephrine reuptake. Guanfacine and clonidine are preferential α_{2A}-adrenoceptor agonists, and clonidine is used in the treatment of hypertension and migraine. Their presynaptic action may reduce norepinephrine effects and create sedation and depression as hazards of therapy. Modafinil's pharmacological actions are multiple and somewhat obscure but include increase of striatal dopamine as well as effects on norepinephrine, glutamate and hypocretin in the brain; it is used for the treatment of narcolepsy and daytime sleepiness.

Table 43.1 summarizes the dose ranges for children and how long an individual dose can be expected to last. The stimulants are notable for their rapid onset and offset and some extended-release preparations have therefore been formulated and are referred to by their proprietary rather than generic names. Adverse effects (including those on the cardiovascular system) and their management in children with ADHD are described in Chapter 55.

Antipsychotics

Antipsychotics have a clear place in the treatment of schizophrenia and bipolar disorder and a more controversial one, in low dose, for a variety of conditions where the control of agitation, anxiety, and aggression is desired. The evidence about their use is extensive for adults, but very scanty for children and adolescents (except for efficacy in severe irritability in autism and /or intellectual disability, where several good-quality trials have received systematic reviews and, recently, approval by regulators). Knowledge about pharmacokinetics and safety is based mostly on analogy with adult effects. All the antipsychotics have pharmacological actions in blocking dopamine receptors and most also act on the serotonin (5HT) receptors. They differ in the details of which dopamine receptors, and which others, receive the blockade.

The first generation of antipsychotics (FGA: chlorpromazine being the standard) coincided with, and facilitated, the social psychiatric effects of normalizing the lives of those with chronic psychoses. They also had a range of unpleasant adverse effects—including those on the extrapyramidal motor system which may have been even more frequent, stigmatizing, and

Table 43.2 Considerations specific to individual second-generation antipsychotics (SGA).

Drug	Receptor actions additional to generic	Other approved indications	Safety considerations
Risperidone, Paliperidone and others	Generic; see text	Irritability in autism	Risperidone has lower risk for seizures than many antipsychotics
Quetiapine	H1 blocker Alpha-1 adrenoreceptor blockade Low D2 binding	Adjunct in major depression	Sedative Hypothyroidism Low rate of EPS Low rate of epilepsy Low rate of hyperprolactinaemia
Amisulpride Low dose	Inhibit Dopamine autoreceptors	Not approved in USA (possibly helpful for negative symptoms)	Agitation
High dose (>400 mg)	Inhibit postsynaptic receptors Antagonises 5HT-7 Little 5HT–1A, 2A, C blockade	(Possibly helpful for depression)	Q-T interval prolonged
Aripiprazole	Partial dopamine agonist	Adjunctive in major depression Irritability in autism	Less metabolic and endocrine risks than most antipsychotics; somewhat more EPS
Olanzapine	Multiple receptor antagonism including muscarinic M3	Alternative to clozapine in refractory psychosis	High efficacy High rates of obesity, metabolic and endocrine problems
Clozapine	Low D2 binding, high D4 Cholinergic and histaminergic antagonism	Refractory psychosis (nonresponse to 2 SGAs)	High efficacy, low EPS High rates of obesity, metabolic and endocrine problems Agranulocytosis, requiring blood counts Seizures, constipation

EPS = extrapyramidal symptoms.

Table 43.3 Antidepressants.

Drug	Metabolites	Dose (mg/day)[a]	Special consideration
Fluoxetine	Norfluoxetine (active, long half-life)	20–40	The standard for treating depression Interacts with many other drugs
Fluvoxamine	Inactive	100–200	Short-acting, and less protein-bound than others so less likely to cause interaction with other protein-bound drugs
Paroxetine	Inactive	20–40	Short-acting and sedative Anticholinergic side effects
Citalopram, Escitalopram	Desmethylcitalopram (possibly active, long half-life)	20–40 10–20	Most selective Few interactions with drugs that are metabolized by P450 Prolongation of Q-T interval
Sertraline	Desmethylsertraline (much less active, long half-life)	50–200	Should be taken with food which increases plasma levels Inhibits dopamine reuptake

[a]Common maintenance dose range. Doses vary: initial dose is usually half the lower dose given above. These figures are only a guide and individual titration should be undertaken. Children younger than 12 may need lower doses and those younger than 6 require detailed specialist consideration.

disabling for young patients. It therefore appeared to be a great advance when a second generation of antipsychotics (SGAs) appeared, with much less propensity to alter motor control. They became the standard for treating first episodes, especially in young people, with risperidone being the most widely used.

There are, however, another set of metabolic adverse effects that are even more prominent than in FGAs: obesity, increases in blood levels of triglycerides, nonhigh-density lipoproteins, cholesterol and glucose (which may amount to Type II diabetes), and endocrine changes such as hyperprolactinemia (which can result in inappropriate lactation for both sexes, and polycystic ovaries and menstrual irregularities in females). Constipation can become a serious problem in developmentally disabled children.

The implications for clinical practice are set out in Chapter 57 for schizophrenia and other psychoses, Chapter 56 for motor tics and Chapter 62 for bipolar disorder.

Most of the SGAs share most of the same good and bad effects. They differ somewhat in the profile of receptors affected, and consequently the clinical actions, requirements for monitoring, and safety profile. Table 43.2 sets out the considerations that are specific to some individual SGAs. Risperidone is taken as the standard and the choice among the other antipsychotics is largely determined by the adverse effects in the individual case. For example, aripiprazole may be preferred in the presence or threat of obesity; quetiapine in hyperprolactinemia, quetiapine or olanzapine plus fluoxetine in depression; clozapine (in spite of adverse effects) in nonresponse to other drugs. The blood levels are determined not only by dose level but also by metabolism in the liver. Different SGAs are broken down by different cytochrome isoenzymes. Interactions with other drugs and food substances which inhibit those enzymes (e.g., some antidepressants) or potentiate their action (e.g., some anticonvulsants) will therefore vary from drug to drug.

Antidepressants

Tricyclics

Tricyclic antidepressants act on several neurotransmitter receptor sites, notably serotonergic and norepinephrinergic. They are effective in reducing ADHD features, but not often used because of toxicity (requiring, *inter alia*, monitoring of ECG). They are also effective in reducing symptoms of obsessive-compulsive disorder, especially if they have strong serotonergic activity (e.g., clomipramine), and they can suppress bedwetting. Curiously, however, they have proved ineffective in treating depression in children (systematic review by Hazell *et al.*, 1995).

Selective serotonin reuptake inhibitors (SSRIs)

Selective SSRIs have small to moderate effect sizes as antidepressants and moderate to good effects in the therapy of obsessions and compulsions and anxiety disorder (see Chapters 60, 61 & 63). Distressing adverse reactions include gastrointestinal symptoms and headaches. They can alter the metabolism of other drugs, notably antipsychotics.

Some differences between the various SSRIs are set out in Table 43.3. The main consideration in practice is that of the risk for "suicidality"—usually, thoughts about self-destruction or the valuelessness of life, and occasionally even self-harming gestures or acts (Hammad *et al.*, 2006). Systematic guidance has been developed by national drug regulators and favors fluoxetine (Chapter 63 and Committee on Safety of Medicines, 2003). In practice fluoxetine is nearly always the first choice and others are reserved for situations where fluoxetine has failed,

or is itself contraindicated (e.g., by intolerance), or is likely to cause hazardous interactions with other drugs.

In conditions other than depression, there is a wider choice of antidepressants. While they all increase serotonergic activity, they interact with many other receptors as well. Citalopram and escitalopram are the most selective for serotonin reuptake, fluoxetine the least. By the same token, fluoxetine is most likely to inhibit the cytochrome P450 family of enzymes that metabolize many drugs in the liver; citalopram and escitalopram the least—and therefore the most suitable to administer in combination with other psychotropics. Fluvoxamine and sertraline are less protein-bound than other SSRIs, and correspondingly less likely to interact with other protein-bound drugs (including some anticonvulsants).

Weight gain and metabolic changes are possible adverse effects, but are least prominent with fluoxetine and sertraline in the adult studies from which most of our information is derived (Hiemke & Härtter, 2000). Citalopram and escitalopram appear particularly likely to give rise to sexual dysfunction (a problem which adolescents often resent and seldom express spontaneously). Sertraline appears least likely to cause insomnia.

All the SSRIs can give rise to discontinuation problems, even the long-acting fluoxetine, and patients and families should be warned to avoid stopping suddenly. Interestingly, the effects are not interchangeable. A person who has not responded to fluoxetine may well respond to any of the other SSRIs, and it is not usually necessary to proceed to a drug with a different pharmacological profile such as venlafaxine (Brent *et al.*, 2008).

Newer antidepressants

A wide range is available: norepinephrine-SSRIs (SNRIs—such as venlafaxine), norepinephrinergic and specific serotonergic antidepressants (NaSSAs—such as mianserin and mirtazepine), selective norepinephrine reuptake inhibitors (such as reboxetine), and norepinephrine-dopamine reuptake inhibitors (such as bupropion). None of them are approved for use in children, but some—especially bupropion and venlafaxine—are in wide use for depression or refractory ADHD. Prescribers should regard them as experimental and monitor with particular care for significant complications such as suicidal thoughts and actions (venlafaxine) and seizures (bupropion).

Monoamine oxidase inhibitors (MAOIs)

Monoamine oxidase inhibitors (MAOIs) were the first antidepressants to be developed and are now little used because of their capacity for dangerous interactions with other drugs and some foods (especially those containing tyramine). If, for instance, they are used after fluoxetine then the latter drug must be withdrawn for at least 5 weeks before the MAOI is given. More selective MAOIs such as selegiline, and reversible ones such as moclobemide, have much less risk and have been used with some success in children for treating ADHD (Trott *et al.*, 1992; Rubinstein *et al.*, 2006).

Drugs used for stabilizing mood

Lithium is a mineral, usually administered as the carbonate or citrate salt, with well-established indications in adults for bipolar mania, prophylaxis of depression and mania, and potentiation of antidepressant drugs. It interferes with ionic transport by neurones and may have a variety of effects on neurone chemistry—including effects on the neurotransmitter glutamate, serotonin release, and nitric oxide (Jope, 1999). Its use in children is complicated by uncertainties about efficacy, the need for close monitoring of blood levels and thyroid and kidney function, and the high rate of adverse events in young children (Hagino *et al.*, 1995). Chapter 62 reviews its antimanic uses.

Anticonvulsants and antipsychotics are also used as mood stabilizers. McClellan *et al.* (2007) review and provide practice parameters for their use in bipolar-I illness affecting children. Divalproex, other valproate preparations, carbamazepine, and perhaps lamotrigine are the best evaluated of the anticonvulsants for this purpose. They do not have a sound evidence base for children and their adverse effects—while less troublesome than those of the second-generation antipsychotics described earlier—are not inconsiderable (see Chapter 62).

Other drugs

Benzodiazepines (and other GABA-A promoters such as zolpidem) are widely used in children, but with little scientific evidence for their value or safety. In the treatment of anxiety, they should be very much subordinate, first to psychological treatment and then to SSRIs (systematic review by Reinblatt & Riddle, 2007). The hazards of chronic use include disinhibition, aggression, cognitive blunting, withdrawal reactions, and dependence.

Single doses (or very short-term use) can nevertheless be useful—for instance, in premedication for dental surgery. Short-acting benzodiazepines (e.g., lorazepam) are advised. They can also be helpful in emergency situations involving great anxiety and/or aggression and may be preferred to antipsychotics (such as olanzapine) when there is the possibility that illegal drugs, other hallucinogens or alcohol have contributed to the crisis. There may also be a rapid effect on catatonic states.

Pregabalin is an anticonvulsant drug that binds to a subunit of the voltage-dependent calcium channel and thereby reduces norepinephrine and glutamate activity. It is an effective anxiolytic and is licensed for this purpose, in adults but not children, and in Europe but not USA. It can be considered for severe cases in young people where SSRIs have failed and is probably to be preferred to benzodiazepines for this purpose.

Hypnotics: Sedative antihistamines, tricyclics, and melatonin all have their advocates (see Chapter 70). Melatonin is a naturally occurring hormone playing a role in the regulation of the sleep-wake cycle and can help children to fall asleep more quickly (rather than extending time spent asleep) (Gringras *et al.*, 2012). Drugs acting as agonists on the melatonin receptor are being developed as treatments for depression and agomelatine has a license, in Europe and for adults, as an adjunctive treatment in atypical depression.

Oxytocin is attracting investigational interest as a promoter of prosocial behavior and empathy.

Drugs affecting endorphin systems (e.g., naltrexone) may also prove to have a role in promoting social behaviors and in moderating pain responses and repetitive self-injury. They are, for the moment, to be observed as experimental.

Dietary interventions
Elimination diets

Substances in the diet can upset behavior either by a toxic effect or by an idiosyncratic effect on predisposed individuals. There has long been concern that food additives can worsen children's behavior and learning and that hyperactivity and irritability in particular can be treated by removing certain colorings (especially tartrazine) and preservatives (especially sodium benzoate) from a child's intake. The possibility came to be regarded as somewhat eccentric and research trials were for the most part inconclusive. In recent years, however, better evidence has emerged. In careful studies such as that by McCann *et al.* (2007), children's behavior was worsened, in the short term in population samples, by mixtures of artificial colorings and preservatives, using randomized double-blind comparison with placebo. The effect was not particularly on children with features of ADHD, nor on children with other evidence of allergy. There was some evidence that histamine degradation gene polymorphisms mediated the effect. The main impact of the research has been on public health rather than clinical psychiatry (Stevenson *et al.*, 2010). In December 2009, the UK government requested food manufacturers to exclude tartrazine from their products, and the issue is under review by the FDA. For the clinician, the key question is whether individual children can be helped if the additives are eliminated from what they eat.

Nigg *et al.* (2012) provided a systematic review and meta-analysis, with the probable conclusion that elimination has a significantly positive effect but that the size of the effect is small. The clearest evidence came from the best quality trials that focused on colorings and used parent ratings. Teachers and observers did not find significant effects, but psychometric tests did find an effect in improving attention. Meta-analysis by Sonuga-Barke *et al.* (2013) had similar conclusions and added that a small effect could still be found by observers not involved in the delivery of the treatment. Small effect sizes in group studies could come from a large effect on a small number of children, or a small effect on many, and the question of how to identify those who will respond is unsolved. Where parents wish to explore the effect of eliminating artificial colors, there is reason for the clinician to support them. (Many families will already have tried before they get as far as a mental health service). Possible adverse effects include an undue restriction of a child's social activities to avoid exposure to additives. Advice should include warning against such restriction, bearing in mind that there is as yet only weak evidence for a helpful effect outside the home.

Elimination of individually identified food substances

A wider range of foods with potentially harmful effects on intolerant individuals has also been proposed. The key evidence comes from studies in which a food has been identified by an open individual trial, and then presented in disguised form, and contrasted with an indistinguishable food known not to provoke an adverse reaction. Randomized controlled trials have received meta-analysis from Sonuga-Barke *et al.* (2013), with the conclusion that there is a statistically significant benefit from the procedure on ratings of behavior—but that the effect is confined to ratings made by parents involved in the administration of the diet.

There are many incriminated foods. The list includes natural foods (e.g., cow's milk, wheat flour, citrus fruit, other fruits, eggs, etc) as well as artificial colorings and preservatives. As a result, the treatment is arduous to deliver and if applied strenuously can result in a seriously distorted diet. One practical approach is with a food diary, linking daily behavior ratings to foods taken and eliminating only those foods linked to deterioration. A full approach, capable of detecting delayed effects, is a period on a very restricted diet (typically, six ingredients only) followed (if problems have disappeared) by a process of introducing new foods, one at a time, to detect the ones that are harmful in the individual case. Such a few-food diet is only appropriate if used as an investigation and for a limited period; it is not recommended as a long-term substitute for normal eating. The advice of a pediatric dietitian, if available, would be very helpful in this rather drastic intervention.

Dietary supplements

Supplementation with long-chain polyunsaturated fatty acids (PUFAs) has the rationale of animal studies, especially on arachidonic acid (AA), eicosapentaenoic acid (EPA), and docosahexaenoic (DHA). Humans lack the enzyme needed to produce these fatty acids and therefore they have to come from the diet. Experimentally induced dietary deficiencies lead to animals showing brain abnormalities, for instance, in functions associated with neural activity such as membrane fluidity, neurotransmission, ion channels, enzyme regulation, gene expression, myelination, and the transport of serotonin. There has therefore been research interest in applications to psychiatry, and trials are accumulating (Freeman *et al.*, 2006). Omega-3 PUFAs (DHA and EPA) appear to have some efficacy in the adjunctive treatment of major depressive disorder (Jazayeri *et al.*, 2008). A systematic review and meta-analysis of trials has indicated a small but statistically significant effect in children with ADHD (Bloch & Qawasmi, 2011). Adverse effects are few, but PUFAs are contraindicated in the presence of bleeding diatheses. Their place in practice is not yet secure.

Families can be advised that PUFAs do not yet command the evidence that can lead to a firm recommendation, and that they should not be preferred to effective medicines; but that the chief disadvantage is only their cost, which is not covered by health insurance or the NHS in the UK. A service may well offer to monitor response, if only to ensure that established therapies are not neglected. Other food supplements—with vitamins and mineral micronutrients—do not have a sound evidence base and are not recommended for routine use (NICE, 2009); but nevertheless are widely used.

Neurotherapies

Electroconvulsive therapy retains a place in adult psychiatry, but is used very little in childhood and adolescence. Nevertheless, it has a role in treating otherwise refractory cases of severe depression, persistent mania and catatonia. Bertagnoli *et al.* (1990) provide a review of reported cases and Shoirah and Hamoda (2011) provide update. The offensive reputation of the treatment in the public mind would make wide consultation and explanation essential. It is usually regarded as an "irreversible" treatment from the perspectives of ethical review and requirements for informed consent. Expert administration would be necessary.

Nonconvulsive electrotherapies include transcranial magnetic stimulation (TMS) and DC current stimulation (TDCS). TMS involves the use of a magnetic coil on the scalp to produce focal currents in the underlying brain and thereby to modify neuronal excitability. It is used as a diagnostic tool in some neurological disorders. It is capable of showing developmental changes in childhood and detecting immaturity. Compared to adults, children have higher thresholds for activating motor cortex, and a previous pulse produces less inhibition of a succeeding one (Garvey & Volker, 2008). It therefore has promise as a diagnostic and monitoring tool for motor disorders and possibly for the inhibitory dysfunction that is observed in ADHD. Repetitive TMS produces enduring changes, is used experimentally to treat depression in adults, and might become a therapeutic tool. Indications and safety are not yet worked out and it should only be used experimentally and in expert centers.

In TDCS, weak currents (app. 1 mA) are applied to the brain via scalp electrodes. The idea is to manipulate nerve cell resting membrane potentials and make them more or less ready to fire. Activation is accompanied by changes in GABA and glutamate and in neuropsychological test performance. At present, they are tools for research only (Utz *et al.*, 2010), but they are of interest for therapies involving improvements of executive function.

Neurofeedback involves the detection of specific brain signals—usually from the EEG—and rapidly informing the child with a light, sound, or change in a video game when the desired signal is present. It has been a controversial intervention for years, with conflicting results from trials, inadequate methodology and excessive unsupported claims for its value. Recently, however, improvements in study design have made for a better and more positive evidence base in the therapy of epilepsy, dyslexia, and especially ADHD. A recent study on ADHD and providing meta-analyses concluded that "While the [unblinded data] on neurofeedback … was promising, evidence of efficacy from blinded assessments is required before they can be recommended as ADHD treatments." (Sonuga-Barke *et al.*, 2013).

Combinations of treatment

There is an increasing trend, at least in the USA, for multiple psychotropic agents to be prescribed to children, sometimes in doses higher than the recommended maxima. This practice is not supported by an evidence base. Polypharmacy has sometimes been held to be wrong in principle. This is too sweeping: one drug with multiple pharmacological actions is not necessarily an advantage over two simpler drugs. It is easier to vary pharmacological actions independently when each action is achieved by a separate drug. In theory, it does not make much sense to combine two pharmacologically similar drugs (e.g., two SSRIs); but our knowledge of pharmacology is not yet precise enough to provide accurate prediction and the wise prescriber goes by empirical evidence about what works. When drugs work in dissimilar ways, there is a clearer rationale for combination. The major consideration in combining drugs becomes the presence of interactions between them and these can be quite complex. Two simple steps are important for the prescriber: the first is to become very familiar with one drug of each main class, know it well (including its interactions), and use it preferentially and the second is to use a manual or a website that lists interactions (e.g., Taylor *et al.*, 2012; Pediatric Formulary Committee, 2012; epocrates.com).

Research and future developments

The next few years are likely to witness emerging trials that will fill some of the evidence gaps noted throughout this chapter. The appearance of new drugs, however, may slow down. Pharmaceutical companies have come to view psychiatric conditions as unpromising, because of their complexity, their heterogeneity without clear segregation of subtypes, the uncertainties about how to stage disorders, the scarcity of good preclinical models, the costly experience of drugs failing to meet modern standards of efficacy and safety, and the reputational damage that companies suffer from past mistakes and antidrug attitudes. Better ways of using existing drugs may result from better monitoring (e.g., from brain imaging) and improved prediction (e.g., from pharmacogenomics). Development of cognitive-enhancing drugs will lead to racetams, nicotine analogues, and many others—to join the existing enhancers such as stimulants, D-cycloserine, and modafinil. Tensions will emerge on drug use outside diagnostic boundaries. Psychiatrists will have much to learn.

References

Academy of Medical Sciences (2008) *Brain Science, Addiction and Drugs*. Academy of Medical Sciences, London. http://www.acmedsci .ac.uk/p99puid126.html

Bertagnoli, M.W. *et al.* (1990) A review of ECT for children and adolescents. *Journal of the American Academy of Child & Adolescent Psychiatry* **29**, 302–307.

Bloch, M.H. & Qawasmi, A. (2011) Omega-3 fatty acid supplementation for the treatment of children with attention-deficit/hyperactivity disorder symptomatology: systematic review and meta-analysis. *Journal of the American Academy of Child & Adolescent Psychiatry* **50**, 991–1000.

Brent, D. *et al.* (2008) Switching to another SSRI or to venlafaxine with or without cognitive behavioural therapy for adolescents with SSRI-resistant depression: the TORDIA randomized controlled trial. *JAMA* **299**, 901–913.

Charach, A. *et al.* (2004) Stimulant treatment over five years: adherence, effectiveness, and adverse effects. *Journal of the American Academy of Child & Adolescent Psychiatry* **43**, 559–567.

Committee on Safety of Medicines (CSM) (2003) Selective serotonin reuptake inhibitors (SSRIs): overview of regulatory status and CSM advice relating to major depressive disorder (MDD) in children and adolescents including a summary of available safety and efficacy data, http://www.mhra.gov.uk/home/idcplg?IdcService=SS_GET_PAGE&ss

Ferrin, M. *et al.* (2012) Evaluation of attitudes towards treatment in adolescents with ADHD. *European Child & Adolescent Psychiatry* **21**, 387–401.

Freeman, M.P. *et al.* (2006) Omega-3 Fatty acids: evidence basis for treatment and future research in psychiatry. *Journal of Clinical Psychiatry* **67**, 1954–1967.

Garvey, M.A. & Volker, M. (2008) Transcranial magnetic stimulation in children. *Clinical Neurophysiology* **119**, 973–984.

Gringras, P. *et al* (2012) Melatonin for sleep problems in children with neurodevelopmental disorders: randomised double masked placebo controlled trial. *British Medical Journal* **345**, e664.

Hagino, O.R. *et al.* (1995) Untoward effects of lithium treatment in children aged four through six years. *Journal of the American Academy of Child & Adolescent Psychiatry* **34**, 1584–1590.

Hammad, T. *et al.* (2006) Suicidality in pediatric patients treated with antidepressant drug. *Archives of General Psychiatry* **63**, 332–339.

Hazell, P. *et al.* (1995) Efficacy of tricyclic drugs in treating child and adolescent depression: a meta-analysis. *British Medical Journal* **310**, 897–901.

Heal, D.J. *et al.* (2012) ADHD: current and future therapeutics. *Current Topics in Behavioral Neurosciences* **9**, 361–390.

Hiemke, C. & Härtter, S. (2000) Pharmacokinetics of selective serotonin reuptake inhibitors. *Pharmacology and Therapeutics* **85**, 11–28.

Jazayeri, S. *et al.* (2008) Comparison of therapeutic effects of omega-3 fatty acid eicosapentaenoic acid and Fluoxetine, separately and in combination, in major depressive disorder. *Ausralian & New Zealand Journal of Psychiatry* **42**, 192–198.

Jope, R.S. (1999) Anti-bipolar therapy: mechanism of action of lithium. *Molecular Psychiatry* **4**, 117–128.

Knellwolf, A.L. *et al.* (2008) Prevalence and patterns of methylphenidate use in French children and adolescents. *European Journal of Clinical Pharmacology* **64**, 311–317.

March, J. *et al.* (2004) Fluoxetine, cognitive-behavioral therapy, and their combination for adolescents With depression: treatment for adolescents with depression study (TADS) randomized controlled trial. *JAMA* **292**, 807–820.

McCann, D. *et al.* (2007) Food additives and hyperactive behaviour in 3-year-old and 8/9-year-old children in the community: a randomised, double-blinded, placebo-controlled trial. *The Lancet* **370**, 1560–1567.

McCarthy, S. *et al.* (2012) The epidemiology of pharmacologically treated attention deficit hyperactivity disorder (ADHD) in children, adolescents and adults in UK primary care. *BMC Pediatrics* **12**, 78.

McClellan, J. *et al.* (2007) Practice parameter for the assessment and treatment of children and adolescents with bipolar disorder. *Journal of the American Academy of Child & Adolescent Psychiatry* **46**, 107–125.

National Institute for Health and Care Excellence (2009) *Attention Deficit Hyperactivity Disorder*. British Psychological Society and The Royal College of Psychiatrists, Leicester & London. www.nice.org.uk/CG72.

National Institute for Health and Care Excellence (2013) *Conduct Disorders and Antisocial Behaviour in Children and Young People: Recognition, Intervention and Management*. British Psychological Society and The Royal College of Psychiatrists, Leicester & London.

Nigg, J.T. *et al.* (2012) Meta-analysis of attention-deficit/hyperactivity disorder or attention-deficit/hyperactivity disorder symptoms, restriction diet, and synthetic food color additives. *Journal of the American Academy of Child & Adolescent Psychiatry* **51**, 86–97.

Olfson, M. *et al.* (2006) National trends in the outpatient treatment of children and adolescents with antipsychotic drugs. *Archives of General Psychiatry* **63**, 679–685.

Paediatric Formulary Committee (2012) *British National Formulary for Children (BNFC 2012-2013)*. British National Formulary Publications, Royal Pharmaceutical Society of Great Britain, London.

Rapoport, J. (2013) Pediatric psychopharmacology: too much or too little? *World Psychiatry* **12**, 118–123.

Reinblatt, S.P. & Riddle, M. (2007) The pharmacological management of childhood anxiety disorders: a review. *Psychopharmacology* **191**, 67–86.

Rubinstein, S. *et al.* (2006) Placebo-controlled study examining effects of selegiline in children with ADHD. *Journal of Child & Adolescent Psychopharmacology* **16**, 404–415.

Seixas, M. *et al.* (2012) Systematic review of national international guidelines on attention-deficit hyperactivity disorder. *Journal of Psychopharmacology* **26**, 753–765.

Shoirah, H. & Hamoda, H.M. (2011) Electroconvulsive therapy in children and adolescents. *Expert Review of Neurotherapeutics* **11**, 127–137.

Simpson, S.H. *et al.* (2006) A meta-analysis of the association between adherence to drug therapy and mortality. *British Medical Journal* **333**, 15.

Singh, I. (2012). *VOICES study: final report*. London, UK [Online]. Available: www.adhdvoices.com [10 Aug 2014].

Sonuga-Barke, E.J.S. *et al.* (2013) Nonpharmacological interventions for ADHD: systematic review and meta-analyses of randomized controlled trials of dietary and psychological treatments. *The American Journal of Psychiatry* **170**, 275–289.

Stevenson, J. *et al.* (2010) The role of histamine degradation gene polymorphisms in moderating the effects of food additives on children's ADHD symptoms. *American Journal of Psychiatry* **167**, 1108–1115.

Taylor, E. (2013) Pediatric psychopharmacology: too much and too little. *World Psychiatry* **12**, 124–125.

Taylor, D. *et al.* (2012) *The Maudsley Prescribing Guidelines in Psychiatry*, 11th edn. Wiley-Blackwell, Oxford.

Trip, A.-M. *et al.* (2009) Large increase of the use of psycho-stimulants among youth in the Netherlands between 1996 and 2006. *British Journal of Clinical Pharmacology* **67**, 466–468.

Trott, G.E. *et al.* (1992) Use of moclobemide in children with ADHD. *Psychopharmacology (Berlin)* **106**, S134–S136.

Utz, K.S. *et al.* (2010) Electrified minds: transcranial direct current stimulation (tDCS) and galvanic vestibular stimulation (GVS) as methods of non-invasive brain stimulation in neuropsychology. *Neuropsychologia* **48**, 2789–2810.

B: Considering and selecting available treatments

CHAPTER 44

Refugee, asylum-seeking and internally displaced children and adolescents

Mina Fazel, Ruth Reed and Alan Stein
Department of Psychiatry, University of Oxford, UK

Introduction

Children forced to flee from their homes because of organized violence, political or religious persecution, or rising ethnic tensions are often exposed to events that place great stress upon their psychological development. These children commonly witness and are subject to extreme violence, lose attachment figures because of family separations or bereavement and invariably leave familiar home and cultural surroundings with resultant disruption to their education and peer relationships. This can lead to different effects on children depending on the nature of their particular experiences, their environment and ongoing support as well as their personal characteristics. Some continue to develop on their pre-existing trajectory, showing remarkable resilience and capacity to survive or even thrive in the face of adversity (Tol *et al.*, 2013). Others increasingly struggle with psychological difficulties under the weight of negative events and circumstances.

There is a misconception that potentially traumatic events are confined to displaced peoples' experiences in their homeland. However, these are often only the beginning of a chain of adverse events. Migration journeys and post-migration experiences are often sources of further distressing occurrences. Achieving settled status in a safe location may take years, or may never be achieved, depending on the legal frameworks and political stability of the resettlement location. During this period and beyond, displaced children and families must make new peer and neighborhood relationships, manage changes in familial roles and master a new language and cultural environment. In high-income countries, they must simultaneously negotiate the asylum processing systems and welfare agencies; in low-resource settings, flight may be followed by years of struggle to meet basic survival needs amid eruptions of organized violence and gender or ethnicity-based attacks. The serious consequences of cumulative adversity for children's mental health have long been established (Rutter, 1999).

Refugee, asylum seeking, and internally displaced children and adolescents are therefore a group of major concern. In addition, an understanding of the way in which their experiences influence them has the potential to contribute to our knowledge of psychological development. Studying the interplay of the many factors highlighted earlier can elucidate processes underlying resilience as well as psychopathology and help focus on potential areas of intervention (see Chapter 27). In this chapter, some background information on these populations is provided, followed by discussion of particular risk and protective factors for psychopathology, highlighting important studies. Finally, there will be a focus on interventions highlighting some that have been evaluated. It should be noted that interventions are important to consider at all levels—individual, family, school, community, and societal.

In 2011, approximately 16 million children, almost half of the total global population of refugees and people in refugee-like situations, were displaced from their homes (UNHCR, 2011). The variation between refugees' background circumstances, country-of-origin, country-of-resettlement, culture and experiences is so great that it should not be assumed that they are a homogeneous group. There are, however, key elements that are almost universally experienced by refugees: loss, uncertainty, fear, and discrimination. Many experience family and community disruption. It is common for the asylum process to last several years after arrival in the country of resettlement. Financial support for asylum-seekers is typically low even in high-income countries, and many report difficulties in accessing services to which they are legally entitled; those in low and middle-income countries (LMIC) are not uncommonly in situations of humanitarian crisis.

Rutter's Child and Adolescent Psychiatry, Sixth Edition.
Edited by Anita Thapar and Daniel S. Pine, James F. Leckman, Stephen Scott, Margaret J. Snowling, Eric Taylor.
© 2015 John Wiley & Sons Ltd. Published 2018 by John Wiley & Sons Ltd.

For those internally displaced, or displaced to neighboring countries, local tensions and economic circumstances may necessitate a series of moves, which means that the children may experience repeated adversity and instability. Many have to live in refugee camps and the instability and greater experience of cumulative adverse events appear to place children in these situations at particularly high risk of psychological difficulty (Reed *et al.*, 2012). Hereafter, the general term "forcibly displaced children" will be used to encompass this population, unless specifically referring to a subgroup.

Research with forcibly displaced children has largely focused on the minority who have resettled in high-income countries (Fazel *et al.*, 2012). There are many challenges to conducting research with refugee populations, especially those living in LMICs including the need for cultural and linguistic adaptation of measures, and culturally differing models of conceptualizing adverse events (Bhui *et al.*, 2003). Moreover, studies of interventions for displaced populations have been hampered by a number of methodological issues (Nickerson *et al.*, 2011). These include small sample sizes, lack of post-treatment and long-term follow-up assessments, a lack of random assignment, the absence of appropriate control conditions or interventions and little treatment manualization. Therefore, only a small number of interventions have been adequately evaluated and those that have been evaluated have shown small to moderate effect sizes. While many of the interventions have had good face validity, these difficulties have limited the conclusions that can be drawn about the best way forward.

Definition of terms and the global refugee situation

People who have moved away from their home locality owing to persecution or organized violence are described as "forcibly displaced" and their situation is often exacerbated by the pressures of extreme poverty or environmental challenges. Those moving within their own national borders are described as "internally displaced." This term is also used for people who have moved owing to natural disasters or severe economic hardship, but in this chapter we use it with reference to those fleeing organized violence. Those who migrate to a different country to escape persecution are typically described by the broad term "refugees," although in many countries "refugee" has a more specific legal meaning denoting someone who has applied for and been granted political asylum. Hence refugees in these contexts have long-term or permanent rights of residence in the host country. An "asylum seeker" is someone who has applied for but not yet been granted refugee status by the host country. A "failed asylum seeker" is someone who has not been successful in their asylum application and, in many countries, has limited access to health or social care, employment or training, state-funded accommodation, financial support, or family reunification. Moreover, they may be at risk of forcible return to their country-of-origin. The 1951 UN Refugee Convention gave the original classification of a refugee (UNHCR, 1951)

and although this definition is now potentially limited (Quinn, 2011), its principle of protection remains for those whose home countries offer limited protection or who are at risk of torture.

More children and adolescents are internally displaced than are displaced across national borders. Of the latter, most remain in front-line states close to their country of origin. The vast majority of the world's forcibly displaced populations are, therefore, displaced from one LMIC to other nearby LMICs.

Unaccompanied and separated children are of particular concern as they are under 18 years, living outside their country of origin and separated from their parents or primary caregivers. Some may be totally alone while others may be living with extended family members. All such separated children are entitled to international protection under a broad range of international and regional legal instruments (Hancilova & Knauder, 2011). However, in practice, they can be subject to conflicting policy agendas: the protection of children and children's rights versus the enforcement of immigration control (Sigona & Hughes, 2012). Despite often experiencing potentially traumatic events in their countries of origin as well as poverty and disrupted education, many experience further harrowing events, abuse and hardship in their journeys to new countries and then have to settle and survive in a new country. Throughout, they lack the physical and psychological support of a trusted adult and this can render them particularly vulnerable. They can fall prey to victimization and trafficking for sexual or labour exploitation (Becker-Blease *et al.*, 2010; Hancilova & Knauder, 2011).

Over the past decade, countries, especially those in the European Union, have been placing increasingly restrictive measures to prevent displaced populations from making asylum claims. Of particular concern is the use of immigration detention facilities that have so far been documented in 60 countries across the globe, both high-income and LMIC (Global Detention Project, 2013, Fazel *et al.*, 2014). Children and adolescents can be detained in many countries for variable lengths of time. In addition, in some countries, children can be separated from their parents when parents are placed in immigration detention.

Prevalence of psychiatric disorder

The main studies that have explored psychiatric morbidity in forcibly displaced populations have focused on the disorders of PTSD, depression and anxiety disorders. Studies have typically (Tousignant *et al.*, 1999; Fazel *et al.*, 2005; Bronstein *et al.*, 2013), although not universally (Rousseau *et al.*, 2000) shown, that forcibly displaced children have substantially higher rates of psychiatric disorder than host populations. This higher prevalence has been demonstrated in systematic reviews for PTSD (Fazel *et al.*, 2005), depression (Bronstein *et al.*, 2013) and anxiety (Bronstein *et al.*, 2013). The range of prevalence estimates for any of these disorders is variable between studies. Part of this variation reflects genuine differences in the balance of risk and protective factors between the populations being studied, as well as methodological differences between studies.

The prevalence estimates for PTSD in forcibly displaced children show wide variation. A systematic review of PTSD in refugee children (Fazel *et al.*, 2005), which excluded self-report questionnaire-based studies, showed a relatively narrow range of 7–17% across the eligible studies. Estimates of 10–25% are common in studies of children displaced to relatively safe high-income settings, those for internally displaced children in LMICs tend to be higher; for example, a study in a camp for internally displaced persons (IDP) in Darfur showed a PTSD prevalence of 75% in adolescents (Hasanović *et al.*, 2006; Morgos *et al.*, 2007). PTSD in forcibly displaced children is also potentially different to that more typically observed in other populations. This is primarily because they might have been subjected to multiple traumatic events that could be different in nature and in the context they were experienced. For example, a child might witness the death of a parent in their home country, followed by exposure to long and frightening migration journeys, possibly unaccompanied. These children might live without the support of their primary caregiver or with caregivers suffering from their own psychological disorders. All are living in a new country and culture where access to services, if these services exist, might be difficult. Moreover, these factors will have a potential impact on the presentation and treatment of other psychological disorders, such as depression and anxiety.

Estimates of depression typically fall in the range of 5–30% (Servan-Schreiber *et al.*, 1998; Tousignant *et al.*, 1999; Hasanović *et al.*, 2006), again tending toward higher proportions in refugee camp situations (Morgos *et al.*, 2007). Estimates for anxiety range from 10–30% (Tousignant *et al.*, 1999; Bronstein *et al.*, 2013). For depression and anxiety, as for PTSD, there is a relative dearth of high quality evidence. There are fewer studies reporting on other psychiatric symptoms, but a study of psychotic adolescents in in-patient units across London reported an over-representation of black African refugees (Tolmac & Hodes, 2004).

These disorders are also likely to be prevalent in any accompanying parents or caregivers (Hollifield *et al.*, 2002; De Jong *et al.*, 2003; Steel *et al.*, 2009). Parental disorders might impact on their children's development (see Chapter 28). A systematic review of 181 studies of adults who had experienced conflict and displacement indicated a weighted prevalence of over 30% for both depression and for PTSD (Steel *et al.*, 2009). Given the dual challenges of socioeconomic adversity and parental psychological difficulties, it is unsurprising that the children of forcibly displaced parents born after arrival in the country of settlement may also be at elevated risk of a range of conditions, including PTSD, depression and psychosis (Sigal and Weinfeld, 2001; Rutter, 2013).

In summary (Table 44.1), although studies commonly find forcibly displaced children and adolescents to be at increased risk of PTSD, depression, and anxiety, there is little evidence to suggest a significantly increased risk of other conditions, such as conduct problems or substance misuse (Sack *et al.*, 1994; Tousignant *et al.*, 1999). In fact, some studies suggest fewer behavioral problems in forcibly displaced families, citing a range of explanatory factors including being involved in a meaningful struggle, respect for one's cultural background and sensitivity to parents' difficulties (Sack *et al.*, 1986; Rousseau and Drapeau, 2003).

Risk and resilience in young refugees

Although forcibly displaced children and families commonly experience a large number of distressing events, it is important not to make assumptions as to the impact of such events on the individual, based on the apparently "objective" severity or number of events. There is huge heterogeneity in individuals' responses to different stressors and adversity (Rutter, 2013). Whether or not they lead to prolonged adverse psychological consequences for the individual depends on a range of factors and on cultural differences in understanding and responding to adversity (Barber, 2013). These include the pre- and post-event context, ascribed meaning and appraisals, prior mental health, prior and subsequent adversity and distressing events, genetic influences and parental and social support (Miller and Rasmussen, 2010; Reed *et al.*, 2012; Tol *et al.*, 2013).

Those working with these children and adolescents must remain alert to all the standard risk factors for psychopathology in children; the unusual events experienced by displaced families should not distract clinicians from other significant past and present risks to children's mental health. On-going serious risks that therefore need to be assessed include child maltreatment, parental conflict and domestic violence, community violence, racially based discrimination, poverty and bullying, as studies have shown a possible increase in incidence in many of these for forcibly displaced populations (Catani *et al.*, 2010; Layne *et al.*, 2010).

The societal context

Post-migration factors, many of which are modifiable, have been shown to alter the risk of developing psychological problems in forcibly displaced children and adolescents (Fazel *et al.*, 2012; Reed *et al.*, 2012). While exile and repatriation are no doubt stressful experiences for children, remaining in a conflict situation without displacement is equally, if not more, detrimental to psychological well-being. In addition, living in refugee camps (Thabet and Vostanis, 1998; Izutsu *et al.*, 2005) or within immigration detention facilities can place psychological health at serious risk (Rothe *et al.*, 2002; Lorek *et al.*, 2009). Detention facilities may expose children to witnessing and experiencing additional potentially traumatic events, including fires, rioting, violence and self-harm attempts by others (Mares *et al.*, 2002), and furthermore may have a serious impact upon parental mental health, impairing the capacity to sensitively parent children with increased needs.

Table 44.1 Some illustrative studies of the prevalence and risk factors for psychiatric disorder in forcibly displaced children and young people.

Study	Year	Sample	Findings
LMIC studies			
Morgos (2007)	2007	331 internally displaced children in camps in southern Darfur	75% met criteria for PTSD, 38% for depression
Mels (2010)	2010	819 adolescents of age 13–21 in the eastern Democratic Republic of Congo (217 internally displaced and 496 previously displaced returnees)	Internally displaced adolescents reported the highest scores for post traumatic symptoms
Paardekooper *et al.* (1999)	1999	316 Sudanese refugees in Uganda compared to 80 local Ugandan children	Sudanese refugee children reported significantly more depressive and post traumatic symptoms and behavioral difficulties than local children
High-income country studies			
Nielsen (2008)	2008	246 children in Danish detention centers	Children with at least 4 relocations had worse mental health
Sujoldzic (2006)	2006	499 adolescent Bosnian refugees in Croatia and Austria compared to 359 internally displaced Bosnians and 424 non-displaced Bosnians	Girls had worse functioning than boys and were more likely to suffer anxiety and depression; discrimination and poor school and neighborhood connectedness was associated with worse functioning, whereas religious commitment was associated with better functioning
Studies of unaccompanied asylum-seeking children (UASC)			
Bronstein *et al.* (2013)	2012	222 Afghan unaccompanied asylum seeking adolescents, age 13–17	35% scored above cut-offs for anxiety and 23% for depression
Bean *et al.* (2007a)	2007	582 unaccompanied refugee children from 48 countries	Psychological distress was higher with increasing age and girls had higher scores for post traumatic and internalizing symptoms: unaccompanied young people had experienced twice as many post traumatic events as accompanied young people

Prolonged insecure asylum status and residential instability are disorientating and distressing for parents and children alike (Bean *et al.*, 2007b; Nielsen *et al.*, 2008), and often give rise to secondary adversities such as parental unemployment, financial strain, social isolation and limited engagement with education or community life. Government policies differ greatly between countries with regards to the detention of child and adult asylum seekers, and the time-frame for the resolution of asylum claims. Attempts to minimize the duration of uncertainty and residential disruption of asylum-seeking families, to avoid the detention of children, their parents and pregnant women, and to abolish the separation of parents and children for the purposes of detaining adults in a family, are important safeguards to prevent deterioration in children's mental health (Fazel *et al.*, 2012).

Consideration must also be given to the impact of the relative privacy and security of accommodation on mental health (Ajduković and Ajduković, 1993; Geltman *et al.*, 2005). For unaccompanied young people, accommodation in centers is associated with poorer functioning than independent accommodation or foster care (Derluyn and Broekaert, 2007). More supported living arrangements are associated with better psychological outcomes (Bean *et al.*, 2007a; Derluyn and Broekaert, 2007; Hodes *et al.*, 2008). Foster care raises additional challenges but same-ethnicity placements appear to confer a protective effect (Porte & Torney-Purta, 1987; Geltman *et al.*, 2005).

The community context

Higher levels of perceived acceptance and connectedness within a community and low levels of racial discrimination have been associated with lower levels of psychological problems (Sujoldžić *et al.*, 2006; Montgomery and Foldspang, 2008). The issue of acculturation has received considerable attention; the construct is difficult to measure, and usually reduced to linguistic competency and time since migration. Overall, the ability to integrate into the host society and acquire the local language while maintaining a sense of one's cultural identity emerges as somewhat protective (Fazel *et al.*, 2012). The importance of the formation and maintenance of social networks within the same ethnic group and some form of religious belief, as well as a sense of connectedness to the neighborhood and school, are linked to positive mental health outcomes (Sujoldžić *et al.*, 2006; Kia-Keating and Ellis, 2007).

Children and young people with friendships have fewer psychological difficulties (Almqvist and Brandell-Forsberg, 1997; Berthold, 2000) and parental support networks also have an indirect positive impact on children (Ekblad, 1993). In some cultural contexts, a large same-ethnicity network may have an adverse rather than protective effect, possibly related to increased social obligations and expectations (Rousseau *et al.*, 1998).

The family context

There is increasing evidence for the importance of good parental functioning in protecting the mental health of young people who have experienced forced displacement (Catani *et al.*, 2010; Walker *et al.*, 2011; Tol *et al.*, 2013) and a large body of work outside refugee studies also attests to the importance of remaining with family or steadfast caregivers. When we consider young people who arrive with their families, the family may appear to be one "constant" in a maelstrom of change and can cushion against external adversities. However, the dramatic changes and shifts that may occur in forced displacement can cause disruptions to family structure and function that can compromise the adequacy of parental caregiving (Walker *et al.*, 2011). At the very time when children are most in need of sensitive parental care to buffer them against the adverse events around them, parents themselves are distressed, preoccupied and over-burdened with the struggle for basic survival needs.

It is, however, well-demonstrated that the presence of parents is nonetheless protective and improves outcome; unaccompanied young people are known to be at increased risk not only of a higher toll of potentially traumatic events during their migration journey, but also of a higher likelihood of significant psychological difficulty after arrival (Hodes *et al.*, 2008; Thabet *et al.*, 2008).

The individual context

The cumulative number of pre-migration adverse events is the strongest predictor of psychological disturbance (Fazel *et al.*, 2012; Reed *et al.*, 2012). These risks are higher with events of greater personal threat (Angel *et al.*, 2001; Geltman *et al.*, 2005). Different patterns of exposure by gender are observed in different contexts, for example, the use of rape as a weapon against girls in refugee camps (Crisp, 2000), or the targeted recruitment of boys as child soldiers (Betancourt *et al.*, 2010b), and stigma and discrimination resulting from these particular types of exposure are major barriers to recovery and social reintegration (Betancourt *et al.*, 2010a). Exposure to post-migration violence is also associated with increased risk (Berthold, 1999). Children who have experienced conflict also experience a wide range of non-conflict related potentially traumatic events, which they may identify as equally or more traumatic, including experiences of domestic and community violence (Panter-Brick *et al.*, 2009).

With regard to gender, girls generally have a higher risk of poor mental health outcomes, especially after puberty (Sujoldžić *et al.*, 2006; Derluyn and Broekaert, 2007; Fazel *et al.*, 2012), in keeping with childhood patterns of anxiety, depressive, and post traumatic symptoms in the general population (Ford *et al.*, 2003). No clear age effects have emerged from the available studies (Reed *et al.*, 2012; Fazel *et al.*, 2012), although studies from countries where a final asylum decision is made at a specific age (typically

around 18 years) commonly show a deterioration in later adolescence, reflecting the approach of this decision point (Bean *et al.*, 2007a, b).

Assessment

Clinicians may be part of a targeted service or only examine such children infrequently. The assessment of such children needs to be carried out with particular sensitivity. In areas with high forcibly displaced populations, there is scope for a group of professionals to work together and develop expertise in advocacy and in addressing other educational and community needs. A careful explanation as to the purposes of the assessment and wish to help the child is important and an initial focus on the here-and-now and less distressing issues can be helpful. As a result of their experiences, such children may be wary of anybody who appears to be in authority, especially if they are asking questions about their past. Furthermore, many may have difficulty talking about past traumatic experiences especially if, for example, it has involved witnessing the killing of loved ones and the experience of torture. The assessment will need to proceed cautiously and at a pace that the child can manage. The assessment needs to include the range of past and current experiences. Figure 44.1 illustrates some of the specific questions that may need to be considered and their relationship to the child's migration experience.

Children and adolescents who have undergone forced displacement will have experienced life in at least two countries. The assessment needs to include positive strengths and qualities, temperament, coping skills and adaptability, language, ethnic and religious identity, and, for accompanied children, key family relationships. Assessment can, therefore, be particularly complex. For simplicity, this is often considered in pre-migration, peri-migration (journey from the country of origin to the new country, including residence in camps) and post-migration phases. Many children can have more complex experiences, including multiple displacements and returns within their own or other countries, being born in camps or in a country of transit, or being held in immigration detention facilities.

Clinicians should expect to obtain information slowly and patchily. In addition, careful attention must be given to risk assessment and child protection issues, particularly for unaccompanied minors. Time should also be allowed for liaison with other statutory and non-statutory agencies supporting the families and young person, in particular those dealing with accommodation, care needs and legal issues around asylum claims.

Other complexities of assessment include:

1 Language and cultural differences. As with any cross-cultural assessment, it is important to gain an understanding of the cultural influence on concepts of: physical and psychological health and illness; the meaning of the distressing events experienced; any stigma attached to the events experienced, resultant symptoms or attitudes to accessing services; the acceptability of treatments and the use of alternative healing practitioners or preparations. Moreover, it should be borne in mind

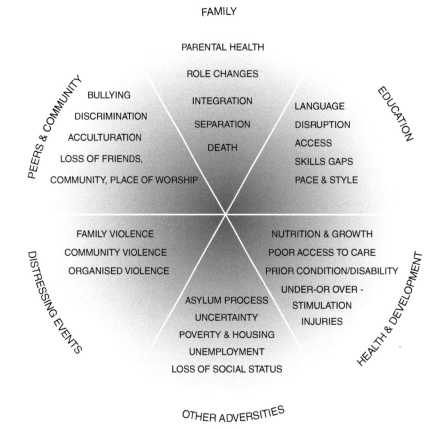

FAMILY

PARENTAL HEALTH

ROLE CHANGES

INTEGRATION

SEPARATION

DEATH

BULLYING

DISCRIMINATION

ACCULTURATION

LOSS OF FRIENDS,

COMMUNITY, PLACE OF WORSHIP

PEERS & COMMUNITY

EDUCATION

LANGUAGE

DISRUPTION

ACCESS

SKILLS GAPS

PACE & STYLE

FAMILY VIOLENCE

COMMUNITY VIOLENCE

ORGANISED VIOLENCE

DISTRESSING EVENTS

NUTRITION & GROWTH

POOR ACCESS TO CARE

PRIOR CONDITION/DISABILITY

UNDER-OR OVER - STIMULATION

INJURIES

HEALTH & DEVELOPMENT

ASYLUM PROCESS

UNCERTAINTY

POVERTY & HOUSING

UNEMPLOYMENT

LOSS OF SOCIAL STATUS

OTHER ADVERSITIES

Figure 44.1 Assessment considerations for forcibly displaced children. Some of the factors described apply only at one phase of the migration process, but it is important to remember that most adverse exposures, such as violence and multiple relocation, can be experienced at any stage of migration.

that family members and young people may be at very different stages of linguistic and cultural adaptation to the host society and may view their cultural identity differently.

2 Use of interpreters. Ensuring the acceptability of a particular interpreter and trying to keep the same interpreter from session to session is ideal. It is important to discuss confidentiality issues with the interpreter before a session, as interpreters might not have health training. It is also essential to have time with the interpreter alone at the end of potentially distressing sessions to discuss confidentiality and ensure that the session has not raised any difficult issues or memories for the interpreter, who might themselves have come from a conflict-affected area. Interpreters from smaller communities or language groups might present difficulties as they can often interpret for the children in multiple contexts. Sharing a language might be indicative of that person coming from the same region but potentially from the "other" side, placing a child at perceived or real risk if the interpreter remains in the session and privy to personal information.

3 Limited availability of information regarding the child's development and current risks, either because of absence of primary caregivers or due to communication difficulties.

4 Misinformation about immigration processes. The children and their families might have been told, by people traffickers and others who helped them enter the country, not to share certain aspects of their background and history with immigration and care organizations. The reasons such people give are often incorrect, potentially exposing them to more difficulties with post-migration authorities.

5 Lack of understanding about the role of the different health and social care agencies involved by children and their families.

6 Use by families of other potential mental health providers including traditional healers and religious leaders.

Interventions

Forcibly displaced children encounter many barriers in accessing health care. The development of interventions to address the needs of forcibly displaced children and adolescents needs to be twofold. General multimodal interventions that concurrently address a number of issues in the environment and social networks need to take place alongside targeted interventions for those with more specific trauma-related needs (Miller and Rasmussen, 2010; Nickerson *et al.*, 2011). This dual strategy approach is supported by a number of reviews exploring interventions for refugee children (Tyrer and Fazel,

2014), war-affected children (Betancourt and Williams, 2008; Jordans et al., 2009) and adults (Nickerson et al., 2011). The available evidence on interventions for forcibly displaced children and adolescents is, however, limited, so general principles and interventions of note are explored in the following sections (see Chapters 36 and 59). There is a scarcity of rigorous studies and the interventions that have been evaluated thus far are different from each other, both in terms of their settings and their specific findings (Jordans, 2009). In the following section, we summarize the key components of these interventions and highlight the areas that are most important.

In LMICs, the resource constraints are considerable and mental health services usually fall far below need, especially when compared to other health care provisions (Patel et al., 2007a). Interventions might need to be delivered in refugee camps and the stigma of having a mental health problem can often impede help-seeking behaviors. Multimodal interventions integrated into other systems of care, such as women's health or primary care, might be more acceptable in these settings, where mental health resources are scarce. Moreover, considerable barriers exist within high-income settings. These include resources, linguistic and cultural barriers, concerns about stigma and confidentiality, and beliefs that having a psychological problem might negatively impact on asylum applications.

Trauma-focused interventions

The best evidence available to date is for trauma-focused interventions. These have mainly been studied when delivered on an individual basis although some interventions have used groups. The settings have ranged from specialized mental health services to schools and refugee camps. These findings are in line with the overall evidence for treatment of PTSD where exposure to the "event" or events is a key feature in effective psychological treatments (see Chapter 59). The majority of studies have been conducted in high-income countries where the best evidence for efficacy lies with cognitive behavioral therapy (CBT), in particular Trauma-Focused CBT (Cohen et al., 2000; Taylor and Chemtob, 2004; Fremont, 2004; Silverman et al., 2008; Tol et al., 2008). In this treatment modality, the fear conditioning is treated as a key etiological agent alongside disturbances in memory processing and cognitive appraisal (Nickerson et al., 2011). CBT facilitates the extinction of this learning by processing the traumatic memories and altering maladaptive appraisals of threat and overcoming avoidance behaviors. For children and adolescents useful techniques include cognitive restructuring, relaxation training, anger management training, teaching coping skills, and grief management (Fremont, 2004).

Other therapeutic treatments for which there is increasing evidence of effectiveness include Narrative Exposure Therapy (NET) (Robjant and Fazel, 2010) and a range of creative-expressive techniques. There is evidence for Eye-Movement Desensitization and Reprocessing in non-refugee children with PTSD (Cloitre, 2009). Studies exploring the use of pharmacotherapy in this population are lacking but given the high prevalence of depression and anxiety, medication may be an adjunct or alternative treatment to psychological therapies and other interventions, depending on treatment availability including supervision, patient preference, comorbidity, and symptom severity.

Multimodal interventions

Multimodal interventions aim to concurrently address issues of psychological functioning, social and cultural adaptation, physical health and ongoing psychosocial difficulties (Nickerson et al., 2011). Although the evidence supporting their use is limited, it is relevant that such programmes offer a range of interventions because forcibly displaced populations can be exposed to diverse stressors and challenges leading to a complex array of psychological reactions.

At the societal level, these interventions aim to influence the wider environment through advocating for more services and stable housing, promoting language proficiency, improving immigration applications, and employment opportunities. The restoration of an enabling/supportive environment for the young person and their family and friends is likely to be key to stabilizing their psychological health (Betancourt and Williams, 2008; Jordans et al., 2009). As Miller points out, a focus on healing the effects of previously experienced war trauma may appear valueless to a child who is currently being beaten or sexually abused at home or in the community (Miller and Rasmussen, 2010) or whose basic survival needs are a day-to-day struggle (Mels et al., 2010).

Multimodal interventions have also tried to address community and school-based needs. Achieving in school, with regard to both education and peer relationships is a key determinant of success and future mental health (Viner et al., 2012). Refugee children can experience specific problems fitting into school because of language and cultural differences as well as bullying and discrimination (Kia-Keating and Ellis, 2007). A systematic review of community and school interventions for forcibly displaced children and adolescents (Tyrer and Fazel, 2014) identified 20 studies in total, of which seven were conducted in refugee camp settings and the rest were mainly school-based interventions in high-income countries. The interventions were a combination of individual, family and group, or classroom interventions and the multimodal interventions used an array of creative art techniques, often in combination with trauma-focused interventions.

Interventions should aim to help strengthen families (Walker et al., 2011). This is because a consistent finding across studies is the importance of parental support for children's mental health (Tol et al., 2013). The studies to elucidate how best this can be performed are limited, but some studies have offered support to parents and siblings and others have focused on the parent–child interaction in therapy. Restoration of social support networks for children and their families is another important aspect of multimodal interventions more generally (Jordans et al., 2010). Although some studies have tried to address these in post-conflict settings, the studies on forcibly displaced children and adolescents are still limited. Moreover, the importance of harnessing cultural resources and extended kin networks are likely to be important (Tingvold et al., 2012).

In summary, the individual psychological needs of these children require addressing using the most effective available interventions (Table 44.2). Moreover, the overall needs of this population need to be considered. If housing or educational needs are not being addressed, for example, if they are living in an unhappy foster home or if they have additional learning difficulties, then a clinical service might need to work to assist all these areas. For the young person, having these different services brought under the umbrella or oversight of one service might be very helpful and so ensuring flexibility in response is likely to be of greatest overall benefit. In addition, many young people find their therapists getting involved in their asylum application supportive and important.

Course and long-term outcomes for young refugees

A 9-year follow-up study of 131 refugees in Denmark (mean age 15.3 years) showed that the long-term effects of pre-migration trauma are mediated by risk and protective factors at the individual, family, and community level (Montgomery and Foldspang, 2008; Montgomery, 2010). Aspects of social life in Denmark and the stresses experienced in exile were more strongly predictive of psychological problems 8–9 years after arrival than traumatic experiences before arrival, highlighting the importance of the post-migration environment. Sack and colleagues' 12-year follow-up study of Cambodian adolescents indicated that post-migration stressors were particularly associated with depression, whereas post-traumatic stress was more closely related to pre-migration events (Sack et al., 1993; Sack et al., 1994). Bean and colleagues noted strong continuity and ongoing high levels of psychopathology at 1-year follow-up in a cohort of 582 unaccompanied minors (Bean et al., 2007b).

There are a number of studies of note from adult populations that can also inform our understanding of the long-term outcomes in children and adolescents exposed to forced displacement or war experiences. A study of adults in four post-conflict settings (Ethiopia, Algeria, Cambodia, and Gaza)

highlighted the range of PTSD prevalence rates across contexts with a diversity of risk factors (De Jong et al., 2001; De Jong et al., 2003). In addition, the study demonstrated that conflict events after age 12 were particularly likely to have an adverse effect, and this could be because of developmental, cognitive, or environmental influences. Another study of Cambodian refugees interviewed two decades after resettlement in the United States of America showed how prolonged the psychological effects of forced displacement can be as 62% fulfilled diagnostic criteria for PTSD and 51% for depression (Marshall et al., 2005). Those who had been displaced in adolescence had better psychological health but these results highlight how both children and their parents can be affected by their experiences for considerable periods of time.

There is limited knowledge regarding the intergenerational repercussions of traumatic events, although second generation refugee children had worse psychological outcomes in a study in rural South Africa (Cortina et al., 2013) and there is evidence from a registry-based study that second-generation refugees have an increased risk of hospital admission for psychotic illness, whereas there was no elevated risk for second generation labor migrants (Rutter, 2013).

Conclusions

The psychological adjustment of a child or adolescent who has been forcibly displaced because of organized violence is likely to be influenced by a number of different factors that may be inter-related or independent. These include the severity of exposure to any potentially traumatic experiences, previous and current family support, the degree and duration of disruption to their life and the amount of social disorganization that ensued and still exists in their environment (Pine et al., 2005). Therefore, when trying to meet the mental health needs of these children, interventions to address distressing memories and family dynamics must take place alongside attempts to address the wider local and regional social, economic, and educational systems disrupted by war. This can seem like an impossible task for the LMIC countries, in which the majority of forcibly displaced children live, given their overall lack of mental health services, especially for young people (Patel et al., 2007b; Chapter 16).

Table 44.2 Examples of randomized controlled trials.

Intervention domain	Study	Year	Sample	Intervention	Findings
Individual therapy	Ertl (2011)	2011	85 Ugandan former child soldiers	Narrative Exposure Therapy-8 sessions conducted in camps	Improvements in PTSD symptoms
School-based	Rousseau (2005)	2005	138 immigrant children in Canada	Creative expression classroom programme over 12 weeks	Beneficial effects on self-esteem
Community-based	Bolton (2007)	2007	Ugandan internally displaced children living in refugee camps	Group Interpersonal Therapy (IPT-G)-16 sessions conducted in camps	IPT-G helped reduce levels of depression, especially in girls and older children

Moreover, while education and employment are likely to be key factors for their long-term mental health (Viner *et al.*, 2012), access to these is a further challenge in LMIC settings.

The main focus of research now lies in the development of appropriate and sustainable interventions (Tol *et al.*, 2009). For LMICs, interventions developed in high-income settings are unlikely to be generalizable to these environments (De Jong *et al.*, 2001). A major development involves understanding how to adapt interventions delivered by clinical health specialists so that they may be carried out by lay or generic workers with limited training (Tol *et al.*, 2012; see Chapter 48). This has been achieved in some studies for adult refugee populations and for children in conflict settings (Robjant & Fazel, 2010). Further research should identify the core skills that are necessary, how training should be conducted and the groups most likely to benefit from such interventions. There is some emerging evidence of differential gender effects, with girls possibly benefiting more from certain interventions (Bolton *et al.*, 2007); research should also seek to identify how to modify interventions to optimize outcomes across all groups. It is also vital that interventions do not undermine natural recovery processes in individuals, families, or communities (Tol *et al.*, 2012). It may be necessary to adapt interventions to make them more culturally sensitive in areas with relatively homogeneous displaced populations, which might be more likely in LMICs. However, in high-income settings, where refugee communities can be highly heterogeneous, they might instead be targeted to the local context rather than a specific cultural group, for example, improving school integration and addressing bullying in a locality where the refugee community suffers discrimination and stigmatization.

Regardless of the setting, learning how best to harness cultural, community, and family resources is essential. Certain policies and practices are overtly detrimental to mental health (Viner *et al.*, 2012) and need to be prevented, such as immigration detention. There are also likely to be benefits of integrating mental health services with other youth health and welfare expertise (Patel *et al.*, 2007b) and delivering a multi-layered care package (Jordans *et al.*, 2010).

While developing emotionally, socially, intellectually, and physically, forcibly displaced children and adolescents face disruption to their family structure, accommodation, cultural and linguistic environment, friendships, and education. Many also suffer bereavements or disappearance of family or friends and struggle with intrusive memories of violence. Despite this, many children nonetheless thrive and develop well, and there is much to be learnt from the processes and factors that promote positive outcomes after extreme adversity. Although there has been encouraging progress in research into refugee mental health, many potentially modifiable factors continue to impact adversely upon children and families' health even after arrival in safe, stable, and well-resourced resettlement countries. There is a clear role for mental health professionals to address barriers to accessing health care, improve the cultural sensitivity and acceptability of services, challenge stigma and prejudice, develop effective interventions and modes of service delivery and advocate for refugees' mental health when local or national policy and practice endangers the fragile balance between risk and resilience.

References

Ajduković, M. & Ajduković, D. (1993) Psychological well-being of refugee children. *Child Abuse and Neglect* **17**, 843–854.

Almqvist, K. & Brandell-Forsberg, M. (1997) Refugee children in Sweden: post-traumatic stress disorder in Iranian preschool children exposed to organized violence. *Child Abuse and Neglect* **21**, 351–366.

Angel, B. *et al.* (2001) Effects of war and organized violence on children: a study of Bosnian refugees in Sweden. *American Journal of Orthopsychiatry* **71**, 4–15.

Barber, B.K. (2013) Annual research review: the experience of youth with political conflict—challenging notions of resilience and encouraging research refinement. *Journal of Child Psychology and Psychiatry* **54**, 461–473.

Bean, T. *et al.* (2007a) Comparing psychological distress, traumatic stress reactions, and experiences of unaccompanied refugee minors with experiences of adolescents accompanied by parents. *Journal of Nervous and Mental Disease* **195**, 288–297.

Bean, T.M. *et al.* (2007b) Course and predictors of mental health of unaccompanied refugee minors in the Netherlands: one year follow-up. *Social Science and Medicine* **64**, 1204–1215.

Becker-Blease, K.A. *et al.* (2010) Disasters, victimization, and children's mental health. *Child Development* **81**, 1040–1052.

Berthold, S.M. (1999) The effects of exposure to community violence on Khmer refugee adolescents. *Journal of Traumatic Stress* **12**, 455–471.

Berthold, S.M. (2000) War traumas and community violence: psychological, behavioral, and academic outcomes among Khmer refugee adolescents. *Journal of Multicultural Social Work* **8**, 15–46.

Betancourt, T.S. & Williams, T. (2008) Building an evidence base on mental health interventions for children affected by armed conflict. *Intervention (Amstelveen, Netherlands)* **6**, 39–56.

Betancourt, T.S. *et al.* (2010a) Past horrors, present struggles: the role of stigma in the association between war experiences and psychosocial adjustment among former child soldiers in Sierra Leone. *Social Science and Medicine* **70**, 17–26.

Betancourt, T.S. *et al.* (2010b) Sierra Leone's former child soldiers: a longitudinal study of risk, protective factors, and mental health. *Journal of the American Academy of Child & Adolescent Psychiatry* **49**, 606–615.

Bhui, K. *et al.* (2003) Cultural adaptation of mental health measures: improving the quality of clinical practice and research. *British Journal of Psychiatry* **183**, 184–186.

Bolton, P. *et al.* (2007) Interventions for depression symptoms among adolescent survivors of war and displacement in northern Uganda. *JAMA* **298**, 519–527.

Bronstein, I. *et al.* (2013) Emotional and behavioural problems amongst Afghan unaccompanied asylum-seeking children: results from a large-scale cross-sectional study. *European Child and Adolescent Psychiatry* **22**, 285–294.

Catani, C. *et al.* (2010) Tsunami, war, and cumulative risk in the lives of Sri Lankan schoolchildren. *Child Development* **81**, 1176–1191.

Cloitre, M. (2009) Effective psychotherapies for posttraumatic stress disorder: a review and critique. *CNS Spectrums* **14**, 32–43.

Cohen, J.A. *et al.* (2000) Treating traumatized children a research review and synthesis. *Trauma, Violence, & Abuse* **1**, 29–46.

Cortina, M. *et al.* (2013) Childhood psychological problems in school settings in rural southern Africa. *PLOS One* **8**, e65041.

Crisp, J. (2000) A state of insecurity: the political economy of violence in Kenya's refugee camps. *African Affairs* **99**, 601–632.

De Jong, J.T.V.M. *et al.* (2001) Lifetime events and posttraumatic stress disorder in 4 postconflict settings. *JAMA* **286**, 555–562.

De Jong, J.T. *et al.* (2003) Common mental disorders in postconflict settings. *Lancet* **361**, 2128–2130.

Derluyn, I. & Broekaert, E. (2007) Different perspectives on emotional and behavioural problems in unaccompanied refugee children and adolescents. *Ethnicity and Health* **12**, 141–162.

Ekblad, S. (1993) Psychosocial adaptation of children while housed in a Swedish refugee camp: aftermath of the collapse of Yugoslavia. *Stress Medicine* **9**, 159–166.

Ertl, V. *et al.* (2011) Community-implemented trauma therapy for former child soldiers in northern Uganda. *JAMA* **306**, 503–512.

Fazel, M. *et al.* (2005) Prevalence of serious mental disorder in 7000 refugees resettled in Western countries: a systematic review. *Lancet* **365**, 1309–1314.

Fazel, M. *et al.* (2012) Mental health of displaced and refugee children resettled in high-income countries: risk and protective factors. *Lancet* **379**, 266–282.

Fazel, M. *et al.* (2014) Detention, denial and death: migration hazards for refugee children. *Lancet Global Health* **2**, e313–e314.

Ford, T. *et al.* (2003) The British child and adolescent mental health survey 1999: the prevalence of *DSM-IV* disorders. *Journal of the American Academy of Child & Adolescent Psychiatry* **42**, 1203–1211.

Fremont, W.P. (2004) Childhood reactions to terrorism-induced trauma: a review of the past 10 years. *Journal of the American Academy of Child & Adolescent Psychiatry* **43**, 381–392.

Geltman, P.L. *et al.* (2005) The "lost boys of Sudan": functional and behavioral health of unaccompanied refugee minors resettled in the United States. *Archives of Pediatrics & Adolescent Medicine* **159**, 585–591.

Global Detention Project (2013) *Global Detention Project* [Online]. Available: http://www.globaldetentionproject.org/countries.html [18 May 2013].

Hancilova, B. & Knauder, B. (2011) Unaccompanied minor asylum-seekers: overview of protection, assistance and promising practices. Budapest: International Organization for Migration.

Hasanović, M. *et al.* (2006) Psychological disturbances of war-traumatized children from different foster and family settings in Bosnia and Herzegovina. *Croatian Medical Journal* **47**, 85–94.

Hodes, M. *et al.* (2008) Risk and resilience for psychological distress amongst unaccompanied asylum seeking adolescents. *Journal of Child Psychology and Psychiatry* **49**, 723–732.

Hollifield, M. *et al.* (2002) Measuring trauma and health status in refugees. *JAMA* **288**, 611–621.

Izutsu, T. *et al.* (2005) Nutritional and mental health status of Afghan refugee children in Peshawar, Pakistan: a descriptive study. *Asia-Pacific Journal of Public Health* **17**, 93–98.

Jordans, M.J. *et al.* (2009) Systematic review of evidence and treatment approaches: psychosocial and mental health care for children in war. *Child and Adolescent Mental Health* **14**, 2–14.

Jordans, M.J. *et al.* (2010) Development of a multi-layered psychosocial care system for children in areas of political violence. *International Journal of Mental Health Systems* **4**, 15.

Kia-Keating, M. & Ellis, B.H. (2007) Belonging and connection to school in resettlement: young refugees, school belonging, and psychosocial adjustment. *Clinical Child Psychology and Psychiatry* **12**, 29–43.

Layne, C.M. *et al.* (2010) Unpacking trauma exposure risk factors and differential pathways of influence: predicting postwar mental distress in Bosnian adolescents. *Child Development* **81**, 1053–1076.

Lorek, A. *et al.* (2009) The mental and physical health difficulties of children held within a British immigration detention center: a pilot study. *Child Abuse & Neglect* **33**, 573.

Mares, S. *et al.* (2002) Seeking refuge, losing hope: parents and children in immigration detention. *Australasian Psychiatry* **10**, 91–96.

Marshall, G.N. *et al.* (2005) Mental health of Cambodian refugees 2 decades after resettlement in the United States. *JAMA* **294**, 571–579.

Mels, C. *et al.* (2010) The psychological impact of forced displacement and related risk factors on Eastern Congolese adolescents affected by war. *Journal of Child Psychology and Psychiatry* **51**, 1096–1104.

Miller, K.E. & Rasmussen, A. (2010) War exposure, daily stressors, and mental health in conflict and post-conflict settings: bridging the divide between trauma-focused and psychosocial frameworks. *Social Science & Medicine* **70**, 7–16.

Montgomery, E. (2010) Trauma and resilience in young refugees: a 9-year follow-up study. *Development and Psychopathology* **22**, 477–489.

Montgomery, E. & Foldspang, A. (2008) Discrimination, mental problems and social adaptation in young refugees. *The European Journal of Public Health* **18**, 156–161.

Morgos, D. *et al.* (2007) Psychosocial effects of war experiences among displaced children in Southern Darfur. *Omega: Journal of Death and Dying* **56**, 229–253.

Nickerson, A. *et al.* (2011) A critical review of psychological treatments of posttraumatic stress disorder in refugees. *Clinical Psychology Review* **31**, 399–417.

Nielsen, S.S. *et al.* (2008) Mental health among children seeking asylum in Denmark–the effect of length of stay and number of relocations: a cross-sectional study. *BMC Public Health* **8**, 293.

Paardekooper, B. *et al.* (1999) The psychological impact of war and the refugee situation on South Sudanese children in refugee camps in Northern Uganda: an exploratory study. *Journal of Child Psychology and Psychiatry* **40**, 529–536.

Panter-Brick, C. *et al.* (2009) Violence, suffering, and mental health in Afghanistan: a school-based survey. *Lancet* **374**, 807–816.

Patel, V. *et al.* (2007a) Treatment and prevention of mental disorders in low-income and middle-income countries. *Lancet* **370**, 991–1005.

Patel, V. *et al.* (2007b) Mental health of young people: a global public-health challenge. *Lancet* **369**, 1302–1313.

Pine, D.S. *et al.* (2005) Trauma, proximity, and developmental psychopathology: the effects of war and terrorism on children. *Neuropsychopharmacology* **30**, 1781–1792.

Porte, Z. & Torney-Purta, J. (1987) Depression and academic achievement among Indochinese refugee unaccompanied minors in ethnic and nonethnic placements. *American Journal of Orthopsychiatry* **57**, 536–547.

Quinn, E. (2011) *The refugee convention sixty years on: relevant or redundant? Working Notes* [Online]. 68:19–25, Available:

http://www.workingnotes.ie/index.php/item/the-refugee-convention-sixty-years-on-relevant-or-redundant.

Reed, R.V. *et al.* (2012) Mental health of displaced and refugee children resettled in low-income and middle-income countries: risk and protective factors. *Lancet* **379**, 250–265.

Robjant, K. & Fazel, M. (2010) The emerging evidence for narrative exposure therapy: a review. *Clinical Psychology Review* **30**, 1030–1039.

Rothe, E.M. *et al.* (2002) Posttraumatic stress disorder among Cuban children and adolescents after release from a refugee camp. *Psychiatric Services* **53**, 970–976.

Rousseau, C. & Drapeau, A. (2003) Are refugee children an at-risk group? A longitudinal study of Cambodian adolescents. *Journal of Refugee Studies* **16**, 67–81.

Rousseau, C. *et al.* (1998) Risk and protective factors in Central American and Southeast Asian refugee children. *Journal of Refugee Studies* **11**, 20–37.

Rousseau, C. *et al.* (2000) Living conditions and emotional profiles of Cambodian, Central American, and Québécois youth. *Canadian Journal of Psychiatry* **45**, 905–911.

Rousseau, C. *et al.* (2005) Evaluation of a classroom program of creative expression workshops for refugee and immigrant children. *Journal of Child Psychology and Psychiatry* **46**, 180–185.

Rutter, M.L. (1999) Psychosocial adversity and child psychopathology. *British Journal of Psychiatry* **174**, 480–493.

Rutter, M. (2013) Annual research review: resilience: clinical implications. *Journal of Child Psychology and Psychiatry* **54**, 474–487.

Sack, W.H. *et al.* (1986) The psychiatric effects of massive trauma on Cambodian children: II. The family, the home, and the school. *Journal of the American Academy of Child Psychiatry* **25**, 377–383.

Sack, W.H. *et al.* (1993) A 6-Year follow-up study of Cambodian refugee adolescents traumatized as children. *Journal of the American Academy of Child and Adolescent Psychiatry* **32**, 431–437.

Sack, W.H. *et al.* (1994) The Khmer adolescent project: I. Epidemiologic findings in two generations of Cambodian refugees. *Journal of Nervous and Mental Disease* **182**, 387–395.

Servan-Schreiber, D. *et al.* (1998) Prevalence of posttraumatic stress disorder and major depressive disorder in Tibetan refugee children. *Journal of the American Academy of Child and Adolescent Psychiatry* **37**, 874–879.

Sigal, J.J. & Weinfeld, M. (2001) Do children cope better than adults with potentially traumatic stress? A 40-year follow-up of Holocaust survivors. *Psychiatry: Interpersonal & Biological Processes* **64**, 69–80.

Sigona, N. & Hughes, V. 2012. No way out, no way in: irregular migrant children and families in the UK. *Research Report ESRC Centre on Migration, Policy and Society.* Oxford: University of Oxford.

Silverman, W.K. *et al.* (2008) Evidence-based psychosocial treatments for children and adolescents exposed to traumatic events. *Journal of Clinical Child & Adolescent Psychology* **37**, 156–183.

Steel, Z. *et al.* (2009) Association of torture and other potentially traumatic events with mental health outcomes among populations exposed to mass conflict and displacement. *JAMA* **302**, 537–549.

Sujoldžić, A. *et al.* (2006) Social determinants of health–a comparative study of Bosnian adolescents in different cultural contexts. *Collegium Antropologicum* **30**, 703–711.

Taylor, T.L. & Chemtob, C.M. (2004) Efficacy of treatment for child and adolescent traumatic stress. *Archives of Pediatrics & Adolescent Medicine* **158**, 786–791.

Thabet, A. & Vostanis, P. (1998) Social adversities and anxiety disorders in the Gaza Strip. *Archives of Disease in Childhood* **78**, 439–442.

Thabet, A. *et al.* (2008) Exposure to war trauma and PTSD among parents and children in the Gaza strip. *European Child & Adolescent Psychiatry* **17**, 191–199.

Tingvold, L. *et al.* (2012) Seeking balance between the past and the present: Vietnamese refugee parenting practices and adolescent well-being. *International Journal of Intercultural Relations* **36**, 260–270.

Tol, W.A. *et al.* (2008) School-based mental health intervention for children affected by political violence in Indonesia. *JAMA* **300**, 655–662.

Tol, W.A. *et al.* (2009) Brief multi-disciplinary treatment for torture survivors in Nepal: a naturalistic comparative study. *International Journal of Social Psychiatry* **55**, 39–56.

Tol, W.A. *et al.* (2012) Outcomes and moderators of a preventive school-based mental health intervention for children affected by war in Sri Lanka: a cluster randomized trial. *World Psychiatry* **11**, 114–122.

Tol, W.A. *et al.* (2013) Annual research review: resilience and mental health in children and adolescents living in areas of armed conflict–a systematic review of findings in low-and middle-income countries. *Journal of Child Psychology and Psychiatry* **54**, 445–460.

Tolmac, J. & Hodes, M. (2004) Ethnic variation among adolescent psychiatric in-patients with psychotic disorders. *British Journal of Psychiatry* **184**, 428–431.

Tousignant, M. *et al.* (1999) The Quebec adolescent refugee project: psychopathology and family variables in a sample from 35 nations. *Journal of the American Academy of Child & Adolescent Psychiatry* **38**, 1426–1432.

Tyrer, R. & Fazel, M. (2014) School and community-based interventions for refugee and asylum seeking children: a systematic review. *PLoS ONE* **9**, e89359.

UNHCR (1951) *Convention Relating to the Status of Refugees,* Geneva.

UNHCR (2011) *UNHCR Statistical Yearbook 2011: Trends in Displacement, Protection and Solutions,* 11th edn. UNHCR, Geneva. Available: http://www.unhcr.org/516282cf5.html [18 May 2013].

Viner, R.M. *et al.* (2012) Adolescence and the social determinants of health. *Lancet* **379**, 1641–1652.

Walker, S.P. *et al.* (2011) Inequality in early childhood: risk and protective factors for early child development. *Lancet* **378**, 1325–1338.

CHAPTER 45

Pediatric consultation and psychiatric aspects of somatic disease

Elizabeth Pinsky[1], Paula K. Rauch[2] and Annah N. Abrams[1]

[1] Child and Adolescent Psychiatry Consultation Service, Massachusetts General Hospital, Boston, MA, USA
[2] Child and Adolescent Psychiatry Consultation Service and Cancer Center Parenting Program, Massachusetts General Hospital, Boston, MA, USA

Introduction

"Pediatric consultation" or "pediatric consultation-liaison" care refer to child psychiatrists or child psychologists who are mental health professionals providing psychological and/or psychiatric care to medically ill children, with special attention to biological, psychological, and social mediators of well-being. In other contexts, "consultation" can refer to school (see Chapter 42) or forensic (see Chapter 49) settings. In this chapter, we refer to the task of the "mental health consultant" as assessment and management of the psychiatric status of the medically ill child, most often in a medical hospital environment.

Mental health consultants assess (i) children with primary psychiatric illnesses leading to medical conditions, (ii) psychiatric manifestations of medical illnesses or treatments, (iii) adjustment to a chronic or life threatening illness, and (iv) differential diagnosis of psycho somatic illness. In addition, the consultant's scope may include working with anxious or challenging parents, providing liaison work with ward staff, offering didactic lectures for medical staff or parents, and advocating with hospital leadership to develop more psychologically attuned standard practices.

The medically ill child's phase of development, temperament, social and cultural context, type and stage of illness, family dynamics, and level of pain and anxiety are among the multitude of contributing factors determining the complexity of clinical care and research in the pediatric consultation population.

History

Adult consultation psychiatry arose in general hospitals during the 1930s, with the recognition that a mind-body dichotomy was an inadequate approach to provide quality medical care and that psychological issues have an impact on medical illness and treatment (Ortiz, 1997). As the integral role of psychological factors was established in adult medical care, similar attention was focused on the needs of children (Work, 1989). While the literature continues to demonstrate benefits of collaboration between child psychiatrists and pediatric staff (Carter *et al.*, 2003; Fritz, 2003), consultation psychiatry by no means exists in every pediatric medical and surgical setting today. Throughout Europe consultation resources are limited, and they are virtually unavailable in many low- and middle-income countries.

In part this is because consultation services require institutional support, especially for otherwise unreimbursed activities such as pediatric and psychiatric clinical collaborations, comprehensive evaluations, and interdisciplinary team meetings. In addition, as the medical care of children, like adults, is moving toward shorter hospital stays and greater utilization of outpatient settings for treatment of chronic and life threatening illness, mental health consultants will be called upon to shift their availability to encompass these outpatient settings.

Consultation service models

Consultation service models will be determined by the size of the patient group served, the illness severity of treatment populations, and the availability of child mental health consultants. In many pediatric medical settings, child psychologists are the primary child mental health consultants with child psychiatrists limited to acting as pediatric psychopharmacologists. Mental health consultants, regardless of their training discipline, need understanding of disease process, medical

Rutter's Child and Adolescent Psychiatry, Sixth Edition.
Edited by Anita Thapar and Daniel S. Pine, James F. Leckman, Stephen Scott, Margaret J. Snowling, Eric Taylor.
© 2015 John Wiley & Sons Ltd. Published 2018 by John Wiley & Sons Ltd.

management of relevant illnesses, and a comprehensive set of psychological interventions (see Chapter 36), including mind-body techniques.

Consultations can be initiated on a case-by-case basis or by protocol or as a mix of each. In the case-by-case model, the pediatrician requests a consultation after assessing an individual patient, while consultation by protocol systematizes psychiatric consultation for children with certain diagnoses or risk factors. Examples of protocol driven consultation include routine consultation to patients who are candidates for transplant, or have been admitted after suicide attempts, or require hospitalization longer than 2 weeks.

"Liaison" care

Arguably, no consultation to a hospitalized child can be provided effectively without the integral "liaison" component addressing concerns arising from members of the treatment team. Work with medically ill children is rewarding, but it can also arouse powerful feelings of sadness, frustration, and helplessness. Pediatric units may seek input from the consultant to address the emotional challenges experienced by the medical team, assist them in their ability to provide the best care for patients and prevent long-term burn out (Levi et al., 2004; Bateman et al., 2012).

Approach to consultation requests

The first task for the consultant when responding to a request is to understand: *what is the consultation question?* While the consultation question is sometimes clear (e.g., is there underlying psychiatric illness; what is the appropriate disposition for a child admitted with self-harming behavior), often it is obscured by affect between care providers or with the family or patient (e.g., why is this family driving us crazy; why can't the medical teams agree on treatment goals). The consultant should speak directly with the consulting pediatrician or staff member, listen to the expressed concerns and ask for elaboration about concerns that appear present but not disclosed. It is important to establish realistic goals and to determine acuity for the initial consultation as early as possible and as part of a step-by-step approach to the consultation (Table 45.1).

The pediatrician or subspecialist with whom the family already has a relationship should inform the parents of the decision to obtain a psychiatric consultation. Psychiatric consultation may be presented as part of the diagnostic process, as a way to help the team understand how the child is feeling, or as a response to the challenges that hospitalization has presented. Some parents and children may be uncomfortable with the idea of psychiatric consultation, and yet appreciate the intervention upon finding the child mental health consultant respectful, knowledgeable, and attuned to the needs of the child and family. Other parents will be resistant, reluctantly agree under some pressure from the referring pediatrician, and perhaps remain ambivalent

Table 45.1 Steps to the consultation.

1. Consult request
   Case-by-case or protocol driven
   Psychiatrist, psychologist, supervised trainee
2. Discussion with consulting team
   What is the consultation question?
   What is the acuity of the request?
   Who will inform the family of the consultation?
3. Review of medical data
   Data specific to the child
   Information specific to the medical illness
4. Interview
   Family and child
   Collateral data: school, existing treatment team
5. Mental status examination
6. Formulation
   Premorbid medical and psychiatric function
   Developmental/age specific perspective
   Illness specific perspective
7. Presentation of recommendations to team

about the benefit of the assessment or come to appreciate its value. Parents who are concerned about stigma around mental health care may be reassured when the consultant is introduced as a member of the multidisciplinary team and a resource for the family to assist their child with adjustment and coping, as opposed to being involved due to concern about psychopathology. For those families who refuse consultation, the consultant may meet with the team in a liaison capacity and assist the team without directly interviewing the child. If the psychiatric consultation is deemed urgent, the pediatrician should seek input from the hospital legal counsel about the appropriate way to proceed within the legal system in which the pediatrician practices.

Prior to meeting with the family and child, the consultant should review relevant medical data, including pediatric and subspecialist notes, laboratory and imaging studies, medication administration reports, and other studies where appropriate. The consultant should also review basic information about any specific medical illness and be familiar with general planned work-up or treatment.

The consultation

Interview of child and family

Depending on the age and circumstances of the child's condition, the consultant will decide whether to meet with the parents first, the child first, or both together. Meeting with older children without a parent present at some point is usually essential. This allows them to voice private concerns and allows for observation of differences in mental status (including mood and affect) with and without family present. Children under six are often more comfortable meeting with the consultant along with a parent. The parents of young children are likely to want time alone with the consultant to share observations and concerns which are not appropriate to share in the child's presence. Similarly, many parents of older children will find it easier to be candid about their worries in the absence of the child.

No child can be understood independently of his or her family. In the initial evaluation, it is therefore essential to assess the family's level of functioning and their ability to support the child in the hospital and through the anticipated treatment and outcome. Parental anxiety and distress are associated with a child's psychological adjustment and capacity to cope (Sawyer et al., 1998; Wagner et al., 2003; Palmer et al., 2011). Asking parents to share the history of the current illness, from the first symptoms through to the present hospital stay, allows the consultant to learn about the parents' experience of the medical care. It is helpful to understand the parents' views of past and present medical caregivers as well as their experience of their own role in the child's medical condition. An assessment of the family should include psychiatric history for each parent and the siblings, and questions about the family's past experiences with illness and loss. Helping the parent differentiate the current medical situation from past experiences helps the parent be more attuned to the child's actual needs.

Siblings are often the forgotten sufferers (Alderfer et al., 2010). The sick child is commonly the object of everyone's attention, while siblings often live with disrupted schedules, less attention, and less emotionally available parents. The consultant can model empathy for siblings and help parents with ways of addressing the needs of their well children.

Difficult parents often cannot bear the feelings of helplessness and vent their anger and frustration on hospital staff by being critical and devaluing (Groves & Beresin, 1999). Pediatric hospital staff members may have a harder time working with some parents than the patient. The consultant can help the team understand the family better and feel more empathy for difficult behaviors.

Collateral sources

The consultant should seek information from other members of the treatment team, including nursing staff and child life specialists, who may offer especially valuable observations. After the initial assessment and with permission from the parents or guardian, the consultant may seek input provided by sources outside of the medical arenas such as an outpatient psychotherapist, school professionals, or members of other involved social agencies such as the department of social services, or the court system.

Formulation: premorbid medical and psychiatric functioning

When the consultant is assessing a hospitalized child, the consultant is seeing only "a snap shot" out of the child's life. Some families will be confronting a new diagnosis or change in the prognosis, while others may have had time to develop an ongoing coping strategy in the face of a chronic illness or a lengthy treatment protocol. Assessment should recognize the potential for wide variation in coping at different points in the unfolding medical experience.

Formulation: conceptions of medical illness across child development

Development is an important lens through which a childhood medical illness can be observed. A full review of the interplay of development and medical illness is beyond the scope of this chapter, but a few key developmental points will be highlighted to illustrate common issues.

Infants and toddlers cannot understand the gravity of a given diagnosis. They live in the moment experiencing the medical condition and treatment according to the physical limitations and discomforts imposed. Infants rely on key caretakers to hold and soothe them and to make the hospital environment feel safe. It is important for the hospital staff to support the infant–parent attachment, and not allow treatments and technologies to interfere with this key emotional milestone. Interventions include supporting breast-feeding mothers and allowing rooming-in by parents.

Very young children (3–6 year olds) are egocentric, that is, they understand all events as occurring in relation to them. They have associative logic, which means that for them any two unrelated things can be understood as if one is causing or explaining the other. The combination of egocentricity and associative logic leads to "magical thinking," the weaving together of fantasy and logic to explain how the young child caused something to happen. In the medical setting, it is frequently the child's misconception that having a "bad illness" means he did something wrong and is being punished. It is helpful to get young children (and often older children as well) to elaborate their understanding of the etiology of their medical conditions to uncover self-blaming misconceptions and correct them.

At this age, children cannot localize a medical condition to a specific body part, so they feel particularly physically vulnerable when ill. Faced with needle sticks, intravenous medication and surgical procedures, they are often fearful. They rely on parents and medical staff to prepare them for procedures so they come to trust that there will not be surprise medical attacks at any moment. The young child is likely to demonstrate the most affect around separations, such as having anxiety about going to sleep at night in his own bed, or wanting a parent to promise to be there when she wakes up from surgery.

Older children (approximately 7–12 years of age) can understand simple, functional explanations of medical conditions. Many will pride themselves on mastering the names of medicines, illness related terminology, and how to use hospital equipment. Children of this age look for simple cause and effect etiologies for illnesses. They can understand viral illnesses being caused by "germs," but are perplexed when there is no clear causal explanation, for example, for why they have cancer without having smoked cigarettes. It is important to explain illness and treatment simply and clearly. In the context of understanding why a treatment plan is being initiated, the medical staff should seek the child's assent to procedures and treatments. This age group is typically rule-bound, and it is troubling to the child that so often medical illness does not follow "the rules" (e.g., she avoids her asthma triggers and has an asthma attack anyway).

Adolescents (13 and older) generally have abstract thinking and thus are able to understand the chance bad luck of having an uncommon, life threatening, or chronic illness with the same cognitive complexity of an adult. That said, teens often do not have the maturity to incorporate the healthy behaviors that they know that they should engage in, into appropriate changes in lifestyle. Turning cognitive understanding into behavioral change is the common battleground of adolescent and authority figure—parent or physician. Consent should be sought from adolescents who have the cognitive ability to comprehend the purpose of treatment and the ramifications of refusing treatment.

Adolescence is a self-conscious time with the emergence of sexual interests and heightened reliance on peer group norms for style and status. Medical illnesses or treatments that affect appearance are particularly difficult such as becoming cushingoid on steroids or bald with chemotherapy. The medical staff is challenged to find ways to respect the teen's age appropriate wish to be more independent in the face of illness that so often increases dependency.

As children with chronic illnesses live into adulthood, the transition to young adulthood and understanding associated issues becomes relevant. Young adults are negotiating intimate relationships, career decisions, independence from parents, and sometimes relocation or parenthood. One challenge that the treatment team and patient may face is whether to transition care from a pediatric setting into an adult setting, which often necessitates a new treatment team. This is a particularly vulnerable time as adolescents are at risk of medication nonadherence increase and of loss to follow-up (Shemesh *et al.*, 2010; Garvey *et al.*, 2012). Some patients may prefer to be on an adult ward or waiting room, but may find it very difficult to leave lifelong caretakers and the pediatric model of care.

Formulation: illness-specific medical perspective

Each medical condition carries its own specific challenges. When the consultant is familiar with common frustrations or limitations imposed by a particular medical illness, they have credibility with a child or parent as they relate what is hardest for them. Routine consultation to the same pediatric unit leads to the consultant becoming familiar with technology, treatment protocols, and terminology, all of which makes it easier for the child and family to tell their medical story and feel understood.

Mental status examination in the hospitalized or medically ill child

Hospitalized children have many reasons to have an altered mental status including delirium, central nervous system (CNS) changes secondary to medical conditions, effects of medications, and trauma. A formal mental status examination should be part of the medical record including observations of appearance, motor function, speech, mood, affect, thought, suicidal ideation, memory, and cognition.

Medically ill children may be developmentally delayed or emotionally immature. It is helpful for the consultant to integrate the information from the mental status examination and premorbid school and developmental information to assist the medical team in understanding the child's ability to comprehend medical information.

Presenting recommendations to the team

After meeting with the child and family for the initial assessment, the consultant will share observations and recommendations with the referring pediatrician, available team members, and write a note in the hospital record. The consultant should attend to the urgency and time frame in which the referring doctor needs assistance. The formulation and recommendations should avoid the use of psychiatric jargon. Clear practical recommendations to improve coping, address behavioral problems, treat primary psychiatric disorders, and maintain safety are most helpful. Sharing an understanding of motivations that may underlie maladaptive behaviors can increase empathy for the child and family, but the consultant should also provide concrete, practical suggestions. One should assume that patients and parents will read the record, as can hospital staff and insurers.

Reasons for consultation: primary psychiatric illnesses

Depression

For a general review of depression please see Chapter 63.

Depression is common in the hospitalized child. It may be a secondary response to the stress of acute or chronic illness, or it may be primary presenting as psychosomatic illness or behavioral problems including self-harm. One barrier to the appropriate treatment of depression in hospitalized children is the misconception that depressed mood and symptoms are an appropriate response to serious illness. Another barrier to treatment is the difficulty of making the diagnosis of depression in a medically ill child given the overlap of somatic symptoms and depressive symptoms (Shemesh *et al.*, 2005). Individual and family therapy, play therapy, behavioral therapy, and medication are useful modalities in the hospital setting (see Chapters 62 and 63). Antidepressants are also being used medically in children and adolescents with preliminary studies reporting benefit (Kersun & Elia, 2007). Selective serotonergic reuptake inhibitors (SSRIs) are typically the first-line agent of choice as they are well tolerated, have limited interactions with other medications, and present a lower risk of intentional or accidental overdose (see Chapter 43).

Anxiety

Anxiety can be preexisting or secondary to the stresses of the medical condition and treatment. Children with preexisting generalized anxiety or specific fear of doctors, needles, and shots are likely to have more difficulty adjusting to medical assessment and treatment. In addition to the discomfort anxiety causes to children and parents, anxiety can interfere with procedures and complicate history taking and symptom assessment.

Age appropriate explanation of medical interventions for older children, and medical play with explanation for younger children, can decrease anxiety. Children from around 6 years of age can learn a variety of coping techniques to help them with anxiety provoking procedures. Many children will respond to distraction, breathing exercises, visualization, or hypnotherapy (Landier & Tse, 2010; Koller & Goldman, 2012).

Clinicians must pay attention to minimizing pain for every child (Greco & Berde, 2005). Effective interventions include preparation, relaxation, distraction, use of anesthetic creams before procedures, and treating chronic and acute pain with analgesics (Fein *et al.*, 2012; Sohn *et al.*, 2012). For young children, all painful procedures should occur in a treatment room and not in the child's bed nor in the playroom. Protecting the child's bed and the playroom as safe havens will eventually help the young child relax in these settings.

Despite quality pain management, relaxation techniques, and preparation for procedures, some children will continue to be too anxious to comply with treatment and may suffer sleep disturbance, nausea, or agitation during the hospital stay or in anticipation of visits to the hospital. Benzodiazepines may be helpful adjuncts to lessen debilitating anxiety. In young children, one must be aware of the potential for benzodiazepines to cause a "paradoxical reaction" with disinhibition and worsening anxiety.

Anorexia nervosa

For a general review of anorexia nervosa please see Chapter 71.

Pediatric hospitalization for anorexia usually occurs when there has been rapid or profound weight loss, cardiovascular abnormalities, electrolyte imbalance, or hypothermia. The goal of hospitalization is medical stabilization with nutritional assessment and treatment, psychological assessment of the child and family, and recommendation for level of psychiatric intervention after medical stabilization. Eating disorder protocols (also referred to as nutritional deficiency protocols) provide established guidelines for inpatient clinical care. The guidelines should include meal plans, weight expectations, and goals of the admission. The protocols are detailed and include restrictions of activity, observation during and after meal times and bathroom privileges only after weight gain has begun (Sylvester & Forman, 2008). Once the child is medically stable, recommendations about disposition can be initiated.

Psychosomatic illness

For a general review of psychosomatic illness please see Chapter 72.

Some children are admitted to pediatric units with intense, persistent somatic complaints such as headaches, abdominal pains, bowel complaints, neurologic symptoms, or fatigue. The pediatricians may suspect that the intensity of the symptoms or the combination of complaints exceeds what can be explained by a medical condition and reflects underlying emotional factors and may thus seek a psychiatric consultation. The pediatrician's assessment that psychological factors are influencing the somatic presentation is usually at odds with the child and parents' understanding of the etiology of the condition. Often the child and parents are viewed as overly invested in an exhaustive medical work-up to prove a purely medical etiology.

Commonly, psychiatric consultation is resisted, because it is viewed as evidence that the medical team either does not believe the symptoms or medical condition to be "real" or is unwilling to fully investigate all the medical possibilities. It is common for the family to seek multiple medical opinions and often to choose the most aggressive specialists. Diagnostic tests may be repeated to satisfy parental demands for action or in an attempt to decrease persistent patient and parental anxiety about undetected serious illness. Parents may overvalue insignificant positive findings from the diagnostic work-ups to vindicate their belief that a yet undiscovered medical etiology exists.

Hospitalization may be an important opportunity for a coordinated care plan addressing psychological and medical issues together. Presenting the consultant's role as one of helping the child cope with chronic symptoms that are interfering with school, peer activities, or family life is less threatening than suggesting that the consultant has been sought because the symptom intensity reflects psychological issues. The child and family must be reassured that the presence of the child mental health consultant will not be associated with reduced access to the medical team, but is truly an adjunct to ongoing medical care. The pediatrician plays the important role of re-examining the child regularly, reassuring the patient and family that no worrying new findings exist and not acquiescing to unnecessary testing.

Nonadherence

Nonadherence with medical treatments is common ranging from estimates of 50% to as high as 88%. Physicians recognize that education and an alliance with parents and children can improve patient adherence rates. More recently care providers are employing text messaging and other behavioral interventions to improve patient adherence with clinic visits and medications (Dowshen *et al.*, 2012; Ting *et al.*, 2012). There are many factors contributing to nonadherence including the medication regimen, family systems, denial, psychiatric illness, and relationships with medical providers.

When consultation is sought for nonadherence, usually it is because of risk to the child's health, escalating conflict in the family, or frustration with inappropriate use of medical resources. The consultant's task is to understand why the child is nonadherent and to work with the team to modify aspects of treatments that trouble the child where possible, while working to help the child and family adopt strategies that support clinically important treatments. Treatable psychiatric disorders need to be identified and addressed. Treatment promoting supports, including disease specific support groups, more frequent meetings with clinicians and psychoeducation groups can be helpful.

Reasons for consultation: emergency consultations

Suicide attempts

For a general review of suicide attempts please see Chapter 64.

The most common emergent consultations relate to the suicidal or self-abusive child. The consultant's first recommendations focus on the child's immediate safety and the child's risk for self harm in the medical unit setting. Once safety has been assured, the consultant can assess the precipitants for the acts of self-harm and recommend appropriate treatment in the hospital and disposition.

Delirium

Delirium is commonly encountered in medically ill children. Also known as acute confusional state, delirium is a syndrome characterized by (i) acute onset and waxing and waning course, (ii) cognitive impairment or confusion, and (iii) disturbance of arousal. Delirium can occur either in the setting of an underlying general medical illness or secondary to substances including medicines or toxins. The mnemonic "I WATCH DEATH" provides an overview of the conditions commonly associated with delirium (Table 45.2); infectious and toxic etiologies (including medications) are the most common in the pediatric population.

The underlying mechanisms of delirium remain poorly understood, but it is thought to represent derangements in multiple neurotransmitter systems, particularly dysregulation of acetylcholine and dopamine. In addition to confusion, symptoms of delirium commonly include hallucinations, delusions, disorganized behavior, disorientation, and disruptions in memory, mood, affect, and the sleep-wake cycle (Turkel *et al.*, 2006). The nature of the disturbance of arousal in delirium varies. Hyperactive delirium is associated with combativeness and agitation. Hypoactive delirium is a state of quiet confusion and is often overlooked as the symptoms do not interfere with delivery of care.

Definitive treatment for the delirious patient is identification and treatment of the underlying cause of the syndrome, while managing symptoms in order to ensure safety for patients and staff. Management incorporates environmental interventions, including reassurance, use of environmental cues, and frequent reorienting to place and familiar people. Pharmacologic interventions can ease distressing symptoms including psychosis and fear as well as decrease agitation. Dopamine blockade is the mainstay of pharmacologic management and for adult patients intravenous haloperidol is the traditional treatment of

Table 45.2 Conditions commonly associated with delirium.

Infectious	Encephalitis, meningitis, syphilis, pneumonia, UTI
Withdrawal	Alcohol, benzodiazepines, sedative-hypnotics
Acute metabolic	Acidosis, alkalosis, electrolyte disturbances, liver or kidney failure
Trauma	Heat stroke, burns, post-operative
CNS pathology	Abscess, hemorrhage, seizure, stroke, tumor, vasculitis, normal pressure hydrocephalus
Hypoxia	Anemia, carbon monoxide poisoning, hypotension, pulmonary embolus, lung or heart failure
Deficiencies	B12, niacin, thiamine
Endocrinopathies	Hyper- or hypoglycemia, hyper- or hypoadrenocorticism, hyper- or hypothyroidism
Acute vascular	Hypertensive encephalopathy or shock
Toxins or drugs	Medications, pesticides, solvents
Heavy metals	Lead, manganese, mercury

Source: I WATCH DEATH (from Stern, T.A. *et al.* (2010) *Massachusetts General Hospital Handbook of General Hospital Psychiatry*, 6th edn, Philadelphia, PA: Saunders.)

choice (Jacobi *et al.*, 2002). Atypical antipsychotics have become increasingly first-line agents for delirious patients who are able to take oral medications (Karnik *et al.*, 2007). Benzodiazepines and diphenhydramine can compound the core symptoms of confusion and disorientation and should usually be avoided in the delirious patient (with the notable exception of delirium that is due to withdrawal from alcohol or benzodiazepines).

The challenging family

Parental behavior may be the reason for an urgent referral to the mental health consultant or to the team social worker. Parents may be refusing essential medical treatment for the child, including threatening to remove an ill child from the hospital against medical advice, or acting bizarrely. The reason for the parental actions may remain unclear, or may be explained by beliefs at odds with standard medical practice, mistrust of the hospital staff, psychiatric illness in the parent, or extreme anxiety. Hostile parents may interfere with critical care by frightening the medical staff.

Often parents who are obstructing needed care for their child are doing so because they are themselves overwhelmed with helplessness and are trying to control what they consider as uncontrollable. By helping the parent to feel that he or she is an essential member of the decision-making process and thus has some control in productive ways, many parents will step out of a combative stance and into a more collaborative one. Specific legal interventions may be implemented when parents prevent a life sustaining treatment and will be determined by legal parameters of the place of practice.

Child abuse

Physical abuse, neglect, and sexual abuse may result in emergent consultation and are discussed elsewhere in this book (see Chapters 29 and 30). In the consultation setting, it is appropriate to restate the importance of suspecting abuse. Without educated suspicion, abuse will often go undetected. Suspicious injuries, implausible or inconsistent stories from caretakers, and inappropriate delay in bringing a child for medical care should raise suspicion, as should caretakers who ascribe the injury to siblings or self-inflicted injuries.

Suspicion of abuse must be reported to the appropriate social agency. When abuse is suspected, the child should be fully examined for other physical signs. It is important to notify authorities of other children known to be in a potential unsafe home. The pediatric unit may serve as a safe haven for a child while allegations are being investigated.

The pediatric unit may also be the setting in which the fabrication of medical illness by a parent or caregiver, widely known as Munchausen Syndrome by Proxy (MSBP), is either identified or investigated. As originally described, symptoms are inflicted on the child (e.g., contamination of a central line to induce bacteremia, asphyxiation to induce cardiac arrest); in variations of MSBP symptoms are exaggerated or elaborated and result in unnecessary medical interventions (hence the increasing use of the broader terminology Pediatric Condition Falsification and/or Medical Child Abuse). In a recent review, Squires and Squires (2010) discuss the "facilitating medical environment;" because of the nature of the abuse in MSBP, medical care providers and the health care system are often unintentional perpetrators of the abuse. The pediatric medical unit may be the primary setting as families or patients seek excessive medical treatment for their reported symptoms/illness. The psychiatric consultant may initially become involved as the medical team grapples with providing appropriate medical treatment when the history and presentation are inconsistent. When the child suffers harm related to these interventions, regardless of caregiver intent, medical child abuse has occurred.

Reasons for consultation: psychological distress in the medically ill children

Children with medical illnesses serious enough to warrant hospitalization are recognized as at increased risk for emotional disorders, with estimates of psychological distress in hospitalized children and adolescents varying from 20% to greater than 35% (Stoppelbein et al., 2005). Those conditions that result in long-term physical disabilities or impact on the CNS pose additional risk (Meyer et al., 2004; Poggi et al., 2005), as may certain symptoms and challenges associated with specific diseases. Official practice parameters released by the American Academy of Child and Adolescent Psychiatry in 2009 offer principles for the assessment, management, and treatment of the medically ill child (DeMaso et al., 2009).

Coping with chronic illness

Chronically ill children should not be defined by their illnesses, that is, there is no typical child with diabetes or classic child with asthma. To the contrary, chronically ill children have the same range of personalities, and coping styles observed in healthy children and are engaged in mastering the developmental milestones and challenges they share with their peers.

Estimates of psychological morbidity associated with chronic illnesses in childhood range from 10% to 30%, which is only slightly higher than the general pediatric population (Barlow & Ellard, 2006). Greater morbidity is associated with multiple hospitalization admissions (Geist, 1977). Other documented risk factors for adaptation to chronic illness include physical disability and brain dysfunction, pain frequency, younger age, poverty, single parent family, and increased psychological symptoms in the parents (Knapp & Harris, 1998). Parental anxiety, anger, sadness, guilt, or blame can impede adjustment (Wagner et al., 2003; Vance & Eiser, 2004).

Specific illnesses present specific challenges, (some are discussed below). That said, innumerable unique factors influence how problematic any given challenge is for an individual child. It is the consultant's job to understand the unique meaning of the illness to the child and family and to assist in the process of adaptation. The consultant will need to ask many questions to elucidate the child's subjective experience of the illness, such as what is the hardest aspect of the illness or treatment from the child's perspective, how does it affect the child's image of himself, and are there specific worries about the future? Inquiries about the impact on peer interactions or favorite activities, areas of conflict between the child and parent in relation to the illness, and the child's perception of the parents' worries may be useful.

Asthma

Asthma is the most common chronic illness of childhood with a pediatric population prevalence of 5–10% and an increasing mortality rate from 1980 to 1998 that appears to have reached a plateau (Akinbami & Schoendorf, 2002). Racial and ethnic disparities account for much of the increase in morbidity (McDaniel et al., 2006). Recent studies have sought to understand the factors that affect adherence, delineate common psychosocial stresses that may act as triggers for asthma attacks, and devise psycho educational programs, combined medical and psychological treatment strategies, and teach stress management skills to improve adherence and decrease morbidity (Self et al., 2005; Peters & Fritz, 2010).

Hospitalization is an opportunity to emphasize education. Clear guidelines on when to call the pediatrician can be established while seeking input from the family about barriers to these contacts. Triggers in the home can be addressed realistically and empathically in light of the exacerbation that led to admission. Common triggers, such as smoking and pets, require a major commitment from family members in order to enact change. School-related issues need to be explored from the perspective of the child (e.g., embarrassment associated with going to the school nurse) and the school (e.g., access to inhalers in the classroom). Strategies to improve parent and child anxiety and to address parent child conflicts around adherence are valuable.

Diabetes

Insulin-dependent diabetes presents special medical challenges associated with control of blood sugars and insulin delivery, as well as special emotional challenges related to the primary role of food as a source of nurturance and soothing. The acute consequences of blood sugar abnormalities include symptomatic hypoglycemia, hyperglycemia, and ketoacidosis and may lead to hospitalization. The long-term sequelae include effects on vision, renal function, and neuropathy. Symptoms associated with hypoglycemia are often difficult for parents to differentiate from common irritability in young children or for older children to recognize as different from anxiety in themselves. This leads to either more frequent blood testing or a tendency to keep the blood sugars at a higher level than the physician would recommend. Some children will have considerable anxiety about hypoglycemia, either in response to an actual episode or arising independently. It is a key to treat anxiety disorders in order to improve adherence as well as recognize emerging eating disorders in the female teenage population as a factor in nonadherence (Jacobson, 1996; Hamilton & Daneman, 2002).

Nonadherence in insulin dependent diabetes can be life threatening. Blood testing (hemoglobin A1C) enables pediatricians to assess the child's adherence over an extended period and may be considered an appropriate factor for protocol driven mental health consultation. Subcutaneous insulin pumps can now deliver a continuous infusion of rapid-acting insulin at both basal and bolus rates, allowing for tighter control of blood sugars when combined with careful tracking of carbohydrate intake. Compared to long-acting insulin regimens, additional benefits that may be especially appealing to adolescents include greater flexibility in meal and activity planning and more discreet delivery of insulin.

Cancer

Childhood cancer presents numerous challenges to adaptation and development, fortunately though most studies suggest that childhood cancer survivors adapt well following treatment (Zeltzer et al., 2009). There are predictable high stress points in the course of an illness that often coincide with hospitalization including diagnosis, onset of treatment, and treatment completion as well as, for some, the time of a recurrence, renewed treatment, and end of life care. Psychological support for the child and parents is particularly beneficial at these critical points. Siblings also benefit from support at the various transitions during the course of the illness (Alderfer et al., 2010).

Diagnosis of a life threatening illness is understandably frightening to parents and older children creating a family crisis. Some children and parents may respond to diagnosis and aspects of treatment by exhibiting symptoms observed in posttraumatic stress syndrome (Stuber et al., 1998; Norberg and Boman, 2008; Phipps et al., 2009). Psychosocial assessment to screen for distress in families of a child with a new diagnosis of cancer can help identify families most at risk (Kazak et al., 2012).

Frequently children and families will face the child's cancer diagnosis with past experiences with cancer in a family member, or close friend, coloring their understanding of what lies ahead for their child. It is helpful to invite the child to share his understanding of the diagnosis as an opportunity to differentiate the child's situation from that of others, while potentially uncovering misconceptions about the illness.

Challenges to psychological adaptation include persistent pain (whether as a result of the cancer or the procedures), persistent debilitating side effects of treatment such as nausea, alteration in body image, school disruptions, compromised peer relationships, interference with ability to engage in favorite activities, or conflicts in the family (Hockenberry et al., 2011; Kurtz & Abrams, 2011). Adolescents may worry about future health status, sexual function and reproductive capacities, and future career choices (Patenaude & Kupst, 2005). This age group benefits from special attention to their specific developmental needs (Abrams et al., 2007).

During the course of cancer treatment, many children develop strong positive relationships with members of the medical team, experience a special closeness with supportive parents, and maintain key preexisting peer friendships while acquiring new friends in the hospital. Many children will report feeling a special sense of purpose for living as a result of the cancer diagnosis and most will be treated with special status as a result of the illness. Resilience and positive life change are also part of the cancer experience (Phipps et al., 2012).

Organ transplantation

Liver, kidney, heart, and lung transplantation are well-established practices in the pediatric population and intestinal transplantation is beginning to be undertaken. Transplantation centers in the United States are required to include psychological assessment in order to receive accreditation. Data on criteria for approval of candidacy for transplant are vague. The serious disease process leading up to transplantation, the risks of surgery, the long-term medical management of organ rejection posttransplantation, the threat to survival, and the vast array of medical treaters involved place these children in the highest of high risk populations. It is noteworthy therefore that the data on adjustment to liver and renal transplantation suggests that overall these children view themselves as healthy and competent (Tong et al., 2011). Not surprisingly, some children and parents are vulnerable to anxiety and experience distress posttransplant. It is therefore important that transplant centers involve mental health consultants and provide emotional support (Shemesh, 2008).

Inflammatory bowel disease

Inflammatory bowel disease (IBD), including Crohn's disease and ulcerative colitis, are distinct disease processes characterized by chronic inflammation of the gastrointestinal tract with relapsing and remitting courses that lead to chronic abdominal pain, bloody diarrhea, and fatigue. Neither Crohn's disease nor ulcerative colitis has a cure, and they are managed through medical and surgical interventions aimed at controlling inflammation. Pain, unpredictability, and functional impairment are only some of the potential challenges posed to the psychosocial development of the child with IBD. Treatment with systemic steroids is a mainstay of IBD regimens during acute flares and may lead to derangements in cognitive function, mood, and behavior, sometimes including severe symptoms such as major depression or psychosis. Additional stressors include adaptation to the physical sequelae of IBD (e.g., short stature, weight loss, weakness, and delayed puberty) as well as physical sequelae of treatment (e.g., steroid-induced acne, visible feeding tubes, and J-pouches) and embarrassment around needing frequent use of public bathrooms—including in the school setting.

Rates of depression among adolescents with IBD vary widely between studies, but have been found to be as high as 25% (Szigethy et al., 2004). Moreover, children with IBD have been found to have increased rates of anxiety as well as decreased psychosocial health, social functioning, and school functioning compared to well-peers (Mackner et al., 2006; Greenley et al., 2010). The mental health consultant is often involved in the care of IBD patients in both inpatient and outpatient settings. Psychosocial interventions (including psychoeducation, school-based services, and support groups), talk therapy (including cognitive behavioral therapy (CBT) and narrative therapy), and psychopharmacology aimed at depression, anxiety and insomnia all have demonstrated efficacy in adults or children with IBD (for review, see Szigethy et al., 2011).

Cystic fibrosis

Cystic fibrosis (CF) is the most common life-limiting genetic disorder among Caucasian populations, affecting 1 in 2500 newborns, or more than 30,000 individuals in the United States and 7000 in the United Kingdom (Davies et al., 2007). CF is a commonly encountered diagnosis in the inpatient pediatric medical setting. Typically diagnosed in infancy or early childhood, CF is caused by a gene defect in the chloride transport protein that leads to complex, multisystem disease, most notably chronic pulmonary inflammation and infection as well as gastrointestinal sequelae including pancreatic insufficiency with malabsorption and failure to thrive. Treatment advances have enabled many children with CF to live well into adulthood, but it remains a chronic and progressive life-limiting illness. Treatment regimens aimed at maintenance of pulmonary and systemic health are very demanding, and typically require strict dietary regimens, multiple medications, vigorous daily physical therapies, and both chronic and acute antibiotics. For many children, periodic exacerbations of pulmonary disease require repeated hospitalizations for "clean-outs," consisting of weeks-long admissions for parenteral antibiotics and aggressive physical therapy.

Despite the staggering demands of the diagnosis on child and family, most children and families living with CF report high quality of life and have rates of psychopathology similar to cohorts of well peers (Szyndler et al., 2005). Nevertheless

a full range of psychiatric problems have been reported in children with CF, and some studies have shown higher rates of psychopathology among children with CF, including anxiety, depression, and eating disorders emerging in adolescence (Quittner et al., 2008; Smith et al., 2010). As with other chronic illnesses, nonadherence is a significant issue for adolescents with CF and needs to be monitored closely.

Neurologic illness

Epilepsy is the most common neurologic disorder of childhood, affecting between 0.5% and 1% of children under age 16 (Shinnar & Pellock, 2002). Epidemiologic investigations around the globe and in both community and hospital-based settings have consistently demonstrated that psychiatric comorbidity is over-represented in pediatric epilepsy, with rates ranging from 33% to 77% (Davies et al., 2003; Plioplys et al., 2007).

Epilepsy is commonly associated with attention deficit hyperactivity disorder (ADHD), depression, anxiety disorders, and autism spectrum disorders (Jones et al., 2008). Rarely, interictal psychotic disorders may occur, or psychosis may be a feature of partial-complex seizure semiology. Some antiepileptic drugs may cause poor concentration, inattention, impulsivity, and/or hyperactivity; others have been associated with depressed mood or mood lability. For children with epilepsy who require pharmacologic management—ideally in combination with cognitive behavioral or other therapy—SSRIs remain first-line for depression and anxiety. Careful attention should be paid to potential interactions with hepatically metabolized anti-epileptic drugs and cytochrome P450 inhibitors, including fluoxetine, paroxetine, and fluvoxamine. For children with comorbid ADHD, there is mounting evidence that methylphenidate treatment is safe in children with epilepsy and clinical guidelines state that benefits outweigh risks (Davis et al., 2010; Koneski et al., 2011).

Encopresis and soiling/wetting

Soiling may be voluntary or involuntary, but is most frequently encountered as encopresis, which is involuntary and paradoxically related to constipation ("overflow incontinence"). Chronic withholding of stool leads to colonic distension and impaction, followed by eventual disruption of normal signals to defecate and leakage around hard impacted stools. Encopresis is generally managed by the pediatrician with a combination of laxatives and behavioral interventions aimed at re-establishing normal bowel habits, including short periods (<5 min) of toilet sitting after meals (to capitalize on the gastrocolic reflex), self-initiated toileting and self-management of cleanliness.

Primary nocturnal enuresis (bedwetting in a child who has never been dry) is extremely common, but can be a significant social stressor and when prolonged is associated with poor self-esteem. Secondary nocturnal enuresis (bedwetting in a child who has been dry for 6 months or more) is sometimes precipitated by psychological stressors. Daytime wetting is more commonly associated with psychological disturbance than nocturnal wetting. These conditions are generally managed by the pediatrician after history and physical examination has ruled-out medical causes, with a nonpunitive approach and options including behavioral interventions (limiting evening liquids, voiding at daytime intervals and/or before bedtime) and sometimes medications (desmopressin acetate, anticholinergic agents, and imipramine) that provide symptomatic control. Bedwetting alarms are the only demonstrated effective strategy for curing nocturnal enuresis, with reported success rates as high as 66–70% (Graham & Levy, 2009).

Children affected by encopresis and enuresis are generally emotionally healthy, but soiling and wetting can be exacerbated in children with anxiety or ADHD, and successful treatment sometimes requires treatment of comorbid psychiatric illness. For these children, assessment of adherence and psychopharmacology aimed at inattention or anxiety can be an essential part of successful treatment and maintenance of remission. Mental health professionals may also be involved for refractory cases of soiling, when constipation is not playing a part or the problem involves voluntary deposition of feces in inappropriate places. Such a pattern is often accompanied by other emotional or behavioral problems.

Dying in the hospital

The death of a child is an enormous tragedy affecting every member of the child's family. There is no way to protect a child or family from the unique pain of the loss of a child, but sensitive care may serve to lessen regrets and support bereavement (Kreicbergs et al., 2004). Attending to pain, anxiety, and privacy/dignity needs is key. Adapting the medical setting to allow parents to nurture the dying child or facilitating a child's return home to die can play a significant role in the family's experience of the death and the subsequent bereavement (Stevenson et al., 2013).

The emotional impact on the medical team deserves careful attention in order to preserve the team's ability to deliver quality care into the future. The grieving process of the staff warrants recognition. Some units will have staff meetings including the child mental health consultant or other facilitator after every death or after those deaths that are most troubling to staff members (Bateman et al., 2012).

Many of the hospital-based pediatric deaths occur in neonatal intensive care units or during infancy. Key to supporting the family of a dying infant is respecting the infant's full status as a loved child. This may include facilitating religious ceremonies such as a naming or christening, creating mementos such as photographs, footprints, or a lock of hair, and creating the most loving situation possible for the moment of dying such as providing a private room and allowing a parent to hold the infant at the time life support is disconnected.

From age 3 years onwards, the child's personal experience of impending death should be considered. The child should be offered developmentally appropriate opportunities to express thoughts and fears associated with dying either with words, drawings, or through play. It is common for even 3 and 4 year olds to verbalize explicit thoughts of joining dead grandparents and seeing angels, but it is also common for dying children to focus only on wanting parents with them at all times, and exhibiting a shift in behavior with more resistance to medical treatment, loss of interest in activities and food, but without any explicit verbalization of an awareness of dying.

Children of all ages, but especially younger children, are likely to take their cues about whether explicit discussion of death is permissible from parents and caregivers. When parents invite this dialog, it is more likely to occur. When parents signal that such discussion would be unbearable, the child is likely either not to speak about dying or to talk with a medical staff member when the parent is not present.

Child mental health consultants may help ready parents for discussions with their dying child. Asking open ended questions about worries, inquiring whether the child has questions that he is afraid to say aloud, or asking if he thinks about peers from the hospital who have died may serve as invitations to begin the dialog. Reminding children that articulating worries does not make them happen may free some children who are worrying silently to speak. Many parents will feel more comfortable embarking on end of life conversations with a child if they are told that they can welcome the child's questions warmly without having specific answers. "I am interested in your ideas." "What got you wondering about that?" "Your good questions deserve good answers. I want to think about that or talk to our minister or the doctor." These are examples of reasonable responses to a child's existential or medical questions. In the role of child mental health consultant, one of the most useful comments in response to questions about death is to tell a child "I don't know what it is like to be dead, because I have never been dead. But, I am always interested to hear children's ideas about it."

Children from age 7 onward may talk about the life experiences that they will not get to enjoy. These discussions challenge a parent's or professional's ability to bear the sadness of facing an untimely death as well as whether to talk directly with a child about their death (Kreicbergs et al., 2004). The child may talk about not getting to attend the fifth grade, never being able to drive a car, or not growing up to be a doctor or a teacher. It is often the specificity of the opportunities lost in the words of a child that is so evocative. There is a sense of privilege that one experiences in listening to children as they face the end of their lives that is as special as it is sad.

Often children will talk about being tired of the fight against the disease and will look to parents for permission to stop treatment. When the surviving family members can support each other in the painful process of letting go of the beloved child, believing that everything that could be done was done, and that further treatment would be unfair to the child, the final phase of dying can seem more peaceful. In the setting of a long battle against an illness, it can be easier to get to this difficult emotional state. In the setting of an acute event with little time for adjustment, or when parental discord interferes with the parents' ability to grieve together, such peace is harder to achieve.

The consultant should encourage hospital staff to follow up with parents 6 months to a year after the death of a child. Parents are appreciative when staff attend memorial services and funerals, write sympathy cards, and make telephone calls (Bedell *et al.*, 2001; MacDonald *et al.*, 2005). Telephone calls provide an opportunity to assess the parents grieving and need for referral as well as help the staff member connect with the family.

Conclusion

Child mental health consultants must stay attuned to the changes in the field of pediatrics. Advances in pharmacology, genomics, and technology offer new hope and new challenges to psychosocial adaptation. Patterns of access to consultation will need to reflect shorter hospital stays and utilization of outpatient venues. New technology, such as telemedicine, may offer novel access to consultative expertise. Research in adherence outcomes, efficacy and quality of life become increasingly important as the financial pressures of modern medicine force the consultant to justify the value of the work.

However, many of the key features of quality consultation will remain unchanged. The consultant will continue to bring to the multidisciplinary medical team the combined expertise of psychodynamic understanding, psychopharmacology, developmental perspective on the meaning of illness, adaptation to trauma, knowledge of psychiatric conditions, behavioral interventions, and CNS influences in medical illness and as a result of medical treatment. The goal will remain to answer the consultation request in a thoughtful, timely fashion that respects the needs of the child, the family and the treatment team while facilitating quality of care and quality of life.

References

Abrams, A.N. *et al.* (2007) Psychosocial issues in adolescents with cancer. *Cancer Treatment Reviews* **33** (7), 622–630.

Akinbami, L.J. & Schoendorf, K.C. (2002) Trends in childhood asthma: prevalence, health care utilization, and mortality. *Pediatrics* **110** (2 Pt 1), 315–322.

Alderfer, M.A. *et al.* (2010) Psychosocial adjustment of siblings of children with cancer: a systematic review. *Psycho-Oncology* **19** (8), 789–805.

Barlow, J.H. & Ellard, D.R. (2006) The psychosocial well-being of children with chronic disease, their parents and siblings: an overview of the research evidence base. *Child: Care, Health and Development* **32** (1), 19–31.

Bateman, S.T. *et al.* (2012) The wrap-up: a unique forum to support pediatric residents when faced with the death of a child. *Journal of Palliative Medicine* **15** (12), 1329–1334.

Bedell, S.E. *et al.* (2001) The doctor's letter of condolence. *The New England Journal of Medicine* **344** (15), 1162–1164.

Carter, B.D. *et al.* (2003) Inpatient pediatric consultation-liaison: a case-controlled study. *Journal of Pediatric Psychology* **28** (6), 423–432.

Davies, S. *et al.* (2003) A population survey of mental health problems in children with epilepsy. *Developmental Medicine and Child Neurology* **45** (5), 292–295.

Davies, J.C. *et al.* (2007) Cystic fibrosis. *BMJ (Clinical Research Ed.)* **335** (7632), 1255–1259.

Davis, S.M. *et al.* (2010) Epilepsy in children with attention-deficit/hyperactivity disorder. *Pediatric Neurology* **42** (5), 325–330.

DeMaso, D.R. *et al.* (2009) Practice parameter for the psychiatric assessment and management of physically ill children and adolescents. *Journal of the American Academy of Child and Adolescent Psychiatry* **48** (2), 213–233.

Dowshen, N. *et al.* (2012) Improving adherence to antiretroviral therapy for youth living with HIV/AIDS: a pilot study using personalized, interactive, daily text message reminders. *Journal of Medical Internet Research* **14** (2), e51.

Fein, J.A. *et al.* (2012) Relief of pain and anxiety in pediatric patients in emergency medical systems. *Pediatrics* **130** (5), e1391–e1405.

Fritz, G.K. (2003) Promoting effective collaboration between pediatricians and child and adolescent psychiatrists. *Pediatric Annals* **32** (6), 383, 387–389.

Garvey, K.C. *et al.* (2012) Health care transition in patients with type 1 diabetes: young adult experiences and relationship to glycemic control. *Diabetes Care* **35** (8), 1716–1722.

Geist, R.A. (1977) Consultation on a pediatric surgical ward: creating an empathic climate. *The American Journal of Orthopsychiatry* **47** (3), 432–444.

Graham, K.M. & Levy, J.B. (2009) Enuresis. *Pediatrics in Review* **30** (5), 165–172.

Greco, C. & Berde, C. (2005) Pain management for the hospitalized pediatric patient. *Pediatric Clinics of North America* **52** (4), 995–1027, vii–viii.

Greenley, R.N. *et al.* (2010) A meta-analytic review of the psychosocial adjustment of youth with inflammatory bowel disease. *Journal of Pediatric Psychology* **35** (8), 857–869.

Groves, J. & Beresin, E. (1999) Difficult patients, difficult families. *New Horizons* **6**, 331–343.

Hamilton, J. & Daneman, D. (2002) Deteriorating diabetes control during adolescence: physiological or psychosocial? *Journal of Pediatric Endocrinology & Metabolism* **15** (2), 115–126.

Hockenberry, M.J. *et al.* (2011) Managing painful procedures in children with cancer. *Journal of Pediatric hematology/oncology* **33** (2), 119–127.

Jacobi, J. *et al.* (2002) Clinical practice guidelines for the sustained use of sedatives and analgesics in the critically ill adult. *Critical Care Medicine* **30** (1), 119–141.

Jacobson, A.M. (1996) The psychological care of patients with insulin-dependent diabetes mellitus. *New England Journal of Medicine* **334** (9), 1249–1253.

Jones, J.E. *et al.* (2008) Psychiatric disorders in children and adolescents who have epilepsy. *Pediatrics in Review / American Academy of Pediatrics* **29** (2), e9–e14.

Karnik, N.S. *et al.* (2007) Subtypes of pediatric delirium: a treatment algorithm. *Psychosomatics* **48** (3), 253–257.

Kazak, A.E. *et al.* (2012) Screening for psychosocial risk in pediatric cancer. *Pediatric Blood & Cancer* **59** (5), 822–827.

Kersun, L.S. & Elia, J. (2007) Depressive symptoms and SSRI use in pediatric oncology patients. *Pediatric Blood & Cancer* **49** (7), 881–887.

Knapp, P.K. & Harris, E.S. (1998) Consultation-liaison in child psychiatry: a review of the past 10 years. *Part II: Research on treatment approaches and outcomes. Journal of the American Academy of Child and Adolescent Psychiatry* **37** (2), 139–146.

Koller, D. & Goldman, R.D. (2012) Distraction techniques for children undergoing procedures: a critical review of pediatric research. *Journal of Pediatric Nursing* **27** (6), 652–681.

Koneski, J.A. *et al.* (2011) Efficacy and safety of methylphenidate in treating ADHD symptoms in children and adolescents with uncontrolled seizures: a Brazilian sample study and literature review. *Epilepsy & Behavior* **21** (3), 228–232.

Kreicbergs, U. *et al.* (2004) Talking about death with children who have severe malignant disease. *The New England Journal of Medicine* **351** (12), 1175–1186.

Kurtz, B.P. & Abrams, A.N. (2011) Psychiatric aspects of pediatric cancer. *Pediatric Clinics of North America* **58** (4), 1003–1023, xii.

Landier, W. & Tse, A.M. (2010) Use of complementary and alternative medical interventions for the management of procedure-related pain, anxiety, and distress in pediatric oncology: an integrative review. *Journal of Pediatric Nursing* **25** (6), 566–579.

Levi, B.H. *et al.* (2004) Jading in the pediatric intensive care unit: implications for healthcare providers of medically complex children. *Pediatric Critical Care Medicine: A Journal of the Society of Critical Care Medicine and the World Federation of Pediatric Intensive and Critical Care Societies* **5** (3), 275–277.

Macdonald, M.E. *et al.* (2005) Parental perspectives on hospital staff members' acts of kindness and commemoration after a child's death. *Pediatrics* **116** (4), 884–890.

Mackner, L.M. *et al.* (2006) Psychosocial functioning in pediatric inflammatory bowel disease. *Inflammatory Bowel Diseases* **12** (3), 239–244.

McDaniel, M. *et al.* (2006) Racial disparities in childhood asthma in the United States: evidence from the National Health Interview Survey, 1997 to 2003. *Pediatrics* **117** (5), e868–e877.

Meyer, W.J. 3rd, *et al.* (2004) Psychological problems reported by young adults who were burned as children. *The Journal of Burn Care & Rehabilitation* **25** (1), 98–106.

Norberg, A.L. & Boman, K.K. (2008) Parent distress in childhood cancer: a comparative evaluation of posttraumatic stress symptoms, depression and anxiety. *Acta Oncologica (Stockholm, Sweden)* **47** (2), 267–274.

Ortiz, P. (1997) General principles in child liaison consultation service: a literature review. *European Child & Adolescent Psychiatry* **6** (1), 1–6.

Palmer, S.L. *et al.* (2011) How parents cope with their child's diagnosis and treatment of an embryonal tumor: results of a prospective and longitudinal study. *Journal of Neuro-Oncology* **105** (2), 253–259.

Patenaude, A.F. & Kupst, M.J. (2005) Psychosocial functioning in pediatric cancer. *Journal of Pediatric Psychology* **30** (1), 9–27.

Peters, T.E. & Fritz, G.K. (2010) Psychological considerations of the child with asthma. *Child and Adolescent Psychiatric Clinics of North America* **19** (2), 319–333, ix.

Phipps, S. *et al.* (2009) Symptoms of post-traumatic stress in children with cancer: does personality trump health status? *Psycho-Oncology* **18** (9), 992–1002.

Phipps, S. *et al.* (2012) Resilience in children undergoing stem cell transplantation: results of a complementary intervention trial. *Pediatrics* **129** (3), e762–e770.

Plioplys, S. *et al.* (2007) 10-year research update review: psychiatric problems in children with epilepsy. *Journal of the American Academy of Child and Adolescent Psychiatry* **46** (11), 1389–1402.

Poggi, G. *et al.* (2005) Brain tumors in children and adolescents: cognitive and psychological disorders at different ages. *Psycho-Oncology* **14** (5), 386–395.

Quittner, A.L. *et al.* (2008) Prevalence and impact of depression in cystic fibrosis. *Current Opinion in Pulmonary Medicine* **14** (6), 582–588.

Sawyer, M.G. *et al.* (1998) Influence of parental and family adjustment on the later psychological adjustment of children treated for cancer. *Journal of the American Academy of Child and Adolescent Psychiatry* **37** (8), 815–822.

Self, T.H. *et al.* (2005) Reducing emergency department visits and hospitalizations in African American and Hispanic patients with asthma: a 15-year review. *The Journal of Asthma: Official Journal of the Association for the Care of Asthma* **42** (10), 807–812.

Shemesh, E. (2008) Assessment and management of psychosocial challenges in pediatric liver transplantation. *Liver Transplantation: Official Publication of the American Association for the Study of Liver Diseases and the International Liver Transplantation Society* **14** (9), 1229–1236.

Shemesh, E. *et al.* (2005) Assessment of depression in medically ill children presenting to pediatric specialty clinics. *Journal of the American Academy of Child and Adolescent Psychiatry* **44** (12), 1249–1257.

Shemesh, E. *et al.* (2010) Adherence to medical recommendations and transition to adult services in pediatric transplant recipients. *Current Opinion in Organ Transplantation* **15** (3), 288–292.

Shinnar, S. & Pellock, J.M. (2002) Update on the epidemiology and prognosis of pediatric epilepsy. *Journal of Child Neurology* **17** (Suppl 1), S4–S17.

Smith, B.A. *et al.* (2010) Depressive symptoms in children with cystic fibrosis and parents and its effects on adherence to airway clearance. *Pediatric Pulmonology* **45** (8), 756–763.

Sohn, V.Y. *et al.* (2012) Pain management in the pediatric surgical patient. *The Surgical Clinics of North America* **92** (3), 471–485, vii.

Squires, J.E. & Squires, R.H. Jr., (2010) Munchausen syndrome by proxy: ongoing clinical challenges. *Journal of Pediatric Gastroenterology & Nutrition* **51** (3), 248–253.

Stern, T.A. *et al.* (2010) *Massachusetts General Hospital Handbook of General Hospital Psychiatry*, 6th edn. Saunders, Philadelphia, PA.

Stevenson, M. *et al.* (2013) Pediatric palliative care in Canada and the United States: a qualitative metasummary of the needs of patients and families. *Journal of Palliative Medicine* **16** (5), 566–577.

Stoppelbein, L. *et al.* (2005) Factor analysis of the pediatric symptom checklist with a chronically ill pediatric population. *Journal of Developmental and Behavioral Pediatrics* **26** (5), 349–355.

Stuber, M.L. *et al.* (1998) Is posttraumatic stress a viable model for understanding responses to childhood cancer? *Child and Adolescent Psychiatric Clinics of North America* **7** (1), 169–182.

Sylvester, C.J. & Forman, S.F. (2008) Clinical practice guidelines for treating restrictive eating disorder patients during medical hospitalization. *Current Opinion in Pediatrics* **20** (4), 390–397.

Szigethy, E. *et al.* (2004) Depressive symptoms and inflammatory bowel disease in children and adolescents: a cross-sectional study. *Journal of Pediatric Gastroenterology & Nutrition* **39** (4), 395–403.

Szigethy, E. *et al.* (2011) Inflammatory bowel disease. *Pediatric Clinics of North America* **58** (4), 903–920, x–xi.

Szyndler, J.E. *et al.* (2005) Psychological and family functioning and quality of life in adolescents with cystic fibrosis. *Journal of Cystic Fibrosis: Official Journal of the European Cystic Fibrosis Society* **4** (2), 135–144.

Ting, T.V. *et al.* (2012) Usefulness of cellular text messaging for improving adherence among adolescents and young adults with systemic lupus erythematosus. *The Journal of Rheumatology* **39** (1), 174–179.

Tong, A. *et al.* (2011) Quality of life of adolescent kidney transplant recipients. *The Journal of Pediatrics* **159** (4), 670–675.e2.

Turkel, S.B. *et al.* (2006) Comparing symptoms of delirium in adults and children. *Psychosomatics* **47** (4), 320–324.

Vance, Y. & Eiser, C. (2004) Caring for a child with cancer—a systematic review. *Pediatric Blood & Cancer* **42** (3), 249–253.

Wagner, J.L. *et al.* (2003) The influence of parental distress on child depressive symptoms in juvenile rheumatic diseases: the moderating effect of illness intrusiveness. *Journal of Pediatric Psychology* **28** (7), 453–462.

Work, H.H. (1989) The "menace of psychiatry" revisited: the evolving relationship between pediatrics and child psychiatry. *Psychosomatics* **30** (1), 86–93.

Zeltzer, L.K. *et al.* (2009) Psychological status in childhood cancer survivors: a report from the childhood cancer survivor study. *Journal of Clinical Oncology: Official Journal of the American Society of Clinical Oncology* **27** (14), 2396–2404.

CHAPTER 46

Mental health and resilience in children and adolescents affected by HIV/AIDS

Theresa S. Betancourt[1], David J. Grelotti[2,3] and Nathan B. Hansen[4]

[1] Department of Global Health and Population, Harvard T.H. Chan School of Public Health, Harvard University, Boston, MA, USA
[2] Department of Psychiatry, University of California, San Diego School of Medicine, La Jolla, CA, USA
[3] Owen HIV Clinic, University of California, San Diego Health System, San Diego, CA, USA
[4] Department of Health Promotion and Behavior, College of Public Health, University of Georgia, Athens, GA, USA

The global impact of HIV/AIDS on children and adolescents

Despite significant advances in prevention and treatment, HIV/AIDS (human immunodeficiency virus/acquired immune deficiency syndrome) continues to exact a hefty toll on the world's children. An estimated 330,000 children under 15 were newly infected with HIV in 2011 (over 90% in sub-Saharan Africa), and 40% of new HIV infections are among adolescents and young adults aged 15 to 24 (UNAIDS, 2012). An estimated 3.4 million children and 5 million adolescents and young adults are living with HIV infection (UNAIDS, 2012; UNICEF, 2012).

In addition to those directly infected, the global HIV/AIDS pandemic has also created considerable strain on families and communities. An estimated 17.1 million children have lost one or both parents to HIV/AIDS (UNICEF, 2012), 88% of whom live in sub-Saharan Africa. In addition, many children live with HIV-infected parents and caregivers. Collectively referred to as orphans and children made vulnerable by HIV/AIDS (OVC), many HIV-affected youth lack: access to health care and educational resources, basic safety and economic security, and attachment figures (Betancourt et al., 2010a).

With the advent of antiretroviral therapy (ART), and increasing global access, HIV is slowly becoming a chronic disease. However, there is a considerable treatment gap in many resource-poor areas, with only 28% of treatment eligible children (compared to 58% of adults) receiving appropriate therapy (UNAIDS, 2012). Without treatment, HIV/AIDS has significant consequences for health and mortality in children. But even with treatment, HIV can impact development and health, including

mental health, and is associated with a number of adverse outcomes for children (Benton, 2011; Rydström et al., 2013).

To date, global health funding to address HIV/AIDS has been largely spent on the delivery of ART, but there is increasing recognition of the importance of mental health (Freeman et al., 2005). However, despite the interrelationship between HIV and mental health, and the impact of mental health on engagement and retention in, and adherence to HIV treatment, the extent to which mental health treatment is delivered as a routine part of HIV care is not clear. In the United States, HIV-infected children and adolescents may be more likely to receive mental health care than HIV-affected youth as a result of receiving their care through multidisciplinary clinics (Mellins et al., 2012). Access to mental health services is far more limited in low- and middle-income countries (LMIC) (Betancourt et al., 2012).

The effects of HIV/AIDS on the social ecology, child development, and mental health

An ecological and biopsychosocial lens illuminates how mental health and well-being are shaped by the interplay between individual, family, community, and societal factors (Masten, 2001; Sapienza & Masten, 2011). Bronfenbrenner stressed how "settings" of development interact to support positive child development, creating a nurturing physical and emotional environment that includes, and extends beyond, the immediate family to peer, school and community settings, and cultural and political belief systems (Bronfenbrenner, 1979).

For children, HIV represents a fundamental alteration of the social ecology which undergirds healthy child development, disrupting factors across all levels (Werner, 1989; Benard, 1995; Cowan *et al.*, 1996; Betancourt *et al.*, 2014). For example, children living with an HIV-positive parent may experience worry, anticipatory loss and uncertainty about the future. Young people also have to cope with secrecy and stigma against families affected by HIV/AIDS (Lin *et al.*, 2010). In addition, children affected by HIV often assume adult roles prematurely. In fact, AIDS-orphans have a nearly twofold risk of HIV infection (Stein *et al.*, 1999; Zhang *et al.*, 2009) and often face financial hardships (Cluver *et al.*, 2009a) and relocation from important social networks (Zhao *et al.*, 2011a).

Resilience is the attainment of competence as well as desirable social and emotional adjustment, despite risks (Rutter, 1985; Luthar, 1993). This definition acknowledges the developmental threats facing children affected by HIV/AIDS, and highlights the physical, social, and individual outcomes relevant to healthy development (Rutter, 2006). As protective processes and factors mitigating the impact of risks have not been well explored, it is important to understand the full range of processes with potential to increase resilient outcomes in HIV/AIDS-affected children and to use this knowledge to develop interventions that may be implemented across different levels of the social ecology (Figure 46.1).

The relationship between HIV and mental health is often described as bidirectional, meaning that the effects of living with HIV/AIDS or having an affected family member can increase risk for mental illnesses such as anxiety and depression. Moreover, poor mental health can lead to behaviors which place individuals at risk for HIV infection (Briere & Jordan, 2004; Cluver *et al.*, 2007, 2012). In families, psychological sequelae related to HIV/AIDS have been associated with parental hopelessness, depression, and risk behaviors such as drug abuse and sexual risk taking (Rochat *et al.*, 2006).

HIV/AIDS amplifies vulnerability to community-level risk factors. HIV/AIDS-related stigma can pose barriers to accessing social supports that typically support families and children in challenging circumstances (Cluver & Orkin, 2009). Lack of community understanding can compromise perceived social equity, work opportunities, and inclusion in religious organizations (Anderson *et al.*, 2008; Rutta *et al.*, 2008). Loss of employment combined with taxing medical expenses can compound other risk factors and drive families into poverty (Silver *et al.*, 2003). Although access to HIV-related health care, including ART, is improving (Perez *et al.*, 2004; Betancourt *et al.*, 2010b), systems of social welfare and protection that support the socio-emotional needs of children made vulnerable

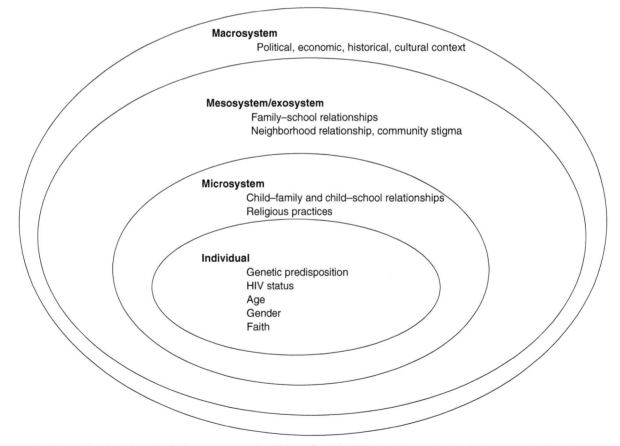

Figure 46.1 The social ecological model of risk and protection for children affected by HIV/AIDS. *Source*: Reprinted with permission from Sage Publications.

by HIV/AIDS remain weak or nonexistent in many low resource settings (UNAIDS, UNICEF, USAID, 2004; UNICEF, 2006).

Brief overview of HIV and child health

As our treatments and interventions are linked to our understanding of HIV virology, readers may benefit from a brief review. HIV is the virus that causes AIDS. The virus invades and infects cells of the body that mediate immunity, most notably CD4+ T-lymphocytes (CD4 cells). HIV replicates within infected cells, or may lie dormant, evading the body's immune system as well as currently available drug treatments.

The amount of CD4 cells in blood samples serves as a proxy for immune status. The absolute number of CD4 cells per cubic millimeter of blood, or CD4 count, is used for children older than 5 years and adults. As CD4 count is not as meaningful clinically in younger children, CD4 percentage is used to assess immune status in children younger than 5 years. A patient's CD4 count and CD4 percentage is related to susceptibility to certain opportunistic infections. AIDS is defined by the presence of an opportunistic infection or the amount of impaired immunity as measured by absolute CD4 count percentage below a certain cutoff.

Currently, there is no cure for HIV. However, antiretroviral therapy (ART) can effectively manage the disease. These drugs are divided into classes based on how they interfere with HIV replication. Single classes of drugs used independently have not proven effective in combating HIV. The use of at least three drugs from two or more drug classes in combination, however, is highly effective. Early initiation of ART is associated with reduced drug resistance, preserved immune functioning, and delayed disease progression. To maintain viral suppression and prevent drug resistance, however, consistent adherence is necessary. It is important to note that, while treatment safety is constantly improving, antiretroviral drugs are highly potent and can have toxicity or unpleasant side-effects (Panel on Antiretroviral Therapy and Medical Management of HIV-Infected Children, 2013). Moreover, the developmental consequences of long-term use of these drugs in children are largely unclear.

Routine HIV testing is recommended for all persons aged 13–64 by the Centers for Disease Control and Prevention (CDC) in areas where HIV prevalence exceeds 0.1% or where the prevalence is unknown. The CDC further recommends annual testing and for all individuals at risk for HIV, even in areas of low HIV prevalence (Branson et al., 2006). The American Academy of Pediatrics has adopted similar guidelines and recommends that pediatricians offer HIV testing at least once by age 16–18 years (Committee on Pediatric AIDS, 2011).

In nations with robust health systems, anyone testing positive for HIV infection will be offered ART and be expected to stay on treatment for life. Evidence continues to accumulate that early treatment is related to improved health outcomes in HIV. Unfortunately, in many LMICs, children are often only eligible for ART if they develop an HIV-related illness or a low CD4 count. However, because of the importance of ART in preventing morbidity and mortality related to HIV encephalopathy, the WHO recommends initiating ART for life in all children under the age of 2 years (World Health Organization, 2010).

HIV is associated with a host of medical conditions. In general, untreated and severely immunocompromised children experience considerable morbidity and mortality as a result of opportunistic infections. With treatment, clinicians have observed decreasing progression to AIDS, hospital admissions and deaths among these children (Judd et al., 2007). However, even treated HIV-infected children suffer sometimes subtle metabolic, cardiovascular, renal, bone, and central nervous system problems as a result of HIV infection, medication side effects, or viral-mediated inflammation (Hazra et al., 2010).

Although a lengthy description of medical comorbidities of the HIV-infected child and adolescent is beyond the scope of this chapter, symptoms of medical illness might be confused for or coexist with psychosomatic complaints. Psychosomatic problems are present in 28% of treated, clinically and immunologically stable HIV-infected children (Nozyce et al., 2006). Psychosomatic complaints have been associated with a variety of factors: medical diagnoses and hospitalizations, perception of parent rejection, stressful life events, conflict, parental distress, school adjustment, younger age, female sex, ethnicity, and drugs and alcohol (Bursch et al., 2008). Clinicians should be aware that somatic symptoms may reflect occult illness related to HIV, so close coordination with medical colleagues is of utmost importance.

Transition from pediatric to adult care has also been an important subject in working with HIV-infected children and adolescents. Many pediatric centers have developed formal approaches to the transition process. Important elements include transition teams, attention to developmental factors, patient education, and skill building. HIV-infected children with depression and/or substance abuse are perceived to have a more difficult transition (Gilliam et al., 2011).

Modes of HIV transmission in children and adolescents

Different modes of HIV transmission are relevant for different age groups. Young children with HIV are often infected perinatally or "vertically" from mother to child. If the mother is infected with HIV, there is an increased risk of transmission to the child at or around the time of birth. Infection may occur during pregnancy, but this is less likely. Fortunately, prevention of mother-to-child transmission (PMTCT) of HIV has been possible through the use of HIV testing and the provision of antiretroviral drugs. Antiretroviral medications provided to HIV-infected mothers also prevent HIV transmission to an uninfected child through breastfeeding, which is critical for areas where formula-feeding is not possible due to lack of safe drinking water.

Sexual contact, especially unprotected sexual intercourse, is a common vector for transmission of HIV. Forty-two percent of HIV-infected youth continue to engage in unprotected sexual intercourse despite knowledge of their HIV status (Tanney *et al.*, 2010), and 65% of sexually active perinatally infected adolescents report unprotected sex (Mellins *et al.*, 2011). Other problematic sexual risk factors include multiple concurrent partners, number of unprotected sexual acts, and unprotected sex with serodiscordant persons. Intravenous drug use, especially sharing needles, is also a common mode of transmission.

HIV and its neurological impact in children and adolescents

HIV is a neurotropic virus which directly and indirectly damages the brain (Dunfee *et al.*, 2006; McArthur & Smith, 2013). HIV crosses the blood–brain barrier, where infection of brain cells leads to the release of cytokines and other agents which have a toxic effect on the brain (Davis *et al.*, 1992; González-Scarano & Martín-García, 2005; Kaul *et al.*, 2006). Chronic, low-grade inflammation as a result of HIV may also have a lasting effect on the brain and cognition (Chang *et al.*, 2011; Garvey *et al.*, 2012).

Unlike in adults, children can experience neurologic disease before clinically significant immunodeficiency (Van Rie *et al.*, 2007). A common neurological sequela of HIV infection in children is HIV encephalopathy. HIV encephalopathy is characterized by acquired microcephaly, developmental delay and/or regression, and motor deficits. Before widespread use of ART, HIV encephalopathy was relatively common, with its greatest incidence before 2 years of age. Antiretroviral treatment has been responsible for prevention of HIV encephalopathy, and treatment of a child with HIV encephalopathy can prevent progression of the illness or death (Patel *et al.*, 2009). However, even with treatment there are a large number of residual symptoms.

Evidence of in utero infection, lack of maternal ART use, and initiation of ART in children after 12 weeks of age are also associated with neurodevelopmental delay. Evidence from resource-poor settings appears to mirror findings from resource-rich areas. Neurodevelopmental deficits using a wide range of assessment tools were reported in 6–40% of HIV-infected children who have never received antiretroviral treatment (Le Doaré *et al.*, 2012).

HIV-exposed but uninfected children from resource-rich settings have no apparent global developmental delay as infants, but subtle deficits in cognitive, motor, language, and behavior may be found in preschool-aged children (Le Doaré *et al.*, 2012). In resource-poor settings such as Africa, HIV-exposed but uninfected children have been shown to have greater cognitive, motor, and expressive language impairment than children with no exposure to HIV (Le Doaré *et al.*, 2012).

In many countries, many HIV-affected children are less likely to be enrolled in or attend school (Monasch & Boerma,

2004; Evans & Miguel, 2007; Mishra *et al.*, 2007), or to be in an appropriate grade for age (Bicego *et al.*, 2003; Zhao *et al.*, 2011b). In China, children affected by HIV had poorer school performance and more behavioral problems when compared to unaffected peers (Tu *et al.*, 2009). Some orphaned children may be less likely to finish school. Children who lost their mothers, double orphans, those living in higher poverty, and girls may be more vulnerable (Guo *et al.*, 2012).

HIV and psychopathology

Multiple studies indicate that children living with and affected by HIV are at risk for a wide range of psychiatric disorders. Among clinically and immunologically stable children aged 2–17 years, behavioral problems, learning problems, attention deficit hyperactivity disorder (ADHD) anxiety, and conduct problems have been reported (Nozyce *et al.*, 2006). Perinatally infected children with HIV and their noninfected, HIV-exposed peers living with an HIV-infected parent also demonstrate high rates of mental health problems (27–69% and 26–70%, respectively) (Williams *et al.*, 2010; Gadow *et al.*, 2010, 2012; Mellins *et al.*, 2012).

Reasons for the high rates of mental disorders in HIV-infected youth and HIV-exposed but uninfected children are not well understood, but a number of potential risk factors are speculated, including genetic factors (many of which may put youth or their parents at risk for HIV infection), HIV disease severity and HIV-related neurocognitive factors, caregiver HIV disease and AIDS-related death, and caregiver psychiatric disorder and/or substance use and other social and environmental factors such as stigma (Bauman & Germann, 2007; Cluver *et al.*, 2008; Doku, 2009; Andrinopoulos *et al.*, 2011; Gadow *et al.*, 2012). Moreover, it must be noted that youth are at increased risk of becoming infected with HIV as a result of mental disorders. In children with HIV infection as a result of engaging in high-risk behaviors, substance abuse is common (Tanney *et al.*, 2010; Mellins *et al.*, 2011). Depressive and anxious symptoms are more common in adolescents engaging in sexual risk behavior (Lehrer *et al.*, 2006). Young men who have sex with men who engage in unprotected anal intercourse and are thus at greater risk of HIV, have higher levels of depression and psychological distress (Perdue *et al.*, 2003).

Although post-traumatic stress disorder (PTSD) is common among adults with HIV, it is unclear how common PTSD is in HIV-infected youth. Trauma-related symptoms are found in many HIV-infected children (Ingerski *et al.*, 2010), and 23.3% of an urban sample of 18–24 year-olds with HIV had PTSD (93% reported the HIV diagnosis as a traumatic event) (Radcliffe *et al.*, 2007). Childhood physical or sexual abuse, intimate partner violence, sexual assault, and other or multiple forms of victimization are all common in men (including young men who have sex with men), women, and transgendered women behaviorally-infected with HIV (Clum *et al.*, 2009; Reisner *et al.*, 2009a; Brennan *et al.*, 2012; Whetten *et al.*, 2012).

The convergence of risk factors, such as substance abuse and violence, working in concert to increase risk of HIV infection led to the idea of *syndemics*, or intersecting epidemics with "mutually enhancing" social, physical, and structural components that interact to increase the vulnerability of a population to a disease (Singer, 2010). It is likely that to be effective, prevention and treatment interventions will have to take into consideration syndemics and the complex biopsychosocial context of HIV.

Mental health and ART adherence

Adherence to ART for life is essential for the effectiveness of HIV treatment regimens, and some of the biggest barriers to adherence are mental health or behavioral problems. In research studies, adherence among study populations of adolescents ranges from 74.5 to 84.0% (Murphy *et al.*, 2005; Williams *et al.*, 2006; Rudy *et al.*, 2010). Children in school, raised by caregivers other than the biological parent, and enrolled in reminder programs and those with less substance use, higher life satisfaction, lower psychological distress, concrete rather than abstract reasoning skills, less sexual risk behavior, simplified drug regimens, and fewer side effects have higher adherence. Similarly, children who have dropped out of school and those with housing instability, fear of HIV stigma and discrimination, poor coping style, substance use, depressive and anxiety symptoms, childhood sexual abuse, prior suicide attempt(s), advanced HIV disease, more negative appraisal of their ability to remain adherent (self-efficacy), and more negative notions of what being adherent would do for them (outcome expectancy) have higher nonadherence. Interventions to improve adherence, such as simplified treatment regimens, text message reminders, education, and counseling, have had modest benefit (Reisner *et al.*, 2009b).

Mental health treatment for children and adolescents with HIV

There is some evidence that HIV-infected children have greater access to mental health treatment than HIV-affected children (Chernoff *et al.*, 2009; Gadow *et al.*, 2012; Mellins *et al.*, 2012). A study in the United States indicated higher rates of special education, psychopharmacology, and behavioral interventions in HIV-infected children (Gadow *et al.*, 2010). Psychiatric treatment may have decreased the prevalence of mental disorders in a longitudinal study of HIV-infected youth (Mellins *et al.*, 2012). However, intervention is needed for both HIV-infected and HIV-affected youth (Malee *et al.*, 2011; Gadow *et al.*, 2012; Mellins *et al.*, 2012).

Although there are very few investigations of mental health treatment in HIV-infected youth, psychiatric treatment, including psychotherapy and psychopharmacology, is common among HIV-infected children and adolescents. Although more systematic studies of treatment effectiveness among HIV-infected and HIV-affected youth are needed, case series and other observational studies suggest similar efficacy and side effect profiles among children and adolescents with HIV who were prescribed antidepressants (Caballero *et al.*, 2005) and stimulants for ADHD (Sirois *et al.*, 2009).

Freudenreich and colleagues surveyed psychiatrists who specialize in the treatment of patients with HIV for their recommendations regarding psychopharmacology and psychotherapy in adults with HIV/AIDS (Freudenreich *et al.*, 2010). One must be mindful of interactions between psychiatric and antiretroviral medication (Thompson *et al.*, 2006). Although this work was not with children, these treatments are generally applicable to children and/or adolescents.

Interestingly, there are also a number of important interactions between HIV medications and illicit substances. Although there is no clear interaction between alcohol, heroin, or cocaine and antiretrovirals, induction of methadone and inhibition of amphetamine and methylenedioxymethamphetamine (MDMA or "ecstasy") has been associated with antiretroviral treatment (Thompson *et al.*, 2006). Moreover, it has been shown that efavirenz, one antiretroviral treatment, is abused for its psychoactive effects (Inciardi *et al.*, 2007), and this form of substance abuse was reported among South African children (Grelotti *et al.*, 2014).

Psychiatric hospitalizations are more common in HIV-infected youth than in the general population and in HIV-exposed but uninfected children (Hein *et al.*, 1995; Gaughan *et al.*, 2004). Mood disorders and behavioral disorders are the most likely reason for hospitalization (Gaughan *et al.*, 2004). In prior studies on this topic, children aware of their HIV status and those who experienced a significant life event were more at risk (Gaughan *et al.*, 2004).

Resilience in children, adolescents, and families affected by HIV/AIDS

The mental health and well-being of children and adolescents affected by HIV/AIDS involves multiple ecological levels—from individual factors, to the family, peer group, and the larger community and culture. Each nested level presents risks (Lazarus & Folkman, 1984; Betancourt & Khan, 2008) as well as sources of potential protection and resilience (Bronfenbrenner, 1979; Ungar, 2011). While the available literature discusses physical, cultural, and community factors influencing the environments in which HIV-infected and -affected children grow and develop, there remains a much greater focus on risk than resilience. Furthermore, strong quantitative studies in diverse cultural settings are lacking.

Individual factors promoting resilience

Research in a variety of settings has documented important associations between coping strategies, mental health, and resilience in HIV-positive and HIV-affected children and adolescents. In a longitudinal investigation of HIV-affected children in the United States, coping self-efficacy was significantly associated with child resilience, and resilient children demonstrated steeper declines in depression over time (Murphy & Marelich, 2008). HIV-infected adolescents in South Africa reported that goal-setting helped them to cope with their diagnosis (Petersen et al., 2010). Negative coping styles have been observed to contribute to poor mental health outcomes. For instance, passive coping (e.g., blaming, wishful thinking, withdrawal, and self-criticism) was more frequently used by adolescents reporting medication-related stressors and was associated with greater depression (Orban et al., 2010).

Self-esteem and hope for the future

Qualitative studies in Rwanda (Betancourt et al., 2011a) and Uganda (Harms et al., 2009) independently categorized perseverance and self-esteem as defining characteristics of resilience. The Rwandan constructs were originally expressed in local terms (*kwigirira, ikizere,* and *kwihangana)* assuaging concerns about imposition of external or Western constructs on these settings. One quantitative study found that non-HIV-affected children scored higher on self-esteem, positive future expectations, hopefulness about the future, and perceived control over the future, compared with children affected by HIV (Fang et al., 2009).

Family-level factors for HIV-affected and HIV-positive children

Positive family processes are a critical source of protection in the mental health of children affected by HIV. Family functioning is often massively disrupted by HIV, increasing fear, blame, conflict, and poor communication. These family processes may raise risks for mental disorders in children directly and indirectly affected by HIV. In particular, the parentification of HIV-affected children increases risks for negative outcomes while positive parental bonds reduce emotional distress in HIV-affected adolescents (Stein et al., 1999; Rotheram-Borus et al., 2005, 2006). Thus, family-based interventions have great promise for assisting HIV-affected children.

Family-based interventions might be most effective if they focus on improving caregiver–child relationships, communication, and parenting in the context of living with HIV. In a qualitative study of HIV-affected children in Rwanda, family unity (*kwizerana)* emerged as an important local resilience promoting construct, comprising indicators such as "living together in harmony," cooperation, mutual respect, and strong communication (Betancourt et al., 2011a). Additionally, a study in New York City observed correlations between positive family functioning, resilience, and lower likelihood of deviant peer affiliation, and substance abuse (Rosenblum et al., 2005). By contrast, child abuse and children's deviant peer affiliation were correlated with less resilient outcomes (Rosenblum et al., 2005).

High levels of parental monitoring combined with positive parent–child relationship have been associated with higher resilience in children (Dutra et al., 2000). The role of both

mothers and fathers has been documented as important to mental health and resilience in HIV/AIDS-affected children (Brook et al., 2002). A father's presence in the home was associated with adaptive coping in HIV-exposed/non-HIV-affected adolescents (Brook et al., 2002). Aspects of the father–child relationship (availability, support, child-centeredness, and satisfaction with the child) and paternal coping strategies increased the likelihood that adolescents themselves would engage in adaptive coping.

Coping in response to parental disease progression

Parental disease progression/impairment has been linked to poor mental health in children. For example, decreases in child resilience have been associated with maternal viral load and disease progression (Murphy & Marelich, 2008). However, in a 6-year longitudinal study of 213 adolescents, while early parentification due to HIV/AIDS was associated with emotional distress, substance use, and conduct problems during the 6 months following death, parentified adolescents actually demonstrated more adaptive coping skills (including positive action and engaging social support) and less alcohol and tobacco use over time as compared to nonparentified HIV-affected adolescents (Stein et al., 2007). Similarly, HIV-affected children in Kenya found that most depicted their role as caregiver in a positive light characterized by independence, problem-solving, and work ethic (Skovdal et al., 2009).

Access to educational resources

A qualitative study of adolescents living with HIV in Brazil found that stigma and lack of social inclusion influenced adolescents' willingness/ability to disclose HIV-status, and interfered with their access to community resources such as education and social support (Ayres et al., 2006). Limited access to HIV information in turn increases adolescents' risk for HIV. Research with Ugandan AIDS-orphans and caregivers found that disclosure and openness were often discussed in the context of resilience and self-efficacy, while silence, secrecy, and stigma contributed to feelings of self-hate, anxiety, hopelessness, and confusion among HIV-affected children (Daniel et al., 2007). Similarly, findings from a mixed-methods study of adolescents in New York City suggest that a stigma-free social context and encouragement of family communication about HIV contributed to promoting adolescent resilience (Pivnick & Villegas, 2000).

Social support

The protective role of social support, including perceived financial, physical, and emotional help from family, friends, and the larger community, has been examined in several studies. For instance, among 703 AIDS-orphaned and nonorphaned children and adolescents in South Africa, perceived social support was associated with lower symptoms of PTSD at all levels of trauma (Cluver et al., 2009b). In the United States, adolescents rated social support and problem solving among the "most helpful" coping strategies; however, these strategies were not widely used (Orban *et al.*, 2010). Similarly, in rural China, tangible support from family predicted less depression and loneliness and more positive social interactions, while emotional support was associated with reduced delinquent behavior (Zhao *et al.*, 2011b).

Peer support

Among HIV-affected adolescents in New York City, positive peer affiliations and community interactions were correlated with less deviant peer affiliations, while peer deviance was associated with older age, community risk factors, and less resilience (Rosenblum *et al.*, 2005). Similarly, among South African AIDS-orphaned children, caregiving, contact with extended family, school/peer support, and positive activities emerged as key protective factors, while negative peer interactions such as bullying and gossip were identified as risks (Cluver & Gardner, 2007). These findings are consistent across multiple studies, indicating that positive interactions with peers and access to elders and psychosocial programs are emotionally beneficial.

Disclosure

Disclosure is an important element in accessing social support. However, protecting the confidentiality of those living with HIV is important to prevent stigma and discrimination. Disclosure should be managed carefully. Most people do not need to know the HIV serostatus of children or adolescents. It is useful for a small number of supportive people, both family and friends, to know the serostatus of the child for support and safety purposes. It is also usually helpful to have peers who are also living with HIV, to whom children, and particularly adolescents, can relate. In families, disclosure of a caregiver's HIV status is also an issue of importance. In recent work in Rwanda, we observed that caregivers often disclosed their HIV status to only certain children or had initiated a conversation without much information, resulting in confusion and anxiety. When children do not understand what it means for parents or caretakers to be living with HIV, misunderstanding and miscommunication can result and contribute to mental health problems such as depression and anxiety.

Among adults, HIV counseling and testing is an important risk-mitigation strategy and is related to safer-sex behaviors among HIV-infected persons (Weinhardt *et al.*, 1999). Despite recommendations that children learn their HIV-status, many children are not informed. Among the issues preventing parents from disclosing are guilt, stigma, and fear of loss. Caregivers reported higher oppositionality, anxiety, and dysthymia in children aware of their HIV status, but only dysthymia remained after adjusting for sex and caregiver factors (Gadow *et al.*, 2010). Children who were aware of their HIV status do report greater anxiety (Gadow *et al.*, 2010). However, as children age, becoming aware of their HIV status and the implications of this for their own and others health is critical for appropriate adherence to treatment and prevention of transmission.

Implications for intervention research and clinical settings

Risk factors associated with HIV and mental health problems occur across each level of the social-ecology; thus, protective factors to build capacities and offset risks at each level are needed. Mental health treatment works; however, the literature on mental health treatment among children and adolescents living with HIV is sparse. While many empirically supported mental health interventions such as cognitive behavioral therapy (CBT) or interpersonal psychotherapy (IPT) exist for children and adolescents in the developed world, few have been adapted to address the context of HIV infection. Furthermore, culturally adapting and delivering interventions in the native language of patients and with clinicians from similar cultural backgrounds increases efficacy (Griner & Smith, 2006).

On the other hand, public health interventions aiming to reduce HIV transmission have rarely addressed mental health issues that contribute to sexual risk behavior and poor adherence to medical care. An exception is the intervention CLEAR ("Choosing Life: Empowerment! Action! Results!"), which specifically targets HIV-positive substance abusing adolescents and young adults (Rotheram-Borus *et al.*, 2004).

Research has shown that individual interventions can have great success in changing high-risk sexual behavior (Malow *et al.*, 2007). A meta-analysis of 98 sexual risk reduction behavioral interventions targeting adolescents revealed that interventions were relatively successful in increasing condom use, reducing incident sexually transmitted infections (STI)s, reducing or delaying penetrative sex, and increasing negotiation skills for sexual safety (Johnson *et al.*, 2011). However, a meta-analysis of 28 interventions for adolescents in South Africa revealed no significant effect on reducing sexual behavior or HIV incidence, and an increase in condom use at last sexual encounter only among males (Michielsen *et al.*, 2010). This suggests that interventions in LMIC may need more adaptation and greater attention to forces that contribute to sexual risk at different levels of the social ecology.

The focus of the majority of interventions for children and adolescents has been on sexual risk reduction among those at risk for HIV. Fewer interventions have focused on those living with or affected by HIV. Among these, individual interventions targeting skill building have been shown to be effective. For Example, participants in the Healthy Choices motivational enhancement intervention were found to have greater reductions in viral load, number of unprotected sexual acts, and less frequent substance abuse (Naar-King *et al.*, 2006, 2010).

Successful Western intervention programs have also been adapted for international purposes. The youth intervention CLEAR (Rotheram-Borus *et al.*, 2004) was culturally adapted for use in Uganda and was associated with greater condom use and fewer sexual partners (Lightfoot *et al.*, 2007). Similarly, a pilot adaptation of an intervention targeting HIV-affected individuals, the Healthy Living Project, was adapted for youth in Kinshasa, Democratic Republic of Congo and showed significant increase in protected sexual acts (Parker *et al.*, 2013). These results suggest that intervention programs can be tailored to meet culturally specific needs of various populations.

Group interventions for children and adolescents living with HIV

Group interventions are the most common type of HIV intervention and have been found to reduce risky health behaviors (Malow *et al.*, 2007). Successful interventions often incorporate theories such as the social action theory and cognitive behavioral theory into their curricula. Groups can offer flexibility and interaction between participants, allowing for opportunities for discussion and role-play on social norms and practices.

An example of a successful group intervention is "Together Learning Choices." (Rotheram-Borus *et al.*, 2001). The intervention comprises of two modules, "Stay Healthy" and "Act Safe," and an optional module, "Being Together." The "Stay Healthy" module discusses coping with HIV, implementing healthy daily routines, and participating in health care decisions; the "Act Safe" module discusses reducing substance abuse and unprotected sex and identifying risk behavior triggers; and the "Being Together" module emphasizes quality of life and improving emotional well-being. The intervention significantly decreased unprotected sexual acts, number of sexual partners, and substance abuse among intervention participants.

Family-based interventions

Negative family dynamics, including intimate partner violence and aggressive parenting, compromise children's ability to establish positive peer or romantic interactions (Capaldi & Clark, 1998; Gilliom *et al.*, 2002). Interventions targeting families made vulnerable by HIV hold great promise (Richter *et al.*, 2005; Betancourt *et al.*, 2011b). For example, *Collaborative HIV Prevention and Adolescent Mental Health* (CHAMP) is a prevention program promoting resilience through educational and skill building activities to increase understanding of HIV, encourage caregiver–child communication, and improve social problem-solving abilities. The CHAMP program was shown through large-scale trials in the United States to be effective and successful adaptations of the program were implemented in South Africa and Trinidad (Baptiste *et al.*, 2006; Bhana *et al.*, 2010).

The *Family Strengthening Intervention* (FSI) for children living in families affected by HIV in Rwanda is prevention oriented and involves the entire family. The FSI is based on the Family-Based

Preventive Intervention (FBPI), one of the earliest programs to adopt an ecological approach to enhancing resilience in the context of chronic family illness (Beardslee, 1998).

Together for Empowerment Activities was designed to improve social support and reduce depression for people living with HIV and their families in China (Li *et al.*, 2011). It emphasizes the interdependence of participants and how relationships among family members can have a positive or a negative impact on an individual's health. Organized into three separate modules broadly covering health, relationships, and personal quality of life, each module is further broken down into a series of small group discussions, family activities, and community activities intended to increase social support for people living with HIV and their families.

Economic strengthening interventions

The loss of parental economic support and the increasing number of orphans in Sub-Saharan Africa create significant economic burden (Ssewamala & Ismayilova, 2009; Ssewamala *et al.*, 2010). The *SUUBI* Project utilizes a family-based economic strengthening model to support children orphaned by HIV in Uganda. Orphans' caregivers are empowered to partner with local organizations, including financial institutions, to save money for the children's postprimary education or to finance the start of a small family business. The intervention works in three parts: workshops in asset-management, peer mentoring, and a child savings account. This intervention led to a decrease in the sexual risk-taking intentions of the children and an observable improvement in school performance (Ssewamala & Ismayilova, 2009).

Community level interventions addressing stigma

For many HIV/AIDS-affected children and families, navigating community stigma remains a very challenging issue. In many settings, social support and social stigma may co-occur. For instance, in Zimbabwe, some children cited family and community support as a positive resource, while others reported experiencing maltreatment from adoptive family members (Wood *et al.*, 2006). Many children expressed a desire to share thoughts and worries, but this went against cultural norms that perseverance and "not breaking down" are the most positive ways to cope.

Community sensitization campaigns and peer-to-peer education have high potential for raising community awareness and combating stigma (Sayson & Meya, 2001). A youth-led community intervention in Tanzania was successful in enhancing positive attitudes toward youth as change agents and spreading HIV risk reduction knowledge (Kamo *et al.*, 2008). Family-based interventions can also contribute to dispelling internalized stigma within the family through open discussion about HIV (Betancourt *et al.*, 2011b, 2013, 2014). Interventions are needed to teach children how to talk to trusted friends and seek support from leadership in the community. Since stigma from peers can be particularly detrimental to children living with and affected by HIV, peer-to-peer support programs and school-based awareness-raising programs have the potential to combat stigma at the level of the school or larger community ecology (Kennedy *et al.*, 2004).

Recommendations

Research on promoting mental health and resilience in children affected by HIV is critically needed, particularly in the global South where the disease burden is high but research attention is limited. Children and adolescents infected with or affected by HIV experience numerous problems, such as internalizing and externalizing behaviors, depression, and poor self-esteem. However, these problems can be attenuated through treatment, supportive programs, and skill development (Funck-Brentano *et al.*, 2005; Rotheram-Borus *et al.*, 2006; Kumakech *et al.*, 2009). Thus, there is need for intervention research that promotes resilience and positive outcomes across all ecological levels.

The development of sustainable and resource efficient HIV and mental health prevention programs is a key research and practice objective. Unfortunately, prevention is rarely perceived as a priority in settings with numerous pressing health care problems. However, in resource limited settings, prevention of mental health problems is critical given limited economic resources, trained mental health care providers, and access to both ART and psychopharmacology medication (Patel *et al.*, 2007a).

A second research and practice objective is to successfully adapt, scale-up, and implement key efficacious interventions in appropriate clinical and community settings (Patel *et al.*, 2007b; Kieling *et al.*, 2011). A number of efficacious interventions have been developed. However, work to implement these interventions and programs with fidelity in practical settings, or to adapt them for LMIC, has been limited to date.

A third research and practice objective is increasing the competence and reach of mental health service systems. This includes task-shifting approaches to train nonspecialists to provide basic mental health services, strengthening programs that train new mental health workers, and building the competence of existing workers to work with children and adolescents in the context of HIV infection (Kakuma *et al.*, 2011). Reach can be increased through integrating mental health care into other child- and adolescent-focused services such as schools, HIV care, pediatric, and primary health care. Finally, efficient use of resources can be obtained through assessment and outcome monitoring, appropriate triage and referral, and stepped-care approaches (Patel *et al.*, 2007b; Beaglehole *et al.*, 2008).

Fourth, culturally appropriate, psychometrically and clinically sound assessment and evaluation approaches for monitoring outcomes, guiding clinical decision-making, and continuous quality improvement are needed, as are efficient and practical approaches to supervision, capacity building, and technical assistance (Beaglehole *et al.*, 2008). This is not limited to LMIC; integrating mental health care into existing HIV services in any setting should include program evaluation and may require technical assistance, developing or adapting measures and benchmarks, and provider and staff training and supervision.

In conclusion, applying a social ecological framework to understanding risk and protective processes in the mental health of children and families affected by HIV/AIDS identified key leverage points for both prevention and intervention in a manner that is holistic, systematic, and responsive to the complex nature of risks and resilience. An important focus for research is to concentrate on modifiable processes that contribute to resilient outcomes. By addressing these gaps in the evidence base, future research can strengthen our understanding of appropriate targets for promoting mental health and resilience in children and families affected by HIV/AIDS.

References

Anderson, M. *et al.* (2008) HIV/AIDS-related stigma and discrimination: accounts of HIV-positive Caribbean people in the United Kingdom. *Social Science & Medicine* **67** (5), 790–798.

Andrinopoulos, K. *et al.* (2011) Health related quality of life and psychosocial correlates among HIV-infected adolescent and young adult women in the US. *AIDS Education and Prevention* **23** (4), 367–381.

Ayres, J.R. *et al.* (2006) Vulnerability, human rights, and comprehensive health care needs of young people living with HIV/AIDS. *American Journal of Public Health* **96** (6), 1001–1006.

Baptiste, D.R. *et al.* (2006) Community collaborative youth-focused HIV/AIDS prevention in South Africa and Trinidad: preliminary findings. *Journal of Pediatric Psychology* **31** (9), 905–916.

Bauman, L.J. & Germann, S. (2007) Psychosocial impact of the HIV/AIDS epidemic on children and youth. In: *Generation at Risk: The Global Impact of HIV/AIDS on Orphans and Vulnerable Children.* (eds G. Foster, *et al.*), pp. 93–133. Cambridge University Press, Cambridge.

Beaglehole, R. *et al.* (2008) Improving the prevention and management of chronic disease in low-income and middle-income countries: a priority for primary health care. *The Lancet* **372** (9642), 940–949.

Beardslee, W.R. (1998) Prevention and the clinical encounter. *American Journal of Orthopsychiatry* **68** (4), 521–533.

Benard, B. (1995) Fostering Resilience in Children. *ERIC/EECE Digest,* EDO-PS-95-9.

Benton, T.D. (2011) Psychiatric considerations in children and adolescents with HIV/AIDS. *Pediatric Clinics of North America* **58** (4), 989–1002.

Betancourt, T.S. & Khan, K.T. (2008) The mental health of children affected by armed conflict: protective processes and pathways to resilience. *International Review of Psychiatry* **20** (3), 317–328.

Betancourt, T.S. *et al.* (2010a) Children affected by HIV/AIDS: SAFE, a model for promoting their security, health, and development. *Psychology, Health & Medicine* **15** (3), 243–265.

Betancourt, T.S. *et al.* (2010b) Family-centred approaches to the prevention of mother to child transmission of HIV. *Journal of the International AIDS Society* **13** (Suppl 2), S2.

Betancourt, T.S. *et al.* (2011a) Nothing can defeat combined hands (Abashize hamwe ntakibananira): protective processes and resilience in Rwandan children and families affected by HIV/AIDS. *Social Science & Medicine* **73** (5), 693–701.

Betancourt, T.S. *et al.* (2011b) Using mixed-methods research to adapt and evaluate a family strengthening intervention in Rwanda. *African Journal of Traumatic Stress* **2** (1), 32–45.

Betancourt, T.S. *et al.* (2012) Global mental health programs for children and families facing adversity: development of a Family Strengthening Intervention in Rwanda. In: *Children and Families Affected by Armed Conflicts in Africa: Implications and Strategies for Helping Professionals in the United States.* (ed J.N. Corbin), pp. 113–142. National Association of Social Workers Press, Washington, DC.

Betancourt, T.S. *et al.* (2013) Annual research review: mental health and resilience in HIV/AIDS-affected children—a review of the literature and recommendations for future research. *Journal of Child Psychology and Psychiatry* **54** (4), 423–444.

Betancourt, T.S. *et al.* (2014) Family-based prevention of mental health problems in children affected by HIV and AIDS: an open trial. *AIDS* **28** (Suppl 3), S359–S368.

Betancourt, T.S. *et al.* (2014) HIV and child mental health: a case-control study in Rwanda. *Pediatrics* **134** (2), e464–472.

Bhana, A. *et al.* (2010) Family-based HIV prevention and intervention services for youth living in poverty-affected contexts: the CHAMP model of collaborative, evidence-informed programme development. *Journal of the International AIDS Society* **13** (Suppl 2), S8.

Bicego, G. *et al.* (2003) Dimensions of the emerging orphan crisis in sub-Saharan Africa. *Social Science & Medicine* **56** (6), 1235–1247.

Branson, B.M. *et al.* (2006) Revised recommendations for HIV testing of adults, adolescents, and pregnant women in health-care settings. *MMWR Recommendations and Reports* Sept. 22, **55** (RR-14), 1–17; quiz CE11-14.

Brennan, J. *et al.* (2012) Syndemic theory and HIV-related risk among young transgender women: the role of multiple, co-occurring health problems and social marginalization. *American Journal of Public Health* **102** (9), 1751–1757.

Briere, J. & Jordan, C.E. (2004) Violence against women: outcome complexity and implications for assessment and treatment. *Journal of Interpersonal Violence* **19** (11), 1252–1276.

Bronfenbrenner, U. (1979) *The Ecology of Human Development: Experiments by Nature and Design.* The Harvard University Press, Cambridge, MA.

Brook, D.W. *et al.* (2002) Coping in adolescent children of HIV-positive and HIV-negative substance-abusing fathers. *Journal of Genetic Psychology* **163** (1), 5–23.

Bursch, B. *et al.* (2008) Psychosocial predictors of somatic symptoms in adolescents of parents with HIV: a six-year longitudinal study. *AIDS Care* **20** (6), 667–676.

Caballero, J. *et al.* (2005) Depression in children with HIV infection: a case series. *The Journal of Pediatric Pharmacology and Therapeutics* **10** (1), 51–60.

Capaldi, D.M. & Clark, S. (1998) Prospective family predictors of aggression toward female partners for at-risk young men. *Developmental Psychology* **34** (6), 1175–1188.

Chang, L. *et al.* (2011) Impact of apolipoprotein E ε4 and HIV on cognition and brain atrophy: antagonistic pleiotropy and premature brain aging. *NeuroImage* **58** (4), 1017–1027.

Chernoff, M. *et al.* (2009) Mental health treatment patterns in perinatally HIV-infected youth and controls. *Pediatrics* **124** (2), 627–636.

Clum, G.A. *et al.* (2009) Adolescent medicine trials network for HIV/AIDS interventions. Child abuse in young, HIV-positive women: linkages to risk. *Qualitative Health Research* **19** (12), 1755–1768.

Cluver, L. & Gardner, F. (2007) Risk and protective factors for psychological well-being of children orphaned by AIDS in Cape Town: a qualitative study of children and caregivers' perspectives. *AIDS Care* **19** (3), 318–325.

Cluver, L. & Orkin, M. (2009) Cumulative risk and AIDS-orphanhood: interactions of stigma, bullying and poverty on child mental health in South Africa. *Social Science & Medicine* **69** (8), 1186–1193.

Cluver, L. *et al.* (2007) Psychological distress amongst AIDS-orphaned children in urban South Africa. *Journal of Child Psychology and Psychiatry* **48** (8), 755–763.

Cluver, L. *et al.* (2008) Effects of stigma on the mental health of adolescents orphaned by AIDS. *Journal of Adolescent Health* **42** (4), 410–417.

Cluver, L. *et al.* (2009a) Poverty and psychological health among AIDS-orphaned children in Cape Town, South Africa. *AIDS Care* **21** (6), 732–741.

Cluver, L. *et al.* (2009b) Posttraumatic stress in AIDS-orphaned children exposed to high levels of trauma: the protective role of perceived social support. *Journal of Traumatic Stress* **22** (2), 106–112.

Cluver, L.D. *et al.* (2012) Persisting mental health problems among AIDS-orphaned children in South Africa. *Journal of Child Psychology and Psychiatry* **53** (4), 363–370.

Committee on Pediatric AIDS (2011) Policy statement: adolescents and HIV infection: the pediatrician's role in promoting routine testing. *Pediatrics* **128** (5), 1023–1029.

Cowan, P.A. *et al.* (1996) Thinking about risk and resilience in families. In: *Stress, Coping, and Resiliency in Children and Families.* (eds E.M. Hetherington & E.A. Blechman), pp. 1–34. Lawrence Erlbaum Associates, Mahwah, NJ.

Daniel, M. *et al.* (2007) Breaching cultural silence: enhancing resilience among Ugandan orphans. *African Journal of AIDS Research* **6** (2), 109–120.

Davis, L.E. *et al.* (1992) Early viral brain invasion in iatrogenic human immunodeficiency virus infection. *Neurology* **42** (9), 1736–1739.

Doku, P. (2009) Parental HIV/AIDS status and death, and children's psychological wellbeing. *International Journal of Mental Health Systems* **3** (1), 26.

Dunfee, R. *et al.* (2006) Mechanisms of HIV-1 neurotropism. *Current HIV Research* **4** (3), 267–278.

Dutra, R. *et al.* (2000) Child resiliency in inner-city families affected by HIV: the role of family variables. *Behaviour Research and Therapy* **38** (5), 471–468.

Evans, D.K. & Miguel, E. (2007) Orphans and schooling in Africa: a longitudinal analysis. *Demography* **44** (1), 35–57.

Fang, X. *et al.* (2009) Parental HIV/AIDS and psychosocial adjustment among rural Chinese children. *Journal of Pediatric Psychology* **34** (10), 1053–1062.

Freeman, M. *et al.* (2005) Integrating mental health in global initiatives for HIV/AIDS. *The British Journal of Psychiatry* **187** (1), 1–3.

Freudenreich, O. *et al.* (2010) Psychiatric treatment of persons with HIV/AIDS: an HIV-psychiatry consensus survey of current practices. *Psychosomatics* **51** (6), 480–488.

Funck-Brentano, I. *et al.* (2005) Evaluation of a peer support group therapy for HIV-infected adolescents. *AIDS* **19** (14), 1501–1508.

Gadow, K.D. *et al.* (2010) Co-occuring psychiatric symptoms in children perinatally infected with HIV and peer comparison sample. *Journal of Developmental & Behavioral Pediatrics* **31** (2), 116–128.

Gadow, K.D. *et al.* (2012) Longitudinal study of emerging mental health concerns in youth perinatally infected with HIV and peer comparisons. *Journal of Developmental & Behavioral Pediatrics* **33** (6), 456–468.

Garvey, L.J. *et al.* (2012) Acute HCV/HIV coinfection is associated with cognitive dysfunction and cerebral metabolite disturbance, but not increased microglial cell activation. *PLoS ONE* **7** (7), 1.

Gaughan, D.M. *et al.* (2004) Psychiatric hospitalizations among children and youths with human immunodeficiency virus infection. *Pediatrics* **113** (6), e544–e551.

Gilliam, P.P. *et al.* (2011) Transition of adolescents with HIV to adult care: characteristics and current practices of the adolescent trials network for HIV/AIDS interventions. *Journal of the Association of Nurses in AIDS Care* **22** (4), 283–294.

Gilliom, M. *et al.* (2002) Anger regulation in disadvantaged preschool boys: strategies, antecedents, and the development of self-control. *Developmental Psychology* **38** (2), 222–235.

González-Scarano, F. & Martín-García, J. (2005) The neuropathogenesis of AIDS. *Nature Reviews Immunology* **5** (1), 69–81.

Grelotti, D.J. *et al.* (2014) Whoonga: potential recreational use of HIV antiretroviral medication in South Africa. *AIDS and Behavior* **18** (3), 511–518.

Griner, D. & Smith, T.B. (2006) Culturally adapted mental health intervention: a meta-analytic review. *Psychotherapy: Theory, Research, Practice, Training* **43** (4), 531–548.

Guo, Y. *et al.* (2012) The impact of HIV/AIDS on children's educational outcome: a critical review of global literature. *AIDS Care* **24** (8), 993–1012.

Harms, S. *et al.* (2009) Conceptions of mental health among Ugandan youth orphaned by AIDS. *African Journal of AIDS Research* **8** (1), 7–16.

Hazra, R. *et al.* (2010) Growing up with HIV: children, adolescents, and young adults with perinatally acquired HIV infection. *Annual Review of Medicine* **61** (1), 169–185.

Hein, K. *et al.* (1995) Comparison of HIV+ and HIV- adolescents: risk factors and psychosocial determinants. *Pediatrics* **95** (1), 96–104.

Inciardi, J.A. *et al.* (2007) Mechanisms of prescription drug diversion among drug-involved club- and street-based populations. *Pain Medicine* **8** (2), 171–183.

Ingerski, L.M. *et al.* (2010) A pilot study comparing traumatic stress symptoms by child and parent report across pediatric chronic illness groups. *Journal of Developmental & Behavioral Pediatrics* **31** (9), 713–719.

Johnson, B.T. *et al.* (2011) Interventions to reduce sexual risk for human immunodeficiency virus in adolescents: a meta-analysis of trials, 1985–2008. *Archives of Pediatrics & Adolescent Medicine* **165** (1), 77–84.

Judd, A. *et al.* (2007) Morbidity, mortality, and response to treatment by children in the United Kingdom and Ireland with perinatally acquired HIV infection during 1996–2006: planning for teenage and adult care. *Clinical Infectious Diseases* **45** (7), 918–924.

Kakuma, R. *et al.* (2011) Human resources for mental health care: current situation and strategies for action. *The Lancet* **378** (9803), 1654–1663.

Kamo, N. *et al.* (2008) Young citizens as health agents: use of drama in promoting community efficacy for HIV/AIDS. *American Journal of Public Health* **98** (2), 201–204.

Kaul, M. *et al.* (2006) HIV-1 coreceptors CCR5 and CXCR4 both mediate neuronal cell death but CCR5 paradoxically can also contribute to protection. *Cell Death and Differentiation* **14**, 296–305.

Kennedy, S.B. *et al.* (2004) Evaluation of HIV/AIDS prevention resources in Liberia: strategy and implications. *AIDS Patient Care & STDs* **18** (3), 169–180.

Kieling, C. *et al.* (2011) Child and adolescent mental health worldwide: evidence for action. *The Lancet* **378** (9801), 1515–1525.

Kumakech, E. *et al.* (2009) Peer-group support intervention improves the psychosocial well-being of AIDS orphans: cluster randomized trial. *Social Science & Medicine* **68** (6), 1038–1043.

Lazarus, R.S. & Folkman, S. (1984) *Psychological Stress and the Coping Process*. Springer, New York, NY.

Le Doaré, K. *et al.* (2012) Neurodevelopment in children born to HIV-infected mothers by infection and treatment status. *Pediatrics* **130** (5), e1326–e1344.

Lehrer, J.A. *et al.* (2006) Depressive symptoms as a longitudinal predictor of sexual risk behaviors among US middle and high school students. *Pediatrics* **118** (1), 189–200.

Li, L. *et al.* (2011) A multilevel intervention for HIV-affected families in China: together for empowerment activities (TEA). *Social Science & Medicine* **73** (8), 1214–1221.

Lightfoot, M.A. *et al.* (2007) Efficacy of a culturally adapted intervention for youth living with HIV in Uganda. *Prevention Science* **8** (4), 271–273.

Lin, X. *et al.* (2010) Perceived HIV stigma among children in a high HIV-prevalence area in central China: beyond the parental HIV-related illness and death. *AIDS Care* **22** (5), 545–555.

Luthar, S. (1993) Methodological and conceptual issues in research on childhood resilience. *Journal of Child Psychology and Psychiatry* **34** (4), 441–453.

Malee, K.M. *et al.* (2011) Mental health functioning among children and adolescents with perinatal HIV infection and perinatal HIV exposure. *AIDS Care* **23** (12), 1533–1544.

Malow, R.M. *et al.* (2007) HIV preventive interventions for adolescents: a look back and ahead. *Current HIV/AIDS Reports* **4** (4), 173–180.

Masten, A.S. (2001) Ordinary magic: resilience processes in development. *American Psychologist* **56** (3), 227–238.

McArthur, J. & Smith, B. (2013) Neurologic complications and considerations in HIV-infected persons. *Current Infectious Disease Reports* **15** (1), 61–66.

Mellins, C.A. *et al.* (2011) Behavioral health risks in perinatally HIV-exposed youth: co-occurrence of sexual and drug use behavior, mental health problems, and nonadherence to antiretroviral treatment. *AIDS Patient Care and STDs* **25** (7), 413–422.

Mellins, C.A. *et al.* (2012) Prevalence and change in psychiatric disorders among perinatally HIV-infected and HIV-exposed youth. *AIDS Care* **24** (8), 953–962.

Michielsen, K. *et al.* (2010) Effectiveness of HIV prevention for youth in sub-Saharan Africa: systematic review and meta-analysis of randomized and nonrandomized trials. *AIDS* **24** (8), 1193–1202.

Mishra, V. *et al.* (2007) Education and nutritional status of orphans and children of HIV-infected parents in Kenya. *AIDS Education and Prevention* **19** (5), 383–395.

Monasch, R. & Boerma, J.T. (2004) Orphanhood and childcare patterns in sub-Saharan Africa: an analysis of national surveys from 40 countries. *AIDS* **18** (Suppl 2), S55–S65.

Murphy, D.A. & Marelich, W.D. (2008) Resiliency in young children whose mothers are living with HIV/AIDS. *AIDS Care* **20** (3), 284–291.

Murphy, D.A. *et al.* (2005) Longitudinal antiretroviral adherence among adolescents infected with human immunodeficiency virus. *Archives of Pediatrics & Adolescent Medicine* **159** (8), 764–770.

Naar-King, S. *et al.* (2006) Healthy choices: motivational enhancement therapy for health risk behaviors in HIV-positive youth. *AIDS Education and Prevention* **18** (1), 1–11.

Naar-King, S. *et al.* (2010) A multisite randomized trial of a motivational intervention targeting multiple risks in youth living with HIV: initial effects on motivation, self-efficacy, and depression. *Journal of Adolescent Health* **46** (5), 422–428.

Nozyce, M.L. *et al.* (2006) A behavioral and cognitive profile of clinically stable HIV-infected children. *Pediatrics* **117** (3), 763–770.

Orban, L.A. *et al.* (2010) Coping strategies of adolescents living with HIV: disease-specific stressors and responses. *AIDS Care* **22** (4), 420–430.

Panel on Antiretroviral Therapy and Medical Management of HIV-infected Children (2013) *Guidelines for the Use of Antiretroviral Agents in Pediatric HIV Infection* [Online]. Available: http://aidsinfo.nih.gov/contentfiles/lvguidelines/pediatricguidelines.pdf [6 Sep 2013].

Parker, L. *et al.* (2013) Feasibility analysis of an evidence-based positive prevention intervention for youth living with HIV/AIDS in Kinshasa, Democratic Republic of the Congo. *AIDS Education & Prevention* **25** (2), 135–150.

Patel, V. *et al.* (2007a) Mental health of young people: a global public-health challenge. *The Lancet* **369** (9569), 1302–1313.

Patel, V. *et al.* (2007b) Treatment and prevention of mental disorders in low-income and middle-income countries. *The Lancet* **370** (9591), 991–1005.

Patel, K. *et al.* (2009) Impact of HAART and CNS-penetrating antiretroviral regimens on HIV encephalopathy among perinatally infected children and adolescents. *AIDS* **23** (14), 1893–1901.

Perdue, T. *et al.* (2003) Depression and HIV risk behavior among Seattle-area injection drug users and young men who have sex with men. *AIDS Education and Prevention* **15** (1), 81–92.

Perez, F. *et al.* (2004) Prevention of mother to child transmission of HIV: evaluation of a pilot programme in a district hospital in rural Zimbabwe. *British Medical Journal* **329** (7475), 1147–1150.

Petersen, I. *et al.* (2010) Psychosocial challenges and protective influences for socio-emotional coping of HIV+ adolescents in South Africa: a qualitative investigation. *AIDS Care* **22** (8), 970–978.

Pivnick, A. & Villegas, N. (2000) Resilience and risk: childhood and uncertainty in the AIDS epidemic. *Culture, Medicine and Psychiatry* **24** (1), 101–136.

Radcliffe, J. *et al.* (2007) Posttraumatic stress and trauma history in adolescents and young adults with HIV. *AIDS Patient Care and STDs* **21** (7), 501–508.

Reisner, S.L. *et al.* (2009a) Stressful or traumatic life events, post-traumatic stress disorder (PTSD) symptoms, and HIV sexual risk taking among men who have sex with men. *AIDS Care* **21** (12), 1481–1489.

Reisner, S.L. *et al.* (2009b) A review of HIV antiretroviral adherence and intervention studies among HIV-infected youth. *Topics in HIV Medicine: A Publication of the International AIDS Society, USA* **17** (1), 14.

Richter, L. *et al.* (2005) *Where the Heart is: Meeting the Psychosocial Needs of Young Children in the Context of HIV/AIDS.* Bernard van Leer Foundation, The Hague, The Netherlands.

Rochat, T.J. *et al.* (2006) Depression among pregnant rural South African women undergoing HIV testing. *JAMA* **295** (12), 1373–1378.

Rosenblum, A. *et al.* (2005) Substance use among young adolescents in HIV-affected families: resiliency, peer deviance, and family functioning. *Substance Use & Misuse* **40** (5), 581–603.

Rotheram-Borus, M.J. *et al.* (2001) Efficacy of a preventive intervention for youths living with HIV. *American Journal of Public Health* **91** (3), 400.

Rotheram-Borus, M.J. *et al.* (2004) Prevention for substance-using HIV-positive young people: telephone and in-person delivery. *Journal of Acquired Immune Deficiency Syndromes (1999)* **37** (Suppl 2), S68.

Rotheram-Borus, M.J. *et al.* (2005) Families living with HIV. *AIDS Care* **17** (8), 978–987.

Rotheram-Borus, M.J. *et al.* (2006) Adolescent adjustment over six years in HIV-affected families. *Journal of Adolescent Health* **39** (2), 174–182.

Rudy, B. *et al.* (2010) Prevalence and interactions of patient-related risks for nonadherence to antiretroviral therapy among perinatally infected youth in the United States. *AIDS Patient Care & STDs* **24** (2), 97–104.

Rutta, E. *et al.* (2008) Prevention of mother-to-child transmission of HIV in a refugee camp setting in Tanzania. *Glob Public Health* **3** (1), 62–76.

Rutter, M. (1985) Resilience in the face of adversity. Protective factors and resistance to psychiatric disorder. *British Journal of Psychiatry* **147** (6), 598–611.

Rutter, M. (2006) Implications of resilience concepts for scientific understanding. In: *Resilence in Children.* (eds B. Lester, *et al.*), Annals of the New York Academy of Sciences vol. 1094, Blackwell, New York.

Rydström, L.L. *et al.* (2013) Experiences of young adults growing up with innate or early acquired HIV infection—a qualitative study. *Journal of Advanced Nursing* **69** (6), 1357–1365.

Sapienza, J.K. & Masten, A.S. (2011) Understanding and promoting resilience in children and youth. *Current Opinion in Psychiatry* **24** (4), 267–273.

Sayson, R. & Meya, A.F. (2001) Strengthening the roles of existing structures by breaking down barriers and building up bridges: intensifying HIV/AIDS awareness, outreach, and intervention in Uganda. *Child Welfare: Journal of Policy, Practice, and Program* **80** (5), 541–550.

Silver, E.J. *et al.* (2003) Factors associated with psychological distress in urban mothers with late-stage HIV/AIDS. *AIDS and Behavior* **7** (4), 421–431.

Singer, M. (2010) Pathogen-pathogen interaction: a syndemic model of complex biosocial processes in disease. *Virulence* **1** (1), 10–18.

Sirois, P.A. *et al.* (2009) Impact of medications prescribed for treatment of attention-deficit hyperactivity disorder on physical growth in children and adolescents with HIV. *Journal of Developmental & Behavioral Pediatrics* **30** (5), 403–412.

Skovdal, M. *et al.* (2009) Young carers as social actors: coping strategies of children caring for ailing or ageing guardians in Western Kenya. *Social Science & Medicine* **69** (4), 587–595.

Ssewamala, F.M. & Ismayilova, L. (2009) Integrating children's savings accounts in the care and support of orphaned adolescents in rural Uganda. *Social Service Review* **83** (3), 453–472.

Ssewamala, F.M. *et al.* (2010) Effect of economic assets on sexual risk-taking intentions among orphaned adolescents in Uganda. *American Journal of Public Health* **100** (3), 483–488.

Stein, J.A. *et al.* (1999) Parentification and its impact on adolescent children of parents with AIDS. *Family Process* **38** (2), 193–208.

Stein, J.A. *et al.* (2007) Impact of parentification on long-term outcomes among children of parents with HIV/AIDS. *Family Process* **46** (3), 317–333.

Tanney, M.R. *et al.* (2010) Multiple risk behaviors among youth living with human immunodeficiency virus in five U.S. cities. *Journal of Adolescent Health* **46** (1), 11–16.

Thompson, A. *et al.* (2006) Psychotropic medications and HIV. *Clinical Infectious Diseases* **42** (9), 1305–1310.

Tu, X. *et al.* (2009) School performance and school behaviour of children affected by acquired immune deficiency syndrome (AIDS) in China. *Vulnerable Children and Youth Studies* **4** (3), 199–209.

UNAIDS (2012) *Report on the Global AIDS Epidemic.* UNAIDS, Geneva, Switzerland.

UNAIDS, UNICEF, USAID (2004) *Children on the Brink 2004: A Joint Report of New Orphan Estimates and a Framework for Action.* United Nations, New York.

Ungar, M. (2011) The social ecology of resilience: addressing contextual and cultural ambiguity of a nascent construct. *American Journal of Orthopsychiatry* **81** (1), 1–17.

UNICEF (2006) *Africa's Orphaned and Vulnerable Generations: Children Affected by AIDS.* UNICEF, UNAIDS, & PEPFAR, New York.

UNICEF (2012) *Statistics by Area / HIV/AIDS* [Online]. Available: http://www.childinfo.org/hiv_aids.html [10 June 2013].

Van Rie, A. *et al.* (2007) Neurologic and neurodevelopmental manifestations of pediatric HIV/AIDS: a global perspective. *European Journal of Paediatric Neurology* **11** (1), 1–9.

Weinhardt, L.S. *et al.* (1999) Effects of HIV counseling and testing on sexual risk behavior: a meta-analytic review of published research, 1985–1997. *American Journal of Public Health* **89** (9), 1397–1405.

Werner, E.E. (1989) High-risk children in young adulthood: a longitudinal study from birth to 32 Years. *American Journal of Orthopsychiatry* **59** (1), 72–81.

Whetten, K. *et al.* (2012) Relationship between trauma and high-risk behavior among HIV-positive men who do not have sex with men (MDSM). *AIDS Care* **24** (11), 1453–1460.

Williams, P.L. *et al.* (2006) Predictors of adherence to antiretroviral medications in children and adolescents with HIV infection. *Pediatrics* **118** (6), e1745–e1757.

Williams, P. *et al.* (2010) Substance use and its association with psychiatric symptoms in perinatally HIV-infected and HIV-affected adolescents. *AIDS and Behavior* **14** (5), 1072–1082.

Wood, K. *et al.* (2006) 'Telling the truth is the best thing': teenage orphans' experiences of parental AIDS-related illness and bereavement in Zimbabwe. *Social Science & Medicine* **63** (7), 1923–1933.

World Health Organization (2010) *Antiretroviral therapy of HIV Infection in Infants and Children: Towards Universal Access. Recommendations for a Public Health Approach: 2010 Revision.* World Health Organization, Geneva.

Zhang, L. *et al.* (2009) 'I felt I have grown up as an adult': caregiving experience of children affected by HIV/AIDS in China. *Child: Care, Health and Development* **35** (4), 542–550.

Zhao, Q. *et al.* (2011a) Household displacement and health risk behaviors among HIV/AIDS-affected children in rural China. *AIDS Care* **23** (7), 866–872.

Zhao, G. *et al.* (2011b) Functions and sources of perceived social support among children affected by HIV/AIDS in China. *AIDS Care* **23** (6), 671–679.

CHAPTER 47

Children with specific sensory impairments

Naomi Dale and Lindsey Edwards
Great Ormond Street Hospital, NHS Foundation Trust, London, UK

Children without vision and hearing, the dominant senses for accessing the environment, face severe disadvantages. Some children follow compensatory developmental trajectories and even develop exceptional abilities; others advance with great difficulty. This chapter describes the impact of visual impairment (VI) and hearing impairment (HI) on child development, with a focus on vulnerable developmental processes and psychiatric risk.

Visual impairment (VI) refers to all degrees of vision reduction, where reduced acuity is defined as vision clarity. For the purposes of international comparison, the US legal definition of blindness is best-corrected visual acuity of less than 6/60, (being able to see at 6 metres what someone with normal vision can see 60 metres away). Snellen notation is now being replaced by the logMar system where logMar 1.0 is equivalent to 6/60. The UK legal definition of blindness is 3/60 or less vision and partial sight as 6/60 to 3/60. Hearing impairment (HI) is defined by the quietest sound that can be heard in decibels across a range of frequencies. According to the UK system, severe hearing loss is the inability to hear sounds quieter than 65-70 decibels (dB) and profound loss at 85-90 dB. Individuals who cannot hear these sounds are unable to hear speech adequately even when using hearing aids.

Visual impairment

The two main types of childhood visual impairment (VI) are *peripheral or ocular* and *cerebral,* although a "mixed" condition is possible. The former arises from abnormalities of the eye globe, retina or anterior optic nerve, and the latter originates in the posterior optic nerve, optic radiations and visual cortex. Peripheral visual disorders can be divided into "simple" or "isolated," where VI is the only impairment, and "complex" or "syndromic," occurring in a wider syndrome. Estimate of the incidence of childhood VI is 4 per 10,000 infants in the first year, rising to 5 per 10,000 at 16 years in the UK (Rahi *et al.*, 2003).

Over three quarters of children with VI in the United Kingdom have additional non ophthalmic disorders including intellectual disability, motor disorders, hearing impairment (HI), epilepsy, autism, attention deficit hyperactivity disorder (ADHD) and health impairments. These reduce to about 20% in children with "simple" congenital VI. Children with cerebral visual disorders have wide ranging visual disturbances and commonly additional brain difficulties. Cerebral vision-processing deficits occur in many conditions: cerebral palsy, Fragile X and Williams syndrome. One in 10 people with intellectual disabilities in the United Kingdom are estimated to have a VI.

Etiology, identification, and visual management

The numerous causes of VI often accompany wider disabilities in high income countries. In the United Kingdom, the most common anatomical sites of origin are cerebral visual pathways (48%), the optic nerve (28%) and the retina (29%). "Isolated" or peripheral visual disorders are associated with prenatal congenital causes, for example, anophthalmia, Leber's amaurosis, corneal anomalies and "complex" syndromic conditions like Joubert syndrome, with increasing knowledge of the genetic anomalies involved. Cerebral visual impairment (CVI) has many causes from prenatal, perinatal, neonatal and childhood factors, including injury, vascular pathology, focal tumors, and infections.

Apart from overt eye defects at birth, parents often first notice that their baby is not looking at them or tracking their movements. Once ophthalmologists and paediatricians have determined the cause of poor visual responses, standard visual function tests are available. Three quarters of childhood visual disorders leading to VI in the United Kingdom are neither preventable nor treatable. For most, treatment provides vision aids for those with sufficient visual capacity. Prompt identification and treatment are essential as infants may have the potential to develop useful vision with interventions applied under 1 year of life. The long-term goal of habilitation is to increase participation in everyday living, regardless of reduced vision abilities.

Rutter's Child and Adolescent Psychiatry, Sixth Edition.
Edited by Anita Thapar and Daniel S. Pine, James F. Leckman, Stephen Scott, Margaret J. Snowling, Eric Taylor.
© 2015 John Wiley & Sons Ltd. Published 2018 by John Wiley & Sons Ltd.

Early family support and intervention

During the early period of diagnosis, parents often feel isolated, confused and distressed. They require support, information and guidance in maximising their baby's development and vision. Parents are dealing with an unfamiliar developmental pathway, and informed guidance will give them normative expectations to anticipate and optimize their infant's next developmental steps. Some early interventions exist, though their effectiveness has not been fully evaluated. The so-called, widely used Oregon method extends the Portage system. The Early Support Developmental Journal for infants with VI, a parent oriented set of materials, provides one of the main intervention frameworks in the United Kingdom and is currently undergoing evaluation (Dale *et al.*, 2007).

Developmental aspects of visual impairment

As much of learning in infancy is vision-based, poor vision can profoundly affect development without intervention. Infants are very reluctant to feel and explore their physical environment, and auditory-directed reaching occurs later than visually directed reaching. Delays in sensorimotor and cognitive development are common, with the greatest vulnerability occurring in profound VI (Dale *et al.*, 2002).

The earliest language milestones are often delayed. Quality of maternal responsiveness, control, and goal setting behaviors are positively related to the young child's advances in language skills, exploration of the environment and sensorimotor development (Hughes *et al.*, 1999). As vocabulary expands, syntax and grammar also begin to normalise. However, language may be more formulaic with expressive ability outstripping semantic understanding. Pragmatic or social use of language can also lag behind, with difficulty in adapting language to the social context including early pronoun use.

Educational attainments

By school years, some children with VI will reach or exceed the verbal IQ of their sighted peers. Growing cognitive capacity can support superior learning in some instances. Nearly three quarters of VI children in the United Kingdom are educated in mainstream settings. Depending on level of vision, children are introduced to Braille or enlarged print (or both) for reading. However, they may struggle to keep up with the mainstream curriculum. By 7 years, Braille readers lag behind their sighted peers in reading and writing (Harris *et al.*, 2012). Children with low vision levels may read enlarged print more slowly. By 13–16 years adolescents may be up to 3 years behind their peers in attainment skills including mathematics though more specialized academic support or helping parents feel confident in supporting their child's reading or mathematics could accelerate progress (e.g., Giesen *et al.*, 2012).

Emotional development and psychological well-being

Following Selma Fraiberg's (1977) seminal work, there was concern about the passivity and self-centredness of the infant with profound VI. However, other work suggests that reciprocity is possible between infants and their parents (e.g., Preisler, 1995). Children can develop secure, albeit at times delayed, attachment, continuing into adulthood (Ardito *et al.*, 2004). However, this process is especially vulnerable when the parent struggles to "tune in" to a more unresponsive baby. The clinical context and support of parents can influence infant bonding (Rahi *et al.*, 2005).

Beyond infancy, the ability to recognize emotions develops slowly though it is debated whether this is part of a general or specific delay (Dyck *et al.*, 2004). In contrast to children with HI, emotional recognition is more vulnerable than emotion understanding and vocabulary, which are more verbally mediated processes.

One of the greater challenges for children with VI is social integration. They may desire friends but lack necessary skills and be restricted from playground activities due to fears of safety or bullying. Adolescents may spend more time alone, have smaller social networks and lower social skills and self esteem—with further risk if the parents are overprotective or the young person is introverted, particularly for boys (Pinquart & Pfeiffer, 2011). However, some young people are resilient, and research suggests that these VI children may exhibit self-esteem that is similar or higher than that in sighted peers (Kef and Deković, 2004; Lifshitz *et al.*, 2007).

Young people with VI face difficulty with everyday tasks. Some studies suggest a lower health-related quality of life (Chadha and Subramanian, 2011), though others find no differences from sighted peers (Wong *et al.*, 2009). A more VI child centered approach is needed to capture the subjective perspective (Rahi *et al.*, 2011). Unfortunately, quality of life may decline with increasing age and greater degree of VI possibly because of unwelcome dependency, increasing isolation and limited employment prospects.

Social processes are particularly vulnerable areas. This can be partly compensated for by parents adapting their interactive routines to ensure that infants enjoy social games and vocal interactions. However, delays in social communication development may continue across the early years, particularly in children with profound VI, and these are greater than in HI.

As infants with VI cannot follow their parent's gaze behaviors or point out things of interest, "joint attention" skills are especially vulnerable (Bigelow, 2003). Even low levels of "form" vision greatly enhance opportunities for object-centred "joint attention" (Dale *et al.*, 2013). Possibly to compensate, parents tend to resort to higher physical and verbal involvement and control of activities which may be more or less adaptive for the child (Moore & McConachie, 1994).

As language skills develop, parents use "mental state" language to help their child understand other people's emotions, beliefs, and intentions (Tadić *et al.*, 2013). The question of whether theory of mind (ToM) is fundamentally limited by lack of vision is strongly debated. Delay occurs in first order "false belief" tasks like the Sally Ann task, which are traditionally visual, with the reported age of acquisition varying from 7 to 12 years (Green *et al.*, 2004; Brambring & Asbrock, 2010). Advanced ToM skills (i.e., awareness that other people have beliefs about beliefs) may possibly emerge more similarly to sighted children, at least in children with a wider range of congenital visual impairment, and appears associated with age and verbal intelligence (Pijnacker *et al.*, 2012).

Neuropsychological processes

School-aged children with VI vary in their "higher order" cognitive processes including attention, working memory, and executive functions. In the clinic context, neuropsychological assessment commonly reveals uneven strengths and weaknesses in school-aged children. For instance, some children are notably weak in tactile or spatial perception, affecting their potential for independent navigation, object manipulation, search strategies, and Braille reading (Gori *et al.*, 2010). Those with the greatest difficulty in attention shifting in the preschool years show more behavioral rigidity and weaker executive function by 6–12 years (Tadić *et al.*, 2009; 2010). Of concern, this subgroup also shows weaker adaptive behavior functioning, which could jeopardize future independent living and employment. In children with cerebral visual impairment, specific weaknesses may be identified in "dorsal stream" processes, such as visual-motor coordination, visual/spatial perception, and visual attention.

Neuroplasticity and brain organization

With the large occipital lobe of the brain under-utilized, the brain migrates nonvisual functions into this area—highlighting the "cross plasticity" of the visual cortex. Behavioral, functional neuroimaging, and electrophysiological studies have shown that adults with congenital blindness activate the visual cortex for Braille reading and other tactile tasks. Auditory motion perception activates visual motion areas of the cortex and semantic linguistic processing occurs in the primary visual cortex (Amedi *et al.*, 2004). Other neural functional networks do not migrate elsewhere and appear amodal; adults with congenital blindness use similar brain regions as sighted adults to reason about mental states (e.g., medial prefrontal cortex) (Bedny *et al.*, 2009). Increased capabilities are found in auditory perception (sound localization, pitch discrimination), speech processing, biographical memory, and associative learning (e.g., Föcker *et al.*, 2012; Withagen *et al.*, 2013). The brain is highly plastic early in life but is more resistant to subsequent experience later on; for instance tactile reorganization does not occur in adults with late onset blindness after 16 years (Sadato *et al.*, 2002).

VI and complexity

Assessment and diagnosis of neurodevelopmental disorders

Even in children with "isolated" peripheral visual disorders, advancing genetic knowledge highlights that ocular genetic mutations (e.g., SOX2) are also expressed in the brain and neurodevelopmental prognosis is variable. Disorder at peripheral or primary visual cortex level may be associated with changes in white matter and "higher" visual processing pathways (Atkinson & Braddick, 2011; Webb *et al.*, 2013). Profound visual impairment is a further risk factor; a third of infants are at risk of regressing or plateauing in their development in their

second year of life, a phenomenon described as "developmental setback." Early behavioral signs emerge between 16 and 27 months, suggesting a critical developmental period. Infants who may have been very responsive in their first year of life show increasing self-directedness, social avoidance, temper tantrums, loss of first words, echolalia or mutism and nonfunctional repetitive actions and stereotypies. These behaviors tend to persist and the chronic disorder generally leads to a later clinical diagnosis of autism. Other risk factors include higher number of brain lesions, male gender, and severe intellectual difficulties (Cass *et al.*, 1994; see review by Sonksen & Dale 2002). Developmental setback is likely to be the most severe manifestation of an autistic spectrum disorder (ASD) in children with VI.

A great clinical challenge to differentiating a chronic ASD in children with VI is that, in the early years, many children with VI show autistic like difficulties. Behavior features like echolalia, self-directed behavior, stereotypies, communicative difficulties, and obsessional restricted interests are common in the preschool period. The long-term outlook for children presenting with ASD features is variable. In some children, the traits reduce significantly as the child develops more adaptive social behavior, language and communication—described as "reversible autism" (Hobson & Lee, 2010). For a substantial subgroup, chronic difficulties persist and it is their continuity and intensity by 4–6 years and older that should alert the clinician to a possible ASD (Absoud *et al.*, 2010) (see Chapter 51). Even milder presentations can have a severe disabling impact in the context of visual impairment.

Current estimates are of 11–20% with clinical autism in heterogeneous populations, with higher incidence in lower IQ and more severe VI—rising to 30% in profound VI (Brown *et al.*, 1997; Fazzi *et al.*, 2007; Mukaddes *et al.*, 2007). Up to 60% of VI children are rated with at least one area of difficulty in social communication/restricted behaviors (Pring & Tadić, 2005; Parr *et al.*, 2010). Careful monitoring across the preschool and primary school years and caution against reaching premature diagnostic conclusions is recommended. Assessment of "higher" vision, intellectual, motor, or ASD impairments in children with vision disorders is very challenging and requires highly specialized expertises in VI and paediatric neurodisability to carry out a differential diagnosis within an "informed" developmental framework (Sargent *et al.*, 2010).

Psychological and psychiatric issues

There is limited knowledge of the prevalence of psychological or psychiatric difficulties in children with VI, but high rates of behavior difficulties (50–70%) have been reported in representative studies (Jan *et al.*, 1977; Tirosh *et al.*, 1998). Of these, anxiety disorders, oppositional disorder with or without attention deficit hyperactivity and avoidant disorder with or without stereotypy are rated most frequently. Some studies find no difference in psychosocial adjustment and well-being between adolescents with VI and their sighted peers, but other studies point to a higher risk of psychological difficulty including depression (Koenes & Karshmer, 2000; Huurre *et al.*, 2001; Pinquart & Pfeiffer, 2013). Risk factors include having additional disabilities, receiving less parental emotional support, being isolated and lacking friends, being female, experiencing bullying, and having lower self-esteem. As in sighted peers, older adolescents are more at risk of psychological difficulties. Higher functioning young people may show considerable resilience, drive, and motivation but raised anxiety and emotional stress are often reported by parents and educators.

Parental well-being and support for parents is an important factor in their ability to cope and support their child; parenting stress and depression and its effects on interaction are likely to be high risk factors. Behavior problems are a high source of stress in parents, especially if the child has high caregiving demands and multiple disabilities (Tröster, 2001).

Young children with VI are often referred to the clinic with behavior difficulties including attention difficulties, temper tantrums, and aggression. Formulations need to account for the impact of VI on behavior and development (and the family) and tailored intervention may include psycho education for parents and teachers, behavioral interventions and strategies to enhance compensatory function and developmental growth. With obsessional interests and self-directed behaviors, parents find it very difficult to influence or help regulate their child's behavior, attention focus, or mood. The shared risk for autism or intellectual disability warrants a full clinical exploration before formulating an intervention plan which draws on principles used for children with autism but adapted for VI. This includes managing the environment, promoting the child's effective communication and supporting their sensory needs.

Anxiety disorders can occur across the age range, particularly in children with ASD tendencies. Young people with VI may be more prone to fears and phobias of potentially harmful situations (Ollendick *et al.*, 1985). Interventions may draw on psycho education, environmental restructuring, goal planning, and behavior modification with parents and educators and also therapeutic approaches including cognitive behavioral therapy (CBT), narrative therapy, or solution-focussed therapy with older children and their families.

Sleep disorders are common in children with VI, with a significant impact on the health of the children and causing distress to their caretakers (see Chapter 70). Sleep hygiene and behavioral approaches may be successful but with unresponsive sleep disorders, improved sleep latency with melatonin has been demonstrated in some cases (Khan *et al.*, 2011). Severe and unpredictable behavior (aggression, self injury, oppositional defiance and temper outbursts) is found in children with combined visual impairment, autism and intellectual disability, and commonly in septo-optic dysplasia with midbrain defects and hypo-pituitarism. A tailored behavioral intervention approach with strategies to support emotion self-regulation is recommended and pharmacological assistance may also be indicated in complex resistant behavior profiles.

Hearing impairment

The two main types of childhood HI are conductive and sensori-neural, although it is possible to have a "mixed" loss. The former, usually resulting from otitis media, may be transient. Permanent conductive hearing loss occurs in many syndromes associated with middle-ear disruptions, such as congenital cholesteatoma. Sensori-neural hearing loss, typically caused by abnormally functioning cochlear hair cells, can be congenital, progressive, or sudden, with an estimated incidence around 1–3 per 1000 live births or 0.3% of all school children (www.patient.co.uk). More than 90% of deaf children are born to two hearing parents. A third hearing disorder is Auditory Neuropathy/Auditory Dys-synchrony (Berlin *et al.*, 2001). The prevalence in children is not known, but it is thought that this condition is present in approximately 1 in 10 children with HI; the children characteristically have poor speech-perception abilities relative to their degree of HI. All types of hearing loss, including as a result of otitis media with infusion, can negatively affect language development. However, less impact occurs in deaf children of deaf parents who are raised within the Deaf culture and use British Sign Language as their means of communication, depending nevertheless on whether the child has additional disabilities or not.

Etiology, identification, and audiological management

The primary cause of permanent HI in children is genetic anomalies, accounting for approximately 60% of cases. In 70–80% of these, HI is the only impairment, for example, Connexin 26 mutation. Up to 30% of genetic HI is syndromic, with over a hundred known syndromes, most associated with sensori-neural hearing loss. Small proportions of childhood HI are due to infections such as toxoplasmosis, bacterial meningitis, cytomegalovirus, and rubella infection, severe prematurity or neonatal complications and ototoxic drugs such as streptomycin. A variety of tests are used in the identification of HI, from shortly after birth (Newborn Screening) through early childhood. Once a permanent HI is confirmed, assistive hearing devices including hearing aids, cochlear implants, and bone-anchored hearing aids aim to optimize access to and clarity of the speech signal. A recent more controversial intervention is a prosthetic auditory brainstem implant as its effectiveness for improving speech and language is unproven (e.g., Goffi-Gomez *et al.*, 2012).

Cochlear implantation is the treatment of choice for severe to profound congenital HI and also for progressive or acquired losses after language has developed. Cochlear implantation (particularly bilateral implantation) has positive effects on speech perception and production, language, and reading skills. Superior outcomes are associated with early implantation, particularly in the first 2 years of life (see Forli *et al.*, 2011 for a review). However, there remains great variability in outcome.

Early family support and intervention

Probably the single largest impact on developmental outcomes for children with HI has been Universal Newborn Hearing Screening, fully implemented across the United Kingdom in 2006. The majority of sensori-neural hearing loss is identified by 2 months of age and amplification or implants should be introduced promptly. Once permanent HI is identified, active involvement of parents in maximizing opportunities for learning through everyday interactions is essential for optimizing speech and language development. Early identification and intervention has been associated with better speech, language, and academic outcomes (e.g., Fulcher *et al.*, 2012).

Possible language interventions range from fully visual-manual to fully auditory-oral, with sign and speech combinations (e.g., sign-supported speech, simultaneous communication, cued speech, and total communication) (Stredler-Brown, 2010). Once an approach has been selected, family members must become proficient in that approach so that the child has access to a complete language model. Effective communication in early childhood is likely to be protective against future emotional and behavioral problems.

Developmental aspects of hearing impairment

Specific cognitive abilities, such as memory and attention, may be adversely affected by HI, and these skills are better predictors of the difficulties of learning language than IQ in children with HI (Marschark & Hauser, 2008).

HI is strongly associated with delays in receptive and expressive language skills and speech intelligibility. Most children with HI have smaller vocabularies and poorer use of grammar than their hearing peers, especially in the early years (e.g., Blamey, 2003). The rate of spoken language development is not strongly dependent on the degree of hearing reduction because other factors such as age of provision of hearing device, educational factors, other abilities and family support are all influential.

Educational attainments

A sound spoken language base is essential for learning to read, therefore many children with HI are at a significant disadvantage. Kyle and Harris (2010) found the gap between the reading scores of HI and hearing children widened from 1-year at 8 years to 3-years at 11 years. Even with the advantage of better access to spoken language afforded by cochlear implants, only a minority (less than 20%) of children with HI have a reading age within 12 months of their chronological age (e.g., Harris & Terlektsi, 2011; Dillon *et al.*, 2012). Much less is known about mathematical achievement but the evidence suggests that it is often significantly compromised (Qi & Mitchell, 2012) and cochlear implants only partly ameliorate the impact of HI. Word-based mathematical problem-solving relies more on reading comprehension and particularly disadvantages children with HI (Edwards *et al.*, 2013).

Emotional development and psychological well-being

Preschool-aged children with HI frequently exhibit high levels of frustration. Toddler tantrums often extend beyond the expected age period for hearing children, particularly when effective age-appropriate communication is lacking and language development is delayed. Some young children with HI

appear excessively shy and avoid interacting with people outside their immediate family. Childhood HI has a significant impact on family communication patterns and dynamics but little is known about the impact on the attachment relationship between mother and infant. Most children do develop close attachment relationships with their parents, and deaf children of deaf parents show similar attachment patterns to hearing children of hearing parents in the Strange Situation Paradigm according to Meadow-Orlans *et al.* (1983). However a higher incidence of avoidant and resistant classifications is observed between deaf children and hearing mother dyads compared with hearing dyads (Spangler, 1987). As in infants with VI, reactions to the diagnosis of HI and degree of support perceived by the parent appear to be important in influencing early bonding with the infant.

In school-aged children with HI, disruptions may occur in the development of empathy and processing of emotions including facial expressions (e.g., Bachara *et al.*, 1980; Ludlow *et al.*, 2010). Consequently many children with HI experience difficulties in establishing and maintaining positive peer relationships. Social competence and the quality of interactions between HI and hearing children are partially dependent on school setting (mainstream versus special education) and are associated with self-esteem and are often negatively impacted by language and communication delays (Antia & Kriemeyer, 2003; Martin *et al.*, 2011). Children with HI are sometimes rejected by their peers and experience victimization or bullying, leading to lowered self-esteem, and emotional and behavioral problems (van Gent *et al.*, 2011; Kouwenberg *et al.*, 2012).

From the earliest days, parent–child interaction shapes the development of prelingual social communicative behaviors such as visual attention and eye contact, joint attention, turn-taking, and the use of facial expressions to support the meaning of verbal information. Research suggests that some, but not all aspects of these early interactions may develop differently in HI children with hearing parents (e.g., Gale & Schick, 2009; Nowakowski *et al.*, 2009).

Development of mentalizing skills in children with HI is significantly delayed, as in those with VI. Children typically fail to pass first order ToM tasks, which are characteristically mastered by hearing 3–4 year olds, until they are aged 13 years and even beyond (e.g., Russell *et al.*, 1998). The ability is strongly related to the language and communicative competency of the child, whether in spoken or sign language; notably, deaf children of deaf parents do not demonstrate such delays (e.g., Meristo *et al.*, 2007). Little or no delay in ToM follows early cochlear implantation when this is associated with improved spoken language proficiency (Remmel & Peters, 2009). Early conversational input about the beliefs and mental states of others is therefore crucial for fostering adaptive social-cognitive development. Unfortunately, parents of deaf children often find it extremely challenging to modify their use of language and communication to meet the changing needs of their child through infancy and childhood. Compensatory strategies such as establishing eye contact before speaking, "scaffolding" the child's attempts at producing spoken words or phrases and using a "sign sandwich" when necessary (saying the target word, signing it, then saying it again) usually need to be explicitly taught to parents by teachers of the deaf or speech and language therapists from the earliest days.

Neuropsychological processes

The "higher-order" cognitive processes comprising executive function abilities are vulnerable in children with HI. Deficits in working memory are consistently found in those with and without cochlear implants (e.g., Pisoni *et al.*, 2008), and deficits in attention control, particularly visual attention and selective attention are common but peripheral attention may be enhanced (Dye *et al.*, 2008). Studies exploring other executive functions generally indicate greater impulsivity and difficulties in problem-solving, sequencing, and planning compared with hearing children (e.g., Hauser *et al.*, 2008; Edwards, 2010; Pisoni *et al.*, 2010). The development of all these functions is closely linked with language skills (e.g., Figueras *et al.*, 2008).

Neuroplasticity and brain organization

In the absence of auditory input, thalamo-cortical areas of the brain and the auditory cortex become utilized by other sensory modalities, particularly the visual modality, showing "cross-modal plasticity" (Bavelier & Neville, 2002; Gordon *et al.*, 2011). In children with HI increased capabilities and compensatory skill in nonauditory modalities have been demonstrated, for example, enhanced tactile accuracy, visual attention, and processing of stimuli in the peripheral visual field (Neville & Lawson, 1987; Bavelier *et al.*, 2000; Levanen & Hamdorf, 2001). In children with normal hearing, synaptic density in the temporal cortex peaks at between 2 and 4 years of age, with HI resulting in delayed synaptogenesis in the auditory cortex (see Kral & Sharma, 2012 for a review). Auditory stimulation is required for normal development of speech perception and language during a "sensitive period" of higher neuronal plasticity up until the age of about 3.5 years. After the age of 7 years, irreversible changes in cortical organization prevent adequate processing of auditory signals. These findings are consistent with the evidence from congenitally deaf children with cochlear implants; early implantation is associated with good spoken language development whereas later implantation may enable the child to detect auditory stimuli but not discriminate complex sounds and only develop limited speech understanding and oral language (Kral & Sharma, 2012).

Hearing impairment and complexity
Assessment and diagnosis of neurodevelopmental disorders

Around 40% of children with HI have additional impairments arising from the underlying syndromic etiology including generalized or specific intellectual disability, visual impairment, autism, ADHD, motor, and health impairments. ASDs are more common among HI than hearing children at around 2–4%, and the prevalence appears to be increasing (Szymanski *et al.*, 2012). Intellectual or learning disability, with its consequent impact on adaptive behavior, affects around 8–10% of children with HI, and specific learning disability a further 8% (http://research.gallaudet.edu/Demographics/annsrvy.php; The Ear Foundation, 2012). Significant neurodevelopmental motor impairments, primarily as a result of cerebral palsy, affect around 14% of deaf children. Rates of attention disorder and hyperactivity are elevated in HI children compared with their hearing peers (Hindley & Kroll, 1998).

In young children with HI great care must be taken to distinguish between ASD and other social communication difficulties that may arise as a result of the impact of HI on language and (preverbal) communication; in the former, there is typically a lack of communicative intent and the presence of restrictive, repetitive and stereotyped patterns of behavior (Edwards & Crocker, 2008a). In the early years, it may be difficult to distinguish between these two forms of communication difficulties. It is common for very young children with HI to actively avoid eye contact or to show restrictive interests in certain toys or activities. While these may be early warning signs of ASD, for many deaf children they are more transient and may reduce with targeted intervention and as more adaptive function emerges. As language develops, these behaviors frequently disappear along with the concerns regarding ASD.

Appropriate diagnosis is most reliably made by multidisciplinary teams with expertise in HI. In children with sensory impairments, cerebral palsy, or other neurodevelopmental impairments, assessment is challenging. Motor or visual disabilities may "mask" relatively well-preserved intellectual abilities, with serious consequences for educational placements and expectations for achievement. Complexity is sometimes used to justify slow progress without identifying other factors, which also need management.

Psychological and psychiatric issues

There is little epidemiological consistency in the reported prevalence of mental health problems with prevalence rates ranging from 11% to 60%; this arises from differences in sampling, assessment method, definitions of "disorder" and criteria for clinical "caseness" (Hindley *et al.*, 1994; Cornes *et al.*, 2006). Further risk factors, such as low language competency, additional disabilities, severe learning difficulty, communication difficulties with family or peers, being bullied, isolation, discrimination, and child abuse, are likely to contribute to emotional and behavioral problems, all of which warrant exploration when assessing psychological or psychiatric disorders clinically (Fellinger *et al.*, 2009; Hogan *et al.*, 2011; van Gent *et al.*, 2011). The overall picture is a higher risk for psychological and psychiatric difficulties in children with HI, though there is considerable individual variation.

Parenting a child with HI is described by mothers as more stressful than parenting a hearing one (Horsch *et al.*, 1997).

However, research suggests that the stresses may vary over time and be related to factors such as behavior problems and language delays (Lederberg & Golbach, 2002; Quittner *et al.*, 2010). Mothers of young children with profound hearing losses have been reported to use physical disciplinary methods for behavioral transgressions more than mothers of hearing children (Knutson *et al.*, 2004).

One of the most common presentations to child mental health services of preschool-aged children with HI is severe noncompliance with adult requests, temper tantrums, and aggressive behavior. Parents typically report that they do not know how to set boundaries and feel helpless in conveying instructions or explanations when the child's language is significantly delayed. Parental attitudes toward childrearing, disability, and personal feelings of guilt or loss may contribute to expectations of the child's appropriate behavior and use of disciplinary strategies. Psychoeducation and behavioral interventions adapted to accommodate the child's communication and language level are effective if implemented in conjunction with support to improve parent–child communication.

School-aged children have an increased referral rate for assessment of ADHD. Delays in language acquisition and deficits in executive function may result in difficulties mastering affect regulation and verbally mediated self-control, with consequent behavioral manifestations of poor attention, impulsivity, and hyperactivity. The assessment and diagnosis of ADHD in children with HI is complicated and controversial; behaviors considered diagnostic in hearing children must be interpreted with caution in those with HI. For example, appearing not to listen when spoken to directly and being distracted by irrelevant visual stimuli are behaviors typical of children with HI; they may not be aware that they are being spoken to or are monitoring what is happening around them visually to compensate for the lack of auditory information (Edwards & Crocker, 2008b). Effective management of these difficulties can usually be achieved through psychoeducation of parents and teachers and behavioral strategies with infrequent necessity for pharmacological treatment.

Anxiety disorders such as obsessive compulsive disorder and social anxiety disorder tend to emerge in older children and adolescents with HI, similar to their hearing peers. High levels of anxiety may be associated with issues around the individual's developing identity and the perception of self as deaf or hearing and their involvement with Deaf culture. Depressive disorders occur more commonly in adolescence and need to be considered in the context of the individual's school setting (whether there is a comparable peer group), emerging personal identity and the ease of communication within the family in terms of communication mode (e.g., Fellinger *et al.*, 2009; Mance & Edwards, 2012).

Assessment and interventions need to take into account the child and family's views regarding communication and treatments such as CBT, family, narrative, or solution-focussed therapy will need to be tailored appropriately.

Professional approaches for management and care

The gold standard for the management of children with VI or HI (or dual sensory impairment) is a multidisciplinary care package, with an integrated service comprising health, education, and social services. The infant and preschool child with VI requires ophthalmology and a peripatetic teacher of the visually impaired and for those with HI the provision of audiology, speech and language therapy, and peripatetic teacher of the deaf. During the early years, the children need access to highly specialized multidisciplinary paediatric teams with expertise in VI or HI and neurodisability, including paediatricians, psychologists, speech and language therapists, occupational therapists, and other clinicians as required. Because of the vulnerabilities of the early years, intervention should promote general development and progress should be closely monitored and reviewed. School-age children continue to need input from the full range of services and on-going support from specialist teachers for VI or HI. Close monitoring of progress from all perspectives will need to continue, with occasional review by multidisciplinary specialist services as required (e.g., at times of education transition). Individualized family centred care, including working with parents in partnership, is known to be the most effective care model for supporting any family with a child with disability.

Assessment of cognition and language

Regular developmental assessments across infancy and preschool years are needed to monitor development and progress. The Reynell Zinkin Scales of Visual Handicap (Reynell & Zinkin, 1978) are the only semi-standardized developmental scales for VI infants (to 5 year olds) and have separate blind, partially sighted, and sighted norms. There is no equivalent for children with HI, although from 2 years of age the Leiter International Performance Scale-Revised is a useful assessment of non verbal reasoning, memory, and attention skills (Roid & Miller, 1997). Auditory/verbal tests and visual/non verbal cognitive tests can be used to assess the child's intellectual level of ability in VI and HI children respectively. Very few standardized tests of intelligence or neuropsychological processes have norms for VI or HI children; test results should, therefore, be interpreted cautiously. The Intelligence Tests for Visually Impaired Children-ITVIC (Dekker *et al.*, 1991) has Dutch norms for children with no or low vision and covers non verbal subtests including haptic and spatial discrimination, memory, and reasoning. Particular challenges occur for testing VI or HI children's language abilities when using standardized language tests, which are pictorial or oral linguistic respectively.

A minority of children with VI have specific difficulties in reading or "braille dyslexia," though the causes are debated (Dodd & Conn, 2000; Greaney & Reason, 2000). Dyslexia is particularly challenging to diagnose in the context of HI as it is difficult to distinguish from the typical or expected impact of HI on the development of literacy skills and is probably under-identified (Edwards, 2010). No specific test of phonological awareness, reading, and spelling is reliable for testing HI children, but some are found to be clinically helpful in describing the difficulties experienced.

Psychological and psychiatric services

In all community and specialized services, holistic positive psychology approaches focussing on normalization, quality of life, self-determination and effective problem solving and coping abilities may assist young people and their families. These protective factors may enhance resilience and self-worth and help overcome the negative self-concept, stigma, and discrimination associated with disability (Wehmeyer, 2013). The richness and diversity of Blind culture and community, such as Blind Sports, and Deaf culture and community with the use of British Sign Language for communication need to be fully recognized.

Nevertheless, the clinician needs to be alert to the full range of possible psychopathology in children and young people with VI or HI, as in sighted peers. Formulation, diagnostic, and treatment approaches draw on the same principles as with a typical child of similar age and intellectual capacity, but need to be informed and tailored to needs arising from the VI or HI.

Access to psychological and psychiatric services comprising professionals with the expertise needed to work with children with VI or HI is still limited. A very small number of highly specialized paediatric services have integrated psychological input for children with VI or HI as part of the specialized developmental vision service or cochlear implant programme respectively. Only a minority of these services include psychologists. The large number of referrals to these services for assistance with behavioral and emotional difficulties highlights the clinical need for specialized provision for supporting children with sensory impairments and their families and educators.

In the absence of support or help from these services, young children may be attended by their local child development team and older children and adolescents may be referred to Child and Adolescent Mental Health Services (CAMHS). In recent years, a small number of specialist Deaf Child and Adolescent Mental Health Services (DCAMHS) have been developed to provide input to deaf children whose primary mode of communication is sign language. Wherever the child is treated, it is essential that their communication abilities and preferences are understood and accommodated, using sign language interpreters if required. Training in deaf awareness and knowledge of the cultural and developmental aspects of deafness are important for working with children with HI and their families. Training in awareness about VI, how to interact with and interpret the socio-emotional responses of the young person (e.g., lack of facial expression, eye contact, and other bodily communications) and knowledge of the developmental and psychological aspects of VI are important for working with children with VI and their families.

Management and intervention may be more complicated compared to those in typically developing children with emotional or behavioral disorders as the child with VI or HI is likely to have more professionals and services already involved in their care.

Global perspective

An estimated 19 million children are visually impaired worldwide. Of these, 12 million children are visually impaired due to refractive errors, a condition that could be easily diagnosed and corrected. Over one million children have an irreversible VI of which nearly a half of these could have been avoidable (Kong *et al.*, 2012). The prevalence of VI is related to the socio economic status of the country, reaching 15 per 10,000 in low income countries, primarily due to diseases and risk factors (measles, vitamin A deficiency and malaria). A rising incidence of retinopathy of prematurity is occurring in middle income countries, such as Latin America and some eastern European countries, as more low weight premature babies survive and more specialized neonatal care is required. In the United Kingdom, children from some ethnic minorities, in particular Pakistani and Bangladeshi groups, are over represented among children with VI. The needs of ethnic minority families with children with VI are harder to establish because they are under represented in health research (Rahi *et al.*, 2005).

Sixty two million children worldwide under the age of 15 years are hearing impaired, with two thirds of those living in low- and middle income countries (Olusanya *et al.*, 2005) with poor health care and lack of prevention for infections such as rubella and meningitis. Limited or no access to hearing aids or cochlear implants, along with cultural beliefs, stigma, and discrimination, result in children failing to develop effective communication or language and thus their exclusion from family and society, with no prospect of employment. A significant number of children from immigrant families in the UK, USA, and other high income countries present to audiological services "late" with undiagnosed HI as a result of lack of screening in their country of origin. The delay in access to appropriate audiological care typically has an irreversible impact on long-term outcomes and the situation is frequently exacerbated by difficulty engaging families with health and educational services, which needs to be addressed as part of a package of care for the child and family.

Useful websites for further information

1. Visual impairment:
   www.rnib.org.uk;
   www.vision2020uk.org.uk
2. Hearing impairment:
   www.ndcs.org.uk;
   www.earfoundation.org.uk

References

Visual impairment

Absoud, M. *et al.* (2010) Developing a schedule to identify social communication difficulties and autism spectrum disorder in young children with visual impairment. *Developmental Medicine & Child Neurology* **53**, 285–288.

Amedi, A. *et al.* (2004) Transcranial magnetic stimulation of the occipital pole interferes with verbal processing in blind subjects. *Nature Neuroscience* **7**, 1266–1270.

Ardito, R.B. *et al.* (2004) Attachment representations in adults with congenital blindness: association with maternal interactive behaviours during childhood. *Psychological Reports* **95**, 263–274.

Atkinson, J. & Braddick, O. (2011) From genes to brain development to phenotypic behavior: "dorsal-stream vulnerability" in relation to spatial cognition, attention, and planning of actions in Williams syndrome (WS) and other developmental disorders. *Progress in Brain Research* **189**, 261–283.

Bedny, M. *et al.* (2009) Growing up blind does not change the neural bases of Theory of Mind. *Proceedings of the National Academy of Sciences* **106**, 11312–11317.

Bigelow, A.E. (2003) The development of joint attention in blind infants. *Development and Psychopathology* **15**, 259–275.

Brambring, M. & Asbrock, D. (2010) Validity of false belief tasks in blind children. *Journal of Autism and Developmental Disorders* **40**, 1471–1484.

Brown, R. *et al.* (1997) Are there "Autistic-like" features in congenitally blind children? *Journal of Child Psychology and Psychiatry* **38**, 693–703.

Cass, H.D. *et al.* (1994) Developmental setback in severe visual impairment. *Archives of Disease in Childhood* **70**, 192–196.

Chadha, R.K. & Subramanian, A. (2011) The effect of visual impairment on quality of life of children aged 3–16 years. *British Journal of Ophthalmology* **95**, 642–645.

Dale, N. *et al.* (2002) Developmental outcome, including setback, in young children with severe visual impairment. *Developmental Medicine & Child Neurology* **44**, 613–622.

Dale, N. *et al.* (2007) Early support developmental journal for children with visual impairment: the case for a new developmental framework for early intervention. *Child: Care, Health and Development* **33**, 684–690.

Dale, N.J. *et al.* (2013) Social communicative variation in 1–3-year-olds with severe visual impairment. *Child: Care, Health and Development* **40**, 158–164.

Dekker, R. *et al.* (1991) Results of the intelligence test for visually impaired children (ITVIC). *Journal of Visual Impairment & Blindness* **65**, 261–267.

Dodd, B. & Conn, L. (2000) The effect of Braille orthography on blind children's phonological awareness. *Journal of Research in Reading* **23**, 1–11.

Dyck, M.J. *et al.* (2004) Emotion recognition/understanding ability in hearing or vision-impaired children: do sounds, sights, or words make the difference? *Journal of Child Psychology and Psychiatry* **45**, 789–800.

The Ear Foundation (2012) *Prevalence of additional disabilities with deafness: a review of the literature.* Report for NDCS.

Fazzi, E. *et al.* (2007) Leber's congenital amaurosis: is there an autistic component? *Developmental Medicine & Child Neurology* **49**, 503–507.

Föcker, J. *et al.* (2012) The superiority in voice processing of the blind arises from neural plasticity at sensory processing stages. *Neuropsychologia* **50**, 2056–2067.

Fraiberg, S. (1977) *Insights from the Blind: Comparative Studies of Blind and Sighted Infants.* Plenum, New York.

Giesen, J.M. *et al.* (2012) Academic supports, cognitive disability and mathematics acheivement for visually impaired youth: a multilevel modeling approach. *International Journal of Special Education* **27**, 1–10.

Gori, M. *et al.* (2010) Poor haptic orientation discrimination in non-sighted children may reflect disruption of cross-sensory calibration. *Current Biology* **20**, 223–225.

Greaney, J. & Reason, R. (2000) Braille reading by children: is there a phonological explanation for their difficulties? *British Journal of Visual Impairment* **18**, 35–40.

Green, S. *et al.* (2004) An investigation of first-order false belief understanding of children with congenital profound visual impairment. *British Journal of Developmental Psychology* **22**, 1–17.

Harris, J. *et al.* (2012) *Sight Impaired at Age Seven: Secondary Analysis of the Millennium Cohort Survey.* RSLB, RNIB and NatCen Social Research, London, UK.

Hobson, R.P. & Lee, A. (2010) Reversible autism among congenitally blind children? A controlled follow-up study. *Journal of Child Psychology and Psychiatry* **51**, 1235–1241.

Hughes, M. *et al.* (1999) Characteristics of maternal directiveness and responsiveness with young children with visual impairments. *Child: Care, Health and Development* **25**, 285–298.

Huurre, T.M. *et al.* (2001) Relationships with parents and friends, self-esteem and depression among adolescents with visual impairments. *Scandinavian Journal of Disability Research* **3**, 21–37.

Jan, J.E. *et al.* (1977) *Visual Impairment in Children and Adolescents.* Grune & Stratton, New York.

Kef, S. & Deković, M. (2004) The role of parental and peer support in adolescents well-being: a comparison of adolescents with and without a visual impairment. *Journal of Adolescence* **27**, 453–466.

Khan, S.A. *et al.* (2011) Therapeutic options in the management of sleep disorders in visually impaired children: a systematic review. *Clinical Therapeutics* **33**, 168–181.

Koenes, S.G. & Karshmer, J.F. (2000) Depression: a comparison study between blind and sighted adolescents. *Issues in Mental Health Nursing* **21**, 269–279.

Kong, L. *et al.* (2012) An update on progress and the changing epidemiology of causes of childhood blindness worldwide. *Journal of American Association for Pediatric Ophthalmology and Strabismus* **16**, 501–507.

Lifshitz, H. *et al.* (2007) Self concept, adjustment to blindness, and quality of friendship among adolescents with visual impairments. *Journal of Visual Impairment and Blindness* **101**, 96–107.

Moore, V. & McConachie, H. (1994) Communication between blind and severely visually impaired children and their parents. *British Journal of Developmental Psychology* **12**, 491–502.

Mukaddes, N.M. *et al.* (2007) Autism in visually impaired individuals. *Psychiatry and Clinical Neurosciences* **61**, 39–44.

Ollendick, T.H. *et al.* (1985) Fears in visually-impaired and normally-sighted youths. *Behaviour Research and Therapy* **23**, 375–378.

Parr, J.R. *et al.* (2010) Social communication difficulties and autism spectrum disorder in young children with optic nerve hypoplasia and/or septo-optic dysplasia. *Developmental Medicine & Child Neurology* **52**, 917–921.

Pijnacker, J. *et al.* (2012) Pragmatic abilities in children with congenital visual impairment: an exploration of non-literal language and advanced theory of mind understanding. *Journal of Autism and Developmental Disorders* **42**, 2440–2449.

Pinquart, M. & Pfeiffer, J.P. (2011) Bullying in German adolescents: attending special school for students with visual impairment. *British Journal of Visual Impairment* **29**, 163–176.

Pinquart, M. & Pfeiffer, J.P. (2013) Change in psychological problems of adolescents with and without visual impairment. *European Child and Adolescent Psychiatry* **23**, 571–578.

Preisler, G.M. (1995) The development of communication in blind and in deaf infants—similarities and differences. *Child: Care, Health and Development* **21**, 79–110.

Pring, L. & Tadić, V. (2005) More than meets the eye: blindness, talent and autism. In: *Autism and Blindness: Research and Reflections.* (ed L. Pring). Whurr, London.

Rahi, J.S. *et al.* (2003) Severe visual impairment and blindness in children in the UK. *The Lancet* **362**, 1359–1365.

Rahi, J.S. *et al.* (2005) Health services experiences of parents of recently diagnosed visually impaired children. *British Journal of Ophthalmology* **89**, 213–218.

Rahi, J.S. *et al.* (2011) Capturing children and young people's perspectives to identify the content for a novel vision-related quality of life instrument. *Ophthalmology* **118**, 819–824.

Reynell, J. & Zinkin, P. (1978) Developmental patterns of visually handicapped children. *Child: Care, Health and Development* **4**, 291–303.

Sadato, N. *et al.* (2002) Critical period for cross-modal plasticity in blind humans: a functional MRI study. *NeuroImage* **16**, 389–400.

Sargent, J. *et al.* (2010) Children with severe brain damage: functional assessment for diagnosis and intervention. In: *Visual Impairment in Children due to Damage to the Brain.* (eds G.N. Dutton & M.C. Bax). MacKeith Press, London.

Sonksen, P.M. & Dale, N. (2002) Visual impairment in infancy: impact on neurodevelopmental and neurobiological processes. *Developmental Medicine & Child Neurology* **44**, 782–791.

Tadić, V. *et al.* (2009) Attentional processes in young children with congenital visual impairment. *British Journal of Developmental Psychology* **27**, 311–330.

Tadić, V. *et al.* (2010) Are language and social communication intact in children with congenital visual impairment at school age? *Journal of Child Psychology and Psychiatry* **51**, 696–705.

Tadić, V. *et al.* (2013) Story discourse and mental state language use between mothers and their school-aged children with and without visual impairment. *International Journal of Language and Communication Disorders* **48**, 679–688.

Tirosh, E. *et al.* (1998) Behavioural problems among visually impaired between 6 months and 5 years. *International Journal of Rehabilitation Research* **21**, 63–70.

Tröster, H. (2001) Sources of stress in mothers of young children with visual impairments. *Journal of Visual Impairment & Blindness* **95**, 623–637.

Webb, E.A. *et al.* (2013) Reduced ventral cingulum integrity and increased behavioural problems in children with isolated optic nerve hypoplasia and mild to moderate or no visual impairment. *PLos One* **8**, e59048.

Withagen, A. *et al.* (2013) Short term memory and working memory in blind versus sighted children. *Research in Developmental Disabilities* **34**, 2161–2172.

Wong, H.-B. *et al.* (2009) Visual impairment and its impact on health-related quality of life in adolescents. *American Journal of Ophthalmology* **147**, 505–511. ,

Hearing impairment

Antia, S.D. & Kriemeyer, K.H. (2003) Peer interactions of deaf and hearing children. In: *Oxford Handbook of Deaf Studies, Language, and Education.* (eds M. Marschark & P.E. Spencer, pp. 164–176). Oxford University Press, New York.

Bachara, G.H. *et al.* (1980) Empathy development in deaf preadolescents. *American Annals of the Deaf* **125**, 38–41.

Bavelier, D. & Neville, H.J. (2002) Cross-modal plasticity: where and how? *Nature Reviews Neuroscience* **3**, 443–452.

Bavelier, D. *et al.* (2000) Visual attention to the periphery is enhanced in congenitally deaf individuals. *Journal of Neuroscience* **20**, RC93, 1–6.

Berlin, C.I. *et al.* (2001) On renaming auditory neuropathy as auditory dys-synchrony. *Audiology Today* **13**, 15–17.

Blamey, P.J. (2003) Development of spoken language by deaf children. In: *The Oxford Handbook of Deaf Studies, Language, and Education. Volume 1.* (eds M. Marschark & P.E. Spencer), pp. 478–490. Oxford University Press, New York.

Cornes, A. *et al.* (2006) Reading the signs: impact of signed versus written questionnaires on the prevalence of psychopathology among deaf adolescents. *Australian and New Zealand Journal of Psychiatry* **40**, 665–673.

Dillon, C.M. *et al.* (2012) Phonological awareness, reading skills and vocabulary knowledge in children who use cochlear implants. *Journal of Deaf Studies and Deaf Education* **17**, 205–226.

Dye, M.W.G. *et al.* (2008) Visual attention in deaf children and adults. In: *Deaf Cognition: Foundations and Outcomes.* (eds M. Marschark & P.C. Hauser), pp. 250–263. Oxford University Press, New York.

Edwards, L. (2010) Learning disabilities in deaf and hard-of-hearing children. In: *The Oxford Handbook of Deaf Studies, Language, and Education. Volume 2.* (eds M. Marschark & P.E. Spencer), pp. 458–472. Oxford University Press, New York.

Edwards, A. *et al.* (2013) The mathematical abilities of children with cochlear implants. *Child Neuropsychology* **19**, 127–142.

Edwards, L. & Crocker, S. (2008a) Disorders of communication. In: *Psychological Processes in Deaf Children with Complex Needs: An Evidence-Based Practical Guide*, pp. 106–131. Jessica Kingsley Publishers, London.

Edwards, L. & Crocker, S. (2008b) Behavioural and emotional disorders. In: *Psychological Processes in Deaf Children with Complex Needs; An Evidence-Based Practical Guide*, pp. 40–60. Jessica Kingsley Publishers, London.

Fellinger, J. *et al.* (2009) Correlates of mental health disorders among children with hearing impairments. *Developmental Medicine and Child Neurology* **51**, 635–641.

Figueras, B. *et al.* (2008) Executive function and language in deaf children. *Journal of Deaf Studies and Deaf Education* **13**, 362–377.

Forli, F. *et al.* (2011) Systematic review of the literature on the clinical effectiveness of the cochlear implant procedure in paediatric patients. *Acta Otorhinolaryngologica Italica* **31**, 281–298.

Fulcher, A. *et al.* (2012) Listen up: children with early identified hearing loss achieve age-appropriate speech/language outcomes by 3 years-of-age. *International Journal of Pediatric Otorhinolaryngology* **76**, 1785–1794.

Gale, E. & Schick, B. (2009) Symbol-infused joint attention and language use in mothers with deaf and hearing toddlers. *American Annals of the Deaf* **153**, 484–503.

Goffi-Gomez, M.V. *et al.* (2012) Auditory brainstem implant outcomes and MAP parameters: report of experiences in adults and children. *International Journal of Pediatric Otorhinolaryngology* **76**, 257–264.

Gordon, K.A. *et al.* (2011) Use it or lose it? Lessons learned from the developing brains of children who are deaf and use cochlear implants to hear. *Brain Topography* **24**, 201–219.

Harris, M. & Terlektsi, E. (2011) Reading and spelling abilities of deaf adolescents with cochlear implants and hearing aids. *Journal of Deaf Studies and Deaf Education* **16**, 24–34.

Hauser, P.C. *et al.* (2008) Development of deaf and hard-of-hearing students' executive function. In: *Deaf Cognition: Foundations and Outcomes.* (eds M. Marschark & P.C. Hauser), pp. 286–308. Oxford University Press, New York.

Hindley, P.A. *et al.* (1994) Psychiatric disorder in deaf and hearing impaired children and young people: a prevalence study. *Journal of Child Psychology and Psychiatry* **35**, 917–934.

Hindley, P.A. & Kroll, L. (1998) Theoretical and epidemiological aspects of attention deficit and overactivity in deaf children. *Journal of Deaf Studies and Deaf Education* **3**, 64–72.

Hogan, A. *et al.* (2011) Communication and behavioural disorders among children with hearing loss increases risk of mental health disorders. *Australian and New Zealand Journal of Public Health* **35**, 377–383.

Horsch, U. *et al.* (1997) Stress experienced by parents of children with cochlear implants compared with parents of deaf children and hearing children. *American Journal of Otology* **18**, S161–S163.

Knutson, J.F. *et al.* (2004) Disciplinary choices of mother of deaf children and mothers of normally hearing children. *Child Abuse and Neglect* **28**, 925–937.

Kouwenberg, M. *et al.* (2012) Peer victimization experienced by children and adolescents who are deaf or hard of hearing. *PLoS One* **7**, e52174.

Kral, A. & Sharma, A. (2012) Developmental neuroplasticity after cochlear implantation. *Trends in Neurosciences* **35**, 111–122.

Kyle, F.E. & Harris, M. (2010) Predictors of reading development in deaf children: a three year longitudinal study. *Journal of Experimental Child Psychology* **107**, 229–243.

Lederberg, A.R. & Golbach, T. (2002) Parenting stress and social support in hearing mothers of deaf and hearing children: a longitudinal study. *Journal of Deaf Studies and Deaf Education* **7**, 330–345.

Levanen, S. & Hamdorf, D. (2001) Feeling vibrations: enhanced tactile sensitivity in congenitally deaf humans. *Neuroscience Letters* **301**, 75–77.

Ludlow, A. *et al.* (2010) Emotion recognition in children with profound and severe deafness: do they have a deficit in perceptual processing? *Journal of Clinical and Experimental Neuropsychology* **32**, 923–928.

Mance, J. & Edwards, L. (2012) Self-perceptions in adolescents with cochlear implants. *Cochlear Implants International* **13**, 93–104.

Marschark, M. & Hauser, P.C. (2008) *Deaf Cognition: Foundations and Outcomes.* Oxford University Press, New York.

Martin, D. *et al.* (2011) Peer relationships of deaf children with cochlear implants: predictors of peer entry and peer interaction success. *Journal of Deaf Studies and Deaf Education* **16**, 108–120.

Meadow-Orlans, K.P. *et al.* (1983) Attachment behaviour of deaf children with deaf parents. *Journal of the American Academy of Child Psychiatry* **22**, 23–28.

Meristo, M. *et al.* (2007) Language access and theory of mind reasoning: evidence from deaf children in bilingual and oralist environments. *Developmental Psychology* **43**, 1156–1169.

Neville, H.J. & Lawson, D. (1987) Attention to central and peripheral visual space in a movement detection task: an event related potential and behavioural study. II. Congenitally deaf adults. *Brain Research* **405**, 268–283.

Nowakowski, M.E. *et al.* (2009) Establishment of joint attention in dyads involving hearing mothers of deaf and hearing children, and its relation to adaptive social behaviour. *American Annals of the Deaf* **154**, 15–29.

Olusanya, B.O. *et al.* (2005) Childhood deafness poses problems in developing countries. *British Medical Journal* **330**, 480–481.

Pisoni, D.B. *et al.* (2008) Efficacy and effectiveness of cochlear implants in deaf infants. In: *Deaf Cognition: Foundations and Outcomes.* (eds M. Marschark & P.C. Hauser), pp. 52–101. Oxford University Press, New York.

Pisoni, D.B. *et al.* (2010) Executive function, cognitive control, and sequence learning in deaf children with cochlear implants. In: *The Oxford Handbook of Deaf Studies, Language, and Education. Volume 2.* (eds M. Marschark & P.E. Spencer), pp. 439–457. Oxford University Press, New York.

Qi, S. & Mitchell, R.E. (2012) Large-scale academic achievement testing of deaf and hard-of-hearing students: past, present and future. *Journal of Deaf Studies and Deaf Education* **17**, 1–18.

Quittner, A.L. *et al.* (2010) Parenting stress among parents of deaf and hearing children: associations with language delays and behaviour problems. *Parenting, Science and Practice* **10**, 136–155.

Remmel, E. & Peters, K. (2009) Theory of mind and language in children with cochlear implants. *Journal of Deaf Studies and Deaf Education* **14**, 218–236.

Russell, P.A. *et al.* (1998) The development of theory of mind in deaf children. *Journal of Child Psychology and Psychiatry* **39**, 903–910.

Roid, G.H. & Miller, L.J. (1997) *Leiter International Performance Scale-Revised.* Stoelting Co, Illinois.

Spangler, Y.H. (1987) *Exploration of the relationship between deaf children's attachment classification in the strange situation and effects of parents' success in grieving and coping.* Dissertation, Los Angeles, CA.

Stredler-Brown, A. (2010) Communication choices and outcomes during the early years: an assessment and evidence-based approach. In: *The Oxford Handbook of Deaf Studies, Language, and Education (Volume 2).* (eds M. Marschark & P.E. Spencer), pp. 292–315. Oxford University Press, New York.

Szymanski, C.A. *et al.* (2012) Deaf children with autism spectrum disorders. *Journal of Autism and Developmental Disorders* **42**, 2027–2037.

Van Gent, T. *et al.* (2011) Self-concept and psychopathology in deaf adolescents: preliminary support for moderating effects of deafness-related characteristics and peer problems. *Journal of Child Psychology and Psychiatry* **52**, 720–728.

Wehmeyer, M.L. (ed) (2013) *The Oxford Handbook of Positive Psychology and Disability.* Oxford University Press, USA.

CHAPTER 48

Assessment and treatment in nonspecialist community health care settings

Tami Kramer and M. Elena Garralda

Academic Unit of Child and Adolescent Psychiatry, Imperial College London, UK

Introduction

Nonspecialist community health-care settings, referred to as primary health-care services, are the first point of contact for families seeking professional attention for health problems. Primary care aims to clarify demand, diagnose disorder, offer information, advice, treatment, and rehabilitation as well as coordinate care with other disciplines and health sectors over time (Boerma, 2006). The place of primary health care in the management of mental health problems has long been recognized, as has the need to enhance its role and build capacity to help reduce the global burden of suffering and impairment caused by mental and behavioral disorders (WHO, 2005). Moreover, the primary care setting offers scope for prevention and early intervention for these disorders. Its role in the field of child and adolescent mental health (CAMH) has been comparatively little documented, but evidence for its potential is slowly accumulating.

This chapter outlines the different structures of nonspecialist community or primary health-care settings across countries, documenting presentations of children and young people with mental health problems in primary care settings and discussing their identification and management by primary care workers. It documents innovative models of mental health service delivery involving partnerships and coordinated care across different health sectors and considers the place of primary health care in the prevention of child mental health disorders. We refer to the setting under consideration predominantly as primary health care and will use the terms general or family practitioners/physicians interchangeably.

Generalist primary health settings

Primary health-care services vary widely across different countries in funding source, setting, staffing provision relative to

the size of the population, and support from specialist services. Services are delivered by a range of physicians, usually general practitioners or family physicians, and/or general and community pediatricians as well as nonphysician health workers, often nurses, health visitors, or public health workers. European pediatric primary care is medically delivered by family practitioners (41%), pediatricians (24%), or a combination of the two (35%), although there has been a recent decline in the number of primary care pediatricians (van Esso et al., 2010). Conversely, in the United States where pediatricians, family physicians, and nurse practitioners provide pediatric primary care, over the last three decades provision by pediatricians has increased (Freed et al., 2010), while in Canada pediatric primary care is provided largely by general practitioners and public health units.

Family practitioners and pediatricians provide different patterns of preventative and curative care (Freed et al., 2004). Family practitioners tend to become involved in prevention and management of physical health problems especially of young children, whereas primary care pediatricians have a broader remit, encompassing the prevention and community management of physical problems, assessing growth and development, child protection, school medicine, behavior problems, and teenage health. It is worth noting, however, that only 40% of countries have community pediatricians and consequently the type and quality of primary care for child mental health problems varies considerably (Katz et al., 2002).

In many low and middle income countries (LMICs), the point of first contact with health services is public health workers, whereas pediatricians provide specialized Western-type medical care (Cheng, 2004). Lay and community or village health workers are trained to offer selected clinical and preventive services as part of "*task shifting*," the practice of delegating tasks to workers with lesser professional and nonprofessional training in order to increase capacity (Bruckner et al., 2011; Fulton et al., 2011). Primary and secondary health care delivery for children in

Rutter's Child and Adolescent Psychiatry, Sixth Edition.
Edited by Anita Thapar and Daniel S. Pine, James F. Leckman, Stephen Scott, Margaret J. Snowling, Eric Taylor.
© 2015 John Wiley & Sons Ltd. Published 2018 by John Wiley & Sons Ltd.

LMICs may also include primary care clinics or health centers, child clinics, school medical services, emergency departments, and ambulatory hospital/outpatient departments. As in higher income countries, funding may be private, insurance based, or part of centrally organized national or regional health services.

In addition to the wide array of different service structures and personnel the level of training given to primary care workers in child and mental health has an impact on provision. Training, however, is quite limited overall. Mean length of specialist pediatric training for family doctors in Europe is 4 months and some have none (van Esso et al., 2010): training in child mental health is even less prevalent. The WHO Child Mental Health Atlas (2005) reported that in only 15% of countries had at least a quarter of their pediatricians received mental health training.

Core roles of primary health care for child and adolescent mental health

As primary care services generally provide the most widespread initial point of contact for health services, they are ideally placed for a role in mental health promotion, prevention, and early intervention. They are also in an ideal position to clarify concerns, signpost help, and refer more severe and complex cases to specialist services. At the same time, they are able to directly offer advice and intervention for milder problems through psycho education and supportive counseling, parenting support, psychotropic medication, and brief cognitive/behavior therapy (see Box 48.1). For children with chronic conditions primary health care has an on going role in monitoring, supporting and coordinating interventions with secondary and tertiary health services, social services, education, and nongovernmental organizations.

The particular scope of the role of primary health care will be determined by local factors and health provision should be shaped accordingly. Disparities in specialist child psychiatric and mental health services are wide, with a higher concentration of services in urban and affluent areas (Morris et al., 2011); poorer and more rural communities frequently having little or no access and being therefore more reliant on primary care. A European survey found that the populations covered by child psychiatrists ranged from 5300 to 52,000 individuals (Remschmidt & van Engeland, 1999). In most countries in Africa, the Eastern Mediterranean, Southeast Asia, and Western Pacific, this range is much broader, of the order of 1 to 4 child psychiatrists per million population. Within countries with

well-developed specialist mental health services, there is an opportunity for primary care to act as a referral gateway to mental health specialists. Where these services are scarce, primary care will act more as a direct source of care with specialists' efforts focussing on supporting primary care providers.

No country has documented fully meeting the need for child and adolescent mental health services (CAMHS) (WHO, 2005). Over the years, this worldwide deficit in provision has resulted in calls to develop the role of primary health care as a means of helping bridge the gap. Primary care has unique strengths as it offers broad direct access, reduced stigma, continuity over time, and knowledge about situations that put children at risk for psychiatric disorders such as families with parental mental illness or substance misuse. Despite this, implementation of programs to increase primary care capacity has been slow. Across most countries, less than 10% of CAMHS are provided by primary care (WHO, 2005).

Child and adolescent mental health problems in nonspecialist primary care settings

Frequency of contact with primary health care

Contact with primary health care is a common experience in childhood and adolescence. Over the course of 1 year, most parents take their children to primary health care services, and work with children has been estimated to occupy a significant proportion of primary care consultations (18% with under 15 year olds in the United Kingdom, 17% in the United States, and 12% in Australia) (Freed et al., 2004; Britt et al., 2008; RCGP, 2008). There are age trends with young preschool children being seen more often than older children, but even so surveys, mainly from high income countries, estimate that as many as 70–90% of young people are in contact with primary care services at least once a year (Tylee et al., 2007), offering a significant potential for intervention.

Modes of presentation

Children and young people present to primary health care for acute complaints as well as health surveillance. The majority of consultations relate primarily to physical concerns. Surveys in various countries have documented that only 1–6% of children and adolescents attending primary care or general pediatric clinics present with primary psychological, behavioral, social, or educational problems (Garralda & Bailey, 1986, 1989; Kramer & Garralda, 1998; Eapen et al., 2004), though other countries

Box 48.1 Key roles in nonspecialist health care settings.

Promotion of mental health and well-being	Early intervention
Prevention of psychiatric disorder and developmental disability	Brief interventions for less severe and complex conditions
First point of contact for concerns	Support and care coordination for chronic conditions
Clarification of concerns	

report higher rates of up to 10% (Haller *et al.*, 2007; Hetlevik *et al.*, 2010). One large survey in the United States demonstrated that 1% of emergency department visits concerned primary mental health presentations and, of those, patients with mood disorders and psychosis were most likely to present more than once.

Other points of contact

Moreover, broad access to children and young people within school provides opportunities for primary health intervention including attention to emotional and behavioral well-being, risk reduction, resilience building, mental health promotion, and access to help for mental health disorders, thus complementing primary health care provision (Table 48.1) (see Chapter 42).

Identification of mental health problems in primary care

Frequency and nature of psychiatric disorder in attenders

There is evidence that psychiatric disorders are present in a considerably higher number of children attending primary health care than may be expected from the overt presenting complaint or from expected disorder rates in the population (Ford *et al.*, 2007). Research interviews with children and parents, following primary care contact, have found psychiatric disorders in one-tenth to one-quarter of children across different countries (Garralda & Bailey, 1986; Costello *et al.*, 1988; Gureje *et al.*, 1994; Eapen *et al.*, 2004), with higher rates in adolescents (40%), (Kramer & Garralda, 1998), schoolchildren attending hospital pediatric outpatients (28%) (Garralda & Bailey, 1989), and children and young people who are frequent service attenders (29% in 7–12 year olds) (Bowman & Garralda, 1993; Vila *et al.*, 2012).

Although the range of psychiatric disorders are represented emotional disorders predominate (Garralda & Bailey, 1986; Kramer & Garralda, 1998), with mild to moderate Diagnostic and Statistical Manual of Mental Disorders (DSM). DSM-IV

defined anxiety disorders in a third of attenders (Burns *et al.*, 1995; Leaf *et al.*, 1996; Chavira *et al.*, 2004). It is likely that the psychiatric disorder contributes to consultations because of the poorer physical well-being of children with emotional disorders and high levels of parental stress about these children (Kramer & Garralda, 1998; Garralda *et al.*, 1999). Mainly, psychiatric symptoms are not mentioned during consultations and go unrecognized.

In the United Kingdom, elevated levels of persistent depressive symptoms (both subsyndromal and diagnosable depressive disorders) have been detected in adolescents attending general practice in both urban and suburban areas reinforcing the relevance of primary care for adolescent depression across socioeconomic groups (Yates *et al.*, 2004; Gledhill & Garralda, 2011, 2013). Depressive symptoms in adolescents attending primary care are associated with increased risk of substance abuse and school problems (Yates *et al.*, 2004; Burns *et al.*, 2004). This and high levels of depressive disorder in young people attending other community health settings, such as sexual health clinics (Fernandez *et al.*, 2009), suggest that identifying psychopathology within primary care will provide the opportunity to address a wide range of psychosocial difficulties.

Within LMICs, however, neuro-psychiatric problems, such as those associated with epilepsy, may be more prominent within clinic-attending populations in line with the increased population levels of brain damage and severe intellectual disability (Patel *et al.*, 2008).

Recognizing need and diagnosing disorder

Attention to mental health problems in primary care is only possible once the problems, their nature, and severity are recognized and any demand for intervention clarified. As a first step, recognition requires either an expression of need by the parent or young person or spontaneous enquiry by the practitioner. However, although parental expression of concern increases clinician recognition (Sayal & Taylor, 2004), and even though many parents believe that it is appropriate to express difficulties with child

Table 48.1 Relative merits of primary health care versus school interventions for mental health problems.

Primary health care	School
Nonstigmatizing	Nonstigmatizing
Confidential	Uncertain confidentiality
Access to most children and young people including school nonattenders	Access to many children and young people
Identification of difficulties dependent on patient expression of concern	Behavioral concerns identified more frequently than emotional difficulties
Practitioners often know family circumstances	Knowledge of family limited
Some doctors specifically trained	Some teachers trained in special needs
Training needs in screening, intervention and referral	Training needs in screening, class management and referral
Setting suitable for individual brief consultations	Setting requires adaptation for individual consultation

behavior to a primary care provider, few with such concerns do so (Horwitz *et al.*, 1998; Ellingson *et al.*, 2004; Sayal & Taylor, 2004). For children under 4 years old, Ellingson *et al.* (2004) demonstrated that whether parents discuss the child's problems was linked to parental worry, perceived low socio-emotional competence in the child, and disruption to family routines.

As children enter adolescence their own readiness to raise concerns is important. Nevertheless, even when adolescents perceive themselves to have serious difficulties, half fail to mention them during the consultation; conversely, practitioners fail to discuss psychological issues even when they perceive them to be present (Martinez *et al.*, 2006). Sayal's (2006) systematic review documented low rates of recognition of both psychiatric disorder and broader psychosocial concerns, with recognition low in sensitivity (15–20% for psychiatric disorder and 50–57% for psychosocial difficulties) but high specificity (84–96%). The higher sensitivity for recognition of psychosocial difficulties over psychiatric disorder might reflect either practitioner's greater awareness of psychosocial problems or their reluctance to use psychiatric diagnostic labels (Iliffe *et al.*, 2008).

Determinants of parental and youth help-seeking

Broad socio-cultural attitudes and values have an impact on decisions to seek help for mental health across population groups. Sayal *et al.*'s (2010) UK qualitative study classified barriers to parental help-seeking for child mental health concerns into parental perceptions of service features (such as difficulty getting appointments and short appointments), fear of the consequences of identification—for example, embarrassment, stigma, and labeling—and being judged a bad parent. The study also identified trust in the service and continuity of care as facilitators of parental help-seeking.

From the perspective of young people themselves, barriers to seeking help include a perceived lack of youth friendly services, stigma, and embarrassment, lack of mental health literacy, a belief that treatment will not help, and a preference for self-reliance (Rickwood *et al.*, 2007; Tylee *et al.*, 2007; Vanheusden *et al.*, 2008; Gulliver *et al.*, 2010). The facilitators of youth help-seeking are less well researched, but include positive past experiences, social support, and encouragement from others, as well as perceptions that doctors are interested in psychosocial issues (Ferrin *et al.*, 2009; Gulliver *et al.*, 2010).

Determinants of practitioner recognition

Practitioner recognition of mental health problems during consultations has been linked to a wide range of factors. These include (i) disorder-related issues such as severity and type of presenting physical symptoms—severe and chronic problems, digestive and ill-defined presentations being more likely to lead to identification of psychiatric morbidity; (ii) socio-demographic, with better recognition in males, 7–14 year olds over younger children, and in the presence of social difficulties such as socioeconomic disadvantage, broken homes, adverse life events, and academic problems; (iii) type of

consultation: well child clinics faring better than acute care visits; and (iv) a variety of other factors, such as the clinician's relationship with the child, parental and young persons' perception of difficulty, young persons' fears, impairment, and previous treatment for psychological problems (Goldberg *et al.*, 1984; Kramer & Garralda, 1998; Brugman *et al.*, 2001; Haller *et al.*, 2009).

Cultural factors and ethnic minority status might also affect recognition. In a Dutch study of well child visits by Crone *et al.* (2010), identification of psychosocial problems by clinicians was lower in children of Turkish and Moroccan descent compared with those of Dutch background.

However, overall, the best predictor of a primary care clinician (PCC) identifying a child's mental health problem is whether parents draw the clinician's attention to them rather than any clinician-initiated procedure (Zuckerbrot *et al.*, 2007).

It follows that important first steps in promoting primary care identification of child mental health problems should consider public education aimed at diminishing stigma and identifying primary care as a source of help, thus enabling parents and adolescents to identify needs and express them during the consultation. These expressions of concern by parents and adolescents will need to be met with practitioner understanding, empathy, and appropriate interventions, informed by adequate knowledge of normal development, emotional and behavioral problems, and evidence-based treatments. Primary care services will need to enhance capacity and interest in the field, and this will only be possible when clinicians feel confident to do so (Sanci *et al.*, 2010).

Systematic screening or case-finding

Use of screening or case finding instruments such as questionnaires has been considered a potentially quick and easy method to improve primary care identification of emotional and behavioral difficulty. Instruments should be brief; easy to administer, score and interpret; have adequate reliability and validity; identify a significant proportion of those with problems; and provide developmentally appropriate and clinically useful information. Case identification should lead to interventions which improve prognosis.

Primary care studies on questionnaires targeting emotional and behavioral symptoms demonstrate reasonable sensitivity, specificity and feasibility across the age range (Zuckerbrot *et al.*, 2007; US Preventive Services Task Force, 2009) as does the alternative approach of brief systematic clinical questioning by clinicians (Rutman *et al.*, 2008; Wintersteen, 2010). However, the implementation of screening programs such as the American Medical Association's Guideline for Adolescent Preventive Screening has had mixed results, and increased screening is also likely to enhance the need for specialist CAMHS (Elster & Kuznets, 1994; Ozer *et al.*, 2009).

Electronic screening

One means of facilitating primary care mental health screening is use of computer or internet-based tools by young people waiting to see the primary care practitioner (PCP) (Stevens *et al.*, 2008; Fein *et al.*, 2010) but further work is required on practical implementation, including the process for feeding results to practitioners and how information is used within the consultation.

At best, however, screening questionnaires or systematic screening questions provide a guide for further enquiry. Importantly, evidence on whether they lead to improved access to effective intervention or to better health outcomes is lacking. Moreover, this depends on whether identified adolescents feel "ready" to accept intervention (Tanielian *et al.*, 2009) and this "readiness" is likely to be linked to cultural factors (Brown *et al.*, 2007). The adult literature shows that screening or case finding for adult depression in primary care shows little or no impact on recognition, management, or outcome of depression (Gilbody *et al.*, 2005), unless this is embedded within a broader program of collaborative care (Gilbody *et al.*, 2006).

Delivering interventions, partnerships, and coordinated care

It is clear that policies aiming to reduce the service gap in meeting the mental health needs of children and young people through improved access to interventions within primary care will only be realized through substantial expansion of primary care provision. Unfortunately, there is a dearth of quality intervention research (Martinez-Castaldi *et al.*, 2008). Nevertheless, descriptions of innovative collaborative approaches have begun to accumulate. They include a focus on complex interventions for specific disorders, broad restructuring of service design and delivery, and incorporation of the collaborative approach found to be effective in the adult population. These approaches will now be summarized following a description of the more traditional models.

Traditional models of service design and delivery

A systematic review of child mental health interventions offered within primary care in the UK (Bower *et al.*, 2001) identified three different types of services: (i) management by specialist mental health professionals in primary care, often referred to as shifted outpatient clinics; (ii) treatments offered by the primary care team; and (iii) consultation liaison models. The review identified few quality studies to support these approaches and highlighted the need for research.

Specialist or shifted mental health clinics

Early work on treatment by specialist staff within primary care included brief interventions (6–12 sessions) and a variety of techniques such as psychiatric evaluation and guidance, nondirective counseling, parent education and counseling, cognitive behavior and family therapies, dynamic therapy, group work, and child education (Bower *et al.*, 2001). More recent evaluations of outreach psychologist, therapy or nurse primary care clinics have yielded mixed results (Day & Davis, 2006; Kolko *et al.*, 2010).

Despite this, in the US "colocation" of mental health specialists within primary care facilities is advocated as a means of improving mental health service utilization through diminishing stigma, while at the same time increasing care coordination and educational exchanges between primary care and specialist practitioners (Williams *et al.*, 2006). Comprehensive coverage of primary care settings of this kind would, however, require high numbers of mental health specialists and is probably not achievable in most regions of the world.

Treatments offered by the primary care team

There has been limited study of the management of child emotional and behavioral difficulties offered by the actual primary care team. Although early work by one general practitioner using preventative interviews with preschool children demonstrated significant improvement in some child outcomes (Cullen, 1976), widespread primary care management of mood or anxiety syndromes (Wren *et al.*, 2005) or attention deficit hyperactivity disorder (ADHD) (Sonuga-Barke *et al.*, 2004) would appear to be uncommon and ineffective. Thus, the impact of the work of PCCs themselves within traditional models of service delivery remains relatively untested and recent work has focused on more complex and collaborative models of care (Table 48.2).

Consultation-liaison

Consultation-liaison, where the specialist acts to support primary care management rather than take responsibility for individual patients (Gask *et al.*, 1997) has traditionally been viewed as a means of increasing the capacity of PCCs to offer mental health services, partly through improving their skills and knowledge.

Table 48.2 Child & adolescent psychiatric problems appropriate for direct primary health care intervention.

Nature of problems	
	Childhood disruptive behavior disorders (including ADHD)
	Somatization
	Anxiety disorders
	Depressive disorders
	Adjustment disorders
Severity of problems	
	Mild-moderate impairment
	Low complexity (e.g., no co morbidity, low family risk)
Treatment needs	
	Psycho,education
	Self-help
	Parenting support/intervention
	Medication
	Brief psychotherapy

CAMHS work in this area has been little documented or evaluated (Neiro-Munoz & Ward, 1998). In a model by Connor et al. (2006), a child psychiatrist or specialist nurse offered telephone consultation during office hours to 139 PCP's. A proportion of cases were then managed within primary care while the rest were referred to the child psychiatrist for assessment within 4 weeks. During the first 18 months, the child psychiatrist offered direct evaluation to half the patients. Time was also spent educating PCP's in case conferences and informal consultations. This model served as a pilot for developing a more complex intervention, the Massachusetts Child Psychiatry Access Project (MCPAP), described later.

In the UK, a survey of all specialist CAMHS in England demonstrated that collaborative work with primary care was significantly associated with well developed 'specialist' provision, and larger sized services (Bradley et al., 2003). This confirms the difficulty for small specialist CAMHS to provide consultation liaison in primary care. Furthermore, future work will need to address the medico legal responsibilities in those cases where PCP's with limited training and experience in the area provide treatment on the advice of specialist clinicians, especially when prescribing psychotropic medications.

Newer models of collaborative care
Disorder specific models
Collaborative care differs from the traditional models described earlier as it is a complex, multifaceted, organizational intervention involving combinations of staff working in new ways, with varied content and intensity (Bower et al., 2006). These programs include the flexible use of consultants, care managers as patient educators, and mental health clinicians working with PCCs. This model has shown effectiveness for adults with depression and anxiety, especially when they have access to an adult psychiatrist.

Adolescent depressive disorders
The use of the collaborative care model in child mental health has been best addressed in adolescent depression. Asarnow et al.'s (2005) quality improvement study (Youth Partners in Care) was the first multisite effectiveness trial for depressed adolescents in primary care. It demonstrated superiority over usual care in reducing depressive symptoms, and increasing both quality of life and satisfaction with care at 6-months posttreatment. The intervention included: (i) expert leader teams at each site; (ii) care managers to support PCCs with evaluation, education, medication and psychosocial treatment, and with linking to specialist mental health services; (iii) training care managers in manualized cognitive behavior therapy (CBT); and (iv) access to participant and clinician choice of treatment. Treatment options included CBT, medication, combined CBT with medication, care manager follow-up, and specialist referral. At 12 and 18 month follow-up, there was a trend for between-group differences, although these were not statistically significant (Asarnow et al., 2009). The sample size in this study was smaller than that in adult studies and

larger samples might be required to demonstrate significant differences.

Of note, the majority of youth in either treatment arm failed to take up any intervention, indicating that universal treatment coverage was far from achieved, and for those that did there were higher rates of uptake for psychotherapy. In light of the known efficacy of medication and combined treatments for adolescent depression (March et al., 2004; Brent et al., 2008), these findings suggest that additional attention to health beliefs and treatment-readiness might be required as part of psycho education.

Within the UK, the TIDY program or Therapeutic Identification of Depression in Young people (Kramer et al., 2012) has been developed incorporating specific training for PCPs. The target is screening and identifying depression, followed by primary care delivered interventions for mild and moderate cases based on cognitive and interpersonal principles. TIDY has been shown to be feasible and acceptable to practitioners (Iliffe et al., 2012; Kramer et al., 2013). Implementation leads to significantly improved rates of depression recognition and provides practitioners with clear guidance on which young people require specialist referral. As this model is less resource intensive than others described earlier it may prove adaptable for lower resource environments. Moreover, it is appropriate for use in subthreshold depression, which is common and persistent among young people in this setting (Gledhill & Garralda, 2013).

Early behavior disorders
Evidence is accumulating on the use of collaborative interventions within primary care for early behavior disorders. Kolko et al. (2012) enhanced their program of colocated nurse provision, with a doctor-led intervention incorporating psychoeducation, parent and child skills training, and ADHD management alongside mental health practitioner delivered psychoeducation compared to enhanced usual care. This intervention was significantly superior in service use and completion, and improved child behaviors and was associated with high pediatrician and parent satisfaction.

Usual care in this study was substantial and it might be argued that the intervention was a specialized package delivered within the primary care setting, therefore not feasible in lower resource settings. The challenge lies in replication with nonspecialist health workers or with lay workers picking up specific tasks as in *task shifting* and as trialed in India with adults (Patel et al., 2010).

However, less complex individual and group parenting interventions, have shown effectiveness when delivered in primary care (Stewart-Brown et al., 2004; Turner & Sanders, 2006; Lavigne et al., 2008), even when delivered by nonspecialist trainers within the voluntary sector (Gardner et al., 2006) and using trained peer facilitators (Day et al., 2012). Manualized self-help programs (Lavigne et al., 2008) and those with telephone support (Reid et al., 2013) have shown similar effectiveness.

Given the success of community-based group parenting programs (see Chapter 37), it would appear appropriate for primary care to have a role in the initial detection and referral of behavioral problems. Thus early treatment of behavior disorders following a stepped approach that starts with self-help and moves onto peer or professionally delivered programs in primary care and to specialist referral for the most complex cases would use resources effectively.

Attention deficit hyperactivity disorder (ADHD)

This stepped care approach is also appropriate for ADHD (Leslie *et al.*, 2004) and may be supplemented with internet resources (Epstein *et al.*, 2011), although it requires specific training for clinicians, as well as resources within primary care for liaison with schools and mental health agencies (Power *et al.*, 2008). Current programs have involved US primary care pediatricians and it is unclear whether medical practitioners in other countries would participate to the same extent.

Broad service redesign and delivery models

Innovative programs that involve change in service design and delivery for the range of child psychiatric problems have been described across a range of countries, predominantly those with higher incomes. They include (i) collaborative care services which incorporate a combination of consultation, coordination and education for primary care providers, and (ii) integrated youth services, combining a broad range of cross-sector provisions incorporating general and mental health, education, or vocational services and social care.

Collaborative care services

Campo *et al.* (2005) described a US collaborative care service illustrating the stepped care approach. The team included an advanced practice nurse located within primary care who performed the initial assessment, triage and psycho education, as well as medication management and brief psychotherapeutic interventions; a social worker who delivered on-site psychotherapy; and a child psychiatrist attending weekly sessions for case reviews, supervision, consultation, and to attend selected children.

Other US collaborative services have been developed (Gabel, 2010; Sarvet *et al.*, 2010; Gabel & Sarvet, 2011; Hilt *et al.*, 2013). PCPs who are central to this approach receive mental health assessment and treatment training. Individual consultation by child and adolescent psychiatrists is provided mainly by telephone but also face-to-face and via video-conferencing with support regarding referral. Similar innovations have been described in other countries, for example, in Finland (Laukkanen *et al.*, 2010) and through the development of primary care child mental health workers in the UK (Macdonald *et al.*, 2004; Hickey *et al.*, 2010).

The MCPAP is the most established of the collaborative care programs. It comprises six regional teams each including a child psychiatrist, a child and family psychotherapist, a care coordinator and, in some teams, an advanced practice registered nurse who works in a role similar to that of the child psychiatrist

(Sarvet *et al.*, 2010). The service is accessed via a telephone hotline and the call is routed to the most relevant MCPAP team member. Over 3 years 353 practices (1341 PCPs) enrolled covering 1.36 million children. A provider survey demonstrated that more felt that they are able to meet patient emotional or behavioral needs (increased from 8% to 63%), more felt that they had received a timely consultation (from 8% to 80%), and perceptions of adequate access to a child psychiatrist rose from 5% to 33%. Similarly, the Partnership Access Line (PAL), in Washington State involves a large rural population with poor access to child psychiatrists (Hilt *et al.*, 2013).

Integrated youth service models

Integrated youth services have been advocated as a means of improving young people's access to and engagement with mental health services. (Tylee *et al.*, 2007; Anderson & Lowen, 2010). Services of this nature include Headspace in Australia with a focus on "youth friendliness" by being accessible; comprehensive, including both physical and mental health provision, and colocated with youth workers, and other social and vocational services (Patulny *et al.*, 2013). However, evidence on efficacy so far is limited to case descriptions and uncontrolled observational studies.

Prevention and early intervention

The widespread, comprehensive, and community-based nature of primary care services, their knowledge of local social and family risk factors for CAMH and well-being puts them in a unique position to contribute to prevention and early intervention and help prevent the development of chronic conditions. However, questions arise about whether preventative programs are best delivered within clinical or community settings and whether they should be universal or selective. Complex research designs with long follow-up are required to demonstrate impacts on health outcomes, harms, and cost-effectiveness (Sanci, 2011) (Box 48.2). (Cross reference Prevention of Mental Disorders and Promotion of Competence—Chapter 17).

Primary prevention

By targeting risk and resilience factors both well care and acute visits present opportunities for primary prevention in children and young people. Examples include family planning programs, pre- and postnatal care including detection and management of maternal depression, promotion of adequate nutrition, information on child safety, and home visiting programs. A range of professionals including general/family practitioners, primary care pediatricians, community pediatricians, advanced practice nurses, health visitors, and community nurses are all in an excellent position to disseminate information on child health, development, behavior, and positive parenting (Bower *et al.*, 2003; Van Cleve *et al.*, 2013).

Box 48.2 Areas for primary prevention and early intervention.

Primary prevention	Parenting programs
Family planning	Iodine and iron deficiency prevention
Antenatal and postnatal care including maternal depression	**Early intervention**
Promoting good nutrition	Parenting programs for early behavior problems
Child safety education	Adolescent health risk screening, counseling, and psycho education
Home visiting	

A study of preventative consultations by one general practitioner aimed to influence parenting during the child's first 4 years; it demonstrated favorable outcomes on behavior at 6-years and even 20-years later (Cullen, 1976; Cullen & Cullen, 1996). However, it is unlikely that many general practitioners or pediatricians are in a position to invest the time required for such interventions. It may be more practical and cost-effective to implement prenatal and infancy home visiting by trained nurses with mothers at high risk of difficulties.

The best researched of home visiting programs for disadvantaged mothers (Olds *et al.*, 1997, 2007) have demonstrated benefits for young, low income, unmarried mothers, and their children in several large randomized controlled trials. (Cross reference Prevention of Mental Disorders and Promotion of Competence—Chapter 17).

By contrast, a far less intensive intervention in Iran—a randomized trial of a parenting intervention to prevent abuse—offering two sessions to mothers attending child monitoring visits in primary care—demonstrated significant change in maternal reported parenting practices (Oveisi *et al.*, 2010). It remains important to establish which elements of such interventions are the minimum required to achieve mental health gains for children.

Within LMICs links have been described between the early cognitive deficits associated with early stunting and living in poverty and impaired academic achievement, a possible mediator of the intergenerational transmission of poverty (Grantham-McGregor *et al.*, 2007). While primary care has a role in early detection of epilepsy and developmental delays, in order to prevent cognitive deficits, Walker *et al.* (2007) encouraged reduction of exposure to four key risk factors: under nutrition, inadequate cognitive stimulation, iodine deficiency, and iron deficiency. They concluded that there is sufficient evidence to warrant interventions for malaria, intrauterine growth restriction, maternal depression, exposure to violence, and exposure to heavy metals as a means of reducing cognitive deficits in children.

Outcomes of programs targeting child development have been mixed (Kieling *et al.*, 2011). A Jamaican trial of psycho-stimulation for stunted children was associated with significantly reduced anxiety, depression, and attention deficits, and enhanced self-esteem at age 17–18, when compared with dietary supplementation (Walker *et al.*, 2006). However, though commonly used, overall there has been so far little evidence of effectiveness of skill training parents in enrichment activities for children with intellectual disability (Kieling *et al.*, 2011). Factors associated with effectiveness of early psycho-stimulation programs across LMICs include: providing services directly to children and skill demonstrations and practice with parent. Disadvantaged, stunted children benefit more than advantaged children, 2–3 year olds fare better than 5–6 year olds and longer exposure results in larger effects (Engle *et al.*, 2007).

As primary care may be the only service that many children access, particularly those under age 3, and in light of the close relationships between physical and mental health and development, the primary setting is well placed to provide preventative interventions. Nevertheless broad implementation to date has been slow (Engle *et al.*, 2007).

Early identification of behavioral problems and suicidal risk in adolescents

In adolescence much morbidity and mortality is associated with risk factors considered preventable and linked with mental health, such as substance use, risky sexual behavior, accidents, and suicide. Accordingly, preventative screening for health risks during primary care wellness visits by adolescents has been advocated as a means of detection and early intervention. Two trials including behavioral counseling for areas of concern identified through screening demonstrated modest effects on behavior (Walker *et al.*, 2002; Ozer *et al.*, 2011). Of note in one study identifying "possible" adolescent depression was associated with significant improvement in mental health scores at 3-months and 1-year follow-up (Walker *et al.*, 2002).

The role of primary care in suicide prevention has been well described (Gould *et al.*, 2003; Mann *et al.*, 2005). Many suicidal young people in the age range 15-34 years have contact with primary care in the month prior to suicide or self-harm (Pfaff *et al.*, 1999; Luoma *et al.*, 2002) and screening for suicidal thoughts has been found to be safe (Gould *et al.*, 2005) and have acceptable sensitivity and specificity (Shaffer *et al.*, 2004). Nevertheless, a US study of pediatricians and family physicians revealed that less than half reported that they routinely screened their adolescent patients for suicide risk (Frankenfield *et al.*, 2000). One-day training for general practitioners in Australia enhanced detection rates of distress and suicidal ideation, but failed to lead to changes in management (Pfaff *et al.*, 2001).

A trial of a computerized screening tool of primary care attenders demonstrated that young people are willing to disclose suicidal thoughts using a computer screen within primary care and that a vulnerable group can be identified and managed (Gardner *et al.*, 2010) within a collaborative system of care.

Building capacity in the front line

Calls to increase primary care capacity to address CAMH are numerous; however, there are few comprehensive national policies or plans. Explicit in such proposals is the prominent need for training, including under- and postgraduate training, and continuing professional development. Dedicated training for pediatricians and general practitioners has been shown to lead to significant self-reported improvements in knowledge, skills, and confidence (Laraque *et al.*, 2009; Kramer *et al.*, 2013).

Exploring the barriers to work in this area has shown that general practitioners spend less time in consultations with young people than adults (Jacobson *et al.*, 1994) and that they have concerns about managing mental health problems within their time constraints (Iliffe *et al.*, 2012). They perceive young people as using primary care impulsively and intermittently, not engaging and being hard to communicate with (Iliffe *et al.*, 2008). They are wary of over-medicalization (Iliffe *et al.*, 2004), and using the word "depression," although they feel more comfortable discussing "social difficulties" (Iliffe *et al.*, 2012). This indicates that training should address attitudinal factors in addition to practical skills. Excellent interpersonal communication skills are required to fulfill the central role of the PCC in overcoming barriers to help-seeking for mental health problems. Chronic care principles have been identified as relevant. A comprehensive toolkit has been developed as part of the Mental Health Gap Intervention Guide (World Health Organization, 2010).

Conclusions and further developments

Child psychiatric disorders are common among children and young people attending primary care, particularly among frequent attenders, although presentations are usually with physical symptoms and the psychiatric problems often go unrecognized. Nevertheless, because of its very nature the primary care setting provides a unique opportunity to help close the gap in service provision for children and adolescents with mental health problems. Initiatives to increase screening and attend to affected children and young people are slowly being described and piloted in primary care.

Future work should address the best use of screening during clinical consultations, consider the adjunctive use of computer or internet-based interventions, explore what contributes to patient readiness for treatment uptake following identification, and the potential harm of false positive identification. Controlled studies with adequate sample sizes are needed to ascertain whether systematic early detection in primary care

leads to better child mental health outcomes in the medium to long term.

Outstanding tasks to be addressed are public education to help diminish stigma and promote primary care as a source of help, helping clinicians facilitate parents' and young people's communication of their concerns during primary care consultations and generally building primary care professional capacity for CAMH.

New collaborative service models to help improve primary care involvement with CAMH need to be tested and piloted beyond their "product champions" and their efficacy rigorously demonstrated in terms of patient outcomes, but also in relation to service access, engagement, satisfaction, and cost.

Central to all these developments is an overall need, likely to be more pronounced in LMICs, to design and evaluate training programs for all frontline workers, whether general health practitioners, child care or education providers, or lay workers in CAMH.

References

Anderson, J.E. & Lowen, C.A. (2010) Connecting youth with health services: systematic review. *Canadian Family Physician* **56**, 778–784.

Asarnow, J.R. *et al.* (2005) Effectiveness of a quality improvement intervention for adolescent depression in primary care clinics: a randomized controlled trial. *JAMA: The Journal of the American Medical Association* **293**, 311–319.

Asarnow, J.R. *et al.* (2009) Long-term benefits of short-term quality improvement interventions for depressed youths in primary care. *American Journal of Psychiatry* **166**, 1002–1010.

Boerma, W.G.W. (2006) *Primary Care in the Driver's Seat? Organisational reform in European Primary Care*. Open University Press, Buckingham.

Bower, P. *et al.* (2001) The treatment of child and adolescent mental health problems in primary care: a systematic review. *Family Practice* **18**, 373–382.

Bower, P. *et al.* (2003) Postal survey of services for child and adolescent mental health problems in general practice in England. *Primary Care Mental Health* **1**, 17–26.

Bower, P. *et al.* (2006) Collaborative care for depression in primary care. Making sense of a complex intervention: systematic review and meta regression. *The British Journal of Psychiatry* **189**, 484–493.

Bowman, F.M. & Garralda, M.E. (1993) Psychiatric morbidity among children who are frequent attenders in general practice. *The British Journal of General Practice* **43**, 6–9.

Bradley, S. *et al.* (2003) Child and adolescent mental health interface work with primary services: a survey of NHS provider trusts. *Child and Adolescent Mental Health* **8**, 170–176.

Brent, D. *et al.* (2008) Switching to another SSRI or to venlafaxine with or without cognitive behavioral therapy for adolescents with SSRI-resistant depression: the TORDIA randomized controlled trial. *JAMA* **299**, 901–913.

Britt, H. *et al.* (2008) General practice activity in Australia 2006–07. General Practice Series no. 21. Canberra: Australian Institute of Health and Welfare. Cat. no. GEP 21.

Brown, J.D. *et al.* (2007) Receiving advice about child mental health from a primary care provider: African American and Hispanic parent attitudes. *Medical Care* **45**, 1076–1082.

Bruckner, T.A. *et al.* (2011) The mental health workforce gap in low-and middle-income countries: a needs-based approach. *Bulletin of the World Health Organization* **89**, 184–194.

Brugman, E. *et al.* (2001) Identification and management of psychosocial problems by preventive childhealth care. *Archives of Pediatrics and Adolescent Medicine* **155**, 462–469.

Burns, B.J. *et al.* (1995) Children's mental health service use across service sectors. *Health Affairs (Millwood)* **14**, 147–159.

Burns, J.J. *et al.* (2004) Depressive symptoms and health risk among rural adolescents. *Pediatrics* **113**, 1313–1320.

Campo, J.V. *et al.* (2005) Pediatric behavioral health in primary care: a collaborative approach. *Journal of the American Psychiatric Nurses Association* **11**, 276–282.

Chavira, D.A. *et al.* (2004) Childhood anxiety disorders in primary care: prevalent but untreated. *Depression and Anxiety* **20**, 155–164.

Cheng, T.L. (2004) Primary care pediatrics: 2004 and beyond. *Pediatrics* **113**, 1802–1809.

Connor, D.F. *et al.* (2006) Targeted child psychiatric services: a new model of pediatric primary clinician—child psychiatry collaborative care. *Clinical Pediatrics* **45**, 423–434.

Costello, E.J. *et al.* (1988) Psychiatric disorders in pediatric primary care. Prevalence and risk factors. *Archives of General Psychiatry* **45**, 1107–1116.

Crone, M.R. *et al.* (2010) Professional identification of psychosocial problems among children from ethnic minority groups: room for improvement. *The Journal of Pediatrics* **156**, 277–284.

Cullen, K.J. (1976) A six-year controlled trial of prevention of children's behavior disorders. *Journal of Pediatrics* **88**, 662–667.

Cullen, K.J. & Cullen, A.M. (1996) Long-term follow-up of the Busselton six-year controlled trial of prevention of children's behavior disorders. *Journal of Pediatrics* **129**, 136–139.

Day, C. & Davis, H. (2006) The effectiveness and quality of routine child and adolescent mental health care outreach clinics. *British Journal of Clinical Psychology* **45**, 439–452.

Day, C. *et al.* (2012) Evaluation of a peer led parenting intervention for disruptive behaviour problems in children: community based randomized controlled trial. *BMJ* **344**, 1107.

Eapen, V. *et al.* (2004) Child psychiatric disorders in a primary care arab population. *The International Journal of Psychiatry in Medicine* **34**, 51–60.

Ellingson, K.D. *et al.* (2004) Parent identification of early emerging child behavior problems: predictors of sharing parental concern with health providers. *Archives of Pediatrics and Adolescent Medicine* **158**, 766–772.

Elster, A.B. & Kuznets, N.J. (1994) *Guidelines for Adolescent Preventive Services*. Williams and Wilkins, Baltimore.

Elster, A.B. & Kuznets, N.J. (2010) Guidelines for adolescent preventive services. Evaluation of the PHQ-2 as a brief screen for detecting major depression among adolescents. *Pediatrics* **125**, 1097.

Engle, P.L. *et al.* (2007) Strategies to avoid the loss of developmental potential in more than 200 million children in the developing world. *The Lancet* **369**, 229–242.

Epstein, J.N. *et al.* (2011) Use of an internet portal to improve community-based pediatric ADHD care: a cluster randomized trial. *Pediatrics* **128**, e1201–e1208.

van Esso, D. *et al.* (2010) Paediatric primary care in Europe: variation between countries. *Archives of Disease in Childhood* **95**, 791–795.

Fein, J.A. *et al.* (2010) Feasibility and effects of a web-based adolescent psychiatric assessment administered by clinical staff in the pediatric emergency department. *Archives of Pediatrics and Adolescent Medicine* **164**, 1112–1117.

Fernandez, V. *et al.* (2009) Depressive symptoms and behavioural health risks in young people attending an urban sexual health clinic. *Child Care Health & Development* **35**, 799–806.

Ferrin, M. *et al.* (2009) Factors influencing primary care attendance in adolescents with high levels of depressive symptoms. *Social Psychiatry and Psychiatric Epidemiology* **10**, 825–833.

Ford, T. *et al.* (2007) Child mental health is everybody's business; the prevalence of contacts with public sectors services by the types of disorder among British school children in a three-year period. *Child and Adolescent Mental Health* **12**, 13–20.

Frankenfield, D.L. *et al.* (2000) Adolescent patients—healthy or hurting?: missed opportunities to screen for suicide risk in the primary care setting. *Archives of Pediatrics and Adolescent Medicine* **154**, 162–168.

Freed, G.L. *et al.* (2004) Which physicians are providing health care to America's children? Trends and changes during the past 20 years. *Archives of Pediatrics and Adolescent Medicine* **158**, 22–26.

Freed, G.L. *et al.* (2010) Research Advisory Committee of the American Board of pediatrics. Perspectives and preferences among the general public regarding physician selection and board certification. *Journal of Pediatrics* **156**, 841–845.

Fulton, B.D. *et al.* (2011) Health workforce skill mix and task shifting in low income countries: a review of recent evidence. *Human Resources for Health* **9**, 1.

Gabel, S. (2010) The integration of mental health into pediatric practice: child and adolescent psychiatrists and pediatricians working together in new models of care. *Journal of Pediatrics* **157**, 848–851.

Gabel, S. & Sarvet, B. (2011) Public-academic partnerships to address the need for child and adolescent psychiatric services. *Psychiatric Services* **62**, 827–829.

Gardner, F. *et al.* (2006) Randomised controlled trial of a parenting intervention in the voluntary sector for reducing child conduct problems: outcomes and mechanisms of change. *Journal of Child Psychology and Psychiatry* **47**, 1123–1132.

Gardner, W. *et al.* (2010) Screening, triage, and referral of patients who report suicidal thought during a primary care visit. *Pediatrics* **125**, 945–952.

Garralda, M.E. & Bailey, D. (1986) Children with psychiatric disorders in primary care. *Journal of Child Psychology and Psychiatry* **27**, 611–624.

Garralda, M.E. & Bailey, D. (1989) Psychiatric disorders in general paediatric referrals. *Archives of Disease in Childhood* **64**, 1727–1733.

Garralda, M.E. *et al.* (1999) Children with psychiatric disorders who are frequent attenders to primary care. *European Child and Adolescent Psychiatry* **8**, 34–44.

Gask, L. *et al.* (1997) Evaluating models of working at the interface between mental health services and primary care. *The British Journal of Psychiatry* **170**, 6–11.

Gilbody, S. *et al.* (2005) Screening and case finding instruments for depression. *Cochrane Database of Systematic Reviews* **19**, CD002792.

Gilbody, S. *et al.* (2006) Collaborative care for depression: a cumulative meta-analysis and review of longer-term outcomes. *Archives of Internal Medicine* **166**, 2314–2321.

Gledhill, J. & Garralda, M.E. (2011) The short-term outcome of depressive disorder in adolescents attending primary care: a cohort study. *Social Psychiatry and Psychiatric Epidemiology* **46**, 993–1002.

Gledhill, J. & Garralda, M.E. (2013) Sub-syndromal depression in adolescents attending primary care: frequency, clinical features and 6 months outcome. *Social Psychiatry and Psychiatric Epidemiology* **48**, 735–744.

Goldberg, I.D. *et al.* (1984) Mental health problems among children seen in pediatric practice: prevalence and management. *Pediatrics* **73**, 278–293.

Gould, M.S. *et al.* (2003) Youth suicide risk and preventative interventions: a review of the past 10 years. *Journal of the American Academy of Child and Adolescent Psychiatry* **42**, 386–405.

Gould, M.S. *et al.* (2005) Evaluating iatrogenic risk of youth suicide screening programs. *JAMA* **293**, 1635–1643.

Grantham-McGregor, S. *et al.* (2007) Developmental potential in the first 5 years for children in developing countries. *Lancet* **369**, 60–70.

Gulliver, A. *et al.* (2010) Perceived barriers and facilitators to mental health help-seeking in young people: a systematic review. *BMC Psychiatry* **10**, 113.

Gureje, O. *et al.* (1994) Psychiatric disorders in a pediatric primary care clinic. *The British Journal of Psychiatry* **165**, 527–530.

Haller, D.M. *et al.* (2007) Toward youth friendly services: a survey of young people in primary care. *Journal of General Internal Medicine* **22**, 775–781.

Haller, D.M. *et al.* (2009) Toward youth friendly services: health competencies for pediatric primary care. *Pediatrics* **124**, 410–421.

Hetlevik, Ø. *et al.* (2010) Young people and their GP: a register-based study of 1717 Norwegian GPs. *Family Practice* **27**, 3–8.

Hickey, N. *et al.* (2010) Developing the primary mental health worker (PMHW) role in England. *Child & Adolescent Mental Health* **15**, 23–29.

Hilt, R.J. *et al.* (2013) The partnership access line: evaluating a child psychiatry consult program in Washington state. *JAMA Pediatrics* **167**, 162–168.

Horwitz, S.M. *et al.* (1998) Identification of psychosocial problems in pediatric primary care: do family attitudes make a difference? *Archives of Pediatrics and Adolescent Medicine* **152**, 367–371.

Iliffe, S. *et al.* (2004) The recognition of adolescent depression in general practice: issues in the acquisition of new skills. *Primary Care Psychiatry* **9**, 51–56.

Iliffe, S. *et al.* (2008) General practitioners' understanding of depression in young people: qualitative study. *Primary Health Care Research & Development* **9**, 269–279.

Iliffe, S. *et al.* (2012) Therapeutic identification of depression in young people: lessons from the introduction of a new technique in general practice. *British Journal of General Practice* **62**, 174–182.

Jacobson, L. *et al.* (1994) Is the potential of teenage consultations being missed?: a study of consultation times in primary care. *Family Practice* **11**, 296–299.

Katz, M. *et al.* (2002) Demography of pediatric primary care in Europe: delivery of care and training. *Pediatrics* **109**, 788–796.

Kieling, C. *et al.* (2011) Child and adolescent mental health worldwide: evidence for action. *The Lancet* **378**, 1515–1525.

Kolko, D.J. *et al.* (2010) Improving access to care and clinical outcome for pediatric behavioral problems: a randomized trial of a nurse administered intervention in primary care. *Journal of Developmental and Behavioral Pediatrics* **31**, 393–404.

Kolko, D. *et al.* (2012) Doctor office collaborative care for pediatric behavioral problems: a preliminary clinical trial. *Archives of Pediatrics and Adolescent Medicine* **166**, 224–231.

Kramer, T. & Garralda, M.E. (1998) Psychiatric disorders in adolescents in primary care. *The British Journal of Psychiatry* **173**, 508–513.

Kramer, T. *et al.* (2012) Recognizing and responding to adolescent depression in general practice: developing and implementing the therapeutic identification of depression in young people (TIDY) programme. *Clinical Child Psychology & Psychiatry* **17**, 482–494.

Kramer, T. *et al.* (2013) Testing the feasibility of therapeutic identification of depression in young people in British general practice. *Journal of Adolescent Health* **52**, 539–545.

Laraque, D. *et al.* (2009) Reported physician skills in the management of children's mental health problems following an educational intervention. *Academic Pediatrics* **9**, 164–171.

Laukkanen, E. *et al.* (2010) A brief intervention is sufficient for many adolescents seeking help from low threshold adolescent psychiatric services. *BMC Health Services Research* **10**, 261–271.

Lavigne, J.V. *et al.* (2008) Treating oppositional defiant disorder in primary care: a comparison of three models. *Journal of Pediatric Psychology* **33**, 449–461.

Leaf, P.J. *et al.* (1996) Mental health service use in the community and schools: results from the four community MECA study—methods for the epidemiology of child and adolescent mental disorders study. *Journal of the American Academy of Child and Adolescent Psychiatry* **35**, 889–897.

Leslie, L. *et al.* (2004) Implementing the AAP attention deficit/hyperactivity disorder diagnostic guidelines in primary care settings. *Pediatrics* **114**, 129–140.

Luoma, J.B. *et al.* (2002) Contact with mental health and primary care providers before suicide: a review of the evidence. *American Journal of Psychiatry* **159**, 909–916.

Macdonald, W. *et al.* (2004) Primary mental health workers in child and adolescent mental health services. *Journal of Advanced Nursing* **46**, 78–87.

Mann, J.J. *et al.* (2005) Suicide prevention strategies: a systematic review. *JAMA* **294**, 2064–2074.

March, J. *et al.* (2004) Fluoxetine, cognitive-behavioral therapy, and their combination for adolescents with depression: treatment for adolescents with depression study (TADS) randomized controlled trial. *JAMA* **292**, 807–820.

Martinez, R. *et al.* (2006) Factors that influence the detection of psychological problems in adolescents attending general practices. *British Journal of General Practice* **56**, 594–599.

Martinez-Castaldi, C. *et al.* (2008) Child versus adult research: the gap in high-quality study design. *Pediatrics* **122**, 52–57.

Morris, J. *et al.* (2011) Treated prevalence of and mental health services received by children and adolescents in 42 low-and-middle-income countries. *Journal of Child Psychology and Psychiatry* **52**, 1239–1246.

Neiro-Munoz, E. & Ward, D. (1998) Side by side. *HSJ* **108**, 26–27.

Olds, D.L. *et al.* (1997) Long-term effects of home visitation on maternal life course and child abuse and neglect. Fifteen-year follow-up of a randomized trial. *JAMA* **278**, 637–643.

Olds, D.L. *et al.* (2007) Programs for parents of infants and toddlers: recent evidence from randomized trials. *Journal of Child Psychology and Psychiatry* **48**, 355–391.

Oveisi, S. *et al.* (2010) Primary prevention of parent–child conflict and abuse in Iranian mothers: a randomized-controlled trial. *Child Abuse & Neglect* **34**, 206–213.

Ozer, E.M. *et al.* (2009) Are adolescents being screened for emotional distress in primary care? *Journal of Adolescent Health* **44**, 520–527.

Ozer, E.M. *et al.* (2011) Does delivering preventive services in primary care reduce adolescent risky behavior? *Journal of Adolescent Health* **49**, 476–482.

Patel, V. *et al.* (2008) Promoting child and adolescent mental health in low and middle income countries. *Journal of Child Psychology and Psychiatry* **49**, 313–334.

Patel, V. *et al.* (2010) Effectiveness of an intervention led by lay health counsellors for depressive and anxiety disorders in primary care in Goa, India (MANAS): a cluster randomised controlled trial. *The Lancet* **376**, 2086–2095.

Patulny, R. *et al.* (2013) Are we reaching them yet? Service access patterns among attendees at the *headspace* youth mental health initiative. *Child and Adolescent Mental Health* **18**, 95–102.

Pfaff, J.J. *et al.* (1999) The role of general practitioners in parasuicide: a western Australia perspective. *Archives of Suicide Research* **5**, 207–214.

Pfaff, J.J. *et al.* (2001) Training general practitioners to recognise and respond to psychological distress and suicidal ideation in young people. *Medical Journal of Australia* **174**, 222–226.

Power, T.J. *et al.* (2008) Managing attention-deficit/hyperactivity disorder in primary care: a systematic analysis of roles and challenges. *Pediatrics* **121**, e65–e72.

Reid, G.J. *et al.* (2013) Randomized trial of distance-based treatment for young children with discipline problems seen in primary health care. *Family Practice* **30**, 14–24.

Remschmidt, H. & van Engeland, H. (eds) (1999) *Child and Adolescent Psychiatry in Europe. Historical Development. Current Situation. Future Perspectives.* Darmstadt, Steinkopff; Springer, New York.

Rickwood, D.J. *et al.* (2007) When and how do young people seek professional help for mental health problems? *Medical Journal of Australia* **187**, S35–S39.

Royal College of General Practitioners (2008) *Weekly Returns Service Annual Prevalence Report 2007.* Birmingham Research Unit. pp 1–89.

Rutman, M.S. *et al.* (2008) Brief screening for adolescent depressive symptoms in the emergency department. *Academic Emergency Medicine* **15**, 17–22.

Sanci, L. (2011) Clinical preventive services for adolescents: facing the challenge of proving "An Ounce of Prevention Is Worth a Pound of Cure". *Journal of Adolescent Health* **49**, 450–452.

Sanci, D. *et al.* (2010) Detecting emotional disorder in young people in primary care. *Current Opinion in Psychiatry* **23**, 318–323.

Sarvet, B. *et al.* (2010) Improving access to mental health care for children: the Massachusetts child psychiatry project. *Pediatrics* **126**, 1191–1200.

Sayal, K. (2006) Annotation: pathways to care for children with mental health problems. *Journal of Child Psychology and Psychiatry* **47**, 649–659.

Sayal, K. & Taylor, E. (2004) Detection of child mental health disorders by general practitioners. *British Journal of General Practice* **54**, 348–352.

Sayal, K. *et al.* (2010) Parental help-seeking in primary care for child and adolescent mental health concerns: qualitative study. *The British Journal of Psychiatry* **197**, 476–481.

Shaffer, D. *et al.* (2004) The Columbia suicide screen: validity and reliability of a screen for youth suicide and depression. *Journal of the American Academy of Child & Adolescent Psychiatry* **43**, 71–79.

Sonuga-Barke, E.J.S. *et al.* (2004) Parent training for pre-school attention deficit/hyperactivity disorder: is it effective as part of routine primary care? *British Journal of Clinical Psychology* **43**, 449–457.

Stevens, J. *et al.* (2008) Trial of computerized screening for adolescent behavioral concerns. *Pediatrics* **121**, 1099–1105.

Stewart-Brown, S. *et al.* (2004) Impact of a general practice based group parenting programme: quantitative and qualitative results from a controlled trial at 12 months. *Archives of Disease in Childhood* **89**, 519–525.

Tanielian, T. *et al.* (2009) Improving treatment seeking among adolescents with depression: understanding readiness for treatment. *Journal of Adolescent Health* **45**, 490–498.

Turner, K.M.T. & Sanders, M.R. (2006) Help when it's needed first: a controlled evaluation of brief, preventive behavioral family intervention in a primary care setting. *Behavior Therapy* **37**, 131–142.

Tylee, A. *et al.* (2007) Youth-friendly primary-care services: how are we doing and what more needs to be done? *Lancet* **369**, 1565–73.

US Preventive Services Task Force (2009) Screening and treatment for major depressive disorder in children and adolescents: US preventive services task force recommendation statement. *Pediatrics* **123**, 1223–1228.

Van Cleve, S.N. *et al.* (2013) Nurse practitioners: integrating mental health in pediatric primary care. *The Journal for Nurse Practitioners* **9**, 243–248.

Vanheusden, K. *et al.* (2008) The use of mental health services among young adults with emotional and behavioural problems: equal use for equal needs? *Social Psychiatry and Psychiatric Epidemiology* **43**, 808–815.

Vila, M. *et al.* (2012) Adolescents who are frequent attenders to primary care: contribution of psychosocial factors. *Social Psychiatry and Psychiatric Epidemiology* **47**, 323–329.

Walker, Z. *et al.* (2002) Health promotion for adolescents in primary care: randomized controlled trial. *British Medical Journal* **325**, 524–530.

Walker, S.P. *et al.* (2006) Effects of psychosocial stimulation and dietary supplementation in early childhood on psychosocial functioning in late adolescence: follow-up of randomised controlled trial. *British Medical Journal* **333**, 472–474.

Walker, S.P. *et al.* (2007) Child development: risk factors for adverse outcomes in developing countries. *The Lancet* **369**, 145–157.

WHO (2005) *Atlas Child and Adolescent Mental Health Resources—Global Concerns: Implications for the Future,* WHO Geneva Switzerland [Online]. Available: http://www.who.int/mental_health/resources/Child_ado_atlas.pdf [05 Aug 2014].

WHO (2010) *mhGAP Intervention Guide for Mental, Neurological and Substance Use Disorders in Non-Specialized Health Settings:*

Mental Health Gap Action Programme (mhGAP), WHO Geneva Switzerland.

Williams, J. *et al.* (2006) Co-location of mental health professionals in primary care settings: three North Carolina models. *Clinical Pediatrics* **45**, 537–543.

Wintersteen, M.B. (2010) Standardized screening for suicidal adolescents in primary care. *Pediatrics* **125**, 938.

Wren, F.J. *et al.* (2005) How do primary care clinicians manage childhood mood and anxiety syndromes? *International Journal of Psychiatry in Medicine* **35**, 1–12.

Yates, P. *et al.* (2004) Depressive symptoms amongst adolescent primary care attenders. Levels and associations. *Social Psychiatry and Psychiatric Epidemiology* **39**, 588–594.

Zuckerbrot, R.A. *et al.* (2007) GLAD-PC Steering Group. Guidelines for adolescent depression in primary care (GLAD-PC): I. Identification, assessment, and initial management. *Pediatrics* **120**, e1299–e1312.

CHAPTER 49

Forensic psychiatry

Susan Young[1] and Richard Church[2]

[1] Centre for Mental Health, Imperial College London, UK
[2] South London and Maudsley NHS Foundation Trust, London, UK

Introduction

Forensic psychiatry is predominantly associated with children's interactions with the criminal and civil law—the assessment and management of mentally disordered offenders, or those at risk of offending, and issues such as mental competency, fitness to testify, reliability of testimony, victimization, and child custody disputes.

This is a complicated area, which may require clinicians to interact with the courts and consider legal aspects of a child's behavior. Typically, forensic psychiatry involves the assessment and management of both clinical and criminogenic factors presenting in mentally disordered offenders. A prominent aspect is the assessment and management of risks toward others, especially violence and other antisocial behavior—whether the individual has actually broken the law or not. Some aspects of forensic psychiatry are described elsewhere in this volume, including the chapters on intellectual disability, children's testimony and child maltreatment.

While there is considerable international variation in the development of adult forensic psychiatric services, there is even greater heterogeneity in forensic child and adolescent psychiatric services, both between countries and within regions of countries. Marked differences exist in the types of services delivered and the degree to which these services are integrated with other judicial or welfare agencies for young people. International standards are clear that whenever juveniles are deprived of their liberty, this should be as a last resort and always within an age-appropriate environment suited to their needs (United Nations, 1990). In this context, there is a requirement for specialized secure psychiatric services for mentally disordered young people who pose very high risks to others (Bailey *et al.*, 1994). In the absence of such specialist resources, mentally unwell young people are often kept in suboptimal settings such as juvenile prisons, secure residential placements, secure mental health wards for adults and potentially fail to receive appropriate treatment.

Aside from secure psychiatric hospitals, forensic child and adolescent mental health teams may also be located in any setting where children are deprived of their liberty. Such teams may have significant roles in running specialized mental health services within institutions, assessing and managing risk and managing continuity in mental health care between the locked institution and other settings including the community. Similar teams work with juvenile offenders serving non custodial sentences in the community and may be linked to primary care services (Callaghan *et al.*, 2003). Such community-based teams typically liaise with a large number of partner agencies and may become involved in the assessment and management of young people who are not necessarily in conflict with the law, but who nonetheless present high risks to themselves or others (Table 49.1).

Juvenile justice systems: a global perspective

General principles of juvenile justice

The United Nations has published extensively on matters related to youth justice. Core principles are enshrined in the United Nations Convention on the Rights of the Child (United Nations, 1990), where Article 37 describes minimum standards in the treatment and punishment of juvenile offenders. More specific guidance is contained in documents such as the Standard Minimum Rules for the Administration of Juvenile Justice ("Beijing Rules") of 1985, Guidelines for the Prevention of Juvenile Delinquency ("Riyadh Guidelines") of 1990 and Rules for the Protection of Juveniles Deprived of their Liberty ("Havana Rules") of 1990. These documents, among many others, describe

Rutter's Child and Adolescent Psychiatry, Sixth Edition.
Edited by Anita Thapar and Daniel S. Pine, James F. Leckman, Stephen Scott, Margaret J. Snowling, Eric Taylor.
© 2015 John Wiley & Sons Ltd. Published 2018 by John Wiley & Sons Ltd.

Table 49.1 Roles for forensic child and adolescent mental health services *(Mental disorder includes mental illnesses, neurodevelopmental disorders, and substance misuse).*

Time/location		Roles for forensic child and adolescent mental health teams
Arrest		Training police officers in identification of mental disorder in juvenile offenders
		Effective police liaison for prompt mental health assessments and transfers to psychiatric healthcare settings as required
Juvenile detention		Screening for mental disorder and substance misuse on entry to establishment
	Effective screening for mental disorder and timely access to mental health and social care services in all settings	Assessment and management of inmates/residents with mental disorder
		Joint working with staff to manage risk and implement care plans
		Liaison with other agencies for continuity of care and support after release
Trial		Assessment of capacity/fitness to be interviewed, plead, testify or stand trial
		Recommendation of any special measures to be implemented during trial
		Opinion on mitigating circumstances and psychiatric defences to alleged offences
Sentencing/disposal		Provision of opinions on: diagnosis of mental disorder, risks, treatment needs, suitability of setting for treatment and management, court-mandated mental health treatment in psychiatric hospital or the community, safeguarding or parenting concerns, social needs or educational requirements.
Secure psychiatric hospital		Provision of age-appropriate secure psychiatric hospital services. Liaison with juvenile prisons, secure residential homes, general children's inpatient units and community services.
Community		Collaboration with youth justice and other community agencies for delivery of mental health care and risk management, delivery of systemic interventions, advocacy for young people and support for protective factors (e.g., education).
Prevention		Collaboration with stakeholders (families, education, healthcare, social services, police and youth justice) in the development of coherent strategies for prevention of juvenile offending, early identification of problems, referral to services and delivery of effective interventions.

ideal standards of juvenile justice that have been implemented to a somewhat inconsistent and limited extent around the world (Goldson & Muncie, 2012).

The degree to which juvenile offenders receive special treatment as juveniles varies across the world, and differences have been highlighted by the growing trend for an international comparative approach (Muncie & Goldson, 2006; Hazel, 2008). Juvenile justice systems have historically been divided into either "welfare" or "justice" models. While "welfare" approaches share a focus on the needs of the child, diagnosis, treatment and more informal procedures, the "justice" approach emphasizes accountability, punishment and procedural formality. In reality, there are elements of both welfare and justice models within most countries. However, there are notable differences in standards of behavior deemed to constitute juvenile offending, the very definition of a youth/juvenile and, particularly significantly, vast differences in the minimum age of criminal responsibility. Many consider that the low age of criminal responsibility of 10 years in England and Wales, and 6 years in several US states, is out of keeping with international norms and criminalizes children at an age that is developmentally inappropriate. The issue continues to be the subject of vigorous debate (Church *et al.*, 2013). Overall, there is a vast array of factors that shape the characteristics of youth justice systems and their development is subject to numerous further influences, not least the prevailing political ideology and media/public responses to significant adverse events.

Youth justice process

The journey of a young person through a welfare or juvenile justice process can include several stages such as arrest, interviews by officials, official statement of alleged offences, entering a plea, giving evidence, an adversarial or inquisitorial process to determine fact, and disposal or sentencing.

Numerous problems can arise during such a process. Firstly, there is evidence to indicate that children are vulnerable to interrogation and to making false confessions. In a self-report study of 10,472 Icelandic youth, of the 18.6% who reported being interrogated by the police, 7.3% reported having made a false confession. Compared to other suspects, the false confessors reported increased anxiety, depression, anger problems, poorer self-esteem, less parental support, more delinquency during the previous year and more delinquency among friends (Gudjonsson *et al.*, 2006). These findings highlight the importance of support during interrogation, such as the practice of having an "appropriate adult" present when a child is interviewed for a suspected offence in the United Kingdom, or having legal representation (see also Chapters 19 and 20).

Juveniles are also vulnerable during court processes if they lack the ability to understand charges, follow proceedings, work with their legal representatives or give evidence in their own defence, either as a result of mental disorder or developmental immaturity. A study of 927 adolescents tested for competence to stand trial concluded that one-third of 11–13 years olds and one-fifth of 14–15 year olds performed as poorly as adults with severe mental illness who would be deemed incompetent to stand trial. Furthermore, defendants under the age of 15 years have been found to be more likely to make poor legal decisions, including choices that reflected compliance with authority (Grisso *et al.*, 2003; Viljoen *et al.*, 2005).

In order to cater for the particular needs of child defendants, the United Nations supports the development of specialized systems for managing children in conflict with the law. This has led to the promotion of juvenile courts; however, many countries lack juvenile justice services or specialist legal provision for juveniles.

Disposal and sentencing

The term "disposal" is used to describe all outcomes following contact with the police. This can include a large number of contacts that are dealt with informally by the police, such as with a warning, in which young people are particularly over represented. When a young person is convicted of having committed an offence, they may be sentenced to serve a term in a locked environment, or they may receive any of a number of community sentences with requirements such as fines, community service, reparation work, parenting orders, curfews, exclusions, electronic monitoring, testing, and treatment for substance misuse or mental health treatment requirements.

While there has been a sustained trend toward reducing the number of incarcerated juveniles, this has not been observed consistently in all communities; black and minority ethnic groups continue to be vastly over represented, especially in North America, Australia and New Zealand. Some countries, such as Sweden, have carefully tailored age-dependent sentencing guidelines, tuned to the developmental immaturity of defendants. In particular, a flexible approach around matching court orders to the individual needs of young offenders may be a particularly beneficial model (Vieira *et al.*, 2009). As part of such individualized sentencing, court orders directing mental health treatment in inpatient or community settings can be a valuable care pathway for managing mentally disordered offenders, if permitted under the local jurisdiction. Specialized youth mental health courts may be a helpful model to support multidisciplinary coordination and avoid protracted justice system involvement (Callahan *et al.*, 2012).

A particularly emotive topic continues to be capital punishment (the death penalty) for juvenile offenders; the practice was outlawed in the United States following a landmark ruling in the US Supreme Court in 2005 (Roper v. Simmons), but continues in a small number of other countries, sometimes upheld by religious laws.

Restorative justice

The restorative justice approach has grown significantly worldwide over the last 30 years, with diverse local implementation in Australia, Canada, Germany, Japan, New Zealand, United Kingdom and United States. A central theme is the bringing together of the victim and perpetrator of an offence for mediation, with elements of both accountability and reintegration. Family group conferences, first developed in New Zealand, are sometimes considered to fall within a restorative justice model. While this approach may not be applicable to all offences, and may not serve to reduce recidivism, it is associated with high user satisfaction for both victims and perpetrators.

A developmental understanding of juvenile delinquency

Juvenile delinquent is a term commonly used to describe a young person who has broken the law. However, the term is often problematic, and an alternative preferred by the United Nations is "children in conflict with the law"—perhaps reflecting changing understanding and attitudes. The distinction between criminological, social and biomedical research has become somewhat blurred in literature regarding the developmental origins and risk factors for juvenile delinquency. Early criminological cohort studies formulated to explore the precursors of crime have had a strong psychosocial component (Farrington & West, 1971) and epidemiological studies of psychiatric disorder in children have included examination of the risk factors for conduct disorder (Rutter *et al.*, 1975), yielding complementary results. The increased prevalence of conduct disorder in urban compared to rural settings was consistent with an increased urban prevalence of risk factors for development of delinquency. As developmental perspectives of delinquency, including evidence on parenting as an important proximal risk factor, were increasingly explored (Patterson *et al.*, 1989), a broader understanding of antisocial behavior by young people emerged within a biomedical framework (Rutter *et al.*, 1998), informed by a growing stream of follow-up data from large cohort studies (see Chapter 65).

The Cambridge Study in Delinquent Development has now followed up 411 males from age 8 to 50 years with repeated personal interviews and criminal record searches. It provides a rich source of information and analysis of risk factors associated with offending. Early predictors at age 8–10 years for subsequent convictions include low family income, poor housing, large family size, school delinquency, having a convicted parent, a delinquent sibling, having a young mother, a depressed mother, poor child-rearing skills, poor supervision and a disrupted family. Individual factors that predicted offending include low non verbal IQ, low verbal IQ, low attainment, high daring, poor concentration, high impulsivity, low popularity, and both troublesome and dishonest behavior (Farrington *et al.*, 2009a). Bullying has also been identified as a significant predictor of subsequent offending and violence (Farrington & Ttofi, 2011).

Findings from the collation of six large longitudinal studies of children (Montreal, Quebec, Christchurch, Dunedin, Pittsburgh, and the US Child Development Project) indicate that while male childhood physical aggression is the most consistent predictor of both violent and non violent offending, early non aggressive conduct problems also increase the risk of later violent offending. Early oppositional behaviors were observed to independently increase the risk of non violent offending (Broidy *et al.*, 2003).

Results from the Edinburgh Study of Youth Transitions and Crime noted similar well-established risk factors for offending, and highlighted the broad range of vulnerabilities and social adversity in juvenile offenders. It proposed that critical moments in early teenage years influenced pathways into or away from offending, with events such as exclusion from school being particularly deleterious. While the authors support diversion strategies to facilitate desistance from offending, they express concern at the risk of labeling and stigmatizing children judged to be at-risk through early identification (McAra & McVie, 2010).

The widely cited dual taxonomy of adolescence-limited and life course persistent offenders (Moffitt, 1993; Moffitt *et al.*, 2002; see Chapters 4 and 65) is not always fully supported by longitudinal data and the original grouping has since been refined, but has been a helpful framework for the analysis of patterns of offending behavior (Farrington *et al.*, 2009b). The life course persistent group is more likely to have neurodevelopmental impairments, difficult temperament, neurological abnormalities, lowered intellectual capacity and hyperactivity. By contrast, the far more common adolescence-limited group tends to display short-lived antisocial behavior with social origins, such as peer influence and intoxication with alcohol and substances.

As parental delinquency is generally accepted to be a significant predictor of juvenile delinquency, it may be no surprise that parental imprisonment is associated with further poor outcomes (Murray *et al.*, 2009). The finding that persistently delinquent individuals are at risk of having delinquent offspring has sometimes been termed the "cycle of violence," supported by evidence that constitutional and environmental risk factors contribute to delinquency, that constitutional risks are amplified by adverse rearing environments (see adoption studies, Chapter 12) and by newer evidence of potential gene–environment interactions.

Increased understanding and consensus around risk factors and protective factors for juvenile delinquency has implications for public health research and implementation of strategies to reduce juvenile offending (Loeber & Farrington, 2000; Hall *et al.*, 2012). The benefits of this are potentially far-reaching; the 14 year follow-up report on the Pittsburgh Youth Study showed that many risk factors known to be associated with delinquent behavior also predicted mental health problems (Loeber *et al.*, 2001), indicating that action to prevent juvenile offending might have wider benefits on the mental health of young people.

The mental health of juvenile offenders

Over the last 15 years, the mental health of juvenile offenders has received increasing attention, with numerous psychiatric morbidity studies conducted across the world. Methodological differences hamper effective comparison of studies, but in general significantly elevated levels of psychiatric morbidity have been observed in juvenile offenders across virtually all categories of mental disorder.

A national study of detained young offenders aged 16–20 years in the United Kingdom found that 13% of remanded males had received support for a mental or emotional problem in the 12 months before coming to prison, compared to 27% of females. Nearly 1 in 10 of sentenced female young offenders reported having had a psychiatric hospital admission in the past. High prevalence of psychiatric disorders in sentenced inmates included personality disorder (88%), any psychosis (10%), mood/anxiety disorders (41% of males and 67% of females), lifetime suicide attempts (20% of males and 33% of females), self-harm (7% for males and 11% for females), hazardous alcohol consumption (70% of males and 51% of females) and drug misuse (70%). The proportion of young people taken into local authority care in their childhood was 35% for remanded females and 42% for remanded males. These results are consistent with other studies that consistently identify much higher rates of mood/anxiety disorders and self-harm in female young offenders than in male. Of note, overall at least 95% of all young offenders were identified as having a mental disorder, with comorbidity observed in 80% (Lader *et al.*, 2000).

High prevalence of mental disorder among juvenile offenders has been replicated in the United States (Atkins *et al.*, 1999; Teplin *et al.*, 2002; Shufelt & Cocozza, 2006), Finland (Sailas *et al.*, 2005), Sweden (Fazel *et al.*, 2008a), Switzerland (Gisin *et al.*, 2012) and several other countries, with further support for high psychiatric comorbidity (Abram *et al.*, 2003). Systematic reviews have noted a wide range of prevalence of overall mental illness in juvenile offenders, invariably far higher than found in the general population (Fazel *et al.*, 2008b; Penner *et al.*, 2011).

Neurodevelopmental disorders

In the last decade, the prevalence and severity of neurodevelopmental disorders in young offenders has received greater scrutiny. A study of incarcerated juvenile offenders in the United States identified average prevalence rates for youth with disabling conditions (including "emotional disturbance") of 33.4%, with 38.6% of these individuals displaying specific learning disabilities and 9.7% mental retardation (Quinn *et al.*, 2005).

A review of neurodisability in young offenders indicated an elevated prevalence of intellectual disability (23–32%, compared to 2–4% of the general population), specific learning disability such as dyslexia (43–57%, compared with 10% of the general population), communication disorders (60–90%, compared with 1–7% of the general population), autism spectrum disorders (15% compared with 0.6–1.2%), traumatic brain injury (65–76% compared with 5–24%), fetal alcohol syndrome (10.9–11.7% compared with 0.1–5%, and attention deficit/hyperactivity disorder (ADHD; 11.7% for males and 18.5 % for females, compared with 1–2% for ICD-10 hyperkinesis or 3–9% for DSM-IV ADHD), (Hughes *et al.*, 2012). Studies of ADHD in young offenders in the United Kingdom and Germany have indicated a higher rate of 43–45% (Rösler *et al.*, 2004; Young *et al.*, 2010). A meta-analysis of the rate of ADHD in young offenders reported a prevalence of 30.1% (Young *et al.*, 2015).

Unmet needs

Despite the known high prevalence of mental disorder, the mental health needs of young offenders are generally not adequately met (Kurtz *et al.*, 1998; Teplin *et al.*, 2005) and even when services are available, may not be accessed equally by offenders of all racial groups (Rawal *et al.*, 2004). The stakes could not be higher: a high suicide rate has been observed in young male prisoners (Fazel *et al.*, 2005) and the elevated general mortality rate of young offenders sentenced to prison is associated with mental disorder (Sailas *et al.*, 2006). Furthermore, while the presence of a psychiatric disorder in detained adolescents alone may not represent a risk factor for serious recidivism (Colins *et al.*, 2011) better mental health services may reduce the risk of future juvenile justice system involvement (Foster *et al.*, 2004).

Building on knowledge of high prevalence of mental disorder, investigative tools such as the Salford Needs Assessment Schedule for Adolescents have been used to highlight the substantial rates of unmet mental health and psychosocial needs for boys in secure care (Kroll *et al.*, 2002; Harrington *et al.*, 2005) and young offenders (Chitsabesan *et al.*, 2006).

The relationship between mental disorder and juvenile offending is not always clear and merits further investigation. Some evidence indicates that juvenile mental health users are more likely to come into conflict with the law, having more arrests than non mental health service users (Rosenblatt *et al.*, 2000). In the case of ADHD (and most likely several other mental disorders), the associated increase in juvenile offending may not be directly related to the disorder but mediated indirectly by comorbidity with conduct disorder, substance misuse and peer delinquency (Gudjonsson *et al.*, 2014).

Forensic psychiatric assessment of juveniles

Principles of assessment

The broad range of needs and risks presented by juvenile offenders puts particular demands on the clinician, with a requirement for a thorough assessment, information from collateral sources, timeliness, clear notes, clear risk assessments, clear management plans, good communication with other disciplines and agencies and arrangements to maintain continuity of care. A clinical history should include a developmental history, with information from multiple sources including family, paediatrics, family doctor, education, social services, youth justice agencies,

police-and not least, from the young person themselves (see Chapters 32–35).

A forensic psychiatric assessment should include consideration of conduct disorder, depressive and anxiety disorders, suicidality and self-injurious behavior, post traumatic stress disorder, substance misuse, psychotic disorders, ADHD, language and communication disorders, cognitive impairment and autism spectrum disorders. The ICD-10 multiaxial diagnostic system for children and adolescents (see Chapter 2) is particularly well suited to this population.

The primary difference from a regular (non forensic) child psychiatric assessment lies in the need to assess criminogenic factors and their association with underlying psychiatric conditions. These factors may include the perception of the circumstances of the antisocial behavior/crime, the role they played in the behavior/alleged offence and that of others, antecedents and consequences of the behavior, their attitude, and beliefs toward the behavior/crime, level of remorse and blame attribution. Obtaining this history may be complicated by many factors, including a reluctance to fully engage in the assessment, a lack of openness and honesty, a tendency to give socially desirable responses, perceived peer pressure and fear of reprisals.

It is not feasible to conduct a comprehensive psychiatric assessment for all juveniles who come into contact with a youth justice system. The practice of screening for mental disorder has therefore been adopted, using instruments such as the Massachusetts Youth Screening Instrument (MAYSI; Grisso *et al.*, 2001) and by embedding mental health screening into youth justice policy and routine practice (Bailey *et al.*, 2006). In the United Kingdom, the Department of Health is introducing the Comprehensive Health Assessment Tool (CHAT) across young offender establishments.

Effective awareness of and screening for anxiety and depression as well as suicidal risk may be particularly important as they are often overlooked in secure environments (Mitchell & Shaw, 2011). This is particularly necessary when assessing females who more commonly present with emotional disorders (see Chapters 58–64). For disruptive and neurodevelopmental disorders, screening by self-rating and informants is helpful for identifying cases requiring further assessment (Young *et al.*, 2010).

A set of healthcare standards for children and young people in secure settings published in the United Kingdom notes the importance of physical and mental health care in this population, including attention to history of vaccinations, nutrition, dental health and continuity in care for ongoing conditions (Royal College of Paediatrics and Child Health, 2013).

Risk assessment

Risk assessment, risk formulation and risk management may be considered to be among the core tasks of forensic child and adolescent psychiatrists. As with general assessment, risk assessment depends on obtaining a good history from multiple sources. The commonly encountered risks associated with juvenile offenders are listed in Table 49.2. Many young offenders are at risk of victimization themselves; a high proportion will

Table 49.2 Types of risks.

Risks to self

Neglect by carer or self-neglect

Abuse (emotional, physical, or sexual, including exposure to domestic violence)

Substance misuse (acute intoxication, longer term harm and withdrawal)

Self-harm (self-cutting, overdoses, burning, insertion, ligatures and suicide attempts)

Exploitation (coercion, financial and sexual)

Vulnerability arising from mental disorder or homelessness

Reprisals from victim or parties linked to victim

Gang-related violence

Risks to others

Violence (pushing, punching, slapping, kicking, biting and strangling)

Use of weapons (blades, firearms, makeshift weapons e.g., chairs, biological weapons e.g., blood or saliva, harmful chemicals e.g., hazardous cleaning materials)

Emotional abuse and bullying (personal, racial, ethnic, religious or sexual themes)

Electronic aggression (cyberbullying, cyberstalking or cyberharassment)

Sexually harmful behavior (exposure, touching, penetration and indecent images)

Stalking

Unsafe fire setting (accidental, impulsive, planning, method, fuel, disabling alarms and blocking exits)

Criminal damage

Theft/burglary

Vehicle offences (no licence, no insurance and "joy riding")

Substance-related offences (possessing, using, selling and trafficking)

Fraud (identity and financial)

Non compliance and breaching community orders

Subversion of security (tampering with alarms, locks, doors and cybersecurity)

Escape from secure setting or abscondsion/running away

Hostage taking (likely targets and demands)

Concerted disorder (coordinated antisocial acts, riots, instigator or follower)

have been subjected to abuse of various forms at the hand of their carers, and these safeguarding risks may require urgent action (see Chapters 29 and 30). Gang membership is known to be an important risk factor for delinquency (see Chapter 12). Gang-related tensions and risks of reprisals following offences may also pose significant risks that authorities must consider. Furthermore, juvenile offenders may be vulnerable to exploitation by others due to neurodevelopmental problems or other mental disorder.

Risk of violence to others

Most risk assessments assess risk of future violence to others. The "risk formulation" is a statement of the risk—a description of the current nature, severity, likelihood and immediacy of an adverse event, combined with an analysis of factors that are likely to modify the risk, and a plan for monitoring or review of risk. In particular, an analysis of past events is essential as past behaviors are the best predictor of future behaviors; important factors include planning, weapons, motivation, intention, discoverability, substance misuse, mental disorder and peer influence.

Three main approaches to risk assessment are generally acknowledged: clinical judgements, actuarial risk assessments

and structured professional judgements. A clinical judgement on risk is a fast but unstructured risk assessment; there are no requirements around the minimum information required, and the quality of the assessment depends very much on the practitioner performing it. Actuarial risk assessments are statistically determined tools that use historical information to predict risks of reoffending; they may be more reliable than clinical judgement and a meta-analysis of their predictive validity indicates some potential benefit (Schwalbe, 2008). However, actuarial tools are rather static; they do not take account of changeable clinical factors and do not indicate points for interventions. Hence, the third method is the most commonly applied in practice, structured professional judgement tools that include items that have been statistically associated with violence. The Structured Assessment of Violence Risk in Youth (SAVRY; Borum *et al.*, 2005) combines historical factors (e.g., history of violence) with dynamic social (e.g., peer delinquency), individual (e.g., substance misuse) and protective factors (e.g., strong commitment to school) that lead very naturally to a risk management plan. For younger children, the gender-specific Early Assessment Risk List (EARL; Augimeri *et al.*, 2010) is also used widely.

The term "violence" encompasses a wide range of acts from slapping to homicide, with or without weapons. A useful distinction is often made between instrumental (planned or proactive) aggression and reactive (affective, defensive or impulsive) aggression. While instrumental aggression is classically associated with low anxiety and psychopathic traits, reactive aggression is associated with angry outbursts, mood dysregulation and disorders such as ADHD. Markers of psychopathy in children and adolescents typically assess behaviors categorized as callous and unemotional, as there have been concerns about applying the term "psychopathy" to juveniles. Callous and unemotional traits are widely accepted as a significant risk factor for violent offending (Farrington and Welsh, 2005) and are now included within the DSM-5 conduct disorder specifier of "limited prosocial emotions." Psychopathy in young people can be assessed using the Psychopathy Checklist Youth Version (PCL:YV; Forth *et al.*, 2003). Some have argued that while useful, the construct of childhood psychopathy deserves greater scrutiny, with more attention to potentially dynamic developmental aspects that may contribute to an individual's apparently callous or unemotional presentation (Cooke *et al.*, 2004; Dawson *et al.*, 2012). See Chapter 68.

Sexually harmful behavior

Tools for assessing risk of sexually harmful behaviour include the Juvenile Sex Offender Assessment Protocol II (J-SOAP-II; Prentky & Righthand, 2003) and Estimate of Risk of Adolescent Sexual Offense Recidivism (ERASOR; Worling & Curwen, 2001). The AIM (Assessment, Intervention, and Moving on) program, based on the Good Lives Model (GLM), has been gaining popularity as an approach that draws on the young person's strengths to undertake a comprehensive assessment and to deliver treatment (Griffin *et al.*, 2008). An appreciation of developmental and gender aspects of sexuality is essential for this sort of assessment. A behavioral analysis approach (i.e., a functional analysis of behavior) may be more suitable for individuals with significant intellectual disability and sexually harmful behavior.

Unsafe fire setting and arson

Unsafe fire setting by adolescents should be considered within a developmental framework (MacKay *et al.*, 2012), with particular attention to intent and planning (Table 49.2). The assessment must include a behavioral analysis of the antecedents and consequences of the behavior in order to gain a comprehensive understanding of the factors and beliefs influencing behavior, so as to identify targets for intervention. Female juvenile fire setters may present increased mental health needs and risks (Hickle & Roa-Sepowitz, 2010). Arson is a legal term and a young person may be convicted of attempted arson even in the absence of actual fire setting.

Emotional abuse and stalking

Emotional abuse, bullying and harassment including stalking (Purcell *et al.*, 2009) may take a variety of forms and themes. Cyberbullying, cyber-harassment and cyberstalking via electronic media are increasingly recognized as a serious form of victimization (Ybarra & Mitchell, 2004; Patchin & Hinduja, 2006; Kiriakidis & Kavoura, 2010) and one that may deserve special attention in risk assessment.

Risk management

It is important to be mindful that the objective of a risk assessment is to generate a risk management plan that has a constructive and applied purpose to reduce risk as opposed to an overarching prediction of the likelihood of reoffending. This will include strategies for reducing and managing risk behavior(s), including the need for specific monitoring, treatment, support, disclosure and consideration of the need for multiagency involvement. It should be integrated into the general care plan for the young person, shared with all relevant professionals and agencies and updated every 6–12 months especially for change in dynamic factors to assess need for physical security (locks, doors, and alarms), operational security (procedures, and protocols) and relational security (good clinical knowledge of the young person and a therapeutic relationship between patients and staff).

Interventions

Principles of intervention

Interventions in criminal justice systems often operate under the risk-need-responsivity (RNR) model, which focuses on the prediction of risk and classification of offenders for treatment (Andrews *et al.*, 1990). This model identifies those presenting highest risks to others as candidates for the most intense

intervention. A contrasting approach known as the GLM (Ward & Brown, 2004) presents a positive, restorative model of rehabilitation based on strengths. This makes for a more customized intervention focused on prosocial ways of meeting the particular physical, social, and psychological needs of an individual. In parallel to these developments, the consideration of juvenile delinquency within a public health approach shifts young people into a biomedical sphere where evidence-based interventions are considered for the primary, secondary and tertiary prevention of juvenile delinquency (Stevens *et al.*, 2006). Primary prevention encompasses universal approaches to prevent crime before it occurs; secondary prevention focuses on those at highest risk of offending; tertiary prevention consists of approaches with young people who have already offended (Table 49.3).

Given the mental health needs in young offenders, support for mental disorders should be included as a central component of any intervention (see individual disorder chapters). Furthermore, the high prevalence of disturbed early attachments and post traumatic stress should be considered in the delivery of appropriate interventions (Kerig *et al.*, 2009). There has been some support for extending the concept of attachment styles into adolescence (Scott *et al.*, 2011) and this may represent a helpful framework for assessing and understanding the interpersonal styles and difficulties of juvenile offenders.

Evidence for early interventions

Findings from the Cambridge Study in Delinquent Development identified four targets for early intervention: (i) low intelligence/attainment, which can be targeted by preschool

---

Table 49.3 A public health model for youth offending.

Primary prevention

Parenting programs
Preschool programs
Day-care programs
School programs
Cognitive skills training
Peer programs
Community programs
Situational crime prevention

Secondary prevention

Family-focused therapies
Mentoring
Therapeutic foster care
Safeguarding of children
Treatment of parental substance misuse

Tertiary prevention

Cooperation between police, social services and mental health
Intensive supervision and surveillance
Assertive treatment of mental disorder
Restorative justice
Victim support

Source: Adapted from Stevens *et al.* (2006).

intellectual enrichment programs; (ii) poor parental child-rearing behavior, which can be targeted by parenting programs as early as pregnancy; (iii) impulsiveness, which can be targeted by cognitive-behavioral skills programs; and (iv) poverty, although there is little evidence to support reduced juvenile delinquency resulting from income maintenance (Farrington et al., 2009a, b). Programs for early family and parent training show beneficial effects on delinquency and problem behaviors (Scott, 2005; Piquero et al., 2008; see Chapter 37); strategies that support children under 10 to improve self-control have also been suggested (Piquero et al., 2010). Many of these treatments overlap with those for conduct disorder (see Chapters 36, 37 and 65). Recently published national guidelines for treatment of antisocial behavior and conduct disorders in the United Kingdom are helpful (National Institute for Health and Care Excellence, 2013).

Systemic interventions

Among the best known interventions for those at risk of juvenile offending is multisystemic therapy (MST) which was developed to be an effective alternative to incarceration (Henggeler et al., 1992). It consists of an intensive set of integrated interventions across multiple systems in the young person's life, following nine treatment principles such as using strengths in the young person's environment as levers for change and promoting responsible behavior in the family. Support for MST in juvenile offending has emerged from independent effectiveness trials (Timmons-Mitchell et al., 2006) and cost-effectiveness analysis (Cary et al., 2013). However, meta-analytic reviews reveal several trials that failed to replicate its effectiveness (Littell et al., 2005). The training requirements, intensity of the work and strict requirements around fidelity to the treatment model can sometimes hamper implementation (see Chapter 50).

Multidimensional treatment foster care (MTFC) was formulated within a social learning model. It uses a foster home as the primary site of therapeutic intervention, encouraging contact with prosocial young people. There are high levels of clinical support, daily contact and points systems for rewards alongside clear consequences for negative behavior. General therapeutic foster care has been suggested as being effective in the prevention of violence (Hahn et al., 2005) although evidence from randomized controlled trials is mixed (see Chapters 50 and 65). Another manifestation of an intensive systemic approach is the "wraparound" process designed to support children and their families (Suter & Bruns, 2009). The meta-analysis by Lipsey (2009) of 548 diverse intervention studies found three factors that predicted success: a "therapeutic" intervention philosophy, serving high risk offenders and good quality implementation.

Psychological and offending behavior programs

Structured programs using a cognitive-behavioral model have been associated with marked reductions in recidivism in high risk detained males (Tong & Farrington, 2006; Garrido et al., 2007). On the other hand, more modest benefits have been reported when delivered in residential settings (Armelius & Andreassen, 2007). Specific cognitive-behavioral programs developed for juvenile delinquents may be more promising and require further evaluation, such as Anger Replacement Training (ART; Glick & Goldstein, 1987) and the revised Reasoning & Rehabilitation (R&R2; Young & Ross, 2007a, b).

For working with perpetrators and victims of sexually harmful behavior, the manualized AIM program has been gaining popularity in the United Kingdom. This includes a repertoire of numerous modules for males, females, young children, children with intellectual disability, schools and foster carers. Based on the GLM, it draws on the young person's strengths to undertake a comprehensive assessment and deliver treatment (Griffin et al., 2008). Clinicians should be alert to the high proportion of juvenile sexual offending that occurs against other children and the higher likelihood of complex needs during the assessment and treatment of females who display sexually harmful behavior (McCartan et al., 2011).

Other psychological interventions with some evidence of effectiveness include school-based programs for social skills and information processing (Wilson & Lipsey, 2006), mentoring (Tolan et al., 2008) and leisure time activities for youth at risk (Danish Crime Prevention Council, 2012). There has also been a rise in programs aiming to tackle and prevent gang-affiliation.

Substance misuse programs for young people are widespread, but meaningful engagement and motivation to change are often an obstacle. The technique of motivational interviewing for treatment of substance misuse (Miller & Rollnick, 1991) is a promising approach that has been applied to juvenile offender populations but requires further investigation (Feldstein & Ginsburg, 2006). Limited data from studies of youth drug courts indicate a modest reduction in recidivism (Mitchell et al., 2012). See Chapter 66.

Special consideration should be given to individuals with neurodevelopmental disorders, who may not find it easy to access the services they require, or may need environmental or procedural modification to help manage their risk or vulnerability. A study looking at the language and communication skills of juvenile offenders found that 66–90% of the sample had below average language skills, with 46–67% of these being in the poor or very poor range, suggesting that these young people may not have the necessary skills to cope with verbally mediated interventions aimed at reducing reoffending (Bryan et al., 2007). Clinicians must therefore be alert to these potential barriers preventing young people from participating in therapeutic programs, particularly in group settings. Intervention by a speech and language therapist may help improve confidence, communication skills and engagement in therapeutic programs (see Chapters 51–57).

Medical interventions

Aside from addressing criminogenic needs, individuals with mental disorder should be treated for psychiatric conditions in the usual way (see chapters for clinical syndromes and personality disorder). For young offenders with severe psychiatric disturbance and complex needs, secure psychiatric hospitals provide a safe and contained setting for intensive assessment, treatment, and management, with a multi disciplinary and multi-agency focus.

Due to the high prevalence of neurodevelopmental disorder, traumatic brain injury and elevated rates of alcohol and substance misuse in young offenders, clinicians may wish to be cautious when prescribing psychotropic medication in view of constitutional sensitivities and interactions with substances. Other challenges include the potential for non concordance with medication, sequestration of tablets for overdose, taking irregular or excessive doses, trading of tablets and potential for abuse. Supervised medication delivered in liquid or orodispersible formulations may sometimes be most appropriate.

Moreover, there may also be a role for the use of pharmacological treatment in the rapid tranquilization of acutely mentally disturbed aggressive young people, as described in established guidelines (Taylor *et al.*, 2012). However, efforts should be made to avoid such a situation by early identification of distress, engaging the patient, establishing a therapeutic rapport and considering environmental modification to help de-escalate a situation. The preferred method of managing severe aggression in young patients varies between countries; the United Kingdom routinely implements physical restraint by staff and seclusion, but there is a degree of reluctance and caution in the use of rapid tranquillization of juveniles and virtually complete avoidance of mechanical restraint. Some other countries use mechanical restraint more liberally, with much less use of seclusion for juveniles.

Unhelpful interventions

Well known but discredited approaches include "Scared Straight" programs in which juveniles at an early stage of offending are exposed to high security prison inmates; there is evidence that this approach may actually increase risk of recidivism, compared to no intervention (Petrosino *et al.*, 2004). Another example is correctional military style boot camps with harsh discipline. Moreover, trying juveniles in adult courts, juvenile curfews and probation are cited as measures that are not effective in preventing juvenile crime (Stevens *et al.*, 2006).

Professional considerations

Whether for criminal or civil proceedings including family, child custody, immigration or mental health law, a psychiatric expert who prepares a report for court must adhere to standards of integrity and professionalism expected by their professional body (see Chapter 19). Depending on the jurisdiction, a forensic psychiatrist may be instructed to provide a report on pretrial issues such as fitness to plead and special measures for effective participation, trial issues such as psychiatric defences and mitigating circumstances, opinions on risk and recommendations on disposal or care pathway. Further information, including practical guidance, is available in specialist textbooks (Bailey & Dolan, 2004; Benedek *et al.*, 2009; Young *et al.*, 2009; Rix, 2011).

Ethical dilemmas facing the forensic psychiatrist

It has been argued that objectivity is almost invariably compromised when a treating practitioner presents medical evidence to court about their patient. This position creates a compelling need for independent experts, who bring not only enhanced objectivity to proceedings but also specialist medicolegal skills and experience. The United States probably provides the best example of where the practice of such "forensicists" has become firmly established and hotly debated. Disagreement has emerged around the extent to which these largely court-bound professionals 'practice medicine' in their advisory role. The Ethics Committee of the American Psychiatric Association has brought some clarity to the matter by stating that "psychiatrists are physicians, and physicians are physicians at all times," affirming the medical responsibility of professionals to patients wherever they practice. Indeed, the duty of care to the patient and the duty to protect the public from harm are often in harmony, as effective treatment and management strategies tend to address both types of risk simultaneously. Furthermore, such a role may be considered as lying outside the professional remit of the treating clinician and/or the treating psychiatrist may simply not have the time or resources to provide specialist advice to courts.

For these and other reasons, it is most likely that independent experts will continue to be required in court proceedings. Measures should therefore be in place to help legal teams and courts appoint appropriately qualified experts, who are competent and clinically active in the relevant field. In cases involving children and adolescents, court experts should demonstrate competence, experience and up-to-date knowledge of working with children. Experts should not stray outside of their area of expertize, for example, by giving 'bedside' estimates of IQ or by interpreting psychological test results when not trained to do so. It is important that effective professional collaborations are developed with other disciplines, for example, with clinical, forensic and/or neuropsychology.

Conclusions

Forensic child and adolescent psychiatry has emerged as a significant clinical subspecialty, straddling the interface between child and adolescent psychiatry, forensic psychiatry, and the law in a clinically and ethically challenging, multidisciplinary and multi-agency setting. This chapter has provided an introduction to this clinical subspecialty with the hope that it will encourage readers from psychiatry and allied disciplines to engage with a vulnerable population of young people whose needs and rights are so often overlooked across the world, and for whom early intervention may be life-changing.

Acknowledgments

The authors thank David Farrington for helpful correspondence that supported the writing of this chapter.

References

Abram, K. *et al.* (2003) Comorbid psychiatric disorders in youth in juvenile detention. *Archives of General Psychiatry* **60**, 1097.

Andrews, D.A. *et al.* (1990) Classification for effective rehabilitation: rediscovering psychology. *Criminal Justice and Behavior* **17**, 19.

Armelius, B.A. & Andreassen, T.H. (2007) Cognitive-behavioral treatment for antisocial behavior in youth in residential treatment. *Campbell Systematic Reviews* 3.

Atkins, D.L. *et al.* (1999) Mental health and incarcerated youth. I: prevalence and nature of psychopathology. *Journal of Child and Family Studies* **8**, 193–204.

Augimeri, L.K. *et al.* (2010) Gender-specific childhood risk assessment tools: early assessment risk lists for boys (EARL-20B) and girls (EARL-21G). In: *Handbook of Violence Risk Assessment*, pp. 43–62.

Bailey, S. & Dolan, M. (eds) (2004) *Adolescent Forensic Psychiatry*. CRC Press.

Bailey, S.M. *et al.* (1994) The first 100 admissions to an adolescent secure unit. *Journal of Adolescence* **17**, 207–220.

Bailey, S. *et al.* (2006) Recent developments in mental health screening and assessment in juvenile justice systems. *Child and Adolescent Psychiatric Clinics of North America* **15**, 391–406.

Benedek, E.P. *et al.* (eds) (2009) *Principles and Practice of Child and Adolescent Forensic Mental Health*. American Psychiatric Association.

Borum, R. *et al.* (2005) Structured assessment of violence risk in youth. In: *Mental Health Screening and Assessment in Juvenile Justice*, pp. 311–323.

Broidy, L.M. *et al.* (2003) Developmental trajectories of childhood disruptive behaviors and adolescent delinquency: a six-site, cross-national study. *Developmental Psychology* **39**, 222.

Bryan, K. *et al.* (2007) Language and communication difficulties in juvenile offenders. *International Journal of Language & Communication Disorders* **42**, 505–520.

Callaghan, J. *et al.* (2003) Primary mental health workers within youth offending teams: a new service model. *Journal of Adolescence* **26**, 185–199.

Callahan, L. *et al.* (2012) A national survey of U.S. juvenile mental health courts. *Psychiatric Services (Washington, D.C.)* **63**, 130–134.

Cary, M. *et al.* (2013) Economic evaluation of multisystemic therapy for young people at risk for continuing criminal activity in the UK. *PloS One* **8**, e61070.

Chitsabesan, P. *et al.* (2006) Mental health needs of young offenders in custody and in the community. *British Journal of Psychiatry* **188**, 534–540.

Church, R. *et al.* (2013) The minimum age of criminal responsibility: clinical, criminological/sociological, developmental and legal perspectives. *Youth Justice* **13**, 99–101.

Colins, O. *et al.* (2011) Psychiatric disorder in detained male adolescents as risk factor for serious recidivism. *Canadian Journal of Psychiatry-Revue Canadienne de Psychiatrie* **56**, 44–50.

Cooke, D.J. *et al.* (2004) Reconstructing psychopathy: clarifying the significance of antisocial and socially deviant behavior in the diagnosis of psychopathic personality disorder. *Journal of Personality Disorders* **18**, 337–357.

Danish Crime Prevention Council (2012). *The effectiveness of mentoring and leisure time activities for youth at risk. A systematic review* [Online]. Available: http://www.dkr.dk/mentoring-and-leisure-time-activities-youth-risk [06 Aug 2014].

Dawson, S. *et al.* (2012) Critical issues in the assessment of adolescent psychopathy: an illustration using two case studies. *International Journal of Forensic Mental Health* **11**, 63–79.

Farrington, D.P. & Ttofi, M.M. (2011) Bullying as a predictor of offending, violence and later life outcomes. *Criminal Behaviour and Mental Health* **21**, 90–98.

Farrington, D.P. & Welsh, B.C. (2005) Randomized experiments in criminology: what have we learned in the last two decades? *Journal of Experimental Criminology* **1**, 9–38.

Farrington, D.P. & West, D.J. (1971) A comparison between early delinquents and young aggressives. *British Journal of Criminology* **11**, 341.

Farrington, D.P. *et al.* (2009a) The development of offending from age 8 to age 50: recent results from the Cambridge study in delinquent development. *Monatsschrift fur Kriminologie und Strafrechtsreform* **92**, 160–173.

Farrington, D.P. *et al.* (2009b) Development of adolescence limited, late-onset and persistent offenders from age 8 to age 48. *Aggressive Behavior* **35**, 150–163.

Fazel, S. *et al.* (2005) Suicides in male prisoners in England and Wales, 1978–2003. *The Lancet* **366**, 1301–1302.

Fazel, M. *et al.* (2008a) Psychopathology in adolescent and young adult criminal offenders (15–21 years) in Sweden. *Social Psychiatry and Psychiatric Epidemiology* **43**, 319–324.

Fazel, S. *et al.* (2008b) Mental disorders amongst adolescents in juvenile detention and correctional facilities: a systematic review and metaregession analysis of 25 surveys. *Journal of the American Academy of Child and Adolescent Psychiatry* **47**, 1010–1019.

Feldstein, S.W. & Ginsburg, J.I. (2006) Motivational interviewing with dually diagnosed adolescents in juvenile justice settings. *Brief Treatment and Crisis Intervention* **6**, 218.

Forth, A.E. *et al.* (2003) *Hare Psychopathy Checklist: Youth Version (PCL: YV)*. Multi-Health Systems, Toronto, Canada.

Foster, E.M. *et al.* (2004) Can better mental health services reduce the risk of juvenile justice system involvement? *American Journal of Public Health* **94**, 859–865.

Garrido, V. *et al.* (2007) Serious (violent or chronic) juvenile offenders: a systematic review of treatment effectiveness in secure corrections. *Campbell Systematic Reviews* 3.

Gisin, D. *et al.* (2012) Mental health of young offenders in Switzerland: recognizing psychiatric symptoms during detention. *Journal of Forensic and Legal Medicine* **19**, 332–336.

Glick, B. & Goldstein, A.P. (1987) Aggression replacement training. *Journal of Counseling & Development* **65**, 356–362.

Goldson, B. & Muncie, J. (2012) Towards a global 'child friendly' juvenile justice? *International Journal of Law, Crime and Justice* **40**, 47–64.

Griffin, H.L. *et al.* (2008) The development and initial testing of the AIM2 framework to assess risk and strengths in young people who sexually offend. *Journal of Sexual Aggression* **14**, 211–225.

Grisso, T. *et al.* (2001) Massachusetts youth screening instrument for mental health needs of juvenile justice youths. *Journal of the American Academy of Child & Adolescent Psychiatry* **40**, 541–548.

Grisso, T. *et al.* (2003) Juveniles' competence to stand trial: a comparison of adolescents' and adults' capacities as trial defendants. *Law and Human Behavior* **27**, 333–363.

Gudjonsson, G.H. *et al.* (2006) Custodial interrogation, false confession and individual differences: a national study among Icelandic youth. *Personality and Individual Differences* **41**, 49–59.

Gudjonsson, G.H. *et al.* (2014) A national epidemiological study of offending and its relationship with ADHD symptoms and associated risk factors. *Journal of Attention Disorders* **18**, 3–13.

Hahn, R.A. *et al.* (2005) The effectiveness of therapeutic foster care for the prevention of violence: a systematic review. *American Journal of Preventive Medicine* **28**, 72–90.

Hall, J.E. *et al.* (2012) Implications of direct protective factors for public health research and prevention strategies to reduce youth violence. *American Journal of Preventive Medicine* **43**, S76–S83.

Harrington, R.C. *et al.* (2005) Psychosocial needs of boys in secure care for serious or persistent offending. *Journal of Child Psychology and Psychiatry* **46**, 859–866.

Hazel, A.N. (2008) *Cross-National Comparison of Youth Justice.* Youth Justice Board, London, UK.

Henggeler, S.W. *et al.* (1992) Family preservation using multisystemic therapy: an effective alternative to incarcerating serious juvenile offenders. *Journal of Consulting and Clinical Psychology* **60**, 953.

Hickle, K.E. & Roa-Sepowitz, D.E. (2010) Female juvenile arsonists: an exploratory look at characteristics and solo and group arson offences. *Legal and Criminological Psychology* **15**, 385–399.

Hughes, N. *et al.* (2012) *Nobody Made the Connection: The Prevalence of Neurodisability in Young People Who Offend.* Office of the Children's Commissioner, London, UK.

Kerig, P.K. *et al.* (2009) Posttraumatic stress as a mediator of the relationship between trauma and mental health problems among juvenile delinquents. *Journal of Youth and Adolescence* **38**, 1214–1225.

Kiriakidis, S.P. & Kavoura, A. (2010) Cyberbullying: a review of the literature on harassment through the internet and other electronic means. *Family & Community Health* **33**, 82–93.

Kroll, L. *et al.* (2002) Mental health needs of boys in secure care for serious or persistent offending: a prospective, longitudinal study. *The Lancet* **359**, 1975–1979.

Kurtz, Z. *et al.* (1998) Children in the criminal justice and secure care systems: how their mental health needs are met. *Journal of Adolescence* **21**, 543–553.

Lader, D. *et al.* (2000) *Psychiatric Morbidity Among Young Offenders in England and Wales.* Office for National Statistics, London.

Lipsey, M.W. (2009) The primary factors that characterize effective interventions with juvenile offenders: a meta-analytic overview. *Victims and Offenders* **4**, 124–147.

Littell, J. *et al.* (2005) *Multisystemic Therapy for Social, Emotional, and Behavioural Problems in Youth Aged 10–17.* Nordic Campbell Center.

Loeber, R. & Farrington, D.P. (2000) Young children who commit crime: epidemiology, developmental origins, risk factors, early interventions, and policy implications. *Development and Psychopathology* **12**, 737–762.

Loeber, R. *et al.* (2001) Male mental health problems, psychopathy, and personality traits: key findings from the first 14 years of the Pittsburgh youth study. *Clinical Child and Family Psychology Review* **4**, 273–297.

MacKay, S. *et al.* (2012) Research and practice in adolescent firesetting. *Criminal Justice and Behavior* **39**, 842–864.

McAra, L. & McVie, S. (2010) Youth crime and justice: key messages from the Edinburgh study of youth transitions and crime. *Criminology and Criminal Justice* **10**, 179–209.

McCartan, F.M. *et al.* (2011) Child and adolescent females who present with sexually abusive behaviours: a 10-year UK prevalence study. *Journal of Sexual Aggression* **17**, 4–14.

Miller, W.R. & Rollnick, S. (1991) *Motivational Interviewing: Preparing People to Change Addictive Behavior.* Guilford Press, New York.

Mitchell, P. & Shaw, J. (2011) Factors affecting the recognition of mental health problems among adolescent offenders in custody. *Journal of Forensic Psychiatry & Psychology* **22**, 381–394.

Mitchell, O. *et al.* (2012) Drug courts' effects on criminal offending for juveniles and adults. *Campbell Systematic Reviews* 8.

Moffitt, T.E. (1993) Adolescence-limited and life-course-persistent antisocial behavior: a developmental taxonomy. *Psychological Review* **100**, 674.

Moffitt, T.E. *et al.* (2002) Males on the life-course-persistent and adolescence-limited antisocial pathways: follow-up at age 26 years. *Development and Psychopathology* **14**, 179–207.

Muncie, J. (2008) The punitive turn in juvenile justice: cultures of control and rights compliance in Western Europe and the USA. *Youth Justice* **8**, 107–121.

Muncie, J. & Goldson, B. (eds) (2006) *Comparative Youth Justice Sage,* London, UK.

Murray, J. *et al.* (2009) Effects of parental imprisonment on child antisocial behaviour and mental health. *Campbell Systematic Reviews* (4).

National Institute for Health and Care Excellence (2013). *Antisocial behaviour and conduct disorders in children and young people: recognition, intervention and management* [Online]. Available: http://guidance.nice.org.uk/cg158 [13 Jun 2013].

Patchin, J.W. & Hinduja, S. (2006) Bullies move beyond the schoolyard a preliminary look at cyberbullying. *Youth Violence and Juvenile Justice* **4**, 148–169.

Patterson, G.R. *et al.* (1989) A developmental perspective on antisocial behavior. *American Psychologist* **44**, 329.

Penner, E.K. *et al.* (2011) Young offenders in custody: an international comparison of mental health services. *International Journal of Forensic Mental Health* **10**, 215–232.

Petrosino, A. *et al.* (2004) 'Scared Straight' and other juvenile awareness programs for preventing juvenile delinquency. *Campbell Systematic Reviews* (2).

Piquero, A.R. *et al.* (2008) Effects of early family/parenting programs on antisocial behavior and delinquency. *Campbell Systematic Reviews* (11).

Piquero, A.R. *et al.* (2010) Self-control interventions for children under age 10 for improving self-control and delinquency and problem behaviors. *Campbell Systematic Reviews* (2).

Prentky, R. & Righthand, S. (2003) *Juvenile Sex Offender Assessment Protocol-II (J-SOAP-II) Manual.* US Department of Justice, Office of Justice Programs, Office of Juvenile Justice and Delinquency Prevention, Washington, DC.

Purcell, R. *et al.* (2009) Stalking among juveniles. *The British Journal of Psychiatry* **194**, 451–455.

Quinn, M.M. *et al.* (2005) Youth with disabilities in juvenile corrections: a national survey. *Exceptional Children* **71**, 339–345.

Rawal, P. *et al.* (2004) Racial differences in the mental health needs and service utilization of youth in the juvenile justice system. *The Journal of Behavioral Health Services & Research* **31**, 242–254.

Rix, K. (2011) *Expert Psychiatric Evidence*. RCPsych Publications.

Rösler, M. *et al.* (2004) Prevalence of attention deficit-/hyperactivity disorder (ADHD) and comorbid disorders in young male prison inmates. *European Archives of Psychiatry and Clinical Neuroscience* **254**, 365–371.

Rosenblatt, J.A. *et al.* (2000) Criminal behavior and emotional disorder: comparing youth served by the mental health and juvenile justice systems. *The Journal of Behavioral Health Services & Research* **27**, 227–237.

Royal College of Paediatrics and Child Health (2013). *Healthcare standards for children and young people in secure settings* [Online]. Available: www.rcpch.ac.uk/cypss [13 June 2013].

Rutter, M. *et al.* (1975) Attainment and adjustment in two geographical areas. I—The prevalence of psychiatric disorder. *The British Journal of Psychiatry* **126**, 493–509.

Rutter, M. *et al.* (1998) *Antisocial Behavior by Young People: A Major New Review*. Cambridge University Press.

Sailas, E.S. *et al.* (2005) Mental disorders in prison populations aged 15–21: national register study of two cohorts in Finland. *BMJ: British Medical Journal* **330**, 1364.

Sailas, E.S. *et al.* (2006) The mortality of young offenders sentenced to prison and its association with psychiatric disorders: a register study. *The European Journal of Public Health* **16**, 193–197.

Schwalbe, C.S. (2008) A meta-analysis of juvenile justice risk assessment instruments predictive validity by gender. *Criminal Justice and Behavior* **35**, 1367–1381.

Scott, S. (2005) Do parenting programmes for severe child antisocial behaviour work over the longer term, and for whom? One year follow-up of a multi-centre controlled trial. *Behavioural and Cognitive Psychotherapy* **33**, 403.

Scott, S. *et al.* (2011) Attachment in adolescence: overlap with parenting and unique prediction of behavioural adjustment. *Journal of Child Psychology and Psychiatry* **52**, 1052–1062.

Shufelt, J.L. & Cocozza, J.J. (2006) *Youth with Mental Health Disorders in the Juvenile Justice System: Results from a Multi-State Prevalence Study*. National Center for Mental Health and Juvenile Justice, Delmar, NY.

Stevens, A *et al.* (2006). *Review of good practices in preventing juvenile crime in the European Union* [Online]. Available: http://www.eucpn .org/library/index.asp [13 Jun 2013].

Suter, J.C. & Bruns, E.J. (2009) Effectiveness of the wraparound process for children with emotional and behavioral disorders: a meta-analysis. *Clinical Child and Family Psychology Review* **12**, 336–351.

Taylor, D. *et al.* (eds) (2012) *The Maudsley Prescribing Guidelines in Psychiatry*. Wiley.com

Teplin, L.A. *et al.* (2002) Psychiatric disorders in youth in juvenile detention. *Archives of General Psychiatry* **59**, 1133.

Teplin, L.A. *et al.* (2005) Detecting mental disorder in juvenile detainees: who receives services. *American Journal of Public Health* **95**, 1773–1780.

Timmons-Mitchell, J. *et al.* (2006) An independent effectiveness trial of multisystemic therapy with juvenile justice youth. *Journal of Clinical Child and Adolescent Psychology* **35**, 227–236.

Tolan, P. *et al.* (2008) Mentoring interventions to affect juvenile delinquency and associated problems. *Campbell Systematic Reviews* (16).

Tong, L.S. & Farrington, D.P. (2006) How effective is the "Reasoning and Rehabilitation" programme in reducing reoffending? A meta-analysis of evaluations in four countries. *Psychology, Crime and Law* **12**, 3–24.

United Nations (1990). *United Nations Convention on the rights of the child* [Online]. Available: http://www.unhchr.ch/html/menu3/b/ k2crc.htm [06 Aug 2014].

Vieira, T.A. *et al.* (2009) Matching court-ordered services with treatment needs. *Criminal Justice and Behaviour* **36**, 385–401.

Viljoen, J.L. *et al.* (2005) Legal decisions of preadolescent and adolescent defendants: predictors of confessions, pleas, communication with attorneys, and appeals. *Law and Human Behavior* **29**, 253–277.

Vizard, E. (2013) Practitioner review: the victims and juvenile perpetrators of child sexual abuse–assessment and intervention. *Journal of Child Psychology and Psychiatry* **54**, 503–515.

Ward, T. & Brown, M. (2004) The good lives model and conceptual issues in offender rehabilitation. *Psychology, Crime & Law* **10**, 243–257.

Wilson, S.J. & Lipsey, M.W. (2006) The effects of school-based social information processing interventions on aggressive behavior: part 1: universal programs. *Campbell Systematic Reviews* (5).

Worling, J.R. & Curwen, T. (2001) Estimate of risk of adolescent sexual offense recidivism (ERASOR; Version 2.0). In: *Juveniles and Children Who Sexually Abuse: Frameworks for Assessment*, pp. 372–397.

Ybarra, M.L. & Mitchell, K.J. (2004) Online aggressor/targets, aggressors, and targets: a comparison of associated youth characteristics. *Journal of Child Psychology and Psychiatry* **45**, 1308–1316.

Young, S.J. & Ross, R.R. (2007a) *R&R2 for ADHD Youths and Adults: A Prosocial Competence Training Program*. Cognitive Centre of Canada, Ottawa (www.cognitivecentre.ca).

Young, S.J. & Ross, R.R. (2007b) *R&R2 for Youths and Adults with Mental Health Problems: A Prosocial Competence Training Program*. Cognitive Centre of Canada, Ottawa (www.cognitivecentre.ca).

Young, S. *et al.* (eds) (2009) *Forensic Neuropsychology in Practice: A Guide to Assessment and Legal Processes*. Oxford University Press, Oxford.

Young, S. *et al.* (2010) Prevalence of ADHD symptoms among youth in a secure facility: the consistency and accuracy of self-and informant-report ratings. *The Journal of Forensic Psychiatry & Psychology* **21**, 238–246.

Young, S. *et al.* (2015) A meta-analysis of the prevalence of attention deficit hyperactivity disorder in incarcerated populations. *Psychological Medicine*, **45**, 247–258.

CHAPTER 50

Provision of intensive treatment: intensive outreach, day units, and in-patient units

Anthony James[1] and Anne Worrall-Davies[2]

[1] Department of Psychiatry, University of Oxford, UK

[2] Adolescent Inpatient Service, Leeds Community Healthcare NHS Foundation Trust, Leeds, UK

Introduction

Intensive community services and inpatient care are essential components of a comprehensive child and adolescent mental health service (CAMHS), particularly for those more severely disturbed children and adolescents and for those at risk of self-harm, suicide, or harm to others. Intensive community services form an increasingly important level of care between outpatient and inpatient services. Often these services can provide more immediate and flexible local care, sometimes on a home basis, to a greater number of children and adolescents. Inpatient care remains an economically costly but essential part of a CAMH service and has become specialized, often dealing with greater complexities and more violent children and adolescents. In this chapter, we present community models of intensive services first, followed by day programs, and inpatient models, to reflect increasing intensity and level of restriction.

Community intensive services
Historical development

Changing philosophical beliefs among health, education, and social care professionals, alongside a growing service user movement, have led to the development of a range of community alternatives to day and residential psychiatric care, sometimes specifically to reduce the need for hospitalization or residential care, sometimes to allow more patient choice, or to promote active involvement in care. These alternatives include multisystemic therapy (MST), treatment foster care (TFC), case management, and home treatment. While MST and TFC were developed specifically for young people, case management and home treatment have been adapted from adult models of care. The diverse development of these services makes comparison between them difficult, and this has proved a limitation to robust controlled studies assessing their relative effectiveness. Two other key factors have limited comparison studies of community services: the "treatment as usual" comparator against which community intensive treatments are measured is often poorly defined and can vary widely from study to study; and at least in early studies, the samples comprised young people not at the highest risk (Mattejat et al., 2001).

Overall principles

Although community intensive models vary widely, they share key characteristics (Smyth & Hoult, 2000; Shepperd et al., 2009; Sjolie et al., 2010; Williamson & Marshall, 2010). Most community intensive services have a defined remit. This may be to prevent hospitalization, as in the case of a home treatment or outreach model, or to prevent delinquency and repeat offending, as in MST or TFC. Operationally, such services are able to respond rapidly (within hours or same working day) and staff are generally available outside the nine-to-five working day, sometimes 24 hours a day, 7 days a week. Low caseloads (typically less than ten cases per fulltime worker) allow flexible working with families and their networks in a range of settings, including the family home, school, and other nonhealth bases such as drop-in centers. Face-to-face or telephone contacts by staff with families are frequent, a minimum three times a week but may be several times a day. Staff undertake assessment, care planning, and treatment delivery to young people and their families, with multidisciplinary team input as and when appropriate. Staff have a detailed knowledge of the services offered by key partner agencies in their locality and will have good relationships with those agencies, which may be statutory, independent, or third sector and reciprocal protocols will exist between them to ensure easy referral pathway.

Evidence for effectiveness of community intensive services is summarized in Table 50.1.

Rutter's Child and Adolescent Psychiatry, Sixth Edition.
Edited by Anita Thapar and Daniel S. Pine, James F. Leckman, Stephen Scott, Margaret J. Snowling, Eric Taylor.
© 2015 John Wiley & Sons Ltd. Published 2018 by John Wiley & Sons Ltd.

Table 50.1 Defining characteristics of specific community intensive services and evidence to support effectiveness.

Service	Defining characteristics	Key evidence for effectiveness
Multi Systemic Therapy (MST)	Strictly manualized treatment program	*Review:* Henggeler & Sheidow (2012): early efficacy studies supported by recent positive findings. (Littell *et al.*, 2009; Pane *et al.*, 2013): improvements not sustained over time
Treatment Foster Care (TFC)	Reliance on trained professional foster caregivers to deliver prescribed interventions	*Systematic review:* Macdonald & Turner, 2008; Leve *et al.* (2009) and Chamberlain *et al.* (2008): clinically meaningful reductions immediately posttreatment in levels of antisocial behavior, although not well sustained at follow-up
Home treatment	Emphasis on preventing hospitalization or reducing length of stay	*Individual studies:* Winsberg *et al.* (1980); Mattejat *et al.* (2001) suggest home treatment as clinically effective as hospitalization
Case management	Emphasis on a single case manager coordinating or delivering treatment	*Meta-analysis:* (Suter & Bruns, 2009): inconclusive findings concerning effectiveness of wraparound
Family preservation services (FPS)	Emphasis on preventing family breakdown Manualized program	*Systematic review:* Shepperd *et al.* (2009): small clinically significant effects postintervention not maintained at 6-month follow-up *Review:* Bowyer, 2009: programs with high model fidelity can mediate the consequences of early adverse life events and abuse *Meta-analyses:* (i) Nelson *et al.* (2009): programs with high model fidelity significantly reduce family breakdown (ii) Lindsey *et al.* (2002). Less evidence of efficacy shown by studies with more robust methodologies
Dialectic Behavior Therapy (DBT)	Manualized program	Review: MacPherson *et al.* (2013) suggests clinical improvements sustained 1 year postintervention

Community intensive services based on specific models

Multisystemic therapy

MST is an intensive approach to working with young offenders presenting with serious antisocial behaviors, at risk of being placed out-of-home. MST clinicians work with the young person in their community and are on call 24 hours a day, 7 days a week, working intensively with caregivers to give them back parental control, to help their child focus on gaining educational and social skills, and to replace maladaptive unstructured activities ("hanging out"). MST has translated successfully globally across a range of cultures including New Zealand, Scandinavia, and the United Kingdom (Ogden and Hagen, 2006; Gustle *et al.*, 2007; Curtis *et al.*, 2009; Wells *et al.*, 2010). MST has systems theory at its base and is a strictly manualized intensive intervention, time-limited to 4 to 6 months.

MST is one of the better-evidenced community intensive treatments for young people, although pooled analyses do not wholly support the strong positive outcomes reported by individual studies and it is not widely available. Henggeler and Sheidow's review (2012) concluded that the positive findings of early efficacy studies had been sustained in more recent research, namely reduction in offending behavior, substance misuse, recidivism, and psychiatric symptoms, and improvements in school attendance and self-reported improvements by young people and their families (Borduin *et al.*, 2009; Letourneau *et al.*, 2009). Three main factors predict positive outcomes: adherence by staff to the MST model, supported through robust clinical supervision and regular professional

development (Schoenwald *et al.*, 2008; Schoenwald *et al.*, 2009), adherence by families to the program, (Henggeler *et al.*, 2009; Boxer, 2011) and treatment of maternal depression (Grimbos and Granic, 2009). However, two systematic reviews (Littell *et al.*, 2009; Pane *et al.*, 2013) showed data that were of mixed quality revealing inconclusive findings. There was no evidence that MST has harmful effects but little to support the effects of MST being well sustained over time. Study sample sizes for both these reviews were small and the effectiveness findings inconsistent.

Treatment foster care

TFC comprises structured intensive therapy for adolescents with severe antisocial and delinquency problems whose birth family placement has broken down. TFC is delivered by specially trained and salaried foster families who look after just one child at a time. They receive robust supervision and support from TFC specialists and mental health practitioners to ensure that the treatment plan is followed and that services are coordinated round the child. Therapeutic work with the child and foster parents is based on "ABC" principles (antecedents, behaviors, and consequences) and follows comprehensive functional analysis of problem behaviors (see Chapters 21 and 37). TFC has translated with some difficulties outside North America, often in an altered format, and with difficulties in recruiting and retaining foster carergivers (Gustle *et al.*, 2007; Chamberlain *et al.*, 2012).

Pooled analyses and a recent study (Green *et al.*, 2014) suggest that the evidence base is less robust than individual studies indicate. Macdonald and Turner's 2008 review of five studies (total of 390 participants) all conducted by TFC program developers found clinically meaningful reductions posttreatment in levels of antisocial behavior, the number of days young people ran away from their placements, and the time they spent in locked settings (Macdonald & Turner, 2008). Young people spent more time in school and had better rates of homework completion and employment posttreatment. Individual studies (Chamberlain *et al.*, 2008; Leve *et al.*, 2009; Biehal *et al.*, 2012) concur, although the improvements may not be sustained postintervention due to re-engagement of young people with delinquent peers and attrition of consistency in parental discipline.

Case management

The case management model originated as assertive outreach in Wisconsin in the late 1960s: a "hospital without walls" for adult patients (Stein and Test, 1980). Case management has been adopted in the United States and United Kingdom, several European countries and Australia. The three main models of case management are assertive outreach, intensive case management, and wraparound. Assertive outreach employs a flexible approach to engaging and working with severely mentally ill young people in their own community, offering a potentially more accessible service than a traditional mental health service provision (Sainsbury, 2001). Intensive case management shares many key features with assertive outreach, but case managers are more likely to "broker" services rather than provide them directly (Werrbach, 1996). Wraparound services deliver an individually tailored package of care with an emphasis on family strengths. Services are provided through teams that link children, families, and foster parents and their support networks with child welfare, health, mental health, education, and the criminal justice services to develop and implement comprehensive support plans (Suter and Bruns, 2009).

The evidence base for case management approaches is small and yields mixed findings. The one meta-analysis of wraparound services (Suter and Bruns, 2009) showed small treatment effects and could not support or refute the effectiveness of wraparound. Individual studies show varied results. Morthorst *et al.* (2012) reported no significant difference in self-harm repetition rates in adolescents randomized post-self harm episode to treatment as usual or assertive outreach at 12-month follow-up. Conversely, young people posttreatment had clinically meaningful improvements (rated on the Children's Global Assessment Scale, the Brief Symptoms Inventory and Health of the Nation Outcome Scales for Children and Adolescents), a twofold reduction in hospitalization rate and twofold increase in fulltime education (Slesnick *et al.*, 2008; Simpson *et al.*, 2010; Rots-de Vries *et al.*, 2011a, b; Chia *et al.*, 2012).

Intensive home treatment

Intensive home treatment delivers rapid assessment of young people with mental illness in crisis and eligible for hospital admission, with the intention of offering comprehensive acute psychiatric care at home (NIMH, 2004). The primary aim is to avoid or shorten hospitalization through reducing psychiatric symptoms and psychosocial problems. The approach is child and family centered; models used include intensive family therapy and solution-focused approaches.

There are only two published, randomized controlled trials (Winsberg *et al.*, 1980; Mattejat *et al.*, 2001) comparing home treatment with inpatient psychiatric admission. A third trial, of the home treatment program across Connecticut, will be reported in 2015 (Woolston, http://clinicaltrials.gov/ct2/show/NCT01567969).

Mattejat *et al.* (2001) reported on 92 young people (mean age 12 years, M:F 2:1) with a range of psychiatric diagnoses including habit disorders, eating disorders, conduct and emotional disorders, and attention deficit hyperactivity disorder (ADHD). Immediately postintervention, the treatment effect sizes for young people allocated to home treatment or hospital admission were similar. However, only 15% of the allocated home treatment group was able to complete the intervention. The remaining 85% needed to be transferred for inpatient treatment because of presence of severe psychosis or a life-threatening eating disorder, severe risk-taking behaviors, or their families lived too far away from the unit for home treatment to be possible logistically. Two to five years later, the observed treatment effects had diminished equally for both groups. However, home treatment remained as effective as inpatient treatment across diagnoses in reducing symptom scores and improving psychosocial functioning. The young person's compliance with the interventions and the therapist skill were the two most important predictors of treatment outcome.

Winsberg *et al.* (1980) evaluated a home treatment intervention for children (5–13 years) with severe emotional and behavioral disorders referred for an inpatient admission, each child spending between 1 and 3 weeks in hospital before randomization to home treatment or further inpatient stay. Intensive home treatment was delivered by case workers supervised by a child psychiatrist, with consultation from an educational psychologist. At 1–3 year follow-up of the entire original sample, 50% of children treated in hospital were living at home compared with 72% of children who had been treated in the community. Parental satisfaction levels with home services and inpatient care did not differ significantly.

Family preservation services

Family preservation services (FPSs) are based on the Homebuilders® model for crisis intervention (Wilmshurst, 2002). This intervention is family focused and community based, aimed at preventing out-of-home placement for children at high risk. Interventions include reframing of problems, anger management, and cognitive behavioral therapy. FPSs have extended into Europe and Australia, but programs are becoming less popular even in the United States because of the lack of robust outcomes evidence. Two reviews and two meta-analyses conclude that the efficacy evidence for FPS is not as robust as that suggested in early studies (Bowyer, 2009). Close adherence of the program to the Homebuilders® model significantly reduces family breakdown but with varying effect sizes from −0.14 to +0.77 across nine studies (Nelson et al., 2009) and the improvements in family functioning and children's emotional problems may not be sustained postdischarge. (Shepperd et al., 2009) The more robust the research study, the less compelling the evidence for FPS's effectiveness (Lindsey et al., 2002). Family-based and program-based factors predict positive outcomes (Berry et al., 2000; Littell & Schuerman, 2002; Ryan & Schuerman, 2004; Bagdasaryan, 2005; Gockel, 2008; Nelson et al., 2009; Tully, 2008). Program-based factors include high intensity of contact (12–15 hours a week), very low caseloads (two families per worker), clear targeting of problems, and a strong therapist-family relationship, perceived as nurturing by families. Family-based factors include presence of two parents in the home, imminent risk of foster placement preintervention when families were highly motivated to change, and absence of parental health problems.

Intensive services based on dialectical behavior therapy

Dialectical behavior therapy (DBT) is an intensive service model based often on the manualized version for adolescents (Miller et al., 2007). It is based on the adult DBT model, which posits emotional dysregulation as a central feature of many psychiatric problems, eating disorders, repeated self-harming behaviors, mood disorders, and emergent borderline personality disorder (Aldao et al., 2010). Empirical theory states that this arises out of an innate biological vulnerability (often observed as impulsive behavior in childhood) plus an "invalidating environment" characterized by negation, punishment, lack of understanding of a child's internal experiences, inconsistent responses, and over-simplification of problem-solving shown by main caregivers. Young people arrive at adolescence not having learned how to regulate emotions (see Chapter 5). A DBT program typically might include weekly individual therapy and weekly groups work in which young people learn and hone skills including how to accept distress and pain, how to manage healthy relationships, adaptive ways to deal with emotional crises; mindfulness meditation, and mentalization. Multifamily work, telephone coaching, outreach strategies, and a weekly consultation team meeting help keep the program on track (James et al., 2008, 2010a).

Outcome research is in the early days. Results of randomized controlled trials of DBT comparing it to other modalities or treatment as usual are awaited. MacPherson et al. (2013) evaluated 18 studies, suggesting that across a range of psychiatric problems and in diverse settings (outpatient through intensive provision) DBT in adolescents shows promising outcome: over 8–12 months follow-up, there were reduced rates of psychiatric symptoms and suicidal ideation and actions.

Day programs (partial hospitalization)

Day programs developed in the 1940s and remain a cornerstone of CAMHS especially in North America, but in many low and middle income countries (LMIC) and developing countries, they are scarce or nonexistent. In the last decade, the development of community-based intensive services has put pressure on day programs to justify their existence and focus their role more tightly.

What do day programs offer?

Partial hospitalization may be categorized by function (Worrall-Davies, 2014). Increasingly, they offer a step-up, step-down support and transition between community CAMHS or an inpatient unit. They may provide a nonresidential option for harm reduction, assessing and treating severe and complex patterns of disruptive, delinquent, or offending behaviors. Some day programs offer neuro developmental assessment and treatment with specialist programs of care for prepubertal children with autism, ADHD, speech and language disorders, or neuropsychiatric conditions. Intensive family work may be offered within 5-day-a-week day program interventions with whole families (Multi-family Therapy model (see Chapter 39)). Finally, problem-specific targeted packages of care may be provided within a day program for specific problems such as eating disorders or psychosis.

Day programs have a number of advantages and disadvantages compared to full inpatient admission. Day services work round young people's school or college timetables, can offer family appointments early or late in the day more easily, and individually tailor interventions to young people's needs. School-aged prepubertal children are rarely admitted to inpatient units so day programs are one option for providing detailed observation, assessment, and treatment. The partial "therapeutic milieu facilitates close liaison with families and schools and increases likelihood of learning transferring across settings. However, traveling each day to and from the day program may be tiring and anxiety-provoking for young people and the costs of travel and loss of income from taking time off work to transport their children may be substantial for families.

Young people attend a day unit typically between 8 and 12 hours up to 5 days a week. Traditionally, programs were timetabled rigidly but nowadays they are usually individually tailored, with young people having opportunities to attend their own school, undergo specialized assessments or individual and family therapy sessions. Therapeutic alliance and milieu are as important as in the inpatient setting as they influence outcomes (Hougaard, 1994; Grizenko, 1997; Green et al., 2001; Green et al., 2007). Robust supervision is needed at individual and group level to hold tight care boundaries, otherwise the staff team may mirror dysfunctional family relationships or parenting difficulties. Policies and procedures must be in place to safely manage aggression, bullying, self-harm or harm to others, and absconding. As in inpatient units, staff must be trained in de-escalation and restraint techniques. Treatment goals should be specific, measurable, and achievable, yet flexible so that they can evolve during treatment. There should be a multiprofessional team plus a core nursing team. Child and adolescent psychiatrists, social workers, clinical child psychologists, speech and language therapists, occupational therapists, physiotherapists, family therapists, child psychotherapists, and teachers all have important roles. The most popular team model is staff working generically, with a flat hierarchy, with task-focused "mini teams" rather than staff working solely within their professional discipline role (Worrall-Davies, in press).

The wide range of partial hospitalization programs makes effectiveness studies difficult to interpret. Furthermore, the necessary evolution of day programs to align with intensive and changing use of inpatient provision of developing community means that efficacy research may not now be as relevant. Recent research has focused on day programs for specific disorders, with mixed findings. The multiple family day treatment model shows promising results with significant symptomatic improvement, low drop-out rates and high family satisfaction with the treatment model (Rockwell et al., 2011). Martin et al. (2013) showed significant reduction in behavioral problems in preschoolers who had failed to respond to evidence-based outpatient treatment (see Chapter 65). The classic Grizenko (1997) study also suggested that day programs for prepubertal children with conduct disorder led to significantly more improvements in behavior, self-esteem, and self-reported mood, compared to those on a waiting list, both at discharge and at 6-month follow-up. Poor parental engagement with treatment predicted further required input from social or health services. One study suggests that a day program for substance abuse in adolescents is as effective as hospitalization in terms of treatment completion rates, reductions in substance use and behavior difficulties, and improved psychosocial functioning (Cornwall and Blood, 1998).

Inpatient services

Historical background and trends

Child and adolescent inpatient services have developed from two broadly differing theoretical concepts: "therapeutic milieu," which aims at effecting personality and behavior change (Bettlelheim, 1955; Kennard, 1983), and a bio-psychosocial model (Cameron, 1949), using a comprehensive approach to assessment and treatment often based in a hospital type setting. Today many facets of these models are incorporated into smaller units with a modified ethos or therapeutic milieu alongside more individual psychosocial and medical treatments. While there was a steady expansion of such services particularly in the 1960s and 1970s, more recently there has been a dramatic change in the delivery of inpatient care. In the United States, as elsewhere, there has been a reduction in the length of stay, a greater number of prior admissions, and a greater severity of those admitted, as judged by the level of general functioning (Meagher et al., 2012). In Germany between 2000 and 2007, inpatient admission rates for children and adolescents increased by 38.1% overall, but with striking variations—conduct disorders rose by 18.1%, hyperkinetic disorder by 111.3%, and both considerably less than depressive disorders 219.6% (Holtmann et al., 2010). In the United States, psychiatric discharges between 1996 and 2007 also increased but more for children (180%) than for adolescents (141%), whereas there was very little change reported for adults (108%) (Blader, 2011). Alongside this, there has been a change in the pattern of diagnoses with a large increase in the United States in admissions of those with early-onset bipolar disorder (see Chapter 62) (Blader and Carlson, 2007; Meagher et al., 2012), which has been reflected to a lesser extent in Germany (Holtmann et al., 2010), but not in the United Kingdom (James, 2010) Moreover, there have been considerable changes in the pattern of clinical care as demonstrated, for instance, by the increased use of antipsychotic medication within the United States only 11.4% receiving antipsychotics on discharge in 1991 compared to 46.7% in 2008 (Meagher et al., 2012). This does not appear to be linked to greater rates of psychosis, but may reflect use of antipsychotics for mood stabilization and possible control of aggression.

There is a steep rise in hospital admissions in the teenage years from 0.2/1000 at 10 years to 2.2/1000 per year at 19 years (James, 2010). These findings alongside the recognition of higher rates of psychiatric disorder in adolescence (Costello et al., 2011) and an increase in the rates of emotional disorders in the 1990s (Maughan et al., 2008), led to a realization of an under-provision of inpatient services in United Kingdom. In 1999, there were 80 adolescent psychiatric units in England and Wales providing 900 beds; this inpatient provision increased by 33% to 1128 beds by 2006 (O'Herlihy et al., 2007). Previously, up to a third of all adolescents in England were admitted to adult wards (James, 2010) or to pediatric wards, half of which were thought to be inappropriate (Worrall et al., 2004).

Types of unit

Inpatient units are general or specialized by function. A major division of inpatient psychiatric services is based upon age and differing developmental needs, particularly those between prepubertal and postpubertal children and adolescents. Child units, often have a greater involvement of parents and family, including in some case the provision to stay, which reflects the finding that compared to adolescents, younger children tend to come from families with higher rates of psychosocial problems (Rice et al., 2002). Adolescence marks a transition for the individual and socially, with the greater influence of peers, and change in schooling and the possibility of leaving home. Such a large transitional period means in practice that general adolescent units often have an informal distinction between the older adolescents (over 16 years) and younger adolescents.

In some countries, particularly those in Scandinavia and Northern Europe, child psychiatric units with an emphasis upon family and parental involvement continue to flourish. Recent surveys in the United States (Blader, 2011) point to a substantial increase in the use of child psychiatric beds, while in the United Kingdom the number of child psychiatric units has decreased substantially (O'Herlihy *et al.*, 2003). The latter may reflect not only the increased provision of community child and adolescent psychiatric services (CAMHS), but also a reluctance to separate children from families.

There are specialized inpatient services for eating disorders. The need for this specialized service may reflect parental or indeed adolescent demands. However, while there is accumulating evidence for better outcomes for eating disorders with specialized community eating disorder services (Gowers *et al.*, 2010), there is no such evidence for an advantage for dedicated adolescent eating disorder units.

Adolescent intensive care units for violent and or persistently disruptive behaviors, as well as serious self-harming behaviors and persistent suicide attempts, are organized on a supra-regional level. While many modern adolescent units may incorporate purpose built intensive care suites, longer-term intensive care is best provided in purposebuilt units where security can be more easily maintained and where there is access to adequate resources including sports facilities. Patients admitted to such units must be under the Mental Health Act or other statutory provisions (see Chapter 19). Severely disturbed adolescents or those who have committed offenses in the context of mental illness may be referred to adolescent forensic inpatient services (see Chapter 49).

Children and adolescents with mild to moderate intellectual disabilities can usually be catered for in general inpatient units with consultation from learning disability services and by employing dually trained staff. Those with severe intellectual disabilities require separate provision because of the specialized needs and communication difficulties (see Chapter 54). Other specialist units include services for children and adolescents with autism.

How are young people admitted to an inpatient unit?

Inpatient beds are a scare and costly resource, and therefore preadmission assessment is often considered as a crucial filtering mechanism. In one study of an Irish adolescent unit (Wilson *et al.*, 2012), 46% of referrals were admitted. Depression and suicidality were the most common reasons for referral. While a majority of admissions occurred within 5 days of referral a significant minority were not admitted until over 20 days after referral. Referrers, however, value the possibility of urgent admissions, and it is possible for a service to be configured to accept urgent referrals (Corrigall & Mitchell, 2002), provided there are good community links.

Types of admission
Emergency
Emergency psychiatric admission is required for a range of conditions, particularly serious suicide risk, risk of harm to others associated with mental illness, acute florid psychosis,

and eating disorders with physical complications among others. Accepting emergencies on a 24 hour basis seven days per week, has only been widely accepted practice in the United Kingdom since 2004 (DOH, 2004), previously one third of all adolescent admissions were admitted in adult wards (James, 2010). In order to ensure the necessary availability of an emergency bed, a well integrated community service, including a psychiatric crisis team with in-reach is necessary.

Planned and respite admissions
Referrals should not be delayed: a well-timed intensive treatment may prevent further deterioration (Green & Worrall-Davies, 2008). Brief respite admissions can also be useful in certain situations where the aim is to maintain an ill child or adolescent in the community as far as possible and to help support a family though a difficult period, particularly those families with a child with learning impairment and behavioral problems. The concern that these types of admissions can engender dependency and undermine a family's ability to cope can be over-played.

Reasons for admission and characteristics of who is admitted
The reasons for admission generally fall into a number of broad categories (Box 50.1).

Among a nationwide birth cohort of Finnish children, 6.2% of males and 4.1% of females between the ages 13 and 24 were admitted to hospital for a primary psychiatric reason. The combination of conduct and emotional symptoms was the strongest predictor for admission in both sexes (Gyllenberg *et al.*, 2010). Admission practices vary between countries, and in England the admission rate (2.2/1000 population at age 19 years) is lower, with schizophrenia, affective disorders, neurotic disorders, and eating disorders being the mostly frequent diagnoses (James, 2010). Eating disorders represent a major use of beds as the length of stay is longer.

It is clear, however, that besides psychiatric illness, social factors play a significant role in who is admitted (Kylmanen *et al.*, 2010). Children in the welfare system are overrepresented in child and adolescent psychiatric units (Laukkanen *et al.*, 2013), reflecting the high rates of psychiatric morbidity in this population (McCann *et al.*, 1996). Indeed, alongside any principal psychiatric problem, adolescent inpatients suffer a multitude of difficulties including educational and social difficulties (Tonge *et al.*, 2008). A high level of family dysfunction is common, and many but not all studies report parental personality or psychological disturbance (Tonge *et al.*, 2008). Not surprisingly then, given the multiple problems that adolescent inpatients suffer, treatment that focuses on only some of these factors is likely to have limited effectiveness.

Assessment
Unfortunately, even in inpatient services standardized assessments of psychopathology are not routinely undertaken.

Box 50.1 Indications for inpatient hospital admission.

To manage risk of self-harm and suicide, violence and harm to others, and medical complications associated with eating disorders. When psychiatric symptomatology is escalating despite the most intensive outpatient treatment available. The need for detailed assessment in complex cases where the formulation is unclear.	Assessment or treatment away from the family. This has become less of an indication with family therapy becoming more available to assess the family *in situ*. For controlled trials of specific interventions and drug regimes (i.e., starting clozapine) and coordination of complex physical investigations such as electroencephalography (EEG) and magnetic resonance imaging (MRI).

This has led to the systematic under-reporting and, therefore, treatment of various disorders such as post traumatic stress disorder (PTSD) (Havens *et al.*, 2012). In one study (Lauth *et al.*, 2008), the introduction of standardized semi-structured instruments such as the Kiddie-Schedule for Affective Disorders and Schizophrenia (K-SADS) (Kaufman *et al.*, 1997) led to the increasing recognition of several main diagnostic categories (depressive, anxiety, bipolar, and disruptive disorders), suggesting that those disorders were likely underreported.

Therapeutic function

Inpatient care encompasses a multitude of functions, including the provision of a broad range of evidence-based therapies such as pharmacotherapy, cognitive behavioral therapy, family therapy, supportive individual counseling, and possibly art and music therapy. There is no evidence that these treatments *per se* are more effectively delivered in an inpatient setting; however, there is a belief that with more intensity and consistency these treatments can be more effective.

Inpatient treatment is not just "residential" care with the provision of on-site therapies. A unit will have its own "milieu or ethos" with some specifically designed, such as behavioral units or those adopting family therapy or indeed psychodynamic approaches. Core elements for "milieu therapy" are consistency, boundaries, limit setting, role modeling led by staff, as well as open group forms for exploration and discussion of day-to-day emotional and psychological issues as they arise. A crucial component of inpatient care is physical and psychological containment (Bion, 1962). Patients will often be admitted following the breakdown of social relationships and appear in a distressed, unsettled, and fragmentary psychological state. The act of physical containment, alongside psychological support with boundaries appears essential to help settle the disorganized and sometimes suicidal patient.

Although difficult to define, the therapeutic "milieu" is often seen by staff as a crucial aspect of the functioning of the unit; it is the setting where multiple split transferences and transference reactions are worked through; that is, relationship patterns are re-enacted and often re-played within staff groups, which can then provide a focus for intervention (Pestalozzi *et al.*, 1998). In order to maintain a therapeutic milieu, it is essential that there is good communication among staff, alongside the ability to be able to reflect not only on the day-to-day business but also the emotional aspects of the work. A coherent therapeutic culture

has been shown to be related to therapeutic outcome (Pfeiffer & Strzelecki, 1990; Green *et al.*, 2007).

Behavioral management

Complex behavioral regimes can be implemented within an inpatient service to underpin a psychological treatment program for a variety of disorders such as obsessive-compulsive disorders (OCDs). However one of the main indications for the use of behavioral regimes is to treat aggression (Dean *et al.*, 2007). Physical aggression during admission is common, occurring in one study in up to 23% of inpatients (Dean *et al.*, 2008). Factors that predict persistent physical aggression include a history of aggression and use of medication at presentation. Persistent aggression is also associated with an increased length of stay, but not necessarily a worse outcome. Broad-based behavioral management programs lead to a reduction in aggression (Dean *et al.*, 2010) emphasizing the importance of an organizational approach to behavioral management. Among inpatient staff exposure to aggression is common—occurring in over 84% in one study (Dean *et al.*, 2010). The impact on staff is considerable with difficulty attending work and other emotional and professional sequelae, highlighting the need for a cohesive staff group and regular training to deal with violence.

Seclusion

Seclusion is defined as the placement of a patient in a specifically designed room in order to de-escalate behaviors, assure physical safety, and achieve behavioral control. Restraint refers to a physical intervention, either through therapeutic holding by a caregiver/staff member, or as in certain countries through mechanical restraining tools. Reasons for seclusion and restraint include threats (73%), agitation (63%), and physical aggression (63%) (Delaney and Fogg, 2005). A recent review showed that the use of both seclusion and restraint are reduced after behavioral interventions or more systematic use of restraint (De Hert *et al.*, 2011) and use of the correct legislation. In some countries, for example, in the United Kingdom, mechanical restraints are very rarely used, while a Finnish study found that mechanical restraint was used in 6.9% of adolescent inpatients (Hottinen *et al.*, 2012).

Restraint in particular can have severe consequences including trauma for the individual, a reactivation of prior traumatic experiences and serious physical side effects, such as asphyxia, aspiration, blunt trauma to the chest, thrombosis, and even death.

One US national study (Nunno *et al.*, 2006) reported 45 fatalities between 1993 and 2003 in child and adolescent psychiatric facilities related to restraints.

In certain cases, aggression or disturbed behavior may be managed by the use of medication. Rapid tranquillization techniques involve the administration of short acting benzodiazepines or antipsychotics intramuscularly or via rapidly absorbed oral preparations. Such procedures are relatively safe provided that there is a clear protocol and regular and frequent physical monitoring by trained staff.

Risk management

The management and reduction of risk of harm to self or others is a crucial function of an inpatient unit. Vital to this process is the detection and quantification of risk. A thorough and detailed history with corroborative evidence is essential. Finely tuned clinical skills can be enhanced in an inpatient setting with a multidisciplinary perspective, which adds an extra dimension—for example, by having both male and female viewpoints. Furthermore, it is possible to assess risk over time, and dynamically, via the interaction with observable stressors within the unit. A major advantage of residential psychiatric care is the possibility of modifying the milieu by various means—varying the level of nursing observations, excluding stressors and gradually re-introducing them.

Clinical skills based upon detailed observation are at the heart of a risk assessment. Routine questionnaires can supplement the risk assessment for self-harm, but cannot replace it. The limited research available indicates that violence toward others, unlike self-directed violence, can be successfully predicted using clinical judgment (Phillips *et al.*, 2012). Semi-structured assessments of violence such as the SAVRY (Structured Assessment of Violence Risk in Youth) have good predictive validity (Singh *et al.*, 2011) and can be recommended.

Does inpatient admission work?

Length of stay

There is trend for shorter admissions but with more complex presentations (Olfson *et al.*, 2005). Shorter admissions have been shown not only to be feasible, but effective. In one study (Swadi & Bobier, 2005), the mean length of admission was 23.7 days for mood disorders, 18.9 days for anxiety disorders, and 46.9 days for major psychoses. Most improvements occurred during the first 3 weeks of admission. Importantly, readmission rates were not elevated. However, longer stays, positive therapeutic alliance and better premorbid family functioning have been found independently to predict better outcome (Green *et al.*, 2007).

Readmission

Readmission occurs in a surprisingly high number of cases—for example, 43% (James *et al.*, 2010). Re-hospitalization is highest during the first 30 days following discharge and remains elevated for 3 months. Medication nonadherence and a history of childhood sexual abuse are associated with readmission (Bobier &

Warwick, 2005). A Danish 10-year follow-up study found that 25% of those re-admitted became "long-term" psychiatric inpatients, particularly those with schizophrenia and affective psychoses (Pedersen & Aarkrog, 2001).

Outcomes and evaluation

The evidence for inpatient care is limited by the fact that as safety is a major driver for use of inpatient services, it is neither feasible nor ethical to conduct randomized controlled trials to evaluate its use. Nevertheless, a meta-analysis of 34 open studies of children and adolescent inpatients highlighted clear clinical improvements for inpatient care (Pfeiffer & Strzelecki, 1990), but poor long-term prognosis has been noted for some early-onset disorders such as psychosis (Healy & Fitzgerald, 2000). A prospective study (Green *et al.*, 2007) found significant and clinically meaningful clinical improvements across all diagnoses, maintained at 1-year follow-up, following an average 16-week admission. The mean cost of admission was £24,100 (UK costs in 2007). Curiously, despite the clinical improvements, which enabled the patients to be subsequently treated within community mental health services (CAMHS), preadmission and postdischarge support costs were similar. This finding for inpatient care contrasts with that from a community study of 56 severely disturbed adolescents in United Kingdom (Clark *et al.*, 2005) whose costs including placement in various residential units amounted to £56,000 per child/adolescent per year—over double that of psychiatric inpatient care with no appreciable change in the level of symptoms or functioning. Direct comparisons may not be possible and while there is evidence pointing clearly to improvements for inpatient psychiatric care, it is evident, nonetheless, that residential care for the severely disturbed children and adolescents is expensive.

Suicide

A prospective study (Kapur *et al.*, 2013) of patients admitted to national health service (NHS) inpatient psychiatric care in England between 1997 and 2008 showed a significant drop ($p < 0.001$) in inpatient suicides from 0.4 to 0.1 per 100,000 population in the 15–24 age range (Kapur, personal communication). Moreover, for all ages, rates fell for the most common suicide methods, particularly suicide by hanging (a 59% reduction). On a unit level, the design of the unit with the removal of ligature points is essential and implementing procedures such as follow-up appointments within 7 days of discharge may contribute to better outcomes.

Cost/benefits

As with all therapies, inpatient care can have side effects. Admission to an inpatient service often involves disruption of family, school, and links with the community. While support and care for the young person can be an important part of the inpatient treatment, patients and families can feel deskilled, possibly because crucial supporting structures within the community and family are lost and patients can become isolated and dependent on hospital care. Additionally admission can be costly personally with parents paying up to £2000 in travel costs to the unit alone (UK costs 2007) (Green *et al.*, 2007).

Discharge and transition to the community

There is some preliminary evidence from adults that the introduction of care coordination (CPA)—the process of coordinating multidisciplinary professional input with the patient, family, and family GP or physician—results in better care with less psychiatric crisis team input, lower rates of readmission and greater satisfaction for both patients and relatives following discharge (Stewart *et al.*, 2012). Curiously, a US and Canadian study found that while only 50% of discharged adolescents received aftercare, those who did were more likely to be re-admitted (Carlisle *et al.*, 2012). Disappointingly, follow-up research shows that only a proportion of inpatients receive the recommended services upon discharge (Green *et al.*, 2007).

Transition points into and out of an inpatient service and the transition of the older adolescent to adult mental health services are vital points in any care pathway because of the increased risk of disruption in continuity of care, disengagement from services, and possibly poorer clinical outcomes, including the risk of suicide. Some young people, such as those with neurodevelopmental disorders and complex needs, are at a greater risk of falling through the care gap during transition to adult services (Singh, 2009). This has led some to argue for the development of youth community services with an upper age range of 25 years. It would not be envisaged that this would extend to residential facilities with the disparate needs of younger adolescents and adults.

Postdischarge is recognized as a risk period. The death rate within 1 year of discharge from an adolescent inpatient service is six times higher than that in the general population of the same age, although the total number of deaths following discharge from NHS child adolescent psychiatric units in England was low at 120 over a 6-year period (1998–2004) (James, 2010). The suicide rate is highest in the year after inpatient admission with a Korean study showing that the standardized mortality ratio (SMR) among former adolescent inpatients was 7.8 (95% CI 4.7, 12.3) for unnatural causes and for suicide, it was 14.2 (95% CI 7.7, 23.7) (Park *et al.*, 2013). Among the different diagnostic groups, patients with personality disorders, schizophrenia, or affective disorders had the highest risk for suicide.

Summary of some key findings

There is accumulating evidence that intensive community programs, partial hospitalization, and day patient programs are effective, but it is not clear which type of program works best for which young people. More research is needed to delineate this. In the global context, community intensive services may be more achievable in the foreseeable future than inpatient units, for financial, geographical, and resource issues, but again care should be taken before embarking on setting up expensive services to establish whether they are effective in the settings they are being conducted in.

Moreover, there is evidence that inpatient care can produce substantial clinical improvement in the short and medium term. Readmissions rates are high (30%) and continued clinical improvement is dependent upon aftercare provision. The longer-term outlook for those with major mental illness, particularly psychosis, is poor in a proportion of cases, but evidence from early intervention services with appropriate inpatient care is encouraging (see Chapter 57).

Final conclusions

There has been an expansion of types of intensive services, some focused on certain patient populations or types of therapy and many of which have evidential support. Further work is needed to determine whether integration of these services with inpatient care can improve clinical outcomes, reduce the number of admissions, length of stay, and reduce costs. The move for shorter hospital stays, but with increased complexity (Olfson *et al.*, 2005) will continue to pose considerable clinical demands.

References

Aldao, A. *et al.* (2010) Emotion-regulation strategies across psychopathology: a meta-analytic review. *Clinical Psychology Review* **30**, 217–237.

Bagdasaryan, S. (2005) Evaluating family preservation services: reframing the question of effectiveness. *Children and Youth Services Review* **27**, 615–635.

Berry, M. *et al.* (2000) Intensive family preservation services: an examination of critical service components. *Child and Family Social Work* **5**, 191–203.

Bettlelheim, B. (1955) *Truants from Life*. Free Press, New York.

Biehal, N. *et al.* (2012) Intensive fostering: an independent evaluation of MTFC in an english setting. *Adoption & Fostering* **36**, 13–26.

Bion, W. (1962) *Learning from Experience*. Heinemann, London.

Blader, J.C. (2011) Acute inpatient care for psychiatric disorders in the United States, 1996 through 2007. *Archives of General Psychiatry* **68**, 1276–1283.

Blader, J.C. & Carlson, G.A. (2007) Increased rates of bipolar disorder diagnoses among U.S. child, adolescent, and adult inpatients, 1996–2004. *Biological Psychiatry* **62**, 107–114.

Bobier, C. & Warwick, M. (2005) Factors associated with readmission to adolescent psychiatric care. *Australian & New Zealand Journal of Psychiatry* **39**, 600–606.

Borduin, C.M. *et al.* (2009) A randomized clinical trial of multisystemic therapy with juvenile sexual offenders: effects on youth social ecology and criminal activity. *Journal of Consulting and Clinical Psychology* **77**, 26–37.

Bowyer, S. (ed) (2009) *Children on the Edge of Care: Intensive Family Preservation Services and Family Intervention Projects*. Research in Practice, Dartington.

Boxer, P. (2011) Negative peer involvement in multisystemic therapy for the treatment of youth problem behavior: exploring outcome and process variables in "real-world" practice. *Journal of Clinical Child & Adolescent Psychology* **40**, 848–854.

Cameron, K. (1949) A psychiatric in-patient department for children. *Journal of Mental Science* **95**, 560–566.

Carlisle, C.E. et al. (2012) Aftercare, emergency department visits, and readmission in adolescents. *Journal of the American Academy of Child and Adolescent Psychiatry* **51**, e4.

Chamberlain, P. et al. (2008) Prevention of behavior problems for children in foster care: outcomes and mediation effects. *Prevention Science* **9**, 17–27.

Chamberlain, P. et al. (2012) Three collaborative models for scaling up evidence-based practices. *Administration and Policy in Mental Health* **39**, 278–290.

Chia, A. et al. (2012) Innovation in practice: effectiveness of specialist adolescent outreach service for at-risk adolescents. *Child and Adolescent Mental Health* **16**, 116–119.

Clark, A.F. et al. (2005) Children with complex problems: needs, costs and predictors over 1 year. *Child and Adolescent Mental Health* **10**, 170–178.

Cornwall, A. & Blood, L. (1998) Inpatient versus day treatment for substance abusing adolescents. *Journal of Nervous and Mental Disease* **186**, 580–582.

Corrigall, R. & Mitchell, B. (2002) Service innovations: rethinking in-patient provision for adolescents: a report from a new service. *Psychiatric Bulletin* **26**, 388–392.

Costello, E.J. et al. (2011) Trends in psychopathology across the adolescent years: what changes when children become adolescents, and when adolescents become adults? *Journal of Child Psychology and Psychiatry* **52**, 1015–1025.

Curtis, N.M. et al. (2009) Dissemination and effectiveness of multisystemic treatment in New Zealand: a benchmarking study. *Journal of Family Psychology* **23**, 119–129.

De Hert, M. et al. (2011) Prevalence and correlates of seclusion and restraint use in children and adolescents: a systematic review. *European Child & Adolescent Psychiatry* **20**, 221–230.

Dean, A.J. et al. (2007) Behavioral management leads to reduction in aggression in a child and adolescent psychiatric inpatient unit. *Journal of the American Academy of Child and Adolescent Psychiatry* **46**, 711–720.

Dean, A.J. et al. (2008) Physical aggression during admission to a child and adolescent inpatient unit: predictors and impact on clinical outcomes. *Australian & New Zealand Journal of Psychiatry* **42**, 536–543.

Dean, A.J. et al. (2010) Exposure to aggression and the impact on staff in a child and adolescent inpatient unit. *Archives of Psychiatric Nursing* **24**, 15–26.

Delaney, K.R. & Fogg, L. (2005) Patient characteristics and setting variables related to use of restraint on four inpatient psychiatric units for youths. *Psychiatric Services* **56**, 186–192.

DOH (2004) *National Service Framework for Children, Young People and Maternity Services: The Mental Health and Psychological Wellbeing of Children and Young People.* (ed D.O. Health). Crown, London, UK.

Gockel, A. (2008) Recreating family: parents identify worker-client relationships as paramount in family preservation programs. *Child Welfare* **87**, 91–113.

Gowers, S.G. et al. (2010) A randomised controlled multicentre trial of treatments for adolescent anorexia nervosa including assessment of cost-effectiveness and patient acceptability - the TOuCAN trial. *Health Technology Assessment* **14**, 1–98.

Green, J. & Worrall-Davies, A. (2008) Provision of intensive treatments: in-patient units, day units and intensive outreach. In: *Rutter's Child and Adolescent Psychiatry.* (eds M. Rutter, et al.), 5th edn. Wiley Blackwell, Oxford.

Green, J. et al. (2001) Health gain and outcome predictors during inpatient and related day treatment in child and adolescent psychiatry. *Journal of the American Academy of Child and Adolescent Psychiatry* **40**, 325–332.

Green, J. et al. (2007) Inpatient treatment in child and adolescent psychiatry—a prospective study of health gain and costs. *Journal of Child Psychology and Psychiatry* **48**, 1259–1267.

Green, J. et al. (2014) Multidimensional treatment foster care for high risk looked after adolescents in England: national evaluation through an RCT and an observational cohort. *British Journal of Psychiatry* **204**, 214–221.

Grimbos, T. & Granic, I. (2009) Changes in maternal depression are associated with MST outcomes for adolescents with co-occurring externalizing and internalizing problems. *Journal of Adolescence* **32**, 1415–1423.

Grizenko, N. (1997) Outcome of multimodal day treatment for children with severe behavior problems: a five-year follow-up. *Journal of the American Academy of Child and Adolescent Psychiatry* **36**, 989–997.

Gustle, L.H. et al. (2007) Blueprints in Sweden. Symptom load in Swedish adolescents in studies of functional family therapy (FFT), multisystemic therapy (MST) and multidimensional treatment foster care (MTFC). *Nordic Journal of Psychiatry* **61**, 443–451.

Gyllenberg, D. et al. (2010) Childhood predictors of later psychiatric hospital treatment: findings from the Finnish 1981 birth cohort study. *European Child & Adolescent Psychiatry* **19**, 823–833.

Havens, J.F. et al. (2012) Identification of trauma exposure and PTSD in adolescent psychiatric inpatients: an exploratory study. *Journal of Traumatic Stress* **25**, 171–178.

Healy, E. & Fitzgerald, M. (2000) A 16-year follow-up of a child inpatient population. *European Child & Adolescent Psychiatry* **9**, 46–53.

Henggeler, S.W. & Sheidow, A.J. (2012) Empirically supported family-based treatments for conduct disorder and delinquency in adolescents. *Journal of Marital & Family Therapy* **38**, 30–58.

Henggeler, S.W. et al. (2009) Mediators of change for multisystemic therapy with juvenile sexual offenders. *Journal of Consulting and Clinical Psychology* **77**, 451–462.

Holtmann, M. et al. (2010) Bipolar disorder in children and adolescents in Germany: national trends in the rates of inpatients, 2000–2007. *Bipolar Disorder* **12**, 155–163.

Hottinen, A. et al. (2012) Mechanical restraint in adolescent psychiatry: a Finnish register study. *Nordic Journal of Psychiatry* **67**, 132–139.

Hougaard, E. (1994) The therapeutic alliance—a conceptual analysis. *Scandinavian Journal of Psychology* **35**, 67–85.

James, A. (2010) Adolescent inpatient psychiatric admission rates and subsequent one-year mortality in England: 1998–2004. *Journal of Child Psychology and Psychiatry* **51**, 1395–1404.

James, A.C. et al. (2008) A preliminary community study of dialectic behavioural therapy (DBT) with adolescent females demonstrating persistent, deliberate self-harm (DSH). *Child and Adolescent Mental Health* **13**, 148–152.

James, A.C. et al. (2010a) A preliminary study of an extension of a community dialectic behaviour therapy (DBT) programme to adolescents in the looked after care system. *Child and Adolescent Mental Health* **16**, 9–13.

James, S. *et al.* (2010) Post-discharge services and psychiatric rehospitalization among children and youth. *Administration and Policy in Mental Health* **37**, 433–445.

Kapur, N. *et al.* (2013) Psychiatric in-patient care and suicide in England, 1997 to 2008: a longitudinal study. *Psychological Medicine* **43**, 61–71.

Kaufman, J. *et al.* (1997) Schedule for affective disorders and schizophrenia for school-age children-present and lifetime version (K-SADS-PL): initial reliability and validity data. *Journal of the American Academy of Child and Adolescent Psychiatry* **36**, 980–988.

Kennard, D. (1983) *An Introduction to Therapeutic Communities.* Routledge & Kegan Paul, London, UK.

Kylmanen, P. *et al.* (2010) Is family size related to adolescence mental hospitalization? *Psychiatry Research* **177**, 188–191.

Laukkanen, M. *et al.* (2013) Does the use of health care and special school services, prior to admission for psychiatric inpatient treatment, differ between adolescents housed by child welfare services and those living with their biological parent(s)? *Community Mental Health Journal* **49**, 528–539.

Lauth, B. *et al.* (2008) Implementing the semi-structured interview Kiddie-SADS-PL into an in-patient adolescent clinical setting: impact on frequency of diagnoses. *Child and Adolescent Psychiatry and Mental Health* **2**, 14.

Letourneau, E.J. *et al.* (2009) Multisystemic therapy for juvenile sexual offenders: 1-year results from a randomized effectiveness trial. *Journal of Family Psychology* **23**, 89–102.

Leve, L.D. *et al.* (2009) Multidimensional treatment foster care as a preventive intervention to promote resiliency among youth in the child welfare system. *Journal of Personality* **77**, 1869–1902.

Lindsey, D. *et al.* (2002) The failure of intensive casework services to reduce foster care placements: an examination of family preservation studies. *Children and Youth Services Review* **24**, 743–775.

Littell, J. & Schuerman, J. (2002) What works best for whom? A closer look at intensive family preservation services. *Children and Youth Services Review* **24**, 673–699.

Littell, J.H. *et al.* (2009) Multisystemic therapy for social, emotional, and behavioral problems in youth aged 10–17. *Cochrane Database of Systematic Reviews* (4), CD004797.

Macdonald, G.M. & Turner, W. (2008) Treatment foster care for improving outcomes in children and young people. *Cochrane Database Systematic Reviews* (1), CD005649.

Macpherson, H.A. *et al.* (2013) Dialectical behavior therapy for adolescents: theory, treatment adaptations, and empirical outcomes. *Clinical Child and Family Psychology Review* **16**, 59–80.

Martin, S.E. *et al.* (2013) Partial hospitalization treatment for preschoolers with severe behavior problems: child age and maternal functioning as predictors of outcome. *Child and Adolescent Mental Health* **18**, 24–32.

Mattejat, F. *et al.* (2001) Efficacy of inpatient and home treatment in psychiatrically disturbed children and adolescents. Follow-up assessment of the results of a controlled treatment study. *European Child & Adolescent Psychiatry* **10**, I71–179.

Maughan, B. *et al.* (2008) Recent trends in UK child and adolescent mental health. *Social Psychiatry and Psychiatric Epidemiology* **43**, 305–310.

McCann, J.B. *et al.* (1996) Prevalence of psychiatric disorders in young people in the care system. *BMJ* **313**, 1529–1530.

Meagher, S.M. *et al.* (2012) Changing trends in inpatient care for psychiatrically hospitalized youth: 1991–2008. *Psychiatric Quarterly* **84**, 159–168.

Miller, A.L. *et al.* (2007) *Dialectical Behaviour Therapy with Suicidal Adolescents.* Guilford Press, New York.

Morthorst, B. *et al.* (2012) Effect of assertive outreach after suicide attempt in the AID (assertive intervention for deliberate self harm) trial: randomised controlled trial. *British Medical Journal* **345**, 12.

Nelson, K. *et al.* 2009 *A ten-year review of family preservation research. Building the evidence base. Casey family programs* [Online]. Available: http://www.casey.org/Resources/Publications/pdf/TenYearReviewFamilyPreservation_FR.pdf [28 Jan 2013].

NIMH (2004) *Crisis Resolution and Home Treatment.* Birmingham City University, Birmingham, UK.

Nunno, M.A. *et al.* (2006) Learning from tragedy: a survey of child and adolescent restraint fatalities. *Child Abuse & Neglect* **30**, 1333–1342.

O'Herlihy, A. *et al.* (2007) Provision of child and adolescent mental health inpatient services in England between 1999–2006. *Psychiatric Bulletin* **31**, 454–456.

Ogden, T. & Hagen, K.A. (2006) Multisystemic treatment of serious behaviour problems in youth: sustainability of effectiveness two years after Intake. *Child and Adolescent Mental Health* **11**, 142–149.

O'Herlihy, A. *et al.* (2003) Distribution and characteristics of in-patient child and adolescent mental health services in England and Wales. *British Journal of Psychiatry* **183**, 547–551.

Olfson, M. *et al.* (2005) National trends in hospitalization of youth with intentional self-inflicted injuries. *American Journal of Psychiatry* **162**, 1328–1335.

Pane, H.T. *et al.* (2013) Multisystemic therapy for child non-externalizing psychological and health problems: a preliminary review. *Clinical Child and Family Psychology Review* **16**, 81–99.

Park, S. *et al.* (2013) Unnatural causes of death and suicide among former adolescent psychiatric patients. *Journal of Adolescent Health* **52**, 207–211.

Pedersen, J. & Aarkrog, T. (2001) A 10-year follow-up study of an adolescent psychiatric clientele and early predictors of readmission. *Nordic Journal of Psychiatry* **55**, 11–16.

Pestalozzi, J. *et al.* (1998) *Psychoanalytic Psychotherapy in Institutional Settings.* Karnac Books, London.

Pfeiffer, S.I. & Strzelecki, S.C. (1990) Inpatient psychiatric treatment of children and adolescents: a review of outcome studies. *Journal of the American Academy of Child and Adolescent Psychiatry* **29**, 847–853.

Phillips, N.L. *et al.* (2012) Risk assessment of self- and other-directed aggression in adolescent psychiatric inpatient units. *Australian and New Zealand Journal of Psychiatry* **46**, 40–46.

Rice, B.J. *et al.* (2002) Differences in younger, middle, and older children admitted to child psychiatric inpatient services. *Child Psychiatry & Human Development* **32**, 241–261.

Rockwell, R.E. *et al.* (2011) An innovative short-term, intensive, family-based treatment for adolescent anorexia nervosa: case series. *European Eating Disorders Review* **19**, 382–367.

Rots-de Vries, C. *et al.* (2011a) Evaluation of an assertive outreach intervention for problem families: intervention methods and early outcomes. *Scandinavian Journal of Caring Sciences* **25**, 211–219.

Rots-de Vries, C. *et al.* (2011b) Psychosocial child adjustment and family functioning in families reached with an assertive outreach intervention. *Scandinavian Journal of Caring Sciences* **25**, 269–276.

Ryan, J.P. & Schuerman, J.R. (2004) Matching family problems with specific family preservation services: a study of service effectiveness. *Children and Youth Services Review* **24**, 347–372.

Sainsbury. 2001 *Mental health topics: assertive outreach* [Online]. Available: http://www.thurrock.gov.uk/socialcare/support/pdf/mental_health_sainsbury.pdf [07 Aug 2014].

Schoenwald, S.K. *et al.* (2008) The international implementation of multisystemic therapy. *Evaluation & the Health Professions* **31**, 211–225.

Schoenwald, S.K. *et al.* (2009) Clinical supervision in treatment transport: effects on adherence and outcomes. *Journal of Consulting and Clinical Psychology* **77**, 410–421.

Shepperd, S. *et al.* (2009) Alternatives to inpatient mental health care for children and young people. *Cochrane Database Systematic Reviews* (2), CD006410.

Simpson, W. *et al.* (2010) The effectiveness of a community intensive therapy team on young people's mental health outcomes. *Child and Adolescent Mental Health* **15**, 217–223.

Singh, S.P. (2009) Transition of care from child to adult mental health services: the great divide. *Current Opinion in Psychiatry* **22**, 386–390.

Singh, J.P. *et al.* (2011) A comparative study of violence risk assessment tools: a systematic review and metaregression analysis of 68 studies involving 25,980 participants. *Clinical Psychology Review* **31**, 499–513.

Sjolie, H. *et al.* (2010) Crisis resolution and home treatment: structure, process, and outcome—a literature review. *Journal of Psychiatric and Mental Health Nursing* **17**, 881–892.

Slesnick, N. *et al.* (2008) Six- and twelve-month outcomes among homeless youth accessing therapy and case management services through an urban drop-in center. *Health Services Research* **43**, 211–229.

Smyth, M.G. & Hoult, J. (2000) The home treatment enigma. *British Medical Journal* **320**, 305–308.

Stein, L. & Test, M.A. (1980) Alternative to mental hospital treatment I. Conceptual model, treatment program, and clinical evaluation. *Archives of General Psychiatry* **37**, 392–397.

Stewart, M.W. *et al.* (2012) Care coordinators: a controlled evaluation of an inpatient mental health service innovation. *International Journal of Mental Health Nursing* **21**, 82–91.

Suter, J.C. & Bruns, E.J. (2009) Effectiveness of the wraparound process for children with emotional and behavioral disorders: a meta-analysis. *Clinical Child and Family Psychology Review* **12**, 336–351.

Swadi, H. & Bobier, C. (2005) Hospital admission in adolescents with acute psychiatric disorder: how long should it be? *Australasian Psychiatry* **13**, 165–168.

Tonge, B.J. *et al.* (2008) Comprehensive description of adolescents admitted to a public psychiatric inpatient unit and their families. *Australian and New Zealand Journal of Psychiatry* **42**, 627–635.

Tully, L. 2008 *Family preservation services. Centre for Parenting & Research Service System Development* [Online]. Available: http://www.community.nsw.gov.au/docswr/_assets/main/documents/research_familypreservation_review.pdf [28 Jan 2013].

Wells, C. *et al.* (2010) Multisystemic therapy (MST) for youth offending, psychiatric disorder and substance abuse: case examples from a UK MST team. *Child and Adolescent Mental Health* **15**, 142–149.

Werrbach, G.B. (1996) Family strengths based intensive child case management. *Families in Society: The Journal of Contemporary Human Services* **77**, 216–226.

Williamson, P. & Marshall, L. (2010) *A review of crisis resolution home treatment services in Scotland* [Online]. Available: http://www.qihub.scot.nhs.uk/media/264761/crisis_resolution_home_treatment_report%20final%20november.pdf [29 Jan 2013].

Wilmshurst, L.A. (2002) Treatment programs for youth with emotional and behavioral disorders: an outcome study of two alternate approaches. *Mental Health Services Research* **4**, 85–96.

Wilson, L.S. *et al.* (2012) Who gets admitted? Study of referrals and admissions to an adolescent psychiatry inpatient facility over a 6-month period. *Irish Journal of Medical Science* **181**, 555–560.

Winsberg, B.G. *et al.* (1980) Home vs hospital care of children with behavior disorders. A controlled investigation. *Archives of General Psychiatry* **37**, 413–418.

Worrall, A. *et al.* (2004) Inappropriate admission of young people with mental disorder to adult psychiatric wards and paediatric wards: cross sectional study of six months' activity. *British Medical Journal* **328**, 867.

Worrall-Davies, A. (2014) Day services. In: *Specialist Mental Health Care for Children and Young People: Hospital and Community Intensive Services.* (eds T. MacDougall & A. Cotgrove). Taylor & Francis, Oxford.

C: Contexts of the clinical encounter and specific clinical situations

PART III

Approaching the clinical encounter

CHAPTER 51

Autism spectrum disorder

Ann Le Couteur[1] and Peter Szatmari[2]

[1]Institute of Health and Society, Newcastle University and Northumberland, Tyne and Wear NHS Foundation Trust, Newcastle upon Tyne, UK
[2]Child and Youth Mental Health Collaborative, Hospital for Sick Children, Centre for Addiction and Mental Health, Division of Child and Adolescent Psychiatry, University of Toronto, Toronto, ON, Canada

Overview

This chapter will provide a comprehensive review of the clinical presentation, etiology, outcome, risk factors, assessment, and treatment associated with autism spectrum disorder (ASD). The term ASD will be used throughout this chapter (consistent with the newly published DSM-5 diagnostic criteria) to report on findings with respect to autism, Asperger syndrome (AS), or pervasive developmental disorder not otherwise specified (PDDNOS). Systematic reviews and meta-analyses have been employed rather than primary studies, to provide summaries of the literature in as unbiased and as comprehensive a way as possible. If several reviews on a topic were available, the most methodologically rigorous reviews were retained or those that contained the highest quality studies (using PRISMA or Preferred Reporting Items for Systematic Reviews and Meta-Analyses as a guide, see Liberati *et al.*, 2009). Individual studies have been used to highlight areas only when a recent systematic review was not available or to contextualize the information, provide historical background, or highlight emerging trends.

Clinical characteristics of ASD

ASD is the term now widely used to describe a neurodevelopmental disorder characterized by impairments in reciprocal social communication and a tendency to engage in repetitive stereotyped patterns of behaviors, interests, and activities. In common with other neurodevelopmental disorders, ASD arises from atypical brain development. Boys outnumber girls, the core features are typically present in early childhood (but may not always be apparent) and the etiology (as yet incompletely understood) is likely to be multi-factorial (see Chapter 3). The clinical presentation can change over time, often in response to the demands of the environment or in the presence of co-occurring conditions. Many individuals with ASD have an early history of apparent regression or a period of lack of progress of language, of cognition more generally, or social behavior in the early preschool period. Overall there is a tendency for core behavioral symptoms to improve over time but some behaviors may persist and present a longer term challenge. Affected individuals often have additional problems with independent daily living skills, motor coordination, sensory sensitivities, sleep and eating problems, mental health difficulties, and behaviors that place themselves and others at risk.

The clinical presentation of ASD is remarkably diverse usually with a combination of some delayed/immature behaviors together with the emergence of more unusual behavioral profiles. Some of the earliest social communication symptoms represent difficulties in joint attention, eye contact, lack of social intention to communicate with others, lack of social imitative play and fascination with sensory stimuli. Symptoms change over time, in some cases becoming more obvious (motor stereotypies, lining up of objects, lack of interest in other children and inability to play cooperatively), in other cases becoming more subtle (difficulties in conversation with others, lack of empathy, emergence of intense circumscribed interests, rigid thinking style, problems with reciprocal friendships). Some symptoms of ASD are an exaggeration of delays observed in typical development (lack of useful speech, limited symbolic, and imaginative play skills) whereas other symptoms are quite distinct and are rarely (or only very transiently) observed in the development of typical children (delayed echolalia and neologisms).

Cognitive difficulties are very common in individuals with ASD although their nature can vary dramatically. Some degree of intellectual disability is found in approximately 25–50% of individuals with ASD depending on ascertainment (Matson & Shoemaker, 2009). With the broadening of the diagnostic criteria for ASD, the proportion of individuals with intellectual

Rutter's Child and Adolescent Psychiatry, Sixth Edition.
Edited by Anita Thapar and Daniel S. Pine, James F. Leckman, Stephen Scott, Margaret J. Snowling, Eric Taylor.
© 2015 John Wiley & Sons Ltd. Published 2018 by John Wiley & Sons Ltd.

disability has declined (Fombonne, 2005) over time. The most common pattern of cognitive profile is poor language and social comprehension but with relative strengths, even "splinter skills" (see Chapters 52 and 53) in visual-spatial abilities (Meyer & Minshew, 2002). Among higher functioning individuals the opposite pattern may also occur, a profile sometimes labeled as a "non verbal learning disability" (Klin et al., 1995; Mayes & Calhoun, 2003). "Hyperlexia," a remarkable ability to read but with little comprehension of content, is sometimes observed in severely disabled individuals (see Chapter 53).

Children with moderate to severe cognitive impairment at earlier developmental stages in the preschool years often present with little or no speech and poor non verbal communication. They also tend to engage in repetitive play with sensory stimuli and can become quite upset by stimuli from the environment such as the texture of certain clothes, some everyday noises and particular foods. With higher functioning or older individuals, speech and language are often present, grammar and vocabulary may be age appropriate, but there remain pragmatic difficulties in the social use of communication. In addition to the sensory interests, higher functioning children and adolescents with ASD often develop intense circumscribed interests that are observed in typically developing children but are pursued in a solitary, non social, manner.

The history of diagnosis and classification

Many terms have been used to refer to children with these complex neurodevelopmental presentations: autism, infantile autism, childhood schizophrenia, childhood psychosis, ASD, atypical autism. With the publication of DSM-III, autism was clearly differentiated from childhood schizophrenia and other psychoses, the term "pervasive developmental disorders" (PDDs) was first introduced and some standardized, reliable criteria became widely available (American Psychiatric Association, 1980). DSM-IV (American Psychiatric Association, 1994) included several subtypes of PDD: autism, AS, PDDNOS, Rett syndrome, and disintegrative disorder. AS referred to individuals with characteristics of autism but without clinically significant cognitive or language delay. PDDNOS referred to individuals with characteristics of autism but not enough to qualify for a diagnosis of either autism or AS. Rett syndrome was a type of PDD that was characterized by a period of normal development and then a very specific set of signs and symptoms (e.g., hand wringing) with developmental regression. Disintegrative disorder was a subtype of PDD characterized by normal development past 36 months of age at which point the clinical presentation of autism would emerge.

Prior to the publication of DSM-5 (2013), a systematic literature review and some commissioned primary research were conducted by the DSM-5 Neurodevelopmental Disorder Working Group. The group concluded that there was insufficient evidence that the clinical distinctions between autism and the other subcategories could be made reliably (Lord et al., 2012a) or that these subcategories differed on important variables with respect to etiology, outcome, or response to treatment. As a result, the subcategories have been eliminated and replaced with the single diagnosis of "ASD" with the opportunity to indicate any coexisting diagnoses [epilepsy, Attention Deficit Hyperactivity Disorder (ADHD), social anxiety disorder], or accompanying intellectual disability or language disorder. DSM-5 has also revised the diagnostic criteria for ASD replacing a triad of impairments with two behavioral domains—social communication and repetitive stereotyped behaviors. Although delays in language acquisition are common in ASD, they are nonspecific and so have been removed from the diagnostic criteria. Each domain includes different groups of symptoms or sub-domains (see Figure 51.1) and can be represented dimensionally depending on the need for intervention and support.

DSM-5 includes stereotyped and repetitive speech within the restricted/repetitive behaviors domain and for the first time sensory reactivity to aspects of the individual's environment has also been included. For an individual to meet criteria for a DSM-5 diagnosis of ASD, evidence of symptoms in all three of the social-communication sub-domains and any two (or more) of the four restricted and repetitive behavior sub-domains is required (see Figure 51.1). For individuals who meet criteria for impaired Social Communication in the absence of restricted and repetitive behaviors, a new diagnostic category of Social Communication Disorder has been included in DSM-5 (see Chapter 52).

The changes published in DSM-5 have generated considerable controversy. Some advocates, clinicians, and researchers have expressed concerns that the revised DSM-5 criteria might under-diagnose individuals who would previously have received an ICD-10/DSM-IV diagnosis of (high functioning) autism or AS (McPartland et al., 2012). To date, recently published data do not support this concern (Frazier et al., 2012; Huerta et al., 2012; Kent et al., 2013). Indeed there is evidence that in addition to equivalent levels of sensitivity, reported higher estimates of specificity suggest an improvement in overall diagnostic accuracy.

Epidemiology

Prevalence rates

Up until the 1980s autism was considered to be a rare disorder affecting approximately 4 per 10,000 children (Fombonne, 2005). With the publication of DSM-III, reported prevalence rates of ASD have steadily risen both in the developed and developing world. Systematic reviews (Fombonne, 2005; Williams et al., 2006; Elsabbagh et al., 2012) suggest a prevalence rate of 1 per 100 in developed countries with a lower rate in developing countries. Very high rates (3%) have been reported in South Korea and Japan (Williams et al., 2006; Kim et al., 2011). These findings will need replication as cultural or measurement issues may have contributed (Elsabbagh et al., 2012).

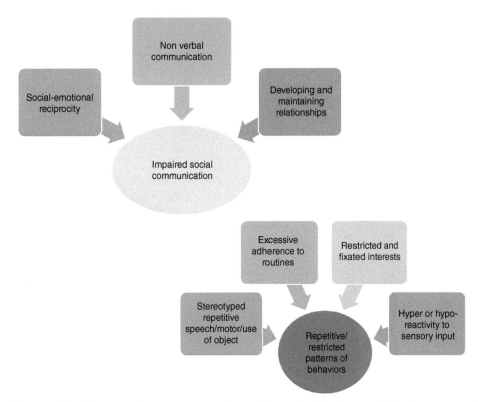

Figure 51.1 The two domains in the DSM-5 1. social-communication and 2. repetitive and restricted patterns of behaviors are shown in the circles. The sub-domains that make up the domains are shown in the squares. *Source*: Reproduced with permission of Rachel Kent and Sarah Carrington, Wales Autism Research Centre, Cardiff University.

There has certainly been an increase in public awareness of ASD, the diagnostic criteria have been broadened and clinicians have a much better understanding of the clinical presentation of ASD in very young children, in those who are higher functioning as well as in adolescents and adults. Moreover, it is true that a diagnosis of ASD can now be made in conjunction with other co-occurring conditions such as a mental health disorder, ADHD, Down syndrome, or the fragile X chromosomal anomaly, a practice that was discouraged within the previous classification systems. In the USA, a rapid increase in the number of children receiving a diagnosis occurred once legislation for special schooling was introduced for autistic children (Gurney *et al.*, 2003). There is also some evidence of "diagnostic substitution" occurring, that is, the prevalence of "mental retardation" is decreasing at roughly the same rate as the prevalence of ASD has been increasing (King & Bearman, 2009). The recent estimates provided by the US Center for Disease Control show considerable variation between states probably as a consequence of significant variation in access to diagnostic services (Center for Disease Control, 2012). Even given these caveats, it is still unclear whether there has been a true increase in prevalence of ASD in recent years.

Although it is well recognized that boys outnumber girls with the disorder, the exact sex ratio is uncertain. Clinic samples tend to report higher ratios (4–6 to 1) of boys versus girls while community samples tend to report lower ratios (2–3 to 1)

(Fombonne, 2005). This has prompted discussion as to whether ASD is under recognized in higher functioning females. It is generally understood that girls with a diagnosis of ASD tend to have lower IQ, more cognitive impairment and fewer repetitive stereotyped behaviors (Amiet *et al.*, 2008). While there is no clear understanding of the male bias in prevalence and difference in presentation, it is also true for other neurodevelopmental disorders and so an ASD-specific explanation may not be required (see Chapter 3).

Population screening

Parents often become concerned about the development of their children at 12–18 months of age but children most commonly do not receive a diagnosis until 4 or 5 years of age (Zwaigenbaum *et al.*, 2009). This represents a significant time lag in access to ASD specific interventions and management of any identified co-occurring problems. These now well replicated findings have given rise to the question as to whether universal screening programmes should be instituted to perhaps reduce the time to diagnosis. However, the American Academy of Pediatrics (AAP) and the UK National Screening Committee do not recommend universal screening. The AAP does suggest that surveillance for ASD should take place at well baby visits at 6, 12, 18, and 24 months (Johnson & Myers, 2007) despite the lack of screening tools with good psychometric properties. It is also true that no randomized control trial of a combined screening and treatment intervention has been conducted to determine whether early screening and earlier age of diagnosis does in fact lead to better long-term outcomes (Al-Qabandi et al., 2011).

Other screening tools have been developed with the aim to be more diagnostic-specific; that is, to have both high sensitivity and specificity. A systematic review by Norris and Lecavalier (2010) examined the sensitivity and specificity of several parent-rated questionnaires and concluded that no screening instrument currently available has sufficient sensitivity and specificity to be used as a diagnostic instrument.

Economic cost

Knapp et al. (2009) suggested that the annual societal cost associated with caring for children with ASD in the United Kingdom is approximately £2.7 billion and nearer £25 billion for adults. In the United States, health care costs per individual with ASD have risen by 20.4% from $4965 in 2000 to $5979 in 2004 (Leslie & Martin, 2007). These figures indicate that among all mental disorders, health care spending in the United States is the highest for individuals with ASD, who had higher physician and outpatient visits as well as greater prescribed medication use when compared to the non ASD paediatric population (Liptak et al., 2006).

Cultural factors

The prevalence of ASD is reported to be lower in countries outside North America, Europe, Japan, and South Korea (Zaroff & Uhm, 2012). This may be attributed to methodological factors which can influence the nature of detection, diagnosis and treatment of ASD (Brown & Rogers, 2003). Currently, there are limited data on the difference in ASD prevalence among various ethnicities and methodological issues have made it difficult to decipher the role of culturally specific influences (see Chapter 16). Zaroff and Uhm (2012) have reported higher rates of ASD among white Americans compared to Hispanic individuals. Likewise, according to Bernier et al. (2010), white Americans receive a diagnosis approximately a year and a half before African-American children and two and a half years before Latino children.

Cognitive and emotional processes

Identifying the cognitive phenotype or profile of ASD is likely to play a critical role in increasing understanding of the underlying brain systems and structures involved in this phenotypically heterogeneous disorder. Understanding these processes may potentially enhance our understanding of how autistic behaviors arise and of the lived "autistic experience" (Charman et al., 2011). Two neuro cognitive models (Theory of Mind (ToM) (Baron-Cohen et al., 1985, 1995) and Executive Dysfunction (Turner, 1999a; Ozonoff & Strayer, 2001) appear related to aspects of the diagnostic criteria for autism/ASD. Subsequent cognitive theories such as Weak Central Coherence (WCC) (Frith, 1989; Happé & Frith, 2006), enhanced perceptual functioning (Mottron et al.,

2006), reduced generalization and enhanced discrimination (Plaisted, 2001) and hyper-systemization (Baron-Cohen et al., 2005) have focussed on different aspects of cognitive functioning. Taking into account the heterogeneity of ASD and the high rates of co-occurring conditions, it is perhaps not surprising that none of these models has provided a satisfactory unitary account of all domains of the ASD behavioral phenotype. Each profile/model has, however, provided useful insights into some of the difficulties experienced by individuals with ASD (see Chapters 3 and 31).

The "ToM" deficit focuses on aspects of the social communication impairments and the inability to impute mental states either to oneself or to others (Baron-Cohen et al., 1985, 1995). The early studies using the false belief task (FBT) identified that individuals with ASD showed deficits in tasks involving mentalizing. However it is now clear that individuals with ASD of higher verbal ability are capable of completing the FBT. A different approach has been used to reconceptualize the ToM deficit as an innate inability to find social meaning in events (Klin et al., 2003)—a problem often reported in individuals with ASD.

Executive function (EF) refers to a range of skills including working memory, capacity to plan, the initiation and monitoring of one's actions, impulse control, capacity to shift set, and inhibition of pre-potent responses. These functions are usually understood to involve the prefrontal cortex (Ozonoff et al., 1991). Executive dysfunction refers to difficulties in any or all of these functions and can be a feature of many clinical conditions. It is unlikely, therefore, that there is a diagnosis specific profile of executive dysfunction in ASD (see Chapter 3). Moreover, findings suggest that the executive control laboratory experimental tasks may capture atypical cognition in ASD rather than EF deficits. Furthermore, inconsistencies have been identified between human administered and computer administered tasks. For ASD subjects, reported impairments in EF may be a consequence of ability rather than of autism (Hill, 2004; Russo et al., 2007 Kenworthy et al., 2008; Sanders et al., 2008; Geurts et al., 2009). However, as with the ToM deficit, these difficulties are reported as common in ASD and may help our understanding of some of the behavioral features of ASD including a lack of ability to generalize learned responses across settings and the presence of repetitive and stereotyped behaviors (Turner, 1999b; Pellicano and Stears, 2011).

The WCC Theory was formulated by Frith (1989) arguing that individuals with autism demonstrated a local processing bias (and thus a WCC). This cognitive style could explain the enhanced performance of children with autism on tasks such as the Embedded Figures Task (EFT) and could account for "islets of ability" such as the superior performance on the Block Design test (Frith & Happé, 1994) that are commonly observed in individuals with ASD. These perceptual abilities might also account for the extreme distress experienced by some children with ASD at small changes in the environment. Research findings (Happé & Frith, 2006) have shown support for this cognitive style across different abilities but have also highlighted inconsistencies. For instance WCC appeared to be a characteristic only of a subset of individuals with ASD, can occur in children with other disorders, and individuals with autism were shown to be able to process at a global level if they are instructed to do so (Plaisted *et al.*, 1999). Happé and Frith (2006) revised the concept of WCC placing increased emphasis on possible superiority of local/detail-focussed processing over more holistic processing which can be overridden with specific situational demands to encourage processing at a global level. This conceptualization is certainly consistent with some of the imaging findings in ASD (see Chapters 11 and 31).

Longitudinal outcome

Diagnostic stability and adult outcome studies

Woolfenden *et al.* (2012) conducted a systematic review of 23 longitudinal studies examining diagnostic stability of children diagnosed with ASD. Using DSM-IV diagnostic criteria, although autistic disorder was found to be a stable diagnosis there was a small percentage of individuals, approximately 15%, in whom the child's symptom profile at follow-up no longer met the diagnostic criteria for an autistic disorder. The pattern of stability was much more variable for those with AS and PDDNOS. Within these two groups only a minority retained their initial diagnosis at follow-up. For some, their profile of skills and difficulties no longer met the diagnostic criteria for any PDD, while for others the diagnostic profile at follow-up was more in keeping with a diagnosis of autistic disorder.

There are surprisingly few prospective longitudinal studies following children with ASD from early childhood to adulthood. It is fortunate that the studies that have been conducted use a common outcome tool (Howlin *et al.*, 2004) that classifies individuals as having an outcome ranging from "very good" to "very poor" (Billstedt *et al.*, 2005; Eaves & Ho, 2008; Farley *et al.*, 2009; Howlin, 2013). These studies report wide variation in outcome with between <5% and 25% having a very good outcome (Levy & Perry, 2011). Overall for many individuals, there is a gradual reduction in autistic symptoms and an improvement in adaptive abilities over time but it is the *variability* in individual outcomes that is most striking. The major predictors of better long-term outcome appear to be higher IQ and the presence of useful speech before 5 years of age, but even within that higher functioning group there is considerable variability (Billstedt *et al.*, 2007; Levy & Perry, 2011). The origin of this variability remains obscure.

Although there is a general trend of improvement, new challenges often appear especially at times of change and transition such as changing educational setting, becoming an adolescent and moving on to young adulthood. Some studies report a deterioration in functioning during adolescence. This may coincide with the development of epilepsy or onset of comorbid psychiatric disorders including anxiety and mood disorders.

Individuals with ASD appear to have higher rates than the general population of ADHD, mood and anxiety disorders, Obsessive Compulsive Disorder (OCD), Tourette's Syndrome, Disruptive Behavior Disorders/Oppositional Defiant Disorder and behaviors that challenge (Matson & Nebel-Schwalm, 2007; Shattuck *et al.*, 2007; Simonoff *et al.*, 2008, 2012; Szatmari & McConnell, 2011; Van Steensel *et al.*, 2011). ADHD and anxiety disorders are probably the two most common comorbid disorders (Szatmari & McConnell, 2011). The specific risk factors and mechanisms associated with the occurrence of these co-occurring disorders have not been determined.

Recent studies have reported the developmental trajectories of adolescents with ASD across the transition into young adulthood (Taylor, 2009). The exit from school can be extremely stressful and lead to a slowing down of overall progress. The issue of transition into adulthood is a serious concern for many individuals with ASD and their families as the lack of resources in adult mental health, social care, and developmental disability provision becomes apparent (Seltzer *et al.*, 2003, 2004; Farley *et al.*, 2009).

There are few data on mortality rates in individuals with ASD but it does appear that mortality is slightly increased (Woolfenden *et al.*, 2012), perhaps a reflection of medical events such as status epilepticus or accidental death associated with epilepsy. This emphasizes the importance of monitoring for seizures during adolescence as a potentially preventable cause of mortality.

Risk factors and possible aetiologic mechanisms

Genetic studies

It was with the publication of the first twin study by Folstein and Rutter (1977) that the importance of genetic factors in ASD was appreciated. Early studies reported that the sibling recurrence risk (the risk that a sibling of a child with autism would also carry this diagnosis) was extremely low, around 2–3% (Szatmari *et al.*, 1998). More recent family studies have used the baby sibling design, in which infant siblings of an older child with autism are followed from birth. A combined analysis of many different samples reported that the sibling recurrence risk is around 19% in siblings followed prospectively from birth (Ozonoff *et al.*, 2011). This much larger estimate probably reflects broader diagnostic criteria for ASD and a longitudinal design (see Chapter 24).

A number of twin and family studies have also reported that sub-threshold autistic like traits occur in the relatives of individuals with ASD more commonly than expected. These traits, termed the "broader autism phenotype" (BAP), are said to occur in upwards of 20% of the parents and siblings of individuals with ASD compared to 5–10% in control families (Le Couteur *et al.*, 1996; Sucksmith *et al.*, 2011). These traits refer to qualitatively similar difficulties in social communication, rigidity, and circumscribed interests but are associated with less impairment and disability compared to individuals with an ASD diagnosis.

A number of recent reviews (Ronald & Hoekstra, 2011; Posthuma & Polderman, 2013) have confirmed that more recent twin studies support a strong genetic contribution to the etiology of ASD although the estimates of heritability vary. These high heritability estimates have encouraged researchers to look for autism susceptibility genes. Systematic reviews of the different linkage studies have identified replication of linkage regions across the genome where susceptibility genes may exist (Trikalinos et al., 2005; Li et al., 2012). However, fine mapping under those linkage peaks has not detected definite evidence of genetic variants that cause ASD. Genome Wide Association Studies (GWAS) have also been considered a fruitful approach to identify the underlying genetic causes of ASD, but generally speaking the majority of reported genetic variants have not been replicated across different studies (Sullivan et al., 2012).

GWAS have relied on the assumption that the genetic variants that cause ASD are relatively common in the population. However, there is an argument that rare genetic variants are more likely to cause most cases of ASD than common variants. ASD has a profound effect on fertility as people with ASD generally do not reproduce and so the likelihood that common variants could act as susceptibility genes with high penetrance is low (Malhotra & Sebat, 2012).

It has been recognized for many years that rare single gene disorders such as fragile X, tuberous sclerosis, neurofibromatosis, and certain chromosomal abnormalities are important examples of rare genetic variants associated with ASD. There are many Mendelian disorders (most often associated with intellectual disability) that are associated with ASD (Abrahams & Geschwind, 2008; Betancur, 2011). In studies with large sample sizes, chromosomal abnormalities at many different loci have also been reported to be associated with ASD. The most common abnormalities involve chromosome 7q and 15q but given that there are so many brain expressed genes it is not surprising that ASD can be associated with abnormalities at many different loci. The well-replicated finding that between 5% and 15% of individuals with ASD have either a single gene disorder or a chromosomal abnormality (Devlin & Scherer, 2012) highlights the importance of general medical screening and genetic testing as part of the diagnostic assessment.

Copy number variants (CNVs) are another important example of genetic variants (see Chapter 24). Rare de novo CNVs have now been reported in an ever-increasing proportion of individuals with ASD. Each occurs in less than 1% of the population of individuals with ASD, but cumulatively may account for 15–20% of the population of individuals with ASD (Devlin & Scherer, 2012). These CNVs tend to be rather large and so are likely to disrupt coding regions of one or more genes.

Many genes carrying CNVs have been reported in ASD. These genes appear to be involved in synaptic plasticity, neuronal development, and chromatin re-modelling. In other words, many of the genes associated with ASD (and with intellectual disability, schizophrenia, ADHD and epilepsy) are involved in maintaining the integrity of the synapse and DNA structure within neurons (see Chapter 24). This provides some evidence that the genes involved in ASD are likely to be part of one or more common pathways. Another outcome of the discovery of CNVs has been the ability to test the function of these genes in animal models where specific loci are "knocked out" or disrupted in some way. This work may lead to the development of new treatment approaches (Crawley, 2012).

Environmental risk factors

The study of environmental risk factors has attracted considerable attention in recent years, especially in the context of gene–environment interactions, but for the most part it has been difficult to identify risk factors that are replicated across studies or to understand the chain of causation that might link a potential risk factor to ASD (see Chapter 23). Many different risk factors have been studied but available systematic reviews have focused on pre- peri- and post natal obstetric complications, exposure to toxins, migration, and parental age.

Pre-, peri-, and post natal complications

Systematic reviews and meta-analyses have addressed the question of whether children with ASD are more likely to be exposed to obstetric complications than the general population (Kolevzon et al., 2007; Gardener et al., 2009; Guinchat et al., 2012). Many obstetric complications have been studied as possibly associated with autism. These include extreme prematurity, hypoxia, bleeding during pregnancy, Caesarean delivery, maternal gestational diabetes, medication use (valproate), breech presentation and neonatal encephalopathy (National Institute for Health and Care Excellence (NICE), 2011). The odds ratios associated with these risk factors tend to be relatively low (less than 3.0) but there is some consistency across the systematic reviews. Using retrospective case-control designs it is still unclear whether the obstetric complications are a true risk factor, represent an outcome associated with a primary abnormality in the fetus, or reflect a methodological artefact.

Environmental chemicals and teratogens, ethnic status and parental age

A systematic review by De Cook et al. (2012) evaluated the role of endocrine disruptors such as bisphenol A (BPA), phthalates, pesticides and hazardous air pollutants (HAPs) in the environment. The authors concluded that there was possibly a positive relationship between exposure to pesticides in the atmosphere and the prevalence of ASD in that region. However, these studies are based on ecological data and are far from providing proof of causality.

Two systematic reviews (Landrigan, 2010; Dufour-Rainfray et al., 2011) discussed the role of maternal use of thalidomide, valproic acid (VPA), ethanol misoprostal, and chlorpyrifos during pregnancy. It appears that individuals who were exposed to thalidomide prenatally were 50 times more likely to have a child with ASD than mothers in the general population (Dufour-Rainfray *et al.*, 2011). VPA, an anti-epileptic drug, is another teratogen and has been shown to increase the prevalence among those exposed by 8–18 times compared to the general population (Dufour-Rainfray *et al.*, 2011). There are mixed results with respect to alcohol intake and autism so no conclusion is possible.

According to Gardener *et al.* (2009), maternal birth abroad is associated with a 28% increased risk, while in Nordic countries the risk associated with immigrant mothers increases to a statistically significant 58%. Dealberto (2011) investigated the association between the prevalence of autism and maternal immigrant status or ethnic origin as it relates to vitamin D insufficiency. Out of the four studies that were reviewed, three reported an increased risk of autism in children from mothers with a different ethnic origin, with one study indicating a greater risk for immigrant mothers from East Asia.

Four reviews (Kolevzon *et al.*, 2007; Gardener *et al.*, 2009; Hultman *et al.*, 2010; Hamlyn *et al.*, 2012) suggest that both advanced maternal and paternal age are risk factors for autism, with paternal age perhaps playing a more significant role. According to Hultman *et al.* (2010) fathers over the age of 50 have the greatest risk of having an offspring with autism compared to fathers below 30 years of age. Gardener *et al.* (2009) estimated that mothers over the age of 30 had a 27% increased risk. Possible biological mechanisms involved in maternal ageing may increase risk for chromosomal imbalances which in turn increases risk for ASD. Older fathers, on the other hand, may experience a higher frequency of point mutations, gene imprinting effects, genetic changes in sperm cells, de novo CNVs, or epigenetic influences that may increase the risk of autism in their offspring (Shelton *et al.*, 2010; Sandin *et al.*, 2012).

Neurotransmitters and neuromodulators

Neurotransmitters have been studied in ASD for over 50 years (see Chapter 3). The most consistent and well-replicated finding has been that 25–50% of children and adolescents with autism have elevated serotonin levels in blood and platelets (McDougle *et al.*, 2005; Lam *et al.*, 2006). However, the relationship between serotonin measured in blood and serotonergic neurotransmission is not well understood. Several studies have reported no difference in CSF levels of 5HIAA (a metabolite of serotonin) between individuals with autism and non autism control groups (Lam *et al.*, 2006). Other researchers have identified differences in whole brain serotonin synthesis capacity in children with autism compared to age-matched non autistic children and also asymmetries of cortical serotonin synthesis in children with autism using neuroimaging (Chugani *et al.*, 1999; Chandana *et al.*, 2005).

Other neurotransmitter systems that have been studied include dopamine, norepinephrine, acetylcholine, oxytocin (OT), endogenous opioids, cortisol, glutamate, and gamma-amino butyric acid (GABA) (McDougle *et al.*, 2005; Lam *et al.*, 2006). There is little replicated research that supports the role of norepinephrine and endogenous opioids in autism. Findings on central dopamine turnover are conflicting, so no conclusion is yet possible. OT and arginine vasopressin (AVP) are important regulators of complex social behaviors (Donaldson & Young, 2008; Heinrichs *et al.*, 2009). There have been some reports of differences in levels of peripheral OT and AVP in children with autism compared to age-matched controls (Modahl *et al.*, 1998; Green *et al.*, 2001; Al-Ayadhi, 2005), but peripheral levels do not necessarily reflect central levels (Bartz &Hollander, 2006). Moreover, GABA abnormalities in blood and platelets have been reported in individuals with autism (Rolf *et al.*, 1993). Post mortem studies have identified widespread decreased number of GABA receptor binding sites (Oblak *et al.*, 2009). Fatemi *et al.* (2009) also suggest widespread decreases in expression of GABA synthetic enzymes and GABA receptors in a variety of brain regions.

Observations of immune system abnormalities in ASD have been noted including fetal protein reactive IgG antibodies in plasma from mothers of children with autism, maternal infection, and dysregulated cytokine signaling (Braunschweig *et al.*, 2012). In addition, inflammation in the brain has been reported in post mortem brain specimens of individuals with ASD, suggesting that this is an area worthy of further investigation (Gesundheit *et al.*, 2013).

Neuropathology findings and post mortem studies

Post mortem studies of brain tissue offer the possibility of studying the functional impact of genetic variants in ASD and understanding, at a microscopic level, some of the structural and functional brain imaging findings. Unfortunately, current studies in this area are hampered by poor tissue quality, small sample sizes and confounding factors such as cause of death (Schumann & Nordahl, 2011). Many different neuropathological changes have been described in post mortem samples including macroencephaly, acceleration and deceleration in brain growth, increased neural packing, decreased cell size in the limbic system and decreased Purkinje cell number in the cerebellum. Abnormalities in organization of the cortical minicolumn, representing the fundamental subunit of vertical cortical organization may underlie the pathology of ASD and result in altered thalamocortical organization, cortical disinhibition and dysfunction of the arousal-modulating system of the brain.

Brain imaging

One of the most widely replicated findings in ASD is the increased head size and brain volume (mainly due to increased volumes in frontal lobes and anterior temporal regions) most notably in the preschool period (Bailey *et al.*, 1993; Courchesne *et al.*, 2007). Neuroimaging methods such as magnetic resonance imaging have identified other abnormalities that appear consistent with some of the proposed social communication and EF deficits identified using psychometric and neuropsychological testing paradigms (Verhoeven *et al.*, 2010; see Chapter 11). A recent meta-analysis of voxel-based global gray matter volumes (using data from 24 independent data sets of adolescent and adult subjects with ASD and healthy controls) has found consistent evidence of reduction in gray matter volumes in the bilateral amygdala-hippocampus complex and the bilateral precuneus and a small increase in gray matter volume in the middle-inferior frontal gyrus (Stanfield *et al.*, 2008). The meta-analysis included studies of adults and adolescents with ASD but only the gray matter volume in the right precuneus was higher in adults than in adolescents with ASD. These findings appear to confirm the crucial involvement of structures linked to social cognition in ASD (Via *et al.*, 2011).

With technological advances, there has been a remarkable increase in studies looking at brain function both during resting states and during specific tasks in individuals with ASD (mostly adults and those who are higher functioning) (see Chapter 11). Studies have focused on brain connectivity between the "social brain" and other regions of the cortex. Systematic reviews and meta-analyses are few but do conclude that there is ineffective integration across brain regions, especially frontal and more posterior cortical regions (Philip et al., 2012). There may be, by contrast, enhanced local connectivity especially in the parietal-occipital regions (Minshew & Keller, 2010) associated with an increased reliance on visual-spatial abilities for visual and verbal reasoning. This work has been extended by more recent work using diffusion tensor imaging to assess white matter integrity. In general, studies show that there are abnormalities in measures of white matter, particularly in those pathways integrating higher order cognitive processes or complex social-emotional processing (Ameis & Szatmari, 2012). A recent meta-analysis has emphasized the role of the superior longitudinal fasciculus, uncinate fasciculus and corpus callosum in understanding the long-distance underconnectivity model of ASD (Aoki *et al.*, 2013).

Assessment

In recent years, a number of evidence-based clinical guidelines and practice parameters have been published in several countries (Le Couteur, 2003; Johnston & Hawken, 2007; Scottish Intercollegiate Guideline Network, 2007; Ministry of Health and Education, 2008; NICE, 2011). Evidence based guidelines, if implemented, are an effective way of disseminating research findings and examples of agreed best practice with the aim to improve and standardize clinical care in community and hospital settings (Davis & Taylor-Vaisey, 1997).

With the increased awareness and recognition that ASDs are relatively common (Centers for Disease Control and Prevention, 2012), there is pressure on local community child health and child and adolescent mental health services to identify and make an appropriate diagnosis as early as possible. The best practice would also recommend the provision of a comprehensive skill- and need-based assessment for the affected individual and their family or carers to inform the development of an individualized education and management plan (see Chapter 32). Timely diagnosis and planning are important for access to effective psychoeducation, interventions, and support (Keenan *et al.*, 2006; see Chapter 32).

Although there are no pathognomonic signs or symptoms of ASD, a number of the national clinical guidelines provide detailed information about the types of signs and symptoms that are commonly observed in preschool, school-aged children and adolescents with a possible ASD (NICE, 2011).

Several authors and guidelines highlight the so-called "Red Flags" for an immediate "fast track" referral of certain "high risk" groups for an ASD specific assessment (Johnson *et al.*, 2007; Allison *et al.*, 2012). For example, a history of loss of speech and early language in a young child under the age of 3 years, is highly suggestive of a possible ASD (Baird *et al.*, 2008; Pickles *et al.*, 2009).

For children with a diagnosis of ASD, review and re-assessment, especially at times of transition (such as starting in education, changing school, onset of adolescence or emerging into early adulthood) are likely to be beneficial either in anticipation of possible change in circumstances or if there is evidence of deterioration, onset of a mental health problem, or a new disorder such as epilepsy. Furthermore, some children and youth may not have been identified or assessed during the early years, but additional developmental, social, and academic pressures or the increased expectations of the school years may lead to symptoms and behaviors that require a multidisciplinary ASD diagnostic assessment at a later stage. All guidelines published in the last decade recommend a multi professional approach for the ASD diagnostic assessment that: responds to the parents'/carers' and when appropriate, the child or youth's concerns; makes the best use of existing information about the child or youth and combines assessment information from a variety of sources. Moreover, these processes reveal the differential diagnosis and identification of any co-occurring condition(s) (see Tables 51.1 and 51.2).

The core components of an ASD diagnostic assessment include:

- an ASD specific developmental history using the framework of published internationally agreed diagnostic criteria (ICD-10; DSM-IV-TR; DSM-5; American Psychiatric Association, 2013; World Health Organization, 1992). Most guidelines indicate that using a published standardized diagnostic instrument may assist this process.
- medical history including a prenatal and perinatal history, identification of any relevant past and/or current health conditions and risk factors such as a history of possible epilepsy, and family history to identify genetic disorders, recognized medical and mental health conditions.

Table 51.1 Differential diagnosis.

Consider the following differential diagnosis for autism and whether specific assessments are needed to help interpret the autism history and observations

- Neurodevelopmental disorders:
  ° Specific language delay or disorder
  ° Intellectual disability or global developmental delay
  ° Developmental coordination disorder (DCD).
- Mental and behavioral disorders:
  ° Attention deficit hyperactivity disorder (ADHD)
  ° Mood disorder
  ° Anxiety disorder
  ° Attachment disorders
  ° Oppositional defiant disorder (ODD)
  ° Conduct disorder
  ° Obsessive compulsive disorder (OCD)
  ° Psychosis.
- Conditions in which there is developmental regression:
  ° Rett syndrome
  ° Epileptic encephalopathy.
- Other conditions:
  ° Severe hearing impairment
  ° Severe visual impairment
  ° Maltreatment
  ° Selective mutism.

National Institute for Health and Care Excellence (2011) CG 128 Autism diagnosis in children and young people: recognition, referral and diagnosis of children and young people on the autism spectrum. Available from http://guidance.nice.org.uk/CG128. *Reproduced with permission.*
Source: Adapted from National Institute for Health and Care Excellence.

Table 51.2 Coexisting conditions.

Consider whether the child or young person may have any of the following as a coexisting condition, and if suspected carry out appropriate assessments and referrals:

- Mental and behavior problems and disorders:
  ° ADHD
  ° Anxiety disorders and phobias
  ° Mood disorders
  ° Oppositional defiant behavior
  ° Tics or Tourette's syndrome
  ° OCD
  ° Self-injurious behavior.
- Neurodevelopmental problems and disorders:
  ° Global delay or intellectual disability
  ° Motor coordination problems or DCD
  ° Academic learning problems, for example, in literacy or numeracy
  ° Speech and language disorder
- Medical or genetic problems and disorders:
  ° Epilepsy and epileptic encephalopathy
  ° Chromosome disorders
  ° Genetic abnormalities, including fragile X
  ° Tuberous sclerosis
  ° Muscular dystrophy
  ° Neurofibromatosis.
- Functional problems and disorders:
  ° Feeding problems, including restricted diets
  ° Urinary incontinence or enuresis
  ° Constipation, altered bowel habit, faecal incontinence, or encopresis
  ° Sleep disturbances
  ° Vision or hearing impairment.

National Institute for Health and Care Excellence (2011) CG 128 Autism diagnosis in children and young people: recognition, referral, and diagnosis of children and young people on the autism spectrum. Available from http://guidance.nice.org.uk/CG128. *Reproduced with permission.*
Source: Adapted from National Institute for Health and Care Excellence.

- physical examination including an assessment for congenital anomalies, any evidence of skin conditions, evaluation of growth, and measurement of head circumference.
- individual ASD specific assessments (through direct interaction and observation usually in more than one setting). Observational assessment may include the use of an ASD-specific tool such as the Autism Diagnostic Observation Schedule (ADOS) (Lord *et al.*, 2000, 2012b) or the Childhood Autism Rating Scale (CARS) (Schopler *et al.*, 1980, 1986).
- other individual assessments depending on the clinical presentation.
- individual assessments such as vision or hearing, cognitive, sensory, perceptual, motor co-ordination, and psychological investigations to complete a skill- and need-based profile (see Chapters 32–35).

The ASD specific developmental history, ASD observational assessments and standardized individual assessments should all be undertaken by clinicians with experience assessing and working with children and youth with ASD across the ability range. A number of ASD rating scales and diagnostic instruments have been developed that can provide structure and high quality standardized information as part of the referral and diagnostic process but these measures should not be used in the absence of sound clinical knowledge of ASD (Charman & Gotham, 2013).

The four most commonly used diagnostic instruments for ASD include three semi-structured instruments for obtaining a developmental history (Autism Diagnostic Interview-Revised (ADI-R)(Lord *et al.*, 1994; Rutter *et al.*, 2003); Diagnostic Interview for Social and Communication Disorders (DISCO) (Leekam *et al.*, 2002; Wing *et al.*, 2002) and Development, Dimensional and Diagnostic Interview (3di) (Skuse *et al.*, 2004) and one observational measure (the ADOS (Lord *et al.*, 2000, 2012b). For details refer to NICE (2011). Although these and other instruments are widely used in research and clinical practice, they cannot be used in isolation, are usually time consuming and require dedicated training. They provide standardized methods for gathering detailed descriptions of behavior that when integrated with sound clinical expertize in the variable presentation of ASD, will inform an individualized management and educational plan for a child or young person with ASD. Furthermore, there are little published data on the psychometric properties of these measures when used in community clinical settings or other models of health-care service configuration. At present there is no evidence to recommend any one measure for universal clinical practice.

All ASD diagnostic assessments should include a physical examination by a medically qualified practitioner (with expertize in ASD) to assess general development taking into account those factors associated with an increased risk of autism/ASD (NICE, 2011; see Chapter 35). The examiner requires the skills and knowledge to consider the differential diagnosis and identify dysmorphic features, developmental regression (such as Rett syndrome, epileptic encephalopathy), specific genetic conditions such as the fragile X chromosomal anomaly, muscular dystrophy, neurofibromatosis, Tuberose sclerosis; medical conditions such as epilepsy, overgrowth syndromes; neurodevelopment disorders (including Developmental Coordination Disorder (DCD); and other conditions (including severe sensory and perceptual difficulties, severe hearing impairment, severe visual impairment and child maltreatment) that may also require further investigations. Other problems such as gastrointestinal symptoms and functional impairments of sleep and eating are also common. Any of these conditions and/or problems may have a substantial adverse impact on the child and family. Identification should lead to referral to the relevant specialist professional.

Any further physical and medical investigation such as genetic testing for specific genetic syndromes or mutations, or use of specific tests (such as electroencephalogram (EEG), magnetic resonance imaging (MRI)) should not be performed routinely but based on clinical indications such as family history, dysmorphology or abnormalities in growth (see Chapter 35). In some parts of the world, comparative genomic hybridization arrays are now recommended within professional clinical best practice guidelines to be used as first line investigations (Manning & Hudgins, 2010; Miller et al., 2010) especially in the presence of intellectual disability or dysmorphology.

Assessment of family strengths and needs and the social and cultural context for the child or young person is important as part of a skill- and need-based assessment (see Chapter 32). Evidence is emerging that the burden of raising a child with ASD is greater in families with a child with ASD compared to children with other mental health and developmental disorders (Dumas et al., 1991; Sivberg, 2002; Abbeduto et al., 2004). A range of factors including severity of ASD and problem behaviors, social support, religion, the family's attitude to the diagnosis (reframing) and psychological acceptance are likely to influence family adaptation to ASD and impact on parent mental health (Taunt & Hastings, 2002; Weiss et al., 2012).

The conclusions of an ASD multidisciplinary assessment should be collated as a profile of the child or young person. The findings should include a best-estimate clinical diagnosis, the identification of any co-occurring conditions and a summary of skills and needs for the child or young person and their family (see Chapter 32).

Treatments

An individualized management plan for the child/youth with ASD and their family or carers needs to be developed. Over time,

intervention plans will change in response to the child's developmental profile, their circumstances and the onset of any additional physical and mental health disorders. Management and support are likely to include a number of different agencies and professionals working collaboratively (NICE, 2013).

The goals of interventions include:
- Reduce the core symptoms and behaviors of ASD.
- Enable an individual to achieve their own potential.
- Treat any co-occurring problems or symptoms that impair developmental progress or cause significant distress for the affected individual and other family members or carers.
- Support the family and those providing the care and interventions for the affected individual through education and specific evidence-based strategies.

There are many different interventions and treatments proposed for ASD and the additional problems that individuals with ASD experience. It is unfortunate that most interventions have not been independently and adequately evaluated. To date, there are few systematic reviews and meta-analyses to inform an evidence-based approach for the management of affected children at different ages. National and professional organizations have published practice guidelines which provide general and specific recommendations usually based on the best clinical practice (Myers et al., 2007; Scottish Intercollegiate Guidelines Network, 2007; Ministry of Health and Education, 2008; AHRQ, 2011; Warren et al., 2011a; NICE, 2013).

Psychosocial and behavioral interventions for the management of core features of ASD

Despite the limited evidence base, there is a growing consensus that early identification and access to specific psychosocial interventions delivered by trained professionals is likely to improve the outcomes for some children with ASD (NICE, 2013). Using recent systematic reviews and meta-analyses published since 2005, Magiati et al. (2012) and Reichow et al. (2012) have identified that early intensive behavioral intervention (EIBI) is the most frequently evaluated intervention in preschool children with ASD. These interventions are largely based on the model of Applied Behavioral Analysis (ABA) principles and other comprehensive behaviorally and developmentally based programmes for young children with ASD such as those developed by Lovaas (1987; McEachin et al., 1993). The evaluation of EIBI and other interventions include "efficacy" trials undertaken in university or specialist clinics under laboratory conditions and some effectiveness studies conducted with parents in community, "real-life," settings. Most studies compare the intervention with treatment as usual or no treatment and do report a positive outcome particularly in communication skills. An increasing number of studies have reported on early interventions such as the Early Start Denver Model (ESDM), Learning Experiences and Alternative Programme for Preschoolers and their Parents (LEAP), Preschool Autism Social-Communication Trial (PACT) and Treatment and Education for Autistic and Related Communication Handicapped Children (TEACCH) (Rogers & Vismara, 2008; Eikeseth, 2009; Dawson et al., 2010;

Green *et al.*, 2010; Virués-Ortega, 2010; Strain & Bovey, 2011; Warren *et al.*, 2011a, b). In contrast to the Lovaas type models, these psychosocial interventions are developmentally orientated, may include principles of ABA and often focus on social communication. For preschool children, the interventions usually involve teaching parents, carers, or teachers strategies to increase joint attention skills and reciprocal communication often through interactive play and action routines (Kasari *et al.*, 2006; Yoder & Stone, 2006; Green *et al.*, 2010; Kaale *et al.*, 2012). The improvements in outcome are usually either in proximal measures specific to the intervention such as joint attention or more general measures of intellectual, language and/or adaptive function. Very few studies assess impact on autism behaviors and no studies to date have investigated longer-term outcomes (Green *et al.*, 2010).

For older school-aged children and young people, a small number of systematic reviews have identified a limited number of studies evaluating interventions, such as social skills training for improving social communication and peer-mediated social communication interventions (Maglione *et al.*, 2012; Reichow *et al.*, 2012). As with preschool children, interventions have been delivered in a variety of contexts including home, clinic settings, and educational/school-based provision. The studies to date are of relatively poor quality and although there is some evidence that greater intensity and longer treatment duration may lead to improved outcome, further research with manualized interventions and appropriate well-validated outcome measures is needed.

The recently published NICE Clinical Guideline (CG) 170 (2013) clinical guidelines development group judged that the social-communication programmes may help address social isolation. There is, however, little evidence for interventions aimed at the core ASD feature of restricted, repetitive behaviors, or sensory sensitivities, either as a direct or indirect outcome. Some psychosocial interventions evaluation studies have included repetitive behaviors and reported either no change or a small treatment effect from parent training and/or antipsychotic medication (Dawson *et al.*, 2010; Green *et al.*, 2010; Scahill *et al.*, 2012). There is evidence (Maglione *et al.*, 2012) that augmentative forms of communication such as the Picture Exchange Communication System (PECS) can improve the communication skills of young children with ASD and should be part of the comprehensive treatment plan, but may not be as effective as originally thought.

Other Interventions for the treatment of core features of ASD

Interventions such as sensory integration therapy (SIT) and auditory integration training (AIT) have been proposed to alleviate hyper- or hypo-sensitivity to certain stimuli (Kadar *et al.*, 2012) and to particular frequencies and sounds (Bettison, 1996). However, systematic reviews indicate that the study designs are of poor quality and the evidence is inadequate to recommend SIT as an evidence-based treatment for ASD (Baranek, 2002; Case-Smith & Arbesman, 2008). For AIT,

systematic reviews (Baranek, 2002; Case-Smith & Arbesman, 2008; Parr, 2008; Sinha *et al.*, 2011) have indicated that the evidence is insufficient to conclude that these are effective treatments for individuals with ASD. Moreover, the reviews highlighted concerns about hearing loss as a result of listening to various sounds of high volume.

Visual therapies, music therapy and use of restricted diets and dietary supplementation such as omega-3 fatty acids, have also been used by families to treat both core ASD symptoms and associated problems such as ADHD-like behaviors, gastrointestinal problems, and sensory disturbances (Baranek, 2002; Gold *et al.*, 2006; Hodgetts & Hodgetts, 2007; Case-Smith & Arbesman, 2008; Parr, 2008; Millward *et al.*, 2009; Buie *et al.*, 2010; James *et al.*, 2011; Sinha *et al.*, 2011). The gluten free, casein free diet (GFCFD) is the most frequently implemented restrictive dietary intervention for individuals with ASD. Three reviews have been published highlighting the poor quality of the studies and the lack of evidence for this intervention (Parr, 2008; Millward *et al.*, 2009; James *et al.*, 2011). With respect to fatty acid supplementation, James *et al.* (2011) concluded that there was no evidence of a difference between individuals with autism who received omega-3 fatty acids and a placebo group. With regard to older adolescents and young adults, a recent systematic review of vocational interventions has reported that despite the small number of studies and the poor quality, there is some evidence that vocational programmes may increase employment success for some individuals with ASD (Dove *et al.*, 2012).

Systematic reviews have also demonstrated some evidence that the use of antipsychotic medications (such as risperidone) can reduce repetitive behaviors in children and adolescents (usually in association with irritability and other behaviors that challenge) though there is some disagreement in the field (RUPP, 2005; Jesner *et al.*, 2007; McPheeters *et al.*, 2011). For example, taking into account the evidence for statistically significant adverse effects associated with antipsychotics (see NICE CG 170, 2013 for an updated review) the NICE clinical guideline development group did not recommend antipsychotic medications for the treatment of core symptoms of ASD. A systematic review by Williams *et al.* (2010) has examined the effectiveness of selective serotonin reuptake inhibitors (SSRIs) in treating symptoms associated with ASD and found that there are no data supporting the use of SSRIs in improving symptoms of individuals with ASD and strong data recording the incidence of adverse effects (see Chapter 43). Finally, there is now sufficient evidence to recommend that certain interventions should not be used to treat core features of ASD. These include long-term chelation therapy, hyperbaric oxygen, and secretin (NICE, 2013).

Management of associated and co-occurring conditions

All published clinical guidelines identify the importance of the early identification and implementation of evidence-based treatment for any recognized medical problems. For the management of commonly occurring conditions such as sleep problems as with other difficulties, a combination of a detailed specific assessment leading to a behavioral management plan to improve sleep hygiene should be implemented before considering the use of medication (NICE, 2013). Systematic reviews by Guenole et al. (2011) and Rossignol and Frye (2011) examined the effects of melatonin in improving sleep disturbances and found that melatonin shortened time to falling asleep but did not necessarily prolong sleep duration (see Chapter 70).

Identification and treatment of co-occurring behavioral and mental health problems

It is now widely recognized that children and young people with ASD have higher rates of co-occurring mental health disorders than individuals in the general population and children with other disabilities (Leyfer et al., 2006; de Bruin et al., 2007; Simonoff et al., 2008, 2012; Joshi et al., 2010; Van Steensel et al., 2011). These include ADHD; other behavioral and mental health problems including Oppositional Defiant Disorder, anxiety, mood disturbance, Obsessive Compulsive Disorder; behaviors that challenge as well as catatonia, a rare but debilitating comorbidity (Wing & Shah, 2000). Most clinical guidelines recommend implementation of evidence-based interventions for the co-occurring disorder but indicate that modifications in the delivery of the intervention may be required to meet the needs of the person with ASD.

For example, children and young people with ASD with good verbal and cognitive skills and comorbid anxiety disorder may have the capacity to engage in a course of cognitive behavior therapy (CBT). There is evidence that a group or individual-based intervention adjusted to the needs of children with ASD can be effective (see Chapters 38 and 60; Sofronoff et al., 2007; Drahota et al., 2011; NICE, 2013). Similarly for the treatment of co-occurring ADHD, a combination of family and school-based behavioral interventions could be instigated and later, if required, supported by a trial of medication. However, the use of stimulants and other recommended second line medications for the treatment of ADHD-like symptoms show that the response rate is lower than for children and adolescents without ASD and with a higher rate of adverse side effects (see Chapter 55; NICE, 2013). SSRI's have also been used to treat OCD, some severe anxiety disorders and mood disorders in ASD but with no real evidence of efficacy (McPheeters et al., 2011; see Chapters 43, 60, 61 and 63).

To anticipate and prevent behaviors that challenge, identifying factors that increase risk such as sensory sensitivities, changing circumstances, physical or mental illness, exploitation, bullying at school, or abuse should always be considered and the necessary actions put in place. A functional behavioral analysis based on a thorough understanding of precipitating circumstances and reinforcing factors needs to be undertaken by staff with an understanding of ASD before medication is initiated (see Chapter 38).

Antipsychotic medication has been used to ameliorate associated symptoms such as aggression and irritability. The evidence appears to be consistent in demonstrating a positive impact on these symptoms (McPheeters et al., 2011; Dove et al., 2012). The starting dose should be low, aiming for the minimum effective dose and carefully monitoring for adverse effects with a plan for regular review and eventual discontinuation (see Chapter 43).

Educational issues

In most countries over recent decades, the emphasis has been on inclusive environments for the education of children with special education needs including ASD (see Chapters 41 and 42). However, education for children with ASD includes both the acquisition of culturally valued skills in settings that promote full participation and the need to learn specific skills and social understanding to "compensate" for their ASD. There is no evidence of the effectiveness of different educational settings, nor how children with ASD experience education in the context of "real-world" classrooms. Furthermore, although some studies have attempted to evaluate interventions for young children, the educational needs of older children and those in post compulsory education, consideration of diversity of need and, most importantly, the views of young people about their experiences of education have all been relatively neglected. The efficacy of one comprehensive programme (TEACCH) that has been incorporated into a wide range of education settings has been reported in one meta-analysis. Moderate to large gains in social behavior and behaviors that challenge has been reported, but much smaller effect sizes exist on more cognitively related outcomes (Virues-Ortega et al., 2013). Social skill interventions and emotional learning programmes are often carried out in schools and there is some evidence of efficacy for these interventions (Reichow & Volkmar, 2010).

Family support

Some studies have shown that family stress can be modified (see Chapter 39) (Dunn et al., 2001; Hastings & Brown, 2002; Benson & Karlof, 2009). The recently published NICE CG170, 2013 report a meta-analysis of three psychosocial intervention studies, which were of small sample sizes with relatively poor methodologies. For this reason, the guideline development group concluded that as there was to date insufficient evidence to recommend interventions for improving parental stress, mental health, or quality of life, the focus of intervention should be the management of behaviors that challenge. The benefits of involving parents as the so-called 'co-therapists' has long been recognized particularly with respect to the maintenance of treatment effects and generalization of learned responses across settings (Schopler et al., 1982; Howlin & Rutter, 1987). However, for parents such therapeutic tasks may also be a source of increased stress. The range of ways to engage with parents includes individual work in the home or clinic, group-based interventions and/or parents taking on the role of parent peers/mentors to help other parents learn new skills.

Transition planning

There is an increasing recognition of the difficulties individuals with ASD have with anticipating and managing change from minor apparently irrelevant changes to larger changes such as moving into a new nursery group or classroom, moving to a larger secondary school, leaving school and going to college or looking for paid employment. As individuals approach early adulthood there is an expectation that they should take on more responsibility for self-management of their own condition. While this is a key issue, there is little literature based on clinical trials evaluating the effectiveness of transition planning interventions (Watson *et al.*, 2011).

Future developments and necessary research

There has been a remarkable increase in the knowledge base for ASD since the first edition of this textbook. Although progress has been made in measurement and diagnostic tools, in understanding prevalence and etiology and in developing evidence-based treatments both for core symptoms and comorbid conditions, much remains to be learned. Throughout the history of ASD research, there has been a tension between understanding autism as a unitary diagnosis at the same time acknowledging the complexity implied by considering autism as a spectrum disorder. Multiple unitary explanations of phenomenology, etiology, and underlying cognitive impairments have encouraged different schools to promote treatments based on separate paradigms of understanding. But the reality is one of complexity and heterogeneity at multiple levels creating major challenges for researchers, families, clinicians, and policy makers alike.

In terms of basic research, new paradigms are needed to uncover not only heterogeneous genetic mechanisms but also the functional impact of those genetic variants, including animal models and imaging studies. Cognitive behavior neuroscience and molecular genetic findings together might identify gene–environment interactions in particular individuals with ASD. Appreciation of this heterogeneity of ASD also has important clinical implications. Personalizing care by identifying effective treatment for each individual at appropriate points in development should be a key priority, working in partnership with young people with ASD and their families/carers. Further research is needed into how individuals with ASD access health and social care services. A key issue will be to identify early risk markers for ASD and co-occurring conditions that are amenable to interventions that could reduce the likelihood of a cascade of further difficulties with the inevitable adverse impacts on later lifetime functioning. Finally, it is not known how best to disseminate training, knowledge, and the best practice about

particular interventions among all professionals in contact with individuals with ASD. Overall the ultimate goal is for a sufficiently accurate evidence base to inform effective intervention planning for every individual with ASD and their family. This evidence base includes an individualized genetic profile, in combination with the identification of relevant environmental and family factors.

Acknowledgments

We would like to thank Sofia Al Balkhi, Laura Fox (Canada) together with Hannah Merrick (Newcastle University), Dr. Hasan Aman (Northumberland. Tyne & Wear NHS Foundation Trust) (UK) for their assistance with the literature searches and Rachael Taylor (UK) for her dedicated administrative support, leading to the completion of this chapter.

We also appreciate the assistance provided by the NICE for their permission to include Tables 51.1 and 51.2 from the NICE CG 128, 2011 and Sarah Carrington & Rachel Kent, Cardiff University for permission to reprint Figure 51.1.

References

Abbeduto, L. *et al.* (2004) Psychological well-being and coping in mothers of youths with autism, down syndrome, or fragile X syndrome. *American Journal on Mental Retardation* **109** (3), 237–254.

Abrahams, B.S. & Geschwind, D.H. (2008) Advances in autism genetics: on the threshold of a new neurobiology. *Nature Reviews Genetics* **9** (5), 341–355.

Agency for Healthcare Research and Quality (AHRQ) (2011) [Online]. Available: http://www.qualityindicators.ahrq.gov/ [08 Aug 2014].

Al-Ayadhi, L.Y. (2005) Altered oxytocin and vasopressin levels in autistic children in Central Saudi Arabia. *Neurosciences (Riyadh, Saudi Arabia)* **10** (1), 47–50.

Allison, C. *et al.* (2012) Toward brief "red flags" for autism screening: the short autism spectrum quotient and the short quantitative checklist in 1,000 cases and 3,000 controls. *Journal of the American Academy of Child & Adolescent Psychiatry* **51** (2), 202–212.

Al-Qabandi, M. *et al.* (2011) Early autism detection: are we ready for routine screening? *Pediatrics* **128** (1), e211–e217.

Ameis, S.H. & Szatmari, P. (2012) Imaging-genetics in autism spectrum disorder: advances, translational impact, and future directions. *Frontiers in Psychiatry* **3**, 46.

American Psychiatric Association (1980) *Diagnostic and Statistical Manual of Mental Disorders* (DSM-III). American Psychiatric Association, Washington, DC.

American Psychiatric Association (1994) *Diagnostic and Statistical Manual of Mental Disorders* (DSM-IV), 4th revised edn. American Psychiatric Association, Washington, DC.

American Psychiatric Association (2013) *Diagnostic and Statistical Manual of Mental Disorders* (DSM-5), 5th edn. American Psychiatric Association, Washington, DC.

Amiet, C. *et al.* (2008) Epilepsy in autism is associated with intellectual disability and gender: evidence from a meta-analysis. *Biological Psychiatry* **64** (7), 577–582.

Aoki, Y. *et al.* (2013) Comparison of white matter integrity between autism spectrum disorder subjects and typically developing individuals: a meta-analysis of diffusion tensor imaging tractography studies. *Molecular Autism* **4** (1), 25.

Bailey, A. *et al.* (1993) Autism and megalencephaly. *Lancet* **341** (8854), 1225–1226.

Baird, G. *et al.* (2008) Regression, developmental trajectory and associated problems in disorders in the autism spectrum: the SNAP study. *Journal of Autism and Developmental Disorders* **38** (10), 1827–1836.

Baranek, G.T. (2002) Efficacy of sensory and motor interventions for children with autism. *Journal of Autism and Developmental Disorders* **32** (5), 397–422.

Baron-Cohen, S. *et al.* (1985) Does the autistic child have a "theory of mind"? *Cognition* **21** (1), 37–46.

Baron-Cohen, S. *et al.* (2005) Sex differences in the brain: implications for explaining autism. *Science* **310** (5749), 819–823.

Baron-Cohen, S. *et al.* (1995) Are children with autism blind to the mentalistic significance of the eyes? *British Journal of Developmental Psychology* **13** (4), 379–398.

Bartz, J. & Hollander, E. (2006) The neuroscience of affiliation: forging links between basic and clinical research on neuropeptides and social behavior. *Hormones and Behavior* **50** (4), 518–528.

Benson, P.R. & Karlof, K.L. (2009) Anger, stress proliferation, and depressed mood among parents of children with ASD: a longitudinal replication. *Journal of Autism and Developmental Disorders* **39** (2), 350–362.

Bernier, R. *et al.* (2010) Psychopathology, families, and culture: autism. *Child and Adolescent Psychiatric Clinics of North America* **19** (4), 855.

Betancur, C. (2011) Etiological heterogeneity in autism spectrum disorders: more than 100 genetic and genomic disorders and still counting. *Brain Research* **1380**, 42–77.

Bettison, S. (1996) The long-term effects of auditory training on children with autism. *Journal of Autism and Developmental Disorders* **26** (3), 361–374.

Billstedt, E. *et al.* (2005) Autism after adolescence: population-based 13-to 22-year follow-up study of 120 individuals with autism diagnosed in childhood. *Journal of Autism and Developmental Disorders* **35** (3), 351–360.

Billstedt, E. *et al.* (2007) Autism in adults: symptom patterns and early childhood predictors. Use of the DISCO in a community sample followed from childhood. *Journal of Child Psychology and Psychiatry* **48** (11), 1102–1110.

Braunschweig, D. *et al.* (2012) Maternal autism-associated IgG antibodies delay development and produce anxiety in a mouse gestational transfer model. *Journal of Neuroimmunology* **252** (1–2), 56–65.

Brown, J.R. & Rogers, S.J. (2003) Cultural issues in autism. In: *Autism Spectrum Disorders: A Research Review for Practitioners*, pp. 209–226. American Psychiatric Association, Washington, DC.

de Bruin, E.I. *et al.* (2007) High rates of psychiatric co-morbidity in PDD-NOS. *Journal of Autism and Developmental Disorders* **37** (5), 877–886.

Buie, T. *et al.* (2010) Evaluation, diagnosis and treatment of gastrointestinal disorders in individuals with ASDs: a consensus report. *Pediatrics* **125** (Suppl 1), S1–S18.

Case-Smith, J. & Arbesman, M. (2008) Evidence-based review of interventions for autism used in or of relevance to occupational therapy. *The American Journal of Occupational Therapy* **62** (4), 416–429.

Centers for Disease Control and Prevention (2012) *CDC 24/7: Saving lives. Protecting people* [Online]. Available: www.cdc.gov [08 Aug 2014].

Chandana, S.R. *et al.* (2005) Significance of abnormalities in developmental trajectory and asymmetry of cortical serotonin synthesis in autism. *International Journal of Developmental Neuroscience* **23** (2), 171–182.

Charman, T. & Gotham, K. (2013) Measurement Issues: Screening and diagnostic instruments for autism spectrum disorders—lessons from research and practise. *Child and Adolescent Mental Health* **18** (1), 52–63.

Charman, T. *et al.* (2011) Defining the cognitive phenotype of autism. *Brain Research* **1380**, 10–21.

Chugani, D.C. *et al.* (1999) Developmental changes in brain serotonin synthesis capacity in autistic and nonautistic children. *Annals of Neurology* **45** (3), 287–295.

Courchesne, E. *et al.* (2007) Mapping early brain development in autism. *Neuron* **56** (2), 399–413.

Crawley, J.N. (2012) Translational animal models of autism and neurodevelopmental disorders. *Dialogues in Clinical Neuroscience* **14** (3), 293.

Davis, D.A. *et al.* (1997) Translating guidelines into practice: a systematic review of theoretic concepts, practical experience and research evidence in the adoption of clinical practice guidelines. *Canadian Medical Association Journal* **157** (4), 408–416.

Dawson, G. *et al.* (2010) Randomized, controlled trial of an intervention for toddlers with autism: the early start Denver model. *Pediatrics* **125** (1), e17–e23.

De Cook, M. *et al.* (2012) Does prenatal exposure to endocrine disrupters induce autism spectrum and attention hyperactivity disorder? Review. *Acta Psychiatrica Scandinavica* **101** (8), 811–818.

Dealberto, M. (2011) Prevalence of autism according to maternal immigrant status and ethnic origin. *Acta Psychiatrica Scandinavica* **123** (5), 339–348.

Devlin, B. & Scherer, S.W. (2012) Genetic architecture in autism spectrum disorder. *Current Opinion in Genetics & Development* **22** (3), 229–237.

Donaldson, Z.R. & Young, L.J. (2008) Oxytocin, vasopressin, and the neurogenetics of sociality. *Science* **322** (5903), 900–904.

Dove, D. *et al.* (2012) Medications for adolescents and young adults with autism spectrum disorders: a systematic review. *Pediatrics* **130** (4), 717–726.

Drahota, A. *et al.* (2011) Effects of cognitive behavioral therapy on daily living skills in children with high-functioning autism and concurrent anxiety disorders. *Journal of Autism and Developmental Disorders* **41** (3), 257–265.

Dufour-Rainfray, D. *et al.* (2011) Fetal exposure to teratogens: evidence of genes involved in autism. *Neuroscience & Biobehavioral Reviews* **35** (5), 1254–1265.

Dumas, J.E. *et al.* (1991) Parenting stress, child behavior problems, and dysphoria in parents of children with autism, Down syndrome, behavior disorders, and normal development. *Exceptionality: A Special Education Journal* **2** (2), 97–110.

Dunn, M.E. *et al.* (2001) Moderators of stress in parents of children with autism. *Community Mental Health Journal* **37** (1), 39–52.

Eaves, L.C. & Ho, H.H. (2008) Young adult outcome of autism spectrum disorders. *Journal of Autism and Developmental Disorders* **38** (4), 739–747.

Eikeseth, S. (2009) Outcome of comprehensive psycho-educational interventions for young children with autism. *Research in Developmental Disabilities* **30** (1), 158–178.

Elsabbagh, M. *et al.* (2012) Global prevalence of autism and other pervasive developmental disorders. *Autism Research* **5** (3), 160–179.

Farley, M.A. *et al.* (2009) Twenty-year outcome for individuals with autism and average or near-average cognitive abilities. *Autism Research* **2** (2), 109–118.

Fatemi, S.H. *et al.* (2009) GABAA receptor down regulation in brains of subjects with autism. *Journal of Autism and Developmental Disorders* **39** (2), 223–230.

Folstein, S. & Rutter, M. (1977) Infantile autism: a genetic study of 21 twin pairs. *Journal of Child Psychology & Psychiatry & Allied Disciplines* **18** (4), 297–321.

Fombonne, E. (2005) Epidemiology of autistic disorder and other pervasive developmental disorders. *Journal of Clinical Psychiatry* **66** (Suppl 10), 3–8.

Frazier, T.W. *et al.* (2012) Validation of proposed DSM-5 criteria for autism spectrum disorder. *Journal of the American Academy of Child and Adolescent Psychiatry* **51** (1), 28–40.

Frith, U. (1989) *Autism: Explaining the Enigma*, pp. 16–26. Blackwell Scientific Publications, Oxford.

Frith, U. & Happé, F. (1994) Autism: beyond "theory of mind". *Cognition* **50** (1), 115–132.

Gardener, H. *et al.* (2009) Prenatal risk factors for autism: comprehensive meta-analysis. *British Journal of Psychiatry* **195** (1), 7–14.

Gesundheit, B. *et al.* (2013) Immunological and autoimmune considerations of autism spectrum disorders. *Journal of Autoimmunity* **44**, 1–7.

Geurts, H.M. *et al.* (2009) The paradox of cognitive flexibility in autism. *Trends in Cognitive Sciences* **13** (2), 74–82.

Gold, C. *et al.* (2006) Music therapy for autistic spectrum disorder. *Cochrane Database of Systematic Reviews* (2), CD004381.

Green, L. *et al.* (2001) Oxytocin and autistic disorder: alterations in peptide forms. *Biological Psychiatry* **50** (8), 609–613.

Green, J. *et al.* (2010) Parent-mediated communication-focused treatment in children with autism (PACT): a randomised controlled trial. *The Lancet* **375** (9732), 2152–2160.

Guenole, F. *et al* (2011) Melatonin for disordered sleep in individuals with autism spectrum disorders: systematic review and discussion. *Sleep Medicine Reviews* **15** (6), 379–387.

Guinchat, V. *et al.* (2012) Pre-, peri-and neonatal risk factors for autism. *Acta Obstetricia et Gynecologica Scandinavica* **91** (3), 287–300.

Gurney, J.G. *et al.* (2003) Analysis of prevalence trends of autism spectrum disorder in Minnesota. *Archives of Pediatrics & Adolescent Medicine* **157** (7), 622.

Hamlyn, J. *et al.* (2012) Modifiable risk factors for schizophrenia and autism-shared risk factors impacting on brain development. *Neurobiology of Disease* **53**, 3–9.

Happé, F. & Frith, U. (2006) The weak coherence account: detail-focused cognitive style in autism spectrum disorders. *Journal of Autism and Developmental Disorders* **36** (1), 5–25.

Hastings, R.P. & Brown, T. (2002) Behavior problems of children with autism, parental self-efficacy, and mental health. *American Journal on Mental Retardation* **107** (3), 222–232.

Heinrichs, M. *et al.* (2009) Oxytocin, vasopressin, and human social behavior. *Frontiers in Neuroendocrinology* **30** (4), 548.

Hill, E.L. (2004) Evaluating the theory of executive dysfunction in autism. *Developmental Review* **24** (2), 189–233.

Hodgetts, S. & Hodgetts, W. (2007) Somatosensory stimulation interventions for children with autism: literature review and clinical considerations. *Canadian Journal of Occupational Therapy* **74** (5), 393–400.

Howlin, P. (2013) *Outcomes in Adults with Autism Spectrum Disorders, Handbook of Autism*, 4th edn. John Wiley & Sons, Hoboken, NJ.

Howlin, P. & Rutter, M. (1987) *Treatment of Autistic Children*. John Wiley & Sons, Chichester.

Howlin, P. *et al.* (2004) Adult outcome for children with autism. *Journal of Child Psychology and Psychiatry* **45** (2), 212–229.

Huerta, M. *et al.* (2012) Application of DSM-5 criteria for autism spectrum disorder to three samples of children with DSM-IV diagnoses of pervasive developmental disorders. *American Journal of Psychiatry* **169** (10), 1056–1064.

Hultman, C.M. *et al.* (2010) Advancing paternal age and risk of autism: new evidence from a population-based study and a meta-analysis of epidemiological studies. *Molecular Psychiatry* **16** (12), 1203–1212.

James, S. *et al.* (2011) Omega-3 fatty acids supplementation for autism spectrum disorders (ASD). *Cochrane Database of Systematic Reviews* (11), CD007992.

Jesner, O.S. *et al.* (2007) Risperidone for autism spectrum disorder. *Cochrane Database of Systematic Reviews* (1), CD005040.

Johnson, C.P. & Myers, S.M. (2007) Identification and evaluation of children with autism spectrum disorder. *Pediatrics* **120** (5), 1183–1215.

Johnson, C.P. *et al.* (2007) Identification and evaluation of children with autism spectrum disorders. *Pediatrics* **120** (5), 1183–1215.

Johnston, S.S. & Hawken, L.S. (2007) Preventing severe problem behavior in young children: the behavior education program. *Journal of Early and Intensive Behavior Intervention* **4** (3), 599–613.

Joshi, G. *et al.* (2010) The heavy burden of psychiatric comorbidity in youth with autism spectrum disorders: a large comparative study of a psychiatrically referred population. *Journal of Autism and Developmental Disorders* **40** (11), 1361–1370.

Kaale, A. *et al.* (2012) A randomized controlled trial of preschool-based joint attention intervention for children with autism. *Journal of Child Psychology and Psychiatry* **53** (1), 97–105.

Kadar, M. *et al.* (2012) Evidence-based practice in occupational therapy services for children with autism spectrum disorders in Victoria, Australia. *Australian Occupational Therapy Journal* **59** (4), 284–293.

Kasari, C. *et al.* (2006) Joint attention and symbolic play in young children with autism: a randomized controlled intervention study. *Journal of Child Psychology and Psychiatry* **47** (6), 611–620.

Keenan, M. *et al.* (2006) *Applied Behaviour Analysis and Autism: Building a Future Together*. Jessica Kingsley Publishers, London.

Kent, R. *et al.* (2013) Diagnosing autism spectrum disorder: who will get a DSM-5 diagnosis?, *Journal of Child Psychology and Psychiatry* **54** (11), 1242–1250.

Kenworthy, L. *et al.* (2008) Understanding executive control in autism spectrum disorders in the lab and in the real world. *Neuropsychology Review* **18** (4), 320–338.

Kim, Y.S. *et al.* (2011) Prevalence of autism spectrum disorders in a total population sample. *American Journal of Psychiatry* **168** (9), 904–912.

King, M. & Bearman, P. (2009) Diagnostic change and the increased prevalence of autism. *International Journal of Epidemiology* **38** (5), 1224–1234.

Klin, A. *et al.* (1995) Validity and neuropsychological characterization of Asperger syndrome: convergence with nonverbal learning disabilities syndrome. *Journal of Child Psychology and Psychiatry* **36** (7), 1127–1140.

Klin, A. *et al.* (2003) The enactive mind, or from actions to cognition: lessons from autism. *Philosophical Transactions of the Royal Society of London. Series B: Biological Sciences* **358** (1430), 345–360.

Knapp, M. *et al.* (2009) Economic cost of autism in the UK. *Autism* **13** (3), 317–336.

Kolevzon, A. *et al.* (2007) Prenatal and perinatal risk factors for autism: a review and integration of findings. *Archives of Pediatrics & Adolescent Medicine* **161** (4), 326.

Lam, K.S.L. *et al.* (2006) Neurochemical correlates of autistic disorder: a review of the literature. *Research in Developmental Disabilities* **27** (3), 254–289.

Landrigan, P.J. (2010) What causes autism? Exploring the environmental contribution. *Current Opinion in Pediatrics* **22** (2), 219–225.

Le Couteur, A. (2003) *National Autism Plan for Children*. National Autistic Society, London.

Le Couteur, A. *et al.* (1996) A broader phenotype of autism: the clinical spectrum in twins. *Journal of Child Psychology and Psychiatry and Allied Disciplines* **37** (7), 785–801.

Leekam, S.R. *et al.* (2002) The Diagnostic Interview for social and communication disorders: algorithms for ICD-10 childhood autism and Wing and Gould autistic spectrum disorder. *Journal of Child Psychology and Psychiatry* **43** (3), 327–342.

Leslie, D.L. & Martin, A. (2007) Health care expenditures associated with autism spectrum disorders. *Archives of Pediatrics & Adolescent Medicine* **161** (4), 350.

Levy, A. & Perry, A. (2011) Outcomes in adolescents and adults with autism: a review of the literature. *Research in Autism Spectrum Disorders* **5** (4), 1271–1282.

Leyfer, O.T. *et al.* (2006) Comorbid psychiatric disorders in children with autism: interview development and rates of disorders. *Journal of Autism and Developmental Disorders* **36** (7), 849–861.

Li, X. *et al.* (2012) Genes associated with autism spectrum disorder. *Brain Research Bulletin* **88** (6), 543–552.

Liberati, A. *et al.* (2009) The PRISMA statement for reporting systematic reviews and meta-analyses of studies that evaluate health care interventions: explanation and elaboration. *Annals of Internal Medicine* **151** (4), W-65–W-94.

Liptak, G.S. *et al.* (2006) Health care utilization and expenditures for children with autism: data from US national samples. *Journal of Autism and Developmental Disorders* **36** (7), 871–879.

Lord, C. *et al.* (1994) Autism diagnostic interview-revised: a revised version of a diagnostic interview for caregivers of individuals with possible pervasive developmental disorders. *Journal of Autism and Developmental Disorders* **24** (5), 659–685.

Lord, C. *et al.* (2000) The autism diagnostic observation schedule—generic: a standard measure of social and communication deficits associated with the spectrum of autism. *Journal of Autism and Developmental Disorders* **30** (3), 205–223.

Lord, C. *et al.* (2012a) A multisite study of the clinical diagnosis of different autism spectrum disorders. *Archives of General Psychiatry* **69** (3), 306–313.

Lord, C. *et al.* (2012b) *Autism Diagnostic Observation Schedule (ADOS2)*, 2nd edn. Western Psychological Services, Los Angeles, CA.

Lovaas, O.I. (1987) Behavioral treatment and normal educational and intellectual functioning in young autistic children. *Journal of Consulting and Clinical Psychology* **55** (1), 3.

Magiati, I. *et al.* (2012) Early comprehensive behaviorally based interventions for children with autism spectrum disorders: a summary of findings from recent reviews and meta-analyses. *Neuropsychiatry* **2** (6), 543–570.

Maglione, M.A. *et al.* (2012) Nonmedical interventions for children with ASD: recommended guidelines and further research needs. *Pediatrics* **130** (Supplement 2), S169–S178.

Malhotra, D. & Sebat, J. (2012) CNVs: harbingers of a rare variant revolution in psychiatric genetics. *Cell* **148** (6), 1223–1241.

Manning, M. & Hudgins, L. (2010) Array-based technology and recommendations for utilization in medical genetics practice for detection of chromosomal abnormalities. *Genetics in Medicine* **12** (11), 742–745.

Matson, J.L. & Nebel-Schwalm, M.S. (2007) Comorbid psychopathology with autism spectrum disorder in children: an overview. *Research in Developmental Disabilities* **28** (4), 341–352.

Matson, J.L. & Shoemaker, M. (2009) Intellectual disability and its relationship to autism spectrum disorders. *Research in Developmental Disabilities* **30** (6), 1107–1114.

Mayes, S.D. & Calhoun, S.L. (2003) Ability profiles in children with autism influence of age and IQ. *Autism* **7** (1), 65–80.

McDougle, C.J. *et al.* (2005) Risperidone for the core symptom domains of autism: results from the study by the autism network of the research units on pediatric psychopharmacology. *American Journal of Psychiatry* **162** (6), 1142–1148.

McEachin, J.J. *et al.* (1993) Long-term outcome for children with autism who received early intensive behavioral treatment. *American Journal of Mental Retardation* **97**, 359–359.

McPartland, J.C. *et al.* (2012) Sensitivity and specificity of proposed DSM-5 diagnostic criteria for autism spectrum disorder. *Journal of the American Academy of Child and Adolescent Psychiatry* **51** (4), 368–383.

McPheeters, M.L. *et al.* (2011) A systematic review of medical treatments for children with autism spectrum disorders. *Pediatrics* **127** (5), e1312–e1321.

Meyer, J.A. & Minshew, N.J. (2002) An update on neurocognitive profiles in Asperger syndrome and high-functioning autism. *Focus on Autism and other Developmental Disabilities* **17** (3), 152–160.

Miller, D.T. *et al.* (2010) Consensus statement: chromosomal microarray is a first-tier clinical diagnostic test for individuals with developmental disabilities or congenital anomalies. *The American Journal of Human Genetics* **86** (5), 749–764.

Millward, C.A. *et al.* (2009) Genetic factors for resistance to diet-induced obesity and associated metabolic traits on mouse chromosome 17. *Mammalian Genome* **20** (2), 71–82.

Ministry of Health and Education (2008) *New Zealand Autism Spectrum Disorder Guidelines*. Ministry of Health, Wellington, New Zealand.

Minshew, N.J. & Keller, T.A. (2010) The nature of brain dysfunction in autism: functional brain imaging studies. *Current Opinion in Neurology* **23** (2), 124.

Modahl, C. *et al.* (1998) Plasma oxytocin levels in autistic children. *Biological Psychiatry* **43** (4), 270–277.

Mottron, L. *et al.* (2006) Enhanced perceptual functioning in autism: an update, and eight principles of autistic perception. *Journal of Autism and Developmental Disorders* **36** (1), 27–43.

Myers, S.M. *et al.* (2007) Management of children with autism spectrum disorders. *Pediatrics* **120** (5), 1162–1182.

National Institute for Health and Care Excellence (2011) *Clinical Guideline 128. Autism: recognition, referral and diagnosis of children and young people on the autism spectrum* [Online]. Available: http//www.nice.org.uk/CG128 [Sept 2011].

National Institute for Health and Care Excellence (2013) *Clinical Guideline. Autism: the management and support of children and young people on the autism spectrum* [Online]. Available: http://guidance.nice.org.uk [08 Aug 2014].

Norris, M. & Lecavalier, L. (2010) Screening accuracy of level 2 autism spectrum disorder rating scales: a review of selected instruments. *Autism* **14** (14), 263–284.

Oblak, A. *et al.* (2009) Decreased GABAA receptors and benzodiazepine binding sites in the anterior cingulate cortex in autism. *Autism Research* **2** (4), 205–219.

Ozonoff, S. & Strayer, D.L. (2001) Further evidence of intact working memory in autism. *Journal of Autism and Developmental Disorders* **31** (3), 257–263.

Ozonoff, S. *et al.* (1991) Executive function deficits in high-functioning autistic individuals: relationship to theory of mind. *Journal of Child Psychology and Psychiatry* **32** (7), 1081–1105.

Ozonoff, S. *et al.* (2011) Recurrence risk for autism spectrum disorders: a baby siblings research consortium study. *Pediatrics* **128** (3), e488–e495.

Parr, J. (2008) Autism. *American Family Physician* **78** (6), 758–760.

Pellicano, E. & Stears, M. (2011) Bridging autism, science and society: moving toward an ethically informed approach to autism research. *Autism Research* **4** (4), 271–282.

Philip, R. *et al.* (2012) A systematic review and meta-analysis of the fMRI investigation of autism spectrum disorders. *Neuroscience & Biobehavioral Reviews* **36** (2), 901–942.

Pickles, A. *et al.* (2009) Loss of language in early development of autism and specific language impairment. *Journal of Child Psychology and Psychiatry and Allied Disciplines* **50** (7), 843–852.

Plaisted, K.C. (2001) Reduced generalization in autism: an alternative to weak central coherence. In: *The Development of Autism: Perspectives from Theory and Research.* (eds J.A. Burack, T. Charman, N. Yirmiya & P.R. Zelazo), pp. 149–169. Lawrence Erlbaum Associates Publishers, Mahwah, NJ, US.

Plaisted, K.C. *et al.* (1999) Children with autism show local precedence in a divided attention task and global precedence in a selective attention task. *Journal of Child Psychology and Psychiatry* **40** (5), 733–742.

Posthuma, D. & Polderman, T.J.C. (2013) What we have learned from recent twin studies about the etiology of neurodevelopmental disorders? *Current Opinion in Neurology* **26** (2), 111–121.

Reichow, B. & Volkmar, F.R. (2010) Social skills interventions for individuals with autism: evaluation for evidence-based practices within a best evidence synthesis framework. *Journal of Autism and Developmental Disorders* **40** (2), 149–166.

Reichow, B. *et al.* (2012) Social skills groups for people aged 6 to 21 with autism spectrum disorders (ASD). *Cochrane Database of Systematic Reviews* (7), CD008511.

Research Units on Pediatric Psychopharmacology Autism Network (RUPP) (2005) Risperidone treatment of autistic disorder: longer-term benefits and blinded discontinuation after 6 months. *American Journal of Psychiatry* **162** (7), 1361–1369.

Rogers, S.J. & Vismara, L.A. (2008) Evidence-based comprehensive treatments for early autism. *Journal of Clinical Child & Adolescent Psychology* **37** (1), 8–38.

Rolf, L.H. *et al.* (1993) Serotonin and amino acid content in platelets of autistic children. *Acta Psychiatrica Scandinavica* **87** (5), 312–316.

Ronald, A. & Hoekstra, R.A. (2011) Autism spectrum disorders and autistic traits: a decade of new twin studies. *American Journal of Medical Genetics Part B-Neuropsychiatric Genetics* **156b** (3), 255–274.

Rossignol, D.A. & Frye, R.E. (2011) Melatonin in autism spectrum disorders: a systematic review and meta-analysis. *Developmental medicine & Child Neurology* **53** (9), 783–792.

Russo, N. *et al.* (2007) Deconstructing executive deficits among persons with autism: implications for cognitive neuroscience. *Brain and Cognition* **65** (1), 77–86.

Rutter, M. *et al.* (2003) *Autism Diagnostic Interview-Revised.* Western Psychological Services, Los Angeles, CA.

Sanders, J. *et al.* (2008) A review of neuropsychological and neuroimaging research in autistic spectrum disorders: attention, inhibition and cognitive flexibility. *Research in Autism Spectrum Disorders* **2** (1), 1–16.

Sandin, S. *et al.* (2012) Advancing maternal age is associated with increasing risk for autism: a review and meta-analysis. *Journal of the American Academy of Child & Adolescent Psychiatry* **51** (5), 477–486.

Scahill, L. *et al.* (2012) Effects of risperidone and parent training on adaptive functioning in children with pervasive developmental disorders and serious behavioral problems. *Journal of the American Academy of Child & Adolescent Psychiatry* **51** (2), 136–146.

Schopler, E. *et al.* (1980) Toward objective classification of childhood autism: childhood autism rating scale (CARS). *Journal of Autism and Developmental Disorders* **10** (1), 91–103.

Schopler, E. *et al.* (1982) Evaluation of treatment for autistic children and their parents. *Journal of the American Academy of Child Psychiatry* **21** (3), 262–267.

Schopler, E. *et al.* (1986) *The Childhood Autism Rating Scale (CARS): For Diagnostic Screening and Classification of Autism.* Irvington, New York.

Schumann, C.M. & Nordahl, C.W. (2011) Bridging the gap between MRI and postmortem research in autism. *Brain Research* **1380**, 175–186.

Scottish Intercollegiate Guidelines Network (2007) *Assessment, diagnosis and clinical interventions for children and young people with autism spectrum disorders* [Online]. Available: http://sign.ac.uk/guidelines/fulltext/98/index.html [08 Aug 2014].

Seltzer, M.M. *et al.* (2003) The symptoms of autism spectrum disorders in adolescence and adulthood. *Journal of Autism and Developmental Disorders* **33** (6), 565–581.

Seltzer, M.M. *et al.* (2004) Trajectory of development in adolescents and adults with autism. *Mental Retardation and Developmental Disabilities Research Reviews* **10** (4), 234–247.

Shattuck, P.T. *et al.* (2007) Change in autism symptoms and maladaptive behaviors in adolescents and adults with an autism spectrum disorder. *Journal of Autism and Developmental Disorders* **37** (9), 1735–1747.

Shelton, J.F. *et al.* (2010) Independent and dependent contributions of advanced maternal and paternal ages to autism risk. *Autism Research* **3** (1), 30–39.

Simonoff, E. *et al.* (2008) Psychiatric disorders in children with autism spectrum disorders: prevalence, comorbidity, and associated factors in a population-derived sample. *Journal of the American Academy of Child & Adolescent Psychiatry* **47** (8), 921–929.

Simonoff, E. *et al.* (2012) Severe mood problems in adolescents with autism spectrum disorder. *Journal of Child Psychology and Psychiatry* **53** (11), 1157–1166.

Sinha, I.P. *et al.* (2011) Using the Delphi technique to determine which outcomes to measure in clinical trials: recommendations for the future based on a systematic review of existing studies. *PLoS Medicine* **8** (1), e1000393.

Sivberg, B. (2002) Family system and coping behaviors a comparison between parents of children with autistic spectrum disorders and parents with non-autistic children. *Autism* **6** (4), 397–409.

Skuse, D. *et al.* (2004) The developmental, dimensional and diagnostic interview (3di): a novel computerized assessment for autism spectrum disorders. *Journal of the American Academy of Child & Adolescent Psychiatry* **43** (5), 548–558.

Sofronoff, K. *et al.* (2007) A randomized controlled trial of a cognitive behavioural intervention for anger management in children diagnosed with Asperger syndrome. *Journal of Autism and Developmental Disorders* **37** (7), 1203–1214.

Stanfield, A.C. *et al.* (2008) Towards a neuroanatomy of autism: a systematic review and meta-analysis of structural magnetic resonance imaging studies. *European Psychiatry* **23** (4), 289–299.

Strain, P.S. & Bovey, E.H. (2011) Randomized, controlled trial of the LEAP model of early intervention for young children with autism spectrum disorders. *Topics in Early Childhood Special Education* **31** (3), 133–154.

Sucksmith, E. *et al.* (2011) Autistic traits below the clinical threshold: re-examining the broader autism phenotype in the 21st century. *Neuropsychology Review* **21** (4), 360–389.

Sullivan, P.F. *et al.* (2012) Genetic architectures of psychiatric disorders: the emerging picture and its implications. *Nature Reviews Genetics* **13** (8), 537–551.

Szatmari, P. & McConnell, B. (2011) Anxiety and mood disorders in individuals with autism spectrum disorder. In: *Autism Spectrum Disorders*. (eds D.G. Amaral, G. Dawson & D.H. Geschwind), pp. 330–338. Oxford University Press, New York.

Szatmari, P. *et al.* (1998) Genetics of autism: overview and new directions. *Journal of Autism and Developmental Disorders* **28** (5), 351–368.

Taunt, H.M. & Hastings, R.P. (2002) Positive impact of children with developmental disabilities on their families: a preliminary study. *Education and Training in Mental Retardation and Developmental Disabilities* **37** (4), 410–420.

Taylor, J.L. (2009) Chapter one-the transition out of high school and into adulthood for individuals with autism and for their families. *International Review of Research in Mental Retardation* **38**, 1–32.

Trikalinos, T.A. *et al.* (2005) A heterogeneity-based genome search meta-analysis for autism-spectrum disorders. *Molecular Psychiatry* **11** (1), 29–36.

Turner, M.A. (1999a) Generating novel ideas: fluency performance in high-functioning and learning disabled individuals with autism. *Journal of Child Psychology and Psychiatry* **40** (2), 189–201.

Turner, M.A. (1999b) Annotation: repetitive behaviour in autism: a review of psychological research. *Journal of Child Psychology and Psychiatry* **40** (6), 839–849.

Van Steensel, F.J.A. *et al.* (2011) Anxiety disorders in children and adolescents with autistic spectrum disorders: a meta-analysis. *Clinical Child and Family Psychology Review* **14** (3), 302–317.

Verhoeven, J.S. *et al.* (2010) Neuroimaging of autism. *Neuroradiology* **52** (1), 3–14.

Via, E. *et al.* (2011) Meta-analysis of gray matter abnormalities in autism spectrum disorder: should Asperger disorder be subsumed under a broader umbrella of autistic spectrum disorder? *Archives of General Psychiatry* **68** (4), 409.

Virués-Ortega, J. (2010) Applied behavior analytic intervention for autism in early childhood: meta-analysis, meta-regression and dose–response meta-analysis of multiple outcomes. *Clinical Psychology Review* **30** (4), 387–399.

Virues-Ortega, J. *et al.* (2013) The TEACCH program for children and adults with autism. A meta-analysis of intervention studies. *Clinical Psychology Review* **33** (8), 940–953.

Warren, Z. *et al.* (2011a) A systematic review of early intensive Intervention for autism spectrum disorders: *Pediatrics* **127** (5), e1303–e1311.

Warren, Z. *et al.* (2011b) *Therapies for Children with Autism Spectrum Disorders*. Comparative Effectiveness. Review No. 26. Agency for Healthcare Research and Quality, Rockville, Maryland.

Watson, R. *et al.* (2011) Models of transitional care for young people with complex health needs: a scoping review. *Child: Care, Health and Development* **37** (6), 780–791.

Weiss, J.A. *et al.* (2012) The impact of child problem behaviours of children with ASD on parent mental health: the mediating role of acceptance and empowerment. *Autism* **16** (3), 261–274.

Williams, J.G. *et al.* (2006) Systematic review of prevalence studies of autism spectrum disorders. *Archives of Disease in Childhood* **91** (1), 8–15.

Williams, K. *et al.* (2010) Selective serotonin reuptake inhibitors (SSRIs) for autism spectrum disorders (ASD). *Cochrane Database of Systematic Reviews* (8).

Wing, L. & Shah, A. (2000) Catatonia in autistic spectrum disorders. *The British Journal of Psychiatry* **176** (4), 357–362.

Wing, L. *et al.* (2002) The diagnostic interview for social and communication disorders: background, inter-rater reliability and clinical use. *Journal of Child Psychology and Psychiatry* **43** (3), 307–325.

Woolfenden, S. *et al.* (2012) A systematic review of the diagnostic stability of autism spectrum disorder. *Research in Autism Spectrum Disorders* **6** (1), 345–354.

World Health Organisation (1992) *The ICD-10 Classification of Mental and Behavioural Disorders*. World Health Organization, Geneva.

Yoder, P. & Stone, W.L. (2006) Randomized comparison of two communication interventions for preschoolers with autism spectrum disorders. *Journal of Consulting and Clinical Psychology* **74** (3), 426.

Zaroff, C.M. & Uhm, S.Y. (2012) Prevalence of autism spectrum disorders and influence of country of measurement and ethnicity. *Social Psychiatry and Psychiatric Epidemiology* **47** (3), 395–398.

Zwaigenbaum, L. *et al.* (2009) Clinical assessment and management of toddlers with suspected autism spectrum disorder: insights from studies of high-risk infants. *Pediatrics* **123** (5), 1383–1391.

CHAPTER 52

Disorders of speech, language, and communication

Courtenay Frazier Norbury[1] and Rhea Paul[2]

[1] Department of Psychology, Royal Holloway, University of London, Surrey, UK
[2] Department of Speech-Language Pathology, College of Health Professions, Sacred Heart University, Fairfield, CT, USA

Introduction

Distinguishing speech, language, and communication

Communication is the transmission of information (a message) between a source and a receiver, using a common signaling system and is an essential function of many social animals, including humans. Honey bees, for example, perform a "dance" when they return to the hive, using movement patterns to indicate the direction and distance of food. Human communication includes body language, gesture, and facial expression to convey messages. Humans have also evolved a unique form of communication that appears to be unshared by other species, *language*. Language is a complex, formal system that makes use of a finite number of units (sounds and words) that can be combined in rule-governed ways to convey an infinite number of meanings. Language, too, can take a variety of forms; it can be written or expressed with manual signs, for example. However, the most widely used form for expressing language is through *speech*. Speech is composed of a relatively small set of sounds, or phonemes, produced by means of articulation of the oral structures (lips, tongue, teeth, and palate), which are used to modify the vibration of air, initiated by the vocal cords, as it passes through the oral cavity, resulting in acoustic patterns we perceive as speech. The sounds of speech are ordered sequentially according to language-specific rules in order to produce words recognized by users of a particular language. The relationship among communication, language, and speech is represented in Figure 52.1. *Communication* is the broadest term, encompassing a wide range of methods of conveying information; *language* is a specific type of communication governed by rules that allow novel combination of elements; *speech* is a particular way of expressing language, through orally produced units of sounds, combined, again, in rule-governed ways.

Disorders of communication can occur at any level within this system, and some communication disorders can affect one level without affecting others. Consider Dana:

Dana is a bright, garrulous 7 year old, who sounds like a much younger child when she talks. She makes lots of errors in her speech, including substituting one sound for another (saying "wabbit" for "rabbit") leaving off sounds (saying "cool" for "school") and syllables ("Saying "mato" for "tomato"), and reversing sounds (saying "pesgetti" for "spaghetti"). The result of these errors is that she is often hard to understand, even though she has lots to say, uses long sentences and understands what others say to her. When people don't understand her, she tries repeating, using gestures and facial expression to repair the communication. She seems very eager to talk and engage with others, despite her occasional frustration at being misunderstood.

Dana is a child with a speech disorder. Her communication (desire to exchange information) and her language (ability to use words and sentences) appear to be developing typically. But Nick is another story:

Nick is a nine-year old boy who can produce sounds clearly, but his language is impaired. He produces short, immature sentences that leave off word endings ("I have two shoe; Mommy help me at the store), uses incorrect forms of words (Me like ice cream; He goed home), and has trouble finding the words he wants to say ("For lunch I had, you know, that spiky thing, yellow inside). Nick likes to play with other children and enjoys talking, but has limited means at his disposal for expressing and elaborating his intentions.

Nick's speech is intact and he, too, is motivated to communicate, but his language disorder disrupts successful communication; he has not acquired the words and the grammatical rules that would allow him to express the ideas he has in an age-appropriate way. His communication style is in sharp contrast to Ben's:

Rutter's Child and Adolescent Psychiatry, Sixth Edition.
Edited by Anita Thapar and Daniel S. Pine, James F. Leckman, Stephen Scott, Margaret J. Snowling, Eric Taylor.
© 2015 John Wiley & Sons Ltd. Published 2018 by John Wiley & Sons Ltd.

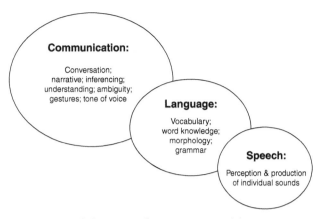

Figure 52.1 Speech, language, and communication and their component skills.

Ben is an extremely bright five-year-old. He uses precise articulation and long, complex sentences to express himself, but he isn't always successful at talking with others. He likes to play with action figures, and narrates long scenes and dialogue from his favorite films and video games. He is reluctant to interact with other children because he is often confused about what they are saying. If they tell a joke he thinks they are laughing at him, because he often doesn't get the punch line. He prefers to interact with adults, but sometimes gets in trouble for not responding the way they want him too. For example, mum might ask, 'can you shut the door' and then gets cross when he replies 'yes' but doesn't actually move to shut the door. He often interrupts adults to talk to them but they can't really follow what he's trying to say because he leaves out important details.

Ben does not have much difficulty with the form of his speech or language. Rather, his ability to use language skills to communicate effectively with other people, or *pragmatics,* is affected. Children who have difficulties with pragmatics and using language for social exchanges may be diagnosed with "social communication disorder." Dana, Nick, and Ben exemplify children with communication disorders that affect one level of communication more or less discretely. Many children with communication disorders, though, have impairments that affect several of these levels and are continuous with a range of neurodevelopmental disorders including specific learning disorders (see Chapter 53), attention deficit hyperactivity disorder (ADHD) (see Chapter 55) and autism spectrum disorder (ASD, see Chapter 51).

In this chapter, we discuss the three major categories of communication disorder—speech, language, and social (pragmatic) communication disorder (SPCD), as defined by the diagnostic and statistical manual of mental disorder (DSM)-V (American Psychiatric Association, 2013). We begin by considering assessment of children with suspected communication disorder. We then outline typologies for the three categories of communication disorder, addressing issues of differential diagnosis within communication disorders and between these and other neurodevelopmental disorders (see also Chapter 3). We focus most on language disorders, as these have the greatest

evidence base and likely impact on mental health, given the limited research base for SPCD that exists currently. Finally, we provide an overview of current intervention approaches for each category of communication disorder.

General principles of assessment

The evaluation of children suspected of communication disorder is generally undertaken by speech-language pathologists or therapists (SLTs), specialists trained in the anatomy, physiology, psychology, linguistics, and pedagogy of communication and its disorders. The general process of assessment often follows the progression depicted in Figure 52.2. The process may begin with a referral from a clinician, such as a health visitor, general practitioner, or child psychiatrist, or with a screening test administered in an educational setting. Although parents may also self-refer, many parents may not suspect a communication disorder at first and may be more focused on a child's problems with behavior regulation, social interaction, or learning in school. While these difficulties can exist without an underlying communication disorder, it is often the case that a problem in speech or language is masked by more obvious trouble in other areas (Cohen *et al.*, 1998)

For any child referred, it is essential to request a thorough hearing assessment by an audiologist as part of the evaluation, in order to rule out hearing impairment as a potential cause of communication disorder. A case history, including questions about the child's feeding, speech, and hearing history will be used to determine whether early problems in sucking, chewing, and swallowing were present, suggesting potential neuromotor involvement. The case history will also address the child's motivation to communicate and interact with others, as well as use of any compensatory strategies, such as gestures or vocalizations. The forms of speech currently available, whether sounds, words, phrases, or sentences will help determine the level at which to begin the formal assessment and the degree to which the child's speech can be understood by familiar and less familiar people, will also be informative. The interviewer will also want to know if the child is able to follow verbal instructions and respond to others, and what language(s) the child is exposed to at home. With regard to older children, the ability to understand a story or joke will also be of interest.

A second tool frequently used by SLTs is an informal conversational sample, in which the child and clinician engage in talk around objects and/or topics of interest to the child and the clinician observes the child's motivation to communicate and the forms and functions the child's communication takes. This observation allows the clinician to estimate the richness of the child's vocabulary, grammatical complexity, ability to retrieve words, and reply to questions. The observation will also reveal important information about the intelligibility and fluency of speech as well as about the volume, quality, and resonance of the voice. If the child is learning more than one language, the

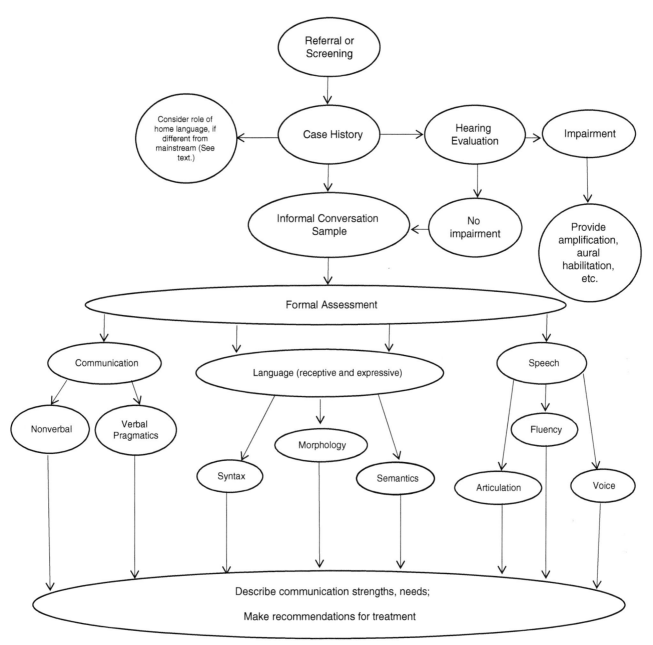

Figure 52.2 Assessment of communication.

clinician may ask parents to interact with the child first in one language and then in the other(s), to observe the child's comfort and fluency in each. Finally, other aspects of development can also be observed, such as the child's play skills, attention capacity, interest in others, motivation to communicate, persistence and frustration tolerance, and so on. These observations can help the clinician determine the forms of interaction that might be most fruitful for a particular child.

The informal speech sample allows the clinician to form a hypothesis about areas of communication strength and weakness. This hypothesis will be tested with the use of formal assessments, such as standardized tests and structured parent questionnaires and interviews, such as those listed in Table 52.1. Each area of hypothesized weakness will be assessed, as schematized in Figure 52.2. These findings will not only provide a working diagnosis, but should also inform the intervention plan (see **Intervention** section in this chapter, and Chapter 41).

Differential diagnosis of speech disorders

Speech sound disorders affect the intelligibility and quality of the oral language produced. DSM-5 (American Psychiatric Association, 2013) *speech sound disorder* and *childhood onset*

Table 52.1 A sample of formal language assessments in common use.

Area	Assessment tool	Age range	Description
Speech: Articulation	*Goldman-Fristoe Test of Articulation—Second Edition* GFTA-2; (Goldman & Fristoe, 2000)	2–21 yr	Can be used with Khan-Lewis Phonological Analysis Yields percentile rank by age score Administration time: 10–15 min for single-word portion
	Photo Articulation Test—Third Edition PAT-3; (Pendergrast et al., 1997)	3–12 yr	Provides means and standard deviations for age
Speech: Fluency	*Test of Childhood Stuttering* (Gillam et al., 2009)	4-12 yr	Uses rapid picture naming, modeled sentences, narration and structured conversation to identify stuttering, judge severity, and monitor progress
Speech: Voice	*Voice Assessment Protocol for Children and Adults* VAP; (Pindzola, 1987)	3-Adult	Systematic evaluation of vocal pitch, loudness, quality, breath features, and speech rate/rhythm
Language: Semantics	*British Picture Vocabulary Scales –Fourth Edition* BPVS-3; (Dunn et al., 2009)	2:6 yr–adult	Receptive vocabulary
	MacArthur Bates Communicative Development Inventory (Fenson et al., 1993)	8-36 mo.	Parent checklist of words understood and said, as well as communicative gestures and early word combinations
Language: Syntax	*Rice-Wexler Test of Early Grammatical Impairment* (TEGI; Rice & Wexler, 2001)	3.0–8.0	Grammatical morphology
	Test for Reception of Grammar-2 (TROG; (D. V. M. Bishop, 2003b)	4-adult	Child matches spoken sentence to one of four pictures to assess understanding of grammatical forms
Communication: Narrative	*The Bus Story Test* (Renfrew, 1991)	3–8	Provides age-equivalent scores for story information value and sentence length
	Test of Narrative Language (Gillam & Pearson, 2004)	5–11	Elicits stories using picture sequences, single pictures and no pictures to measure the ability to answer literal and inferential comprehension questions and narrative discourse
Communication: Pragmatics	*Test of Pragmatic Language—Second Edition* TOPL-2; (Phelps-Terasaki & Phelps-Gunn, 2006)	6–18 yr	Comprehensive assessment of student's abilities to use pragmatic language effectively
	Children's Communication Checklist-2 (Bishop, 2003a, b)	4–16 yr	Parent report of language and pragmatic behaviors with normative scores
Omnibus	*Clinical Evaluation of Language Fundamentals—Fourth Edition* CELF-4UK; (Semel et al., 2006)	3–6 yr	Concepts, syntax, semantics, morphology
	Preschool Language Scale—Fourth Edition UK PLS-4; (Zimmerman et al., 2009)	Birth–7:11 yr	Language precursors; expressive and receptive semantics, syntax, morphology, integrative thinking, auditory comprehension
	Test for Auditory Comprehension of Language—Third Edition TACL-3; (Carrow-Woodfolk, 1998)	3–9:11 yr	Receptive aspects of: word classes and relations, grammatical morphemes, elaborated sentence constructions
	Test of Language Development—Fourth Edition: Primary TOLD-4:P; (Hammill & Newcomer, 2008)	4–8:11 yr	Receptive and expressive semantics and syntax
	Woodcock Language Proficiency Battery—Revised (Woodcock, 1991)	2–adult yr	Oral language, vocabulary, antonyms and synonyms, reading and writing

Source: Adapted from various sources

fluency disorder. We will briefly describe the clinical presentation of each and discuss differential diagnosis. Intervention procedures typically applied to this class of disorders are outlined in the Intervention section of this chapter.

Speech sound disorder

All human languages make use of a small set of speech sounds, called *phonemes*, to encode meaning. For example, British English uses only 24 consonants and 20 vowels in combination to produce the tens of thousands of words. Children make mistakes when they first start to talk, often leaving out some of the sounds required in adult words (Saying "pay" for *play*, for example), substituting known sounds for some of the more difficult sounds in language (saying "wabbit" for *rabbit*), or distorting some sounds, for example, lisping. In typical development, most of these errors resolve by 4–5 years of age, but for some children they persist for longer than normal. For most children, these persistent errors make them sound immature when they talk, although they can make themselves understood. For others, speech may be mostly unintelligible to people outside the family.

For most children with speech sound disorder, no physical cause is obvious. Instead, the disorder is thought to have its roots in the child's difficulty in learning to "sort out" the sounds of the ambient language into their appropriate categories. As these categories differ from language to language, it should not be surprising that some children find this difficult. For example, compare this problem to the one Japanese speakers have when they try to distinguish the words, *rice* and *lice*. While the beginning consonants in these words are clearly different to English speakers, Japanese speakers do not have separate categories for the sounds [r] and [l]; only one approximant sound is used in their language. As a result, Japanese speakers have a great deal of difficulty either hearing or producing the distinction between the two words.

Prevalence, prognosis, causes, and correlates of speech disorders

Shriberg *et al.* (1999) estimated the prevalence of speech sound disorders in 6-year-old children at 3.8%. Rates for younger children are much higher, with some studies reporting rates of 15.6% in 3-year-old children (Shriberg *et al.*, 1999; Campbell *et al.*, 2003a, b), but the rate decreases with age, to an overall rate of 1% at school age (McKinnon *et al.*, 2007). Speech sound disorder of unknown origin accounts for the vast majority of these cases. Although the origin of speech sound disorder is unknown, it has been found to run in families, (Newbury & Monaco, 2010) and high rates of comorbidity with both language and literacy disorders are observed, particularly in children whose delays persist to school age (Pennington & Bishop, 2009)

Children with speech sound disorder who receive intervention in the preschool or primary grades generally have a good prognosis for speech normalization. Shirberg *et al.* (1994)

reported that normalization is achieved by most preschoolers even with moderate to severe speech sound delays by 8 years of age, although children with the more severe delays are likely to retain speech sound distortions beyond this age.

Assessment of speech sound disorders

Gordon-Brannan and Weiss (2007) reported levels of intelligibility for children that serve as a benchmark for the assessment of speech. At age 2, 50% of what a child says should be understood by people outside the family; at 3, 75% should be intelligible, and at 4, 100% should be understood, though some errors may still occur that do not impact intelligibility to a great extent. Children who fail to meet these basic intelligibility benchmarks should be referred for assessment. By 8 years of age, all errors should have resolved and children aged 8 and over who have any speech errors, even on only one or two sounds, should be evaluated. Although these residual errors may not impact intelligibility, they do call attention to speech and may result in teasing or other social consequences that can impact development.

Assessment of speech generally consists of both standardized testing (Table 52.1) and analysis of spontaneous speech. An SLT will generally administer a test to determine the child's speech sound accuracy and the types of speech errors made, whether substitutions, omissions, or distortions of sounds. A sample of spontaneous speech is used to determine the level of intelligibility, by computing the number of intelligible versus unintelligible words. It will also provide a phonetic inventory or a list of all sounds produced, in order to identify any missing sounds that need to be taught. Finally, clinicians use speech samples to identify patterns of error that go beyond a single sound. For example, children often leave off final sounds in words, regardless of what the sound is, or they reduce clusters of consonants to a single consonant, again without regard to the particular consonants in the cluster (e.g., star → tar). These assessments determine whether intervention is warranted and help to specify the targets of intervention. Assessment for motor speech disorders is similar, although the focus will be on intelligibility rather than on identification of specific speech sound errors.

Childhood onset fluency disorder

Disorders of fluency are characterized by interruptions in the flow of speech with atypical rate, rhythm, and repetitions in sounds, syllables, words, and phrases. This may be accompanied by excessive tension, struggle behavior, and secondary mannerisms, such as eye blinking or arm movements, which give the impression of struggle.

Prevalence, prognosis, causes, and correlates

Dysfluency is quite common in preschool children and is associated with early difficulties in language formulation (Bloodstein, 2006). Seventy-five percent of dysfluent preschoolers recover without intervention (Yairi & Ambrose, 1999), although prognosis for full recovery after age 7 is more guarded. The prevalence of dysfluency in the general school-aged population is between 0.3% and 1% (McKinnon *et al.*, 2007). The behaviors indicative of persistent dysfluency in preschoolers (Campbell *et al.*, 2003a, b) are:

- Frequent part-word repetitions
- Physical tension and struggle
- Signs of frustration
- Delays in other aspects of speech and language development

The disorder is more prevalent, and more likely to be persistent, in males (Prasse & Kikano, 2008). Over 60% of people who stutter present with concurrent speech and language disorders, the most common of which is speech sound disorder (SSD) (Newbury & Monaco, 2010). Although there are emotional and psychological components to dysfluency, risk for the disorder is also genetically influenced (Kraft & Yairi, 2012).

Assessment and Intervention

Assessment of dysfluency typically has two goals: to describe the dysfluency itself and to assess the impact of the dysfluency on communication and daily living. Description will usually involve analyzing a sample of spontaneous speech and calculating the types and frequency of disruptions. Assessment of the impact of the disorder is usually accomplished through interviews with the client or caregiver. Baseline data from both of these assessments are used to monitor progress throughout the course of intervention.

Intervention for dysfluency generally falls into one of four classes (Ramig & Pollard, 2010):

- *Fluency Shaping.* This method teaches strategies for reducing the occurrence of stuttered speech, which include building from single word to longer utterances while maintaining fluency, management of the breath stream, and reducing the rate of speech.
- *Stuttering Modification.* Rather than attempting to eliminate stuttering, this method aims to modify stuttering so it is less conspicuous and to desensitize the client to the stress of dysfluency.
- *Use of Electronic Devices.* It has long been known that delayed auditory feedback reduces stuttering, leading to the development of compact devices that resemble hearing aids and deliver delayed auditory feedback. These devices have been reported to show some efficacy for some people who stutter (Pollard *et al.*, 2009), but the effect is only present while the device is worn.
- *Parent-implemented.* For young children, parents are often taught techniques to help the child reduce dysfluency.

Voice disorders

Voice disorders are not described in DSM-5, but can be associated with various developmental conditions. Voice disorders are characterized by the abnormal production and/or absences of vocal quality, pitch, loudness, resonance, and/or duration, which is inappropriate for an individual's age and/or sex. In some cases, voice disorders severely limit communication, when, for example, the speaker is unable to generate adequate volume to make himself heard or when abnormal growths on the vocal folds interfere with the vibration that underlies speech. In other cases, though, voice disorders do not preclude communication; instead they distract the listener and call attention to the form of the communication rather than its message. In children, voice disorders generally fall into two broad classes: vocal strain and resonance disorders.

Shouting, the use of unnatural pitch (to sound older or more masculine), perpetual loud talking (to be heard above siblings or classmates), or singing (in choir) can lead to vocal strain, as can excessive throat clearing associated with compulsive disorders such as Tourette's syndrome. Vocal strain can lead to the development of vocal nodules, polyps, or contact ulcers, which may require surgical intervention. Many resonance disorders are caused by malformations of the speech mechanism. Children with cleft palate, who may lack the tissue and musculature to separate the oral and nasal cavities, allowing air to leak into the nose during speech, often show hypernasal resonance. Muscular weakness, such as that observed in cerebral palsy, can also affect these functions. In addition, many children with ASDs exhibit hypernasal speech, without any structural or known neuromuscular abnormalities.

Prevalence, prognosis, causes, and correlates

McKinnon *et al.* (2007) estimate the prevalence of voice disorders in children to be 0.12%, although estimates among preschool children are as high as 3.9% (Duff *et al.*, 2004). Vocal strain is observed in children without comorbid disabilities. Resonance disorders, on the other hand, usually accompany a variety of conditions including cerebral palsy, Down syndrome, cleft palate, ASDs and, less frequently, language disorders.

Assessment and Intervention

In the case of resonance disorders, the amount of airflow from the nose during speech is sometimes measured, for example, by means of nasometry, a device that computes the percentage of nasal acoustic energy out of the total energy (oral plus nasal) produced in an utterance. For children with vocal strain, training in vocal hygiene is usually effective in preventing further difficulties, although once polyps or nodules develop, surgical intervention may be necessary. Resonance disorders due to dysmorphology such as cleft palate are typically treated with surgery to correct the malformation, followed by speech-language therapy to address residual errors. For children with resonance disorders of nonanatomical origin, particularly in children with ASD, the voice problem is usually more resistant to treatment.

Language disorder

Diagnostic criteria

DSM-5 defines language disorder as persistent difficulties in the acquisition and use of language across modalities (i.e., spoken, written, sign language, and/or other symbol systems) and may involve comprehension or production deficits in one or more of the following: (i) vocabulary (word knowledge and use), (ii) sentence structure (the ability to put words and word endings together to form sentences based on the rules of grammar and morphology), (iii) discourse (the ability to use vocabulary and connect sentences to explain or describe a topic or series of events or have a conversation) (American Psychiatric Association, 2013). The particular features of language disorder at each of these levels are detailed in the following sections.

Vocabulary

Children with language disorders are slow to acquire first words. Even when basic vocabulary is learned, children with language disorders often have more limited vocabularies than their peers (McGregor et al., 2013). They tend to rely on nonspecific words (*thingy*) and have difficulty acquiring words with abstract meanings, multiple senses, and figurative uses. In addition, word finding is often affected. Children may even have difficulty retrieving words they know and resort to circumlocutions or imprecise terms such as "whatsit."

Grammar and Morphology

Children with language disorders are also generally slow to produce first word combinations. While children typically produce their first multi-word utterances at 18–24 months, those with language disorders are often 2 1/2 to 4 years old before word combinations appear. Once sentences are used, children with language disorders produce shorter utterances than their peers throughout the preschool period. They tend to be delayed in their acquisition of grammatical morphology, the markers added on to words that denote meanings such as plural (two book*s*) and possessive forms (Rhea'*s* book). In English, they have particular difficulty with word endings that mark tense (help*ed*) and subject-verb agreement (He run*s*), use of pronouns (*Me* want ice cream), and often omit auxiliary verbs (She *is* reading; He *can* help), and articles (*the* cake, *a* book; *an* apple). During the school years, children with language disorders continue to use simpler sentences and make more grammatical errors than peers.

Discourse

Three genres of discourse have been studied in children with language disorders: conversation, narrative, and exposition. *Conversational* discourse, the verbal exchange between interlocutors, can be a relative strength for many children with language disorders. By school age, many have mastered enough basic vocabulary and sentence structure to maintain basic conversations, although they may still make errors and are less able to produce complex forms than peers.

Narrative is defined as a primarily monologic discourse, involving the relation of a sequence of events enacted by an agent in which plans and goals play a role (Stein & Glenn, 1979). Narratives typically have a prescribed structure with a conventional beginning, middle, and end, although this structure varies somewhat from culture to culture. Narrative performance is a strong prognostic indicator of persistent language impairment (Stothard et al., 1998) and academic success (Fey et al., 2004) and is thought to form the bridge between basic oral language and the more literate language styles encountered in print (Westby, 2004).

Expository discourse is the language used to explain, describe, compare, and otherwise present factual material, for example, the type of formal language used in educational settings. Unlike narrative, expository structures are more varied and less reliable as a guide to comprehension. As a result, children with language impairments are particularly weak in this kind of discourse (Nippold et al., 2008). Expository deficits are especially likely to impact academic performance, as most material presented in school, either orally or in writing, makes use of expository structures.

Assessment of language

Deficits in language production are often obvious to adult listeners. Children who mispronounce words, leave words out of sentences, make grammatical errors, or produce very sparse speech are more likely to be noticed by parents and teachers. Other children may experience more subtle deficits in grammatical complexity and language comprehension, which may go unnoticed (Zhang & Tomblin, 2000). There is a high degree of comorbidity between language disorders and a range of other psychiatric and learning conditions, including attention deficits, learning disabilities, and conduct disorders (Im-Bolter & Cohen, 2007), although language impairments in children referred for psychiatric disturbance are frequently undiagnosed, in as many as 40% of cases (Cohen et al., 1998). For these reasons, school-aged children referred for or suspected of psychiatric or learning disorders should be assessed for language disorder.

Preschool assessment

Assessment of language skills in preschoolers typically involves some standardized testing using measures like those in Table 52.1. In addition, a sample of spontaneous speech, collected in a play interaction with a clinician, parent, or peer, can reveal the child's functional communication skills, as well as the kinds of errors made in natural speech. For children who are extremely reticent to talk, some elicited production tasks may be used, such as allowing the child to "talk" for a puppet, or using a game format such as "I spy" to elicit speech. Parent and teacher reports also provide important information, and several standardized report forms are available including the Vineland Adaptive Behavior Scales (Sparrow et al., 2005) and the Children's Communication Checklist-2 (Bishop, 2003a).

School-aged assessment

Standardized testing and parent/teacher report are used to identify language disorders and the impact on academic attainment in older children and adolescents. Test scores are often used to qualify young people for special educational services. Assessment of both language comprehension and production in this case is crucial. In addition, the conversations of young people with language disorder may sound normal to the casual listener, so it is often necessary to use more demanding contexts to assess their spontaneous speech. Samples of narrative language, elicited by asking students to tell a story from a set of pictures or recount a personal or traditional story have been shown to be sensitive to language deficits at school age (Boudreau, 2007). For adolescents, assessment of curriculum-based expository text is an especially relevant area both in terms of the comprehension of factual material and the ability to produce clear, cohesive arguments. Both narrative and expository deficits, when identified, serve as important intervention targets for school-aged students.

Differential diagnosis and common comorbidities

When a child presents with language impairment, the clinician needs to establish whether there are any factors present that may causally influence language difficulties or whether the language impairment is part of a recognized syndrome. Some common co-occurring conditions are considered in the following sections.

Auditory problems

Hearing should always be assessed by an audiologist in a child presenting with language disorder. Universal neonatal hearing screening means that it is unusual to find a previously undetected sensorineural hearing loss in an older child. It is, however, much more common to find conductive hearing losses in young children with language impairment, though the causal relationship with mild-moderate conductive hearing losses is debatable (see Chapter 47). Epidemiological studies have questioned whether otitis media with effusion, which can cause conductive hearing loss of up to 40 dB, is a major etiological factor in language disorder (Paradise *et al.*, 2003). Such prospective studies have revealed that many young children may have prolonged episodes of otitis media and hearing loss with little or no impact on verbal skills.

Diagnosis of central auditory processing deficits (APDs) is also fraught with controversy. One difficulty with diagnosis is that APD is typically assessed using verbal materials (e.g., listening to speech in noise), thus one cannot be sure if poor performance reflects a primary language disorder, or a genuine auditory problem (Moore, 2011). The diagnosis of APD as opposed to a diagnosis of language disorder, ADHD, or dyslexia may depend more on the referral route than the presenting symptoms (Moore *et al.*, 2013). To resolve this difficulty, better assessment methods and inter-disciplinary diagnosis and management are needed to ensure an appropriate diagnosis and management plan.

Low nonverbal cognitive ablities

Both DSM-IV and ICD-10 required a discrepancy between verbal and nonverbal abilities, usually of 1SD, for a diagnosis of language disorder. However, recent evidence has questioned the validity of this distinction. First, language skills and nonverbal reasoning skills tend to be highly correlated; children with the most severe language disorders also tend to have greater deficits in nonverbal reasoning (Conti-Ramsden *et al.*, 2012). Second, there is no evidence that children with discrepant versus equivalent abilities are etiologically distinct (Bishop, 1994). Finally, there is limited evidence to indicate that lower nonverbal IQ limits response to intensive language intervention (Bowyer-Crane *et al.*, 2011). For these reasons, nonverbal IQ restrictions do not feature in DSM-5 criteria.

Acquired epileptic aphasia (AEA)

Acquired epileptic aphasia (AEA), also known as Landau-Kleffner syndrome, is a rare cause of language disorder which is often misdiagnosed and is associated with epileptiform electroencephalographic abnormalities, though overt seizures are uncommon. The typical presentation is one of language regression after a period of normal language development. Language comprehension is severely affected and deafness may be suspected, but ruled out by a hearing test. Language regression is not a feature of typical language disorder (Pickles *et al.*, 2009), thus evidence of language regression should prompt neurological evaluation for possible AEA. Because children once spoke normally, differential diagnosis will center on selective mutism and ASD (see Chapter 51). These distinctions are further complicated by the fact that although many children with AEA have relatively selective problems with language, a significant minority may have more pervasive developmental and behavioral disturbances (Stefanatos, 2011). Sleep electroencephalogram (EEG) is necessary to document EEG abnormalities and confirm the appropriate diagnosis. Some children, particularly those with onset after age 6, can make a good recovery, but the prognosis for those with preschool onset is often poor. When receptive language deficits persist for more than a few weeks, it is crucial to provide children with alternative modes of communication, such as sign language (Deonna & Roulet-Perez, 2010). While pharmacological interventions may be effective, there is wide variation in response to treatment and a paucity of controlled clinical trials to advocate their widespread use (Stefanatos, 2011).

Specific learning disorders

There is little doubt that language disorder places children at greatly increased risk for reading impairments, contributing to lower educational attainments (Catts *et al.*, 2002; Snowling *et al.*, 2001). The particular profile of literacy skill will depend in part on the child's profile of language impairment; however, children with deficits in language comprehension have particularly poor literacy outcomes. For example, in a longitudinal study of children attending language units at age 7, 67% of children with predominantly expressive language impairments and 88% of children with comprehension deficits had literacy impairments at age 11 (Botting *et al.*, 2006). In addition to reading impairments, children with language disorders have pronounced difficulties with many aspects of arithmetic, including count sequences and simple computation, though they may have a sound understanding of arithmetic principles (Donlan *et al.*, 2007). Approximately 1/3 of children with language disorder also meet criteria for Developmental Co-ordination Disorder (Flapper & Schoemaker, 2013) (see Chapter 53).

Selective mutism

Selective mutism may be considered when there is a consistent failure to speak in social situations where speaking is expected (e.g., school) despite clear evidence that the child does speak in other situations (e.g., home). Most children with selective mutism also meet criteria for social phobia (Keeton & Budinger, 2012), prompting inclusion of selective mutism among the anxiety disorders in DSM-5 (see Chapter 60). Prevalence rates vary substantially depending on the setting, but suggest that selective mutism is rare, with prevalence estimates of .11% in clinical settings (Carlson *et al.*, 1994) to 2.0% in population surveys (Kopp & Gillberg, 1997). Selective mutism is more common in immigrant and bilingual communities (Elizur & Perednik, 2003).

The fact that children can speak in certain settings suggests that language impairment cannot fully account for the child's reticence to speak. Nevertheless, studies have consistently found that children with selective mutism have lower scores on standardized measures of language relative to peers and children with social anxiety/phobia (Manassis *et al.*, 2003). Indeed, approximately 50% of children with selective mutism meet diagnostic criteria for language disorder in one or more domains (Steinhausen & Juzi, 1996; Kristensen, 2000).

Treatment approaches aim to lower the anxiety that a child has for speaking in certain situations and increase the contexts in which the child may speak comfortably. In general, behavioral treatments, cognitive-behavioral therapy, and/or play therapy will be the first choice of intervention, though at present there are no randomized controlled trials to support any particular treatment approach. Controlled trials have examined pharmacological approaches to manage selective mutism, specifically through the use of SSRIs such as fluoxetine (Dummit *et al.*, 1996; March *et al.*, 2007). Such studies have shown marginal improvements in parent ratings of child anxiety, but many children remain symptomatic after medication. Selective mutism is persistent, with a remission rate of only 58% 13 years after first referral, and high rates of phobia and social anxiety, as well as increased risk for other psychiatric disorder (substance abuse and depression) even in resolved cases (Steinhausen *et al.*, 2006).

Psychiatric disorders, including ADHD

A recent meta-analysis confirmed that language impairment significantly increases risk for social and emotional difficulties in late childhood and adolescence (Yew & O'Kearney, 2013). Children with language disorders are more than 1.5 times more likely to meet criteria for ADHD relative to TD (typically developing) peers and more than twice as likely to experience general externalizing symptoms. Snowling *et al.* (2006) investigated adolescent outcomes for a clinically referred sample of children with language impairment. The authors reported that diagnoses of ADHD were more common in children with expressive language impairments, whereas social impairments were more common in those with receptive language difficulties.

The high rates of comorbidity observed in language disorder raises obvious questions about causal relationships. Our ability to answer these questions is hampered by a paucity of studies that measure common comorbidities early in development and follow children prospectively. One notable exception is the Ottowa Longitudinal Study, in which language disorder at 5 years of age was one of the strongest predictors of psychiatric outcome at age 12 (Beitchman *et al.*, 1996). However, this study does not elucidate the mechanism of association. The assumption is that language disorder predisposes children to adverse outcome because of the important role language plays in behavior regulation. A child with limited language comprehension may find it challenging to delay gratification, think through another person's motivations or predict the likely consequences of present actions. Another possibility is that the role of language impairment on behavioral outcome is mediated by the experience of academic failure. For example, Tomblin *et al.* (2000) found that risk for psychiatric disturbance was increased when language disorder was accompanied by literacy impairments and was much lower in those children experiencing academic success. The association was less evident when children were assessed prior to learning to read, suggesting that it is the sense of school failure that exacerbates the risk. However, it is also possible that the neurobiological factors that confer risk for language disorder are at least shared with other developmental disorders.

Prevalence

Prevalence figures vary dramatically depending on the diagnostic criteria employed, with estimates ranging from 2% (Weindrich *et al.*, 2000) to 31% (Jessup *et al.*, 2008) of children at school entry. There is no indication that figures vary systematically from country to country; differences in prevalence rates across countries likely reflect variation in diagnostic criteria and availability of services. However, there are few studies regarding the prevalence of language disorder in non-Western European communities.

The most commonly cited prevalence estimate is 7.4% (95% confidence interval 6.3–8.5%), taken from a study of kindergarten children in Iowa (Tomblin *et al.*, 1997). These children had non verbal IQ scores within the normal range, but scored more than 1.25SD below the normative mean on two out of five composite language scores, including receptive and expressive language, vocabulary, sentence grammar, and narrative. Intriguingly, only 29% had been identified by parents or teachers as having language concerns, and only half met the same criteria for language impairment 1 year later. These findings suggest the need to incorporate measures of functional impact to complement test scores; this may include measures of scholastic achievement or impact on family life and friendships. Moreover, these findings suggest that the features that lead to children being identified as having language concerns may be different to those identified on standardized tests (Bishop & Hayiou-Thomas, 2008). In general, the child starting school with pronounced speech errors or speaking only in short, simple phrases is likely to attract attention, whereas poor comprehension, limited vocabulary, and lack of sophisticated grammar are easier to miss.

As with many other neurodevelopmental disorders, more males than females are affected with language disorder, though again, the rates vary from study to study. For instance, Tomblin *et al.* (1997) reported a gender ratio of 1.33:1 boys to girls in their epidemiological study; by contrast, ratios in clinically referred samples can be as high as 3.8:1 (Robinson, 1991).

Causal models and risk factors

Cognitive theories of language disorder have attempted to explain why language may be disproportionately impaired relative to other developmental achievements. In the past, theories have suggested that the grammatical deficits that characterize language disorder occurred because of a "selective" deficit in dedicated cortical structures that sub-serve language (van der Lely, 2005). However, our recognition that grammatical deficits are rarely "all or nothing," coupled with our understanding of the developing brain means that a strong version of this hypothesis is no longer tenable. Increasingly, theories attempt to elucidate general cognitive processes that if faulty (or inefficient) could render language acquisition unduly challenging. These theories are outlined below.

Auditory perceptual

Auditory accounts have revealed that children with language disorder have difficulties perceiving sounds that are presented rapidly, are of brief duration, and therefore are not perceptually salient. Such deficits could conceivably lead to problems perceiving and categorizing meaningful phonemic contrasts, leading to problems with language learning. Furthermore, many grammatical contrasts in English are signaled with unstressed phonemes of brief duration occurring in a rapidly changing speech stream; thus a general impairment in temporal or perceptual processing may lead to highly selective impairments in grammatical processing (Joanisse & Seidenberg, 2003). Despite an intuitively attractive account, research has demonstrated that auditory deficits are neither necessary nor sufficient to cause language disorder. Notably, while auditory deficits are more common in children with language disorders, not all children are affected and some children with auditory deficits do not have any language difficulties (Bishop *et al.*, 1999). In addition, intervention studies have indicated that improving auditory skills does not confer improvements to other aspects of language or literacy, calling the causal relationship into question (Cohen *et al.*, 2005; McArthur *et al.*, 2008).

Limited processing capacity

Leonard (1998) argued that perceptual deficits may be more detrimental to language development in the context of a system that has limited capacity to hold information in store while processing perceptually challenging input. Evidence for a limited capacity system stems from poor performance on tasks of working memory and phonological short-term memory (Montgomery *et al.*, 2010). Measures of working memory typically require children to make true/false judgments about simple statements such as "balls are round" and "pumpkins are purple" (the processing component) and then recall the last words of each statement: for example, "round" and "purple" (the capacity component). The argument is that there is a trade-off between processing and capacity, such that when processing demands increase, capacity for recall is reduced and vice versa. On this view, children with language disorders would be expected to have greater difficulty processing sentences of increasing length and complexity, which is the typical profile seen. Similarly, repeating nonwords is thought to index phonological short-term memory, which, in turn, supports the development of vocabulary. Children with language disorders tend to have difficulties repeating nonwords, particularly as syllable length increases ("hampent; blonterstaping"). This in turn is thought to support vocabulary development as acquiring new words depends on the ability to retain novel sound sequences in memory.

While there is little doubt that children with language disorders have substantial verbal memory deficits, the direction of causation is debatable. These theories take a bottom-up view of language processing but there is also evidence for top-down influences on task performance. For example, the more "word-like" nonwords are (i.e., "trumpetine") the easier they are to remember, suggesting that existing vocabulary knowledge influences nonword repetition abilities. However, even when word-likeness is strictly controlled, there is limited longitudinal evidence that repetition skills predict later vocabulary outcomes (Melby-Lervag *et al.*, 2012). Similarly, verbal working memory tasks are essentially complex language tasks, making poor performance in children with language disorders difficult to interpret (Baird *et al.*, 2010). However, findings of working memory deficits outside the verbal domain lend credence to the view that domain-general cognitive processes contribute to language difficulties (Bavin *et al.*, 2005).

Procedural deficit hypothesis

Ullman and Pierpont (2005) made a distinction between procedural memory systems, which are important for rule-based learning (such as grammar) and declarative memory systems, which underlie knowledge-based learning (such as vocabulary). They hypothesized that language disorder resulted from a primary deficit in procedural memory systems, in the context of relatively intact declarative systems. The appeal of this theory is that it makes explicit connections between brain and behavior, has the potential to explain deficits outside the language system that are also contingent on procedural learning (such as motor sequencing) and is developmentally attractive in its emphasis on re-organization and compensation. Several recent investigations have noted that children with language disorder are impaired on measures of implicit learning, which tap procedural memory systems (Evans *et al.*, 2009; Lum *et al.*, 2012) and that performance on these learning measures is correlated with language scores (Misyak *et al.*, 2010). However, impairments in learning are not limited to procedural memory systems (Lum *et al.*, 2010) and extend to declarative memory impairments involved in learning facts and associations.

The conclusions from theoretical studies of the cognitive basis of language disorder are that there is unlikely to be a single cognitive factor that can cause the variety of language profiles seen. Instead, multiple cognitive risk factors are present, which act in concert to determine the severity and course of language disorder.

Etiology of language disorders
Genetic basis of language disorder
It is well documented that genetic factors contribute to susceptibility for language disorder. The disorder is highly heritable and shows strong familial aggregation (Conti-Ramsden *et al.*, 2007; see also Chapter 24). Furthermore, twin studies have consistently reported that monozygotic twins have greater concordance rates for language disorder than dizygotic twins, suggesting that much of this aggregation is influenced by genetic factors (Hayiou-Thomas, 2008). There is a strong consensus that the genetic mechanisms at play are multifactorial in nature, consisting of complex interactions between common genetic risk variants and environmental factors (Newbury & Monaco, 2010).

Initial excitement was generated by the discovery that a mutation to the FOXP2 gene resulted in a severe form of verbal dyspraxia and language impairment (Lai *et al.*, 2001). While subsequent research has indicated that such mutations are unlikely to be responsible for the majority of cases of language disorder, there has been considerable interest in the downstream targets of this regulatory gene. In particular, common genetic variants of *CNTNAP2* are associated with poor performance across a range of language measures (Vernes *et al.*, 2008). Intriguingly, this gene has also been implicated in many other neurodevelopmental disorders, pointing to possible shared mechanisms for language impairment across disparate diagnostic categories (Newbury & Monaco, 2010).

Further progress in identifying candidate risk genes may rely on refining clinical phenotypes and identifying particular phenotypic traits that may be heritable across diagnostic boundaries. For example, the *ATP2C2* and *CMIP* genes on chromosome 16 have been identified as having common variants that are associated with performance on tests of nonword repetition (Newbury *et al.*, 2009). The mechanisms by which this association emerges are not currently well understood; however, it is clear that the majority of genes implicated in language disorder are involved in early neurobiological development of brain regions important for language development (Rice, 2012).

An important message to emerge from this line of research is that such genetic influences are not deterministic, but can increase risk for language disorder in probabilistic fashion (see Chapter 24).

Neurobiology
Most children with language disorder do not show obvious brain abnormalities on structural imaging. Instead, like genetics, subtle neurobiological risks act in a probabilistic fashion. Imaging studies of language disorder are few and often yield conflicting results, perhaps due to variations across studies in age of participants, the diagnostic criteria employed and the possible presence of comorbid conditions. Leonard *et al.* (2006) identified seven anatomical variables that increased risk for oral language impairments versus written word decoding difficulties. These included: total size of cerebral hemispheres, asymmetry of the planum temporale, rightward cerebral asymmetry, summed leftward planar and parietal asymmetry, the first Heschl's gyrus on the left, the size of an anomalous second Heschl's gyrus, and rightward cerebellar anterior lobe asymmetry. Individuals with language disorders (and reading comprehension deficits) had strongly negative anatomical risk indices, suggesting smaller cerebral and auditory cortex and more symmetrical brain structures than typically developing peers. Despite the promise of identifying neural signatures of language disorder, Leonard and colleague urge caution in the use of neuroimaging for diagnosis and treatment planning, stating "a negative anatomical risk index is not sufficient for the development of oral language deficits. There is clearly a complex interplay between genetic, environmental, educational, and neurobiological factors in the development of reading and language phenotypes (pp. 3339)."

Environmental factors
There is little evidence that environmental factors alone are sufficient to cause language disorders in all but the most extreme circumstances. However, environmental factors may be implicated in early language delay and may have a role in mediating the developmental course and impact of language disorders on the child's well-being. For example, twin studies have shown that the quality of early mother–children interactions (i.e., the extent to which they elaborate utterances, link their talk to the child's attentional focus, invite the child to comment or take part in the interaction) predicts variation in language abilities at 36 months (Thorpe *et al.*, 2003). Maternal education and socio economic status have also long been associated with child language development, with children from disadvantaged backgrounds experiencing protracted rates of language acquisition and less success on structured measures of language competence (Letts *et al.*, 2013). Furthermore, recent evidence suggests that neural differences in regional brain volume in the hippocampus and amygdala align with SES status (Noble *et al.*, 2012), possibly resulting from qualitative differences in linguistic input and exposure to stress.

On the other hand, prospective, population studies of risk for language disorder report that although environmental factors may increase risk, the amount of variance explained in language outcome is relatively small (Reilly *et al.* 2010). Furthermore, SES and maternal education levels are at least partially genetically influenced (Oliver *et al.*, 2005). In other words, a mother may have limited educational experience or poor career prospects because of her own language limitations. Nevertheless, early language delay in the context of environmental disadvantage should alert clinicians and educators of the need to monitor linguistic progress carefully.

Distinguishing difference from disorder

In multicultural societies, it can often be difficult to determine whether a child has language disorder, or simply has had limited exposure to the mainstream language or dialect. Standardized testing can complicate this problem, since the words, sentence types, and format of the test may be unfamiliar to child, even when his/her basic language learning capacity is intact. For this reason, other methods of assessment that tap underlying language learning abilities may be used to assess children with English as an additional language. These measures, thought to serve as clinical markers of impairment (Conti-Ramsden, 2003), include repetition of nonwords (which rely on phonological memory and encoding skills thought to underlie word learning), fast mapping, (in which children are taught and asked to retain meanings of nonsense or unfamiliar words), and rapid automatic naming (such as saying all the days of the week in rapid sequence). These more process-oriented tasks can be helpful in determining whether a child has normal language-learning capacity and simply needs more exposure to master English, or needs more focused intervention for language disorder.

Longitudinal outcomes

Long-term prospective studies of children with language disorder converge on very similar findings; language disorder is a remarkably stable diagnosis from school entry (Law *et al.*, 2008; Conti-Ramsden *et al.*, 2012), with the primary difference in language outcomes between children being initial severity. For most aspects of language, growth is linear, with no differences between children with language disorder and their typical peers in rate of growth (Rice, 2013). For aspects of grammar (especially morphosyntax), growth is curvilinear, with a plateau for typical children around the age of four, while children with language disorder lag behind their peers by some 2 years (Rice, 2013).

Educational outcomes are the most vulnerable for children with language disorder; even for those children with apparently resolved language difficulties at age 5, their statutory examination grades are lower than those of age-matched peers (Snowling *et al.*, 2001). Those with persistent language disorder have worse outcome, with nonverbal IQ and literacy skills accounting for independent variance in achievement (Conti-Ramsden & Durkin, 2012). These longitudinal studies have also reported that those who continue into education post-18 are more likely to follow vocational and training courses rather than pursue University education. Furthermore, young people with language disorder are far more likely than peers to not be in education, employment or training at 19 years of age (Conti-Ramsden & Durkin, 2012).

Early longitudinal studies of boys with severe receptive language disorders at school-age reported a number of adverse social outcomes, including difficulties with independent living, maintaining close romantic relationships and participating in social activities (Howlin *et al.*, 2000). More recent studies report similar, though less severe, social difficulties in adults with language disorder (Whitehouse *et al.*, 2009). All studies report persistent language and literacy difficulties into adulthood. Differences in outcome between cohorts may reflect differences in initial severity, the extent to which language comprehension is affected, and differences in the stability of educational experience, which tends to be more variable for children with language disorder.

Social (pragmatic) communication disorders

The introduction of SPCDs to DSM-5 is in part inspired by the changes to diagnostic criteria for ASD and in part recognition of the fact that many children present in clinic with pronounced difficulties using language for social purposes. As illustrated by the third case history presented in the introduction, these *social communication* difficulties may include a poor understanding of speaker intentions and the verbal and nonverbal cues that signal those intentions, difficulty interpreting the environmental context and societal expectations, and problems integrating these skills with structural aspects of language to achieve successful communication. In addition, children may also have difficulties with *pragmatic* aspects of language, which center more on how children infer meaning or resolve ambiguities by integrating the surrounding language with their prior knowledge and experience.

Nosologies of developmental disorders have included children with social and pragmatic communication deficits for more than 30 years, though the diagnostic status of these children has often been controversial. For instance, Rapin and Allen (1983) first described "semantic-pragmatic deficit syndrome" as a constellation of symptoms including: verbosity, comprehension deficits for connected speech, word finding deficits, atypical word choices, unimpaired phonology and syntax, inadequate conversation skills, speaking aloud to no one in particular, poor topic maintenance, and answering beside the point of a question. Rapin and Allen used this as a descriptive term that was most commonly applied to the communication profiles of children with ASD, but also observed in many other developmental disorders. Bishop and Rosenbloom (1987) considered "semantic-pragmatic disorder" to represent a distinct subgroup of children who occupied a diagnostic space between ASD and specific language impairment. Later research established that semantic deficits did not reliably co-occur with pragmatic difficulties, and the term "pragmatic language impairment" became more widespread (Bishop, 1998). Typically, these labels have been used to identify deficits in social communication and/or pragmatic language abilities in the context of relatively age appropriate phonology and grammar. However, many children identified with pragmatic deficits using standardized instruments such as the Children's Communication Checklist (Bishop, 2003a, b) have structural language impairments (Norbury et al., 2004) and pragmatic deficits may also be evident in other neurodevelopmental conditions, such as Williams syndrome (cf. Laws & Bishop, 2004).

As a new disorder, there is limited research concerning the causes, consequences or developmental course of affected children with SPCD. Thus, this section will focus on diagnostic criteria, assessment and differential diagnosis, and consideration of common comorbidities. Although it is now conceptualized as a discrete disorder, it is crucial to bear in mind that social-pragmatic deficits can occur in other neurodevelopmental disorders (e.g., ADHD) and are a key diagnostic feature of ASD.

Diagnostic criteria and limitations

Diagnostic criteria for SPCD include four key aspects of deficit, all of which must be present for diagnosis. These include: using communication for social purposes such as greeting or exchanging information; changing communication to match context or the needs of the listener; following rules for conversation or storytelling, such as turn taking; and understanding what is not explicitly stated and nonliteral or ambiguous meanings of language (American Psychiatric Association, 2013). The criteria go on to specify that these communication deficits occur in the absence of a restricted repertoire of interests and behaviors; in other words children receiving a diagnosis of SPCD must not also meet criteria for ASD, even though the two groups may exhibit similar patterns of social communication behavior. DSM-5 further stipulates that although social and pragmatic difficulties may co-occur with intellectual and language impairments, they should not be caused by those impairments. It is far from clear how that distinction is to be made. Furthermore, as noted earlier, diagnostic criteria for Language Disorder also include deficits in discourse, thus complicating differential diagnosis of these two disorders.

A major challenge for the new diagnosis is that currently, no gold standard, culturally validated instruments exist with which to measure social-pragmatic communication. In part, this is because social communication by definition occurs in dyadic exchanges, making them notoriously difficult to measure in a standardized way. The structure provided by the test situation makes it difficult to capture social communication problems that may arise in everyday situations where the rules of engagement are less explicit and highly dynamic (Volden et al., 2009).

The proposed criteria require that deficits in both conversational skills and pragmatic language (i.e., inferencing and understanding linguistic ambiguities) are required for diagnosis. There is emerging evidence that these difficulties might dissociate; for instance, experimental measures of inferencing ability and ambiguity resolution have found few differences between individuals with ASD and typically developing peers, providing the individuals with ASD had age-appropriate grammar and vocabulary (Brock et al., 2008; Pijnacker et al., 2009). Thus it would appear that social communication deficits may be evident in children who are indistinguishable from TD peers on measures of pragmatic language functioning.

Autism spectrum disorder and SPCD

A key diagnostic distinction will need to be made between SPCD and ASD and ASD and Communication Disorders more generally (Norbury, 2014). Diagnosis of ASD is fully described in Chapter 51, so here we focus on particular areas of diagnostic difficulty. A major challenge is that many children with ASD have clinically significant language disorders, with recent population studies indicating that almost half of school-aged children with ASD will have language abilities significantly below chronological and mental age expectations (Loucas et al., 2008). In addition, by definition children with ASD also have deficits in social communication, which overlap with diagnostic features of SPCD. There is considerable controversy about the causal relationships between the language and communication deficits that frequently accompany ASD and the core social and behavioral features of the disorder, with some evidence for distinct genetic influences (Happe & Ronald, 2008).

The key differentiation would appear to be the presence of restricted and repetitive interests and behaviors. Previous reports of "pragmatic language impairment" suggested that there were children who experienced substantial pragmatic language deficits but did not meet threshold criteria for restrictive interests and repetitive behaviors (Bishop & Norbury, 2002). However, the majority of children included in the study by Bishop and Norbury (2002) were rated as having speech abnormalities associated with autism, used stereotyped language and a significant minority was reported to have unusual sensory interests. Changes to DSM-5 include the reclassification of stereotyped language as a repetitive behavior, rather than a communication symptom, and include sensory interests. Thus, many of the children studied by Bishop and Norbury (2002) may meet new DSM-5 criteria for ASD. The few studies that have attempted to determine how many children currently diagnosed with ASD would meet new criteria for SPCD have produced mixed results; however, Huerta et al. (2012) reported that only 1.5% of their participant pool met social-communication criteria for ASD but did not meet threshold criteria for restrictive and repetitive behaviors (RRIBs).

In the absence of a gold standard assessment of SPCD, we recommend that as a first step, children presenting at child and adolescent mental health or psychiatric services should be evaluated for possible social communication and pragmatic language impairments. The Children's Communication Checklist-2 (Bishop, 2003a, b) is a commonly used and well-validated parent report instrument that identifies children with social and pragmatic language difficulties in both clinical (Norbury *et al.*, 2004) and community contexts (Ketelaars *et al.*, 2009). The checklist does not provide a categorical diagnosis, but Norbury *et al.* (2004) suggested that negative scores on the Social-Interaction Deviance Composite were more common in those who had social-pragmatic deficits that were out of step with their overall level of language. Children scoring between 0 and 7 were those that tended to have both social-pragmatic and structural (i.e., grammar, vocabulary, and phonological) communication disorders. These children should then be evaluated for ASD: the presence of restricted and repetitive interests and behaviors, rigid routines, unusual sensory interests, and stereotyped language would suggest that a diagnosis of ASD was more appropriate than that of SPCD (see Chapter 51). Those children who do not meet criteria for ASD should be referred to an SLT for a more detailed examination of language and social communication. At present, it is far from clear how Language Disorders and SPCD can be meaningfully distinguished; many children with language impairments struggle with discourse, narrative and pragmatic aspects of language. Therefore, it is best to characterize an individual child's profile of communicative strength and need, and plan intervention to meet those needs, regardless of diagnostic label.

Intervention

General principles of intervention

Intervention goals may vary according to the age and needs of the child. Most randomized controlled trials focus on normalization of the developmental trajectory, as measured by change in scores on standardized assessments. In contrast, many clinicians and educators may focus on teaching discrete new language forms, providing the child with strategies to minimize the impact of communication disorder, or modifying the environment (especially parent–child interaction techniques) in order to improve communication despite speech or language weaknesses. Whatever the ultimate goal, selection of a treatment approach should be based on sound evidence that it is effective, as discussed in Chapter 41.

Speech sound disorders

Williams *et al.* (2010) give an overview of contemporary approaches to intervention which generally fall into three categories: (i) those that focus on the practice, generalization, and maintenance of correct sound production; (ii) those that embed sound production practice in a larger context including sound perception, integration of sounds into grammatical production (producing /s/ as a plural ending rather than as simply a sound), or the understanding of sounds as units within words that can be represented by letters (referred to as *phonological awareness*, often used to improve reading readiness); and (iii) those that

focus on motor movements rather than sounds themselves. Law *et al.* (2004) reported in a meta-analysis that treatments such as these were effective for speech sound disorders, although the number of studies meeting criteria for inclusion in the analysis was small. The one exception is the use of nonspeech oral exercises (e.g., blowing whistles) without speech practice to improve speech production, which is not considered an evidence-based approach. For children with the most severe forms of speech sound disorder, communication often involves the multimodalities, such as signs, pictures, or electronic communication aids, to expand the child's opportunities for successful communication.

Language disorders

There is a dearth of well-designed, randomized controlled trials with which to evaluate interventions for children with clinically significant language disorders. The range of treatments provided by SLTs in the United Kingdom, along with a systematic assessment of the quality of the evidence base supporting each intervention was recently summarized by (Law *et al.*, 2012) and forms a searchable database: https://www.thecommunicationtrust.org.uk/schools/what-works.aspx.

The few, randomized controlled trials that exist suggest that interventions which target underlying processes, such as auditory processing, are generally not effective in changing language profiles (Strong *et al.*, 2011). Interventions delivered by highly specialist SLTs that target semantic skills (Ebbels *et al.*, 2012) or particular grammatical forms (Ebbels *et al.*, 2007) in school-aged children with persistent and severe language disorder can be effective, though sample sizes have been small and there is a need for further replication. In contrast to much research in this field, Bowyer-Crane *et al.*, (2008) evaluated interventions that were delivered by trained (and well-supported) teaching assistants. Mainstream school children with poor oral language skills at school entry were randomly allocated to either an oral language intervention that focused on developing vocabulary and narrative skills or a phonology with reading intervention that focused on developing phonological skills and letter-sound correspondences. The children received individual and group sessions three times a week over 20 weeks. In contrast to the phonology with reading intervention, those in the oral language intervention improved significantly on measures of bespoke vocabulary and expressive grammar (see Chapter 41). While these results are highly encouraging, replication in children with more severe language impairments is urgently needed. In general, language comprehension deficits are extremely resistant to change (Boyle *et al.*, 2010) and such children are likely to require on-going support for their language disorder.

Social (pragmatic) communication disorder

There is a paucity of good quality intervention research for children with SPCD, in part hampered by inconsistencies in diagnostic labels, lack of agreement concerning diagnostic criteria and valid instruments for measuring change (Gerber *et al.*,

2012). Adams *et al.* (2012) reported the first randomized controlled trial of the Social Communication Intervention Project, an individualized intervention approach that targets development in three areas: social understanding and social interaction; verbal and nonverbal pragmatic skills, including conversation; and language processing, including narrative, inferencing, and developing word knowledge. In the trial, 88 children with SPCD were randomly assigned to receive the intervention or treatment as usual. The treatment group received 20 sessions of intensive intervention by a highly specialist SLT. No significant treatment effects were observed for the primary outcome measure (the *Clinical Evaluation of Language Fundamentals -4UK*, Semel *et al.*, 2006) or a test of narrative expression. However, significant treatment effects were reported for parent and teacher ratings of conversational competence, pragmatic language skill, and classroom learning.

The study is promising in demonstrating that observable differences in social communication behavior can be achieved after a period of intensive intervention, though for the most part, raters were not blind to the treatment status of individual children. However, study participants were extremely heterogeneous, varying from the 3rd to the 95th centile on all measures of structural language, nonverbal reasoning, and ASD symptomatology, making it difficult to ascertain for whom intervention is most likely to be effective. In addition, the primary outcome measure bore little relationship to the treatment content or treatment aims and was unlikely to be sensitive enough to show change. Given the complexities of social communication and pragmatic language, it is likely that these children will require on-going support as they get older and the complexity of social communication and language increases.

Conclusions

This chapter has focused on children with speech, language, and SPCDs. Such disorders are highly comorbid with other neurodevelopmental disorders and are often present in children referred solely for psychiatric assessment. Furthermore, speech, language, and communication skills are highly predictive of academic and employment outcomes, and critical to the cognitive and social development of children, whatever their primary diagnosis. For that reason, clinicians should be alert to these aspects of development so that appropriate referrals and assessments can be made, in order to facilitate the most appropriate avenues for education and intervention.

Acknowledgments

Work on this chapter was supported by a grant from the Wellcome Trust (WT094836AIA) to CFN and a Autism Center of Excellence grant # P50 MH81756 from the U.S. National Institute of Mental Health to RP.

References

Adams, C. *et al.* (2012) The Social Communication Intervention Project: a randomized controlled trial of the effectiveness of speech and language therapy for school-age children who have pragmatic and social communication problems with or without autism spectrum disorder. *International Journal of Language & Communication Disorders* **47** (3), 233–244.

American Psychiatric Association (2013) *Diagnostic and Statistical Manual of Mental Disorders*, 5th: DSM-5 edn. American Psychiatric Association, Washington, DC.

Baird, G. *et al.* (2010) Memory impairment in children with language impairment. *Developmental Medicine & Child Neurology* **52** (6), 535–540.

Bavin, E. *et al.* (2005) Spatio-visual memory of children with specific language impairment: evidence for generalised processing problems. *International Journal of Language and Communication Disorders* **40** (3), 319–332.

Beitchman, J.H. *et al.* (1996) Seven-year follow-up of speech/language impaired and control children: psychiatric outcome. *Journal of Child Psychology and Psychiatry* **37** (8), 961–970.

Bishop, D.V.M. (1994) Is specific language impairment a valid diagnostic category? Genetic and psycholinguistic evidence. *Philosophical Transactions of the Royal Society of London B: Biological Sciences* **346** (1315), 105–111.

Bishop, D.V.M. (1998) Development of the children's communication checklist (CCC): a method for assessing qualitative aspects of communicative impairment in children. *Journal of Child Psychology and Psychiatry* **39** (6), 879–891.

Bishop, D.V.M. (2003a) *Children's Communication Checklist*, 2nd edn. Psychological Corporation (Pearson), London.

Bishop, D.V.M. (2003b) *Test for Reception of Grammar-2*. Psychological Corporation (Pearson), London.

Bishop, D.V.M. & Hayiou-Thomas, M.E. (2008) Heritability of specific language impairment depends on diagnostic criteria. *Genes, Brain and Behavior* **7** (3), 365–372.

Bishop, D.V.M. & Norbury, C.F. (2002) Exploring the borderlands of autistic disorder and specific language impairment: a study using standardised diagnostic instruments. *Journal of Child Psychology and Psychiatry* **43** (7), 917–929.

Bishop, D.V.M. & Rosenbloom, L. (1987) Childhood language disorders: classification and overview. In: *Language Development and Disorders*. (eds W. Yule & M. Rutter). MacKeith Press, London.

Bishop, D.V.M. *et al.* (1999) Auditory temporal processing impairment: neither necessary nor sufficient for causing language impairment in children. *Journal of Speech Language and Hearing Research* **42** (6), 1295–1310.

Bloodstein, O. (2006) Some empirical observations about early stuttering: a possible link to language development. *Journal of Communication Disorders* **39** (3), 185–191.

Botting, N. *et al.* (2006) Associated reading skills in children with a history of specific language impairment (SLI). *Reading and Writing* **19** (1), 77–98.

Boudreau, D. (2007) Narrative abilities in children with language impairments. In: *Child Language Disorders from a Developmental Perspective: Essays in Honor of Robin Chapman.* (ed R. Paul). Lawrence Erlbaum, Mahwah, N.J.

Bowyer-Crane, C. *et al.* (2008) Improving early language and literacy skills: differential effects of an oral language versus a phonology with reading intervention. *Journal of Child Psychology and Psychiatry* **49** (4), 422–432.

Bowyer-Crane, C. *et al.* (2011) The response to intervention of children with SLI and general delay. *Learning Disabilities: A Contemporary Journal* **9** (2), 5–19.

Boyle, J. *et al.* (2010) Intervention for mixed receptive-expressive language impairment: a review. *Developmental Medicine & Child Neurology* **52** (11), 994–999.

Brock, J. *et al.* (2008) Do individuals with autism process words in context? Evidence from language-mediated eye-movements. *Cognition* **108** (3), 896–904.

Campbell, T.F. *et al.* (2003a) Risk factors for speech delay of unknown origin in 3-year-old children. *Child Development* **74** (2), 346–357.

Campbell, T.C. *et al.* (2003b) Disorders of language, phonology, fluency, and voice: indicators for referral. In: *Handbook of Pediatric Otolaryngology.* (eds C.D. Bluestone & S.E. Stool), 4th edn, pp. 1773–1788. W.B. Saunders Co., Philadelphia.

Carlson, J.S. *et al.* (1994) Prevalence and treatment of selective mutism in clinical-practice - a survey of child and adolescent psychiatrists. *Journal of Child and Adolescent Psychopharmacology* **4** (4), 281–291.

Carrow-Woodfolk, E. (1998) *Test for the Auditory Comprehension of Language (TACL-3)*: PRO-Ed.

Catts, H.W. *et al.* (2002) A longitudinal investigation of reading outcomes in children with language impairments. *Journal of Speech, Language and Hearing Research* **45** (6), 1142–1157.

Cohen, N.J. *et al.* (1998) Language, achievement, and cognitive processing in psychiatrically disturbed children with previously identified and unsuspected language impairments. *Journal of Child Psychology and Psychiatry* **39** (6), 865–877.

Cohen, W. *et al.* (2005) Effects of computer-based intervention through acoustically modified speech (FastForWord) in severe mixed receptive-expressive language impairment: outcomes from a randomised controlled trial. *Journal of Speech, Language and Hearing Research* **48** (3), 715–729.

Conti-Ramsden, G. (2003) Processing and linguistic markers in young children with specific language impairment (SLI). *Journal of Speech, Language and Hearing Research* **46** (5), 1029–1037.

Conti-Ramsden, G. & Durkin, K. (2012) Postschool educational and employment experiences of young people with specific language impairment. *Language, Speech, and Hearing Services in Schools* **43** (4), 507–520.

Conti-Ramsden, G. *et al.* (2007) Familial loading in specific language impairment: patterns of differences across proband characteristics, gender and relative type. *Genes, Brain and Behavior* **6** (3), 216–228.

Conti-Ramsden, G. *et al.* (2012) Developmental trajectories of verbal and nonverbal skills in individuals with a history of specific language impairment: from childhood to adolescence. *Journal of Speech, Language and Hearing Research* **55** (6), 1716–1735.

Deonna, T. & Roulet-Perez, E. (2010) Early-onset acquired epileptic aphasia (Landau-Kleffner syndrome, LKS) and regressive autistic disorders with epileptic EEG abnormalities: the continuing debate. *Brain Development* **32** (9), 746–752.

Donlan, C. *et al.* (2007) The role of language in mathematical development: evidence from children with specific language impairments. *Cognition* **103** (1), 23–33.

Duff, M.C. *et al.* (2004) Prevalence of voice disorders in African American and European American preschoolers. *Journal of Voice* **18** (3), 348–353.

Dummit, S.E. *et al.* (1996) Fluoxetine treatment of children with selective mutism: an open trial. *Journal of the American Academy of Child and Adolescent Psychiatry* **35** (5), 615–621.

Dunn, L.M. *et al.* (2009) *British Picture Vocabulary Scale*, 3rd edn. Granada, London.

Ebbels, S.H. *et al.* (2007) Intervention for verb argument structure in children with persistent SLI: a randomized control trial. *Journal of Speech Language and Hearing Research* **50** (5), 1330–1349.

Ebbels, S.H. *et al.* (2012) Effectiveness of semantic therapy for word-finding difficulties in pupils with persistent language impairments: a randomized control trial. *International Journal of Language & Communication Disorders* **47** (1), 35–51.

Elizur, Y. & Perednik, R. (2003) Prevalence and description of selective mutism in immigrant and native families: a controlled study. *Journal of the American Academy of Child and Adolescent Psychiatry* **42** (12), 1451–1459.

Evans, J.L. *et al.* (2009) Statistical learning in children with specific language impairment. *Journal of Speech, Language and Hearing Research* **52** (2), 321–335.

Fenson, L. *et al.* (1993) *MacArthur Bates Communicative Development Inventories.* Paul Brookes Publishing, Baltimore, MD.

Fey, M.E. *et al.* (2004) Oral and written story composition skills of children with language impairment. *Journal of Speech, Language and Hearing Research* **47** (6), 1301–1318.

Flapper, B.C. & Schoemaker, M.M. (2013) Developmental coordination disorder in children with specific language impairment: co-morbidity and impact on quality of life. *Research in Developmental Disabilities* **34** (2), 756–763.

Gerber, S. *et al.* (2012) Language use in social interactions of school-age children with language impairments: an evidence-based systematic review of treatment. *Language, Speech, and Hearing Services in Schools* **43** (2), 235–249.

Gillam, R. & Pearson, N.A. (2004) *Test of Narrative Language*. PRO-Ed, Austin, TX.

Gillam, R. *et al.* (2009) *Test of Childhood Stuttering*. PRO-Ed.

Goldman, R. & Fristoe, M. (2000) *Goldman-Fristoe Test of Articulation—2*. Pearson, San Antonio, TX.

Gordon-Brannan, M. & Weiss, C. (2007) *Clinical Management of Articulatory and Phonologic Disorders*. Lippincott, Williams, & Wilkin, Baltimore, MD.

Hammill, D. & Newcomer, P. (2008) *Test of Language Development: Primary*, 4th edn. Pearson, San Antonio, TX.

Happe, F. & Ronald, A. (2008) The 'fractionable autism triad': a review of evidence from behavioural, genetic, cognitive and neural research. *Neuropsychology Review* **18** (4), 287–304.

Hayiou-Thomas, M.E. (2008) Genetic and environmental influences on early speech, language and literacy development. *Journal of Communication Disorders* **41** (5), 397–408.

Howlin, P. *et al.* (2000) Autism and developmental receptive language disorder--a follow-up comparison in early adult life. II: social, behavioural, and psychiatric outcomes. *Journal of Child Psychology and Psychiatry* **41** (5), 561–578.

Huerta, M. *et al.* (2012) Application of DSM-5 criteria for autism spectrum disorder to three samples of children with DSM-IV diagnoses of pervasive developmental disorders. *American Journal of Psychiatry* **169** (10), 1056–1064.

Im-Bolter, N. & Cohen, N.J. (2007) Language impairment and psychiatric comorbidities. *Pediatric Clinics of North America* **54** (3), 525–542, vii.

Jessup, B. *et al.* (2008) Prevalence of speech and/or language impairment in preparatory students in northern Tasmania. *International Journal of Speech-Language Pathology* **10** (5), 364–377.

Joanisse, M.F. & Seidenberg, M.S. (2003) Phonology and syntax in specific language impairment: evidence from a connectionist model. *Brain and Language* **86** (1), 40–56.

Keeton, C.P. & Budinger, M.C. (2012) Social phobia and selective mutism. *Child and Adolescent Psychiatric Clinics of North America* **21** (3), 621.

Ketelaars, M.P. *et al.* (2009) Screening for pragmatic language impairment: the potential of the children's communication checklist. *Research in Developmental Disabilities* **30** (5), 952–960.

Kopp, S. & Gillberg, C. (1997) Selective mutism: a population-based study: a research note. *Journal of Child Psychology and Psychiatry and Allied Disciplines* **38** (2), 257–262.

Kraft, S.J. & Yairi, E. (2012) Genetic bases of stuttering: the state of the art, 2011. *Folia Phoniatrica Et Logopaedica* **64** (1), 34–47.

Kristensen, H. (2000) Selective mutism and comorbidity with developmental disorder/delay, anxiety disorder, and elimination disorder. *Journal of the American Academy of Child and Adolescent Psychiatry* **39** (2), 249–256.

Lai, C.S. *et al.* (2001) A forkhead-domain gene is mutated in a severe speech and language disorder. *Nature* **413** (6855), 519–523.

Law, J. *et al.* (2004) The efficacy of treatment for children with developmental speech and language delay/disorder: a meta-analysis. *Journal of Speech, Language and Hearing Research* **47** (4), 924–943.

Law, J. *et al.* (2008) Characterizing the growth trajectories of language-impaired children between 7 and 11 years of age. *Journal of Speech, Language and Hearing Research* **51** (3), 739–749.

Law, J., *et al.* (2012). *What Works: Interventions for Children and Young People with Speech, Language and Communication Needs: Technical Annex.* (DFE-RR247-BCRP10a). London.

Law, G. & Bishop, D.V.M. (2004). Pragmatic language impairment and social deficits in Williams syndrome: a comparison with Down's syndrome and specific language impairment. *International Journal of Language and Communication Disorders* **39**, 45–64.

van der Lely, H. (2005) Domain specific cognitive systems: insights from grammatical SLI. *Trends in Cognitive Sciences* **9** (2), 53–59.

Leonard, L.B. (1998) *Children with Specific Language Impairment.* MIT Press, Cambridge, MA.

Leonard, C. *et al.* (2006) Individual differences in anatomy predict reading and oral language impairments in children. *Brain* **129** (Pt 12), 3329–3342.

Letts, C. *et al.* (2013) Socio-economic status and language acquisition: children's performance on the new Reynell developmental language scales. *International Journal of Language & Communication Disorders* **48** (2), 131–143.

Loucas, T. *et al.* (2008) Autistic symptomatology and language ability in autism spectrum disorder and specific language impairment. *Journal of Child Psychology and Psychiatry* **49** (11), 1184–1192.

Lum, J.A. *et al.* (2010) Procedural and declarative memory in children with and without specific language impairment. *International Journal of Language & Communication Disorders* **45** (1), 96–107.

Lum, J.A. *et al.* (2012) Working, declarative and procedural memory in specific language impairment. *Cortex* **48** (9), 1138–1154.

Manassis, K. *et al.* (2003) Characterizing selective mutism: is it more than social anxiety? *Depress Anxiety* **18** (3), 153–161.

March, J.S. *et al.* (2007) A randomised controlled trial of venlafaxine ER versus placebo in pediatric social anxiety disorder. *Biological Psychiatry* **62** (10), 1149–1154.

McArthur, G.M. *et al.* (2008) Auditory processing deficits in children with reading and language impairments: can they (and should they) be treated? *Cognition* **107** (3), 946–977.

McGregor, K.K. *et al.* (2013) Children with developmental language impairment have vocabulary deficits characterized by limited breadth and depth. *International Journal of Language & Communication Disorders* **48** (3), 307–319.

McKinnon, D.H. *et al.* (2007) The prevalence of stuttering, voice, and speech-sound disorders in primary school students in Australia. *Language, Speech, and Hearing Services in Schools* **38** (1), 5–15.

Melby-Lervag, M. *et al.* (2012) Nonword-repetition ability does not appear to be a causal influence on children's vocabulary development. *Psychological Science* **23** (10), 1092–1098.

Misyak, J.B. *et al.* (2010) On-line individual differences in statistical learning predict language processing. *Frontiers in Psychology* **1**, 31.

Montgomery, J.W. *et al.* (2010) Working memory and specific language impairment: an update on the relation and perspectives on assessment and treatment. *American Journal of Speech-Language Pathology* **19** (1), 78–94.

Moore, D.R. (2011) The diagnosis and management of auditory processing disorder. *Language, Speech, and Hearing Services in Schools* **42** (3), 303–308.

Moore, D.R. *et al.* (2013) Evolving concepts of developmental auditory processing disorder (APD): a British Society of Audiology APD special interest group 'white paper'. *International Journal of Audiology* **52** (1), 3–13.

Newbury, D.F. & Monaco, A.P. (2010) Genetic advances in the study of speech and language disorders. *Neuron* **68** (2), 309–320.

Newbury, D.F. *et al.* (2009) CMIP and ATP2C2 modulate phonological short-term memory in language impairment. *American Journal of Human Genetics* **85** (2), 264–272.

Nippold, M.A. *et al.* (2008) Expository discourse in adolescents with language impairments: examining syntactic development. *American Journal of Speech-Language Pathology* **17** (4), 356–366.

Noble, K.G. *et al.* (2012) Neural correlates of socioeconomic status in the developing human brain. *Developmental Science* **15** (4), 516–527.

Norbury, C.F. (2014) Social (Pragmatic) Communication Disorder—conceptualization, evidence and clinical implications. *Journal of Child Psychology and Psychiatry* **55** (3), 204–216.

Norbury, C.F. *et al.* (2004) Using a parental checklist to identify diagnostic groups in children with communication impairment: a validation of the Children's Communication Checklist-2. *International Journal of Language & Communication Disorders* **39** (3), 345–364.

Oliver, B.R. *et al.* (2005) Predicting literacy at age 7 from preliteracy at age 4. *Psychological Science* **16** (11), 861–865.

Paradise, J.L. *et al.* (2003) Otitis media and tympanostomy tube insertion during the first three years of life: developmental outcomes at the age of four years. *Pediatrics* **112** (2), 265–277.

Pendergrast, K. *et al.* (1997) *Photo Articulation Test - 3*. Pro-Ed.

Pennington, B.F. & Bishop, D.V. (2009) Relations among speech, language, and reading disorders. *Annual Review of Psychology* **60**, 283–306.

Phelps-Terasaki, D. & Phelps-Gunn, T. (2006) *Test of Pragmatic Language-2*. Ann Arbor Publishers, Northumbria.

Pickles, A. *et al.* (2009) Loss of language in early development of autism and specific language impairment. *Journal of Child Psychology and Psychiatry* **50** (7), 843–852.

Pijnacker, J. *et al.* (2009) Pragmatic inferences in high-functioning adults with autism and Asperger syndrome. *Journal of Autism and Developmental Disorders* **39** (4), 607–618.

Pindzola, R. (1987) *Voice Protocol for Children and Adults*. PRO-Ed.

Pollard, R. *et al.* (2009) Effects of the speechEasy on objective and perceived aspects of stuttering: a 6-month, phase I clinical trial in naturalistic environments. *Journal of Speech Language and Hearing Research* **52** (2), 516–533.

Prasse, J.E. & Kikano, G.E. (2008) Stuttering: an overview. *American Family Physician* **77** (9), 1271–1276.

Ramig, C. & Pollard, R. (2010) Stuttering and other disorders of fluency. In: *Human Communication Disorders: An Introduction*. (eds N.B. Anderson & G.H. Shames), 8th edn, pp. 164–201. Allyn & Bacon, New York.

Rapin, I. & Allen, D. (1983) Developmental language disorders: nosological considerations. In: *Neuropsychology of Language, Reading and Spelling*. (ed U. Kirk). Academic Press, New York.

Reilly, S. *et al.* (2010) Predicting language outcomes at 4 years of age: findings from early language in victoria study. *Pediatrics* **126** (6), e1530–e1537.

Renfrew, C. (1991) *The Bus Story Test*. Speechmark Publishing, Oxford.

Rice, M.L. (2012) Toward epigenetic and gene regulation models of specific language impairment: looking for links among growth, genes, and impairments. *Journal of Neurodevelopmental Disorders* **4** (1), 27.

Rice, M.L. (2013) Language growth and genetics of specific language impairment. *International Journal of Speech Language Pathology* **15** (3), 223–233.

Rice, M.L. & Wexler, K. (2001) *Rice/Wexler Test of Early Grammatical Impairment*. Psychological Corporation (Pearson), London.

Robinson, R.J. (1991) Causes and associations of severe and persistent specific speech and language disorders in children. *Developmental Medicine and Child Neurology* **33** (11), 943–962.

Semel, E. *et al.* (2006) *Clinical Evaluation of Language Fundamentals-4UK*. Psychological Corporation (Pearson), London.

Shriberg, L.D. *et al.* (1994) Developmental phonological disorders III: long term speech-sound normalization. *Journal of Speech and Language and Hearing Research* **35**, 1151–1177.

Shriberg, L.D. *et al.* (1999) Prevalence of speech delay in 6-year-old children and comorbidity with language impairment. *Journal of Speech, Language and Hearing Research* **42** (6), 1461–1481.

Snowling, M. *et al.* (2001) Education attainments of school leavers with a preschool history of speech-language impairments. *International Journal of Language & Communication Disorders* **36** (2), 173–183.

Snowling, M.J. *et al.* (2006) Psychosocial outcomes at 15 years of children with a preschool history of speech-language impairment. *Journal of Child Psychology and Psychiatry* **47** (8), 759–765.

Sparrow, S. *et al.* (2005) *Vineland Adaptive Behavior Scales*, 2nd edn. Pearson, San Antonio, TX.

Stefanatos, G. (2011) Changing perspectives on Landau-Kleffner syndrome. *Clinical Neuropsychology* **25** (6), 963–988

Stein, N.L. & Glenn, C.G. (1979) An analysis of story comprehension in elementary school children. In: *New Directions in Discourse Processing II*. (ed R. Freedle). Ablex, Norwood, N.J.

Steinhausen, H.C. & Juzi, C. (1996) Elective mutism: an analysis of 100 cases. *Journal of the American Academy of Child and Adolescent Psychiatry* **35** (5), 606–614.

Steinhausen, H.C. *et al.* (2006) A long-term outcome study of selective mutism in childhood. *Journal of Child Psychology and Psychiatry* **47** (7), 751–756.

Stothard, S.E. *et al.* (1998) Language-impaired preschoolers: a follow-up into adolescence. *Journal of Speech, Language and Hearing Research* **41** (2), 407–418.

Strong, G.K. *et al.* (2011) A systematic meta-analytic review of evidence for the effectiveness of the 'Fast ForWord' language intervention program. *Journal of Child Psychology and Psychiatry* **52** (3), 224–235.

Thorpe, K. *et al.* (2003) Twins as a natural experiment to study the causes of mild language delay: II: family interaction risk factors. *Journal of Child Psychology and Psychiatry* **44** (3), 342–355.

Tomblin, J.B. *et al.* (1997) Prevalence of specific language impairment in kindergarten children. *Journal of Speech, Language and Hearing Research* **40** (6), 1245–1260.

Tomblin, J.B. *et al.* (2000) The association of reading disability, behavioral disorders, and language impairment among second-grade children. *Journal of Child Psychology and Psychiatry* **41** (4), 473–482.

Ullman, M.T. & Pierpont, E.I. (2005) Specific language impairment is not specific to language: the procedural deficit hypothesis. *Cortex* **41** (3), 399–433.

Vernes, S.C. *et al.* (2008) A functional genetic link between distinct developmental language disorders. *The New England Journal of Medicine* **359** (22), 2337–2345.

Volden, J. *et al.* (2009) Brief report: pragmatic language in autism spectrum disorder: relationships to measures of ability and disability. *Journal of Autism and Developmental Disorders* **39** (2), 388–393.

Weindrich, D. *et al.* (2000) Epidemiology and prognosis of specific disorders of language and scholastic skills. *European Child & Adolescent Psychiatry* **9** (3), 186–194.

Westby, C. (2004) 21st century literacy for a diverse world. *Folia Phoniatrica Et Logopaedica* **56** (4), 254–271.

Whitehouse, A.J. *et al.* (2009) Adult psychosocial outcomes of children with specific language impairment, pragmatic language impairment and autism. *International Journal of Language & Communication Disorders* **44** (4), 511–528.

Williams, A.L. *et al.* (2010) *Intervention for Speech Sound Disorders*. Paul H. Brookes Publishing Co., Baltimore, MD.

Woodcock, R. (1991) *Woodcock Language Proficiency Battery-Revised*. Riverside Publishing Company, Meadows, IL.

Yairi, E. & Ambrose, N.G. (1999) Early childhood stuttering I: persistency and recovery rates. *Journal of Speech, Language and Hearing Research* **42** (5), 1097–1112.

Yew, S.G. & O'Kearney, R. (2013) Emotional and behavioural outcomes later in childhood and adolescence for children with specific language impairments: meta-analyses of controlled prospective studies. *Journal of Child Psychology and Psychiatry* **54** (5), 516–524.

Zhang, X.Y. & Tomblin, J.B. (2000) The association of intervention receipt with speech-language profiles and social-demographic variables. *American Journal of Speech-Language Pathology* **9** (4), 345–357.

Zimmerman, I.L. *et al.* (2009) *Pre-School Language Scales - 4UK*. Psychological Corporation (Pearson), London.

CHAPTER 53

Disorders of reading, mathematical and motor development

Margaret J. Snowling[1] and Charles Hulme[2]

[1]Department of Experimental Psychology and St John's College, University of Oxford, UK
[2]Division of Psychology and Language Sciences, University College London, UK

Learning difficulties can occur in the context of global delays in development or where there are more circumscribed deficits in the cognitive processes that underpin learning and school achievement. However, recent conceptualizations of what for many years were considered *specific* or *selective* impairments of reading (dyslexia), writing (dysgraphia) or arithmetic (dyscalculia) now emphasize their frequent co-occurrence with other developmental cognitive disorders including communication impairments, attention disorders (ADHD, attention deficit hyperactivity disorder) and developmental coordination disorder (DCD) (Hulme & Snowling, 2009). Similarly, DSM-5 (American Psychiatric Association, 2013) groups together under a single overarching diagnosis, reading disorders, mathematical disorders, and disorders of written expression as specific learning disorder (SLD). In DSM-5, SLD is placed under the broader category of neurodevelopmental disorders since their impact on neurobiological development is early and probably heavily influenced by genetic risk factors (see Chapter 3). However, as we will argue, the classification of all of these learning difficulties together is not optimal, given what is known of their distinct causes and the need for different treatments to address them.

In this chapter we focus on reading disorders, mathematics disorders, and motor learning disorders, describing their nature and what is known of their causes, before offering advice regarding their management. These disorders are all relatively common and compromise children's learning not only in specific domains but also more generally across the curriculum. Moreover, there is a growing body of evidence of close connections between language skills and educational attainments, at least in part because oral language is the foundation for learning to read which, in turn, provides access to the curriculum. In practice, learning disorders are properly the domain of educators rather than of psychiatrists. Arguably, the new DSM-5 criteria are

more aligned with educational practice than previous versions since the medical model is de-emphasized. According to DSM-5 the diagnosis of SLD requires "difficulties learning and using academic skills...for at least 6 months despite the provision of interventions that target those difficulties." The difficulties should affect one or more of: "word reading, understanding the meaning of what is read, spelling, written expression, number sense, calculation (arithmetic), or mathematical reasoning... The learning difficulties are not better accounted for by intellectual disabilities, uncorrected visual or auditory acuity, other mental or neurological disorders, psychosocial adversity, lack of proficiency in the language of instruction or inadequate educational instruction." As we shall argue, however, this definition ignores important dissociations between disorders (for example, there are many children with reading disorders without mathematics disorder, and vice versa). Considering SLDs as a single category blurs the key distinctions between the different disorders in this category that are crucial to understanding their causes and developing theoretically motivated interventions.

Definitions and diagnosis

Conceptual issues

SLDs can be described at several different levels of explanation. While clinicians tend to focus on their behavioral manifestations, much research examines their distal causes (genetic and environmental) as well as proximal causes at the cognitive level. Hulme and Snowling (2009) outlined a unified framework for considering the causes of developmental disorders of language and learning. Within this framework the development of any given disorder can be seen as depending on the interplay of genetic and environmental risk factors which influence brain development. Critically, however, they argued that it is

Rutter's Child and Adolescent Psychiatry, Sixth Edition.
Edited by Anita Thapar and Daniel S. Pine, James F. Leckman, Stephen Scott, Margaret J. Snowling, Eric Taylor.

important to identify factors at a cognitive level of explanation that play a causal role in the development of a given disorder. For example, in the case of dyslexia, phonological problems (deficits in how speech sounds are represented in the brain) appear to play a major role in the genesis of reading problems; additional cognitive impairments increase the risk (see Figure 53.1). Identifying causal factors at a cognitive level is important, as it leads directly to ideas for treatments that target the underlying deficits responsible for the development of a disorder.

We used the term "causal risk factors" because these risk factors operate probabilistically rather than deterministically to influence development. This means that an individual may be "at risk" but not actually develop a disorder. Here the concept of a cognitive risk factor is useful. By cognitive risk factor we refer to what Bearden and Freimer (2006), referred to as an "endophenotype," a marker of a disorder which is related to the disorder but present in unaffected as well as affected relatives. Cognitive "endophenotypes" are conceived of as heritable risk factors (or processes) that combine to cause learning disorders but seldom cause diagnosed conditions when they occur in isolation (Bishop, 2006).

A related conceptual issue which confronts the clinician is where to set the boundary between "typical" development and a learning disorder. It is now well established that cognitive and language skills are continuous traits, ranging from weak to strong in the population. It follows that there is no clear cut-off between "normal" and "impaired"; this is perhaps well illustrated by findings from prospective longitudinal studies of children at family risk of dyslexia by virtue of having an affected parent (e.g., Pennington & Lefly, 2001; Snowling *et al.*, 2003). In terms of literacy outcomes, these studies show that children

at family risk do less well in reading and spelling than children from families with no such history. Interestingly, however, there is a step-wise pattern, such that children at family risk who do not fulfill criteria for dyslexia fall midway in terms of their literacy and literacy-related skills between children at family risk who are dyslexic and typical readers. Thus, dyslexia, like other neurodevelopmental disorders, is a dimensional problem, not a clear-cut category.

Related to the issue of cut-offs for "SLDs," the role of IQ in their definition continues to be debated. Stanovich and Siegel (1994) argued that the core deficit in reading difficulty is a phonological deficit which is sufficient to explain the reading problem and the construct of IQ is therefore not needed. Accordingly the "discrepancy definition" has fallen from favor and DSM-5 makes no explicit reference to this.

A final issue is how to conceptualize the frequent co-occurrence of different SLDs. Many children with dyslexia, for example, have language impairments, symptoms of inattention, and problems of motor coordination (see Snowling, 2009 for a review on changing concepts of dyslexia). It appears that shared genetic risk factors play an important role in explaining the comorbidities that exist between different SLDs.

In summary, key issues for theories of SLDs are the nature of the cognitive mechanisms that are affected and the risk factors that underlie their development.

Disorders of reading and writing

Normal literacy development: a framework

In order to appreciate the causes of disorders of reading and writing, it is important first to consider the process of learning to read, arguably a challenge for all children. According to the Simple View of Reading (Gough & Tunmer, 1986), reading comprehension is the product of decoding (the ability to translate text into speech) and linguistic comprehension. If decoding skills are limited, text comprehension will suffer, and if language skills are weak, a child will read without understanding.

In all alphabetic orthographies (writing systems), reading requires the ability to translate written words into their pronunciations (decoding). An important finding in recent years has been that the predictors of individual differences in learning to read appear to be similar across different alphabetic languages. Alphabetic orthographies differ in the regularity or consistency with which letters in printed words map onto the phonemes in spoken words. English is the least consistent orthography in terms of its spelling-to-sound consistency, French and Danish are intermediate, and other orthographies such as Finnish are very highly consistent. The phonological consistency of an orthography influences how easy it is to learn to read it and learning to read in English is notoriously difficult. Nevertheless, recent evidence indicates that there are three key predictors of individual differences in learning to read that have similar importance in all alphabetic orthographies so far studied:

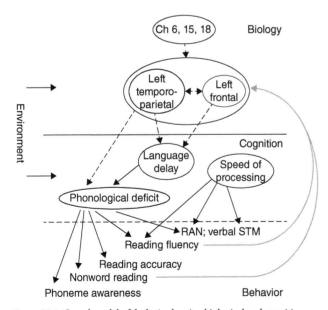

Figure 53.1 Causal model of dyslexia showing biological and cognitive levels of explanation. *Source*: Reproduced with permission of Wiley. *Notes*: Ch-chromosomes; RAN-rapid automatized naming; STM- short term memory.

letter–sound knowledge, phoneme awareness (the ability to reflect on the sound structure of spoken words), and rapid automatized naming (RAN; performance on a test requiring the rapid naming of sets of letters, digits or objects) (Caravolas *et al.*, 2012). In everyday life, children with reading (decoding) difficulties are likely to have had difficulty learning not only letter names and sounds but also numbers and color names. These children have word-finding difficulties and find playing rhyming games or "I-Spy" difficult.

Beyond decoding, the goal of reading is comprehension. Decoding is the first step to comprehension and in the early years of learning to read, children's resources are directed to decoding. However, to comprehend text, broader language skills, including vocabulary and grammatical skills, are required and individual differences in these skills predict individual differences in reading comprehension after basic decoding accuracy is controlled (e.g., Muter *et al.*, 2004). In addition, higher-level skills, such as inference-making, are important for some aspects of text comprehension (Cain, 2010).

Reading and spelling difficulties

There are two different, commonly occurring forms of reading disorder in children: dyslexia refers to children who have difficulty learning to decode (i.e., in mastering the relationships between the spelling patterns of words and their pronunciations). These children typically read aloud inaccurately and slowly and experience additional problems with spelling. The other major form of reading difficulty is reading comprehension impairment. These children show a contrasting pattern to children with dyslexia in that they can read aloud accurately and fluently but have difficulty understanding what they have read. Children with reading comprehension impairment tend to go unnoticed in the classroom and tend not to come to the attention of clinical or educational services.

Dyslexia

The most widely accepted definition of dyslexia is that of the International Dyslexia Association: "a specific learning disability characterized by difficulties learning to read and write despite adequate cognitive ability, motivation, access to instruction, and intact sensory mechanisms" (Lyon *et al.*, 2003). Building on this conceptualization, a draft DSM-5 definition of "dyslexia" was welcomed by the field when put out for consultation in 2011, though much debate ensued (e.g., Snowling & Hulme, 2012). Unfortunately, the published DSM-5 does not have a separate entry for dyslexia though it is included in the descriptive text; a welcome addition is that problems in reading for meaning are listed separately from problems of word reading (decoding).

Problems of decoding, usually referred to as "dyslexia," are a bottleneck to reading comprehension; however, the nature of the difficulties change with age. Early on in development, children with dyslexia have difficulty learning letter names and sounds. Later the problem is with "phonics," literally the translation of print into sound. In adolescence and adulthood, reading may be

accurate but fluency is usually affected and a slow reading rate will affect performance in formal settings such as examinations. Alongside reading difficulties are problems of spelling, initially in producing a phonetically acceptable transcription of target words and later, in English and to a lesser extent in other languages, with the many irregularities of the orthographic system.

Dyslexia is typically diagnosed when a person has severe difficulties with reading accuracy as assessed by a well-standardized test. Given that reading skills have a continuous distribution in the population, the cut-off point for defining "dyslexia" is arbitrary. Estimates of its prevalence in English-speaking countries range from 3% to 10% of school-aged children. In the classic epidemiological studies of Rutter and colleagues (Rutter & Maughan, 2005 for a review), prevalence rates were more than double in an inner city area compared with the Isle of Wight, suggesting that social factors play a key role in risk for reading disability. Boys are more likely to be referred for reading difficulties than girls and this is not simply a matter of referral bias because sex ratios of between 1.5:1 and 3:1 boys to girls have been reported in large-scale community studies (Rutter *et al.*, 2004).

In a recent test standardization of the *York Assessment of Reading for Comprehension* (*YARC*; Snowling *et al.*, 2009; Stothard *et al.*, 2010) a number of different criteria for the classification of decoding difficulties/dyslexia were tested. Taking account of the prevalence estimates from previous epidemiological surveys, a standard score of 77.5 (1.5 SDs below the mean, around 7% of the population) was taken as indicative of dyslexia and a standard score cut-off of 70 (2 SDs below the mean, around 2% of the population) as severe dyslexia.

From a large subsample of children attending state-funded primary and secondary schools in England, 10.5% of the primary school sample obtained a standard score below 77.5 and 3.9% below 70 in single word reading. Similarly, within the secondary school sample, 8.1% had moderate decoding difficulties and 3.9% severe. More boys than girls were affected at primary school and the proportion of pupils with English as an additional language was significantly higher among poor decoders than in the remainder of the sample. Decoding difficulties were also more common among children from socially deprived areas, underlining the fact that social and cultural factors influence the prevalence of reading difficulties.

Importantly, data from this standardization sample also showed that even when word-level decoding skills are poor, reading comprehension can be intact. Thus, 3.3% of the poor decoders in primary and 4.9% in secondary school showed a significant discrepancy between good reading comprehension (from the prose reading task) and poor reading accuracy (16–41 standard score points), a profile sometimes associated with discrepancy-defined dyslexia.

Typically, the spelling difficulties of people with dyslexia are more severe and more resistant to remediation than their reading difficulties (Romani *et al.*, 2005). Such problems may be seen as a direct consequence of difficulties in mastering the mappings between orthography (spelling patterns) and phonology (the sounds of words). However, in a minority of cases there are dissociations between reading and spelling skills; some children with adequate reading skills have poor spelling skills and vice versa (Moll & Landerl, 2009).

Problems of reading comprehension

As noted above, reading comprehension impairment is a distinct disorder from dyslexia. Children with reading comprehension impairment can decode and spell words accurately but have problems understanding what they read. Informal observations suggest that these children often read rather quickly and their processing of text is superficial; they do not appear to monitor what they read and may not self-correct, accepting what is termed "a low standard of coherence" for text that they are reading.

Data from the YARC standardization (op. cit.) revealed that 5.3% of the primary sample and 5% of the secondary school sample had single word reading which was at the age-expected level with reading comprehension below a standard score of 77.5. Reading comprehension impairment is therefore quite a common disorder which often goes undetected. It has been suggested that the gender imbalance for reading comprehension problems is more even than for decoding difficulties though evidence is sparse.

Many children with reading comprehension impairment have wide-ranging oral language impairments coupled with good phoneme awareness (it is these phonological skills that account for their ability to decode normally). They also experience higher-level language difficulties, including problems with inferencing and with figurative language use, and in text-related processes such as comprehension monitoring and knowledge of story structure (Cain, 2010). Other problems may include poor working memory and problems making inferences and clinically the profile is often seen in combination with ADHD.

Many children with autism spectrum disorders (ASDs) resemble poor comprehenders in that they learn to read well but fail to understand what they read (Brown et al., 2013). The term "hyperlexia" is often used to describe their reading profile. Notwithstanding this, there is considerable variability in the reading profile of children with ASD (Nation et al., 2006; White et al., 2006a) and, just as for typical readers, oral language skills are a good predictor of individual differences in reading in these children. Indeed, in line with the Simple View, impairments in word recognition as well as in oral language comprehension constrain the development of reading comprehension.

Language learning impairments

In recent years, there has been a growing tendency to collapse together disorders of reading (primarily dyslexia) with disorders of speech and language development, reflecting the clinical impression of considerable behavioral overlap between these disorders and their effects on academic performance. Given that reading builds on a foundation in oral language

skills, children who come to school with poorly developed speech and language skills are at high risk of reading disorders (see Chapter 52). The term "language learning impairment" is increasingly used to describe these children who may have varied problems with literacy but who may not fulfill traditional diagnostic criteria. Among this group are children with a history of language delay, children with specific language impairment and children with speech–sound disorders. However, as we shall see, the nature of the risk depends on a number of factors including the pervasiveness and persistence of the speech–language impairment (Pennington & Bishop, 2009; Peterson et al., 2009).

Causal models and risk factors

Phonological deficits in dyslexia

The predominant cognitive explanation of dyslexia is that it arises from a phonological deficit; that is, a problem in processing the speech sounds of spoken words (Vellutino et al., 2004). Phonological skills provide support for verbal short-term memory and more broadly the learning of verbal information. Early manifestations are difficulties with the development of phonological memory, phonological awareness, and phonological learning. These in turn affect the acquisition of letter-knowledge, one of the first signs that a child is at risk of reading problems. Problems with word recognition ensue together with phonological decoding deficits, seen most clearly when attempting to read novel words.

Arguably, the phonological deficit theory does not fully account for the reading problems found in children with dyslexia. Wolf and Bowers (1999) distinguished between disabled readers with deficits in phonological awareness and those with deficits in naming speed measured by RAN (a task requiring the rapid naming of familiar objects, colors, etc.); they also identified a subgroup with deficits in both processes. It is important to understand more fully how RAN is related to the process of learning to read, since performance in RAN is a better marker of who will go on to have reading problems among children with communication impairments than are measures of phonological skill (Bishop et al., 2009).

In recent years, there has been considerable interest in the relationship between RAN and reading (Kirby et al., 2010). One hypothesis is that RAN taps processing speed and this accounts for its relationship particularly with reading fluency. This hypothesis is interesting in view of the fact that slow processing speed is a shared risk factor between dyslexia and the ADHD-inattentive subtype (McGrath et al., 2011); however, the relationship between RAN and learning to read cannot simply be explained in terms of a general processing speed factor. RAN taps the automaticity of naming and, given that object naming is subserved by similar left hemisphere brain circuits to those involved in reading (Price & McCrory, 2005), this leads to the hypothesis that RAN taps a brain circuit involved in establishing the visual–verbal mappings that are critical to learning to read (Lervåg & Hulme, 2009) and somehow compromised in dyslexia.

Sensory impairments in dyslexia

A large body of research has assessed whether reading difficulties are associated with low-level impairments of sensory and perceptual processing. Investigations have examined putative impairments in visual, auditory, and motor domains as explanations for different manifestations of dyslexia (White *et al.*, 2006b).

Visual deficits

Although most people with reading difficulties have normal visual acuity, there is a raised incidence of abnormalities on psychophysical tasks assessing motion processing which have been related to a deficit within the magnocellular division of the visual system (Lovegrove *et al.*, 1986). However, evidence is mixed and it has been suggested that group differences may be related to uncontrolled differences in IQ (e.g., Hulslander *et al.*, 2004). Some people with dyslexia are also reported to experience visual stress following long periods of reading (sometimes referred to as Meares–Irlen Syndrome or Scotopic Sensitivity); symptoms include reports of text jumping around on the page, headaches and eye strain. However, it has proved difficult to validate these subjective experiences and although the use of colored lenses or filters to reduce visual stress is recommended by some practitioners, there is no evidence for the efficacy of such treatments as a way of improving reading performance.

Auditory deficits

A hypothesis that has attracted considerable research is that the phonological deficit in dyslexia stems from a deficit in basic auditory processing (Tallal, 1980). A recent meta-analysis has shown that frequency discrimination is the auditory processing task most often impaired in dyslexia (Hämäläinen *et al.*, 2013). However, typically only 30–40% of people with dyslexia show auditory impairments, suggesting it may be a co-occurring feature rather than a cause of the disorder.

The direct investigation of speech perception in dyslexia has produced mixed findings. Evidence comes primarily from performance on categorical perception tasks (e.g., identifying synthetic speech sounds as [ka] or [ga]). As a group, children with dyslexia show fuzzy boundaries between different phonemes, constituting a categorical speech perception deficit (but it should be noted that such difficulties are more marked if children have concomitant language impairments (Joanisse *et al.*, 2000; see Chapter 52).

Overall, evidence for the involvement of perceptual problems in dyslexia is equivocal; findings suggest that neither auditory nor visual deficits are necessary or sufficient causes of dyslexia

(Ramus *et al.*, 2003; White *et al.*, 2006b). However, in the absence of longitudinal data, it remains possible that a sensory deficit early in development (that may resolve by the time children are diagnosed as having reading problems) may play a causal role in the etiology of the disorder (Bishop, 2006).

Language delays and difficulties as precursors of reading difficulties

Prospective studies starting in the very early stages of learning to read suggest that children who go on to be poor comprehenders show weaknesses in basic language skills, including weaknesses in vocabulary knowledge, grammar, and syntax from an early age (Catts *et al.*, 2005; Nation *et al.*, 2010). Furthermore, strong evidence for the role of vocabulary impairments in the etiology of reading comprehension comes from a randomized controlled trial of an oral language impairment intervention for poor comprehenders. Gains in these children's reading comprehension skills some 11 months after the intervention ceased were mediated by gains in vocabulary knowledge (Clarke *et al.*, 2011). Similarly, Fricke *et al.* (2013) showed that boosting children's oral language at school entry had positive effects on reading comprehension some 12 months later (Fricke *et al.*, 2013).

Bishop and Snowling (2004) reviewed studies of the relationship between reading and language impairments and proposed that in order to understand these inter-relationships it is important to take a two-dimensional view accounting for both phonological and broader oral language skills (see Figure 53.2). Within this model, the risk of word-level decoding deficits is related to phonological skills (that vary from good to poor) and the risk of reading comprehension deficits is related to language skills beyond phonology (grammar and vocabulary again varying from good to poor). This two-dimensional model has direct implications for the assessment and management of children's reading difficulties and suggests that concerns over whether

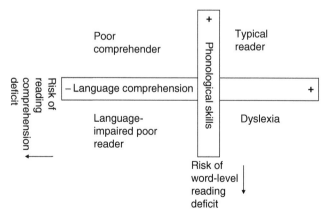

Figure 53.2 A two-dimensional model of the relationship between dyslexia and language impairment. *Source*: Adapted from American Psychological Association.

a particular child fulfills the diagnostic criteria for a specific reading disorder may be of little importance—there are continuous variations in reading skills in the general population and children with either decoding or reading comprehension problems will benefit from appropriate educational interventions that need to be tailored to individual children's needs.

Thus, children who enter school with poorly developed phonological skills (poor phonological awareness, phonological memory, or naming skills) are at risk of decoding difficulties, while children with broader language impairments are at risk of reading comprehension problems. The "type" of reading impairment they display will depend upon their cognitive skills and language weaknesses as well as the interventions they receive, both formally in school and informally in the home environment. Children with clinically diagnosed specific language impairment generally have pervasive reading disorders with both processes affected (see Chapter 52).

Attentional difficulties and reading disorders

It is not unreasonable to think that problems with attention could cause children's reading problems. However, although measures of self-regulation do account for variance in children's early reading skills, many children with ADHD learn to read without difficulty; moreover, medical interventions to improve functioning in ADHD do not lead to improvements in reading skill (Gittelman & Feingold, 1983) (see Chapter 55).

Despite this, dyslexia and ADHD often co-occur and epidemiological findings suggest that their comorbidity is attributable to inattention and not hyperactivity (Carroll *et al.*, 2005); moreover, evidence from twin studies suggests that the disorders are associated with a common risk factor, namely slow processing speed as measured by RAN (McGrath *et al.*, 2011). Beyond dyslexia, it is thought that some children with attention problems have reading comprehension difficulties; although there is limited research evidence it would seem that these are attributable to problems with working memory and the executive control of attention, which is required to build up a coherent memory representation of a text as it is processed.

Etiology of reading difficulties

Genetic basis of dyslexia and related disorders

Prospective studies following the development of children born to parents with dyslexia confirm a heightened risk of literacy impairment in "dyslexic" families (e.g., Snowling *et al.*, 2003; Lyytinen *et al.*, 2006). However, families share environments as well as genes and twin studies can be helpful in disentangling genetic and environmental influences on reading behavior.

Twin studies of dyslexia find that the proportion of variance attributable to genetic factors (heritability) is significant (Pennington & Olson, 2005; Scerri & Schulte-Korne, 2010) and the heritability of reading difficulties appears to be higher among those with higher IQ (Wadsworth *et al.*, 2010). However, some of the shared genetic variance between twins may be due to gene–environment correlation (Rutter, 2005). For example, the home literacy background provided by more literate parents may foster reading skills and shared reading in the early years has been shown to confer a longer term benefit for children's reading comprehension (Senechal & Lefevre, 2001). Moreover, better readers seek out more literary experiences and print exposure is lower among children with dyslexia than their unaffected siblings (Snowling *et al.*, 2007).

Studies of the molecular basis of genetic influences on reading have used a variety of methods (Grigorenko, 2005, for review). Genetic linkage studies have identified several loci which may contribute to dyslexia, including chromosome regions 15q21, 6p21, 2p, 3p, 18p11, 1p, and Xq27 (Scerri & Schulte-Korne, 2010). Some candidate genes have been mapped within these linkage regions, including DCDC2 and KIAA0319 on 6p and DYX1C1 on 15q21, which have all been replicated in independent studies (Paracchini, 2011). It is important to remember, however, that these genetic influences are associated with reading across the population and are not dyslexia-specific. Moreover, all the genes involved have small effects; much current research is directed toward trying to understand the impact of these genes on neurodevelopment.

To date, there is no comparable analysis of reading comprehension difficulties. However, work on the genetic basis of specific language impairment suggesting linkage to chromosomes 16 and 18 is likely to be relevant (Monaco, 2007).

Brain bases of dyslexia

The majority of children with specific reading difficulties do not show any structural brain abnormalities, but early neurodevelopmental abnormalities appear to be involved (Galaburda, 1994).

Findings from functional brain-imaging studies indicate that children and adults with dyslexia typically show less activity than controls in left hemisphere reading networks in temporo-parietal cortex when reading (Shaywitz *et al.*, 2004; Price & McCrory, 2005; Richlan, 2012). Moreover, a recent study suggested that greater right prefrontal activation during a phonological reading task (in turn indicative of better white-matter organization) significantly predicted reading outcomes in dyslexia whereas behavioral measures including tests of reading and language did not. Together the findings identify right prefrontal brain mechanisms that may be critical for reading improvement in dyslexia and may be indicative of the ability to develop compensatory mechanisms (Hoeft *et al.*, 2011). However, at present, such information cannot inform treatment of reading difficulties.

Social and environmental influences on reading development and disorder

Home and school background

It is important not to overlook the critical role of the environment in shaping a child's reading development (Phillips & Lonigan, 2005). Evidence indicates that reading disorders show a strong social gradient that is not entirely attributable to differences in phonological skills or general intellectual abilities (Hecht *et al.*, 2000) and poor readers often come from large families, where later-born children may face delays in language development. One aspect of delayed language development is poor vocabulary, which in turn appears to be related to later developing deficits in phoneme awareness (Carroll *et al.*, 2003). Parental educational level is also an influence on literacy skills, which may reflect differences in the amount and quality of literacy-related activities delivered to children at home (White-hurst & Lonigan, 1998). More specifically, parental teaching of print concepts has been found to be associated with better reading outcomes early in development when decoding is primary, whereas shared reading as a literary experience appears more important later for reading comprehension (Senechal & Lefevre, 2001).

Traditional definitions of dyslexia excluded children whose reading failure was caused by "inadequate opportunity to learn," but how to interpret this is unclear. Comparisons of children from the same catchment area attending different schools have emphasized that schooling can make a substantial difference to reading achievement (Rutter & Maughan, 2002). Equally, school experience can differ markedly between good and poor readers.

Cross-linguistic manifestations of reading disorders

Aside from the home and school environment, an important macro-environmental influence on reading development is the language in which a child learns. The reading and spelling symptoms of dyslexia vary across orthographies; in languages such as German or Finnish which are more regular than English, reading difficulties are identified by slow rates of reading (few reading errors occur), whereas in English, poor reading and spelling accuracy are the primary behavioral markers of dyslexia. Recent research in scripts with large character sets indicates that learning the basic symbol set is protracted and poor readers have difficulty in mastering it (Nag & Snowling, 2010; for akshara in an alphasyllabic script; McBride-Chang *et al.*, 2011 for Chinese). Parents may be concerned about the literacy skills of children with bilingual or multilingual backgrounds. The evidence available suggests that learning to decode in one language facilitates learning in a second language (at least if they are both alphabetic); however, reading comprehension depends upon the children having proficient language skills in the language they read in (Melby-Lervåg & Lervåg, 2014).

Summary

As might be expected for a complex trait such as reading, the etiology of reading disorders is varied and depends on both genetic and environmental factors. It is critical to distinguish between problems with decoding and problems of reading comprehension. Some children carry a genetic risk of dyslexia but whether or not they are classified as dyslexic depends upon the particular language and school context in which they learn and the other skills (or deficits) they bring to the task of reading. In keeping with this, there is currently a move away from single-deficit toward multi-factorial models that explain the nature and causes of dyslexia. This point was first made forcibly by Pennington (2006) who argued that the etiology of complex disorders, such as dyslexia, involves the interaction of multiple risk and protective factors, genetic or environmental, which alter the development of cognitive function and thereby produce the behavioral symptoms that define these disorders. It follows from this that comorbidity between disorders is to be expected because of shared risk factors.

Problems of numeracy

Problems in learning basic mathematical skills (Mathematics Disorder) is another form of SLD that is relatively common. In order to understand such problems it is important to first briefly consider evidence about the typical development of these skills.

The typical development of number skills and arithmetic

There is evidence from studies of preverbal human infants and nonhuman animals that some form of "approximate number sense" exists in the absence of language. For example, 6-month-old infants can discriminate between arrays of 16 versus 32 dots, but not between arrays of 16 versus 24 dots (Xu & Spelke, 2000). It has been suggested that this approximate number sense forms the basis of more refined forms of number representation seen in older children, though this proposal remains controversial.

One critical skill for mastering basic arithmetic skills is counting. The ability to count typically begins to develop in the preschool years but shows an extended period of development over the early school years (5–10 years of age) with the accuracy and speed of counting showing steady improvements with age. Counting depends upon understanding a set of abstract "how to count" principles (Gelman & Gallistel, 1978) but also requires verbal skills. Once at school, children are taught arithmetic formally, and master (in roughly the following order) addition (beginning with single-digit addition before moving on to deal with multidigit numbers), subtraction, multiplication, and division. Usually, fractions, proportions, and percentages are introduced after arithmetical operations dealing with whole numbers have been mastered.

Definition, classification, and prevalence of mathematical difficulties

DSM-IV identified a condition referred to as Mathematics Disorder, but as noted earlier, DSM-5 conflates this condition with a range of other educational difficulties, under the category of SLDs. An alternative term that is sometimes used for this disorder is dyscalculia. While comorbidities between mathematics disorder and reading and other disorders are certainly common, it seems a backward step to not separate such different problems which have separable cognitive causes and require different forms of educational interventions (see Chapter 41).

Mathematics disorder has typically been defined as a difficulty in learning mathematics which is out of line with other aspects of a child's development (particularly IQ). In practice, most studies of this disorder have focussed on children in the 7- to 11-year-old range, and the problems leading to a diagnosis of mathematics disorder are difficulties with basic arithmetic skills, rather than difficulties with higher-level mathematical skills such as algebra and geometry.

The incidence of mathematics difficulties is less well documented than for reading difficulties. Perhaps the best estimates of prevalence come from a UK study by Lewis et al. (1994) which used a simple cut-off approach to defining difficulties among 9- to 10-year-old children. They reported that only 1.3% of children showed specific difficulty in maths (standard score less than 85) in the presence of normal nonverbal ability and reading (at or above standard score of 90 on both). However, another 2.3% had both reading and maths problems defined in an analogous way. This study reported an equal incidence of maths difficulties in boys and girls, in contrast to the higher incidence of reading difficulties among boys that they (and other studies) reported.

The behavioral profile of children with mathematics disorder

The typical profile of children with mathematics disorder is that they show patterns of performance on simple arithmetic tasks that are characteristic of much younger, typically developing children. The pattern of problems with arithmetic seen in such children will vary as a function of age. Children with arithmetic difficulties initially experience problems learning to count. Once the formal teaching of arithmetic begins, these children show delays in mastering addition and subtraction, and they may tend to rely on the "count-on" strategy when solving simple addition problems for longer than typically developing children (Geary, 2004).

With more complex addition problems, children with mathematics disorder tend to guess more often and less accurately than their peers (Geary et al., 2004). Although they use the same strategies as age-matched controls, they differ in the speed and skill of strategy execution, can retrieve fewer number facts from memory, are poor at monitoring their counting, and poor at detecting computational errors (Geary, 2004). It is plausible to argue that problems in counting lead children with mathematics disorder to produce incorrect answers to arithmetic problems frequently, and these errors in turn may lead to the creation of inaccurate representations for the solutions to problems that are stored in memory.

Cognitive explanations of arithmetic difficulties

There has been a growing interest in the last 10 years in trying to identify the cognitive impairments that cause mathematics disorder. Four areas of difficulty have been suggested: problems with number (magnitude) representation; counting problems; number–fact storage problems, and working memory/executive impairments. We will consider each in turn.

Deficits in number (magnitude) representation

Dehaene (1997) has argued that the basis of numerical cognition is an innate "approximate number sense" (ANS)—a preverbal system involving the ability to understand physical magnitudes and numerical quantities. It has been suggested that the ANS is a basic building block for the later cultural construction of abstract, symbolic number concepts which in turn underpin the development of arithmetic skills. In this view, a deficit in the ANS may be a basic cause of the problems in learning arithmetic seen in children with mathematics disorder.

The ANS is a system that serves to represent magnitudes and numerosities in an abstract analog code. The precision of coding within the ANS is typically assessed by tasks that measure the accuracy and speed of discriminating groups of objects on the basis of their numerosity (Piazza et al., 2010). The difficulty of such discriminations varies in proportion to the ratio between the numerosities to be judged. The precision of ANS coding increases with age: 6-month-old infants can distinguish 8 from 16 objects but not 8 from 12 objects, while most adults can distinguish 9 from 10 objects without counting. There are also reported to be large individual differences in the precision of the ANS within an age group (Castronovo & Göbel, 2012).

If variations in the precision of coding within the ANS are a cause of the difficulties with arithmetic seen in Mathematics Disorder, we would expect variations in the functioning of this system to predict individual differences in arithmetic performance. Most of the evidence relevant to this idea comes from concurrent studies which have yielded mixed findings (e.g., Sasanguie et al., 2012).

Such concurrent correlations are inherently ambiguous with regard to questions of cause and effect, and longitudinal studies potentially provide more powerful evidence. Here again however, evidence is at best mixed, with some studies reporting significant longitudinal correlations between earlier ANS skills and later arithmetic performance (Mazzocco *et al.*, 2011; Libertus *et al.*, 2013) while other studies have failed to find such an effect (Fuhs & McNeil, 2013). Furthermore, it may be that learning arithmetic leads to improvements in the precision of coding in the ANS and in line with this possibility, Piazza *et al.* (2013) found that the precision of coding in the ANS was greater in participants who had received formal education compared with those who had not.

There is evidence that children with arithmetic problems are less accurate than age-matched control children at comparing the magnitudes represented by Arabic digits (Landerl *et al.*, 2004; Rouselle & Noel, 2007). However, in two of these studies, the children with mathematics disorder were just as fast and accurate in making physical size judgements or judging numerosities. Hence, these children's difficulties in comparing the magnitudes of digits do not seem to align with a problem with the functioning of an ANS system, and may instead reflect difficulties in learning associations between verbal symbols and magnitudes.

In summary, while deficits in an approximate number sense system are a possible cause of problems learning arithmetic, to date evidence for this suggestion is at best weak.

Deficits in counting

Counting is a fundamental skill for learning to perform arithmetic. Learning basic addition usually begins with children counting to compute the answer (What is $4 + 2$? Response 4...5...6 (the answer)). It is well established that children with mathematics disorder find learning to count hard and these children frequently make errors when counting arrays of objects. Furthermore counting is typically slower in children with mathematics disorder than in age-matched control children (Passolunghi & Siegel, 2001; Landerl *et al.*, 2004). It appears that problems in learning to count are a likely contributory cause to the problems seen in children with mathematics disorder, though longitudinal studies of the relationship between early counting skills and later arithmetic skills are badly needed.

Number fact storage deficits

Children with mathematics disorder have problems storing number bonds in memory (remembering that $4 + 2 = 6$). This is demonstrated by the observation that when presented with relatively simple sums they are likely to calculate answers by counting rather than retrieving the answer directly from memory. As noted earlier, one interpretation of this effect is that repeated errors in calculating the answers to simple problems result in "noisy" information being stored in memory. It is also possible, however, that these children have specific problems in storing numerical information in long-term memory. Evidence from acquired disorders of arithmetic following brain

damage suggests that number facts may be stored in a partially independent system, from verbal long-term memory. It remains a possibility that this memory system fails to develop adequately in children with mathematics disorder (see Hulme & Snowling, 2009).

Working memory deficits

The term "working memory" refers to the ability to store and process information at the same time (Melby-Lervåg & Hulme, 2013). During calculation, subcomponents of an arithmetic problem must be held in temporary storage while processing proceeds. With multidigit problems, it is necessary to monitor the calculation process, to inhibit numbers from the initial calculation and to hold in mind the products of different steps in the calculation. Thus, arithmetic skills carry both simple and complex working memory demands and also tap executive function. It is therefore not surprising that working memory deficits are associated with arithmetic difficulties. Children with arithmetic difficulties perform poorly on complex working memory tasks, such as backward digit span (which has an executive component) and counting span, but typically perform normally on simple tests of verbal short-term or phonological memory unless the task has a numerical component.

Executive deficits

A body of evidence implicates executive deficits in arithmetic disability (Hulme & Snowling, 2009 for review). These include impairments on the "Trail Making" task where children were required to connect alternating sequences of numbers and letters (e.g., 1–A, 2–B) or numbers and colors (e.g., 1–yellow, 1–pink, 2–yellow, 2–pink) and on several aspects of the Wisconsin Card Sorting Test, notably perseveration. It has been proposed that such difficulties impair their ability to shift psychological set, plan action, and judge the reasonableness of answers—all skills that are involved in mathematics. However, such difficulties may be attributable to comorbidities with other disorders (e.g., ADHD) that have not been controlled for in these studies.

Summary

To summarize, the nature of mathematics disorder is much less well understood than reading difficulties, and this reflects the fact that much less is known about the mechanisms of mathematical skills and their development. Mathematical skills depend upon a complex interplay between nonverbal and verbal cognitive systems, and mathematical skills are arguably more diverse and more complex than reading skills. It seems likely from a cognitive perspective that mathematical difficulties result from a number of underlying cognitive deficits. Possible deficits include impairments in an approximate number sense system located in parietal brain areas, as well as verbal systems that interact with this system. Further progress in this area is likely to depend upon longitudinal studies that attempt to focus on more well-defined arithmetical skills.

Etiology of mathematics disorder

Genetic effects

There is evidence indicating substantial genetic and environmental influences on the development of mathematical skills generally, and more specifically on the development of mathematics difficulties. There is good evidence that mathematical difficulties tend to run in families but this may reflect either shared environment or genetic effects. In a large-scale UK twin study, Kovas et al. (2005) found evidence for substantial heritability for normal variations in mathematical skills. There were substantial overlaps between the genes responsible for arithmetic and general intelligence, and arithmetic and reading, though the degree of overlap was far from perfect, suggesting that there are specific genetic effects on the development of arithmetic skills.

There are very few studies that have directly assessed possible genetic influences on mathematical difficulties (as opposed to normal variations in mathematical skills). In a study with a large sample (Oliver et al., 2004), the heritability of mathematical difficulties was assessed by selecting children in the bottom 15% of the population on teacher ratings of children's mathematical abilities. This study yielded a high group heritability estimate for mathematical difficulties of 0.65. These results are compatible with the same genetic influences operating to produce the group deficits in mathematics as well as the range of individual differences in mathematical skills observed within the population as a whole (Plomin & Kovas, 2005; see Chapter 24). It has also been reported that the comorbidity between mathematical and reading difficulties is in part due to common genetic influences operating on both disorders (Knopik et al., 1997).

Brain bases of arithmetic disorders

The neural substrate of the ANS system appears to depend critically upon bilateral areas of the horizontal intra-parietal sulcus (HIPS). Dehaene et al. (2003) have proposed that there are three parietal circuits for numerical processing. Problems in the development of such brain systems may be fundamental to the problems observed in children with mathematical difficulties, though as yet direct evidence for this is lacking. Consistent with the idea of mathematical difficulties being associated with parietal dysfunction, Isaacs et al. (2001) reported a specific reduction in gray matter in the left HIPS in a group of adolescents with mathematical difficulties (without reading problems) who had been born prematurely, compared to a control group without mathematical difficulties who had been born equally prematurely. This difference in the left HIPS was only found for children with problems with calculation, and not for another group of children who had problems with mathematical reasoning. Also, several studies have shown parietal deficits in Turner syndrome, a syndrome associated with arithmetic deficits.

Developmental coordination disorder (DCD)

Nature, classification, and incidence of DCD

DCD, sometimes referred to as "developmental dyspraxia," is a disorder of motor skill learning. An earlier term used to refer to this group is developmental apraxia and agnosia, capturing the central role of perceptual disorders in the clinical profile of these children. DCD is included here because problems with motor skills can adversely affect children's educational achievements and self-esteem.

The criterion for diagnosis of DCD from DSM-5 is as follows: "Motor performance that is substantially below expected levels, given the person's chronologic age and previous opportunities for skill acquisition. The poor motor performance may manifest as coordination problems, poor balance, clumsiness, dropping or bumping into things; marked delays in achieving developmental motor milestones (e.g., walking, crawling, sitting) or in the acquisition of basic motor skills (e.g., catching, throwing, kicking, running, jumping, hopping, cutting, coloring, printing, writing)." Additionally, such difficulties need to be of a severity such that they interfere with "daily living or academic achievement" and they should not be due to a general medical condition (e.g., cerebral palsy, hemiplegia, or muscular dystrophy). It is notable that this definition has moved away from specifying a discrepancy between motor skills and IQ (as was the case in DSM-IV). A diagnosis of DCD should preferably be made using a standardized test of motor skill though parent and teacher rating scales exist that are also useful (Wilson, 2005; Chambers & Sugden, 2006). DCD is commonly comorbid with other developmental disorders (see Hulme & Snowling, 2009) such as language impairment (Hill, 2001) and autism and the overlap with attention problems is high (Gillberg, 1999).

Population estimates of the incidence of DCD vary widely (from 5% to 18%) and these estimates depend both on the tests and the cut-offs used for diagnosis. It has been reported that there is a ratio of at least two boys to each girl with DCD (Wright & Sugden, 1996), though data on gender ratios may be hard to interpret because some of the tasks used to assess motor skills are gender-biased (e.g., throwing a ball) and there is little agreement among professionals about diagnostic criteria. The symptoms of DCD can vary considerably and may include gross motor difficulties, such as problems running, hopping, jumping, catching a ball and balancing, and fine motor difficulties including a lack of manual dexterity, difficulty in doing up buttons and laces, in dressing and in using eating utensils. Speech–motor skills can be affected and problems of pencil control are widespread.

A mistaken view is that children with DCD grow out of their clumsiness; follow-up studies are rare but evidence suggests that such children remain less physically competent throughout adolescence (Gillberg & Gillberg, 1989) and the difficulties they have at secondary school include problems with handwriting and the presentation of work, and difficulties in science, art, design, and technology (Losse et al., 1991). However, the coupling between motor impairments and academic achievement may not be causal and is likely mediated by comorbidities and/or psychosocial problems.

Explanations of developmental coordination disorder

The normal development of motor skills appears to be heavily dependent on maturational changes which nevertheless are subject to environmental influences (particularly with respect to the timing of motor skill development). Perceptual processes appear to play a critical role in adult motor skills and in their development. The control of movements depends upon inputs from the vestibular system (responsible for balance), proprioception (awareness of the positions of body parts), and kinaesthesis (awareness of body movements). Most crucially, however, most motor actions depend on visual information to initiate and guide movements. It has been proposed that guidance of our movements in space depends upon a sensorimotor map that serves to translate visually perceived locations to spatially appropriate action patterns (Held & Hein, 1963). Deficits in this sensorimotor map have been proposed as a unifying cognitive explanation for many of the problems seen in motor control in children with DCD (see Hulme & Snowling, 2009). Problems in the development of such a system may depend upon a range of perceptual problems, but most prominently deficits in visual perception.

Visual perceptual deficits

Strong evidence exists for an association between visual perceptual problems and motor disorders (in the absence of problems with visual acuity), with the greatest deficiency being observed in visuo-spatial tasks, regardless of whether they have a motor component (see Hulme & Snowling, 2009). It could be argued that a deficit in the visual perception of spatial information will inevitably lead to problems in the guidance of movements and problems in "calibrating" and "re-calibrating" the sensorimotor map during development. Clinically, occupational therapists often use visual perceptual training programs with these children (Cermak & Larkin, 2002).

Balance and postural control

More proximal causes of DCD have been proposed in balance and postural control, movement planning and preparation, and execution and feedback processes (Geuze, 2005). In addition, limitations of memory and attention and reduced muscle strength may play a role. It should be noted that in principle some of these difficulties might arise as a consequence of the perceptual impairments discussed above.

Etiology

There is evidence that low birth weight or prematurity increases the risk of developing DCD (Jongmans et al., 1996), suggesting

links with neurodevelopmental immaturity. Furthermore, a careful clinical examination may reveal neurological symptoms such as choreiform movements of unsupported limbs in such children. More generally, the comorbidity of DCD with impairments of reading and language, as well as with ADHD and autism spectrum disorder, suggests shared genetic risk with these other developmental disorders (see Chapter 3). Behavior genetic evidence (Martin et al., 2006) indicates a substantial heritable influence on both DCD and ADHD, as well as a substantial shared genetic influence on both disorders.

Longitudinal outcome of learning disorders

Relatively little is known about the adolescent and adult outcomes of children with SLDs although some evidence is available with regard to dyslexia. For some individuals, difficulties of learning in school leads to a downward spiral of disengagement, low attainment, and poor career prospects, with associated mental health issues. It is however, not known how common this clinical picture is. Here we summarize briefly the current state of knowledge, with a particular emphasis on reading disorders.

Cognitive and educational outcomes

There is stability in literacy skills from an early stage and although there has been discussion of "compensated" dyslexia, most poor readers continue to have problems of reading fluency, spelling, and phonological awareness into adulthood (Bruck, 1992). Furthermore it is likely that the effects of reduced reading experience are cumulative, causing differences in reading competence to become magnified over time. A follow-up of the literacy outcomes of preschool children with speech–language impairments at school-leaving age showed that educational achievements were strongly predicted by literacy skills (Snowling et al., 2006), underlining the importance of literacy to later attainments across the curriculum. In a long-term follow-up from the Isle of Wight Study, Maughan et al. (2009) reported that poor reading at school-leaving age was associated with a correlation of over 0.9 between spelling in adolescence and spelling at age 46 years. These individuals had typically spent careers in jobs which did not require literacy skills.

Psychosocial and mental health outcomes

There is a dearth of information regarding the psychosocial outcomes of children with SLDs. It is generally thought that learning disorders have a negative impact on emotional and behavioral development and an association between dyslexia and self-esteem has been reported. Snowling et al. (2007) reported that adolescents with dyslexia were rated by parents as having more emotional difficulties (but not social difficulties or conduct problems) than children at family risk without dyslexia. The same adolescents perceived themselves to be less academic than their peers (which of course was true) but no different in terms of social or athletic ability.

There is evidence of a link between reading difficulties and both conduct problems (Maughan *et al.*, 1996) and depression and anxiety (Maughan *et al.*, 2003). However, the processes responsible for these outcomes are not understood and comorbidities likely complicate the picture. For example, disruptive behavior at school may be the result of attention problems which are comorbid with poor reading and may interfere generally with school engagement. Maughan *et al.* (1996) followed 127 poor readers from the age of 10 years into early adulthood. There was a tendency for reading difficulties to be associated with poor attention and over-activity, which in turn placed poor readers at risk of behavior problems. However, behavior problems at 14 years reflected earlier behavior problems rather than reading difficulties and social adversity was found to increase the risk of antisocial behavior among girls but not among boys (for whom increased rates of offending were associated with poor school attendance).

As young adults, about 25% of this sample remained severely impaired in reading (Maughan & Hagell, 1996). Nonetheless, relatively positive self-reports suggested that many had gained employment in which there were restricted literacy demands and their reading problems were no longer of functional significance. In the majority of areas, those with a history of specific reading difficulties were functioning comparably to peers. However, young women with a history of specific reading retardation were at increased risk of psychiatric disorder, particularly depression, possibly related to a high rate of relationship breakdown. Male poor readers, in contrast, had more difficulty in gaining independence. However, these difficulties were the consequence of comorbid difficulties with peer relationships rather than reading problems.

In a study of 289 9- to 15-year-olds identified as having specific literacy difficulties from a representative sample of some 5000 UK children, Carroll *et al.* (2003) reported that children with reading difficulties are at increased risk of attention problems, conduct disorder, anxiety disorders, and depressed mood. However, they argued that the mediating mechanisms differ. The association between literacy difficulties and behavior problems was mediated by inattention (rather than hyperactivity), whereas the link with heightened levels of anxiety was direct. A similar conclusion was reached from a twin study of literacy difficulties by Willcutt and Pennington (2000). These investigators reported an increased risk of attention and conduct difficulties in probands as well as co-twins; however, anxiety was reported only in those with reading difficulties, suggesting that such difficulties may arise as the result of stresses associated with educational difficulties. Regarding the link between poor reading and low mood, Willcutt and Pennington (2000) reported heightened levels of depression in girls, mediated by ADHD, whereas Carroll *et al.* (2003) found that self-reported low mood was more common in boys than girls, and primarily in the 11- to 12-year-old age group.

Other learning difficulties

Relatively little attention has been paid to the outcomes of specific learning difficulties other than reading. Some evidence suggests that the psychosocial outcomes of children with DCD can be reasonably good, with low self-esteem restricted to the motor domain (Losse *et al.*, 1991). However, Skinner and Piek (2001) found that children and adolescents with significant movement problems had lower self-worth and higher levels of anxiety than controls. Similarly, Dewey *et al.* (2002) reported that children with DCD experienced social problems and displayed a relatively high level of somatic complaints based on parent report.

Although it is generally believed that SLDs can cause psychosocial problems, the evidence for this view is sparse. A reasonable conclusion is that the majority of children with specific difficulties in literacy and numeracy are relatively free of mental health problems but there may be more variability among those with motor disorders, perhaps because of the comorbidities associated with this condition.

Clinical implications

Children with SLDs will rarely be referred to child psychiatrists unless such difficulties have contributed to emotional or behavioral difficulties. However, it may be easy to miss a specific learning difficulty in a child with a mental health problem. Here we outline an approach to assessment, beginning with a set of questions a clinician might ask about educational progress before outlining the components of a comprehensive assessment battery.

In DSM-5, SLD is diagnosed via clinical review of an individual's developmental, medical, educational, and family history, reports of test scores and teacher observations, and response to academic interventions. Risk signs evident from the history include late talking, speech difficulties, delayed motor development, and a slow start in learning the names of colors, letters, and numbers. A family history of reading or maths difficulties, or an affected older sibling, is a noteworthy sign. In the case of DCD, tell-tale signs will include significant problems with gross and fine motor coordination and often balance. Speech–motor skills are sometimes, but not usually, affected.

Most clinicians will have access to educational data and school reports and a simple questionnaire asking for teacher ratings of reading, spelling, and maths can be very helpful. Teacher ratings of children's progress are available in UK schools and have been validated against objective tests (Snowling *et al.*, 2011). At the time of writing, parents in England also have access to their child's scores on a statutory Phonics Screening Check given to all Year 1 (6-year-old) children. For school-age children there are easily accessible standardized questionnaires for completion by parents and teachers for assessing DCD (e.g., *Developmental Coordination Disorder Questionnaire*; Green *et al.*, 2005). The *Strengths and Difficulties Questionnaire* (Goodman, 1997) can provide information on attention control. Documentation of whether a child's additional learning needs are recognized, the history of interventions received including speech and language therapy, and any special support currently in place is important. Some simple tests may also aid in determining whether the child needs further assessment. For dyslexia, these might include asking the child to repeat some difficult words, such as "preliminary," "philosophical," and "statistical," and some nonwords ("bagmivishent," "turnadulatical") to assess whether they do less well than might be expected for their age; and to complete a short reading test, such as the *Test of Word Reading Efficiency* (TOWRE–2; Wagner *et al.*, 2011) which takes only 90 seconds and provides a very useful tool. Together, the findings will enable the clinical team to decide:

(i) Does the child's school have sufficient resources to support the child without further educational assessment?

(ii) Should the child be referred directly to a specialist teacher who can offer tuition?

(iii) Should the child be referred for a comprehensive educational assessment (see below)?

(iv) Is there need for additional assessment, for example, referral to a speech and language therapist (see Chapter 52) or in the case of motor incoordination, to a physiotherapist or occupational therapist?

Diagnostic assessment

If a referred child has significant academic difficulties or has dyspraxic tendencies affecting physical coordination and handwriting, the most appropriate strategy is to refer this child to an agency within the school system for assessment.

Ideally a psychological assessment should be hypothesis-driven (see Chapter 34). In practice, to provide a comprehensive picture of a child's learning problems and teaching needs, it should include an assessment of general cognitive ability, single-word reading and spelling, reading comprehension, expressive writing, and number skills (see Figure 53.3). The Wechsler scales provide tools for comprehensive assessment of these skills (*WISC–IV*; Wechsler, 2004; *WIAT–II*; Wechsler, 2005). Measures of phonological awareness, Rapid Naming and verbal short-term memory are often included because of their value as concurrent predictors of dyslexia. The assessment will have more value if it proceeds to assess the reading strategies the child is using and the nature of spelling errors, with a view to prescribing appropriate intervention and an in-depth investigation of oral language skills may be appropriate (Snowling & Stackhouse, 2006).

In the past, such assessments were the domain of educational psychologists; however, now it is often a teacher with specialist qualifications who would undertake such assessments, replacing IQ testing with assessment of language and/or nonverbal reasoning. Given the substantial overlap between reading difficulties and difficulties with mathematics, an assessment of arithmetic and mathematical reasoning using standardized tests should ideally be part of a comprehensive assessment (see Figure 53.3).

A number of different practitioners, including physiotherapists, occupational therapists, specialist teachers, and pediatricians, play a role in the assessment of DCD. It is generally agreed that such assessments should incorporate the evaluation of a range of movements as well as the impact of motor difficulties on everyday skills and psychosocial functioning. Individually administered tests of gross and fine motor

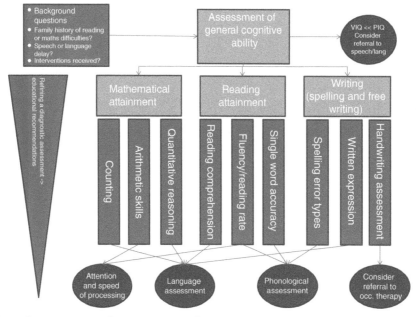

Figure 53.3 Diagram outlining the steps in a comprehensive assessment of SLD.

skills, incorporating ball skills, manipulative skills and balance are commonly used (Henderson *et al.*, 2007) and parent- and teacher-completed checklists and self-report questionnaires can be useful (Green *et al.*, 2005; Chambers & Sugden, 2006). It is also recommended that prior to an intervention program, physical fitness should be assessed.

Communicating findings

Given the dimensional nature of SLDs, it can be difficult for clinicians to provide parents with the answer to the question foremost in their mind: "Is my child dyslexic?" or perhaps "Does my child have dyscalculia?" Current practice varies considerably, and it is important for clinicians to be aware that the label dyslexia may be used differently by different agencies.

Clinicians need to provide as much feedback as possible to families, emphasizing the dimensional nature of SLDs and the comorbidities between them. The diagnostic report is critical and ideally it should outline recommendations for educational management, intervention, and advice on monitoring and review of progress.

Management of specific learning disorders

Here we will focus on principles which guide the management of dyslexia and related disorders. An extensive review of evidence on treatments for dyslexia, reading comprehension impairment, language disorders, and mathematics disorder is given in Chapter 41.

Children with speech–language difficulties are at high risk of dyslexia, especially if speech production deficits persist to school age (Bishop & Snowling, 2004). Such children should receive appropriate support during the preschool period, including speech and language therapy, and parental assistance with the development of pre-literacy skills will be helpful. However, it is important to be mindful that many children with language learning impairments may make a good start in learning to read but fail later as literacy demands increase. Careful monitoring of high-risk children is therefore advisable throughout the primary school years.

Theoretical knowledge of the relationship between phonological skills and learning to read, and phonological deficits in dyslexia has led to the development of effective reading intervention programmes that promote these skills in the context of reading (see Chapter 41). It is important to emphasize, however, that children with dyslexia can respond very slowly even to the most effective teaching approach. Because of the intractable nature of the disorder in some cases, some families turn to alternative or complementary therapies. However, for children who do not respond to conventional treatments, the best advice at the present time is to consider more intensive therapies, including placement in special units. In addition, information technologies have a lot to offer. Ideally, students

with dyslexia should be taught to become fluent keyboard users, with special instruction in the use of a spell-checker. In addition, some children with dyslexia can use voice-recognition technology as an aid to written work. In formal assessments and examinations, people with dyslexia should normally be eligible for special arrangements. The most common arrangement is extra time in written examinations. If the student has particularly poor reading and writing skills, then they may be allowed someone to read the questions to them, an amanuensis (scribe) or use of a keyboard.

In contrast to what is known about how to teach word-level reading skills, far less is known about how to promote reading comprehension effectively (Duff & Clarke, 2011; see Chapter 41). Since reading comprehension impairments stem from oral language weaknesses, the collaborative practice of speech and language therapists with teachers is likely to provide useful strategies for these children to learn.

Conclusions and future directions

Understanding of the nature and causes of children's reading difficulties is well advanced as is knowledge about appropriate interventions. In this domain, cognitive models of reading acquisition have had a positive effect on progress. Although less is known about children's arithmetic difficulties, the influence of cognitive models is beginning to improve methods of assessment and intervention. An advantage of the cognitive approach to SLDs is that it makes contact with what is known about typical development; furthermore, an understanding of the cognitive risk factors for disorders can foster understanding of links between genes, brain, and behavior. Future research is needed to understand the causes and treatments of motor impairments and to better understand how comorbidity changes the nature, developmental course, and outcomes of SLDs.

References

American Psychiatric Association (2013) *Diagnostic & Statistical Manual (DSM-5)*. American Psychiatric Association, Washington, DC.

Bearden, C.E. & Freimer, N.B. (2006) Endophenotypes for pscyhiatric disorders: ready for primetime? *Trends in Genetics* **22**, 306–313.

Bishop, D.V.M. (2006) Developmental cognitive genetics: how psychology can inform genetics and vice versa. *Quarterly Journal of Experimental Psychology* **59**, 1153–1168.

Bishop, D.V.M. & Snowling, M.J. (2004) Developmental dyslexia and specific language impairment: same or different? *Psychological Bulletin* **130**, 858–888.

Bishop, D.V.M. *et al.* (2009) Children who read accurately despite language impairment: who are they and how do they do it? *Child Development* **80**, 593–605.

Brown, H.M. *et al.* (2013) A meta-analysis of the reading comprehension skills of individuals on the autism spectrum. *Journal of Autism and Developmental Disorders* **43**, 932–955.

Bruck, M. (1992) Persistence of dyslexics' phonological awareness deficits. *Development Psychology* **28**, 874–886.

Cain, K. (2010) *Reading Development and Difficulties*. Wiley-Blackwell, Chichester.

Caravolas, M. *et al.* (2012) Common patterns of prediction of literacy development in different alphabetic orthographies. *Psychological Science* **23**, 678–686.

Carroll, J. *et al.* (2003) The development of phonological awareness in pre-school children. *Developmental Psychology* **39**, 913–923.

Carroll, J. *et al.* (2005) Literacy difficulties and psychiatric disorders: evidence for co-morbidity. *Journal of Child Psychology & Psychiatry* **46**, 524–532.

Castronovo, J. & Göbel, S.M. (2012) Impact of high mathematics education on the number sense. *PLoS ONE* **7**, e33832.

Catts, H.W. *et al.* (2005) Are specific language impairment and dyslexia distinct disorders? *Journal of Speech, Hearing and Language Research* **48**, 1378–1396.

Cermak, S.A. & Larkin, D. (2002) *Developmental Coordination Disorder*. Delmar Thompson Learning, Albany, New York.

Chambers, M. & Sugden, D. (2006) *Early Years Movement Skills: Description, Diagnosis and Intervention*. John Wiley & Sons, Chichester, Sussex.

Clarke, P.J. *et al.* (2011) Ameliorating children's reading comprehension difficulties: a randomised controlled trial. *Psychological Science* **21**, 1106–1116.

Dehaene, S. (1997) *The Number Sense: How the Mind Creates Mathematics*. Oxford University Press, New York.

Dehaene, S. *et al.* (2003) Three parietal circuits for number processing. *Cognitive Neuropsychology* **20**, 487–506.

Dewey, D. *et al.* (2002) Developmental coordination disorder: associated problems in attention, learning, and psychosocial adjustment. *Human Movement Science* **21**, 905–918.

Duff, F.J. & Clarke, P.J. (2011) Practitioner review: reading disorders—what are effective interventions and how should they be implemented and evaluated? *Journal of Child Psychology & Psychiatry* **52**, 3–12.

Fricke, S. *et al.* (2013) Efficacy of language intervention in the early years. *Journal of Child Psychology and Psychiatry* **54**, 280–290.

Fuhs, M.W. & McNeil, N.M. (2013) ANS acuity and mathematics ability in preschoolers from low-income homes: contributions of inhibitory control. *Developmental Science* **16**, 136–148.

Galaburda, A. (1994) Developmental dyslexia and animal studies: at the interface between cognition and neurology. *Cognition* **50**, 133–149.

Geary, D.C. (2004) Mathematics and learning disabilities. *Journal of Learning Disabilities* **37**, 4–15.

Geary, D.C. *et al.* (2004) Strategy choices in simple and complex addition: contributions of working memory and counting knowledge for children with mathematical disability. *Journal of Experimental Child Psychology* **88**, 121–151.

Gelman, R. & Galistel, C.R. (1978) *The Child's Understanding of Number*. Harvard University Press, Cambridge, Mass.

Geuze, R.H. (2005) Motor impairment in DCD and activities of daily living. In: *Children with Developmental Coordination Disorder*. (eds D. Sugden & M. Chambers), pp. 19–46. Whurr, London.

Gillberg, C. (1999) *Clinical Child Neuropsychiatry*. Cambridge University Press, Cambridge.

Gillberg, I. & Gillberg, C. (1989) Children with preschool minor neurodevelopmental disorders IV: behaviour and school achievement at age 13. *Developmental Medical Child Neurology* **31**, 520–531.

Gittelman, R. & Feingold, I. (1983) Children with reading disorders—I. Efficacy of reading remediation. *Journal of Child Psychology and Psychiatry* **24**, 167–191.

Goodman, R. (1997) The strengths and difficulties questionnaire. *Journal of Child Psychology & Psychiatry* **38**, 581–586.

Gough, P.B. & Tunmer, W.E. (1986) Decoding, reading and reading disability. *Remedial and Special Education* **7**, 6–10.

Green, D. *et al.* (2005) Is questionnaire-based screening part of the solution to waiting lists for children with developmental coordination disorder? *British Journal of Occupational Therapy* **68**, 2–10.

Grigorenko, E.L. (2005) A conservative meta-analysis of linkage and linkage-association studies of developmental dyslexia. *Scientific Studies of Reading* **9**, 285–316.

Hamäläinen, J. *et al.* (2013) Basic auditory processing deficits in dyslexia: review of behavioral and event-related potential/field evidence. *Journal of Learning Disabilities* **46**, 413–427.

Hecht, S.A. *et al.* (2000) Explaining social class differences in growth of reading skills from beginning kindergarten through fourth grade: the role of phonological awareness, rate of access, and print knowledge. *Reading and Writing* **12**, 99–127.

Held, R. & Hein, A. (1963) Movement produced stimulation in the development of visually guided reaching. *Journal of Comparative and Physiological Psychology* **56**, 872–876.

Henderson, S.E. *et al.* (1992) *Movement Assessment Battery for Children*. Psychological Corporation, London.

Henderson, S.E. *et al.* (2007) *Movement ABC-2: Pearson Assessment*. Pearson.

Hill, E.L. (2001) Non-specific nature of specific language impairment: a review of the literature with regard to concomitant motor impairments. *International Journal of Language & Communication Disorders* **36**, 149–171.

Hoeft, F. *et al.* (2011) Neural systems predicting long-term outcome in dyslexia. *Proceedings of National Academic Science USA* **108**, 361–366.

Hulme, C. & Snowling, M. (2009) *Developmental Disorders of Language, Learning and Cognition*. Wiley-Blackwell, Chichester.

Hulslander, J. *et al.* (2004) Sensory processing, reading, IQ and attention. *Journal of Experimental Child Psychology* **88**, 274–295.

Isaacs, E. *et al.* (2001) Calculation difficulties in children of very low birth weight: a neural correlate. *Brain* **124**, 1701–1707.

Joanisse, M.F. *et al.* (2000) Language deficits in dyslexic children: speech perception, phonology and morphology. *Journal of Experimental Child Psychology* **77**, 30–60.

Jongmans, M. *et al.* (1996) How local is the impact of a specific learning difficulty on premature children's evaluation of their own self-competence. *Journal of Child Psychology & Psychiatry* **37**, 565–568.

Kirby, J.R. *et al.* (2010) Naming speed and reading: from prediction to instruction. *Reading Research Quarterly* **45**, 341–362.

Knopik, V. *et al.* (1997) Comorbidity of mathematics and reading deficits: evidence for a genetic etiology. *Behavior Genetics* **27**, 447–453.

Kovas, Y. *et al.* (2005) 'Generalist genes' and mathematics in 7-year-old twins. *Intelligence* **33**, 473–489.

Landerl, K. *et al.* (2004) Developmental dyscalculia and basic numerical capacities: a study of 8- to 9-year-old students. *Cognition* **93**, 99–125.

Lervåg, A. & Hulme, C. (2009) Rapid automatized naming (RAN) taps a mechanism that places constraints on the development of early reading fluency. *Psychological Science* **20**, 1040–1048.

Lewis, C. *et al.* (1994) The prevalence of specific arithmetic difficulties and specific reading difficulties in 9- to 10-year old boys and girls. *Journal of Child Psychology and Psychiatry* **35**, 283–292.

Libertus, M.E. *et al.* (2013) Is approximate number precision a stable predictor of math ability? *Learning and Individual Differences* **25**, 126–133.

Losse, A. *et al.* (1991) Clumsiness in children – do they grow out of it? A 10-year follow-up study. *Developmental Medical Child Neurology* **33**, 55–68.

Lovegrove, W. *et al.* (1986) The theoretical and experimental case for a visual deficit in specific reading disability. *Cognitive Neuropsychology* **3**, 225–267.

Lyon, G.R. *et al.* (2003) A definition of dyslexia. *Annals of Dyslexia* **53**, 1–14.

Lyytinen, H. *et al.* (2006) Trajectories of reading development; a follow-up from birth to school age of children with and without risk for dyslexia. *Merrill-Palmer Quarterly* **52**, 514–546.

Martin, N.C. *et al.* (2006) DCD and ADHD: a genetic study of their shared aetiology. *Human Movement Science* **25**, 110–124.

Maughan, B. & Hagell, A. (1996) Poor readers in adulthood: psychosocial functioning. *Development and Psychopathology* **8**, 457–476.

Maughan, B. *et al.* (1996) Reading problems and antisocial behaviour: developmental trends in comorbidity. *Journal of Child Psychology and Psychiatry* **37**, 405–418.

Maughan, B. *et al.* (2003) Reading problems and depressed mood. *Journal of Abnormal Child Psychology* **31**, 219–229.

Maughan, B. *et al.* (2009) Persistence of literacy problems: spelling in adolesence and at mid-life. *Journal of Child Psychology & Psychiatry* **50**, 893–901.

Mazzocco, M.M. *et al.* (2011) Preschoolers' precision of the approximate number system predicts later school mathematics performance. *PLoS ONE* **6**, e23749.

McBride-Chang, C. *et al.* (2011) Early predictors of dyslexia in Chinese children: familial history of dyslexia, language delay, and cognitive profiles. *Journal of Child Psychology and Psychiatry* **52**, 204–211.

McGrath, L.M. *et al.* (2011) A multiple deficit model of reading disability and attention-deficit/hyperactivity disorder: searching for shared cognitive deficits. *Journal of Child Psychology and Psychiatry* **52**, 547–557.

Melby-Lervåg, M. & Hulme, C. (2013) Is working memory training in children effective? A meta-analytic review. *Developmental Psychology* **49**, 270–291.

Melby-Lervåg, M. & Lervåg, A. (2014) Reading comprehension and its underlying components in second-language learners: a meta-analysis of studies comparing first- and second-language learners. *Arne Psychological Bulletin* **140**, 409–433.

Moll, K. & Landerl, K. (2009) Double dissociation between reading and spelling deficits. *Scientific Studies of Reading* **13**, 359–382.

Monaco, A.P. (2007) Multivariate linkage analysis of specific language impairment (SLI). *Annals of Human Genetics* **71**, 660–673.

Muter, V. *et al.* (2004) Phonemes, rimes, vocabulary, and grammatical skills as foundations of early reading development: evidence from a longitudinal study. *Developmental Psychology* **40**, 665–681.

Nag, S. & Snowling, M. (2010) Cognitive profiles of poor readers of Kannada. *Reading and Writing* **24**, 615–622.

Nation, K. *et al.* (2006) Patterns of reading ability in children with autism. *Journal of Autism and Developmental Disorders* **36**, 911–919.

Nation, K. *et al.* (2010) A longitudinal investigation of early reading and language skills in children with poor reading comprehension. *Journal of Child Psychology and Psychiatry* **51**, 1031–1039.

Oliver, B. *et al.* (2004) A twin study of teacher-reported mathematics performance and low performance in 7-year-olds. *Journal of Educational Psychology* **96**, 504–517.

Paracchini, S. (2011) Dissection of genetic associations with language-related traits in population-based cohorts. *Journal of Neurodevelopmental Disorders* **3**, 365–373.

Passolunghi, C.M. & Siegal, L.S. (2001) Short-term memory, working memory, and inhibitory control in children with difficulties in arithmetic problem solving. *Journal of Experimental Child Psychology* **80**, 44–57.

Pennington, B.F. (2006) From single to multiple deficit models of developmental disorders. *Cognition* **101**, 385–413.

Pennington, B.F. & Bishop, D.V.M. (2009) Relations among speech, language, and reading disorders. *Annual Review of Psychology* **60**, 283–306.

Pennington, B.F. & Lefly, D.L. (2001) Early reading development in children at family risk for dyslexia. *Child Development* **72**, 816–833.

Pennington, B.F. & Olson, R.K. (2005) Genetics of Dyslexia. In: *The Science of Reading: A Handbook.* (eds M.J. Snowling & C. Hulme), pp. 453–472. Blackwell, Oxford.

Peterson, R. *et al.* (2009) What influences literacy outcome in children with speech sound disorder. *Journal of Speech, Language, & Hearing Research* **52**, 1175–1188.

Phillips, B.M. & Lonigan, C.J. (2005) Social correlates of emergent literacy. In: *The Science of Reading: A Handbook.* (eds M.J. Snowling & C. Hulme), pp. 173–187. Blackwell, Oxford.

Piazza, M. *et al.* (2010) Developmental trajectory of number acuity reveals a severe impairment in developmental dyscalculia. *Cognition* **116**, 33–41.

Piazza, M. *et al.* (2013) Education enhances the acuity of the nonverbal approximate number system. *Psychological Science* **24**, 1037–1043.

Plomin, R. & Kovas, Y. (2005) Generalist genes and learning disabilities. *Psychological Bulletin* **131**, 592–617.

Price, C.J. & McCrory, E. (2005) Functional brain imaging studies of skilled reading and developmental dyslexia. In: *The Science of Reading: A Handbook.* (eds M.J. Snowling & C. Hulme), pp. 473–496. Blackwell, Oxford.

Ramus, F. *et al.* (2003) Theories of developmental dyslexia: insights from a multiple case study of dyslexic adults. *Brain* **126**, 1–25.

Richlan, F. (2012) Developmental dyslexia: dysfunction of a left hemisphere reading network. *Frontiers in Human Neuroscience* **6**, 1–5.

Romani, C. *et al.* (2005) Spelling disorders. In: *The Science of Reading: A Handbook.* (eds M.J. Snowling & C. Hulme), pp. 431–448. Blackwell, Oxford.

Rouselle, L. & Noel, M.-P. (2007) Basic numerical skills in children with mathematics learning disabilities: a comparison of symbolic versus non-symbolic number comparison. *Cognition* **102**, 361–395.

Rutter, M. (2005) *Genes and Behavior.* Blackwell, Oxford.

Rutter, M. & Maughan, B. (2002) School effectiveness findings 1979-2002. *Journal of School Psychology* **40**, 451–475.

Rutter, M. & Maughan, B. (2005) Dyslexia: 1965-2005. *Behavioural and Cognitive Psychotherapy* **33**, 389–402.

Rutter, M. *et al.* (2004) Sex differences in developmental reading disability: new findings from 4 epidemiological studies. *JAMA* **291**, 2007–2012.

Sasanguie, D. *et al.* (2012) Approximate number sense, symbolic number processing, or number–space mappings: what underlies mathematics achievement? *Journal of Experimental Child Psychology* **114**, 418–431.

Scerri, T.S. & Schulte-Korne, G. (2010) Genetics of developmental dyslexia. *European Child and Adolescent Psychiatry* **19**, 179–197.

Senechal, M. & LeFevre, J.A. (2001) Storybook reading and parent teaching: links to language and literacy development. *New Directions for Child and Adolescent Development* **92**, 39–52.

Shaywitz, B.A. *et al.* (2004) Development of left occipito-temporal systems for skilled reading in children after a phonologically-based intervention. *Biological Psychiatry* **55**, 926–933.

Skinner, R.A. & Piek, J.P. (2001) Psychosocial implications of poor motor coordination in children and adolescents. *Human Movement Science* **20**, 73–94.

Snowling, M.J. (2009) Changing concepts of dyslexia: nature, treatment and co-morbidity. *Journal of Child Psychology & Psychiatry* **53**, e1–e3.

Snowling, M.J. & Hulme, C. (2012) The nature and classification of reading disorders: a commentary on proposals for DSM-5. *Journal of Child Psychology & Psychiatry* **53**, 593–607.

Snowling, M.J. & Stackhouse, J. (eds) (2006) *Dyslexia, Speech and Language: A Practitioner's Handbook*, 2nd edn. Whurr, London.

Snowling, M.J. *et al.* (2003) Family risk of dyslexia is continuous: individual differences in the precursors of reading skill. *Child Development* **74**, 358–373.

Snowling, M.J. *et al.* (2006) Psycho-social outcomes at 15 years of children with a pre-school history of speech-language impairment. *Journal of Child Psychology & Psychiatry* **47**, 759–765.

Snowling, M. *et al.* (2007) Outcomes in adolescence of children at family-risk of dyslexia, *Journal of Child Psychology & Psychiatry*, **48**, 609–618.

Snowling, M.J. *et al.* (2009) *YARC York Assessment of Reading for Comprehension*. GL Publishers, Passage Reading.

Snowling, M.J. *et al.* (2011) Identification of children at risk of dyslexia: the validity of teacher judgements using 'Phonic Phases'. *Journal of Research in Reading* **34**, 157–170.

Stanovich, K.E. & Siegel, L.S. (1994) The phenotypic performance profile of reading-disabled children: a regression-based test of the phonological-core variable-difference model. *Journal of Educational Psychology* **86**, 24–53.

Stothard, S.E. *et al.* (2010) *YARC York Assessment of Reading for Comprehension (Secondary)*. GL Assessment.

Tallal, P. (1980) Auditory-temporal perception, phonics and reading disabilities in children. *Brain and Language* **9**, 182–198.

Vellutino, F.R. *et al.* (2004) Specific reading disability (dyslexia): what have we learned in the past four decades? *Journal of Child Psychology & Psychiatry* **45**, 2–40.

Wadsworth, S.J. *et al.* (2010) Differential genetic etiology of reading difficulties as a function of IQ: an update. *Behavior Genetics* **40**, 751–758.

Wagner, R. *et al.* (2011) *Test of Word Reading Efficiency; Second Edition (TOWRE-2)*. Pro-Ed, Austin, Texas.

Wechsler, D. (2004) *Wechsler Intelligence Scale for Children® – Fourth UK Edition (WISC-IV^{UK})*. Harcourt Assessment, London.

Wechsler, D. (2005) *Wechsler Individual Achievement Test – Second UK Edition (WIAT-II^{UK})*. Harcourt Assessment, London.

White, S. *et al.* (2006a) A double dissociation between sensorimotor impairments and reading disability: a comparison of autistic and dyslexic children. *Cognitive Neuropsychology* **23**, 748–761.

White, S. *et al.* (2006b) The role of sensorimotor impairments in dyslexia: a multiple case study of dyslexic children. *Developmental Science* **9**, 237–269.

Whitehurst, G.J. & Lonigan, C.J. (1998) Child development and emergent literacy. *Child Development* **69**, 848–872.

Willcutt, E. & Pennington, B. (2000) Psychiatry co-morbidity in children and adolescents with reading disability. *Journal of Child Psychology & Psychiatry* **41**, 1039–1048.

Wilson, P. (2005) Practitioner review: approaches to assessment and treatment of children with DCD: an evaluative review. *Journal of Child Psychology & Psychiatry* **46**, 806–823.

Wolf, M. & Bowers, P.G. (1999) The double-deficit hypothesis for the developmental dyslexias. *Journal of Educational Psychology* **91**, 415–438.

Wright, H. & Sugden, D. (1996) A two-step procedure for the identification of children with developmental coordination disorder in Singapore. *Developmental Medical Child Neurology* **38**, 1099–1105.

Xu, F. & Spelke, E.S. (2000) Large number discrimination in 6-month-old infants. *Cognition* **74**, B1–B11.

CHAPTER 54
Intellectual disability

Emily Simonoff

Department of Child and Adolescent Psychiatry, Institute of Psychiatry, Psychology and Neuroscience, King's College London, UK
National Institute for Health Research (NIHR) Biomedical Research Centre for Mental Health, King's College London, UK

Terminology and classification

Intellectual disability (ID) refers to the presence of global and impairing deficits in intellectual functioning which commence in early life and persist with development. ID is a descriptive diagnosis with many identified causes. Over the past century, terminology has varied widely including "mental retardation" and, in the United Kingdom, both "learning disability" and "learning difficulties." The changes reflect attempts by professionals and advocates to change social attitudes toward people with ID, who experience high levels of stigma and discrimination, and where each name has eventually become a term of abuse.

Diagnostic criteria for ID have included two mandatory elements: substantially below average intellectual function, as measured on tests of intelligence (IQ) and significant impairment in adaptive functioning. The recently published DSM-5 criteria maintain this framework, with significantly reduced IQ usually (but allowing for some variance) of two or more standard deviations below average, that is, below 70. However, the concept of functional impairment is more clearly specified. In earlier classifications, both DSM and ICD, this criterion was considered problematic to operationalize because of its vagueness and the lack of agreed measures of adaptive function. However, in recent years, several reliable and valid measures have been developed, which quantify adaptive functioning in different domains. DSM-5 places greater emphasis on the measurement of functioning in relation to communication, social skills, personal independence, and school or work functioning. As with previous classifications, there is a requirement that the impairments were evident during childhood or adolescence, explicitly excluding acquired brain injury. While the latter makes good sense with respect to etiological differences, it can become a barrier to accessing services for people with an acquired condition who are functioning in the ID range, as services sometimes use rigid inclusion criteria, requiring an ID diagnosis.

The degree of ID is subclassified according to the extent of impairment, which should reflect a combination of IQ and level of adaptive functioning. The boundaries are not firmly fixed and serve as a guide. Mild ID is associated with IQ of 50–69, moderate 35–49, severe ID 20–35, and profound ID below 20. In contrast to clinicians, researchers often distinguish only two groups, referred to as mild (IQ 50–69) and severe ID (IQ below 50), discussed below under the two-group theory.

While adaptive function correlates moderately well with IQ at a group level (Papazoglou et al., 2013), there are considerable individual differences. In general, people with autism spectrum disorders (ASDs) perform more poorly on measures of adaptive functioning than would be expected on the basis of their IQ (Charman et al., 2011). Genetic syndromes show different relationships between IQ and adaptive function, both cross-sectionally and over time. For example, children with both Fragile X and Williams Syndrome have greater discrepancies between IQ and adaptive function than those with neurofibromatosis type 1 (NF1) and the former two also show age-related relative decline in adaptive function while NF1 does not (Fisch et al., 2007). Individual circumstances may also influence the level of adaptive function with family stress and adversity associated with poorer functioning (Koskentausta et al., 2007) and engagement in daily living activities appropriate for developmental level associated with enhanced functioning (Felce & Emerson, 2001).

From a clinical perspective, the requirement for impairment in adaptive function in ID is consistent with diagnostic criteria for other mental disorders which also require impact on functioning. However, from a research perspective, the coupling of the two criteria limits the ability of researchers to explore the factors associated with variation in adaptive behavior in people of subaverage IQ. Until recently, there has also been a paucity of brief measures suitable for use in research studies and these have often defined the population of study on the basis of IQ alone.

Epidemiology of intellectual disability

Level of IQ is a key criterion in defining ID; because IQ tests are designed to be normally distributed with a mean of 100 and standard deviation of 15, on this basis alone, 2.3% of the population would be expected to have IQ <70. In fact, one recent meta-analysis showed that studies report prevalence rates ranging from 3.31 to 156.03/1000 population (Maulik *et al.*, 2011). While variation across populations is expected, the wide range cannot be accurate and is almost certainly due to methodological flaws. IQ is a truly continuously distributed trait and any threshold will be arbitrary; there are no "gold standards" or biomarkers for ID. Therefore, operational definitions that combine IQ with impairment in adaptive function and produce a prevalence rate in Western countries that is in the region of 2–3% are the best practical solution at present, although scientifically unsatisfactory. However, a number of factors are known to influence reported prevalence. The first is mode of *ascertainment,* where there are large and consistent differences in reported prevalence rates according to whether ascertainment is via whole population screening, leading to higher rates, or by the use of registers of preidentified cases. There is less variation for severe ID (IQ <50) and an earlier summary reported rates ranging from 3 to 7/1000 while comparable rates for mild ID (IQ 50–69) ranged from 5 to 80/1000 (Roeleveld *et al.*, 1997). This reflects the fact that people with severe ID are more likely to be included in administrative registers and that mode of ascertainment is less crucial for this group.

Second, studies using IQ as the sole criterion report higher rates than those also including adaptive function (Maulik *et al.*, 2011). Studies employing more systematic ascertainment strategies are also more likely to base their definition on cognitive criteria alone and these effects are difficult to disentangle. Third, studies of children and adolescents report substantially higher rates than those of adults. This finding is confounded with both mode of ascertainment and method of assessment, but other factors such as selective mortality may play a role. When applying definitions that include adaptive function, it is possible that people with milder cognitive impairments are most adversely affected during their education and that appropriate adult employment lessens the impact on functioning. Milder levels of ID may not be recognized, however, before school-age, and cognitive testing in children under 6 years is unreliable (Anastasi & Urbina, 1997).

Fourth, higher rates of ID are also found in low- and medium-compared with high-income countries, with a meta-analysis reporting comparative rates of 16.41, 15.94, and 9.21/1000, for low- medium- and high-income countries respectively (Maulik *et al.*, 2011). Many of the studies undertaken in low-income countries have significant methodological flaws, including

the use of nonstandardized and nonspecific assessments that may identify other types of disability. This raises the issue of "culture-fair" tests of intelligence, which aim to be less reliant on prior experience and learning. Cognitive assessments not only need to be standardized for the population in which they are used but also need to take into consideration the cognitive characteristics that are associated with successful independent functioning. In the past, it has been argued strongly that people living in agrarian and rural societies, exposed to different educational practices, need different cognitive skills than those living in high-income, industrialized societies. With increasing globalization, there will be greater consistency in the cognitive skills associated with good adult functioning. However, variation in exposure to formal education, as opposed to underlying ability, remains an important factor influencing performance on cognitive tests. Despite the limitations in interpretation imposed by methodological considerations, rates of ID are greater in more impoverished countries.

Factors influencing the prevalence of intellectual disability

Severity

As highlighted above, mild ID is more common than severe (IQ <50) forms of the disorder, with the former accounting for about 85% of all ID. This is predicted from the normal distribution of the IQ scores. However, rates of severe ID may be greater than would be expected, because of an increase in pathological causes of ID. In some respects, this is a tautological question, as the test standardization is based on the distribution of test scores. Furthermore, IQ scores at the extreme lower end are not precise and many standard tests do not provide scores below IQ of 40.

Sex

The available studies are consistent in finding about a 20% male excess for severe ID (Roeleveld *et al.*, 1997). Reasons include the role of X-linked genetic disorders, including fragile X and many other, less common disorders. Greater male vulnerability to adverse environmental experiences is also cited. In mild ID, the aggregate data also suggest a male excess, but the ratio varies considerably across studies and those with more complete ascertainment are less likely to demonstrate a male preponderance (Roeleveld *et al.*, 1997; Simonoff *et al.*, 2006).

Socioeconomic factors

Various indices of socioeconomic adversity in developed countries are associated with mild ID (Drews *et al.*, 1995; Leonard and Wen 2002; Emerson *et al.*, 2006) but less so or not at all with severe ID (Broman *et al.*, 1987; Roeleveld *et al.*, 1997). Studies in developing countries have identified a relationship to both mild and severe ID (Gustavson, 2005) which is at least partly due to increased exposure to risk factors such as obstetric adversity, environmental toxins, and poor schooling (Brooks-Gunn & Duncan, 1997). In high-income countries, raising a child with

ID is associated with significant direct and opportunity costs, as demonstrated for autism (Knapp *et al.*, 2009). What is less clear is whether genetic risk factors are also at play. Hence, parental socioeconomic disadvantage may also index intellectual impairment in parents, which increases the risk of ID in their offspring. However, even if this were the case, the effects of poverty on children are themselves undesirable.

Ethnicity

Attempts to disentangle ethnicity from related risk factors for ID have proved highly controversial. Studies in the United States (Croen *et al.*, 2001) and Australia (Australian Institute of Health and Welfare & O'Rance, 2007) show that ethnic minorities are more likely to be affected, and the relationship is largely with mild ID. However, when prevalence rates are adjusted for indices of social disadvantage, maternal education, maternal age, birth order, and economic status, the risk associated with minority status is reduced or eliminated (Yeargin-Allsopp *et al.*, 1995). Ethnic groups vary in their genetic makeup, and this could contribute to differences in prevalence rates, although the variation is likely to be small. Furthermore, studies from different countries report higher rates in minority and/or socially deprived groups, whatever the ethnic origin, suggesting that a particular ethnic makeup is not a primary explanation. However, consanguinity, which occurs more commonly in certain ethnic groups, is a cause of recessive genetic disorders that are associated with ID.

Higher rates in low- and middle-income countries

A multitude of factors are likely responsible for higher rates in low and middle income countries. The lack of available antenatal screening increases the burden of genetic disorders and poor antenatal care contributes to high rates of obstetric complications, with one study suggesting that more than half the cases of ID were potentially preventable through improvement in these two elements alone (Dave *et al.*, 2005). Poor nutrition, exposure to environmental toxins, and pre- and postnatal infections also play a significant role.

Causes of intellectual disability

The two-group theory of ID was first proposed by Lewis (1933) and Penrose (1938, 1939) and subsequently elaborated by Zigler and colleagues (Zigler, 1967). It distinguishes between "pathological" and "sociocultural/familial" mechanisms as discrete causes of ID, and links these to severe versus mild ID. Pathological causes included relatively rare medical-genetic and extreme environmental events that almost invariably lead to ID. In contrast, the sociocultural/familial form of ID was postulated to be caused by common adverse family- and socially based risk factors, including low parental IQ, lack of environmental stimulation, and social deprivation. Pathological causes were also thought to cause severe ID (IQ <50), while sociocultural/familial factors were associated with mild ID and

borderline intelligence. It is helpful clinically to differentiate individuals based on the severity of intellectual impairment, in determining investigations, planning interventions, and guiding longer-term prognosis. However, the dichotomy is overrestrictive in applying a threshold to a truly continuous trait. This is especially the case in terms of causation. People with genetic disorders, such as Down syndrome and Fragile X, vary in IQ from average ability to severe impairment, and the same applies for those experiencing severe environmental adversity such as prematurity. Similarly, families with high rates of ID and socioenvironmental adversity may have members with severe as well as mild ID (Broman *et al.*, 1987). However, despite the limitations of the two-group theory, causes and severity of ID are linked and it is often helpful to consider different etiologies in the context of the degree of intellectual impairment, as well as other factors such as associated physical, cognitive, and behavioral features.

Genetic factors

Twin and adoption studies consistently indicate that intelligence in the general population is moderately heritable (Calvin *et al.*, 2012; Nisbett *et al.*, 2012; see Chapter 24). Several twin studies have examined intelligence at the extreme low end of the general population, including mild ID. Two of these report heritabilities that are similar to those seen in the rest of the IQ range (Cherny *et al.*, 1992; Thompson *et al.*, 1993), while the third, conducted in preschool children, suggests a somewhat higher heritability in the low end of the distribution (Spinath *et al.*, 2004). These findings suggest that inherited genetic factors are at least as important in determining intelligence in people with borderline intelligence and mild ID as in the rest of the population, although of course the level of intelligence is different.

Two large family studies of ID suggested that mild, but not severe, ID aggregates in families of affected individuals (Reed, 1965; Nichols & Broman, 1974). However, a further study of mild ID indicated that recurrence risk depended on whether other family members were affected, increasing the recurrence rate to ~35% (Bundey *et al.*, 1989). Recent research has focussed on identifying individual genetic risk factors and their mechanisms.

Chromosomal anomalies are variations from the usual diploid set of chromosomes or segments of chromosomes. They are typically identified by cytogenetic analysis, which can identify abnormalities in chromosomal segments down to a resolution of 5–10 mega bases (mB). Chromosomal anomalies identified with cytogenetic methods account for ~15% of severe ID (Ropers, 2010). Down syndrome (trisomy 21) is the most common chromosomal anomaly causing ID, occurring in about 1.5 per 1000 pregnancies (Siffel *et al.*, 2004). Like other chromosomal anomalies, Down syndrome is significantly associated with advanced maternal age, with a 6.5-fold increase in incidence among women over 35 years (Siffel *et al.*, 2004).

Sex chromosome anomalies are the most common group of chromosomal anomalies in live-born infants. The most frequent are Klinefelter syndrome (XXY), Turner syndrome (XO) and XYY syndrome. Aggregate prevalence is about 2–5 per 1000 with Klinefelter syndrome the most common (Maeda *et al.*, 1991). Most people with sex chromosomal anomalies have IQs that are in the low normal/borderline range but occasionally mild ID. Speech/language problems are common as are social and behavioral difficulties (Leggett *et al.*, 2010).

Mutations in all forms of Mendelian inheritance are causes of ID. Common *autosomal dominant* disorders include NF1, Noonan syndrome, and tuberous sclerosis. Autosomal dominant disorders are characteristically passed from one generation to the next; therefore these causes are typically characterized either by high rates of new mutations, for example, tuberous sclerosis, or a highly variable phenotype, for example, neurofibromatosis. In addition to these well-recognized disorders, new genetic methods such as mutation screening targeted at genes known to be involved in cognitive function, have provided the technological basis to identify novel heterozygous (and therefore presumably dominant) genetic mutations associated with nonsyndromic ID (Ropers, 2010).

Autosomal recessive causes of ID are often associated with more severe forms of ID; those that were first recognized often involved inborn errors of metabolism, such as phenylketonuria or homocystinuria, identified through biochemical investigations. Recently, the use of single nucleotide polymorphism (SNP)-based arrays has identified regions of homozygosity. This technique has been used to study families with nonsyndromic autosomal recessive ID, including those with consanguinity, and has led to the identification of a number of new causative mutations (Ropers, 2010).

Current estimates suggest that *X-linked* genetic disorders account for 10–12% of all ID in males; at least, 91 X-linked genes have been identified (Ropers, 2008). Fragile X syndrome is the most common cause of X-linked ID, but its pattern of inheritance is complex, involving intergenerational expansion in the FMR1 gene causing the mutation, so that familial inheritance is not typical of X-linked inheritance (Loesch & Hagerman, 2012). Fragile X occurs in about one in 5000 males and females can also be affected (Coffee *et al.*, 2009). Individuals with a repeated sequence of DNA (three nucleotides, called trinucleotide repeats) in the "premutation" range may present with a milder condition that includes premature ovarian failure, a neurodegenerative disorder in older adults, and fragile X-associated tremor/ataxia (Hagerman *et al.*, 2004). Other forms of X-linked ID are very heterogeneous and are therefore broadly classified into the syndromic forms, in which there is a recognizable and fairly consistent physical and behavioral phenotype, and the nonsyndromic forms, which are more variable and may not include features beyond ID (Chiurazzi *et al.*, 2008; Ropers, 2008).

Advances in molecular genetic methods have identified much smaller duplications and deletions of chromosomal regions, well below the resolution of light microscopy. Using these techniques, the underlying "*microdeletion*" was identified for Williams (deletion of 7q11.23) and Smith-Magenis syndromes (deletion of 17p12) (Mefford *et al.*, 2012). Subsequently, much smaller deletions and duplications, referred to as copy number variants (CNVs), have been identified in ID. With the current molecular genetic techniques, CNVs are thought to be causal in about 15% of children presenting with developmental delay and it is now proving useful to review patients with previously idiopathic ID, as genetic abnormalities are now revealed in a substantial minority (Mefford *et al.*, 2012). However, some CNVs will represent normal variation rather than a pathogenic mutation and this proportion will only increase as the techniques detect smaller variations. CNVs are more likely to be pathogenic when larger in size, when replicated across unrelated individuals with ID/developmental disorder, and when they occur *de novo* in a child whose parents are unaffected with ID. Craniofacial dysmorphisms often characterize the population in whom CNVs are identified (Ropers, 2010).

Imprinted disorders are ones in which the parental origin of the genetic abnormality alters the phenotype. Prader–Willi and Angelman syndromes are both due to abnormalities in the chromosomal region 15q11-13 but with very different phenotypes. The absence of a paternally derived copy of this region, whether through deletion or uniparental disomy, causes Prader–Willi syndrome, typically with mild ID. In contrast, Angelman syndrome, with severe to profound ID, is caused by deletion of the maternal region or a mutation in the UBE3A gene. Finally, a maternal duplication in this region is reported in 1–3% of patients with autism (Hogart *et al.*, 2010).

Other medical disorders associated with ID

A host of disorders that affect brain structure or function are associated with ID (see Chapter 31). Epilepsy is more common in people with ID and is related to its severity, occurring in about 7% of children with mild ID versus 35% with severe ID (Airaksinen *et al.*, 2000). Cerebral palsy and meningo-encephalitis are other medical causes. By definition, ID is diagnosed when impairment in cognitive function occurs during the "developmental period," leaving some ambiguity about the diagnostic classification of low IQ among those with early exposure to insults such as acquired brain injuries and exposures to toxins. However, these are important conditions to note from a public health perspective as they represent tractable targets in reducing low IQ.

Environmental factors

There is wide variation across countries in which environmental risks are most common. Premature birth and the impact of hypoxia continue to be a risk factor in all societies. In those with good neonatal care, cognitive outcomes are generally good for those born at 32 weeks gestation or later, while those who were very preterm or of very low birth weight are at increased risk of low IQ and ID (Marlow, 2004; Aylward, 2005). In low- and middle-income countries, obstetric complications currently account for about 10% of severe ID (Lundvall *et al.*, 2012). The care of high-risk neonates is constantly improving and outcome studies are by definition out of date, but in general as survival and major morbidity have improved, more subtle developmental problems have become more obvious. These include not only ID but also educational difficulties often related to specific cognitive impairments (Hutchinson *et al.*, 2013). The role of milder "obstetric suboptimality" as a causal risk factor is less clear; the observation that infants with Down and Prader–Willi syndromes have increased rates of obstetric complications highlights the role of fetal characteristics in the pregnancy. Obstetric problems are also seen when there has been poor antenatal care, which may arise from factors associated with immigrant status, social deprivation, and maternal ID/mental disorder.

Certain maternal infections during pregnancy, including toxoplasmosis, cytomegalovirus, rubella, and herpes, are well-recognized causes of infant morbidities, which include ID. Prenatal exposure to toxins is an important and potentially preventable risk. In societies where alcohol is freely available, this is the leading toxin cause of ID; fetal alcohol syndrome (FAS) occurs in 0.5–3 per 1000 births (May & Gossage, 2001) and accounts for as much as 3% of ID (O'Leary *et al.*, 2013). However, rates of FAS and FAS spectrum disorder also vary widely and diagnostic practice is a key factor. Rates are lower when the dual criteria of physical stigmata, such as the classical facies, and a history of heavy prenatal alcohol use are applied, than when only a history of heavy alcohol use in pregnancy is applied. The physical features are variable and sometimes subtle; it is likely that there is underdiagnosis under the former practice and overdiagnosis in the latter. Congenital hypothyroidism is detected with routine screening in one in 3000 pregnancies in high-income countries and is associated with both low IQ and ID (Grosse *et al.*, 2011). Newborn screening is important but suffers from false positive results (Buyukgebiz, 2006). Exposure to heavy metals such as arsenic and mercury during pregnancy and/or infancy is also associated with ID (McDermott *et al.*, 2012) while childhood lead exposure is a risk factor for low IQ and ID (Needleman *et al.*, 1990; Nevin, 2009). All these risk factors are considerably increased in low-income countries and will contribute to the increased rate of ID.

As described above, socioeconomic adversity is associated with increased rates of ID, but the mechanisms are complex and bidirectional. Severe and chronic social deprivation is a direct cause, as exemplified by the poor early institutional rearing experienced by the English Romanian adoptees (Rutter *et al.*, 2004). Grantham-McGregor and colleagues demonstrated the beneficial medium- and long-term effects of early childhood psychosocial stimulation on growth-retarded infants and children from several low-income countries, including Jamaica and Bangladesh (Gardner *et al.*, 2005; Walker *et al.*, 2006; Walker *et al.*, 2010). Interestingly, psychosocial stimulation was more effective than nutritional supplementation in improving both cognition and behavior (Gardner *et al.*, 2005; Walker *et al.*, 2006).

Biology-environmental interplay

As with other behavioral and cognitive phenotypes, many risk factors for ID increase susceptibility but are not deterministic. Hence, genetic mutations that are risk factors for ID can be inherited as well as occurring *de novo* in a child with ID. Zinc supplementation for malnourished children was most effective in improving cognition and coordination when administered alongside psychosocial stimulation (Gardner *et al.*, 2005). Similarly, the effects of prenatal alcohol exposure are not invariant, as demonstrated by a small (and statistically nonsignificant) twin study showing concordance for FAS among all five pairs of MZ but only seven of 11 DZ twin pairs (Streissguth & Dehaene, 1993). The same applies to preterm birth, where there is wide variability in cognitive outcomes (Moore *et al.*, 2012). The IQ of boys with Fragile X syndrome is significantly influenced by the quality of their home environment (Dyer-Friedman *et al.*, 2002). Clearly, a better understanding of the environmental mediators and moderators of biological risk has the potential to improve interventions for high-risk groups.

Assessment and diagnosis of intellectual disability

Early identification of ID provides the possibility for children to receive appropriate support from education, health, and social services. Parents often find a diagnosis aids their understanding of their child, especially if strengths as well as impairments are identified. Furthermore, if a genetic cause for ID is identified, it may influence family planning. In general, severe ID is identified early in life, while mild ID may not be recognized, particularly in the absence of additional medical problems. Therefore, clinicians should be alert to more subtle indicators, such as school nonattendance, poor academic performance, and immaturity of interests and behavior. School reports with information about attainments as well as behavior can be helpful. A common clinical error is to misattribute these warning signs to other factors, such as adverse early experiences, family stress, or other risk factors, and to fail to consider ID.

History

The history should consider intellectual development, to establish that the present level of functioning is consistent with that at an earlier age and that there is no history of regression. The gap between the achievements of a child with average intelligence and one with ID becomes more obvious with age, and parents of children with mild ID are often only aware of differences when their child starts school. Loss of skills or stasis in development during the first 3 years is common in autism, and indeed almost pathognomonic (Pickles *et al.*, 2009). However, a clear history of loss of skills after the age of 3 years should trigger referral to a pediatric neurologist for further investigation.

The history should also elicit any risk factors for ID, genetic, other medical, or environmental. A three-generation family history, including ID, and neurological and specific developmental disorders, should be obtained. ID may not have been formally diagnosed in relatives and questions should include difficulties with routine scholastic attainments and extra support required at school. The obstetric history should include prescribed and recreational drugs, alcohol and tobacco use, physical trauma, as well as any other indicators of suboptimality. A full medical history for the child should identify any neurological, neuromuscular or brain-based conditions such as epilepsy, cerebral palsy, or muscular dystrophy. General health problems are both more common in people with ID and also more likely to be overlooked (Allerton *et al.*, 2011). Enquiry should establish that hearing and vision have been assessed.

Educational history should identify the type of school attended and any additional academic and pastoral support received. Liaison with schools will ensure that academic and social support and expectations are appropriate. For older adolescents, plans for extended education and training (post statutory leaving age) should be identified.

Psychological assessment

In making the diagnosis of ID, a careful cognitive assessment is required. In the busy clinic, a pragmatic alternative may be to first undertake brief cognitive screening administered by a wide range of professionals. Care should be taken to ensure assessment is valid; with more behaviorally disturbed children, flexibility in approach is important. However, only a very small proportion of children are truly "untestable." Even when the diagnosis of ID is clear from the history and observation, a cognitive assessment at some stage is recommended because establishing cognitive level and strengths within the profile is often important in planning educational strategies and behavioral management.

The diagnosis of ID should only be given once low IQ and impairment in adaptive function are both established. The latter is often evident from the history and presentation. In other cases where it is less apparent, a structured review should focus on everyday functioning in the domains of communication, conceptual understanding, motor skills, self-care, and independence. Several standardized measures will quantify these characteristics (Sparrow *et al.*, 1984; Harrison & Oakland, 2003).

Physical examination and investigations

The role of the child psychiatrist in undertaking a physical examination and organizing appropriate investigations varies across health care systems. Regardless of local arrangements, child and adolescent mental health services may be the first to identify the presence of ID and will have responsibility for arranging for examination and investigations. A comprehensive physical examination is required, both to look for stigmata of underlying cause of ID and also to identify co-occurring health problems. Screening for impairments in hearing and vision should be undertaken in early childhood and repeated if there is suspicion of a problem. The presence of several dysmorphic features, particularly craniofacial dysmorphisms, are suggestive of an underlying genetic etiology (Caliskan *et al.*, 2005; Toriello, 2008). Common skin abnormalities of note include café au lait spots in neurofibromatosis and areas of depigmentation, detected by Wood's lamp, in tuberous sclerosis. Delayed motor coordination with some degree of clumsiness is common and may represent a nonspecific developmental immaturity. However, focal neurological signs suggest an additional condition that warrants further investigation. The diagnosis of epilepsy should be made by a specialist, on clinical grounds rather than on the basis of the electroencephalogram (EEG), which frequently reveals nonspecific abnormalities in people with ID (National Institute for Health and Care Excellence, 2012).

There is increasing consensus that genetic testing should be undertaken routinely in people with ID (Morrow, 2010; Ropers, 2010; Mefford *et al.*, 2012). The technology employed for such assessments is changing on an almost annual basis. Hence, at the time of writing, the favored technique is array comparative genome hybridization (array CGH), which picks up major chromosomal abnormalities as well as many CNVs. However, this is likely in the near future to be superseded by more sensitive measures. Genetic testing should be performed in conjunction with the regional specialist genetics center, to ensure the appropriate investigations and interpretation of any findings (see Chapter 24). Furthermore, the utility of retesting people in whom genetic tests were previously negative should be reviewed with specialist colleagues (Baker *et al.*, 2012b; Rauch *et al.*, 2012). Positive findings from genetic testing may not only identify risks for other family members but may also highlight associated features of a genetic syndrome where early intervention may be helpful, such as the more subtle cardiac problems in Noonan syndrome and 22q deletion syndrome.

Other universally agreed investigations, where no cause of ID has been established, include a full blood count, urea and electrolytes, creatine kinases, lead, thyroid function, urate, ferritin, and biotinidase (McDonald *et al.*, 2006). Recommendations regarding other investigations are less consistent. The rate of diagnostically meaningful findings from routine MRI scanning is 1% or less (McDonald *et al.*, 2006); it is recommended as a routine investigation in the United States (Michelson *et al.*, 2011) but not the United Kingdom (McDonald *et al.*, 2006). Routine metabolic screening is not recommended but should be considered in selected groups, including those from highly inbred populations or where there is parental consanguinity, an affected sibling, episodic de-compensation, suggestive dysmorphic features, ophthalmic abnormalities, and failure of growth (Shevell, 2008).

Longitudinal course of intellectual disability

Although ID typically involves a life-persistent diminution in cognitive function, there is considerable variability in the course and adaptive outcomes of individuals. Children who have experienced significant environmental deprivation may show substantial intellectual gains with appropriate environmental stimulation, including placement in typical families (Beckett *et al.*, 2006; Walker *et al.*, 2010). Across the population, while the broad aspects of a child's intellectual ability may be apparent in early childhood, prediction of later IQ from tests performed under the age of 6 years is poor (Anastasi & Urbina, 1997) and it is often best to wait until the child is in mid- to late-childhood to discuss long-term plans with parents and carers.

Over and above the age-related widening gap in cognition and skills, several disorders, including Down syndrome, fragile X and Williams syndrome, show a relative decline in IQ from childhood through adolescence and early adult life, including Alzheimer dementia in Down syndrome (Fisch *et al.*, 2007). NF1 is different, with cognitive skills continuing along the same trajectory. In contrast, one longitudinal assessment showed that adolescents with either autism or with Down syndrome continued to acquire new functional skills into the mid-20s (Hastings & Beck, 2004; Smith *et al.*, 2012a). Several tentative lessons emerge. First, the developmental pattern of cognitive ability may be disorder-specific. Second, daily living skills can continue to develop into adult life among those with ID. Third, trajectories for cognition and daily living skills may not run in parallel, and divergence may depend on the individual disorder.

Mortality is increased among those with severe to profound ID, with an overall excess of 2.5- to 3-fold (Tyrer & McGrother, 2009) and most common in early adulthood (Tyrer *et al.*, 2007). Central nervous system disorders, congenital anomalies, and mental disorders including dementia are particular risk factors, but most causes are increased in people with ID.

Behavioral phenotypes

The term "behavioral phenotype" refers to a relatively predictable set of behavioral and sometimes cognitive characteristics that occur in individuals with a known genetic abnormality (see Chapter 31). The individual features of behavioral phenotypes may be common or rare; what distinguishes these conditions is the typical *combination* of features and their association with a particular condition. This is useful for clinicians in predicting behaviors and preventing negative consequences, such as compulsive overeating with severe obesity in Prader–Willi syndrome. From the other direction, observing a characteristic pattern of behaviors may provoke specific genetic testing, leading to a diagnosis that is relevant to other family members. It should be noted that no behavioral phenotype is invariant; for example, schizophreniform psychosis occurs in only ~25% of people with 22q deletion syndrome (formerly referred to as velocardiofacial syndrome) (Murphy, 2005); however, no other single risk factor is so strongly associated with psychosis. Researchers are particularly interested in behavioral phenotypes because of the light they can shed on the biological pathways involved in gene-cognition-behavior links. Table 54.1

describes the most well-known behavioral phenotypes and their underlying etiology.

Mental disorders in children and adolescents with intellectual disability

Prevalence rates for psychiatric disorders in children and adolescents with ID are consistently increased 3- to 5-fold (Einfeld *et al.*, 2011). The entire range of psychiatric disorders is increased in ID (Dekker *et al.*, 2002; Emerson, 2003). However, the two greatest increases occur for children with ASD, of whom about 50% have ID (Charman *et al.*, 2011) and for attention deficit hyperactivity disorder (ADHD) where 15–20% have ID (Emerson, 2003; Simonoff *et al.*, 2007). Emotional and behavioral problems are roughly equally increased (about threefold) according to parent reports, but teacher ratings detect fewer emotional (about twofold increase) than behavioral problems (about threefold increase) (Dekker *et al.*, 2002; Emerson, 2003; Simonoff *et al.*, 2007).

Differences in psychiatric presentation among children with ID

As the degree of intellectual impairment increases, the risk for both ASD and ADHD increases (Gillberg *et al.*, 1986; Simonoff *et al.*, 2007). At the same time, differentiating specific psychiatric disorders becomes more difficult (Gillberg *et al.*, 1986) and eliciting a history and/or mental state that fulfills diagnostic criteria can be problematic. First, it may be difficult to identify symptoms that require the behavior to be inappropriate for developmental age, such as ASD or ADHD, in those with severe or profound ID. Second, the mental state is more difficult to examine in people with severe communication impairments, and informants may have limited insight into internal experiences. Third, some disorders include symptoms that require higher cognitive processes, such as hopelessness and helplessness in depression. For all these reasons, there has been a movement for a separate psychiatric classification with modified criteria for people with severe to profound ID and at least one system has been proposed for adults (Royal College of Psychiatrists, 2001).

The syndrome of "behavior that challenges": a distinct condition?

Although alternative classification systems have not gained widespread acceptance, terms such as "behavior that challenges" or "maladaptive behavior" are frequently used to describe a syndrome of problematic behavior that is relatively specific to people with ID and associated neurodevelopmental disorders such as ASD. Behavior that challenges refers to aggression directed at others or self, severe temper tantrums, destruction of property, and high levels of noncompliance. The lack of consensus regarding operational criteria hinders prevalence estimates, but most population-based studies report rates of ~10% in

Table 54.1 Behavioral phenotypes.

Name of condition	Genetic abnormality	Behavioral/cognitive features	Physical and other features
Down syndrome (Trisomy 21)	Additional chromosome 21 (95% of cases) or chromosomal translocation causing partial trisomy (~4%) or chromosomal mosaicism (~1%)	Wide IQ variation from low average to severe ID, mainly mild to moderate ID. Wide variety of behavior (in contrast to previous view of very sociable personality) Relative strength in social communication. Alzheimer disease in mid-to-late adulthood. Epilepsy in 5–10%	Classical dysmorphic features include epicanthal folds, upward-slanting palpebral fissures, Brushfield spots, and palmar crease

Wide and variable range including cardiac and gastrointestinal congenital anomalies, hearing loss secondary to impaired nasopharyngeal structures

Mild growth retardation. Increased rates of leukemia, hypothyroidism and altered immune function |
| Rett syndrome | X-linked mutation in MECP2 gene, affecting girls only as lethal in males | Normal early development with abnormalities beginning toward end of first year; some autistic symptoms, compulsive hand movements, hyperventilation. Often stabilizes in mid-to-late childhood with no further progression, bruxisms

Profound ID | Deceleration of head growth leading to microcephaly, short stature. Constipation and gastro-oesophageal reflux, prolonged QT interval on ECG, spasticity, seizures, ataxia |
| Lesch–Nyhan syndrome | X-linked mutation in hypoxanthine–guanine phosphoribosyltransferase gene | Low average to mild ID is typical, severe self-injurious behavior, typically compulsive biting of fingers and lips | Spastic cerebral palsy, choereoathetois, uric acid urinary stones |
| Cornelia de Lange syndrome | Marked genetic heterogeneity: 50% of cases with mutation in NIPBL gene but also cases with mutations in X-linked SMC1A gene, SMC3, CDLS4, RAD21, and HDAC8 (also X-linked). All involved in two systems pathways | Typically severe ID but variable IQ into normal range

Self-injurious behavior

Communication relatively impaired compared to adaptive function | Multiple and variable abnormalities but typical facial features include low anterior hairline, arched eyebrows, anteverted nares, maxillary prognathism, long philtrum, thin lips, and "carp" mouth

Prenatal and postnatal growth retardation

Ptosis, nystagmus and high myopia

Microcephaly

Gastro-oesophageal reflux in ~60%, hypothesized to be a cause of behavior that challenges |
| Fragile X Syndrome | X-linked expanding trinucleotide repeat in FMR1 gene, affecting males more commonly but also females

Fragile X tremor/ataxia syndrome caused by smaller size of expanded trinucleotide repeat | Variable level of ID, typically moderate to severe but including mild and borderline

Variable behavioral manifestations include hyperactivity and ADHD, poor eye contact and autistic features | Notable features include long face, large ears, and prominent jaw and macroorchidism, typically postpubertally |

Table 54.1 (*continued*)

Name of condition	Genetic abnormality	Behavioral/cognitive features	Physical and other features
Prader–Willi Syndrome	Caused by deletion or disruption of a gene or several genes on paternal chromosome 15 or maternal uniparental of same region. Overlapping clinical phenotype in chromosome 15q11-q13 duplication syndrome	Mild ID/borderline IQ. Excessive appetite in which food-seeking behavior can cause behavior that challenges. Excessive daytime sleepiness with sleep architecture abnormalities. Delayed motor milestones and speech difficulties. Skin-picking	Features include diminished fetal activity, neonatal hypotonia, subsequent obesity, muscular hypotonia, short stature, hypogonadotropic hypogonadism, and small hands and feet Depigmentation compared to family members
Angelman syndrome	~70% maternal deletions involving chromosome 15q11.2-q13 (same region as Prader-Willi); ~ 2% paternal uniparental disomy, 2–3% result from imprinting defects. Some of the remaining due to UBE3A gene mutations. protein ligase E3A gene (UBE3A; mutations in the MECP2 gene can present a similar phenotype)	Usually severe to profound ID with absence of speech, episodic paroxysmal laughter	Features include ataxia, hypotonia, epilepsy, unusual large mandible and open-mouthed expression revealing the tongue Frequent depigmentation relative to family members
22q deletion syndrome (previously Velocardiofacial Syndrome)	Deletion involving chromosome 22q11	Mild ID to borderline IQ is typical Childhood features include ADHD, autistic features. Mood swings are also common In adolescence/adulthood, ~25% develop schizophreniform psychosis	Highly variable but main features include cleft palate and cardiac anomalies. Typical facies involve marrow palpebral fissures, square nasal root. Less frequent features include microcephaly, short stature, slender hands and digits, minor auricular anomalies, and inguinal hernia
Smith-Magenis Syndrome	Deletion in chromosome 17p11	Severe ID is usual, often with additional speech delay. Typically includes severe self-injurious behavior, disruptive/aggressive outbursts, sleep disturbance, possibly with absence of REM sleep, hyperactivity, and ADHD may occur	Common features include broad flat face, brachycephaly, midface hypoplasia, prognathism, hoarse voice, and peripheral neuropathy
Williams syndrome	Deletion in chromosome 7q11.	Moderate ID to borderline IQ. Language acquisition delayed but subsequent superficially good expressive language with high sociability but a failure of social flexibility. Often anxious despite friendliness	Supravalvular aortic stenosis is common, Distinctive facies involve broad forehead, medial eyebrow flare, periorbital fullness, strabismus, stellate iris pattern, flat nasal bridge, malar flattening, full cheeks and lips, long smooth philtrum, pointed chin, wide mouth and dental deformities. Infantile hypercalcaemia is frequent as is a harsh, brassy voice

people with ID (Emerson *et al.*, 2001; McClintock *et al.*, 2003). It is not associated with other features of oppositional defiant or conduct disorder, such as spiteful or vindictive behavior, stealing or truanting. Furthermore, unlike oppositional defiant or conduct disorder, it does not appear to be associated with family adversity and rather shows person-specific correlates, including male sex, lower adaptive functioning, poor communication skills, a diagnosis of ASD and physical conditions causing pain (Emerson *et al.*, 2001; McClintock *et al.*, 2003). Furthermore, self-injury occurring in the context of behavior that challenges typically lacks the intentions associated with suicidal behavior or deliberate self-harm and often includes stereotypies, for example, head-banging, and/or sensory, for example, picking or biting elements.

Clinicians find the term useful because it highlights the need for different types of assessment and interventions. Applied behavior analysis (ABA) conceptualizes behavior that challenges in relation to learning theory, with maladaptive behaviors arising for a host of reasons but being reinforced, often inadvertently. While this is an important viewpoint, others are equally important. Certain genetic conditions, such as Prader–Willi and Cornelia de Lange syndromes, are particularly prone to show such behavior and the pattern of aggression/self-injury may vary, highlighting the role of biological factors (Petty & Oliver, 2005; Arron *et al.*, 2011). Recent research has expanded the causes of behavior that challenges to implicate a wide range of psychiatric disorders such as ADHD, anxiety, depression, and psychosis (Moss *et al.*, 2000; Tsiouris *et al.*, 2011), subdiagnostic traits such as low mood (Hayes *et al.*, 2011), poor impulse control (Burbidge *et al.*, 2010), and repetitive/stereotyped behaviors (Oliver *et al.*, 2012). Any condition causing pain or discomfort may cause behavior that challenges, including chronic physical disorders, acute infection or inflammation, and adverse effects of treatments (McGuire *et al.*, 2010; Oliver & Richards, 2010).

Risk factors for psychiatric disorders in ID

Several mechanisms are involved in explaining the increased risk for psychiatric disorders in children with ID. First, a number of risk factors are *shared* between ID and psychiatric disorder, contributing to their co-occurrence. *Genetic* risk factors have been linked to autism, ADHD, and ID. Twin studies of general population samples report moderate genetic correlations between lower IQ and ADHD (Kuntsi *et al.*, 2004) and somewhat smaller between low IQ and ASD traits (Hoekstra *et al.*, 2009). Molecular genetic studies have identified the same CNVs in samples selected for ADHD, ASD, and/or ID (Morrow, 2010; Williams *et al.*, 2010; Mefford *et al.*, 2012). A host of *medical* adversities, such as epilepsy, cerebral palsy, and acquired brain injury, that affect brain structure and/or function predispose to both ID and psychiatric disorder. In both these cases, it is likely that the shared risk factors are having their effects primarily if not exclusively directly at the level of brain function, with ID

and psychiatric disorder being pleiotropic effects of the same risk factors/insults.

With respect to emotional and behavioral disorders, the greater family-based psychosocial adversity, indexed by reduced parental educational qualifications, lower socioeconomic status, and family poverty, partially but not fully accounts for the higher rate of psychiatric problems (Emerson & Hatton, 2007c; Emerson *et al.*, 2010a). As with medical/genetic factors, these psychosocial factors are known to be present before or shortly after the child's birth and therefore are unlikely to be caused by ID. However, the direction of effect is less clear with respect to the increased psychopathology (Dekker & Koot, 2003) and physical symptoms of stress reported in parents of children with ID (Smith *et al.*, 2012b). Some studies indicate parental psychiatric disorder is largely accounted for by family psychosocial adversity (Emerson *et al.*, 2010b) while others report that child behavior problems are a strong predictor of maternal distress (Hastings & Beck, 2004; Totsika *et al.*, 2011).

ID itself may increase the risk of psychiatric disorder. Decreased ability to communicate personal needs, understand the environment, and respond flexibly to varying situations may cause anxiety or oppositional, noncompliant behavior. Exposure to a range of additional adversities is increased in ID, including physical illness (Emerson & Hatton, 2007a), high parental expressed emotion (Beck *et al.*, 2004), peer relationship problems (Larkin *et al.*, 2012), and negative life events (Dekker and Koot, 2003; Owen *et al.*, 2004), including abuse and neglect (Horner-Johnson & Drum, 2006). The direction of effects among these associations, however, is poorly understood, and it is possible that some adversities are increased in response to difficult behavior, although this exposure may further increase behavioral problems.

Assessment of psychiatric disorders in people with ID

Many aspects of assessment and treatment overlap with those discussed in relation to individual disorders and what follows are the particular considerations that are distinctive in children with ID. Assessment should place developmental considerations at the core. It is essential to have a good understanding of a child's cognitive function, level and style of communication, and adaptive function to contextualize the patterns of behavior and emotions. If a formal cognitive assessment has not previously been undertaken, it should ordinarily be completed at this stage. The parent/carer's understanding of the child's level of functioning, the pattern and complexity of communication with the child, and the appropriateness of the educational placement should be identified. Enquiry about psychiatric symptoms should elicit specific descriptions, as many of the behaviors may be atypical. Emotional symptoms may be more difficult to identify when the child's communication ability is significantly impaired, and in such instances, observable features of emotional disorders should be a prime focus. As in other populations, accounts of behavior in different contexts and a personal interview and/or direct observation of the child are essential. Judgments about the presence of symptoms should be made in the context of developmental (rather than chronological) age.

While the assessment should aim to identify psychiatric disorders as treatment targets, it should not exclude other causes of disturbed behavior, as described under behavior that challenges. The assessment should ascertain the presence of eating/feeding and sleeping problems, the role of coexisting physical disorders, especially brain-based disorders such as epilepsy, but also conditions that may cause pain, the presence of parental learning problems/ID and parental stress, psychosocial adversity, and support from statutory and voluntary services.

Assessing behavior in its context

A key element in the evaluation of behavior that challenges is the assessment of triggers or precipitants and reinforcement of maladaptive behaviors. Applied behavioral analysis is a rigorous, detailed, and quasi-experimental approach used by trained specialists, in the context of learning theory to understand the causes and modify the environment in order to reduce maladaptive behavior. In contrast, functional behavior assessment is a fundamental skill for all clinicians working in the field, to generate hypotheses about triggers and consequences that may provoke and reinforce behaviors. This involves obtaining a history of the antecedents and context, a detailed description of the behaviors and the response of others, both immediate and longer-term. Different behaviors should be evaluated separately. Information should include the effect of different settings, whether the onset was acute or insidious, and the relation to environmental changes or life events, whether there has been a change over time and, if so, whether it has been gradual or abrupt. When behavioral changes are sudden, particular consideration should be given to environmental changes, life events, physical conditions causing pain, and adverse effects of medication.

Assessment measures for psychiatric symptoms and disorders in ID

Many questionnaires and interviews designed for children of average ability are suitable in their *content* for children with mild ID. However, almost none of these has been normed on populations with ID and therefore use of the scores and cut-offs may not be valid (Simonoff *et al.*, 2013a). Standardized questionnaires may either exaggerate symptoms, for example, in children whose level of ID has not been recognized, or provide an underestimate, for example, when completed in specialist settings where most children have psychiatric problems. Therefore, they should be seen as an aid to comprehensive data-gathering and should not be used to rule in/exclude diagnosis.

In children with severe to profound ID, measures developed for the general population are often not suitable and instruments designed specifically for use in populations with ID are preferred. Several are widely used (Aman, 1986) and the Developmental Behavior Checklist in particular is both comprehensive in coverage and provides norms and subscales for the population with ID (Einfeld, 1995). Standardized child psychiatric diagnostic interviews, most commonly used in research, have not been modified for children with ID, although the Kiddie-SADS has been altered for people with ASD (Leyfer *et al.*, 2006). In general, the interviewer-based measures are sufficiently flexible to have face validity for populations with ID but will not include ID-specific behaviors. Typically developing younger children often have difficulty understanding key concepts in standardized interviews (Breton *et al.*, 1995) and this applies to a wider age range of people with ID, so informants are used more extensively. Strategies employed in assessing younger children (e.g., simpler language, visual prompts, checking understanding of concepts) are appropriate here. Tools specific for people with ID include the suite of measures comprising the Psychiatric Assessment Schedule for Adults with Developmental Disorders (PAS-ADD) (Moss *et al.*, 1998); these are designed to identify psychiatric conditions in adults, including affective and psychotic disorders. While intended for use with adults, their structure is useful in gathering accounts about behaviors that may indicate a severe mental disorder.

Other measures are available to assess behavior that challenges. The Challenging Behavior Interview measures the range, severity, and frequency of such behaviors (Oliver *et al.*, 2003). Both the Aberrant Behavior Checklist and Developmental Behavior Checklist have reported scores and subscales that are associated with behaviors that challenge (Einfeld & Tonge, 2002; Aman *et al.*, 2010). Other measures such as the Questions about Behavioral Function (Matson *et al.*, 1999) structure the functional behavioral assessment that aims to identify triggers for and consequences of behavior that challenges, which may increase its frequency or severity.

Differential diagnosis

There are two particular considerations with respect to differential diagnosis in people with ID. Developmental age should be considered in deciding whether symptoms are present, as behaviors may be abnormal for chronological but not for developmental age. On the other hand, care should be taken not to inappropriately ascribe psychiatric symptoms to ID itself, the well-documented process of "diagnostic overshadowing" (Jopp & Keys, 2001). This is best achieved by gaining careful accounts with behavioral descriptions and avoiding attributions.

Physical examination and investigations

If ID has not previously been diagnosed, the examination should include those elements that may identify an underlying cause, which may also shed light on psychopathology. With respect to behavior that challenges, examination should look for possible causes of pain and adverse drug effects, such as akathisia or Parkinsonism. If treatment will involve pharmacotherapy, it is timely to evaluate for any physical contraindications, as people with ID are more likely to have congenital anomalies and other conditions that may limit therapeutic options.

Intervention

Most clinical trials have excluded those with ID, leaving a small evidence base. Treatment planning should ordinarily therefore follow recommendations for children of average ability. Behavioral interventions for challenging behavior, based on ABA principles, are often effective (Brosnan & Healy, 2011), although there is a very limited evidence base exploring when they should be used in combination with other approaches such as pharmacology (Brosnan & Healy, 2011). Psychological interventions for the emotional disorders in those with mild-to-moderate ID have not been adequately evaluated; using first principles, modifications should simplify language, reduce the need for abstract thinking, include visual materials, and review progress more regularly. Greater involvement of parents/carers is often helpful. In children with severe to profound ID or developmental age under about 7 years, behavioral interventions that are delivered by parents/carers and other adults are likely to be more effective. Principles should include clearly described, visually depicted expectations and reinforcers that are activated immediately when the behavior occurs, usually with short-term effects. It is important to identify reinforcers for the individual child, rather than relying on more generally used rewards and sanctions. For behaviors that occur in multiple settings, it is essential that a consistent approach is adopted in all domains.

Parents' needs should be addressed as there is a likely reciprocal relationship between child psychopathology and parental mental health and stress (Baker et al., 2012a; Smith et al., 2012b). Psychoeducation should be standard. The potential negative impact on siblings should also be considered (Neece et al., 2010). Parents report wanting support, which may be provided by specific parent groups, and respite care, particularly when their child has mental health problems (Douma et al., 2006).

With respect to pharmacotherapy, there is a small but consistent evidence base for treatment of ADHD in children with ID (Aman et al., 2003; Simonoff et al., 2013b) reporting reduced but significant effect sizes and higher rates of adverse effects. Medication should therefore commence at low doses with slow increases and frequent monitoring for both positive and adverse effects, wherever possible using rating scales. Children with ASD may be particularly sensitive to adverse effects but nevertheless can also experience benefit (Research Units on Pediatric Psychopharmacology (RUPP) Autism Network, 2005; Simonoff et al., 2013b). Most of the trials assessing the use of antipsychotics in ASD include children with ID (Aman et al., 2005; Marcus et al., 2009); although the results have not been stratified for IQ, it is reasonable to consider that risperidone

and aripiprazole can significantly improve irritable, aggressive behavior in this group. One trial comparing risperidone alone and with parent training showed that the combined intervention led to the use of lower doses of medication and slightly greater behavioral improvement than risperidone alone (Scahill et al., 2012). The results need replication and generalization to other treatments, but provide an appealing model for multimodal intervention. In the absence of an evidence base for pharmacological interventions in other disorders, clinicians should use the principles described above for stimulants.

As multiple psychiatric problems/disorders are frequent in people with ID, polypharmacy (the excessive use of multiple medications) is common (Holden et al., 2004; Haw & Stubbs, 2005; Tobi et al., 2005). However, it should be avoided whenever possible because of the increased susceptibility to adverse drug effects. Several steps may help minimize the use of multiple drugs. First, the target symptoms should be carefully identified, prioritized for treatment, and linked to an underlying psychiatric disorder or evidence-based intervention. Second, baseline information on severity, frequency, and duration should be obtained, using either a standardized or bespoke measure. Regular monitoring of change should use the same scale, along with a systematic enquiry about adverse effects. If no or inadequate response occurs, compliance should first be checked and consideration given to whether the dose can be increased. In evaluating possible adverse effects, the clinician needs to balance up the increased susceptibility of this population against variation in the client's behavior; certain potential adverse effects, such as irritability, aggression, and mood changes, may reflect variation in the child's behavior for other reasons. When treatment response remains inadequate despite therapeutic doses, the diagnostic hypothesis should be reviewed before initiating an alternative medication.

Other nonspecific elements of intervention for children with ID include enhancement of communication, adaptive function, and social skills, which, in adults, can improve community participation (Woolf et al., 2010). These are often best undertaken in the school setting. The suitability of the educational placement should be considered, with a view to whether it is meeting both academic and emotional/behavioral needs, and whether the school is able to support the recommended interventions. Arrangements vary both locally and nationally, but all children with ID and a psychiatric disorder should have additional educational support. The overwhelming majority of children with severe/profound ID will be best placed in specialist schools catering for their educational and mental health needs.

Input from social services and the voluntary sector should also be addressed in the management plan. The needs of children and their families for respite care vary widely but families should be aware of the range of options. Often, voluntary organizations, including disorder-specific societies, offer a range of information and support for both parents and children. Social care and voluntary agencies may also help by increasing access to community activities for children and young people with ID.

Mental health services for children and adolescents with ID

The successful delivery of mental health services for children and adolescents with ID depends not only on the expertise of mental health clinicians within that service but also on the configuration of supporting health, education, and social services. Different models operate across and within national boundaries (Anagnostopoulos & Soumaki, 2011; Ispanovic-Radojkovic & Stancheva-Popkostadinova, 2011, Kwok *et al.*, 2011; Lin & Lin, 2011) and there is an absence of research that identifies preferred service models. However, some principles can be distilled to guide service organization. First, the rights of people with disability to equal access to services (among other rights) has been established in a large number of documents, including the Human Rights Act (1998) and the World Report on Disability (Emerson, 2012), as well as national documents such as the United Kingdom's National Service Framework (Department of Health, 2004). Second, approximately 15% of the child and adolescent population with mental disorders have ID, most of which are mild (Emerson & Hatton, 2007b), constituting a significant minority of those requiring provision. Furthermore, in many (but not all) countries, children and adolescents with mild ID attend mainstream schools and the links that services have with local schools would equally apply to children with ID. Third, the population requiring highly specialist mental health services are those with significant communication problems, severe or profound ID, unusual behavioral phenotypes and significant behavior that challenges, which is a much smaller group. Fourth, the effective function of mental health services for this population requires collaborative relationships with services in physical health, education, and social services, as well as adult mental health (both with respect to transitional arrangements for adolescents and also to provide services for parents). Fifth, consideration should be given to the accessibility of inpatient psychiatric units with the professional skills and appropriate environment to assess and treat patients with significant levels of ID. In units without these qualities, children and adolescents are often misdiagnosed, for example, as having a psychotic disorder when their communication is idiosyncratic or difficult to understand. Sixth, while there are no agreed standards, the mental health services should include professionals from a range of backgrounds and trained to work with children and adolescents with ID; psychiatry and psychology and psychiatric nursing/behavior therapy are essential for outpatient care and there should be access to team members who have the skills to work with families and speech/language and occupational therapists. In terms of wider relationships, mental health services should develop links with paediatricians, clinical geneticists, physiotherapists, specialist teachers/educational psychologists and social workers. Seventh, the model of care often practiced in mental health services, in which treatment for an episode of illness is followed by discharge, may not be optimal for children with ID, whose mental health problems can be chronic. Some children and their families may benefit from predictable reviews, even if these are infrequent. Eighth, in a climate of inclusion and de-institutionalization, day and residential education and care in specialist settings should not be viewed necessarily as indicating a failure of services; rather the focus should be on reducing behavioral and psychiatric disorder and optimizing well-being and quality of life for the child and family. Specialist care may be the best choice for children with significant ID and/or behavior that challenges, when both child and family-wide outcomes are considered (Brown *et al.*, 2011).

Special issues in mental health and ID

Children and adolescents with ID and the criminal justice system

The literature on prevalence of ID among adult prisoners is generally of low quality and mixed in its findings (Fazel *et al.*, 2008); in contrast, one birth cohort study clearly demonstrates increased criminality among adults with ID (Hodgins, 1992). Systematic studies of young people in the criminal justice system report that youth with IQs in the mild ID and borderline range are overrepresented (Farrington & Loeber, 2000; Herrington, 2009), although rates of identification vary widely (Hodgins, 1992; Sondenaa *et al.*, 2008; see Chapter 49). It appears that those with more severe ID are protected by greater levels of community supervision, a reduced range of activities and social interaction, and also by intervention from carers when they come into contact with the criminal justice system (Lyall *et al.*, 1995). Factors associated with ID that probably increase the likelihood of juvenile offending include behavioral problems and autistic symptoms (Douma *et al.*, 2007; Geluk *et al.*, 2012), as well as the increased likelihood of detection.

Young people with ID are also more likely to be the victims of crime (Petersilia, 2001) and other forms of maltreatment (Horner-Johnson & Drum, 2006; Turner *et al.*, 2011). Furthermore, they are perceived as poor witnesses and as being more suggestible (Gudjonsson & Henry, 2003; Manzanero *et al.*, 2012), and this may influence the willingness of authorities to prosecute.

Parents with ID and their parenting

With changing attitudes to disability, de-institutionalization, and the Human Rights Act, many societies now recognize the desire of adults with ID to become parents and are beginning to investigate their needs and those of their children (O'Keeffe & O'Hara, 2008). Estimated rates of ID among parents vary widely and formal identification is likely to prove an underestimate (Department of Health and Department for Education and Skills, 2007; Weiber *et al.*, 2011), Most research involves families who have come to the attention of services, so generalizability of the findings is uncertain. These studies indicate increased risk of neglect among children (Feldman, 2002). Parents with ID have high rates of psychopathology and previous childhood abuse and trauma (McGaw *et al.*, 2007) and these factors are linked to professional concern about their parenting (McGaw *et al.*, 2010; Azar *et al.*, 2012; see Chapter 28). Mothers with ID may also be more prone to have antisocial (often without ID) male partners (McGaw *et al.*, 2010).

Once concerns have reached the judicial system, children are more likely to be removed from their birth parents and subsequently placed for adoption (Booth & Booth, 2004). Recent modifications of parent training programs to meet the needs of parents with ID have been evaluated and early results are promising (Coren *et al.*, 2010; see Chapter 37).

Future developments and necessary research

Research and clinical advances in ID have lagged behind those in other areas of child and adolescent psychiatry. There has been a tendency to assume "one size fits all" and that clinical advances in other areas can be directly applied to children with ID; where the evidence is available, this is not at all the case. Substantial work is required in all domains to reach the same level of care for this population, but key priorities can be identified.

Prevention of ID and service development in low- and middle-income countries

While considerable progress has been made in high-income countries in prevention and early intervention to reduce the incidence of ID, many of these advances have not been translated into care in poorer countries, which are actually less well-equipped to support people with ID. However, research suggests that such programs, for example, to provide genetic screening and improve obstetric optimality, can be delivered and are successful in reducing ID (Dave *et al.*, 2005). Research should focus on effective and cost-effective prevention strategies.

Improved tools for assessing mental disorder in ID and quantifying outcome

There are few available validated measures of psychopathology for those with ID, which limits other clinical and scientific advances. The problem is most acute in relation to self-report measures, for unusual behaviors, and in measuring outcomes. Furthermore, many of the currently available measures do not map well to recognized mental disorders and therefore are not helpful in guiding intervention. Efforts should include developing and modifying instruments that are aligned with recognized conditions and allow evaluation of treatment response. As diagnostic and predictive biomarkers become available, these may be particularly useful in populations with ID and therefore need evaluation in this group.

Interventions trialed for children and adolescents with ID

The current state of affairs, in which the accruing literature on treatment efficacy and effectiveness excludes people with ID, is unacceptable, given that this group represents 15% of the mental health burden. Pharmacological trials indicate significantly reduced effect sizes for conventional interventions in children with ID but the reasons for this are unclear. More experimental approaches to pharmacological trials (e.g., different treatments) can help understand this phenomenon. Psychological interventions need modification and robust testing (including blinded outcome measures).

New technologies and ID

Developments in computer technology make the software increasingly flexible and easy to use. The modification and development of software for people with ID could enhance their communication, promote independence and adaptive function, and complement educational methods.

Treating ID: how far away are we?

The genetic advances over the past two decades in identifying causes of ID have been immense. The gap is closing between gene identification, understanding of function, and intervention and promising early work with animal models will eventually translate into treatments for humans. Although ID is especially challenging for intervention, this area holds promise for conditions caused by single mutations.

References

Airaksinen, E.M. *et al.* (2000) A population-based study on epilepsy in mentally retarded children. *Epilepsia* **41**, 1214–1220.

Allerton, L.A. *et al.* (2011) Health inequalities experienced by children and young people with intellectual disabilities: a review of literature from the United Kingdom. *Journal of Intellectual Disabilities* **15**, 269–278.

Aman, M. (1986) *Aberrant Behavior Checklist - Community*. Slosson Educational Publications, Inc., New York.

Aman, M.G. *et al.* (2003) Methylphenidate treatment in children with borderline IQ and mental retardation: analysis of three aggregated studies. *Journal of Child & Adolescent Psychopharmacology* **13**, 29–40.

Aman, M.G. *et al.* (2005) Acute and long-term safety and tolerability of risperidone in children with autism. *Journal of Child & Adolescent Psychopharmacology* **15**, 869–884.

Aman, M.G. *et al.* (2010) Line-item analysis of the Aberrant Behavior Checklist: results from two studies of aripiprazole in the treatment of irritability associated with autistic disorder. *Journal of Child & Adolescent Psychopharmacology* **20**, 415–422.

Anagnostopoulos, D.C. & Soumaki, E. (2011) Perspectives of intellectual disability in Greece: epidemiology, policy, services for children and adults. *Current Opinion in Psychiatry* **24**, 425–430.

Anastasi, A. & Urbina, S. (1997) *Psychological Testing*. Prentice Hall, Upper Saddle River, New Jersey.

Arron, K. *et al.* (2011) The prevalence and phenomenology of self-injurious and aggressive behaviour in genetic syndromes. *Journal of Intellectual Disability Research* **55**, 109–120.

Australian Institute of Health and Welfare & O'Rance, L. (2007) Intellectual disability in Australia's Aboriginal and Torres Strait Islander peoples. *Journal of Intellectual & Developmental Disability* **32**, 222–225.

Aylward, G.P. (2005) Neurodevelopmental outcomes of infants born prematurely. *Journal of Developmental & Behavioral Pediatrics* **26**, 427–440.

Azar, S.T. *et al.* (2012) Intellectual disabilities and neglectful parenting: preliminary findings on the role of cognition in parenting risk. *Journal of Mental Health Research in Intellectual Disabilities* **5**, 94–129.

Baker, J.K. *et al.* (2012a) Behaviour problems, maternal internalising symptoms and family relations in families of adolescents and adults with fragile X syndrome. *Journal of Intellectual Disability Research* **56**, 984–995.

Baker, K. *et al.* (2012b) Genetic investigation for adults with intellectual disability: opportunities and challenges. *Current Opinion in Neurology* **25**, 150–158.

Beck, A. *et al.* (2004) Mothers' expressed emotion towards children with and without intellectual disabilities. *Journal of Intellectual Disability Research* **48**, 628–638.

Beckett, C. *et al.* (2006) Do the effects of early severe deprivation on cognition persist into early adolescence? Findings from the English and Romanian adoptees study. *Child Development* **77**, 696–711.

Booth, T. & Booth, W. (2004) Findings from a court study of care proceedings involving parents with intellectual disabilities. *Journal of Policy and Practice in Intellectual Disabilities* **1**, 179–181.

Breton, J.J. *et al.* (1995) Do children aged 9 through 11 years understand the DISC Version 2.25 questions? *Journal of the American Academy of Child and Adolescent Psychiatry* **34**, 946–954.

Broman, S. *et al.* (1987) *Retardation in Young Children: A Developmental Study of Cognitive Deficit*. Lawrence Erlbaum Associates, Hillsdale, NJ.

Brooks-Gunn, J. & Duncan, G.J. (1997) The effects of poverty on children and youth. *Future of Children* **7**, 55–71.

Brosnan, J. & Healy, O. (2011) A review of behavioral interventions for the treatment of aggression in individuals with developmental disabilities. *Research in Developmental Disabilities* **32**, 437–446.

Brown, R.I. *et al.* (2011) Family life and the impact of previous and present residential and day care support for children with major cognitive and behavioural challenges: a dilemma for services and policy. *Journal of Intellectual Disability Research* **55**, 904–917.

Bundey, S. *et al.* (1989) The recurrence risk for mild idiopathic mental retardation. *Journal of Medical Genetics* **26**, 260–266.

Burbidge, C. *et al.* (2010) The association between repetitive behaviours, impulsivity and hyperactivity in people with intellectual disability. *Journal of Intellectual Disability Research* **54**, 1078–1092.

Buyukgebiz, A. (2006) Newborn screening for congenital hypothyroidism. *Journal of Pediatric Endocrinology* **19**, 1291–1298.

Caliskan, M.O. *et al.* (2005) Subtelomeric chromosomal rearrangements detected in patients with idiopathic mental retardation and dysmorphic features. *Genetic Counseling* **16**, 129–138.

Calvin, C.M. *et al.* (2012) Multivariate genetic analyses of cognition and academic achievement from two population samples of 174,000 and 166,000 school children. *Behavior Genetics* **42**, 699–710.

Charman, T. *et al.* (2011) IQ in children with autism spectrum disorders: data from the SNAP project. *Psychological Medicine* **41**, 619–627.

Cherny, S.S. *et al.* (1992) Differential heritability across levels of cognitive ability. *Behavior Genetics* **22**, 153–162.

Chiurazzi, P. *et al.* (2008) XLMR genes: update 2007. *European Journal of Human Genetics* **16**, 422–434.

Coffee, B. *et al.* (2009) Incidence of fragile X syndrome by newborn screening for methylated FMR1 DNA. *American Journal of Human Genetics* **85**, 503–514.

Coren, E. *et al.* (2010) Parent training support for intellectually disabled parents. *Cochrane Database of Systematic Reviews* **6**, CD007987.

Croen, L.A. *et al.* (2001) The epidemiology of mental retardation of unknown cause. *Pediatrics* **107**, e86.

Dave, U. *et al.* (2005) A community genetics approach to population screening in India for mental retardation – a model for developing countries. *Annals of Human Biology* **32**, 195–203.

Dekker, M.C. & Koot, H.M. (2003) DSM-IV disorders in children with borderline to moderate intellectual disability II: child and family predictors. *Journal of American Academy of Child and Adolescent Psychiatry* **42**, 923–931.

Dekker, M.C. *et al.* (2002) Emotional and behavioral problems in children and adolescents with and without intellectual disability. *Journal of Child Psychology & Psychiatry & Allied Disciplines* **43**, 1087–1098.

Department of Health (2004) *Disabled Child Standard, National Service Framework for Children, Young People and Maternity Services*. Department of Health, London.

Department of Health and Department for Education and Skills (2007) *Good practice Guidance on Working with Parents with an Intellectual Disability*. DH/DfES, London.

Douma, J.C. *et al.* (2006) Supporting parents of youths with intellectual disabilities and psychopathology. *Journal of Intellectual Disability Research* **50**, 570–581.

Douma, J.C. *et al.* (2007) Antisocial and delinquent behaviors in youths with mild or borderline disabilities. *American Journal of Mental Retardation* **112**, 207–220.

Drews, C.D. *et al.* (1995) Variation in the influence of selected sociodemographic risk factors for mental retardation. *American Journal of Public Health* **85**, 329–334.

Dyer-Friedman, J. *et al.* (2002) Genetic and environmental influences on the cognitive outcomes of children with fragile X syndrome. *Journal of the American Academy of Child & Adolescent Psychiatry* **41**, 237–244.

Einfeld, S.L. (1995) The developmental behavior checklist: the development and validation of an instrument to assess behavioral and emotional disturbance in children and adolescents with mental retardation. *Journal of Autism and Developmental Disorders* **25**, 81–104.

Einfeld, S.L. & Tonge, B.J. (2002) *Manual for the Developmental Behaviour Checklist*. University of New South Wales and Monash University, Sydney.

Einfeld, S.L. *et al.* (2011) Comorbidity of intellectual disability and mental disorder in children and adolescents: a systematic review. *Journal of Intellectual & Developmental Disability* **36**, 137–143.

Emerson, E. (2003) Prevalence of psychiatric disorders in children and adolescents with and without intellectual disabilities. *Journal of Intellectual Disability Research* **47**, 51–58.

Emerson, E. (2012) The World report on disability. *Journal of Applied Research in Intellectual Disabilities* **25**, 495–496.

Emerson, E. & Hatton, C. (2007a) Contribution of socioeconomic position to health inequalities of British children and adolescents with intellectual disabilities. *American Journal of Mental Retardation* **112**, 140–150.

Emerson, E. & Hatton, C. (2007b) Mental health of children and adolescents with intellectual disabilities in Britain. *British Journal of Psychiatry* **191**, 493–499.

Emerson, E. & Hatton, C. (2007c) Poverty, socio-economic position, social capital and the health of children and adolescents with intellectual disabilities in Britain: a replication. *Journal of Intellectual Disability Research* **51**, 866–874.

Emerson, E. *et al.* (2001) The prevalence of challenging behaviors: a total population study. *Research in Developmental Disabilities* **22**, 77–93.

Emerson, E. *et al.* (2006) Socio-economic position, household composition, health status and indicators of the well-being of mothers of children with and without intellectual disabilities. *Journal of Intellectual Disability Research* **50**, 862–873.

Emerson, E. *et al.* (2010a) The mental health of young children with intellectual disabilities or borderline intellectual functioning. *Social Psychiatry & Psychiatric Epidemiology* **45**, 579–587.

Emerson, E. *et al.* (2010b) Socioeconomic circumstances and risk of psychiatric disorders among parents of children with early cognitive delay. *American Journal on Intellectual & Developmental Disabilities* **115**, 30–42.

Farrington, D.P. & Loeber, R. (2000) Epidemiology of juvenile violence. *Child & Adolescent Psychiatric Clinics of North America* **9**, 733–748.

Fazel, S. *et al.* (2008) The prevalence of intellectual disabilities among 12,000 prisoners - a systematic review. *International Journal of Law & Psychiatry* **31**, 369–373.

Felce, D. & Emerson, E. (2001) Living with support in a home in the community: predictors of behavioral development and household and community activity. *Mental Retardation & Developmental Disabilities Research Reviews* **7**, 75–83.

Feldman, M.A. (2002) *Children of Parents with Intellectual Disabilities.* Kluwer Academic/Plenum Publishers, New York, NY.

Fisch, G.S. *et al.* (2007) Studies of age-correlated features of cognitive-behavioral development in children and adolescents with genetic disorders. *American Journal of Medical Genetics Part A* **143A**, 2478–2489.

Gardner, J.M. *et al.* (2005) Zinc supplementation and psychosocial stimulation: effects on the development of undernourished Jamaican children. *American Journal of Clinical Nutrition* **82**, 399–405.

Geluk, C.A. *et al.* (2012) Autistic symptoms in childhood arrestees: longitudinal association with delinquent behavior. *Journal of Child Psychology & Psychiatry & Allied Disciplines* **53**, 160–167.

Gillberg, C. *et al.* (1986) Psychiatric disorders in mildly and severely mentally retarded urban children and adolescents: epidemiological aspects. *British Journal Of Psychiatry* **149**, 68–74.

Grosse, S.D. *et al.* (2011) Prevention of intellectual disability through screening for congenital hypothyroidism: how much and at what level? *Archives of Disease in Childhood* **96**, 374–379.

Gudjonsson, G.H. & Henry, L. (2003) Child and adult witnesses with intellectual disability: the importance of suggestibility. *Legal and Criminological Psychology* **8**, 241–252.

Gustavson, K.-H. (2005) Prevalence and aetiology of congenital birth defects, infant mortality and mental retardation in Lahore, Pakistan: a prospective cohort study. *Acta Paediatrica* **94**, 769–774.

Hagerman, R.J. *et al.* (2004) Fragile-X-associated tremor/ataxia syndrome (FXTAS) in females with the FMR1 premutation. *American Journal of Human Genetics* **74**, 1051–1056.

Harrison, P. & Oakland, T. (2003) *Adaptive Behavior Assessment System ® (ABAS) Oxford.* Pearson.

Hastings, R.P. & Beck, A. (2004) Practitioner review: stress intervention for parents of children with intellectual disabilities. *Journal of Child Psychology and Psychiatry* **45**, 1338–1349.

Haw, C. & Stubbs, J. (2005) A survey of off-label prescribing for inpatients with mild intellectual disability and mental illness. *Journal of Intellectual Disability Research* **49**, 858–864.

Hayes, S. *et al.* (2011) Low mood and challenging behaviour in people with severe and profound intellectual disabilities. *Journal of Intellectual Disability Research* **55**, 182–189.

Herrington, V. (2009) Assessing the prevalence of intellectual disability among young male prisoners. *Journal of Intellectual Disability Research* **53**, 397–410.

Hodgins, S. (1992) Mental disorder, intellectual deficiency, and crime. Evidence from a birth cohort. *Archives of General Psychiatry* **49**, 476–483.

Hoekstra, R.A. *et al.* (2009) Association between extreme autistic traits and intellectual disability: insights from a general population twin study. [Erratum appears in *British Journal of Psychiatry.* 2010;197(1):77]. *British Journal of Psychiatry* **195**, 531–536.

Hogart, A. *et al.* (2010) The comorbidity of autism with the genomic disorders of chromosome 15q11.2-q13. *Neurobiology of Disease* **38**, 181–191.

Holden, B. *et al.* (2004) Psychotropic medication in adults with mental retardation: prevalence, and prescription practices. *Research in Developmental Disabilities* **25**, 509–521.

Horner-Johnson, W. & Drum, C.E. (2006) Prevalence of maltreatment of people with intellectual disabilities: a review of recently published research. *Mental Retardation & Developmental Disabilities Research Reviews* **12**, 57–69.

Hutchinson, E.A. *et al.* (2013) School-age outcomes of extremely preterm or extremely low birth weight children. *Pediatrics* **131**, e1053–e1061.

Ispanovic-Radojkovic, V. & Stancheva-Popkostadinova, V. (2011) Perspectives of intellectual disability in Serbia and Bulgaria: epidemiology, policy and services for children and adults. *Current Opinion in Psychiatry* **24**, 419–424.

Jopp, D.A. & Keys, C.B. (2001) Diagnostic overshadowing reviewed and reconsidered. *American Journal of Mental Retardation* **106**, 416–433.

Knapp, M. *et al.* (2009) Economic cost of autism in the UK. *Autism* **13**, 317–336.

Koskentausta, T. *et al.* (2007) Risk factors for psychiatric disturbance in children with intellectual disability. *Journal of Intellectual Disability Research* **51**, 43–53.

Kuntsi, J. *et al.* (2004) Co-occurrence of ADHD and low IQ has genetic origins. *American Journal of Medical Genetics* **124B**, 41–47.

Kwok, H. *et al.* (2011) Perspectives of intellectual disability in the People's Republic of China: epidemiology, policy, services for children and adults. *Current Opinion in Psychiatry* **24**, 408–412.

Larkin, P. *et al.* (2012) Interpersonal sources of conflict in young people with and without mild to moderate intellectual disabilities at transition from adolescence to adulthood. *Journal of Applied Research in Intellectual Disabilities* **25**, 29–38.

Leggett, V. *et al.* (2010) Neurocognitive outcomes of individuals with a sex chromosome trisomy: XXX, XYY or XXY: a systematic review. *Developmental Medicine & Child Neurology* **52**, 119–129.

Leonard, H. & Wen, X. (2002) The epidemiology of mental retardation: challenges and opportunities in the new millennium. *Mental Retardation & Developmental Disabilities Research Reviews* **8**, 117–134.

Lewis, E.O. (1933) Types of mental deficiency and their social significance. *Journal of Mental Science* **79**, 293–304.

Leyfer, O.T. *et al.* (2006) Comorbid psychiatric disorders in children with autism: interview development and rates of disorders. *Journal of Autism and Developmental Disorders* **36**, 849–861.

Lin, L.P. & Lin, J.D. (2011) Perspectives on intellectual disability in Taiwan: epidemiology, policy and services for children and adults. *Current Opinion in Psychiatry* **24**, 413–418.

Loesch, D. & Hagerman, R. (2012) Unstable mutations in the FMR1 gene and the phenotypes. *Advances in Experimental Medicine & Biology* **769**, 78–114.

Lundvall, M. *et al.* (2012) Aetiology of severe mental retardation and further genetic analysis by high-resolution microarray in a population-based series of 6- to 17-year-old children. *Acta Paediatrica* **101**, 85–91.

Lyall, I. *et al.* (1995) Offending by adults with learning disabilities and the attitudes of staff to offending behaviour: implications for service development. *Journal of Intellectual Disability Research* **39**, 501–508.

Maeda, T. *et al.* (1991) A cytogenetic survey of 14,835 consecutive liveborns. *Jinrui Idengaku Zasshi [Japanese Journal of Human Genetics]* **36**, 117–129.

Manzanero, A.L. *et al.* (2012) Effects of presentation format and instructions on the ability of people with intellectual disability to identify faces. *Research in Developmental Disabilities* **33**, 391–397.

Marcus, R.N. *et al.* (2009) A placebo-controlled, fixed-dose study of aripiprazole in children and adolescents with irritability associated with autistic disorder. *Journal of the American Academy of Child & Adolescent Psychiatry* **48**, 1110–1119.

Marlow, N. (2004) Neurocognitive outcome after very preterm birth. *Archives of Disease in Childhood Fetal & Neonatal Edition* **89**, F224–F228.

Matson, J.L. *et al.* (1999) A validity study on the Questions About Behavioral Function (QABF) Scale: predicting treatment success for self-injury, aggression, and stereotypies. *Research in Developmental Disabilities* **20**, 163–175.

Maulik, P.K. *et al.* (2011) Prevalence of intellectual disability: a meta-analysis of population-based studies. *Research in Developmental Disabilities* **32**, 419–436.

May, P.A. & Gossage, J. (2001) Estimating the prevalence of fetal alcohol syndrome: a summary. *Alcohol Research & Health. The Journal of the National Institute on Alcohol Abuse & Alcoholism* **25**, 159–167.

McClintock, K. *et al.* (2003) Risk markers associated with challenging behaviours in people with intellectual disabilities: a meta-analytic study. *Journal of Intellectual Disability Research* **47**, 405–416.

McDermott, S. *et al.* (2012) When are fetuses and young children most susceptible to soil metal concentrations of arsenic, lead and mercury? *Spatial and Spatio-Temporal Epidemiology* **3**, 265–272.

McDonald, L. *et al.* (2006) Investigation of global developmental delay. *Archives of Disease in Childhood* **91**, 701–705.

McGaw, S. *et al.* (2007) Prevalence of psychopathology across a service population of parents with intellectual disabilities and their children. *Journal of Policy and Practice in Intellectual Disabilities* **4**, 11–22.

McGaw, S. *et al.* (2010) Predicting the unpredictable? Identifying high-risk versus low-risk parents with intellectual disabilities. *Child Abuse & Neglect* **34**, 699–710.

McGuire, B.E. *et al.* (2010) Chronic pain in people with an intellectual disability: under-recognised and under-treated? *Journal of Intellectual Disability Research* **54**, 240–245.

Mefford, H.C. *et al.* (2012) Genomics, intellectual disability, and autism. *New England Journal of Medicine* **366**, 733–743.

Michelson, D.J. *et al.* (2011) Evidence report: genetic and metabolic testing on children with global developmental delay: report of the Quality Standards Subcommittee of the American Academy of Neurology and the Practice Committee of the Child Neurology Society. *Neurology* **77**, 1629–1635.

Moore, T. *et al.* (2012) Neurological and developmental outcome in extremely preterm children born in England in 1995 and 2006: the EPICure studies. *British Medical Journal* **345**, e7961.

Morrow, E.M. (2010) Genomic copy number variation in disorders of cognitive development. *Journal of the American Academy of Child & Adolescent Psychiatry* **49**, 1091–1104.

Moss, S. *et al.* (1998) Reliability and validity of the PAS-ADD checklist for detecting psychiatric disorders in adults with intellectual disability. *Journal of Intellectual Disability Research* **42**, 173–183.

Moss, S. *et al.* (2000) Psychiatric symptoms in adults with learning disability and challenging behaviour. *British Journal of Psychiatry* **177**, 451–456.

Murphy, K.C. (2005) Annotation: velo-cardio-facial syndrome. *Journal of Child Psychology & Psychiatry & Allied Disciplines* **46**, 563–571.

National Institute for Health and Care Excellence. (2012). *The Epilepsies: The Diagnosis and Management of the Epilepsies in Adults and Children in Primary and Secondary Care NICE Clinical Guideline 137.* NICE, London.

Neece, C.L. *et al.* (2010) Impact on siblings of children with intellectual disability: the role of child behavior problems. *American Journal on Intellectual & Developmental Disabilities* **115**, 291–306.

Needleman, H.L. *et al.* (1990) The long-term effects of exposure to low doses of lead in childhood. *New England Journal of Medicine* **322**, 83–88.

Nevin, R. (2009) Trends in preschool lead exposure, mental retardation, and scholastic achievement: association or causation? *Environmental Research* **109**, 301–310.

Nichols, P.L. & Broman, S.H. (1974) Familial resemblance in infant mental development. *Developmental Psychology* **10**, 442–446.

Nisbett, R.E. *et al.* (2012) Intelligence: new findings and theoretical developments. *American Psychologist* **67**, 130–159.

O'Keeffe, N. & O'Hara, J. (2008) Mental health needs of parents with intellectual disabilities. *Current Opinion in Psychiatry* **21**, 463–468.

O'Leary, C. *et al.* (2013) Intellectual disability: population-based estimates of the proportion attributable to maternal alcohol use disorder during pregnancy. *Developmental Medicine & Child Neurology* **55**, 271–277.

Oliver, C. & Richards, C. (2010) Self-injurious behaviour in people with intellectual disability. *Current Opinion in Psychiatry* **23**, 412–416.

Oliver, C. *et al.* (2003) Assessing the severity of challenging behaviour: psychometric properties of the Challenging Behaviour Interview. *Journal of Applied Research in Intellectual Disabilities* **16**, 53–61.

Oliver, C. *et al.* (2012) The association between repetitive, self-injurious and aggressive behavior in children with severe intellectual disability. *Journal of Autism & Developmental Disorders* **42**, 910–919.

Owen, D.M. *et al.* (2004) Life events as correlates of problem behavior and mental health in a residential population of adults with developmental disabilities. *Research in Developmental Disabilities* **25**, 309–320.

Papazoglou, A. *et al.* (2013) Sensitivity of the BASC-2 Adaptive Skills Composite in detecting adaptive impairment in a clinically referred sample of children and adolescents. *The Clinical Neuropsychologist* **27**, 386–395.

Penrose, L.S. (1938) *A Clinical and Genetic Study of 1280 Cases of Mental Defect (The Colchester Study)*. Medical Research Council, London.

Penrose, L.S. (1939) Intelligence test scores of mentally defective patients and their relatives. *British Journal of Psychology* **30**, 1–18.

Petersilia, J.R. (2001) Crime victims with developmental disabilities: a review essay. *Criminal Justice and Behavior* **28**, 655–694.

Petty, J. & Oliver, C. (2005) Self-injurious behaviour in individuals with intellectual disabilities. *Current Opinion in Psychiatry* **18**, 484–489.

Pickles, A. *et al.* (2009) Loss of language in early development of autism and specific language impairment. *Journal of Child Psychology and Psychiatry* **50**, 843–852.

Rauch, A. *et al.* (2012) Range of genetic mutations associated with severe non-syndromic sporadic intellectual disability: an exome sequencing study. *Lancet* **380**, 1674–1682.

Reed, E.W. (1965) *Mental Retardation: A Family Study*. W.B. Saunders, Philadelphia.

Research Units on Pediatric Psychopharmacology (RUPP) Autism Network (2005) Randomized, controlled, crossover trial of methylphenidate in pervasive developmental disorders with hyperactivity. *Archives of General Psychiatry* **62**, 1266–1274.

Roeleveld, N. *et al.* (1997) The prevalence of mental retardation: a critical review of recent literature. *Developmental Medicine and Child Neurology* **39**, 125–132.

Ropers, H.H. (2008) Genetics of intellectual disability. *Current Opinion in Genetics & Development* **18**, 241–250.

Ropers, H.H. (2010) Genetics of early onset cognitive impairment. *Annual Review of Genomics & Human Genetics* **11**, 161–187.

Royal College of Psychiatrists (2001) *DC-LD: Diagnostic Criteria for Psychiatric Disorders for Use with Adults with Learning Disabilities/Mental Retardation*. Royal College of Psychiatrists, London.

Rutter, M. *et al.* (2004) Are there biological programming effects for psychological development? Findings from a study of Romanian adoptees. *Developmental Psychology* **40**, 81–94.

Scahill, L. *et al.* (2012) Effects of risperidone and parent training on adaptive functioning in children with pervasive developmental disorders and serious behavioral problems. *Journal of the American Academy of Child and Adolescent Psychiatry* **51**, 136–146.

Shevell, M. (2008) Global developmental delay and mental retardation or intellectual disability: conceptualization, evaluation, and etiology. *Pediatric Clinics of North America* **55**, 1071–1084.

Siffel, C. *et al.* (2004) Prenatal diagnosis, pregnancy terminations and prevalence of Down syndrome in Atlanta. *Birth Defects Research* **70**, 565–571.

Simonoff, E. *et al.* (2006) The Croydon Assessment of Learning study: prevalence and educational identification of mild mental retardation. *Journal of Child Psychology & Psychiatry* **47**, 828–839.

Simonoff, E. *et al.* (2007) ADHD symptoms in children with mild intellectual disability. *Journal of the American Academy of Child & Adolescent Psychiatry* **46**, 591–600.

Simonoff, E. *et al.* (2013a) The persistence and stability of psychiatric problems in adolescents with autism spectrum disorders. *Journal of Child Psychology & Psychiatry* **54**, 186–194.

Simonoff, E. *et al.* (2013b) Randomized controlled double-blind trial of optimal dose methylphenidate in children and adolescents with severe attention deficit hyperactivity disorder and intellectual disability. *Journal of Child Psychology and Psychiatry* **54**, 527–535.

Smith, L.E. *et al.* (2012a) Developmental trajectories in adolescents and adults with autism: the case of daily living skills. *Journal of the American Academy of Child & Adolescent Psychiatry* **51**, 622–631.

Smith, L.E. *et al.* (2012b) Daily health symptoms of mothers of adolescents and adults with fragile x syndrome and mothers of adolescents and adults with autism spectrum disorder. *Journal of Autism & Developmental Disorders* **42**, 1836–1846.

Sondenaa, E. *et al.* (2008) Forensic issues in intellectual disability. *Current Opinion in Psychiatry* **21**, 449–453.

Sparrow, S. *et al.* (1984) *Vineland Adaptive Behavior Scales*. Circle Pines, Minnesota, American Guidance Services.

Spinath, F.M. *et al.* (2004) Substantial genetic influence on mild mental impairment in early childhood. *American Journal of Mental Retardation* **109**, 34–43.

Streissguth, A.P. & Dehaene, P. (1993) Fetal alcohol syndrome in twins of alcoholic mothers: concordance of diagnosis and IQ. *American Journal of Medical Genetics* **47**, 857–861.

The Stationery Office (1998) *Human Rights Act*. The Stationery Office, London.

Thompson, L.A. *et al.* (1993) Differential heritability across groups differing in ability, revisited. *Behavior Genetics* **23**, 331–336.

Tobi, H. *et al.* (2005) Drug utilisation by children and adolescents with mental retardation: a population study. *European Journal of Clinical Pharmacology* **61**, 297–302.

Toriello, H.V. (2008) Role of the dysmorphologic evaluation in the child with developmental delay. *Pediatric Clinics of North America* **55**, 1085–1098.

Totsika, V. *et al.* (2011) Behavior problems at 5 years of age and maternal mental health in autism and intellectual disability. *Journal of Abnormal Child Psychology* **39**, 1137–1147.

Tsiouris, J. *et al.* (2011) Association of aggressive behaviours with psychiatric disorders, age, sex and degree of intellectual disability: a large-scale survey. *Journal of Intellectual Disability Research* **55**, 636–649.

Turner, H.A. *et al.* (2011) Disability and victimization in a national sample of children and youth. *Child Maltreatment* **16**, 275–286.

Tyrer, F. & McGrother, C. (2009) Cause-specific mortality and death certificate reporting in adults with moderate to profound intellectual disability. *Journal of Intellectual Disability Research* **53**, 898–904.

Tyrer, F. *et al.* (2007) Mortality in adults with moderate to profound intellectual disability: a population-based study. *Journal of Intellectual Disability Research* **51**, 520–527.

Walker, S. *et al.* (2006) Effects of psychosocial stimulation and dietary supplementation in early childhood on psychosocial functioning in late adolescence: follow-up of a randomised controlled trial. *British Medical Journal* **333**, 472–474.

Walker, S.P. *et al.* (2010) The effect of psychosocial stimulation on cognition and behaviour at 6 years in a cohort of term, low-birthweight Jamaican children. *Developmental Medicine & Child Neurology* **52**, e148–e154.

Weiber, I. *et al.* (2011) Children born to women with intellectual disabilities - 5-year incidence in a Swedish county. *Journal of Intellectual Disability Research* **55**, 1078–1085.

Williams, N.M. *et al.* (2010) Rare chromosomal deletions and duplications in attention-deficit hyperactivity disorder: a genome-wide analysis. *The Lancet* **376**, 1401–1408.

Woolf, S. *et al.* (2010) Adaptive behavior among adults with intellectual disabilities and its relationship to community independence. *Intellectual & Developmental Disabilities* **48**, 209–215.

Yeargin-Allsopp, M. *et al.* (1995) Mild mental retardation in black and white children in metropolitan Atlanta: a case-control study. *American Journal of Public Health* **85**, 324–328.

Zigler, E. (1967) Familial mental retardation: a continuing dilemma. *Science* **155**, 292–298.

CHAPTER 55

ADHD and hyperkinetic disorder

Edmund J.S. Sonuga-Barke[1,2] and Eric Taylor[3]

[1] Department of Psychology, University of Southampton, Southampton, UK

[2] Department of Experimental Clinical and Health Psychology, Ghent University, Belgium

[3] Department of Child and Adolescent Psychiatry, Institute of Psychiatry, Psychology and Neuroscience, King's College London, UK

Diagnosis

The key concept underlying the diagnoses of attention deficit/ hyperactivity disorder (ADHD) and hyperkinetic disorder (HKD) is that of maladaptively high levels of inattention, over-activity, and impulsiveness. These problems occur in different combinations in different individuals, and with different levels and types of associated problems. They are descriptions of behavior, not explanations.

Presentations, therefore, vary a great deal. A "classical" presentation would be of the full picture without other problems. A child presents because of disorganized behavior in which *inattention* describes a lack of attention to detail, a short attention span in unmotivating situations, forgetfulness, distractibility in situations requiring focus on a task, and a slapdash attitude. *Overactivity* describes an excess of movement in situations requiring calm, such as the classroom, family meals, or visits to church or relatives. *Impulsiveness* refers to action without reflection, so affected people are accident-prone, impatient, intrusive on the activities of other people, and hasty (and therefore inept) in making decisions.

The results are manifold. Difficulties in personal relationships, school achievement, discipline, and emotional life can all appear (see section "Longitudinal Course"). Clinical presentations are, therefore, with a wide range of difficulties, and one of the clinical skills required is to recognize the ADHD pattern underlying the surface presentation.

Historical evolution of the concept

The prehistory of ADHD is the formulations of mental disorder in childhood that stressed lack of control and wildly disruptive behavior and presumed roots in the individual's constitution (Crichton, 1798; Haslam, 1809). The idea developed into "a defective organization in those parts of the body which are occupied by the moral faculties of the mind" (Rush, 1812). George

Frederick Still (1902) described disorders of "moral control," in which aggressive, defiant, and overemotional conduct was attributed to constitutional failures of inhibitory volition. With hindsight, this is often claimed as a first description of ADHD; and indeed problems in sustaining attention were included in Still's descriptions; but there is no evidence from contemporary citations that he influenced other clinical scholars before the 1970s. Rather, a neurological tradition described "hyperkinetic syndrome" or "Kramer-Pollnow syndrome" (Neumärker, 2005), and a "minimal brain damage" (MBD) syndrome, so that hyperactive behavior became part of the picture of the "brain-injured child" (Strauss & Lehtinen, 1947). The idea of MBD was largely abandoned as it became clear that there was no unique syndrome of brain damage and that it was not legitimate to infer brain damage on the basis of hyperactive (or other) symptomatology alone (Rutter *et al.*, 1970).

The idea of a syndrome in which activity and attention problems were central may be attributable in part to the rise of medication. Early trials of amphetamines described the outcomes as better school performance and relaxation (Bradley, 1937; Cutler *et al.*, 1940; Bender & Cottington, 1942); as the description of drug effects became more refined, overactivity and inattentiveness took over as key outcomes (Eisenberg *et al.*, 1963). Emotional over-reactiveness was often included in descriptions of minimal brain dysfunction (e.g., Clements, 1966), until the very influential DSM-III codified the key problems as inattentiveness (IA), hyperactivity (HA) and impulsiveness (Imp).

Diagnostic schemes

Current differences between schemes reflect the disparate historical origins of the concept. DSM-IIIR, -IV, -IV(TM), and DSM-5 have tweaked the criteria of DSM-III, but maintained a tradition of description based on adding the criteria that are met, and applying a cut-off validated by the scores of young people who have been diagnosed in US practice. ICD-9 and ICD-10

Rutter's Child and Adolescent Psychiatry, Sixth Edition.
Edited by Anita Thapar and Daniel S. Pine, James F. Leckman, Stephen Scott, Margaret J. Snowling, Eric Taylor.
© 2015 John Wiley & Sons Ltd. Published 2018 by John Wiley & Sons Ltd.

have relied rather on providing a description of the condition, as a prototype to which clinicians fit cases on the basis of symptom pattern. ICD-10 calls the condition "HKD," requires the combination of IA and HA-Imp, and has strict requirements for pervasiveness of symptoms. The result is that HKD is a subtype nested within ADHD, accounting for about a quarter of cases, and characterized by more neurodevelopmental alterations in motor and language development than other forms of ADHD (Taylor *et al.*, 1991), a more marked response to methylphenidate compared with placebo (Taylor *et al.*, 1987), and a less satisfactory response to behavioral treatment than to medication (Santosh *et al.*, 2005). HKD does not, however, seem to be a separate condition, either genetically or in course over time.

It is clear that the defining behaviors cluster together; a systematic review and meta-analysis concluded that their association with each other is indeed strong enough to sustain ADHD as a valid concept (National Institute for Health and Care Excellence (NICE), 2009). It is less clear how their structure is best described.

Dimensions, categories, and subtypes
Dimensions
Parent and teacher rating scales have found that levels of hyperactivity and inattentiveness are continuously distributed in the population, without any sign of a discontinuity at the extreme (e.g., Taylor *et al.*, 1991). Factor analytic studies have (of course) found dimensions. An innovative approach has come from the comparison of different types of factor structure. Toplak *et al.* (2009) contrasted two models of confirmatory factor analysis and two bifactor models, all applied to the same data set of parent and self-report interviews for adolescents. The best fit came from allowing both a unitary component across all ADHD symptoms and two distinct factors of inattention and hyperactivity-impulsivity.

The separation of dimensions of inattentiveness and overactive impulsiveness has clinical and scientific value. A systematic review and meta-analysis of 546 studies by Willcutt *et al.* (2012) concludes that there is "overwhelming" support for the distinction, not only from the internal, statistical correlations of symptoms, but also from stability over time, and the differential prediction of external associations. HA-Imp predicts selectively to aggression, rejection by peers and accidents; IA to poor academic function, shy and passive social behavior in children, and lower life satisfaction in adults. The distinction is not absolute; the dimensions are correlated with each other; but they deserve separate attention in clinical assessment. The correlation between inattentiveness and impulsiveness can mostly be attributed to their having genetic influences in common (McLoughlin *et al.*, 2007).

A dimensional way of thinking allows the balance of components to be assessed, and related problems brought in. As instance, emotional lability and irritability are very common features—and were part of the diagnosis until DSM-III removed them as criteria—but carry extra implications about clinical profile and family history (Sobanski *et al.*, 2010) and should contribute to a diagnostic formulation.

Categories and subtypes
By contrast with the validity of dimensions, the categorical subtypes of DSM-IV—predominantly inattentive, predominantly hyperactive, and combined—have fared less well. They show only modest differences between themselves, and they are unstable over time (Lahey & Willcutt, 2010). Such differences as there are do not suggest that the DSM-IV subtypes add any extra predictive validity to that which is achieved by dimensions. The DSM-5 downgrades them from "subtypes" to "presentations".

The weakness of the subtypes may come—not from the absence of categorical dysfunctions in nature—but from poor operational definition. A "predominantly inattentive" subtype, for instance, is defined partly by having fewer than six symptoms of hyperactivity-impulsiveness (American Psychiatric Association, 2000). Five symptoms, however, still imply a substantial load of impulsive behavior. Many children characterized as predominantly inattentive might more realistically be seen as showing a mild form of a combined subtype. Some studies, based on questionnaire ratings rather than DSM criteria, have identified a group of inattentive children with a more rigorously defined absence of impulsive or hyperactive features—for instance, scoring less than one standard deviation above the population mean (Taylor *et al.*, 1991; Warner-Rogers *et al.*, 2000). This "restrictive inattentive" type is not disruptive or aggressive. Indeed, affected children may be dreamy and rather inert, but muddled, disorganized, and impersistent in the classroom. They often show neurocognitive problems, but of a rather mixed kind, including working memory problems, poor spatial skills, language delay, poor motor coordination, and even (but not necessarily) a low IQ. Such a group has not found its way into the DSM-5 or ICD-10 classifications, because of a lack of adequate scientific study.

There are practical advantages to a category of ADHD (see Chapter 2). It helps clinicians who must make binary decisions such as whether or not to refer or to medicate, and it helps people who suffer from the condition, their families, and the public at large to understand the nature of the condition. Most clinicians in most countries will find it useful to use a mixture of categorical and dimensional approaches. The first step in assessment will probably be to define the presence or absence of ADHD; but a fuller analysis should quantify the levels of severity of inattentiveness and hyperactivity/impulsivity separately—together with the levels of associated problems, functional impairment, impact on others, other strengths and weaknesses (e.g., athletic ability), peer acceptance, and risk, as indicated in Chapter 32.

Clinical assessment

A range of screening questionnaires is available (see Chapter 33). Some were developed to monitor response to therapy (e.g., Conners' Teacher and Parent Rating Scales) and subsequently refined statistically (Conners, 2008). (Modifications, such as the IOWA Conners, selected items from the most relevant subscales). Some other scales came from an epidemiological tradition (e.g., the Strengths and Difficulties Questionnaire (SDQ), which modified the Rutter A(2) and B(2) Scales (Goodman, 1997) and the longer Child Behavior Problems Checklist (Achenbach & Edelbrock, 1983)). Other scales were developed from DSM-III or DSM-IV criteria, such as the ADHD Rating Scale (DuPaul, 1991), the Vanderbilt Rating Scale (Wolraich *et al.*, 2003), and the SNAP-IV scale (Swanson *et al.*, 2005). Others again were developed for specific purposes, for example, to describe the range of behaviors that can occur in different situations (Barkley, 1991).

Many of these rating scales have similar strengths and weaknesses. Test–retest reliability is typically around 0.7; most give a discrimination between cases and controls at around two standard deviations, separating the means of ADHD and control populations; all are sensitive to the effects of medication. Free access from the internet is available for the SNAP-IV and SWAN (www.adhd.net) and the SDQ (www.sdqinfo.org). Most consist of items, reflecting DSM descriptions, each of which is scored for intensity (e.g., SNAP, DBD, Conners) or frequency (Vanderbilt, DuPaul [as above]), which are then summed to give a dimensional score. The distribution of scores on most scales is far from normal: there is a J-shaped distribution with a great excess of cases at the lowest levels. One consequence is that the scales are not suitable for parametric analyses (though often submitted to them); another is that a cut-off score based on a standard deviation criterion will identify more cases than may be intended. The SWAN scale was therefore developed with a wider range of scores for each item (e.g., "far above average" as well as "far below average") to yield a more Gaussian distribution (Swanson *et al.*, 2005). It is likely to be helpful in describing the full range in the population. All scales, used as a population screen, are liable to overidentify cases at the extreme. The questionnaires are best seen as a first stage of screening, not as defining casehood.

Indeed, screening in the general population is not yet established as a valuable clinical procedure (e.g., Tymms & Merrell, 2006). The limitations of population screening are likely to include not only an overidentification of cases, but also harmful effects of identification on stigma and teachers' expectations; a lack of community agencies to respond to screen-positive cases; and the risk that impaired children who are not detected will go without service.

Referral to services

Prevalence estimates in many countries outside the United States (see later, *Epidemiology* section) make it plain that most cases of ADHD are never diagnosed. In the United Kingdom, most parents do discuss their concerns with education services, but this does not lead to referral even to primary health care (Sayal *et al.*, 2006). For those parents who do seek help from

primary care, much depends on their health literacy. If they complain of hyperactivity, an appropriate referral follows; if their complaint is of behavior or learning problems in general terms, then hyperactivity, impulsiveness, and inattention are not diagnosed even if present (Sayal *et al.*, 2002). A systematic screen, applied selectively for children with problems presenting to primary health care and remedial education services—using the rating scales described above—is therefore a promising way of improving recognition, and assisting specialist referral, in countries where recognition is incomplete.

At mental health and pediatric services, the course of assessment will follow the outline of Chapter 32. Parental interview, report from teachers, and examination and observation of child are the recommended means of eliciting behavior. Multiple informants are useful because affected children will still vary across contexts. Research interviews are systematic and encourage comprehensive coverage, but are usually too lengthy and focused to be feasible in clinical practice. It remains important to ask for details of behavior in specific situations rather than for generalized ratings of problems (such as "impulsiveness"), which are vulnerable to imperfect knowledge of what is typical.

Problems and pitfalls in diagnosis
Cut-offs

The continuous distribution of ADHD symptoms in the population makes for uncertainty about where to place the division between normal variation and psychopathology. For research purposes, where replicability is key, it is sensible to follow the international conventions: at least six out of the nine inattentiveness criteria, and/or at least six out of nine hyperactive-impulsive. These remain the standard for childhood and adolescent diagnosis in DSM-5.

For clinical purposes, however, an unintelligent addition of criteria is not always best. For instance, a child with five out of nine inattentiveness criteria and five out of nine hyperactive-impulsive does not get an ADHD diagnosis, while one with no inattentiveness and six out of nine hyperactive-impulsive does receive a diagnosis (HA-IMP presentation)—in spite of a lower load of ADHD symptoms.

Developmental appropriateness

Symptoms need to be considered in the light of what is appropriate to different ages and levels of development. "Hyperactivity," for example, may be a whirlwind in the preschool period, fidgetiness in adolescence, and subjective restlessness in adulthood. Diagnosticians need to build up sufficient experience of attention and activity at different ages, both in typically developing children and in differing forms of psychopathology, that they can recognize when a child's attention and activity are deviating from what is expected. Indeed, this should be an important aspect of professional training. A short cut is to accept the judgment of other professionals, especially experienced teachers, about what is atypical. There will, however, be times when those judgments are misleading—for example, are colored by the rater's relationship with the child.

Misdiagnosis is particularly easy for children with intellectual disability (see Chapter 54). The diagnosis can be missed by attributing all the problems to a low IQ, or overrecognized by treating the cognitive problems of intellectual disability as evidence for ADHD. There are two styles of coping with this problem: the first is to refer the child's level of difficulty to that of others at similar levels of intellectual delay. This distributional approach, however, risks overlooking the probability that ADHD features are *disproportionately* common in people with immature brains. A second approach is to refer the child's level of difficulty to those of ordinary children whose chronological age corresponds to the developmental age of the child being assessed.

Diagnosis in adult life

Inattention and impulsiveness often persist into adult life; some people are not diagnosed in childhood; therefore some people will present for the first time as adults. The number of DSM symptoms tends to diminish, but impairment persists (and DSM-5 requires 5 rather than 6 symptoms to be present).

Self-report can be more accurate than in childhood, but the report of people who know the person well remains crucially important. Furthermore, evidence about childhood status needs to be sought—from parents, siblings, school reports, and a reconstruction of biography. It is rare for ADHD features to appear for the first time in adulthood, and when they do, they suggest other psychopathology such as substance misuse, early dementia, mania, or encephalopathy. Diagnosis therefore requires evidence of ADHD symptoms in childhood – but not necessarily of impairment from them. The retrospective dating of onset is often imprecise, and DSM-5 therefore requires only the presence of symptoms before the age of 12 years.

Sources of information: conflicts

If there is disagreement between sources, the diagnostician should make a judgment about the reasons. Perhaps an inexperienced parent is making ratings without knowledge of what to expect from children, or in a way that is colored by their relationship. Perhaps a teacher is overstating problems in order to obtain help for the child, or understating because of fear that the child may be medicated. Alternatively, the problem behaviors may indeed be situation-specific, directing attention to the qualities of the situation, including domestic conflict or inappropriate school expectations.

Differential diagnosis

The presence of ADHD or HKD should be recognized even in the presence of other psychiatric conditions. Some conditions, however, may masquerade as ADHD by reproducing some of its features.

Other forms of overactivity can be distinguished. Manic overactivity is goal-directed, rather than the disorganized pattern of ADHD. Children in the spectrum of autism may show a driven, stereotyped pattern of overactivity that can be extreme and worsened by anti-hyperactivity medication. Children with multiple tics may appear to show impulsive overactivity until it is appreciated—sometimes by prolonged observation—that the activity level is composed solely of a large number of sudden, repetitive movements.

Other forms of inattentiveness can also be separated. Learning disorders may be accompanied by reluctance to engage in academic tasks, but (unlike that of ADHD) it is often specific to tasks that are unduly difficult for the individual.

Other forms of disruptive behavior may also need to be distinguished. Insomnia may produce an irritable child who is not engaging in classroom activity, but (unlike ADHD) it is accompanied by daytime sleepiness, and the problems do not disappear when the insomnia is relieved. Oppositional behavior alone may be responsible for a child's appearance of not listening and task refusal, and in young children it can be hard to distinguish from impulsive behavior, so the absence of inattention is a helpful guide when the problem is oppositionality without ADHD.

Other forms of emotional dysregulation need consideration. Emotional dysregulation is also a feature of bipolar disorder. The ADHD pattern is distinguished from bipolar in that it is not episodic but a persisting trait, and by the absence of the euphoria and grandiosity that characterize the episodes of mania (see Chapter 62).

All these conditions that can masquerade as ADHD may also be coexistent with ADHD. The key for the diagnostician is, therefore, to discern whether the disorganized pattern of ADHD behavior is also present, and to make the additional diagnosis (or diagnoses) as necessary.

This process of differential diagnosis is to be distinguished from the confusion that may come from a different etiology. Brain syndromes, such as fragile-X or tuberous sclerosis may well be responsible for ADHD features. Both the neurological condition and the ADHD should then be recognized. More subtly, severe neglect in early childhood is probably a cause of attention and activity abnormalities (see section "Risk Factors"), and if ADHD is present in such a child, then it should still be diagnosed. A social worker identifying a neglect syndrome and a physician diagnosing ADHD in the same child may both be right.

Coexistent disorders

Other neurodevelopmental phenotypes are frequently present. Autism spectrum conditions, for example, affect about one-third of children with diagnosed ADHD (Reiersen *et al.*, 2007). Twin studies suggest that about half of the genetic influences are common to both disorders (Ronald *et al.*, 2008). Motor problems, specific learning difficulties, and tics are also common (and see Chapter 3).

Disruptive mood dysregulation disorder, in which a persisting trait of dysphoric and irritable mood is accompanied by extreme outbursts of temper or aggression, is usually accompanied by dyscontrol of activity and attention. It is therefore better seen as a coexistent, rather than as a differential disorder: the question for formulation is not either/or but which component should be tackled first.

Oppositional and conduct problems, anxiety and social immaturity often emerge in the course of development (see section "Longitudinal Course"). When oppositional and conduct problems are present together with ADHD, then the ADHD is likely to have come first; the ADHD carries the same implications of neurocognitive delays and responsiveness to stimulant drugs as does ADHD alone; and genetic influences inferred from twin studies are for the most part common to both (Taylor, 2010). A variant of the gene coding for catechol-*o*-methyl transferase (COMT) is associated only with the combined condition, not with either ADHD or conduct problems alone, which could imply that the combined condition is genetically partially distinct (Caspi, 2008). Nevertheless, for clinical purposes, one can proceed on the basis that ADHD functions as a risk factor for the development of conduct problems, and can be treated separately.

Epidemiology

Prevalence

ADHD is remarkable for the great disparity in rates of given diagnosis in different parts of the world. Estimates gathered by Hinshaw *et al.* (2011) of children who were medicated because of ADHD varied from around 60 per 1000 school-age children in the United States, through 10–30 per 1000 in Canada, to 3 per 1000 in the United Kingdom and less than 1 in Brazil and China. Estimates from other surveys suggested 9 per 1000 in Germany and 1.8 per 1000 in France (Taylor, 2013).

Figures for the rates of diagnoses, as given in practice, are not usually gathered systematically, and are often hard to interpret, but the picture is one of marked variation by country. Even within the United States, administrative prevalence rates vary greatly with the Centers for Disease Control and Prevention (2010) reporting rates varying from 62/1000 (in California) to 156/1000 (North Carolina) on the basis of parents reporting whether their child had ever received the diagnosis. Skounti *et al.* (2007) summarized results of 39 community surveys from various countries (1992–2005); the reported rates for school-age children varied from 22 to 178 per 1000. The highest rates came from the United States, Spain, and Germany, and from studies based on single-source ratings (e.g., teacher only).

Polanczyk *et al.* (2007) made a systematic review of all prevalence studies reporting rates of DSM or ICD diagnoses for people under the age of 18. Worldwide, the average rate was 53/1000; it varied greatly (from 10 to 190/1000) but the main reasons for variation were in the diagnostic criteria used, the source of information used, and whether impairment was included in the criteria. Geographical differences, after allowing for the above,

were minor and only significant in discriminating between North America on the one hand and Africa and the Middle East on the other. In one set of studies, comparing 7-year-olds in London, England and Hong Kong, the "local" definition—based on questionnaires from teachers and parents—yielded a much higher prevalence in Hong Kong; while the "international" definition—based on interviews and tests—yielded a somewhat higher prevalence in London (Luk, 1996).

The implication is that cultures vary only a little in the true prevalence of activity and attention problems—but vary greatly in the impact that these problems have on the concerns of adults who know the children and are responsible for their welfare. Correspondingly, the rates of children diagnosed in practice have been rising in most countries: in the United States, from 78 per 1000 in 2003 to 95/1000 in 2007 (Centers for Disease Control and Prevention, 2010). At both points, rates were higher when the family's primary language was English, or when they had Medicaid cover for health care. The gender ratio was 2.8:1.

Risk factors

ADHD risk is made up of many interacting genetic and environmental factors, and is mediated by multiple brain networks—with different individuals affected in different ways and at different times and to different degrees by these factors. There is good evidence for ADHD dimensionality and against the notion that there is a causal discontinuity when one reaches pathological levels of inattention and impulsiveness (review by Coghill & Sonuga-Barke (2012)). A developmental perspective is necessary. Figure 55.1 gives a simplified picture of multiple early influences (genetic and prenatal) interacting with later (genetic and social and physical environmental) risk and protective processes to create a spectrum of disease liability.

Genetic influences

It is pretty clear that genetic influences are involved. The strongest evidence comes from studies comparing the similarity of monozygotic and dizygotic twins: genetic influences account for 70–90% of the variance in different studies, on the (reasonable) assumption that environmental factors influence both twins more or less equally. Data from research has not, however, established an unequivocally causative role for individual genetic variants (Thapar *et al.*, 2012). Several molecular genetic variants are known to be associated, but their effects are small and the causal pathways are not established.

Some of the best evidence for specific genetic influences comes from recent findings of an increased rate of *de novo* and inherited chromosomal deletions and/or local duplications (so-called copy number variants—CNVs) in ADHD (Williams *et al.*, 2010; Williams *et al.*, 2012). The sites involved appear diverse, but different genes may converge on shared biological processes (Stergiakouli *et al.*, 2012).

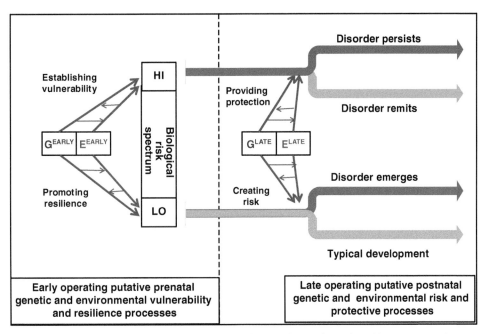

Figure 55.1 ADHD pathogenesis: developmental psychopathology schematic showing the way that early and late operating risks act together to determine continuities and discontinuities in disorder paths.

Meta-analysis of candidate gene studies has established associations with genes regulating brain neurochemistry, especially in the dopamine (DA) system (e.g., D4 and the dopamine transporter (DAT1); Faraone *et al.*, 2005) and other neuromodulator systems such as serotonin and norepinephrine; Oades *et al.*, 2008). Linkage studies have not found replicable disease susceptibility loci for ADHD (Arcos-Burgos *et al.*, 2004). Hypothesis-free genome-wide association studies, which tag a very large number of markers of common genetic variants in very large samples, have confirmed an overall genetic contribution to ADHD (Stergiakouli *et al.*, 2012) but have so far failed to identify genome-wide substantial effects for individual markers. To date, therefore, most of the heritability is unexplained. Five of the best established genetic variants—serotonin 1b receptor, serotonin transporter, DA D4 and D5 receptors, and the DAT—have been estimated to account for only 3.2% of the variance in symptoms of ADHD, and 4.2% of the heritability (Kuntsi *et al.*, 2006). The advice given to families should still be that genetic influences are strong. The risk of ADHD occurring in other first-degree family members (such as brothers and sisters) is raised about fivefold. Nevertheless, the scientific difficulty in specifying the precise influences responsible makes genetic counseling inexact for affected families. We only recommend investigation of chromosomes and DNA for individual patients when there are specific reasons—such as a phenotype suggesting a large gene effect (e.g., Williams syndrome), or the presence of many affected family members, or the existence of other neurodevelopmental problems (e.g., intellectual disability) that are enough in themselves to indicate genetic evaluation (see Chapter 54).

Environmental influences

Genetic and environmental influences are profoundly intertwined for ADHD and need to be considered jointly (see Chapter 24). Several, potentially harmful factors in the early environment are reliably associated with ADHD, but none is unequivocally established as a cause (Thapar *et al.*, 2012). The developmental pathways involved can be complex. Genetic factors can influence both the exposure to environmental risks (G–E correlation) and the susceptibility of the individual to them (G–E interaction; see Chapter 24).

Prenatal associations include maternal smoking during pregnancy (in contrast, see Thapar *et al.*, 2009), maternal alcohol consumption, and use of non-prescribed drugs of abuse, prescribed drugs such as anticonvulsants and anxiolytics, maternal stress, and maternal hypothyroidism.

Perinatal associations include low birth weight, prematurity, and obstetric complications.

In postnatal life, associations include an inadequate diet, iodine deficiency and major B vitamin deficiencies, iron and lead poisoning, high exposure to industrially contaminated areas, old paint, and soft-water areas where lead water pipes are common.

Some artificial food colorings and preservatives have been implicated as risk factors by contrasting them with inert substances in a community-based randomized double-blind trial (McCann *et al.*, 2007): as a consequence the implicated coloring has been regulated in the UK and Europe. Exposure to insecticides, such as dichlorodiphenyltrichloroethane (DDT), has been implicated in animal models but has not been confirmed clinically (Mariussen & Fonnum, 2006).

Social environmental effects include exposure to extremely depriving institutional environments (Stevens *et al.*, 2008). More ordinary variations in family environment may also be implicated as influences on developmental course rather than initiating factors. ADHD elicits negative, intrusive, and harsh responses from parents, which then influence the later emergence of comorbid social and emotional problems (Taylor *et al.*, 1996).

Various medical illnesses are also risks for the development of poor concentration, irritable mood, and problems of conduct. In young children, eczema and sleep problems are common reasons for the upsets, and successful treatments of these primary problems will often relieve the mental problems too (see Chapter 70).

A narrow disease model of ADHD has led to genetic factors typically being thought of as operating in a rather fixed way across the lifespan. By contrast, our developmental model of ADHD pathogenesis makes a distinction between early and late operating genetic effects (see Figure 55.1). Greven *et al.* (2011) demonstrated, using longitudinal twin data, that patterns of stability and change in ADHD symptoms were the result of both stable genetic influences and newly appearing influences emerging at different points across the life span. Environmental influences too need to be appraised in relation to their timing. There is, for instance, evidence from the English Romanian Adoptees study that at least 6 months institutional deprivation is required before the risk of ADHD rises, while later catch-up can be achieved for many deprived children once exposed to normal family environments (Stevens *et al.*, 2008).

Clinical implications

Knowledge of risks has advanced to the point where it can inform advice to patients and their families. The understanding that there are genetic influences often comes as a liberation from personal guilt. Parents are vulnerable to societal views that their parenting failures have produced the features of ADHD, and can be freed by good advice to use their problem-solving and coping skills. It is also important to avoid any impression that genetic influences imply an unalterable course. Parents and teachers can have a major influence for good on their children's ability to cope with ADHD.

Parents have sometimes been led to give undue weight to single events in the history. Minor obstetric complications are seldom "the cause," any more than minor infractions of health advice in pregnancy (such as low levels of alcohol intake). In many countries, there is a public view that broad social factors are responsible—for instance, rises in television viewing or internet use. It is therefore worth noting that shared environmental factors appear to play very little part.

Prevention programs, however, do not yet have a comprehensive rationale. It certainly makes sense for clinicians to support good services for maternal health in pregnancy and to include mental health in that remit; to know their community's

exposure to lead or deficiency in iodine and include screening for their effects when it is cost-effective; to support nutrition programs (including psychological enrichment); to detect and refer learning difficulties when they are present; and to end exposure to depriving institutional care; but none of these desirable approaches rely solely on ADHD risk for their justification (see Chapter 3).

Pathogenesis

ADHD and brain structure

Structural alterations in multiple brain systems have been implicated in ADHD (Sonuga-Barke & Fairchild, 2012). Group comparisons with controls find significantly smaller brains in ADHD (Castellanos *et al.*, 2002) with cerebellum, corpus callosum, striatal—for example, caudate nucleus, putamen and globus pallidus (Ellison-Wright *et al.*, 2008) – and frontal regions—for example, dorso-lateral prefrontal cortex (DLPFC) (Valera *et al.*, 2007) – especially affected. Reduced thickness of cortex, especially DLPFC, is evident (Batty *et al.*, 2010). There is also evidence of altered patterns of cortical folding—effects perhaps related to early environmental influences (Wolosin *et al.*, 2009). Diffusion tensor imaging suggests alterations in white matter integrity in a range of key fiber pathways thought to subserve cognitive functions implicated in ADHD (van Ewijk *et al.*, 2012). Key regions in the reward and emotion processing networks such as the ventral striatum and the amygdala may also be implicated (Plessen *et al.*, 2006).

The few studies that have examined developmental changes in brain structure have demonstrated a degree of continuity in ADHD effects (Castellanos *et al.*, 2002). Recent analyses have supported the notion of a delayed developmental trajectory in ADHD rather than a fixed deficit. Remission of symptoms is associated in some studies with a relative normalization of brain structure and function (Shaw *et al.*, 2010).

ADHD and brain chemistry

The hypothesis that ADHD is based on dopamine (DA) dysregulation is supported by genetic, imaging, and pharmacological studies (Oades *et al.*, 2005). Positron emission tomographic studies have produced mixed results with some supporting the view that ADHD is associated with low tonic levels of DA, with phasic levels varying according to task demands (reviewed by Prince, 2008). This is supported by the clinical observation that some DA agonists (e.g., methylphenidate, amphetamine) reduce ADHD symptoms, probably through an increase of extracellular DA (Pliszka, 2005). DA neurons innervate the brain networks (see below) implicated in ADHD deficits. A DA hypothesis is further supported by the genetic studies implicating DA genes (see above) and by studies using animal models with pharmacological lesions and gene knockouts of catecholamine systems (Madras *et al.*, 2005). It must however be added that other neurochemicals, such as norepinephrine and serotonin (Oades *et al.*, 2008), are implicated in ADHD, that some effective medications (e.g., imipramine) have little DA effect, and the interactions between neurotransmitters are complex (Olijslagers *et al.*, 2006).

ADHD and brain function

Brain function is altered in ADHD in multiple networks subserving a range of neuropsychological functions, often mapping on to the structural effects reported above. Simple models of ADHD as a disorder of executive function have been replaced by a model of pathophysiological heterogeneity.

Executive function is altered in several domains (Willcutt *et al.*, 2005), especially in inhibitory-based interference control processes (Barkley, 1997) and in working memory (Rapport *et al.*, 2008), but also in planning and attentional flexibility (Willcutt *et al.*, 2005). Functional imaging studies provide evidence to suggest that inhibitory-based deficits are linked to hypoactivation in prefrontal cortex (Rubia *et al.*, 2005) and the dorsal striatum (Vaidya *et al.*, 2005).

Altered motivational and reward-related processes are also implicated in ADHD. Functional magnetic resonance imaging (fMRI) studies implicate hypoactivation in the ventral striatum/nucleus accumbens and the orbito-frontal cortex in response to cues of anticipated rewards (e.g., Plichta *et al.*, 2009). One of the most consistent findings in this domain is that ADHD individuals respond differently to delayed reward (e.g., Marco *et al.*, 2009). This may be due to altered signaling of future rewards and higher rate of decay of the value of those rewards as suggested in models by Sagvolden *et al.* (2005). Alternatively, it has been suggested that ADHD is associated with delay aversion (a negative affective state induced by delay cues and imposition) and that escape from delay is a primary motivator for ADHD behavior (Sonuga-Barke *et al.*, 2010).

A third network attracting increasing attention in ADHD research is the so-called default mode network. This is one of a number of resting state networks centered on the mid-line structures—the medial prefrontal cortex and the posterior cingulate cortex/precuneus, which in optimal conditions are active during rest and deactivate during the transition to task performance (Raichle & Snyder, 2007). During rest, these regions are important for introspective thought and self-awareness but persistence or emergence of activity within this network during task performance is associated with intra-individual variability and intermittent errors thought to reflect attentional lapses This network shows reduced connectivity in ADHD during rest (Fair *et al.*, 2010) and reduced attenuation during rest-to-task transitions: both effects that can be normalized with stimulant medication (e.g., Liddle *et al.*, 2011).

The research on reward and delay has highlighted the context-dependent nature of ADHD deficits. An alternative perspective on this issue is provided by the state regulation model. This is based on the cognitive energetic framework of Saunders which integrates energetic factors such as arousal, activation, and effort into information processing. According to this model ADHD children are hypothesized to have particular difficulties in regulating their psycho-physiological state during periods of under- or over-activation/arousal and are therefore less capable of effectively allocating effort to regulate suboptimal states (Sergeant, 2005).

ADHD is probably not a single neurobiological entity but rather an umbrella term covering a range of different pathophysiological profiles. Each deficit (i.e., executive, reward/delay, default mode, and cognitive-energetic) affects only a minority of cases. In one recent study, distinctive groups of ADHD were affected selectively by either executive function problems, delay aversion, or timing problems (Sonuga-Barke *et al.*, 2010). Psychological changes may map on to development: Halperin *et al.* (2008) found that patients who showed a persistent pattern of disorder between childhood and adolescence could be distinguished from those who remitted on the basis of the integrity of their executive or effortful control processes, a finding which the authors argue is consistent with the idea that recovery from ADHD is associated with emergence of well-functioning executive control functions. The frequency of brain changes in people with ADHD, and their continuity over time, have contributed to the reclassification in DSM-5 of ADHD as a "neurodevelopmental disorder"; see Chapter 3.

Longitudinal course

Referral for ADHD is most common in middle childhood when the symptoms of ADHD, their neuropsychological correlates, and associated clinical features start to impact negatively on everyday function across a range of psychological domains and social and educational arenas (von Stauffenberg & Campbell, 2007). Because of this, the 8-year-old boy struggling to work alone at school, disruptive at home, and experiencing difficulty making friends because of his overbearing and reactive style of interaction is in many minds the ADHD archetype. Longitudinal studies, however, make clear that these patterns of impairment nearly always have their roots early on in the preschool period (Sonuga-Barke & Halperin, 2010) and very often persist across the life span in one form or another (Biederman *et al.*, 2012).

Preschool

Accounts of ADHD in the preschool period highlight the early emergence of extreme overactivity, noncompliance, and a tendency to temper outbursts linked to emotion dysregulation, in children with already established temperamental reactivity (Campbell *et al.*, 2000). This early behavioral pattern is usually already linked with a range of neuropsychological deficits and intellectual delay (Schoemaker *et al.*, 2012). The existence in ADHD preschoolers of social and pragmatic language problems may make the differential early diagnosis of autism challenging (Mandell *et al.*, 2007). These impairment patterns can be compounded by parenting that is disorganized and ineffective within chaotic family environments, sometimes reflecting genetic similarity of parent and child (Mokrova *et al.*, 2010). This early appearing constellation of ADHD-related features may be described as risk markers or a prodromal state of the later clinical condition. Psychometric studies, however, suggest that the ADHD diagnosis has validity and utility by the age of 3 or 4 (Riddle *et al.*, 2013). At this age, the predominantly hyperactive/impulsive subtype is more prevalent than the inattentive subtype—probably because evidence of attention deficits is not so apparent in the contexts in which infants and young children operate (Lahey *et al.*, 2005).

Middle childhood

Community-based and longitudinal studies highlight symptomatic and diagnostic continuity between preschool and school (e.g., Lee *et al.*, 2008). Children meeting the criteria for ADHD in preschool are likely to go on to have ADHD in middle childhood, while many new cases are diagnosed. School entry may be seen as the first major life transition of particular significance for children with ADHD. Children diagnosed after this will rarely be true *de novo* cases, but more likely cases where histories of subclinical symptoms and/or impairment are exacerbated by the new challenges in the academic and social environment and associated increased demands for self-regulation and effective attention management (Sonuga-Barke *et al.*, 2005). Failure to adapt to this new and challenging environment may lead children with ADHD to fall behind in their studies, and get into trouble at school and at home (Lahey & Willcutt, 2010). There can be great difficulty creating and maintaining strong and positive relationships outside the home (Mrug *et al.*, 2002). At the same time, coercive cycles of interaction with parents and siblings within the home often develop (Lifford *et al.*, 2009). Typical patterns of comorbidity, especially aggression and noncompliance, become more apparent during these middle-child years (Kadesjö & Gillberg, 2003).

Adolescence

The next major pinch point in the ADHD life journey occurs during the transition from childhood to adolescence. Once again longitudinal study suggests strong continuities between these two developmental periods with the persistence of disorder in the majority of cases (Barkley *et al.*, 1990). The disorder seems to be especially persistent in children with comorbid conduct problems. While overall levels of overt hyperactivity may start to recede, impulsiveness and inattention continue to constrain adolescent adjustment and healthy development (Willoughby, 2003). There is a risk of low self-esteem and distorted self concept, perhaps a product of dysfunctional family and peer relationships and school and social failure in childhood; and these can lead on to low mood and feeling of worthlessness (Drabick *et al.*, 2006; Edbom *et al.*, 2006).

Educational underachievement is common and the risk for the emergence of delinquency and early onset substance use disorder is increased (Molina & Pelham, 2003). ADHD may increase the risk of suicidal ideation and behaviors during adolescence, especially where there are co-occuring mood disorders (Chromis-Tuscano *et al.*, 2010).

Adult life

The next crucial developmental transition is from adolescence to adulthood. Once again continuities in disorder are evident, but levels of overt ADHD symptoms appear to reduce further, often replaced by feelings of internal agitation and restlessness that in turn further the risks of anxiety and depression (Adler, 2004). Levels of impairment across a range of outcomes and reduced quality of life remain stubbornly problematic, especially in the case where ADHD in childhood was accompanied by conduct problems (Kessler *et al.*, 2006).

Adulthood brings new challenges and new opportunities for people with ADHD. There is an increased need for self-organization, in budgeting, paying bills on time, remembering appointments, finding lost objects, maintaining personal appearance, and meeting deadlines. In personal relationships, good timing is no less important; and calmness in the face of provocation is often needed in many kinds of personal and business negotiations. Impulsive decision making can have worse consequences than in childhood, with more opportunity to destroy one's life through risky behavior. All these can make inattention and impulsiveness more handicapping than they were in childhood, and are responsible for some apparently *de novo* presentations.

On the other hand, adulthood brings more opportunities for managing one's life. Choice of career may take one into walks of life where rapid changes of activity are necessary and valued (e.g., sales, trading, and some kinds of performing arts). Delegation of routine and tedious tasks may be possible in teams; a partner may take over some of the organizational tasks of everyday life. An increasing capacity to understand one's condition brings the possibility of a happier relationship to it.

Heterogeneity

While it is helpful to think of ADHD as having a characteristic developmental phenotype that can be charted across the life span, the idea that there is a single trajectory runs counter to what we know of the complexity of ADHD developmental psychopathology (as illustrated in Figure 55.1) and the heterogeneity within disorders (see Chapter 3). Multiple ADHD developmental phenotypes exist, each marked by different temporal patterns of symptoms and impairment, leading to different ages of onset, persistence, acceleration, elaboration, and adjustment—and, for some, recovery. Some children may have an early onset and severe form which accelerates during middle childhood to become associated with substantial comorbidity during adolescence but remits as the person enters adulthood. For others, ADHD problems may be later in onset but persist long into adult life. Although little is currently known about the genetic and environmental factors and underlying neurobiological processes that might shape these different developmental pathways, there are some interesting examples of environmental buffering from the literature (Sonuga-Barke & Halperin, 2010). For instance, parental responsiveness and tolerance, perhaps promoted by parent-focused interventions, may protect against the development of conduct problems in children with ADHD (Taylor, 1999). Actual (through remission) or functional (through the development of coping) recovery is perhaps more common than we might suspect and a study of the factors that would predict such an optimal outcome is urgently required.

Treatment

Treatment should begin with careful and responsive advice and explanation (see "Clinical Implications"). Extended courses of "psychoeducation" can have beneficial effects on parental ratings of hyperactivity (Ferrin & Taylor, 2011) as well as on their intended target of assisting people to cope with the problems imposed.

Specific treatments have been widely researched and reviewed. Drug trials especially provide a substantial evidence base. National guidelines generally agree on the forms of intervention that should be used, and that both psychological and pharmacological therapies should be available (Seixas et al., 2012), but differ on the important question of indications. North American guidelines suggest either that both forms of treatment should be used, according to clinical judgment (American Academy of Child and Adolescent Psychiatry, 2007); or that medication is primary, with psychosocial interventions an important adjunct (American Academy of Pediatrics, 2011). By contrast, guidelines for England, Wales, and Northern Ireland (NICE, 2009), Scotland (Scottish Intercollegiate Guidelines Network, 2009), and Europe (Taylor et al., 2004) give priority to psychosocial interventions (especially parent training) in all but severe cases, with medication as a second line of intervention.

The differences between countries arise for several reasons, partly cultural and partly professional. Prendergast et al. (1988) compared the practices of US and UK clinicians in diagnosing the same bank of case vignettes and videotapes: in comorbid cases, the US clinicians gave priority to the component of ADHD, the British to that of oppositionality and conduct problems.

Medication

Central nervous stimulants (methylphenidate, dexamfetamine and lisdexamfetamine) and atomoxetine are licensed in many countries. Bupropion, guanfacine, clonidine, and modafinil are also in widespread use as alternative antihyperkinetics, in spite of not being approved in Europe. Some preparations

of methylphenidate are available in North America, but not widely elsewhere—for instance, a transdermal preparation and a dextro-enantiomer. Chapter 43 summarizes the pharmacology of the main drugs available, their dose ranges and durations of action, and their legal status.

Central nervous stimulants

CNS stimulants are usually the first choice of medication, and methylphenidate is usually the first choice of stimulant. Dexamfetamine is at least as powerful—probably more so—but its safety is less well established. The prodrug lisdexamfetamine has been recently introduced (and may have advantages related to its longer duration of action).

All show beneficial effects in reducing parent-, teacher-, and self-ratings of hyperactive, impulsive and inattentive behaviors. Effect sizes are, in general, large (meta-analysis by Banaschewski et al., 2006). Quality of life ratings also tend to improve; many tests of cognitive function show changes toward becoming more normal; no tests of cognitive function are known to deteriorate. With careful attention to administration and monitoring, the majority of treated children should reach a good level of social function.

Safety

Adverse effects can also occur. Serious adverse effects are rare in trials (Aagaard & Hansen, 2011). This might underestimate the hazards in real life, but a review of adverse effects, from surveillance programs as well as trials, has come to a similar conclusion—that adverse effects are for the most part minor, readily managed symptomatically, and do not persist when the drug is stopped (Graham et al., 2011). Table 55.1 indicates recommended monitoring, symptomatic management, and "second-line" actions when the problems do not resolve or are severe.

The rare, severe problems that can be encountered in practice are not necessarily the result of medication, and referral to an appropriate specialist is usually appropriate. Increases in blood pressure are considered hazardous when they exceed the 95th centile for the population, corrected for age and sex, and should lead to immediate dose reduction or discontinuation. Further management should be between cardiology and psychiatry, preferably with psychiatry leading. Most alternative medications are just as likely as the stimulants to cause raised blood pressure, so the choice for persisting hypertension will be between dose reduction or discontinuation and the addition of clonidine (or guanfacine) which tend to lower the blood pressure. The choice will depend largely on the severity and impact of the ADHD itself.

Arrhythmias, or risky changes in the electrocardiogram (ECG), will naturally call for a cardiological evaluation before treatment. Indeed, some authorities recommend ECG evaluation for all children before beginning therapy, as would be the case for imipramine (which is effective for ADHD, but not included in these recommendations because of its

Table 55.1 Management of adverse effects of medication.

	Monitoring	Symptomatic	Second line
Appetite loss and growth reduction	Growth charts	Altering intake through day. Modifying times of doses. Dose reduction. Drug holiday	Alternate antihyperkinetics or nondrug therapy
Sleep problems	Parent report Pre- and post-medication	Altering dose regime (either reducing or increasing evening cover) Sleep hygiene Melatonin	Replace with Atomoxetine Alternative antihyperkinetics or agreed nondrug therapy
Blood pressure increase	Measurement and plotting on age charts: every 6 months when treatment is stable	Dose reduction Clonidine	24-hour recording Specialist referral if over 95th centile
Tachycardia	Pretreatment history and examination Measurement when BP recorded	ECG evaluation Dose reduction	Specialist referral
Substance misuse	Tablet count Enquiry at psychiatric review	Psychoeducation Motivational interview	Replace with Atomoxetine
Mood change	Psychiatric review	Consider alternative antihyperkinetic	Add Fluoxetine or mood stabilizer

potential for cardiotoxicity). For stimulants and atomoxetine, however—which do not prolong conduction times—the purpose would be to detect the presence of a congenitally prolonged Q-Tc interval and therefore a risk that an arrhythmia might be precipitated if the heart rate were increased by the drug. In our view, the frequency of this congenital anomaly (approximately 1 in 2000 children) is not great enough to make a routine ECG cost-effective. Rather, there should be a clinical evaluation before treatment to detect any suspicion of cardiac problems—including a history of undue breathlessness or syncope on exertion, a cardiac murmur on examination, or a family history of sudden death in young family members—with ECG if risk factors are present.

Substance misuse figures strongly in the worries of families about drug treatment. The stimulants are controlled drugs, and can be misused to obtain euphoria if they are taken intravenously or by inhalation. In these circumstances the drug should be stopped at once and permanently. Oral administration, however, does not lead to euphoria. Absorption from the gut leads to a much slower onset and offset of DA increase in the striatum, by comparison with the addictive drugs that increase DA, such as cocaine (Volkow *et al.*, 2001). Extended-release preparations (such as Oros-methylphenidate and lisdexamfetamine) are very hard to abuse, since they do not support rapid increases in blood level.

While misuse for recreation is rare, diversion by selling or giving tablets to others is not uncommon. The main current misuse is by students who do not have ADHD but value the effects of stimulants in improving concentration on study and counteracting fatigue. Modafinil has a similar niche. Cognitive enhancement such as this raises issues for society at large, about the acceptability of such attempts at self-improvement by people without disorders.

Supposed risks have sometimes been given scare coverage by the media and in the professional press. The risk for sudden cardiac death is probably no higher than in the general population—though it is so rare that millions of treated cases will be needed to rule out the possibility completely—and such data are being accumulated in current research (Graham *et al.*, 2011). Brain damage has not been found: MRI suggests that those who have been given stimulants, by comparison with unmedicated ADHD, show a more normal pattern of age-related maturation (Nakao *et al.*, 2011). Cancer, in the Danish National Registries, was not associated with use of stimulants (Steinhausen & Helenius, 2013).

Dosage

Chapter 43 provides the usual range of doses but individuals vary in their requirements both for overall quantity and for timing of doses. Prescription begins at the lower end of the range, and builds up (e.g., by 10 mg daily each week) to the level giving optimal combination of benefits and adverse effects. Some young people require, and can take safely, doses above the normal range. Where there is only a small response, and no adverse effects have appeared, then doses up to the equivalent of 100 mg of methylphenidate in a day have been regarded as reasonable by NICE (2009) but require careful monitoring.

Immediate-release versus extended-release treatment

In the initial phase of dosage adjustment, immediate-release stimulants allow for frequent adjustments of timing and dose. This does however assume the possibility of close monitoring with adequate professional time and good cooperation (e.g., from teachers). Furthermore, the transfer to extended-release may not be straightforward. When close titration is not possible, then we advise using extended-release treatments from the start and adjusting dose (and, if necessary, preparation) to give the best profile of action through the day—taking into account the desirability of monitoring action into the evening to allow for satisfactory family relationships and successful homework, yet of not interfering with sleep.

In the longer term, meta-analytic comparison of those taking immediate-release with extended-release preparations does not suggest major superiority for one or the other (Punja *et al.*, 2013). Limited evidence favors long-acting for parent ratings, quick-acting for teacher ratings (Banaschewski *et al.*, 2006). This could indicate the extent to which parent ratings are driven by behavior in the evenings, and the risk that prescribers relying solely on parent reports may go to higher dose levels than is optimal for school. Teachers may then be concerned that children are over-treated and lacking in spontaneity.

Atomoxetine

Atomoxetine is also an effective drug. Its beneficial effects are similar to those of the stimulants (reviewed by Hanwella *et al.*, 2011), but the time course of action is longer. The effect size is somewhat smaller than for methylphenidate in meta-analyses of controlled trials (Banaschewski *et al.*, 2006), but it may be underestimated because of the restricted length of most trials. The manufacturers indicate that the full effects may take 6–8 weeks to appear, but clinical experience suggests that it may take longer and there may still be improvements up to 12 weeks. This prolonged process of establishing effect can have both strengths and weaknesses: some families will give up prematurely if the early changes are insufficiently striking. On the other hand, there are benefits for some in a medication whose effects do not fluctuate greatly during the day.

Adverse effects over the longer term are in general similar to those of the stimulants (Hanwella *et al.*, 2011). Suicidal thinking emerged as a complication from reviews of the trial data, and families should be warned of the need to take seriously and report any expression of self-destructive thoughts. The drug is however much less likely than the stimulants to cause insomnia; it reduces rather than increases tics; it does not give rise to euphoria and is not a controlled drug. It may well be the first choice of medication when those additional problems are present or expected. It is still effective in cases which do not respond to stimulants, and is regarded as the best approach in those cases. It can then be given together with methylphenidate for the transitional period while its effect is building up.

Nonpharmacological therapies

Given the current limitations of, and constraints on, pharmacological treatments, the availability of effective nonpharmacological treatments is imperative. These may involve psychological therapies and/or dietary modifications. Their value as distinct from pharmacological approaches is especially important for those patients and/or practitioners who are resistant to the use of medicines for ADHD. The use of psychological and dietary treatments has been advocated as part of multimodel packages (Taylor *et al.*, 2004), with these recommendations based on published reviews (Arns *et al.*, 2009; Fabiano *et al.*, 2009; Bloch & Qawasmi, 2011; Nigg *et al.*, 2012).

Dietary interventions involve both supplements to address putative deficiencies (minerals, vitamins, and fatty acids) and exclusions (of artificial food colors and preservatives; or a wider range of foods to which children may be idiosyncratically intolerant). They are not specific to ADHD and they are described more fully in Chapter 43.

Psychological interventions are also various. Parent training is the most commonly employed. It comes in a range of different forms (see Chapter 37) and some are recommended for use with ADHD children specifically (Thompson *et al.*, 2009; Webster-Stratton *et al.*, 2011). Modifications for ADHD may include psycho-educational modules about the nature of the condition (Montoya *et al.*, 2011); and/or an increased focus on the clarity and directness of communication (e.g., eye contact and short and clear messages) (Sonuga-Barke *et al.*, 2001). In some cases parent training is integrated with school-focused approaches employing teachers (Sayal *et al.*, 2012). A number have a special focus on improving the parent-child relationship and emphasis on increasing enjoyment in interactions (Griggs & Mikami, 2011).

More recently, parenting approaches have started to include elements that aim to strengthen self-regulatory abilities thought to be deficient in children with ADHD in the form of specific games and tasks (Halperin & Healey, 2011). They are recommended for ADHD children through middle childhood, and thought to be especially valuable for preschool children (Halperin *et al.*, 2012). Specific behavioral approaches can be valuable in targeting particular areas of difficulty such as social relationships (Corkum *et al.*, 2010) and organizational skills (Abikoff *et al.*, 2012). With some adaptation, they can be useful in adolescence (Sibley *et al.*, 2012). In adolescence and adulthood, approaches incorporate elements of cognitive behavior therapy to help support functional, and reduce dysfunctional, responses to daily social and practical challenges, increase problem solving, and develop self-control (Safren, 2006).

Other nonpharmacological approaches that might be valuable include intensive computerized training of attention, inhibition, and working memory, and neurofeedback. Computerized training approaches typically work on the principle that underlying deficits in brain networks and associated cognitive processes can be remediated by structured exposure to repeated cognitive tasks in which task difficulty is continuously titrated so as to challenge but not overwhelm an individual's abilities (Klingberg *et al.*, 2005). Packages often require extended treatment programs before improvements can be seen and therefore require a significant investment from families. A range of different neurofeedback packages are available—these employ adaptive reward-based techniques using brain visualization to improve attention via cortical self-regulation (Arns *et al.*, 2009).

For many of these psychological approaches there are insufficient well designed trials published to allow one to say whether they represent empirically-based treatments for ADHD, but isolated trials have provided positive results. A recent meta-analysis of randomized controlled trials challenged the existing evidence for the efficacy of some of these treatments (Sonuga-Barke *et al.*, 2013). The investigation, which was confined to studies at ages 3–18 years in ADHD populations and using ADHD outcomes, separated outcomes into those made by people close to the intervention (e.g., parents delivering treatment) and those made by blinded investigators—either direct observations or made by raters (e.g., teachers) working in different settings from those where the intervention was made. Dietary interventions in general seemed to be helpful even when the probably blinded outcome was considered—although the effects were modest. For diets eliminating artificial colors and additives, the effect size (which in all cases was the standardized mean difference (SMD) between treated groups and controls) was 0.32 for the "open" raters, 0.42 for the "blind." For diets eliminating a wider range of foodstuffs (usually, but not invariably, those suggested by individual testing for intolerance), the SMD calculation for the "open" raters was difficult to interpret because of great heterogeneity among studies. "Blind" ratings yielded a 0.51 SMD (but with wide confidence intervals and not statistically significant). Essential fatty acid supplements (e.g., fish oil to provide omega-3 polyunsaturated fatty acids), gave SMDs for "open" raters of 0.21, and for "blind" 0.16.

The psychological treatments gave a rather different picture. For cognitive training procedures, such as working memory training and attention training, SMD for "open" raters was 0.64, for "blind" raters 0.24. For neurofeedback the relevant figures were 0.59 for the most proximal raters and 0.29 for the "blind." For behavioral interventions, (typically parent- or teacher-mediated training to increase desired /reduce undesired behaviors) SMD for "open" raters was 0.40, which dropped dramatically to 0.02 for probably blinded ratings. In summary, statistical significance was found in a wide variety of therapies. The effect sizes, however, are rather small by comparison with those of drugs. Furthermore, for the psychological interventions they are critically dependent upon using outcomes provided by people who are aware that the child received the active therapy and were often heavily invested in its delivery and outcomes.

In the meta-analyses described above, only the elimination of artificial colorings and giving of fish oil had statistically significant effects upon blinded outcomes; the effect of the latter intervention was modest or very small.

The NICE and EAGG recommendation—for parent training to be the front line for most children—could therefore be seen as overstating the case. The NICE analysis did concur in finding much smaller effects of parent training on teacher ratings than on parent ratings. This could reflect an inflated estimate of change at home resulting from nonblind raters. It could, however, also represent a problem of generalization from home to school rather than a failure to have an effect; and blind raters during direct observation in the home might be insensitive to real therapeutic actions. Even if the effects were only on short term and localized to changes in parental perception, they could still prove to be valuable—especially for situations where the ADHD problems are specifically intra-familial. If they lead to more generally sympathetic rearing environments in the longer term, this could cut the risk of the development of comorbid disorders such as ODD and anxiety/depression. The effects of the interventions on ODD and other comorbidities, or on parental behavior and expectations, were not studied in these meta-analyses.

The challenge for the future is to bring our growing knowledge of the pathophysiological basis of ADHD to the process of therapeutic innovation to allow us to develop more effective nonpharmacological treatments for the benefit of patients and their families. Given the somewhat disappointing nature of some of these results, it has been suggested that efforts relating to non-pharmacological treatments for ADHD should be focused on the development of early identification and intervention in the preschool period when the disorder and its underlying causes may be more amenable to environmental influence (Halperin *et al.*, 2012).

Choice of initial treatment approaches

Both pharmacological and psychological approaches should be available for children and their families, and clinicians should be able to give advice about diet and exercise. Medication is more efficacious than psychological approaches, but carries some physical hazards. The decision about whether to begin with either or both needs to be made on an individual basis. It would be useful to be able to predict which children will do better with which treatment approach. A randomized, 14-month comparison of behavioral and medication approaches favored the latter (The MTA Cooperative Group, 1999). Intensive medication was superior to intensive behavior therapy in reducing core ADHD features, and behavior therapy added little to medication. Longer term follow-up yielded a different emphasis: improvements were maintained, but there seemed to be no superiority of any of the intensive treatments—either to each other or to routine community treatment (Molina *et al.*, 2009). One should note that the later outcome came after both randomization and intensive interventions had ended. The apparent equivalence of treatments probably reflected both the ending of intensive therapeutic efforts after the 14-month outcome, and the effectiveness of self-selection of individual families for the treatment approach that suited them best. Both possibilities emphasize the importance of including families in the choice of therapy.

Individual prediction of drug responsiveness from laboratory measures has not been very powerful—certainly less informative than a short medication trial (Ferrin & Taylor, 2011). A reanalysis of the MTA study, however, did suggest that children meeting the ICD-10 criteria for 'HKD' showed a much greater superiority, of intensive medication to intensive behavioral work, than was the case for other children with milder levels of ADHD symptoms (Santosh *et al.*, 2005). The most severely affected children are also the most likely to benefit from the help of medication.

Treatment of refractory cases

Some children will fail to respond even to a combination of behaviorally oriented parent training and trials of stimulants and atomoxetine. The reasons for poor response should then be analyzed (see Figure 55.2). Sometimes the standard treatment has not been optimally delivered and is worth a more strenuously supervised trial. Sometimes the persisting problems are the comorbid features and need managing in their own right. Sometimes the case features of impulsiveness, overactivity, and inattention have not responded to full standard therapy, and will require a more intensive and specialist approach, such as higher doses of standard drugs, off-label use of alternative antihyperkinetic drugs (see Chapter 43), management of side-effects that have limited the therapy (Table 55.1), or intensive behavioral work with child or family. Sometimes a full assessment of drugs is needed, even requiring in-patient admission.

Treatment in comorbidity

Figure 55.2 includes some actions to be taken when other problems are present. For the most part, the treatment of the ADHD itself is unaltered, albeit with particular attention in monitoring to avoid worsening the coexistent condition. For children with autism and other neurological problems, dosage titration may need to be frequent, and primarily against

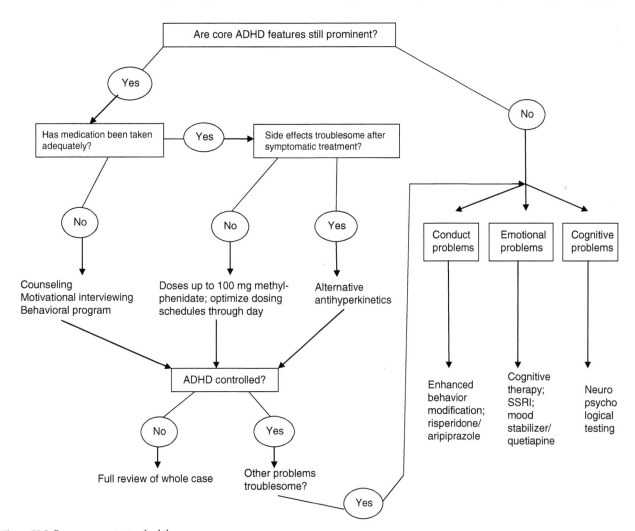

Figure 55.2 Poor response to standard therapy.

adverse effects (see Chapter 51). Substance misuse presents particular difficulties. Occasional cannabis use is not necessarily a contraindication to stimulants—there seem to be few interactions—but addicted patients with ADHD need to be managed by someone expert in both. Stimulant and other drugs may well help the ADHD, but should not be expected to be effective for established substance misuse.

Long-term treatment

ADHD is a risk for later mental health and for health problems such as accidents. A systematic review by Shaw *et al.* (2012) has found evidence for adverse outcomes being more common in ADHD than in unaffected people, and less common in those who have been treated than for people with ADHD who have not.

There have now been enough trials of treatment in adults to be confident that medication is still effective, and that cognitively based therapies and learning coping skills are promising; a systematic review is provided by the Canadian Agency for Drugs and Technologies in Health (2011). It is less clear what degree of continuation of therapy is needed. There is a little evidence that adults with continuing symptoms make a better adjustment if their ADHD is controlled with medication. Lichtenstein *et al.* (2012), for instance, find less offending during periods of medication than in periods of abstinence.

In the absence of definitive evidence, an individualized approach is recommended. Periodic periods off medication (e.g., 2 weeks every 2 years) will make it clear whether a drug is still desirable. (There should still be an option for returning to medication subsequently if necessary.) Patients should become increasingly knowledgeable about medication effects through their adolescence. Most do so and become intelligent consumers (Singh *et al.*, 2005). Existential questions are raised by the power of the therapies, and patients are often taxed to understand whether their 'real self' is that with ADHD or that when ADHD is controlled. The consequences include decision making about whether to take the medication at all—or only when environmental demands for attention and self-control are high. Responsive discussion with a knowledgeable professional is greatly valued by most people with ADHD, who share with other forms of disability the need to make a balance between overcoming its continuing problems and living within the limitations that it imposes.

References

Aagaard, L. & Hansen, E.H. (2011) The occurrence of adverse drug reactions reported for attention deficit hyperactivity disorder (ADHD) medications in the pediatric population: a qualitative review of empirical studies. *Neuropsychiatric Disease and Treatment* 7, 729–744.

Abikoff, H. *et al.* (2012) Remediating organizational functioning in children with ADM: immediate and long-term effects from a randomized controlled trial. *Journal of Clinical Psychiatry* 81, 113–128.

Achenbach, T.M. & Edelbrock, C.S. (1983) *Manual for the Child Behaviour Checklist and Revised Behaviour Profile.* University of Vermont Department of Psychiatry, Burlington.

Adler, L.A. (2004) Clinical presentations of adult patients with ADHD. *Journal of Clinical Psychiatry* 65, 8–11.

American Academy of Child and Adolescent Psychiatry (2007) Practice parameter for the assessment and treatment of children and adolescents with attention-deficit/hyperactivity disorder. *Journal of the American Academy of Child and Adolescent Psychiatry* 46, 894–921.

American Academy of Pediatrics (2011) ADHD: clinical practice guideline for the diagnosis, evaluation, and treatment of attention-deficit/hyperactivity disorder in children and adolescents. *Pediatrics* 128, 1007–1022.

American Psychiatric Association (2000) *Diagnostic and Statistical Manual of Mental Disorders* (4th ed), Text Revision. American Psychiatric Association, Washington, DC.

Arcos-Burgos, M. *et al.* (2004) Attention-deficit/hyperactivity disorder in a population isolate: linkage to loci at 4q13.2, 5q33.3, 11q22, and 17p11. *American Journal of Human Genetics* 75, 998–1014.

Arns, M. *et al.* (2009) Efficacy of neurofeedback treatment in ADHD: the effects on inattention, impulsivity and hyperactivity: a meta-analysis. *Clinical EEG Neuroscience* 40, 180–189.

Banaschewski, T. *et al.* (2006) Long-acting medications for the hyperkinetic disorders: a systematic review and European treatment guideline. *European Child & Adolescent Psychiatry* 15, 476–495.

Barkley, R.A. (1991) *Attention-Deficit Hyperactivity Disorder: A Clinical Workbook.* Guilford Press, New York.

Barkley, R.A. (1997) Behavioral inhibition, sustained attention, and executive functions: constructing a unifying theory of ADHD. *Psychological Bulletin* 121, 65–94.

Barkley, R.A. *et al.* (1990) The adolescent outcome of hyperactive-children diagnosed by research criteria. 1. An 8-year prospective follow-up study. *Journal of the American Academy of Child and Adolescent Psychiatry* 29, 546–557.

Batty, M.J. *et al.* (2010) Cortical gray matter in attention-deficit/hyperactivity disorder: a structural magnetic resonance imaging study. *Journal of the American Academy of Child and Adolescent Psychiatry* 49, 229–238.

Bender, L. & Cottington, F. (1942) The use of amphetamine sulphate (Benzedrine) in child psychiatry. *American Journal of Psychiatry* 99, 116–121.

Biederman, J. *et al.* (2012) Adult outcome of attention-deficit/hyperactivity disorder: a controlled 16-year follow-up study. *Journal of Clinical Psychiatry* 73, 941–950.

Bloch, M.H. & Qawasmi, A. (2011) Omega-3 fatty acid supplementation for the treatment of children with attention-deficit/hyperactivity disorder symptomatology: systematic review and meta-analysis. *Journal of American Academy of Child Adolescent Psychiatry* 50, 991–1000.

Bradley, C. (1937) The behaviour of children receiving Benzedrine. *American Journal of Psychiatry* 94, 577–585.

Campbell, S.B. *et al.* (2000) Early externalizing behaviour problems: toddlers and preschoolers at risk for later maladjustment. *Development and Psychopathology* 12, 467–488.

Canadian Agency for Drugs and Technologies in Health (2011) *Pharmacological and Non-Pharmacological Therapies for Adults with Attention-Deficit/Hyperactivity Disorder: Systematic Review and Meta-Analysis of Clinical Evidence.* Health Technology Assessment

Database: http://www.crd.york.ac.uk/crdweb/ShowRecord.asp?Link From=OAI&ID=32011001514

Caspi, A. (2008) A replicated molecular genetic basis for sub-typing antisocial behavior in children with attention-deficit/hyperactivity disorder. *Archives of General Psychiatry* **65**, 203–210.

Castellanos, F.X. et al. (2002) Developmental trajectories of brain volume abnormalities in children and adolescents with attention-deficit/hyperactivity disorder. *JAMA* **288**, 1740–1748.

Centers for Disease Control and Prevention (2010) Increasing prevalence of parent-reported attention-deficit/hyperactivity disorder among children—United States, 2003 and 2007. *CDC Morbidity and Mortality Weekly Report* November 12, 2010 www.cdc.gov/mmwr/preview/mmwrhtml

Chromis-Tuscano, A. et al. (2010) Very early predictors of adolescent depression and suicide attempts in children with Attention-Deficit/Hyperactivity Disorder. *Archives of General Psychiatry* **67**, 1044–1051.

Clements, SD. (1966) *Minimal Brain Dysfunction in Children: Terminology and Identification, Phase One of a Three-Phase Project*. NINDB Monograph No. 3. US Department of Health, Education and Welfare, Public Health Service publication no. 1415, Washington.

Coghill, D. & Sonuga-Barke, E.J.S. (2012) Annual research review: categories versus dimensions in the classification and conceptualization of child and adolescent mental disorders – implications of recent empirical study. *Journal of Child Psychology and Psychiatry* **53**, 469–489.

Conners, C.K. (2008) *Conners' Rating Scales*, 3rd edn. Multi Health Systems, Toronto.

Corkum, P. et al. (2010) Evaluation of a school-based social skills program for children with attention-deficit/hyperactivity disorder. *Child and Family Behavior Therapy* **32**, 139–151.

Crichton, A. (1798) *An Inquiry Into the Nature and Origin of Mental Derangement*. T. Cadell & W. Davies, London.

Cutler, M. et al. (1940) The effect of Benzedrine on mentally deficient children. *American Journal of Mental Deficiency* **45**, 59–68.

Drabick, D.A.G. et al. (2006) Co-occurrence of conduct disorder and depression in a clinic-based sample of boys with ADHD. *Journal of Child Psychology and Psychiatry* **47**, 766–774.

DuPaul, G.J. (1991) Parent and teacher ratings of ADHD symptoms: psychometric properties in a community-based sample. *Journal of Clinical Child Psychology* **20**, 245–253.

Edbom, T. et al. (2006) Long-term relationships between symptoms of Attention Deficit Hyperactivity Disorder and self-esteem in a prospective longitudinal study of twins. *Acta Paediatrica* **95**, 650–657.

Eisenberg, L. et al. (1963) A psychopharmacologic study in a training school for delinquent boys. *American Journal of Orthopsychiatry* **33**, 431–447.

Ellison-Wright, I. et al. (2008) Structural brain change in Attention Deficit Hyperactivity Disorder identified by meta-analysis. *BMC Psychiatry* **8**, 51.

Fabiano, G.A. et al. (2009) A meta-analysis of behavioral treatments for attention-deficit/hyperactivity disorder. *Clinical Psychology Review* **29**, 129–140.

Fair, D.A. et al (2010) Atypical default network connectivity in youth with attention-deficit/hyperactivity disorder. *Biological Psychiatry* **68**, 1084–1091.

Faraone, S.V. et al. (2005) Molecular genetics of attention-deficit/hyperactivity disorder. *Biological Psychiatry* **57**, 1313–1323.

Ferrin, M. & Taylor, E. (2011) Child and caregiver issues in the treatment of ADHD: education, adherence and treatment choice. *Future Neurology* **6**, 399–413.

Goodman, R. (1997) The strengths and difficulties questionnaire: a research note. *Journal of Child Psychology and Psychiatry* **38**, 581–586.

Graham, J. et al. (for the European Guidelines Group) (2011) European guidelines on managing adverse effects of medication for ADHD. *European Child & Adolescent Psychiatry* **20**, 17–37.

Greven, C.U. et al. (2011) A longitudinal twin study on the association between inattentive and hyperactive-impulsive ADHD symptoms. *Journal of Abnormal Child Psychology* **39**, 623–632.

Griggs, M.S. & Mikami, A.Y. (2011) Parental attention-deficit/hyperactivity disorder predicts child and parent outcomes of parental friendship coaching treatment. *Journal of the American Academy of Child and Adolescent Psychiatry* **50**, 1236–1246.

Halperin, J.M. & Healey, D.M. (2011) The influences of environmental enrichment, cognitive enhancement and physical exercise on brain development: can we alter the developmental trajectory of ADHD? *Neuroscience and Biobehavioral Reviews* **35**, 621–634.

Halperin, J.M. et al. (2008) Neuropsychological outcome in adolescents/young adults with childhood ADHD: profiles of persisters, remitters and controls. *Journal of Child Psychology and Psychiatry* **49**, 958–966.

Halperin, J.M. et al. (2012) Preventive interventions for ADHD: a neuro developmental perspective. *Neurotherapeutics* **9**, 531–541.

Hanwella, R. et al. (2011) Comparative efficacy and acceptability of methylphenidate and atomoxetine in treatment of attention deficit hyperactivity disorder in children and adolescents: a meta-analysis. *BMC Psychiatry* **11**, 176.

Haslam, J. (1809) *Observations on Madness and Melancholy including Practical Remarks on these Diseases together with Cases*. J. Callow, London.

Hinshaw, S.P. et al. (2011) International variation in treatment procedures for ADHD: social context and recent trends. *Psychiatric Services* **62**, 459–464.

Kadesjö, B. & Gillberg, C. (2003) The comorbidity of ADHD in the general population of Swedish school-age children. *Journal of Child Psychology and Psychiatry* **42**, 487–492.

Kessler, R.C. et al. (2006) The prevalence and correlates of adult ADHD in the United States: results from the National Comorbidity Survey Replication. *American Journal of Psychiatry* **163**, 716–723.

Klingberg, T. et al. (2005) Computerized training of working memory in children with ADHD: a randomized, controlled trial. *Journal of the American Academy of Child and Adolescent Psychiatry* **44**, 177–186.

Kuntsi, J. et al. (2006) The IMAGE project: methodological issues for the molecular genetic analysis of ADHD. *Behavioral Brain Function* **2**, 27.

Lahey, B.B. & Willcutt, E.G. (2010) Predictive validity of a continuous alternative to nominal subtypes of attention-deficit/hyperactivity disorder for DSM-V. *Journal of Clinical Child and Adolescent Psychology* **39**, 761–775.

Lahey, B.B. et al. (2005) Instability of the DSM-IV subtypes of ADHD from preschool through elementary school. *Archives of General Psychiatry* **62**, 896–902.

Lee, S.S. et al. (2008) Few preschool boys and girls with ADHD are well-adjusted during adolescence. *Journal of Abnormal Child Psychology* **36**, 373–383.

Lichtenstein, P. et al. (2012) Medication for attention deficit-hyperactivity disorder and criminality. *New England Journal of Medicine* **367**, 2006–2014.

Liddle, E.B. et al. (2011) Task-related default mode network modulation and inhibitory control in ADHD: effects of motivation and methylphenidate. *Journal of Child Psychology and Psychiatry* **52**, 761–771.

Lifford, K.J. et al. (2009) Parent-child hostility and child ADHD symptoms: a genetically sensitive and longitudinal analysis. *Journal of Child Psychology and Psychiatry* **50**, 1468–1476.

Luk, S.-L. (1996) Cross-cultural aspects. In: *Hyperactivity Disorders of Childhood*. (ed S. Sandberg), pp. 350–381. Cambridge University Press, Cambridge.

Madras, B.K. et al. (2005) The dopamine transporter and attention-deficit/hyperactivity disorder. *Biological Psychiatry* **57**, 1397–1409.

Mandell, D.S. et al. (2007) Disparities in diagnoses received prior to a diagnosis of Autism Spectrum Disorder. *Journal of Autism and Developmental Disorders* **37**, 1795–1802.

Marco, R. et al. (2009) Delay and reward choice in ADHD: an experimental test of the role of delay aversion. *Neuropsychology* **23**, 367–380.

Mariussen, E. & Fonnum, F. (2006) Neurochemical targets and behavioral effects of organohalogen compounds: an update. *Critical Reviews in Toxicology* **36**, 253–289.

McCann, D. et al. (2007) Food additives and hyperactive behaviour in 3-year-old and 8/9-year-old children in the community: a randomised, double-blinded, placebo-controlled trial. *The Lancet* **370**, 1560–1567.

McLoughlin, G. et al. (2007) Genetic support for the dual nature of attention deficit hyperactivity disorder: substantial genetic overlap between the inattentive and hyperactive-impulsive components. *Journal of Abnormal Child Psychology* **35**, 999–1008.

Mokrova, I. et al. (2010) Parental ADHD symptomology and ineffective parenting: the connecting link of home chaos. *Parenting-Science and Practice* **10**, 119–135.

Molina, B.S.G. & Pelham, W.E. (2003) Childhood predictors of adolescent substance use in a longitudinal study of children with ADHD. *Journal of Abnormal Psychology* **112**, 497–507.

Molina, B.S. et al. (2009) The MTA at 8 years: prospective follow-up of children treated for combined-type ADHD in a multisite study. *Journal of American Academy of Child and Adolescent Psychiatry* **48**, 484–500.

Montoya, A. et al. (2011) Is psychoeducation for parents and teachers of children and adolescents with ADHD efficacious? A systematic literature review. *European Psychiatry* **26**, 166–175.

Mrug, S. et al. (2002) Relationships and peer-oriented interventions new directions. *Child and Adolescent Development* **91**, 51–78.

Nakao, T. et al. (2011) Gray matter volume abnormalities in ADHD: voxel-based meta-analysis exploring the effects of age and stimulant medication. *American Journal of Psychiatry* **168**, 1154–1163.

National Institute for Health and Care Excellence (2009) *Attention Deficit Hyperactivity Disorder*. British Psychological Society and The Royal College of Psychiatrists, Leicester & London.

Neumärker, K.-J. (2005) The Kramer-Pollnow Syndrome: a contribution on the life and work of Franz Kramer and Hans Pollnow. *History of Psychiatry* **16**, 435–451.

Nigg, J.T. et al. (2012) Meta-analysis of attention-deficit/hyperactivity disorder or attention-deficit/hyperactivity disorder symptoms, restriction diet, and synthetic food color additives. *Journal of the American Academy of Child and Adolescent Psychiatry* **51**, 86–97.

Oades, R.D. et al. (2005) The control of responsiveness in ADHD by catecholamines: evidence for dopaminergic, noradrenergic and interactive roles. *Developmental Science* **8**, 122–131.

Oades, R.D. et al. (2008) The influence of serotonin- and other genes on impulsive behavioral aggression and cognitive impulsivity in children with attention-deficit/hyperactivity disorder (ADHD): findings from a family-based association test (FBAT) analysis. *Behavioral and Brain Functions* **4**, 48.

Olijslagers, J.E. et al. (2006) Modulation of midbrain dopamine neurotransmission by serotonin, a versatile interaction between neurotransmitters and significance for antipsychotic drug action. *Current Neuropharmacology* **4**, 59–68.

Plessen, K.J. et al. (2006) Hippocampus and amygdale morphology in attention-deficit/hyperactivity disorder. *Archives of General Psychiatry* **63**, 795–807.

Plichta, M.M. et al. (2009) Neural hyporesponsiveness and hyperresponsiveness during immediate and delayed reward processing in adult attention-deficit/hyperactivity disorder. *Biological Psychiatry* **65**, 7–14.

Pliszka, S.R. (2005) The neuropsychopharmacology of attention-deficit/hyperactivity disorder. *Biological Psychiatry* **57**, 1385–1390.

Polanczyk, G. et al. (2007) The worldwide prevalence of ADHD: a systematic review and metaregression analysis. *American Journal of Psychiatry* **164**, 942–948.

Prendergast, M. et al. (1988) The diagnosis of childhood hyperactivity: a U.S.-U.K. cross-national study of DSM-III and ICD-9. *Journal of Child Psychology & Psychiatry & Allied Disciplines* **29**, 289–300.

Prince, J. (2008) Catecholamine dysfunction in attention-deficit/ hyperactivity disorder: an update. *Journal of Clinical Psychopharmacology* **28**, S39–S45.

Punja, S. et al. (2013) Long-acting versus short-acting methylphenidate for paediatric ADHD: a systematic review and meta-analysis of comparative efficacy. *BMJ Open* **15**, 3.

Raichle, M.E. & Snyder, A.Z. (2007) A default mode of brain function: a brief history of an evolving idea. *NeuroImage* **37**, 1083–1090.

Rapport, M.D. et al. (2008) Working memory deficits in boys with attention-deficit/hyperactivity disorder (ADHD): the contribution of central executive and subsystem processes. *Journal of Abnormal Child Psychology* **36**, 825–837.

Reiersen, A.M. et al. (2007) Autistic traits in a population-based ADHD twin sample. *Journal of Child Psychology and Psychiatry* **48**, 464–472.

Riddle, M. et al. (2013) The Preschool ADHD Treatment Study (PATS) 6-year follow-up. *Journal of the American Academy of Child and Adolescent Psychiatry* **52**, 264–272.

Ronald, A. et al. (2008) Evidence for overlapping genetic influences on autistic and ADHD behaviours in a community twin sample. *Journal of Child Psychology and Psychiatry* **49**, 535–542.

Rubia, K. et al. (2005) Abnormal brain activation during inhibition and error detection in medication-naive adolescents with ADHD. *American Journal of Psychiatry* **162**, 1067–1075.

Rush, B. (1812) *Medical Inquiries and Observations Upon the Diseases of the Mind*, pp. 1962. Macmillan-Hafner Press, New York.

Rutter, M. et al. (1970) *A Neuropsychiatric Study in Childhood*. Clinics in Developmental Medicine, Nos. 35/36. S.I.M.P with Heinemann, London.

Safren, S.A. (2006) Cognitive-behavioral approaches to ADHD treatment in adulthood. *Journal of Clinical Psychiatry* **67**, 46–50.

Sagvolden, T. *et al.* (2005) A dynamic developmental theory of attention-deficit/hyperactivity disorder (ADHD) predominantly hyperactive/ impulsive and combined subtypes. *Behavioral and Brain Science* **28**, 397–419.

Santosh, P.J. *et al.* (2005) Refining the diagnoses of inattention and over-activity syndromes: a reanalysis of the Multimodal Treatment study of ADHD based on ICD-10 criteria for hyperkinetic disorder. *Clinical Neuroscience Research* **5**, 307–331.

Sayal, K. *et al.* (2002) Pathways to care in children at risk of attention-deficit hyperactivity disorder. *British Journal of Psychiatry* **181**, 43–48.

Sayal, K. *et al.* (2006) Barriers to the identification of children with attention deficit/hyperactivity disorder. *Journal of Child Psychology & Psychiatry* **47**, 744–750.

Sayal, K. *et al.* (2012) Protocol evaluating the effectiveness of a school-based programme for parents of children at risk of ADHD. *British Medical Journal Open* **2**, 5.

Schoemaker, K. *et al.* (2012) Executive function deficits in preschool children with ADHD and DBD. *Journal of Child Psychology and Psychiatry* **53**, 111–119.

Scottish Intercollegiate Guidelines Network (2009) *Management of Attention Deficit and Hyperkinetic Disorders in Children and Young People.* SIGN, Edinburgh.

Seixas, M. *et al.* (2012) Systematic review of national international guidelines on attention-deficit hyperactivity disorder. *Journal of Psychopharmacology* **26**, 753–765.

Sergeant, J.A. (2005) Modeling attention-deficit/hyperactivity disorder: a critical appraisal of the cognitive-energetic model. *Biological Psychiatry* **57**, 1248–1255.

Shaw, P. *et al.* (2010) Childhood psychiatric disorders as anomalies in neurodevelopmental trajectories. *Human Brain Mapping* **31**, 917–925.

Shaw, M. *et al.* (2012) A systematic review and analysis of long-term outcomes in ADHD: effects of treatment and non-treatment. *BMC Medicine* **10**, 99.

Sibley, M.H. *et al.* (2012) Treatment Response to an Intensive Summer Treatment Program for Adolescents With ADHD. *Journal of Attention Disorders* **16**, 443–448.

Singh, I. *et al.* (2005) Will the "real boy" please behave: dosing dilemmas for parents of boys with ADHD. *American Journal of Bioethics* **5**, 34–47.

Skounti, M. *et al.* (2007) Variations in prevalence of attention deficit hyperactivity disorder worldwide. *European Journal of Pediatrics* **166**, 117–123.

Sobanski, E. *et al.* (2010) Emotional lability in children and adolescents with Attention Deficit/Hyperactivity Disorder (ADHD): clinical correlates and familial prevalence. *Journal of Child Psychiatry and Psychology* **51**, 915–923.

Sonuga-Barke, E.J.S. & Fairchild, G. (2012) Neuroeconomics of attention-deficit/hyperactivity disorder: differential influences of medial, dorsal and ventral prefrontal brain networks on suboptimal decision making. *Biological Psychiatry* **72**, 126–133.

Sonuga-Barke, E.J.S. & Halperin, J.M. (2010) Developmental phenotypes and causal pathways in attention deficit/hyperactivity disorder: potential targets for early intervention? *Journal of Child Psychology and Psychiatry* **51**, 368–389.

Sonuga-Barke, E.J.S. *et al.* (2001) Parent-based therapies for preschool attention deficit/hyperactivity disorder: a randomized, controlled trial with a community sample. *Journal of the American Academy of Child & Adolescent Psychiatry* **40**, 402–408.

Sonuga-Barke, E.J.S. *et al.* (2005) Varieties of preschool hyperactivity: multiple pathways from risk to disorder. *Developmental Science* **8**, 141–150.

Sonuga-Barke, E.J.S. *et al.* (2010) Beyond the dual pathway model: evidence for the dissociation of timing, inhibitory and delay-related impairments in attention-deficit/hyperactivity disorder. *Journal of the American Academy of Child and Adolescent Psychiatry* **49**, 345–355.

Sonuga-Barke, E.J.S. *et al.* (2013) Nonpharmacological interventions for ADHD: systematic review and meta-analyses of randomized controlled trials of dietary and psychological treatments. *The American Journal of Psychiatry* **170**, 275–289.

Steinhausen, H.-C. & Helenius, D. (2013) The association between medication for attention-deficit/hyperactivity disorder and cancer. *Journal Of Child And Adolescent Psychopharmacology* **23**, 208–213.

Stergiakouli, E. *et al.* (2012) Investigating the contribution of common genetic variants to the risk and pathogenesis of ADHD. *American Journal of Psychiatry* **169**, 186–194.

Stevens, S.E. *et al.* (2008) Inattention/over activity following early severe institutional deprivation: presentation and associations in early adolescence. *Journal of Abnormal Child Psychology* **36**, 385–398.

Still, G.F. (1902) The Goulstonian lectures on some abnormal psychical conditions in children. *The Lancet* **1**, 1008–1012, 1077–1082, 1163–1168.

Strauss, A.A. & Lehtinen, L.E. (1947) *Psychopathology and Education of the Brain-Injured Child.* Grune & Stratton, New York.

Swanson, J. *et al.* (2005) *Categorical and Dimensional Definitions and Evaluations of Symptoms of ADHD: The SNAP and the SWAN Rating Scales.* Available at: http://www.adhd.net/SNAP SWAN.pdf

Taylor, E. (1999) Developmental neuropsychopathology of attention deficit and impulsiveness. *Development and Psychopathology* **11**, 607–628.

Taylor, E. (2010) Comorbidity in neurodevelopmental disorders: the case of attention-deficit-hyperactivity disorder. In: *Comorbidities in Developmental Disorders.* (eds M. Bax & C. Gillberg). Mac Keith Press, London.

Taylor, E. (2013) Uses and misuses of treatments for ADHD. The second Birgit Olsson lecture. *Nordic Journal of Psychiatry* **68**, 236–242.

Taylor, E. *et al.* (1987) Which boys respond to stimulant medication? A controlled trial of methylphenidate in boys with disruptive behaviour. *Psychological Medicine* **17**, 121–143.

Taylor, E. *et al.* (1991) *The Epidemiology of Childhood Hyperactivity.* Maudsley Monograph No. 33. Oxford University Press, Oxford.

Taylor, E. *et al.* (1996) Hyperactivity and conduct problems as risk factors for adolescent development. *Journal of the American Academy of Child & Adolescent Psychiatry* **35**, 1213–1226.

Taylor, E. *et al.* (2004) European clinical guidelines for hyperkinetic disorder: first upgrade. *European Child and Adolescent Psychiatry* **13**, 17–130.

Thapar, A. *et al.* (2009) Prenatal smoking might not cause attention-deficit/hyperactivity disorder: evidence from a novel design. *Biological Psychiatry* **66**, 722–727.

Thapar, A. *et al.* (2012) What causes attention deficit hyperactivity disorder? *Archives of Disease in Childhood* **97**, 260–265.

The MTA Cooperative Group (1999) A 14-month randomized clinical trial of treatment strategies for attention-deficit/hyperactivity disorder. *Archives of General Psychiatry* **56**, 1073–1086.

Toplak, M.E. *et al.* (2009) The unity and diversity of inattention and hyperactivity/impulsivity in ADHD: evidence for a general factor with separable dimensions. *Journal of Abnormal Child Psychology* **37**, 1137–1150.

Tymms, P. & Merrell, C. (2006) The impact of screening and advice on inattentive, hyperactive and impulsive children. *European Journal of Special Needs Education* **21**, 321–337.

Vaidya, C.J. *et al.* (2005) Altered neural substrates of cognitive control in childhood ADHD: evidence from functional magnetic resonance imaging. *American Journal of Psychiatry* **162**, 1605–1613.

Valera, E.M. *et al.* (2007) Meta-analysis of structural imaging findings in attention-deficit/hyperactivity disorder. *Biological Psychiatry* **61**, 1361–1369.

Van Ewijk, H. *et al.* (2012) Diffusion tensor imaging in attention deficit/hyperactivity disorder: a systematic review and meta-analysis. *Neuroscience and Biobehavioral Reviews* **36**, 1093–1106.

Volkow, N.D. *et al.* (2001) Therapeutic doses of oral methylphenidate significantly increase extracellular dopamine in the human brain. *Journal of Neuroscience* **21** (RC121), 1–5.

Von Stauffenberg, C. & Campbell, S.B. (2007) Predicting the early developmental course of symptoms of attention deficit hyperactivity disorder. *Journal of Applied Developmental Psychology* **28**, 536–552.

Warner-Rogers, J. *et al.* (2000) Inattentive behavior in childhood: epidemiology and implications for development. *Journal of Learning Disabilities* **33**, 520–536.

Webster-Stratton, C.H. *et al.* (2011) Combining parent and child training for young children with ADHD. *Journal of Clinical Child and Adolescent Psychology* **40**, 191–203.

Willcutt, E.G. *et al.* (2005) Validity of the executive function theory of attention-deficit/hyperactivity disorder: a meta-analytic review. *Biological Psychiatry* **57**, 1336–1346.

Willcutt, E.G. *et al.* (2012) Validity of DSM-IV attention deficit/ hyperactivity disorder symptom dimensions and subtypes. *Journal of Abnormal Psychology* **121**, 991–1010.

Williams, N. *et al.* (2010) Rare chromosomal deletions and duplications in attention-deficit hyperactivity disorder: a genome-wide analysis. *Archives of Disease in Childhood* **97**, 260–265.

Williams, N. *et al.* (2012) Genome-wide analysis of copy number variants in attention deficit hyperactivity disorder: the role of rare variants and duplications at 15q13.3. *American Journal of Psychiatry* **169**, 195–204.

Willoughby, M.T. (2003) Developmental course of ADHD symptomatology during the transition from childhood to adolescence: a review with recommendations. *Journal of Child Psychology and Psychiatry* **44**, 88–106.

Wolosin, S.M. *et al.* (2009) Abnormal cerebral cortex structure in children with ADHD. *Human Brain Mapping* **30**, 175–184.

Wolraich, M.L. *et al.* (2003) Psychometric properties of the Vanderbilt ADHD diagnostic parent rating scale in a referred population. *Journal of Pediatric Psychology* **28**, 559–568.

CHAPTER 56

Tic disorders

James F. Leckman[1,2] and Michael H. Bloch[2]

[1] Child Study Center and the Departments of Psychiatry, Pediatrics and Psychology, Yale University, New Haven, CT, USA
[2] Child Study Center and the Department of Psychiatry, Yale University, New Haven, CT, USA

Introduction

Tic disorders are transient or chronic conditions associated with difficulties in self-esteem, family life, social acceptance, or school or job performance that are directly related to the presence of motor and/or phonic tics. Although tic symptoms have been reported since antiquity, systematic study of individuals with tic disorders dates only from the 19th century with the reports of Itard (1825) and Gilles de la Tourette (1885). Gilles de la Tourette described nine cases characterized by motor "incoordinations" or tics, "inarticulate shouts accompanied by articulated words with echolalia [automatic repetition of words or made by another person] and coprolalia [sudden vocalization of obscene or socially inappropriate speech]." In addition to identifying the cardinal features of severe tic disorders, his report noted an association between tic disorders and obsessive-compulsive (OC) symptoms, as well as the hereditary nature of the syndrome in some families.

In addition to tics, individuals with tic disorders may present with a broad array of behavioral difficulties, including disinhibited speech or conduct, impulsivity, distractibility, motoric hyperactivity, and obsessive compulsive symptoms (Leckman *et al.*, 2013). Scientific opinion has been divided on how broadly to conceive the spectrum of maladaptive behaviors associated with Tourette's syndrome (TS) (Shapiro *et al.*, 1988). This controversy is fueled in part by the frustration that parents and educators encounter when they attempt to divide an individual child's repertoire of problem behaviors into those that are "Tourette-related" and those that are not. Population-based epidemiological studies and family-genetic studies have begun to clarify these issues, but much work remains to be done.

In this chapter, a presentation of the phenomenology and classification of tic disorders precedes a review of the etiology, neurobiological substrates, assessment, and management of these conditions. The general perspective that will be presented is that TS and related disorders are associated with multiple genetic and environmental (epigenetic) mechanisms that interact over the course of development to produce a distinctive range of complex syndromes of varying severity.

Phemonenology of tics and diagnosis of tic disorders

Phenomenology of tics

A *tic* is a sudden, repetitive movement, gesture, or utterance that typically mimics some aspect or fragment of normal behavior (Leckman *et al.*, 2013). Individual tics rarely last more than a second. Individual tics can occur singly or together in an orchestrated pattern. They vary in their intensity or forcefulness. Motor tics vary from simple abrupt movements such as eye blinking, head jerks, or shoulder shrugs to more complex, apparently purposive behaviors such as facial expressions or gestures of the arms or head. In extreme cases, these movements can be obscene (copropraxia) or self-injurious, for example, hitting or biting. Phonic or vocal tics can range from simple throat clearing sounds to more complex vocalizations and speech. In severe cases, coprolalia (obscene or socially unacceptable speech) is present.

By the age of 10 years, most individuals with tics are aware of premonitory urges that may either be experienced as a focal perception in a particular body region where the tic is about to occur (like an itch or a tickling sensation) or as a mental awareness (Leckman *et al.*, 1993). Most patients also report a fleeting sense of relief after a bout of tics has occurred. These premonitory and consummatory phenomena contribute to an individual's sense that tics are a habitual, yet partially intentional, response to unpleasant stimuli. Indeed, most adolescent and adult subjects describe their tics as either "voluntary" or as having both voluntary and involuntary aspects. In contrast,

Rutter's Child and Adolescent Psychiatry, Sixth Edition.
Edited by Anita Thapar and Daniel S. Pine, James F. Leckman, Stephen Scott, Margaret J. Snowling, Eric Taylor.
© 2015 John Wiley & Sons Ltd. Published 2018 by John Wiley & Sons Ltd.

many young children are oblivious to their tics and experience them as wholly involuntary movements or sounds. Most tics can also be suppressed for brief periods of time. The warning given by premonitory urges may contribute to this phenomenon.

Clinicians characterize tics by their anatomical location, number, frequency, and duration. The intensity or "forcefulness" of the tic can also be an important characteristic. Finally, tics vary in terms of their "complexity." Complexity usually refers to how simple or involved a movement or sound is, ranging from brief, meaningless, abrupt fragments (simple tics) to ones that are longer, more involved, and seemingly more goal-directed in character (complex tics). Each of these elements has been incorporated into clinician rating scales that have proved to be useful in monitoring tic severity (Leckman *et al.*, 1989).

Diagnostic categories

Diagnostic categories provide a common basis for discussion and are an essential tool in epidemiological and clinical research. Several widely used diagnostic classifications currently include sections on tic disorders. These include both the *Diagnostic and Statistical Manual—Fifth Edition* (*DSM-5*) classification system published by the American Psychiatric Association (2013), and the *International Classification of Disease and Related Health Problems—10th Revision* (*ICD-10*) criteria by the World Health Organization (1996). Although differences exist, these classification schemes are broadly congruent, with each containing three major categories: TS or its equivalent; persistent (chronic) motor or vocal tic disorder (CMT or CVT) or its equivalent; and transient tic disorder or its equivalent. However, the *ICD-10* and *DSM-5* diagnostic groupings suffer from uncertainties about how best to categorize conditions that potentially encompass a broad range of symptoms that wax and wane in severity. Since the current nosological boundaries are set by convention and clinical practice, they may not reflect true etiological differences.

Transient tic disorder

Almost invariably a disorder of childhood, transient tic disorder is usually characterized by one or more simple motor tics that wax and wane in severity over weeks to months. The anatomical distribution of these tics is usually confined to the eyes, face, neck, or upper extremities. Transient phonic tics, in the absence of motor tics, can also occur, though more rarely. The age of onset is typically 3–10 years. Boys are at greater risk. The initial presentation may be unnoticed. Family practitioners, pediatricians, allergists, and ophthalmologists are typically the first to see the child. Missed diagnoses are common, particularly as the symptoms may have completely disappeared by the time of the consultation.

Persistent (chronic) motor or vocal tic disorder

This chronic condition can be observed among children and adults. As with other tic disorders, this condition is characterized by a waxing and waning course and a broad range of symptom severity. Chronic simple and complex motor tics are the most common manifestations. A majority of tics involve the eyes, face, head, neck, and upper extremities. Although some children may display other developmental difficulties such as attention deficit hyperactivity disorder (ADHD), the disorder is not incompatible with an otherwise normal course of childhood. This condition can also appear as a residual state, where a predictable repertoire of tic symptoms may be seen only during periods of heightened stress or fatigue.

Tourette's syndrome (combined vocal and multiple motor tic disorder)

The most severe tic disorder is best known by the eponym, "Gilles de la Tourette's Syndrome." Typically the disorder begins in early childhood with transient bouts of simple motor tics such as eye blinking or head jerks. These tics may initially come and go, but eventually they become persistent and begin to have adverse effects on the child and the family. The repertoire of motor tics can be vast, incorporating virtually any voluntary movement by any portion of the body (Leckman *et al.*, 2013). Although some patients have a "rostral-caudal" progression of motor tics (head, neck, shoulders, arms, and torso), this course is not predictable. As the syndrome develops, complex motor tics may appear. Typically, they accompany simple motor tics. Often they have a "camouflaged" or purposive appearance, for example, brushing hair away from the face with an arm, and can only be distinguished as tics by their repetitive character. They can involve dystonic movements. In a small fraction of cases (<5%), complex motor tics have the potential to be self-injurious. These self-injurious symptoms may be relatively mild, for example, slapping or tapping, or quite dangerous, for example, punching one side of the face, biting a wrist or gouging eyes to the point of blindness. On average, phonic tics begin 1–2 years after the onset of motor symptoms and are usually simple in character, for example, throat clearing, grunting, and squeaks. More complex vocal symptoms such as echolalia (repeating another's speech), palilalia (repeating one's own speech), and coprolalia occur in a minority of cases. Other complex phonic symptoms include dramatic and abrupt changes in rhythm, rate, and volume of speech.

Epidemiology

Children are 5–12 times more likely to be identified as having a tic disorder than adults. As with other neurodevelopmental disorders, including autism and ADHD, boys are more commonly affected with tic behaviors than girls (see Chapter 3). However, the reported male–female ratio varies considerably from 1:1 to 10:1 across epidemiological studies (Scahill *et al.*, 2013). Once thought to be rare, current estimates of the prevalence of TS vary 100-fold, from 2.9 per 10,000 (Caine *et al.*, 1988) to 299 per 10,000 (Mason *et al.*, 1998). More recently, Khalifa and von Knorring (2003, 2005) studied a total population of 4479 Swedish children aged 7–15 years. Twenty-five were identified as having TS, yielding a prevalence estimate of 5.6 per 1000 pupils. Similar findings have been reported in Denmark and China (Jin *et al.*, 2005; Kraft *et al.*, 2012). Methodological differences (parent-report vs direct observation in the classroom) and threshold differences (chronic motor disorder is much more common that a full case of TS) likely account for some of the reported variation in prevalence rates and possibly the male–female ratio estimates.

Clinical course

Motor and phonic tics tend to occur in bouts. Their frequency ranges from nonstop bursts that are virtually uncountable (>100 tics per minute) to rare events that occur only a few times a week (Peterson & Leckman, 1998). Single tics may occur in isolation, or there may be orchestrated combinations of motor and phonic tics that involve multiple muscle groups. The forcefulness of motor tics and the volume of phonic tics can also vary from behaviors that are not noticeable (a slight shrug or a hushed guttural noise) to strenuous displays (arm thrusts or loud barking) that are frightening and exhausting. During periods of waxing tic symptoms, clinicians may find themselves under extreme pressure to intervene medically. While such interventions may be warranted, it is often the case that the tic symptoms will wane substantially within a few weeks (Figure 56.1).

By the age of ten, most children and adolescents have some awareness of the premonitory urges that frequently precede both motor and vocal tics (Leckman *et al.*, 1993; Woods *et al.*, 2005). These urges add to the subjective discomfort associated with having a tic disorder. They may also contribute to an individual's ability to suppress their tics for longer periods of time.

The factors that determine the degree of disability and handicap versus resiliency are largely unknown. They are likely to include the presence of additional developmental, mental, and behavioral disorders; the level of support and understanding from parents, peers, and educators; and the presence of special abilities (as in sports) or personal attributes (intelligence, social abilities, and personality traits). The behavioral and emotional

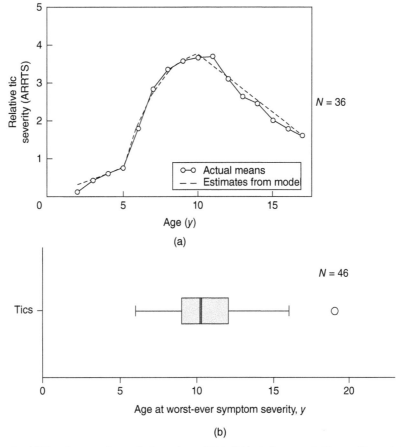

Figure 56.1 Course of tic severity. (a) Plot of average tic severity in a cohort of 36 individuals from ages 2–18 years. Tics typically have an onset between ages 4 and 6 years, reach their worst between ages 10 and 12 years, and then decline in severity throughout adolescence. In the ARRTS (Annual Rating of Relative Tic Severity), parents rate the tic symptoms of their children on a six-point ordinal scale (absent [0], least severe, mild, moderate, severe, and most severe [6]). (b) Box plot representing age when tic symptoms were at their worst. Age (years) is represented for all 46 subjects with Tourette's syndrome in a prospective longitudinal study (Bloch *et al.*, 2006). The mean ± SD worst-ever tic severity score using the Yale Global Tic Severity Scale (0–50) was 31.6 ± 7.7 (range, 15–48) at a mean ± SD age of 10.6 ± 2.6 years (range, 6–19 years). *Source*: Reproduced with permission of Wiley.

problems that frequently complicate TS range from impulsive, "disinhibited," and immature behavior to compulsive touching or sniffing. At present, there are no clear dividing lines between these disruptive behaviors and complex tics on the one hand and comorbid conditions of ADHD and obsessive-compulsive disorder (OCD) on the other (Leckman *et al.*, 2013).

Although children with TS can be loving and affectionate, maintaining age-appropriate social skills is particularly difficult for many of them (Dykens *et al.*, 1990; Cath & Ludolph, 2013). Whether this is due to the stigmatizing effects of the tics, the patients' own uneasiness, or some more fundamental difficulty linked to the neurobiology of this disorder is unknown.

Relatively few cross-sectional or longitudinal studies of tic disorders have been performed (Leckman *et al.*, 1998; Bloch *et al.*, 2006a). These studies indicate that tic disorders tend to improve in late adolescence and early adulthood (Bloch, 2013). In many instances, the phonic symptoms become increasingly rare or may disappear altogether, and the motor tics may be reduced in number and frequency. Complete remission of both motor and phonic symptoms has also been reported. In contrast, adulthood is also the period when the most severe and debilitating forms of tic disorder can be seen. The factors that influence the continuity of tic disorders from childhood to adolescence to adulthood are not well understood but likely involve the interaction of normal maturational processes occurring in the central nervous system (CNS) with the neurobiological mechanisms responsible for TS, the exposure to cocaine, other CNS stimulants, androgenic steroids, and the amount of emotional trauma and distress experienced by affected individuals during childhood and adolescence. In addition, tic disorders may be etiologically separable so that some of these factors, such as activation of the immune system or exposure to heat stress, may influence the clinical course for some individuals but not for others. Other factors, such as psychological stress often associated with the negative and stigmatizing interactions with others (parents, teachers, peers, and other people in the environment) who do not understand the involuntary nature of tics, may have a more uniform impact.

The natural history of TS has clear implications for the treatment of individuals with this condition. Children with tics have a substantial probability of improvement of their tic symptoms during adolescence and young adulthood. Given the ephemeral nature of tics in many children, pharmacological treatment should be conservative and focused on reducing functional impairment. Parents, teachers, and peers can benefit from psychoeducational interventions.

Clinical assessment

Assessment instruments

The complex motor, vocal, and behavioral phenotype of TS presents a unique challenge to measurement. Although the visible and audible nature of core TS symptoms allows direct observation, their waxing and waning character, even over the course of the day, presents challenges to the clinician. A variety of clinician-, parent-, and self-report rating instruments are available for tics and associated symptoms, for use in clinical practice and/or research settings (Cavanna & Pansaon Piedad, 2013). The Yale Global Tic Severity Scale (YGTSS) is the most widely used measure of tic severity in TS and other tic disorders (Leckman *et al.*, 1989). It is based on a semistructured interview of symptoms over the past week, where the clinician is asked to document the patient's motor and phonic tics. The motor and vocal tics are rated separately, based on their number, frequency, intensity, complexity, and interference from 0 (no tic symptoms) to 5 (severe). The tic severity subscore consists of the motor and phonic tic severity scores. This is added to the impairment subscore, which rates the severity of functional impairment from 0 to 50, to produce the total score (0–100). In addition to the YGTSS, the Premonitory Urge for Tics Scale (PUTS) is being increasingly used to characterize individuals with tic disorders. The PUTS is a relatively brief self-report scale designed to quantify the premonitory sensory urges that frequently precede motor and vocal tics (Woods *et al.*, 2005). The PUTS contains 10 descriptions of somatic sensations. The severity of these urges is rated on a 4-point ordinal scale ranging from 1 (not at all true) to 4 (very much true). A wide range of psychometrically validated clinician- and self-rated measures for OC, ADHD, depressive, and anxiety symptoms are also available (see Chapters 33, 55, 60, 61, and 63) and they are commonly used in assessing individuals with TS and other tic disorders. As noted in Chapter 33, the potential differences between information gathered from clinicians and patients should always be considered if the assessment is to be considered comprehensive and accurate.

Comorbid conditions

The past decade has seen a renewed emphasis on the range of neurological and psychiatric symptoms seen in patients with TS (Leckman & Cohen, 1998; Martino & Leckman, 2013). In both clinical and epidemiological samples TS alone is the exception rather than the rule (Khalifa & von Knorring, 2005, 2006; Scahill *et al.*, 2013). Symptoms associated with ADHD and OCD have received the most attention. It is also becoming clear that the more severe the tic disorder, the greater the likelihood of detecting coexisting conditions, even in representative, population-based samples (Scahill *et al.*, 2013).

Both clinical and epidemiological studies vary according to setting and established referral patterns, but it is not uncommon to see reports of 30–50% of children with TS diagnosed with comorbid ADHD (Khalifa & von Knorring, 2006). TS has the highest rate of ADHD relative to the other lesser variants of tic disorders. Although the etiological relationship between TS and ADHD is in dispute, it is clear that those individuals with both TS and ADHD are at a much greater risk for a variety of untoward outcomes (Dykens *et al.*, 1990; Carter *et al.*, 2000;

Peterson *et al.*, 2001; Sukhodolsky *et al.*, 2003, 2005). They are often regarded as less likeable, more aggressive, and more withdrawn than their classmates (Stokes *et al.*, 1991).

More than 40% of individuals with TS experience recurrent OC symptoms (Leckman *et al.*, 1994, 1997; Khalifa & von Knorring, 2005; Ferrão *et al.*, 2013). Genetic, neurobiological, and treatment response studies suggest that there may be qualitative differences between tic-related forms of OCD and cases of OCD in which there is no personal or family history of tics. Specifically, tic-related OCD has a male preponderance, an earlier age of onset, a poorer level of response to standard anti-obsessional medications, and a greater likelihood of first-degree family members with a tic disorder (Hounie *et al.*, 2006). Symptomatically the most common OC symptoms encountered in TS patients are obsessions concerning a need for symmetry or exactness, repeating rituals, counting compulsions, and ordering/arranging compulsions (Leckman *et al.*, 1997). Also, OC symptoms, when present in children with TS, appear more likely to persist into adulthood than the tics themselves (Bloch *et al.*, 2006a).

The co-occurrence of *depression* and *anxiety* symptoms with TS are commonplace and may reflect the cumulative psychosocial burden of having tics or shared etiological factors or both (Cath & Ludolph, 2013). Antecedent depressive symptoms do predict modest increases in tic severity (Lin *et al.*, 2007). However, this study also documented that future depression severity is more closely associated with antecedent worsening of psychosocial stress and OC symptoms than it is with future measures of tic severity.

Children with a range of neurodevelopmental disorders are at increased risk for tic disorders. Kurlan and colleagues (1994) reported a fourfold increase in the prevalence of tic disorders among children in special educational settings in a single school district in upstate New York. These children did not have an intellectual disability but did have significant specific learning problems, and/or other speech or physical impairments. Children with autism and other pervasive developmental disorders are also at higher risk for developing TS (Baron-Cohen *et al.*, 1999; Cath & Ludolph, 2013). However, in many instances the tics go unrecognized and regarded as stereotypies.

A number of medical and neurological disorders have a higher prevalence in children with TS. These include asthma and allergic disorders, streptococcal infections, as well as restless legs syndrome, and migraine and tension headaches (Lespérance *et al.*, 2004; Chang *et al.*, 2011; Ghosh *et al.*, 2012; Murphy, 2013). The etiological basis for these associations is yet to be elucidated.

Prognosis and quality of life

Prospective cohort studies have fairly consistently shown that most children with TS will improve during adolescence (range: 67–96%) (Bloch, 2013). Current research indicates that estimates of current tic severity have limited value in terms of long-term prognosis. Although lifetime histories of comorbid ADHD and OCD symptoms are associated with poorer

adulthood psychosocial functioning in patients with TS, the presence of these comorbid symptoms in childhood has not been found to be associated with higher levels of severity in adulthood (Bloch *et al.*, 2006b; Gorman *et al.*, 2010). However, initial studies do suggest that poor performance on standardized tests of fine-motor coordination (dominant hand, Purdue Pegboard test) and smaller caudate nucleus volumes (using volumetric MRIs) are associated with more severe tic symptoms in adulthood (Bloch *et al.*, 2005; Bloch *et al.*, 2006b).

Over the past two decades, several studies have documented that many children, adolescents, and adults with TS may have a reduced *Quality of Life* (Elstner *et al.*, 2001; Sukhodolsky *et al.*, 2013). Cavanna and colleagues (2008) developed the Gilles de la Tourette's Syndrome-Quality of Life Scale. The relative contribution of tics versus other co-occurring conditions to impairments in adaptive functioning is an active area of research. In a recent study, 50 children with "pure" TS had a higher quality of life than did individuals with TS, ADHD, and OCD (Eddy *et al.*, 2012). Careful clinical evaluation is required to understand profiles of strengths and weaknesses in adaptive functioning and to disentangle the relative contributions of tics and co-occurring disorders from other problems with peers, academic functioning, or family life. Whenever possible, clinical interviews should be supplemented by collecting standardized ratings of adaptive functioning.

Risk factors

Genetic risk factors

Twin and family studies provide evidence that genetic factors are involved in the vulnerability to TS and related disorders (Pauls & Leckman, 1986; Fernandez & State, 2013). The concordance rate for TS among monozygotic twin pairs is greater than 50% while the concordance of dizygotic twin pairs is about 10% (Price *et al.*, 1985). If cotwins with chronic motor tic disorder are included, these concordance figures increase to 77% for monozygotic and 30% for dizygotic twin pairs. These differences in the concordance of monozygotic and dizygotic twin pairs indicate that genetic factors play an important role in the etiology, but the fact that concordance for monozygotic twins is less than 100% also indicates that nongenetic factors are critical in determining the nature and severity of the clinical syndrome.

Other studies indicate that first-degree family members of probands with TS are at substantially higher risk for having TS, chronic motor tic disorder, and OCD than unrelated individuals (Pauls *et al.*, 1991). The rates are substantially higher than might be expected by chance in the general population, and greatly exceed the rates for these disorders among the relatives of individuals with other psychiatric disorders except OCD.

The pattern of vertical transmission among family members has led several groups of investigators to test specific genetic hypotheses. While not definitive, segregation analyses could not rule out autosomal transmission (Pauls & Leckman, 1986). However, subsequent efforts to identify susceptibility genes within large multigenerational families or using affected sibling pair or genome-wide association designs have met with limited success (Fernandez & State, 2013). The one exception is the report by Ercan-Sencicek et al. (2010) that described a two-generation family with nine affected members with TS. They eventually identified a rare functional mutation in the gene encoding L-histidine decarboxylase, the rate-limiting enzyme in histamine biosynthesis.

In addition, a number of cytogenetic abnormalities have been reported in TS families (State et al., 2003; Cuker et al., 2004). Verkerk and colleagues (2003) reported the disruption of the contactin-associated protein 2 gene on chromosome 7. This gene encodes a membrane protein located at nodes of Ranvier of axons that may be important for the distribution of the K(+) channels, which would affect signal conduction along myelinated neurons. In addition, using a candidate gene approach identified by chromosomal anomalies, Abelson et al. (2005) identified and mapped a de novo chromosome 13 inversion in a patient with TS. The gene SLITRK1 was found to be expressed in multiple neuroanatomical areas implicated in TS neuropathology.

Microarray technologies that can detect submicroscopic structural variation have revealed extensive copy number variation (CNV) throughout the human genome (Conrad et al., 2010) and provided new opportunities for genome-wide studies of such variation in TS and other neurodevelopmental disorders. Initial CNV studies have identified multiple rare variants in TS and hypothesized an overlap of risk with autism and other neurodevelopmental disorders (Sundaram et al., 2010; Fernandez et al., 2012). Further studies are needed to clarify the importance of these variants.

In sum, there are a number of promising leads in the field of genetics. For example, several lines of evidence suggest that histaminergic neurotransmission modulates dopamine release (Ferrada et al., 2008). The technology is now available to explore the role of variations in noncoding RNA as well as the impact of epigenetic modifications of DNA methylation and chromatin remodeling on patterns of gene expression that may be due in part to environmental adversity.

Perinatal risk factors

Twin studies, despite their small size and number, have consistently demonstrated that nongenetic factors play a role in the pathogenesis of TS (Fernandez & State, 2013). Among the risk factors most consistently documented, adverse perinatal problems and infectious and immunological events have been the most consistently implicated.

The most straightforward method of investigating the potential role of perinatal complications in the pathogenesis of TS is to compare the frequencies of these events in children with TS (or tics in general) to a matched group of healthy control children. A number of such case–control studies have been published

(Hoekstra, 2013). In a pioneering study, Pasamanick and Kawi (1956) reviewed the hospital obstetrical records of a cohort of 83 children of normal intelligence diagnosed as "tiqueurs" at Johns Hopkins Medical Center and compared these with the obstetrical records of the very next newborn reported from the same hospital as the child with tics, matched by race, sex, and maternal age group. The percentage of mothers of children with tics with one or more complications was 33.3%, compared with 17.6% for the controls; the percentage of those with two or more complications in the tic group was 7.8% versus only 2.0% in the healthy controls. Subsequently a number of associations have been reported, including advanced paternal age, severe maternal psychosocial stress during pregnancy, severe nausea and/or vomiting during the first trimester, maternal smoking during pregnancy, more and earlier prenatal care visits, delivery complications, and low Apgar score at 5 min after birth (Hoekstra, 2013). Maternal smoking during pregnancy and low birth weight are risk factors for the presence of comorbid ADHD in individuals with a tic disorder. Older paternal age, maternal use of coffee, cigarettes, or alcohol during pregnancy and forceps deliveries are risk factors for the presence of comorbid OCD in individuals with a tic disorder.

A number of fundamental questions remain in this area of research, including whether or not there is a real cause–effect relationship between perinatal adversities and tic disorders (see Chapters 9 and 12). If this can be documented, it will be important to determine what the pathogenic mechanisms are by which perinatal adversities lead to chronic tics over the course of CNS development. Other related questions pertain to the potential presence of critical periods in brain development and the role of genetic risk factors or the possible involvement of epigenetic alterations leading to enduring changes in the levels of gene expression in specific brain regions.

Gender-specific endocrine factors

Males are more frequently affected with TS than females (Shapiro et al., 1988), but male-to-male transmission within families rules out the presence of an X-linked vulnerability gene. This observation has led to the hypothesis that androgenic steroids act at key developmental periods to influence the natural history of TS and related disorders (Peterson et al., 1992). These developmental periods include the prenatal period when the brain is being formed, adrenarche when adrenal androgens first appear at age 5–7 years, and puberty. Androgenic steroids may be responsible for these effects or they may act indirectly through estrogens formed in key brain regions by the aromatization of testosterone (see Chapters 3 and 9).

The importance of gender differences in expression of associated phenotypes is also clear, given the observation that women are more likely than men to develop OC symptoms without concomitant tics (Pauls et al., 1991), and that boys with TS are much more likely than girls to display ADHD and disruptive behaviors.

Surges in testosterone and other androgenic steroids during critical periods in fetal development are involved in the production of long-term functional augmentation of subsequent hormonal challenges (as in adrenarche and during puberty) and in the formation of structural CNS dimorphisms (Goy *et al.*, 1988; Sikich & Todd, 1988). Sexually dimorphic brain regions include portions of the amygdala (and related limbic areas) and the hypothalamus (including the medial preoptic area that mediates the body's response to thermal stress) (Boulant, 1981). These regions contain high levels of androgen and estrogen receptors and influence activity in the basal ganglia both directly and indirectly. Indeed, a proportion of patients with TS appear to be uniquely sensitive to thermal stress and when their core body temperature increases and they begin to sweat, their tics increase (Lombroso *et al.*, 1991). It is also of note that some of the neurochemical and neuropeptidergic systems implicated in TS and related disorders, such as dopamine, serotonin, and the opioids, are involved with these regions and appear to be regulated by sex-specific factors.

Further support for a role for androgens comes from anecdotal reports of tic exacerbation following androgen use (Leckman & Scahill, 1990) and from trials of antiandrogens in patients with severe TS and/or OCD (Peterson *et al.*, 1998b). In the most rigorous study to date, Peterson and colleagues (1998b) found that the therapeutic effects of the antiandrogen, flutamide, were modest in magnitude and these effects were short-lived, possibly because of physiologic compensation for androgen receptor blockade.

Psychosocial stress

Tic disorders have long been identified as "stress-sensitive" conditions. Typically, symptom exacerbations follow in the wake of stressful life events. As noted by Shapiro and colleagues (1988), these events need not be adverse in character. However, clinical experience suggests that in some instances a vicious cycle is initiated in which attempts to suppress the symptoms by punishment and humiliation lead to a further exacerbation of symptoms and further increase in stress in the child's interpersonal environment. Unchecked, this vicious cycle can lead to the most severe manifestations of TS. Prospective longitudinal studies have shown that patients with TS experience more stress than matched healthy controls (Findley *et al.*, 2003) and that antecedent stress may play a role in subsequent tic exacerbation (Lin *et al.*, 2007, 2010). Increases in depressive symptoms have also emerged as a significant predictor of future tic severity.

In addition to the effects of stress, anxiety, and depression, premorbid stress may also act as a sensitizing agent in the pathogenesis of TS among vulnerable individuals (Leckman *et al.*, 1984). It is likely that the immediate family environment, for example, parental discord, and the coping abilities of family members play some role (Leckman *et al.*, 1990), and this may lead to a sensitization of stress-responsive biological systems such as the hypothalamic–pituitary–adrenal axis (Chappell *et al.*, 1994, 1996; Leckman *et al.*, 1995).

Antecedent infections and immune responses

The relationship between antecedent infections and immune responses has been an object of interest for clinical and basic researchers for centuries (Kushner, 1999). For example, Sydenham's chorea is known to be an autoimmune disorder following group A beta-hemolytic streptococcus (GABHS) infections (Dale & Brilot, 2012). Among the clinical manifestations of Sydenham's chorea, OCD as well as motor and vocal tics are not uncommon (Mercadante *et al.*, 2000). In addition to GABHS, *Mycoplasma pneumoniae, Borrelia burgdorferi*, as well as viral agents such as varicella zoster, have all been reported as potential causes of "postinfectious tourettism" in anecdotal reports as well as in larger observational clinical series (Murphy, 2013).

It has been proposed that Pediatric Autoimmune Neuropsychiatric Disorder Associated with Streptococcal (*PANDAS*) infection represents a distinct clinical entity, and includes Sydenham's chorea and some cases of TS and OCD (Swedo *et al.*, 1998) (see also Chapter 61). The most compelling evidence of an etiological link between these disorders and GABHS infection comes from a study that found an increased proportion of GABHS infections (odds ratio = 13.6) within the preceding 12 months in children newly diagnosed with TS compared to well-matched controls (Mell *et al.*, 2005). The PANDAS hypothesis is also indirectly supported by the presence of high levels of antistreptococcal antibodies in some patients with TS (Cardona & Orefici, 2001; Church *et al.*, 2003; Martino *et al.*, 2011). Animal model systems have also been developed that provide proof of concept for PANDAS (Yaddanapudi *et al.*, 2010; Brimberg *et al.*, 2012). Thus far, however, prospective longitudinal studies have provided little support for the idea that GABHS infections induce future tic exacerbations (Kurlan *et al.*, 2008; Leckman *et al.*, 2011). These findings have led in part to a reformulation of the PANDAS concept, with a greater emphasis now being placed on the overnight onset of OCD as the cardinal feature of pediatric acute-onset neuropsychiatric syndrome (*PANS*) (Swedo *et al.*, 2012). The PANS concept also removes the requirement for an antecedent GABHS infection. Ideally, this will allow investigators to identify similar cohorts of children and to explore a range of possible etiological factors.

There is also a growing literature that suggests possible systemic alterations of circulating levels of proinflammatory cytokines, immunoglobulins, and immune cells in TS (Martino, 2014). For example, there is preliminary evidence of decreased numbers of regulatory T-cells during periods of tic exacerbation (Kawikova *et al.*, 2007). A number of genes related to both cell- and antibody-mediated immune responses have been reported to be overexpressed in peripheral blood (Lit *et al.*, 2007, 2009). Preliminary postmortem studies also support the presence of neuroinflammatory processes in some adults with severe persistent TS (Morer *et al.*, 2010).

Finally, it should be noted that neuroimmunology is an emerging area of scientific discovery. For example, although microglia are the resident macrophages of the brain, and act as the first and main form of active immune defense in CNS, it is also clear that microglia and the proteins that they produce are not synonymous with inflammation. Indeed, microglia appear to play an important and ongoing role in surveying and shaping neuronal circuit structure and function over the lifespan (Wake et al., 2013). In addition, some "proinflammatory" cytokines, proteins of the innate immune system, and components of the major histocompatibility complex, complement proteins, and various T- and B-cell receptors play essential roles in the establishment and modulation of synaptic connections during development (Yirmiya & Goshen, 2011). These effects occurring over the course of neural development set the stage for a deeper understanding of the neuroanatomy and circuit anomalies seen in TS and other neurodevelopmental disorders.

Pathophysiology

Neural circuits

Investigators interested in procedural learning, habit formation, and internally and externally guided motor control have focused their attention on multisynaptic cortico-striato-thalamo-cortical (CSTC) circuits or loops that link the cerebral cortex with several subcortical regions (Graybiel & Canales, 2001). As a result, the most widely accepted neuroanatomical model of TS proposes a regional imbalance of the direct versus the indirect pathway (Figure 56.2) within one or more of these CSTCs (Albin & Mink, 2006). In the direct pathway, an excitatory glutamatergic signal projects to the striatum, sending an inhibitory γ-aminobutyric acid (GABA)-ergic signal to the internal part of the globus pallidus. This signal results in a decreased inhibition (disinhibition) of the thalamus and thus an increased excitatory effect on the prefrontal cortex. In the indirect pathway, the striatum projects an inhibitory signal to the external part of the globus pallidus and the subthalamic nucleus, sending an excitatory signal to the internal part of the globus pallidus. The net effect is an increased inhibition of the thalamus and decreased excitation on the prefrontal cortex. It is hypothesized that the direct pathway functions as a self-reinforcing positive feedback loop and contributes to the initiation and continuation of behaviors, whereas the indirect pathway provides a mechanism of negative feedback, which is important for the inhibition of behaviors and in switching between behaviors. Based on postmortem studies, as well as structural and functional neuroimaging studies, it appears that an imbalance between these frontal–striatal circuits might mediate tic symptomatology as well as that of related disorders.

Neuropathology

Although neuropathological studies of postmortem TS brains are few in number, a recent stereological study indicates that there is a marked alteration in the number and density of at least two classes of interneurons (parvalbumin-positive fast-spiking

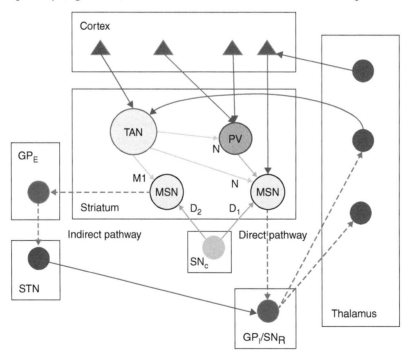

Figure 56.2 Cortico-striato-thalamo-cortical circuitry in Tourette's syndrome. Red, excitatory glutamatergic neurons; blue, GABAergic inhibitory neurons; green, cholinergic tonically active interneurons (TANs); orange, dopaminergic neurons. Parvalbumin fast-spiking GABAergic interneurons (PVs, parvalbumins) mediate the cortical feed-forward inhibition upon medium spiny neurons (MSNs) of the striatopallidal direct pathway, resulting in inhibition of voluntary movements. Cholinergic TANs enhance the responsiveness of MSNs of the striatonigral indirect pathway, resulting in movement suppression. PVs and TANs are diminished in number in the brains of adults with severe, persistent Tourette's syndrome (see text). The volume of the striatum, particularly the caudate nuclei, is smaller in both children and adults with Tourette's syndrome. Receptors include: M1 and nicotinic (N) cholinergic receptors; D_1 and D_2 dopamine receptors. *Source*: Adapted with permission from Vaccarino et al. (2013).

GABAergic interneurons and cholinergic tonically active neurons) in the caudate and putamen (Kalanithi *et al.*, 2005; Kataoka *et al.*, 2010). Most recently, Lennington *et al.* (2014) reported on the results of a whole transcriptome analyses of the basal ganglia of 9 adults with TS. They found a down regulation of striatal interneuron transcripts associated with cholinergic and GABAergic interneurons. They also observed a marked increase in immune-related genes, consistent with activation of microglia in the striatum. Further studies are needed to confirm and extend these findings. A key question concerns whether these alterations are causal or simply a consequence of having lifelong TS (Leckman *et al.*, 2006).

Structural brain imaging

Volumetric magnetic resonance imaging (MRI) studies of basal ganglia in individuals with TS are largely consistent with these postmortem results—with the finding of a slight reduction in caudate volume (Hyde *et al.*, 1995; Peterson *et al.*, 2003). For example, in a study of 154 subjects with TS and 130 healthy controls, Peterson *et al.* (2003) found a significant decrease in the volume of the caudate nucleus in both children and adults. Although there was no correlation between symptom severity and caudate volumes in this cross-sectional study, Bloch *et al.* (2005) found an inverse correlation between caudate volumes measured in childhood and tic severity rated in early adulthood.

Cortical thinning in sensorimotor cortices has also been detected in children and adults with TS, with a negative correlation between thickness and orofacial tic severity (Sowell *et al.*, 2008). Several portions of the brain, including the prefrontal cortex, the corpus callosum, amygdala, and hippocampus have been proposed to constitute a network of neural adaptation to the presence of tics, a network in which compensatory changes help to suppress or modulate the severity of tic symptoms (Plessen *et al.*, 2009). Recently, Bansal *et al.* (2012) employed a semisupervised learning algorithm to identify spatial patterns of variation in the morphology of the cerebral cortex and other brain regions that were specifically associated with TS. Regional volumes and surface features morphology of the right hippocampus and the right globus pallidus provided the best sensitivity and specificity.

Functional brain imaging

There are a growing number of studies using functional magnetic resonance imaging (fMRI) to study individuals with TS. In one of the first, Peterson *et al.* (1998a) compared brain activity during blocks of time during which tics were voluntarily suppressed or not suppressed. During tic suppression, prefrontal cortical, thalamic, and basal ganglia areas were activated. These activations were inversely correlated with tic severity (i.e., lower activation was associated with higher tic severity). This suggests that a greater ability of basal ganglia to suppress cortical activity might be linked with decreased tic severity, and is in agreement with single photon emission-computed tomography (SPECT) and positron emission tomography (PET) studies that

suggest involvement of the basal ganglia in TS (Braun *et al.*, 1995). More recently, Kumar *et al.* (2014) has documented activated microglia-mediated neuroinflammation in the caudate nuclei bilaterally using PET adolescents with TS. This finding is consistent with the whole transcriptome findings reported by Lennington *et al.* (2014). Bohlhalter *et al.* (2006) studied the neural correlates of tics and associated urges using an event-related fMRI protocol. On the basis of synchronized video/audio recordings, fMRI activities were analyzed 2 s before and at tic onset. A brain network of paralimbic areas including the anterior cingulate and insular cortex, supplementary motor area, and parietal operculum was found to be activated before tic onset. In contrast, at the beginning of tic action, significant fMRI activities were found in sensorimotor areas including superior parietal lobule bilaterally and cerebellum. Similar results were reported by Hampson (2009) who found that the spatiotemporal pattern of coactivation was similar for both the healthy controls and the TS subjects. However, the timing and magnitude of the activation in the supplementary motor area differed in the TS, perhaps reflecting the importance of this region in relation to the premonitory sensory urges.

Resting-state functional connectivity has also been studied in adolescents and adults with TS (Church *et al.*, 2009). Results demonstrated widespread functional immaturity in both the frontoparietal and the cingulo-opercular networks. In addition, a number of anomalous connections, not seen in age-match peers, were also identified, primarily in the frontoparietal network. These findings are consistent with studies using diffusion tensor imaging that again reveal altered interhemispheric connectivity in individuals with TS (Neuner *et al.*, 2010).

Neurophysiology

Noninvasive *in vivo* neurophysiological research in TS has led to several areas of significant progress. The first concerns the use of a startle paradigm to measure inhibitory deficits by monitoring the reduction in startle reflex magnitude. Swerdlow *et al.* (2001) have confirmed and extended earlier findings indicating that patients with TS have deficits in sensory gating across a number of sensory modalities. Prepulse inhibition abnormalities have been observed across a variety of neuropsychiatric populations, including schizophrenia, OCD, Huntington's disease, nocturnal enuresis, ADHD, Asperger's syndrome, and TS, suggesting that some final common pathways mediate abnormal prepulse inhibition in all of these conditions. With respect to TS, these deficits are consistent with the idea that there is diminished ability to appropriately manage or "gate" sensory inputs to motor programs, which are released as tics (Swerdlow & Sutherland, 2006; Zebardast *et al.*, 2013). A second advance has been the investigation of motor system excitability by means of single and paired pulse transcranial magnetic stimulation. Studies of groups of patients with TS have indicated that the cortical silent period (a period of decreased excitability following stimulation) is shortened. This intracortical excitability is frequently seen in children with ADHD comorbid with a tic disorder (Ziemann *et al.*, 1997; Moll *et al.*, 1999). This heightened level of cortical excitability may be related to a reduction in the number of GABAergic interneurons in the cortex. Third, Serrien *et al.* (2005) identified similar sensorimotor-frontal connections involved in the acute suppression of involuntary tics as evidenced by increased EEG coherence in the α frequency band (8–12 Hz) during suppression of voluntary movements in individuals with TS and healthy subjects during a Go-NoGo task. This finding, taken with the functional findings from Peterson *et al.* (1998a), suggests that the frontal lobes may play a key role in tic suppression, and coherence in the α band may be part of this process. The combination of imaging techniques with real-time neurophysiological techniques, such as electroencephalography or magnetoencephalography, may help to determine whether any abnormalities seen in brain imaging contribute to the production of tics or whether they constitute a compensatory response (Llinas *et al.*, 2005; Leckman *et al.*, 2006).

Neurotransmitter systems

Extensive immunohistochemical studies of the basal ganglia have demonstrated the presence of a wide spectrum of classic neurotransmitters, neuromodulators, and neuropeptides. The most compelling data have implicated central dopaminergic systems in the pathobiology of TS (Albin & Mink, 2006). Of the various dopaminergic hypotheses proposed, an alteration of the tonic-phasic neurotransmitter release system appears most viable (Singer, 2013). However, it remains highly likely that TS patients exhibit dysfunction in several neurotransmitter systems, including serotonergic, glutamatergic, GABAergic, cholinergic, and possibly histaminergic pathways.

Treatment

Tic disorders are frequently chronic, if not lifelong, conditions. Continuity of care is desirable and should be considered before embarking on a course of treatment. Usual clinical practice focuses initially on educational and supportive interventions. Pharmacological treatments are typically held in reserve. Given the waxing and waning course of the disorders, it is likely that whatever is done (or not done) will lead in the short term to some improvement in tic severity. The decision to employ psychoactive medications is usually made after the educational and supportive interventions have been in place for a period of months and it is clear that the tic symptoms are persistently severe and are themselves a source of impairment in terms of self-esteem, relationships with the family or peers, or school performance.

Educational and supportive interventions

Educational activities are among the most important interventions available to the clinician (Lebowitz and Scahill, 2013). They should be undertaken first, not only with children with TS but also with those with milder presentations. Although the efficacy of these educational and supportive interventions has not been rigorously assessed, they appear to have positive effects by reshaping familial expectations and relationships (Cohen *et al.*, 1988). This is particularly true when the family and others have misconstrued the tic symptoms as being intentionally provocative. Families also find descriptions of the natural history comforting in that the disorders tend not to be relentlessly progressive and usually improve during adulthood. This information often contradicts the impressions gained from the available lay literature on TS that typically focuses on the most extreme cases. Armed with this knowledge, patients and family members and others can begin to understand why waiting before beginning medical treatment makes sense. If a child is in the midst of a bad period of tics, it is likely that whether or not a new medication is prescribed, the tics will improve in the near future. This insight will also help children and their families realize why at times in the past their medications have suddenly stopped working. These dialogs can be relieving and can interrupt a vicious cycle of recrimination that leads to further tic exacerbation and it can help parents shift the focus from blame to problem solving.

By educating the educators, clinicians can make significant progress toward securing for the child a positive and supportive environment in the classroom (Pruitt & Packer, 2013). If possible, teachers need to respond to outbursts of tics with grace and understanding. Repeatedly scolding a child for his tics can be counterproductive. The child may develop a negative attitude to authority figures and may be reluctant to attend school, and classmates may feel freer to tease the child. If tics interfere with a student's ability to receive information in the classroom, it is imperative to find alternative ways to present the material. By helping the student find a way to function even during periods of severe tics, teachers model problem-solving skills that will foster future self-esteem. It is also important for teachers to know that in unstructured settings such as the cafeteria, gym, playground, and school bus, peers who tease or taunt tend to take advantage of the lack of adult supervision. The assignment of a paraprofessional aide to accompany the student can be remarkably beneficial—particularly in situations where there is a history of teasing. Other useful strategies that teachers may consider include providing short breaks out of the classroom to let the tics out in private, allowing students with severe tics to take tests in private so that a child does not have the pressure to suppress tics during the test period, and being flexible with regard to scheduling so that the child is not expected to make an oral presentation at a point when the tics are severe (Bronheim, 1991). A compendium of educational accommodations is available at: http://www.tourettesyndrome.net/.

Educated peers are equally important. Many clinicians actively encourage children, families, and teachers to help educate peers and classmates about TS. It is remarkable what can be tolerated in the classroom and on the playground when teachers and peers simply know what the problem is and learn to disregard it.

Finally, it is important for clinicians to determine the family's awareness of and potential interest in advocacy organizations such as the Tourette Action (www.tourettes-action.org.uk/); Tourette's Syndrome Association (www.tsa-usa.org/); the International Obsessive Compulsive Foundation (http://www.ocfoundation.org/); and the Children and Adults with Attention Deficit Disorder (http://www.chadd.org/). These organizations have made a positive contribution to the lives of many patients and their families by providing support and information. They can also be a valuable outlet for families—to advance research and raise the general level of awareness among health care professionals, educators, and the public at large.

Behavioral, cognitive, and other psychotherapeutic treatments

The presence of premonitory urges and the characteristic suppressibility of tic symptoms may have broad implications for behavioral interventions and treatment. Prior to seeking professional consultation, many families will have experimented with a variety of *ad hoc* behavioral approaches on their own. It is useful to elicit information concerning these efforts and their sequelae.

A variety of cognitive and behavioral approaches have been used with TS (Capriotti & Woods, 2013). Although success with various techniques such as assertiveness training, biofeedback, massed practice, time-out, hypnosis, and differential reinforcement has been reported, most of these studies have involved small numbers of poorly characterized participants with no replication. To date, only Habit Reversal Training, also known as Comprehensive Behavioral Intervention for Tics (C-BIT), has been shown to be efficacious in two large multisite clinical trials involving both children and adults with TS (Piacentini et al., 2010; Wilhelm et al., 2012). Medium effect sizes were found in both the pediatric (ES = 0.68) and the adult (ES = 0.57) trials. C-BIT is now considered to be the first-line treatment for children above the age of 9 years.

C-BIT includes a number of techniques: awareness training, self-monitoring, contingency management, inconvenience review, relaxation, and competing responses. For example, awareness training includes: (i) response description, that is, the patient is trained to describe tic occurrences in detail and to re-enact tic movements while looking in a mirror; (ii) response detection, where the therapist helps the patient's ability to detect tics; (iii) an early warning procedure, in which the patient is taught to become aware of the earliest signs of tic occurrence (such as the premonitory urge); and (iv) situation awareness training in which situations that make tics more likely are identified. When the patient is able to detect the tic and related urges, he or she is instructed to invoke a Competing Response at each occurrence of the tic or the urge and to hold it until the urge passes. Historically, a Competing Response involved a voluntary act that is physically incompatible with production of a particular motor or vocal tic, for example, humming instead of making a vocal tic or slightly tilting one's head to the left when the tic involves a sudden tilt to the right. More recent applications have been less strict, deemphasizing tensing of opposite muscles and occasionally selecting unrelated alternative behaviors.

Researchers are also now exploring the possibility of adding acceptance-based cognitive components to Habit Reversal Training to enhance treatment outcomes. In this intervention, a standard Habit Reversal Training was integrated with a TS-specific version of Acceptance and Commitment Therapy (ACT; Franklin et al., 2011). In general, ACT aims to improve patients' functioning by offering exercises to distance patients from distressing cognitions/urges and other distressing emotions. As applied to TS, ACT focuses on teaching skills to behave flexibly in the presence of (i) uncomfortable premonitory urges, (ii) emotional distress associated with the tics (e.g., embarrassment about occurrence of tics in public or when meeting someone new or recalling past events), and/or (iii) cognitive symptoms associated with comorbid psychiatric conditions such as OCD and ADHD. Future trials are needed to determine whether the presence of ADHD has a negative impact on the treatment outcomes following CBIT.

Exposure and Response Prevention is another promising behavioral treatment for chronic tics (Piacentini & Chang, 2006). As applied to tics, Exposure and Response Prevention focuses on exposure to the premonitory urges. Exposure to the urge occurs by having the patient suppress the tics for long periods of time while the therapist "coaches" him or her through the process (Verdellen et al., 2008). Unlike C-BIT, Exposure and Response Prevention does not teach specific strategies for inhibiting tics. Larger randomized clinical trials are needed to establish the relative efficacy of Exposure and Response Prevention to C-BIT.

Some individuals with TS, or at least many clinically referred patients, report disruptive behavioral symptoms characterized by sudden and unpredictable anger, irritability, temper outbursts, self-injurious behavior, and aggression. In many cases, these symptoms are intertwined with each other and with OCD and ADHD symptoms. Children with this type of disruptive behavior are a difficult-to-treat population, as they are noncompliant almost by definition. Antecdotally, the use of Functional Behavioral Analysis has been of value in some cases.

Pharmacological treatments

The decision whether or not to use medication is based on the level of symptoms and the clinical presentation of the individual case. Given the waxing and waning of tic symptoms, it is best to withhold psychotropic medications until the tics, even at their best, are a significant source of impairment. Many cases of TS can be successfully managed without medication. When patients present with coexisting ADHD, OCD, depression, or bipolar illness, it is often better to treat these comorbid conditions first, as successful treatment of these disorders will often diminish tic severity.

Pharmacotherapy of tics

A wide variety of therapeutic agents are now available to treat tics (Singer, 2010; Roessner & Rothenberger, 2013). The goal should be to use as little medication as possible to render the tics more "tolerable." Efforts to stop the tics completely risk overmedication. Each medication should be selected on the basis of expected efficacy and potential side effects.

Clonidine and guanfacine are potent α2-receptor agonists that are thought to function by stimulating postsynaptic α-2A receptors on dendritic spines of the prefrontal cortical pyramidal cells and by increasing the functional connectivity of the prefrontal cortical networks (Arnsten, 2010). Initial randomized trials of clonidine had mixed results. A subsequent trial involving 136 subjects with chronic tics or TS confirmed clonidine's efficacy in the treatment of tics with comorbid ADHD (Tourette's Syndrome Study Group, 2002). A recent meta-analysis of six randomized, placebo-controlled trials demonstrated that α-2 agonists had a medium effect size (ES = 0.68) in reducing tic symptoms in trials in which participants also had ADHD. However, in the absence of ADHD, the efficacy of these agents was small (ES = 0.15) and nonsignificant (Weisman et al., 2012). Although this finding calls into question existing treatment guidelines for TS that recommend α-2 agonists as first-line pharmacological treatment of tics (Singer, 2010), the available studies for review were few in number and sample sizes were small. Consequently, firm conclusions cannot be drawn due to the less than adequate state of current evidence. Guanfacine is generally preferred to clonidine because it is less sedating and not associated with rebound hypertension following withdrawal. Guanfacine is generally started at a dose of 0.5 mg at night and then gradually increased by 0.5 mg roughly weekly to TID dosing with a maximum dose being 4 mg daily (Singer, 2010; Roessner & Rothenberger, 2013). Unfortunately, guanfacine is not widely available outside the United States.

Classic dopamine D_2 receptor antagonists remain the most predictably effective tic-suppressing agents in the short term. Documentation of haloperidol's effectiveness in the early 1960s was a landmark in the history of TS as it called into question the prevailing view that tics were psychogenic in origin. The most widely used typical D_2 receptor antagonists are haloperidol, pimozide, fluphenazine, and tiapride. Tiapride is not presently available in the United States but is widely used in the United Kingdom and continental Europe. Favorable data from double-blind clinical trials are available for three of these agents (haloperidol, pimozide, and tiapride) (Eggers et al., 1988; Shapiro et al., 1989; Sallee et al., 1997; Tourette's Syndrome Study Group, 1999). Potential side effects associated with typical neuroleptics include acute dystonia, sedation, depression, school and social phobias, weight gain, and tardive dyskinesia. Consequently, long-term experience has not been particularly favorable, so the "reflexive" use of these agents should be avoided.

To avoid the extrapyramidal side effects associated with typical neuroleptics, atypical neuroleptics, such as risperidone, olanzapine, ziprasidone, and aripiprazole have been used to treat tic symptoms. These agents have potent 5-HT2 blocking effects as well as more modest blocking effects on dopamine D_2. Four randomized controlled trials have shown that risperidone was superior to placebo (Bruggeman et al., 2001; Dion et al., 2002; Gaffney et al., 2002; Scahill et al., 2003). Doses ranging from 1.5 to 3.5 mg/day were effective and neurological side effects were rare. However, a number of adverse effects are commonly associated with the use of these agents (weight gain, lipid metabolism abnormalities, sedation, and sleep disturbance).

Open label pilot studies are available for medications such as tetrabenazine and benzodiazepines. Tetrabenazine is a nonantipsychotic dopamine antagonist, approved as an investigational drug; it may be useful but more study is needed (Singer, 2010; Roessner & Rothenberger, 2013). The benzodiazepines, such as clonazepam, are used as anxiolytics and occasionally used as an adjunctive treatment for tics, though they have not been well studied (Scahill et al., 2006; Singer, 2010). Common side effects with benzodiazepine use include sedation, ataxia, short-term memory problems, disinhibition, depression, and addiction. Given these drawbacks, clonazepam is not used widely to treat TS. The use of botulinum toxin injections to temporarily weaken muscles associated with severe motor or vocal tics also appears effective (Jankovic, 1994; Kwak et al., 2000), and in some cases the recurrent use of botulinum can significantly reduce the premonitory urges associated with both motor and vocal tics in the regions injected. There is also some evidence to support the use of Δ-9-tetrahydrocannabinol (Δ-9-THC) in the treatment of TS (Curtis et al., 2009).

Pharmacotherapy of coexisting ADHD

The stimulants methylphenidate, D-amphetamine, and mixtures of D- and L-amphetamine are first-line agents for the medical management of ADHD (Brown et al., 2005). However, the use of stimulants in ADHD associated with a tic disorder remains controversial. Many patients with both ADHD and a preexisting tic disorder will do well on stimulants. For example, in one large-scale multicenter, randomized, double-blind clinical trial with 136 children with ADHD and a chronic tic disorder, significant improvements in ADHD symptoms occurred for subjects assigned to clonidine alone and those assigned to methylphenidate alone; however, the greatest benefit was seen in those children receiving both medications (Tourette's Syndrome Study Group, 2002). Compared with placebo, the greatest benefit occurred with combination. Clonidine appeared to be most helpful for impulsivity and hyperactivity, while methylphenidate appeared to be most helpful for inattention. The proportion of individuals reporting a worsening of tics was no higher in those treated with methylphenidate (20%) than those being administered clonidine alone (26%) or placebo (22%). Sedation was common with clonidine treatment (28% reported moderate or severe sedation), but otherwise the drugs were tolerated well, with no evidence of cardiac toxicity. This trial did not support prior recommendations to avoid methylphenidate in these children because of concerns of worsening tics; however, data from clinical case reports and controlled studies indicate that some children with ADHD will exhibit tics *de novo* when exposed to a stimulant. In particular, supratherapeutic doses of dextroamphetamine should be avoided. In sum, methylphenidate offers the greatest and most immediate improvement of ADHD symptoms and typically does not worsen tic symptoms (Bloch *et al.*, 2009). As noted above, α-2 agonists can also improve ADHD symptoms although patience is required as the beneficial effects are not immediate (Weisman *et al.*, 2012). Atomoxetine, selective norepinephrine reuptake inhibitor, has also been found to reduce ADHD symptoms in children with comorbid tics (Bloch *et al.*, 2009).

Pharmacotherapy of coexisting OCD

The presence of a comorbid tic disorder may predict a poorer outcome in the acute treatment of pediatric-onset OCD. In contrast to cognitive behavioral therapy with Exposure and Response Prevention outcomes, which are not differentially impacted, co-occurring tic disorders appear to impact adversely the outcome of medication management of pediatric OCD (McDougle *et al.*, 1993; March *et al.*, 2007). Consequently, children and adolescents with OCD and a comorbid tic disorder should begin treatment with Exposure and Response Prevention alone or the combination of Exposure and Response Prevention plus a serotonin reuptake inhibitor (SSRI). In adult subjects, controlled clinical trials have also shown that addition of small doses of classical (haloperidol) or atypical neuroleptics (risperidone) can increase the response to SSRIs (Bloch *et al.*, 2006b). The dosage level of the SSRI may also be an important consideration, particularly for older adolescents. In adults with OCD, higher doses are more efficacious than low or medium doses (Bloch *et al.*, 2010). However, the relevance of this observation to younger children and individuals with comorbid tics is unknown.

Pharmacotherapy of cooccurring aggressive behavior (rage attacks)

The management of co-occurring aggressive symptoms and explosive outbursts has not been fully addressed in randomized clinical trials. Preliminary data support the use of aripiprazole in such cases (Budman *et al.*, 2008).

Future directions

Along with a deepening appreciation of the clinical phenomenology and natural history, recent progress in genetics, neuroanatomy, systems neuroscience, and functional *in vivo* neuroimaging has set the stage for major advances in our understanding of TS and related neurodevelopmental disorders (Leckman, 2012). Many mysteries remain, including why there is such a high rate of cooccurring neurodevelopmental disorders in individuals with TS, particularly those with complex motor and vocal tics, relative to individuals with just chronic motor tics. Although TS is etiologically heterogeneous, recent genetic studies have provided important leads including the suggestion that histaminergic neurotransmission may be a key factor for some families and pharmacological modulation of this system might be beneficial more broadly (Bloch *et al.*, 2011; Fernandez *et al.*, 2012).

The natural history of TS also remains a puzzle (Bloch and Leckman, 2009). What is the neurobiological basis of the usual tic improvement during the second decade of life? Longitudinal studies of the trajectories of brain growth are currently under way to discover how the structure of the TS brain may change over time. These studies have the potential to determine how the regional connectivity may change depending on the course and outcome of the disorder. They may also help explain aspects of the sensorimotor gating abnormalities seen in some individuals with TS (Zebardast *et al.*, 2013).

In addition, a deeper understanding of the role of the immune system in TS and related disorders is urgently needed (Kumar *et al.*, 2014; Lennington *et al.*, 2014; Martino *et al.*, 2014). Key controversies in this area include whether a subset of cases with sudden onset (overnight) of OCD and tics are caused by postinfectious autoimmune processes that parallel what is seen in other movement disorders such as Sydenham's chorea.

The development of C-BIT has been a major advance for the field. Now the challenge is to understand the neural mechanisms underlying this treatment and how best to train a sufficient number of practitioners to ensure access to this intervention. In our estimation, efforts to increase acceptance and reduce stigma are important avenues for the future. Despite these therapeutic advances, we are still in need of ideal antitic medications that work quickly, effectively, and with few side effects. For interventions currently in use, it will be important to determine the relative long-term benefits of behavioral interventions when combined with drugs.

Acknowledgments

We are indebted to the Yale Tourette's Syndrome; Obsessive-Compulsive Disorder; and Trichotillomania Research Group. Portions of the research described in this review were supported by grants from the National Institutes of Health: MH18268, MH49351, MH30929, HD03008, NS16648, and RR00125, as well as by the Tourette's Syndrome Association.

References

Abelson, J.F. *et al.* (2005) Sequence variants in SLITRK1 are associated with Tourette's syndrome. *Science* **310**, 317–320.

Albin, R.L. & Mink, J.W. (2006) Recent advances in Tourette's syndrome research. *Trends in Neurosciences* **29**, 175–182.

American Psychiatric Association (2013) *Diagnostic and Statistical Manual of Mental Disorders, (5th ed)* (DSM-5). American Psychiatric Association, Washington, DC.

Arnsten, A.F. (2010) The use of alpha-2A adrenergic agonists for the treatment of attention-deficit/hyperactivity disorder. *Expert Review of Neurotherapeutics* **10**, 1595–1605.

Bansal, R. *et al.* (2012) Anatomical brain images alone can accurately diagnose chronic neuropsychiatric illnesses. *PLoS ONE* **7**, e50698.

Baron-Cohen, S. *et al.* (1999) The prevalence of Gilles de la Tourette's syndrome in children and adolescents with autism. *Journal of Child Psychology and Psychiatry* **40**, 213–218.

Bloch, M.H. (2013) Clinical course and adult outcome in Tourette's syndrome. In: *Tourette's Syndrome.* (eds D. Martino & J.F. Leckman), pp. 107–119. Oxford University Press, Oxford.

Bloch, M.H. & Leckman, J.F. (2009) Clinical course of Tourette's syndrome. *Journal of Psychosomatic Research* **67**, 497–501.

Bloch, M.H. *et al.* (2006a) A systematic review: antipsychotic augmentation with treatment refractory obsessive-compulsive disorder. *Molecular Psychiatry* **11**, 622–632.

Bloch, M.H. *et al.* (2005) Caudate volumes in childhood predict symptom severity in adults with Tourette's syndrome. *Neurology* **65**, 1253–1258.

Bloch, M.H. *et al.* (2010) Meta-analysis of the dose-response relationship of SSRI in obsessive-compulsive disorder. *Molecular Psychiatry* **15**, 850–855.

Bloch, M.H. *et al.* (2009) Meta-analysis: treatment of attention-deficit/hyperactivity disorder in children with comorbid tic disorders. *Journal of the American Academy of Child Psychiatry* **48**, 884–893.

Bloch, M.H. *et al.* (2006b) Adulthood outcome of tic and obsessive-compulsive symptom severity in children with Tourette's syndrome. *Archives of Pediatric and Adolescent Medicine* **160**, 65–69.

Bloch, M.H. *et al.* (2011) Recent advances in Tourette's syndrome. *Current Opinion in Neurology* **24**, 119–125.

Bohlhalter, S. *et al.* (2006) Neural correlates of tic generation in Tourette's syndrome: an event-related functional MRI study. *Brain* **129**, 2029–2037.

Boulant, J.A. (1981) Hypothalamic mechanisms in thermoregulation. *Federation Proceedings* **40**, 2843–2850.

Braun, A.R. *et al.* (1995) The functional neuroanatomy of Tourette's syndrome: an FDG-PET Study. II: relationships between regional cerebral metabolism and associated behavioral and cognitive features of the illness. *Neuropsychopharmacology* **13**, 151–168.

Brimberg, L. *et al.* (2012) Behavioral, pharmacological, and immunological abnormalities after streptococcal exposure: a novel rat model of Sydenham chorea and related neuropsychiatric disorders. *Neuropsychopharmacology* **37**, 2076–2087.

Bronheim, S. (1991) An educator's guide to Tourette's syndrome. *Journal of Learning Disabilities* **24**, 17–22.

Brown, R.T. *et al.* (2005) Treatment of attention-deficit/hyperactivity disorder: overview of the evidence. *Pediatrics* **115**, e749–e757.

Bruggeman, R. *et al.* (2001) Risperidone versus pimozide in Tourette's disorder: a comparative double-blind parallel-group study. *Journal of Clinical Psychiatry* **62**, 50–56.

Budman, C.L. *et al.* (2008) Aripiprazole in children and adolescents with Tourette's disorder with and without explosive outbursts. *Journal of Child and Adolescent Psychopharmacology* **18**, 509–515.

Caine, E.D. *et al.* (1988) Tourette's syndrome in Monroe County school children. *Neurology* **38**, 472–475.

Capriotti, M.R. & Woods, D.W. (2013) Cognitive-behavioral treatment for tics. In: *Tourette's Syndrome.* (eds D. Martino & J.F. Leckman), pp. 503–523. Oxford University Press, Oxford.

Cardona, F. & Orefici, G. (2001) Group A streptococcal infections and tic disorders in an Italian pediatric population. *Journal of Pediatrics* **138**, 71–75.

Carter, A.S. *et al.* (2000) Social and emotional adjustment in children affected with Gilles de la Tourette's syndrome: associations with ADHD and family functioning. Attention Deficit Hyperactivity Disorder. *Journal of Child Psychology and Psychiatry* **41**, 215–223.

Cath, D.C. & Ludolph, A.G. (2013) Other psychiatric comorbidies in Tourette's syndrome. In: *Tourette's Syndrome.* (eds D. Martino & J.F. Leckman), pp. 74–106. Oxford University Press, Oxford.

Cavanna, A.E. & Pansaon Piedad, J.C. (2013) Clinical rating instruments in Tourette's syndrome. In: *Tourette's Syndrome.* (eds D. Martino & J.F. Leckman), pp. 411–438. Oxford University Press, Oxford.

Cavanna, A.E. *et al.* (2008) The Gilles de la Tourette's syndrome-quality of life scale (GTS-QOL): development and validation. *Neurology* **71**, 1410–1416.

Chang, Y.T. *et al.* (2011) Correlation of Tourette's syndrome and allergic disease: nationwide population-based case-control study. *Journal of Developmental and Behavioral Pediatrics* **32**, 98–102.

Chappell, P. *et al.* (1996) Elevated cerebrospinal fluid corticotropin-releasing factor in Tourette's syndrome: comparison to obsessive compulsive disorder and normal controls. *Biological Psychiatry* **39**, 776–783.

Chappell, P.B. *et al.* (1994) Enhanced stress responsivity of Tourette's syndrome patients undergoing lumbar puncture. *Biological Psychiatry* **36**, 35–43.

Church, A.J. *et al.* (2003) Tourette's syndrome: a cross sectional study to examine the PANDAS hypothesis. *Journal of Neurology, Neurosurgery and Psychiatry* **74**, 602–607.

Church, J.A. *et al.* (2009) Control networks in paediatric Tourette's syndrome show immature and anomalous patterns of functional connectivity. *Brain* **132**, 225–238.

Cohen, D.J. *et al.* (1988) Family functioning and Tourette's Syndrome. In: *Tourette's Syndrome and Tic Disorders.* (eds D.J. Cohen, R.D. Brunn & J.F. Leckman), pp. 179. John Wiley & Sons, New York.

Conrad, D.F. *et al.* (2010) Origins and functional impact of copy number variation in the human genome. *Nature* **464**, 704–712.

Cuker, A. *et al.* (2004) Candidate locus for Gilles de la Tourette's syndrome/obsessive compulsive disorder/chronic tic disorder at 18q22. *American Journal of Medical Genetics, Section A* **130**, 37–39.

Curtis, A. *et al.* (2009) Cannabinoids for Tourette's syndrome. *Cochrane Database Systematic Reviews*: **4**, CD006565.

Dale, R.C. & Brilot, F. (2012) Autoimmune basal ganglia disorders. *Journal of Child Neurology* **27**, 1470–1481.

Dion, Y. *et al.* (2002) Risperidone in the treatment of Tourette's syndrome: a double-blind, placebo-controlled trial. *Journal of Clinical Psychopharmacology* **22**, 31–39.

Dykens, E. *et al.* (1990) Intellectual, academic, and adaptive functioning of Tourette's syndrome children with and without attention deficit disorder. *Journal of Abnormal Child Psychology* **18**, 607–615.

Eddy, C.M. *et al.* (2012) The effects of comorbid obsessive-compulsive disorder and attention-deficit hyperactivity disorder on quality of life in Tourette's syndrome. *Journal of Neuropsychiatry and Clinical Neuroscience* **24**, 458–462.

Eggers, C. *et al.* (1988) Clinical and neurobiological findings in children suffering from tic disease following treatment with tiapride. *European Archives of Psychiatry and Neurological Sciences* **237**, 223–229.

Elstner, K. *et al.* (2001) Quality of life (QOL) of patients with Gilles de la Tourette's syndrome. *Acta Psychiatrica Scandavanic* **103**, 52–59.

Ercan-Sencicek, A.G. *et al.* (2010) L-histidine decarboxylase and Tourette's syndrome. *New England Journal of Medicine* **362**, 1901–1908.

Fernandez, T.V. *et al.* (2012) Rare copy number variants in Tourette's syndrome disrupt genes in histaminergic pathways and overlap with autism. *Biological Psychiatry* **71**, 392–402.

Fernandez, T.V. & State, M.W. (2013) Genetic susceptibility in Tourette's syndrome. In: *Tourette's Syndrome.* (eds D. Martino & J.F. Leckman), pp. 137–155. Oxford University Press, Oxford.

Ferrada, C.S. *et al.* (2008) Interactions between histamine H3 and dopamine D2 receptors and the implications for striatal function. *Neuropharmacology* **55**, 190–197.

Ferrão, Y.A. *et al.* (2013) The phenomenology of obsessive-compulsive disorder in Tourette's syndrome. In: *Tourette's Syndrome.* (eds D. Martino & J.F. Leckman), pp. 50–73. Oxford University Press, Oxford.

Findley, D.B. *et al.* (2003) Development of the Yale Children's Global Stress Index (YCGSI) and its application in children and adolescents with Tourette's syndrome and obsessive-compulsive disorder. *Journal of the American Academy of Child and Adolescent Psychiatry* **42**, 450–457.

Franklin, M.E. *et al.* (2011) Habit reversal training and acceptance and commitment therapy for Tourette's syndrome: a pilot project. *Journal of Developmental and Physical Disabilities* **23**, 49–60.

Gaffney, G.R. *et al.* (2002) Risperidone versus clonidine in the treatment of children and adolescents with Tourette's syndrome. *Journal of the American Academy of Child and Adolescent Psychiatry* **41**, 330–336.

Ghosh, D. *et al.* (2012) Headache in children with Tourette's syndrome. *Journal of Pediatrics* **161**, 303–307.

Gilles De La Tourette, G. (1885) Etude sur affection nerveuse caractérisée par de l'incoordination motrice accompagnée d'écholalie et coprolalie. *Archive Neurologie* **9**, 158–200.

Gorman, D.A. *et al.* (2010) Psychosocial outcome and psychiatric comorbidity in older adolescents with Tourette's syndrome: controlled study. *British Journal of Psychiatry* **19**, 36–44.

Goy, R.W. *et al.* (1988) Behavioral masculinization is independent of genital masculinization in prenatally androgenized female rhesus macaques. *Hormones and Behavior* **22**, 552–571.

Graybiel, A.M. & Canales, J.J. (2001) The neurobiology of repetitive behaviors: clues to the neurobiology of Tourette's syndrome. *Advances in Neurology* **85**, 123–131.

Hampson, M. (2009) Brain areas coactivating with motor cortex during chronic motor tics and intentional movements. *Biological Psychiatry* **65**, 594–599.

Hoekstra, P.J. (2013) Perinatal adversities and Tourette's syndrome. In: *Tourette's Syndrome.* (eds D. Martino & J.F. Leckman), pp. 156–167. Oxford University Press, Oxford.

Hounie, A.G. *et al.* (2006) Obsessive-compulsive disorder in Tourette's syndrome. *Advances in Neurology* **99**, 22–38.

Hyde, T.M. *et al.* (1995) Cerebral morphometric abnormalities in Tourette's syndrome: a quantitative MRI study of monozygotic twins. *Neurology* **45**, 1176–1182.

Itard, J.M.G. (1825) Memoire sur quelques fonctions involuntaries ses appareils de la locomotion de la prehension et de la voix. *Archives Générales de Médecine* **8**, 385–407.

Jankovic, J. (1994) Botulinum toxin in the treatment of dystonic tics. *Movement Disorders* **9**, 347–349.

Jin, R. *et al.* (2005) Epidemiological survey of Tourette's syndrome in children and adolescents in Wenzhou of P.R. China. *European Journal of Epidemiology* **20**, 925–927.

Kalanithi, P.S. *et al.* (2005) Altered parvalbumin-positive neuron distribution in basal ganglia of individuals with Tourette's syndrome. *Proceedings of the National Academy of Sciences U S A* **102**, 13307–13312.

Kataoka, Y. *et al.* (2010) Decreased number of parvalbumin and cholinergic interneurons in the striatum of individuals with Tourette's syndrome. *Journal of Comparative Neurology* **518**, 277–291.

Kawikova, I. *et al.* (2007) Decreased number of regulatory T cells suggests impaired immune tolerance in children with Tourette's syndrome. *Biological Psychiatry* **61**, 273–278.

Khalifa, N. & von Knorring, A.L. (2003) Prevalence of tic disorders and Tourette's syndrome in a Swedish school population. *Developmental Medicine and Child Neurology* **45**, 315–319.

Khalifa, N. & von Knorring, A.L. (2005) Tourette's syndrome and other tic disorders in a total population of children: clinical assessment and background. *Acta Paediatrica* **94**, 1608–1614.

Khalifa, N. & von Knorring, A.L. (2006) Psychopathology in a Swedish population of school children with tic disorders. *Journal of the American Academy of Child and Adolescent Psychiatry* **45**, 1346–1353.

Kraft, J.T. *et al.* (2012) Prevalence and clinical correlates of tic disorders in a community sample of school-age children. *European Child and Adolescent Psychiatry* **21**, 5–13.

Kumar, A. *et al.* (2014) Evaluation of basal ganglia and thalamic inflammation in children with pediatric autoimmune neuropsychiatric disorders associated With streptococcal infection and Tourette's syndrome: a positron emission tomographic (PET) study using 11C-[R]-PK11195. *Journal of Child Neurology.* First published online August 12, 2014.

Kurlan, R. *et al.* (2008) Streptococcalinfection and exacerbations of childhood tics and obsessive-compulsive symptoms: a prospective blinded cohort study. *Pediatrics* **121**, 1188–1197.

Kurlan, R. *et al.* (1994) Tourette's syndrome in a special education population: a pilot study involving a single school district. *Neurology* **44**, 699–702.

Kushner, H.I. (1999) *A Cursing Brain? The Histories of Tourette's Syndrome.* Harvard University Press, Cambridge, MA.

Kwak, C.H. *et al.* (2000) Botulinum toxin in the treatment of tics. *Archives of Neurology* **57**, 1190–1193.

Lebowitz, E.R. & Scahill, S. (2013) Psychoeducational interventions: what every parent and family member needs to know. In: *Tourette's Syndrome.* (eds D. Martino & J.F. Leckman), pp. 487–502. Oxford University Press, Oxford.

Leckman, J.F. (2012) Tic disorders. *British Medical Journal* **344**, d7659.

Leckman, J.F. & Cohen, D.J. (1998) *Tourette's Syndrome-Tics, Obsessions, Compulsions. Developmental Psychopathology and Clinical Care.* John Wiley & Sons, New York.

Leckman, J.F. *et al.* (1984) The pathogenesis of Gilles de la Tourette's syndrome. A review of data and hypothesis. In: *Movement Disorders.* (eds A.B. Shah, N.S. Shah & A.G. Donald). Plenum, New York.

Leckman, J.F. *et al.* (1990) Perinatal factors in the expression of Tourette's syndrome: an exploratory study. *Journal of the American Academy of Child and Adolescent Psychiatry* **29**, 220–226.

Leckman, J.F. *et al.* (1995) Cerebrospinal fluid biogenic amines in obsessive compulsive disorder, Tourette's syndrome, and healthy controls. *Neuropsychopharmacology* **12**, 73–86.

Leckman, J.F. *et al.* (2013) Phenomenology of tics and sensory urges. In: Tourette's Syndrome. (eds D. Martino & J.F. Leckman), pp. 3–25. Oxford University Press, Oxford.

Leckman, J.F. *et al.* (1997) Symptoms of obsessive-compulsive disorder. *American Journal of Psychiatry* **154**, 911–917.

Leckman, J.F. *et al.* (2011) Streptococcal upper respiratory tract infections and exacerbations of tic and obsessive-compulsive symptoms: a prospective longitudinal study. *Journal of the American Academy of Child and Adolescent Psychiatry* **50**, 108–118.

Leckman, J.F. *et al.* (1989) The Yale Global Tic Severity Scale: initial testing of a clinician-rated scale of tic severity. *Journal of the American Academy of Child and Adolescent Psychiatry* **28**, 566–573.

Leckman, J.F. & Scahill, L. (1990) Possible exacerbation of tics by androgenic steroids. *New England Journal of Medicine* **322**, 1674.

Leckman, J.F. *et al.* (2006) Tourette's syndrome: a relentless drumbeat. *Journal of Child Psychology and Psychiatry* **47**, 537–550.

Leckman, J.F. *et al.* (1993) Premonitory urges in Tourette's syndrome. *American Journal of Psychiatry* **150**, 98–102.

Leckman, J.F. *et al.* (1994) "Just right" perceptions associated with compulsive behavior in Tourette's syndrome. *American Journal of Psychiatry* **151**, 675–680.

Leckman, J.F. *et al.* (1998) Course of tic severity in Tourette's syndrome: the first two decades. *Pediatrics* **102**, 14–19.

Lennington, J.B. *et al.* (2014) Transcriptome analysis of the human striatum in Tourette's syndrome. *Biological Psychiatry*. First published online July 24, 2014.

Lespérance, P. *et al.* (2004) Restless legs in Tourette's syndrome. *Movement Disorders* **19**, 1084–1087.

Lin, H. *et al.* (2007) Psychosocial stress predicts future symptom severities in children and adolescents with Tourette's syndrome and/or obsessive-compulsive disorder. *Journal of Child Psychology and Psychiatry* **48**, 157–166.

Lin, H. *et al.* (2010) Streptococcal upper respiratory tract infections and psychosocial stress predict future tic and obsessive-compulsive symptom severity in children and adolescents with Tourette's syndrome and obsessive-compulsive disorder. *Biology Psychiatry* **67**, 684–691.

Lit, L. *et al.* (2009) Age-related gene expression in Tourette's syndrome. *Journal of Psychiatric Research* **43**, 319–330.

Lit, L. *et al.* (2007) A subgroup of Tourette's patients overexpress specific natural killer cell genes in blood: a preliminary report. *American Journal of Medical Genetics B* **144B**, 958–963.

Llinas, R. *et al.* (2005) Rhythmic and dysrhythmic thalamocortical dynamics: GABA systems and the edge effect. *Trends in Neurosciences* **28**, 325–333.

Lombroso, P.J. *et al.* (1991) Exacerbation of Gilles de la Tourette's syndrome associated with thermal stress: a family study. *Neurology* **41**, 1984–1987.

March, J.S. *et al.* (2007) Tics moderate treatment outcome with sertraline but not cognitive-behavior therapy in pediatric obsessive-compulsive disorder. *Biological Psychiatry* **61**, 344–347.

Martino, D. *et al.* (2014) The role of immune mechanisms in Tourette's syndrome. *Brain Research* May 15, 2014 [Epub ahead of print].

Martino, D. & Leckman, J.F. (eds) (2013) *Tourette's Syndrome.* Oxford University Press, Oxford.

Martino, D. *et al.* (2011) The relationship between group A streptococcal infections and Tourette's syndrome: a study on a large service-based cohort. *Developmental Medicine and Child Neurology* **53**, 951–957.

Mason, A. *et al.* (1998) The prevalence of Tourette's syndrome in a mainstream school population. *Developmental Medicine and Child Neurology* **40**, 292–296.

Mcdougle, C.J. *et al.* (1993) The efficacy of fluvoxamine in obsessive-compulsive disorder: effects of comorbid chronic tic disorder. **13**, 354–358.

Mell, L.K. *et al.* (2005) Association between streptococcal infection and obsessive-compulsive disorder, Tourette's syndrome, and tic disorder. *Pediatrics* **116**, 56–60.

Mercadante, M.T. *et al.* (2000) The psychiatric symptoms of rheumatic fever. *American Journal of Psychiatry* **157**, 2036–2038.

Moll, G.H. *et al.* (1999) Deficient motor control in children with tic disorder: evidence from transcranial magnetic stimulation. *Neuroscience Letters* **272**, 37–40.

Morer, A. *et al.* (2010) Elevated expression of MCP-1, IL-2 and PTPR-N in basal ganglia of Tourette's syndrome cases. *Brain and Behavioral Immunology* **24**, 1069–1073.

Murphy, T.Y. (2013) Infections and tic disorders. In: *Tourette's Syndrome.* (eds D. Martino & J.F. Leckman), pp. 168–201. Oxford University Press, Oxford.

Neuner, I. *et al.* (2010) White-matter abnormalities in Tourette's syndrome extend beyond motor pathways. *NeuroImage* **51**, 1184–1193.

Pasamanick, B. & Kawi, A. (1956) A study of the association of prenatal and paranatal factors with the development of tics in children; a preliminary investigation. *Journal of Pediatrics* **48**, 596–601.

Pauls, D.L. & Leckman, J.F. (1986) The inheritance of Gilles de la Tourette's syndrome and associated behaviors. Evidence for autosomal dominant transmission. *New England Journal of Medicine* **315**, 993–997.

Pauls, D.L. *et al.* (1991) A family study of Gilles de la Tourette's syndrome. *American Journal of Human Genetics* **48**, 154–163.

Peterson, B.S. & Leckman, J.F. (1998) The temporal dynamics of tics in Gilles de la Tourette's syndrome. *Biological Psychiatry* **44**, 1337–1348.

Peterson, B.S. *et al.* (1992) Steroid hormones and CNS sexual dimorphisms modulate symptom expression in Tourette's syndrome. *Psychoneuroendocrinology* **17**, 553–563.

Peterson, B.S. *et al.* (2001) Prospective, longitudinal study of tic, obsessive-compulsive, and attention-deficit/hyperactivity disorders in an epidemiological sample. *Journal of the American Academy of Child and Adolescent Psychiatry* **40**, 685–695.

Peterson, B.S. *et al.* (1998a) A functional magnetic resonance imaging study of tic suppression in Tourette's syndrome. *Archives of General Psychiatry* **55**, 326–333.

Peterson, B.S. *et al.* (2003) Basal Ganglia volumes in patients with Gilles de la Tourette's syndrome. *Archives of General Psychiatry* **60**, 415–424.

Peterson, B.S. *et al.* (1998b) A double-blind, placebo-controlled, crossover trial of an antiandrogen in the treatment of Tourette's syndrome. *Journal of Clinical Psychopharmacology* **18**, 324–331.

Piacentini, J.C. & Chang, S.W. (2006) Behavioral treatments for tic suppression: habit reversal training. *Advances in Neurology* **99**, 227–233.

Piacentini, J.C. *et al.* (2010) Behavior therapy for children with Tourette's disorder: a randomized controlled trial. *JAMA* **303**, 1929–1937.

Plessen, K.J. *et al.* (2009) Imaging evidence for anatomical disturbances and neuroplastic compensation in persons with Tourette's syndrome. *Journal of Psychosomatic Research* **67**, 559–573.

Price, R.A. *et al.* (1985) A twin study of Tourette's syndrome. *Archives of General Psychiatry* **42**, 815–820.

Pruitt, S.K. & Packer, L.E. (2013) Information and support for educators. In: *Tourette's Syndrome.* (eds D. Martino & J.F. Leckman), pp. 636–655. Oxford University Press, Oxford.

Roessner, V. & Rothenberger, A. (2013) Pharmacological treatment of tics. In: *Tourette's Syndrome.* (eds D. Martino & J.F. Leckman), pp. 524–552. Oxford University Press, Oxford.

Rothenberger, A. & Roessner, V. (2013) The phenomenology of attention deficit/hyperactivity disorder in Tourette's syndrome. In: *Tourette's Syndrome.* (eds D. Martino & J.F. Leckman), pp. 26–49. Oxford University Press, Oxford.

Sallee, F.R. *et al.* (1997) Relative efficacy of haloperidol and pimozide in children and adolescents with Tourette's disorder. *American Journal of Psychiatry* **154**, 1057–1062.

Scahill, L. *et al.* (2013) The prevalence of Tourette's syndrome and its relationship to clinical features. In: *Tourette's Syndrome.* (eds D. Martino & J.F. Leckman), pp. 121–133. Oxford University Press, Oxford.

Scahill, L. *et al.* (2006) Contemporary assessment and pharmacotherapy of Tourette's syndrome. *NeuroRx* **3**, 192–206.

Scahill, L. *et al.* (2003) A placebo-controlled trial of risperidone in Tourette's syndrome. *Neurology* **60**, 1130–1135.

Serrien, D.J. *et al.* (2005) Motor inhibition in patients with Gilles de la Tourette's syndrome: functional activation patterns as revealed by EEG coherence. *Brain* **128**, 116–125.

Shapiro, A.K. *et al.* (1988) *Gilles de la Tourette's Syndrome*, 2nd edn. Raven Press, New York.

Shapiro, E. *et al.* (1989) Controlled study of haloperidol, pimozide and placebo for the treatment of Gilles de la Tourette's syndrome. *Archives of General Psychiatry* **46**, 722–730.

Sikich, L. & Todd, R.D. (1988) Are the neurodevelopmental effects of gonadal hormones related to sex differences in psychiatric illnesses? *Psychiatric Developments* **6**, 277–309.

Singer, H.S. (2010) Treatment of tics and Tourette's syndrome. *Current Treatment Options in Neurology* **12**, 539–561.

Singer, H.S. (2013) The neurochemistry of Tourette's syndrome. In: *Tourette's Syndrome.* (eds D. Martino & J.F. Leckman), pp. 276–300. Oxford University Press, Oxford.

Sowell, E.R. *et al.* (2008) Thinning of sensorimotor cortices in children with Tourette's syndrome. *Nature Neuroscience* **11**, 637–639.

State, M.W. *et al.* (2003) Epigenetic abnormalities associated with a chromosome 18(q21-q22) inversion and a Gilles de la Tourette's syndrome phenotype. *Proceedings of the National Academy of Sciences of the United States of America (PNAS)* **100**, 4684–4689.

Stokes, A. *et al.* (1991) Peer problems in Tourette's disorder. *Pediatrics* **87**, 936–942.

Sukhodolsky, D.G. *et al.* (2005) Adaptive, emotional, and family functioning of children with obsessive-compulsive disorder and comorbid attention deficit hyperactivity disorder. *American Journal of Psychiatry* **162**, 1125–1132.

Sukhodolsky, D.G. *et al.* (2013) Social and adaptive functioning in Tourette's syndrome. In: *Tourette's Syndrome.* (eds D. Martino & J.F. Leckman), pp. 468–484. Oxford University Press, Oxford.

Sukhodolsky, D.G. *et al.* (2003) Disruptive behavior in children with Tourette's syndrome: association with ADHD comorbidity, tic severity, and functional impairment. *Journal of the American Academy of Child and Adolescent Psychiatry* **42**, 98–105.

Sundaram, S.K. *et al.* (2010) Tourette's syndrome is associated with recurrent exonic copy number variants. *Neurology* **74**, 1583–1590.

Swedo, S.E. *et al.* (2012) From research subgroup to clinical syndrome: modifying the PANDAS criteria to describe PANS (pediatric acute-onset neuropsychiatric syndrome). *Pediatrics and Therapeutics* **2**, 2–8.

Swedo, S.E. *et al.* (1998) Pediatric autoimmune neuropsychiatric disorders associated with streptococcal infections: clinical description of the first 50 cases. *American Journal of Psychiatry* **155**, 264–271.

Swerdlow, N.R. *et al.* (2001) Tactile prepuff inhibition of startle in children with Tourette's syndrome: in search of an "fMRI-friendly" startle paradigm. *Biological Psychiatry* **50**, 578–585.

Swerdlow, N.R. & Sutherland, A.N. (2006) Preclinical models relevant to Tourette's syndrome. *Advances in Neurology* **99**, 69–88.

Tourette's Syndrome Study Group (1999) Short-term versus longer-term pimozide therapy in Tourette's syndrome: a preliminary study. *Neurology* **52**, 874–877.

Tourette's Syndrome Study Group (2002) Treatment of ADHD in Children with tics. A randomized controlled trial. *Neurology* **58**, 527–536.

Vaccarino, F.M. *et al.* (2013) Cellular and molecular pathology in Tourette's syndrome. In: *Tourette's Syndrome.* (eds D. Martino & J.F. Leckman). Oxford University Press, Oxford.

Verdellen, C.W. *et al.* (2008) Habituation of premonitory sensations during exposure and response prevention treatment in Tourette's syndrome. *Behavior Modification* **32**, 215–227.

Verkerk, A.J. *et al.* (2003) CNTNAP2 is disrupted in a family with Gilles de la Tourette's syndrome and obsessive compulsive disorder. *Genomics* **82**, 1–9.

Wake, H. *et al.* (2013) Microglia: actively surveying and shaping neuronal circuit structure and function. *Trends in Neuroscience* **36**, 209–217.

Weisman, H. *et al.* (2012) Systematic review: pharmacological treatment of tic disorders - efficacy of antipsychotic and alpha-2 adrenergic agonist agents. *Neuroscience and Biobehavioral Reviews* **37**, 1162–1171.

Wilhelm, S. *et al.* (2012) Randomized trial of behavior therapy for adults with Tourette's syndrome. *Archives of General Psychiatry* **69**, 795–803.

Woods, D.W. *et al.* (2005) Premonitory Urge for Tics Scale (PUTS): initial psychometric results and examination of the premonitory urge phenomenon in youths with tic disorders. *Journal of Developmental and Behavioral Pediatrics* **26**, 397–403.

World Health Organization (1996) *Multiaxial Classification of Child and Adolescent Disorders: The ICD-10 Classification of Mental and Behavioral Disorders in Children and Adolescents*, pp. 43–45. World Health Organization, Cambridge University Press, Cambridge.

Yaddanapudi, K. *et al.* (2010) Passive transfer of streptococcus-induced antibodies reproduces behavioral disturbances in a mouse model of pediatric autoimmune neuropsychiatric disorders associated with streptococcal infection. *Molecular Psychiatry* **15**, 712–726.

Yirmiya, R. & Goshen, I. (2011) Immune modulation of learning, memory, neural plasticity and neurogenesis. *Brain and Behavioral Immunology* **25**, 181–213.

Zebardast, N. *et al.* (2013) Brain mechanisms for prepulse inhibition in adults with Tourette's syndrome: initial findings. *Psychiatry Research: Neuroimaging* **214**, 33–41.

Ziemann, U. *et al.* (1997) Decreased motor inhibition in Tourette's disorder: evidence from transcranial magnetic stimulation. *American Journal of Psychiatry* **154**, 1277–1284.

CHAPTER 57

Schizophrenia and psychosis

Chris Hollis and Lena Palaniyappan

Division of Psychiatry and Applied Psychology, Institute of Mental Health, University of Nottingham, UK

Introduction

Schizophrenia is a particularly devastating psychiatric disorder. Although extremely rare before the age of 10, the incidence of schizophrenia rises steadily through adolescence to reach its peak in early adult life. Early-onset schizophrenia (EOS) arising in childhood and adolescence is now accepted to be clinically and biologically continuous with the adult-onset disorder. The most striking differences associated with early-onset appear to be the greater clinical severity, more frequent and more pronounced early neurodevelopment abnormalities, and poorer treatment response.

The current concept of EOS evolved from a different perspective held during much of the 20th century. Until the early 1970s the term childhood schizophrenia was applied to children who would now be diagnosed with autism. Until the 1990s, there was doubt about the validity of diagnosing schizophrenia in children and younger adolescents. However, in DSM-III and ICD-9 the separate category of childhood schizophrenia was removed, and the same diagnostic criteria for schizophrenia were applied across the age range. Good evidence for the validity of the diagnosis in childhood and adolescence comes from follow-up studies of young people diagnosed with schizophrenia that show a high level of diagnostic stability into adult life and poorer outcomes compared to nonschizophrenic psychoses (Hollis, 2000a). Furthermore, studies of brain structure and function in people diagnosed with schizophrenia have shown very similar types of abnormalities, regardless of the age of onset (Hollis & Rapoport, 2011).

Clinical features

Schizophrenia is characterized by psychotic symptoms. These include:

1 **Hallucinations:** These are sensory perceptions in the absence of external stimuli. Auditory hallucinations are by far the most common type of hallucination in schizophrenia. Typically their content is threatening, derogatory, or commanding. Auditory hallucinations are classified according to their form: voices addressing the patient directly (second person); voices discussing or commenting on the patient's actions in the third person (third person or running commentary); and voices speaking the patient's thoughts aloud (thought echo).

2 **Delusions:** These are false beliefs, incompatible with the patient's social, religious, or educational background, arising from an incorrect inference about external reality and not amenable to reason. Paranoid delusions (belief one is persecuted), delusions of reference (belief that events or people's behavior refer to oneself), or delusions of control (belief that one's own thoughts, emotions, or movements are controlled by external forces), are particularly common in schizophrenia.

3 **Passivity phenomena:** These include the experience of one's own thoughts becoming automatically available to others (thought broadcast); alien thoughts being inserted into one's mind (thought insertion); and the experience of one's thoughts being removed from one's mind (thought withdrawal).

4 **Disordered thought and speech**: This may present as incoherent speech (loosening of associations), neologisms, or a paucity of content and ideas (poverty of speech).

5 **Reduced or inappropriate emotional reactivity and lack of volition:** People with schizophrenia may demonstrate reduced emotional expression (flattened affect) or incongruous emotional reactions, lack of drive and initiative, and social withdrawal.

6 **Motor abnormalities:** These phenomena may include posturing, mannerisms, stereotypies, and catatonic immobility or excitement.

Symptoms in schizophrenia and psychosis can be seen as either representing an excess or distortion of normal function (positive symptoms) or a reduction or loss of normal function (negative symptoms). Positive symptoms include

Rutter's Child and Adolescent Psychiatry, Sixth Edition.
Edited by Anita Thapar and Daniel S. Pine, James F. Leckman, Stephen Scott, Margaret J. Snowling, Eric Taylor.
© 2015 John Wiley & Sons Ltd. Published 2018 by John Wiley & Sons Ltd.

hallucinations, delusions, passivity phenomena, thought disorder, disorganized behavior, and inappropriate affect. Negative symptoms include poverty of thought and speech, blunted affect, impaired volition, and social withdrawal. Liddle (1987) showed that symptoms in chronic schizophrenia cluster into three syndromes: psychomotor poverty (negative symptoms); reality distortion (hallucinations and delusions); and disorganization (bizarre behavior, inappropriate affect, and disorganized thought).

A wide variety of anomalous perceptual experiences may occur at the onset of psychosis, leading to a sense of fear or puzzlement which may constitute a delusional mood and herald a full psychotic episode. These anomalous experiences may include the sense that familiar places and people and their reactions have changed in some subtle way, creating a breakdown between perception and memory (e.g., for familiar places and people) and associated affective responses. For example, a young person at the onset of illness may study his/her reflection in the mirror for hours because it looks strangely unfamiliar, or misattribute threatening intent to an innocuous comment, or experience family members or friends as being unfamiliar, leading to a secondary delusional belief that they have been replaced by doubles or aliens. In summary, some clinical phenomena in schizophrenia can be understood in terms of a loss of normal contextualization and coordination of cognitive and emotional processing. The disconnection between perception, memory, and affective response parallels neurobiological descriptions (see section "Neurobiology").

The clinical phases of schizophrenia

Premorbid social and developmental impairments

EOS is associated with poor premorbid functioning and early developmental delays (Alaghband-Rad et al., 1995; Hollis, 1995, 2003). Similar developmental and social impairments in childhood have been reported in adult-onset schizophrenia, but premorbid impairments appear to be more common and severe in the early-onset form of disorder. In the Maudsley Study (Hollis, 2003), just over 20% of cases of adolescent schizophrenia had significant early delays in either language or motor development. In contrast, language and motor developmental delays occur in about 10% of individuals who develop schizophrenia in adult life (Jones et al., 1994). Impaired sociability occurs in about a third of EOS cases (Hollis, 2003). Premorbid IQ in EOS averages mid to low 80s, some 10–15 points lower than in the adult form of the disorder (Alaghband-Rad et al., 1995; Hollis, 2000b). Around one-third of EOS cases have an IQ below 70, with the whole distribution of IQ shifted down compared to both adolescent affective psychoses and adult schizophrenia (Hollis, 2000b).

Cannon et al. (2002) reported a specific association between adult schizophreniform disorder and childhood neurodevelopmental impairments. During childhood, the adult schizophreniform group when compared to controls had poorer motor skills (0.3 SD), increased neurological signs (OR = 4.6), lower IQ scores (0.4 SD), and poorer receptive language skills (0.2–0.6 SD), findings consistent with genetic/neurodevelopmental perspectives. The premorbid phenotype does not just represent nonspecific psychiatric disturbance. Looking backward from schizophrenia to early impairment, subtle problems of language, cognition, attention, and social relationships are typical, while conduct problems are rare. However, looking forward from childhood impairments to later schizophrenia, prediction is much weaker. In addition, premorbid social and behavioral difficulties are not unique to schizophrenia and do occur in other psychoses and overlap with features of neurodevelopmental disorders (e.g., autism spectrum disorder (ASD) and attention deficit hyperactivity disorder (ADHD)).

Premorbid psychopathology

Many diagnoses, including ADHD, conduct disorder, anxiety, depression, and ASD, may precede EOS (Schaeffer & Ross, 2002) and adult schizophrenia (Kim-Cohen et al., 2003). However, specificity is not sufficiently strong to aid early identification. More promising research has demonstrated a strong link between self-reported psychotic symptoms in childhood and later schizophrenia. In the Dunedin cohort (Poulton et al., 2000), self-reported psychotic symptoms at age 11 increased the risk of schizophreniform disorder at age 26 but not other psychiatric diagnoses (OR = 16.4). Of those with "strong" psychotic symptoms at age 11, 70% developed schizophrenic symptoms by age 26, and 25%, schizophreniform disorder. While none of these met criteria for a diagnosis of schizophrenia during adolescence, it appears that isolated or attenuated psychotic symptoms (Poulton et al., 2000) in combination with developmental impairment (Cannon et al., 2002) constitute an important high-risk premorbid phenotype.

Prodromal symptoms and onset of psychosis

People who develop schizophrenia typically enter a prodromal phase with a gradual but marked decline in social and academic functioning. An insidious deterioration prior to onset of psychosis is typical of the presentation of schizophrenia in children and adolescents (Werry et al., 1994), and is more common in schizophrenia than in affective psychoses (Hollis, 1999). The prodrome is characterized by nonspecific behavioral changes including social withdrawal, declining school performance, uncharacteristic and odd behavior and ideas, eccentric interests, change in affect, and unusual and bizarre perceptual experiences.

At risk mental states

In recent years there has been a growing emphasis on early detection and intervention. This focus has stimulated an interest in prospectively identifying, and potentially intervening in, so called "at risk mental states" (ARMS) which may precede the onset of the disorder. Unlike the "prodrome" which is a retrospective concept, ARMS describe the clinical characteristics of those thought to be at greatest risk of transition to psychosis or schizophrenia.

ARMS, sometimes also known as "ultra high risk" (UHR) states, are characterized by help-seeking behavior and the presence of attenuated positive symptoms of schizophrenia, brief-limited intermittent psychotic symptoms (BLIPS), or a combination of familial risk indicators with recent functional deterioration. The risk for schizophrenia emerging over a 12-month period is increased in these individuals with between 1 in 5 to 1 in 10 expected to develop a schizophrenia spectrum disorder (Ruhrmann et al., 2010; Fusar-Poli et al., 2012). However, prediction of schizophrenia based on ARMS is modest given that the majority of those identified do not become psychotic. Furthermore, transition rates are lower in young people than adults (Fusar-Poli et al., 2012). Most young people identified with ARMS have a mixture of other mental health problems (e.g., depression, anxiety, substance misuse disorder, and emerging personality disorder) requiring a range of targeted interventions. ARMS may be best viewed as a diagnostically neutral but evolving clinical phase associated with a variety of outcomes rather than a diagnostic category specifically related to schizophrenia. Finally, the potential use of a clinical label that conveys a future risk of psychosis or schizophrenia raises ethical issues and may itself be perceived as stigmatizing. Given the low rate of transition to psychosis, any interventions used must benefit (and not harm) the majority of young people (false-positives) who do not develop psychosis.

Diagnosis of schizophrenia in childhood and adolescence

The two dominant diagnostic systems and International Classification of Diseases (DSM and ICD) have slightly different definitions for schizophrenia, though both require the clear evidence of psychosis (in the absence of predominant affective symptoms) with minimum duration criteria. The reader should refer to the original manuals (DSM-5 and ICD-10) when making diagnoses in clinical or research practice.

Although the same diagnostic criteria apply across the age range, there are developmental variations in phenomenology, with early-onset cases of schizophrenia characterized by a more insidious onset, negative symptoms, hallucinations in different modalities, and fewer systematized or persecutory delusions (Werry et al., 1994). EOS is characterized by greater disorganization (incoherence of thought and disordered sense of self) and more negative symptoms, while in later-onset cases there is a higher frequency of systematized and paranoid delusions (Hafner & Nowotny, 1995).

Course and outcome

Course and prognosis

EOS typically runs a chronic course. Hollis (1999) found that only 12% of patients with schizophrenia were in full remission at discharge from first episode compared to 50% of cases with affective psychoses. The short-term outcome for schizophrenia presenting in early life is worse than for first-episode adult patients (Robinson et al., 1999). If full recovery does occur, then it is most likely within the first 3 months of onset of psychosis. In the Maudsley study, adolescent first-onset patients who were still psychotic after 6 months had only a 15% chance of achieving full remission at follow-up (mean length of follow-up 11.5 years) while over half of all cases that made a full recovery had active psychotic symptoms for less than 3 months (Hollis, 1999).

A number of long-term follow-up studies of EOS describe a typically chronic, unremitting long-term course with severely impaired functioning in adult life (Werry et al., 1991; Hollis, 2000a; Fleischhaker et al., 2005). However, a recent follow-up study from the "EPPIC, Early Psychosis Prevention and Intervention Centre" early intervention psychosis programme in Australia (Amminger et al., 2011) challenges the finding of worse outcome in EOS and reports fewer positive symptoms and better social outcomes for schizophrenia-spectrum disorder with onset at <18 years. A possible explanation is that a lower threshold for recognition and diagnosis of psychosis in EPPIC may have led to inclusion of a larger proportion of good outcome cases than other clinical samples. Several common themes emerge from these studies. First, the generally poor outcome of EOS conceals considerable heterogeneity. About one-fifth of patients have a good outcome with only mild impairment, while at the other extreme about a third of patients are severely impaired requiring intensive social and psychiatric support. Second, after the first few years of illness there is little evidence of further progressive decline. Third, EOS, typically, has a worse outcome than either early-onset affective psychoses or adult-onset schizophrenia. Fourth, social functioning, in particular the ability to form friendships and love relationships, appears to be very impaired in EOS. Taken together, these findings confirm schizophrenia presenting in childhood and adolescence lies at the extreme end of a continuum of phenotypic severity.

The predictors of poor outcome in adolescent-onset psychoses include premorbid social and cognitive impairments (Hollis, 1999; Fleischhaker et al., 2005), a prolonged first psychotic episode (Schmidt et al., 1995), extended duration of untreated psychosis, and the presence of negative symptoms (Hollis, 1999). Premorbid functioning and negative symptoms at onset provide better prediction of long-term outcome than categorical diagnosis (Hollis, 1999; Fleischhaker et al., 2005).

Mortality

The risk of premature death is increased in EOS. In the Maudsley follow-up study (Hollis, 1999), there were nine deaths out of the

106 cases (8.5%), corresponding to a 12-fold increase in the risk of death compared to an age and sex-matched general UK population over the same period. Of the nine deaths in the cohort, three suffered violent deaths, two died from self-poisoning, and three had unexpected deaths due to previously undetected physical causes (cardiomyopathy and status epilepticus) and were possibly associated with high-dose antipsychotic medication.

Epidemiology

Incidence and prevalence
Self-reported psychotic symptoms have a high prevalence in children and adolescents, with a meta-analysis of population-based studies suggesting rates of 17% in children aged 9–12 years and 7.5% among adolescents aged 13–18 years (Kelleher et al., 2012). Horwood et al. (2008) reported a 6-month prevalence in 11-year-old children of 13.7% for "suspected or definite" psychotic-like symptoms (the figure included in the meta-analysis by Kelleher et al., 2012). This was reduced to 5.6% when only "definite" symptoms were included. While non-clinical psychotic symptoms are relatively common in children and fall in prevalence during adolescence, psychotic disorders are extremely rare in children and increase in incidence and prevalence throughout adolescence.

Clinically defined schizophrenia has an incidence of 15.2 per 100,000, point prevalence of 4 in 1000 with conspicuous geographical variations in the incidence and prevalence rates (McGrath et al., 2008). While it is generally agreed that the onset of schizophrenia before the age of 12 is very rare, good, population-based incidence figures for EOS are lacking. At present, no data are available to comment on the geographical variations or time trends in the rates of EOS. Studies of clinical samples suggest that <1% of all reported cases with schizophrenia have an onset before age 10, and 4% before age 15 (Remschmidt et al., 1994). Using hospital admission data of an epidemiologically defined sample, the prevalence of DSM-III schizophrenia in children and adolescents was calculated as 0.23%, with half of the prevalent cases younger than 16 years of age (Gillberg, 2000).

Sex differences
Females have a delayed onset of schizophrenia (~1.5 years) compared to males (Eranti et al., 2013) and show a distinct later peak (>age 35 years). This is reflected in the epidemiology of childhood-onset cases, wherein males are over-represented in many clinical studies (Russell et al., 1989). However, other studies of predominantly adolescent-onset schizophrenia have described an equal sex ratio (Werry et al., 1994; Hollis, 2000a). The interpretation of these studies is complicated by the possibility of referral biases. The finding of an equal sex distribution with adolescent-onset is intriguing as it differs from the consistent male predominance (ratio 1.4:1) reported in the overall incidence of schizophrenia (McGrath et al., 2008).

Genetic risk factors

Schizophrenia is very highly heritable (80%) (Gejman et al., 2011), though in most patients the illness is sporadic with no family history of psychosis (Yang et al., 2010). Existing genetic data suggest that multiple genetic variants of varying frequencies (common to rare variants) contribute (Sullivan et al., 2012). Subgroups with strong Mendelian segregation have not been found.

Common variants
To date, the most consistent finding from schizophrenia Genome Wide Association Studies (GWAS; see Chapter 24) implicates a role for major histocompatibility complex (MHC) on chromosome 6, microRNA MIR137 (a noncoding RNA implicated in synaptic potentiation and axonal guidance signaling) (Wright et al., 2013), TCF4 (a neuronal transcription factor associated with Pitt–Hopkins syndrome), CSMD1 (CUB and Sushi Multiple Domains 1, a complement cascade controlling gene), and NGRN (a calmodulin-binding protein kinase that modulates NMDA receptor signaling) (Stefansson et al., 2009; Ripke et al., 2011). Of note, none of the candidate genes (NRG1, COMT, DISC1, DTNBP1, BDNF, and G72 (DAOA)) implicated from pre-GWAS genetic studies has survived the rigorous approach undertaken by the GWAS. The use of an explicit polygenic model that uses a low statistical threshold in GWAS has indicated that several hundreds of common variants confer the susceptibility to develop schizophrenia, adding support to the common-disease common-variant model (Purcell et al., 2009). While all the selected individual loci that survive genome-wide significance could explain only 3% of the heritability (Purcell et al., 2009; Lee et al., 2012), polygenic discovery sets explain up to 30% of the heritability of schizophrenia.

Rare variants
The contribution of rare variants has received significant support with the discovery of structural variations in the genome (copy number variants (CNVs); see Chapter 24). Several studies report a significant increase in the net burden of CNVs among patients with schizophrenia, compared to controls (OR = 1.15) (Stone et al., 2008). A CNV deletion at 22q11.21 (associated with velocardiofacial syndrome) is present in nearly 1% of patients with schizophrenia (Ivanov et al., 2003), and is one of the largest individual risk factors for the development of schizophrenia (20–25% risk), trumped only by the risk of having an identical twin with schizophrenia (Gejman et al., 2011). Other replicated CNVs include deletions at 1q21.1, 2p16.3 (NRXN1) and 3q29. Unlike common variants implicated in schizophrenia, individual CNVs are associated with higher risk ratios (individual OR = 3–25), though several healthy subjects also carry a number of CNVs (Sullivan et al., 2012). As a result, the overall positive predictive value of CNVs (≈12%) remains much lower than that required for diagnostic clinical use (Levinson et al., 2011). Most CNVs discovered so far appear nonspecific to

schizophrenia, and are seen in other disorders such as autistic spectrum disorders (ASD) or mental retardation (see Chapter 3). Such pleiotropic effects are also noted among the Single Nucleotide Polymorphisms (SNP). Pooled GWAS data from five major psychiatric disorders (schizophrenia, bipolar disorder, ASD, ADHD, and major depression) suggest that a common cross-disorder genetic risk may be conferred by intronic SNPs at 3p21, 10q24 and CACNA1C, CACNB2 genes coding for alpha-1C and beta-2 subunits of voltage-dependent calcium channels at 12p13 and 10p12, respectively (Cross-Disorder Group of the Psychiatric Genomics Consortium, 2013).

Genetic data exclusive to EOS is limited. The true familial risk of EOS is not known. But existing evidence suggests that the candidate genes originally implicated in adult onset cases (G72, DTNBP1, COMT, NRG1) may have a higher penetrance in EOS (Addington & Rapoport, 2009). In the NIMH sample EOS, a high proportion (10%) showed cytogenetic abnormalities, including 5% with 22q11 deletion (Sporn et al., 2004b). Further, younger onset patients have higher net burden of CNVs compared to adult-onset cases, or parental controls (28% in EOS, 13% in parental controls, OR = 2.6), with a disproportionate representation of genes from signaling networks controlling neurodevelopment and synaptic function (Walsh et al., 2008; Rapoport et al., 2012). The rate of CNV burden is further pronounced (~53%) if the EOS sample is selected for the presence of speech and social or motor developmental problems (Addington & Rapoport, 2009). Interestingly, the presence of sex chromosome anomalies in EOS are significantly higher than that found in adult cases or in the general population (Addington & Rapoport, 2009). At least a portion of the hidden heritability related to sex chromosomes is not detected by current GWAS (Hickey & Bahlo, 2011).

A number of identified SNPs from schizophrenia GWAS are intronic, while the CNVs are of very large size; as a result, locating the causally important genes is challenging. Consequently, the present knowledge of causal pathways bridging the genetic loci with the observable features of schizophrenia is limited. Nevertheless, a large body of evidence indicates that the bulk of the genetic variants implicated in schizophrenia affect brain development, possibly converging on synaptic functions (Rapoport et al., 2012).

Environmental risk factors

Advanced paternal age

Advanced paternal age at the time of birth has a significant association with later risk of schizophrenia, especially in sporadic cases (population attributable risk of paternal age >30 = 10%), independent of maternal age, social class, family history, and birth complications (Malaspina et al., 2001a). Spermatogonial stem cells undergo constant replication and in the presence of diminished DNA repair mechanisms in advanced age, the likelihood of de novo mutations is amplified (Crow, 2003).

Pregnancy and birth complications

Obstetric complications (OCs) have long been implicated as a risk factor in schizophrenia, with support from the meta-analytic literature (Cannon et al., 2002), though the pooled effect is small (OR = 2.0). Specific OCs such as abnormal presentation and cesarean birth have been reported as more common in patients with onset of schizophrenia <22 years of age (Verdoux et al., 1997) but findings are inconsistent (Ordoñez et al., 2005; Margari et al., 2011). Insofar as there is a significant association, it seems likely that OCs are *consequences* rather than *causes* of abnormal neurodevelopment (Goodman, 1988). This view is supported by the finding that people with schizophrenia have smaller head size at birth than controls (McGrath & Murray, 1995), which is a likely consequence of either defects in genetic control of neurodevelopment or earlier environmental factors such as viral exposure.

Role of infection/inflammation

Many studies have investigated the relationship between prenatal influenza and schizophrenia with inconsistent results from ecological studies (Selten et al., 2010) though seroepidemiological studies suggest a significant trend, especially if the exposure is in the first trimester (Brown, 2011). A twofold increase in risk of schizophrenia in offspring has been observed in association with increased maternal levels of IgG antibodies to Toxoplasma gondii (Mortensen et al., 2007). Though the exact causal mechanism is unknown, animal models of maternal immune activation suggest cytokine-mediated disruption of neurodevelopment that expresses as postpubertal disruption in neurotransmitter functions (Meyer et al., 2009). Childhood viral infections also show an association with adult schizophrenia (RR = 2.1), though it is unclear if this is a cause or consequence of schizophrenia-related deficits (Khandaker et al., 2012).

Prenatal famine

Severe maternal intrauterine nutritional deficiency may increase the risk for schizophrenia in adult life. Evidence of a twofold increase for schizophrenia in children born to the most malnourished mothers comes from studies of the 1944–1945 Dutch Hunger Winter and the Chinese Famine of 1959–1961 (Susser et al., 1996; St Clair et al., 2005). Several micronutrient deficiencies including folate, iron, and vitamin D have been hypothesized to mediate this association.

Cannabis and schizophrenia

A meta-analysis of four well-conducted longitudinal population-based studies from Sweden (Swedish conscript cohort), the Netherlands (NEMESIS), and New Zealand (Dunedin and Christchurch cohorts) concluded that, at an individual level, cannabis confers an overall twofold increased risk for later schizophrenia, varying in a dose-dependent fashion (Arseneault et al., 2004). In the Dunedin cohort, the association was strongest for the youngest cannabis users (after controlling for prior psychotic symptoms) with 10.3% of the cannabis users at age 15 developing schizophreniform disorder at age 26 (Arseneault *et al.*, 2002). So far, cannabis use has not been directly implicated in EOS—possibly because of the relatively lower prevalence of cannabis use in younger adolescents and a short duration between exposure and psychotic outcome; an average delay of 7–8 years has been observed between the first exposure to cannabis and the onset of psychotic symptoms (Stefanis *et al.*, 2013). However, cannabis use is associated with an average of 2.7 years earlier onset of psychotic symptoms (Large *et al.*, 2011).

Psychosocial risks

Migration and social class
Migration and social class are both associated with variation in the incidence of schizophrenia. First- and second-generation migrants have a significantly (RR = 2.7 in first generation, RR = 4.5 in second generation) inflated risk of schizophrenia (Cantor-Graae & Selten, 2005), especially if immigration occurs at a younger age. The relative risk is highest in migrants from developing countries and where the majority population is black. Adjustment for social class reduces, but does not eliminate, the effects of migration. Migrants living in deprived inner cities are exposed to a range of psychosocial adversities including increased exposure to drugs, discriminatory experiences, violence, and crime. Notably, the degree of urbanicity during upbringing (March *et al.*, 2008) and living in regions with low density of members of own ethnic group (Boydell *et al.*, 2001) are also associated with elevated risk of schizophrenia, while the evidence for a link with social class is inconsistent and fraught with confounders (Brown, 2011). The mechanisms linking social adversity to psychosis are unclear—but one suggestion is that experience of social defeat and isolation increases liability to dopamine dysregulation and cognitive distortions (Broome *et al.*, 2005).

Childhood abuse and neglect
A putative link between childhood trauma and psychotic symptoms in adult life has been noted in population-based surveys (Janssen *et al.*, 2004; Bebbington *et al.*, 2011). While strong claims have been made for this link, the evidence to date remains inconclusive, with most studies supporting the link having serious methodological weaknesses (Morgan *et al.*, 2006), and the reported associations are for nonspecific psychotic symptoms rather than clinically defined schizophrenia.

Gene–environment interactions

Genotype–environment (G–E) interplay is often suspected to underlie a significant portion of schizophrenia heritability. For example, a number of genetic factors linked to schizophrenia can increase the risk of fetal hypoxia, which can in turn increase the risk of schizophrenia (Schmidt-Kastner *et al.*, 2012). Traumatic brain injury, which is associated with an elevated risk of schizophrenia (OR = 2.06), is more common in individuals with high familial loading for schizophrenia (Malaspina *et al.*, 2001b). Some of the apparent interactions may arise from genetic differences in exposure to particular environment (G–E correlations). Another aspect to consider is the epigenetic influence of environmental factors that can "instruct" (activate or silence) gene expression. Overall methylation patterns of several hundreds of genes expressed in the prefrontal cortex, including those involved in GABA and glutamatergic transmission, are abnormal in schizophrenia (Pidsley & Mill, 2011). With individual genetic loci being increasingly clarified through genome-wide searches, seeking specific G–E effects presents great promise in the near future.

Neurobiology

The concept of schizophrenia as a neurodevelopmental disorder has been a dominant explanatory model over several decades. The original notion was that of a "fixed" lesion occurring in early development but only manifesting as later psychosis following maturation (Murray & Lewis, 1987; Weinberger, 1987), or a pathological "lesion" that primarily emerges due to disturbed "late" maturational processes (Feinberg, 1982). In particular, the "late" neurodevelopmental model proposes that *excessive* synaptic and/or dendritic elimination occurring during adolescence produces aberrant neural connectivity (McGlashen & Hoffman, 2000). A third viewpoint, the neurodevelopmental "risk" model, proposes that early and/or late brain pathology acts as a risk factor rather than a sufficient cause, so that its effects can only be understood in the light of an individual's exposure to other risk and protective factors (Hollis & Taylor, 1997). This latter formulation provides a probabilistic model of the onset of schizophrenia in which aberrant brain development is expressed primarily as neuro cognitive impairments that interact with environmental risk factors to produce psychotic symptoms.

The current notion posits that several deviant maturational trajectories in brain development beginning early in fetal life are set in motion by genetic and environmental factors, and continue to be shaped by influences that occur during developmentally critical time periods, and culminate in and continue beyond the clinical expression of schizophrenia. Aberrant brain connectivity, both at a synaptic microscale, and a larger scale involving distributed brain networks, is considered as a crucial mechanism for the manifestation of symptoms.

Cross-sectional structural changes
Cross-sectional structural neuroimaging studies of adult schizophrenia have repeatedly demonstrated a reduction in total gray matter (GM) volume, especially focussed on bilateral

insula, anterior cingulate cortex, thalamus and superior temporal cortex, irrespective of the stage of illness. While some of these changes are reflective of factors related to disease severity rather than the diagnostic status, frontoinsular and temporal changes are consistently noted in meta-analytic studies (Ellison-Wright *et al.*, 2008; Glahn *et al.*, 2008) and appear to be related to clinical symptoms such as hallucinations (Palaniyappan *et al.*, 2012), making them one of the most robust structural findings besides ventricular enlargement (Sayo *et al.*, 2012) in schizophrenia. The brain changes reported in EOS appear to be very similar to those described in adult schizophrenia, supporting the idea of an underlying neurobiological continuity (Rapoport & Gogtay, 2011). EOS patients have a higher rate of developmental brain abnormalities than controls (Nopoulos *et al.*, 1998).

Volumetric changes are associated with a number of surface anatomical properties such as thickness, surface area, and gyrification (Palaniyappan & Liddle, 2012). Increased gyral curvature and a reduction in sulcal curvature along with sulcal thinning affecting frontal, temporal and parietal lobes is noted in EOS (White *et al.*, 2003). In adolescent-onset cases, both thickness and surface area reduction have been noted in prefrontal and superior temporal cortex (Voets *et al.*, 2008; Janssen *et al.*, 2009).

Apart from changes in GM structure, diffusion tensor studies have observed significant disruption in WM integrity. The nature of WM changes are much more heterogeneous than GM changes in adults (Melonakos *et al.*, 2011) though most common changes are localized to (i) a left frontal region that involves fibers connecting frontal lobe, thalamus and cingulate gyrus and (ii) a left temporal region that involves fibers connecting frontal lobe, insula, hippocampus–amygdala, temporal and occipital lobe (Ellison-Wright & Bullmore, 2009). In EOS, there is a more widespread, albeit less consistent, reduction in WM integrity (Samartzis *et al.*, 2014). Along with GM changes, the disruptions in WM integrity add a strong case for the existence of structural dysconnectivity in schizophrenia.

Progressive structural changes

There is evidence of progressive ventricular enlargement and volume reductions after the onset of schizophrenia affecting the whole brain, with frontal lobe showing somewhat greater reduction in EOS (Kempton *et al.*, 2010; Olabi *et al.*, 2011). Significant insights have been gained from the NIMH EOS cohort (see Figure 57.1). Progressive GM reduction of comparable magnitude to the EOS cohort has also been noted in the first 2 years after the onset of illness in adolescents with schizophrenia (Arango *et al.*, 2012). At present, it is difficult to distinguish if any of the progressive morphometric changes are due to antipsychotic medications, though this is suggested by long-term follow up of adult samples (Ho *et al.*, 2011).

Progressive changes do not appear to be triggered entirely by the onset of illness; specific changes precede the onset (Pantelis *et al.*, 2003). Meta-analysis of studies comparing high-risk individuals who later develop psychosis from high-risk individuals without this transition indicates a consistent reduction in prefrontal, insular, cingulate, and cerebellar volumes before the onset of psychosis (Fusar-Poli *et al.*, 2011). In particular progressive changes in superior temporal and frontoinsular regions appear to predict the emergence of psychosis in those at a high risk (Takahashi *et al.*, 2009a, b) and the surface anatomical development of these regions continue to deviate in the initial

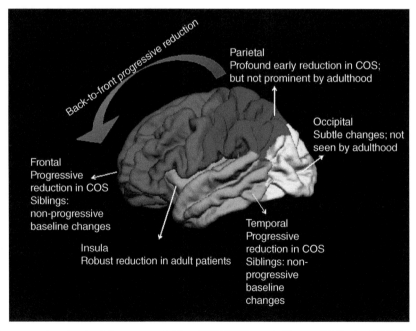

Figure 57.1 Summary of key gray matter structural changes reported from NIMH EOS sample (Rapoport & Gogtay, 2011). In addition, ventricular enlargement at baseline and slower growth rates of (especially right hemispheric) white matter are also noted. COS: Childhood-onset schizophrenia.

stages of schizophrenia in adolescents (Palaniyappan *et al.*, 2013).

Present evidence suggests that a disruption of the developmental trajectories during the critical periods preceding and immediately after the onset of illness contribute to the diverse changes in the GM structure that characterize schizophrenia (Figure 57.1).

Functional imaging

A consistent picture has emerged from a group of task-based functional magnetic resonance imaging (fMRI) studies that suggests that patients show inefficiency in recruiting brain regions when engaging in specific cognitive tasks. This is most apparent in tasks that require prefrontal recruitment, wherein increased recruitment of brain regions often not directly relevant to the cognitive task (e.g., increased recruitment of medial frontal regions during executive tasks) is notable alongside a significant reduction in the dorsolateral prefrontal recruitment when the task demands increase further (Glahn *et al.*, 2005). In the absence of external task demands ("resting state"), patients show abnormal time-based correlations among brain regions that form large-scale brain networks. This dysconnectivity is observed in both within-network and cross-network interactions (Pettersson-Yeo *et al.*, 2011), and are also noted in EOS (Alexander-Bloch *et al.*, 2010; Zhou *et al.*, 2010).

Oscillatory activity is thought to be a fundamental aspect of cortical neuronal coordination. A number of studies suggest that synchronous oscillations in the gamma range (30–80 Hz) are abnormal in patients, and this may be linked to the deficits in prefrontal GABAergic interneurons (Uhlhaas & Singer, 2010). In EOS, abnormalities in evoked oscillatory activity have been noted, especially in the theta and gamma frequencies (Wilson *et al.*, 2008; Haenschel *et al.*, 2009). Adolescence appears to be a crucial period for oscillation-related cortical plasticity (Uhlhaas *et al.*, 2009). The emergence of novel methods such as MEG to study the oscillatory activity has the potential to study the moderating effect of developmental changes on the various stages of development of schizophrenia.

Neuropathology

The prominent neuropathology in schizophrenia involves a region-specific (dorsolateral prefrontal cortex, layer 3 pyramidal cells) reduction in dendritic spines and synapses with increased neuronal density and decreased intraneuronal space (Glantz & Lewis, 2000). Parvalbumin expressing GABAergic interneurons show the most consistent and substantial deficits in the frontal cortex. However, early postmortem findings of aberrant neuronal migration have not been replicated (Beasley *et al.*, 2002); so the developmental timing of these core neuropathological features remains unclear.

A number of postmortem studies in schizophrenia observe a lack of a typical glial response expected in the presence of an explicit pathological insult (Schnieder & Dwork, 2011), but several lines of evidence converge to suggest abnormalities in the metabolic and synthetic activities of the glial cells such as abnormal glutamate homeostasis and myelin production (Katsel *et al.*, 2011; Takahashi *et al.*, 2011). Glial pathology is an active area of investigation at present.

There is a recent resurgence of interest in the links between inflammation and schizophrenia, as discussed in the earlier sections. Circulating cytokine levels are altered in patients with schizophrenia. Interleukin (IL)-1β, IL-6, and transforming growth factor-β are elevated during relapses and also during first episode but are normalized with antipsychotic treatment. In contrast, certain cytokines such as IL-12, interferon-γ, tumor necrosis factor-α, and soluble IL-2 receptor remain elevated despite antipsychotic treatment (Miller *et al.*, 2011). Though there is no direct evidence implicating immunological insults in this context, two PET studies that have noted increased microglial activation (van Berckel *et al.*, 2008; Doorduin *et al.*, 2009) suggest that focal neuro inflammation is a feature of schizophrenia, at least in a subset of patients. In line with this, early treatment trials of both anti-inflammatory (e.g., NSAIDs as add-on treatments (Sommer *et al.*, 2012)) and antibiotic agents (e.g., minocycline for negative symptoms (Chaudhry *et al.*, 2012)) have been found to be promising, though these beneficial effects could be mediated via mechanisms unrelated to inflammation.

Neurochemistry

Schizophrenia is an illness that affects almost all of the major neurotransmitter systems. At present, more is known about aberrations in the dopaminergic system than in other neurotransmitters; striatal presynaptic dopamine synthetic capacity is increased at least in a subset of patients with schizophrenia from an early stage of illness (Howes *et al.*, 2012). Glutamate/GABA abnormalities are also being increasingly appreciated from postmortem and magnetic resonance spectroscopy (MRS) studies. An excess of glutamate in the medial prefrontal cortex is noted in early stages of schizophrenia, though in later stages, reduced levels are noted (Marsman *et al.*, 2011). GABA/glutamatergic system is a strong suspect for mediating cognitive dysfunction in schizophrenia, providing a promising therapeutic target for a symptom domain that is clearly resistant to dopaminergic interventions.

Neuropsychology of schizophrenia

The pattern of cognitive deficits

Cognitive deficits form a core feature linked to functional outcome and recovery. A prominent aspect is the presence of a broad performance deficit. Patients with EOS show notable reduction in IQ, with nearly one-third showing IQ levels below 70 in some studies (Hollis, 2000b). This deficit does not appear to be progressive, but stabilizes after the early stage of the illness (Gochman *et al.*, 2005). The largest effect size of cognitive deficits reported in EOS so far pertain to the domain of executive functions (Rhinewine *et al.*, 2005), and along with processing speed deficits, explain a large portion of the variance in everyday living skills in patients (Puig *et al.*, 2012). A reduction in processing speed is often claimed to be the central factor explaining a number of other cognitive abnormalities in patients (Dickinson *et al.*, 2007). Verbal memory deficits are also prominent, with deficits somewhat more pronounced in EOS cases (Kravariti *et al.*, 2003). Despite the widespread nature of cognitive deficits, "over learned" rote language and simple perceptual skills are unimpaired in EOS. These observations are consistent with the notion that both a broad deficit affecting various cognitive domains and specific deficits affecting some but not all cognitive domains are present in schizophrenia (Gold *et al.*, 2009).

The course of cognitive deficits

When do these cognitive deficits appear? Dunedin cohort participants (observed from the age of 3–32), who developed adult schizophrenia, exhibited static cognitive deficits that emerge early and remain stable on tests indexing verbal and visual knowledge acquisition, reasoning, and conceptualization. In contrast, a developmental lag pattern (slower gain relative to healthy comparison subjects) was noted on tests indexing processing speed, attention, visual-spatial problem solving ability, and working memory. Interestingly, there was no evidence of progressive cognitive deterioration in children destined to develop schizophrenia at a later stage (Reichenberg *et al.*, 2010).

Do these deficits show progressive deterioration after illness onset? A decline in IQ from childhood through adolescence preceding the onset of schizophrenia in adult life has been reported in a large population-based cohort (Reichenberg *et al.*, 2005). There is some tentative evidence for a small decline in IQ following the onset of EOS (Alaghband-Rad *et al.*, 1995), followed by a stabilization of cognitive function (Gochman *et al.*, 2005). In adolescent-onset cases, while several cognitive functions

remain stable, a decline in verbal memory (Frangou *et al.*, 2008; Øie *et al.*, 2010), along with lack of age-related improvement in learning and processing speed (Øie *et al.*, 2010), is seen. This longitudinal pattern appears to be different from the changes seen in children with ADHD (Øie *et al.*, 2010). However, another follow-up study did not find evidence for declining verbal memory over a 2-year period (Cervellione *et al.*, 2007).

In summary, patients with EOS show consistent impairments in IQ, processing speed, verbal memory and measures of attention, albeit with notable heterogeneity. A number of these deficits show a well-established relationship between younger age of onset and the severity of cognitive impairment (Rajji *et al.*, 2009). Overall, there is little evidence for persisting progressive decline in any of the specific cognitive domains after the illness onset (Table 57.1).

Assessment

The assessment of a child or adolescent with possible schizophrenia should include a detailed history, mental status, risk assessment (including self-harm and suicidal risk) and physical examination (see Chapters 32 and 35). In addition, a baseline psychometric assessment is desirable. A detailed understanding of specific cognitive deficits in individual cases can be particularly helpful in guiding education and rehabilitation. In the physical examination, particular attention should be given to detecting clinical features that may betray an underlying genetic syndrome (e.g., 22q11 velocardiofacial syndrome). The neurological examination should focus on abnormal involuntary movements and other signs of extrapyramidal dysfunction. Spontaneous, abnormal involuntary movements have been detected in a proportion of drug-naïve first-episode schizophrenic or schizophreniform

Table 57.1 Comparison of early-onset and adult-onset schizophrenia.

	Early onset schizophrenia versus adult onset schizophrenia
Epidemiology	Clinically defined early-onset schizophrenia is rare (<4% of all cases) though higher rates of self-reported psychotic symptoms occur in children and adolescents.
Neurocognition	More severe impairments in association with earlier onset. No significant variations in the cognitive domains affected (IQ, processing speed, verbal memory, and executive functions show largest deficits in both groups).
Brain structure	Spatial distribution of defects comparable in both groups. More prominent progressive changes in early onset group.
Genetics	Higher penetrance of candidate genes, higher burden of structural variations, and sex chromosome anomalies in early-onset group.
Risk factors	Most environmental/psychosocial risk factors common across the two groups, though the proportion of overall risk attributable to specific factors vary in accordance with age-specific prevalence rates for the risk factors (e.g., cannabis use is less frequent in children).
Phenomenology	Clinical symptoms common across the two groups. No unique features noted in the early-onset group, though more insidious onset, negative symptoms, hallucinations in different modalities, and a fewer systematized delusions are reported.
Course	More chronic course associated with earlier onset.
Outcome	Poorer long-term functional outcome associated with earlier onset.

patients, as well as in those receiving typical antipsychotics (Gervin *et al.*, 1998).

Developmental issues

The cognitive level of the child will influence its ability to understand and express complex psychotic symptoms such as passivity phenomena, thought alienation, and hallucinations. In younger children careful distinctions have to be made between developmental immaturity and psychopathology. For example, distinguishing true hallucinations from normal subjective phenomena like dreams and communication with imaginary friends may be difficult for young children. Developmental maturation can also affect the localization of hallucinations in space. Internal localization of hallucinations is more common in younger children and makes these experiences more difficult to subjectively differentiate from inner speech or thoughts (Garralda, 1984). Formal thought disorder may also appear very similar to the pattern of illogical thinking and lose associations seen in children with immature language development. Negative symptoms can appear very similar to non-psychotic language and social impairments and can also be easily confused with anhedonia and depression.

Differential diagnosis

Psychotic symptoms in children and adolescence are diagnostically nonspecific, occurring in a wide range of functional psychiatric and organic brain disorders. A summary of physical investigations that may be considered in children and adolescents with suspected schizophrenia is listed in Table 57.2. Referral for a neurological opinion is recommended if neurodegenerative disorder is suspected (see below).

Affective and "atypical" psychoses

Because significant affective symptoms also occur in about one-third of first-episode patients with schizophrenia, it may be impossible to make a definitive diagnosis on the basis of a single cross-sectional assessment. In DSM-5 the distinction between schizophrenia and affective psychoses is determined by the relative predominance and temporal overlap of psychotic symptoms (hallucinations and delusions) and affective symptoms (elevated or depressed mood). Given the difficulty in applying these rules with any precision, there is a need to identify other features to distinguish between schizophrenia and affective psychoses. Irrespective of the presence of affective symptoms, the most discriminating symptoms of schizophrenia are an insidious onset and the presence of negative symptoms (Hollis, 1999). Similarly, complete remission from a first psychotic episode within 6 months of onset is the best predictor of a diagnosis of affective psychosis (Hollis, 1999).

Autistic spectrum and developmental language disorders

Some children with ASD have social and cognitive impairments that overlap closely with the premorbid phenotype described in schizophrenia (see Chapter 51). While children on the autistic spectrum can develop psychotic symptoms in adolescence (Volkmar & Cohen, 1991), adult follow-up suggests no increased risk of schizophrenia (Hutton *et al.*, 2008). However, an increased risk for psychosis has been noted in the adult follow-up of childhood developmental receptive language disorders (Clegg *et al.*, 2005). In the NIMH EOS sample, 19 cases (25%) had a lifetime diagnosis of ASD; 1 had autism, two had Asperger's Syndrome and 16 had PDD–NOS (Sporn *et al.*, 2004a). The EOS–ASD subgroup did not differ from the rest of the EOS sample on a range of measures including age of onset, IQ, response to medications and familial schizotypy. However, the rate of cortical GM loss was greater in the ASD group. While some children on the autistic spectrum can show a clear progression into classic schizophrenia, others show a more episodic

Table 57.2 Physical investigations in child and adolescent-onset psychoses.

Investigation	Target disorder
Urine drug screen	Drug-related psychosis (amphetamines, ecstasy, cocaine, LSD and other psychoactive compounds)
EEG	Complex partial seizures/TLE
MRI brain scan	Ventricular enlargement, structural brain anomalies (e.g., cavum septum pellucidum)
	Enlarged caudate (typical antipsychotics)
	Demyelination (metachromatic leukodystrophy)
	Hypodense basal ganglia (Wilson's disease)
Serum copper and caeruloplasmin/Urinary copper	Wilson's disease
Arylsulfatase A (white blood cell)	Metachromatic leukodystrophy
Karyotype/cytogentics (FISH)	Sex chromosome aneuploides, velocardiofacial syndrome (22q11 microdeletion)
Anti-NMDA IgG antibodies	NMDA receptor encephalitis (acute psychosis with headaches, speech disorder, and dyskinesia)

EEG, electroencephalogram; FISH, fluorescent *in situ* hybridization; LSD, lysergic acid diethylamine; MRI, magnetic resonance imaging; TLE, temporal lobe epilepsy; NMDA, *N*-methyl D-aspartate.

pattern of psychotic symptoms without the progressive decline in social functioning and negative symptoms characteristic of EOS. Often it is possible to distinguish between schizophrenia and ASD only by taking a careful developmental history that details the age of onset and pattern of autistic impairments in communication, social reciprocity, and interests/behaviors.

Multidimensionally impaired syndrome

"Multidimensionally impaired (MDI) syndrome" is a label applied to children who have brief, transient, psychotic symptoms, emotional lability, poor interpersonal skills, normal social skills, and multiple deficits in information processing (Kumra et al., 1998a). The diagnostic status of this group remains to be fully resolved (see discussion of ARMS). Short-term follow-up suggests that they do not develop full-blown schizophrenic psychosis. However, they have an increased risk of schizophrenia-spectrum disorders among first-degree relatives and the neurobiological findings (e.g., brain morphology) are similar to those noted in EOS (Kumra et al., 1998a).

Epilepsy

Psychotic symptoms can occur in temporal and frontal lobe partial seizures. A careful history is usually sufficient to reveal an aura followed by clouding of consciousness and the sudden onset of brief ictal psychotic phenomena accompanied often by anxiety, fear, derealization, or depersonalization. However, longer lasting psychoses associated with epilepsy can occur in clear consciousness during postictal or interictal periods (Sachdev, 1998). In epileptic psychoses, hallucinations, disorganized behavior and persecutory delusions predominate, while negative symptoms are rare. Children with complex partial seizures may also have increased illogical thinking and use fewer linguistic-cohesive devices which can resemble formal thought disorder (Caplan et al., 1992).

Epilepsy and schizophrenia may co-occur in the same individual, so that the diagnoses are not mutually exclusive. The onset of epilepsy almost always precedes psychosis unless seizures are secondary to antipsychotic medication. In a long-term follow-up of 100 children with temporal lobe epilepsy, 10% developed schizophrenia in adult life (Lindsay et al., 1979). An EEG should be performed if a seizure disorder is considered in the differential diagnosis or arises as a side effect of antipsychotic treatment. Ambulatory EEG monitoring and telemetry with event recording may be required if the diagnosis remains in doubt.

Neurodegenerative disorders

Rare neurodegenerative disorders with onset in late childhood and adolescence can mimic schizophrenia. The most important examples are Wilson's disease (hepato-lenticular degeneration) and metachromatic leukodystrophy. These disorders usually involve significant extrapyramidal symptoms (e.g., tremor, dystonia, and bradykinesia) or other motor abnormalities (e.g., unsteady gait) and a progressive loss of skills (dementia) that can aid the distinction from schizophrenia.

Suspicion of a neurodegenerative disorder is one of the clearest indications for brain magnetic resonance imaging (MRI) in adolescent psychoses. Adolescents with schizophrenia show relative GM reduction with white matter (WM) sparing. In contrast, metachromatic leukodystrophy is characterized by frontal and occipital WM destruction and demyelination. In Wilson's disease, hypodense areas are seen in the basal ganglia, together with cortical atrophy and ventricular dilatation. The pathognomonic Kayser–Fleisher ring in Wilson's disease begins as a greenish-brown crescent-shaped deposit in the cornea above the pupil (this is most easily seen during slit lamp examination). In Wilson's disease there is increased urinary copper excretion, and reduced serum copper and serum caeruloplasmin levels. The biochemical marker for metachromatic leukodystrophy is reduced arylsulfatase-A (ASA) activity in white blood cells. This enzyme deficiency results in a deposition of excess sulfatides in many tissues including the central nervous system (CNS).

Drug psychoses

Illicit drug use is increasingly common among young people, so the frequent co-occurrence of drug use and psychosis is to be expected. Psychotic symptoms can occur as a direct pharmacological effect of intoxication with stimulants, hallucinogens, cannabis, and ketamine. The psychotic symptoms associated with drug intoxication are usually short-lived and resolve within a few days of abstinence from the drug. These drugs can have surprisingly long half-lives with cannabinoids still measurable up to 6 weeks after a single dose. Psychotic symptoms in the form of "flashbacks" can also occur after cessation from chronic cannabis and lysergic acid diethylamide (LSD) abuse. These phenomena are similar to alcoholic hallucinosis and typically involve transient, vivid, auditory hallucinations occurring in clear consciousness.

Other investigations

Whether any physical investigations should be viewed as routine is debatable. However, it is usual to obtain a full blood count and biochemistry including liver and thyroid function and a drug screen. The high yield of cytogenetic abnormalities reported in EOS (Nicholson et al., 1999) suggest the value of cytogenetic testing including karyotyping for sex chromosome aneuploidies and fluorescent in situ hybridization (FISH) for 22q11DS (velocardiofacial syndrome).

At present the clinical value of a structural MRI scan lies in detecting suspected underlying brain disorders rather than being of diagnostic value in schizophrenia. However, with the use of sophisticated statistical approaches that enable individual-level classification (e.g., machine learning), structural MRI is increasingly being appreciated as a tool with a promise to become a part of regular diagnostic workup for psychosis in the near future.

Assessment interviews and rating scales

The DSM and ICD definitions of schizophrenia do not provide symptom definitions but structured diagnostic investigator-based interviews that cover child and adolescent psychotic disorders (see Chapter 33) have detailed glossaries that can be particularly useful.

Rating scales give quantitative measures of psychopathology and functional impairment. Scales to assess psychotic symptoms include the Scale for Assessment of Positive Symptoms (SAPS) (Andreasen, 1984), the Scale for Assessment of Negative Symptoms (SANS) (Andreasen, 1983), and the Positive and Negative Syndrome Scale (PANSS) (Kay et al., 1987). The 30-item Kiddie-PANSS (Positive and Negative Syndrome Scale) has been developed for use in children and adolescents, and contains three subscales: positive syndrome, negative syndrome, and general psychopathology (Fields et al., 1994). The Children's Global Assessment Scale (C-GAS) provides a rating of functional impairment on a 0–100 scale (Shaffer et al., 1983). These scales can be used to record the longitudinal course of illness and treatment response. The Kiddie Formal Thought Disorder Story Game and Kiddie Formal Thought Disorder Scale (Caplan et al., 1989) are research instruments produced for the assessment of thought disorder in children. Assessments of extrapyramidal symptoms and involuntary movements can be made using the Abnormal Involuntary Movements Scale (AIMS) (Rapoport et al., 1985) and the Simpson–Angus Neurological Rating Scale (Simpson & Angus, 1970).

Treatment approaches

General principles

While antipsychotic drugs remain the cornerstone of treatment in child and adolescent schizophrenia, all young patients with schizophrenia require a multimodal treatment package that includes pharmacotherapy, family and individual counseling, education about the illness, and provision to meet social and educational needs (National Institute for Health and Care Excellence (NICE), 2013).

Interventions targeting "at risk mental states" (ARMS)

Recent studies have examined the feasibility of detecting and treating individuals with "ARMS" (see above) to prevent transition to psychosis. To date, there have been nine randomized controlled trials (RCTs) in ARMS, which have reported findings regarding prevention or delay of transition to psychosis in young people. Stafford et al. (2013) reported a meta-analysis of those studies, using antipsychotic medication and/or CBT or complex psychosocial interventions. Risperidone and olanzapine were no more effective than a psychological intervention or placebo in preventing transition to psychosis or in reducing psychotic symptoms. Furthermore, olanzapine treatment resulted in significant weight gain. In contrast, CBT reduced the rate of transition to psychosis at 12 months relative to supportive counselling (RR 0.54), but did not significantly improve psychosocial functioning (Stafford et al., 2013). Amminger et al.

(2010) reported a 12-week RCT in which intake of omega-3 polyunsaturated fatty acids resulted in a significantly lower transition rate compared to placebo. At 12-month follow-up, 2 of 41 individuals (4.9%) in the omega-3 treatment group developed psychosis compared with 11 of 40 (27.5%) on placebo. There was also a significant reduction in positive and negative symptoms and improved general functioning.

Based on this evidence, the UK NICE clinical guideline for schizophrenia and psychosis in children and young people (CG155) recommended that antipsychotic medication should not be used in young people with transient or attenuated psychotic symptoms with the aim of preventing transition to psychosis (NICE, 2013). The NICE Guideline supports the use of psychosocial interventions (family intervention and/or individual CBT) in children and young people with transient or attenuated psychotic symptoms (subthreshold for a diagnosis of schizophrenia or psychosis), as well as evidence-based treatments targeted at associated anxiety disorders, depression, emerging personality disorder, or substance misuse.

Treatments for schizophrenia and psychosis
Pharmacological

While the efficacy of antipsychotics is broadly similar in children, young people, and adults, the young show a greater sensitivity to a range of antipsychotic-related adverse events, including extrapyramidal side effects (EPS), treatment resistance with traditional antipsychotics (Kumra et al., 1998b), and weight gain, obesity, and metabolic syndrome with the newer atypical antipsychotics (Correll et al., 2009). The pharmacology of antipsychotic drugs and management of adverse effects is discussed in Chapter 43.

Although the number of RCTs of antipsychotics in children and young people (<18 years) with schizophrenia remains small, in recent years there have been trials reported for aripiprazole (Findling et al., 2008), risperidone (Haas et al., 2009), olanzapine (Kryzhanovskaya et al., 2009), and paliperidone (Singh et al., 2011). Taken together, antipsychotics show a small but significant effect (ES = 0.3) in reducing psychotic symptoms (NICE, 2013). While antipsychotics do not differ significantly in terms of efficacy, differences in side effects are notable; weight gain is greatest with olanzapine (with up to 8 kg gain reported in the first 12 weeks of treatment), intermediate with clozapine, quetiapine, and risperidone and least with aripiprazole (Correll et al., 2009). EPS are greater with "typical" antipsychotics such as haloperidol and higher dose (>4 mg) risperidone than with quetiapine or olanzapine. Aripiprazole may cause akathisia at higher doses. Sedation is greater with olanzapine, clozapine, quetiapine, and haloperidol than with risperidone (Toren et al., 2004) and aripiprazole. Hyperprolactinaemia is greatest with risperidone, amisulpride, and haloperidol and least with quetiapine and aripiprazole (aripiprazole may lower prolactin levels from baseline).

Clozapine has been shown in randomized double blind head-to-head trials to be superior to haloperidol (Kumra et al.,

1996) and olanzapine (Shaw *et al.*, 2006) for EOS. Clozapine's use is restricted under license in the United Kingdom to treatment-resistant schizophrenia defined as follows: (i) nonresponse with at least two antipsychotics (drawn from different classes and at least one being an atypical) each used for at least 4–6 weeks, and/or (ii) significant adverse effects with conventional antipsychotics. Adverse effects of clozapine include weight gain, sedation, hypersalivation, and reduced seizure threshold. The risk of blood dyscrasias on clozapine is effectively managed by mandatory routine blood monitoring.

Baseline investigations and monitoring

Before starting treatment with antipsychotic medication, a physical examination should include height, weight (BMI, body mass index), and cardiovascular system examination, including pulse and blood pressure, and a neurological examination for evidence of abnormal movements. Baseline laboratory investigations include full blood count, liver function and electrolytes, prolactin, fasting blood glucose, HbA$_{1C}$, and plasma lipids. The NICE (2013) guidance recommends that weight be measured weekly for the first 6 weeks of treatment, again at 12 weeks and thereafter 6-monthly and pulse, blood pressure, prolactin, fasting blood glucose, HbA$_{1C}$ and lipids should be repeated at 12 weeks and thereafter 6-monthly.

Pharmacological interventions: summary

Choice of antipsychotic medication is determined primarily by side effect profile, given broadly similar efficacy of antipsychotics. The greater sensitivity of children and young people to adverse effects of antipsychotics means that the benefit to risk ratio may be lower than in adults. Drug choice should be a collaborative exercise, tailored to the needs and preferences of the young person and the family. In children and young people naive to antipsychotics, atypical drugs are preferred as they minimize the risk of acute dystonic reactions that are common with high-potency conventional antipsychotics (e.g., haloperidol) in young people. Antipsychotics should be started below the usual dose range for adults and titrated slowly upwards against clinical response and side effects to determine the minimum effective dose. Short-term use of benzodiazepines (e.g., lorazepam) is preferable to high-dose antipsychotics in the management of severe behavioral disturbance associated in acute psychosis. The recommended order of treatment for first-episode schizophrenia in children and adolescents is: atypical as first line; if inadequate response, change to a different atypical or conventional antipsychotic; if response is still inadequate or side effects are intolerable, then initiate clozapine. Antipsychotic medication is usually maintained for at least 2 years after a first episode of schizophrenia, with formal review of medication, including physical health, conducted at least annually (NICE, 2013).

Psychosocial intervention
Cognitive behavior therapy (CBT)

In contrast to the adult literature, there is a much smaller and weaker evidence base to support CBT and family interventions in EOS. The NICE Guideline for schizophrenia and psychosis (NICE, 2013) identified only six RCTs ($N = 460$) comparing individual CBT with a control intervention in children and young people with mean age 25 years and younger (Power *et al.*, 2003; Haddock *et al.*, 2006; Mak *et al.*, 2007; Jackson *et al.*, 2008; Jackson *et al.*, 2009; Edwards *et al.*, 2011). There were no studies of CBT where all participants were <18 years. Three of the studies (Power *et al.*, 2003; Jackson *et al.*, 2008; Edwards *et al.*, 2011) were conducted in a specialist EPPIC in Australia. All participants in these studies received the relatively intensive "treatment as usual" (TAU) offered by EPPIC. Taken together, these studies found no benefit of CBT compared to control interventions for psychotic symptoms (Jackson *et al.*, 2008; Edwards *et al.*, 2011), depression/suicidality (Power *et al.*, 2003; Edwards *et al.*, 2011), or social adjustment (Jackson *et al.*, 2008). Haddock *et al.* (2006) reported an interaction with age, so that for young people <age 21, results were better for supportive counselling compared to CBT or wait-list control, while in contrast, for young people age >21, outcomes were superior for CBT.

These results are intriguing as they suggest that for young people (<21 years) CBT may be relatively less effective as an intervention for schizophrenia than in adults. Reasons for this apparent lack of benefit of CBT in EOS may include (i) methodological weaknesses and small numbers of young people included in these studies and (ii) the early phase of the illness and primary outcomes chosen. The strongest evidence for CBT in adults with schizophrenia is for treatment-resistant positive symptoms (Turkington & Kingdon, 2000), while in trials in young people, CBT has been evaluated in the acute phase of the illness. (iii) Greater cognitive impairments and/or illness severity in young people may moderate the effectiveness of unmodified CBT interventions developed for adults with schizophrenia.

Family intervention

The UK NICE Guideline for schizophrenia and psychosis in children and young people identified only two RCTs ($N = 158$) comparing family intervention with an active control in young people aged <25 years. Both studies were conducted with young people in remission for psychosis and compared family CBT with individual CBT (Linszen *et al.*, 1996; Gleeson *et al.*, 2009). Family intervention was no more effective than an active control in reducing the number of participants who relapsed. In summary, family intervention in young people with schizophrenia fails to show the clear benefits for relapse prevention (Number Needed to Treat of 4; see Chapter 14) reported in adults (NICE, 2013).

Psychosocial interventions: summary

For both CBT and family interventions, the evidence from a small number of RCTs in young people (mean age <age 25), so far fails to replicate benefits seen from the much larger body of evidence in adults. The NICE (2013) guideline concluded that there were insufficient good quality studies in children and young people to draw firm clinical recommendations from this evidence base. NICE reasoned that as there was no *a priori* reason to treat EOS differently from adults, psychosocial interventions (family intervention and/or individual CBT) that have been shown to be effective in adults should be offered in conjunction with antipsychotic medication to children and young people. However, it is recommended that CBT manuals developed for adults should be adapted for use with children and young people.

Organization of treatment services

From the early 2000s onwards in the United Kingdom and other Western countries, Early Intervention in Psychosis (EIP) services covering ages 14–35 have been developed that provide rapid assessment and intervention for the first 3 years following onset of psychosis. Children and adolescents under the age of 18 may be assessed and treated either in a generic child and adolescent mental health service (CAMHS) or in a 14–35 EIP service. The drawbacks of these parallel mental health services for children and young people are that generic CAMHS may lack specific psychosis expertise and the range of interventions typically found in EIP services. Generic CAMHS services are usually unable to provide the mix of assertive outreach, early intervention and crisis resolution services that have developed in EIP teams. Meanwhile, EIP services may lack CAMHS expertise around developmental issues, differential diagnosis of neurodevelopmental disorders, and in delivering family interventions.

The UK NICE (2013) guideline supported rapid referral of children and young people with suspected psychosis from primary care to a consultant psychiatrist with training in child and adolescent mental health (either in CAMHS or an EIP service). The assessment and accurate diagnosis of psychosis and schizophrenia in children and young people can be complex and clinically challenging because it has to take into account developmental factors and the potential differential diagnoses and comorbid conditions arising in children and young people, which differ from adults. In the United Kingdom, CAMHS input to EIP teams is limited and models of joint working have been proposed (Tiffin & Hudson, 2007). There is emerging evidence that the EIP model of working has health economic benefits compared to generic CAMHS, principally because of reduced in-patient utilization for psychosis treatment (McCrone *et al.*, 2013). Ideally, CAMHS trained staff should be embedded in EIP services and take the lead for assessment and management of young people between the ages of 14 and 17 (NICE, 2013).

Conclusions

There has been a dramatic growth in our understanding of the neurobiological underpinnings and clinical course of schizophrenia presenting in childhood and adolescence. Recent findings from genetics suggest pleiotropic mechanisms underlie the dimensional overlaps between neurodevelopmental disorders, rather than finding specific genes for different disorders. Neuroimaging research has uncovered the importance of dysfunctional coordination of brain networks. It is now clear that adult-based diagnostic criteria have validity in this age group and the disorder has clinical and neurobiological continuity with schizophrenia in adults. EOS is a severe variant of the adult disorder associated with greater premorbid impairment, a higher familial risk, and more severe clinical course and poorer outcome. The poor outcome of children and adolescents with schizophrenia has highlighted the need for more trials recruiting young people <18 years to increase the evidence base for effective early intervention strategies and treatments for young people with psychosis and schizophrenia.

References

Addington, A. & Rapoport, J.L. (2009) The genetics of childhood-onset schizophrenia: when madness strikes the prepubescent. *Current Psychiatry Reports* **11**, 156–161.

Alaghband-Rad, J. *et al.* (1995) Childhood-onset schizophrenia: the severity of premorbid course. *Journal of the American Academy of Child and Adolescent Psychiatry* **34**, 1273–1283.

Alexander-Bloch, A.F. *et al.* (2010) Disrupted modularity and local connectivity of brain functional networks in childhood-onset schizophrenia. *Frontiers in Systems Neuroscience* **4**, 147.

Amminger, G.P. *et al.* (2010) Long-chain omega-3 fatty acids for indicated prevention of psychotic disorders: a randomized, placebo-controlled trial. *Archives of General Psychiatry* **67**, 146–154.

Amminger, G.P. *et al.* (2011) Outcome in early-onset schizophrenia revisited: findings from the early psychosis prevention and intervention centre long-term follow-up study. *Schizophrenia Research* **131**, 112–119.

Andreasen, N.C. (1983) *Scale for the Assessment of Negative Symptoms (SANS)*. University of Iowa, Iowa City.

Andreasen, N.C. (1984) *Scale for the Assessment of Positive Symptoms (SAPS)*. University of Iowa, Iowa City.

Arango, C. *et al.* (2012) Progressive brain changes in children and adolescents with first-episode psychosis. *Archives of General Psychiatry* **69**, 16–26.

Arseneault, L. *et al.* (2002) Cannabis use in adolescence and risk for adult psychosis: longitudinal prospective study. *British Medical Journal* **325**, 1212–1213.

Arseneault, L. *et al.* (2004) Causal association between cannabis and psychosis: examination of the evidence. *British Journal of Psychiatry* **184**, 110–117.

Beasley, C.L. *et al.* (2002) Density and distribution of white matter neurons in schizophrenia, bipolar disorder and major depressive disorder: no evidence for abnormalities of neuronal migration. *Molecular Psychiatry* **7**, 564–570.

Bebbington, P. *et al.* (2011) Childhood sexual abuse and psychosis: data from a cross-sectional national psychiatric survey in England. *British Journal of Psychiatry* **199**, 29–37.

Boydell, J. *et al.* (2001) Incidence of schizophrenia in ethnic minorities in London: ecological study into interactions with environment. *British Medical Journal* **323**, 1336–1338.

Broome, M.R. *et al.* (2005) What causes the onset of psychosis? *Schizophrenia Research* **79**, 23–34.

Brown, A.S. (2011) The environment and susceptibility to schizophrenia. *Progress in Neurobiology* **93**, 23–58.

Cannon, M. *et al.* (2002) Evidence for early childhood, pan-developmental imparment specific to schizophreniform disorder: results from a longitudinal birth cohort. *Archives of General Psychiatry* **59**, 449–456.

Cantor-Graae, E. & Selten, J.-P. (2005) Schizophrenia and migration: a meta-analysis and review. *The American Journal of Psychiatry* **162**, 12–24.

Caplan, R. *et al.* (1989) The Kiddie Formal Thought Disorder Scale (K-FTDS): clinical assessment reliability and validity. *Journal of the American Academy of Child and Adolescent Psychiatry* **28**, 408–416.

Caplan, R. *et al.* (1992) Formal thought disorder in paediatric complex partial seizure disorder. *Journal of Child Psychology and Psychiatry* **33**, 1399–1412.

Cervellione, K.L. *et al.* (2007) Neurocognitive deficits in adolescents with schizophrenia: longitudinal stability and predictive utility for short-term functional outcome. *Journal of the American Academy of Child and Adolescent Psychiatry* **46**, 867–878.

Chaudhry, I.B. *et al.* (2012) Minocycline benefits negative symptoms in early schizophrenia: a randomised double-blind placebo-controlled clinical trial in patients on standard treatment. *Journal of Psychopharmacology* **26**, 1185–1193.

Clegg, J. *et al.* (2005) Developmental language disorders – a follow-up in later adult life: cognitive, language and psychosocial outcomes. *Journal of Child Psychology and Psychiatry* **46**, 128–149.

Correll, C.U. *et al.* (2009) Cardiometabolic risk of second-generation antipsychotic medications during first-time use in children and adolescents. *JAMA* **302**, 1765–1773.

Cross-Disorder Group of the Psychiatric Genomics Consortium (2013) Identification of risk loci with shared effects on five major psychiatric disorders: a genome-wide analysis. *The Lancet* **381**, 1371–1379.

Crow, J.F. (2003) Development. There's something curious about paternal-age effects. *Science* **301**, 606–607.

Dickinson, D. *et al.* (2007) Overlooking the obvious: a meta-analytic comparison of digit symbol coding tasks and other cognitive measures in schizophrenia. *Archives of General Psychiatry* **64**, 532–542.

Doorduin, J. *et al.* (2009) Neuroinflammation in schizophrenia-related psychosis: a PET study. *Journal of Nuclear Medicine* **50**, 1801–1807.

Edwards, J. *et al.* (2011) Randomized controlled trial of clozapine and CBT for first-episode psychosis with enduring positive symptoms: a pilot study. *Schizophrenia Research and Treatment* **2011**, 8.

Ellison-Wright, I. & Bullmore, E. (2009) Meta-analysis of diffusion tensor imaging studies in schizophrenia. *Schizophrenia Research* **108**, 3–10.

Ellison-Wright, I. *et al.* (2008) The anatomy of first-episode and chronic schizophrenia: an anatomical likelihood estimation meta-analysis. *American Journal of Psychiatry* **165**, 1015–1023.

Eranti, S.V. *et al.* (2013) Gender difference in age at onset of schizophrenia: a meta-analysis. *Psychological Medicine* **43**, 155–167.

Feinberg, I. (1982) Schizophrenia: caused by a fault in programmed synaptic elimination during adolescence? *Journal of Psychiatric Research* **17**, 319–334.

Fields, J.H. *et al.* (1994) Assessing positive and negative symptoms in children and adolescents. *American Journal of Psychiatry* **151**, 249–253.

Findling, R.L. *et al.* (2008) A multiple-centre, randomised, double-blind, placebo-controlled study of oral aripiprazole for treatment of adolescents with schizophrenia. *American Journal of Psychiatry* **165**, 1432–1441.

Fleischhaker, C. *et al.* (2005) Long-term course of adolescent schizophrenia. *Schizophrenia Bulletin* **31**, 769–780.

Frangou, S. *et al.* (2008) The Maudsley early onset schizophrenia study: cognitive function over a 4-year follow-up period. *Schizophrenia Bulletin* **34**, 52–59.

Fusar-Poli, P. *et al.* (2011) Neuroanatomical maps of psychosis onset: voxel-wise meta-analysis of antipsychotic-naive VBM studies. *Schizophrenia Bulletin* **38**, 1297–1307.

Fusar-Poli, P. *et al.* (2012) Predicting psychosis: meta-analysis of transition outcomes in individuals at high clinical risk. *Archives of General Psychiatry* **69**, 220–229.

Garralda, M.E. (1984) Hallucinations in children with conduct and emotional disorders; I. The clinical phenomena. *Psychological Medicine* **14**, 589–596.

Gejman, P.V. *et al.* (2011) Genetics of schizophrenia: new findings and challenges. *Annual Review of Genomics and Human Genetics* **12**, 121–144.

Gervin, M. *et al.* (1998) Spontaneous abnormal involuntary movements in first-episode schizophrenia and schizophreniform disorder: baseline rate in a group of patients from an Irish catchment area. *American Journal of Psychiatry* **155**, 1202–1206.

Gillberg, C. (2000) Epidemiology of early onset schizophrenia. In: *Schizophrenia in Children and Adolescents*. Cambridge Child and Adolescent Psychiatry. Cambridge University Press.

Glahn, D.C. *et al.* (2005) Beyond hypofrontality: a quantitative meta-analysis of functional neuroimaging studies of working memory in schizophrenia. *Human Brain Mapping* **25**, 60–69.

Glahn, D.C. *et al.* (2008) Meta-analysis of gray matter anomalies in schizophrenia: application of anatomic likelihood estimation and network analysis. *Biological Psychiatry* **64**, 774–781.

Glantz, L.A. & Lewis, D.A. (2000) Decreased dendritic spine density on prefrontal cortical pyramidal neurones in schizophrenia. *Archives of General Psychiatry* **57**, 65–73.

Gleeson, J.F. *et al.* (2009) A randomized controlled trial of relapse prevention therapy for first-episode psychosis patients. *Journal of Clinical Psychiatry* **70**, 477–486.

Gochman, P.A. *et al.* (2005) IQ stabilization in childhood-onset schizophrenia. *Schizophrenia Research* **77**, 271–277.

Gold, J.M. *et al.* (2009) Turning it upside down: areas of preserved cognitive function in schizophrenia. *Neuropsychology Review* **19**, 294–311.

Goodman, R. (1988) Are complications of pregnancy and birth causes of schizophrenia? *Developmental Medicine and Child Neurology* **30**, 391–406.

Haas, M. *et al.* (2009) A 6-week, randomized, double-blind, placebo-controlled study of the efficacy and safety of risperidone in adolescents with schizophrenia. *Journal of Child and Adolescent Psychopharmacology* **19**, 611–621.

Haddock, G. *et al.* (2006) Influence of age on outcome of psychological treatments in first-episode psychosis. *The British Journal of Psychiatry* **188**, 250–254.

Haenschel, C. *et al.* (2009) Cortical oscillatory activity is critical for working memory as revealed by deficits in early-onset schizophrenia. *The Journal of Neuroscience* **29**, 9481–9489.

Hafner, H. & Nowotny, B. (1995) Epidemiology of early-onset schizophrenia. *European Archives of Psychiatry and Clinical Neuroscience* **245**, 80–92.

Hickey, P.F. & Bahlo, M. (2011) X chromosome association testing in genome wide association studies. *Genetic Epidemiology* **35**, 664–670.

Ho, B.C. *et al.* (2011) Long-term antipsychotic treatment and brain volumes: a longitudinal study of first-episode schizophrenia. *Archives of General Psychiatry* **68**, 128–137.

Hollis, C. (1995) Child and adolescent (juvenile onset) schizophrenia: a case control study of premorbid developmental impairments. *British Journal of Psychiatry* **166**, 489–495.

Hollis C. (1999) *A study of the course and adult outcomes of child and adolescent-onset psychoses*. PhD Thesis, University of London.

Hollis, C. (2000a) The adult outcomes of child and adolescent-onset schizophrenia: diagnostic stability and predictive validity. *American Journal of Psychiatry* **157**, 1652–1659.

Hollis, C. (2000b) Adolescent schizophrenia. *Advances in Psychiatric Treatment* **6**, 83–92.

Hollis, C. (2003) Developmental precursors of child- and adolescent-onset schizophrenia and affective psychoses: diagnostic specificity and continuity with symptom dimensions. *British Journal of Psychiatry* **182**, 37–44.

Hollis, C. & Rapoport, J. (2011) Child and adolescent schizophrenia. In: *Schizophrenia*. (eds D. Weinberger & P. Harrison), 3rd edn, pp. 24–46. John Wiley & Sons, London.

Hollis, C. & Taylor, E. (1997) Schizophrenia: a critique from the developmental psychopathology perspective. In: *Neuorodevelopment and Adult Psychopathology*. (eds M.S. Keshervan & R.M. Murray), pp. 213–233. Cambridge University Press, Cambridge.

Horwood, J. *et al.* (2008) IQ and non-clinical psychotic symptoms in 12-year olds: results from the ALSPAC birth cohort. *British Journal of Psychiatry* **193**, 185–191.

Howes, O.D. *et al.* (2012) The nature of dopamine dysfunction in schizophrenia and what this means for treatment. *Archives of General Psychiatry* **69**, 776–786.

Hutton, J. *et al.* (2008) New-onset psychiatric disorders in individuals with autism. *Autism* **12**, 373–390.

Ivanov, D. *et al.* (2003) Chromosome 22q11 deletions, velo-cardio-facial syndrome and early-onset psychosis. Molecular genetic study. *British Journal of Psychiatry* **183**, 409–413.

Jackson, H.J. *et al.* (2008) Acute-phase and 1-year follow-up results of a randomized controlled trial of CBT versus befriending for first-episode psychosis: the ACE project. *Psychological Medicine* **38**, 725–735.

Jackson, C. *et al.* (2009) Improving psychological adjustment following a first episode of psychosis: a randomised controlled trial of cognitive therapy to reduce post psychotic trauma symptoms. *Behaviour Research and Therapy* **47**, 454–462.

Janssen, I. *et al.* (2004) Childhood abuse as a risk factor for psychotic experiences. *Acta Psychiatrica Scandinavica* **109**, 38–45.

Janssen, J. *et al.* (2009) Gyral and sulcal cortical thinning in adolescents with first episode early-onset psychosis. *Biological Psychiatry* **66**, 1047–1054.

Jones, P. *et al.* (1994) Child development risk factors for adult schizophrenia in the British, 1946 birth cohort. *The Lancet* **344**, 1398–1402.

Katsel, P. *et al.* (2011) Astrocyte and glutamate markers in the superficial, deep, and white matter layers of the anterior cingulate gyrus in schizophrenia. *Neuropsychopharmacology* **36**, 1171–1177.

Kay, S.R. *et al.* (1987) The Positive and Negative Syndrome Scale (PANSS) for schizophrenia. *Schizophrenia Bulletin* **13**, 261–276.

Kelleher, I. *et al.* (2012) Prevalence of psychotic symptoms in childhood and adolescence: a systematic review and meta-analysis of population-based studies. *Psychological Medicine* **42**, 1857–1863.

Kempton, M.J. *et al.* (2010) Progressive lateral ventricular enlargement in schizophrenia: a meta-analysis of longitudinal MRI studies. *Schizophrenia Research* **120**, 54–62.

Khandaker, G.M. *et al.* (2012) Childhood infection and adult schizophrenia: a meta-analysis of population-based studies. *Schizophrenia Research* **139**, 161–168.

Kim-Cohen, J. *et al.* (2003) Prior juvenile diagnosis in adults with mental disorder: developmental follow-back of a prospective longitudinal cohort. *Archives of General Psychiatry* **60**, 709–717.

Kravariti, E. *et al.* (2003) The Maudsley early onset schizophrenia study: cognitive function in adolescents with recent onset schizophrenia. *Schizophrenia Research* **61**, 137–148.

Kryzhanovskaya, L. *et al.* (2009) Olanzapine versus placebo in adolescents with schizophrenia: a 6-week, randomized, double-blind, placebo-controlled trial. *Journal of the American Academy of Child and Adolescent Psychiatry* **48**, 60–70.

Kumra, S. *et al.* (1996) Childhood-onset schizophrenia: a double blind clozapine-haloperidol comparison. *Archives of General Psychiatry* **53**, 1090–1097.

Kumra, S. *et al.* (1998a) Case series: spectrum of neuroleptic-induced movement disorders and extrapyramidal side-effects in childhood-onset schizophrenia. *Journal of the American Academy of Child and Adolescent Psychiatry* **37**, 221–227.

Kumra, S. *et al.* (1998b) "Multidimensionally impaired disorder": is it a variant of very early-onset schizophrenia? *Journal of the American Academy of Child and Adolescent Psychiatry* **37**, 91–99.

Large, M. *et al.* (2011) Cannabis use and earlier onset of psychosis: a systematic meta-analysis. *Archives of General Psychiatry* **68**, 555–561.

Lee, S.H. *et al.* (2012) Estimating the proportion of variation in susceptibility to schizophrenia captured by common SNPs. *Nature Genetics* **44**, 247–250.

Levinson, D.F. *et al.* (2011) Copy number variants in schizophrenia: confirmation of five previous findings and new evidence for 3q29 microdeletions and VIPR2 duplications. *The American Journal of Psychiatry* **168**, 302–316.

Liddle, P. (1987) The symptoms of chronic schizophrenia: a re-examination of the positive-negative dichotomy. *British Journal of Psychiatry* **151**, 145–151.

Lindsay, J. *et al.* (1979) Long-term outcome of children with temporal lobe seizures. II. Marriage, parenthood and sexual indifference. *Developmental Medicine and Child Neurology* **21**, 433–440.

Linszen, D. *et al.* (1996) Treatment, expressed emotion and relapse in recent onset schizophrenic disorders. *Psychological Medicine* **26**, 333–342.

Mak, G.K.L. *et al.* (2007) A pilot study on psychological interventions with Chinese young adults with schizophrenia. *Hong Kong Journal of Psychiatry* **17**, 17–23.

Malaspina, D. *et al.* (2001a) Advancing paternal age and the risk of schizophrenia. *Archives of General Psychiatry* **58**, 361–367.

Malaspina, D. *et al.* (2001b) Traumatic brain injury and schizophrenia in members of schizophrenia and bipolar disorder pedigrees. *American Journal of Psychiatry* **158**, 440–446.

March, D. *et al.* (2008) Psychosis and place. *Epidemiologic Reviews* **30**, 84–100.

Margari, F. *et al.* (2011) Familial liability, obstetric complications and childhood development abnormalities in early onset schizophrenia: a case control study. *BMC Psychiatry* **11**, 60.

Marsman, A. *et al.* (2011) Glutamate in schizophrenia: a focused review and meta-analysis of 1H-MRS studies. *Schizophrenia Bulletin* **39**, 120–129.

McCrone, P. *et al.* (2013) The economic impact of early intervention in psychosis services for children and adolescents. *Early Intervention Psychiatry* **7**, 368–373.

McGlashen, T.H. & Hoffman, R.E. (2000) Schizophrenia as a disorder of developmentally reduced synaptic connectivity. *Archives of General Psychiatry* **57**, 637–648.

McGrath, J. & Murray, R. (1995) Risk factors for schizophrenia: from conception to birth. In: *Schizophrenia.* (eds S.R. Hirsch & D.R. Weinberger), pp. 187–205. Blackwell Science, Oxford.

McGrath, J. *et al.* (2008) Schizophrenia: a concise overview of incidence, prevalence, and mortality. *Epidemiologic Reviews* **30**, 67–76.

Melonakos, E. *et al.* (2011) Voxel-based morphometry (VBM) studies in schizophrenia--can white matter changes be reliably detected with VBM? *Psychiatry Research* **193**, 65–70.

Meyer, U. *et al.* (2009) A review of the fetal brain cytokine imbalance hypothesis of schizophrenia. *Schizophrenia Bulletin* **35**, 959–972.

Miller, B.J. *et al.* (2011) Meta-analysis of cytokine alterations in schizophrenia: clinical status and antipsychotic effects. *Biological Psychiatry* **70**, 663–671.

Morgan, C. *et al.* (2006) Child abuse and psychosis [comment]. *Acta Psychiatrica Scandinavica* **113**, 238, author reply 238–239.

Mortensen, P.B. *et al.* (2007) Toxoplasma gondii as a risk factor for early-onset schizophrenia: analysis of filter paper blood samples obtained at birth. *Biological Psychiatry* **61**, 688–693.

Murray, R.M. & Lewis, S.W. (1987) Is schizophrenia a neurodevelopmental disorder? *British Medical Journal (Clinical Research Ed.)* **295**, 681–682.

National Institute for Health and Care Excellence (2013) *Psychosis and Schizophrenia in Children and Young People: Recognition and Management. CG155.* National Institute for Health and Care Excellence, London.

Nicholson, R.M. *et al.* (1999) Clinical and neurobiological correlates of cytogenetic abnormalities in childhood-onset schizophrenia. *American Journal of Psychiatry* **156**, 1575–1579.

Nopoulos, P.C. *et al.* (1998) Frequency and severity of enlarged septi pellucidi in childhood-onset schizophrenia. *American Journal of Psychiatry* **155**, 1074–1079.

Øie, M. *et al.* (2010) Neurocognitive decline in early-onset schizophrenia compared with ADHD and normal controls: evidence from a 13-year follow-up study. *Schizophrenia Bulletin* **36**, 557–565.

Olabi, B. *et al.* (2011) Are there progressive brain changes in schizophrenia? A meta-analysis of structural magnetic resonance imaging studies. *Biological Psychiatry* **70**, 88–96.

Ordoñez, A.E. *et al.* (2005) Lack of evidence for elevated obstetric complications in childhood onset schizophrenia. *Biological Psychiatry* **58**, 10–15.

Palaniyappan, L. & Liddle, P.F. (2012) Differential effects of surface area, gyrification and cortical thickness on voxel based morphometric deficits in schizophrenia. *NeuroImage* **60**, 693–699.

Palaniyappan, L. *et al.* (2012) Structural correlates of auditory hallucinations in schizophrenia: a meta-analysis. *Schizophrenia Research* **137** (1–3), 169–173.

Palaniyappan, L. *et al.* (2013) Gyrification of Broca's region is anomalously lateralized at onset of schizophrenia in adolescence and regresses at 2 year follow-up. *Schizophrenia Research* **147**, 39–45.

Pantelis, C. *et al.* (2003) Neuroanatomical abnormalities before and after onset of psychosis: a cross-sectional and longitudinal MRI comparison. *The Lancet* **361**, 281–288.

Pettersson-Yeo, W. *et al.* (2011) Dysconnectivity in schizophrenia: where are we now? *Neuroscience and Biobehavioral Reviews* **35**, 1110–1124.

Pidsley, R. & Mill, J. (2011) Epigenetic studies of psychosis: current findings, methodological approaches, and implications for postmortem research. *Biological Psychiatry* **69**, 146–156.

Poulton, R. *et al.* (2000) Children's self-reported psychotic symptoms and adult schizophreniform disorder: a 15-year longitudinal study. *Archives of General Psychiatry* **57**, 1053–1058.

Power, P.J. *et al.* (2003) Suicide prevention in first episode psychosis: the development of a randomised controlled trial of cognitive therapy for acutely suicidal patients with early psychosis. *Australian and New Zealand Journal of Psychiatry* **37**, 414–420.

Puig, O. *et al.* (2012) Processing speed and executive functions predict real-world everyday living skills in adolescents with early-onset schizophrenia. *European Child & Adolescent Psychiatry* **21**, 315–326.

Purcell, S.M. *et al.* (2009) Common polygenic variation contributes to risk of schizophrenia and bipolar disorder. *Nature* **460**, 748–752.

Rajji, T.K. *et al.* (2009) Age at onset and cognition in schizophrenia: meta-analysis. *The British Journal of Psychiatry* **195**, 286–293.

Rapoport, J.L. & Gogtay, N. (2011) Childhood onset schizophrenia: support for a progressive neurodevelopmental disorder. *International Journal of Developmental Neuroscience: The Official Journal of the International Society for Developmental Neuroscience* **29**, 251–258.

Rapoport, J.L. *et al.* (1985) Rating scales and assessment instruments for use in paediatric psychopharmacology research. *Psychological Bulletin* **21**, 713–1111.

Rapoport, J.L. *et al.* (2012) Neurodevelopmental model of schizophrenia: update 2012. *Molecular Psychiatry* **17**, 1228–1238.

Reichenberg, A. *et al.* (2005) Elaboration on premorbid intellectual performance in schizophrenia: premorbid intellectual decline and risk for schizophrenia. *Archives of General Psychiatry* **62**, 1297–1304.

Reichenberg, A. *et al.* (2010) Static and dynamic cognitive deficits in childhood preceding adult schizophrenia: a 30-year study. *The American Journal of Psychiatry* **167**, 160–169.

Remschmidt, H.E. *et al.* (1994) Childhood-onset schizophrenia: history of the concept and recent studies. *Schizophrenia Bulletin* **20**, 727–745.

Rhinewine, J.P. *et al.* (2005) Neurocognitive profile in adolescents with early-onset schizophrenia: clinical correlates. *Biological Psychiatry* **58**, 705–712.

Ripke, S. *et al.* (2011) Genome-wide association study identifies five new schizophrenia loci. *Nature Genetics* **43**, 969–976.

Robinson, D. *et al.* (1999) Predictors of relapse following a first episode of schizophrenia or schizoaffective disorder. *Archives of General Psychiatry* **56**, 241–247.

Ruhrmann, S. *et al.* (2010) Prediction of psychosis in adolescents and young adults at high risk: results from the Prospective European Prediction of Psychosis Study. *Archives of General Psychiatry* **67**, 241–251.

Russell, A.T. *et al.* (1989) The phenomena of schizophrenia occurring in childhood. *Journal of the American Academy of Child and Adolescent Psychiatry* **28**, 399–407.

Sachdev, P. (1998) Schizophrenia-like psychosis and epilepsy: the status of the association. *American Journal of Psychiatry* **155**, 325–336.

Samartzis, L. *et al.* (2014) White matter alterations in early stages of schizophrenia: a systematic review of diffusion tensor imaging studies. *Journal of Neuroimaging: Official Journal of the American Society of Neuroimaging* **24**, 101–110.

Sayo, A. *et al.* (2012) Study factors influencing ventricular enlargement in schizophrenia: a 20 year follow-up meta-analysis. *NeuroImage* **59**, 154–167.

Schaeffer, J.L. & Ross, R.G. (2002) Childhood-onset schizophrenia: premorbid and prodromal diagnostic and treatment histories. *Journal of the American Academy of Child & Adolescent Psychiatry* **41**, 538–545.

Schmidt, M. *et al.* (1995) Course of patients diagnosed as having schizophrenia during first episode occurring under age 18 years. *European Archives of Psychiatry and Clinical Neuroscience* **245**, 93–100.

Schmidt-Kastner, R. *et al.* (2012) An environmental analysis of genes associated with schizophrenia: hypoxia and vascular factors as interacting elements in the neurodevelopmental model. *Molecular Psychiatry* **17**, 1194–1205.

Schnieder, T.P. & Dwork, A.J. (2011) Searching for neuropathology: gliosis in schizophrenia. *Biological Psychiatry* **69**, 134–139.

Selten, J.-P. *et al.* (2010) Schizophrenia and 1957 pandemic of influenza: meta-analysis. *Schizophrenia Bulletin* **36**, 219–228.

Shaffer, D. *et al.* (1983) The children's global assessment scale (CGAS). *Archives of General Psychiatry* **40**, 1228–1231.

Shaw, P. *et al.* (2006) Childhood-onset schizophrenia: a double-blind, randomized clozapine-olanzapine comparison. *Archives of General Psychiatry* **63**, 721–730.

Simpson, G. & Angus, J.S.W. (1970) A rating scale for extrapyramidal side effects. *Acta Psychiatrica Scandinavica* **212**, 9–11.

Singh, J. *et al.* (2011) A randomized, double-blind study of paliperidone extended-release in treatment of acute schizophrenia in adolescents. *Biological Psychiatry* **70**, 1179–1187.

Sommer, I.E. *et al.* (2012) Nonsteroidal anti-inflammatory drugs in schizophrenia: ready for practice or a good start? A meta-analysis. *The Journal of Clinical Psychiatry* **73**, 414–419.

Sporn, A.L. *et al.* (2004a) Pervasive developmental disorder and childhood-onset schizophrenia: co-morbid disorder or phenotypic variant of a very early onset illness? *Biological Psychiatry* **55**, 989–994.

Sporn, A.L. *et al* (2004b) 22q11 deletion syndrome in childhood-onset schizophrenia: an update. *Molecular Psychiatry* **9**, 225–226.

St Clair, D. *et al.* (2005) Rates of adult schizophrenia following prenatal exposure to the Chinese famine of 1959-1961. *JAMA* **294**, 557–562.

Stafford, M.R. *et al.* (2013) Early interventions to prevent psychosis: systematic review and meta-analysis. *BMJ* **346**, f185.

Stefanis, N.C. *et al.* (2013) Age at initiation of cannabis use predicts age at onset of psychosis: the 7- to 8-year trend. *Schizophrenia Bulletin* **39**, 251–254.

Stefansson, H. *et al.* (2009) Common variants conferring risk of schizophrenia. *Nature* **460**, 744–747.

Stone, J.L. *et al.* (2008) Rare chromosomal deletions and duplications increase risk of schizophrenia. *Nature* **455**, 237–241.

Sullivan, P.F. *et al.* (2012) Genetic architectures of psychiatric disorders: the emerging picture and its implications. *Nature Reviews Genetics* **13**, 537–551.

Susser, E. *et al.* (1996) Schizophrenia after prenatal famine. Further evidence. *Archives of General Psychiatry* **53**, 25–31.

Takahashi, T. *et al.* (2009a) Insular cortex gray matter changes in individuals at ultra-high-risk of developing psychosis. *Schizophrenia Research* **111**, 94–102.

Takahashi, T. *et al.* (2009b) Progressive gray matter reduction of the superior temporal gyrus during transition to psychosis. *Archives of General Psychiatry* **66**, 366–376.

Takahashi, N. *et al.* (2011) Linking oligodendrocyte and myelin dysfunction to neurocircuitry abnormalities in schizophrenia. *Progress in Neurobiology* **93**, 13–24.

Tiffin, P.A. & Hudson, S. (2007) An early intervention service for adolescents. *Early Intervention in Psychiatry* **1**, 112–218.

Toren, P. *et al.* (2004) Benefit-risk assessment of atypical antipsychotics in the treatment of schizophrenia and comorbid disorders in children and adolescents. *Drug Safety* **27**, 1135–1156.

Turkington, D. & Kingdon, D. (2000) Cognitive-behavioural techniques for general psychiatrists in the management of patients with psychoses. *British Journal of Psychiatry* **177**, 101–106.

Uhlhaas, P.J. & Singer, W. (2010) Abnormal neural oscillations and synchrony in schizophrenia. *Nature Review Neuroscience* **11**, 100–113.

Uhlhaas, P.J. *et al.* (2009) The development of neural synchrony reflects late maturation and restructuring of functional networks in humans. *Proceedings of the National Academy of Sciences of the United States of America* **106**, 9866–9871.

Van Berckel, B.N. *et al.* (2008) Microglia activation in recent-onset schizophrenia: a quantitative (R)-[11C]PK11195 positron emission tomography study. *Biological Psychiatry* **64**, 820–822.

Verdoux, H. *et al.* (1997) Obstetric complications and age at onset in schizophrenia: an international collaborative meta-analysis of individual patient data. *The American Journal of Psychiatry* **154**, 1220–1227.

Voets, N.L. *et al.* (2008) Evidence for abnormalities of cortical development in adolescent-onset schizophrenia. *NeuroImage* **43**, 665–675.

Volkmar, F.R. & Cohen, D.J. (1991) Comorbid association of autism and schizophrenia. *American Journal of Psychiatry* **148**, 1705–1707.

Walsh, T. *et al.* (2008) Rare structural variants disrupt multiple genes in neurodevelopmental pathways in schizophrenia. *Science (New York, N.Y.)* **320**, 539–543.

Weinberger, D.R. (1987) Implications of normal brain development for the pathogenesis of schizophrenia. *Archives of General Psychiatry* **44**, 660–669.

Werry, J.S. *et al.* (1991) Childhood and adolescent schizophrenia, bipolar and schizoaffective disorders: a clinical and outcome study.

Journal of the American Academy of Child and Adolescent Psychiatry **30**, 457–465.

Werry, J.S. *et al.* (1994) Clinical features and outcome of child and adolescent schizophrenia. *Schizophrenia Bulletin* **20**, 619–630.

White, T. *et al.* (2003) Gyrification abnormalities in childhood- and adolescent-onset schizophrenia. *Biological Psychiatry* **54**, 418–426.

Wilson, T.W. *et al.* (2008) Cortical gamma generators suggest abnormal auditory circuitry in early-onset psychosis. *Cerebral Cortex (New York, N.Y.: 1991)* **18**, 371–378.

Wright, C. *et al.* (2013) Potential impact of miR-137 and its targets in schizophrenia. *Frontiers in Behavioral and Psychiatric Genetics* **4**, 58.

Yang, J. *et al.* (2010) Sporadic cases are the norm for complex disease. *European Journal of Human Genetics* **18**, 1039–1043.

Zhou, B. *et al.* (2010) Brain functional connectivity of functional magnetic resonance imaging of patients with early-onset schizophrenia. *Zhong nan da xue xue bao. Yi xue ban = Journal of Central South University Medical Sciences* **35**, 17–24.

A: Neurodevelopmental

CHAPTER 58

Disorders of attachment and social engagement related to deprivation

Charles H. Zeanah and Anna T. Smyke

Department of Psychiatry and Behavioral Sciences, Tulane University School of Medicine, New Orleans, LA, USA

Although attachment disorders have been described in the literature for nearly 75 years and have been defined by specified criteria in psychiatric nosologies for more than three decades, they have been studied systematically only recently. More than 90% of the research related to understanding attachment disorders has appeared in the past decade. Controversies remain, but there is a growing consensus at least about the manifestations of the disorders in early childhood.

The purpose of this chapter is to review what is known about reactive attachment disorder (RAD) and disinhibited social engagement disorder (DSED), especially in the context of severe deprivation, and in light of emerging research. Although different or more expanded versions of attachment disorders have been proposed by some (Zeanah & Boris, 2000; van IJzendoorn & Bakermans-Kranenburg, 2002; Minnis *et al.*, 2006) these alternative approaches are less well studied, and we have focused our review primarily on the traditional conceptualization of the disorders, as defined in contemporary nosologies.

Definitions

The term "attachment" itself has been used variably to refer to different constructs, and this has led to confusion in the literature. Bowlby, who developed attachment theory, asserted that attachment referred to the young child's strong disposition "to seek proximity to and contact with a specific figure and to do so in certain situations, notably when ... frightened, tired, or ill. The disposition to behave in this way is an attribute of the child, an attribute which changes only slowly over time and which is unaffected by the situation of the moment" (Bowlby, 1982, p. 371). Therefore, we describe attachment as a tendency for human infants to seek comfort, support, nurturance, and protection preferentially from one or more caregivers. This is

sometimes referred to as "focused," "preferred," "selective," or "discriminated" attachment between child and parent. Because the parent–child attachment relationship is asymmetrical, the young child is the seeker and the adult caregiver/parent is the provider in the attachment relationship. Therefore, it is the parent's job to support the child and not vice versa (see also Chapter 6).

The tendency to approach an adult is believed to be stimulated by increased levels of negative arousal, accompanied by emotions such as distress, fear, frustration, and hurt. These increase the child's motivation to seek support and comfort from someone they have learned is reliably available to provide it. In attachment terms, the child seeks and receives a feeling of security from the physical closeness and emotional availability of a trusted adult caregiver.

A significant challenge to the definition of disordered attachment, however, is the very ubiquity of attachment in young children. Under species-typical rearing conditions, virtually all children form attachments to their caregivers. In children with clinical disturbances of a variety of types, attachment formation or expression may be compromised. Thus, an important question is when the disturbed attachment is the primary problem, in which case it comprises an attachment disorder, and when disturbed attachment is merely an associated feature of some other disorder. An appreciation of the development of attachment under usual circumstances provides a useful foundation from which to begin to answer this question.

Development of attachment

Parents' affiliative feelings for their infants often begin prenatally. Studies have indicated that parents are willing to describe a sense of who the baby is and assert that they have a relationship with

Rutter's Child and Adolescent Psychiatry, Sixth Edition.
Edited by Anita Thapar and Daniel S. Pine, James F. Leckman, Stephen Scott, Margaret J. Snowling, Eric Taylor.

the baby even before the baby is born (Zeanah *et al.*, 1985; Benoit *et al.*, 1997). The birth of the infant usually intensifies feelings of affection, and the newborn's physical attributes, called "babyishness" (Lorenz 1943), are known to draw the attention, interest, and even affection of adults (Stern, 1977).

Although most parents report feeling attached at birth or even before, infants are not born attached to their caregivers. The tendency for selective seeking of comfort is not apparent in the first 6 months after birth. Instead, attachment emerges gradually over the first year of life. By 2–3 months of age, social engagement behaviors emerge, with responsive smiling and cooing and more sustained eye-to-eye contact between infants and adult caregivers. Of note, these behaviors are readily displayed toward both familiar and unfamiliar adults until about 7 or 8 months of age. Two new infant behaviors become apparent at that point: stranger wariness and separation protest. Stranger wariness describes an apparent discomfort with unfamiliar adults and preferentially turning to those caregivers the child knows and trusts. Separation protest refers to the infant's tendency to protest separation from familiar caregivers. Although individual differences in the intensity and expression of these behaviors are clear, they may be considered universal. When these behaviors appear, the infant is said to be "attached" to one or more caregivers. The phases in the development of attachment that correspond to these behavioral changes, which are modified slightly from Bowlby's (1982) original formulation, are described in Table 58.1.

From a clinical perspective, we emphasize that two conditions appear to be necessary for infants to form attachments to adult caregivers. First, infants must have a significant amount of interaction on a regular basis with the caregiver. Infants can neither develop nor sustain attachments to adults with whom they have contact for only a few hours a week, although they may have positive social and playmate relationships with considerably less contact time. Second, they must attain a cognitive age of 7–9 months before the kind of preference seeking that defines attachment is present.

By the end of the first year of life, it is possible to assess the quality of the young child's attachment to a particular caregiver. Usually, this is accomplished by means of a laboratory paradigm known as the Strange Situation Procedure (Ainsworth *et al.*, 1978). Alternating episodes of separations and reunions between a young child and a familiar caregiver and an unfamiliar adult or stranger, the procedure yields classification of a young child's pattern of attachment to the caregiver with whom he or she is assessed as secure, insecure/avoidant, insecure/resistant, or disorganized. It is important to note that these classifications are not diagnoses and should be considered risk and protective factors that are probabilistically related to clinical disorders. Although secure attachment may confer protection for young children in high-risk environments (McGoron *et al.*, 2012), major risks for psychopathology appear to be associated with disorganized or other aberrant attachments (Green & Goldwyn, 2002; Zeanah *et al.*, 2011).

Table 58.1 Development of attachment in early childhood.

Age	Phase	Characteristics
Newborn—2 months	Limited discrimination	Ability to discriminate among different caregivers is limited and preferences are not readily observable
2–8 months	Discrimination with limited preference	Clearly discriminates different caregivers as evident by different patterns of interacting but usually engages readily with strangers and familiar caregivers
8–12 months	Focused attachment	Begins when separation protest and stranger wariness appear. Infant becomes notably more wary of interacting with strangers and protests readily if he or she anticipates or experiences separation from a preferred caregiver (i.e., attachment figure). In typical rearing circumstances, infants attach to more than one caregiver and demonstrate a hierarchy of preferences evident when stressed, fatigued or frightened
12–20 months	Secure base	Independent ambulation ushers in increasing exploratory forays away from the attachment figure, alternating with returns in which proximity is sought. Different patterns of attachment reflect differences in balance between exploration and secure base behavior
20 months and beyond	Goal corrected partnership	Attachment relationship shifts from nearly complete dependency on the caregiver to one in which the toddler becomes aware that others, including the caregiver, have intentions and wishes different from their own

Attachment classifications and psychopathology

Infant behaviors in the presence of the parent or caregiver suggesting fearfulness, freezing, or other contradictory attachment behaviors (e.g., initial approach followed by avoidance while in close contact with the caregiver) during the Strange Situation Procedure are indices of a disorganized attachment classification. Although disorganized attachment has a prevalence of 14% in low-risk samples (van IJzendoorn *et al.*, 1999), it is as high as 75–80% in maltreated and institutionalized samples (Carlson *et al.*, 1989; Vorria *et al.*, 2003; Zeanah *et al.*, 2005). Furthermore, disorganized attachment is associated with various disturbances in caregiving behavior, including frightening/frightened behavior, as well as antagonism, role confusion, withdrawal, and contradictory cues (Lyons-Ruth *et al.*, 1999; Schuengel *et al.*, 1999). As some children reach preschool age, disorganization is transformed into controlling/punitive or solicitous/caregiving behaviors directed toward the parent, though in some high-risk preschool samples, disorganized behaviors remain evident (Smyke *et al.*, 2010).

Of the various attachment classifications, disorganized attachment has the strongest links to subsequent psychopathology, including social difficulties, role-inappropriate parent–child interactive behavior, peer rejection and poor social adjustment, aggression, and disruptive behavior in middle childhood, in addition to emotional problems, low self-esteem, and dissociative disorders in adolescence (Green & Goldwyn, 2002).

Most descriptions of attachment as a clinical disorder have derived from studies of the effects on social and emotional development in young children who have experienced severe deprivation, such as that associated with institutional rearing. Because of that, we turn next to a brief review of the association between institutional care and attachment disorders and consider how studies of institutionalized children informed psychiatric nosologies.

Historical considerations

Institutional care and deprivation

Maternal deprivation and the material deprivation that often accompanies it have long been recognized as important risk factors to development in humans (Chapin, 1915; Spitz, 1945; Bowlby, 1965; Rutter, 1981), primates (Suomi *et al.*, 1976; O'Connor & Cameron, 2006) and rodents (Zhang *et al.*, 2002; Hofer, 2006). For the past 50 years, children raised in institutions have been studied to assess the risks associated with this atypical rearing environment because it has been associated with deprivation. A series of small-scale descriptive studies began to raise questions about the consequences of institutionalization in the 1940s. Early studies focused on behavioral and cognitive manifestations of the effects of poor rearing environments (Goldfarb, 1945; Levy, 1947). In addition to disturbances of growth, cognitive development, and language, these studies also documented that children who had been institutionalized during the first 3 years of life demonstrated consistently greater levels of problem behaviors, including feeding and sleeping difficulties, aggressive behavior and hyperactivity, and excessive attention-seeking and sociability with strangers when compared with children in foster care.

A recent resurgence in studies of children adopted or fostered out of Romanian and other institutions has demonstrated some significant problems across a range of outcomes, including disturbed attachment (Chisholm, 1998; Vorria *et al.*, 2003; The St. Petersburg—USA Orphanage Research Team, 2008; Dobrova-Krol *et al.*, 2010; Rutter *et al.*, 2010; Bakermans-Kranenburg *et al.*, 2011; Smyke *et al.*, 2012). These findings have elaborated many important features of the disorders which had been defined descriptively by previous studies of children living in conditions of deprivation.

Tizard's study
Barbara Tizard's (1977) landmark study deconstructed the institutional experience by largely removing the material deprivation often associated with institutional care and focusing selectively on the variable of caregiver—child relationship. She described the cognitive and socioemotional development of a group of children who experienced varying lengths of institutional care in residential nurseries in Great Britain in the early 1970s. Caregiver to child ratios in these nurseries were substantially better than those found in older studies of institutions (Goldfarb, 1945; Provence & Lipton, 1962). Children were maintained in small, mixed age groups, in a stimulating environment which included books, toys, and instruction (Tizard, 1977).

Three groups of children with histories of early institutional rearing were studied at age 4 years: 24 children who were adopted between 2 and 4 years of age, 15 children who were returned to their biological families (often despite marked ambivalence on the part of their parents), and 26 children who remained institutionalized between 2 and 4 years of age (Tizard, 1977). By age 4, this latter group had experienced an average of 50 different caregivers who had cared for the child for at least a week. Of these 26 children who remained in the residential nurseries, 8 had developed a preferred attachment, 8 were withdrawn and unresponsive, and 10 were indiscriminate, attention-seeking, and socially superficial (Tizard & Rees, 1975). The latter two groups displayed behaviors that had been described in some earlier studies and formed the basis of RAD and disinhibited attachment (DA) disorder in ICD-10 (World Health Organization, 1992).

An important contribution of this landmark study is that much of the material and even social privation that is evident in studies of children in other institutional settings (such as the contemporary studies of children raised in Romanian, Ukranian, or Russian institutions) were not present. Because these residential nurseries were better staffed, had smaller groups of children, and included adequate material resources, this study permitted isolating the effects of the variable of interest for attachment disorders, that is, children's opportunity to form selective attachments to caregivers. Because caregivers were explicitly discouraged from forming attachments to children (or encouraging children to attach to them), the Tizard study showed that this particular caregiving condition was linked clearly to the phenotypes that we now call attachment disorders.

Attachment disorders in nosologies

RAD of Infancy first appeared in the DSM-III (American Psychiatric Association, 1980). Disordered social and emotional development was a hallmark of the disorder, which also included failure to thrive. Inexplicably, there also was a requirement that the disorder be manifest prior to 8 months of age; that is, prior to the age at which preferred attachment ordinarily emerges (Zeanah, 1996).

Subsequent versions of the DSM removed this requirement and made the age of onset below 5 years of age. However, in DSM-IV (American Psychiatric Association, 1994), a specified etiology was included: the child's signs of disturbed attachment were in response to "pathogenic care." ICD-10 (World Health Organization, 1992) criteria were generally consistent with DSM criteria. ICD-10 criteria do not specify pathogenic care, but they do caution against making the diagnosis in the absence of a history of maltreatment.

Interestingly, all revisions in criteria in nosologies through DSM-IV (American Psychiatric Association, 1994) and ICD-10 (World Health Organization, 1992) occurred in the absence of systematic research of the disorders. Two other sets of criteria for disorders of attachment have been published since 2000, the Research Diagnostic Criteria-Preschool Age (RDC-PA; AACAP Task Force on Research Diagnostic Criteria: Infancy and Preschool Age, 2003) and the Diagnostic Classification: 0-3R (Zero to Three, 2005). These descriptions differed from DSM-IV-TR (American Psychiatric Association, 2000) and ICD-10 by focusing more explicitly on disturbed attachment behaviors rather than disturbed social behaviors more generally. The DSM-5 criteria (American Psychiatric Association, 2013) including defining two distinct disorders were based primarily on research in the last decade. Chapter 7 discusses more generally how classifications of early childhood disorders are made in different nosologies.

Clinical disorders of attachment: the phenotypes

Attachment disorders, which have been assessed both continuously and categorically, describe a constellation of aberrant attachment behaviors and other social behavioral anomalies in early childhood which are believed to result from the child having limited opportunities to form selected attachments. Historically, attachment disorders have been linked to deprivation or social neglect. The diagnosis is excluded in the presence of autistic spectrum disorders to distinguish them from social abnormalities associated with those disorders. Although attachment classifications are relationship-specific for the young child, signs of attachment disorders must be evident across situations and relationships.

Two clinical patterns of attachment disorders have been described:

1 An emotionally withdrawn/inhibited pattern, in which the child exhibits limited or absent seeking or responding to comfort when distressed, and a variety of aberrant social and emotional behaviors, such as lack of responsiveness and reciprocity, reduced positive affect, and emotion regulation difficulties. In both ICD-10 and DSM-5, this is called RAD. Evidence suggests that this disorder represents absence of preferred attachment in children who are old enough to have formed them. In keeping with this formulation, institutionalized children showed moderately high convergence between observer rated absence of attachment behaviors with familiar caregivers and caregiver reports of RAD (Zeanah et al., 2005).

2 An indiscriminately social/disinhibited pattern, in which the child exhibits lack of expectable selectivity in seeking comfort, support, and nurturance, with lack of social reticence with unfamiliar adults, including a willingness to "go

off" with strangers and a violation of expected verbal and social boundaries with relative strangers. In ICD-10 (World Health Organization, 1992), this is called disinhibited attachment disorder (DAD) and in DSM-5 (American Psychiatric Association, 2013), this is called DSED. The essence of this disorder is indiscriminate social behavior in children who are expected developmentally to show some degree of stranger wariness.

Reactive attachment disorder

Core features of RAD include lack of social and emotional responses, an absence or near-absence of attachment behaviors even in times of stress, and serious problems of emotion regulation. In addition, RAD includes a paucity of positive emotional responses and bouts of fear or irritability that are seemingly unprovoked, or at least out of proportion to the situation. Social and emotional reciprocal interactions are absent or at least severely dampened. Cognitive and language delays, though not core features, are often associated with RAD because the conditions of neglect believed to lead to this pattern of attachment disorder are also associated with developmental delays.

These signs have been described in young children with a history of severe maltreatment (Zeanah et al., 2004) and those being raised in institutions (Smyke et al., 2002; Zeanah et al., 2005). Interestingly, they have been much less noted in children adopted out of institutions (Chisholm, 1998; Rutter et al., 2010).

Disinhibited social engagement disorder/disinhibited attachment disorder

Core behavioral features of this disorder in young children include inappropriate approach to unfamiliar adults, a lack of wariness of strangers, failure to check back with a caregiver in unfamiliar settings, and a readiness to accompany a stranger, and wander away from a familiar caregiver. Indiscriminate behavior also may be associated with lack of appropriate verbal and physical boundaries, so that children may interact with strangers intrusively and aggressively and may even seek out physical contact (O'Connor & Zeanah, 2003).

For example, some investigators have referred to "indiscriminately friendly" behavior (Chisholm, 1998; Tarullo et al., 2011), but others have suggested that these terms imply more than is actually known about the nature of the child's behavior (O'Connor & Zeanah, 2003). Some children exhibit passive lack of reticence and willingness to accompany a stranger, but this may be quite distinct from children who eagerly accompany a stranger without even checking back with their putative attachment figure. Other behaviors subsumed under this description include lack of initial reticence around unfamiliar adults (e.g., sitting in the lap of an unfamiliar adult at an initial meeting), actively choosing to approach an unfamiliar adult over an attachment figure in times of need, failing to monitor the whereabouts of the attachment figure in unfamiliar settings, displaying inappropriate social boundaries (e.g., making eye contact for too long or asking overly personal questions on initial meeting), or verbally or physically aggressive engagement of unfamiliar adults. These behaviors are not experienced as sociable or friendly by those on the receiving end, and they are not always indiscriminately demonstrated (O'Connor & Zeanah, 2003). Because of this heterogeneity, more precise delineation of behaviors subsumed by this term is indicated.

Still, measurement of the construct has been reasonably consistent across studies. For example, comparing three different caregiver interview measures of indiscriminate behavior, Zeanah and colleagues (2002) showed substantial convergence across measures. Subsequent studies have shown concordance between interviews and observational measures (O'Connor et al., 2003; Gleason et al., 2011a; Oliveira et al., 2012).

Middle childhood and adolescence

Less is known about the measurement of attachment in middle childhood than early childhood. There is no gold standard comparable to the Strange Situation Procedure, and the observable behaviors used to index attachment are less apparent in middle childhood. Not surprisingly, this means defining disordered attachment in this age group is challenging.

Minnis and colleagues have conducted a series of studies relying on combinations of parent report, standardized observations, and structured psychiatric interviews identifying RAD in school-aged children (Millward et al., 2006; Minnis et al., 2006; Minnis et al., 2007; Minnis et al., 2009). Nevertheless, their measures of RAD differ in important ways from the way RAD is defined in early childhood. There was no requirement for "pathogenic care" and an amalgam of disinhibited/indiscriminate behaviors and inhibited/emotionally withdrawn behaviors were included. Therefore, it is likely that the phenotype being described is not the same as the one described in early childhood, since they differ in important respects.

Indiscriminate behavior, on the other hand, has been described and studied in several different populations of children longitudinally from early to middle childhood and has been defined reasonably similarly across studies (Tizard & Hodges, 1978; Bruce et al., 2009; Smyke et al., 2012).

The most careful and intentional examination of the DSED phenotype in middle childhood to date was the English and Romanian Adoptees Study (Rutter et al., 2007a, b). They used a combination of an examiner-based interview of parents when children were 6 and 11 years old and observed interactions with an unfamiliar adult. A factor analysis suggested that two internally consistent composites best summarized the data: violation of boundaries and physical contact. They found significant convergence in these measures of indiscriminate behavior, suggesting a cohesive construct across middle childhood.

In adolescence, Hodges and Tizard (1989) reported no relationship between indiscriminate behavior with unfamiliar adults at age 8 and age 16 years. However, they did report that children who had shown indiscriminate behavior at age 8, tended to be indiscriminate with peers at age 16. Rutter and colleagues (Kreppner et al., 2010) reported the persistence of DA into

adolescence as part of their examination of deprivation-specific psychological (DSP) patterns. They noted the changing clinical picture as they tracked DA from early childhood, where specific behavioral patterns were more defined, to adolescence. They developed measures to assess DA in a way which reflected issues associated with the emerging developmental tasks of adolescence, including difficulties with social boundaries and behaviors which appeared flirtatious to others but were not thought to be so by the previously institutionalized young person. On the other hand, they noted that at times the intrusive and outgoing social style exhibited by some of their subjects had seemed to become a relative social strength in interaction with peers. Nonetheless, symptoms of DA appeared to persist in close to 70% of children who had exhibited DA signs earlier on (Kreppner et al., 2010).

Differential diagnosis

RAD shares some features with autistic spectrum disorders, including disturbances in emotion regulation and impaired or absent social and emotional reciprocity. In addition, children with either disorder may have cognitive delays or stereotypies. However, children with RAD should not have a selective impairment in pretend play, repetitive preoccupations, or language abnormalities other than delays. Further, they should have a history of seriously adverse caregiving. Because RAD and cognitive delays are associated with severe deprivation, meaning social neglect warranting intervention by child protection or institutional rearing (Zeanah et al., 2006), RAD also may be confused with intellectual disability. Young children with RAD should be distinguishable from children with intellectual disability because the latter group has social and emotional behaviors that are consistent with their developmental age, whereas children with RAD show clear evidence of deviance in their social responsiveness and regulation of emotion. Clearly, both conditions may co-occur.

DSED may share features of attention deficit/hyperactivity disorder, particularly impulsivity. Both ADHD and DSED have been reported as sequelae of institutional rearing, and they have both been defined as deprivation specific behavior patterns in postinstitutional children (see Rutter et al., 2010). Roy and colleagues (Roy et al., 2004) found that school-age children with a history of institutional rearing had high levels of both DA behavior and inattention/hyperactivity, as well as a strong association between the two. In addition to lack of selectivity in relationships with caregivers, the children also showed lack of selectivity with peers, echoing the findings of Hodges and Tizard (1989) with adolescents who had formerly been indiscriminate with caregivers. Less clear has been whether the social impulsivity of DSED is related to the cognitive and behavioral impulsivity of ADHD. In children with histories of institutional or other challenging rearing environments, impulse control difficulties are apparent in some children who exhibit indiscriminate behavior (Bruce *et al.,* 2009; Pears *et al.,* 2010), but it is clear that DSED and ADHD may be distinguished clinically (Gleason *et al.,* 2011a). A child with DSED without ADHD will not show inattention/distractibility or restless/overactive behavior in situations demanding quiet and focused behavior. In addition, there is no reason to expect impulsivity beyond social impulsivity in a child with DSED only. For children with ADHD who also demonstrate social impulsivity, both diagnoses may be appropriate if full criteria for DSED are evident. Willingness to accompany unfamiliar adults, on the other hand, is not a part of the ADHD phenotype, unless the child's attention is drawn to some specific activity (e.g., joining a game or throwing a ball).

Prevalence

There is a consensus that these disorders are rare, even though there have been no careful epidemiological studies of their prevalence in community samples. When diagnostic criteria are applied, both RAD and DSED are unusual in populations attending outpatient clinics and more likely to be detected in extreme populations, that is, in young children who have experienced severe deprivation (Chisholm, 1998; Smyke *et al.,* 2002; O'Connor *et al.,* 2003; Boris *et al.,* 2004; Zeanah *et al.,* 2004). In a sample of 300 children aged 2–5, recruited from pediatric clinics in Durham, North Carolina, Egger *et al.* (2006) found no cases of attachment disorders using DSM-IV or the RDC-PA criteria (Boris & Zeanah, 2005). In a similarly designed study in Bucharest, Romania, Gleason and colleagues (Gleason *et al.,* 2011b), also found no cases of RAD.

Several recent studies of clinic-referred and high-risk children have assessed signs of disordered attachment using structured interviews and observational assessments. These studies have found that, even among maltreated children, few met criteria for attachment disorders, with the exception of some maltreated children in foster care (Boris *et al.,* 2004; Zeanah *et al.,* 2004; Oosterman & Schuengel, 2007). In a sample of 12- to 30-month-old children living in institutions in Bucharest, Romania, 10% met criteria for RAD and 24% for DSED (Zeanah, 2006). Thus, although signs of the disorder may be common in extreme populations, a minority of children seem to reach the threshold of disorder.

Etiology

Together with posttraumatic stress disorder, RAD and DSED are among the few psychiatric disorders in which the etiology is specified as one of the diagnostic criteria. A requirement of DSM-5 is that the child has experienced extremes of insufficient caregiving, such as serious social neglect or deprivation (i.e., persistent lack of having basic emotional needs for comfort, stimulation, and affection met), repeated changes of primary caregivers that limit opportunities to form stable attachments, or rearing in institutions that limit opportunities to form selective attachments. Although DSED has been described in children with parents who have psychiatric disorders (see Chapter 28), and many children in foster care have parents with these disorders or serious substance use disorders, we caution against using parent characteristics other than caregiving behavior to identify extremes of insufficient care. It is the seriously deficient caregiving and not the feature associated with it that should be identified. In ICD-10, clinicians are cautioned about making the diagnosis in the absence of a history of maltreatment.

In the Bucharest Early Intervention Project (BEIP), signs of RAD assessed by caregiver report and caregiving quality assessed by coding naturalistic interactions when children were living in institutions were compared. Quality of caregiving, defined by caregiver sensitivity, stimulation of development, positive regard toward child, absence of detachment, absence of flat affect, and absence of intrusiveness, was inversely related to signs of RAD (Zeanah *et al.,* 2005). This finding cannot address the direction of effects, but it does illustrate the grossly insufficient care associated with this disorder. For children in the same study with signs of DSED, no relationship with caregiving quality was found (Zeanah *et al.,* 2005).

Understanding the link with grossly insufficient care is especially important for indiscriminate behavior for at least three reasons. First, the boundaries between highly sociable children and children exhibiting pathologically indiscriminate behavior are not completely delineated. Second, some children with ADHD seem to be socially as well as cognitively and behaviorally impulsive, and this makes delimiting what is indiscriminate behavior challenging. Third, children with congenital abnormalities may exhibit high levels of indiscriminate behavior. Children with Williams syndrome, for example, have been reported to show high levels of indiscriminate behavior, even with more than adequate caregiving (Järvinen-Pasley *et al.,* 2010). Williams syndrome is caused by a microdeletion on chromosome 7q11.23, and is characterized by a tendency for affected individuals to approach persons they do not know and interact with them verbally. Parents of young children with Williams syndrome expend much effort to monitor their children's whereabouts and teach them to refrain from approaching strangers. Compared with nonaffected individuals, they are unable to distinguish threatening faces and consider them just as trustworthy as nonthreatening faces (Järvinen-Pasley *et al.,* 2010).

One study has explored vulnerability factors in children exposed to deprivation. In the BEIP, Drury and colleagues (Drury *et al.,* 2012) demonstrated that children with either the s/s genotype of a serotonin transporter gene variant (5HTTLPR) or BDNF val66met met allele carriers demonstrated the lowest levels of indiscriminate behavior in young children in foster care, but the highest levels in the care as usual (CAU) group who experienced more prolonged institutional rearing. Children with both "plasticity genotypes" had the most signs of indiscriminate behavior at 54 months if they were randomized to CAU, while those with both plasticity genotypes randomized to the foster care intervention had the fewest signs at 54 months.

These specific results need to be replicated before they are accepted, but they demonstrate an approach to delineating individual differences in vulnerability to environmental risk.

Course of the disorders

Based upon the results from several longitudinal studies, however, it seems clear that RAD and DSED generally have different courses.

Studies of children adopted out of institutions have not reported evidence of RAD following adoption (Tizard & Hodges, 1978; Chisholm, 1998; O'Connor *et al.*, 2003). Furthermore, in the BEIP, the first randomized controlled trial to evaluate an intervention for attachment disorders, children who were being raised in institutions were assessed between 11 and 30 months of age for signs of RAD. Half were randomized to a foster care intervention and half to CAU (continued institutional rearing). Follow-ups were conducted at 30, 42, 54, and 96 months of age. Signs of RAD in the group removed from institutions and placed in foster care dropped to the level of never institutionalized children by 30 months and remained low at every subsequent assessment age (Smyke *et al.*, 2012). For children in the CAU group, signs of the disorder slowly decreased over time, but they were always significantly greater than the intervention group. Further, the slow decline of signs of the disorder were accounted for completely by children who were placed in families—either reintegrated with their own biological families or placed into government sponsored foster care (Smyke *et al.*, 2012). In other words, over a 6-year period, there was no significant reduction in signs of RAD for children who remained in institutions. This latter finding is important, as it represents preliminary evidence of persistence of the disorder in children who remain in an adverse caregiving environment. These results indicate that signs of RAD are eliminated by placement of children into families where they receive at least adequate care. Less clear is what the long-term sequelae of RAD in early childhood may be in adolescence or adulthood.

In contrast, there is reasonably clear evidence demonstrating that indiscriminate behavior persists over time—sometimes even after improvements in the caregiving environment. This was demonstrated originally in the work of Tizard and colleagues, who showed that young children who had been indiscriminate with caregivers at age 4 were more likely to have serious peer disturbances at 16 years, including superficial and even indiscriminate behavior with peers (Hodges & Tizard, 1989). Subsequent studies of children adopted into Canada and the UK from Romanian institutions have also demonstrated a tendency for indiscriminate behavior to persist even after the child forms attachments to the adopted family (Chisholm, 1998; O'Connor *et al.*, 2003). In fact, of those children adopted into the UK from Romanian institutions who had high levels of indiscriminate behavior at age 6, more than half continued to show high levels at age 11 (Rutter *et al.*, 2007a). Furthermore,

in the BEIP, indiscriminate behavior persisted in children who had been reared in institutions (Smyke *et al.*, 2012).

Clinical assessment

In keeping with recent trends in the assessment of early childhood psychopathology (delCarmen-Wiggins & Carter, 2004), attachment disorders are best identified through a combination of caregiver interview and observed interactions. In our view, there are no gold standard interviews nor observational paradigms of interactions between parents and children that must be included, but several useful approaches have been described.

Interviews
Structured interviews specifically focused on the child's attachment behaviors and signs of disordered attachment (O'Connor *et al.*, 1999; Smyke *et al.*, 2002; Boris *et al.*, 2004; Zeanah *et al.*, 2005) are more likely to be useful than interviews that are less specifically focused. At least two structured psychiatric interviews, the Psychiatric Assessment Preschool Age (Egger & Angold, 2004) and the Diagnostic Infant/Preschool Assessment (Scheeringa & Haslett, 2010) include modules on attachment disorders. These approaches are able to characterize attachment disorders both categorically and continuously.

Observations
Potentially clinically useful observations of parent and child together include procedures designed specifically to examine attachment behaviors (O'Connor *et al.*, 2003; Boris *et al.*, 2004; Oliveira *et al.*, 2012), or those in which other aspects of parent–child interaction are also assessed (Zeanah *et al.*, 2000). It is generally useful to include in the observation some degree of distress that is likely to activate the child's need for the attachment figure. Conventionally, this has involved brief separations followed by reunions, but other approaches such as a novel (i.e., scary) toy also have been used (Boris *et al.*, 2004). Although the Strange Situation Procedure was not designed for clinical assessments, in some circumstances it may be helpful (Zeanah *et al.*, 2011). The Circle of Security Intervention, for example, includes review of videotaped recordings of a child's Strange Situation behavior with the parent as a part of the intervention (Hoffman *et al.*, 2006). Although systematic observations of the child's behavior in paradigms designed to elicit attachment behaviors are often clinically valuable, naturalistic observations of a child's attachment behaviors also may yield important data.

Interventions

Studies of interventions for RAD and DSED are limited. Intervention efforts to date have been guided by the principle that enhancing the caregiving environment will ameliorate signs of attachment disorder. Smyke *et al.* (2002), for example, studied signs of RAD and DSED in young children being raised in a large institution for young children in Bucharest. This institution had implemented a pilot unit designed to reduce the number of caregivers responsible for each child. In fact, compared to the more standard units, which included large numbers of rotating caregivers, on the pilot unit no more than four caregivers were responsible for each child on the day and evening shifts. Caregivers on the pilot unit reported that children had significantly fewer signs of both RAD and DSED. Importantly, this reduction was evident even though the ratio of caregivers to children remained at 1:12 on the pilot unit (the same as on the standard units).

Studies of young children adopted out of institutions are also useful to examine because they represent such a dramatic change in caregiving environments. Two longitudinal studies of young children adopted out of Romanian institutions are particularly instructive. A longitudinal study of young children adopted into Canada from Romanian institutions used parent reports of attachment and indiscriminate behavior. They found significant increases in attachment to adoptive parents during the first several years following adoption, although indiscriminate behavior persisted in a minority of children (Chisholm, 1998). Another longitudinal study of children adopted from Romanian institutions into families in the UK assessed signs of disordered attachment from parent reports at ages 4, 6, 11, and 15 (O'Connor & Rutter, 2000; O'Connor *et al.*, 2003; Rutter *et al.*, 2007a; Rutter *et al.*, 2010). They reported little change in the numbers of children with high levels of indiscriminate behaviors between 4 and 6 years, but some decline by age 11 years (O'Connor & Rutter, 2000; Rutter *et al.*, 2007a). To date, however, there has been no demonstration that quality of care in adoptive homes is inversely related to signs of indiscriminate behavior in children.

In summary, findings from studies of children living in institutions and those adopted out of institutions suggest that signs of DSED are remediated by enhanced caregiving only in some children. It is unclear whether this represents individual differences among children or partial remediation with persistence in those most severely affected initially. To date, adoption studies have not included assessments of children in the institutions prior to adoption, making it difficult to explain individual differences in response.

The only contemporary intervention study that included assessments of children's attachment prior to removal from institutions and placement in an enhanced caregiving environment is the BEIP, described earlier. Results of this study indicate that foster care leads to significant reductions in signs of RAD in young children who had signs of the disorder when they were living in institutions (Smyke *et al.*, 2012).

At this stage, clinicians must be guided by data indicating that secure attachment is fostered by caregivers who are emotionally available and sensitively responsive, who know and value the child as an individual, and who place the needs of the child ahead of their own needs. Preliminary data indicate that psychoeducational approaches involving training parents to respond sensitively to their child (Juffer *et al.*, 2005) and to understand their own and their child's attachment pattern (Hoffman *et al.*, 2006) have been shown to promote attachment security in the child. These interventions are reasonable starting points for developing an evidence base about intervening in disordered attachments.

Conclusions

Our understanding of attachment disorders has deepened considerably in the past decade as a result of a number of systematic studies of children with histories of severe neglect or institutional rearing. These studies have affirmed the reliable identification of both RAD and DSED. They also have supported the link between extremes of inadequate caregiving and these disorders. Further, they have demonstrated that the specific "pathogen" is any environment in which young children have limited opportunities to form selective attachments, as happens in cases of severe social neglect or in settings in which the child lacks regular and consistent contact with an emotionally involved caregiver (e.g., institutional settings or frequent changes in foster care).

Although RAD and DSED arise from similar conditions of risk, they have different correlates and different courses. In particular, placement in enhanced caregiving environments seems to lead to rapid and complete elimination of signs of RAD, but DSED remains persistent in some children, apparently for years.

However, a number of questions remain to be addressed. First, not enough is known about individual vulnerabilities to the disorder – in particular, why such phenomenologically distinct syndromes arise from similar conditions of risk. Genetic polymorphisms, temperamental dispositions, and differential caregiving experiences should all be examined. In addition, the relationship between the two types of disorder—if any—needs to be clarified. Second, why some children with indiscriminately social/DA disorder seem to respond to enhanced caregiving and others do not is unclear. Third, the specific components of enhanced caregiving that are crucial for amelioration of signs of the disorder are unclear. This is especially important, given the heterogeneity of outcomes in postadoption studies. Fourth, the putative social cognitive abnormalities that characterize indiscriminate behavior need to be delineated. It seems reasonable that such abnormalities are the most concerning aspect of the disorder from the standpoint of functional impairment. Finally, the underlying neurobiology of these disorders is largely unexplored. The phenomenological similarities and differences between indiscriminate behavior and Williams syndrome may suggest hypotheses about the neural substrate of DSED. Answers to these questions will assist clinicians concerned with helping children recover from the long-term effects of early adversity.

References

AACAP Task Force on Research Diagnostic Criteria: Infancy and Preschool Age (2003) Research diagnostic criteria for infants and preschool children: the process and empirical support. *Journal of the American Academy of Child and Adolescent Psychiatry* **42**, 1504–1512.

Ainsworth, M. *et al.* (1978) *Patterns of Attachment*. Erlbaum, Hillsdale, NJ.

American Psychiatric Association (1980) *Diagnostic and Statistical Manual of Mental Disorders*, 3rd edn. American Psychiatric Association, Washington, DC.

American Psychiatric Association (1994) *Diagnostic and Statistical Manual of Mental Disorders*, 4th edn. American Psychiatric Association, Washington, DC.

American Psychiatric Association (2000) *Diagnostic and Statistical Manual of Mental Disorders, Text Revision*, 4th edn. American Psychiatric Association, Washington, DC.

American Psychiatric Association (2013) *Diagnostic and Statistical Manual of Mental Disorders*, 5th edn. American Psychiatric Association, Washington, DC.

Bakermans-Kranenburg, M. *et al.* (2011) Attachment and emotional development in institutional care: characteristics and catch-up. In: *Children without Permanent Parental Care: Research, Practice, and Policy*. (eds R.B. McCall, M.H. van IJzendoorn, F. Juffer, V.K. Groza & C.J. Groark). Monographs of the Society for Research in Child Development, Serial No. 301, **76**, pp. 62–91.

Benoit, D. *et al.* (1997) Mothers' representations of their infants assessed prenatally: stability and association with infants' attachment classifications. *Journal of Child Psychology, Psychiatry and Allied Disciplines* **38**, 307–313.

Boris, N. & Zeanah, C. (2005) Reactive attachment disorder. In: *Kaplan & Sadock's Comprehensive Textbook of Psychiatry*. (eds B.J. Sadock & V.A. Sadock), 8th edn, pp. 3248–3254. Williams and Wilkins, Philadelphia.

Boris, N. *et al.* (2004) Comparing criteria for attachment disorders: establishing reliability and validity in high-risk samples. *Journal of the American Academy of Child and Adolescent Psychiatry* **43**, 568–577.

Bowlby, J. (1965) *Child Care and the Growth of Love*. Penguin, London.

Bowlby, J. (1982) *Attachment and Loss*, 2nd edn. Vol. 1. Attachment. Basic Books, New York.

Bruce, B. *et al.* (2009) Disinhibited social behavior among internationally adopted children. *Development and Psychopathology* **21**, 157–171.

Carlson, V. *et al.* (1989) Finding order in disorganization: lessons from research on maltreated infants' attachments to their caregivers. In: *Child Maltreatment: Theory and Research on the Causes and Consequences of Child Abuse and Neglect*. (eds D. Cicchetti & V. Carlson), pp. 494–528. Cambridge University Press, New York.

del Carmen-Wiggins, R. & Carter, A. (2004) *Handbook of Infant, Toddler, and Preschool Mental Health Assessment*. Oxford University Press, New York.

Chapin, H. (1915) Are institutions for infants necessary? *JAMA* **64**, 1–3.

Chisholm, K. (1998) A three year follow-up of attachment and indiscriminate friendliness in children adopted from Romanian orphanages. *Child Development* **69**, 1092–1106.

Dobrova-Krol, N. *et al.* (2010) The importance of quality of care: effects of perinatal HIV infection and early institutional rearing on preschoolers' attachment and indiscriminate friendliness. *Journal of Child Psychology and Psychiatry* **51**, 1368–1376.

Drury, S. *et al.* (2012) Genetic sensitivity to the caregiving context: the influence of 5httlpr and BDNF val66 met on indiscriminate social behavior. *Physiology and Behavior* **106**, 728–735.

Egger, H. & Angold, A. (2004) The Preschool Age Psychiatric Assessment (PAPA): a structured parent interview for diagnosing psychiatric disorders in preschool children. In: *Handbook of Infant, Toddler, and Preschool Mental Health Assessment*. (eds R. DelCarmenWiggins & A. Carter), pp. 223–243. Oxford University Press, New York.

Egger, H. *et al.* (2006) Test-retest reliability of the Preschool Age Psychiatric Assessment (PAPA). *Journal of the American Academy of Child and Adolescent Psychiatry* **45**, 538–549.

Gleason, M. *et al.* (2011a) Validity of evidence-derived criteria for reactive attachment disorder: indiscriminately social/disinhibited and emotionally withdrawn/inhibited types. *Journal of American Academy of Child and Adolescent Psychiatry* **50**, 216–231.

Gleason, M. *et al.* (2011b) Epidemiology of psychiatric disorders in very young children in a Romanian pediatric setting. *European Journal of Child and Adolescent Psychiatry* **20**, 527–535.

Goldfarb, W. (1945) Effects of psychological deprivation in infancy and subsequent stimulation. *American Journal of Psychiatry* **102**, 18–33.

Green, J. & Goldwyn, R. (2002) Annotation: attachment disorganization and psychopathology: new findings in attachment research and their potential implications for developmental psychopathology in childhood. *Journal of Child Psychology and Psychiatry* **43**, 835–846.

Hodges, J. & Tizard, B. (1989) Social and family relationships of ex-institutional adolescents. *Journal of Child Psychology, Psychiatry, and Allied Disciplines* **30**, 77–97.

Hofer, M. (2006) Psychobiological roots of early attachment. *Current Directions in Psychological Science* **15**, 84–88.

Hoffman, K. *et al.* (2006) Changing toddlers' and preschoolers' attachment classifications: the Circle of Security intervention. *Journal of Consulting and Clinical Psychology* **74**, 1017–1026.

van IJzendoorn, M. & Bakermans-Kranenburg, M. (2002) Disorganized attachment and the dysregulation of negative emotions. In: *Emotion Regulation and Developmental Health: Infancy and Early Childhood*. (eds B. Zuckerman, A. Lieberman & N. Fox), pp. 159–179. Johnson and Johnson Pediatric Institute, Somerville, NJ.

van IJzendoorn, M. *et al.* (1999) Disorganized attachment in early childhood: meta-analysis of precursors, concomitants, and sequelae. *Development and Psychopathology* **11**, 225–249.

Järvinen-Pasley, A. *et al.* (2010) Affiliative behavior in Williams syndrome: social perception and real-life social behavior. *Neuropsychologia* **48**, 2110–2119.

Juffer, F. *et al.* (2005) Enhancing children's socio-emotional development: a review of intervention studies. In: *Handbook of Research Methods in Developmental Science*. (ed D.M. Teti), pp. 213–232. Oxford, Blackwell.

Juffer, F. *et al.* (2007) *Promoting Positive Parenting: An Attachment-Based Intervention*. Lawrence Erlbaum, Mahwah, NJ.

Kreppner, J. *et al.* (2010) Developmental course of deprivation-specific psychological patterns: early manifestations, persistence to age 15, and clinical features. In: *Deprivation-Specific Psychological Patterns: Effects of Institutional Deprivation*. (eds M. Rutter, *et al.*). Monographs of the Society for Research in Child Development, Serial No. 295, vol. **75**, pp. 79–101.

Levy, R. (1947) Effects of institutional vs. boarding home care on a group of infants. *Journal of Personality* **15**, 233–241.

Lorenz, K. (1943) Die angeborenen Formen möglicher Erfahrung. *Zeitschrift für Tierpsychologie* **5**, 235–409.

Lyons-Ruth, K. *et al.* (1999) Maternal frightened, frightening, or atypical behavior and disorganized attachment patterns. In: *Atypical Attachment in Early Childhood Among Children at Developmental Risk.* (eds K. Lyons-Ruth, E. Bronfman, E. Parsons, J. Vondra & D. Barnett). Monographs of the Society for Research in Child Development, Serial No. 258, vol. **64**, pp. 67–96.

McGoron, L. *et al.* (2012) Recovering from early deprivation: attachment mediates effects of caregiving on psychopathology. *Journal of the American Academy of Child and Adolescent Psychiatry* **51**, 683–693.

Millward, R. *et al.* (2006) Reactive attachment disorder in looked-after children. *Emotional and Behavioural Difficulties* **11**, 273–279.

Minnis, H. *et al.* (2006) Reactive attachment disorder: a theoretical model beyond attachment. *European Journal of Child and Adolescent Psychiatry* **15**, 336–342.

Minnis, H. *et al.* (2007) Genetic, environmental and gender influences on attachment disorder behaviours. *British Journal of Psychiatry* **190**, 490–495.

Minnis, H. *et al.* (2009) An exploratory study of the association between reactive attachment disorder and attachment narratives in early school-age children. *Journal of Child Psychology and Psychiatry* **50**, 931–942.

O'Connor, T. & Cameron, J. (2006) Translating research findings on early experience to prevention: animal and human evidence on early attachment relationships. *American Journal of Prevention Medicine* **31**, S175–S181.

O'Connor, T. & Rutter, M. (2000) Attachment disorder behavior following early severe deprivation: extension and longitudinal follow-up. *Journal of the American Academy of Child and Adolescent Psychiatry* **39**, 703–712.

O'Connor, T. & Zeanah, C. (2003) Assessment strategies and treatment approaches. *Attachment and Human Development* **5**, 223–244.

O'Connor, T. *et al.* (1999) Attachment disturbances and disorders in children exposed to early severe deprivation. *Infant Mental Health Journal* **20**, 10–29.

O'Connor, T. *et al.* (2003) Child-parent attachment following early institutional deprivation. *Development and Psychopathology* **15**, 19–38.

Oliveira, P. *et al.* (2012) Indiscriminate behavior observed in the strange situation among institutionalized toddlers: relations to caregiver report and to early family risk. *Infant Mental Health Journal* **33**, 187–196.

Oosterman, M. & Schuengel, C. (2007) Autonomic reactivity of children to separation and reunion with foster parents. *Journal of the American Academy of Child and Adolescent Psychiatry* **46**, 1196–1203.

Pears, K. *et al.* (2010) Indiscriminate friendliness in maltreated foster children. *Child Maltreatment* **15**, 64–75.

Provence, S. & Lipton, R. (1962) *Infants in Institutions.* International Universities Press, New York.

Roy, P. *et al.* (2004) Institutional care: associations between overactivity and lack of selectivity in social relationships. *Journal of Child Psychology and Psychiatry* **45**, 866–873.

Rutter, M. (1981) *Maternal Deprivation Reassessed*, 2nd edn. Penguin Books, Harmondsworth, UK.

Rutter, M. *et al.* (2007a) Effects of profound early institutional deprivation: an overview of findings from a UK longitudinal study of Romanian adoptees. *European Journal of Developmental Psychology* **4**, 332–350.

Rutter, M. *et al.* (2007b) Early adolescent outcomes for institutionally-deprived and non-deprived adoptees. I. Disinhibited attachment. *Journal of Child Psychology and Psychiatry* **48**, 17–30.

Rutter, M. *et al.* (2010). Deprivation-specific psychological patterns: effects of institutional deprivation. *Monographs of the Society for Research in Child Development* **75**, Serial No. 295.

Scheeringa, M. & Haslett, N. (2010) The reliability and criterion validity of the Diagnostic Infant and Preschool Assessment: a new diagnostic instrument for young children. *Child Psychiatry and Human Development* **41**, 299–312.

Schuengel, C. *et al.* (1999) Frightening maternal behavior linking unresolved loss and disorganized infant attachment. *Journal of Consulting and Clinical Psychology* **67**, 54–63.

Smyke, A. *et al.* (2002) Disturbances of attachment in young children. I. The continuum of caretaking casualty. *Journal of the American Academy of Child and Adolescent Psychiatry* **41**, 972–982.

Smyke, A. *et al.* (2010) Placement in foster care enhances quality of attachment among young institutionalized children. *Child Development* **81**, 212–223.

Smyke, A. *et al.* (2012) A randomized controlled trial comparing foster care and institutional care for children with signs of reactive attachment disorder. *American Journal of Psychiatry* **169**, 508–514.

Spitz, R.A. (1945) Hospitalism: an inquiry into the genesis of psychiatric conditions in early childhood. *Psychoanalytic Study of the Child* **1**, 53–74.

Stern, D. (1977) *The First Relationship: Mother and Infant.* Harvard University Press, Cambridge, MA.

Suomi, S. *et al.* (1976) Effects of maternal and peer separation on young monkeys. *Journal of Child Psychology and Psychiatry* **17**, 101–112.

Tarullo, A. *et al.* (2011) Atypical EEG power correlates with indiscriminately friendly behavior in internationally adopted children. *Developmental Psychology* **47**, 417–431.

The St. Petersburg—USA Orphanage Research Team (2008) The effects of early social-emotional and relationship experience on the development of young orphanage children. *Monographs of the Society for Research in Child Development*, **73**, vii–295, Serial No. 291.

Tizard, B. (1977) *Adoption: A Second Chance.* Open Books, London.

Tizard, B. & Hodges, J. (1978) The effect of early institutional rearing on the development of eight year old children. *Journal of Child Psychology and Psychiatry* **19**, 99–118.

Tizard, B. & Rees, J. (1975) The effect of early institutional rearing on the behaviour problems and affectional relationships of four-year-old children. *Journal of Child Psychology and Psychiatry* **16**, 61–73.

Vorria, P. *et al.* (2003) Early experiences and attachment relationships of Greek infants raised in residential group care. *Journal of Child Psychology and Psychiatry* **44**, 1208–1220.

World Health Organization (1992) *ICD-10 Classifications of Mental and Behavioural Disorders: Clinical Descriptions and Diagnostic Guidelines.* World Health Organization, Geneva. Cambridge University Press, Cambridge, UK.

Zeanah, C. (1996) Beyond insecurity: a reconceptualization of attachment disorders of infancy. *Journal of Consulting and Clinical Psychology* **64**, 42–52.

Zeanah, C. (2006) *Bucharest Early Intervention Project: Psychiatric Outcomes.* Presented at the American Association for Advancement of Science Annual Meeting, St. Louis, MO.

Zeanah, C. & Boris, N. (2000) Disturbances and disorders of attachment in early childhood. In: *Handbook of Infant Mental Health*. (ed C.H. Zeanah), 2nd edn, pp. 353–368. Guilford Press, New York.

Zeanah, C. *et al.* (1985) Prenatal perception of infant personality: a preliminary investigation. *Journal of the American Academy of Child Psychiatry* **24**, 204–210.

Zeanah, C. *et al.* (2000) Infant-parent relationship assessment. In: *Handbook of Infant Mental Health*. (ed C.H. Zeanah), 2nd edn, pp. 222–235. Guilford Press, New York.

Zeanah, C. *et al.* (2002) Disturbances of attachment in young children. II. Indiscriminate behavior and institutional care. *Journal of the American Academy of Child and Adolescent Psychiatry* **41**, 983–989.

Zeanah, C. *et al.* (2004) Reactive attachment disorder in maltreated toddlers. *Child Abuse and Neglect* **28**, 877–888.

Zeanah, C. *et al.* (2005) Attachment in institutionalized and noninstitutionalized Romanian children. *Child Development* **76**, 1015–1028.

Zeanah, C. *et al.* (2006) Orphanages as a developmental context for early childhood. In: *Blackwell Handbook of Early Childhood Development*. (eds K. McCartney & D. Phillips), pp. 224–254. Blackwell Publishing, Malden, MA.

Zeanah, C. *et al.* (2011) Practitioner review: clinical applications of attachment theory and research for infants and young children. *Journal of Child Psychology and Psychiatry* **52**, 819–833.

Zero to Three (2005) *Diagnostic Classification: 0-3R: The Diagnostic Classification of Mental Health and Developmental Disorders of Infancy and Early Childhood*, revised edn. Zero to Three Press, Washington, DC.

Zhang, L. *et al.* (2002) Maternal deprivation increases cell death in the infant rat brain. *Developmental Brain Research* **133**, 1–11.

CHAPTER 59

Post traumatic stress disorder

William Yule and Patrick Smith

Institute of Psychiatry, Psychology and Neuroscience, Kings's College London, UK

Characteristics and diagnosis of the condition

The diagnosis of posttraumatic stress disorder (PTSD) was first conceptualized in response to observations of Vietnam war veterans presenting with what came to be recognized as a particular pattern of symptoms in three clusters—intrusive recollections of a traumatic event; emotional numbing and avoidance of reminders of that event; and physiological hyperarousal. In retrospect, similar patterns were noted as reactions in earlier wars, and in prospect, the criteria were adapted, partly operationalized and applied to adult civilians. Next, the diagnosis was applied to children who had experienced an "event outside the range of usual human experience ... that would be markedly distressing to almost anyone" (American Psychiatric Association, 1987).

Thus, it was argued that there were certain types of stressful experiences that were very severe and/or unusual and that there was a distinctive form of stress reaction to these. PTSD was classified as an anxiety disorder, but many argued that it should be included as a dissociative disorder, and more recently it has been recognized as a disorder of memory. It was increasingly described as "a normal reaction to an abnormal situation," and so, logically, it was queried whether it should be regarded as a psychiatric disorder at all (O'Donohue & Eliot, 1992). Far from being "abnormal," exposure to traumatic events is all too common in childhood and adolescence (Giaconia et al., 1995; Costello et al., 2002). PTSD usually occurs in only a minority of those exposed to trauma (Copeland et al., 2007). Comorbidity with other disorders is the norm rather than the exception (Bolton et al., 2000). Even if it were regarded as a normal reaction, it causes substantial impairment in sufficient cases to be regarded as a disorder.

While adult studies suggest that PTSD is predominantly an anxiety disorder, it differs from other anxiety disorders in important ways. Thus, Foa et al. (1989) showed that the trauma suffered violated more of the patients' safety assumptions than did events giving rise to other forms of anxiety. There was a much greater generalization of fear responses in the PTSD groups, and, unlike other anxious patients, they reported far more frequent reexperiencing of the traumatic event. Indeed, it is this internal, subjective experience that seems most to mark out PTSD from other disorders (Jones & Barlow, 1992). Given that exposure to traumatic events is common (Kessler et al., 1995), and that only a minority of exposed individuals go on to develop the disorder (e.g. McFarlane, 2005), the argument is therefore made that PTSD is an "abnormal reaction" that involves a complex interaction of biological, psychological, and social causes (Yehuda & McFarlane, 1995): exposure to trauma is insufficient to explain the development of the disorder. Current biopsychosocial and cognitive models (see later) are paying increasing attention to factors underlying individual differences in response to traumatic events. Concern has been expressed that there are other forms of stress reactions to chronic stressors as experienced in repeated physical or sexual abuse (see Chapters 27–30). While these are important debates that will alter the views taken on PTSD, here we will concentrate on acute conditions as manifested in children and adolescents.

Manifestations of stress reactions in children and adolescents

Immediately following a very frightening experience, children are likely to be very distressed, tearful, frightened, and in shock. They need protection and safety. They need to be reunited with their families wherever possible. Clinical experience, surveys, and clinical descriptive studies quoted below show that the main manifestations of stress reactions are as follows.

Rutter's Child and Adolescent Psychiatry, Sixth Edition.
Edited by Anita Thapar and Daniel S. Pine; James F. Leckman, Stephen Scott, Margaret J. Snowling, Eric Taylor.
© 2015 John Wiley & Sons Ltd. Published 2018 by John Wiley & Sons Ltd.

Starting almost immediately, most children are troubled by *repetitive, intrusive thoughts* about the accident. Such thoughts can occur at any time, but particularly when the children are otherwise quiet, as when they are trying to drop off to sleep. At other times, the thoughts and vivid recollections are triggered off by reminders in their environment. Vivid, dissociative *flashbacks* are uncommon. In a flashback, the child reports that he or she is reexperiencing the event, as if it were happening all over again. It is almost a dissociated experience. *Sleep disturbances* are very common, particularly in the first few weeks. Fears of the dark and bad dreams, nightmares, and waking through the night are widespread (and often manifest outside the developmental age range in which they normally occur).

Separation difficulties are frequent, even among teenagers. For the first few days, children may not want to let their parents out of their sight, even reverting to sleeping in the parental bed. Many children become much more *irritable and angry* than previously, both with parents and peers.

Although child survivors experience a pressure to talk about their experiences, paradoxically they also find it very *difficult to talk* with their parents and peers. Often they do not want to upset the adults, and so parents may not be aware of the full extent of their children's suffering. Peers may hold back from asking what happened in case they upset the child further; the survivor often feels this as a rejection.

Children report a number of cognitive changes. Many experience difficulties in *concentration*, especially in school work. Others report *memory* problems, both in mastering new material and in remembering old skills such as reading music. They become very *alert to danger* in their environment, being adversely affected by reports of other disasters.

Survivors have learned that life is very fragile. This can lead to a loss of faith in the future or a sense of foreshortened future, or a premature awareness of their own mortality. Their priorities change. Some feel they should live each day to the full and not plan far ahead. Others realize they have been overconcerned with materialistic or petty matters and resolve to rethink their values. Their "assumptive world" has been challenged (Janoff-Bulman, 1985).

Not surprisingly, many develop *fears* associated with specific aspects of their experiences. They avoid situations they associate with the disaster. Many experience "survivor guilt"—about surviving when others died; about thinking they should have done more to help others; about what they themselves did to survive.

Adolescent survivors report significantly high rates of *depression*, some becoming clinically depressed, having suicidal thoughts and taking overdoses in the year after a disaster. A significant number become very *anxious* after accidents, although the appearance of panic attacks is sometimes considerably delayed. Some children may have been bereaved and may develop *traumatic grief* reactions.

In summary, children and adolescents surviving a traumatic event may show a wide range of symptoms which tend to cluster around signs of reexperiencing the traumatic event, trying to avoid dealing with the emotions that this gives rise to, and a range of signs of increased physiological arousal. In a substantial minority, this cluster of symptoms will amount to a diagnosable PTSD. Just as in adults, a broad range of adverse outcomes is common (Bolton *et al.*, 2000; Pine & Cohen, 2002): there may be considerable overlap of symptoms with depression, generalized anxiety, or pathological grief reactions although whether this indicates the presence of mixed disorders or comorbidity of separate disorders remains to be clarified.

However, this has implications for assessment. It is not sufficient to enquire solely about symptoms of PTSD. Symptoms of anxiety, depression, and grief need also to be formally investigated. Nor are self-completed questionnaires measuring these aspects sufficient to make a diagnosis. They have an important role, but sensitive clinical interviews with the child and separately with the parents remain the cornerstone of good assessment.

Developmental aspects

Considerable debate remains as to whether the very young child's limited cognitive development is protective against developing a chronic posttraumatic stress reaction. Certainly, until recently, the diagnostic criteria in both of the major classification schemes were not appropriate for preschool children.

Some community surveys of trauma-exposed children reported very low rates of PTSD diagnosis according to DSM-IV criteria. None of the very young children exposed to the September 11 attacks in New York and studied by Saigh *et al.* (2011) met criteria. Are the children very resilient or are the criteria developmentally insensitive?

In a series of studies, Scheeringa and colleagues (Scheeringa *et al.*, 1995, 2001, 2003, 2006) examined the phenomenology reported in published cases of trauma in infants and young children and evolved an alternative set of criteria for diagnosing PTSD in very young children. This alternative algorithm (PTSD-AA) reduces the threshold for diagnosis by dropping the required number of avoidance symptoms (the most difficult to elicit in young children) and reformulating other criteria in more developmentally appropriate terms.

The DSM-5 criteria for "PTSD-Preschool subtype" closely match the research criteria developed by Scheeringa. De Young *et al.* (2011) examined children aged 1–6 following burns and found that the PTSD-AA and DSM-5 identified nearly identical children. At 1 month post trauma, both methods diagnosed 25% as having PTSD, and this is considerably more than the incidence of 5% yielded by DSM-IV criteria.

Cultural issues

Traumatic events such as wars and natural disasters happen globally, but especially in low and middle income countries where mental health services are often least developed. There is continuing debate about how best to meet mental health needs in differing cultures. The validity of Western frameworks for assessment and intervention needs to be constantly reviewed.

PTSD presents very similarly in many different cultures, but ways of intervening may need to be modified. For example, very similar stress reactions have been reported in children across all continents where studies have been undertaken (in Europe: Giannopoulou *et al.*, 2006; North America: Pynoos *et al.*, 2008; Central America: Arroyo, 1997; the Middle East: Thabet & Vostanis, 1999; Southeast Asia: Neuner *et al.*, 2006; Australasia: Bryant *et al.*, 2007; and elsewhere: Perrin *et al.*, 2000).

If PTSD "transcends cultural barriers" (Sack *et al.*, 1997), then similar underlying factor structures should be found if similar self-completed screening questionnaires are measuring the same construct (Smith *et al.*, 2003). To date, this has been the case in Cambodia (Sack *et al.*, 1997, 1998), Croatia (Dyregrov *et al.*, 1996) and Bosnia (Smith *et al.*, 2003). Large-scale studies in China have also replicated the same underlying factors (Ma *et al.*, 2011) indicating that stress reactions are indeed more similar than different across cultures.

It might be argued that the use of questionnaires constrains the way children can express their reactions. Open-ended interviewing and ethnographic methods, however, come to the same conclusion. Bolton (2001) found that the postgenocide symptoms reported by Rwandan youth were very close to those described in DSM-IV for both PTSD and depression.

Thus, the evidence at present is that posttraumatic stress reactions are not culture bound.

Impact of disorder on functioning

Given that PTSD affects mood, memory, and learning, it is surprising how few studies are reported on the effect of trauma on academic attainment. Tsui (1990; reported in Yule & Gold, 1993) found that adolescent girls who survived the sinking of the cruise ship "Jupiter" showed a marked decline in academic attainments a year later when compared with peers of matched ability who had not gone on the cruise. Broberg *et al.* (2005) found that 2 years after a devastating discotheque fire, adolescents reported significant effects on school attainment. Only 17% reported no impact on schooling while nearly a quarter had had to repeat a year or even dropped out of education. More generally, community violence was reported to have significant adverse effects on the educational attainment of adolescents. Those who developed severe PTSD scored significantly lower grade point averages than those with moderate PTSD. Fortunately, their attainment responded to treatment of their PTSD (Saltzman *et al.*, 2001). Dyregrov (2004) indicates how PTSD reactions can interfere with learning, self control and peer relationships within school and advises that schools be better prepared to help traumatized children.

Differential diagnosis

Differential diagnosis should not be difficult, provided clinicians take a good trauma history as part of their normal screening procedures (Greenwald, 2005). Without this, it could be possible to misidentify intrusive phenomena as hallucinations or delusions. Similarly, poor concentration and difficulty learning might be confused with Attention Deficit Hyperactivity Disorder (ADHD). In general, differential diagnosis is more complicated following multiple exposure but appears more straightforward following single-incident trauma.

Assessment

In contrast to other child mental health complaints, the traumatic event is likely to be well known (other than sexual or physical abuse). Therefore, when a referral is made, the clinician can gather together considerable detail of the incident in the form of press reports, photographs, videos, and even architectural drawings. This can greatly help the child recall details of the experience and places it in context.

The initial assessment should involve a brief joint parent and child meeting to describe the interview process. This is followed by asking parents and child separately to complete standardized, self-report measures, and then conduct separate parent and child interviews. Children will frequently reveal details of what happened and how they reacted during their interview, details of which the parents are unaware. Indeed, parents and children frequently avoid discussing the incident for fear of upsetting each other. This is why it is vital to get the child's own account when the parent is not present. All clinicians and researchers need to have a good understanding of children's development to be able to assist them express their inner distress.

A great deal can be achieved in this first session. The therapist aims to engage the child and parents in therapy as well as assess problems for planning treatment. All too often, children are referred long after the traumatic event and will have built-up patterns of avoiding discussing the trauma. The child often feels that the reactions are out of control and so the therapist must show that the child can get control over small aspects, such as deciding whether the child or parents are interviewed first. Every opportunity is taken even at this early stage to normalize the child's reactions—not dismissing them, but getting across the message that they are frequent and well understood. The information is used to set treatment goals and the child and parents are given the rationale for trauma-focused cognitive behavioral therapy (CBT) which is outlined.

It is very rare to find a child presenting with only PTSD. Separation anxiety, depression, bereavement reactions, fears, and so on may be present. Thus, it is important that the early assessment enquires about this whole range of problems. To cut down on the time involved, the clinician can use a variety of self-completed questionnaires with children aged over 7 or 8 years of age, and parallel ones completed by their parents.

Effective social support is key to good prognosis. Mental health problems in parents can greatly interfere with the support they can give the child. This is especially true when parent and child have been in the same incident. Thus, a careful evaluation of the parents' adjustment is needed. Where the traumatic incident has involved personal violence, it is important to assess the extent of any ongoing risk to the child.

No specific physical investigations are necessary. Increasingly, there is evidence (reviewed later) that a number of peri- and posttraumatic factors influence the development and course of PTSD. It is already possible to measure children's cognitive distortions, and further diagnostic tools will become available in the near future. Thus, at an early stage of assessment it will be possible to identify key issues that will be targeted in therapy. In general, what is needed is for clinicians to obtain much better trauma histories and pay attention to the ways in which children react to the traumatic event (Greenwald, 2005).

Epidemiology

Estimates of the incidence of PTSD in trauma-exposed children vary enormously, partly as a result of differing methodologies, and partly as a result of different types of traumatic event. Studies of the mental health of child refugees from war torn countries find the incidence to be close to 67%. Sexual abuse results in high rates of PTSD (Salmon & Bryant, 2002), as does witnessing violence (Margolin & Gordis, 2000). In various studies of the effects of traffic accidents, rates of 15–30% are reported (e.g. Stallard et al., 2004). A study of 200 adolescent survivors of the sinking of the cruise ship "Jupiter" (Yule et al., 2000) reported an incidence of PTSD of 51%. Most cases manifested within the first few weeks with delayed onset being rare. Following a nightclub fire in Gothenburg, 25% of the 275 adolescent survivors met DSM-IV criteria for PTSD 18 months after the fire (Broberg et al., 2005). This appears fairly constant across developmental levels. In other words, significantly increased demands will be made at all levels of primary and secondary child and adolescent mental health services following major traumatic events.

Most epidemiological studies have been of older adolescents and adults. For example, Giaconia et al. (1995) report a lifetime prevalence of 6% in a community sample of older adolescents. More recently, Merikangas et al. (2010) report a lifetime prevalence of 5% using data collected from adolescents (up to 18 years old) in the United States National Comorbidity Survey—Adolescent Supplement. A national sample of eighth grade Danish students estimated a 9% lifetime prevalence (Elklit, 2002). By contrast, the British National Survey of Mental health of over 10,000 children and adolescents (Meltzer et al., 2003) report that only 0.4% of 11–15-year-olds were diagnosed with PTSD, with girls showing twice the rate of boys. Below age 10, it was scarcely registered. This lower rate is, of course, a point prevalence estimate and is bound to be lower than a lifetime prevalence estimate. Moreover, the screening instrument was not specifically developed to screen for PTSD. The implication is that while the numbers of children and adolescents experiencing PTSD at any one point in time may be as low as 1%, this is still a significant level of morbidity in any community.

Most teachers will hardly ever encounter a child who suffers from it. When they do, they may be ill-prepared to deal with it. In addition, professionals in primary care frequently underestimate how often PTSD does occur in children (Ehlers et al., 2009). However, it is important for all service providers and planners to remember the difference between incidence and prevalence. While the point prevalence and lifetime prevalence may appear low, the incidence following a particular disaster may overwhelm local services.

Large-scale disasters such as the attacks in New York on September 11, the London underground on July 7 and Hurricane Katrina result in many children being exposed directly and indirectly to the traumatic event. Such incidents require a different clinical response from the usual individual referral. Indeed, communities and schools should have emergency plans in place that allow quick response and appropriate care of those exposed. In turn, this argues for better screening of large numbers. Appropriate early screening does not mean that inappropriate early intervention is undertaken. Rather it permits a rational and efficient "screen and treat" approach to ensure that those most affected receive help (Brewin et al., 2010a). As Mollica et al. (2004) argued, few communities have tried and trusted procedures in place to deal with the mental health consequences of complex emergencies. Agencies such as WHO and NCPTSD have suggested ways of responding, although these have not always been evidence-based.

Longitudinal outcome

Data from numerous adult studies show that there is substantial natural recovery from PTSD in the initial months after the trauma. Many individuals recover from PTSD without treatment, and the steepest decline in rates of PTSD is usually seen in the first year. This still leaves a substantial minority—roughly a third—who are likely to develop a chronic disorder which may persist for years if left untreated (National Institute for Health and Care Excellence (NICE), 2005).

A similar picture is emerging from prospective follow-up studies of children. For example, Meiser-Stedman et al. (2005) found that among young survivors of assaults and traffic accidents, nearly one in five met criteria for acute stress disorder (ASD) 2–4 weeks after the event. When reinterviewed at 6 months posttrauma, the rate of PTSD was 12%. The question remains: What factors distinguish those children who will recover spontaneously from those who will go on to develop a chronic reaction requiring treatment?

There have been very few long-term follow-up studies of children who developed PTSD. The 5–7-year follow-up study of adolescents who survived the sinking of the cruise ship "Jupiter" found that 15% still met criteria for PTSD long after the event (Yule *et al.*, 2000).

A 33-year follow-up of the children who survived the Aberfan land-slide disaster found that 29% of those traced and interviewed still met criteria for PTSD (Morgan *et al.*, 2003). Exposure to trauma in childhood is also associated with a broad range of adverse psychiatric outcomes in adulthood. For example, in a large epidemiological study ($N = 43,000$ adults), physical abuse in childhood was associated with increased lifetime prevalence of ADHD, PTSD, bipolar disorder, panic disorder, substance abuse, generalized anxiety, and major depression after the age of 18 (Sugaya *et al.*, 2012). Similarly, Copeland *et al.* (2013) found that young adults who had been victims of bullying in childhood were at increased risk of anxiety disorders, depression, and suicidality. Childhood trauma is also associated with psychotic symptoms in adulthood (e.g. Aas *et al.*, 2011; Aresenault *et al.*, 2011; Heins *et al.*, 2011) and with conduct problems (e.g. Jaffee *et al.*, 2005). The effects of life-threatening traumatic events in childhood can be severe and very long-lasting.

Risk factors

The established finding that only a minority of trauma-exposed young people will develop a persistent PTSD has led to the search for risk factors. Findings from such research have potential for practical clinical application. For example, identification of fixed markers (such as severity of trauma exposure, or gender) may be useful in identifying children most at risk so that services can be directed to them; identification of causal risk factors (such as cognitive misappraisals) may help to define targets for therapeutic intervention.

Early studies investigated whether the severity of exposure to trauma was associated with later pathology. There is now good evidence for a significant exposure–response relationship among children exposed to single-event trauma (e.g. Pynoos *et al.*, 1987), war (e.g. Gupta *et al.*, 1996; Smith *et al.*, 2002) and mass disaster (e.g. La Greca *et al.*, 2010). In a series of large-scale studies of children exposed to hurricanes, La Greca and colleagues (2010) have shown that this relationship is not straightforward: in addition to a direct link between exposure and PTSD, exposure also predisposes to further life events and disrupts social support, which in turn influence persistent PTS symptoms. A recent meta-analysis (of 96 studies; total $N = 74,000$) of children exposed to disaster (Furr *et al.*, 2010) found a medium effect size ($r = 0.33$) of exposure severity, measured by proximity to the event, on PTS symptoms. In sum, there is a significant relationship between the "objective" level of trauma exposure and later adjustment across a broad range of trauma types. However, the strength of this relationship is generally modest.

In this context, researchers have investigated additional factors that may be associated with the development of persistent PTSD. Trickey *et al.*'s (2012) meta-analysis of risk factors provides a helpful and timely account of this rapidly growing area. Using data from $k = 64$ studies (total $N = 32,000$ children and adolescents aged 6–18 years) which included a broad range of trauma types, population effect size estimates were derived for 25 potential risk factors for PTSD. In line with two key meta-analyses of risk factors in adults (Brewin *et al.*, 2000b; Ozer *et al.*, 2003), it was found that peri- and posttraumatic factors showed larger effect sizes on persistent PTSD than pretrauma demographic factors and the severity of exposure. Specifically, fixed markers such as age, gender, and ethnicity showed negligible to small effects ($\rho = 0.03$–0.15). Objective trauma severity showed a small to medium effect ($\rho = 0.29$). Peri-traumatic variable risk factors such as fear and the perception of life threat during the event showed large effects ($\rho = 0.36$). A number of posttrauma variable risk factors also yielded large effect sizes, including cognitive factors (thought suppression, blaming others, distraction; $\rho = 0.47$–0.70); social and family factors (social withdrawal, poor family functioning; $\rho = 0.38$–0.46) and psychological factors (severity of initial PTSD symptoms and comorbid psychological problems; $\rho = 0.40$–0.64). Some caution is needed in interpreting these findings, given the relatively small number of included participants for some variables. However, in terms of clinical application, it is encouraging that the largest effects were found for variable risk factors that can in principle be targeted and modified in therapy.

For example, in line with clear predictions from cognitive models of the disorder (Ehlers and Clark, 2000), subjective appraisals appear to have a central role in maintaining PTSD in older children and adolescents. Both Furr *et al.*'s (2010) and Trickey *et al.*'s (2012) meta-analyses found perceived life threat to be at least as important as objective trauma severity in maintaining PTS symptoms. The role of subjective appraisal has been directly tested in a number of carefully designed prospective longitudinal follow-up studies of children exposed to single-event trauma such as assaults and accidents. Building on earlier work (Ehlers *et al.*, 2003; Bryant *et al.*, 2007; Meiser-Stedman *et al.*, 2007, 2009a, b; Salmon *et al.*, 2007), Nixon *et al.* (2010) recently found that the initial unhelpful appraisals of hospitalized injured children accounted for around 30% of the variance in PTS symptoms 6 months later. Misappraisals also appear important in the adjustment of children who have been repeatedly maltreated, abused or neglected (Leeson & Nixon, 2011). Cross-cultural evidence for the role of unhelpful trauma-related appraisals was also found in a very large study of the effects on children of the Wenchuan earthquake in China (Ma *et al.*, 2011). Finally, analog studies with adults using the trauma film paradigm have found that manipulating such appraisals using computerized training can ameliorate intrusive recollections (Woud *et al.*, 2012), implying that cognitive misappraisals are a causal risk factor. Indeed, an earlier randomized controlled trial (RCT) of trauma-focused cognitive behavioral therapy (TF-CBT) for young people with PTSD (Smith *et al.*, 2007) found that the effect of therapy was partially mediated by changes in unhelpful appraisals.

Family functioning and parental mental health posttrauma both show significant associations with children's PTS symptoms in a number of studies. At least 25 studies have established that poor parental mental health (depression, anxiety, and PTSD) correlates with child PTS symptoms, showing a medium effect size overall (Trickey *et al.*, 2012). In a prospective study of young attendees at an emergency department, Meiser-Stedman *et al.* (2006) found that parental depression was related to child PTS in the acute posttrauma period and 6 months later. Parental worry mediated the relationship between parental depression and child adjustment. Family functioning has been measured in various ways, for example using the Family Functioning Questionnaire, the Family Environment Scale, indices of Expressed Emotion, or *ad hoc* measures. Although there are far fewer studies of family functioning than parental mental health, initial effect size estimates are larger for family functioning than for parental mental health, and more research is needed. The mechanisms underlying these familial associations remain unclear. In part, they may derive from a complex interaction between parents and children who can become locked into cycles of not talking about the event for fear of upsetting each other. That is, carers and children may negatively reinforce each other for avoiding processing their traumatic memories, and this is likely to maintain the symptoms of both.

Social support may be highly relevant in the maintenance and resolution of PTSD (Pine & Cohen, 2002) but has been insufficiently studied in children. Trickey *et al.* (2012) estimated a medium effect size of social support on PTSD, but this was based on just four studies. La Greca *et al.* (2010) have shown in a large longitudinal study how social support may mediate the effect of trauma exposure on PTS symptoms among hurricane-exposed adolescents in the United States. McDermott *et al.* (2012) used a cross-sectional design to show that a related construct—social connectedness—was related to PTSD among children exposed to a cyclone in Australia.

Genetically informative studies of adults have established that PTSD risk is modestly heritable, but such findings have yet to be reliably replicated in children and adolescents. First, adult twin studies find evidence for some degree of heritability of risk for exposure to trauma, probably via genetic effects on personality (Stein *et al.*, 2002). Second twin studies of adults report heritability estimates of PTSD to be around 30% for males (True *et al.*, 1993), with higher estimates for females (Sartor *et al.*, 2011), and a striking degree of overlap in heritability of PTSD and depression in trauma-exposed adults (Sartor *et al.*, 2012). Third, molecular genetic studies have focused on candidate genes implicated in the dopaminergic, serotonergic, and noradrenergic systems, as well as on markers of the hypothalamic–pituitary–adrenal (HPA) axis (see Koenen *et al.* (2009) for a review). For example, a higher incidence of the short allele in the promoter region (5-HTTLPR) of the serotonin transporter gene (SLC6A4) was found in adults with PTSD compared to controls (Lee *et al.*, 2005). The same variant has been found to increase risk for PTSD when social support is low (Kilpatrick *et al.*, 2007) and is associated with poorer treatment response to trauma-focused CBT (Bryant *et al.*, 2010). Further research with children and adolescents is needed.

Pathological risk processes

Physiological processes

Trauma exposure activates a neurobiological stress response in humans. It is proposed that traumatic stress activates the locus ceruleus and the sympathetic nervous system (SNS), resulting in increased heart rate, blood pressure, metabolic rate, alertness, and circulating catecholamines (adrenaline, noradrenaline, and dopamine). The locus ceruleus also stimulates the HPA axis, resulting in release of corticotropin-releasing factor (CRF or CRH) from the hypothalamus. This stimulates the pituitary to secrete adreno-corticotropin, which in turn promotes cortisol release from the adrenal gland, further stimulating the SNS. Cortisol then supresses the HPA axis (acting via negative feedback inhibition on the hypothalamus, pituitary, and hippocampus), which leads to homeostasis. Investigation of these two major stress systems—the catecholamine system and the HPA axis—has been the focus of research with children and young people.

There is evidence for disruption to the catecholamine system in traumatized children with symptoms of PTSD. For example, after traffic accidents, children with PTSD show higher morning noradrenaline at 1 and 6 months posttrauma (Pervanidou *et al.*, 2007). Children with abuse-related PTSD also show higher 24-hour urinary adrenaline or noradrenaline (De Bellis *et al.*, 1999a, b). In line with a sensitized adrenergic response, Scheeringa *et al.* (2004) found that preschool children with PTSD showed increased heart rate in response to trauma reminders, compared to nontraumatized controls. Follow-up studies of hospitalized injured children have shown that children who go on to develop PTSD have higher heart rates at admission (Kassam-Adams *et al.*, 2005; Bryant *et al.*, 2007; de Young *et al.*, 2011).

Alteration in functioning of the HPA axis appears to differ according to time since exposure, and to whether the child has recently been exposed to further stress or trauma. In acutely traumatized children, there is evidence for hypersecretion of cortisol (e.g. Weems & Carrion, 2007), whereas young people with chronic PTSD show lower resting baseline levels of cortisol (e.g. Goenjian *et al.*, 2003), although findings are mixed (see Kirsch *et al.* (2011) for a recent review). Chronically maltreated children show a blunted cortisol reactivity to psychosocial stress (MacMillan *et al.*, 2009; Ouellet-Morin *et al.*, 2011), and lower cortisol responses are in turn associated with greater social and behavioral problems (Ouellet-Morin *et al.*, 2011). The suggestion is that compensatory downregulation of the HPA axis occurs in children with chronic PTSD, leading to an increasingly maladaptive response over time.

Consistent with disruption to the HPA axis, reductions in the volume of the hippocampus have been reported in children with

PTSD relative to nonexposed controls (Carrion *et al.*, 2010). This is consistent with convincing meta-analytic evidence for reduced hippocampal volume in adults with PTSD (Woon & Hedges, 2011). However, several studies have reported significantly larger hippocampal volume in children with PTSD (e.g. Tupler and de Bellis, 2006), and further imaging research is needed.

The neural basis of emotional processing in trauma-exposed children has been investigated using fMRI methods. McCrory *et al.* (2013) found increased right amygdala activation in response to preattentively presented emotional faces (angry and happy) among maltreated children, compared to matched controls. This enhanced neural response implies differences in very early (preconscious) processing of affect among maltreated children relative to healthy controls.

Cognitive processes and models

Cognitive models of anxiety predict attention bias toward threat among anxious individuals. Experimental investigations using the dot-probe task have generally (although not always) demonstrated attention bias toward threat in anxious children (e.g. Taghavi *et al.*, 1999; Roy *et al.*, 2008; see Chapter 60). Since hypervigilance for danger characterizes the phenomenology of PTSD, it is predicted that attention bias to threat can be demonstrated experimentally among children with PTSD. However, findings are mixed. For example, relative to healthy controls, young people with PTSD have shown attention *toward* threat (e.g. Moradi *et al.*, 1999), *away* from threat (Pine *et al.*, 2005), or no bias (Dalgleish *et al.*, 2003). A recent very large community study ($N = 1774$; Salum *et al.*, 2013) found attention bias toward threat in young people with high internalizing symptoms (including PTSD), alongside bias away from threat in young people with phobic disorders. Interpretation of discrepant findings is limited by sampling and methodological differences between studies (Dalgleish *et al.*, 2005), and further work is needed to investigate attentional vigilance and avoidance in PTSD (Schechter *et al.*, 2012).

Higher order cognitive processes including memory and appraisals are fundamental to cognitive models of PTSD. Under Ehlers and Clark's (2000) cognitive model, persistent PTSD is maintained by the disjointed nature of the trauma memory; misappraisals of the trauma and its sequelae and maladaptive coping strategies. The applicability to children of cognitive models of PTSD has been tested in a series of carefully designed prospective studies. There is now considerable evidence from independent research groups that the initial unhelpful appraisals of trauma-exposed children account for substantial variance in PTSD symptoms 6 months later (see page above). As predicted by cognitive models, the particular characteristics of trauma memories—specifically their degree of disorganization—have recently been found to distinguish trauma-exposed children with ASD from those without ASD (Salmond *et al.*, 2011). Consistent with cognitive models, unhelpful coping strategies (such as thought suppression, rumination, cognitive avoidance) are strongly related to PTSD symptom severity in both

cross-sectional and longitudinal studies (e.g. Meiser-Stedman *et al.*, 2005; Stallard and Smith, 2007). This has clear implications for treatment (see page below).

Brewin and colleagues' (Brewin *et al.*, 1996; Brewin, 2001) dual representation theory of PTSD proposes that there are two types of trauma memory, stored in different representational formats: verbally accessible memory (VAM) supports ordinary autobiographical memories; situationally accessible memory (SAM) supports specific trauma-related dreams and flashbacks. An update to this structural model (Brewin *et al.*, 2010b) describes a contextual memory system and a sensory memory system, and specifies how each system has a distinct neural basis. Recent fMRI work with adults has supported the prediction from dual representational theory that VAMs are associated with activity in the dorsal visual stream rather than the medial temporal lobe (Whalley *et al.*, 2013), but this remains untested with children and young people.

Treatment

There is an increasing number of RCTs of treatments for PTSD (or subthreshold posttraumatic stress symptoms) in children and adolescents. A number of expert reviews and systematic reviews summarize this published evidence (Feeny *et al.*, 2004; Stallard, 2006; Silverman *et al.*, 2008; Gillies *et al.*, 2012; Forman-Hoffman *et al.*, 2013). Recent professional guidelines also utilize the RCT evidence and provide expert clinical consensus when trial evidence is lacking (American Academy of Child and Adolescent Psychiatry, 2010; NICE, 2005). All published international guidelines and reviews recommend trauma-focused cognitive behavioral therapy (TF-CBT) for children and young people with PTSD. Other treatments are available but none is as thoroughly evaluated as TF-CBT. An overview of the current evidence base is provided below.

Early interventions

While prevention is seen as better than cure, in respect of PTSD this has to be seen as preventing the occurrence of traumatic events or children's exposure to them. Early intervention would be attractive if it could be shown that it prevented later development of PTSD or other disorders. Critical incident stress debriefing was originally developed by Mitchell (1983) to prevent traumatic stress reactions in fire-fighters. These were people who worked and trained together, and use was made of the dynamics and support of the existing group. At some point, other professionals extended debriefing to civilian survivors of traumatic incidents, and also to children. Thus, a single, one-off intervention subsumed under the heading "debriefing" was born. However, subsequent studies with trauma-exposed adults generally found that debriefing is not very effective in preventing later PTSD, although the survivors appreciated being offered help. Several RCTs of single-session debriefing, delivered universally to all trauma-exposed children and young people, have now been carried out (Stallard & Salter, 2003; Stallard *et al.*, 2006; Kenardy *et al.*, 2008; Zehnder *et al.*, 2010). None of them has demonstrated that debriefing prevents PTSD. There is evidence from work with trauma-exposed adults that debriefing may be harmful in that it slows down natural recovery (Mayou *et al.*, 2000). While there is no evidence that debriefing is harmful to children, it is now widely agreed that such one-off, brief, individually administered interventions do not help reduce later PTSD.

Given the lack of evidence for single-session debriefing, alternative approaches to early intervention have been trialed recently. Rather than single-session intervention for everyone exposed to trauma, multiple-session early interventions for symptomatic children have been tested using a "screen and intervene" model. For example, Kassam-Adams *et al.* (2011) report that a screen-and-intervene approach was feasible to implement within a pediatric hospital setting. Berkowitz *et al.* (2011) report positive RCT findings for an early intervention screen-and-intervene approach for children (7–17 years old) exposed to a variety of traumatic events. A four-session intervention, the Child and Family Traumatic Stress Intervention (CFTSI), was flexibly delivered to parents and symptomatic children in the first 2 months posttrauma, and included psychoeducation, techniques to improve family communication and behavioral and cognitive skills teaching (coping enhancement). Postintervention, and at 6-month follow-up, there were significant and meaningful improvements in PTSD among those in the CFTSI group.

These studies show that although universal single-session early interventions have not been helpful, screen-and-intervene approaches appear feasible and promising. In reality, it often takes several weeks to implement an early intervention program. That is not to say that one should do nothing in the first few days posttrauma. Parents and teachers need better guidance on what to say to children early on, and how to say it, so that any normal healing processes are not compromised. The WHO Inter Agency Standing Committee (2007) and the US National Child Traumatic Stress Network (Brymer *et al.*, 2006) have issued guidance for "Psychological First Aid." Both emphasize the need for good social support to child survivors and families in the first few weeks, although these interventions have yet to be empirically tested (Yule, 2008).

Trauma-focused CBT (TF-CBT) for persistent PTSD

Systematic reviews of interventions for children with PTSD are in good agreement that, as with adults, TF-CBT is currently the best supported treatment. Components of TF-CBT include psycho education about PTSD, developing a trauma narrative, identifying and updating problematic meanings and missappraisals, dropping unhelpful cognitive, and behavioral avoidance, *in vivo* exposure to reminders, behavioral activation, arousal management (e.g. learning relaxation skills) and work with parents.

PTSD and single-event traumas

To date, a small number of randomized controlled trials of psychological interventions with children who developed PTSD symptoms as a result of single-event traumas have been reported (Chemtob *et al.*, 2002; Stein *et al.*, 2002; Smith *et al.*, 2007; Gilboa-Schechtman *et al.*, 2010; Nixon *et al.*, 2012).

Group-based CBT in schools has been shown to be effective. After Hurricane Iniki hit Hawaii, all elementary school children were screened for serious stress reactions and the high-risk group of 248 children were randomly assigned to one of three treatments (Chemtob *et al.*, 2002). This consisted of four sessions delivered either individually or in groups. The specially developed, manualized treatment had many elements in common with other CBT approaches. Both individual and group treatment had equally good results but more children dropped out of individual than group treatment. Stein *et al.* (2002) report an RCT in which 61 children who had been exposed to violence were given 10 sessions of group CBT and compared with 65 children who were allocated to a delayed intervention condition. At 3 months posttreatment, the treated group had significantly lower scores on the Child PTSD Symptom Scale (CPSS) (Foa *et al.*, 2000). Significant differences were also found on measures of depression and psychosocial dysfunction. Teacher-rated behavioral difficulties did not reflect improvement. The delayed treatment group then made significant PTSD improvement following treatment. In both these studies, children were recruited from school-based screening rather than from clinic-referred children. Not all participants had diagnoses of PTSD.

More recent RCTs have shown individual TF-CBT and Prolonged Exposure to be highly effective in treating PTSD following single-incident trauma. For example, Smith *et al.* (2007) compared TF-CBT to a Wait List comparison condition for $N = 24$ children who developed clinician-validated PTSD following assault or RTA. Treatment was adapted from Ehlers and Clark's cognitive therapy treatment protocol, based on Ehlers and Clark's (2000) model of PTSD, and included a variety of components which were aimed at reducing known maintaining factors (see above). Posttreatment, 11 of the 12 young people who received TF-CBT no longer met criteria for PTSD compared with 5 of the 12 on the wait list. Treated children also showed significant reductions in symptoms of depression and anxiety. Improvements remained at 6-month follow-up. As predicted, therapeutic gains in the TF-CBT group were partially mediated via changes in maladaptive cognitions.

Therapeutic exposure to the trauma memory is a key component of most forms of TF-CBT. Two recent RCTs have tested whether such exposure is really essential. Gilboa-Schechtman *et al.* (2010) directly compared 12–15 sessions of prolonged exposure with 15–18 sessions of psychodynamic therapy in a randomized controlled trial (RCT) for adolescents ($N = 38$). Both treatments were associated with reductions in PTSD and depression at posttreatment and at follow-up. Prolonged exposure was superior to psychodynamic therapy in reducing PTSD symptoms and depression symptoms at posttreatment and at

6-month follow-up. Of the adolescents who completed the treatment, 87% (prolonged exposure) and 47% (psychodynamic therapy) were free of PTSD diagnosis posttreatment. Results imply that exposure to the trauma memory is an important component of effective treatment.

In contrast, the RCT by Nixon et al. (2012) showed that a form of cognitive therapy which explicitly precluded exposure was highly efficacious for adolescents suffering from PTSD. Thirty-three adolescents who had developed PTSD (or sub-syndromal PTSD symptoms) after exposure to single-incident trauma such as road traffic accidents and assaults were included. One group had nine sessions of cognitive therapy (including anxiety management, cognitive restructuring, and working with parents); the other group had nine sessions of TF-CBT (including the same components as well as imaginal and *in vivo* exposure). In the cognitive therapy arm, 90% of completers ($N = 10$) and 56% of the intention-to-treat samples ($N = 16$) were diagnosis-free at posttreatment. In the CBT arm, 91% of completers ($N = 11$) and 65% of the intention-to-treat samples ($N = 17$) were diagnosis free at posttreatment. Differences between cognitive therapy and TF-CBT were not significant. Results of this RCT imply that exposure to the trauma memory through imaginal reliving is not necessary for therapeutic effect, and that techniques of modifying trauma-related misappraisals and dysfunctional beliefs may be equally effective. An earlier study (Smith et al., 2007) found that changes in trauma-related misappraisals mediated the effect of TF-CBT (relative to a waiting list control condition) on PTSD symptoms. The relative contribution of exposure techniques and cognitive techniques to symptom reduction is not yet clear, but it may be that their careful integration is important to successful outcome. Although TF-CBT is a powerful treatment, further investigations of mediators and moderators will help to refine and enhance future protocols.

Thus, TF-CBT has been found effective for treating stress reactions after single-incident traumas. Moreover, it has been shown that it improves anxiety and depression as well. The effects appear to last and it seems to be effective when delivered in groups as well as individually. However, as Forman-Hoffman et al. (2013) point out in their comparative effectiveness review, the evidence remains small, sample sizes in published RCTs are small to modest and further work is needed.

Trauma-focused-CBT with preschool children
TF-CBT has been successfully adapted to help young, 3-to-6-year-old children, suffering PTSD (Scheeringa et al., 2011). Adaptions include greater parental involvement, more emphasis on behavioral management training and relaxation techniques, use of visual aids (e.g. cartoons for psych-education), and imaginative use of drawing and playing to complete imaginal reliving. Scheeringa et al. (2011) undertook a randomized trial with 64 children given either a 12-session manualized TF-CBT or placed on a waiting list for 12 weeks. Interestingly, TF-CBT reduced

PTSD with large effect size, but did not immediately reduce depression, separation anxiety, or oppositional disorders. These were found to improve after the waiting group received treatment and the gains on PTSD increased at 6-month follow-up. Thus therapy based on TF-CBT principles, suitably adapted to young children's development, is feasible to deliver and appears effective with preschool children.

PTSD and child sexual abuse
In recent years, many of the reactions children develop to sexual abuse have been formulated as part of a spectrum of post-traumatic stress reactions (see Chapter 30). This has resulted in a number of therapeutic trials of CBT to treat these reactions, including full PTSD. Most published RCTs of TF-CBT report outcomes for children traumatized by sexual abuse. For example, of 21 studies included in Silverman et al.'s (2008) review of evidence-based psychosocial treatment, 11 were concerned with sexual abuse. TF-CBT is now a well-established treatment for PTSD that has arisen following sexual abuse (Silverman et al., 2008).

Ramchandani and Jones (2003) report a systematic review of RCTs treating a range of psychological symptoms in sexually abused children. They identified 12 RCTs—3 investigating Group CBT; 6 investigating individual CBT; 1 of adding group therapy to a family therapy intervention; and 2 comparing individual (non-CBT) therapy with group therapy. The dependent (outcome) measures were very varied, and only four studies looked at recognized, specific measures of PTSD. Nevertheless, TF-CBT was recommended as the treatment of choice for PTSD in sexually abused children.

In the largest study to date, Cohen et al. (2004) carried out a multisite RCT of TF-CBT compared to child-centered therapy for symptoms of PTSD and other problems in $N = 229$ sexually abused children (8–14 years old). TF-CBT was associated with significant and clinically meaningful improvements in PTSD symptoms, as well as depression, anxiety, and externalizing problems. Treatment gains were maintained at 6- and 12-month follow-up. These findings were in line with previous RCTs from Cohen's group and others (Cohen & Mannarino, 1996, 1997, 1998; Deblinger et al., 1996, 2001, 1997; King et al., 2000), which provide convincing evidence of the efficacy of TF-CBT across a variety of settings.

The relative importance of exposure-based therapy components was investigated recently by Deblinger et al. (2011) in an evaluation of TF-CBT for children who developed PTSD symptoms following sexual abuse. They tested directly whether the development of a trauma narrative was necessary for symptom reduction. About 210 children (4–11 years old) and their parents were randomized to one of four conditions: eight sessions with or without a trauma narrative component, or 16 sessions with or without a trauma narrative. Consistent with their earlier studies, they report a large effect for TF-CBT across all treatment conditions (effect size across all outcome measures and all treatment arms, $d = 0.94$) However, children allocated to the conditions that included a trauma narrative component reported less fear associated with thinking or talking about the abuse, and less general anxiety, compared with children in the conditions that did not include a trauma narrative component. Many of the children in the trauma narrative conditions reported that talking about the abuse specifically was the most important part of therapy. In contrast, parents assigned to the 16-session, no trauma narrative condition reported greater increases in effective parenting practices and fewer externalizing child behavioral problems. This study is therefore an important step toward the delivery of psychological therapies that are tailored toward young children's specific profile of posttrauma difficulties.

Mannarino *et al.* (2012) reported 6- and 12-month follow-up of 158 children (4–11 years) treated by TF-CBT after child sexual abuse. The study contrasted a variant of their version of TF-CBT with or without a module on trauma narrative. It was found that the initial gains in both groups were maintained. Initial higher levels of internalizing and depressive symptoms predicted those whose PTSD did not improve.

The immediate and long-term psychological effects of childhood sexual abuse are many, varied and serious (see Chapter 30). The studies reviewed by Ramchandani and Jones (2003), and Silverman *et al.* (2008) strongly indicate that TF-CBT is currently the treatment of choice, although there is clearly a great need for further RCTs. As Feeny *et al.* (2004) note, child survivors of sexual abuse may present a different symptom picture to that of children exposed to single-incident traumas and so generalization of findings to those may be problematic (see also American Academy of Child and Adolescent Psychiatry, 2010).

Other approaches to treatment

Eye movement desensitization and reprocessing (EMDR)

Eye movement desensitization and reprocessing (EMDR) was discovered by chance by Shapiro (2001) and has been applied with good results with adults (NICE, 2005). EMDR is an empirical treatment with little theoretical underpinning. The detailed protocols for treatment include a careful history and ensuring that the patient can have a break if the intrusions during treatment prove too frightening. Essentially, the child is asked to focus on a traumatic memory while simultaneously following the moving fingers of the therapist. This "dual attention" task is thought to help the child confront the frightening memory and so "process" the emotional reaction to that memory. There is some controversy about the active components of treatment in EMDR. For example, dismantling studies (e.g. Pitman *et al.*, 1996) have not provided evidence for a cardinal role for saccadic eye movements. The overlap between treatment components of CBT and EMDR (e.g. therapeutic exposure) have led some to suggest that the mechanisms of change may be broadly similar in both approaches.

Two case series illustrate the use of EMDR with children. Hensel (2009) reported a consecutive series of 36 children aged 1 year 9 months to 18 years. About 32 received an average of three EMDR sessions and reduction in distress both immediately after treatment and at follow-up. Ribchester *et al.* (2010) used EMDR with 11 children who developed PTSD after road traffic accidents. None met criteria for PTSD on standardized assessments after an average of only 2.4 sessions. Significant improvements in PTSD, anxiety, and depression were found both immediately after treatment and at follow-up. Treatment was associated with a significant trauma-specific reduction in attentional bias on the modified Stroop task, with results apparent both immediately after therapy and at follow-up. This case series suggests that EMDR may produce reductions in attentional bias and so indicates ways of tapping the processes behind the change in posttraumatic stress.

DeRoos *et al.* (2004) reported an RCT involving 52 children following the 2000 Enschede (Netherlands) fireworks disaster. Both EMDR and CBT produced significant lowering of stress symptoms, with EMDR doing slightly better in fewer sessions. Ahmad *et al.* (2007) similarly reported significantly lower stress scores after EMDR, relative to wait list in an RCT involving 33 children diagnosed with PTSD. Kemp *et al.* (2010) report a pilot RCT involving 13 children receiving four sessions of EMDR compared with 14 children on a 6-week wait list control. EMDR was significantly better than the comparison condition, and treatment gains were maintained at 12-month follow-up.

While the NICE (2005) report found good evidence from RCTs with adults to be able to make a firm recommendation that it be available to patients in the UK NHS, the evidence base with children remains less robust. Even despite the lack of theoretical basis for EMDR, it appears that it can work very quickly and so should be considered as a possible treatment for children.

Narrative exposure therapy (NET)

Arising in part from South American methods of helping victims of torture and in part from a thoroughgoing analysis of the neurobiology of autobiographical memory and ways of completing fragmented memories, Schauer *et al.* (2004) have developed Narrative Exposure Therapy and used it in RCTs with adult refugees in the Sudan (Neuner *et al.*, 2004). It has now been evaluated as a treatment for PTSD in war-affected children in Sri Lanka (Onyut *et al.*, 2005; Schauer *et al.*, 2005; Neuner *et al.*, 2006), child soldiers in Uganda (Ertl *et al.*, 2011) and for refugee children who settled in Germany (Ruf *et al.*, 2010). NET is associated in these RCTs with significant improvements in PTSD symptoms and functioning, relative to wait list controls and active comparison conditions. The technique has the advantage that children who have experienced multiple trauma can discuss memories of all of them. The disadvantage is that as the intervention is at present only given individually, it is difficult to reach many of the child survivors of conflicts. To date, there are no published RCTs other than those undertaken by the developers of the model.

Structured writing

Pennebaker (1995) has long demonstrated that writing about emotional events in structured ways can have very positive effects. Typically, participants are asked to write about their emotions for brief periods, usually 3–6 times for 15 min on each occasion (see review by Frattaroli (2006) of 146 emotional disclosure studies). Van der Oord *et al.* (2010) included a structured writing component within a broader treatment approach. Children typed their story into a computer (or were helped to do so). A case series of 23 children (8–18 years) received an average of 5.5 sessions of cognitive behavioral writing therapy (CBWT) and showed significant reductions in stress reactions at 6-month follow-up, indicating that CBWT is a promising technique.

Kalantari *et al.* (2012) used the Children and War Foundation's Writing for Recovery manual in an RCT of 61 bereaved Afghani adolescents. They followed the structured emotional writing protocol for six sessions of 15 min each. The treated group showed a highly significant drop in scores on the Child Traumatic Grief Inventory, indicating that this promises to be an effective group intervention for bereaved children and adolescents after disasters.

Medication

Despite the paucity of proper trials on children by pharmaceutical companies in developing psychotropic drugs, many children are indeed prescribed such medication (often by general practitioners rather than child specialists) following traumas. Given the recent disclosures that trials of selective serotonin reuptake inhibitors (SSRIs) increased the risk of self-harm in depressed adolescents, one's confidence in the use of medication with children is not great. Indeed, the NICE (2005) Guideline Development Group found no study that met its stringent criteria. Medication is not recommended as a treatment for PTSD in children in the United Kingdom (NICE, 2005). Guidelines from the American Association for Child and Adolescent Psychiatry (AACAP, 2010) recommend that SSRIs, and other medications may be considered in the treatment of PTSD.

Contingency planning/school-based interventions after mass incidents

When trauma affects a large number of children at once, as in an accident at school, then a public health approach to dealing with the emergency is required (Pynoos *et al.*, 1995). Schools need to plan ahead not only to deal with large-scale disasters, but also to respond to the needs of children after threatening incidents that affect only a few of them. There are now a number of texts written especially for schools to help them develop contingency plans to deal with the effects of a disaster (Johnson, 1993; Klingman, 1993; Yule & Gold, 1993).

There is a small but growing literature suggesting that TF-CBT can be effective when delivered by education professionals in schools, or by community-based clinicians for patients referred via standard clinical pathways. For example, in the aftermath of Hurricane Katrina, Jaycox *et al.* (2010) screened nearly 700 schoolchildren and identified 195 with elevated symptoms of PTSD. These children were then invited either to participate in a school-based group CBT program or to attend a local mental health clinic and receive TF-CBT. While both treatments were effective in reducing PTSD symptoms, TF-CBT showed marginally better outcomes. However, there was a high dropout rate and no intention to treat analysis was reported. Importantly, 98% of the children who were offered the school-based program accepted treatment, and 91% completed treatment. In contrast, only 37% of children offered TF-CBT at the clinic started treatment, and only 9% completed. Thus, treatment location as opposed to treatment type appeared to have a large influence on treatment uptake, and some families asked for the TF-CBT to be delivered at the school. School-based treatment may be more convenient and/or less stigmatizing for some families.

Most developed countries have well-established plans to deal with major civil emergencies. Increasingly, these include a psychosocial or mental health component and it is advisable for child and adolescent mental health services to be involved in the planning (Canterbury & Yule, 1999). UN agencies are increasingly prepared to meet the mental health needs of children after war and major disasters (Machel, 2001) and again mental health services need to collaborate with other agencies to meet such needs. In considering the need to plan for "Mental Health in Complex Emergencies," Mollica *et al.* (2004) argued that all countries should develop plans to meet mental health sequelae of disasters. Since most disasters occur in developing countries, it is vital that appropriate assessment and intervention tools are developed that are culturally appropriate. It is also essential that such interventions are properly evaluated. Research is essential, not a luxury and that message needs to be accepted by nongovernmental organizations (NGOs) responding to disasters. Given that disasters happen with great frequency, then by planning ahead, proper consideration can be given to the ethical aspects of intervening soon after a crisis. Unless one does evaluate early interventions responsibly, significant resources are wasted and survivors suffer unnecessarily.

The Children and War Foundation has developed measures that can be used in large-scale emergencies as well as manuals for helping groups of children (Yule *et al.*, 2013). Case series and RCTs demonstrate that the Teaching Recovery Techniques manual produces significant decline in stress reactions. Notably, Barron *et al.* (2012) and Quota *et al.* (2012) both worked with traumatized children in Palestine and produced worthwhile improvements, despite the ongoing nature of the war there.

The World Health Organization and the Inter Agency Standing Committee (IASC) have produced guidance on how and when to intervene after disasters. These have achieved considerable agreement across many NGOs, but interrater agreement is not the same as validity and much more evidence is required before such guidelines can be accepted at face value (Yule, 2008). Fortunately, there are now a number of reviews that indicate empirical approaches to developing better interventions after wars and disasters (see, for example, Peltonen & Punamaki, 2010; Betancourt, 2011; Panter-Brick *et al.*, 2011; Tol *et al.*, 2011; Jordans *et al.*, 2011). Together, these initiatives should result in a fundamental rethink on how countries respond to children affected by wars and disasters and so result in much less distress.

Conclusions and recommendations

Considerable progress has been made in the past 25 years in understanding the nature of posttraumatic stress reactions in young people. There are now a number of empirically validated interventions both for individuals and groups. Cognitive models are proving a fertile source for understanding the mechanisms that give rise to serious and chronic reactions. It is better realized that whereas the point prevalence of full PTSD may be relatively small in child populations, the incidence following particular traumatic events can be so high as to overwhelm local mental health resources.

More recently, there has been greater emphasis on understanding stress reactions in young children, but much remains to be done. There is a paucity of well-designed studies of stress reactions in children and as the long-term consequences are better understood, the need for greater investment in research in this area is all too apparent.

References

Aas, M. *et al.* (2011) Childhood trauma and cognitive function in first-episode affective and non-affective psychosis. *Schizophrenia Research* **129**, 12–19.

Ahmad, A. *et al.* (2007) EMDR treatment for children with PTSD: results of a randomized controlled trial. *Nordic Journal of Psychiatry* **61**, 349–354.

American Psychiatric Association (1987) *Diagnostic and Statistical Manual of Mental Disorders (Third Edition Revised).* American Psychiatric Association, Washington, DC.

Arroyo, W. (1997) Central American children. In: *Transcultural Child Development: Psychological Assessment and Treatment.* (eds G. Johnson-Powell, J. Yamamoto, G. Wyatt & W. Arroyo), pp. 80–91. John Wiley & Sons, USA.

Arseneault, L. *et al.* (2011) Childhood trauma and children's emerging psychotic symptoms: a genetically sensitive longitudinal cohort study. *American Journal of Psychiatry* **168**, 65–72.

Barron, I. *et al.* (2012) Randomized control trial of a CBT trauma recovery program in Palestinian schools. *Journal of Loss and Trauma* **18**, 306–321.

Berkowitz, S. *et al.* (2011) The Child and Family Traumatic Stress Intervention: secondary prevention for youth at risk of developing PTSD. *Journal of Child Psychology and Psychiatry* **52**, 676–685.

Betancourt, T.S. (2011) Attending to the mental health of war-affected children: the need for longitudinal and developmental research perspectives. *Journal of the American Academy of Child and Adolescent Psychiatry* **50**, 323–325.

Bolton, P. (2001) Cross-cultural validity and reliability testing of a standard psychiatric assessment instrument without a gold standard. *Journal of Nervous and Mental Disease* **189**, 238–242.

Bolton, D. *et al.* (2000) The long-term psychological effects of a disaster experienced in adolescence: II: general psychopathology. *Journal of Child Psychology and Psychiatry* **41**, 513–523.

Brewin, C.R. (2001) A cognitive neuroscience account of posttraumatic stress disorder and its treatment. *Behaviour Research and Therapy* **39**, 373–393.

Brewin, C.R. *et al.* (1996) A dual representation theory of post-traumatic stress disorder. *Psychological Review* **103**, 670–686.

Brewin, C. *et al.* (2000) Meta-analysis of risk factors for posttraumatic stress disorder in trauma exposed adults. *Journal of Consulting and Clinical Psychology* **68**, 748–766.

Brewin, C.R. *et al.* (2010a) Outreach and screening following the 2005 London bombings: usage and outcomes. *Psychological Medicine* **40**, 2049–2057.

Brewin, C.R. *et al.* (2010b) Intrusive images in psychological disorders: characteristics, neural mechanisms, and treatment implications. *Psychological Review* **117**, 210–232.

Broberg, A. *et al.* (2005) The Goteborg discotheque fire: posttraumatic stress, and school adjustment as reported by the primary victims 18 months later. *Journal of Child Psychology and Psychiatry* **46**, 1279–1286.

Bryant, R. *et al.* (2007) A prospective study of appraisals in childhood posttraumatic stress disorder. *Behaviour Research and Therapy* **45**, 2502–2507.

Bryant, R. *et al.* (2010) Preliminary evidence of the short allele of the serotonin transporter gene predicting poor response to cognitive behavior therapy in posttraumatic stress disorder. *Biological Psychiatry* **67**, 1217–1219.

Brymer, M., *et al.* (National Child Traumatic Stress Network and National Center for PTSD), *Psychological First Aid: Field Operations Guide: 2nd Edition,* July 2006. Available on www.nctsn.org and www.ncptsd.va.gov.

Canterbury, R. & Yule, W. (1999) Debriefing and crisis intervention, Chapter 11 in Yule, W. In: *Post Traumatic Stress Disorder,* pp. 221–238. John Wiley & Sons, Chichester.

Carrion, V. *et al.* (2010) Reduced hippocampal activity in youth with posttraumatic stress symptoms: an fMRI study. *Journal of Pediatric Psychology* **35**, 559–569.

Chemtob, C.M. *et al.* (2002) Psychosocial intervention for postdisaster trauma symptoms in elementary school children: a controlled community field study. *Archives of Pediatrics and Adolescent Medicine* **156**, 211–216.

Cohen, J.A. & Mannarino, A.P. (1996) A treatment outcome study for sexually abused preschool children: initial findings. *Journal of the American Academy of Child and Adolescent Psychiatry* **34**, 42–50.

Cohen, J.A. & Mannarino, A.P. (1997) A treatment study for sexually abused preschool children: outcome during a one-year follow-up. *Journal of the American Academy of Child and Adolescent Psychiatry* **36**, 1228–1235.

Cohen, J.A. & Mannarino, A.P. (1998) Interventions for sexually abused children: initial treatment outcome findings. *Child Maltreatment* **3**, 17–26.

Cohen, J.A. *et al.* (2004) A multisite, randomized controlled trial for children with sexual abuse-related PTSD symptoms. *Journal of American Academy of Child and Adolescent Psychiatry* **43**, 393–402.

Copeland, W.E. *et al.* (2007) Traumatic events and posttraumatic stress disorder in childhood. *Archives of General Psychiatry* **64**, 577–584.

Copeland, W. *et al.* (2013) Adult psychiatric outcomes of bullying and being bullied by peers in childhood and adolescence. *JAMA Psychiatry* **70**, 419–426.

Costello, E.J. *et al.* (2002) The prevalence of potentially traumatic events in childhood and adolescence. *Journal of Traumatic Stress* **15**, 99–12.

Dalgleish, T. *et al.* (2003) Patterns of processing bias for emotional information across clinical disorders: a comparison of attention, memory, and prospective cognition in children and adolescents with depression, generalized anxiety, and PTSD. *Journal of Clinical Child and Adolescent Psychology* **32**, 10–21.

Dalgleish, T. *et al.* (2005) Cognitive aspects of posttraumatic stress reactions and their treatment in children and adolescents: an empirical review and some recommendations. *Behavioural and Cognitive Psychotherapy* **33**, 459–486.

De Bellis, M.D. *et al* (1999a) Developmental traumatology part 1: biological stress systems. *Biological Psychiatry* **45**, 1259–1270.

De Bellis, M.D. *et al.* (1999b) Developmental traumatology part 2: brain development. *Biological Psychiatry* **45**, 1271–1284.

Deblinger, E. *et al.* (1996) Sexually abused children suffering posttraumatic stress symptoms: initial treatment outcome findings. *Child Maltreatment* **1**, 310–321.

Deblinger, E. *et al.* (2001) Comparative efficacies of supportive and cognitive behavioral group therapies for young children who have been sexually abused and their nonoffending mothers. *Child Maltreatment: Journal of the American Professional Society on the Abuse of Children* **6**, 332–343.

Deblinger, E. *et al.* (2011) Trauma-focused cognitive behavioural therapy for children: impact of trauma narrative and treatment length. *Depression and Anxiety* **28**, 67–75.

Dyregrov, A. (2004) Educational consequences of loss and trauma. *Educational and Child Psychology* **21**, 77–84.

Dyregrov, A. *et al.* (1996) Factor analysis of the Impact of Event Scale with children in war. *Scandinavian Journal of Psychology* **37**, 339–350.

Ehlers, A. & Clark, D.M. (2000) A cognitive model of posttraumatic stress disorder. *Behaviour Research and Therapy* **38**, 319–345.

Ehlers, A. *et al.* (2003) Cognitive predictors of posttraumatic stress disorder in children: results of a prospective longitudinal study. *Behaviour Research and Therapy* **41**, 1–10.

Ehlers, A. *et al.* (2009) Low recognition of posttraumatic stress disorder in primary care. *London Journal of Primary Care* **2**, 36–42.

Elklit, A. (2002) Victimization and PTSD in a Danish national youth probability sample. *Journal of the American Academy of Child & Adolescent Psychiatry* **41**, 174–181.

Ertl, V. *et al.* (2011) Community-implemented trauma therapy of former child soldiers in Northern Uganda. A randomized controlled trial. *JAMA* **306**, 503–512.

Feeny, N.C. *et al.* (2004) Posttraumatic stress disorder in youth: a critical review of the cognitive and behavioral treatment outcome literature. *Professional Psychology: Research and Practice* **35**, 466–476.

Foa, E.B. *et al.* (1989) Behavioral/cognitive conceptualizations of post-traumatic stress disorder. *Behavior Therapy* **20**, 155–176.

Foa, E.B. *et al.* (2000) The child PTSD symptom scale: a preliminary examination of its psychometric properties. *Journal of Clinical Child Psychology* **30**, 376–384.

Forman-Hoffman, V. *et al.* (2013) Comparative effectiveness of interventions for children exposed to nonrelational traumatic events. *Pediatrics* **131**, 526–539.

Frattaroli, J. (2006) Experimental disclosure and its moderators: a meta analysis. *Psychological Bulletin* **132**, 823–865.

Furr, J. *et al.* (2010) Disasters and youth: a meta-analytic examination of posttraumatic stress. *Journal of Consulting and Clinical Psychology* **78**, 765–780.

Giaconia, R.M. *et al.* (1995) Traumas and posttraumatic stress disorder in a community population of older adolescents. *Journal of the American Academy of Child and Adolescent Psychiatry* **34**, 1369–1380.

Giannopoulou, I. *et al.* (2005) Post-traumatic stress reactions of children and adolescents exposed to the Athens 1999 earthquake. *European Psychiatry* **21**, 160–166.

Gilboa-Schechtman, E. *et al.* (2010) Prolonged exposure versus dynamic therapy for adolescent ptsd: a pilot randomized controlled trial. *Journal of The American Academy of Child and Adolescent Psychiatry* **49**, 1034–1042.

Gillies, D. *et al.* (2012) Psychological therapies for the treatment of post-traumatic stress disorder in children and adolescents. *Cochrane Database of Systematic Reviews*, CD006726.

Goenjian, A. *et al.* (2003) Hypothalamic-pituitary-adrenal activity among Armenian adolescents with PTSD symptoms. *Journal of Traumatic Stress* **16**, 319–323.

Greenwald, R. (2005) *Child Trauma Handbook: A Guide for Helping Trauma-Exposed Adolescents.* Haworth Press, New York.

Gupta, L., *et al.* (1996). *Trauma, exposure, and psychological reactions to genocide among Rwandan refugees.* Paper presented at the 12th Annual Convention of the International Society for Traumatic Stress Studies (November), San Fancisco, CA.

Heins, M. *et al.* (2011) Childhood trauma and psychosis: a case-control and case-sibling comparison across different levels of genetic liability, psychopathology, and type of trauma. *American Journal of Psychiatry* **168**, 1286–1294.

Hensel, T. (2009) EMDR with children and adolescents after single-incident trauma. *Journal of EMDR Practice and Research* **3**, 2–9.

Inter Agency Standing Committee (2007) *IASC Guidelines on Mental Health and Psycho-Social Support in Emergency Settings.* IASC, Geneva.

Jaffee, S. *et al.* (2005) Nature x nurture: genetic vulnerabilities interact with physical maltreatment to promote conduct problems. *Development and Psychopathology* **17**, 67–84.

Janoff-Bulman, R. (1985) The aftermath of victimization: rebuilding shattered assumptions. In: *Trauma and its Wake.* (ed C.R. Figley). Brunner/Mazel, New York.

Jaycox, L.H. *et al.* (2010) Children's mental health following Hurricane Katrina: a field trial of trauma-focused psychotherapies. *Journal of Traumatic Stress* **23**, 223–231.

Johnson, K. (1993) *School Crisis Management: A Team Training Guide.* Hunter House, Alameda, CA.

Jones, J.C. & Barlow, D.H. (1992) A new model of posttraumatic stress disorder. In: *Posttraumatic Stress Disorder: A Behavioral Approach to Assessment and Treatment.* (ed P.A. Saigh), pp. 147–165. Macmillan, New York.

Jordans, M.J.D. *et al.* (2011) Mental health interventions for children in adversity: pilot-testing a research strategy for treatment selection in low-income countries. *Social Science and Medicine* **73**, 456–466.

Kalantari, M. *et al.* (2012) Efficacy of writing for recovery on traumatic grief symptoms of Afghani refugee bereaved adolescents. *Omega* **65**, 139–150.

Kassam-Adams, N. *et al.* (2005) Heart rate and posttraumatic stress in injured children. *Archives of General Psychiatry* **62**, 335–340.

Kassam-Adams, N. *et al.* (2011) A pilot randomized controlled trial assessing secondary prevention of traumatic stress integrated into pediatric trauma care. *Journal of Traumatic Stress* **24**, 252–259.

Kemp, M. *et al.* (2010) A wait-list controlled pilot study of eye movement desensitization and reprocessing (EMDR) for children with post-traumatic stress disorder (PTSD) symptoms from motor vehicle accidents. *Clinical Child Psychology and Psychiatry* **15**, 5–25.

Kenardy, J. *et al.* (2008) Information provision intervention for children and their parents following pediatric accidental injury. *European Child & Adolescent Psychiatry* **175**, 316–325.

Kessler, R.C. *et al.* (1995) Post-traumatic stress disorder in the National Comorbidity Survey. *Archives of General Psychiatry* **52**, 1048–1060.

Kilpatrick, D. *et al.* (2007) The serotonin transporter genotype and social support and moderation of posttraumatic stress disorder and depression in hurricane-exposed adults. *American Journal of Psychiatry* **164**, 1693–1699.

King, N.J. *et al.* (2000) Treating sexually abused children with post-traumatic stress symptoms: a randomized clinical trial. *Journal of the American Academy of Child and Adolescent Psychiatry* **39**, 1347–1355.

Kirsch, V. *et al.* (2011) Psychophysiological characteristics of PTSD in children and adolescents: a review of the literature. *Journal of Traumatic Stress* **24**, 146–154.

Klingman, A. (1993) School-based intervention following a disaster, Chapter 10. In: *Children and Disasters.* (ed C.F. Saylor), pp. 187–210. Plenum, New York.

Koenen, K. *et al.* (2009) Gene-environment interaction in posttraumatic stress disorder: an update. *Journal of Traumatic Stress* **22**, 416–426.

La Greca, A.M. *et al.* (2010) Hurricane related exposure experiences and stressors, other life events, and social support: concurrent and prospective impact on children's persistent posttraumatic stress symptoms. *Journal of Consulting and Clinical Psychology* **78**, 794–805.

Lee, H. *et al.* (2005) Influence of the serotonin transporter promoter gene polymorphism on susceptibility to posttraumatic stress disorder. *Depression and Anxiety* **21**, 135–139.

Leeson, F.J. & Nixon, R.D.V. (2011) The role of children's appraisals on adjustment following psychological maltreatment: a pilot study. *Journal of Abnormal Child Psychology* **39**, 759–771.

Ma, X. *et al.* (2011) Risk indicators for posttraumatic stress disorder in adolescents exposed to the 5.12 Wenchuan earthquake in China. *Psychiatry Research* **189**, 385–391.

Machel, G. (2001) *The Impact of War on Children: A Review of Progress Since the 1996 United Nations Report on the Impact of Armed Conflict on Children.* Hurst & Co, London, UK.

MacMillan, H. *et al.* (2009) Cortisol response to stress in female youths exposed childhood maltreatment: results of the Youth Mood Project. *Biological Psychiatry* **66**, 62–68.

Mannarino, A.P. *et al.* (2012) Trauma-focused cognitive-behavioral therapy for children: sustained impact of treatment 6 and 12 months later. *Child Maltreatment* **17**, 231–241.

Margolin, G. & Gordis, E.B. (2000) The effects of family and community violence on children. *Annual Review of Psychology* **51**, 445–479.

Mayou, R.A. *et al.* (2000) A three- year follow-up of psychological debriefing for road traffic accident survivors. *British Journal of Psychiatry* **176**, 589–593.

McCrory, E. *et al.* (2013) Amygdala activation in maltreated children during pre-attentive emotional processing. *British Journal of Psychiatry* **202**, 269–276.

McDermott, B. *et al.* (2012) Social connectedness: a potential aetiological factor in the development of child posttraumatic stress disorder. *Australian and New Zealand Journal of Psychiatry* **46**, 109–117.

McFarlane, A. (2005) Psychiatric morbidity following disasters: epidemiology, risk and protective factors. In: *Disasters and Mental Health.* (eds J. Lopez-Ibor, G. Christodoulou, M. Maj, N. Sartorius & A. Okasha), pp. 37–63. John Wiley & Sons, New York.

Meiser-Stedman, R. *et al.* (2005) Acute stress disorder and posttraumatic stress disorder in children and adolescents involved in assaults or motor vehicle accidents. *American Journal of Psychiatry* **162**, 1381–1383.

Meiser-Stedman, R. *et al.* (2006) The role of the family in child and adolescent posttraumatic stress following attendance at an emergency department. *Journal of Pediatric Psychology* **31**, 397–402.

Meiser-Stedman, R. *et al.* (2007) Diagnostic, demographic, memory quality and cognitive variables associated with acute stress disorder in children and adolescents. *Journal of Abnormal Psychology* **16**, 65–79.

Meiser-Stedman, R. *et al.* (2009a) Maladaptive cognitive appraisals mediate the evolution of posttraumatic stress reactions: a 6-month follow-up of child and adolescent assault and motor vehicle accident survivors. *Journal of Abnormal Psychology* **118**, 778–787.

Meiser-Stedman, R. *et al.* (2009b) Development and validation of the Child Post-Traumatic Cognitions Inventory (CPTCI). *Journal of Child Psychology and Psychiatry* **50**, 432–440.

Meltzer, H. *et al.* (2003) Mental health of children and adolescents in Great Britain. *International Review of Psychiatry* **15**, 185–187.

Merikangas, K. *et al.* (2010) Lifetime prevalence of mental disorders in US adolescents: results from the national co-morbidity survey replication adolescent supplement (NCS-A). *Journal of the American Academy of Child and Adolescent Psychiatry* **49**, 980–989.

Mitchell, J.T. (1983) When disaster strikes … the critical incident stress debriefing. *Journal of Emergency Medical Services* **8**, 36–39.

Mollica, R.F. *et al.* (2004) Mental health in complex emergencies. *The Lancet* **364**, 2058–2067.

Moradi, A. *et al.* (1999) The performance of children and adolescents with PTSD on the Stroop colour naming task. *Psychological Medicine* **29**, 415–534.

Morgan, L. *et al.* (2003) The Aberfan disaster: 33-year follow-up of survivors. *British Journal of Psychiatry* **182**, 532–536.

National Institute for Health and Care Excellence (2005) *Post Traumatic Stress Disorder: The Management of PTSD in Adults and Children in Primary and Secondary Care (Clinical Guideline 26).* Gaskell and the British Psychological Society, London.

Neuner, F. *et al.* (2004) A comparison of narrative exposure therapy, supportive counseling, and psychoeducation for treating posttraumatic stress disorder in an African refugee settlement. *Journal of Consulting and Clinical Psychology* **72**, 579–587.

Neuner, F. *et al.* (2006) Post-tsunami stress: a study of posttraumatic stress disorder in children living in three severely affected regions in Sri Lanka. *Journal of Traumatic Stress* **19**, 339–347.

Nixon, R.D.V. *et al.* (2010) Predictors of posttraumatic stress in children following injury: the influence of appraisals, heart rate, and morphine use. *Behaviour Research and Therapy* **48**, 810–815.

Nixon, R.D.V. *et al.* (2012) A randomized trial of cognitive behaviour therapy and cognitive therapy for children with post traumatic stress disorder following single-incident trauma. *Journal of Abnormal Child Psychology* **40**, 327–337.

O'Donohue, W. & Eliot, A. (1992) The current status of post-traumatic stress disorder as a diagnostic category: problems and proposals. *Journal of Traumatic Stress* **5**, 421–439.

Onyut, L. *et al.* (2005) Narrative exposure therapy as a treatment for child war survivors with posttraumatic stress disorder: two case reports and a pilot study in an African refugee settlement. *BMC Psychiatry* **5**, 7.

Silverman, W. *et al.* (2008) Evidence-based psychosocial treatments for children and adolescents exposed to traumatic events. *Journal of Clinical Child and Adolescent Psychology* **37**, 2008, 156–183.

Ouellet-Morin, I. *et al.* (2011) A discordant monozygotic twin design shows blunted cortisol reactivity among bullied children. *Journal of the American Academy of Child & Adolescent Psychiatry* **50**, 574–582.

Ozer, E. *et al.* (2003) Predictors of posttraumatic stress disorder and symptoms in adults: a meta-analysis. *Psychological Bulletin* **129**, 52–73.

Panter-Brick, C. *et al.* (2011) Mental health and childhood adversities: a longitudinal study of Kabul, Afghanistan. *Journal of the American Academy of Child and Adolescent Psychiatry* **50**, 349–363.

Peltonen, K. & Punamaki, T.-L. (2010) Preventive interventions among children exposed to trauma of armed conflict: a literature review. *Aggressive Behavior* **36**, 95–116.

Pennebaker, J.W. (ed) (1995) *Emotion, Disclosure, and Health.* American Psychological Association, Washington, DC.

Perrin, S. *et al.* (2000) Practitioner review: the assessment and treatment of PTSD in children and adolescents. *Journal of Child Psychology & Psychiatry* **41**, 277–289.

Pervanidou, P. *et al.* (2007) The natural history of neuroendocrine changes in pediatric posttraumatic stress disorder (PTSD) after motor vehicle accidents: progressive divergence of noradrenaline and cortisol concentrations over time. *Biological Psychiatry* **62**, 1095–1102.

Pine, D.S. & Cohen, J. (2002) Trauma in children and adolescents: risk and treatment of psychiatric sequelae. *Biological Psychiatry* **51**, 519–531.

Pine, D.S. *et al.* (2005) Attention bias to threat in maltreated children: Implications for vulnerability to stress related psychopathology. *American Journal of Psychiatry* **162**, 291–296.

Pitman, R.K. *et al.* (1996) Emotional processing during eye movement desensitization and reprocessing therapy of Vietnam veterans with chronic post traumatic stress disorder. *Comprehensive Psychiatry* **37**, 419–429.

Pynoos, R.S. *et al.* (1987) Life threat and posttraumatic stress in school age children. *Archives of General Psychiatry* **44**, 1063.

Pynoos, R.S. *et al.* (1995) Strategies of disaster interventions for children and adolescents. In: *Extreme Stress and Communities: Impact and Intervention.* (eds S.E. Hobfoll & M. deVries). Kluwer, Dordrecht, Netherlands.

Pynoos, R. *et al.* (2008) The National Child Traumatic Stress Network: collaborating to improve the standard of care. *Professional Psychology: Research and Practice* **39**, 389–395.

Quota, S.R. *et al.* (2012) Intervention effectiveness among war affected children: a cluster randomized control trial on improving mental health. *Journal of Loss and Trauma* **25**, 288–298.

Ramchandani, P. & Jones, D.P.H. (2003) Treating psychological symptoms in sexually abused children: from research findings to service provision. *British Journal of Psychiatry* **183**, 484–490.

Ribchester, T. *et al.* (2010) EMDR for childhood PTSD after road traffic accidents: attentional, memory and attributional processes. *Journal of EMDR Practice and Research* **4**, 138–147.

deRoos, C. et al. (2004) *EMDR versus CBT for disaster-exposed children: a controlled study*, Poster presented at ISTSS 20th Annual Meeting, New Orleans, November.

Roy, A.M. *et al.* (2008) Attention bias towards threat in pediatric anxiety disorders. *Journal of the American Academy of Child and Adolescent Psychiatry* **47**, 1189–1196.

Ruf, M. *et al.* (2010) Narrative exposure therapy for 7- to 16-year-olds: a randomized controlled trial with traumatized refugee children. *Journal of Traumatic Stress* **23**, 437–445.

Sack, W. *et al.* (1997) Does PTSD transcend cultural barriers? A study from the Khmer Adolescent refugee project. *Journal of the American Academy of Child & Adolescent Psychiatry* **36**, 49–54.

Sack, W. *et al.* (1998) Psychometric properties of the Impact of Events Scale in traumatized Cambodian refugee youth. *Personality and Individual Differences* **25**, 57–67.

Saigh, P.A. *et al.* (2011) The psychological adjustment of a sample of New York City preschool children 8–10 months after September 11, 2001. *Psychological Trauma* **3**, 109–116.

Salmon, K. & Bryant, R. (2002) Posttraumatic stress disorder in children: the influence of developmental factors. *Clinical Psychology Review* **22**, 163–188.

Salmon, K. *et al.* (2007) The role of maladaptive appraisals in child acute stress reactions. *British Journal of Clinical Psychology* **46**, 203–210.

Salmond, C. *et al.* (2011) The nature of trauma memories in acute stress disorder in children and adolescents. *Journal of Child Psychology and Psychiatry* **52**, 560–570.

Saltzman, W. *et al.* (2001) Trauma- and grief-focussed intervention for adolescents exposed to community violence: results of a schoolbased screening and group treatment protocol. *Group Dynamics* **5**, 291–303.

Salum, G.A. *et al.* (2013) Threat bias in attention orienting: evidence of specificity in a large community-based study. *Psychological Medicine* **43**, 733–745.

Sartor, C.E. *et al.* (2011) Common genetic and environmental contributions to post-traumatic stress disorder and alcohol dependence in young women. *Psychological Medicine* **41**, 1497–1505.

Sartor, C. *et al.* (2012) Common heritable contributions to low-risk trauma, high-risk trauma, posttraumatic stress disorder, and major depression. *Archives of General Psychiatry* **69**, 293–299.

Schauer, E. *et al.* (2004) Narrative exposure therapy in children: a case study. *Intervention: International Journal of Mental Health, Psychosocial Work & Counselling in Areas of Armed Conflict* **2**, 18–32.

Schauer, M. *et al.* (2005) *Narrative Exposure Therapy: A Short-Term Intervention for Traumatic Stress Disorders After War, Terror, or Torture.* Hogrefe & Huber Publishers, Ohio, USA.

Schechter, T. *et al.* (2012) Attention biases, anxiety, and development—toward or away from threats or rewards? *Depression and Anxiety* **29**, 282–294.

Scheeringa, M.S. *et al.* (1995) Two approaches to the diagnosis of postttraumatic stress disorder in infancy and early childhood. *Journal of the American Academy of Child and Adolescent Psychiatry* **34**, 191–200.

Scheeringa, M. *et al.* (2001) Toward establishing procedural, criterion, and discriminant validity for PTSD in early childhood. *Journal of the American Academy of Child and Adolescent Psychiatry* **40**, 52–60.

Scheeringa, M. *et al.* (2003) New findings on alternative criteria for PTSD in preschool children. *Journal of the American Academy of Child and Adolescent Psychiatry* **42**, 561–570.

Scheeringa, M.S. *et al.* (2004) Heart period and variability findings in preschool children with posttraumatic stress symptoms. *Biological Psychiatry* **55**, 685–691.

Scheeringa, M. *et al.* (2006) Factors affecting the diagnosis and prediction of PTSD symptomatology in children and adolescents. *American Journal of Psychiatry* **163**, 644–651.

Scheeringa, M.S. *et al.* (2011) Trauma-focused cognitive-behavioral therapy for posttraumatic stress disorder in three-through six year-old children: a randomized clinical trial. *Journal of Child Psychology and Psychiatry* **52**, 853–860.

Shapiro, F. (2001) *Eye Movement Desensitization and Reprocessing: Basic Principles, Protocols and Procedures*, 2nd edn. Guilford Press, New York.

Smith, P. *et al.* (2002) War exposure among children from Bosnia-Hercegovina: psychological adjustment in a community sample. *Journal of Traumatic Stress* **15**, 147–156.

Smith, P. *et al.* (2003) Principal components analysis of the impact of event scale with children in war. *Personality and Individual Differences* **34**, 315–322.

Smith, P. *et al.* (2007) A randomised controlled trial of cognitive behaviour therapy for PTSD in children and adolescents. *Journal of American Academy of Child and Adolescent Psychiatry* **46**, 1051–1061.

Stallard, P. (2006) Psychological interventions for post traumatic stress reactions in children and young people: a review of randomised controlled trials. *Clinical Psychology Review* **26**, 895–911.

Stallard, P. & Salter, E. (2003) Psychological debriefing with children and young people following traumatic events. *Clinical Child Psychology and Psychiatry* **8**, 445–457.

Stallard, P. & Smith, E. (2007) Appraisals and cognitive coping styles associated with chronic post-traumatic symptoms in child road traffic accident survivors. *Journal of Child Psychology and Psychiatry* **48**, 194–201.

Stallard, P. *et al.* (2004) Posttraumatic stress disorder following road traffic accidents: a second prospective study. *European Child & Adolescent Psychiatry* **13**, 172–178.

Stallard, P. *et al.* (2006) A randomised controlled trial to determine the effectiveness of an early psychological intervention with children involved in road traffic accidents. *Journal of Child Psychology and Psychiatry* **47**, 127–134.

Stein, M.B. *et al.* (2002) Genetic and environmental influences on trauma exposure and posttraumatic stress disorder symptoms: a twin study. *American Journal of Psychiatry* **159**, 1675–1681.

Sugaya, L. *et al.* (2012) Child physical abuse and adult mental health: a national study. *Journal of Traumatic Stress* **25**, 384–392.

Taghavi, R. *et al.* (1999) Biases in visual attention in children and adolescents with clinical anxiety and mixed anxiety-depression. *Journal of Abnormal Child Psychology* **27**, 215–223.

Thabet, A. & Vostanis, P. (1999) Post-traumatic stress reactions in children of war. *Journal of Child Psychology and Psychiatry* **40**, 385–391.

Tol, W. *et al.* (2011) Mediators and moderators of a psychosocial intervention for children affected by political violence. *Journal of Consulting and Clinical Psychology* **78**, 818–828.

Trickey, D. *et al.* (2012) A meta-analysis of risk factors for post traumatic stress disorder in children and adolescents. *Clinical Psychology Review* **32**, 122–138.

True, W. *et al.* (1993) A twin study of genetic and environmental contributions to liability for posttraumatic stress symptoms. *Archives of General Psychiatry* **50**, 257–264.

Tsui, E. (1990). *Effects of a disaster on children's academic attainment.* Unpublished Master's thesis, University of London (Quoted in Yule and Gold, 1993).

Tupler, L. & De Bellis, M. (2006) Segmented hippocampal volume in children and adolescents with posttraumatic stress disorder. *Biological Psychiatry* **59**, 523–529.

Van der Oord, S.K. *et al.* (2010) Treatment of post-traumatic stress disorder in children using cognitive behavioural writing therapy. *Clinical Psychology and Psychotherapy* **17**, 240–249.

Weems, C. & Carrion, V. (2007) The association between PTSD symptoms and salivary cortisol in youth: the role of time since the trauma. *Journal of Traumatic Stress* **20**, 903–907.

Whalley, M. *et al.* (2013) An fMRI investigation of posttraumatic flashbacks. *Brain and Cognition* **81**, 151–159.

Woon, F. & Hedges, D.W. (2011) Gender does not moderate hippocampal volume deficits in adults with posttraumatic stress disorder: a meta-analysis. *Hippocampus* **21**, 243–252.

Woud, M. *et al.* (2012) Ameliorating intrusive memories of distressing experiences using computerized reappraisal training. *Emotion* **12**, 778–784.

Yehuda, R. & McFarlane, A.C. (1995) Conflict between current knowledge about posttraumatic stress disorder and its original conceptual basis. *American Journal of Psychiatry* **152**, 1705–1713.

de Young, A.C. *et al.* (2011) Prevalence co-morbidity and course of trauma reactions in young burn injured children. *Journal of Child Psychology and Psychiatry* **53**, 56–63.

Yule, W. (2008) IASC guidelines, generally welcome but ... . *Intervention* **6**, 248–251.

Yule, W. & Gold, A. (1993) *Wise Before the Event: Coping with Crises in Schools.* Calouste Gulbenkian Foundation, London.

Yule, W. *et al.* (2000) The long-term psychological effects of a disaster experienced in adolescence: I: the incidence and course of post traumatic stress disorder. *Journal of Child Psychology and Psychiatry* **41**, 503–511.

Yule, W. *et al.* (2013) Children and war: the work of the Children and War Foundation. *European Journal of Psychotraumatology* **4**, 18424.

Zehnder, D. *et al.* (2010) Effectiveness of a single-session early psychological intervention for children after road traffic accidents: a randomised controlled trial. *Child and Adolescent Psychiatry and Mental Health* **4**, 7.

CHAPTER 60

Anxiety disorders

Daniel S. Pine[1] and Rachel G. Klein[2]

[1] Section on Development and Affective Neuroscience, National Institute of Mental Health (NIMH) Intramural Research Program, Bethesda, MD, USA
[2] The Child Study Center at New York University Langone Medical Center, Department of Child and Adolescent Psychiatry, New York University School of Medicine, NY, USA

Introduction

The chapter reviews anxiety disorders, which include specific phobias, separation anxiety disorder, social anxiety disorder, generalized anxiety disorder, panic disorder, and agoraphobia. The first four anxiety disorders are unique in at least one respect. The features that define them represent aspects of normal development, raising questions on the boundary between normal and pathological anxiety.

Fear and anxiety play important roles in functioning, and have major evolutionary significance; they enable the awareness of danger, and prepare the individual to avoid threat. The term *fear* refers to a state elicited by an immediately present specific object or situation that is capable of harm or danger. *Anxiety* resembles fear but occurs in situations that are not acutely dangerous, but which are experienced as such. Although adaptive, fear and anxiety may become pathological when they are provoked by objects or situations that are not legitimately harmful or threatening or when they limit the person's functioning.

Diagnosis

Boundaries between normal and pathological anxiety are not clear-cut, and there is no defining point at which we can aver that pathology begins. Clearly, extreme anxiety is readily recognized as abnormal in the same way that extreme intellectual disability is readily distinguished from normal intelligence. For milder expressions of anxiety, however, decisions are more difficult, since anxiety is adaptive in some contexts or developmental periods. The dilemma is not inconsequential because the identification of pathological anxiety calls for the development and delivery of effective treatments, as well as efforts to prevent, and hopefully cure, the disorders. Distinguishing pathological from normal anxiety requires the clinician to recognize a departure from anxiety's adaptive role in functioning, ultimately based on judgments about the presence of clinically meaningful avoidance or distress.

At any age, anxiety is pathologic when it interferes with adaptive behavior. Parents and clinicians are often quick to recognize markedly impairing anxiety that causes significant avoidance, but anxiety may be pathological under other circumstances, even without the presence of manifest functional impairment, if anxiety causes clinically significant distress. It is useful to consider a child's ability to recover from anxiety, and to remain anxiety-free, when the anxiety provoking situation is absent or removed, since failure to modify appropriately one's responses to changing circumstances is a hallmark of psychopathology.

Nosology

A major shift occurred in 1980, with the publication of DSM-III, which introduced several anxiety disorders. There have been objections to having multiple anxiety disorders in nosology, because of inadequately clear definitional boundaries among the disorders. In the future, the hope is that distinctions among anxiety disorders will be informed by data on outcome (Pine *et al.*, 1998, 2001), genetics, or psychobiology (Pine & Cohen, 2002). This was not yet possible for the DSM-5 and ICD-11. DSM-IV, which appeared in 1994, eliminated two DSM-III pediatric anxiety disorders, avoidant disorder and overanxious disorder. This change reflected the principle that common diagnostic standards should be applied from childhood through adulthood, with age-relevant clinical examples, an approach that remains in DSM-5. ICD-10 and DSM-IV were broadly similar but differed in the handling of comorbidity and in the placement of obsessive compulsive disorder (OCD) and posttraumatic stress disorder (PTSD); DSM-5 brings greater alignment with the ICD. Both ICD-11 and DSM-5 place OCD and PTSD outside the anxiety disorders. Otherwise, there have been only minor changes in the anxiety disorders.

Rutter's Child and Adolescent Psychiatry, Sixth Edition.
Edited by Anita Thapar and Daniel S. Pine, James F. Leckman, Stephen Scott, Margaret J. Snowling, Eric Taylor.
© 2015 John Wiley & Sons Ltd. Published 2018 by John Wiley & Sons Ltd.

Specific conditions
Specific phobia
This diagnosis is defined by marked, unreasonable fear of specific objects or situations that do not pose actual danger, such as various animals or situations. Although unreasonable fears are common, they are diagnosable only when they cause distress or avoidance, severe enough to interfere with normal activities. Phobic disorders may begin at any age, but onset is typically in childhood, and usually do not persist through adolescence and adulthood (Fyer, 1998; Pine *et al.*, 1998).

Separation anxiety disorder
Relative to other anxiety disorders, separation anxiety disorder has an unusually skewed age distribution, typically occurring before the age of 18 and usually, but not always, remitting before adulthood. While separation anxiety is part of normal early-childhood development, separation anxiety *disorder* reflects pathology, which interferes with functioning. Typically, the child avoids activities that require ordinary separation from caretakers, such as play dates in friends' homes. Children with separation anxiety disorder may display symptoms that defy logic. For example, a child who attends school comfortably may face extreme distress when attending a social gathering without a parent. Clinical descriptions of "school phobia" typically do not, strictly speaking, identify children with a phobia. Such children often suffer from an extreme form of separation anxiety. Though unusual, separation anxiety may be episodic, with periods of impairing anxiety that remit, and may reoccur. Strikingly, severe separation anxiety may develop in children and adolescents who, previously, had not evidenced concerns about separation.

Social anxiety disorder
In social anxiety disorder, the classic presentation involves concerns about being perceived as acting foolish or stupid. Some children may fail to report these concerns. The diagnosis is then based on observations that these children appear self-conscious and uncomfortable in social settings. To be diagnosed, children must experience discomfort with peers, not only with adults, and anxiety cannot be due to impaired capacity for socialization, as occurs in autism spectrum disorders. This aspect of classification can complicate diagnosis, as children with autism spectrum disorders may receive the diagnosis of social anxiety disorder, provided their anxiety in social situations can be distinguished from the dysfunction they exhibit due to impaired socialization.

Generalized anxiety disorder
Generalized anxiety disorder is characterized by a variety of worries. Children often worry about their ability to succeed, often related to schoolwork, appearance, or future, and because of their self-doubt, they strive for perfection. The age-of-onset is poorly understood, with the available evidence placing peak onset in late adolescence or early adulthood. Relative to other anxiety disorders, generalized anxiety disorder is more likely to occur with other psychopathology, to the point where the disorder rarely occurs on its own. The relationship with other anxiety disorders and with major depressive disorder is particularly robust (Costello *et al.*, 2002; Kessler *et al.*, 2002).

Panic disorder
Panic disorder is characterized by the repeated experience of unprovoked, spontaneous, panic attacks, consisting of fear of impending doom or danger to oneself, accompanied by physical symptoms. Panic disorder is rare before puberty. Typically, the disorder begins with an initial spontaneous panic attack, occurring around late adolescence. Most individuals suffer only a few instances of spontaneous panics. Progression to recurring attacks and eventual full-blown panic disorder is the exception, but when it happens, this typically occurs by early adulthood (Pine *et al.*, 1998).

Agoraphobia
Agoraphobia refers to extreme fear and avoidance of independent travel. In DSM-IV, agoraphobia was an aspect of panic disorder, because it typically develops in individuals with panic disorder. ICD-10 did not follow this convention, nor does DSM-5. Since panic disorder is rare in prepubertal children, minimal work examines pediatric agoraphobia, which is believed also to be rare. Children with separation anxiety, for example, may fear traveling on their own.

Developmental fluctuations
Across cultures, there are similar age-related fluctuations in fears and anxiety. This consistency suggests that age-related changes in anxiety represent a core aspect of human development (Ollendick *et al.*, 1996; Ingman *et al.*, 1999). However, beyond this research on typical fears, cross-cultural differences in the rates of anxiety disorders have not been addressed sufficiently. When it does occur, the onset of pathological anxiety mimics developmental fluctuations in normal fears that are observed across cultures. Thus, fears of animals regularly begin in early childhood, so do specific phobias. Fears of separation also first manifests in early childhood, and separation anxiety disorder exhibits a particular high prevalence in children only a few years beyond this developmental stage (Pine *et al.*, 1998). Similarly, social concerns typically emerge as part of normal adolescent development (Ollendick & Hirshfeld-Becker, 2002), virtually coinciding with a rise in the incidence of social anxiety disorder.

Rates of anxiety, as well as the expression of anxiety, vary across development. Changes may reflect children's changing capacities with cognitive maturation, the effects of changing social contexts, which expose children to novel forms of stress, or rapid changes in biology that occur at puberty. For example, developmental manifestations of social anxiety change from a pattern of "high reactivity" during infancy (Fox *et al.*, 2005), to "behavioral inhibition" in childhood, and ultimately to social anxiety disorder in adolescence (Clauss & Blackford, 2012).

Comorbidity

Comorbidity is an important clinical feature since it has been shown to entail relatively greater dysfunction. Although comorbidity is less apparent in community-based, than clinically based, studies, there is strong comorbidity across anxiety disorders in both settings. Elevated rates of co-occurring anxiety disorders raise the question whether the anxiety disorders represent distinct conditions, as opposed to variable expressions of underlying anxiety vulnerability.

There is unanimous agreement that major depression in adolescence is highly comorbid with anxiety disorders, with anxiety typically preceding the mood disorder. The strength of this relationship rivals virtually all others in developmental psychopathology (Angold *et al.*, 1999; Costello *et al.*, 2002; Costello *et al.*, 2004). Since depression is much rarer than anxiety disorders, especially in preadolescents, it follows that, among those with anxiety, the overlap with depression is not great, and that comorbidity increases with age. Some clinical studies report comorbidity between anxiety and attention deficit hyperactivity disorder (ADHD), but population-based studies do not confirm this relationship (Angold *et al.*, 1999). While some have reported comorbidity between current anxiety disorders and substance abuse or conduct disorder, these associations also are weak (Kaplow *et al.*, 2001; Rutter *et al.*, 2006). Moreover, longitudinal findings raise questions on the nature of the relationship between anxiety and either substance abuse or conduct disorder, since anxiety predicts better outcome in some children with conduct problems (Pine *et al.*, 2000). It may be that children with conduct and anxiety disorders represent a distinct clinical subgroup of conduct disorder. Although studies have not linked anxiety and learning disorders in children, it behooves clinicians to rule out learning problems, particularly in children who present with school-based anxiety.

Assessment

Efforts to systematically assess pediatric anxiety benefit from a proliferation of instruments, including paper and pencil scales, as well as multiple diagnostic interviews. Because several reviews summarize these (Brooks & Kutcher, 2003; Seligman *et al.*, 2004; Silverman & Ollendick, 2005), only an overview is provided.

Rating scales

Rating scales serve many purposes. They may screen large groups or facilitate the collection of data relatively efficiently for large studies of genetic and environmental correlates. Early rating scales, which anteceded DSM-III and ICD-10, comprised factors such as worry, physiological anxiety, and fear of bodily harm. Other scales, such as the Children's Behavior Checklist (CBCL) (Achenbach, 1991), generate a nonspecific factor of emotional disturbance, called an "internalizing" factor. In general, these scales appear to assess constructs distinct from those assessed by newer scales. One major important clinical challenge is to differentiate between anxiety and depression based on scale scores, a challenge reflected by the single, unitary factor scale in the CBCL. The meaning of self-ratings of anxiety is further complicated by the finding that children's self-ratings often correlate poorly with parent ratings, or with symptoms of anxiety obtained from clinical interviews (RUPP, 2003). Anxiety scales may provide overall estimates of anxiety levels, but they do not provide diagnoses of specific anxiety disorder. Clinicians would be unwise to rely on scales for differential diagnosis.

Growing interest in anxiety disorders has spurred the development of more diagnostically relevant child- and parent-rated measures. Recent scales parallel the clinical definitions of anxiety disorders by providing specificity of content, so that items correspond to the clinical criteria provided in the DSM. In this vein, several scales have been devised. The Multidimensional Anxiety Scale for Children (MASC) (March *et al.*, 1997; March & Sullivan, 1999) and the Self Report for Child Anxiety Related Disorders (SCARED) (Birmaher *et al.*, 1997) have been used in many studies. They possess strong psychometric properties, and they are sensitive to treatment effects, rendering them useful in treatment studies and clinical monitoring. The Pediatric Anxiety Rating Scale (PARS) has emerged as the standard clinician-rated measure in most clinical trials and is particularly useful for assessing progress during treatment.

Diagnostic interviews

Several interviews exist, each devised to meet different purposes. The highly structured Diagnostic Interview Schedule for Children (DISC) was developed for use in epidemiological studies, to be administered by individuals without clinical training (Shaffer *et al.*, 2000), or by a computer. Support for the clinical utility is mixed, with some research documenting agreement with clinicians (Schwab-Stone *et al.*, 1996), but other studies finding unduly high rates of disorders and questionable validity (March *et al.*, 2000). The Child and Adolescent Psychiatric Assessment (CAPA) (Angold & Costello, 2000), with excellent psychometric properties, also was developed for use in epidemiological studies. Relative to the DISC, the CAPA requires more training, and has not been used as widely. The Kiddie-Schedule for Affective Disorder and Schizophrenia (K-SADS) was developed for use by clinicians, and allows full latitude of inquiry. Multiple versions exist (Kaufman *et al.*, 1997; Kaufman *et al.*, 2000), but differences are small. The Diagnostic Interview for Children and Adolescents (DICA) (Reich, 2000) is a highly structured clinical interview that has been used in various ways, including in semistructured, flexible, formats. The Anxiety Disorders Interview Schedule for Children (ADIS) was designed for clinicians. It was originally limited to the assessment of anxiety, but has been expanded to include other major disorders (Silverman *et al.*, 2001).

All of these interviews demonstrate modest to adequate test-retest reliability. The major factor informing selection concerns the availability and training of clinicians for implementation. Without highly trained clinicians, the DISC or CAPA seem the best options. Although diagnostic interviews were conceived for research purposes, they may be useful to clinicians by providing comprehensive coverage of psychopathology and are useful teaching tools.

Epidemiology

Prevalence

Most studies (Table 60.1) find that anxiety disorders are the most common pediatric mental disorders and more frequent in girls than boys. Importantly, epidemiological studies confirm that child and adolescent anxiety disorders are associated with significant impairment. Studies have followed the same individuals over extended periods of time, enabling identification of typical age of onsets and incidence (Costello *et al.*, 2004; Costello *et al.*, 2005; Copeland *et al.*, 2009; Beesdo *et al.*, 2010). In childhood, phobias and separation anxiety disorder are most prevalent, diminishing in adolescence, when social anxiety disorder becomes salient. Rates of generalized anxiety disorder generally increase later in adolescence, and panic disorder is rare before this time period.

For 6-to-12-month prevalence, anxiety disorders range from 1.8% in New Zealand (Anderson *et al.*, 1987) to 23.5% in Holland (Verhulst *et al.*, 1997), reflecting large cross-study differences. Prospective studies find much higher lifetime rates of anxiety and other disorders than studies using a single assessment with retrospective recall to estimate lifetime prevalence (Angold *et al.*, 1996; Costello *et al.*, 2003; Jaffee *et al.*, 2005).

Developmental factors may explain some cross-study differences. For example, studies finding relatively high rates of separation anxiety disorder tend to include young children, whereas those that include older children find high rates of social phobia. Nevertheless, there is marked variation even for studies performed in similar populations (e.g., two studies from Germany [Essau *et al.*, 1999; Wittchen *et al.*, 1999]). Methodological differences are likely to account for such findings. Because there is large variation in prevalence in similar cultures, it is difficult to determine how, and whether, cultural factors are influential.

Could secular changes affect rates of anxiety disorders? This possibility cannot be ruled out, but does not seem to account for discrepancies across studies, since there is no evidence suggesting time-dependent changes in young people. Similarly, could different methods for generating diagnoses, such as combining reports from different informants or relying on a single informant, contribute to cross-study differences? The low rate of informant agreement in most studies makes this a reasonable possibility. Rates of anxiety disorders consistently vary across studies as a function of the reporting source, be it children or parents, and whether their reports are combined or not (Anderson *et al.*, 1987).

Longitudinal outcome

The high proportion of affected children and their impairment has fostered concern about the long-term consequences of childhood anxiety disorders. Most anxiety assessments generate only moderate test-retest reliability. Since reliability places an upper limit on associations, outcome findings may represent lower-bound estimates of stability. Anxiety has a particularly early onset, compared to other emotional disorders such as major depression. A major source of data on early risk manifestations derives from studies of temperament, especially behavioral inhibition.

Inhibited temperament and psychopathology

Kagan and colleagues (Kagan, 1994; Kagan *et al.*, 2001) first called attention to the relationship between childhood temperament and later anxiety disorders. They identified highly reactive infants, who, as toddlers, were behaviorally inhibited and reacted with apprehension to novelty. These children are defined as high reactive during infancy and as behaviorally inhibited during toddlerhood. Studies of associations with psychopathology have been conducted in thousands of children. Inhibited temperament has been consistently linked to anxiety disorders, including separation anxiety disorder, social anxiety, and phobias, though some have reported associations with depression (Caspi *et al.*, 1996). The most compelling relationship is with social anxiety disorder. Based on the data from seven longitudinal studies, inhibited children face sevenfold increased odds of developing social anxiety disorder, relative to their uninhibited peers (Clauss & Blackford, 2012).

Stability of anxiety disorders

The clearest information about diagnostic stability emerges from community-based studies, which have obtained multiple assessments across development. The first, from Dunedin, New Zealand (Anderson *et al.*, 1987), conducted multiple assessments, from age 11 through adulthood (McGee *et al.*, 1992; Feehan *et al.*, 1993; Kim-Cohen *et al.*, 2003; Poulton *et al.*, 2009). In the first follow-up, a composite index of any mood or anxiety disorder at age 11 predicted later anxiety at age 15 for girls, but not boys (McGee *et al.*, 1992). Similar sex differences were obtained in two other prospective population studies (Costello *et al.*, 1999; Rueter *et al.*, 1999). The latter found that anxiety symptoms also predicted major depression. More recent follow-ups from the Dunedin sample, as well as others, document a pattern of moderate longitudinal continuity of anxiety disorders, but little evidence of gender-specificity or concordance between specific anxiety disorders during childhood and adulthood (Lewinsohn *et al.*, 1997; Bittner *et al.*, 2004; Copeland *et al.*, 2009; Beesdo *et al.*, 2010). Other work finds longitudinal specificity of social anxiety disorder across adolescence, but not of separation anxiety disorder (Hayward *et al.*, 1998). Perhaps the strongest evidence of long-term diagnostic specificity derives from the New York longitudinal study, which

Table 60.1 Prevalence (%) of anxiety disorders in children, adolescents, and adults followed prospectively.

Location	Authors	N	Age in years	Interview	Time frame	Rates (%)					
						Any	SiPh	SAD	OAD	SoPh	PD
New Zealand											
Dunedin	Anderson et al. (1987)[a]	785	11	DISC-C[b]	12 mos[c]	1.8–7.5	0–2.4	0.06–3.5	0.05–2.9	0–0.9	–
					12 mos[d]	3.6[e]	1.7	1.9	2.5	0.4	
	McGee et al. (1990)[a]	943	15	DISC-C	12 mos[f]	10.7[e]	3.6	2.0	5.9	1.1	–
	Kim-Cohen et al. (2003)[a]	976	26	DIS	12 mos[f]	26.1[e]	7.1	–	5.5[g]	10.7	3.9
Christchurch	Fergusson et al. (1993)	986	15	DISC-P	12 mos[f]	3.9	1.3	0.1	0.6	0.7	
		965		DISC-C	12 mos[f]	10.8	5.1	0.5	2.1	1.7	
	Goodwin et al. (2004)	969	16–18	M-CIDI[h,i]	12 mos[f]	18.4	9.6	–	2.7[g]	7.5	–
		957	18–21	M-CIDI[h,i]	12 mos[f]	14.6	6.5	–	1.8[g]	6.7	–
Germany											
Manheim	Esser et al. (1990)	191	13	Graham/Rutter[j-1]	6 mos	5.8	–	–	–	–	–
Munich	Reed and Wittchen (1998)[a]	3021	14–24	M-CIDI[m,h]	12 mos	–	–	–	–	–	0.6
					Lifetime	–	–	–	–	–	0.8
	Wittchen et al. (1999)[a]	925	14–17	M-CIDI[m,h]	12 mos	–	–	–	–	3.0	–
					Lifetime	–	–	–	–	4.0	–
Bremen	Essau et al. (1999)	1035	12–17	M-CIDI[m,h]	Lifetime	–	–	–	–	1.6	–
UK London ‡	Kramer and Garralda (1998)	131	13–17	K-SADS[h,o]	12 mos	5.3	–	–	3.1	1.5	0.8
Holland	Verhulst et al. (1997)	312/780[p]	13–18	DISC-C	6 mos	10.5	4.5	1.4	1.8	3.7	0.2
				DISC-P		16.5	9.2	0.6	1.5	6.3	0.3
				DISC[q]		23.5	12.7	1.8	3.1	9.2	0.4
				DISC[l]		5.3	–	–	–	–	–
						4.4					
Puerto Rico	Bird et al. (1988)	386/777[m]	4–16	DISC[l]	6 mos	7.0	2.6	4.7	–	–	–
							1.3	2.1	–	–	–
USA											
Pennsylvania	Costello et al. (1988)[a]	300/789[p]	7–11	DISC-C	12 mos	10.5	6.7	4.1	2.0	1.0	–
				DISC-P	12 mos	6.5	3.0	0.4	2.8	0	–
	Benjamin et al. (1990)[a]	300/789[kp]	7–11	DISC[f]	12 mos	15.4	9.1	4.1	4.6	1.0	–
New York State	Pine et al. (1998)	776	9–18	DISC[f]	12 mos	–	11.6	8.6	14.3	8.4	0.0
		760	11–20	DISC[f]	12 mos	–	5.9	3.7	8.0	9.9	0.0
		716	17–26	DISC[f]	12 mos	–	22.1	–	5.0[g]	5.6	0.1
Nationwide	Kessler et al. (2012)	10,148	13–17	CIDI	12 mos	24.9	15.8	1.6	1.1[g]	8.2	1.9
Nationwide	Magee et al. (1996)	1765	15–24	CIDI[h,i]	Lifetime	–	10.8	–	–	14.9	–
Nationwide	Merikangas et al. (2010)	3042	8–15	DISC[r]	12 mos	0.7	–	–	0.3[g]	–	0.4
North Carolina	Costello et al. (1996)	1015	9, 11, 13	CAPA[h,s]	3 mos	5.7	0.3	3.5	1.4	0.6	0.03
	Costello et al. (2003)	1420	9–16	CAPA[h,s]	3 mos	2.4	–	–	–	–	–
Georgia, New Haven, New York, Puerto Rico	Shaffer et al. (1996)	1285	9–17	DISC-P[t,u]	6 mos	21.0	11.7	2.5	4.3	7.9	–
				DISC-C[u]		23.7	11.2	3.1	5.4	8.5	
				DISC[l]		18.5	9.5	4.1	8.0	8.2	–
						13.9	6.8	3.5	6.5	6.6	
				DISCS		20.5	3.3	5.8	7.7	7.6	–

Table 60.1 (*continued*)

Location	Authors	N	Age in years	Interview	Time frame	Rates (%)					
						Any	SiPh	SAD	OAD	SoPh	PD
Oregon	Lewinsohn *et al.* (1998)	1709	15.5	KSADS	12 mos	2.8	1.3	0.2	0.5	0.9	0.3
Virginia	Simonoff *et al.* (1997)	2762 (twins)	8–16	CAPA[s,v]	3 mos	–	21.2	7.2	10.8	8.4	–
							4.4	1.5	4.4	2.5	

[a]Same cohort within site.

[b]DISC-C and DISC-P, Diagnostic Interview Schedule for Children, Child and Parent Version.

[c]Rates vary depending on diagnostic criteria based on DISC-C, and parent and teacher ratings, for example, diagnostic criteria met (i) by two of three sources or by one source and symptoms confirmed by at least one other source; (ii) by one source but no other source confirms symptoms; (iii) by combining symptoms from all three sources.

[d]Percent meeting diagnostic criteria applying same standards as at age 15 in McGee *et al.* (1992).

[e]Rates calculated from papers: SAD, separation anxiety disorder; OAD, overanxious disorder; SiPh, simple phobia; SoPh, social phobia; PD, panic disorder.

[f]Percent meeting criteria based on DISC-C plus parent ratings.

[g]Generalized anxiety disorder.

[h]Diagnosis based on interview with adolescent.

[i]CIDI, Composite International Diagnostic Interview.

[j]Interview by Rutter & Graham (1968).

[k]Includes anxiety and mood disorders.

[l]*Top line*: percent meeting diagnostic criteria on parent OR child interview *and* had a C-GAS <61; *bottom line*: percent meeting diagnostic criteria on parent OR child interview *and* had a C-GAS between 61 and 70.

[m]M-CIDI, Munich modification of CIDI.

[n]Adolescents in primary care clinics.

[o]K-SADS, Kiddie Schedule for Affective Disorders and Schizophrenia.

[p]Two-stage study: *N* in stage 2/*N* in Stage 1.

[q]Percent meeting diagnostic criteria based on interview with parent OR child.

[r]DISC-IV (Shaffer *et al.*, 2000).

[s]CAPA, Child and Adolescent Psychiatric Assessment.

[t]DISC Version 2.3 (Shaffer *et al.*, 1996).

[u]Percent meeting diagnostic criteria only for symptom number, age-of-onset, and duration.

[v]*Top line*: percent meeting diagnostic criteria; *bottom line*: percent meeting diagnostic criteria *and* impairment criteria.

found distinct longitudinal patterns for the course of pediatric separation anxiety disorder, social phobia, and specific phobia from adolescence into early adulthood (Pine *et al.*, 1998). In contrast, there was little stability of overanxious disorder (replaced by Generalized Anxiety Disorder in the DSM-IV and DSM-5), from early to late adolescence (Pine *et al.*, 1998).

Beyond community-based studies, a prospective longitudinal study of offspring of referred parents with major depression or panic disorder found that specific phobias and overanxious disorder, but not separation anxiety disorder, incurred a two-to-four increase of major depression at follow-up (Weissman *et al.*, 1997). In such high-risk studies, the children's comorbidity and outcome patterns are expected to be relatively free of referral biases, but they do not eliminate referral biases of parents (Breslau *et al.*, 1987). Other findings from clinical samples (Klein, 1995; Last *et al.*, 1997; Aschenbrand *et al.*, 2003) confirm the generally good outcome for most youth with anxiety disorders, although a minority may experience significant negative psychiatric outcomes (Klein, 1995), Also, these clinical studies provide some support for a connection between separation anxiety disorder and later-onset panic disorder.

In conclusion, longitudinal studies point to several clinical observations. There is only moderate stability in pediatric anxiety, so that most affected children will be free of anxiety disorders in adulthood. However, since most adults with anxiety disorders, as well as those with mood disorders, will have had a childhood history of anxiety disorders, childhood anxiety disorders do increase risk.

Risk factors

Due to referral biases, epidemiological studies are the best source of information about risk. However, when there is inconsistent or insufficient data, we also note findings from clinical studies. In epidemiological reports, girls have higher rates than boys of most anxiety disorders, occurring as early as age six (Lewinsohn *et al.*, 1997). Anxiety also may have greater long-term impact in girls than boys (McGee *et al.*, 1992; Costello *et al.*, 1999), but findings are not unanimous (Pine *et al.*, 1998).

Social stress

Anxiety has been linked to a range of life events, but there is little consensus regarding influential environmental factors. These include economic disadvantage, stressful life events, family dysfunction, single-parent households, and low parental education. However, relationships are neither strong nor consistent. The lack of relationships between anxiety and social factors is not due to the inability of environmental features to relate to pediatric mental disorders, since they play a clear role in conduct disorder (McGee *et al.*, 1992). Thus, a recent study, using a quasi-experimental design, found stronger effects of poverty and its associated stresses on children's behavior problems than anxiety symptoms (Costello *et al.*, 2010). Differing stresses may relate differentially to child psychopathology. For example, stress related to social disadvantages has been shown to be associated with behavior problems, not anxiety disorders. In contrast, it may be that stress, in the form of loss, is associated with anxiety symptoms. Although epidemiological studies have the advantage of minimizing referral biases, they typically include relatively small numbers of children with any single disorder, and these are often relatively mild. As a result, it is also helpful to consider data from clinically referred samples of severe cases.

The considerable effort that has been made to examine associations between children's anxiety disorders and aspects of their family social environment, such as parenting, has yielded inconsistent results, whether from community- or clinic-based studies. Some research suggests that parental behaviors represent nonspecific correlates of psychopathology in children: they relate to many forms of dysfunction, including anxiety, mood, and behavior disorders, and are not specific to anxiety disorders (Wood *et al.*, 2003). Moreover, parenting behaviors may have indirect effects, through interactions with genetic influences or/and children's temperament (Lewis-Morrarty *et al.*, 2012), which complicates attempts to relate parenting behavior to children's anxiety.

Despite inconsistency in findings, interest in environmental influences persists for two reasons. First, as reviewed below, basic research demonstrates strong developmental plasticity in responses to threats in rodents and nonhuman primates (Gross & Hen, 2004). Such findings generate interest concerning whether, and how, adverse social experiences may shape children's responses to threats through changes in brain function. Second, from a clinical perspective, anxiety disorders are associated with traumatic experiences (Steinberg & Avenevoli, 2000; Pine & Cohen, 2002). Some children may develop PTSD, but others may develop an anxiety disorder. Anxiety's consistent association with trauma raises the possibility of an association across a range of mild-to-more-severe environmental adversity.

Some studies find associations between adverse life events and pediatric anxiety, with the overall pattern suggesting modest associations (Eley & Stevenson, 2000; Hankin & Abramson, 2001; Williamson *et al.*, 2005). Few studies have been longitudinal, and most have determined life events through retrospective recall, thus raising the possibility that life events represent correlates rather than causes of anxiety. However, one longitudinal study found that adverse life events during adolescence predicted risk for anxiety 4 years later, especially generalized anxiety disorder in females (Pine *et al.*, 2002). Finally, there may be particularly potent effects from stressors that interact with a child's underlying vulnerability. For example, children with underlying anxiety have been reported to face particularly high risk for social anxiety disorder when exposed to stressful peer relationships, that is, bullying (Crawford & Manassis, 2011).

Stress reactivity

There is great variability in children's reactivity to stress, suggesting that underlying vulnerability may interact with stress exposure. Stress vulnerability has been indexed by physiological responses. For example, elevated heart rates after trauma have been linked to risk for PTSD (Kassam-Adams *et al.*, 2005). Similarly, there are associations reported among children's internalizing symptoms, children's physiologic response to a stressor, and marital conflict (Obradovic *et al.*, 2011). Reactions to various forms of stress have been examined, charted with many physiological parameters, including heart rate, cortisol level, skin conductance, and blinking rate. While some evidence of increased stress reactivity does emerge in anxiety, no clear and consistent strong associations emerge with specific forms of stress or particular physiological parameters.

Efforts have been made to quantify vulnerability to stress using questionnaires and personality inventories. A link has been reported between stress-reactivity tendencies and later anxiety disorders among children followed longitudinally (Pine *et al.*, 2001). Similarly, the Children's Anxiety Sensitivity Index (CASI), devised to assess the child's response to anxiety, may predict risk for anxiety symptoms. However, such measures may reflect current symptoms of anxiety disorders rather than vulnerability (Mannuzza *et al.*, 2002). Little data document associations between these or other stress vulnerability measures in currently healthy children and future anxiety disorders.

Medical conditions

Various medical conditions have been viewed as risk factors for anxiety disorders, operating during various phases of development. During the perinatal period, this includes overt neurological injury, febrile seizures, low birth weight, exposure to toxins, and minor neurological soft signs (Shaffer *et al.*, 1985; Breslau, 1995; Whitaker *et al.*, 1997; Breslau & Chilcoat, 2000; Breslau *et al.*, 2000; Vasa *et al.*, 2002). However, as is the case for other risk factors, relationships are neither strong nor consistent. Relative to behavior disorders, pediatric anxiety is less consistently associated with overt neurological injury and brain trauma (Gerring *et al.*, 2002). In fact, some forms of injury may even be protective (Vasa *et al.*, 2004). Like other risks, medical factors likely interact with children's underlying vulnerabilities to place them at risk for anxiety (Shaffer *et al.*, 1985).

Of all physiological factors associated with childhood anxiety disorders, the strongest evidence is for the role of respiratory dysregulation. Recurrent experiences that produce dyspnea incur risk for pediatric anxiety disorders (Slattery *et al.*, 2002; Goodwin *et al.*, 2003); Asthma, for one, confers risk for two specific anxiety states: separation anxiety disorder and panic attacks. Similarly, cigarette smoking during adolescence, which has deleterious effects on respiratory function, also predicts future panic attacks but not social anxiety (Johnson *et al.*, 2000). The same is not generally the case for illicitly abused substances, which exhibit broader associations with anxiety (Rutter *et al.*, 2006). These findings are consistent with considerable research implicating respiratory dysfunction in childhood separation anxiety disorder and adult panic disorder.

Pathophysiology

Genetics

Research on familial aggregation has examined genetic transmission at the level of diagnostic concordance, that is, family and genetically informative studies. Other research examines concordance of intermediate phenotypes and associations with specific genes.

Family studies

Multiple studies, appearing in Table 60.2, have reported an association between parental psychopathology and childhood anxiety disorders. These so-called "top-down" studies evaluate offspring of parents with anxiety disorders. A handful of so-called "bottom-up" studies have ascertained parents of children with anxiety disorders.

A major question concerns the diagnostic specificity of transmission of anxiety disorders. Are they associated with parental anxiety disorders exclusively, or also with major depression (Middeldorp *et al.*, 2005)? The weight of the evidence from studies in Table 60.2 indicates that both parental anxiety and depression predispose children to develop anxiety disorders. Another question concerns the concordance between specific anxiety disorders in parents and offspring. Do anxiety disorders breed true? Here, the evidence is mixed. Some work supports specificity of concordance. For example, a specific, consistent association has been found between parental panic disorder and separation anxiety disorder in offspring. (Capps *et al.*, 1996; Biederman *et al.*, 2001; Biederman *et al.*, 2004). Moreover, separation anxiety disorder accompanied by respiratory dysregulation has a specific association with parental panic disorder (Roberson-Nay *et al.*, 2010), consistent with other data (Klein, 1993). At the same time, others find little transgenerational specificity (Biederman *et al.*, 2004).

Genetically informative designs

Attempts to quantify environmental and genetic components traditionally use twin and adoption studies. However, only twin studies have been conducted on pediatric anxiety disorders.

Twin studies with adults suggest that genetic factors account for approximately 40% of the risk for anxiety, with the remaining variance mostly attributed to nonshared environmental factors (Hettema *et al.*, 2001; Hettema *et al.*, 2005). Moreover, in adults, there is evidence of both unique and shared

liabilities across specific disorders. Thus, adult generalized anxiety disorder and major depressive disorder have been found to share an underlying genetic substrate, differing largely in contributions from nonshared environmental factors. Studies of depressive symptoms in adolescents report comparable associations, namely, that the same set of genes predispose to anxiety before puberty, and to depression after puberty (Silberg *et al.*, 1999; Silberg *et al.*, 2001). There is other evidence of disorder-specific genetic risk for a few features of adult anxiety disorders. For example, in adults, there appears to be distinct genetic risk for panic disorder, phobias, generalized anxiety disorder, and major depression (Hettema *et al.*, 2005). At the same time, other evidence suggests that all forms of adult anxiety result from a complex mix of genetic influences, including both disorder-specific, and disorder-unique, liability factors (Middeldorp *et al.*, 2005).

Early studies generated divergent estimates of heritability, related to methodological differences (Eley & Stevenson, 1999; Topolski *et al.*, 1999; Eley *et al.*, 2003; Eley *et al.*, 2004; Bolton *et al.*, 2006). However, recent approaches have begun to overcome methodological difficulties. The most extensive research has been with separation anxiety disorder. Eighteen cohorts have generated heritability estimates generally consistent with findings on adult anxiety disorders (Scaini *et al.*, 2012). Other work has examined the heritability of scale scores on broad-band scales (Lamb *et al.*, 2010) or of behavioral inhibition (Goldsmith & Lemery, 2000). For both, genetic factors account for about 30–40% of the variance, with nonshared environmental factors accounting for much of the remaining variance, as in adults. Novel findings also emerge from longitudinal studies of twins using brief anxiety-symptom rating scales. They suggest that the underlying genetic architecture of pediatric anxiety transforms with development, potentially reflecting time-sensitive activation, and suppression of specific genetic factors, potentially interacting with environmental risk (Kendler *et al.*, 2008).

Symptomatic expression may represent a downstream manifestation of genetically-based perturbations in neural function. The term "endophenotype" refers to the heritable component of a phenotype, believed to be more closely linked to neural function than the disorder itself (Gottesman & Gould, 2003). In the entire field of mental health, there is only weak support for a few possible endophenotypes. In pediatric anxiety disorders, three have received moderate support: behavioral inhibition, autonomic function (Grillon *et al.*, 1997; Merikangas *et al.*, 1999), and respiratory dysfunction (Battaglia *et al.*, 2009; Roberson-Nay *et al.*, 2010).

Molecular genetics

Perspectives on psychiatric genetics have advanced to the point where most mental disorders, including pediatric anxiety disorders, are viewed as so-called "complex disorders." The complexity is related to the panoply of genetic and nongenetic factors, each making small contributions to the phenotype. One approach has attempted to link specific genetic polymorphisms

Table 60.2 Anxiety in children as a function of parental psychopathology.

Top-down studies		Odds ratio between parental psychopathology and anxiety disorders in offspring versus normal controls
Author	**Parental diagnosis (N of offspring)**	
Weissman et al. (1984)	MDD and PD (19) (mothers)	10.4*
	MDD (23) (mothers)	2.3
Turner et al. (1987)	OCD or AGO (16)	7.2*
	Dysthymia (14)	5.5*
Rende et al. (1995)	MDD (164)	2.2 T1*; 2.9 T2*
	No MDD (68)	0.92 T1; 0.92 T2
Warner et al. (1995)	MDD (32)	2.5*
	MDD and PD (60)	1.1
	PD (17)	2.3*
Capps et al. (1996)	AGO (16)	3.9*
Beidel and Turner (1997)	AD (28)	5.4*
	MDD (24)	5.7*
	AD and MDD (29)	5.4*
Merikangas et al. (1999)	AD, AGO, and OAD (36)	2.5
Biederman et al. (2001)		(≥two anxiety disorders)
	PD and MDD (141)	8.2*
	MDD (46)	4.3
	PD (26)	8.8*
	No PD or MDD (99)	–
McClure et al. (2001)	Anxiety, no MDD (40 in mother)	3.1* (anxiety in child)
	MDD, no anxiety (248 in mother)	1.6 (anxiety in child)
	Anxiety and MDD (110 in mother)	3.6* (anxiety in child)
Biederman et al. (2004)		(≥two anxiety disorders)
	PD and MDD (56)	2.3* (anxiety in child, PD in parent)
	MDD (132)	1.3 (anxiety in child, MDD in parent)
	PD (55)	
	No PD or MDD (491)	
Pine et al. (2005)	PD and MDD (41)	4.9* (anxiety in child, PD in parent)
	MDD (53)	
	PD (24)	4.8* (anxiety child, MDD in parent)
	No PD or MDD (26)	
Bottom-up studies		Odds ratio between parental psychopathology and anxiety disorders in offspring versus normal controls
Author	Children's diagnoses (N of mothers)	
Last et al. (1991)	SAD (19)	With PD in parents
		1.4 (SAD in child)
	OAD (22)	4.2* (OAD in child)
	OAD and SAD (17)	10.7* (OAD & SAD in child)
Lieb et al. (2000)	SoPh (n = 58)	With SoPh in child
		4.7* (parent SoPh)
		3.5* (parent other anxiety)
		3.6* (parent depression)
Beesdo et al. (2010)	GAD (106)	3.8* (parent–child GAD)
	Other anxiety (732)	1.8* (parent non-GAD anxiety, child GAD)
	Depressive disorders (686)	1.8* (parent depressive disorder, child GAD)

Parental diagnoses: MDD, OCD, AGO, PD, = major depression, obsessive compulsive disorder, agoraphobia, panic disorder.
Offspring diagnoses: OAD, GAD, SAD, AD = overanxious disorder, generalized anxiety, separation anxiety, anxiety disorder including PD, OCD, or social phobia.
T1, time one; T2, 2-year follow-up.
*95% confidence interval of odds ratio excludes 1.0 (i.e., statistically significant at $p \leq 0.05$)

to neural and cognitive dysfunction in anxiety disorders, but this has not generated consistent findings (Pine *et al.*, 2010). Some findings suggest that genetic perturbations predispose to psychopathology through their interaction with environmental risk (see Chapters 23–25). For example, adults with two specific alleles and high stress exposure are reported to be at relatively elevated risk for major depressive disorder (Caspi *et al.*, 2003). However, there is controversy about the robustness of these associations (reviewed elsewhere in this volume), and about approaches used for testing interactions with specific genes. A final set of studies has used other techniques with inconclusive results (McGrath *et al.*, 2012; Sakolsky *et al.*, 2012).

Psychobiology
Neural circuitry in animals

Advances in animal research have led to the view that differences in anxiety states reflect individual differences in neural function (Gross & Hen, 2004). Animal models have been useful because there is strong cross-species conservation in the brain circuitry of fear and anxiety states. Perhaps the best understood phenomena are learned fears, which can be modeled by the so-called "fear-conditioning" experiment, where an aversive stimulus, such as a shock or air-puff, is paired with a neutral stimulus, such as a light or tone. Figure 60.1 illustrates the format of the fear-conditioning experiment in a rodent.

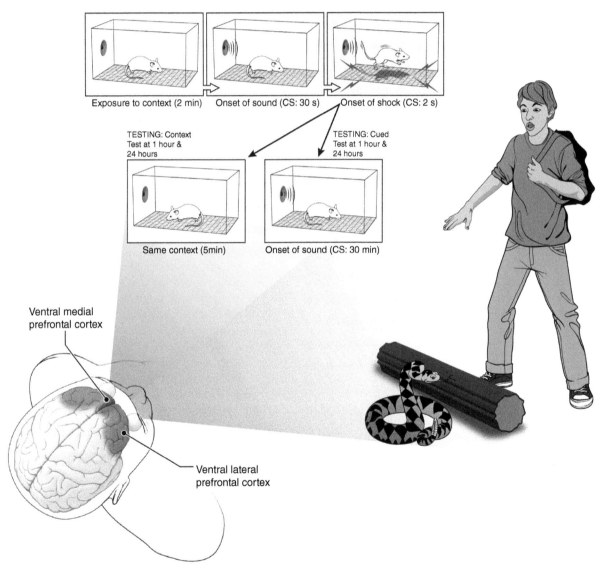

Exposure to context (2 min) Onset of sound (CS: 30 s) Onset of shock (CS: 2 s)

TESTING: Context
Test at 1 hour &
24 hours

TESTING: Cued
Test at 1 hour &
24 hours

Same context (5min) Onset of sound (CS: 30 min)

Ventral medial
prefrontal cortex

Ventral lateral
prefrontal cortex

Figure 60.1 This figure shows two specific behaviors that have been studied in animals and extended through brain imaging research to children. One of these behaviors involves fear conditioning, when a neutral stimulus acquires the capacity to evoke fear, and extinction, when subsequent learning allows the organism to no longer treat the conditioned stimulus as dangerous. The other behavior involves attention orienting, when a threat in the environment captures attention. Brain imaging research links fear conditioning to a brain circuit involving the amygdala and the ventro-medial portion of the prefrontal cortex (PFC). Similarly, studies of the amygdala and ventro-lateral PFC functions link clinical anxiety to perturbed attention to threat.

Following conditioning, the formerly neutral stimulus provokes fear, through changes in neural circuitry involving the amygdala, which is a bilateral collection of individual nuclei located within the brain's medial temporal lobes (LeDoux, 2000). Once fear is established, some individuals retain it, while others do not—the fear has become extinguished. The failure to extinguish might reflect the failure of an active neural process leading to a tendency to maintain anxiety. Consequently, there is considerable interest in the process of extinction, which is mediated by specific sectors of the frontal cortex (Quirk & Gehlert, 2003). This process is also illustrated in Figure 60.1, when the conditioned stimulus is repeatedly presented without the aversive stimulus.

Unlearned fears that develop without prior experience are regulated by distinct, but related, neural circuits from the circuits that regulate conditioning and extinction (Davis, 1998). Unlike learned fears, unlearned fears may not extinguish, suggestive of distinct neural circuitry. Much like work on extinction, research on unlearned fear may be particularly clinically relevant, because most clinical anxiety involves fear about circumstances that arise independent of previous learning.

Neural development and fear

Functioning of the mature fear circuit in rodents reflects long-term influences of the early life rearing environment. Much work in rodents shows that rearing effects occur during specific points in development. Interference with normal maternal care, specifically early in development, lowers the threshold for engaging the fear circuit (Meaney, 2001). Work in nonhuman primates demonstrates at least some comparable associations (Suomi, 2003), with some evidence of unique developmental effects (Amaral, 2002).

Human physiology and neural circuitry

The peripheral physiologic measure best understood in humans, in terms of neuroanatomical detail, is the startle reflex. At least in some circumstances, the same neural circuit involved in fear conditioning in rodents is thought to mediate augmentation of this reflex in humans. Individual differences in anxiety have been related to startle abnormalities in various samples, including in children and adult anxiety disorders (Grillon, 2002; Grillon & Baas, 2003), and in asymptomatic children of parents with an anxiety disorder (Grillon et al., 1997, 1998) or major depression (Grillon et al., 2005).

Despite cross-species parallels, reservations about clinical relevance remain. Overall, observed associations with clinical indices are marginal, at best, for either startle or skin conductance response (SCR) (Lissek et al., 2005). Beyond measures related to conditioning, the most developed physiologic line of research has examined associations between respiratory dysregulation and panic disorder (Klein, 1993). Much like a well-lit room for a rodent, respiratory stimulants represent unlearned, fear-inducing, stimuli for air-breathing organisms, including humans. A wealth of studies suggests that

sensitivity to respiratory stimulants (such as carbon dioxide [CO_2]) identifies individuals with a diathesis for anxiety closely related to spontaneous panic attacks. Sensitivity to CO_2 has been found in children with separation anxiety disorder, but not social anxiety disorder, and especially in children with the combination of separation anxiety disorder and parental panic disorder (Roberson-Nay et al., 2010). These associations tend to be found more consistently than with measures of startle or SCR. Nevertheless, even for such respiratory measures, the findings remain of minimal clinical significance at the current time.

Recent work in rodents suggests that the amygdala directly detects CO_2 and produces fear behaviors. In an experiment of nature in humans, the role of the amygdala in response to CO_2 was examined in three individuals with a very rare condition, the Urbach–Wiethe syndrome, which produces both specific bilateral amygdala lesions, and the inability to experience some types of normal fears. It was expected that, in the absence of a functioning amygdala, subjects would not experience fear when exposed to 35% CO_2. Unexpectedly, all three responded with severe fear, approximating panic. Therefore, it appears that fear reactions to CO_2 are regulated by a circuit that does not encompass the amygdala. Such findings are consonant with the view that neural mechanisms, leading to panic disorder, differ from those in conditioned fears and phobias, and that panic attacks are not simply expressions of exaggerated fear. This topic has received much attention, primarily focused on research in adults, where panic disorder typically is expressed.

Human cognition and anxiety

Threats receive priority for cognitive processing, relative to neutral stimuli, as is reflected in several psychological processes, most consistently attention and memory. In animals, the effect can be studied using brain lesions or neurophysiologic recordings, and in humans using performance on laboratory paradigms. While a range of cognitive processes have been explored, the data most consistently link individual differences in attention to differences in anxiety (Pine et al., 2009). Therefore, this area is selectively summarized.

In animals, threats have been shown to disrupt strategic control of attention or attention orienting (Davis & Whalen, 2001). Two procedures have been used most consistently in humans to probe threat-related effects on attention. In one procedure, the so-called emotional-Stroop test, increases in latency emerge when naming the colors of "threat" words compared to "neutral" words (Williams et al., 1996). In the other procedure, the so-called "dot-probe test," reaction time to a spatial probe is quantified depending on how close the probe is to "threat" words or pictures (Mogg & Bradley, 1998; Bar-Haim et al., 2007). Both tests find relatively consistent associations with anxiety in children and adults. The circuitry mediating these behaviors has been mapped in humans and other mammals, as illustrated in Figure 60.1, adjacent to the schematic fear conditioning experiment. For attention, the figure displays the capacity of natural threats, such as the snake in the figure, to capture attention. This circuitry is thought to be supported by multiple components, including a component in ventro-lateral prefrontal cortex (PFC) that becomes engaged very rapidly after a threat is encountered. Because this attention response can be deployed very rapidly, even outside of awareness, special techniques might be needed to change such attention responding. For example, novel work in this area uses computer-based cognitive training to reduce attention bias in healthy and anxious children and adults (Eldar *et al.*, 2012). Thus, research on attention in anxiety may one day become clinically relevant.

Imaging

Most brain imaging studies in anxious children rely on one of two imaging procedures: neuromorphometry, which measures brain structure, and functional magnetic resonance imaging (fMRI), which measures changes in blood flow in various brain regions, during various cognitive processes. Only a handful of imaging studies examine anxious children. While morphometry studies have demonstrated perturbations in amygdala volume as a function of anxiety in children and adults (Blackford & Pine, 2012), some studies find increased volume whereas others find decreased volume in anxious relative to nonanxious individuals. Other findings are similarly inconclusive.

Functional imaging studies have used fMRI in children with anxiety disorders, as well as related phenotypes, such as behavioral inhibition. Here, consistent findings emerge for the amygdala, expressed as increased response in anxiety relative to healthy individuals for various fear producing stimuli (Pine *et al.*, 2009), as well as in the PFC and striatum (Blackford & Pine, 2012). Thus, findings link perturbations in distributed neural circuits to individual differences in anxiety.

Given cross-species conservation of brain-behavior relationships for fear, there is interest in using fMRI to extend studies in animal models to children and adolescents in a way that is clinically relevant. This research, referred to as "translational" or "clinical" neuroscience, attempts to connect work in animals and humans, as illustrated in Figure 60.1. This figure shows two types of behaviors for which relevant circuitry has been mapped in animals, and for which brain imaging studies are now extending to children and adolescents.

One of these behaviors is shown for a rodent, in the top left-hand corner of the figure, illustrating the expression of fear conditioning. In humans, the circuitry of this process is depicted in the lower left-hand corner of the figure, in blue shading. This circuitry connects the amygdala to the ventro-medial portion of the PFC, as illustrated in the schematic depiction of the child in Figure 60.1. Understanding the relationship between fear expression and brain function has led to interest in the possibility of developing novel pharmacological, computer-based, or psychotherapeutic treatments that target specific circuitry, including the amygdala-PFC circuit involved in conditioning. However, this area is in its infancy, and means for achieving this clinical goal have not yet been defined.

Figure 60.1 also shows a second, potentially clinically relevant behavior. The figure depicts a boy, as he walks in a wooded area, appearing in the lower right corner of the figure, encountering a snake. The figure conveys that dangerous stimuli, such as snakes, capture the boy's attention. As noted above, there has been considerable work mapping the brain circuitry of this attention capture. Like extinction, this behavior also involves a brain circuit connecting the amygdala and PFC. However, whereas extinction involves ventro-medial aspects of the PFC, the capture of attention by threats is thought to involve ventro-lateral aspects of the PFC. In Figure 60.1, this component of the PFC is illustrated in green, and conveys the role of this circuit in regulating attention capture. Much like work on ventro-medial PFC function, interest in ventro-lateral PFC function in anxiety also relates to the pursuit of novel treatments. However, this goal is complicated by the fact that changes in brain circuitry involve a huge number of neurons, whose extraordinary speed of function may prove difficult to capture through currently available techniques.

Treatment

Evidence of suffering experienced by children with anxiety disorders, coupled with findings of long-term effects on functioning, highlights the need for effective treatments. This summary is limited to replicated, large controlled studies that provide evidence of efficacy, and excludes claims of efficacy from case studies. However, the discussion of treatment, unlike other sections of this chapter, includes some observations from clinical experience. In this instance, reference to clinical experience is designed to inform about the use of treatments, which have been shown to be effective.

Although it is parents who seek help for their child, they are frequently unaware of multiple aspects of the child's disorder and its functional ramifications. Therefore, regardless of treatment modality, therapists need to assist parents in understanding the child's condition in all its aspects, as well as how treatment is expected to proceed.

The treatment of anxiety disorders is privileged insofar as several effective approaches, psychotherapeutic and psychopharmacological, have been documented. Many studies include multiple anxiety disorders, typically generalized anxiety disorder, separation anxiety disorder, and social phobia; only a few are restricted to one diagnosis. As a result, clinicians are on reasonably solid ground when extrapolating data on therapeutics to children with any of these anxiety disorders.

Some interventions, such as cognitive behavior therapy (CBT), were originally implemented in anxiety disorders based on a theoretical model of anxiety; others, such as selective serotonin reuptake inhibitor (SSRI) medications, followed from demonstrated efficacy in adults. However, for both, decisions on clinical utility ultimately rest on results of well-conducted randomized controlled trials. Independent of the results from such trials, there are national differences in attitudes toward psychiatric treatment of children, which affect practice. Generally, psychopharmacology is widely accepted in the US, but not universally so, for treating children's psychiatric disorders including anxiety disorders. It is much less so in Europe. However, negative views of psychopharmacological treatment are not based on empirical data establishing the better efficacy or less extreme adverse consequences of one approach versus another, but more likely on beliefs about medication. For example, some individuals view the use of medication as stigmatizing or as defining a child as sick. Others have raised concerns about medications' harmful effects on development. Chapter 43 discusses these issues in depth. Regardless, while more research is needed on various aspects of medications, at the current time, data do not support such concerns with regard to pediatric anxiety disorders. Moreover, as reviewed below, the available data document additive effects with the use of medication and psychotherapy, over either alone, in anxious children. As a result, both treatments clearly have a role in the management of pediatric anxiety disorder.

Psychotherapy

CBT is the best-studied psychotherapy. It is based on various theoretical concerns. One of these concerns follows from the notion that distorted cognitions underlie anxiety symptoms. Consequently, a key aspect of CBT focuses on the child's thought processes, aiming to replace negative beliefs with realistic, neutral, thoughts. The goal is to enable children to abandon irrational thinking about their fears and develop more realistic evaluations.

A second concern relates to avoidance. When children are encouraged to confront their fears and no longer avoid them, they can learn to overcome their fears. Consequently, a second aspect of CBT focuses on reducing avoidance and facilitating children's exposure to feared situations.

Eventually, in virtually all treatments that adopt a CBT approach, a systematic program of gradual exposure to feared situations is implemented, typically using similar components. These may include psycho-education about anxiety, instructing the child to understand his condition, relaxation training, identifying the physical symptoms of one's anxiety, teaching of cognitive strategies for coping, and cognitive restructuring. These components are usually implemented early. Next, children are helped to undergo graded exposure during which they are expected to use their newly learned strategies while receiving self-reinforcement as well as encouragement from the therapist and parents. Of note, not all CBT treatments actively include the family's involvement. However, because parent involvement is important in most cases to facilitate the child's exposure to feared situations, active involvement of families is expected even for forms of CBT that do not explicitly stipulate family involvement. For example, it is difficult to appreciate how a child with severe separation anxiety can receive optimal therapeutic assistance without considerable parental involvement. Some children may have difficulty articulating their thoughts and

even their fears. In such situations, more effort will be deployed on systematic gradual exposure, to eliminate behavioral avoidance, than on self-monitoring of thought processes. Because a main source of anticipatory anxiety is due to the uncertainty of what may happen, it is helpful to involve anxious children in the process of selecting how to implement exposures to feared situations, so children are fully cognizant of what is expected of them (the "what if" worry, characteristic of anxious children, is thereby minimized).

A major positive feature of CBT is the availability of treatment manuals. These provide a useful guide for treating individual children. Moreover, treatment manuals allow comparisons across studies using different variants of CBT. Many studies have compared CBT to other conditions, most often a no-treatment or wait-list control. Because wait-list controls are inadequate to control for many nonspecific effects of CBT, a far more informative approach involves a comparison with an active attention control (psychotherapy without specific content). Very few studies have included attention controls.

A recent relatively large multisite study found that 12 weeks of intensive CBT was superior to a pill placebo, with marked improvement rates of 59.7% versus 23.7%, respectively (Walkup et al., 2008). Problematically, pill placebo and psychotherapy contrasts cannot be blinded, nor equivalent in professional attention. As a result, in such designs, the true advantage of the psychotherapy cannot be confirmed, since one might assume a greater expectation of benefit to accrue in an unblinded psychotherapy context than in a blinded medication/pill placebo contrast.

Although specific phobias, separation, social, and generalized anxiety disorders all are anxiety disorders, they have different behavioral consequences; these are typically targeted by treatment tailoring. In this spirit, some treatments have been developed specifically for social anxiety. Social Effectiveness Therapy for Children (SET-C), one such treatment, is a clinic-based group psychotherapy for social anxiety, focused on the behavioral, rather than cognitive aspects of social anxiety. It provides the context of a social group, which is often anxiety provoking for those with social anxiety disorder, relying on *in vivo* exposure to feared social situations as a central treatment component. SET-C places particularly strong emphasis on behavioral exposure to enhance extinction, and to social skills training, rather than distorted thinking, which is more strongly emphasized in other studies of CBT.

Evidence shows that most youngsters who suffer from anxiety disorders are not referred for treatment. Various strategies have been used to reach such children; one is incorporated in schools to identify and treat unidentified children. For example, a school-based group intervention for socially anxious adolescents has been developed, utilizing principles of SET-C. This intervention, administered directly in high schools, has been shown to be effective, compared to a nonspecific control treatment (Masia-Warner et al., 2007). Such school-based treatments have the great advantage of allowing for intervening in the setting in which consequences of social anxiety are most deleterious. Other approaches capitalize on increased access that might be possible through computers and social media. For example, internet-delivered CBT has been developed (Khanna & Kendall, 2008). Evidence of efficacy for children with anxiety disorders has not yet been documented.

At this time, we do not know which components of effective treatments produce benefit. Moreover, from a clinical perspective, high rates of remission for a range of treatments, including placebo, suggest that there may be merit to postponing specific formal intervention for a couple of weeks, while monitoring the child's progress.

CBT has been examined for potential preventative effects. Some forms of prevention target children already affected with some relatively mild levels of anxiety or with behavioral inhibition, a potential precursor of more severe anxiety. In these studies, children receive CBT in attempts to prevent the development of full-blown anxiety disorders. Results suggest that CBT reduces anxiety symptoms in such children (Rapee et al., 2005). However, since the children already have some levels of anxiety symptoms, the interventions only apply to an affected, select group of children.

Pharmacotherapy

SSRIs have extensive documentation of safety and efficacy in adult anxiety disorders (specific phobias are exceptions). From a number of controlled studies, the consensus is that SSRIs are highly effective in a variety of pediatric anxiety disorders. The large multisite study, noted earlier, of CBT, sertraline (up to 200 mg/day), combined CBT-sertraline, or placebo, found significant benefit for each mono-therapy over placebo (improvement rates: CBT, 59.7%; sertraline, 54.9%; placebo, 23.7%), and significant superiority for combined treatment (80.7%) over each mono-therapy (Walkup et al., 2008). The contrast between sertraline and placebo in this study is fully blinded, but not the other contrasts, complicating straightforward interpretation of treatment differences. Other findings show efficacy of 6–8 weeks of fluoxetine, paroxetine, sertraline, or fluvoxamine over placebo, in anxious children.

The SSRIs have similar side effect profiles, the most troublesome being behavioral disinhibition (the child becomes ornery, impulsive, or oppositional). Therefore, it seems wise to initiate treatment with a short acting SSRI, and possibly switch to a long-acting formulation, if indicated, such as when compliance is deficient or when the clinician has concerns about potential withdrawal effects. The superiority of combined SSRI and CBT treatment over either mono-therapy fosters questions about the clinical scenarios for which combined treatment is likely to be optimal. Because studies have not addressed this question, we rely on clinical experience. For example, based on clinical observations, there are children who, with behavioral treatment, are able to enter situations they avoided before treatment, but they do so under duress, and still feel anxious. In such instances, addition of an SSRI often reduces residual anxiety. Similarly,

in other scenarios, children may be extremely anxious, to the point where they cannot even begin to initiate exposure therapy. Here, initiation of an SSRI may reduce the child's anxiety in the feared situations to the point where he/she can begin systematic exposure. Based on clinical observations, SSRIs are especially efficacious for anxiety experienced while in the feared situations, but less so for anticipatory anxiety. Consequently, even with a good response to an SSRI, children may retain significant anticipatory anxiety, but not so high so as to preclude exposure, which, in turn, facilitates extinction of anticipatory anxiety. Some clinicians hold that it is advisable to start with behavioral treatment, since it quickly becomes apparent whether it is likely to be helpful, followed by medication, when indicated, for maximal improvement. Thus, based on the literature, one should not settle for less than an excellent response until combined treatment has been attempted.

Summary

Multiple findings demonstrate the clinical importance of child and adolescent anxiety disorders. These include their relatively high prevalence; their associated functional limitations; the fact that they put children at risk for later depression; and their moderately significant continuity with anxiety disorders in adulthood. Epidemiological data generate divergent prevalence rates, with an overall 5-to-10% prevalence in the general population, with girls being overrepresented. Long-term stability has been found for anxiety disorders as a group, but limited evidence of differential outcomes has emerged for particular anxiety disorders. Importantly, childhood anxiety disorders generally have not been found to predict adult psychopathology other than anxiety and depression.

Identification of antecedents of childhood anxiety disorders would facilitate attempts to help children at risk and prevent the development of full-blown anxiety disorders. Early inhibited temperament is one of the few replicated antecedents, acting as a moderate risk factor, particularly for social anxiety disorder. A modest influence for genetic transmission has been found. Nonshared environmental factors appear to play a relatively greater role, but their nature and mechanism of action remain poorly understood. As a result, there is little promise in the targeting of particular environmental factors for prevention or clinical management of childhood anxiety disorders.

Models of brain circuits that regulate fear in animals are being investigated in children. Early studies demonstrate some cross-species similarities. However, it is difficult to disentangle cause and effect, since most imaging studies acquire data at one time point. At this time, the best documented biological feature is for separation anxiety disorder, consisting of respiratory dysregulation, as indexed by hypersensitivity to breathing CO_2 enriched air, which induces perturbations that appear similar to those found in adults with panic disorder.

Treatment of anxiety disorders encompasses psychotherapeutic and psychopharmacological interventions, specifically CBT, behavioral therapy, and SSRIs. Treatment studies of anxious children, with few exceptions, have included multiple anxiety disorders, except for studies of children with social anxiety, exclusively.

References

Achenbach, T.M. (1991) *Manual for the Child Behavior Checklist and 1991 Child Behavior Profile*. Department of Psychiatry, University of Vermont, Burlington, VT.

Amaral, D.G. (2002) The primate amygdala and the neurobiology of social behavior: implications for understanding social anxiety. *Biological Psychiatry* **51** (1), 11–17.

Anderson, J. et al. (1987) DSM-III disorders in preadolescent children: prevalence in a large sample from the general population. *Archives of General Psychiatry* **44** (1), 69–76.

Angold, A. & Costello, E.J. (2000) The child and adolescent psychiatric assessment (CAPA). *Journal of the American Academy of Child and Adolescent Psychiatry* **39** (1), 39–48.

Angold, A. et al. (1996) Precision, reliability and accuracy in the dating of symptom onsets in child and adolescent psychopathology. *Journal of Child Psychology and Psychiatry* **37** (6), 657–664.

Angold, A. et al. (1999) Comorbidity. *Journal of Child Psychology and Psychiatry* **40** (1), 57–87.

Aschenbrand, S.G. et al. (2003) Is childhood separation anxiety disorder a predictor of adult panic disorder and agoraphobia? A seven-year longitudinal study. *Journal of the American Academy of Child and Adolescent Psychiatry* **42** (12), 1478–1485.

Bar-Haim, Y. et al. (2007) Threat-related attentional bias in anxious and non-anxious individuals: a meta-analytic study. *Psychological Bulletin* **133** (1), 1–24.

Battaglia, M. et al. (2009) A genetically informed study of the association between childhood separation anxiety, sensitivity to $CO_{(2)}$, panic disorder, and the effect of childhood parental loss. *Archives of General Psychiatry* **66** (1), 64–71.

Beesdo, K. et al. (2010) Incidence and risk patterns of anxiety and depressive disorders and categorization of generalized anxiety disorder. *Archives of General Psychiatry* **67** (1), 47–57.

Beidel, D.C. & Turner, S.M. (1997) At risk for anxiety: I. Psychopathology in the offspring of anxious parents. *Journal of the American Academy of Child & Adolescent Psychiatry* **36** (7), 918–924.

Benjamin, R.S. et al. (1990) Anxiety disorders in a pediatric sample. *Journal of Anxiety Disorders* **4** (4), 293–316.

Biederman, J. et al. (2001) Patterns of psychopathology and dysfunction in high-risk children of parents with panic disorder and major depression. *The American Journal of Psychiatry* **158** (1), 49–57.

Biederman, J. et al. (2004) Does referral bias impact findings in high-risk offspring for anxiety disorders? A controlled study of high-risk children of non-referred parents with panic disorder/agoraphobia and major depression. *Journal of Affective Disorders* **82** (2), 209–216.

Bird, H. et al. (1988) Estimates of the prevalence of childhood maladjustment in a community survey in Puerto Rico: the use of combined measures. *Archives of General Psychiatry* **45** (12), 1120–1126.

Birmaher, B. et al. (1997) The Screen for Child Anxiety Related Emotional Disorders (SCARED): scale construction and psychometric characteristics. *Journal of the American Academy of Child and Adolescent Psychiatry* **36** (4), 545–553.

Bittner, A. et al. (2004) What characteristics of primary anxiety disorders predict subsequent major depressive disorder? *Journal of Clinical Psychiatry* **65** (5), 618–626.

Blackford, J.U. & Pine, D.S. (2012) Neural substrates of childhood anxiety disorders: a review of neuroimaging findings. *Child and Adolescent Psychiatric Clinics of North America* **21** (3), 501–525.

Bolton, D. et al. (2006) Prevalence and genetic and environmental influences on anxiety disorders in 6-year-old twins. *Psychological Medicine* **36** (3), 335–344.

Breslau, N. (1995) Psychiatric sequelae of low birth weight. *Epidemiologic Reviews* **17** (1), 96–106.

Breslau, N. & Chilcoat, H.D. (2000) Psychiatric sequelae of low birth weight at 11 years of age. *Biological Psychiatry* **47** (11), 1005–1011.

Breslau, N. et al. (1987) Searching for evidence on the validity of generalized anxiety disorder: psychopathology in children of anxious mothers. *Psychiatry Research* **20** (4), 285–297.

Breslau, N. et al. (2000) Neurologic soft signs and low birthweight: their association and neuropsychiatric implications. *Biological Psychiatry* **47** (1), 71–79.

Brooks, S.J. & Kutcher, S. (2003) Diagnosis and measurement of anxiety disorder in adolescents: a review of commonly used instruments. *Journal of Child and Adolescent Psychopharmacology* **13** (3), 351–400.

Capps, L. et al. (1996) Fear, anxiety and perceived control in children of agoraphobic parents. *Journal of Child Psychology and Psychiatry* **37** (4), 445–452.

Caspi, A. et al. (1996) Behavioral observations at age 3 years predict adult psychiatric disorders. Longitudinal evidence from a birth cohort. *Archives of General Psychiatry* **53** (11), 1033–1039.

Caspi, A. et al. (2003) Influence of life stress on depression: moderation by a polymorphism in the 5-HTT gene. *Science* **301** (5631), 386–389.

Clauss, J.A. & Blackford, J.U. (2012) Behavioral inhibition and risk for developing social anxiety disorder: a meta-analytic study. *Journal of the American Academy of Child and Adolescent Psychiatry* **51** (10), 1066–1075, e1061.

Copeland, W.E. et al. (2009) Childhood and adolescent psychiatric disorders as predictors of young adult disorders. *Archives of General Psychiatry* **66** (7), 764–772.

Costello, E. et al. (1988) Psychiatric disorders in pediatric primary care: prevalence and risk factors. *Archives of General Psychiatry* **45** (12), 1107–1116.

Costello, E. et al. (1996) The Great Smoky Mountains Study of youth: functional impairment and serious emotional disturbance. *Archives of General Psychiatry* **53** (12), 1137–1143.

Costello, E.J. et al. (1999) Adolescent outcomes of childhood disorders: the consequences of severity and impairment. *Journal of the American Academy of Child and Adolescent Psychiatry* **38** (2), 121–128.

Costello, E et al. (2002) Development and natural history of mood disorders. *Biological Psychiatry* **52** (6), 529–542.

Costello, E.J. et al. (2003) Prevalence and development of psychiatric disorders in childhood and adolescence. *Archives of General Psychiatry* **60** (8), 837–844.

Costello, E.J. *et al.* (2004) Developmental epidemiology of anxiety disorders. In: *Phobic and Anxiety Disorders in Children and Adolescents.* (ed T.H. Ollendick), pp. 61–91. Oxford University Press, New York.

Costello, E.J. *et al.* (2005) The developmental epidemiology of anxiety disorders: phenomenology, prevalence, and comorbidity. *Child and Adolescent Psychiatric Clinics of North America* **14** (4), 631–648, vii.

Costello, E.J. *et al.* (2010) Association of family income supplements in adolescence with development of psychiatric and substance use disorders in adulthood among an American Indian population. *JAMA* **303** (19), 1954–1960.

Crawford, A.M. & Manassis, K. (2011) Anxiety, social skills, friendship quality, and peer victimization: an integrated model. *Journal of Anxiety Disorders* **25** (7), 924–931.

Davis, M. (1998) Are different parts of the extended amygdala involved in fear versus anxiety? *Biological Psychiatry* **44** (12), 1239–1247.

Davis, M. & Whalen, P.J. (2001) The amygdala: vigilance and emotion. *Molecular Psychiatry* **6** (1), 13–34.

Eldar, S. *et al.* (2012) Attention bias modification treatment for pediatric anxiety disorders: a randomized controlled trial. *The American Journal of Psychiatry* **169** (2), 213–220.

Eley, T.C. & Stevenson, J. (1999) Exploring the covariation between anxiety and depression symptoms: a genetic analysis of the effects of age and sex. *Journal of Child Psychology and Psychiatry* **40** (8), 1273–1282.

Eley, T.C. & Stevenson, J. (2000) Specific life events and chronic experiences differentially associated with depression and anxiety in young twins. *Journal of Abnormal Child Psychology* **28** (4), 383–394.

Eley, T.C. *et al.* (2003) A twin study of anxiety-related behaviours in pre-school children. *Journal of Child Psychology and Psychiatry* **44** (7), 945–960.

Eley, T.C. *et al.* (2004) Heart-beat perception, panic/somatic symptoms and anxiety sensitivity in children. *Behaviour Research and Therapy* **42** (4), 439–448.

Essau, C. *et al.* (1999) Frequency and comorbidity of social phobia and social fears in adolescents. *Behaviour Research and Therapy* **37** (9), 831–843.

Esser, G. *et al.* (1990) Epidemiology and course of psychiatric disorders in school-age children—results of a longitudinal study. *Journal of Child Psychology and Psychiatry* **31** (2), 243–263.

Feehan, M. *et al.* (1993) Mental health disorders from age 15 to age 18 years. *Journal of the American Academy of Child and Adolescent Psychiatry* **32** (6), 1118–1126.

Fergusson, D.M. *et al.* (1993) Prevalence and comorbidity of DSM-III-R diagnoses in a birth cohort of 15 year olds. *Journal of the American Academy of Child & Adolescent Psychiatry* **32** (6), 1127–1134.

Fox, N.A. *et al.* (2005) Behavioral inhibition: linking biology and behavior within a developmental framework. *Annual Review of Psychology* **56**, 235–262.

Fyer, A.J. (1998) Current approaches to etiology and pathophysiology of specific phobia. *Biological Psychiatry* **44** (12), 1295–1304.

Gerring, J.P. *et al.* (2002) Clinical predictors of posttraumatic stress disorder after closed head injury in children. *Journal of the American Academy of Child and Adolescent Psychiatry* **41** (2), 157–165.

Goldsmith, H.H. & Lemery, K.S. (2000) Linking temperamental fearfulness and anxiety symptoms: a behavior-genetic perspective. *Biological Psychiatry* **48** (12), 1199–1209.

Goodwin, R.D. *et al.* (2003) Asthma and panic attacks among youth in the community. *Journal of Asthma* **40** (2), 139–145.

Goodwin, R.D. *et al.* (2004) Association between anxiety disorders and substance use disorders among young persons: results of a 21-year longitudinal study. *Journal of Psychiatric Research* **38** (3), 295–304.

Gottesman, I.I. & Gould, T.D. (2003) The endophenotype concept in psychiatry: etymology and strategic intentions. *The American Journal of Psychiatry* **160** (4), 636–645.

Grillon, C. (2002) Associative learning deficits increase symptoms of anxiety in humans. *Biological Psychiatry* **51** (11), 851–858.

Grillon, C. & Baas, J. (2003) A review of the modulation of the startle reflex by affective states and its application in psychiatry. *Clinical Neurophysiology* **114** (9), 1557–1579.

Grillon, C. *et al.* (1997) Startle modulation in children at risk for anxiety disorders and/or alcoholism. *Journal of the American Academy of Child and Adolescent Psychiatry* **36** (7), 925–932.

Grillon, C. *et al.* (1998) Fear-potentiated startle in adolescent offspring of parents with anxiety disorders. *Biological Psychiatry* **44** (10), 990–997.

Grillon, C. *et al.* (2005) Families at high and low risk for depression: a three-generation startle study. *Biological Psychiatry* **57** (9), 953–960.

Gross, C. & Hen, R. (2004) The developmental origins of anxiety. *Nature Reviews Neuroscience* **5** (7), 545–552.

Hankin, B.L. & Abramson, L.Y. (2001) Development of gender differences in depression: an elaborated cognitive vulnerability-transactional stress theory. *Psychological Bulletin* **127** (6), 773–796.

Hayward, C. *et al.* (1998) Linking self-reported childhood behavioral inhibition to adolescent social phobia. *Journal of the American Academy of Child and Adolescent Psychiatry* **37** (12), 1308–1316.

Hettema, J.M. *et al.* (2001) A review and meta-analysis of the genetic epidemiology of anxiety disorders. *The American Journal of Psychiatry* **158** (10), 1568–1578.

Hettema, J.M. *et al.* (2005) The structure of genetic and environmental risk factors for anxiety disorders in men and women. *Archives of General Psychiatry* **62** (2), 182–189.

Ingman, K.A. *et al.* (1999) Cross-cultural aspects of fears in African children and adolescents. *Behaviour Research and Therapy* **37** (4), 337–345.

Jaffee, S.R. *et al.* (2005) Cumulative prevalence of psychiatric disorder in youths. *Journal of the American Academy of Child and Adolescent Psychiatry* **44** (5), 406–407.

Johnson, J.G. *et al.* (2000) Association between cigarette smoking and anxiety disorders during adolescence and early adulthood. *JAMA* **284** (18), 2348–2351.

Kagan, J. (1994) *Galen's Prophecy.* Basic Books, New York, NY.

Kagan, J. *et al.* (2001) Temperamental contributions to the affect family of anxiety. *The Psychiatric Clinics of North America* **24** (4), 677–688.

Kaplow, J.B. *et al.* (2001) The prospective relation between dimensions of anxiety and the initiation of adolescent alcohol use. *Journal of Clinical Child Psychology* **30** (3), 316–326.

Kassam-Adams, N. *et al.* (2005) Heart rate and posttraumatic stress in injured children. *Archives of General Psychiatry* **62** (3), 335–340.

Kaufman, J. *et al.* (1997) Schedule for Affective Disorders and Schizophrenia for School-Age Children-Present and Lifetime Version (K-SADS-PL): initial reliability and validity data. *Journal of the American Academy of Child and Adolescent Psychiatry* **36** (7), 980–988.

Kaufman, J. *et al.* (2000) K-Sads-Pl. *Journal of the American Academy of Child and Adolescent Psychiatry* **39** (10), 1208.

Kendler, K.S. *et al.* (2008) A longitudinal twin study of fears from middle childhood to early adulthood: evidence for a developmentally dynamic genome. *Archives of General Psychiatry* **65** (4), 421–429.

Kessler, R.C. *et al.* (2002) The effects of co-morbidity on the onset and persistence of generalized anxiety disorder in the ICPE surveys. International Consortium in Psychiatric Epidemiology. *Psychological Medicine* **32** (7), 1213–1225.

Kessler, R.C. *et al.* (2012) Composite International Diagnostic Interview screening scales for DSM-IV anxiety and mood disorders. *Psychological Medicine* **43** (2), 1625–1637.

Khanna, M.S. & Kendall, P.C. (2008) Computer-assisted CBT for child anxiety: the Coping Cat CD-ROM. *Cognitiive Behavioral Practice* **15** (2), 159–165.

Kim-Cohen, J. *et al.* (2003) Prior juvenile diagnoses in adults with mental disorder: developmental follow-back of a prospective-longitudinal cohort. *Archives of General Psychiatry* **60** (7), 709–717.

Klein, D.F. (1993) False suffocation alarms, spontaneous panics, and related conditions. An integrative hypothesis. *Archives of General Psychiatry* **50** (4), 306–317.

Klein, R.G. (1995) Is panic disorder associated with childhood separation anxiety disorder? *Clinical Neuropharmacology* **18**, S7–S14.

Klein, D.F. (1996) Panic disorder and agoraphobia: hypothesis hothouse. *Journal of Clinical Psychiatry* **57** (Suppl 6), 21–27.

Kramer, T. & Garralda, M.E. (1998) Psychiatric disorders in adolescents in primary care. *The British Journal of Psychiatry* **173** (6), 508–513.

Lamb, D.J. *et al.* (2010) Heritability of anxious-depressive and withdrawn behavior: age-related changes during adolescence. *Journal of the American Academy of Child and Adolescent Psychiatry* **49** (3), 248–255.

Last, C.G. *et al.* (1991) Anxiety disorders in children and their families. *Archives of General Psychiatry* **48** (10), 928–934.

Last, C.G. *et al.* (1997) Anxious children in adulthood: a prospective study of adjustment. *Journal of the American Academy of Child and Adolescent Psychiatry* **36** (5), 645–652.

LeDoux, J.E. (2000) Emotion circuits in the brain. *Annual Review of Neuroscience* **23**, 155–184.

Lewinsohn, P.M. *et al.* (1997) Lifetime comorbidity among anxiety disorders and between anxiety disorders and other mental disorders in adolescents. *Journal of Anxiety Disorders* **11** (4), 377–394.

Lewinsohn, P.M. *et al.* (1998) Gender differences in anxiety disorders and anxiety symptoms in adolescents. *Journal of Abnormal Psychology* **107** (1), 109–117.

Lewis-Morrarty, E. *et al.* (2012) Maternal over-control moderates the association between early childhood behavioral inhibition and adolescent social anxiety symptoms. *Journal of Abnormal Child Psychology* **40** (8), 1363–1373.

Lieb, R. *et al.* (2000) Parental psychopathology, parenting styles, and the risk of social phobia in offspring: a prospective-longitudinal community study. *Archives of General Psychiatry* **57** (9), 859–866.

Lissek, S. *et al.* (2005) Classical fear conditioning in the anxiety disorders: a meta-analysis. *Behaviour Research and Therapy* **43** (11), 1391–1424.

Magee, W. *et al.* (1996) Agoraphobia, simple phobia, and social phobia in the national comorbidity survey. *Archives of General Psychiatry* **53** (2), 159–168.

Mannuzza, S. *et al.* (2002) Anxiety sensitivity among children of parents with anxiety disorders: a controlled high-risk study. *Journal of Anxiety Disorders* **16** (2), 135–148.

March, J.S. & Sullivan, K. (1999) Test-retest reliability of the Multidimensional Anxiety Scale for children. *Journal of Anxiety Disorders* **13** (4), 349–358.

March, J.S. *et al.* (1997) The Multidimensional Anxiety Scale for Children (MASC): factor structure, reliability, and validity. *Journal of the American Academy of Child and Adolescent Psychiatry* **36** (4), 554–565.

March, J.S. *et al.* (2000) Anxiety as a predictor and outcome variable in the multimodal treatment study of children with ADHD (MTA). *Journal of Abnormal Child Psychology* **28** (6), 527–541.

Masia-Warner, C. *et al.* (2007) Treating adolescents with social anxiety disorder in school: an attention control trial. *Journal of Child Psychology and Psychiatry* **48** (7), 676–686.

McClure, E. *et al.* (2001) Parental anxiety disorders, child anxiety disorders, and the perceived parent–child relationship in an Australian high-risk sample. *Journal of Abnormal Child Psychology* **29** (1), 1–10.

McGee, R.O.B. *et al.* (1990) DSM-III disorders in a large sample of adolescents. *Journal of the American Academy of Child & Adolescent Psychiatry* **29** (4), 611–619.

McGee, R. *et al.* (1992) DSM-III disorders from age 11 to age 15 years. *Journal of the American Academy of Child and Adolescent Psychiatry* **31** (1), 50–59.

McGrath, L.M. *et al.* (2012) Bringing a developmental perspective to anxiety genetics. *Development and Psychopathology* **24** (4), 1179–1193.

Meaney, M.J. (2001) Maternal care, gene expression, and the transmission of individual differences in stress reactivity across generations. *Annual Review of Neuroscience* **24**, 1161–1192.

Merikangas, K.R. *et al.* (1999) Vulnerability factors among children at risk for anxiety disorders. *Biological Psychiatry* **46** (11), 1523–1535.

Merikangas, K.R. *et al.* (2010) Prevalence and treatment of mental disorders among US children in the 2001–2004 NHANES. *Pediatrics* **125** (1), 75–81.

Middeldorp, C.M. *et al.* (2005) The co-morbidity of anxiety and depression in the perspective of genetic epidemiology. A review of twin and family studies. *Psychological Medicine* **35** (5), 611–624.

Mogg, K. & Bradley, B.P. (1998) A cognitive-motivational analysis of anxiety. *Behaviour Research and Therapy* **36** (9), 809–848.

Obradovic, J. *et al.* (2011) The interactive effect of marital conflict and stress reactivity on externalizing and internalizing symptoms: the role of laboratory stressors. *Development and Psychopathology* **23** (1), 101–114.

Ollendick, T.H. & Hirshfeld-Becker, D.R. (2002) The developmental psychopathology of social anxiety disorder. *Biological Psychiatry* **51** (1), 44–58.

Ollendick, T.H. *et al.* (1996) Fears in American, Australian, Chinese, and Nigerian children and adolescents: a cross-cultural study. *Journal of Child Psychology and Psychiatry* **37** (2), 213–220.

Pine, D.S. & Cohen, J.A. (2002) Trauma in children and adolescents: risk and treatment of psychiatric sequelae. *Biological Psychiatry* **51** (7), 519–531.

Pine, D.S. *et al.* (1998) The risk for early-adulthood anxiety and depressive disorders in adolescents with anxiety and depressive disorders. *Archives of General Psychiatry* **55** (1), 56–64.

Pine, D.S. *et al.* (2000) Social phobia and the persistence of conduct problems. *Journal of Child Psychology and Psychiatry* **41** (5), 657–665.

Pine, D.S. *et al.* (2001) Adolescent fears as predictors of depression. *Biological Psychiatry* **50** (9), 721–724.

Pine, D.S. *et al.* (2002) Adolescent life events as predictors of adult depression. *Journal of Affective Disorders* **68** (1), 49–57.

Pine, D.S. *et al.* (2005) Face-emotion processing in offspring at risk for panic disorder. *Journal of the American Academy of Child & Adolescent Psychiatry* **44** (7), 664–672.

Pine, D.S. *et al.* (2009) Challenges in developing novel treatments for childhood disorders: lessons from research on anxiety. *Neuropsychopharmacology* **34** (1), 213–228.

Pine, D.S. *et al.* (2010) Imaging-genetics applications in child psychiatry. *Journal of the American Academy of Child and Adolescent Psychiatry* **49** (8), 772–782.

Poulton, R. *et al.* (2009). Continuity and etiology of anxiety disorders: are they stable across the life course? In: *Stress-Induced and Fear Circuitry Disorders: Refining the Research Agenda for DSM-V*. (eds. G. Andrews *et al.*). pp. 105–124. American Psychiatric Association, Washington, DC.

Quirk, G.J. & Gehlert, D.R. (2003) Inhibition of the amygdala: key to pathological states? *Annals of the New York Academy of Sciences* **985**, 263–272.

Rapee, R.M. *et al.* (2005) Prevention and early intervention of anxiety disorders in inhibited preschool children. *Journal of Consulting and Clinical Psychology* **73** (3), 488–497.

Reed, V. & Wittchen, H.U. (1998) DSM-IV panic attacks and panic disorder in a community sample of adolescents and young adults: how specific are panic attacks? *Journal of Psychiatric Research* **32** (6), 335–345.

Reich, W. (2000) Diagnostic interview for children and adolescents (DICA). *Journal of the American Academy of Child and Adolescent Psychiatry* **39** (1), 59–66.

Rende, R. *et al.* (1995) Sibling resemblance for psychiatric disorders in offspring at high and low risk for depression. *Journal of Child Psychology and Psychiatry* **36** (8), 1353–1363.

Roberson-Nay, R. *et al.* (2010) Carbon dioxide hypersensitivity in separation-anxious offspring of parents with panic disorder. *Biological Psychiatry* **67** (12), 1171–1177.

Rueter, M.A. *et al.* (1999) First onset of depressive or anxiety disorders predicted by the longitudinal course of internalizing symptoms and parent-adolescent disagreements. *Archives of General Psychiatry* **56** (8), 726–732.

Rupp, A.S.G. (2003) The Pediatric Anxiety Rating Scale (PARS): development and psychometric properties. *Journal of the American Academy of Child and Adolescent Psychiatry* **42**, 13–21.

Rueter, M. & Graham, P. (1968) The reliability and validity of the psychiatric assessment of the child: I. Interview with the child. *British Journal of Psychiatry* **114**, 563–579.

Rutter, M. *et al.* (2006) Continuities and discontinuities in psychopathology between childhood and adult life. *Journal of Child Psychology and Psychiatry* **47** (3–4), 276–295.

Sakolsky, D.J. *et al.* (2012) Genetics of pediatric anxiety disorders. *Child and Adolescent Psychiatric Clinics of North America* **21** (3), 479–500.

Scaini, S. *et al.* (2012) Genetic and environmental contributions to separation anxiety: a meta-analytic approach to twin data. *Depression and Anxiety* **29** (9), 754–761.

Schwab-Stone, M.E. *et al.* (1996) Criterion validity of the NIMH Diagnostic Interview Schedule for Children Version 2.3 (DISC-2.3). *Journal of the American Academy of Child and Adolescent Psychiatry* **35** (7), 878–888.

Seligman, L.D. *et al.* (2004) The utility of measures of child and adolescent anxiety: a meta-analytic review of the Revised Children's Manifest Anxiety Scale, the State-Trait Anxiety Inventory for Children, and the Child Behavior Checklist. *Journal of Clinical Child & Adolescent Psychology* **33** (3), 557–565.

Shaffer, D. *et al.* (1985) Neurological soft signs. Their relationship to psychiatric disorder and intelligence in childhood and adolescence. *Archives of General Psychiatry* **42** (4), 342–351.

Shaffer, D. *et al.* (1996) The NIMH Diagnostic Interview Schedule for Children Version 2.3 (DISC-2.3): description, acceptability, prevalence rates, and performance in the MECA study. *Journal of the American Academy of Child & Adolescent Psychiatry* **35** (7), 865–877.

Shaffer, D. *et al.* (2000) NIMH diagnostic interview schedule for children version IV (NIMH DISC-IV): description, differences from previous versions, and reliability of some common diagnoses. *Journal of the American Academy of Child and Adolescent Psychiatry* **39** (1), 28–38.

Silberg, J. *et al.* (1999) The influence of genetic factors and life stress on depression among adolescent girls. *Archives of General Psychiatry* **56** (3), 225–232.

Silberg, J.L. *et al.* (2001) Genetic and environmental influences on the temporal association between earlier anxiety and later depression in girls. *Biological Psychiatry* **49** (12), 1040–1049.

Silverman, W.K. & Ollendick, T.H. (2005) Evidence-based assessment of anxiety and its disorders in children and adolescents. *Journal of Clinical Child & Adolescent Psychology* **34** (3), 380–411.

Silverman, W.K. *et al.* (2001) Test-retest reliability of anxiety symptoms and diagnoses with the Anxiety Disorders Interview Schedule for DSM-IV: child and parent versions. *Journal of the American Academy of Child and Adolescent Psychiatry* **40** (8), 937–944.

Simonoff, E. *et al.* (1997) The Virginia twin study of adolescent behavioral development: influences of age, sex, and impairment on rates of disorder. *Archives of General Psychiatry* **54** (9), 801–808.

Slattery, M.J. *et al.* (2002) Relationship between separation anxiety disorder, parental panic disorder, and atopic disorders in children: a controlled high-risk study. *Journal of the American Academy of Child and Adolescent Psychiatry* **41** (8), 947–954.

Steinberg, L. & Avenevoli, S. (2000) The role of context in the development of psychopathology: a conceptual framework and some speculative propositions. *Child Development* **71** (1), 66–74.

Suomi, S.J. (2003) Gene-environment interactions and the neurobiology of social conflict. *Annals of the New York Academy of Sciences* **1008**, 132–139.

Topolski, T.D. *et al.* (1999) Genetic and environmental influences on ratings of manifest anxiety by parents and children. *Journal of Anxiety Disorders* **13** (4), 371–397.

Turner, S.M. *et al.* (1987) Psychopathology in the offspring of anxiety disorders patients. *Journal of Consulting and Clinical Psychology* **55** (2), 229–235.

Vasa, R.A. *et al.* (2002) Anxiety after severe pediatric closed head injury. *Journal of the American Academy of Child and Adolescent Psychiatry* **41** (2), 148–156.

Vasa, R.A. *et al.* (2004) Neuroimaging correlates of anxiety after pediatric traumatic brain injury. *Biological Psychiatry* **55** (3), 208–216.

Verhulst, F.C. *et al.* (1997) The prevalence of DSM-III-R diagnoses in a national sample of Dutch adolescents. *Archives of General Psychiatry* **54** (4), 329–336.

Walkup, J.T. *et al.* (2008) Cognitive behavioral therapy, sertraline, or a combination in childhood anxiety. *New England Journal of Medicine* **359** (26), 2753–2766.

Warner, V. *et al.* (1995) Offspring at high and low risk for depression and anxiety: mechanisms of psychiatric disorder. *Journal of the American Academy of Child & Adolescent Psychiatry* **34** (6), 786–797.

Weissman, M.M. *et al.* (1984) Psychopathology in the children (ages 6–18) of depressed and normal parents. *Journal of the American Academy of Child Psychiatry* **23** (1), 78–84.

Weissman, M.M. *et al.* (1997) Offspring of depressed parents. 10 years later. *Archives of General Psychiatry* **54** (10), 932–940.

Whitaker, A.H. *et al.* (1997) Psychiatric outcomes in low-birth-weight children at age 6 years: relation to neonatal cranial ultrasound abnormalities. *Archives of General Psychiatry* **54** (9), 847–856.

Williams, J.M. *et al.* (1996) The emotional Stroop task and psychopathology. *Psychological Bulletin* **120** (1), 3–24.

Williamson, D.E. *et al.* (2005) Stressful life events in anxious and depressed children. *Journal of Child and Adolescent Psychopharmacology* **15** (4), 571–580.

Wittchen, H.-U. *et al.* (1999) Social fears and social phobia in a community sample of adolescents and young adults: prevalence, risk factors and co-morbidity. *Psychological Medicine* **29** (2), 309–323.

Wood, J.J. *et al.* (2003) Parenting and childhood anxiety: theory, empirical findings, and future directions. *Journal of Child Psychology and Psychiatry* **44** (1), 134–151.

CHAPTER 61

Obsessive compulsive disorder

Judith L. Rapoport[1] and Philip Shaw[2]

[1]Child Psychiatry Branch, National Institute of Mental Health, Bethesda, MD, USA

[2]Social and Behavioral Research Branch, and Head, Neurobehavioral Clinical Research Section, National Human Genome Research Institute, Bethesda, MD, USA

Definition: the concept and current issues

Obsessive-compulsive disorder (OCD) was once considered rare in childhood, but recent advances in diagnosis and treatment have led to the recognition that the disorder is a common cause of distress for children and adolescents. OCD is characterized by the presence of obsessions (unwanted, repetitive, or intrusive thoughts) and compulsions (unnecessary repetitive behaviors or mental activities). Because the obsessive-compulsive thoughts and rituals are usually recognized by the child as nonsensical, they are often kept hidden for as long as possible—from both parents and practitioners. This secrecy may have contributed to the fact that until the 1980s OCD was unfamiliar to most child psychiatrists, even though classic descriptions of the disorder featured cases with childhood presentation (Janet, 1903). The recognition that OCD was more common in adults than previously believed, and retrospective reports that one-half to one-third of adult subjects had their onset in childhood or adolescence, focused the attention of the child psychiatric community on this chronic and often disabling disorder (Karno et al., 1988; Karno & Golding, 1991).

Until the mid-19th century, obsessive-compulsive phenomena were considered to be a variant of insanity. However, as the disorder was better defined, it came into focus as one of the neuroses. The descriptions of repetitive unwanted thoughts or rituals, often characterized by magical thinking and usually kept private by the sufferer, were relatively constant observations in those early reports. Debate about core deficits and the relative importance of volitional intellectual and emotional impairments (all of which are in some way abnormal in OCD) have flourished for over 100 years (Berrios, 1989).

Freud (1906, 1958) speculated about the similarity between obsessive-compulsive phenomena, children's games, and religious rites. Although psychoanalytic theory is empirically unproved and has not been shown to be effective in the treatment of OCD, the broad questions raised by Freud about continuity and discontinuity within individual development and OCD, as well as with regard to secular and religious rituals, and cross-cultural studies linking cleanliness and "purity" remain fascinating issues. In addition, the association between certain neurological disorders, such as Tourette's disorder (see Chapter 56), and OCD, supported by current imaging research, has led to possible localization of brain circuits mediating obsessive-compulsive behaviors as well as mechanisms for behavioral encoding. Over the past decade, interest in these general questions, as well as the possibility of unique pediatric subgroups of OCD, has generated a wealth of clinical and translational research (Apter et al., 1996; Fitzgerald et al., 1999; Graybiel & Rauch, 2000a). Key issues which appear throughout this chapter are the degree to which at least some cases with childhood onset represent a distinct subtype (e.g., patients with Tourette's/tics and/or patients with a possible infectious trigger or pediatric autoimmune neuropsychiatric disorders associated with streptococcal infections, PANDAS), the extent to which there is continuity with normal development, as well as the relationship between OCD and several other disorders now seen as part of an OCD spectrum such as body dysmorphic disorder or tricotillomania. The placement of this chapter within the emotional disorders remains warranted because of the comorbidity and familiality of mood and anxiety disorders in OCD patients (Bienvenu et al., 2012).

Epidemiology

Epidemiological studies provide a lifetime prevalence of around 1.9–3.3% (Karno et al., 1988; Karno & Golding, 1991)—see Table 61.1. Using the Diagnostic Interview Schedule (DIS), a structured interview designed for lay interviewers, lifetime prevalence rates without DSM-III exclusions ranged from 1.9% to 3.3% across sites. Even with DSM-III exclusions, the rates were 1.2–2.4%. These rates were 25–60 times greater than had been estimated on the basis of clinical populations. The mean age of onset across the sites ranged from 20 to 25 years with 50%

Rutter's Child and Adolescent Psychiatry, Sixth Edition.
Edited by Anita Thapar and Daniel S. Pine, James F. Leckman, Stephen Scott, Margaret J. Snowling, Eric Taylor.
© 2015 John Wiley & Sons Ltd. Published 2018 by John Wiley & Sons Ltd.

Table 61.1 Community studies of OCD prevalence in children and adolescents.

Study	Sample	Ascertainment and evaluation	Prevalence (%)
Flament et al. (1988)	5596 students grades 9–12 (United States)	Initial screening with Leyton, epidemiological version; 356 screen-positive students then evaluated using semistructured interview by clinicians	1.0 and 1.9 (wt. current and lifetime, respectively)
Zohar et al. (1992)	562 consecutive army recruits, ages 16–17 yrs (Israel)	Short semistructured interview by a child psychiatrist	3.6 (point)
Reinherz et al. (1993)	384 mostly 18-yr-olds (United States)	Structured interview by trained interviewers with research or clinical experience	1.3, 1.3, 2.1 (1-mo, 6-mo, and lifetime, respectively)
Lewinsohn et al. (1993)	1710 14–18-yr-olds (United States)	Semistructured interview mostly by trained, clinically experienced interviewers	0.06, 0.53 (current and lifetime, respectively)
Valleni-Basile et al. (1994)	3283 (mostly) 12–15-yr-olds (United States)	3283 screened; 488 mother–child pairs then given semistructured interview by psychiatric nurses	2.95 (wt. current)
Douglass et al. (1995)	930 18-yr-olds from a birth cohort followed since birth (New Zealand)	Structured interview by trained mental health interviewers	4.0 (1 yr)
Apter et al. (1996)	861 consecutive army recruits, ages 16–17 (Israel)	Initial screening by an OCD self-report questionnaire followed by a structured interview by a child psychiatrist	2.3 (lifetime)
Wittchen et al. (1998)	3021 14–24-yr olds (Germany)	Semistructured interview by clinical interviewers and trained professional health research interviewers	0.6 and 0.7 (1 yr and lifetime, respectively)
Rapoport et al. (2000)	NIMH MECA four-site sample of caretaker–child dyads of 1285 9–17-yr-olds (United States)	Structured interview by trained interviewers	0.3, 2.5, 2.7 (parent report, child report, and total, respectively)

Note: wt. = weighted to reflect sampling design

developing symptoms in childhood or adolescence (Karno & Golding, 1991), providing further support for the retrospective accounts of the frequent pediatric onset of this disorder (Black, 1974). More recent cross-cultural studies with adults have been supportive of similar rates of between 1.9 and 2.5 percent prevalence across widely differing cultures (Horwath & Weissman, 2000). Higher rates are found using DSM-IV than with ICD-10, with only 64% agreement between the two systems (Andrews et al., 1999). As about a half of adult patients report onset after adolescence or childhood, the similar rates for adult and child populations suggest that some pediatric patients must remit. This apparent discrepancy from the chronic nature of most pediatric OCD studied clinically has not been resolved (see discussion later), but may reflect in part that adult cases are typically identified using only one informant, whereas childhood cases are frequently diagnosed on the basis of two informants (the child and parent).

Epidemiological studies of OCD focusing on children and adolescents (see review by Zohar, 1999) and one recent additional study examined the results of a large four-site community survey in the United States (the National Institute of Mental Health [NIMH] Methods for the Epidemiology of Child and Adolescent Mental Disorders [MECA] Study) (Rapoport et al., 2000). The lifetime prevalence across eight studies (from these two articles combined) indicates relative consistency with a

lifetime prevalence from 0.7% to 2.9%. Males have an earlier onset than females, contributing to a striking preponderance of males in most pediatric samples (Geller et al., 1998). The variance in prevalence rates is likely to reflect differences in study design, particularly whether clinicians or nonclinicians conducted interviews. Additionally, prevalence estimates may also be sensitive to the diagnostic tools employed. Structured interviews in particular may yield false positives when given to children who are apt to misinterpret the questions (Breslau, 1987).

There is increasing reliance on standardized interviews and rating scales for both the study and clinical management of OCD. The most commonly used tools, the Diagnostic Interview for Children and Adolescents (Herjanic & Campbell, 1977; Herjanic & Reich, 1982) and the Schedule for Affective Disorder and Schizophrenia for School-Age Children (Kaufman et al., 1997), have sections on OCD. In addition, there are several rating scales in general use, including the child version of the Leyton Obsessional Inventory (Berg et al., 1989) and the Yale–Brown Obsessive Compulsive Scale (Y-BOCS) (Goodman et al., 1989a, b) and a Children's Y-BOCS (CY-BOCS) adapted for 5–8-year-olds (Scahill et al., 1997). Sensory phenomena such as getting things "just right" have been a valid and reliable auxiliary measure for OCD using the Sao Paulo Sensory Phenomena Scale (Rosario et al., 2009).

Diagnostic issues

Continuity with normal development

The boundaries of diagnosis are complex in any disorder, and this is clearly the case with OCD. Individual "habits" that are typical of OCD are extremely common across populations.. For example, in one Israeli study, only 18% of the sample endorsed no obsessive-compulsive symptoms at all, while a longitudinal population study found 21–25% of children and adults endorsed specific obsessions or compulsions (Fullana *et al.*, 2009). Moreover, many ritualistic and "magical" behaviors are part of normal development (Leonard, 1989). As is the case with many disorders, family genetic studies seem to indicate that heritability of obsessive-compulsive symptoms may extend across the entire range of severity, and similarly twin studies support the model of OCD as the extreme of a continuously distributed trait with biological continuity between normal and abnormal behaviors (Jonnal *et al.*, 2000). However, there is evidence from a pediatric sample that symptom levels below the level needed for a categorical diagnosis of OCD predict later onset OCD, and are associated with help seeking for other mental disorders, particularly depression (Berg *et al.*, 1989; Fullana *et al.*, 2009).

The importance of informant history

Secrecy appears to be a hallmark of childhood onset OCD. The children recognize that their symptoms are nonsensical and are embarrassed by them, so they go to great lengths to hide them. Hand-washing might be disguised as more frequent voiding and rituals are carried out in private, so that children are often symptomatic for months before their parents are aware of a problem. Teachers and peers typically are aware only for cases with greater severity. As with Tourette's disorder, children may expend effort controlling their behaviors in public and "let go" when at home. This partial voluntary control of symptoms often baffles and angers parents. Because of the variable degree and timing of control of symptoms, the nature of the informant has particularly important influence on recognition and diagnosis of OCD. As shown for the MECA data (Rapoport *et al.*, 2000), only 0.3% were identified by parents while 2.5% were identified through self-report from the child, with only one overlapping case.

Issues with DSM-5 diagnosis

OCD is defined in both ICD-10 and DSM-5 as repetitive intrusive thoughts and/or rituals that are unwanted and which interfere significantly with function or cause marked distress. The severity criteria avoid confusion of OCD with many childhood habits that are part of normal development. Both the content and relative insight into the unreasonableness of the thoughts/behaviors differentiate OCD from other disorders.

While clinical experience suggests that the adult criteria can be applied to childhood cases, there are several important caveats. Both DSM-5 and ICD-10 state that compulsions are designed to neutralize or prevent some dreaded event or according to rules that must be applied rigidly. The concept of "rules applied rigidly" is particularly useful for childhood OCD. While some children may not be willing or able to verbalize their obsessive thoughts, long-term contact has demonstrated that about 40% of children do not in fact have obsessive thoughts; they steadfastly report the presence of only compulsive rituals (dictated by rigid rules) accompanied by a vague sense of discomfort if the rituals are not carried out (Swedo *et al.*, 1989). At least a third of pediatric patients report that certain stimuli trigger their rituals and that avoidance of the trigger "protects" them from the obsessive-compulsive symptoms (Karno *et al.*, 1988). The degree of insight needed for the diagnosis is also in dispute as some patients, at least some of the time, "believe" their obsessive thoughts. DSM-5 diagnostic criteria now includes a subtype coding for the "belief" in the necessity for these thoughts/behaviors.

Due to the exclusion of either false positives or milder cases, rates of OCD tended to be lower with DSM-IV than earlier versions of the DSM, with a 12-month prevalence rate of 0.6% being reported in a recent study (Crino *et al.*, 2005). Estimates of lifetime prevalence appear to be less affected by the changes in diagnostic criteria (Angst *et al.*, 2004; Swedo *et al.*, 2004). There are several important differences between the ICD-10 and DSM-5 criteria, such as whether exclusions are made based on comorbid psychotic disorders, such as schizophrenia. DSM-5 allows patients to receive a diagnosis of OCD even in the presence of schizophrenias (American Psychiatric Association, 1994) in light of convincing evidence of coexistence with schizophrenia (Byerly *et al.*, 2005; Poyurovsky & Koran, 2005).

Obsessive compulsive spectrum disorders

The longstanding question of the importance of other disorders involving over focused interfering behaviors termed "obsessive compulsive spectrum disorders," and their relationship to OCD and to anxiety disorders, has led to an important reconceptualization of these disorders and a new umbrella category in DSM-5: obsessive-compulsive and related disorders. This grouping does not affect "caseness" but indicates that the OC spectrum disorders appear to be related. Spectrum disorders include body dysmorphic disorder, trichotillomania (hair pulling disorder), excoriation (skin picking), all of interest for pediatric populations, and hoarding disorder. The phenomenological similarities are often striking. For example, similar to OCD, body dysmorphic disorder and skin picking are characterized by over focused ideation and anxiety arousing concerns. Some of these disorders, for example, hoarding disorder, differ not only in content but also in the perceived ego-syntonic nature of the behaviors. The diagnosis of OCD is only given if symptoms are not accounted for by these spectrum disorders. The relationship between OCD and these other disorders is complex. A neurobiological overlap with OCD is suggested by the increased rate of subclinical OCD features in relatives of those with spectrum disorder (Bienvenu *et al.*, 2000) and clinical comorbidity and familiality of these spectrum disorders for OCD probands (Bienvenu *et al.*, 2012). The majority of spectrum disorder patients do *not* have comorbid OCD (Phillips *et al.*, 2010), and body dysmorphic disorder is only comorbid with OCD in about one-third of patients, and their insight is more limited. Hoarding disorder, a new diagnosis for DSM-5, is only comorbid with OCD in 20% of cases. The extent to which hoarding is a clinical problem in childhood is unclear but hoarding is most probably of greater interest for adults (Mataix-Cols *et al.*, 2012). There are also several studies which have suggested some efficacy for serotonin reuptake inhibiting drugs in the treatment of these disorders (Keuthen *et al.*, 2005; Saxena *et al.*, 2007), although there are notable negative treatment trials (Karno *et al.*, 1988; Christenson *et al.*, 1991; Hollander & Wong, 1995; Hollander, 1996; Hollander *et al.*, 2003). We will consider later the overlap between the neural substrates of OCD and the spectrum disorders.

Children with disorders that are less obviously related to OCD, such as autism spectrum disorders (ASDs), frequently exhibit a compulsive need for sameness but lack other features such as ego-dystonicity (the individual's sense that the content of his symptoms are alien and unlike his normal self). Disorders such as anorexia nervosa, pyromania, pathological gambling disorder, and substance abuse disorder overlap with OCD principally in that their symptoms involve overfocused ideation but are neither comorbid for OCD probands, nor is there increase in their families (Bienvenu *et al.*, 2012). There continues to be debate about classification of OCD as an anxiety disorder. However, depression and anxiety are major comorbidities with OCD, and there is evidence from family studies that OCD segregates with anxiety and mood disorders (Hanna *et al.*, 2011; Bienvenu *et al.*, 2012). The placement of OCD and related disorders as a separate category within anxiety disorders in DSM-5 may be a sensible compromise for the present.

Obsessive-compulsive personality disorder (OCPD) is defined by preoccupation with orderliness, perfectionism, and mental control at the expense of flexibility, openness, and efficiency. Generally these behaviors are not seen as ego dystonic in OCPD, but in practice the two disorders can be confused. OCPD has not been studied in pediatric populations but developmental studies would be of great interest.

Unique childhood onset subtypes

This leads to a related question as to whether OCD with very early onset represents an important subtype of the disorder or possibly a different disorder altogether. There is some evidence that at the very least, early age of onset represents a more familial form of the disorder, particularly for pediatric cases with ordering compulsions (Leckman *et al.*, 2009). In one study, no patient with adult onset of OCD had a first-degree relative with OCD (Nestadt *et al.*, 2000). Additionally, very early onset OCD is more frequently associated with tics and/or Tourette's disorder (Grados *et al.*, 2001; Chabane *et al.*, 2004). Moreover, family studies have found that tic disorders are more likely to occur in patients who have relatives with OCD than in patients who lack a familial loading for OCD (Pauls *et al.*, 1995).This is partially addressed by the addition in DSM-5 of a tic-related subtype specifier for OCD (American Psychiatric Association, 2013).

The postulation of a postinfectious subgroup of pediatric OCD came about as a result of early reports of the association of OCD with Sydenham's chorea (Osler, 1894; Freeman *et al.*, 1965). This supported converging evidence of basal ganglia involvement in the etiology and/or maintenance of OCD (Wise & Rapoport, 1989). One example of a postinfectious subgroup has been identified by research at the NIMH, which identified a group of pediatric patients in whom symptom onset or exacerbations are triggered by streptococcal infections; the subgroup is identified by the acronym PANDAS (pediatric autoimmune neuropsychiatric disorders associated with streptococcal infections) (Swedo *et al.*, 2004). This group of patients appears to have an unusually abrupt onset of symptoms, typically has an abnormal neurologic examination during exacerbations (particularly tic or choreiform movements, which are discussed in Chapter 56), comorbidities including separation anxiety and attention deficit hyperactivity disorder (ADHD) like symptoms, and tends to have a better outcome. The disorder is thought to arise through a process of molecular mimicry, with the group A ß-hemolytic streptococcus (*Streptococcus pyogenes*) (GABHS) evoking antibodies that are capable of cross-reacting with specific areas of the human brain (e.g., the basal ganglia) to produce neuropsychiatric and behavioral symptoms. Moreover, the group showed response to immunotherapy (Perlmutter *et al.*, 1999a). However, there remains controversy around the diagnosis, particularly in view of some studies failing to detect elevated levels of autoantibodies in those otherwise meeting criteria for PANDAS (Singer *et al.*, 2005). More recently there has been a proposal to broaden the category to pediatric acute onset neuropsychiatric syndrome or PANS (Swedo *et al.*, 2012) or similarly childhood acute neuropsychiatric symptoms or CANS (Singer *et al.*, 2012), which is defined by abrupt onset rather than etiology and must include OCD or food restriction and other concurrent psychiatric symptoms.

Clinical presentation

Childhood onset OCD has been documented as early as age 2 but more typically begins later in childhood or early adolescence (American Psychiatric Association, 1994). In general, the symptoms of OCD in children mirror those in adult patients and are summarized in Table 61.2. Thus, obsessions on the

Table 61.2 Presenting symptoms in 70 consecutive children and adolescents with primary obsessive compulsive disorder.

Reported symptoms at initial interview	N	%
Obsessions		
Concerns with dirt, germs, and environmental toxins	28	40
Something terrible happening (e.g., death of loved one)	17	24
Symmetry, order, or exactness	12	17
Scrupulosity (religious obsessions)	9	13
Concern or disgust with bodily waste or secretions	6	8
Lucky or unlucky numbers	6	8
Forbidden, aggressive, or perverse sexual thoughts, images, or impulses	3	4
Fear of harming others or self	3	4
Concern with household items	2	3
Intrusive nonsense sounds, words, or music	1	1
Compulsions		
Excessive or ritualized hand-washing, showering, bathing, or grooming	60	85
Repeating rituals (e.g., going in and out of the door)	36	51
Checking (e.g., doors, locks, stoves)	32	46
Miscellaneous rituals (e.g., writing, moving, speaking)	18	26
Rituals to remove contact with contaminants	16	23
Touching	14	20
Measures to prevent harm to self or others	11	16
Ordering or arranging	12	17
Counting	13	18
Hoarding/collecting rituals	8	11
Rituals of cleaning household or inanimate objects	4	6

As multiple obsessions and compulsions are possible, the total thus exceeds 70.
Source: Based on Swedo *et al.* (1989).

themes of contamination, danger to self or others (such as fears that parents will be harmed), symmetry or moral issues are common; typical compulsions include washing, checking, and repeating—particularly until the child experiences a feeling of "getting it just right" (Despert, 1955; Thomsen, 1991; Masi *et al.*, 2005). Most children have a combination of obsessions and rituals, and pure obsessives are rare compared with the more frequent pure ritualizers. Children with an early age at onset (below age 6) usually begin their rituals or obsessions in an easily recognizable fashion, such as excessive hand-washing or ritualized checking and repeating. In some cases, however, the clinical presentation is altered by the child's developmental immaturity. For example, one 6-year-old boy, who was compelled to draw zeros repetitively, had started at age 3 to circle manhole covers on city streets. His tantrums when the circling was interrupted, his subjective distress during the behavior, and his lack of other psychosocial abnormalities or disorders (such as autism or pervasive developmental disorder) led to the diagnosis of OCD. Another child, who presented at age 7 with clinically significant checking compulsions, had been evaluated previously at 3 years of age when he developed a "compulsion" to walk only on the edges of the floor tiles. Cleaning rituals in children too young to reach the water faucet can present as excessive hand-wiping or licking.

Approximately one-third of pediatric patients report that certain stimuli trigger their rituals and that avoidance of the trigger "protects" them from the obsessive-compulsive symptoms (Swedo *et al.*, 1989). These phenomena have been viewed from an ethological perspective, with the compulsions conceptualized as "fixed action patterns" released by key environmental stimuli (Modell *et al.*, 1989; Wise & Rapoport, 1989). These triggers are of particular interest for treatment as they often determine the key approach during behavioral desensitization, namely, exposure with response prevention (see below).

Course and natural history

Epidemiological studies indicate that over 50% of adults with OCD report that their symptoms started during childhood or adolescence, with males generally having earlier onset than females (Rasmussen & Tsuang, 1984). A single epidemiological study of OCD in a group of 18-year-olds suggested that past depression and substance abuse were predictive of onset of OCD (Douglass *et al.*, 1995). There may also be a prodromal phase: parents of nearly half of the NIMH sample revealed that their children had displayed "micro episodes of OCD" years before developing full-blown symptoms. During these episodes, excessive rigidity and repetitive rituals (e.g., wearing the same clothes for a month, refusal to take a different path through the house) were a source of concern, albeit briefly.

A prospective epidemiological survey of 976 children, initially assessed between the ages of 1 and 10 years and then 8, 10, and 15 years later, delineated predictors of OCD symptoms (Peterson *et al.*, 2001). In prospective analyses, tics in childhood and early adolescence predicted an increase in OCD symptoms in late adolescence and early adulthood, whereas ADHD symptoms in adolescence predicted more OCD symptoms in early adulthood.

The clinical course of the disorder indicates some developmental influence on symptoms over time. In a clinic sample, this sensitivity to developmental stage was found first in symptom profile, with the presenting obsessions and compulsions changing over time in 90% of the NIMH pediatric patients (Rettew *et al.*, 1992). Most children began with a single obsession or compulsion and continued with this for months to years, and then gradually acquired different obsessions or rituals. Although the primary symptom would change (e.g., from counting to washing and then checking), some earlier symptoms often remained problematic, although to a lesser degree. The nature of the compulsive rituals also changed over time. A study of adolescents demonstrated that counting and symmetry were most prominent during grade school years, but were replaced by washing rituals during early and midadolescence (Maina *et al.*, 1999).

The outcome of OCD may also have a similar relationship to developmental stage. In their longitudinal epidemiological study of tics, OCD, and ADHD described above, Peterson and colleagues found in prospective analyses that both younger and older adolescents with OCD were more likely to develop depressive and ADHD symptoms. Early adolescents with OCD, however, were especially likely to develop more anxiety and simple phobias in later adolescence. Epidemiological studies of adults suggest that spontaneous remissions occur in as many as one-third of patients (Karno & Golding, 1990). A recent prospective study of 591 adult subjects assessed patients at six time-points between age 20 and 40 (Angst *et al.*, 2004). While OCD was chronic in 60% of the cases, there was considerable improvement over time, even in those who continued to meet diagnostic criteria. It is often argued that pediatric cases will have a more chronic course, and a recent meta-analysis of studies based on sixteen independent samples (521 OCD participants) followed for a mean of 11.2 years indicated earlier age of onset to be a poor prognosis factor, along with comorbid psychiatric illness and poor initial treatment response (Stewart *et al.*, 2004). Overall, there was a 41% persistence for full and 60% for full or subthreshold OCD. A small study in which 45 of 62 pediatric OCD cases were recontacted a mean of 9 years later in early adulthood found 44% remitted in agreement with earlier studies (Bloch *et al.*, 2009). Poorer outcome was associated with absence of tics, more severe baseline symptoms, and female gender, as well as poor visuospatial and fine motor skills (Bloch *et al.*, 2009, 2011). A second clinic-based study found a similar 41% persistence rate of OCD in a group of children followed up over a mean of 5 years (Micali *et al.*, 2010). The pathways determining clinical outcome are complex, and any one single developmental variable, such as age of onset, is likely to account for only a modest amount of the overall variance in final outcome. OCD patients with comorbid tics or Tourette's have a waxing and waning course (Bloch *et al.*, 2006). In patients with comorbid Tourette's and OCD, tics generally start to improve around age 10, while the obsessive-compulsive symptoms typically continue for several more years. PANDAS are also characterized as relapsing/remitting in relation to streptococcal infection (Leonard *et al.*, 1999).

Associated disorders

Both epidemiological (Karno & Golding, 1991) and clinical (LaSalle *et al.*, 2004) studies indicate broad and complex comorbidity for OCD, similar to that seen for other major Axis I disorders. The patterns of comorbidity among childhood onset cases are generally comparable to those for adult samples, but with tic disorders and specific developmental disorders appearing more frequently in the pediatric populations. In the NIMH sample, only 25% of the pediatric subjects had OCD as a single diagnosis (Swedo *et al.*, 1989). Tic disorders (30%), major depression (26%), and specific developmental disabilities (17%) were the most common comorbidities, and there were also high rates of simple phobias (17%), overanxious disorder (16%), adjustment disorder (11%), attention deficit

disorder (10%), conduct disorder (7%), separation anxiety disorder (7%), and enuresis/encopresis (4%). While our own experience with comorbid bipolar disorder is limited, other groups find increased bipolar comorbidity in severely affected pediatric OCD cases (Masi *et al.*, 2004). This broad comorbidity remains to be explained (for this and other disorders) and is not accounted for by any of the etiological models discussed later. Obsessive Compulsive Personality Disorder rates are elevated in adults with OCD (25–32%); however, comorbidity of OCPD with other psychiatric disorders is quite broad, with particularly high rates for Major Depressive Disorder (see review in Phillips *et al.* (2010)).

Case illustrations

Case 1

A 14-year-old boy, whose symptoms had begun gradually, recalls at a very early age having to wash his hands repetitively. He was unable to associate an obsessive thought with this ritual, but he felt compelled to perform it. By age 6, he had developed an obsessive fear of tornadoes. He would repeatedly check the sky for clouds, listen to all weather reports, and query his mother about approaching storms. The tornado obsession faded over time and was replaced by a generalized fear of harm coming to himself or his family. He responded with extensive rituals to protect himself and his family. Particularly at times of separating, such as bedtime or leaving for school, the patient would be compelled to repeat actions perfectly or to check repetitively. When asked how many times he would have to repeat an action, he replied, "It depends. The number isn't always the same, I just have to do it right." When asked how he knew when it was right, he said, "I don't know, it just feels right." As the patient entered puberty, he became obsessed with acquired immunodeficiency syndrome (AIDS) and was convinced he would acquire it through his mouth. He began spitting in an effort to cleanse his mouth and would spit every 15–20 s. In addition, he began extensive washing rituals. Despite these cleansing and washing compulsions, his personal appearance was slovenly and dirty. He never tied his shoelaces because they had touched the ground and were "contaminated"; if he tied them, his hands would be "dirty" and he would have to wash until they were "clean" again. Remarkably, although his family was aware that "something had been wrong for a long time," most of the content of his obsessions was kept secret. This case illustrates the contamination concerns common to adolescents, as well as the variety and evolution of obsessive-compulsive symptoms during development.

Case 2

A 16-year-old girl had symptoms that began abruptly, shortly after the onset of menses. She called herself "a prisoner of my own mind." Her obsessions centered around a fear of harm to her parents. She was plagued by recurrent thoughts of her mother dying in a car accident, her father being killed by an intruder, or both her parents dying of burns received in a house fire. Always a light sleeper, she began to get up during the night to check. She spent hours checking that the doors were locked, that the coffee pot was unplugged, and that the family dog was safely ensconced in the garage. Despite her obsessions about fire, however, she did not check the smoke detector, an excellent example of the irrationality of this superficially rational disorder. This patient involved her family in her rituals. Her mother made a checklist that the daughter carried to school, and both parents had to check the 24 items on the list, signing that they had done so. At night she would wake her father to help her check. The family involvement was so profound that behavioral treatment could only take place after a period of family counseling in which the parents were helped to separate from their daughter's illness.

The differential diagnosis: distinguishing OCD from other disorders

The broad comorbidity of OCD and an array of associated features make the diagnosis in theory seem difficult; in practice, however, it is usually more straightforward. The diagnosis of OCD must be made only if the "obsessive worries" are true obsessions, rather than symptoms of another disorder such as depressive ruminations or phobic avoidance. For example, when OCD is comorbid with bulimia or anorexia, the content of the obsessions or compulsions must be typical for OCD, for example, washing, arranging, counting, and repeating, and not be solely overfocused ideas about food or diet. Depressive ruminations and psychotic preoccupations are also distinguished by the negative content (e.g., everyone dislikes me, I fail at everything). Phobic disorders are not only distinguished by the content of the preoccupation (more often heights, spiders, the dark, etc.), but also by the absence of discomfort when the patient is not confronted with the phobic object. It may be more difficult to separate the obsessional concerns of OCD from the fears and worries of generalized anxiety disorder (Brown et al., 1993). Comorbidity of OCD and anxiety disorders is common, so assigning specific symptoms to a specific disorder may be less important than identifying the presence of OCD in a child presenting with generalized anxiety or separation anxiety disorder.

ASD can be differentiated from OCD by its lack of ego-dystonicity and, in addition, by the content of the preoccupations. For example, in ASD, concerns about danger or contamination occur only rarely, while these are common among children with OCD. Autistic patients also may exhibit obsessive-compulsive symptoms, but these occur within the context of cognitive and psychosocial abnormalities and should not be confused with symptoms of OCD.

The differential diagnosis from Tourette's disorder is problematic, and the two disorders are linked by several neurobiological features. Distinguishing between a compulsion or a tic may be difficult, given the presence of premonitory urges before tics and the complexity of some motor tics (Miguel et al., 2000). Some 20–80% of patients with clear Tourette's disorder have been reported to have obsessive-compulsive symptoms or OCD, while 24–67% of children with primary OCD have been observed to have comorbid tics (Leonard et al., 1992; Zohar et al., 1992). Tics are seen most often in younger patients, those with acute illness, and in males. Preliminary impressions are that compulsions associated with Tourette's disorder may be more likely to involve symmetry, rubbing, touching, or staring and blinking rituals than washing and cleaning (Baer, 1994; Leckman et al., 1994). Additionally, aggressive and/or sexual thoughts or rituals have been reported as more frequent in patients with tics and OCD than in those with OCD alone (Despert, 1955; Thomsen, 1991; Masi et al., 2005). However, although some features distinguish the two disorders, the overlapping clinical profiles and family studies provide partial support for the speculation that some cases of OCD and Tourette's may be alternate forms of the same disorder. Any Tourette/OCD formulation, however, is likely to be oversimplified but both tic disorders and OCD may be symptoms of basal ganglia-frontal circuitry dysfunction for which genetic, toxic, traumatic, and infectious agents can be etiologic. In particular, the working model of PANDAS involves the origin of both the tics and OCD through an autoimmune response to GABHS.

Theories of etiology

OCD is caused by a combination of biological and psychological factors, with both genetic and environmental influences.

Biological factors

Genetics
OCD is a highly heritable disorder, particularly when it has a childhood onset. Twin studies comparing monozygotic and dizygotic twins find genetic factors to account for around 45–65% of the variance in obsessive compulsive symptoms in children, compared to between estimates of 27–47% for adult onset symptoms (van Grootheest et al., 2005). Similarly, family studies find a 10-fold increase in rates of OCD among relatives of children with OCD, compared to a doubling of rates of OCD among relatives of those with adult-onset OCD (Pauls, 2010). A population-based study similarly showed a stepwise decrease in the risk of having OCD among relatives of OCD probands as the degree of relatedness fell (Mataix-Cols et al., 2013). Thus, while first-degree relatives had around a four- to fivefold increase in risk, it fell to around a twofold increase in second-degree relatives, and even lower in third-degree relatives. The genetic contribution to OCD is increased when there is comorbid tic

disorder, leading to suggestions that this combination might represent a distinct genetic subtype (Hanna *et al.*, 2005).

Initial searches for the specific causative genes focused on genetic variants (or polymorphisms) within genes coding for neurotransmitters implicated in OCD. A meta-analysis of over 100 such studies confirmed an association between OCD and polymorphisms within serotonergic genes (the serotonin transporter and one of the receptor subtypes) and a trend to association with variants within the glutamate transporter gene (Taylor, 2012).

Genome-wide linkage studies try to link genetic variation with OCD and two such studies have examined the families of children with the disorder (Willour *et al.*, 2004; Hanna *et al.*, 2005). They converged to find a region on chromosome 9 to be linked with OCD, which contains many genes, including the glutamate transporter gene. The next phase of genomic studies will involve sequencing of either the entire genome or just its coding regions (exome). Initial steps in this direction have been made with sequencing of the glutamatergic transporter gene and finding that "errors" of coding are increased in those with OCD (Wang *et al.*, 2010). Strategies to accelerate genomic discovery include studying subtypes of OCD, such as those with hoarding disorder, or examining the dimensions of the disorder (Samuels *et al.*, 2002; Hasler *et al.*, 2007).

Twin studies also emphasize the importance of the environment in the etiology of OCD, with around 42–55% of the variance of OC symptoms being explained by nonshared environmental factors (Hudziak *et al.*, 2004). Little is known however of the specific factors at play. In a longitudinal study of children with OCD and controls, psychosocial stressors affecting a child, as reported by parents, predicted later depressive and OC symptom severity (Lin *et al.*, 2007). These environmental factors included self-evaluation of daily stressors and long-term contextual threat. The family environment may also contribute to OCD, particularly the ways in which family members take part in the performance of rituals and help relatives avoid anxiety-provoking situations. Such familial accommodation is associated with OCD symptom severity and its reduction is associated with symptom improvement, a point we will return to as we consider treatment (Lebowitz *et al.*, 2012). Given the evidence of the importance of environmental factors in the etiology and course of OCD, more research is needed in this area to complement ongoing genomic studies.

Neural basis

OCD is remarkable in the consistency of support for a conceptual model which links a disorder characterized by endless, repetitive thoughts and actions with uncontrolled activity of parallel, discrete loops within the brain. These loops connect the basal ganglia, prefrontal cortex—particularly the orbitofrontal and anterior cingulate regions—and thalamus, the so-called cortico-striato-thalamocortical (CSTC) loops—see Figure 61.1 (Alexander *et al.*, 1986; Rapoport & Wise, 1988; Modell *et al.*, 1989; Saxena *et al.*, 2001; Kopell *et al.*, 2004).

Several CSTCs have been assumed to be of particular importance in OCD, based on clinical, imaging, and lesion studies. The first "direct" pathway is in essence a positive feedback loop that results in the initiation and continuation of thought and action. It is counterbalanced by an "indirect" pathway that acts as a check on the activation of the direct pathway. The direct pathway starts with a glutamatergic signal to the striatum which in turn sends an inhibitory GABA-ergic signal to the globus pallidus. This results in a disinhibition of the thalamus which is fed forward to the prefrontal cortex, particularly, orbitofrontal regions. The indirect pathway differs in that the striatum projects an inhibitory signal to the globus pallidus, which increases inhibition on the thalamus and thus decreases prefrontal cortical activation. While there are multiple neurotransmitters involved in this circuit, including substance P and GABA, there are also serotonergic projections to this component from the dorsal raphe to the ventral striatum. These projections are speculated to be inhibitory.

One model holds that OCD arise from primary striatal dysfunction within these loops. This causes deficits in thalamic filtering and in turn increases orbitofrontal cortical activity (Graybiel & Rauch, 2000b). By this reasoning, implicit information in no longer filtered at a striatal level but intrudes into consciousness. A refinement of this model argues for an imbalance between the direct and indirect CTSC loops (Saxena *et al.*, 1998; Mataix-Cols & van den Heuvel, 2006). Thus, OC symptoms emerge when an aberrant positive feedback loop develops in the first circuit, which is inadequately modulated by the output from the second circuit.

The implication of abnormal activity in CSTCs is supported to some degree by findings of structural anomalies within these circuits in children with OCD, although there are some inconsistencies in the findings (for a review see Menzies *et al.* 2008; Radua *et al.*, 2010). Functional imaging studies also find evidence of dysfunction within CTSC. For example, striatal dysfunction results in abnormal interactions between the dorsal striatum and prefrontal cortical region. This leads to impaired cognitive control and decreased cognitive flexibility, reflected by the ability to adapt to changing task demands. Studies of children with OCD find reduced activation of the dorsolateral prefrontal cortical regions supporting cognitive flexibility and hypoactivation of the right caudate, a direct demonstration of CTSC dysfunction (Woolley *et al.*, 2008; Britton *et al.*, 2010; Rubia *et al.*, 2011). Others have emphasized the role of the orbitofrontal cortex in cognitive control and flexible responding, conceptualizing the failure to resist obsessions and compulsions in OCD as stemming from its dysfunction. In one study, both young adults with OCD and their unaffected siblings showed decreased activation of the lateral orbitofrontal cortex during a task which required them to alter behavior in response to negative feedback. The centrality of the orbitofrontal cortical dysfunction in OCD has derived considerable support from repeated demonstration in adults that symptom provocation is accompanied by increased orbitofrontal cortical activity

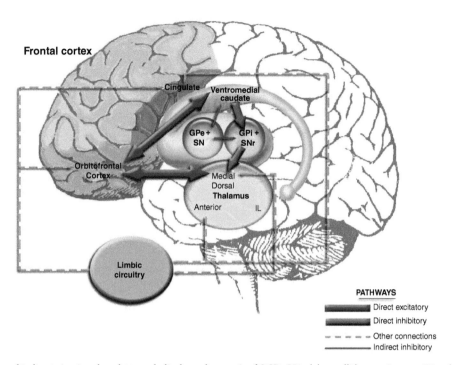

Figure 61.1 The direct and indirect circuitry thought to underlie the pathogenesis of OCD. GPi, globus pallidus pars interna; GPe, globus pallidus pars externa; SNr, substantia nigra pars reticulata. In the DIRECT pathway (thick arrows), the frontal cortex projects to the caudate and then to the GPi/SN complex which provides the main output of the basal ganglia. This in turn projects to the thalamus and finally back to the frontal cortex. The pathway has two excitatory and two inhibitory projections and thus is a net positive feedback loop. This circuit is balanced by the INDIRECT pathway (in thin arrows) which has a net inhibitory effect. This differs in its projection from the caudate to the GPe/SN complex (which also receives direct frontal input) before relaying onto the output station of the basal ganglia (the GPi/SNr complex). Interactions with the limbic system occur at several points and have been increasingly recognized in view of deficits in emotional processing and the anxiety prominent in OCD.

(Menzies *et al.*, 2008). However, in the only study to provoke symptoms among children, the opposite pattern of decreased orbitofrontal activation was found (Gilbert *et al.*, 2009).

A second model of OCD views the disorder as the result of overactivation of a system designed to monitor performance completion, leading to a constant feeling that an action is "not just right" which thus creates a need to correct perceived mistakes (Aouizerate *et al.*, 2004). A range of tasks assessing aspects of performance monitoring, error detection, and response to conflicts have converged to show hyperactivity in the anterior cingulate in adults with OCD (van Veen & Carter, 2002; Ursu *et al.*, 2003; Fitzgerald *et al.*, 2005; Maltby *et al.*, 2005). In pediatric OCD such anterior cingulate hyperactivation was reported in two of three studies examining brain activity during tasks of monitoring performance and detecting errors (Fitzgerald *et al.*, 2010; Huyser *et al.*, 2011; Rubia *et al.*, 2011). One of these studies further suggested that this hyperactivation might be more pronounced in adolescence rather than childhood (Huyser *et al.*, 2011).

How specific are these neural substrate to OCD? Similar anomalous interaction between the striatum and prefrontal cortex is also held to be important in ADHD, tic, and other impulse control disorders (see Castellanos & Tannock, 2002; Marsh *et al.*, 2009).

Some degree of overlap is perhaps inevitable, but there are several unique features in the OCD model outlined above, most importantly, the emphasis on an imbalance of the direct and indirect pathways in OCD and the prominence given to glutaminergic neurotransmission.

Neurochemistry

Monoaminergic neurotransmitters which extensively project from the brain stem to regions within the fronto-striato-thalamic circuitry may contribute to the pathogenesis of OCD. OCD symptoms are frequently exacerbated by serotonin agonists (such as *meta*-chlorophenylpiperazine), and the serotonin reuptake inhibitors are the most effective therapeutic agents (Gross-Isseroff *et al.*, 2004). Abnormalities of serotonergic transmission in OCD are suggested by imaging studies of central serotonin receptors using specific ligands which have demonstrated a reduction in 5-HT synthesis in the ventral prefrontal cortex and caudate in 11 treatment-naïve pediatric subjects, which partially normalized following successful treatment (Simpson *et al.*, 2003). Inconsistent findings on the levels of central serotonin transporter availability may be partly attributable to developmental effects, as reports of an increase of central serotonin transporter availability (indexed by the binding profiles of a ligand thought to bind to the transporter) was found only in those with child- but not adult-onset OCD (Pogarell *et al.*, 2003; Simpson *et al.*, 2003; Stengler-Wenzke *et al.*, 2004). There are less consistent findings for the dopaminergic system, with mixed results concerning changes in peripheral dopaminergic markers and the provocation of obsessive symptoms by dopamine agonists (Denys *et al.*, 2004b). PET neuroimaging studies, however, have demonstrated higher caudate dopamine transporter densities in tandem with lower concentrations of the dopamine D2 receptor, consistent with receptor down-regulation resulting from higher synaptic concentrations of striatal dopamine in adults with OCD (Denys *et al.*, 2004a; van der Wee *et al.*, 2004). Glutamate is the major excitatory neurotransmitter in the fronto-striatal circuitry, and magnetic resonance spectroscopy has demonstrated elevation in levels of glutamate and glutamine in the thalamus of treatment-naïve children with OCD, with a reduction in symptoms occurring in tandem with normalization of the glutamatergic marker (Rosenberg *et al.*, 2000). A decrease in glutamate levels in the anterior cingulate has also been found, although this may not be specific to OCD as it was also seen in children with major depression (Rosenberg *et al.*, 2004). There is, thus, some direct support for anomalous serotonergic neurotransmission and more indirect and somewhat inconsistent evidence of abnormal dopaminergic and glutamatergic signaling.

Treatment approaches

Psychological treatment

The cornerstone of psychological therapies for children is exposure and response prevention (ERP), and its efficacy has been demonstrated in multiple open studies and two randomized controlled trials (Barrett *et al.*, 2004; POTS, 2004). A hierarchy of increasingly intense anxiety-provoking situations that trigger obsessional thinking is constructed and subjects are exposed gradually to these situations and encouraged to refrain from engaging in compulsive behaviors (March & Mulle, 1998). Gradually, the patient progresses through the hierarchy so that situations can be tolerated with minimal anxiety, thus attaining an ever-decreasing urge to engage in compulsions. In clinical practice, and in all controlled studies, ERP is usually combined with other behavioral techniques, such as anxiety management training and extinction (e.g., instructing parents not to give reassurance when a child compulsively seeks it). This makes it difficult to disentangle the relative therapeutic importance of each element. Frequently, cognitive components are added, such as normalizing intrusive thoughts and reappraising notions of personal responsibility. Again, the necessity of these cognitive components is unclear in children as there are no controlled trials comparing these approaches. Tailoring therapy to the symptom profile of the child may be helpful. For example, ERP may be ideal for younger children as it has been shown to be effective in those under 11 and may be particularly helpful for symptoms such as contamination fears and symmetry rituals

(Barrett *et al.*, 2003). By contrast, cognitive approaches may be more suited to the child with obsessional moral guilt or pathological doubt.

The involvement of the family in treatment is essential. Psycho education can help the family to avoid both punitive responses and the alternative family accommodation that can occur if the family becomes enmeshed in rituals. Coercive and disruptive behaviors, and attacks of rage are associated with family accommodation. These disruptive behaviors are often associated with family attempts to limit OCD symptom expression. Behavioral management of these episodes can be critical to successful treatment (Lebowitz *et al.*, 2011; Storch *et al.*, 2012).

While the efficacy of behavior therapy (BT) with ERP as a core component is accepted, the most efficient and efficacious method of providing this treatment is less clear. A randomized controlled study demonstrated that such family-based cognitive behavioral therapy may be equally efficacious when conducted either with individual families or in a group setting (Barrett *et al.*, 2004). The degree of personal contact with the therapist continues to be an important issue given the cost of more intense programs. At one extreme lie computer-based delivery systems, including web camera-based treatment with minimal therapist contact time (Kenwright *et al.*, 2005; Storch *et al.*, 2010). There is also some initial evidence that self-help interventions with no therapist involvement at all are acceptable and effective (Robinson *et al.*, 2012). At the other extreme are highly intensive day or in-patient treatment programs. Only one trial has directly compared once weekly with daily therapy; no significant difference in outcome was found, although this study was not randomized and thus conclusions are limited (Franklin *et al.*, 1998). A meta-analysis suggested that while more therapist-intensive approaches were more efficacious, even those involving relatively little therapist contact time (less than 10 hours) were also effective (National Institute for Health and Care Excellence, 2005). While CBT is a robust frontline treatment overall, about 30% of pediatric populations have little or no response. Poor response is associated with diminished insight, family accommodation, and comorbidity (depression, Tourette's disorder, and cognitive deficits) (Storch *et al.*, 2010). Family accommodation is of particular importance and is worth measuring, monitoring, and tracking in clinical care (Lebowitz *et al.*, 2012). In practice, the severity of the symptom profile, the complexity of comorbidity, and resources available within the family and local health care services are likely to determine the treatment intensity. Many countries also have self-help groups which provide a valuable source of support and information, as well as act as advocates for those living with the disorder.

Pharmacotherapy

There is a relative abundance of randomized controlled trials demonstrating the efficacy of clomipramine and selective serotonin reuptake inhibitors—SSRIs (sertraline, fluoxetine, paroxetine and fluvoxamine)—in the acute phase treatment of childhood OCD, reviewed in Table 61.3.

Table 61.3 Controlled studies of medication in the treatment of pediatric OCD.

Study	Design	Participants	Interventions	Outcomes
Clomipramine				
Deveaugh-Geiss et al. (1992)	RCT, 8 weeks	N = 60, mean age = 14	Clomipramine versus placebo	Mean reduction in Yale–Brown Obsessive Compulsive Scale score of 37% compared to 8% in the placebo group. Sustained at 1 year
Greist et al. (1990)	RCT, 8 weeks	N = 16, mean age = 15	Clomipramine versus placebo	1 (73%) improved, 5 (33%) improved by more than 50%, and none worsened. Only 2 (12.5%) of the 16 placebo-treated patients improved, 1 (6%) by more than 50%; two (13%) worsened
Flament et al. (1985)	Cross-over, 5 weeks in each treatment	N = 27, mean age = 14	Clomipramine versus placebo	Clomipramine significantly more effective than placebo in reduction on all symptom scores
Leonard et al. (1989)	Cross-over, 5 weeks in each treatment (DB) and 2 weeks on placebo (single-blind SB)	N = 49, mean age = 14	Clomipramine versus desipramine versus placebo	Clomipramine significantly more effective than desipramine in symptom reduction. Higher rate of relapse when desipramine was substituted for clomipramine
SSRIs				
POTS (2004)	RCT, DB 12 weeks	N = 112, mean age = 12	CBT versus CBT + sertraline versus sertrlaine	Combined treatment also proved superior to CBT alone and to sertraline alone which did not differ from each other. CBT alone was associated with (nonsignificantly) higher rates of remission than sertraline
March et al. (1998)	RCT, DB 10 weeks	N = 189, mean age =13	Sertraline versus placebo	Sertraline produced significantly greater improvement in CY-BOCS. Based on CGI-I ratings at end point, 42% of patients receiving sertraline and 26% of patients receiving placebo were very much or much improved. Neither age nor sex predicted response to treatment
Geller et al. (2001)	RCT, DB 13 weeks	N = 103, mean age=11	Fluoxetine versus placebo	Fluoxetine produced significantly greater improvement in CY-BOCS (fall of 9.5 points compared to 5.2 for placebo)
Liebowitz et al. (2002)	RCT, DB 12 weeks	N = 43, mean age = 13	Fluoxetine versus placebo	No significant difference at 8 weeks; but by 16 weeks, fluoxetine was associated with greater reduction in CY-BOCS (9.74 points) than was placebo (4.14 points)
Riddle et al. (1992)	Cross-over DB 16 weeks	N = 14, mean age = 12	Fluoxetine versus placebo	CY-BOCS total score decreased 44% (N = 7, p = 0.003) after the initial 8 weeks of fluoxetine treatment, compared with a 27% decrease (N = 6, p = 0.13) after placebo
Geller et al. (2004)	RCT, BD 10 weeks	N = 207, mean age = 11	Paroxetine versus placebo	Paroxetine produced significantly greater improvement in CY-BOCS (fall of 8.78 points compared to 5.34 points in placebo group)
Riddle et al. (2001)	RCT, DB 10 weeks followed by 1-year open label extension	N = 120, mean age = 13	Fluvoxamine versus placebo	The CY-BOCS total score decreased 44% after the initial 8 weeks of fluoxetine treatment, compared with a 27% decrease after placebo

Note: RCT = randomized clinical trial; DB = double-blind; SD = single-blind

A meta-analysis of 12 studies of SRIs and clomipramine found all medications to be superior to placebo and found that clomipramine showed superiority over all the SRIs which did not differ from one another (Geller *et al.*, 2003). However, clomipramine is associated with several adverse side effects, including potential arhythmogenic effects.

Although generally well tolerated, SSRIs are associated with a range of side effects, with nausea, headache, and agitation being common to all in this class. There are widespread concerns about adverse somatic effects of medication in children, and reports of increase suicidal ideation. In some cases, however CBT is not possible to implement without concomitant medication, or not

effective. Moreover in many countries the cost of CBT and/or unavailability of this treatment may also be a limiting factor.

Depression is highly comorbid with OCD, and the treatment of this combination is often challenging. Two studies have found that adding imipramine (Foa *et al.*, 1992) or SRIs (Abramowitz *et al.*, 2000) either before or during ERP may be effective for alleviating depressive symptoms but did not potentiate ERP. There are case reports supporting the use of cognitive therapeutic techniques to increase motivation and compliance in the depressed patient to help them engage with difficult exposure assignments (Abramowitz, 2004).

In children, low initial doses with slow upward titration is the rule. In adults, higher doses are clearly associated with improved treatment efficacy without significant increase in adverse events (Bloch & Leckman, 2010) but this has not been systematically studied for pediatric populations. Patients should be made aware of the common side effects and the need for a 12-week treatment trial. Partial or complete failure to respond to the first SRI should prompt treatment with BT and consideration of another SRI. Use of augmenting agents for youths with treatment-resistant OCD is discussed below.

Combination treatment

How do pharmacological and psychological treatments compare? The best current evidence comes from the Pediatric OCD Treatment (POTS) multicenter study which randomized 112 children to either sertraline, cognitive behavioral therapy (CBT), the treatments combined, or pill placebo for 12 weeks (POTS, 2004). All active treatments were superior to pill placebo. Combined treatment also proved superior to CBT alone and to sertraline alone, which did not differ from each other. Site differences emerged for CBT and sertraline but not for combined treatment, suggesting that combined treatment is less susceptible to setting-specific variations, and, given this generalizability, combined treatment may be the option of choice. Notably, there was no evidence of treatment-emergent suicidality. Much smaller studies similarly found that a combination of BT (based on enterprise resource planning (ERP)) and fluvoxamine was superior to medication alone, both in short-term response and at a follow-up period of 1 year (Neziroglu et al., 2000). A direct comparison of BT with clomipramine in 22 children found a nonsignificant superiority for psychotherapy (de Haan et al., 1998). Overall, it is clear that while medication alone is effective and generally safe and well tolerated, CBT may have the edge in terms of a first-line treatment, particularly when combined with an SSRI or clomipramine. Double-blind trials of D-cycloserine augmentation of CBT in pediatric OCD subjects have yielded mixed results, with one study finding benefit over placebo, and one not (Storch et al., 2010; Farrell et al., 2013).

Augmenting strategies for partial responders

Up to 50% of children will show only a partial response to initial SRI treatment (Geller et al., 1998). The POTS study mentioned earlier found that around 60% of children receiving CBT alone, 46% receiving combined CBT and SRI, and approximately 80% receiving SRI alone do not fully remit (POTS, 2004). For adults showing such suboptimal response to an SRI, several trials have shown a significant reduction of obsessive symptoms in patients with either adjunctive haloperidol or risperidone (McDougle et al., 2000; Li et al., 2005). In treatment-resistant adult OCD patients, second-generation antipsychotics such as quetiapine have been reported to be effective augmenting agents (Kordon et al., 2008) Other treatment strategies in adults include augmentation with clonazepam or oral morphine or combining two SRIs, (for a review see Walsh and McDougle,

2004). There are some case reports demonstrating the potential for the use of each of these strategies in children, although there are no controlled studies to guide the clinician in this complex field (Leonard et al., 1994; Lombroso et al., 1995; Figueroa et al., 1998). Clearly, the side effects of each augmenting agent need to be considered, particularly the risk of tardive dyskinesia with haloperidol, metabolic side effects of risperidone, or other antipsychotic agents, and risk of tolerance and dependence with clonazepam. Recent double-blind studies of N-acetylecycsteine (NAC), an antioxidant precursor to glutathione, have shown significant benefit using 1200–2400 mg/day, in adult patients with OCD, as well as with trichotillomania or skin picking (Afshar et al., 2012). The actions are poorly understood but NAC has been shown to alter neurotransmitters including glutamate.

In spite of the major advances in drug treatment, at least 10% of the OCD population remains severely affected. In adults, for extreme cases there is an option for neurosurgical procedures, which are aimed at disrupting the CSTC loops either through creating a permanent lesion through excision or through repetitive deep brain stimulation (Greenberg et al., 2003). Such physical therapies are not appropriate for children; less invasive alternatives such as transcranial magnetic stimulation, while giving insight into the abnormal responsivity of the motor cortex in OCD (Gilbert et al., 2004), have not proved effective in the treatment of adults and remain untested in children (Martin et al., 2003).

Maintenance treatment

OCD is frequently a chronic disorder and long-term maintenance therapy should be anticipated, with the current recommendation being a minimum treatment period of 6 months following full remission. The need for such maintenance was illustrated by an 8-month study of 26 children and adolescents with severe OCD who had received clomipramine for a mean of 17 months; a 2-month double-blind desipramine-substitution phase resulted in 89% of the substituted (versus 18% of the non-substituted) subjects relapsing during the substitution phase (Leonard et al., 1991).

Immunomodulatory treatments

Based on the observation that some childhood onset OCD patients had onset apparently related to infection with GABHS, a subgroup of children were proposed who were hypothesized to have an autoimmune based form of the disorder—PANDAS (Swedo et al., 2004). As a partial test of this model, two treatments were examined. A controlled treatment trial of intravenous immunoglobulin was carried out, together with an open trial of plasmaphoresis (Perlmutter et al., 1999b). Both treatments were effective in lessening of symptom severity for children with infection-triggered OCD and tic disorders. Penicillin or azithromycin prophylaxis of sufficient intensity to decrease streptococcal infections was also found to decrease neuropsychiatric symptom exacerbations among children in the

PANDAS subgroup (Snider *et al.*, 2005). This study is limited by the absence of a placebo control, particularly as a previous placebo-controlled trial using penicillin prophylaxis was negative (Garvey *et al.*, 1999). These fascinating findings have yet to be replicated but raise the possibility of the prevention of OCD in at least a subset of children with the disorder.

Conclusions

Public awareness of OCD has increased greatly over recent years, allowing this once "secret" disorder to be more readily recognized both by families and mental health professionals. Functional neuroimaging studies increasingly inform and refine models of the pathogenesis of the disorder, and are being matched by neuroanatomic imaging studies which allow a delineation of structural change at an ever-decreasing level of resolution. While candidate gene studies have provided some validation of the implication of monoaminergic anomalies in the disorder, the application of new technologies to scan the entire genome is likely to provide novel insights into the genetics of OCD. Of most practical importance, though, are the strengthening of the evidence base for treatment through recent large-scale double-blind trials and the renewed interest in the management of those with treatment-resistant symptoms. The strides in understanding the neurobiology of the disorder are thus matched by definitive demonstrations of treatment efficacy in children, and make it all the more important that children, parents, and health care professionals remain aware of the disorder and the availability of effective treatments.

References

Abramowitz, J.S. (2004) Treatment of obsessive-compulsive disorder in patients who have comorbid major depression. *Journal of Clinical Psychology* **60**, 1133–1141.

Abramowitz, J.S. *et al.* (2000) Effects of comorbid depression on response to treatment for obsessive-compulsive disorder. *Behavior Therapy* **31**, 517–528.

Afshar, H. *et al.* (2012) N-acetylcysteine add-on treatment in refractory obsessive-compulsive disorder: a randomized, double-blind, placebo-controlled trial. *Journal of Clinical Psychopharmacology* **32**, 797–803.

Alexander, G. *et al.* (1986) Parallel organization of functionally segregated circuits linking basal ganglia and cortex. *Annual Review of Neuroscience* **9**, 357–381.

Andrews, G. *et al.* (1999) Classification in psychiatry: ICD-10 versus DSM-IV. *British Journal of Psychiatry* **174**, 3–5.

Angst, J. *et al.* (2004) Obsessive-compulsive severity spectrum in the community: prevalence, comorbidity, and course. *European Archives of Psychiatry and Clinical Neuroscience* **254**, 156–164.

Aouizerate, B. *et al.* (2004) Pathophysiology of obsessive-compulsive disorder: a necessary link between phenomenology, neuropsychology, imagery and physiology. *Progress in Neurobiology* **72**, 195.

American Psychiatric Association (1994) *Diagnostic and Statistical Manual of Mental Disorders.* American Psychiatric Association, Washington, DC.

American Psychiatric Association (2013) *Diagnostic and Statistical Manual of Mental Disorders*, 5th edn. American Psychiatric Association, Washington, DC.

Apter, A. *et al.* (1996) Obsessive-compulsive characteristics: from symptoms to syndrome. *Journal of the American Academy of Child and Adolescent Psychiatry* **35**, 907–912.

Baer, L. (1994) Factor analysis of symptom subtypes of obsessive compulsive disorder and their relation to personality and tic disorders. *Journal of Clinical Psychiatry* **55**, 18–23.

Barrett, P. *et al.* (2003) Behavioral avoidance test for childhood obsessive-compulsive disorder: a home-based observation. *American Journal of Psychotherapy* **57**, 80–100.

Barrett, P. *et al.* (2004) Cognitive-behavioral family treatment of childhood obsessive-compulsive disorder: a controlled trial. *Journal of the American Academy of Child & Adolescent Psychiatry* **43**, 46–62.

Berg, C.Z. *et al.* (1989) Childhood obsessive compulsive disorder: a two-year prospective follow-up of a community sample. *Journal of the American Academy of Child & Adolescent Psychiatry* **28**, 528–533.

Berrios, G.E. (1989) Obsessive-compulsive disorder: its conceptual history in France during the 19th century. *Comprehensive Psychiatry* **30**, 283–295.

Bienvenu, O.J. *et al.* (2000) The relationship of obsessive-compulsive disorder to possible spectrum disorders: results from a family study. *Biological Psychiatry* **48**, 287–293.

Bienvenu, O. *et al.* (2012) Is obsessive-compulsive disorder an anxiety disorder, and what, if any, are spectrum conditions? A family study perspective. *Psychological Medicine* **42**, 1.

Black, A. (1974) The natural history of obsessional neurosis. In: *Obsessional States.* (ed H. Beech). Methuen, London.

Bloch, M.H. & Leckman, J.F. (2010) Obsessive-compulsive anxiety disorders in childhood. *Encyclopedia of Psychopharmacology* (ed I.P. Stolerman), 914–918 Springer, New York.

Bloch, M. *et al.* (2006) Adult outcome of tic and obsessive-compulsive severity in children with Tourette's syndrome. *Archives of Pedatric and Adolescent Medicine* **160**, 65–69.

Bloch, M.H. *et al.* (2009) Predictors of early adult outcomes in pediatric-onset obsessive-compulsive disorder. *Pediatrics* **124**, 1085–1093.

Bloch, M.H. *et al.* (2011) Poor fine-motor and visuospatial skills predict persistence of pediatric-onset obsessive-compulsive disorder into adulthood. *Journal of Child Psychology and Psychiatry* **52**, 974–983.

Breslau, N. (1987) Inquiring about the bizarre: false positives in Diagnostic Interview Schedule for Children (DISC) ascertainment of obsessions, compulsions, and psychotic symptoms. *Journal of the American Academy of Child & Adolescent Psychiatry* **26**, 639–644.

Britton, J.C. *et al.* (2010) Cognitive inflexibility and frontal-cortical activation in pediatric obsessive-compulsive disorder. *Journal of the American Academy of Child & Adolescent Psychiatry* **49**, 944–953.

Brown, T.A. *et al.* (1993) Diagnostic and symptom distinguishability of generalized anxiety disorder and obsessive-compulsive disorder. *Behavior Therapy* **24**, 227–240.

Byerly, M. *et al.* (2005) Obsessive compulsive symptoms in schizophrenia: frequency and clinical features. *Schizophrenia Research* **76**, 309–316.

Castellanos, F.X. & Tannock, R. (2002) Neuroscience of attention-deficit/hyperactivity disorder: the search for endophenotypes. *Nature Review Neuroscience* **3**, 617–628.

Chabane, N. *et al.* (2004) Early-onset obsessive-compulsive disorder: a subgroup with a specific clinical and familial pattern? *Journal of Child Psychology and Psychiatry* **46**, 881–887.

Christenson, G.A. *et al.* (1991) A placebo-controlled, double-blind crossover study of fluoxetine in trichotillomania. *American Journal of Psychiatry* **148**, 1566–1571.

Crino, R. *et al.* (2005) The changing prevalence and severity of obsessive-compulsive disorder criteria from DSM-III to DSM-IV. *The American Journal of Psychiatry* **162**, 876–882.

De Haan, E. *et al.* (1998) Behavior therapy versus clomipramine for the treatment of obsessive-compulsive disorder in children and adolescents. *Journal of the American Academy of Child & Adolescent Psychiatry* **37**, 1022–1029.

Denys, D. *et al.* (2004a) Low level of dopaminergic D2 receptor binding in obsessive-compulsive disorder. *Biological Psychiatry* **55**, 1041–1045.

Denys, D. *et al.* (2004b) The role of dopamine in obsessive-compulsive disorder: preclinical and clinical evidence. *Journal of Clinical Psychiatry* **65**, 11–17.

Despert, J.L. (1955) Differential diagnosis between obsessive-compulsive neurosis and schizophrenia in children. In: *Psychopathology of Childhood.* (eds P.H. Hoch & J. Zubin). Grune and Stratton, New York.

Deveaugh-Geiss, J. *et al.* (1992) Clomipramine hydrochloride in childhood and adolescent obsessive-compulsive disorder--a multicenter trial. *Journal of the American Academy of Child & Adolescent Psychiatry* **31**, 45–49.

Douglass, H.M. *et al.* (1995) Obsessive-compulsive disorder in a birth cohort of 18-year-olds: prevalence and predictors. *Journal of the American Academy of Child and Adolescent Psychiatry* **34**, 1424–1431.

Farrell, L.J. *et al.* (2013) Difficult to treat pediatric obsessive-compulsive disorder: feasibility and preliminary results of a randomized pilot trial of D-cyloserine augmented behavior therapy. *Depression and Anxiety* **30**, 723–731.

Figueroa, Y. *et al.* (1998) Combination treatment with clomipramine and selective serotonin reuptake inhibitors for obsessive-compulsive disorder in children and adolescents. *Journal of Child & Adolescent Psychopharmacology* **8**, 61–67.

Fitzgerald, K.D. *et al.* (1999) Neurobiology of childhood obsessive-compulsive disorder. *Child & Adolescent Psychiatric Clinics of North America* **8**, 533–575.

Fitzgerald, K.D. *et al.* (2005) Error-related hyperactivity of the anterior cingulate cortex in obsessive-compulsive disorder. *Biological Psychiatry* **57**, 287–294.

Fitzgerald, K.D. *et al.* (2010) Altered function and connectivity of the medial frontal cortex in pediatric obsessive-compulsive disorder. *Biological Psychiatry* **68**, 1039–1047.

Flament, M.F. *et al.* (1985) Clomipramine treatment of childhood obsessive-compulsive disorder. A double-blind controlled study. *Archives of General Psychiatry* **42**, 977–983.

Flament, M.F. *et al.* (1988) Obsessive compulsive disorder in adolescence: an epidemiological study. *Journal of the American Academy of Child & Adolescent Psychiatry* **27**, 764–771.

Foa, E.B. *et al.* (1992) Treatment of depressive and obsessive-compulsive symptoms in OCD by imipramine and behaviour therapy. *British Journal of Clinical Psychology* **31**, 279–292.

Franklin, M.E. *et al.* (1998) Cognitive-behavioral treatment of pediatric obsessive-compulsive disorder: an open clinical trial. *Journal of the American Academy of Child & Adolescent Psychiatry* **37**, 412–419.

Freeman, J.M. *et al.* (1965) The emotional correlates of Sydenham's chorea. *Pediatrics* **35**, 42–49.

Freud, S. (1906) Obsessive actions and religious practices. In: *The Standard Edition of the Complete Psychological Works of Sigmund Freud.* (ed J.A. Strachey). Hogarth Press, London.

Freud, S. (1958) The disposition to obsessional neurosis (1913). In: *The Standard Edition of the Complete Psychological Works of Sigmund Freud.* (ed J.A. Strachey). Hogarth Press, London.

Fullana, M. *et al.* (2009) Obsessions and compulsions in the community: prevalence, interference, help-seeking, developmental stability, and co-occurring psychiatric conditions. *American Journal of Psychiatry* **166**, 329–336.

Garvey, M.A. *et al.* (1999) A pilot study of penicillin prophylaxis for neuropsychiatric exacerbations triggered by streptococcal infections. *Biological Psychiatry* **45**, 1564–1571.

Geller, D.A. *et al.* (1998) Obsessive-compulsive disorder in children and adolescents: a review. *Harvard Review of Psychiatry* **5**, 260–273.

Geller, D.A. *et al.* (2003) Which SSRI? A meta-analysis of pharmacotherapy trials in pediatric obsessive-compulsive disorder. *American Journal of Psychiatry* **160**, 1919–1928.

Geller, D.A. *et al.* (2004) Paroxetine treatment in children and adolescents with obsessive-compulsive disorder: a randomized, multicenter, double-blind, placebo-controlled trial. *Journal of the American Academy of Child & Adolescent Psychiatry* **43**, 1387–1396.

Gilbert, D.L. *et al.* (2004) Association of cortical disinhibition with tic, ADHD, and OCD severity in Tourette's syndrome. *Movement Disorders* **19**, 416–425.

Gilbert, A.R. *et al.* (2009) Neural correlates of symptom dimensions in pediatric obsessive-compulsive disorder: a functional magnetic resonance imaging study. *Journal of the American Academy of Child and Adolescent Psychiatry* **48**, 936–944.

Goodman, W.K. *et al.* (1989a) The Yale-Brown Obsessive Compulsive Scale. II. Validity. *Archives of General Psychiatry* **46**, 1012–1016.

Goodman, W.K. *et al.* (1989b) The Yale-Brown Obsessive Compulsive Scale. I. Development, use, and reliability. *Archives of General Psychiatry* **46**, 1006–1011.

Grados, M.A. *et al.* (2001) The familial phenotype of obsessive-compulsive disorder in relation to tic disorders: the Hopkins OCD family study. *Biological Psychiatry* **50**, 559–565.

Graybiel, A.M. & Rauch, S.L. (2000a) Toward a neurobiology of obsessive-compulsive disorder. *Neuron* **28**, 343–347.

Graybiel, A.M. & Rauch, S.L. (2000b) Toward a neurobiology review of obsessive-compulsive disorder. *Neuron* **28**, 343.

Greenberg, B.D. *et al.* (2003) Neurosurgery for intractable obsessive-compulsive disorder and depression: critical issues. *Neurosurgery Clinics of North America* **14**, 199–212.

Greist, J.H. *et al.* (1990) Clomipramine and obsessive compulsive disorder: a placebo-controlled double-blind study of 32 patients. *Journal of Clinical Psychiatry* **51**, 292–297.

Gross-Isseroff, R. *et al.* (2004) Serotonergic dissection of obsessive compulsive symptoms: a challenge study with m-chlorophenylpiperazine and sumatriptan. *Neuropsychobiology* **50**, 200–205.

Hanna, G.L. *et al.* (2005) A family study of obsessive-compulsive disorder with pediatric probands. *American Journal of Medical Genetics Part B: Neuropsychiatric Genetics* **134**, 13–19.

Hanna, G.L. *et al.* (2011) Major depressive disorder in a family study of obsessive-compulsive disorder with pediatric probands. *Depression and Anxiety* **28**, 501–508.

Hasler, G. *et al.* (2007) Familiality of factor analysis-derived YBOCS dimensions in OCD-affected sibling pairs from the OCD Collaborative Genetics Study. *Biological Psychiatry* **61**, 617–625.

Herjanic, B. & Campbell, W. (1977) Differentiating psychiatrically disturbed children on the basis of a structured interview. *Journal of Abnormal Child Psychology* **5**, 127–134.

Herjanic, B. & Reich, W. (1982) Development of a structured psychiatric interview for children: agreement between child and parent on various symptoms. *Journal of Abnormal Child Psychology* **10**, 307–324.

Hollander, E. (1996) Obsessive-compulsive disorder-related disorders: the role of selective serotonergic reuptake inhibitors. *International Clinical Psychopharmacology* **11**, 75–87.

Hollander, E. & Wong, C.M. (1995) Body dysmorphic disorder, pathological gambling, and sexual compulsions. *Journal of Clinical Psychiatry* **56**, 7–12; discussion 13.

Hollander, E. *et al.* (2003) Obsessive-compulsive behaviors in parents of multiplex autism families. *Psychiatry Research* **117**, 11–16.

Horwath, E. & Weissman, M.M. (2000) The epidemiology and cross-national presentation of obsessive-compulsive disorder. *The Psychiatric Clinics of North America* **23**, 493–507.

Hudziak, J.J. *et al.* (2004) Genetic and environmental contributions to the Child Behavior Checklist Obsessive-Compulsive Scale: a cross-cultural twin study. *Archives of General Psychiatry* **61**, 608.

Huyser, C. *et al.* (2011) Developmental aspects of error and high-related brain activity in pediatric obsessive-compulsive disorder: a fMRI study with a Flanker task before and after CBT. *Journal of Child Psychology and Psychiatry* **52**, 1251–1260.

Janet, P. (1903) *Les Obsessions et la Psychiatrie Vol. 1.* Felix Alan, Paris.

Jonnal, A.H. *et al.* (2000) Obsessive and compulsive symptoms in a general population sample of female twins. *American Journal of Medical Genetics* **96**, 791–796.

Karno, M. & Golding, J. (1990) Obsessive-compulsive disorder. In: *Psychiatric Disorders in America: The Epidemiological Catchment Area Study.* (eds L. Robins & D.A. Regier). Free Press, New York.

Karno, M. & Golding, J.M. (1991) Obsessive compulsive disorder. In: *Psychiatry Disorders in America.* (eds L.N. Robins & D.A. Regier). The Free Press, New York.

Karno, M. *et al.* (1988) The epidemiology of obsessive-compulsive disorder in five US communities. *Archives of General Psychiatry* **45**, 1094–1099.

Kaufman, J. *et al.* (1997) Schedule for Affective Disorders and Schizophrenia for School-Age Children-Present and Lifetime Version (K-SADS-PL): initial reliability and validity data. *Journal of the American Academy of Child and Adolescent Psychiatry* **36**, 980–988.

Kenwright, M. *et al.* (2005) Brief scheduled phone support from a clinician to enhance computer-aided self-help for obsessive-compulsive disorder: randomized controlled trial. *Journal of Clinical Psychology* **61**, 1499–1508.

Keuthen, N.J. *et al.* (2005) Advances in the conceptualization and treatment of body-focused repetitive behaviors. *Obsessive Compulsive Disorder Research* **1**, 1–29.

Kopell, B.H. *et al.* (2004) Deep brain stimulation for psychiatric disorders. *Journal of Clinical Neurophysiology* **21**, 51–67.

Kordon, A. *et al.* (2008) Quetiapine addition to serotonin reuptake inhibitors in patients with severe obsessive-compulsive disorder: a double-blind, randomized, placebo-controlled study. *Journal of Clinical Psychopharmacology* **28**, 550–554.

Lasalle, V.H. *et al.* (2004) Diagnostic interview assessed neuropsychiatric disorder comorbidity in 334 individuals with obsessive-compulsive disorder. *Depression and Anxiety* **19**, 163–173.

Lebowitz, E.R. *et al.* (2011) Coercive and disruptive behaviors in pediatric obsessive–compulsive disorder. *Depression and anxiety* **28**, 899–905.

Lebowitz, E.R. *et al.* (2012) Family accommodation in obsessive-compulsive disorder. *Expert Review of Neurotherapeutics* **12**, 229–238.

Leckman, J.F. *et al.* (1994) Tic-related vs. non-tic-related obsessive compulsive disorder. *Anxiety* **1**, 208–215.

Leckman, J.F. *et al.* (2009) Symptom dimensions and subtypes of obsessive-compulsive disorder: a developmental perspective. *Dialogues in Clinical Neuroscience* **11**, 21.

Leonard, H.L. *et al.* (1989) Childhood rituals and superstitions: developmental and cultural perspective. In: *Obsessive-Compulsive Disorder in Children & Adolescents.* (ed J.L. Rapoport). American Psychiatric Association, Washington, DC.

Leonard, H.L. *et al.* (1989) Treatment of obsessive-compulsive disorder with clomipramine and desipramine in children and adolescents. A double-blind crossover comparison. *Archives of General Psychiatry* **46**, 1088–1092.

Leonard, H.L. *et al.* (1991) A double-blind desipramine substitution during long-term clomipramine treatment in children and adolescents with obsessive-compulsive disorder. *Archives of General Psychiatry* **48**, 922–927.

Leonard, H.L. *et al.* (1992) Tics and Tourette's disorder: a 2- to 7-year follow-up of 54 obsessive-compulsive children. *The American Journal of Psychiatry* **149**, 1244–1251.

Leonard, H.L. *et al.* (1994) Clonazepam as an augmenting agent in the treatment of childhood-onset obsessive-compulsive disorder. *Journal of the American Academy of Child & Adolescent Psychiatry* **33**, 792–794.

Leonard, H.L. *et al.* (1999) Postinfectious and other forms of obsessive-compulsive disorder. *Child and Adolescent Psychiatric Clinics of North America* **8**, 497–511.

Lewinsohn, P.M. *et al.* (1993) Adolescent psychopathology: I. Prevalence and incidence of depression and other DSM-III-R disorders in high school students. *Journal of Abnormal Psychology* **102**, 133–144.

Li, X. *et al.* (2005) Risperidone and haloperidol augmentation of serotonin reuptake inhibitors in refractory obsessive-compulsive disorder: a crossover study. *Journal of Clinical Psychiatry* **66**, 736–743.

Liebowitz, M.R. *et al.* (2002) Fluoxetine in children and adolescents with OCD: a placebo-controlled trial. *Journal of the American Academy of Child & Adolescent Psychiatry* **41**, 1431–1438.

Lin, H. *et al.* (2007) Psychosocial stress predicts future symptom severities in children and adolescents with Tourette's syndrome and/or obsessive-compulsive disorder. *Journal of Child Psychology and Psychiatry* **48**, 157–166.

Lombroso, P.J. *et al.* (1995) Risperidone treatment of children and adolescents with chronic tic disorders: a preliminary report. *Journal of the American Academy of Child and Adolescent Psychiatry* **34**, 1147–1152.

Maina, G. *et al.* (1999) Obsessive-compulsive syndromes in older adolescents. *Acta Psychiatrica Scandinavica* **100**, 447–450.

Maltby, N. *et al.* (2005) Dysfunctional action monitoring hyperactivates frontal-striatal circuits in obsessive-compulsive disorder: an event-related fMRI study. *NeuroImage* **24**, 495–503.

March, J.S. & Mulle, K. (1998) *OCD in Children and Adolescents: A Cognitive-Behavioral Treatment Manual.* Guilford Press, New York.

March, J.S. *et al.* (1998) Sertraline in children and adolescents with obsessive-compulsive disorder: a multicenter randomized controlled trial, *JAMA* **280**, 1752–1756. [erratum appears in *JAMA* 283].

Marsh, R. *et al.* (2009) Functional disturbances within frontostriatal circuits across multiple childhood psychopathologies. *The American Journal of Psychiatry* **166**, 664.

Martin, J.L. *et al.* (2003) Transcranial magnetic stimulation for the treatment of obsessive-compulsive disorder. *Cochrane Database of Systematic Reviews* (3), CD003387.

Masi, G. *et al.* (2004) Obsessive-compulsive bipolar comorbidity: focus on children and adolescents. *Journal of Affective Disorders* **78**, 175–183.

Masi, G. *et al.* (2005) A naturalistic study of referred children and adolescents with obsessive-compulsive disorder. *Journal of the American Academy of Child and Adolescent Psychiatry* **44**, 673–681.

Mataix-Cols, D. & Van Den Heuvel, O.A. (2006) Common and distinct neural correlates of obsessive-compulsive and related disorders. *The Psychiatric Clinics of North America* **29**, 391.

Mataix-Cols, D. *et al.* (2012) The London field trial for hoarding disorder. *Psychological Medicine* **10**, 1–11.

Mataix-Cols, D. *et al.* (2013) Population-based, multigenerational family clustering study of obsessive-compulsive disorder. *JAMA Psychiatry (Chicago, Ill.)* **70**, 1–9.

McDougle, C.J. *et al.* (2000) A double-blind, placebo-controlled study of risperidone addition in serotonin reuptake inhibitor-refractory obsessive-compulsive disorder. *Archives of General Psychiatry* **57**, 794–801.

Menzies, L. *et al.* (2008) Integrating evidence from neuroimaging and neuropsychological studies of obsessive-compulsive disorder: the orbitofronto-striatal model revisited. *Neuroscience & Biobehavioral Reviews* **32**, 525–549.

Micali, N. *et al.* (2010) Long-term outcomes of obsessive-compulsive disorder: follow-up of 142 children and adolescents. *The British Journal of Psychiatry* **197**, 128–134.

Miguel, E.C. *et al.* (2000) Sensory phenomena in obsessive-compulsive disorder and Tourette's disorder. *Journal of Clinical Psychiatry* **61**, 150–156; quiz 157.

Modell, J.G. *et al.* (1989) Neurophysiologic dysfunction in basal ganglia/limbic striatal and thalamocortical circuits as a pathogenetic mechanism of obsessive-compulsive disorder. *Journal of Neuropsychiatry and Clinical Neuroscience* **1**, 27–36.

Nestadt, G. *et al.* (2000) A family study of obsessive-compulsive disorder. *Archives of General Psychiatry* **57**, 358–363.

Neziroglu, F. *et al.* (2000) The effect of fluvoxamine and behavior therapy on children and adolescents with obsessive-compulsive disorder. *Journal of Child & Adolescent Psychopharmacology* **10**, 295–306.

National Institute for Health and Care Excellence (2005) *Obsessive-Compulsive Disorder: Clinical Guidelines 31.* National Institute for Health and Care Excellence.

Osler, W. (1894) *On Chorea and Choreiform Affections.* Taylor & Francis.

Pauls, D.L. (2010) The genetics of obsessive-compulsive disorder: a review. *Dialogues in Clinical Neuroscience* **12**, 149.

Pauls, D.L. *et al.* (1995) A family study of obsessive-compulsive disorder. *The American Journal of Psychiatry* **152**, 76–84.

Perlmutter, S.J. *et al.* (1999a) Therapeutic plasma exchange and intravenous immunoglobulin for obsessive-compulsive disorder and tic disorders in childhood. *The Lancet* **354**, 1153–1158.

Perlmutter, S.J. *et al.* (1999b) Therapeutic plasma exchange and intravenous immunoglobulin for obsessive-compulsive disorder and tic disorders in childhood. *The Lancet* **354**, 1153–1158.

Peterson, B.S. *et al.* (2001) Prospective, longitudinal study of tic, obsessive-compulsive, and attention-deficit/hyperactivity disorders in an epidemiological sample. *Journal of the American Academy of Child & Adolescent Psychiatry* **40**, 685–695.

Phillips, K.A. *et al.* (2010) Should an obsessive-compulsive spectrum grouping of disorders be included in DSM-V? *Depression and Anxiety* **27**, 528–555.

Pogarell, O. *et al.* (2003) Elevated brain serotonin transporter availability in patients with obsessive-compulsive disorder. *Biological Psychiatry* **54**, 1406–1413.

POTS (2004) Cognitive-behavior therapy, sertraline, and their combination for children and adolescents with obsessive-compulsive disorder: the Pediatric OCD Treatment Study (POTS) randomized controlled trial. *JAMA* **292**, 1969–1976.

Poyurovsky, M. & Koran, L.M. (2005) Obsessive-compulsive disorder (OCD) with schizotypy vs. schizophrenia with OCD: diagnostic dilemmas and therapeutic implications. *Journal of Psychiatric Research* **39**, 399–408.

Radua, J. *et al.* (2010) Meta-analytical comparison of voxel-based morphometry studies in obsessive-compulsive disorder vs other anxiety disorders. *Archives of General Psychiatry* **67**, 701.

Rapoport, J.L. & Wise, S.P. (1988) Obsessive-compulsive disorder: evidence for basal ganglia dysfunction. *Psychopharmacology Bulletin* **24**, 380–384.

Rapoport, J.L. *et al.* (2000) Childhood obsessive-compulsive disorder in the NIMH MECA study: parent versus child identification of cases. Methods for the Epidemiology of Child and Adolescent Mental Disorders. *Journal of Anxiety Disorders* **14**, 535–548.

Rasmussen, S.A. & Tsuang, M.T. (1984) The epidemiology of obsessive compulsive disorder. *Journal of Clinical Psychiatry* **45**, 450–457.

Reinherz, H.H.Z. *et al.* (1993) Prevalence of psychiatric disorders in a community population of older adolescents. *Journal of the American Academy of Child & Adolescent Psychiatry* **32**, 369–377.

Rettew, D.C. *et al.* (1992) Obsessions and compulsions across time in 79 children and adolescents with obsessive-compulsive disorder. *Journal of the American Academy of Child and Adolescent Psychiatry* **31**, 1050–1056.

Riddle, M.A. *et al.* (1992) Double-blind, crossover trial of fluoxetine and placebo in children and adolescents with obsessive-compulsive disorder. *Journal of the American Academy of Child & Adolescent Psychiatry* **31**, 1062–1069.

Riddle, M.A. *et al.* (2001) Fluvoxamine for children and adolescents with obsessive-compulsive disorder: a randomized, controlled, multicenter trial. *Journal of the American Academy of Child & Adolescent Psychiatry* **40**, 222–229.

Robinson, S. *et al.* (2012) The feasibility and acceptability of a cognitive-behavioural self-help intervention for adolescents with obsessive-compulsive disorder. *Behavioural and Cognitive Psychotherapy* **1**, 1–6.

Rosario, M.C. *et al.* (2009) Validation of the University of Sao Paulo sensory phenomena scale: initial psychometric properties. *CNS Spectrums* **14**, 315–323.

Rosenberg, D.R. *et al.* (2000) Decrease in caudate glutamatergic concentrations in pediatric obsessive-compulsive disorder patients taking paroxetine. *Journal of the American Academy of Child & Adolescent Psychiatry* **39**, 1096–1103.

Rosenberg, D.R. *et al.* (2004) Reduced anterior cingulate glutamatergic concentrations in childhood OCD and major depression versus healthy controls. *Journal of the American Academy of Child & Adolescent Psychiatry* **43**, 1146–1153.

Rubia, K. *et al.* (2011) Disorder specific dysfunctions in patients with attention, deficit/hyperactivity disorder compared to patients with obsessive-compulsive disorder during interference inhibition and attention allocation. *Human Brain Mapping* **32**, 601–611.

Samuels, J. *et al.* (2002) Hoarding in obsessive compulsive disorder: results from a case-control study. *Behaviour Research and Therapy* **40**, 517–528.

Saxena, S. *et al.* (1998) Neuroimaging and frontal-subcortical circuitry in obsessive-compulsive disorder. *British Journal of Psychiatry* **35**, 26–37.

Saxena, S. *et al.* (2001) Brain-behavior relationships in obsessive-compulsive disorder. *Seminars in Clinical Neuropsychiatry* **6**, 82–101.

Saxena, S. *et al.* (2007) Paroxetine treatment of compulsive hoarding. *Journal of Psychiatric Research* **41**, 481.

Scahill, L. *et al.* (1997) Children's Yale-Brown obsessive compulsive scale: reliability and validity. *Journal of the American Academy of Child & Adolescent Psychiatry* **36**, 844–852.

Simpson, H.B. *et al.* (2003) Serotonin transporters in obsessive-compulsive disorder: a positron emission tomography study with [(11)C]McN 5652. *Biological Psychiatry* **54**, 1414–1421.

Singer, H.S. *et al.* (2005) Serum autoantibodies do not differentiate PANDAS and Tourette's syndrome from controls. *Neurology* **65**, 1701–1707.

Singer, H.S. *et al.* (2012) Moving from PANDAS to CANS. *Journal of Pediatrics* **160**, 725.

Snider, L.A. *et al.* (2005) Antibiotic prophylaxis with arithromycin or penicillin for childhood-onset neuropsychiatric disorders. *Biological Psychiatry* **57**, 788–792.

Stengler-Wenzke, K. *et al.* (2004) Reduced serotonin transporter availability in obsessive-compulsive disorder (OCD). *European Archives of Psychiatry & Clinical Neuroscience* **254**, 252–255.

Stewart, S.E. *et al.* (2004) Long-term outcome of pediatric obsessive-compulsive disorder: a meta-analysis and qualitative review of the literature. *Acta Psychiatrica Scandinavica* **110**, 4–13.

Storch, E.A. *et al.* (2010) A preliminary study of D-cycloserine augmentation of cognitive-behavioral therapy in pediatric obsessive-compulsive disorder. *Biological Psychiatry* **68**, 1073.

Storch, E.A. *et al.* (2012) Rage attacks in pediatric obsessive-compulsive disorder: phenomenology and clinical correlates. *Journal of the American Academy of Child & Adolescent Psychiatry* **51**, 582–592.

Swedo, S. *et al.* (1989) Obsessive-compulsive disorder in children and adolescents. Clinical phenomenology of 70 consecutive cases. *Archives of General Psychiatry* **46**, 335–341.

Swedo, S. *et al.* (2004) The pediatric autoimmune neuropsychiatric disorders associated with streptococcal infection (PANDAS) subgroup: separating fact from fiction. *Pediatrics* **113**, 907–911.

Swedo, S. *et al.* (2012) From research subgroup to clinical syndrome: modifying the PANDAS criteria to describe PANS (Pediatric Acute-onset Neuropsychiatric Syndrome). *Pediatrics & Therapeutics* **2**, 1000113.

Taylor, S. (2012) Molecular genetics of obsessive-compulsive disorder: a comprehensive meta-analysis of genetic association studies. *Molecular Psychiatry* **18**, 799–805.

Thomsen, P.H. (1991) Obsessive-compulsive symptoms in children and adolescents. A phenomenological analysis of 61 Danish cases. *Psychopathology* **24**, 12–18.

Ursu, S. *et al.* (2003) Overactive action monitoring in obsessive-compulsive disorder: evidence from functional magnetic resonance imaging. *Psychological Science* **14**, 347–353.

Valleni-Basile, L.A. *et al.* (1994) Frequency of obsessive-compulsive disorder in a community sample of young adolescents. *Journal of the American Academy of Child & Adolescent Psychiatry* **33**, 782–791.

Van Der Wee, N.J. *et al.* (2004) Enhanced dopamine transporter density in psychotropic-naive patients with obsessive-compulsive disorder shown by [123I]beta-CIT SPECT. *American Journal of Psychiatry* **161**, 2201–2206.

Van Grootheest, D.L.S. *et al.* (2005) Twin studies on obsessive-compulsive disorder: a review. *Twin Research and Human Genetics* **8**, 450–458.

Van Veen, V. & Carter, C.S. (2002) The anterior cingulate as a conflict monitor: fMRI and ERP studies. *Physiology & Behavior* **77**, 477–482.

Walsh, K.H. & Mcdougle, C.J. (2004) Pharmacological augmentation strategies for treatment-resistant obsessive-compulsive disorder. *Expert Opinion on Pharmacotherapy* **5**, 2059–2067.

Wang, Y. *et al.* (2010) A screen of SLC1A1 for OCD-related alleles. *American Journal of Medical Genetics Part B: Neuropsychiatric Genetics* **153**, 675–679.

Willour, V.L. *et al.* (2004) Replication study supports evidence for linkage to 9p24 in obsessive-compulsive disorder. *American Journal of Human Genetics* **75**, 508–513.

Wise, S.P. & Rapoport, J.L. (1989) Obsessive compulsive disorder: is it a basal ganglia dysfunction?. In: *Obsessive-Compulsive Disorder in Children and Adolescents*. American Psychiatric Association, Washington, DC.

Wittchen, H.U. *et al.* (1998) Prevalence of mental disorders and psychosocial impairments in adolescents and young adults. *Psychological Medicine* **28**, 109–126.

Woolley, J. *et al.* (2008) Brain activation in paediatric obsessive-compulsive disorder during tasks of inhibitory control. *British Journal of Psychiatry* **192**, 25–31.

Zohar, A.H. (1999) The epidemiology of obsessive-compulsive disorder in children and adolescents. *Child and Adolescent Psychiatric Clinics of North America* **8**, 445–460.

Zohar, A.H. *et al.* (1992) An epidemiological study of obsessive-compulsive disorder and related disorders in Israeli adolescents. *Journal of the American Academy of Child and Adolescent Psychiatry* **31**, 1057–1061.

CHAPTER 62

Bipolar disorder in childhood

Ellen Leibenluft[1] and Daniel P. Dickstein[2,3]

[1] Section on Bipolar Spectrum Disorders, Emotion and Development Branch, National Institute of Mental Health, Bethesda, MD, USA
[2] PediMIND Program, Bradley Hospital, East Providence, RI, USA
[3] Division of Child Psychiatry, Department of Psychiatry and Human Behavior, Alpert Medical School of Brown University, Providence, RI, USA

Introduction

Bipolar disorder (BD) is among the most impairing childhood psychiatric illnesses. In the last two decades, there has been a marked upsurge in knowledge about childhood-onset BD.

In this chapter, we first review data on the *characteristics and diagnosis* of childhood-onset BD, including its phenomenology, distinction from typical development, impact on functioning, and differential diagnosis. We then describe *assessment* of BD, including comorbid psychopathology such as attention deficit hyperactivity disorder (ADHD). Then, we discuss its *epidemiology, longitudinal course, and risk factors,* before summarizing recent data about the *pathophysiology* and *treatment* of childhood-onset BD. We conclude by predicting *future directions* for research and clinical care for childhood-onset BD.

Characteristics and diagnosis of the condition

Phenomenology

At its core, BD is a mood disorder involving a change from baseline normal mood to elevated, expansive, or irritable mood plus concomitant behavioral changes (section "Diagnosis in DSM, ICD, elsewhere"). Some forms of BD also require depressive episodes.

Distinction between normal and pathological

Episodes of mania and depression differ from normal fluctuations in mood and behavior because they last longer, are associated with other symptoms (e.g., "B" symptoms of mania or neurovegetative dysfunction in depression), and cause impairment, including disruptions of peer, occupational/educational, and family function.

Cultural issues

Relatively little is known about cultural differences in the phenomenology of childhood-onset BD. More such studies are needed, evaluating the impact of culture on the expression and treatment of BD.

Diagnosis in DSM, ICD, elsewhere

In the Diagnostic and Statistical Manual 5th edition (DSM-5), a diagnosis of BD is based on the presence of manic, hypomanic, and major depressive episodes (American Psychiatric Association, 2013). A manic episode involves elevated, expansive, or irritable mood that should be different than the child's baseline mood. Concomitant with the mood change additional symptoms should include decreased need for sleep, increased goal-directed activity [e.g., persistently practicing singing all day long and ignoring other activities], and flight of ideas [e.g., thoughts jumping from topic to topic without logical connection]. The duration of the mood change plus associated symptoms must be at least seven days or require hospitalization for a manic episode, or four to seven days for a hypomanic episode.

Importantly, the mood and activity changes need to represent an episode—that is, a clear period of altered function by comparison with the young person's usual state. It should be clear that they are present throughout the day and occur nearly every day during the episode. The associated features also need to have appeared (or worsened) during the episode, and do not reflect simply the ordinary condition of the young person. Episodicity is therefore an important part of the definition: an episode should last for at least a week to constitute a manic period (and may last for much longer). A hypomanic episode is a period lasting a shorter time—4–7 days of these mood and activity changes and associated features.

Rutter's Child and Adolescent Psychiatry, Sixth Edition.
Edited by Anita Thapar and Daniel S. Pine, James F. Leckman, Stephen Scott, Margaret J. Snowling, Eric Taylor.
© 2015 John Wiley & Sons Ltd. Published 2018 by John Wiley & Sons Ltd.

A major depressive episode consists of depressed mood or decreased interest or pleasure most of the day, nearly every day during a 2-week period, representing a change from previous functioning, and accompanied by additional symptoms, for example, recurrent thoughts of death and inability to experience pleasure ["anhedonia"]. DSM-5 has a child-specific modification allowing irritable, rather than depressed, mood to fulfill the mood criterion for a major depressive episode. A mixed episode is diagnosed when full criteria are met for both a manic and major depressive episode for at least 1 week (see also Chapter 63). If irritability is the only mood change, the diagnostician should remember that it is not very specific to mania (see Chapter 5) and care is needed in assessment.

DSM-5 recognizes three types of BD, based on lifetime history of episode type: type I requires at least one manic episode (no major depressive episode required), type II requires at least one hypomanic episode plus at least one major depressive episode; and "not otherwise specified" (BD-NOS) includes patients whose symptoms do not meet criteria for a specific type of BD, including but not limited to patients whose symptoms do not satisfy duration criteria for a manic or hypomanic episode.

Three issues make establishing the diagnosis of BD difficult in children: (i) duration of a manic episode, (ii) the role of irritability versus euphoria in defining a manic episode, and (iii) overlap with other illnesses, including ADHD. Changes from DSM-IV to DSM-5 are meant to address these issues.

Regarding duration, DSM-5 has a substantive change from DSM-IV-TR in now requiring that irritable or euphoric mood in mania/hypomania should last "most of the day nearly every day" akin to DSM-IV and DSM-5 specifications of a major depressive episode. This language applies regardless of the patient's age—that is, to children and to adults equally. This change is designed to refute prior assertions that BD in children or adolescents is a chronic illness, with fluctuations between all three mood states often occurring within a single day (e.g., "ultradian cycling") (Geller et al., 1998; Biederman et al., 2004). Instead, this promotes the classical view that BD in both children and adults is an episodic illness, with distinct periods (days to weeks) of mania, depression, and euthymia (Leibenluft et al., 2003; Birmaher et al., 2006).

Second, euphoric mood is unique to mania, but it is not necessary for the diagnosis in DSM-5, which allows irritable mood to fulfill this criterion. Irritability and euphoria are weighted differently, so that three associated "B" symptoms are required if the mood is primarily euphoric, and four if the mood is primarily irritable. Moreover, irritability is a diagnostic criterion not only for mania, but also for several other disorders including generalized anxiety disorder, the child-specific modified criterion for a major depressive episode, and oppositional defiant disorder (ODD). Irritability is also an associated symptom for disorders including autism-spectrum disorders and ADHD (American Psychiatric Association, 2000). Unlike DSM-IV, DSM-5 has attempted to clarify how irritability differs among disorders. For example, in DSM-5, irritability in

mania must occur simultaneously with "B" symptom changes (e.g., decreased need for sleep).

The third DSM-related factor leading to potential confusion is the overlap between some of the associated features of mania and those of ADHD. For example, how does one distinguish pressured speech in mania from talking excessively and blurting out answers in ADHD? How to distinguish distractibility in mania from distractibility in ADHD? Unlike DSM-IV, DSM-5 builds on work by Geller et al. who found that five symptoms best distinguished children with BD from those with ADHD [(i) elation, (ii) grandiosity, (iii) hypersexuality, (iv) flight of ideas/increased goal-directed activity, and (v) decreased need for sleep], to now require that these "B" symptoms only count toward a diagnosis of mania if they are present during the episode of mood and activity/energy change (Geller et al., 2002a, b).

In contrast, ICD-10's approach to BD is more conservative than that of the DSM. Specifically, it requires elation in a manic or hypomanic episode, as well as two or more episodes of hypomania, mania, or depression to establish the diagnosis of bipolar affective disorder. With regard to children specifically, the UK's National Institute for Health and Care Excellence (NICE) BD guidelines state that the same criteria should be used to diagnose BD in children as in adults, except that (i) mania must be present (not just hypomania), (ii) euphoria must be present most days, most of the time for at least 7 days, and (iii) consistent with ICD-10, while irritability can be helpful in making a diagnosis of BD if it is severe, episodic, uncharacteristic, and results in functional impairment, it should not be considered a core diagnostic criterion (NICE, 2006).

Impact of the disorder on functioning

BD in childhood is associated with significant morbidity and mortality, including high rates of psychiatric inpatient hospitalization (more than 52–74% hospitalized at least once), suicidal ideation (70–85%), and suicide attempts (30–65%) (Axelson et al., 2006; DelBello et al., 2007; Algorta et al., 2011a).

Differential diagnosis

The differential diagnosis for childhood-onset BD includes any disorder involving euphoria, irritability, or depression as well as psychosis. This includes substance intoxication and substance-related mood or psychotic disorders. It also includes primary medical problems including toxidromes (e.g., anticholinergic ingestion resulting in psychosis/mania), thyroid abnormalities (e.g., hypothyroidism/depression, or hyperthyroidism/mania), or seizure disorders (temporal lobe epilepsy).

In particular, we note the new DSM-5 diagnosis "Disruptive Mood Dyregulation Disorder" (DMDD) that should be considered in the differential of children with functionally impairing irritability. Unlike BD, DMDD involves chronic, severe irritability characterized by (i) frequent temper outbursts out of proportion to the situation and child's developmental

Table 62.1 Severe mood dysregulation (SMD) diagnostic criteria.

Inclusion criteria

1 Age 7–17 years, with symptom onset before age 12.

2 Abnormal mood (specifically, anger or sadness) present at least half of the day most days and of sufficient severity to be noticeable by others (e.g., parents, teachers, or peers).

3 Hyperarousal, as defined by ≥3: insomnia, agitation, distractibility, racing thoughts or flight of ideas, pressured speech, or intrusiveness.

4 Compared to peers, the child exhibits markedly increased reactivity to negative emotional stimuli manifest verbally or behaviorally—that is, temper tantrums out of proportion to the inciting event and/or child's developmental stage—occurring >3 times/week during past 4 weeks.

5 Symptoms are present for ≥12 months without ≥2 months symptom-free.

6 Symptoms are severe in ≥1 setting and mild in a second setting.

Exclusion criteria

1 Child has any "cardinal" BD symptoms: elevated/expansive mood, grandiosity, or episodically decreased need for sleep.

2 Distinct episodes ≥4 days.

3 Individual meets diagnostic criteria for schizophrenia, schizophreniform disorder, schizoaffective illness, pervasive developmental disorder, or post-traumatic stress disorder.

4 Individual meets criteria for substance use disorder in the past 3 months.

5 IQ < 80.

6 Symptoms are direct physiological effect of drug of abuse or general medical/neurological condition.

level, manifest verbally or physically, and occurring frequently (e.g., three or more times per week) and (ii) persistently irritable or angry mood (Table 62.1).

DMDD was added to the DSM nosology based on work demonstrating that children with chronic irritability represent a unique population compared to those with episodic euphoria. Specifically, Leibenluft et al. operationalized criteria for severe mood dysregulation (SMD) (Table 62.1) to determine if children with chronic irritability differ from those with classic BD and episodic euphoria ("narrow-phenotype BD" [NP-BD] (American Psychiatric Association, 2000; Leibenluft et al., 2003). In contrast to other DSM disorders where irritability is not operationalized clearly, SMD criteria define it as temper outbursts (i.e., markedly increased reactivity to negative emotional stimuli manifest verbally or behaviorally) and an abnormally sad or angry baseline mood (i.e., present most days, most of the time).

Over the past decade, over 150 NP-BD and 200 SMD youths have been studied. Both SMD and NP-BD youths do not differ on initial evaluation in impairment, number of psychiatric medications, and number of psychiatric hospitalizations. Prospectively, only one of 84 SMD subjects (1.2%) experienced a (hypo)manic or mixed episode during a median 28.7 months of follow-up, whereas 58 of 93 NP-BD participants (62.4%) experienced such an episode (Stringaris et al., 2010a).

Brotman et al. (2006) conducted a post hoc analysis of data from the Great Smokey Mountain Study (GSMS), a longitudinal, population-based community survey. The lifetime prevalence of SMD among children 9–19 years old ($N = 1420$) in the first wave was 3.3% (Brotman et al., 2006). Children who met SMD criteria during the first wave (mean age 10.6 ± 1.4 years) were more likely to be diagnosed with a depressive disorder during young adulthood than those who never met SMD criteria (mean age 18.3 ± 2.1 years; OR 7.2, CI 1.3–38.8, $p = 0.02$) (Brotman et al., 2006). This suggests that SMD in childhood is associated with unipolar depression, rather than BD, later in life.

This aligns with another study of 631 participants whose parents were interviewed when participants were in early adolescence (mean age $= 13.8 \pm 2.6$ years) and who were themselves interviewed 20 years later (mean age $= 33.2 + 2.9$ years). While irritability in adolescence predicted MDD (odds ratio $= 1.33$, 95% CI $= 1.00$–1.78]), generalized anxiety disorder (OR $= 1.72$, 95% CI $= 1.04$–2.87), and dysthymia (OR $= 1.81$, 95% CI $= 1.06$–3.12) at 20-year follow-up, it did not predict BD in adulthood (Stringaris et al., 2009). Other longitudinal studies confirm the association between irritability (often in the form of ODD) and subsequent unipolar depression and/or anxiety disorders, rather than BD (Copeland et al., 2009; Rowe et al., 2010).

Disentangling the differential diagnosis of BD in children requires a careful psychiatric history with the children and their primary caretakers; screening for medical or substance-related conditions; collateral sources of information (e.g., teachers, primary care doctor, other mental health providers); and repeat assessments.

In general, unlike anxiety disorders, irritability in mania is not the result of worry or fear. Distinguishing whether a child has primary BD, primary ADHD, or both is complicated (see Section "Diagnosis in DSM, ICD, elsewhere"). Although psychosis can accompany either mania or depression, psychosis unaccompanied by mania or depression suggests either schizophrenia or schizoaffective disorder.

Summary

Recent nosological changes in DSM-5 align with prior research that uses the same diagnostic techniques as in adult studies and confirms that BD in childhood involves episodes of euphoria (in addition to irritability) and clearly defined episodes meeting DSM-IV duration criteria (Findling et al., 2001; Birmaher et al., 2006; Dickstein et al., 2007). However, children with BD do tend to cycle more frequently than adults with BD, and all studies agree that childhood-onset BD is a very impairing illness, leaving affected children symptomatic much of the time.

Assessment

Core aspects

Assessing a child for BD requires determining whether a child has had episodes of mania and depression. Once episodes are identified, the interviewer must determine if the features associated with mania or depression (e.g. sleep and activity changes, increased distractibility, etc.—the "B" criteria of

DSM-5) occurred concurrent with mood changes. If the family cannot identify distinct episodes, then the appropriateness of the diagnosis of BD is called into question.

Euphoria should exceed that which a typically developing child experiences in a very exciting situation, such as going to Disneyland, and true grandiosity should be distinguished from developmentally appropriate fantasy or oppositional behavior. Grandiosity or euphoria should represent a distinct change from the child's usual level of function, and should occur at the same time as other manic symptoms (e.g., decreased need for sleep, increased goal-directed activity). Decreased need for sleep should be differentiated from more typical insomnia, whereby youth would prefer to sleep and may nap during the day.

When possible, clinicians should see a child when the parent states that the child is exhibiting manic behavior. A longitudinal approach may be required, with data from multiple informants including parents and other significant caregivers, such as teachers, and with the child seen repeatedly over time. Prospective daily mood ratings and commonly available technology may help, including cell phone camera recordings of manic or depressive behavior, so that clinicians and parents can achieve a shared understanding of target behaviors and symptoms.

Clinicians must balance concerns about over- and underdiagnosis of BD. A longitudinal approach is required, because children who initially present with one diagnosis, such as unipolar depression or ADHD, might subsequently develop mania. Careful follow-up is particularly warranted in youth with a family history of BD.

Comorbid illnesses should be diagnosed only if symptoms are present when the patient is not in an acute mood episode. For example, a child with BD should be diagnosed with ADHD only if ADHD symptoms are present when he/she is euthymic or subsyndromally ill. Family history of BD in a first-degree relative raises concern about BD in the child; however, children should be diagnosed and treated on the basis of their own clinical presentation. For example, in the Course and Outcome of Bipolar Youth (COBY) study, a prospective study of children with BD types I, II, and NOS, most children with BD had first-degree relatives with unipolar major depression or anxiety, and not BD (Axelson et al., 2006).

Common pitfalls and how to avoid them

The most common pitfall in assessing a child for the presence of BD occurs when the child exhibits for no episodes of mania, despite concerning symptoms, such as severe irritability. This raises questions about the most appropriate course of action. The answer to such questions is to treat the child, not for BD, but for diagnoses that are clearly present. BD can remain on the differential diagnosis for ongoing longitudinal assessment if suspicion remains. Another common pitfall occurs when trying to determine if an irritable outburst is part of typical development, mania, or another disorder. However, mania has a specific duration plus concomitant mood change and other "B" symptoms, whereas irritable/temper outbursts do not.

Use of rating scales, diagnostic interviews, and standardized observations

Currently there are no well-validated rating scales that are sensitive and specific to BD, in children. Galanter and colleagues' comparison of six research diagnostic interviews highlights the problems associated with the standardized assessment tools currently available (Galanter et al., 2012). These authors reported considerable variation in how each interview conceptualized the mood criterion, whether the symptoms had to represent a change from the patient's usual state, and whether B-symptoms had to co-occur with the A (mood) symptoms (Young et al., 1978). With regard to parent-rated questionnaires, Faraone et al. found that the Child Behavior Checklist (CBCL) "juvenile BD phenotype" (i.e., T-scores greater than 70 on the attention problems, aggression, and anxiety/depression subscales) had acceptable sensitivity and specificity in identifying BD (Faraone et al., 2005). However, other studies indicate that the CBCL does not specifically identify BD youths (Hazell et al., 1999; Boomsma et al., 2006; Youngstrom et al., 2005; Volk & Todd, 2007). Based on this nonspecificity, Althoff et al. (2012) have suggested that this be renamed the CBCL "dysregulation profile."

This is an important and active area of investigation. For example, in $N = 2252$ US youths presenting either at an urban academic medical center ($N = 813$) or urban community mental health center ($N = 1439$), the 10-item version of the Parent-report General Behavior Inventory (PGBI-10M) discriminated childhood-onset BD from other diagnoses better than chance (AUROC = 0.79) (Freeman et al., 2012). However, the PGBI-10M requires further investigation and should not be used routinely to screen children for mania.

Coexisting problems: ADHD, anxiety, ODD/CD, and learning disabilities

Comorbidity is the rule rather than the exception in childhood BD. Across studies, more than 70% of children with BD also have ADHD. Anxiety disorders range from 14–76%, ODD from 46–80%, and conduct disorder from 12–41% (Wozniak et al., 1995; Geller et al., 2002a; Harpold et al., 2005; Axelson et al., 2006). Substance abuse disorders have received little attention, although one study found that 32% of adolescents with BD ($N = 57$) had substance use disorder (Wilens et al., 2004). It is possible that referral bias may affect these data, with clinical samples involving sicker children resulting in elevated rates of comorbidity. However, the question remains as to whether these are truly comorbid psychiatric disorders—that is, fully present in their own right—or if they represent using a separate label to capture the same symptoms. In clinical care and research studies, the truest assessment of comorbid psychopathology comes from examining a period of euthymia to determine if symptoms of co-occurring disorders are present when symptoms of mania and/or depression abate.

Family and school context

Multiple impairments have been reported in the families of BD youth, including decreased family function and maternal warmth, and increased expressed emotion, conflict, and family stress (Esposito-Smythers et al., 2006; Miklowitz & Scott, 2009; Algorta et al., 2011b). A variety of neurocognitive deficits have been found in children with BD and associations have been demonstrated with academic difficulties (Pavuluri et al., 2006).

Physical investigations

Currently there is no laboratory test or scan that is diagnostic of BD. Selective laboratory studies may be warranted to exclude medical conditions from the differential diagnosis, particularly hyperthyroidism and substance intoxication/ingestion.

Summary and conclusions

Assessing children for BD requires integrating information from many sources to assess specific diagnostic symptoms and whether they are developmentally appropriate and/or functionally impairing. A longitudinal perspective is particularly important in ensuring the presence of episodes.

Epidemiology

Incidence and prevalence

Broadly, epidemiological studies demonstrate that childhood-onset BD is not so rare, with prevalence being less than that of ADHD (3.7%) but more than either panic disorder or generalized anxiety disorder (0.7%) or eating disorders (0.1%) (Merikangas et al., 2010). However, methodological differences among studies—for example, whether children alone or children and parents were assessed and/or whether BD-NOS was included or not—may falsely make it appear that most BD cases start in childhood.

A recent meta-analysis of epidemiological studies of children and adolescents with BD published from 1985 to 2007, including 16,222 youths from six US studies and six non-US studies, found that the overall rate of BD was 1.8% (range 1.1–3.0%). Importantly, they found no significant difference in mean rates between US and non-US studies. However, studies using broad definitions of BD, including BD-NOS, did report the highest prevalence estimates, and the US studies had a wider range of rates. Controlling for study methodological issues, they did not find a significant increase in rates of childhood-onset BD over time between 1985 and 2007 (Van Meter et al., 2011).

As expected, the prevalence of BD increases from childhood to adulthood. For example, Merikangas et al. (2012) conducted a cross-sectional survey of 10,123 US adolescents which showed that 2.5% met criteria for lifetime BD-I or BD-II, with a nearly twofold increase in mania comparing 13–14-year-olds to 17–18-year-olds. However, this study used a modified version of the Composite International Diagnostic Interview administered to adolescents, without corroboration from parental informants, which may result in overdiagnosis (Merikangas et al., 2012). Lewinsohn's longitudinal studies corroborate this finding, with 1.1% of adolescents (N = 1507) meeting criteria for BD when both parents' and childrens' reports were assessed, while 2.1% of a subset reassessed using only individual report at age 24 (N = 893) did so (Lewinsohn et al., 1995; Lewinsohn et al., 2000).

These data align with those of prior cross-national epidemiologic studies of adults showing a lifetime prevalence of 1–3% for BD (Weissman et al., 1996; Kessler et al., 2005). Two large epidemiologic studies of BD adults report a median onset age of 18 (Christie et al., 1988) or 25 (Kessler et al., 2005) years. However, studies indicate that BD age of onset is not distributed normally, with two studies (Bellivier et al., 2003; Lin et al., 2006) each reporting three peaks of onset age. Early onset may be familial or associated with a strong family history of BD (Kennedy et al., 2005; Lin et al., 2006). However, these data are subject to recall bias since they are retrospective recalls of BD-onset, rather than prospective data collected from children.

Global and time variations

Despite the abovementioned meta-analysis by Van Meter et al. suggesting similar rates of BD among US and non-US child studies, we know little about global differences in morbidity, mortality, and service utilization resulting from BD in children and adolescents.

Methodological questions

While epidemiological studies with standardized assessments of BD have shown relative stability in BD among children and adolescents over time, clinical studies suggest that increasing numbers of children are being diagnosed with BD. For example, the percentage of minors discharged from psychiatric hospitals in the United States with a diagnosis of BD has surged from less than 10% in the mid-1990s to more than 20% in the mid-2000s (Blader & Carlson, 2007). Another study demonstrated a 40-fold rise in the incidence of US outpatient visits assigned the diagnosis of BD during a similar period, from 25/100,000 in 1993–1994 to 1003/100,000 in 2002–2003 (Moreno et al., 2007). This phenomenon may not be restricted to the United States, with one study showing that rates of under-19-year-olds admitted to German psychiatric hospitals increased 68.5% between 2000 and 2007, an increase which exceeded that for other diagnoses (Holtmann et al., 2010).

Public health implications

From a public health perspective, the inconsistency between epidemiological data suggesting relative stability in rates of children and adolescents diagnosed with BD and clinical data suggesting increasing numbers of youth globally being diagnosed with BD supports the need for more specific tools that clinicians can employ to effectively diagnose mania and BD. Without them, we run the risk of over, under, and misdiagnosis and potentially incorrect or suboptimal treatment of children and adolescents.

Summary

Inconsistencies between epidemiological and clinical samples highlight the need for the development of assessment tools that can be used in research and in the clinic to evaluate children for BD.

Longitudinal outcome

Methodological factors

Longitudinal studies are clearly needed to determine what happens to children with BD as they become adolescents and ultimately adults. Specifically, there is a need to have samples of BD youths with distinct episodes of mania and hypomania satisfying DSM criteria for BD-I and II, as well as for those with BD-NOS. It also includes the need for comparative studies of BD youths versus those with chronic nonepisodic irritability. However, as illustrated below, variations in how researchers conceptualize the illness may shape their data.

For example, COBY is a longitudinal study of children with BD type I or II, or BD not otherwise specified (BD-NOS). COBY used DSM-IV definitions for BD-I and II. They also operationalized criteria for BD-NOS: (A) clinically relevant BD symptoms of euphoric or irritable mood lasting a minimum of 4 hours within a 24 hour period; (B) at least 2 "B" symptoms if the mood was primarily euphoric (three if primarily irritable), and (C) at least four cumulative lifetime days meeting these criteria. COBY's focus was thus on children with episodes of mania of varying duration.

The COBY study found that at intake, BD-I ($N = 255$), BD-II ($N = 30$), and BD-NOS ($N = 153$) participants did not differ in age of onset, duration of illness, rates of comorbid disorders, suicidal ideation, or manic symptoms during the most serious episode. Elevated and/or expansive mood was found in 91.8% of BD-I and 81.9% of BD-NOS participants. BD-I participants had more severe manic symptoms, greater overall functional impairment, and higher rates of psychiatric hospitalization, psychosis, and suicide attempts than those with BD-NOS (Axelson et al., 2006). However, 4-year longitudinal follow-up data indicate that BD-NOS participants had significantly longer mean time to recovery from the index episode and significantly longer mean time to recurrence. Thus, COBY data indicate that children do have episodes of mania including both euphoria and irritability (Hunt et al., 2013). Moreover, COBY has shown that BD can be reliably diagnosed in children and adolescents, its impairment is similar across BD-I, II, and NOS, and with time, progressive numbers of BD-NOS participants develop more distinct episodes consistent with BD-I or II.

Another example of a longitudinal BD study is that conducted by Barbara Geller's group at Washington University in St. Louis. Taken as a whole, her data align with that of the COBY study

in indicating that mania may start in childhood (mean age of onset $= 7.4 \pm 3.5$) and that youth with BD suffer from recurrent manic and/or depressive symptoms. Specifically, a 4-year study of 86 children with DSM-IV bipolar I disorder (manic or mixed) with at least 1 cardinal symptom (elation and/or grandiosity) to ensure differentiation from ADHD showed that participants spent $56.9\% \pm 28.8\%$ of total weeks with mania or hypomania (unipolar or mixed), and $47.1\% \pm 30.4\%$ of total weeks with major or minor depression and dysthymia (unipolar or mixed) (Geller et al., 2004b).

As described earlier (section "Differential Diagnosis"), Leibenluft et al. at NIMH also conducted a longitudinal study focusing on two groups of children: (i) "narrow-phenotype pediatric BD" (NP-BD) and (ii) SMD. Taken as a whole, data from over 150 NP-BD participants also shows that BD may start early in childhood and result in considerable impairment. Moreover, parents of NP-BD youths were significantly more likely to have BD themselves than were parents of SMD youths (Brotman et al., 2007). Prospective data showed that only one of 84 SMD subjects (1.2%) experienced a (hypo)manic or mixed episode during a median 28.7 months of follow-up, whereas 58 of 93 NP-BD participants (62.4%) experienced such a (hypo)manic or mixed episode (Stringaris et al., 2010b).

Summary

Longitudinal prospective studies are in early stages of seeing how BD youths develop into adults. Data suggest that episodic and chronic irritability in children predict different outcomes in adulthood, and that children with BD continue to experience considerable symptomatology and impairment.

Risk factors

Family studies

Those with a first-degree relative with BD are at an approximately 10-fold increased risk for BD, compared to those without such a history (Hodgins et al., 2002; Smoller & Finn, 2003). The psychopathology among such at-risk children is of considerable interest. Six studies with $N > 50$ have assessed children of adults with BD (Grigoroiu-Serbanescu et al., 1989; Carlson & Weintraub, 1993; Chang et al., 2000; Wals et al., 2001; Henin et al., 2005; Hillegers et al., 2005). All find very high rates of psychopathology in these young people, with 44–63% meeting criteria for at least one DSM-IV-TR diagnosis, including ADHD, anxiety, MDD, and/or BD.

Twin and adoption studies

Twin studies suggest that the heritability of BD in adults is greater than 60%, with greater concordance for BD in monozygotic (60–70%) than dizygotic twins (20–30%) (Smoller & Finn, 2003).

With respect to gene/environment interactions and their relationship to the neural pathology of BD, Van der Schot et al.

found that genetic risk to develop BD was related to decreased gray matter density in the right medial frontal gyrus, precentral gyrus, and insula, and decreased white matter density in the superior longitudinal fasciculi ($N = 232$ participants, including $N = 49$ BD twin pairs – 16% monozygotic concordant, 31% monozygotic discordant, 8% dizygotic concordant, 45% dizygotic discordant) and $N = 67$ healthy twin pairs (58% monozygotic, 42% dizygotic) (van der Schot et al., 2010)).

Molecular genetic studies

The genetics of BD are complex and rapidly evolving, but several themes emerge. First, BD is due to multiple genes, not a single gene (Kelsoe, 2003). Second, the genes conferring risk for BD and those implicated in schizophrenia may overlap, as indicated by genome-wide association studies (GWAS) (Priebe et al., 2012; Craddock & Sklar, 2013; Cross-Disorder Group of the Psychiatric Genomics Consortium et al., 2013a, b). Third, many genes implicated in BD mediate cell signaling, including via calcium or cell growth, for example, brain-derived neurotrophic factor (BDNF) (Geller et al., 2004a). Fourth, data implicating copy number variants (CNVs) are less robust than other disorders, such as autism.

Clinical prodromes/risk factors

Several longitudinal community-based studies have queried which childhood or adolescent diagnoses are associated with increased risk for later BD. A 10-year longitudinal study by Tijssen suggests that progression from symptoms of BD to full-blown BD was predicted by symptom persistence—that is, the longer symptoms exist, the more they progress (Tijssen et al., 2010). Studies following depressed children into late adolescence or early adulthood find that prepubertal MDD is associated with increased risk for BD (Harrington et al., 1990; Kovacs et al., 1994; Rao et al., 1995; Weissman et al., 1999). However, the prevalence of BD ranged widely, perhaps because of small sample sizes or because of differences in patient characteristics (e.g., inpatients vs outpatients). Positive family history, psychosis, and rapid symptom onset may predict BD (Strober & Carlson, 1982; Geller et al., 1994). COBY study data indicate that after 5 years of longitudinal follow-up, 45% (63/140) of BD-NOS patients had converted to either BD type I (32/63) or type II (31/63), with the strongest predictor of conversion being first- or second-degree family history of mania or hypomania (Axelson et al., 2011). Clinic-based follow-up studies of children with ADHD do not consistently support an elevated risk for developing BD by adulthood (Mannuzza et al., 1998; Hazell et al., 2003).

Summary and conclusions

Although BD is clearly heritable, there is no single risk gene, nor is there a matrix of risk factors that is as yet clinically applicable. Ongoing and future work, directed at understanding the brain/behavior/gene interplay responsible for mania, depression, and euthymia, including work focused on understanding full-blown categorical illness as well as the dimensional symptoms underlying these disorders, may prove more fruitful to identifying such biobehavioral markers of BD risk than BD itself as a categorical diagnosis.

Pathophysiology

Neural circuitry: computerized behavioral tasks and neuroimaging

Affective neuroscience—the study of brain/behavior interactions underlying emotion and neuropsychiatric disorders—has greatly advanced our pathophysiological understanding of BD in children and adolescents. With respect to structural magnetic resonance imaging (MRI), the most replicated finding in childhood-onset BD is significantly decreased amygdala volume, compared to controls (Blumberg et al., 2003; DelBello et al., 2004; Chang et al., 2005; Dickstein et al., 2005; Pfeifer et al., 2008; Hajek et al., 2009); data in BD adults are less consistent (Altshuler et al., 1998). Ongoing work is evaluating potential development, gender, medication, and comorbidity effects on structural MRI alterations.

With respect to cognitive and emotional processes, using both out-of-scanner tasks and functional MRI (fMRI), studies have demonstrated that BD youths have aberrant functioning in at least four processes: emotional face processing, response inhibition, frustration, and cognitive flexibility.

Face processing deficits are perhaps the most robustly demonstrated alteration in BD youths. Specifically, BD youths make significantly more errors categorizing emotional faces than both typically developing children (TDC) without psychopathology and those with anxiety disorders (Guyer et al., 2007) and youths with primary ADHD, especially on low-intensity happy faces (Seymour et al., 2013). Similar deficits have been identified in youths at familial risk for BD (Brotman et al., 2008). fMRI studies from several groups indicate that BD youths have abnormal prefrontal cortex (PFC)–amygdala–striatal neural activation compared with healthy subjects when viewing faces with happy, angry, or neutral emotions (Rich et al., 2006; Pavuluri et al., 2007; Kalmar et al., 2009). Finally, studies suggest that different neural mechanisms mediate face processing deficits in children and adolescents with either BD or SMD (Rich et al., 2008; Brotman et al., 2010; Thomas et al., 2013).

Response inhibition is linked to distractibility and impulsivity. Leibenluft et al. found that, compared to controls, BD youths had a reduced striatal "error signal" during failed motor inhibition (Leibenluft et al., 2007), a deficit which might contribute to the patients' inability to inhibit effectively. Another study found that BD youths had greater neural activation than TDCs in the right DLPFC during no-go versus go trials, suggesting greater reliance on cognitive control areas to maintain adequate behavioral performance (Singh et al., 2010).

Tasks using rigged feedback to induce frustration are particularly relevant to advancing what is known about irritability in children and adolescents, given that irritability may be part of both disorders. For example, Rich *et al.* found altered P3 EEG amplitude in BD versus both SMD and TDC participants using a task with rigged feedback, reflecting impairments in executive attention in the BD group. In contrast, regardless of condition, SMD youths had lower N1 amplitude than either BD or TDC participants, reflecting impairments in the initial stage of attention (Rich *et al.*, 2007). In a separate study using magnetoencephalography to identify aberrant brain activity during this frustration task, (after negative feedback,) BD participants had greater superior frontal gyrus activation and decreased insula activation than SMD and TDCs, while SMD participants had greater anterior cingulate cortex and medial frontal gyrus activation than TDCs (Rich *et al.*, 2011).

Cognitive flexibility—defined as the ability to adapt one's thinking and behavior in response to changing rewards and punishments—is relevant to BD because clinical features of BD may reflect specific alterations in how reward inaccurately shapes behavior—that is, hyper-hedonia in mania (e.g., excessive involvement in pleasurable activities with high potential for painful consequences) and hypo-hedonia in depression (e.g., anhedonia) (Cools *et al.*, 2002). Cognitive flexibility can be studied using reversal learning tasks. In these, subjects use trial-and-error learning to determine first, that an object is initially rewarded, and then, that this stimulus/reward relationship had switched, so that the previously rewarded object is now punished and vice versa. BD youths have impaired cognitive flexibility and reversal learning compared to TDC controls and SMD youths (Dickstein *et al.*, 2004; Gorrindo *et al.*, 2005; Dickstein *et al.*, 2007; Dickstein *et al.*, 2010a). FMRI studies have shown that BD youths had the opposite neural response as TDC participants during reversal learning (Dickstein *et al.*, 2010b).

Neurochemistry: magnetic resonance spectroscopy (MRS)

Magnetic resonance spectroscopy (MRS) research in BD has focused on *N*-acetyl asparatate (NAA), an intra-neuronal marker whose levels are decreased in neuropathology, and myo-inositol (mI), an intracellular second messenger, thought to be overabundant in mania, whose levels are decreased by lithium (Moore *et al.*, 1999; Silverstone *et al.*, 2002).

Youth with familial BD (Chang *et al.*, 2003), and adults with BD (Winsberg *et al.*, 2000), have significantly decreased NAA in the dorsolateral PFC compared to controls. Studies also indicate that BD youths have increased ACC mI compared to healthy controls or youth with intermittent explosive disorder (Davanzo *et al.*, 2003), with mI levels being responsive to lithium treatment (Davanzo *et al.*, 2001). Together, these MRS studies suggest that BD youths may be characterized by specific neurochemical alterations that respond to psychopharmacological treatment; future work in this area may ultimately inform such treatment.

Diffusion tensor imaging (DTI)

Diffusion tensor imaging (DTI) studies have shown disrupted white matter integrity in tracts connecting the PFC as indexed by decreased fractional anisotropy (FA) among BD versus TDC youths (Adler *et al.*, 2006). Children with BD and those at risk for BD by virtue of having a first-degree relative with BD had decreased FA versus controls in the superior longitudinal fasciculus bilaterally, suggesting that this might be a trait marker of BD (Frazier *et al.*, 2007). However, others have suggested that these changes might not be specific to BD, as similar alterations have been shown in youths with primary ADHD (Pavuluri *et al.*, 2009).

Summary

In sum, research has demonstrated brain/behavior alterations in children and adolescents with BD, including structural and functional alterations in fronto-temporo-striatal circuits mediating behaviors such as face processing, response inhibition, response to frustration, and cognitive flexibility. Ongoing work is needed to determine the specificity of these brain and behavior alterations, and thus identify if they are useful targets for diagnostic biomarkers or for novel treatments or treatment monitoring.

Treatment

General approach

The past decade has witnessed the publication of several double-blind randomized placebo-controlled trials (RCTs) for antimanic agents in children and adolescents. Current data preclude designating any psychopharmacologic or psychotherapeutic treatment as having "strong" evidentiary support. Given the paucity of pediatric data, clinicians often rely on data from adult BD despite ongoing controversy about phenomenological differences in children with BD versus adults with BD. Hence, where appropriate, we summarize briefly the most relevant adult data. Nevertheless, caution is urged in basing treatment on adult data, since youth may respond differently than adults, as in major depression.

Clinicians should focus treatment on the most acute and disabling aspects of BD—for example, acute mania, depression, psychosis, substance abuse, and suicidality (Figure 62.1). Later treatment addresses other problems—for example, comorbid anxiety, ADHD, substance abuse, and deficient social skills. Treatment decisions require collaboration among physicians, patients, and families to identify target symptoms, educate about side effects, and evaluate each treatment's efficacy. Daily ratings of target symptoms by parents and/or patients allow treatment to be based upon prospective, rather than retrospective, data. Moreover, patient safety, including functional impairment, suicidal thoughts, and treatment-emergent side effects, must be evaluated continuously. This includes considerations of level of care required to manage the patient safely, though there are no universal standards for inpatient versus outpatient care.

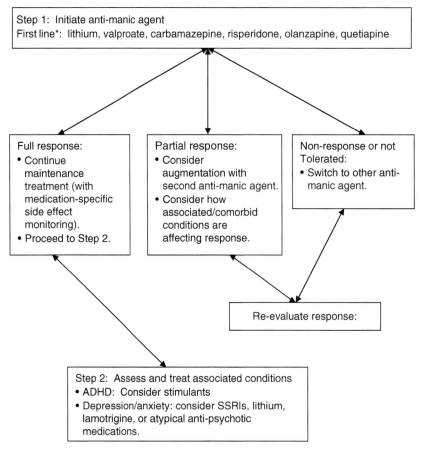

Figure 62.1 Psychopharmacology algorithm. *First-line agents based upon present data in childhood-onset BD. *Source*: Modified from/see also: Kowatch *et al.* (2005).

Furthermore, clinicians must consider common issues affecting children and adolescents, including substance use and pregnancy. Most antimanic and antidepressant agents are metabolized by the liver. Thus, any other medication or drug of abuse also metabolized by the liver, including alcohol, may influence treatment response and side effect risk. Regarding pregnancy, certain antimanic agents, including antiepileptic drugs (e.g., valproate) and lithium, have known adverse effects on the developing fetus. Thus, clinicians must discuss these risks with their patients, as well as potential alternatives to medication and the need for contraception.

Ideally, medication trials should last at least 6–8 weeks, with one new agent added at a time. However, this approach may not be feasible in acutely manic or psychotic patients. Physicians should assess continuously the need for each medication to determine whether any can be discontinued. Moreover, symptoms do not typically resolve on medication alone; rather, comprehensive treatment usually requires both psychopharmacology and psychotherapy. Finally, treatment must address the phase of a child's illness, since acute and maintenance interventions differ.

Psychopharmacology for pediatric bipolar disorder

Pharmacotherapy of mania

Currently available antimanic medications intended to reduce symptoms of, and to prevent the occurrence of, hypo/mania include: (i) lithium, (ii) second-generation antipsychotic medications (SGAs), and (iii) antiepileptic medications (AEDs, for example, valproate and carbamazepine) (see Figure 62.1). Recent RCTs support the following conclusions: (i) SGAs are effective, and potentially superior to other antimanic agents, in the treatment of BD. However, such medications are associated with significant side effects, most notably impairing weight gain and metabolic abnormalities; (ii) lithium's role in BD children is less clear than in BD adults, though further study is warranted, given studies showing its efficacy in pediatric patients with extreme aggression; and (iii) AEDs may be less efficacious than other antimanic agents for children with BD. The lack of a "silver bullet" or single best antimanic agent complicates efforts to select any one agent as a first-line treatment and again emphasizes the importance of thorough discussions with patients and their families. For an individual, a step-wise approach is often needed, involving trying different antimanic agents if initial attempts are unsuccessful. The treatment of acute mania may require augmentation with anxiolytic medications short-term. We focus our discussion on efficacy and the most important side effects, but for dosing guidelines and a more thorough discussion of side effects, see Kowatch *et al.* (2005), Correll *et al.* (2006).

Second-generation antipsychotic medications (SGAs)

SGAs have the strongest efficacy data in BD youths; however, there are concerns about side effects, such as substantial weight gain and metabolic syndrome, and about potential over prescription to children in general (Andrade *et al.*, 2011). Risperidone, aripiprazole, and quetiapine have FDA indications to treat mania or mixed states associated with BD in 10–17-year-olds.

Aripiprazole was evaluated in a 4-week double-blind placebo-controlled RCT of $N = 296$ 10–17-year-olds currently in a mixed or manic episode. At either 10 mg/day or 30 mg/day, aripiprazole was better than placebo in reducing manic symptoms (Findling *et al.*, 2009). A second study found that after 16 weeks of open treatment, 4–9-year-olds with BD ($N = 96$) randomized to remain on aripiprazole were more likely to remain without a mood episode versus those switched to placebo ($N = 30$ per group; weeks without mood episode 6.14 + 11.8 on aripiprazole, 2.29 + 0.38 on placebo) (Findling *et al.*, 2012).

Studies of risperidone include a study of 10–17-year-olds with BD type I currently manic or mixed randomized to receive risperidone 0.5–2.5 mg/day ($N = 50$), 3–6 mg/day ($N = 61$), or placebo ($N = 58$) for 3 weeks. Both risperidone groups showed significant reductions in mania compared to placebo (Haas *et al.*, 2009). Other studies have compared the clinical and neural outcome of BD youths treated with risperidone versus divalproex (Depakote), showed that neither treatment was clearly superior, although this may have been a type II error, given small sample size ($N = 24$ total). They did find that risperidone may have reduced mania faster (Pavuluri *et al.*, 2011a).

A particular concern is the association of SGA with "metabolic syndrome"—that is, extreme and rapid weight gain and endocrine abnormalities, including diabetes mellitus. A study of $N = 338$ children aged 4–19 years treated for a median of 10.8 weeks with SGAs, showed that weight increased by a mean of 8.5 kg for olanzapine, 6.1 kg with quetiapine, 5.3 kg with risperidone, and 4.4 kg with aripiprazole, versus 0.2 kg in an untreated group. Increases were also noted in total cholesterol, triglycerides, and nonhigh-density lipoprotein (Correll *et al.*, 2009). Children treated with SGAs have a greater risk of developing diabetes (3.23/1000) than those receiving antidepressants (1.86/1000) or no treatment (0.76/1000) (Andrade *et al.*, 2011). Patients should be monitored routinely for weight, height, and body mass index, and fasting glucose and lipid panel every 6 months. Finally, for SGAs, firm conclusions on the risk of tardive dyskinesia are not possible because of the lack of long-term data (Ghaemi *et al.*, 2006).

Lithium

Support for lithium's efficacy in childhood-onset BD is mixed. Efficacy and safety data place it in the middle of the three categories of medications typically used in childhood-onset BD—ahead of AEDs but weaker than SGAs. Moreover, lithium has an FDA indication for the treatment of mania in patients as young as 12 years, but it was "grandfathered" in and would not be granted on the basis of current standards. Nevertheless, in BD adults, there is robust evidence for lithium's efficacy in adult acute mania (Bowden *et al.*, 2005), long-term prophylaxis (Bowden *et al.*, 2003), and reduction of suicide risk (Cipriani *et al.*, 2005). Thus, it may be reasonable to prescribe lithium for individual BD youths, especially those who do not respond to SGAs.

The largest and most recent data set about lithium comes from the Treatment of Early Age Mania (TEAM) study of $N = 279$ children aged 6–15 years with type I BD randomized to receive 8 weeks of either lithium, risperidone, or divalproex sodium. Lithium was not significantly better in treating mania than divalproex, and resulted in higher discontinuation rate than risperidone (Geller *et al.*, 2012). However, one wonders if atypical features of this sample may reduce its generalizability to typical childhood-onset BD cases. Specifically, the average age of mania onset was 5.2 ± 2.6 years, and their average mania duration 4 years—translating into the fact that most were in a continuous state of a manic or mixed episode. Another RCT study failed to find a significant difference between adolescents ($N = 108$) whose acute mania was initially stabilized with open lithium treatment, and who were then randomized to either continue lithium or switch to placebo during a double-blind discontinuation study (Kafantaris *et al.*, 2004).

Adult studies suggest that optimal lithium levels are between 0.6 and 1.0 mEq/l for acute mania and down to 0.4 mEq/s for maintenance treatment, but this has not been tested rigorously in youth (Gelenberg *et al.*, 1989). Of note, an MRS study showed that BD youth ($N = 9$) had lower brain/serum lithium concentrations than BD adults ($N = 18$) (Moore *et al.*, 2002), suggesting that BD youths may require higher doses of lithium to achieve the same brain concentration of lithium as adults. However, the clinical implications of this finding have not been studied systematically.

Antiepileptic drugs (AEDs)

Relative to lithium or SGAs, support for the therapeutic efficacy of the AEDs in childhood-onset BD is weakest. However, safety data for AEDs (largely gleaned from studies of pediatric epilepsy) is generally strong, with the exception of questions regarding acute hepatic or pancreatic failure and possible adverse effects on female gonadal function (see below) (de Silva *et al.*, 1996).

Data from two RCTs fail to demonstrate the benefits of AEDs in childhood-onset BD (Wagner *et al.*, 2006, 2009). While open-label trials, most of them small, document some evidence of benefit for carbamazepine, valproate, or lamotrigine, in the absence of a placebo control these studies can provide only weak support for efficacy (Wagner *et al.*, 2002; Chang *et al.*, 2006).

Adult studies of AEDs have shown efficacy for acute and maintenance antimanic treatment in adults, leading to FDA indications for both valproate and a long-acting form of carbamazepine, (Pope *et al.*, 1991). Lamotrigine is another AED with an FDA indication for BD in adults, although data suggest that it is more effective as a maintenance treatment, preventing depressive and manic relapse, than for acute mania (Bowden *et al.*, 2003).

Valproate has a black-box FDA warning due to the possibility of acute, life-threatening hepatic failure and pancreatitis, both of which are more common in those on multiple medications or less than 2 years old (Grauso-Eby *et al.*, 2003). Therefore, any patient taking valproate who develops the acute onset of nausea, vomiting, or acute abdominal pain should receive prompt medical evaluation. Also, irregular menses and polycystic ovary syndrome (PCOS; i.e., polycystic ovarian morphology, increased serum testosterone or luteinizing hormone, and irregular menses) may be associated with valproate use, particularly in young women (McIntyre *et al.*, 2003).

Lamotrigine also has an FDA black-box warning for children younger than 16 due to potential for two different life-threatening rashes, Stephens-Johnson syndrome and toxic epidermal necrolysis. More benign rashes are common, and a meta-analysis found that increased risk for such rashes was associated with patient age less than 12 years or coadministration of medications that inhibit hepatic metabolism (e.g., valproate) (Calabrese *et al.*, 2002).

Pharmacotherapy of depression in childhood-onset BD

The lack of RCT data to guide medication treatment of depression or anxiety in BD youths is problematic. Data suggest that (i) BD youths spend a considerable amount of time struggling with depression and/or anxiety; (ii) BD youths often receive SSRIs to augment their antimanic treatment without the induction of mania; (iii) there is some suggestion that the risk of antidepressant-induced mania is higher in prepubertal children than in older adolescents or adults (Martin *et al.*, 2004), and (iv) in adult BD, it is unclear whether SSRI antidepressants or lithium are preferable in the treatment of adult bipolar depression (Thase, 2007). Specifically Martin *et al.* used nationally representative pharmacy data to show that among 87,920 5–29-year-olds, 5.4% ($N = 4781$) experienced manic conversion during a median of 41 weeks of follow-up. This was more common in prepubertal children than older adolescents or adults (number needed to harm [NNH] = 10 10–14-year olds vs 23 in 15–29-year-olds) and also more common after exposure to tricyclic antidepressants than SSRIs.

In BD adults with depression, RCTs demonstrate efficacy for lamotrigine, quetiapine, and the combination of olanzapine plus fluoxetine (Calabrese *et al.*, 2005; Tohen *et al.*, 2005).

Pharmacotherapy of ADHD in childhood-onset BD

There is a similar lack of evidence-based guidance to treat ADHD among children with BD. Although concerns have been raised about the possibility of ADHD-medication-induced mania, large numbers of phenomenology studies show that these agents are commonly used without such exacerbation (Carlson *et al.*, 2000). One double-blind crossover RCT in children with childhood-onset BD and ADHD found that, once mania remitted on valproate, amphetamine salts plus valproate was more effective in reducing ADHD symptoms than placebo plus valproate, without exacerbating mania ($N = 30$) (Scheffer *et al.*, 2005). Thus, clinicians treating youth with BD and comorbid ADHD should treat the patient's mania, and then consider psychostimulant treatment.

Psychotherapy for pediatric bipolar disorder

When combined with pharmacotherapy, several types of psychotherapy show promise in treating childhood-onset BD. Family-focused psychoeducational therapy (FFT) includes psycho education, communication enhancement, and problem-solving skills. When administered for 21 sessions over 9 months to BD youths after an index mood episode, FFT resulted in faster recovery and fewer weeks depressed versus those randomized to receive only three family sessions focused on relapse prevention. However, there was no significant difference in rates of recovery from mania or time to recurrence of mania or depression (Miklowitz *et al.*, 2008). Multifamily psychoeducational groups are designed to increase parents' knowledge about BD and ability to obtain services. Multifamily psychoeducational groups administered in eight 90-min sessions have shown greater reduction in the mood severity index, a combination of the Young mania rating scale and Children's Depression Rating Scale, than those receiving a wait-list control (Fristad *et al.*, 2009). Cognitive behavioral therapy (CBT) with family involvement was associated with significant symptom reduction in an open trial of $N = 34$ BD youths (Pavuluri *et al.*, 2004). More RCTs are needed to document efficacy and of head-to-head comparisons.

Summary

The treatment of childhood-onset BD requires a comprehensive approach to meet the complex needs of the disorder, with targeted pharmacotherapy and psychotherapy. Ongoing work is evaluating the neural mechanism and outcome of treatment. Important unknowns requiring additional study include (i) how to address anxiety, ADHD, and depression associated with BD; (ii) which agent to use for a particular patient; and (iii) what are the moderators/mediators of treatment response?

Future developments and necessary research

Hopefully, the future will bring greater pathophysiological understanding of childhood-onset BD. New diagnostic criteria in DSM-5 will undoubtedly shape clinical and research work on mood and behavioral disorders in children, including BD and DMDD. Additional advances are likely to come from (i) longitudinal studies of BD youths now becoming young adults and (ii) novel treatments.

Longitudinal studies come of age

Several studies have continued to prospectively follow these participants who are coming of age—entering young adulthood. These longitudinal studies are crucial in understanding what happens to these BD youths when they grow up to answer questions such as: How does the phenomenology of their illness change (duration and frequency of episodes; identifying risks for developing manic and depressive episodes)? What will their pattern of healthcare utilization be (treatment seeking, settings, and costs of care)? How will the brain/behavior interactions underlying BD change as these children with BD become adults with BD?

Novel treatments

Some have expressed concern about the future of novel medication treatments for neuropsychiatric disorders, including BD, given pharmaceutical industry reports about the dearth of novel compounds in the pipeline to be available clinically, reduction of number of companies providing such agents, or reduction in funding mechanisms available to study such agents. However, the future may not be so bleak, as novel approaches, including pharmacoimaging or pharmacogenomics (Pavuluri et al., 2011b), result in a more personalized treatment approach, as an individual's biology is factored into determinations of what treatment is most likely to result in improvement, or least likely to result in side effects, akin to what is currently done in treating cancer, although this is clearly a long way off.

The future will likely require such a union of affective neuroscience techniques and treatment studies. Beyond traditional treatment targets of mania and depression, enhancing cognitive function via nonpharmacological options is an important target for interventions research, given that cognitive impairments in those with psychopathology are strongly linked to functioning at school, work, home, and social relationships (Martinez-Aran et al., 2004). This approach, known as cognitive remediation, has shown great promise in adults with disorders, including schizophrenia (McGurk et al., 2007), and in children with ADHD (Shalev et al., 2007).

In sum, while much is known about BD in children and adolescents, there is ample work for the current and future generations of child mental health clinicians and researchers.

References

Adler, C.M. et al. (2006) Evidence of white matter pathology in bipolar disorder adolescents experiencing their first episode of mania: a diffusion tensor imaging study. *The American Journal of Psychiatry* **163** (2), 322–324.

Algorta, G.P. et al. (2011a) Suicidality in pediatric bipolar disorder: predictor or outcome of family processes and mixed mood presentation? *Bipolar Disorders* **13** (1), 76–86.

Algorta, G.P. et al. (2011b) Suicidality in pediatric bipolar disorder: predictor or outcome of family processes and mixed mood presentation? *Bipolar Disorders* **13** (1), 76–86.

Althoff, R.R. et al. (2012) Temperamental profiles of dysregulated children. *Child Psychiatry and Human Development* **43** (4), 511–522.

Altshuler, L.L. et al. (1998) Amygdala enlargement in bipolar disorder and hippocampal reduction in schizophrenia: an MRI study demonstrating neuroanatomic specificity. *Archives of General Psychiatry* **55** (7), 663–664.

American Psychiatric Association (2000) *Diagnostic and Statistical Manual of Mental Disorders 4th Edition Text Revision (DSM-IV-TR)*. American Psychiatric Association, Washington, DC.

American Psychiatric Association (2013) *American Psychiatric Association: Diagnostic and Statistical Manual of Mental Disorders*, 5th edn. American Psychiatric Association, Washington, DC.

Andrade, S.E. et al. (2011) Antipsychotic medication use among children and risk of diabetes mellitus. *Pediatrics* **128** (6), 1135–1141.

Axelson, D. et al. (2006) Phenomenology of children and adolescents with bipolar spectrum disorders. *Archives of General Psychiatry* **63** (10), 1139–1148.

Axelson, D.A. et al. (2011) Course of subthreshold bipolar disorder in youth: diagnostic progression from bipolar disorder not otherwise specified. *Journal of the American Academy of Child and Adolescent Psychiatry* **50** (10), 1001–1016.

Bellivier, F. et al. (2003) Age at onset in bipolar I affective disorder: further evidence for three subgroups. *American Journal of Psychiatry* **160** (5), 999–1001.

Biederman, J. et al. (2004) Further evidence of unique developmental phenotypic correlates of pediatric bipolar disorder: findings from a large sample of clinically referred preadolescent children assessed over the last 7 years. *Journal of the Affective Disorders* **82** (Suppl 1), S45–S58.

Birmaher, B. et al. (2006) Clinical course of children and adolescents with bipolar spectrum disorders. *Archives of General Psychiatry* **63** (2), 175–183.

Blader, J.C. & Carlson, G.A. (2007) Increased rates of bipolar disorder diagnoses among U.S. child, adolescent, and adult inpatients, 1996-2004. *Biological Psychiatry* **62** (2), 107–114.

Blumberg, H.P. et al. (2003) Amygdala and hippocampal volumes in adolescents and adults with bipolar disorder. *Archives of General Psychiatry* **60** (12), 1201–1208.

Boomsma, D.I. et al. (2006) Longitudinal stability of the CBCL-juvenile bipolar disorder phenotype: a study in Dutch twins. *Biological Psychiatry* **60** (9), 912–920.

Bowden, C.L. *et al.* (2003) A placebo-controlled 18-month trial of lamotrigine and lithium maintenance treatment in recently manic or hypomanic patients with bipolar I disorder. *Archives of General Psychiatry* **60** (4), 392–400.

Bowden, C.L. *et al.* (2005) A randomized, double-blind, placebo-controlled efficacy and safety study of quetiapine or lithium as monotherapy for mania in bipolar disorder. *Journal of Clinical Psychiatry* **66** (1), 111–121.

Brotman, M.A. *et al.* (2008) Facial emotion labeling deficits in children and adolescents at risk for bipolar disorder. *American Journal of Psychiatry* **165** (3), 385–389.

Brotman, M.A. *et al.* (2007) Parental diagnoses in youth with narrow phenotype bipolar disorder or severe mood dysregulation. *American Journal of Psychiatry* **164** (8), 1238–1241.

Brotman, M.A. *et al.* (2010) Amygdala activation during emotion processing of neutral faces in children with severe mood dysregulation versus ADHD or bipolar disorder. *American Journal of Psychiatry* **167** (1), 61–69.

Brotman, M.A. *et al.* (2006) Prevalence, clinical correlates, and longitudinal course of severe mood dysregulation in children. *Biological Psychiatry* **60** (9), 991–997.

Calabrese, J.R. *et al.* (2005) A randomized, double-blind, placebo-controlled trial of quetiapine in the treatment of bipolar I or II depression. *American Journal of Psychiatry* **162** (7), 1351–1360.

Calabrese, J.R. *et al.* (2002) Rash in multicenter trials of lamotrigine in mood disorders: clinical relevance and management. *Journal of Clinical Psychiatry* **63** (11), 1012–1019.

Carlson, G.A. *et al.* (2000) Stimulant treatment in young boys with symptoms suggesting childhood mania: a report from a longitudinal study. *Journal of Child Adolescent Psychopharmacology* **10** (3), 175–184.

Carlson, G.A. & Weintraub, S. (1993) Childhood behavior problems and bipolar disorder--relationship or coincidence? *Journal of Affective Disorders* **28** (3), 143–153.

Chang, K. *et al.* (2003) Decreased N-acetylaspartate in children with familial bipolar disorder. *Biological Psychiatry* **53** (11), 1059–1065.

Chang, K. *et al.* (2005) Reduced amygdalar gray matter volume in familial pediatric bipolar disorder. *Journal of American Academy of Child Adolescent Psychiatry* **44** (6), 565–573.

Chang, K. *et al.* (2006) An open-label study of lamotrigine adjunct or monotherapy for the treatment of adolescents with bipolar depression. *Journal of American Academy of Child and Adolescence Psychiatry* **45** (3), 298–304.

Chang, K.D. *et al.* (2000) Psychiatric phenomenology of child and adolescent bipolar offspring. *Journal of American Academy of Child and Adolescence Psychiatry* **39** (4), 453–460.

Christie, K.A. *et al.* (1988) Epidemiologic evidence for early onset of mental disorders and higher risk of drug abuse in young adults. *American Journal of Psychiatry* **145** (8), 971–975.

Cipriani, A. *et al.* (2005) Lithium in the prevention of suicidal behavior and all-cause mortality in patients with mood disorders: a systematic review of randomized trials. *American Journal of Psychiatry* **162** (10), 1805–1819.

Cools, R. *et al.* (2002) Defining the neural mechanisms of probabilistic reversal learning using event-related functional magnetic resonance imaging. *Journal of Neuroscience* **22** (11), 4563–4567.

Copeland, W.E. *et al.* (2009) Childhood and adolescent psychiatric disorders as predictors of young adult disorders. *Archives of General Psychiatry* **66** (7), 764–772.

Correll, C.U. *et al.* (2009) Cardiometabolic risk of second-generation antipsychotic medications during first-time use in children and adolescents. *JAMA* **302** (16), 1765–1773.

Correll, C.U. *et al.* (2006) Recognizing and monitoring adverse events of second-generation antipsychotics in children and adolescents. *Child & Adolescent Psychiatric Clinics of North America* **15** (1), 177–206.

Craddock, N. & Sklar, P. (2013) Genetics of bipolar disorder. *The Lancet* **381** (9878), 1654–1662.

Cross-Disorder Group of the Psychiatric Genomics Consortium *et al.* (2013a) Genetic relationship between five psychiatric disorders estimated from genome-wide SNPs. *Nature Genetics* **45** (9), 984–994.

Cross-Disorder Group of the Psychiatric Genomics Consortium *et al.* (2013b) Identification of risk loci with shared effects on five major psychiatric disorders: a genome-wide analysis. *The Lancet* **381** (9875), 1371–1379.

Davanzo, P. *et al.* (2001) Decreased anterior cingulate myo-inositol/creatine spectroscopy resonance with lithium treatment in children with bipolar disorder. *Neuropsychopharmacology* **24** (4), 359–369.

Davanzo, P. *et al.* (2003) Proton magnetic resonance spectroscopy of bipolar disorder versus intermittent explosive disorder in children and adolescents. *American Journal of Psychiatry* **160** (8), 1442–1452.

de Silva, M. *et al.* (1996) Randomised comparative monotherapy trial of phenobarbitone, phenytoin, carbamazepine, or sodium valproate for newly diagnosed childhood epilepsy. *The Lancet* **347** (9003), 709–713.

DelBello, M.P. *et al.* (2007) Twelve-month outcome of adolescents with bipolar disorder following first hospitalization for a manic or mixed episode. *American Journal of Psychiatry* **164** (4), 582–590.

DelBello, M.P. *et al.* (2004) Magnetic resonance imaging analysis of amygdala and other subcortical brain regions in adolescents with bipolar disorder. *Bipolar Disorders* **6** (1), 43–52.

Dickstein, D.P. *et al.* (2010a) Impaired probabilistic reversal learning in youths with mood and anxiety disorders. *Psychological Medicine* **40** (7), 1089–1100.

Dickstein, D.P. *et al.* (2010b) Altered neural function in pediatric bipolar disorder during reversal learning. *Bipolar Disorders* **12** (7), 707–719.

Dickstein, D.P. *et al.* (2005) Frontotemporal alterations in pediatric bipolar disorder: results of a voxel-based morphometry study. *Archives of General Psychiatry* **62** (7), 734–741.

Dickstein, D.P. *et al.* (2007) Cognitive flexibility in phenotypes of pediatric bipolar disorder. *Journal of American Academy of Child and Adolescence Psychiatry* **46** (3), 341–355.

Dickstein, D.P. *et al.* (2004) Neuropsychological performance in pediatric bipolar disorder. *Biological Psychiatry* **55** (1), 32–39.

Esposito-Smythers, C. *et al.* (2006) Child comorbidity, maternal mood disorder, and perceptions of family functioning among bipolar youth. *Journal of American Academy of Child and Adolescence Psychiatry* **45** (8), 955–964.

Faraone, S.V. *et al.* (2005) The CBCL predicts DSM bipolar disorder in children: a receiver operating characteristic curve analysis. *Bipolar Disorder* **7** (6), 518–524.

Findling, R.L. *et al.* (2001) Rapid, continuous cycling and psychiatric co-morbidity in pediatric bipolar I disorder. *Bipolar Disorder* **3** (4), 202–210.

Findling, R.L. *et al.* (2009) Acute treatment of pediatric bipolar I disorder, manic or mixed episode, with aripiprazole: a randomized, double-blind, placebo-controlled study. *Journal of Clinical Psychiatry* **70** (10), 1441–1451.

Findling, R.L. *et al.* (2012) Double-blind, randomized, placebo-controlled long-term maintenance study of aripiprazole in children with bipolar disorder. *Journal of Clinical Psychiatry* **73** (1), 57–63.

Frazier, J.A. *et al.* (2007) White matter abnormalities in children with and at risk for bipolar disorder. *Bipolar Disorders* **9** (8), 799–809.

Freeman, A.J. *et al.* (2012) Portability of a screener for pediatric bipolar disorder to a diverse setting. *Psychological Assessment* **24** (2), 341–351.

Fristad, M.A. *et al.* (2009) Impact of multifamily psychoeducational psychotherapy in treating children aged 8 to 12 years with mood disorders. *Archives of General Psychiatry* **66** (9), 1013–1021.

Galanter, C.A. *et al.* (2012) Variability among research diagnostic interview instruments in the application of DSM-IV-TR criteria for pediatric bipolar disorder. *Journal of American Academy of Child Adolescent Psychiatry* **51** (6), 605–621.

Gelenberg, A.J. *et al.* (1989) Comparison of standard and low serum levels of lithium for maintenance treatment of bipolar disorder. *New England Journal of Medicine* **321** (22), 1489–1493.

Geller, B. *et al.* (1994) Rate and predictors of prepubertal bipolarity during follow-up of 6- to 12-year-old depressed children. *Journal of American Academy of Child and Adolescence Psychiatry* **33** (4), 461–468.

Geller, B. *et al.* (2004a) Linkage disequilibrium of the brain-derived neurotrophic factor Val66Met polymorphism in children with a prepubertal and early adolescent bipolar disorder phenotype. *The American Journal of Psychiatry* **161** (9), 1698–1700.

Geller, B. *et al.* (2004b) Four-year prospective outcome and natural history of mania in children with a prepubertal and early adolescent bipolar disorder phenotype. *Archives of General Psychiatry* **61** (5), 459–467.

Geller, B. *et al.* (2012) A randomized controlled trial of risperidone, lithium, or divalproex sodium for initial treatment of bipolar I disorder, manic or mixed phase, in children and adolescents. *Archives of General Psychiatry* **69** (5), 515–528.

Geller, B. *et al.* (1998) Prepubertal and early adolescent bipolarity differentiate from ADHD by manic symptoms, grandiose delusions, ultra-rapid or ultradian cycling. *Journal of Affective Disorders* **51** (2), 81–91.

Geller, B. *et al.* (2002a) DSM-IV mania symptoms in a prepubertal and early adolescent bipolar disorder phenotype compared to attention-deficit hyperactive and normal controls. *Journal of Child and Adolescent Psychopharmacology* **12** (1), 11–25.

Geller, B. *et al.* (2002b) Phenomenology of prepubertal and early adolescent bipolar disorder: examples of elated mood, grandiose behaviors, decreased need for sleep, racing thoughts and hypersexuality. *Journal of Child and Adolescent Psychopharmacology* **12** (1), 3–9.

Ghaemi, S.N. *et al.* (2006) Extrapyramidal side effects with atypical neuroleptics in bipolar disorder. *Progress in Neuro-Psychopharmacology and Biological Psychiatry* **30** (2), 209–213.

Gorrindo, T. *et al.* (2005) Deficits on a probabilistic response-reversal task in patients with pediatric bipolar disorder. *American Journal of Psychiatry* **162** (10), 1975–1977.

Grauso-Eby, N.L. *et al.* (2003) Acute pancreatitis in children from Valproic acid: case series and review. *Pediatric Neurology* **28** (2), 145–148.

Grigoroiu-Serbanescu, M. *et al.* (1989) Psychopathology in children aged 10-17 of bipolar parents: psychopathology rate and correlates of the severity of the psychopathology. *Journal of Affective Disorders* **16** (2–3), 167–179.

Guyer, A.E. *et al.* (2007) Specificity of facial expression labeling deficits in childhood psychopathology. *Journal of Child Psychology and Psychiatry* **48** (9), 863–871.

Haas, M. *et al.* (2009) Risperidone for the treatment of acute mania in children and adolescents with bipolar disorder: a randomized, double-blind, placebo-controlled study. *Bipolar Disorders* **11** (7), 687–700.

Hajek, T. *et al.* (2009) Amygdala volumes in mood disorders–meta-analysis of magnetic resonance volumetry studies. *Journal of Affective Disorders* **115** (3), 395–410.

Harpold, T.L. *et al.* (2005) Examining the association between pediatric bipolar disorder and anxiety disorders in psychiatrically referred children and adolescents. *Journal of Affective Disorders* **88** (1), 19–26.

Harrington, R. *et al.* (1990) Adult outcomes of childhood and adolescent depression. I. Psychiatric status. *Archives of General Psychiatry* **47** (5), 465–473.

Hazell, P.L. *et al.* (2003) Manic symptoms in young males with ADHD predict functioning but not diagnosis after 6 years. *Journal of American Academy of Child and Adolescent Psychiatry* **42** (5), 552–560.

Hazell, P.L. *et al.* (1999) Confirmation that Child Behavior Checklist clinical scales discriminate juvenile mania from attention deficit hyperactivity disorder. *Journal of Paediatric Child Health* **35** (2), 199–203.

Henin, A. *et al.* (2005) Psychopathology in the offspring of parents with bipolar disorder: a controlled study. *Biological Psychiatry* **58** (7), 554–561.

Hillegers, M.H. *et al.* (2005) Five-year prospective outcome of psychopathology in the adolescent offspring of bipolar parents. *Bipolar Disorders* **7** (4), 344–350.

Hodgins, S. *et al.* (2002) Children of parents with bipolar disorder. A population at high risk for major affective disorders. *Child and Adolescent Psychiatric Clinics of North America* **11** (3), 533–553, ix.

Holtmann, M. *et al.* (2010) Bipolar disorder in children and adolescents in Germany: national trends in the rates of inpatients, 2000-2007. *Bipolar Disorders* **12** (2), 155–163.

Hunt, J.I. *et al.* (2013) Irritability and elation in a large bipolar youth sample: relative symptom severity and clinical outcomes over 4 years. *Journal of Clinical Psychiatry* **74** (1), e110–e117.

Kafantaris, V. *et al.* (2004) Lithium treatment of acute mania in adolescents: a placebo-controlled discontinuation study. *Journal of the American Academy of Child and Adolescent Psychiatry* **43** (8), 984–993.

Kalmar, J.H. *et al.* (2009) Relation between amygdala structure and function in adolescents with bipolar disorder. *Journal of the American Academy of Child and Adolescent Psychiatry* **48** (6), 636–642.

Kelsoe, J.R. (2003) Arguments for the genetic basis of the bipolar spectrum. *Journal of Affective Disorders* **73** (1–2), 183–197.

Kennedy, N. *et al.* (2005) Incidence and distribution of first-episode mania by age: results from a 35-year study. *Psychological Medicine* **35** (6), 855–863.

Kessler, R.C. *et al.* (2005) Prevalence, severity, and comorbidity of 12-month DSM-IV disorders in the National Comorbidity Survey Replication. *Archives of General Psychiatry* **62** (6), 617–627.

Kovacs, M. *et al.* (1994) Childhood-onset dysthymic disorder. Clinical features and prospective naturalistic outcome. *Archives of General Psychiatry* **51** (5), 365–374.

Kowatch, R.A. *et al.* (2005) Treatment guidelines for children and adolescents with bipolar disorder. *Journal of the American Academy of Child and Adolescent Psychiatry* **44** (3), 213–235.

Leibenluft, E. *et al.* (2003) Defining clinical phenotypes of juvenile mania. *American Journal of Psychiatry* **160** (3), 430–437.

Leibenluft, E. *et al.* (2007) Neural circuitry engaged during unsuccessful motor inhibition in pediatric bipolar disorder. *American Journal of Psychiatry* **164** (1), 52–60.

Lewinsohn, P.M. *et al.* (1995) Bipolar disorders in a community sample of older adolescents: prevalence, phenomenology, comorbidity, and course. *Journal of American Academy of Child and Adolescence Psychiatry* **34** (4), 454–463.

Lewinsohn, P.M. *et al.* (2000) Bipolar disorder during adolescence and young adulthood in a community sample. *Bipolar Disorders* **2** (3 Pt 2), 281–293.

Lin, P.I. *et al.* (2006) Clinical correlates and familial aggregation of age at onset in bipolar disorder. *American Journal of Psychiatry* **163** (2), 240–246.

Mannuzza, S. *et al.* (1998) Adult psychiatric status of hyperactive boys grown up. *The American Journal of Psychiatry* **155** (4), 493–498.

Martin, A. *et al.* (2004) Age effects on antidepressant-induced manic conversion. *Archives of Pediatrics and Adolescent Medicine* **158** (8), 773–780.

Martinez-Aran, A. *et al.* (2004) Cognitive impairment in euthymic bipolar patients: implications for clinical and functional outcome. *Bipolar Disorders* **6** (3), 224–232.

McGurk, S.R. *et al.* (2007) A meta-analysis of cognitive remediation in schizophrenia. *American Journal of Psychiatry* **164** (12), 1791–1802.

McIntyre, R.S. *et al.* (2003) Valproate, bipolar disorder and polycystic ovarian syndrome. *Bipolar Disorders* **5** (1), 28–35.

Merikangas, K.R. *et al.* (2012) Mania with and without depression in a community sample of US adolescents. *Archives of General Psychiatry* **69** (9), 943–951.

Merikangas, K.R. *et al.* (2010) Prevalence and treatment of mental disorders among US children in the 2001-2004 NHANES. *Pediatrics* **125** (1), 75–81.

Miklowitz, D.J. *et al.* (2008) Family-focused treatment for adolescents with bipolar disorder: results of a 2-year randomized trial. *Archives of General Psychiatry* **65** (9), 1053–1061.

Miklowitz, D.J. & Scott, J. (2009) Psychosocial treatments for bipolar disorder: cost-effectiveness, mediating mechanisms, and future directions. *Bipolar Disorders* **11** (Suppl 2), 110–122.

Moore, C.M. *et al.* (2002) Brain-to-serum lithium ratio and age: an in vivo magnetic resonance spectroscopy study. *American Journal of Psychiatry* **159** (7), 1240–1242.

Moore, G.J. *et al.* (1999) Temporal dissociation between lithium-induced changes in frontal lobe myo-inositol and clinical response in manic-depressive illness. *American Journal of Psychiatry* **156** (12), 1902–1908.

Moreno, C. *et al.* (2007) National trends in the outpatient diagnosis and treatment of bipolar disorder in youth. *Archives of General Psychiatry* **64** (9), 1032–1039.

National Institute for Health and Care Excellence (2006) *Bipolar Disorder: The Management of Bipolar Disorder in Adults, Children, and Adolescents in Primary and Secondary Care.* National Institute for Health and Care Excellence, London.

Pavuluri, M.N. *et al.* (2004) Child- and family-focused cognitive-behavioral therapy for pediatric bipolar disorder: development and preliminary results. *Journal of American Academy of Child and Adolescence Psychiatry* **43** (5), 528–537.

Pavuluri, M.N. *et al.* (2007) Affective neural circuitry during facial emotion processing in pediatric bipolar disorder. *Biological Psychiatry* **62** (2), 158–167.

Pavuluri, M.N. *et al.* (2006) Impact of neurocognitive function on academic difficulties in pediatric bipolar disorder: a clinical translation. *Biological Psychiatry* **60** (9), 951–956.

Pavuluri, M.N. *et al.* (2011a) Double-blind randomized trial of risperidone versus divalproex in pediatric bipolar disorder: fMRI outcomes. *Psychiatry Research* **193** (1), 28–37.

Pavuluri, M.N. *et al.* (2011b) Double-blind randomized trial of risperidone versus divalproex in pediatric bipolar disorder: fMRI outcomes. *Psychiatry Research* **193** (1), 28–37.

Pavuluri, M.N. *et al.* (2009) Diffusion tensor imaging study of white matter fiber tracts in pediatric bipolar disorder and attention-deficit/ hyperactivity disorder. *Biological Psychiatry* **65** (7), 586–593.

Pfeifer, J.C. *et al.* (2008) Meta-analysis of amygdala volumes in children and adolescents with bipolar disorder. *Journal of the American Academy of Child and Adolescent Psychiatry* **47** (11), 1289–1298.

Pope, H.G. Jr. *et al.* (1991) Valproate in the treatment of acute mania. A placebo-controlled study. *Archives of General Psychiatry* **48** (1), 62–68.

Priebe, L. *et al.* (2012) Genome-wide survey implicates the influence of copy number variants (CNVs) in the development of early-onset bipolar disorder. *Molecular Psychiatry* **17** (4), 421–432.

Rao, U. *et al.* (1995) Unipolar depression in adolescents: clinical outcome in adulthood. *Journal of American Academy Child and Adolescence Psychiatry* **34** (5), 566–578.

Rich, B.A. *et al.* (2011) Different neural pathways to negative affect in youth with pediatric bipolar disorder and severe mood dysregulation. *Journal of Psychiatric Research* **45** (10), 1283–1294.

Rich, B.A. *et al.* (2008) Face emotion labeling deficits in children with bipolar disorder and severe mood dysregulation. *Development and Psychopathology* **20** (2), 529–546.

Rich, B.A. *et al.* (2007) Different psychophysiological and behavioral responses elicited by frustration in pediatric bipolar disorder and severe mood dysregulation. *American Journal of Psychiatry* **164** (2), 309–317.

Rich, B.A. *et al.* (2006) Limbic hyperactivation during processing of neutral facial expressions in children with bipolar disorder. *Proceedings of the National Academy of Sciences of the United States of America* **103** (23), 8900–8905.

Rowe, R. *et al.* (2010) Developmental pathways in oppositional defiant disorder and conduct disorder. *Journal of Abnormal Psychology* **119** (4), 726–738.

Scheffer, R.E. *et al.* (2005) Randomized, placebo-controlled trial of mixed amphetamine salts for symptoms of comorbid ADHD in pediatric bipolar disorder after mood stabilization with divalproex sodium. *American Journal of Psychiatry* **162** (1), 58–64.

Seymour, K.E. *et al.* (2013) Emotional face identification in youths with primary bipolar disorder or primary ADHD. *Journal of American Academy of Child and Adolescence Psychiatry* **52** (5), 537–546.

Shalev, L. *et al.* (2007) Computerized progressive attentional training (CPAT) program: effective direct intervention for children with ADHD. *Child Neuropsychology* **13** (4), 382–388.

Silverstone, P.H. *et al.* (2002) Chronic treatment with both lithium and sodium valproate may normalize phosphoinositol cycle activity in bipolar patients. *Human Psychopharmacology* **17** (7), 321–327.

Singh, M.K. *et al.* (2010) Neural correlates of response inhibition in pediatric bipolar disorder. *Journal of Child and Adolescent Psychopharmacology* **20** (1), 15–24.

Smoller, J.W. & Finn, C.T. (2003) Family, twin, and adoption studies of bipolar disorder. *American Journal of Medical Genetics Part C: Seminars in Medical Genetics* **123** (1), 48–58.

Stringaris, A. *et al.* (2010a) Pediatric bipolar disorder versus severe mood dysregulation: risk for manic episodes on follow-up. *Journal of the American Academy of Child and Adolescent Psychiatry* **49** (4), 397–405.

Stringaris, A. *et al.* (2010b) Pediatric bipolar disorder versus severe mood dysregulation: risk for manic episodes on follow-up. *Journal of the American Academy of Child and Adolescent Psychiatry* **49** (4), 397–405.

Stringaris, A. *et al.* (2009) Adult outcomes of youth irritability: a 20-year prospective community-based study. *American Journal of Psychiatry* **166** (9), 1048–1054.

Strober, M. & Carlson, G. (1982) Bipolar illness in adolescents with major depression: clinical, genetic, and psychopharmacologic predictors in a three- to four-year prospective follow-up investigation. *Archives of General Psychiatry* **39** (5), 549–555.

Thase, M.E. (2007) STEP-BD and bipolar depression: what have we learned? *Current Psychiatry Reports* **9** (6), 497–503.

Thomas, L.A. *et al.* (2013) Elevated amygdala responses to emotional faces in youths with chronic irritability or bipolar disorder. *Neuroimage Clinics* **2**, 637–645.

Tijssen, M.J. *et al.* (2010) Prediction of transition from common adolescent bipolar experiences to bipolar disorder: 10-year study. *British Journal of Psychiatry* **196** (2), 102–108.

Tohen, M. *et al.* (2005) Olanzapine versus lithium in the maintenance treatment of bipolar disorder: a 12-month, randomized, double-blind, controlled clinical trial. *American Journal of Psychiatry* **162** (7), 1281–1290.

van der Schot, A.C. *et al.* (2010) Genetic and environmental influences on focal brain density in bipolar disorder. *Brain* **133** (10), 3080–3092.

Van Meter, A.R. *et al.* (2011) Meta-analysis of epidemiologic studies of pediatric bipolar disorder. *Journal of Clinical Psychiatry* **72** (9), 1250–1256.

Volk, H.E. & Todd, R.D. (2007) Does the Child Behavior Checklist juvenile bipolar disorder phenotype identify bipolar disorder? *Biological Psychiatry* **62** (2), 115–120.

Wagner, K.D. *et al.* (2006) A double-blind, randomized, placebo-controlled trial of oxcarbazepine in the treatment of bipolar disorder in children and adolescents. *American Journal of Psychiatry* **163** (7), 1179–1186.

Wagner, K.D. *et al.* (2009) A double-blind, randomized, placebo-controlled trial of divalproex extended-release in the treatment of bipolar disorder in children and adolescents. *Journal of American Academy of Child Adolescence and Psychiatry* **48** (5), 519–532.

Wagner, K.D. *et al.* (2002) An open-label trial of divalproex in children and adolescents with bipolar disorder. *Journal of American Academy of Child and Adolescent Psychiatry* **41** (10), 1224–1230.

Wals, M. *et al.* (2001) Prevalence of psychopathology in children of a bipolar parent. *Journal of American Academy of Child and Adolescence Psychiatry* **40** (9), 1094–1102.

Weissman, M.M. *et al.* (1996) Cross-national epidemiology of major depression and bipolar disorder. *JAMA* **276** (4), 293–299.

Weissman, M.M. *et al.* (1999) Children with prepubertal-onset major depressive disorder and anxiety grown up. *Archives of General Psychiatry* **56** (9), 794–801.

Wilens, T.E. *et al.* (2004) Risk of substance use disorders in adolescents with bipolar disorder. *Journal of American Academy of Child and Adolescence Psychiatry* **43** (11), 1380–1386.

Winsberg, M.E. *et al.* (2000) Decreased dorsolateral prefrontal N-acetyl aspartate in bipolar disorder. *Biological Psychiatry* **47** (6), 475–481.

Wozniak, J. *et al.* (1995) Mania-like symptoms suggestive of childhood-onset bipolar disorder in clinically referred children. *Journal of American Academy of Child and Adolescent Psychiatry* **34** (7), 867–876.

Young, R.C. *et al.* (1978) A rating scale for mania: reliability, validity and sensitivity. *British Journal of Psychiatry* **133**, 429–435.

Youngstrom, E. *et al.* (2005) Bipolar diagnoses in community mental health: Achenbach child behavior checklist profiles and patterns of comorbidity. *Biological Psychiatry* **58** (7), 569–575.

CHAPTER 63

Depressive disorders in childhood and adolescence

David Brent[1] and Fadi Maalouf[2]

[1] Child and Adolescent Psychiatry, Western Psychiatric Institute, University of Pittsburgh, PA, USA
[2] Child and Adolescent Psychiatry Program, Department of Psychiatry, American University of Beirut, Lebanon

Clinical picture

Phenomenology and classification

Depressive disorders are all characterized by persistent, impairing sadness, anhedonia, or irritability that is relatively unresponsive to pleasurable activities and interactions, and attention from other people.

Depressive disorders are classified on the basis of severity, chronicity, presence of mania, and seasonality. To qualify, according to DSM-5, the patient must experience functional impairment related to a change in mood. This mood change cannot better be explained by another condition, for example, medical disorder or substance abuse. ICD-10 does not formally require functional impairment, but describes it as a frequent accompaniment of depression based on severity (World Health Organization, 2010). In DSM-5, major depressive disorder is characterized by at least 2 weeks of persistent change in mood, nearly every day, manifested by either depressed or irritable mood, or loss of interest or pleasure and at least four additional symptoms of depression: changes in appetite or weight, sleep, psychomotor activity, decreased energy, feelings of worthlessness or guilt, difficulty thinking or concentrating, or recurrent thoughts of death or suicidal ideation, plans, or attempts. Chronic depression involves depressive symptomatology that lasts for at least 12 months. Other specified depressive disorder is used for patients whose depressive symptoms are impairing but do not meet duration or number of symptom requirements, such as those with brief recurrent depression, with recurrent symptoms of duration shorter than 2 weeks, or a longer depressive episode that is impairing with fewer than the required number of symptoms for major depressive disorder.

Changes from DSM-IV to DSM-5

Dysthymic disorder, a chronic and intermittent depressive disorder lasting at least 1 year, is now subsumed under persistent depressive disorder.

A newly introduced condition, "disruptive mood dysregulation disorder" (DMDD), is characterized by severe persistent irritability with temper outbursts occurring at least three times weekly in youth at least aged 6 and with onset prior to age 10 (American Psychiatric Association, 2013). DMDD shows extremely high diagnostic overlap with oppositional and mood disorders, and further research is required to clarify if DMDD is distinct from its commonly co-occurring, related conditions (Axelson, 2013; Copeland et al., 2013); see Chapter 62.

The bereavement exclusion for major depression has been dropped, meaning that bereaved patients who meet criteria for major depression within the first 2 months of a loss can be diagnosed accordingly. This change is consistent with findings that the phenomenology, course, and risk factors for depression associated with bereavement are similar to those whose depression is unrelated to bereavement and that the highest risk period for bereaved individuals to become depressed is immediately after the loss (Bridge et al., 2003; Hamdan et al., 2012).

Differential diagnosis

The most important differential diagnosis is between unipolar and bipolar depression. However, manic symptoms do not necessarily mean that the patient has bipolar disorder, as only 25% of youth with clinically significant mania in one clinical epidemiological study meet criteria for bipolar spectrum disorder (Findling et al., 2010). Depression may also present with psychotic features, typically of depressive, self-deprecatory, or paranoid content. With regard to the latter, the main differential is between prodromal symptoms of schizophrenia, and can often only be determined through longitudinal follow-up. Major depression that occurs in the fall and remits in the spring, characterized by hypersomnia, fatigue, and carbohydrate craving is categorized as seasonal affective disorder.

Rutter's Child and Adolescent Psychiatry, Sixth Edition.
Edited by Anita Thapar and Daniel S. Pine, James F. Leckman, Stephen Scott, Margaret J. Snowling, Eric Taylor.
© 2015 John Wiley & Sons Ltd. Published 2018 by John Wiley & Sons Ltd.

Anxiety disorders are often associated with significant dysphoria that is relieved if the anxiogenic situation (e.g., separation, social situations) is eliminated. The social withdrawal of depression should be differentiated from social avoidance due to anxiety.

Altered concentration is not only a symptom of depression, but is a key feature of attention deficit hyperactivity disorder (ADHD). ADHD usually has an earlier onset than depression and is often associated with impulsivity and hyperactivity. Children with ADHD frequently become demoralized due to peer rejection and difficulties at school, but in contrast to depression, the symptomatic presentation of ADHD (e.g., inattention) does not become worse with changes in mood.

Irritability is a prominent symptom of conduct (CD) and oppositional defiant disorder (ODD). In the absence of other mood symptoms, irritability is more likely to be due to the behavioral disorder than depression. However, high levels of irritability in childhood predict depression and anxiety in adulthood (Stringaris *et al.*, 2009; see Chapter 5).

Substance abuse can mimic mood disorders by disrupting sleep, concentration, motivation, and appetite; moreover these conditions frequently co-occur with mood disorders in clinical practice. A careful history and, when warranted, a drug toxicology screen can help detect this important and serious condition.

Patients with eating disorders often show lassitude and dysphoria, which can in part be attributed to poor nutritional status. A diagnosis of current depression in an eating disordered patient should not be made until adequate nutritional status has been restored.

Some medical conditions (e.g., hypothyroidism, mononucleosis, anemia, sleep apnea) may mimic depressive symptoms, particularly fatigue, low energy, and low motivation.

Comorbidity

Between 40% and 90% of youth with depressive disorders also have other psychiatric disorders (Angold *et al.*, 1999). Comorbidity may result from shared etiology, or as a cause or consequence of depression. Anxiety is frequently a precursor of, and shares a genetic diathesis with, depression (Middeldorp *et al.*, 2005). ADHD and depression are also often comorbid, but attentional symptoms should only be counted toward depression if they worsen in association with changes in mood. Comorbidity between depression and behavioral disorders and substance abuse may be attributable to shared family risk factors, such as abuse, exposure to family violence and discord, and parental substance abuse (Harrington, 2000). ODD may predispose to depression via difficulty with emotion regulation and tendency to negative affectivity (Hipwell *et al.*, 2011; Burke, 2012). Longitudinal studies suggest that while the relationship between depression and substance abuse is bidirectional, substance abuse is more likely to lead to depression than *vice versa* (Boden & Fergusson, 2011; Horwood *et al.*, 2012).

Assessment

Self- and parent-report questionnaires are useful for screening for depression and monitoring treatment response and are time-efficient. The Mood and Feelings Questionnaire (MFQ) is the only self- and parent-reported scale validated for both children and adolescents and comes in a 37-item and 13-item form, the latter of which is useful for screening for depression (Wood *et al.*, 1995; Thapar & McGuffin, 1998). The Children's Depression Inventory (CDI) was developed as a downward extension of the Beck Depression Inventory (BDI), has self-, parent-, and teacher-report forms, is highly correlated with other measures of depression, and discriminates depression from anxiety and disruptive disorders (Timbremont *et al.*, 2004). The Patient Health Questionnaire-2, consisting of two items (low mood and anhedonia) has been validated as a screen for depression in adolescents, as has the longer nine-item version (Richardson *et al.*, 2010). Three other measures with good psychometric properties that have been used to screen for depression and to monitor treatment effects are the Center for Epidemiologic Studies-Depression Scale (CES-D; although it lacks a suicide ideation item), the BDI, and the Reynolds Adolescent Depression Scale (RADS-2). In a comparison of the CES-D and BDI using item-response theory, the CES-D performed better in lower ranges of symptomatology, whereas the BDI performed better at higher ranges of symptomatology (Olino *et al.*, 2012). A newly developed eight-item self-report, the Patient Reported Outcome Management Information System (PROMIS), showed better performance than either the CES-D or the BDI over the full range of symptomatology, although it has not been used in treatment studies (Olino *et al.*, 2013). The RADS-2 shows strong psychometric properties, including treatment sensitivity (March *et al.*, 2004; Osman *et al.*, 2010). The Preschool Feelings Checklist is one parent-report instrument validated for preschool depression (Luby *et al.*, 2004).

Interview-rated assessments, while more labor-intensive, can integrate reports from parents and youth, and permit the ascertainment of the temporal sequence, course, and functional significance of different symptoms. The interviewer can determine the extent to which a specific symptom should be attributed to the diagnosis of depression in the face of comorbidity (e.g., if a patient has preexisting ADHD, to determine if concentration problems should be attributed to depression) (see also Chapter 32). The most common interview used in research studies in child and adolescent depression is the semistructured Schedule for Affective Disorders and Schizophrenia for School-Age Children-Present and Lifetime version (K-SADS-PL) (Kaufman *et al.*, 1997). Several other instruments have good psychometric properties, and may be more appropriate for epidemiological studies, because they are either briefer or fully structured.

The most commonly used continuous, interview-based measure of depressive symptomatology is the Children's Depression Rating Scale-Revised (CDRS-R), a 17-item assessment that has been shown to have good reliability and treatment sensitivity (Mayes *et al.*, 2010).

Descriptive epidemiology

Prevalence

The point prevalence of depressive disorders is 1–2% in preschool and older prepubertal children and 3–8% in adolescents, with the lifetime prevalence by the end of adolescence of around 20% (Lewinsohn *et al.*, 1998; Costello *et al.*, 2003). One-year and 1-month prevalence estimates of major depressive disorder in adolescents in the National Comorbidity Survey Replication are 8.2% and 2.6%, respectively (Kessler *et al.*, 2012). Studies conducted in countries of lower or middle income report higher point prevalences of clinically significant depressive symptomatology (10–13% in boys and 12–18% for girls) (Ruchkin *et al.*, 2006; Alyahri & Goodman, 2008).

Age, gender, and puberty

The dramatic female predominance in depression that first emerges with puberty may be mediated by increases in estradiol and testosterone (Angold *et al.*, 1998). Adolescent-onset depressive disorder has a higher risk of recurrent mood disorder into adulthood as compared to depression of prepubertal onset, and shows a greater degree of heritability (Shanahan *et al.*, 2011). Earlier onset of puberty may increase the risk of depression in girls, perhaps mediated by an increased risk of conduct disorder. The dramatic neurodevelopmental remodeling of prefrontal and limbic structures involved in social attribution, emotion regulation, and reward response that occurs in adolescence may contribute to increased vulnerability to depression, as well as increased rates of sleep disruption, and alcohol and drug use (Hayward *et al.*, 1997; Dahl, 2004; Andersen & Teicher, 2008; Boden & Fergusson, 2011; Casey *et al.*, 2011; Shanahan *et al.*, 2011; Horwood *et al.*, 2012).

Course and outcome

Episode length and recovery

The duration for depressive episodes ranges between 3 and 6 months for community samples, and between 5 and 8 months for referred samples (Birmaher *et al.*, 2002), with around 1 in 5 depressed adolescents showing evidence of depression of duration two years or greater (Lewinsohn *et al.*, 1998; Birmaher *et al.*, 2000).

Risk for recurrence

The risk for recurrent depression after an initial episode ranges from 30% to 70% within the first 2 years, and is higher in those with chronic depression, subsyndromal symptoms, comorbidity, and family conflict (Birmaher *et al.*, 2002; Emslie *et al.*, 2008). The continuity between adolescent and adult depression may be partly mediated by comorbid ODD, anxiety, and substance abuse (Copeland *et al.*, 2009).

Bipolar disorder

The risk of bipolar disorder in early-onset depression is estimated to be around 10–20% (Geller *et al.*, 2001), with elevated risk in patients who present with hypomania in response to treatment, psychotic features, hypersomnia (in some studies), and a family history of bipolar disorder (Strober & Carlson, 1982; Geller *et al.*, 2001).

Suicidal behavior and health risk behaviors

Suicidal behavior is a common sequela of early onset depression, and the mortality due to suicide is elevated at least 10-fold compared to nondepressed youth (Bridge *et al.*, 2006). Risk factors for suicidal behavior among depressed youth include greater severity and chronicity of depression, current ideation with a plan or a history of a suicide attempt, a history of nonsuicidal self-injury, insomnia, comorbid anxiety, conduct or substance abuse disorders, high levels of impulsive aggression, greater hopelessness, family history of suicidal behavior, abuse, family conflict, and lack of support (Bridge *et al.*, 2006; Wilkinson *et al.*, 2011; Nock *et al.*, 2013). Depression is associated with multiple health risk behaviors, including obesity (Hasler *et al.*, 2005; Katon *et al.*, 2010), and like suicidal behavior, predisposing factors to health risk behaviors include continued depression, comorbidity, low connection with parents, family discord, and history of abuse (Fergusson & Woodward, 2002; Lewinsohn *et al.*, 2003; Shanahan *et al.*, 2011).

Models of depression

We employ a stress-diathesis perspective for this review of risk factors for depression, that is, depression is most likely to develop in those with a vulnerability—defined by family history, cognitive bias, emotion dysregulation, fearfulness, or irritability, in concert with the experience of stressors—such as family conflict, child maltreatment, or peer victimization (Wilkinson & Goodyer, 2011).

Vulnerability factors for depression
Genetic

Twin studies demonstrate that depressive symptoms have a greater concordance among monozygotic than among dizygotic twins, with a heritability of around 40%, that vulnerability to depression may be cotransmitted with anxiety, and that adolescent-onset depression is more heritable than preadolescent onset depression (Thapar & Rice, 2006). In addition, a number of characteristics that predispose to depression, such as cognitive bias and difficulty with emotion regulation, appear to be familially transmitted (Su *et al.*, 2010; Owens *et al.*, 2012).

"Top-down" studies show a two- to fourfold increased risk of depressive disorder in the offspring of depressed parents

(Weissman, 2006). Greater family loading, such as depression in two generations and increased rates of parental and child anxiety disorders, were associated with an increased risk and earlier onset of depression (Weissman, 2006).

A mega-analysis of genome-wide association studies, comprising 9420 major depression cases and 18,759 controls, found no association between any gene and major depression, but did find 15 single-nucleotide polymorphisms (SNPs) associated with either major depression or bipolar disorder, all located in a 248 kg interval 3p21.1 (Ripke *et al.*, 2013).

The most frequently reported candidate gene variant associated with depression is a less functional allelic variant of the serotonin transporter gene (5HTTLPR), which is associated with early-onset depression, in the presence of stressful life events, a history of abuse, or peer victimization (Caspi *et al.*, 2010). However, the strength and consistency of these findings has been variable (see Chapter 24; Risch *et al.*, 2009). This genetic variant has been shown to be related to biological correlates of depression and anxiety, namely, negative information processing bias (Owens *et al.*, 2012), hypersecretion of cortisol in response to a social stressor (Gotlib *et al.*, 2008), and increased amygdala reactivity to emotional faces (Hariri *et al.*, 2002).

Cognitive distortion and rumination

The cognitive theory for depression is that depression is caused by biased attention to negative emotional cues, thereby reinforcing depressive symptomatology. Individuals with a negative inferential style are more likely to show growth in depressive symptoms; moreover, there is a bidirectional relationship in which cognitive distortions lead to stress generation, which in turn fuels growth in cognitive distortion over time (Gotlib & Joormann, 2010; Hankin, 2012). Rumination, or the tendency to dwell excessively on emotionally upsetting material, predicts the onset and growth of depressive symptomatology and is more prominent as a risk factor in girls (Hankin, 2012).

Emotion regulation

Emotion regulation, which is the ability to achieve emotional equilibrium in the face of perturbation, has been hypothesized to be a core deficit predisposing to depression (Kovacs & Lopez-Duran, 2010). Consistent with the cognitive theory of depression, individuals with emotion regulation difficulties are less able to shift attention away from negative emotion-laden, ruminative cognitions. Both self-report and laboratory assessment of emotion regulation (e.g., persistence in the face of frustration, decreased heart rate variability) are related to growth in children's internalizing and depressive symptoms (Kovacs & Lopez-Duran, 2010).

Fear and anxiety

Both fearfulness and anxiety disorders *per se,* especially social anxiety, are associated with an increased risk of depression, consistent with a shared genetic diathesis between anxiety and depression (Pine *et al.*, 1998, 2001; Middeldorp *et al.*, 2005; Beesdo *et al.*, 2007).

Behavioral disorders and irritability

The rates of depression are increased both in patients with attention deficit disorder hyperactivity (ADHD) and their parents (Faraone & Biederman, 1997). Depression may ensue as a consequence of rejection from peers, teachers, and parents, and due to poor emotion regulation characteristic of ADHD (Seymour *et al.*, 2012). The relationship between ODD and depression may be mediated by the dimension of ODD associated with negative affect and irritability, whereas the link between CD and depression may be because CD results in the generation of stressful life events (e.g., arrests) that may be depressogenic (Fergusson *et al.*, 2003; Stringaris *et al.*, 2009; Hipwell *et al.*, 2011; Burke, 2012).

Sleep

Subjective sleep complaints are a more prominent component of early-onset depression than objective findings (Forbes & Dahl, 2012). However, decreased REM latency, increased REM density, and decreased sleep efficiency have been reported to be associated with depressive onset, recurrence, and persistence in some studies (Rao *et al.*, 2009). Insomnia has been shown to have a bidirectional relationship with the onset and growth of depressive symptoms (Gregory *et al.*, 2009; Cousins *et al.*, 2011). In specific, sleep deprivation results in increased mood lability and greater attention to negative emotional cues (Soffer-Dudek *et al.*, 2011; Dagys *et al.*, 2012).

Comorbid medical illness

Poor physical health is associated with adolescent depression, in part due to interference with activities that are enjoyable or enhance a sense of mastery (Lewinsohn *et al.*, 1998). There are also systemic effects of chronic illness, particularly those that involve the central nervous system (e.g., epilepsy, migraine) or that affect the inflammatory system (e.g., inflammatory bowel disease, asthma), as well as depressogenic effects from some of the treatments (e.g., corticosteroids, interferon) (Lewinsohn *et al.*, 1998; Szigethy *et al.*, 2010; Hoppe & Elger, 2011; Bruti *et al.*, 2012; Goodwin *et al.*, 2012).

Environmental risk factors
Parental depression and family discord

Adoption studies show that maternal depression is not only a genetic, but also an environmental risk factor for both externalizing disorders, and for depression (Tully *et al.*, 2008). Conversely, treatment of maternal depression can result in symptomatic improvement in youth, in both externalizing and internalizing symptoms (Brent *et al.*, 1998; Gunlicks & Weissman, 2008; Swartz *et al.*, 2008). The impact of maternal depression may be mediated by family discord and expressed emotion directed toward the child, which in turn predicts onset, persistence, and recurrence in at-risk subjects (Silk *et al.*, 2009).

Child maltreatment

Physical or sexual abuse, neglect, and exposure to domestic violence are potent risk factors for the onset and recurrence of depression. Abuse may be more likely to lead to depression in those at increased genetic risk (e.g., family history of depression) (Kaufman *et al.*, 2006; Caspi *et al.*, 2010).

Peer victimization

Both bullies and their victims have higher rates of depression than controls (Zwierzynska *et al.*, 2013). Peer victimization can have long-lasting effects on increasing depressive symptomatology, may be mediated by increasing negative cognitions and may be more common in those with a high cortisol response to a laboratory-based social stressor (Rudolph *et al.*, 2011; Sinclair *et al.*, 2012; Zwierzynska *et al.*, 2013).

Sexual minority status

Sexual minority youth (i.e., lesbian, gay, bisexual, or transgendered) are about three times more likely to have depression as heterosexual youth, and these effects appear to be mediated by peer victimization (Marshal *et al.*, 2011; Burton *et al.*, 2013), and may also be accounted for by parental rejection, assault, and higher rates of abuse (Friedman *et al.*, 2011).

Bereavement

Parental or peer bereavement is associated with a threefold increased risk for depression even after controlling for other preexisting risk factors, and appears phenomenologically similar to nonbereavement-related depression (Bridge *et al.*, 2003; Hamdan *et al.*, 2012). The increased risk is greatest immediately after the death, and is more likely in those with a previous history of depression, who lost a close friend rather than an acquaintance, and who lost a mother rather than father (Bridge *et al.*, 2003; Brent *et al.*, 2009a).

Resilience

Higher intelligence, a warm and supportive relationship with parents, more adaptive emotion regulation skills, and a problem-focused coping style can protect at-risk youth from developing depression (Yap *et al.*, 2008; Brent *et al.*, 2009a; Wetter & Hankin, 2009).

Neurobiology of depression

Hypothalamic pituitary adrenal axis

A meta-analytic review found that pediatric depression was associated with dexamethasone suppression test nonsuppression, higher levels of basal cortisol, and an increased cortisol response to social stressors (Lopez-Duran *et al.*, 2009). High nocturnal urinary cortisol predicts depressive recurrences, especially in youth exposed to life stressors (Rao *et al.*, 2009).

Inflammation

Inflammation may play a role in the pathophysiology of depression, through neurotoxicity and interference with serotonin metabolism (Mills *et al.*, 2013), with increased levels of interleukin factor 6 (IL-6) and C-reactive protein (CRP) in depressed youth (Mills *et al.*, 2013). Prospective studies link early adversity, inflammatory markers, and depressive symptoms (Danese *et al.*, 2008, 2009; Miller & Cole, 2012), although some studies show that inflammation is a consequence rather than a precursor of depression (Copeland *et al.*, 2012). Some posit that inflammatory processes found in depression may account for the high rate of cardiometabolic illness in depression (Mills *et al.*, 2013).

Neurocircuitry of depression

The current neural model of depression is consistent with studies implicating cognitive bias and emotion regulation in the pathogenesis of depression. Neuroimaging studies in pediatric depression find alterations in circuits related to biased information processing, for example, with greater attendance to negative emotional cues, less ability to use prefrontal cortical resources to dampen limbic activation to negative emotional cues, and impaired ability to experience positive affect and reward (Hulvershorn *et al.*, 2011). These characteristics are present both in youth at risk for depression as well as depressed youth.

Structural studies

Cortical thinning of the lateral half of the right hemisphere and medial aspect of the left, as well as bilateral hypoplasia of frontal and parietal white matter, have been reported as a familially transmitted phenotype for depression (Peterson & Weissman, 2011). Small hippocampal volume has been identified as a risk factor for depression, especially in interaction with early-life adversity (Rao *et al.*, 2010). Contradictory findings about amygdala size and depression may be explained by the impact of antidepressant medication on subcortical structures (Hamilton *et al.*, 2008; Hulvershorn *et al.*, 2011).

Biased information processing
Peripheral neurocognitive studies

A bias toward sad (vs happy) words on the affective go/no go task was found in acutely depressed but not remitted depressed youth (Maalouf *et al.*, 2012a). Depressed youth respond faster to sad faces as compared to healthy controls and are more easily distracted by negative emotional stimuli while performing cognitive tasks (Ladouceur *et al.*, 2005, 2006).

fMRI studies

Depressed youth, compared to controls, show greater reactivity to negative emotional stimuli in the amygdala, dorsal anterior cingulate cortex (ACC), and insula, and show less reactivity in the dorsolateral prefrontal cortex (DLPFC) to negative stimuli and when performing higher order cognitive tasks (Roberson-Nay *et al.*, 2006; Monk *et al.*, 2008; Halari *et al.*, 2009; Hulvershorn *et al.*, 2011).

Studies of resting state connectivity are consistent with the above-noted findings, supporting the view that the diathesis for depression involves diminished prefrontal cortical modulation of limbic activity. Depressed youth and youth at risk for depression, compared to controls, have diminished connectivity between the amygdala and DLPFC (Luking *et al.*, 2011). Depressed adolescents, and even depressed preschoolers, show evidence of difficulty in emotion processing, with decreased functional connectivity in a subgenual ACC-based neural network (Cullen *et al.*, 2009; Gaffrey *et al.*, 2010). Two studies using diffusion tensor imaging (DTI) in depression have found decreased fractional anisotropy (FA) in the uncinate fasciulus, a white matter tract connecting the ventral prefrontal regions (including the subgenual ACC and ventromedial PFC) with the amygdala (Cullen *et al.*, 2010; Huang *et al.*, 2011).

Positive affect and reward processing

Attenuated positive affect, rather than just excess negative affect, may also be a risk factor for early onset depression (Olino *et al.*, 2011). The interaction of high negative emotionality and low positive emotion predicted growth in anhedonic symptoms, although this relationship was buffered by the experience of supportive relationships (Wetter & Hankin, 2009). Low positive affect, even in positive contexts, is also found in youth at increased familial risk for depression (McMakin *et al.*, 2011).

fMRI studies demonstrate that, in response to a reward decision-making task, depressed adolescents exhibit a blunted response in the striatum, ACC, caudate, and orbito-frontal cortex during reward anticipation and reward outcome, compared to controls (Forbes & Dahl, 2012), suggesting a decreased emotional response to a reward. In addition, in a similar reward task, high-risk subjects show less activation in the right insula compared to a low-risk control group (Gotlib *et al.*, 2010).

Treatment

Overview

Treatment of depression is divided into three stages: (i) acute treatment (first 2–3 months); (ii) consolidation (subsequent 3–6 months), and (iii) continuation (continuing treatment for 12+ months). The goal of acute treatment is to achieve a response, usually defined as at least a 50% decline in depressive symptoms and a global rating of improved or very much improved. Consolidation involves either continuation of the same treatment, or adjusting the treatment to address residual symptoms in order to achieve remission. The type and intensity of treatment depends on severity, and so we provide definitions of mild, moderate, and severe depression in Table 63.1. The magnitude of the effect for treatments are reports with an effect size (*d*), or number needed to treat (NNT), which is the inverse of the difference in response between drug and placebo, so that the smaller the NNT, the greater the treatment effect. The number needed to harm (NNH) is an analogous metric for

Table 63.1 Levels of severity of depression.

Level of severity	Number and type symptoms	Impairment
Mild	≤4, no suicidal ideation or psychosis	Able to function in most ways, but takes more effort
Moderate	5–6, suicidal ideation	Impairment in at least one domain
Severe	7, imminent suicidal risk, could have psychosis, mixed features	Unable to function adequately, with impaired self-care

adverse events. Table 63.2 summarizes findings from recent, large clinical trials.

Acute treatment

Many patients with mild depression respond to assessment and education alone (Birmaher *et al.*, 2007). For moderate-to-severe depression, evidence-based treatments are cognitive behavior therapy (CBT), antidepressant medication, and interpersonal psychotherapy (IPT), or combinations of medication and psychotherapy. For more detailed discussions of psychosocial treatments and CBT specifically, see Chapters 36 and 38.

CBT

CBT focuses on identifying cognitive distortions that may lead to depressed mood and also utilizes problem solving, behavior activation (BA), and emotion regulation skills to help manage and combat depression, with an average of 8–16 sessions. BA helps the patient to identify and participate in activities that are likely to lead to pleasure or mastery and can help relieve depressive symptoms (Lewinsohn *et al.*, 1998). A meta-analysis shows that CBT shows a small to moderate effect on depression, relative to alternative treatments ($d = 0.35$) (Weisz *et al.*, 2006). CBT performs better than supportive, family, and relaxation therapies in acute trials, although these alternative treatments catch up during longer-term follow-up (Wood *et al.*, 1996; Brent *et al.*, 1997; Birmaher *et al.*, 2000). In a community-based effectiveness trial comparing CBT to treatment as usual, CBT produced similar outcomes as treatment as usual, but with fewer sessions, less use of other services, and greater parental satisfaction (Weisz *et al.*, 2009). In the Treatment of Adolescent Depression Study (TADS), a multicenter study that randomized 439 depressed adolescents to CBT alone, fluoxetine alone, CBT with fluoxetine, or pill-placebo, by 12 weeks, CBT alone did not perform better than placebo, and was inferior to medication alone or medication in combination with CBT (March *et al.*, 2004). However, by 18 weeks, the CBT alone group had similar outcomes to the other active treatments (March *et al.*, 2007). Naturalistic data suggest that an adequate response may require at least nine sessions (Kennard *et al.*, 2014). Mediational analyses support that CBT works via the relief of cognitive distortions,

Table 63.2 Summary of some of the more recent clinical trials in adolescent depression.

Study	Sample	Outcome	Primary findings (% outcome)	Predictors/moderators of poorer response
Treatment of Adolescent Depression Study (TADS)	439 youth 12–18 yrs. with MDD Mean CDRS-R = 60 Suicidal = 29% Comorbid = 60%. Randomized to FL, CBT+FL, CBT, PL	CGI-I≤2	Wks / FL / CBT+FL / CBT / PL 12 / 61 / 71 / 43 / 35 18 / 69 / 85 / 65 / — 36 / 81 / 86 / 81 / —	**Predictors:** severity, chronicity, hopelessness, suicidal ideation **Moderator (of CBT):** lower income, sexual abuse, family discord, severity, low cognitive distortion **Predictors of suicidal events:** Highest in FL, predicted by baseline ideation, slower response Fastest response in CBT+FL, and highest rate of early remission at 12 weeks (37% vs. 17–23%)
Adolescent Depression Antidepressant and Psychotherapy Trial (ADAPT)	208 youth 11–17 yrs., ≥4 DSM-IV depressive symptoms Mean CDRS-R = 59 Suicidal = 66.3% Comorbid = 89% Randomized to FL, CBT+ FL	CGI-I≤2	Wks / FL / CBT+FL 12 / 44 / 42 28 / 61 / 53	**Predictors of nonresponse:** OCD symptoms, suicidal ideation, severity **Predictors of suicidal events:** Family dysfunction, high ideation, NSSI
Treatment of SSRI-Resistant Depression in Adolescents	334 youth 12–18 yrs., MDD and did not response to adequate trial with an SSRI Mean CDRS-R=59 Suicidal = 58% Comorbid = 52% Randomized to new SSRI, new SSRI+CBT, VLX, VLX+CBT	CGI-I≤2 and CDRS-R % change from baseline ≥50%	Wks / SSRI / CBT+SSRI / VLX / VLX+CBT 12 / 39 / 55 / 42 / 54 24 / 58 / 54 / 53 / 58 48 / 56 / 54 / 58 / 54 72 / 62 / 54 / 59 / 54	**Correlates:** Drug and Alcohol use, manic symptoms, adherence, drug levels **Predictors:** Severity, family conflict, NSSI **Moderators** (of combined): (negative):abuse history; (positive): comorbidity **Predictors of suicidal events:** drug and alcohol use, slow response, high ideation, family conflict, NSSI
Primary Care-Based Effectiveness Trial	152 youth with depression, 11–17 yrs, CDRS-R=35	Absence of depression diagnosis	Wks / SSRI+UC / CBT+SSRI 12 / 72 / 77 26 / 82 / 89 52 / 94 / 89	Significant difference favoring combined treatment on SF-12 Lower dose of SSRI in combined group

Abbreviations: A-LIFE, Adolescent Longitudinal Interval Follow-Up Evaluation; CBT, Cognitive Behavior Therapy; CDRS-R, Children's Depression Rating Scale-Revised; CGI-I-Clinical Global Impressions-Improvement Subscale; FL, fluoxetine; MDD, major depressive disorder; NSSI, nonsuicidal self-injury; OCD, obsessive compulsive disorder; PL, placebo; SF-12, mental component, quality of life; SSRI, selective serotonin reuptake inhibitor; UC, usual care; VLX, venlafaxine; wks, weeks.

although one naturalistic study suggests that problem-solving and social skills training are also "active ingredients" (Kaufman et al., 2005; Kennard et al., 2014). In patients with higher rates of comorbidity and high levels of cognitive distortion, CBT, either alone, or in combination with medication, outperforms other psychotherapies or medication monotherapy. However, for patients with a history of abuse or current parental depression, CBT is no better, and sometimes worse, than alternative treatments (Brent et al., 1998; Curry et al., 2006; Asarnow et al., 2009).

With regard to Internet-based CBT interventions, one brief intervention with a 4 to 5 session problem-solving therapy for adolescents with depressive symptoms did not show a difference compared to a waitlist control condition, but a larger trial using a more extensive intervention ("Master Your Mood") in youth aged 16–25 showed a substantial difference in outcome, favoring the intervention over a waitlist control condition (NNT = 3; $d = 0.94$) (Hoek et al., 2012; van der Zanden et al., 2012). One RCT with a computerized CBT tested the effects of the intervention versus a waitlist control in youth excluded from mainstream education and with significant depressive symptomatology, and found highly significant effects on remission as rated by clinical interview (NNT = 3) and self-reported depression (Fleming et al., 2012).

IPT

IPT conceptualizes depression as being related to loss, role conflict, and interpersonal discord. Accordingly, IPT aims to help depressed individuals decrease interpersonal conflicts by teaching interpersonal problem-solving skills and helping to modify dysfunctional communication and relational patterns (see Chapter 40). In the modification of IPT for adolescents (IPT-A), parent–child dyadic sessions focus on relief of parent–child conflict, an important contributor to the onset and persistence of early-onset depression. In clinical trials, IPT was delivered in 10–16 sessions, and performed better than supportive clinical management and usual care (Klomek & Mufson, 2006). IPT has not been tested against pill-placebo or medication only, but, in the two trials comparing CBT and IPT for depressed adolescents by the same research group, one trial favored IPT and the other, CBT (Rossello & Bernal, 1999; Rossello et al., 2008). IPT is especially effective compared to clinical management or usual care for depressed adolescents who have poorer interpersonal functioning, high levels of interpersonal conflict with parents, higher depressive severity, and comorbid anxiety (Gunlicks & Weissman, 2008; Young et al., 2009; Gunlicks-Stoessel et al., 2010).

Other psychotherapies with at least one RCT

Family-based attachment therapy (FBAT), which focuses on fostering a positive and supportive relationship between parents and teens, has been shown in two studies to be superior to either a waitlist control or a brief clinical management intervention; a larger trial for suicidal adolescents is now being conducted with a stronger comparator treatment to learn if the effects of ABFT are specific to the treatment or are due to a greater number of sessions in ABFT (Diamond et al., 2002, 2010).

Mentalization-based treatment (MBT) is a year-long individual psychodynamically derived intervention, with monthly family sessions that enhance the capacity of patients and their parents to understand actions in terms of thoughts and feelings, and thus improve agency and self control. MBT, compared to usual care, resulted in significantly greater improvements in self-harm and depressive symptoms, in self-harming adolescents with borderline personality disorder and depressive symptomatology (Rossouw & Fonagy, 2012).

Medication monotherapy

Fluoxetine is the only agent recommended for use in adolescents by the National Institute for Health and Care Excellence (NICE) guidelines, and approved by the US Food and Drug Administration (FDA) for both preadolescent and adolescent depression. It shows the strongest treatment effects of any antidepressant for depressed youth (NNT = 5), although it is unclear if this is attributable to the medication or to the quality of these studies (Bridge et al., 2007). Escitalopram is approved by the FDA for the treatment of adolescent depression, and is the pharmacologically active isomer in citalopram. Sertraline has also been reported to be superior to placebo, although the NNT was 10 (Bridge et al., 2007). Paroxetine is now not recommended for the treatment of pediatric depression because the aggregate trial data do not support efficacy (Bridge et al., 2007). Also, tricyclic antidepressants are not efficacious against child or adolescent depression (Hazell et al., 2002). While there have been no head-to-head comparisons of antidepressants for the acute treatment of adolescent depression, the efficacy of citalopram was found to be similar to that of fluoxetine, and both SSRIs were similar in efficacy to venlafaxine for treatment-resistant depression (Brent et al., 2008). One critique of pediatric antidepressant trials has been the high placebo response (49%) (Bridge et al., 2007). Studies that recruited from fewer sites and enrolled more severely ill participants had lower placebo response rates and were more likely to find significant differences between drug and placebo (Bridge et al., 2009).

Clinical severity, poor sleep, comorbidity, and family conflict predict a poorer response to SSRIs (Emslie et al., 1998; Curry et al., 2006; Asarnow et al., 2009; Emslie et al., 2012). Nonadherence and lower drug concentration have also been associated with a lower response rate to SSRIs (Sakolsky et al., 2011; Woldu et al., 2011). Certain symptom clusters, such as anhedonia and subsyndromal manic symptoms, may also make response to treatment (medication with or without CBT) less likely (Maalouf et al., 2012b; McMakin et al., 2012).

While the risk for a suicidal event (defined as an increase in suicidal ideation or an actual suicide attempt) is increased in those treated with an antidepressant compared to placebo, its incidence is rare, with an NNH of 112, meaning that 11 times as many adolescent patients benefit from an antidepressant than would experience a suicidal event (Bridge et al., 2007). The risk of a suicidal adverse event is elevated 1.58-fold in drug versus placebo, with a risk difference of around 1% (Bridge et al., 2007; Hetrick et al., 2012). This finding is confined to those under the age of 25 (Stone et al., 2009). Suicidal events tend to occur within the first 3–5 weeks and are most common in those who do not respond to antidepressant treatment, experience family conflict, have a history of nonsuicidal self-injury, and use of drugs or alcohol (Brent et al., 2009b; Vitiello et al., 2009; Wilkinson & Goodyer, 2011).

The concern about the association between SSRIs and suicidal events resulted in the FDA issuing a "Black Box Warning," which has been linked to a decline in prescriptions for antidepressants and even the diagnosis of depression in American adolescents (Libby *et al.*, 2009). Pharmacoepidemiological studies, which encompass a broader and more representative sample of treated adolescents than clinical trials, show that a suicide attempt is much more common *prior* to initiation of an antidepressant than afterward, (Simon & Savarino, 2007), that greater use of antidepressants is associated with a decline in suicide rates, and that a decrease in use of antidepressants can be associated with an increase in the youth suicide rate (Gibbons *et al.*, 2005; Ludwig *et al.*, 2009). A recent meta-analysis of trials of fluoxetine examined the impact of medication on depression and suicidal events (Gibbons *et al.*, 2012). Both adolescents and adults showed a decrease in depressive symptoms relative to placebo, but only the adults also showed a decline in suicidal events, suggesting that for adolescents, antidepressant treatment alone may not be sufficient to reduce suicidal ideation, a finding consistent with the TADS study (March *et al.*, 2004, 2007).

Depressed children and adolescents show an increased risk for mania or hypomania when treated with antidepressants, with one meta-analysis finding that 9.8% of antidepressant-treated youth experienced mania or hypomania versus 0.45% of those exposed to placebo, for an NNH = 37 (Offidani *et al.*, 2013). A pharmacoepidemiological study of youth exposed to antidepressants reported a lower rate of mania or hypomania, 5.4%, and found that children and younger adolescents were more likely to have pharmacologically induced mania or hypomania than older adolescents (Martin *et al.*, 2004).

The only two non-SSRI antidepressants with some support for efficacy in adolescent depression are nefazodone and venlafaxine. Nefazodone was examined in only one study, and although the generic compound is still available, the drug is no longer marketed because of an increased risk of hepatoxicity (Bridge *et al.*, 2007). Post-hoc analyses of two clinical trials found that venlafaxine was more efficacious than placebo for adolescent, but not preadolescent, depression, and was as efficacious as fluoxetine and citalopram for treatment-resistant depression (Emslie *et al.*, 2007; Brent *et al.*, 2008).

One small clinical trial in prepubertal and early adolescent depressed patients found that omega-3 was superior to placebo in the acute treatment of depression, but this has never been replicated (Nemets *et al.*, 2006). Although open-label studies suggest that bupropion is efficacious in treating depressed adolescents, particularly with comorbid ADHD, its efficacy has never been studied in a clinical trial (Daviss *et al.*, 2001).

Bright light

Bright light for 1 hour daily has been shown to reduce depressive symptoms in children and adolescents with seasonal affective disorder in a randomized crossover design (Swedo *et al.*, 1997). In addition, randomized trials support the use of bright light as a monotherapy for adolescents with mild depressive symptoms, and as an add-on to medication treatment in depressed adolescents in order to accelerate antidepressant response (Niederhofer & von Klitzing, 2011, 2012).

Combination of medication and CBT

The TADS study found that the combination of CBT and fluoxetine was associated with the most rapid and complete response during acute treatment (March *et al.*, 2004; Kennard *et al.*, 2006). In the Adolescent Depression and Psychotherapy (ADAPT) study, the addition of CBT to fluoxetine did not improve outcome over fluoxetine alone (Goodyer *et al.*, 2007). The ADAPT sample may have been less likely to respond to psychotherapy because potential participants were screened out if they responded to a brief psychosocial intervention, and in contrast to TADS, participants with psychotic symptoms were allowed into the study. The addition of CBT to medication monotherapy provided in primary care was not superior to medication management alone, although measures of self-reported symptoms favored the combination (Clarke *et al.*, 2005). In a recent meta-analysis of studies of primary adolescent depression, combination treatment was found to be superior to antidepressants alone with regard to improvement of functional status (Dubicka *et al.*, 2010), but not with respect to the outcomes of response, remission, or occurrence of suicidal events. However, a Cochrane review that included clinical trials of depressed children and adolescents with depression with or without substance abuse (and therefore included studies of CBT that had a substance abuse focus) found that combination treatment was more likely to result in remission (NNT = 12), and was protective against suicidal events (NNT = 7) (Cox *et al.*, 2012a).

Continuation and maintenance

Placebo-controlled continuation trials in depressed adolescents support the continued use of an antidepressant for at least 6 months after the achievement of remission, with those patients with residual depressive symptoms more likely to relapse (Emslie *et al.*, 2008). A Cochrane review found that the likelihood of relapse was 41% in those maintained on an antidepressant versus 67% in those on placebo (OR = 0.34, NNT = 4) (Cox *et al.*, 2012b). The addition of a wellness-oriented CBT to fluoxetine during the continuation phase resulted in an even lower risk of relapse or recurrence compared to medication continuation alone (Kennard *et al.*, 2014). A quasi-experimental study also supports the utility of monthly CBT booster sessions in preventing depressive relapse (Kroll *et al.*, 1996).

Treatment-resistant depression

In the Treatment of SSRI-Resistant Depression in Adolescents (TORDIA), 334 adolescents who had not responded to an adequate trial to an SSRI antidepressant were randomized to one of four conditions using a balanced 2 × 2 design: switch to another SSRI (paroxetine, fluoxetine, or citalopram), switch to venlafaxine, switch to another SSRI plus CBT, or switch to venlafaxine plus CBT. The 12-week response rate was similar in the two medication conditions, although the rate of side effects, and some secondary symptoms (anxiety, self-reported depression, suicidal ideation) were higher in the venlafaxine group, and the response was better for combined treatment compared to medication monotherapy (Brent *et al.*, 2008; Vitiello *et al.*, 2011). By 24 weeks, response and remission rates had converged across groups (Emslie *et al.*, 2010).

Prevention

A systematic review of school-based prevention and early intervention programs for depression (see Chapters 17 and 42) found support for CBT-based interventions, with the largest effects in those programs that had an indicated (evidence of some depressive risk) as compared to a universal frame, and with smaller effects if there was an attention control group, as compared to no intervention (Calear & Christensen, 2010). While indicated interventions have larger effects, a Cochrane review found some evidence to support the efficacy of both universal and targeted interventions to prevent the onset of depression, especially in the first 12 months of follow-up (Merry *et al.*, 2011). One large indicated prevention trial randomized 316 youth with at least one depressed parent and some evidence of subsyndromal depression to either the Coping With Depression group intervention or usual care, and showed a lower risk for depressive onset in those who received the experimental treatment at 8 (NNT = 9) and 33 months after the intervention;

current parental depression at the time of randomization was a negative moderator of intervention effect (Garber *et al.*, 2009; Beardslee *et al.*, 2013). A family group CBT intervention for offspring of depressed parents also showed a lower rate of onset of depression in the experimental treatment even 24 months after the intervention (Compas *et al.*, 2011), with the effects mediated by changes in positive parenting skills and the youths' secondary control coping (Compas *et al.*, 2010). An RCT compared a cognitive behavior (CB), interpersonal therapy-adolescent skills (IPT-AST) and a no-treatment control for high school students, and found that both CB and IPT-AST were efficacious in reducing depressive symptoms (*d*'s 0.37 and 0.26, respectively), especially in those with high depressive symptoms at intake (*d*'s 0.89 and 0.84) (Horowitz *et al.*, 2007).

Clinical approach to depressed youth

Initial assessment and management

The clinical management of depression involves several significant evaluative and therapeutic steps: determination of level of care, development of a safety plan, assessment of comorbidity and psychosocial stressors, and prioritization for treatment, and then matching available treatments to the patient and family needs and preferences (see Table 63.3). This approach is consistent with both the American Academy of Child and

Table 63.3 Initial approach to the depressed child or adolescent.

Clinical assessment/intervention	Specific guidelines
Determine level of care	• Higher level of care if threat to self or others, failure to respond to less intensive treatment, poor functional status
Develop safety plan	• Develop internal and interpersonal strategies for coping with suicidal urges • Restrict access to lethal agents
Careful diagnostic assessment, assess comorbidity and set treatment priorities	• Rule out bipolar disorder and seasonal affective disorder • Acuity and contribution to functional status may be particularly salient for some conditions such as eating disorders, substance abuse, or parental depression that must be addressed in order to succeed with treatment of depression.
Rule out medical contributors to depression	• For chronic or treatment resistant depression, obtain screening laboratory tests for anemia, hypothyroidism, occult inflammatory processes • Review medications
Assess and address psychosocial stressors that may lead to treatment resistance	• High levels of family conflict, parental depression, history of abuse, same sex attraction, peer victimization all may interfere with otherwise credible treatments and may need to be prioritized in order to have a successful outcome
Match patient to available treatments	• Explain risks and benefits of psychotherapy and medication • For mild depression, may provide education, support, and follow-up • For moderate depression, reasonable to start with monotherapy, although combination may provide quicker and better functional outcomes • For more severe depression, medication, preferably with psychotherapy, will yield the fastest and more complete recovery

Adolescent Psychiatry (AACAP) and NICE guidelines (NICE, 2005; Birmaher *et al.*, 2007).

Risk assessment and treatment planning

The first determination in the assessment of a depressed child or adolescent is whether the child can safely be treated as an outpatient. All depressed patients, but especially those with current or recent suicidal ideation or attempt, should develop a safety plan with the clinician and family to cope with suicidal urges (Birmaher *et al.*, 2007; Stanley *et al.*, 2009). Patients who say that they cannot adhere to a safety plan, or show a clinical presentation that makes it unlikely for patient adherence (e.g., mixed state, psychotic, alcohol/drug dependence) are likely to need more intensive treatment than weekly outpatient treatment, up to and including inpatient care. While hospitalization for high-risk youth is considered standard-of-care, there has not been an empirical demonstration that hospitalization, compared to a lower level of care, actually prevents suicide or suicidal behavior. Other clinical indications for a higher level of care would be lack of progress in a less intensive treatment and/or functional impairment that makes participation in daily activities (e.g. school) impossible. As a general framework, clinicians need to consider the following hierarchy of priorities: (i) life-threatening issues (e.g., suicidality, homicidality, exposure to domestic violence, intravenous drug use); (ii) therapy-threatening issues (hopelessness about treatment, chronically depressed parent who is unable to bring the child for treatment); and (iii) symptom- and functionally oriented treatment.

Patient and family education

Because depression is often a chronic and recurrent illness, the clinician should establish a long-term partnership with the patient and family. This can be achieved by providing the patient and family with all the requisite information about depression and its treatment, and then making treatment decisions collaboratively (Brent *et al.*, 2011). As described in Table 63.4, education focuses on depression as an illness, recognition and monitoring of depressive symptomatology, knowing risks and benefits of different treatments, and, if symptom relief is achieved, development of a plan to prevent relapse and recurrence.

Table 63.4 Psychoeducation: key points for parents and patients.

1 Depression is an illness and not the fault of the patient or family.
2 How to recognize and monitor depressive symptoms, and detect early relapse and recurrence.
3 Modal course, in order to have reasonable expectations for pace and extent of recovery.
4 Analyze risks and benefits of different treatment options, in order to make an informed decision.
5 How to collaborate in development of a plan for relapse prevention, continuation, and maintenance treatment.

Family, social, and individual context

Depressed children and adolescents who are clinically referred often have parents who have active psychiatric difficulties, most commonly depression, anxiety, or substance abuse. These difficulties may make it very difficult for the family to adhere to treatment recommendations, and may contribute to a suboptimal clinical response in the child. Treatment of maternal depression, for example, has been shown to lead to symptomatic improvement in offspring (Gunlicks & Weissman, 2008). Abuse, exposure to family violence, or high levels of criticism or discord must be addressed because of safety issues for the child as well as the negative impact of these factors on duration and recurrence of depressive episodes. When parents are unable to provide the necessary support for treatment, they sometimes are willing to allow involvement of adult surrogates, such as older siblings, other relatives, or close friends who may temporarily step in and help with transportation and even monitoring of treatment response.

Due to decreased energy, concentration, and motivation, depressed children and adolescents often fall behind in school, which in turn leads to a sense of failure, increased anxiety, and a tendency to give up and disconnect from school. There also may be specific school-related stressors that contribute to depressive symptomatology, such as being the target of bullying or cumulative academic problems (Shamseddeen *et al.*, 2011). Therefore, the clinician should assess the depressed child's current school function, identify any school-related stressors, and, if the patient has fallen behind academically, develop a plan, in conjunction with the school, for a reduced workload and a plan for catching up that is mutually acceptable to school, family, and student.

With regard to individual context, it is important to identify and prioritize comorbid health risk behaviors or psychiatric disorders that are likely to be life-threatening or disruptive to therapy. Life-threatening behavior, like intravenous drug use, aggressive criminal behavior, or nonadherence with care for a serious chronic illness should be addressed prior to treatment of depression, even recognizing that depression may be contributing to these problems. Higher priority to targeting comorbid conditions over depression should be given if these symptoms are causing the greatest functional impairment and if the treatment of depression is not likely to be successful unless these other conditions are addressed first. For example, the treatment of a patient with both depression and ADHD, whose main difficulties are decreased motivation, suicidal ideation, and hopelessness, should probably initially focus on the depression, whereas a patient with similar comorbidity, whose depression emerges secondary to school and peer failure due to impulsivity and inattention, should probably have the ADHD addressed first.

Initial treatment approach

The first intervention for mild depression should be family education, supportive counseling, case management, and problem-solving, since there is evidence that a substantial proportion of mildly depressed adolescents will respond to these relatively nonspecific interventions (Renaud et al., 1998; Goodyer et al., 2007; Bridge et al., 2009).

For moderate depression, the NICE guidelines recommend use of CBT, IPT, or family therapy prior to the use of medication, whereas the AACAP guidelines recommend CBT, IPT, or medication as first-line treatments. The NICE guidelines also indicate that antidepressants should never be used without psychotherapy, whereas the AACAP guidelines indicate that while the combination treatment may be preferable, medication monotherapy is an acceptable alternative under certain conditions (NICE, 2005; Birmaher et al., 2007). The rationale for the AACAP stance is that there are not enough qualified therapists to require initial treatment with CBT or IPT, some adolescents do not wish to participate in psychotherapy, and in the only head-to-head comparison of psychotherapy and medication, fluoxetine was greatly superior to CBT over the first 12 weeks (March et al., 2004). With regard to the NICE recommendation requiring that pharmacotherapy always be combined with pharmacotherapy, while there is evidence from TADS that combination results in the fastest response and from TORDIA that combination is better than monotherapy for treatment resistant depression, one meta-analysis found that combination treatment did not improve depression and protect against suicidal events relative to medication monotherapy (Dubicka et al., 2010). Therefore, we tend to favor the AACAP, more flexible approach over that recommended by NICE (and for full disclosure, the senior author helped to draft the AACAP guidelines).

For more persistent or severe depression, one of the three empirically validated treatments, SSRI medication, CBT, or IPT, or preferably, combination of medication and psychotherapy is indicated, dependent on availability and patient preference. As noted above, those with more severe depression are more likely to benefit from antidepressants, a history of abuse may interfere with CBT outcome, and those with high levels of parent-child conflict and difficulties with social functioning may do particularly well with IPT. Whatever the choice of initial treatment, the patient's progress should be reassessed in 4–6 weeks. If the patient has shown a substantial decrease in depressive symptoms and improvement in functioning, then continuing with the same treatment is reasonable, but if the patient has not responded, then a change in strategy is indicated. If the patient is currently receiving psychotherapy only, consideration should be given to adding medication; if the patient is receiving medication monotherapy, consideration is to be given to either increasing the medication dosage and/or adding psychotherapy. Also, patients should be reassessed with regard to comorbidity, presence of mania, and psychosocial stressors that may be contributing to treatment resistance. Relative contraindications for use of antidepressant medication are a history of mania or hypomania, in which case mood stabilization should be undertaken prior to the use of antidepressants, and for those with a strong family history of bipolar disorder, it may be safer to begin with psychotherapy for the same reasons. Patients with a history of seasonal depression should be given a trial of bright light, and those with psychotic symptoms, although not carefully studied in this age group, are thought most likely to benefit from the combination of an antidepressant and an antipsychotic.

Given that the most evidence for efficacy exists for fluoxetine, this should be a first-line medication. For those who have failed to respond to fluoxetine, cannot tolerate it, or for some reason do not wish to take it, use of one of the other SSRIs for which there is some evidence of efficacy is warranted. Current clinical recommendations are to begin with half the usual initial target dose (e.g., 10 mg fluoxetine) for 1 week, to determine if the patient can tolerate the medication, and then increase to 20 mg for the next 3 weeks. If the patient is still depressed, then one can continue to increase the dosage around every 4 weeks because it takes around that amount of time to tell if an increase is going to be helpful. While the NICE guidelines state that increasing the dosage of an SSRI is not likely to be helpful, there are modest data to the contrary (Heiligenstein et al., 2006; Sakolsky et al., 2011). Most patients who respond to fluoxetine achieve symptomatic relief at 20–80 mg of fluoxetine. Once symptomatic relief has been achieved, treatment should continue a minimum of 6–12 months in order to prevent relapse as per both AACAP and NICE guidelines.

Sleep difficulties are common in depression and may be made worse with antidepressant treatment. Behavioral approaches to the management of sleep difficulties (see Chapter 70), and use of melatonin, shown to be efficacious in other patient populations, should be considered early in treatment, given the moderation of antidepressant response by insomnia (Emslie et al., 2012).

Approach to residual symptoms

Often, even in patients who respond, there are still residual symptoms of depression, such as sleep difficulties, anhedonia, irritability, and fatigue (Vitiello et al., 2011). The clinician should rule out medical causes (e.g., sleep disorder, anemia, and hypothyroidism) and possible contribution of comorbid conditions (e.g., substance abuse). Sleep difficulties can be targeted with CBT approaches, which in preliminary studies have been shown to be efficacious in youth (Clarke & Harvey, 2012). Although not studied in youth with depression, clinical trials in youth with ADHD and autism spectrum disorder support the use of melatonin to aid in difficulty falling asleep (Cummings, 2012). Expert clinical practice (although without supporting empirical evidence) supports augmentation with bupropion and/or recommendation of vigorous exercise and BA for those with residual fatigue or anhedonia (Birmaher et al., 2007; Hughes et al., 2007).

Treatment-resistant depression

First, it should be confirmed that the patient has already had an adequate trial of treatment, has the right diagnosis, and indeed has not shown evidence of a response. Second, one should make sure that the patient does not have untreated comorbid conditions that would make treatment response unlikely (e.g., substance abuse, anorexia, etc.). Third, one should rule out that psychosocial stressors likely to contribute to a continuing depression (e.g., parental depression and peer victimization) are not present and have not previously been addressed.

After considering these three important points, patients who have not responded to an adequate trial with an SSRI should be switched to a second SSRI, with the addition of CBT (Brent *et al.*, 2008). Algorithms based on expert opinion recommend that if two consecutive trials with SSRI antidepressants do not result in a treatment response, a switch to another class of antidepressant (e.g., venlafaxine, bupropion) is to be considered. If patients have shown a partial response to one agent (e.g., an SSRI), algorithms recommend augmentation with an antipsychotic, bupropion or lithium, but there are no empirical studies in youth. Open treatment of adolescents with treatment-resistant depression with transcranial magnetic stimulation suggests that this intervention is feasible, safe, and possibly efficacious, supporting further study in clinical trials (Croarkin *et al.*, 2010). Electroconvulsive therapy (ECT) has not been studied systematically in child and adolescent mood disorders, but naturalistic studies suggest that the best responses are in youth with catatonia, bipolar depression, or psychotic depression (Walter & Rey, 2003). Clinical guidelines recommend that ECT be considered after a depressed patient has not responded to psychotherapy and three medication trials, with demonstrated adherence (Birmaher *et al.*, 2007).

Future clinical and research challenges

Depression in childhood and adolescence is a complex and debilitating disease that frequently has a lifelong, chronic, recurrent course. In this concluding section, we focus on the unknowns of youth depression and suggest several key areas for future investigation.

1 **Identify clinically useful early biomarkers that predict treatment response and adverse events.** There is some evidence in adult depression that changes in gene expression related to neurotrophic and inflammatory genes, as well as serum levels of these proteins, may predict treatment response (Mamdani *et al.*, 2011). Identification of early markers that will predict a successful course of treatment could improve fit to treatment and avoid lengthy, unsuccessful medication trials. In addition, studies of gene expression and micro-RNA levels could help identify novel therapeutic targets. fMRI, although useful for clinical research, may be impractical for clinical applications, but it would be useful to identify neurocognitive neurosignatures associated with treatment response to antidepressants and/or psychotherapy. The identification of markers to predict the development of mania or of suicidal events, in concert with markers that predict treatment response, could be useful in personalizing and optimizing treatment.

2 **Identify methods to accelerate initial treatment response.** The risk for suicidal events and nonresponse is much higher in those patients who show a slow and incomplete response to initial treatment. Identification of psychotherapeutic methods (e.g., targeting sleep or anhedonia) or somatic interventions (e.g., bright light, ketamine) to accelerate treatment response in more severely depressed patients could be life saving.

3 **Neurobiological effects of early adversity and developing optimal treatments.** A high proportion of clinically referred depressed youth have a history of early adversity and this history confers a risk for a poorer response to treatment (Nanni *et al.*, 2012). A better understanding of the neurobiological effects of early adversity is needed in order to translate that understanding into effective interventions for depressed youth with a history of adversity.

4 **Research on the use of social media, technology (e.g., smartphones), and online material for the identification, prevention, and treatment of depression.** This area of research will be increasingly important, given the growth in use of technology, increased pressure on health care providers to cut costs, and demonstration of the efficacy of Internet interventions.

References

Alyahri, A. & Goodman, R. (2008) The prevalence of DSM-IV psychiatric disorders among 7-10 year old Yemeni schoolchildren. *Social Psychiatry and Psychiatric Epidemiology* **43**, 224–230.

American Psychiatric Association (2013) *Diagnostic and Statistical Manual of Mental Disorders: DSM-V*, 5th edn. American Psychiatric Association, Washington, DC.

Andersen, S.L. & Teicher, M.H. (2008) Stress, sensitive periods and maturational events in adolescent depression. *Trends in Neurosciences* **31**, 183–191.

Angold, A. *et al.* (1998) Puberty and depression: the roles of age, pubertal status and pubertal timing. *Psychological Medicine* **28**, 51–61.

Angold, A. *et al.* (1999) Comorbidity. *Journal of Child Psychology and Psychiatry* **40**, 57–87.

Asarnow, J.R. *et al.* (2009) Treatment of selective serotonin reuptake inhibitor-resistant depression in adolescents: predictors and moderators of treatment response. *Journal of the American Academy of Child and Adolescent Psychiatry* **48**, 330–339.

Axelson, D. (2013) Taking disruptive mood dysregulation disorder out for a test drive. *The American Journal of Psychiatry* **170**, 136–139.

Beardslee, W. *et al.* (2013) Prevention of depression in at-risk adolescents: longer-term effects. *JAMA Psychiatry* **70**, 1161–1170.

Beesdo, K. *et al.* (2007) Incidence of social anxiety disorder and the consistent risk for secondary depression in the first three decades of life. *Archives of General Psychiatry* **64**, 903–912.

Birmaher, B. *et al.* (2000) Clinical outcome after short-term psychotherapy for adolescents with major depressive disorder. *Archives of General Psychiatry* **57**, 29–36.

Birmaher, B. *et al.* (2002) Course and outcome of child and adolescent major depressive disorder. *Child & Adolescent Psychiatric Clinics of North America* **11**, 619–637.

Birmaher, B. *et al.* (2007) Practice parameter for the assessment and treatment of children and adolescents with depressive disorders. *Journal of the American Academy of Child and Adolescent Psychiatry* **46**, 1503–1526.

Boden, J.M. & Fergusson, D.M. (2011) Alcohol and depression. *Addiction* **106**, 906–914.

Brent, D.A. *et al.* (1997) A clinical psychotherapy trial for adolescent depression comparing cognitive, family, and supportive therapy. *Archives of General Psychiatry* **54**, 877–885.

Brent, D.A. *et al.* (1998) Predictors of treatment efficacy in a clinical trial of three psychosocial treatments for adolescent depression. *Journal of the American Academy of Child and Adolescent Psychiatry* **37**, 906–914.

Brent, D. *et al.* (2008) Switching to another SSRI or to venlafaxine with or without cognitive behavioral therapy for adolescents with SSRI-resistant depression: the TORDIA randomized controlled trial. *JAMA* **299**, 901–913.

Brent, D. *et al.* (2009a) The incidence and course of depression in bereaved youth 21 months after the loss of a parent to suicide, accident, or sudden natural death. *The American Journal of Psychiatry* **166**, 786–794.

Brent, D.A. *et al.* (2009b) Predictors of spontaneous and systematically assessed suicidal adverse events in the treatment of SSRI-resistant depression in adolescents (TORDIA) study. *The American Journal of Psychiatry* **166**, 418–426.

Brent, D.A. *et al.* (2011) *Treating Depressed and Suicidal Adolescents: A Clinician's Guide.* Guilford Press, New York.

Bridge, J.A. *et al.* (2003) Major depressive disorder in adolescents exposed to a friend's suicide. *Journal of the American Academy of Child and Adolescent Psychiatry* **42**, 1294–1300.

Bridge, J.A. *et al.* (2006) Adolescent suicide and suicidal behavior. *Journal of Child Psychology and Psychiatry* **47**, 372–394.

Bridge, J.A. *et al.* (2007) Clinical response and risk for reported suicidal ideation and suicide attempts in pediatric antidepressant treatment: a meta-analysis of randomized controlled trials. *JAMA* **297**, 1683–1696.

Bridge, J.A. *et al.* (2009) Placebo response in randomized controlled trials of antidepressants for pediatric major depressive disorder. *The American Journal of Psychiatry* **166**, 42–49.

Bruti, G. *et al.* (2012) Migraine and depression: bidirectional co-morbidities? *Neurological Sciences* **33**, S107–S109.

Burke, J.D. (2012) An affective dimension within oppositional defiant disorder symptoms among boys: personality and psychopathology outcomes into early adulthood. *Journal of Child Psychology and Psychiatry* **53**, 1176–1183.

Burton, C.M. *et al.* (2013) Sexual minority-related victimization as a mediator of mental health disparities in sexual minority youth: a longitudinal analysis. *Journal of Youth and Adolescence* **42**, 394–402.

Calear, A.L. & Christensen, H. (2010) Systematic review of school-based prevention and early intervention programs for depression. *Journal of Adolescence* **33**, 429–438.

Casey, B. *et al.* (2011) Braking and accelerating of the adolescent brain. *Journal of Research on Adolescence* **21**, 21–33.

Caspi, A. *et al.* (2010) Genetic sensitivity to the environment: the case of the serotonin transporter gene and its implications for studying complex diseases and traits. *The American Journal of Psychiatry* **167**, 509–527.

Clarke, G. & Harvey, A.G. (2012) The complex role of sleep in adolescent depression. *Child and Adolescent Psychiatric Clinics of North America* **21**, 385–400.

Clarke, G. *et al.* (2005) A randomized effectiveness trial of brief cognitive-behavioral therapy for depressed adolescents receiving antidepressant medication. *Journal of the American Academy of Child and Adolescent Psychiatry* **44**, 888–898.

Compas, B.E. *et al.* (2010) Coping and parenting: mediators of 12-month outcomes of a family group cognitive-behavioral preventive intervention with families of depressed parents. *Journal of Consulting and Clinical Psychology* **78**, 623–634.

Compas, B.E. *et al.* (2011) Family group cognitive-behavioral preventive intervention for families of depressed parents: 18- and 24-month outcomes. *Journal of Consulting and Clinical Psychology* **79**, 488–499.

Copeland, W.E. *et al.* (2009) Childhood and adolescent psychiatric disorders as predictors of young adult disorders. *Archives of General Psychiatry* **66**, 764–772.

Copeland, W.E. *et al.* (2012) Cumulative depression episodes predict later C-reactive protein levels: a prospective analysis. *Biological Psychiatry* **71**, 15–21.

Copeland, W.E. *et al.* (2013) Prevalence, comorbidity, and correlates of DSM-5 proposed disruptive mood dysregulation disorder. *The American Journal of Psychiatry* **170**, 173–179.

Costello, E.J. *et al.* (2003) Prevalence and development of psychiatric disorders in childhood and adolescence. *Archives of General Psychiatry* **60**, 837–844.

Cousins, J.C. *et al.* (2011) The bidirectional association between daytime affect and nighttime sleep in youth with anxiety and depression. *Journal of Pediatric Psychology* **36**, 969–979.

Cox, G.R. *et al.* (2012a) Psychological therapies versus antidepressant medication, alone and in combination for depression in children and adolescents. *Cochrane Database of Systematic Reviews* **11**, CD008324.

Cox, G.R. *et al.* (2012b) Interventions for preventing relapse and recurrence of a depressive disorder in children and adolescents. *Cochrane Database of Systematic Reviews* **11**, CD007504.

Croarkin, P.E. *et al.* (2010) The emerging role for repetitive transcranial magnetic stimulation in optimizing the treatment of adolescent depression. *The Journal of ECT* **26**, 323–329.

Cullen, K.R. *et al.* (2009) A preliminary study of functional connectivity in comorbid adolescent depression. *Neuroscience Letters* **460**, 227–231.

Cullen, K.R. *et al.* (2010) Altered white matter microstructure in adolescents with major depression: a preliminary study. *Journal of the American Academy of Child and Adolescent Psychiatry* **49**, 173.

Cummings, C. (2012) Melatonin for the management of sleep disorders in children and adolescents. *Paediatrics & Child Health* **17**, 331–336.

Curry, J. *et al.* (2006) Predictors and moderators of acute outcome in the Treatment for Adolescents with Depression Study (TADS). *Journal of the American Academy of Child and Adolescent Psychiatry* **45**, 1427–1439.

Dagys, N. *et al.* (2012) Double trouble? The effects of sleep deprivation and chronotype on adolescent affect. *Journal of Child Psychology and Psychiatry* **53**, 660–667.

Dahl, R.E. (2004) Adolescent brain development: a period of vulnerabilities and opportunities. Keynote address. *Annals of the New York Academy of Sciences.* **1021**, 1–22.

Danese, A. *et al.* (2008) Elevated inflammation levels in depressed adults with a history of childhood maltreatment. *Archives of General Psychiatry* **65**, 409–415.

Danese, A. *et al.* (2009) Adverse childhood experiences and adult risk factors for age-related disease: depression, inflammation, and clustering of metabolic risk markers. *Archives of Pediatrics and Adolescent Medicine* **163**, 1135–1143.

Daviss, W.B. *et al.* (2001) Bupropion sustained release in adolescents with comorbid attention-deficit/hyperactivity disorder and depression. *Journal of the American Academy of Child and Adolescent Psychiatry* **40**, 307–314.

Diamond, G.S. *et al.* (2002) Attachment-based family therapy for depressed adolescents: a treatment development study. *Journal of the American Academy of Child and Adolescent Psychiatry* **41**, 1190–1196.

Diamond, G.S. *et al.* (2010) Attachment-based family therapy for adolescents with suicidal ideation: a randomized controlled trial. *Journal of the American Academy of Child and Adolescent Psychiatry* **49**, 122–131.

Dubicka, B. *et al.* (2010) Combined treatment with cognitive-behavioural therapy in adolescent depression: meta-analysis. *British Journal of Psychiatry* **197**, 433–440.

Emslie, G.J. *et al.* (1998) Fluoxetine in child and adolescent depression: acute and maintenance treatment. *Depression and Anxiety* **7**, 32–39.

Emslie, G.J. *et al.* (2007) Venlafaxine ER for the treatment of pediatric subjects with depression: results of two placebo-controlled trials. *Journal of the American Academy of Child and Adolescent Psychiatry* **46**, 479–488.

Emslie, G.J. *et al.* (2008) Fluoxetine versus placebo in preventing relapse of major depression in children and adolescents. *The American Journal of Psychiatry* **165**, 459–467.

Emslie, G.J. *et al.* (2010) Treatment of Resistant Depression in Adolescents (TORDIA): week 24 outcomes. *The American Journal of Psychiatry* **167**, 782–791.

Emslie, G.J. *et al.* (2012) Insomnia moderates outcome of serotonin-selective reuptake inhibitor treatment in depressed youth. *Journal of Child and Adolescent Psychopharmacology* **22**, 21–28.

Faraone, S.V. & Biederman, J. (1997) Do attention deficit hyperactivity disorder and major depression share familial risk factors? *Journal of Nervous and Mental Disease* **185**, 533–541.

Fergusson, D.M. & Woodward, L.J. (2002) Mental health, educational, and social role outcomes of adolescents with depression. *Archives of General Psychiatry* **59**, 225–231.

Fergusson, D.M. *et al.* (2003) Deviant peer affiliations and depression: confounding or causation? *Journal of Abnormal Child Psychology* **31**, 605–618.

Findling, R.L. *et al.* (2010) Characteristics of children with elevated symptoms of mania: the Longitudinal Assessment of Manic Symptoms (LAMS) study. *Journal of Clinical Psychiatry* **71**, 1664–1672.

Fleming, T. *et al.* (2012) A pragmatic randomized controlled trial of computerized CBT (SPARX) for symptoms of depression among adolescents excluded from mainstream education. *Behavioural and Cognitive Psychotherapy* **40**, 529–541.

Forbes, E.E. & Dahl, R.E. (2012) Research review: altered reward function in adolescent depression: what, when and how? *Journal of Child Psychology and Psychiatry* **53**, 3–15.

Friedman, M.S. *et al.* (2011) A meta-analysis of disparities in childhood sexual abuse, parental physical abuse, and peer victimization among sexual minority and sexual nonminority individuals. *American Journal of Public Health* **101**, 1481–1494.

Gaffrey, M.S. *et al.* (2010) Subgenual cingulate connectivity in children with a history of preschool-depression. *Neuroreport* **21**, 1182–1188.

Garber, J. *et al.* (2009) Prevention of depression in at-risk adolescents: a randomized controlled trial. *JAMA* **301**, 2215–2224.

Geller, B. *et al.* (2001) Bipolar disorder at prospective follow-up of adults who had prepubertal major depressive disorder. *The American Journal of Psychiatry* **158**, 125–127.

Gibbons, R.D. *et al.* (2005) The relationship between antidepressant medication use and rate of suicide. *Archives of General Psychiatry* **62**, 165–172.

Gibbons, R.D. *et al.* (2012) Suicidal thoughts and behavior with antidepressant treatment: reanalysis of the randomized placebo-controlled studies of fluoxetine and venlafaxine. *Archives of General Psychiatry* **69**, 580–587.

Goodwin, R.D. *et al.* (2012) Asthma and mental health among youth: etiology, current knowledge and future directions. *Expert Review of Respiratory Medicine* **6**, 397–406.

Goodyer, I. *et al.* (2007) Selective serotonin reuptake inhibitors (SSRIs) and routine specialist care with and without cognitive behaviour therapy in adolescents with major depression: randomised controlled trial. *BMJ* **335**, 142.

Gotlib, I.H. & Joormann, J. (2010) Cognition and depression: current status and future directions. *Annual Review of Clinical Psychology* **6**, 285–312.

Gotlib, I.H. *et al.* (2008) HPA axis reactivity: a mechanism underlying the associations among 5-HTTLPR, stress, and depression. *Biological Psychiatry* **63**, 847–851.

Gotlib, I.H. *et al.* (2010) Neural processing of reward and loss in girls at risk for major depression. *Archives of General Psychiatry* **67**, 380–387.

Gregory, A.M. *et al.* (2009) The direction of longitudinal associations between sleep problems and depression symptoms: a study of twins aged 8 and 10 years. *Sleep* **32**, 189–199.

Gunlicks, M.L. & Weissman, M.M. (2008) Change in child psychopathology with improvement in parental depression: a systematic review. *Journal of the American Academy of Child and Adolescent Psychiatry* **47**, 379–389.

Gunlicks-Stoessel, M. *et al.* (2010) The impact of perceived interpersonal functioning on treatment for adolescent depression: IPT-A versus treatment as usual in school-based health clinics. *Journal of Consulting and Clinical Psychology* **78**, 260–267.

Halari, R. *et al.* (2009) Reduced activation in lateral prefrontal cortex and anterior cingulate during attention and cognitive control functions in medication-naive adolescents with depression compared to controls. *Journal of Child Psychology and Psychiatry* **50**, 307–316.

Hamdan, S. *et al.* (2012) The phenomenology and course of depression in parentally bereaved and non-bereaved youth. *Journal of the American Academy of Child and Adolescent Psychiatry* **51**, 528–536.

Hamilton, J.P. *et al.* (2008) Amygdala volume in major depressive disorder: a meta-analysis of magnetic resonance imaging studies. *Molecular Psychiatry* **13**, 993–1000.

Hankin, B.L. (2012) Future directions in vulnerability to depression among youth: integrating risk factors and processes across multiple levels of analysis. *Journal of Clinical Child and Adolescent Psychology* **41**, 695–718.

Hariri, A.R. *et al.* (2002) Serotonin transporter genetic variation and the response of the human amygdala. *Science* **297**, 400–403.

Harrington, R. (2000) Childhood depression: is it the same disorder?. In: *Childhood Onset of "Adult" Psychopathology: Clinical and Research Advances*. (ed J. Rapoport), pp. 223–243. American Psychiatric Association, Washington, DC.

Hasler, G. *et al.* (2005) Depressive symptoms during childhood and adult obesity: the Zurich Cohort Study. *Molecular Psychiatry* **10**, 842–850.

Hayward, C. *et al.* (1997) Psychiatric risk associated with early puberty in adolescent girls. *Journal of the American Academy of Child and Adolescent Psychiatry* **36**, 255–262.

Hazell, P. *et al.* (2002) Tricyclic drugs for depression in children and adolescents. *Cochrane Database Systemic Reviews* **3**, CD002317.

Heiligenstein, J.H. *et al.* (2006) Fluoxetine 40-60 mg versus fluoxetine 20 mg in the treatment of children and adolescents with a less-than-complete response to nine-week treatment with fluoxetine 10-20 mg: a pilot study. *Journal of Child and Adolescent Psychopharmacology* **16**, 207–217.

Hetrick, S.E. *et al.* (2012) Newer generation antidepressants for depressive disorders in children and adolescents. *Cochrane Database of Systematic Reviews* **11**, CD004851.

Hipwell, A.E. *et al.* (2011) Impact of oppositional defiant disorder dimensions on the temporal ordering of conduct problems and depression across childhood and adolescence in girls. *Journal of Child Psychology and Psychiatry* **52**, 1099–1108.

Hoek, W. *et al.* (2012) Effects of Internet-based guided self-help problem-solving therapy for adolescents with depression and anxiety: a randomized controlled trial. *PLoS ONE* **7**, e43485.

Hoppe, C. & Elger, C.E. (2011) Depression in epilepsy: a critical review from a clinical perspective. *Nature Reviews Neurology* **7**, 462–472.

Horowitz, J.L. *et al.* (2007) Prevention of depressive symptoms in adolescents: a randomized trial of cognitive-behavioral and interpersonal prevention programs. *Journal of Consulting and Clinical Psychology* **75**, 693–706.

Horwood, L.J. *et al.* (2012) Cannabis and depression: an integrative data analysis of four Australasian cohorts. *Drug and Alcohol Dependence* **126**, 369–378.

Huang, H. *et al.* (2011) White matter changes in healthy adolescents at familial risk for unipolar depression: a diffusion tensor imaging study. *Neuropsychopharmacology* **36**, 684–691.

Hughes, C.W. *et al.* (2007) Texas Children's Medication Algorithm Project: update from Texas Consensus Conference Panel on medication treatment of childhood major depressive disorder. *Journal of the American Academy of Child and Adolescent Psychiatry* **46**, 667–686.

Hulvershorn, L.A. *et al.* (2011) Toward dysfunctional connectivity: a review of neuroimaging findings in pediatric major depressive disorder. *Brain Imaging and Behavior* **5**, 307–328.

Katon, W. *et al.* (2010) Depressive symptoms in adolescence: the association with multiple health risk behaviors. *General Hospital Psychiatry* **32**, 233–239.

Kaufman, J. *et al.* (1997) Schedule for Affective Disorders and Schizophrenia for School-Age Children-Present and Lifetime Version (K-SADS-PL): initial reliability and validity data. *Journal of the American Academy of Child and Adolescent Psychiatry* **36**, 980–988.

Kaufman, J. *et al.* (2006) Brain-derived neurotrophic factor-5-HTTLPR gene interactions and environmental modifiers of depression in children. *Biological Psychiatry* **59**, 673–680.

Kaufman, N.K. *et al.* (2005) Potential mediators of cognitive-behavioral therapy for adolescents with comorbid major depression and conduct disorder. *Journal of Consulting and Clinical Psychology* **73**, 38–46.

Kennard, B. *et al.* (2006) Remission and residual symptoms after short-term treatment in the Treatment of Adolescents with Depression Study (TADS). *Journal of the American Academy of Child and Adolescent Psychiatry* **45**, 1404–1411.

Kennard, B.D. *et al.* (2014) Cognitive-behavioral therapy to prevent relapse in pediatric responders to pharmacotherapy for major depressive disorder. *Journal of the American Academy of Child and Adolescent Psychiatry* **47**, 1395–1404.

Kennard, B.D. *et al.* (2014) Sequential treatment with fluoxetine and relapse-prevention CBT to improve outcomes in pediatric depression. *The American Journal of Psychiatry* **171**, 1083–1090.

Kessler, R.C. *et al.* (2012) Prevalence, persistence, and sociodemographic correlates of DSM-IV disorders in the National Comorbidity Survey Replication Adolescent Supplement. *Archives of General Psychiatry* **69**, 372–380.

Klomek, A.B. & Mufson, L. (2006) Interpersonal psychotherapy for depressed adolescents. *Child & Adolescent Psychiatrics Clinics of North America* **15**, 959–975.

Kovacs, M. & Lopez-Duran, N. (2010) Prodromal symptoms and atypical affectivity as predictors of major depression in juveniles: implications for prevention. *Journal of Child Psychology and Psychiatry* **51**, 472–496.

Kroll, L. *et al.* (1996) Pilot study of continuation cognitive-behavioral therapy for major depression in adolescent psychiatric patients. *Journal of the American Academy of Child and Adolescent Psychiatry* **35**, 1156–1161.

Ladouceur, C.D. *et al.* (2005) Altered emotional processing in pediatric anxiety, depression, and comorbid anxiety-depression. *Journal of Abnormal Child Psychology* **33**, 165–177.

Ladouceur, C.D. *et al.* (2006) Processing emotional facial expressions influences performance on a Go/NoGo task in pediatric anxiety and depression. *Journal of Child Psychology and Psychiatry* **47**, 1107–1115.

Lewinsohn, P.M. *et al.* (1998) Major depressive disorder in older adolescents: prevalence, risk factors, and clinical implications. *Clinical Psychology Review* **18**, 765–794.

Lewinsohn, P.M. *et al.* (2003) Psychosocial functioning of young adults who have experienced and recovered from major depressive disorder during adolescence. *Journal of Abnormal Psychology* **112**, 353–363.

Libby, A.M. *et al.* (2009) Persisting decline in depression treatment after FDA warnings. *Archives of General Psychiatry* **66**, 633–639.

Lopez-Duran, N.L. *et al.* (2009) Hypothalamic-pituitary-adrenal axis dysregulation in depressed children and adolescents: a meta-analysis. *Psychoneuroendocrinology* **34**, 1272–1283.

Luby, J.L. *et al.* (2004) The Preschool Feelings Checklist: a brief and sensitive screening measure for depression in young children. *Journal of the American Academy of Child and Adolescent Psychiatry* **43**, 708–717.

Ludwig, J. *et al.* (2009) Anti-depressants and suicide. *Journal of Health Economics* **28**, 659–676.

Luking, K.R. *et al.* (2011) Functional connectivity of the amygdala in early-childhood-onset depression. *Journal of the American Academy of Child and Adolescent Psychiatry* **50**, 1027–1041, e3.

Maalouf, F.T. *et al.* (2012a) Bias to negative emotions: a depression state-dependent marker in adolescent major depressive disorder. *Psychiatry Research* **198**, 28–33.

Maalouf, F.T. *et al.* (2012b) Do sub-syndromal manic symptoms influence outcome in treatment resistant depression in adolescents? A latent class analysis from the TORDIA study. *Journal of Affective Disorders* **138**, 86–95.

Mamdani, F. *et al.* (2011) Gene expression biomarkers of response to citalopram treatment in major depressive disorder. *Translational Psychiatry* **1**, e13.

March, J. *et al.* (2004) Fluoxetine, cognitive-behavioral therapy, and their combination for adolescents with depression: Treatment for Adolescents With Depression Study (TADS) randomized controlled trial. *JAMA* **292**, 807–820.

March, J.S. *et al.* (2007) The Treatment for Adolescents With Depression Study (TADS): long-term effectiveness and safety outcomes. *Archives of General Psychiatry* **64**, 1132–1143.

Marshal, M.P. *et al.* (2011) Suicidality and depression disparities between sexual minority and heterosexual youth: a meta-analytic review. *Journal of Adolescent Health* **49**, 115–123.

Martin, A. *et al.* (2004) Age effects on antidepressant-induced manic conversion. *Archives of Pediatrics and Adolescent Medicine* **158**, 773–780.

Mayes, T.L. *et al.* (2010) Psychometric properties of the Children's Depression Rating Scale-Revised in adolescents. *Journal of Child and Adolescent Psychopharmacology* **20**, 513–516.

McMakin, D.L. *et al.* (2011) Affective functioning among early adolescents at high and low familial risk for depression and their mothers: a focus on individual and transactional processes across contexts. *Journal of Abnormal Child Psychology* **39**, 1213–1225.

McMakin, D.L. *et al.* (2012) Anhedonia predicts poorer recovery among youth with selective serotonin reuptake inhibitor treatment-resistant depression. *Journal of the American Academy of Child and Adolescent Psychiatry* **51**, 404–411.

Merry, S.N. *et al.* (2011) Psychological and educational interventions for preventing depression in children and adolescents. *Cochrane Database Systemic Reviews* **12**, CD003380.

Middeldorp, C.M. *et al.* (2005) The co-morbidity of anxiety and depression in the perspective of genetic epidemiology: a review of twin and family studies. *Psychological Medicine* **35**, 611–624.

Miller, G.E. & Cole, S.W. (2012) Clustering of depression and inflammation in adolescents previously exposed to childhood adversity. *Biological Psychiatry* **72**, 34–40.

Mills, N.T. *et al.* (2013) Research review: the role of cytokines in depression in adolescents: a systematic review. *Journal of Child Psychology and Psychiatry* **54**, 816–835.

Monk, C.S. *et al.* (2008) Amygdala and nucleus accumbens activation to emotional facial expressions in children and adolescents at risk for major depression. *The American Journal of Psychiatry* **165**, 90–98.

Nanni, V. *et al.* (2012) Childhood maltreatment predicts unfavorable course of illness and treatment outcome in depression: a meta-analysis. *The American Journal of Psychiatry* **169**, 141–151.

National Institute for Health and Care Excellence (2005) Depression in children and young people: identification and management in primary, community and secondary care. *NICE Clinical Guideline*, **28**.

Nemets, H. *et al.* (2006) Omega-3 treatment of childhood depression: a controlled, double-blind pilot study. *The American Journal of Psychiatry* **163**, 1098–1100.

Niederhofer, H. & Von Klitzing, K. (2011) Bright light treatment as add-on therapy for depression in 28 adolescents: a randomized trial. *Primary Care Companion for CNS Disorder* **13**.

Niederhofer, H. & Von Klitzing, K. (2012) Bright light treatment as mono-therapy of non-seasonal depression for 28 adolescents. *International Journal of Psychiatry in Clinical Practice* **16**, 233–237.

Nock, M.K. *et al.* (2013) Prevalence, correlates, and treatment of lifetime suicidal behavior among adolescents: results from the National Comorbidity Survey Replication Adolescent Supplement. *JAMA Psychiatry* **70**, 300–310.

Offidani, E. *et al.* (2013) Excessive mood elevation and behavioral activation with antidepressant treatment of juvenile depressive and anxiety disorders: a systematic review. *Psychotherapy and Psychosomatics* **82**, 132–141.

Olino, T.M. *et al.* (2011) Developmental trajectories of positive and negative affect in children at high and low familial risk for depressive disorder. *Journal of Child Psychology and Psychiatry* **52**, 792–799.

Olino, T.M. *et al.* (2012) Measuring depression using item response theory: an examination of three measures of depressive symptomatology. *International Journal of Methods in Psychiatric Research* **21**, 76–85.

Olino, T.M. *et al.* (2013) Comparisons across depression assessment instruments in adolescence and young adulthood: an item response theory study using two linking methods. *Journal of Abnormal Child Psychology* **41**, 1267–1277.

Osman, A. *et al.* (2010) Reynolds Adolescent Depression Scale-Second Edition: a reliable and useful instrument. *Journal of Clinical Psychology* **66**, 1324–1345.

Owens, M. *et al.* (2012) 5-HTTLPR and early childhood adversities moderate cognitive and emotional processing in adolescence. *PLoS ONE* **7**, e48482.

Peterson, B.S. & Weissman, M.M. (2011) A brain-based endophenotype for major depressive disorder. *Annual Review of Medicine* **62**, 461–474.

Pine, D.S. *et al.* (1998) The risk for early-adulthood anxiety and depressive disorders in adolescents with anxiety and depressive disorders. *Archives of General Psychiatry* **55**, 56–64.

Pine, D.S. *et al.* (2001) Adolescent fears as predictors of depression. *Biological Psychiatry* **50**, 721–724.

Rao, U. *et al.* (2009) Risk markers for depression in adolescents: sleep and HPA measures. *Neuropsychopharmacology* **34**, 1936–1945.

Rao, U. *et al.* (2010) Hippocampal changes associated with early-life adversity and vulnerability to depression. *Biological Psychiatry* **67**, 357–364.

Renaud, J. *et al.* (1998) Rapid response to psychosocial treatment for adolescent depression: a two-year follow-up. *Journal of the American Academy of Child and Adolescent Psychiatry* **37**, 1184–1190.

Richardson, L.P. *et al.* (2010) Evaluation of the PHQ-2 as a brief screen for detecting major depression among adolescents. *Pediatrics* **125**, e1097–e1103.

Ripke, S. *et al.* (2013) A mega-analysis of genome-wide association studies for major depressive disorder. *Molecular Psychiatry* **18**, 497–511.

Risch, N. *et al.* (2009) Interaction between the serotonin transporter gene (5-HTTLPR), stressful life events, and risk of depression: a meta-analysis. *JAMA* **301**, 2462–2471.

Roberson-Nay, R. *et al.* (2006) Increased amygdala activity during successful memory encoding in adolescent major depressive disorder: an FMRI study. *Biological Psychiatry* **60**, 966–973.

Rossello, J. & Bernal, G. (1999) The efficacy of cognitive-behavioral and interpersonal treatments for depression in Puerto Rican adolescents. *Journal of Consulting and Clinical Psychology* **67**, 734–745.

Rossello, J. *et al.* (2008) Individual and group CBT and IPT for Puerto Rican adolescents with depressive symptoms. *Cultural Diversity & Ethnic Minority Psychology* **14**, 234–245.

Rossouw, T.I. & Fonagy, P. (2012) Mentalization-based treatment for self-harm in adolescents: a randomized controlled trial. *Journal of the American Academy of Child and Adolescent Psychiatry* **51**, 1304–1313.

Ruchkin, V. *et al.* (2006) Depressive symptoms and associated psychopathology in urban adolescents: a cross-cultural study of three countries. *Journal of Nervous and Mental Disease* **194**, 106–113.

Rudolph, K.D. *et al.* (2011) Individual differences in biological stress responses moderate the contribution of early peer victimization to subsequent depressive symptoms. *Psychopharmacology* **214**, 209–219.

Sakolsky, D.J. *et al.* (2011) Antidepressant exposure as a predictor of clinical outcomes in the Treatment of Resistant Depression in Adolescents (TORDIA) study. *Journal of Clinical Psychopharmacology* **31**, 92–97.

Seymour, K.E. *et al.* (2012) Emotion regulation mediates the relationship between ADHD and depressive symptoms in youth. *Journal of Abnormal Child Psychology* **40**, 595–606.

Shamseddeen, W. *et al.* (2011) Treatment-resistant depressed youth show a higher response rate if treatment ends during summer school break. *Journal of the American Academy of Child and Adolescent Psychiatry* **50**, 1140–1148.

Shanahan, L. *et al.* (2011) Child-, adolescent- and young adult-onset depressions: differential risk factors in development? *Psychological Medicine* **41**, 2265–2274.

Silk, J.S. *et al.* (2009) Expressed emotion in mothers of currently depressed, remitted, high-risk, and low-risk youth: links to child depression status and longitudinal course. *Journal of Clinical Child and Adolescent Psychology* **38**, 36–47.

Simon, G.E. & Savarino, J. (2007) Suicide attempts among patients starting depression treatment with medications or psychotherapy. *The American Journal of Psychiatry* **164**, 1029–1034.

Sinclair, K.R. *et al.* (2012) Impact of physical and relational peer victimization on depressive cognitions in children and adolescents. *Journal of Clinical Child and Adolescent Psychology* **41**, 570–583.

Soffer-Dudek, N. *et al.* (2011) Poor sleep quality predicts deficient emotion information processing over time in early adolescence. *Sleep* **34**, 1499–1508.

Stanley, B. *et al.* (2009) Cognitive-behavioral therapy for suicide prevention (CBT-SP): treatment model, feasibility, and acceptability. *Journal of the American Academy of Child and Adolescent Psychiatry* **48**, 1005–1113.

Stone, M. *et al.* (2009) Risk of suicidality in clinical trials of antidepressants in adults: analysis of proprietary data submitted to US Food and Drug Administration. *BMJ* **339**, b2880.

Stringaris, A. *et al.* (2009) Adult outcomes of youth irritability: a 20-year prospective community-based study. *The American Journal of Psychiatry* **166**, 1048–1054.

Strober, M. & Carlson, G. (1982) Bipolar illness in adolescents with major depression: clinical, genetic, and psychopharmacologic predictors in a three- to four-year prospective follow-up investigation. *Archives of General Psychiatry* **39**, 549–555.

Su, S. *et al.* (2010) Common genes contribute to depressive symptoms and heart rate variability: the Twins Heart Study. *Twin Research and Human Genetics* **13**, 1–9.

Swartz, H.A. *et al.* (2008) Brief interpersonal psychotherapy for depressed mothers whose children are receiving psychiatric treatment. *The American Journal of Psychiatry* **165**, 1155–1162.

Swedo, S.E. *et al.* (1997) A controlled trial of light therapy for the treatment of pediatric seasonal affective disorder. *Journal of the American Academy of Child and Adolescent Psychiatry* **36**, 816–821.

Szigethy, E. *et al.* (2010) Inflammatory bowel disease. *Child & Adolescent Psychiatric Clinics of North America* **19**, 301–318, ix.

Thapar, A. & Mcguffin, P. (1998) Validity of the shortened Mood and Feelings Questionnaire in a community sample of children and adolescents: a preliminary research note. *Psychiatry Research* **81**, 259–268.

Thapar, A. & Rice, F. (2006) Twin studies in pediatric depression. *Child & Adolescent Psychiatric Clinics of North America* **15**, 869–881, viii.

Timbremont, B. *et al.* (2004) Assessing depression in youth: relation between the Children's Depression Inventory and a structured interview. *Journal of Clinical Child and Adolescent Psychology* **33**, 149–157.

Tully, E.C. *et al.* (2008) An adoption study of parental depression as an environmental liability for adolescent depression and childhood disruptive disorders. *The American Journal of Psychiatry* **165**, 1148–1154.

Van Der Zanden, R. *et al.* (2012) Effectiveness of an online group course for depression in adolescents and young adults: a randomized trial. *Journal of Medical Internet Research* **14**, e86.

Vitiello, B. *et al.* (2009) Suicidal events in the Treatment for Adolescents With Depression Study (TADS). *Journal of Clinical Psychiatry* **70**, 741–747.

Vitiello, B. *et al.* (2011) Long-term outcome of adolescent depression initially resistant to selective serotonin reuptake inhibitor treatment: a follow-up study of the TORDIA sample. *Journal of Clinical Psychiatry* **72**, 388–396.

Walter, G. & Rey, J.M. (2003) Has the practice and outcome of ECT in adolescents changed? Findings from a whole-population study. *The Journal of ECT* **19**, 84–87.

Weissman, M.M. (2006) Recent advances in depression across the generations. *Epidemiology and Psychiatry Society* **15**, 16–19.

Weisz, J.R. *et al.* (2006) Effects of psychotherapy for depression in children and adolescents: a meta-analysis. *Psychological Bulletin* **132**, 132–149.

Weisz, J.R. *et al.* (2009) Cognitive-behavioral therapy versus usual clinical care for youth depression: an initial test of transportability to community clinics and clinicians. *Journal of Consulting and Clinical Psychology* **77**, 383–396.

Wetter, E.K. & Hankin, B.L. (2009) Mediational pathways through which positive and negative emotionality contribute to anhedonic symptoms of depression: a prospective study of adolescents. *Journal of Abnormal Child Psychology* **37**, 507–520.

Wilkinson, P.O. & Goodyer, I.M. (2011) Childhood adversity and allostatic overload of the hypothalamic-pituitary-adrenal axis: a vulnerability model for depressive disorders. *Development and Psychopathology* **23**, 1017–1037.

Wilkinson, P. *et al.* (2011) Clinical and psychosocial predictors of suicide attempts and nonsuicidal self-injury in the Adolescent Depression Antidepressants and Psychotherapy Trial (ADAPT). *The American Journal of Psychiatry* **168**, 495–501.

Woldu, H. *et al.* (2011) Pharmacokinetically and clinician-determined adherence to an antidepressant regimen and clinical outcome in the

TORDIA trial. *Journal of the American Academy of Child and Adolescent Psychiatry* **50**, 490–498.

Wood, A. *et al.* (1995) Properties of the Mood and Feelings Questionnaire in adolescent psychiatric outpatients: a research note. *Journal of Child Psychology and Psychiatry* **36**, 327–334.

Wood, A. *et al.* (1996) Controlled trial of a brief cognitive-behavioural intervention in adolescent patients with depressive disorders. *Journal of Child Psychology and Psychiatry* **37**, 737–746.

World Health Organization (2010) *ICD-10: International Statistical Classification of Diseases and Related Health Problems*, 10th edn. World Health Organization, Geneva, Switzerland.

Yap, M.B. *et al.* (2008) Interaction of parenting experiences and brain structure in the prediction of depressive symptoms in adolescents. *Archives of General Psychiatry* **65**, 1377–1385.

Young, J.F. *et al.* (2009) Mother-child conflict and its moderating effects on depression outcomes in a preventive intervention for adolescent depression. *Journal of Clinical Child and Adolescent Psychology* **38**, 696–704.

Zwierzynska, K. *et al.* (2013) Peer victimization in childhood and internalizing problems in adolescence: a prospective longitudinal study. *Journal of Abnormal Child Psychology* **41**, 309–323.

B: Emotional

CHAPTER 64

Suicidal behavior and self-harm

Keith Hawton[1], Rory C. O'Connor[2] and Kate E.A. Saunders[1]

[1]Department of Psychiatry, University of Oxford, UK
[2]Suicidal Behaviour Research Laboratory, Institute of Health and Wellbeing, University of Glasgow, UK

Many young people consider suicide or self-harm at some point in their lives. Some carry out nonsuicidal acts of self-harm, while fewer make suicide attempts. A small minority will die, either intentionally or unintentionally. There is a continuum of suicidality but there are also two main points at which discontinuity exists. First, of those who have suicidal ideas only a small proportion engage in some form of self-harm. This represents an important behavioral threshold. Second, some individuals engage in self-harm once, never to repeat, while others carry out multiple acts of self-harm (some repeating many times).

Definitions of terms

Suicide ideation is defined as thoughts about an act of self-harm or suicide, including wishing to kill oneself, making plans of when, where, and how to carry out the act, and having thoughts about the impact of one's self-harm or suicide on others. *Self-harm* is defined as any form of nonfatal self-poisoning or self-injury (such as cutting, taking an overdose, hanging, self-strangulation, and running into traffic), regardless of motivation or the degree of intention to die. *Suicide* includes deaths resulting directly from acts of self-harm. Official verdicts in the United Kingdom, and many other countries, are currently determined by the coroner and are classified using ICD-10 (World Health Organisation, 1996). To reach a verdict of suicide a coroner needs to be satisfied that the act was self-inflicted and that death was the intended outcome. However, strict adherence to these criteria may result in underestimation of the true extent of suicide (Gosney & Hawton, 2007).

In Section 3 (conditions requiring further study) of DSM-5, nonfatal self-harming behavior is classified into diagnostic categories of nonsuicidal self-injury (NSSI) and suicidal behavior disorder. NSSI is defined as repeated physical self-damage or self-injury that is not accompanied by suicidal intent or ideation,

and includes cutting, burning, stabbing, or excessive rubbing. NSSI is performed with the expectation that the injury produced will be minor to moderate and will not be life-threatening. "Suicidal behavior disorder" is applied to individuals with recent acts of self-harm, which they say involved any degree of suicidal intent (American Psychiatric Association, 2013). We prefer to use the term "self-harm" to cover all nonfatal acts and then to define dimensions of the behavior, including methods used, suicidal intent and other motives, and dangerousness/lethality (Kapur *et al.*, 2013a). We believe that self-cutting and other types of self-mutilation should be seen not as diagnoses but as part of the continuum of self-harming phenomena, because they can sometimes lead on to both suicide attempts and death by suicide.

Population prevalence of suicide, suicidal ideation, and self-harm

Suicide

Reported rates of suicide deaths among children and adolescents around the world vary considerably as can be seen in Table 64.1. Some of this diversity may reflect differences in definition as outlined above, and the cultural and legal mores that surround this issue. Generally, more males than females die by suicide in all countries for which data are published, with the exception of China and, possibly, India (Aaron *et al.*, 2004). In several countries, rates of suicide are higher in indigenous or aboriginal populations, particularly among young people. For example, First Nations people in the United States (US Department of Health and Human Services, 2004), Metis and Inuit in Canada (Kirmayer *et al.*, 1996), Australian Aborigines (Tatz, 2001), and New Zealand Maori (Ministry of Health, 2005) are overrepresented in suicide statistics. Historically, the rate of suicide among Black people in the United States has been considerably lower than White people (Bingham *et al.*, 1994); however, from 1980 to 1995

Rutter's Child and Adolescent Psychiatry, Sixth Edition.
Edited by Anita Thapar and Daniel S. Pine, James F. Leckman, Stephen Scott, Margaret J. Snowling, Eric Taylor.
© 2015 John Wiley & Sons Ltd. Published 2018 by John Wiley & Sons Ltd.

Table 64.1 Male and female suicide rates for children, adolescents, and young adults for selected countries (World Health Organization, 2014).

Country	Year	Male age-specific rate per 100,000 population		Female age-specific rate per 100,000 population	
		5–14 years	15–24 years	5–14 years	15–24 years
Australia	2006	0.4	12.2	0.1	3.5
Austria	2010	0.5	17.5	0.2	2.8
Belgium	2005	0.2	15.3	0.0	4.2
Canada	2004	0.8	17.0	0.6	4.8
China	1999	0.9	5.4	0.8	8.6
Denmark	2006	0.3	7.7	0.3	3.0
Finland	2009	0.0	26.4	0.3	8.7
France	2007	0.4	9.9	0.2	2.9
Germany	2010	0.6	10.1	0.2	2.9
Ireland	2009	1.0	24.1	0.3	6.8
Italy	2008	0.1	5.2	0.1	1.2
Japan	2009	0.6	20.4	0.4	9.8
Lithuania	2009	1.7	41.3	1.2	6.3
Netherlands	2009	0.6	7.5	0.2	2.4
New Zealand	2007	0.3	22.6	0.3	7.6
Norway	2009	0.3	16.0	1.0	5.9
Russian Federation	2006	2.8	43.7	1.1	7.4
Spain	2008	0.1	5.3	0.1	1.2
Sweden	2010	0.2	13.6	0.4	5.1
United Kingdom	2009	0.1	7.9	0.1	2.1
United States	2005	1.0	16.1	0.3	3.5

Comparison of male age-specific rate per 100,000 population versus female age-specific rate per 100,000. Population years vary by country because of availability of data.
Source: Reproduced with permission of World Health Organization.

there was a dramatic increase in suicide deaths among Black youth (Joe & Kaplan, 2001).

Youth suicide rates in the United Kingdom and in several other Western countries declined during the late 1990s and early 2000s following a period in which rates in young males had been rising alarmingly. The recent worldwide economic recession may have reversed this pattern in many countries (Chang *et al.*, 2013). It should be noted that official statistics markedly underestimate the true rates of suicide, especially in children and adolescents, with some apparent suicide deaths being recorded as open verdicts, accidents, or misadventure (Gosney & Hawton, 2007). In the United Kingdom, the rate of suicide and undetermined deaths for adolescents aged 15–19 years in 2011 was 6.6 per 100,000 in males and 3.1 per 100,000 in females (The Office for National Statistics, 2013). Undetermined verdicts are not used for 10–14-year-olds.

Suicidal ideation and self-harm

A systematic review of the prevalence of suicidal phenomena in adolescents based on community and school-based studies in several countries demonstrated that averaging across studies nearly one in five adolescents reported having thought about suicide in the previous year. The mean lifetime prevalence of self-harm was 13%, with 6% self-harming in the previous 12 months. Rates of suicidal thoughts and actual self-harm were far higher among females than males (Evans *et al.*, 2005b).

In the United Kingdom, studies have been conducted on the prevalence of suicidal ideation and self-harm in the community (Hawton *et al.*, 2002; O'Connor *et al.*, 2009b). In a school-based study of 6020 students in England, 15% reported thoughts of self-harm (which had not been acted on) in the preceding year. This was much more common among females (22%) than males (9%). Seven percent had self-harmed in the past year. Self-harm was more frequent among females (11%) than males (3%) (Hawton *et al.*, 2002). There were similar findings in a study employing the same methodology in Scotland (O'Connor *et al.*, 2009b). In contrast, in a large national study of suicidal phenomena among children and adolescents of 5–15 years, based on parental report, only 1% of 5- to 10-year-olds had ever tried to harm, hurt, or kill themselves, rising to 2% among those aged 11–15 years (Meltzer *et al.*, 2001). Parents are often unaware of self-harm acts by their offspring (Meltzer *et al.*, 2001; Huey *et al.*, 2004; Sourander *et al.*, 2006b), especially where self-cutting is involved.

In an international comparative study, again using the same methodology as Hawton *et al.* (2002), rates of self-harm in adolescents in the United Kingdom, Australia, Belgium, Ireland, and Norway were similar, but were considerably lower in the Netherlands and Hungary (Madge *et al.*, 2008).

There appear to be some differences between rates of self-harm in children and adolescents of different ethnic groups. Hispanic youth, particularly females, in the United States (Canino & Roberts, 2001) and Maori youth in New Zealand

(Adolescent Health Research Group, 2005) show higher rates than their contemporaries. In the United Kingdom, self-harm appears to be less common among Asian (7%) and Black (7%) girls than White girls (12%) but similar among Asian and White males (3%); (Hawton *et al.*, 2002). More recent studies have reported similar or lower rates of self-harm among Asian youth (Bhugra & Bhui, 2007).

Methods of suicide and self-harm by gender and international differences

There is significant variation between cultures in the methods most commonly used for suicide. The preferred methods of suicide in any given country may have an impact on suicide rates, given that some methods are potentially more lethal than others. In addition, deaths involving a certain method may increase or decrease depending on the availability of that method (Hawton, 2005). Firearms are the most common method of suicide in young people in the United States, but account for a relatively small number of deaths in the United Kingdom, New Zealand, and Australia, where availability is strictly regulated. Substitution of methods relies on both the acceptability and availability of alternative methods. Increasing rates of hanging in young people suggest that it has become a more acceptable method of suicide (Centre for Disease Control and Prevention, 2010).

Charcoal burning has spread from Hong Kong to Taiwan and Japan: the apparent increased acceptability, cultural meaning, and preference for methods of suicide such as this require further research, including the likely role of the media, especially the Internet (Biddle *et al.*, 2013).

In India, in contrast with other countries, hanging is a more frequent method of suicide in girls (57%) than boys (50%), whereas poisoning is slightly more common in boys (50%) than girls (37%) (Lalwani *et al.*, 2004). The use of toxic pesticides in agrarian communities such as in China, India (Prasad *et al.*, 2006), and Sri Lanka (Eddleston *et al.*, 2005a) means that a similar method (self-poisoning) is associated with much higher mortality in these countries than in countries where analgesics and other medications are the most frequently used substances for self-poisoning. The medical management of pesticide poisoning is difficult and a lack of adequate medical services and distances to hospitals in developing countries may elevate death rates (Eddleston *et al.*, 2005b).

At the community level, the most common methods of self-harm in the United Kingdom and many other countries are cutting and overdose (Hawton *et al.*, 2002). However, only a minority of young people engaging in self-harm in the community go to hospital. In studies based on presentations to general hospitals in the United Kingdom, the majority of adolescents had harmed themselves by taking an overdose, self-poisoning with analgesics being particularly common (Hawton *et al.*, 2012b).

Puberty and self-harm

Self-harm increases rapidly during the early teenage years. The female to male gender ratio is particularly high at this time, especially around age 13–15 years. In a survey of 12–15-year-olds in schools in Australia and the United States, the onset of self-harm was found to be related to pubertal phase, especially late or completed puberty, rather than chronological age. This was particularly marked in girls and for self-cutting (Patton *et al.*, 2007). The association of self-harm with puberty and affective symptoms may be related to emerging evidence of a period of particular neurodevelopmental vulnerability around this time, with increased risk of emotional disorders (Blakemore, 2008), risk-taking behaviors, and susceptibility to negative social cues, including ostracism and the expectations of others.

Motives for self-harm

Both adolescents who present to hospital following self-harm (Hawton *et al.*, 1982) and those who are identified through community surveys to have self-harmed (Rodham *et al.*, 2004) choose a wide variety of motives (or reasons) to explain their acts. These include both motives about dealing with intolerable distress (e.g., to die, to escape) and motives related to influencing the behavior or attitudes of other people (e.g., to get someone to change their mind). They also very often choose multiple motives. Differences have been found between adolescents who cut themselves and those who take overdoses, with those who cut themselves more often saying that the behavior was related to tension reduction or self-punishment (Rodham *et al.*, 2004).

Risk factors associated with suicidal phenomena in young people

An overall model of suicidal behavior can help the clinician or researcher conceptualize the main contributory factors identified in a wide range of research studies (Figure 64.1). This can also provide a framework to support formulations and treatment planning. In such a model (Hawton *et al.*, 2012c), suicidal behaviors are viewed as the endpoint of a complex interplay between genetic, biological, psychological, psychiatric, and social risk factors which combine to increase the likelihood of self-harm or suicide (Figure 64. 1). The risk factors associated with fatal and nonfatal suicide behaviors among adolescents have been reviewed recently by Hawton *et al.* (2012c) and Hamza *et al.* (2012).

Family history and genetic influences on suicidal behavior

Research consistently indicates that a family history of suicidal behavior is associated with increased risk for suicide deaths (Brent *et al.*, 1994; Gould *et al.*, 1996; Agerbo *et al.*, 2002) and for nonfatal self-harm and suicidal ideation by adolescents (Roy *et al.*, 1997; Hawton *et al.*, 2002; Mittendorfer-Rutz *et al.*, 2008). Having a suicidal family member may suggest to adolescents that suicide is a possible solution to overwhelming psychological pain (Roy *et al.*, 1997), although the detrimental effects of living

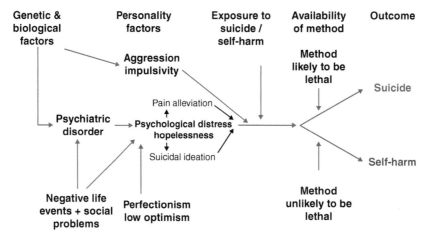

Figure 64.1 Pathway model illustrating key risk factors for adolescent self-harm and suicide. *Source*: Reproduced with permission of Elsevier.

with a parent who has undiagnosed or undertreated mental health problems are also significant (see Chapter 28). More work is required to clarify the extent to which suicidal behavior can be considered as a construct that is transmitted through families independently of the established association with familial risk of depression, impulsivity, and other psychopathology (Brent & Mann, 2005). The risk in these families is not entirely accounted for by the increased rates of psychiatric disorder. Twin studies have shown that the concordance for fatal and nonfatal suicidal behavior is higher among monozygotic than dizygotic twins (Roy, 1993; Tidemalm *et al.*, 2011). Impulsive aggression also shows heritable influences and contributes to suicidal behavior (for a review see Brent & Mann, 2005). The clustering of suicidal behavior in families cannot be explained entirely by behavioral imitation (Brent & Mann, 2005). Importantly, adoption studies have shown elevated rates of suicide among the biological relatives of adoptees who die by suicide compared with those of nonsuicidal adoptees (Roy *et al.*, 1997), including biological siblings of adoptees compared with their adopted siblings (Petersen *et al.*, 2013). Adoption studies also show the importance of environmental influences (Wilcox *et al.*, 2012).

Deviations in the serotonin system are one of the most robust neurobiological findings associated with suicidal behavior (Asberg & Forslund, 2000). The relationship between serotonin dysregulation and suicidal behavior may reflect poor impulse control, which is observed in suicidal, violent, and impulsive behaviors. Dysregulation of serotonin function may predispose a person experiencing stressful events to react impulsively (Mann *et al.*, 2001).

The main focus of interest in the genetic studies of suicidal behavior has been on three gene types: trytophan hydroxylase (TPH), serotonin transporter (SERT), located on chromosome 17, and serotonin A receptor genes. Serotonin transporter polymorphisms, particularly the "short" allele of the promoter variant 5HTTLPR, have been associated with suicidal behavior in adults with psychiatric disorder and in particular violent attempts (Lin & Tsai, 2004) but results are

inconsistent. More recent studies in adults have explored a model of anxiety and stress responses underpinning suicidal behavior, with particular focus on cannabinoid receptors (CB1), corticotropin-releasing hormone (CRH), glucocorticoid receptors, and gamma-aminobutyric acid (GABA) (Bondy *et al.*, 2006). Despite the interest in this area, to date there are relatively few replicated findings or meta-analyses, particularly in children and adolescents.

Psychological characteristics

Psychological characteristics associated with suicidal ideation and behavior include hopelessness (Evans *et al.*, 2004; Taliaferro *et al.*, 2012), dichotomous (all or nothing) thinking, negative biases in future judgment (Pfeffer, 2000; Williams & Pollock, 2000; O'Connor, 2011), and an external locus of control (Kienhorst *et al.*, 1992). Impaired social problem solving is another contributory factor (Speckens & Hawton, 2005; Arie *et al.*, 2008; Labelle *et al.*, 2013). Impaired decision making is also associated with suicide attempts in adolescents (Bridge *et al.*, 2012).

New theoretical models also offer considerable promise in terms of better understanding the psychological processes that underpin suicidal behavior (Joiner, 2005; Van Orden *et al.*, 2010; O'Connor, 2011; O'Connor *et al.*, 2013). Extending the stress-diathesis explanations, the interpersonal model of suicide (Joiner, 2005) and the integrated motivational-volitional model (O'Connor, 2011) suggest that the extent to which individuals feel defeated or trapped, and the degree to which they consider themselves to be a burden on others and that they do not belong, are associated with suicidal behaviors. These models also highlight the importance of distinguishing the factors which are associated with whether an individual actually engages in suicidal behavior (enactor) from those which relate to suicidal thinking only (ideation only). For example, adolescents who self-harm are more impulsive and are more likely to know others who have self-harmed compared to those who have had thoughts of self-harm but have never engaged in self-harm (O'Connor *et al.*, 2012).

Certain personality characteristics such as impulsivity, aggression, neuroticism, perfectionism, irritability, and trait anxiety may act as intermediate factors that are relatively independent from major psychiatric disorders (Bridge et al., 2006). Perfectionism may be particularly risky among those young people who believe that others have excessively high expectations of them (Hewitt et al., 1997; O'Connor, 2007; O'Connor et al., 2009b; Roxborough et al., 2012). Trait optimism protects against self-harm (O'Connor et al., 2009a). Social connectedness, peer attachment, and effective problem-solving skills may also offer protection (Speckens & Hawton, 2005; Hall-Lande et al., 2007).

Poor physical health related to psychological problems

Poor physical health and many chronic illnesses are associated with increased risk for suicidal ideation (Suris et al., 1996) and self-harm (Evans et al., 2004). Furthermore, depressed adolescents commonly present with psychosomatic complaints such as headaches, loss of energy, chest pain, abdominal pain, or other physical symptoms.

Family factors

Longitudinal community studies have shown that difficulties in parent–child relationships, including those related to early attachment problems, perceived low levels of parental caring and communication are related to increased risk of suicide and suicide attempts among children and adolescents (Fergusson & Lynskey, 1995, Fergusson et al., 2000; Ackard et al., 2006); similar observations have been made in clinical samples (Lessard & Moretti, 1998; Pfeffer, 2000). Several reviews have concluded that adolescents from families that have experienced parental separation or divorce are at increased risk of suicide behavior, particularly among females (e.g., (Brent et al., 1994; Gould et al., 1996; Beautrais, 2001). Unsurprisingly, it seems that conflict between parents, both before and after their relationship ends, has a detrimental impact on children.

Childhood sexual and physical abuse are strongly associated with suicide attempts and NSSI in community and clinical samples of adolescents (Beautrais, 2001; Evans et al., 2005a; Taliaferro et al., 2012; Isohookana et al., 2013). In addition, childhood sexual abuse is associated with adult suicide attempts (Perez-Fuentes et al., 2013). Parental history of childhood sexual abuse is also associated with an increased risk of suicide attempts among offspring (Brent et al., 2002).

Peers, including the influence of peer suicidal behaviors and suicide clusters

Peers can have extremely important roles in both self-harm and suicide. As noted below, relationship problems may be a common precipitant, especially in older adolescents. Self-harm can have a "contagious" quality in adolescents and exposure to self-harm by peers appears to be a key risk factor for self-harm (Hawton et al., 2010; Madge et al., 2011). This particularly applies to females and to self-cutting. Suicides can occur in clusters (i.e., related in time and place) in young people (Haw et al., 2013). It has been estimated that 1% of suicides in young people occur in clusters. However, with the massive proliferation of electronic communication the potential for clusters of suicides (not necessarily geographically close) may have increased.

Sexual orientation

Gay, lesbian, and bisexual young people are at increased risk of engaging in self-harm and suicide attempts (King et al., 2008; Haas et al., 2011), with estimates of risk ranging between two and six times that of heterosexual young people (Gould et al., 2003). It is not yet clear whether increased rates of death by suicide are related to sexual orientation (Gould et al., 2003). However, gay, lesbian, and bisexual youth are more likely to experience risk factors associated with suicide, particularly mental health difficulties (King et al., 2008).

Environmental factors
School dropout

Several reviews of studies of young suicide attempters (Beautrais et al., 1996; Evans et al., 2004) and those who die by suicide (Gould et al., 1996) have indicated that more have had school-based difficulties and/or have dropped out of school than have nonsuicidal adolescents. Dropping out of school has been shown to be a risk factor for suicide attempts in Western and non-Western countries (Daniel et al., 2006; Donald et al., 2006; Tang et al., 2009). Children and adolescents who remain in school but have special educational needs appear to have higher rates of suicidal phenomena than their peers without such needs (Meltzer et al., 2001; Denny et al., 2003).

Proximal risk factors/life stressors

Psychological autopsy studies suggest that, compared with controls, young people who die by suicide experience higher rates of exposure to recent stressful life events such as rejection, conflict, or loss following the breakup of a relationship (Marttunen et al., 1993; Brent et al., 1996; Beautrais, 2001; Donald et al., 2006), and disciplinary or legal crises (Marttunen et al., 1998). Bullying, in particular, is associated with poor mental health, suicide ideation, and all types of self-harm (see Chapter 26). There has been recent concern about suicides by young people allegedly bullied by peers via text messaging and social networking sites, so-called "cyberbullying" (Brunstein Klomek et al., 2010; Hawton et al., 2012c). This issue requires urgent research attention.

Another proximal stressor is becoming intoxicated: a short-term solution that many adolescents engage in following crises—but which leads to impaired judgment and decreased inhibition, and hence to suicidal behavior (Apter & Freudenstein, 2000).

Asylum seeking and cultural factors

Refugees and asylum seekers face particular psychosocial stressors that are likely to have an impact on young people and their families. Unemployment, social isolation, and the difficulties involved in applying for asylum experienced by parents are factors that, together with the high rates of depression, anxiety, and posttraumatic stress disorder (PTSD) in this population, may lead to suicidal behavior (Sultan and O'Sullivan, 2001; Keller *et al.*, 2003; Fazel *et al.*, 2005). Indeed, research in the Netherlands showed higher rates of suicide and suicide attempts among asylum seekers compared to the reference population (Goosen *et al.*, 2011). Racial discrimination is another factor which ought to be considered when evaluating risk of suicidal behavior. Research from the United States suggests that perceived discrimination is associated with suicide attempts in young adults (mean age 18.8 years) from different ethnic backgrounds (Gomez *et al.*, 2011). It is also important to consider cultural background when assessing risk of suicide and self-harm (Langhinrichsen-Rohling *et al.*, 2009). For example, among adolescents from East-Asian backgrounds, the shame of failing to meet familial expectations may be a precursor to suicidal behavior (Zane & Mak, 2003; Goldston *et al.*, 2008). Cultural influences may also adversely affect help-seeking. For example, help-seeking for mental health problems may be culturally stigmatized, so even in cultures where the gravity of the problem is acknowledged, cultural influences may constrain the young person from seeking help (Freedenthal & Stiffman, 2007).

Psychiatric disorders associated with self-harm and suicide

Many studies have demonstrated high rates of mental illness in adolescents engaging in both fatal and nonfatal suicidal behavior and rates are of similar magnitude to that seen in adult populations (for reviews see Evans *et al.*, 2004; Hawton *et al.*, 2013b; Figure 64.2). Although mental illness is present in many children and adolescents who engage in suicidal behaviors, clearly not all people who experience mental illness engage in suicidal behavior, so it may be a strong precursor but not a complete explanation.

In a systematic review of psychological autopsy studies (Cavanagh *et al.*, 2003) results of seven studies of adolescents or young adults suggested that 47–74% of suicides examined were attributable to a mental disorder, of which affective disorders made the greatest contribution. This review also highlighted that comorbidity, particularly comorbidity of mental disorder and substance abuse, made a strong contribution to the risk of suicide. An earlier review (Marttunen *et al.*, 1994) indicated that antisocial behavior was present in 43–73% of suicide deaths in adolescents, often in combination with depressive symptoms and/or substance abuse. Several more recent psychological autopsy studies (Houston *et al.*, 2001; Portzky *et al.*, 2005; Fortune *et al.*, 2007) suggest an interaction between mental illness, substance abuse, and interpersonal problems (and, for some, antisocial behaviors). In a case–control study of young people who had died by suicide, serious suicide attempters and a nonsuicidal control group, the same risk factors of mood disorder,

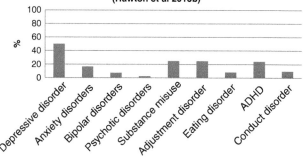

Figure 64.2 Prevalence of mental disorders in children and adolescents attending general hospitals following self-harm.

requirement for psychiatric care, educational disadvantage, and stressful life events were associated with both death by suicide and serious attempts (Beautrais, 2003).

Depression is the most common mental health disorder reported in psychological autopsy studies of young people dying by suicide (see Chapter 63) The course of depression across adolescence also appears to influence suicidality. In a longitudinal study of 193 children and adolescents, persistent depression was associated with significantly higher rates of suicidal ideation and suicide attempts. Depressed females were more likely to experience recurrent episodes, while males tended to experience more persistent mood disorder (Dunn & Goodyer, 2006).

Bipolar disorder (see Chapter 62) is associated with elevated rates of suicide attempts, with the lifetime prevalence ranging from 20% (Strober *et al.*, 1995) to 44% (Lewinsohn *et al.*, 2003). In the only prospective study exploring risk of suicide attempts among youth with bipolar disorder, persistent depressive symptoms, active substance misuse, mixed affective states, and a family history of depression were all found to predict significant risk of suicidal behavior (Goldstein *et al.*, 2012).

Anxiety (see Chapter 60) and subdiagnostic anxiety symptoms were found to be associated with an increase in suicidality in a study of 12,395 adolescents from 11 different countries (Balazs *et al.*, 2013).

Substance abuse disorders, including cigarette smoking, are associated with increased risk of self-harm (Evans *et al.*, 2004; Moran *et al.*, 2012) and suicide (see Chapter 66). Clinically, it can be difficult to establish if substance abuse precedes or follows the mental health difficulties and suicidal phenomena. Adolescence is a period when both suicidal behavior and substance misuse increase and poor impulse control is a risk factor for both (Hawton *et al.*, 2012c).

Psychotic disorders make a relatively small contribution to the overall youth suicide rate. Self-harm, however, is common in the pretreatment phase of first-episode psychosis (Challis *et al.*, 2013) and was present in nearly three-quarters of those presenting to services for the first time (Harvey *et al.*, 2008), the majority describing the act as a means of responding to the distress of their symptoms rather than as a direct result of command or passivity experiences. Depression, early age of onset, substance misuse, and duration of untreated symptoms are risk factors for self-harm in first-episode psychosis (Challis *et al.*, 2013).

Antisocial behavior is a risk factor for self-harm among females although, perhaps surprisingly, the relationship is less clear for males (Evans *et al.*, 2004). Many of the risk factors for conduct disorder are also risk factors for self-harm, including family disruption, childhood abuse, personal and familial substance abuse, and negative life events (Apter & Freudenstein, 2000).

Eating disorders and poor body image are associated with suicidal phenomena (Brausch & Gutierrez, 2009) and some consider starvation to be a form of suicidal behavior that obviates the need for other methods. Suicide risk in anorexia nervosa has been estimated to be 2–15% and 0.4–2% for bulimia nervosa, with higher rates among adolescent males than females with eating disorders (Dancyger & Fornari, 2005).

Attention deficit/hyperactivity disorder has a modestly elevated risk for fatal and nonfatal suicidal behavior, particularly in males, mediated by comorbid conditions, notably depression, conduct disorder, and substance abuse, with the risk considerably raised in young people with all three conditions (James *et al.*, 2004). A recent review of 25 studies on ADHD and suicidality also concluded that there was a positive relationship between the two phenomena (Impey & Heun, 2012).

Personality disorders in adolescence are described in Chapter 67; they are associated with suicidal ideation and attempted suicide as well as self-injury in adolescents.

Exposure to suicide and self-harm in the media, the Internet, and music

It is now well recognized that certain types of media reports and portrayals of suicide and self-harm can increase the risk of suicidal behavior (for review see Pirkis & Norderntoft, 2011). The greatest influence is probably on methods used for suicide and self-harm and seems to be particularly marked in young people. Such effects are more likely where media reporting or portrayal is dramatic, features details of a specific method of suicide, is on television, and is repeated (Stack, 2003; Pirkis & Norderntoft, 2011).

Many children appear to learn about suicide from television (Mishara, 1999), but with the proliferation of new media the relative influences of different modalities need detailed exploration. Some people may respond quickly to media presentations of suicide, acting impulsively or putting previous thoughts about suicide into action, while others may make a more considered response (Schmidtke & Hafner, 1988). Thus, in addition to potential immediate changes in suicidal behavior, media influences may also have longer term effects, by changing attitudes, providing information about methods of suicidal behavior, or planting the idea that suicide is an appropriate response to problems. It may also influence suicidal behavior through provoking images which may act as powerful drivers of behavior, especially when an individual is depressed and having suicidal thoughts.

There has been increasing concern about Internet sites dealing with suicide and their potential negative influence on adolescent suicidal behavior (Collings *et al.*, 2011). The provision of interactive experiences and the development of "online communities" mean that the Internet may have a unique role in influencing suicidal behavior and/or providing peer support and possibly helping prevent suicidal behavior (Daine *et al.*, 2013). Some researchers have highlighted the increased risk that may be associated with Internet use, especially sites that promote suicide methods (Biddle *et al.*, 2008) and also social networking sites (Dunlop *et al.*, 2011).

Few studies have been conducted in this area. In a large community study, depressed young people, especially boys, were heavier users of the Internet, more likely to access the Internet at school, and more likely to use chat rooms and interact with peers they saw infrequently in person, and also strangers (Ybarra *et al.*, 2005). A study of online postings to message boards focusing on self-injurious behavior by young people aged 12–20 years suggested that online interactions provide important social support to users. However, these interactions may also normalize or encourage self-injurious behavior (Whitlock *et al.*, 2006; Daine *et al.*, 2013). The Internet may also provide considerable opportunities for suicide prevention. For example, 6 months after a school-based presentation promoting the use of a website for young people experiencing emotional difficulties, 45% of students said they had visited the website (Nicholas *et al.*, 2004).

While concern has been raised about the possible influence of music (especially certain types of popular music) on suicidal phenomena among children and adolescents, this has received very limited attention in the research literature.

Availability of means for self-harm/suicide

Whether or not a young person engages in self-harm will be influenced by availability of acceptable methods to use. The danger or relative lethality of available methods will also strongly influence the outcome (i.e., whether death is more or less likely). Children and adolescents who die by suicide in the United Kingdom are most likely to have used hanging or self-poisoning.

Suicide is more likely where dangerous means such as firearms (Brent *et al.*, 1991) or pesticides (Eddleston *et al.*, 2005b) are readily available. A major current concern is the increase in hanging or other means of self-suffocation seen in young people of both genders in many countries. Hanging is a readily accessible method as well as having a high rate of lethality (Hawton *et al.*, 1999a). The reasons for the spread in acceptability of hanging and the increased use of this method are not known, but the fact that it is happening in many countries suggests a universal influence, with media portrayal of suicide being a likely candidate (Biddle *et al.*, 2013).

Outcome following self-harm

Repetition of self-harm

Some young people who harm themselves do so on only one occasion. However, during adolescence, many repeat the behavior, often on several occasions. Self-harm that is repeated in adolescence usually ceases by early adulthood (Moran *et al.*, 2012). Persistence is more likely in females than males. Conceptually, the first act of self-harm is different from all those that follow it in that once an adolescent has actually engaged in self-harm, s/he crosses an important behavioral threshold. This seems to reduce the barriers to subsequent self-harm, both nonfatal and fatal. Thus a history of previous self-harm increases the risk of future acts in both clinical and general populations (Gould *et al.*, 2003; Evans *et al.*, 2004). The greatest risk of repetition is in the first year following self-harm, especially the first few months.

Risk estimates for self-harm repetition that involves representation to hospital are between 5% and 15% per year (Bridge *et al.*, 2006), but these are likely to be under estimates as they exclude self-harm which did not receive clinical attention. The risk of repetition remains high for many years after an episode of self-harm. For example, in a 10-year follow-up, Gibb *et al.* (2005) reported that 28% of those admitted for a suicide attempt had been readmitted, with the highest risk in the first 2 years. Repetition rates appear to be similar in the two genders (Gibb *et al.*, 2005; Hawton *et al.*, 2012a).

Depression is a key factor associated with repetition of self-harm in adolescents (Hawton *et al.*, 1999b). Self-reported self-harm at age 12 years predicts suicidal ideation and self-harm at 15 years (Sourander *et al.*, 2006a). Concerns about sexual orientation, history of sexual abuse, family self-harm, anxiety, and self-esteem are also associated with short-term self-harm repetition (O'Connor *et al.*, 2009a). In one study, self-harm in adolescents ceased within 3 years, but those who continued to self-harm into adulthood were characterized by higher rates of psychopathology and adversity in both childhood and adulthood (Harrington *et al.*, 2006); and, in a further study, by anxiety, at least for females (Rudd *et al.*, 2004).

Suicide following self-harm

Follow-up of adolescents who self-harm and present to hospital suggests that the risk of suicide is low in under-15-year-olds (Hawton & Harriss, 2008; Hawton *et al.*, 2012a). However, in older adolescents the risk increases considerably. It is greater in males than females, in those who are repeaters of self-harm and, importantly, in those who cut themselves compared to those who take overdoses (Hawton *et al.*, 2012a). The last point is contrary to the beliefs of many clinicians. The method used for suicide is usually different to the method used for self-harm, death often being due to hanging, at least in the United Kingdom (Hawton *et al.*, 2012a). The risk of suicide following self-harm which does not result in clinical attention is not known.

A history of self-harm is one of the most powerful and clinically relevant predictors of eventual suicide. Most studies find elevated risk of overall mortality following self-harm (Goldacre & Hawton, 1985; Suominen *et al.*, 2004; Gibb *et al.*, 2005). In one follow-up study of 15- to 24-year-olds who had presented to hospital following an episode of self-harm, the overall number of deaths from all causes was 3%, four times higher than expected. This was mainly because of an excess number of suicides (2%), which were 10 times more frequent than expected. The main risk factors for suicide were male gender, previous self-harm, prior psychiatric history, and high suicide intent (Hawton & Harriss, 2007).

Psychosocial adjustment

Aside from repetition of self-harm and occurrence of suicide we know relatively little about the overall outcome of adolescents who self-harm, especially in terms of psychosocial adjustment, describe poor problem solving, impaired peer relationships, and repeated separations in later life for young people who had presented to services following self-harm in adolescence. However, such a negative outcome is certainly not the norm. In an early study of 50 consecutive self-harm patients who presented to a general hospital, those who were classified as having "acute" problems were nearly all doing well even after only a month, whereas many of those with longer term problems, especially if combined with behavioral problems, were doing less well in general after a month (Hawton *et al.*, 1982). In a long-term follow-up of adolescents who took overdoses and then participated in a randomized controlled trial of a brief family intervention (Harrington *et al.*, 1998), after 3 years 70% of the patients were no longer self-harming. Half had used adult mental health services (especially for depression), and among those who continued to self-harm in adulthood, childhood adversity (e.g., sexual abuse) was prevalent and psychiatric disorders, especially depression, common (Harrington *et al.*, 2006). In a Norwegian follow-up study the majority of those who self-harmed as adolescents experienced depressive, anxiety, or personality disorders 8–10 years later (Groholt & Ekeberg, 2009).

Impact of suicide on peers, school and relatives

While there is recognition that self-harm can have a contagious quality in that exposure to self-harm by peers is one of the most important factors associated with adolescents starting to self-harm (Hawton *et al.*, 2002), little is known about other impacts of self-harm on peers. School staff often react with a sense of panic to discovering that pupils are self-harming. Helpful guidance for schools on how to deal with self-harm is available (Hawton *et al.*, 2006). An important but often neglected aspect of self-harm by children and adolescents is the impact this has on their families. There has been little research on the nature, duration, and significance of effects on parents and other carers. Wagner and colleagues (Wagner *et al.*, 2000) in the United States showed that parental reaction to suicidal behavior may include anger, fear, sadness, and frustration, with parents being intimidated by the intensity of suicidal behavior. They may adopt greater restrictiveness in parenting styles, or alternatively abandon responsibility for their child to someone else. How parents respond may depend on the degree of suicidal intent involved in the act and whether self-harm was the first episode or repeat (Wagner *et al.*, 2000). In a pilot study in Ireland a group support program for parents and carers of young people who had self-harmed seemed to reduce their distress and increase satisfaction with care (Power *et al.*, 2009).

Clinical assessment

All young people who express suicidal thoughts or harm themselves should receive a psychosocial assessment (American Academy of Child and Adolescent Psychiatry, 2001; National Collaborating Centre for Mental Health, 2004, 2011). This should be focused on identifying problems, risk, protective factors, mental illness, and gaining an understanding of the suicidal process for the individual concerned. Assessment can also form a therapeutic intervention in itself. It is extremely difficult for clinicians to predict accurately the risk of their patient dying by suicide or of engaging in nonfatal suicidal behavior, so risk management rather than quantification should be the priority. A psychosocial assessment should form the basis of future clinical management and establishing treatment goals. In adults, having an assessment has been associated with reduced rates of repetition (Bergen *et al.*, 2010; Kapur *et al.*, 2013b). The fact that many adolescents spend very little, if any, time planning their self-harm (Rodham *et al.*, 2004), and that being intoxicated is often associated with many such acts, compounds this issue (Esposito-Smythers *et al.*, 2010). A core task of an assessment is to establish an interactive and dynamic therapeutic relationship and to be part of a response to the young person's distress that offers some hope for a better future.

The assessment of children and adolescents following self-harm is influenced by a range of process and service issues. At a process level, the assessment of adolescents can present particular challenges, as young people are often ambivalent about their suicidality and fluctuating mood states can make it difficult to get clear information, particularly retrospectively. Current guidelines emphasize standards of care and note that several studies have suggested that some staff responsible for medical care have, or are perceived by self-harm patients as having, negative attitudes toward those who harm themselves (Saunders *et al.*, 2012). They may also not recognize the complex relationships between self-harm and mental illness (Friedman *et al.*, 2006). Poor continuity of care requiring frequent repetition of their "story" (Dower *et al.*, 2000) and negative expectations about postdischarge therapy (Rotheram-Borus *et al.*, 1996) contribute to dissatisfaction among some adolescents who have

self-harmed. In a study of adolescent self-harm patients, those who were more satisfied with hospital management and subsequent therapy appeared to have better therapeutic outcomes (Burgess *et al.*, 1998).

In recent years there has been a drive toward the use of screening tools to help guide management. While these may be helpful in reminding clinicians about relevant risk factors, their predictive power is very low and they should not be used as an alternative to psychosocial assessment (National Collaborating Centre for Mental Health, 2011).

The content of a full psychosocial assessment is outlined in Table 64.2. An adjunct to standard assessment has recently been developed with the aim of improving patient attendance and engagement with treatment. Specifically, Ougrin and colleagues (Ougrin *et al.*, 2011) have developed and evaluated a tailored therapeutic manualized assessment approach to adolescents who have self-harmed, in which, following a standard psychosocial assessment, the assessing clinician and the adolescent jointly construct a diagram depicting roles in relation to other

Table 64.2 Areas to cover during psychosocial assessment of adolescents who have self-harmed.

History of recent difficulties
Circumstances of the self-harm (before, during, and after)
Alcohol (had it been consumed?) within 6 hours, at time of attempt (i.e., as part of the act)
Motives/reasons for self-harm
Suicidal intent
Other motives/reasons
Evidence of preplanning
History of previous self-harm
Exposure to self-harm/suicide by others
Media influences—looking at Internet, Facebook, and so on
Psychiatric history
Physical health
Family background
Family history, including self-harm and suicide
Personal and social history and current social circumstances
Interpersonal relationships
• Bullying (including cyberbullying)
• Abuse (physical, sexual, and emotional)
• Domestic violence
Offending behavior
Mental state
Risk of future self-harm/suicide
• Suicidal ideation (give details)
• Hopelessness/thoughts of the future
• Risk factors
• Protective factors
• Risk of repetition of self-harm
• Access to means
What help would patient like
Availability of support
Problem solving and coping skills
Problem list
Agree to further actions and aftercare

Table 64.3 Major components of the Therapeutic Assessment.

1 Take standard psychosocial history and assessment
2 Take 10-min break
3 Jointly construct a diagram (based on cognitive analytic therapy) which consists of three elements
  (a) Identification of reciprocal roles
  (b) Identification of the "core pain"
  (c) Identification of the maladaptive procedures
4 Identify the target problem
5 Assess motivation for change and employ motivational interviewing techniques if required
6 Search for ways of breaking the previously identified vicious cycles ("exits"), using a range of cognitive (e.g., future-oriented reflexive questioning) and behavioral (e.g., relaxation) techniques, as appropriate
7 Summarize the above issues in an understanding letter

Source: Adapted from Ougrin *et al.* (2010).

people, core pain, and "maladaptive procedures," identify a target problem and potential ways of breaking vicious circles that have been identified, and then describe the diagram and exits in an "understanding letter," which is shared with the family (see Table 64.3). The therapeutic assessment aims to develop a joint understanding of the difficulties experienced by the young person, to increase motivation for change, to instil hope and to explore alternatives to self-harm (Ougrin *et al.*, 2010). In a randomized controlled trial, adolescents receiving this enhanced assessment were considerably more likely to attend for treatment and to have a greater number of treatment sessions than those who had standard assessment only. There were, however, no differences in measures of psychosocial assessment at follow-up (Ougrin *et al.*, 2011).

Treatments for adolescents who have self-harmed

In a substantial number of adolescents, the crisis associated with self-harm may resolve quite quickly and only supportive care for the adolescent and their family will be required. However, many adolescents will need more intensive therapy, especially in view of the poor longer term outcomes found (as described earlier). There have been surprisingly few randomized evaluations of treatments for children and adolescents who have harmed themselves.

Brief psychological therapy
Problem-solving/cognitive behavior therapy, delivered over 2–10 treatment sessions, appears to be effective in adults in terms of reducing repetition of self-harm and also improving other outcomes compared with treatment as usual (National Collaborating Centre for Mental Health, 2011). Currently, however, there is no evidence of benefits of this with adolescents.

Family therapy
Given the high incidence of family problems in adolescents who self-harm, family therapy, which focuses on the relationships, roles and communication patterns between family members (see Chapter 39), would seem a logical treatment approach for adolescents who self-harm. In a trial in which a brief structured home-based intervention with adolescents who had self-poisoned and their families was compared with treatment as usual, after treatment the nondepressed adolescents in the home-based group had less suicidal ideation than controls, but the home-based intervention was no more effective for depressed adolescents (Harrington *et al.*, 2000).

Group therapy
Group therapy approaches are often used in child and adolescent mental health services. In a preliminary trial in the United Kingdom in which 63 adolescents with a history of repeated self-harm were assigned to group therapy plus treatment as usual (TAU) or TAU only, although there was no apparent effect on depression, group attendees were less likely to repeat self-harm, used fewer routine services and had better school attendance than those who received TAU (Wood *et al.*, 2001). In a similar study in Australia, however, adolescents assigned to the group therapy condition actually repeated self-harm more than those in the control group (Hazell *et al.*, 2009). Finally, in an elegant large-scale trial in the United Kingdom, no differences in outcome were found on a range of measures between those assigned to group therapy plus TAU compared to those in the TAU group (Green *et al.*, 2011). The contradictory results of the first two studies and the definitive negative findings in the much larger third trial probably indicate that group therapy is not a useful approach in this population.

Dialectical behavior therapy
Dialectical behavior therapy (DBT) is a therapeutic approach that focuses on the management of emotional states and interpersonal relationships and which was originally developed for adults with borderline personality disorder and repetitive self-harm. There is growing interest in using this approach in briefer format with adolescents who are multiple repeaters of self-harm, with promising initial results (James *et al.*, 2008).

Hospitalization
The decision to treat adolescents following self-harm in an in-patient setting is usually based on risk of further self-harm and suicide, and severity of psychiatric disorder (Olfson *et al.*, 2005). It may also be influenced by other factors including concerns about litigation, characteristics of the individual and their family (Spooren *et al.*, 1997), the experience and training of the mental health clinician (Morrissey *et al.*, 1995), and the availability of in-patient beds.

However, there is no evidence to suggest that hospitalization prevents young people, particularly those with prior self-harm, mood disorder, and substance abuse, from future self-harm or dying by suicide (Gould *et al.*, 2003). Furthermore, prior hospitalization for any injury, not just self-harm, is associated with increased risk of suicidal behaviors (Agerbo *et al.*, 2002; Bridge *et al.*, 2006), although this may be related to severity of psychopathology and other risk factors.

Two studies have attempted to address these issues. In the first, conducted in the United States, 289 adolescents were randomly allocated to receive social network intervention plus TAU, or TAU alone, following psychiatric hospitalization. There was a reduction in suicidal ideation and parent-reported functional impairment at 6 months follow-up in those assigned to social network intervention, but no effects on repetition of self-harm or emotional symptoms (King *et al.*, 2006). In the second study, 286 adolescents were assigned to rapid response outpatient follow-up or TAU following presentation to an emergency department in Canada. The results showed psychiatric hospitalizations can be prevented using the rapid response model of care (Greenfield *et al.*, 2002).

Treatments for adolescents with specific psychiatric disorders

Further information about reducing suicidality in adolescents comes from studies of treatment focused specifically on individuals with psychiatric disorders.

Medication

Chapter 63 reviews the debate about the use of antidepressant medications in the treatment of children and adolescents with depression and the question of whether selective serotonin reuptake inhibitors (SSRIs) increase the risk of suicidal behaviors in some young people. It supports the position of the American Academy of Child and Adolescent Psychiatry that SSRIs should be available for selected cases. There do not appear to have been any trials in which medication has been evaluated in the treatment of adolescents who have self-harmed.

Cognitive behavior therapy combined with antidepressant

Cognitive behavior therapy (CBT) is the principal treatment for adolescent depression and affective disorders and targets depressive thoughts and behavior patterns (see Chapters 38 and 63). In a large randomized controlled trial, 439 patients aged 12–17 with major depressive disorder (MDD) were randomly allocated to one of four treatment conditions, each lasting 12 weeks: (i) Fluoxetine alone; (ii) CBT alone; (iii) CBT with fluoxetine; or (iv) Placebo. The CBT treatment consisted of 15×1 hour sessions. Patients treated in all conditions showed a reduction in suicide ideation across the trial, those treated with CBT plus fluoxetine showing the greatest improvement (March *et al.*, 2004). However, in two similar trials, CBT combined with an SSRI antidepressant was not superior to the antidepressant alone with regard to suicidality (Melvin *et al.*, 2006; Goodyer *et al.*, 2007).

Multisystemic therapy

Multisystemic therapy (MST) was developed to treat delinquent youth, targeting the systems in which the young people live. MST includes parenting skills, family therapy and educational attainment. In a randomized controlled trial, young people aged 10–17 were assigned to MST or hospitalization following a psychiatric emergency. MST was significantly more effective in reducing youth-reported repetition of suicide attempts (Huey *et al.*, 2004).

Issues of access to treatment and engagement in treatment

Whereas many adolescents may be offered care following an episode of self-harm, only small proportions are successfully engaged in ongoing treatment. Treatment retention for nonhospitalized adolescents is generally below 50% (Van Heeringen *et al.*, 1995; Brent, 1997), and can be as low as 20%, with significant and rapid dropout from treatment (King *et al.*, 1997).

Several studies have investigated mechanisms to improve effectiveness of treatment, including green-card passes to admission to hospital (Cotgrove *et al.*, 1995), enhanced emergency department protocols (Rotheram-Borus *et al.*, 2000; Spirito, 2002), enhanced CBT interventions (Rotheram-Borus *et al.*, 1994), and skills-based interventions (Donaldson *et al.*, 2005). However, to date such efforts have largely been unsuccessful and new therapeutic approaches need to be developed and evaluated (Burns *et al.*, 2005; Ougrin *et al.*, 2012).

Many young people who engage in self-harm do not seek help for their problems. If they do, it is most likely to be from friends and family rather than professionals (De Leo and Heller, 2004; Hawton *et al.*, 2006). There are also gender differences, with distressed young men being less likely to seek help of any kind and those who seek help from their general practitioner (GP) showing more severe symptoms than their female counterparts when they do (Biddle *et al.*, 2004). High school students at highest risk of suicide were found to be more likely to endorse isolative coping strategies such as believing you should be able to sort out your problems on your own and less likely to endorse strategies such as getting advice from friends (Gould *et al.*, 2004).

Prevention of self-harm and suicide by children and adolescents

Approaches to prevention can be divided into those measures that focus on a specific group, for example those with depression (at-risk populations), or measures that target all young people (population-based measures).

School-based interventions

School-based interventions take different forms, including skills-training, gatekeeper training, and screening programs, as well as whole-school approaches (Lake & Gould, 2011). Prevention programs that are aimed at students as helpers, not as victims, are based on evidence that adolescents turn to their peers for support rather than discussing their problems with adults (Beautrais *et al.*, 1998; Hawton *et al.*, 2006). This approach often raises concerns that not all peer confidants communicate with adults about friends whose problems cause them particular concern (Bennett *et al.*, 2003) and that young males in particular do not respond to troubled peers in helpful ways (Kalafat *et al.*, 1993; Hazell & King, 1996). In recent years, there has been growth in skills-based programs in schools, targeting the development of problem solving, coping, and cognitive skills (Gould *et al.*, 2003). Such classroom-based training offers some promise, as it has been associated with improved coping with distress and a reduction in suicide ideation (Thompson *et al.*, 2001), but caution is required as it may be associated with reduced school connectedness and increased high-risk behaviors (Cho *et al.*, 2005). Culturally specific skills-based interventions have also been developed (Lafromboise & Lewis, 2008). A school-based gatekeeper training program in the United States called Signs of Suicide showed fewer suicide attempts in the intervention group compared with controls, and a modest improvement in students' knowledge and attitudes about depression and suicide. However, no improvement in help-seeking was observed (Aseltine & DeMartino, 2004; Aseltine *et al.*, 2007). A randomized controlled trial of a school-based depression prevention program also showed positive results (Merry *et al.*, 2004).

Case-finding strategies have been employed in some schools, particularly in the United States, in an effort to reduce suicide by early detection of young people at high risk (Scott *et al.*, 2010). Although there is some evidence that screening programs can be effective at identifying at-risk young people (Scott *et al.*, 2009), they place considerable burden on school resources, yield false positives, and given the fluctuating nature of suicidal ideation, one-off screening can also give rise to false negatives (Lake and Gould, 2011; Hawton *et al.*, 2012c). Engagement in treatment following identification remains a significant issue (Shaffer & Craft, 1999; Shaffer & Pfeffer, 2001). Data from the Colombia Teen Screen program indicates that 19% of "at risk" young people refused a referral, 25% did not attend the first appointment, and 17% attended one session only (Shaffer, 2003). There are also difficulties with some schools accepting this approach for various reasons, including lack of staff resources and concerns that asking students about suicide will give them ideas about harming themselves. However, in a randomized controlled trial, depressed adolescents and previous attempters reported lower levels of distress and suicidality following a screening questionnaire that included specific questions about suicidal behaviors compared with their counterparts who were not asked those questions. This study also demonstrated that asking about suicide does not "put the idea into a young person's head" for those who would not ordinarily be thinking about this issue (Gould *et al.*, 2005). Finally, whole-school approaches are likely to be important as they "set the tone" for a school, and

they can change the school ethos around mental health but, as yet, their effect on reducing suicide is yet to be established. An obvious difficulty with any school-based program is the fact that high-risk individuals, particularly school dropouts and those with high rates of absenteeism, will not be reached using this approach (Burns & Patton, 2000).

Reducing access to methods of suicide

The strategy of restricting access by the general population to certain methods of suicide is a widely practiced public health initiative and an effective method of preventing suicide (Hawton, 2005).

In most studies, this results in an overall reduction in suicide deaths. Methods of suicide used by young people vary significantly across different countries. Where self-poisoning with medication is common, reducing availability through restricting pack sizes may be effective (Hawton *et al.*, 2013a). Restricting access to firearms has been a significant focus of suicide prevention in the United States (Brent, 2001), Austria (Etzersdorfer *et al.*, 1992), and Canada (Littman, 1983). Because of the extensive problem of suicide by pesticide ingestion in rural areas of developing countries, prevention of suicide by safer storage of products is also receiving attention (Pearson *et al.*, 2011).

Crisis centers and hotlines

Crisis centers and hotlines offering direct counseling or links to mental health services are conceptually popular. Overall, research suggests that such services tend to be used by young White females, with less impact on young men (de Anda & Smith, 1993). In one US study, high school students had more negative attitudes toward hotlines when compared to other formal sources of help (Gould *et al.*, 2006). The most common reasons for nonuse related to feelings of self-reliance and shame. Beautrais *et al.* (1998) reported that 14% of serious suicide attempters had used a telephone crisis line in the year prior to their attempt. There is little evidence of beneficial effects on rates of suicide (Burns & Paton, 2000), although this would be difficult to demonstrate.

Internet sources of help

Because of the hugely increased use of the Internet and other electronic means of communication, especially by young people, attention is focusing on the use of the Internet, social media, and mobile phones as means of providing help for distressed adolescents (Pirkis & Norderntoft, 2011). While this method of help provision is in its infancy, it is likely to be a major source of support and help for young people in the future, including those not in contact with clinical services.

In view of the negative influences of the Internet and other media, voluntary national guidelines for media reporting have been formulated. Website optimization, whereby sites committed to provision of help appear high on sites accessed in relation to distress or suicidal ideation, may be helpful. National governments need to continue to work with Internet service providers to this end.

Conclusions, future clinical and research directions

In recent years, considerable advances have been made in understanding the prevalence, causes, and course of adolescent suicidal behavior and self-harm. There is general consensus that good clinical management requires a comprehensive and compassionate approach to clinical assessment and this assessment should take into consideration psychiatric, psychological, social, and cultural factors. Despite the welcome advances in identifying those at risk, a number of clinical and research challenges remain. The evidence base in respect of what works to reduce self-harm or prevent suicide remains weak. Moreover, little is known about how best to respond to different subgroups of young people at risk (e.g., those with high vs low suicidal intent). Also, given the growth of new media and the powerful effect of such social influences on the enactment of all forms of self-harm, a more in-depth understanding of how these factors increase the occurrence of self-harm and suicide is urgently required.

Acknowledgment

The authors thank Sarah Fortune for her very substantial contribution to the preparation of this chapter in the previous edition of the book.

References

Aaron, R. *et al.* (2004) Suicides in young people in rural southern India. *Lancet* **363**, 1117–1118.

Ackard, D.M. *et al.* (2006) Parent-child connectedness and behavioral and emotional health among adolescents. *American Journal of Preventive Medicine* **30**, 59–66.

Adolescent Health Research Group (2005) *New Zealand Youth: A Profile of Their Health and Wellbeing: Maori Report*. University of Auckland, Auckland.

Agerbo, E. *et al.* (2002) Familial, psychiatric, and socioeconomic risk factors for suicide in young people: nested case-control study. *British Medical Journal* **325**, 74.

American Academy of Child & Adolescent Psychiatry (2001) Summary of the practice parameters for the assessment and treatment of children and adolescents with suicidal behavior. *Journal of the American Academy of Child and Adolescent Psychiatry* **40**, 495–499.

American Psychiatric Association (2013) *Diagnostic and Statistical Manual of Mental Disorders*, 5th edn. American Psychiatric Association, Washington, DC.

Apter, A. & Freudenstein, O. (2000) Adolescent suicidal behaviour: psychiatric population. In: *The International Handbook of Suicide and Attempted Suicide*. (eds K. Hawton & C. Van Heeringen). John Wiley & Sons, Chichester.

Arie, M. *et al.*, (2008) Autobiographical memory, interpersonal problem solving, and suicidal behavior in adolescent inpatients. *Comprehensive Psychiatry* **49**, 22–9.

Asberg, M. and Forslund, K. (2000) Neurobiological aspects of suicide behaviour. *International Review of Psychiatry* **12**, 62–74.

Aseltine, R.H. Jr. & Demartino, R. (2004) An outcome evaluation of the SOS Suicide Prevention Program. *American Journal of Public Health* **94**, 446–451.

Aseltine, R.H. Jr. *et al.* (2007) Evaluating the SOS suicide prevention program: a replication and extension. *BMC Public Health* **7**, 161.

Balazs, J. *et al.* (2013) Adolescent subthreshold-depression and anxiety: psychopathology, functional impairment and increased suicide risk. *Journal of Child Psychology and Psychiatry* **54**, 670–677.

Beautrais, A.L. (2001) Suicides and serious suicide attempts: two populations or one? *Psychological Medicine* **31**, 837–845.

Beautrais, A. (2003) Suicide in New Zealand II: a review of risk factors and prevention. *New Zealand Medical Journal* **116**, U461.

Beautrais, A.L. *et al.* (1996) Risk factors for serious suicide attempts among youths aged 13 through 24 years. *Journal of the American Academy of Child and Adolescent Psychiatry* **35**, 1174–1182.

Beautrais, A.L. *et al.* (1998) Psychiatric illness in a New Zealand sample of young people making serious suicide attempts. *New Zealand Medical Journal* **111**, 44–8.

Bennett, S. *et al.* (2003) Problematising depression: young people, mental health and suicidal behaviours. *Social Science and Medicine* **57**, 289–299.

Bergen, H. *et al.* (2010) Psychosocial assessment and repetition of self-harm: the significance of single and multiple repeat episode analyses. *Journal of Affective Disorders* **127**, 257–265.

Bhugra, D. & Bhui, K. (2007) *Textbook of Cultural Psychiatry*. Cambridge University Press, Cambridge.

Biddle, L. *et al.* (2004) Factors influencing help seeking in mentally distressed young adults: a cross-sectional survey. *British Journal of General Practice* **54**, 248–253.

Biddle, L. *et al.* (2008) Suicide and the internet. *British Medical Journal* **336**, 800–802.

Biddle, L. *et al.* (2013) Information sources used by the suicidal to inform choice of method. *Journal of Affective Disorders* **136**, 702–709.

Bingham, C.R. *et al.* (1994) An analysis of age, gender and racial differences in recent national trends of youth suicide. *Journal of Adolescence* **17**, 53–71.

Blakemore, S.J. (2008) The social brain in adolescence. *Nature Reviews Neuroscience* **9**, 267–277.

Bondy, B. *et al.* (2006) Genetics of suicide. *Molecular Psychiatry* **11**, 336–351.

Brausch, A.M. & Gutierrez, P.M. (2009) The role of body image and disordered eating as risk factors for depression and suicidal ideation in adolescents. *Suicide and Life-Threatening Behavior* **39**, 58–71.

Brent, D.A. *et al.* (1994) Familial risk factors for adolescent suicide: a case-control study. *Acta Psychiatrica Scandinavica* **89**, 52–8.

Brent, D. (1997) The aftercare of adolescents with deliberate self-harm. *Journal of Child Psychology & Allied Disciplines* **38**, 277–286.

Brent, D. (2001) Firearms and suicide. *Annals of the New York Academy of Sciences* **932**, 225–240.

Brent, D.A. & Mann, J.J. (2005) Family genetic studies, suicide, and suicidal behavior. *American Journal of Medical Genetics Part C: Seminars in Medical Genetics* **133C**, 13–24.

Brent, D.A. *et al.* (1991) The presence and accessibility of firearms in the homes of adolescent suicides. A case-control study. *JAMA* **266**, 2989–2995.

Brent, D. *et al.* (1996) A test of the diathesis stress model of adolescent depression in friends and acquaintances of adolescent suicide victims. In: *Severe Stress and Mental Disturbance of Children.* American Psychiatric Association, Washington, DC.

Brent, D.A. *et al.* (2002) Familial pathways to early-onset suicide attempt: risk for suicidal behavior in offspring of mood-disordered suicide attempters. *Archives of General Psychiatry* **59**, 801–807.

Bridge, J.A. *et al.* (2006) Adolescent suicide and suicidal behavior. *Journal of Child Psychology and Psychiatry* **47**, 372–394.

Bridge, J.A. *et al.* (2012) Impaired decision making in adolescent suicide attempters. *Journal of the American Academy of Child and Adolescent Psychiatry* **51**, 394–403.

Brunstein Klomek, A. *et al.* (2010) The association of suicide and bullying in childhood to young adulthood: a review of cross-sectional and longitudinal research findings. *Canadian Journal of Psychiatry* **55**, 282–288.

Burgess, S. *et al.* (1998) Adolescents who take overdoses: outcome in terms of changes in psychopathology and the adolescents' attitudes to care and to their overdose. *Journal of Adolescence* **21**, 209–218.

Burns, J.M. & Patton, G.C. (2000) Preventive interventions for youth suicide: a risk factor-based approach. *The Australian and New Zealand Journal of Psychiatry* **34**, 388–407.

Burns, J. *et al.* (2005) Clinical management of deliberate self-harm in young people: the need for evidence-based approaches to reduce repetition. *The Australian and New Zealand Journal of Psychiatry* **39**, 121–128.

Canino, G. & Roberts, R.E. (2001) Suicidal behavior among Latino youth. *Suicide and Life-Threatening Behavior* **31**, 122–131.

Cavanagh, J.T. *et al.* (2003) Psychological autopsy studies of suicide: a systematic review. *Psychological Medicine* **33**, 395–405.

Centre for Disease Control and Prevention (2010) Youth risk behaviour surveillance - United States, Pfeffer, CR 2009. In: *Surveillance Summaries.*

Challis, S. *et al.* (2013) Systematic meta-analysis of the risk factors for deliberate self-harm before and after treatment for first-episode psychosis. *Acta Psychiatrica Scandinavica* **127**, 442–454.

Chang, S.-S. *et al.* (2013) Impact of 2008 global economic crisis on suicide: time: trend study in 54 countries. *British Medical Journal* **347**, f5239.

Cho, H. *et al.* (2005) Evaluation of a high school peer group intervention for at-risk youth. *Journal of Abnormal Child Psychology* **33**, 363–374.

Collings, S.C. *et al.* (2011) *Media Influences on Suicidal Behaviour: An Interview Study of Young People in New Zealand.* National Centre of Mental Health Research, Information and Development, Auckland.

Cotgrove, A. *et al.* (1995) Secondary prevention of attempted suicide in adolescence. *Journal of Adolescence* **18**, 569–577.

Daine, K. *et al.* (2013) The power of the web: a systematic review of studies of the influence of the internet on self-harm and suicide in young people. *PLoS ONE* **8**, e77555.

Dancyger, I.F. & Fornari, V.M. (2005) A review of eating disorders and suicide risk in adolescence. *Scientific World Journal* **5**, 803–811.

Daniel, S.S. *et al.* (2006) Suicidality, school dropout, and reading problems among adolescents. *Journal of Learning Disabilities* **39**, 507–514.

De Anda, D. & Smith, M.A. (1993) Differences among adolescent, young adult and adult callers of suicide help lines. *Social Work* **181**, 421–428.

De Leo, D. & Heller, T.S. (2004) Who are the kids who self-harm? An Australian self-report school survey. *Medical Journal of Australia* **181**, 140–144.

Denny, S.J. *et al.* (2003) Comparison of health-risk behaviours among students in alternative high schools from New Zealand and the USA. *Journal of Paediatrics and Child Health* **39**, 33–39.

Donald, M. *et al.* (2006) Risk and protective factors for medically serious suicide attempts: a comparison of hospital-based with population-based samples of young adults. *The Australian and New Zealand Journal of Psychiatry* **40**, 87–96.

Donaldson, D. *et al.* (2005) Treatment for adolescents following a suicide attempt: results of a pilot trial. *Journal of the American Academy of Child and Adolescent Psychiatry* **44**, 113–120.

Dower, J. *et al.* (2000) *Pathways to Care for Young People Who Present with Non-Fatal Deliberate Self-Harm.* School of Population Health, University of Queensland, Queensland.

Dunlop, S.M. *et al.* (2011) Where do youth learn about suicides on the Internet, and what influence does this have on suicidal ideation? *Journal of Child Psychology and Psychiatry* **52**, 1073–1080.

Dunn, V. & Goodyer, I.M. (2006) Longitudinal investigation into childhood- and adolescence-onset depression: psychiatric outcome in early adulthood. *British Journal of Psychiatry* **188**, 216–222.

Eddleston, M. *et al.* (2005a) Differences between organophosphorus insecticides in human self-poisoning: a prospective cohort study. *The Lancet* **366**, 1452–1459.

Eddleston, M. *et al.* (2005b) Epidemiology of intentional self-poisoning in rural Sri Lanka. *British Journal of Psychiatry* **187**, 583–584.

Esposito-Smythers, C. *et al.* (2010) Clinical and psychosocial correlates of non-suicidal self-injury within a sample of children and adolescents with bipolar disorder. *Journal of Affective Disorders* **125**, 89–97.

Etzersdorfer, E. *et al.* (1992) Newspaper reports and suicide. *New England Journal of Medicine* **327**, 502–503.

Evans, E. *et al.* (2004) Factors associated with suicidal phenomena in adolescents: a systematic review of population-based studies. *Clinical Psychology Review* **24**, 957–979.

Evans, E. *et al.* (2005a) Suicidal phenomena and abuse in adolescents: a review of epidemiological studies. *Child Abuse and Neglect* **29**, 45–58.

Evans, E. *et al.* (2005b) The prevalence of suicidal phenomena in adolescents: a systematic review of population-based studies. *Suicide and Life-Threatening Behavior* **35**, 239–250.

Fazel, M. *et al.* (2005) Prevalence of serious mental disorder in 7000 refugees resettled in western countries: a systematic review. *The Lancet* **365**, 1309–1314.

Fergusson, D.M. & Lynskey, M.T. (1995) Childhood circumstances, adolescent adjustment, and suicide attempts in a New Zealand birth cohort. *Journal of the American Academy of Child and Adolescent Psychiatry* **34**, 612–622.

Fergusson, D.M. *et al.* (2000) Risk factors and life processes associated with the onset of suicidal behaviour during adolescence and early adulthood. *Psychological Medicine* **30**, 23–39.

Fortune, S. *et al.* (2007) Suicide in adolescents: using life charts to understand the suicidal process. *Journal of Affective Disorders* **100**, 199–210.

Freedenthal, S. & Stiffman, A.R. (2007) "They might think I am crazy" Young American Indians' reasons for not seeking help. *Journal of Adolescent Research* **22**, 58–77.

Friedman, T. *et al.* (2006) Predictors of A&E staff attitudes to self-harm patients who use self-laceration: influence of previous training and experience. *Journal of Psychosomatic Research* **60**, 273–277.

Gibb, S.J. *et al.* (2005) Mortality and further suicidal behaviour after an index suicide attempt: a 10-year study. *The Australian and New Zealand Journal of Psychiatry* **39**, 95–100.

Goldacre, M. and Hawton, K. (1985) Repetition of self-poisoning and subsequent death in adolescents who take overdoses. *British Journal of Psychiatry*, **146**, 395–398.

Goldstein, T.R. *et al.* (2012) Predictors of prospectively examined suicide attempts among youth with bipolar disorder. *Archives of General Psychiatry* **69**, 1113–1122.

Goldston, D.B. *et al.* (2008) Cultural considerations in adolescent suicide prevention and psychosocial treatment. *American Psychologist* **63**, 14–31.

Gomez, J. *et al.* (2011) Acculturative stress, perceived discrimination, and vulnerability to suicide attempts among emerging adults. *Journal of Youth and Adolescence* **40**, 1465–1476.

Goodyer, I. *et al.* (2007) Selective serotonin reuptake inhibitors (SSRIs) and routine specialist care with and without cognitive behaviour therapy in adolescents with major depression: randomised controlled trial. *British Medical Journal* **335**, 142.

Goosen, S. *et al.* (2011) Suicide death and hospital-treated suicidal behaviour in asylum seekers in the Netherlands: a national registry-based study. *BMC Public Health* **11**, 484.

Gosney, H. & Hawton, K. (2007) Inquest verdicts: youth suicides lost. *Psychological Bulletin* **31**, 203–205.

Gould, M.S. *et al.* (1996) Psychosocial risk factors of child and adolescent completed suicide. *Archives of General Psychiatry* **53**, 1155–1162.

Gould, M.S. *et al.* (2003) Youth suicide risk and preventive interventions: a review of the past 10 years. *Journal of the American Academy of Child and Adolescent Psychiatry* **42**, 386–405.

Gould, M.S. *et al.* (2004) Teenagers' attitudes about coping strategies and help-seeking behavior for suicidality. *Journal of the American Academy of Child and Adolescent Psychiatry* **43**, 1124–1133.

Gould, M.S. *et al.* (2005) Evaluating iatrogenic risk of youth suicide screening programs: a randomized controlled trial. *JAMA* **293**, 1635–1643.

Gould, M.S. *et al.* (2006) Teenagers' attitudes about seeking help from telephone crisis services (hotlines). *Suicide and Life-Threatening Behavior* **36**, 601–613.

Green, J.M. *et al.* (2011) Group therapy for adolescents with repeated self harm: randomised controlled trial with economic evaluation. *British Medical Journal* **342**, d682.

Greenfield, B. *et al.* (2002) A rapid-response outpatient model for reducing hospitalization rates among suicidal adolescents. *Psychiatric Services* **53**, 1574–1579.

Groholt, B. & Ekeberg, O. (2009) Prognosis after adolescent suicide attempt: mental health, psychiatric treatment, and suicide attempts in a nine-year follow-up study. *Suicide and Life-Threatening Behavior* **39**, 125–136.

Haas, A.P. *et al.* (2011) Suicide and suicide risk in lesbian, gay, bisexual, and transgender populations: review and recommendations. *Journal of Homosexuality* **58**, 10–51.

Hall-Lande, J.A. *et al.* (2007) Social isolation, psychological health, and protective factors in adolescence. *Adolescence* **42**, 265–286.

Hamza, C.A. *et al.* (2012) Examining the link between nonsuicidal self-injury and suicidal behavior: a review of the literature and an integrated model. *Clinical Psychology Review* **32**, 482–495.

Harrington, R. *et al.* (1998) Randomized trial of a home-based family intervention for children who have deliberately poisoned themselves. *Journal of the American Academy of Child and Adolescent Psychiatry* **37**, 512–518.

Harrington, R. *et al.* (2000) Deliberate self-poisoning in adolescence: why does a brief family intervention work in some cases and not others? *Journal of Adolescence* **23**, 13–20.

Harrington, R. *et al.* (2006) Early adult outcomes of adolescents who deliberately poisoned themselves. *Journal of the American Academy of Child and Adolescent Psychiatry* **45**, 337–345.

Harvey, S.B. *et al.* (2008) Self-harm in first-episode psychosis. *British Journal of Psychiatry* **192**, 178–184.

Haw, C. *et al.* (2013) Suicide clusters: a review of risk factors and mechanisms. *Suicide and Life-Threatening Behavior* **43**, 97–108.

Hawton, K. & Harriss, L. (2007) Deliberate self-harm in young people: characteristics and subsequent mortality in a 20-year cohort of patients presenting to hospital. *Journal of Clinical Psychiatry* **68**, 1574–1583.

Hawton, K. & Harriss, L. (2008) Deliberate self-harm by under 15-year olds: characteristics, trends and outcome. *Journal of Child Psychology and Psychiatry* **49**, 441–448.

Hawton, K. *et al.* (1982) Motivational aspects of deliberate self-poisoning in adolescents. *British Journal of Psychiatry* **141**, 286–291.

Hawton, K. *et al.* (1999a) Suicide in young people. Study of 174 cases, aged under 25 years, based on coroners' and medical records. *British Journal of Psychiatry* **175**, 271–276.

Hawton, K. *et al.* (1999b) Repetition of deliberate self-harm by adolescents: the role of psychological factors. *Journal of Adolescence* **22**, 369–378.

Hawton, K. *et al.* (2002) Deliberate self harm in adolescents: self report survey in schools in England. *BMJ* **325**, 1207–1211.

Hawton, K. *et al.* (2005) Schizophrenia and suicide: systematic review of risk factors. *British Journal of Psychiatry* **187**, 9–20.

Hawton, K. *et al.* (2006) *By Their Own Young Hand: Deliberate Self-Harm and Suicidal Ideas in Adolescents*. Jessica Kingsley, London.

Hawton, K. *et al.* (2010) How adolescents who cut themselves differ from those who take overdoses. *European Child and Adolescent Psychiatry* **19**, 513–523.

Hawton, K. *et al.* (2012a) Repetition of self-harm and suicide following self-harm in children and adolescents: findings from the Multicentre Study of Self-harm in England. *Journal of Child Psychology and Psychiatry* **53**, 1212–1219.

Hawton, K. *et al.* (2012b) Epidemiology and nature of self-harm in children and adolescents: findings from the multicentre study of self-harm in England. *European Child and Adolescent Psychiatry* **21**, 369–377.

Hawton, K. *et al.* (2012c) Self-harm and suicide in adolescents. *The Lancet* **379**, 2373–2382.

Hawton, K. *et al.* (2013a) Long term effect of reduced pack sizes of paracetamol on poisoning deaths and liver transplant activity in England and Wales: interrupted time series analyses. *BMJ* **346**, f403.

Hawton, K. *et al.* (2013b) Psychiatric disorders in patients presenting to hospital following self-harm: a systematic review. *Journal of Affective Disorders* **151**, 821–830.

Hazell, P. & King, R. (1996) Arguments for and against teaching suicide prevention in schools. *The Australian and New Zealand Journal of Psychiatry* **30**, 633–642.

Hazell, P.L. *et al.* (2009) Group therapy for repeated deliberate self-harm in adolescents: failure of replication of a randomized trial.

Journal of the American Academy of Child and Adolescent Psychiatry **48**, 662–670.

Hewitt, P.L. *et al.* (1997) Perfectionism and suicide ideation in adolescent psychiatric patients. *Journal of Abnormal Child Psychology* **25**, 95–101.

Houston, K. *et al.* (2001) Suicide in young people aged 15-24: a psychological autopsy study. *Journal of Affective Disorders* **63**, 159–170.

Huey, S.J. Jr. *et al.* (2004) Multisystemic therapy effects on attempted suicide by youths presenting psychiatric emergencies. *Journal of the American Academy of Child and Adolescent Psychiatry* **43**, 183–190.

Impey, M. & Heun, R. (2012) Completed suicide, ideation and attempt in attention deficit hyperactivity disorder. *Acta Psychiatrica Scandinavica* **125**, 93–102.

Isohookana, R. *et al.* (2013) Adverse childhood experiences and suicidal behavior of adolescent psychiatric inpatients. *European Child and Adolescent Psychiatry* **22**, 13–22.

James, A. *et al.* (2004) Attention deficit hyperactivity disorder and suicide: a review of possible associations. *Acta Psychiatrica Scandinavica* **110**, 408–415.

James, A.C. *et al.* (2008) A preliminary community study of dialectical behaviour therapy (DBT) with adolescent females demonstrating persistent deliberate self-harm (DSH). *Child and Adolescent Mental Health* **13**, 148–152.

Joe, S. & Kaplan, M.S. (2001) Suicide among African American men. *Suicide and Life-Threatening Behavior* **31**, 106–121.

Joiner, T. (2005) *Why People Die by Suicide.* Harvard University Press, Boston.

Kalafat, J. *et al.* (1993) The relationship of bystander intervention variables in adolescents' responses to suicidal peers. *Journal of Primary Prevention* **13**, 231–244.

Kapur, N. *et al.* (2013a) Non-suicidal self-injury v. attempted suicide: new diagnosis or false dichotomy? *British Journal of Psychiatry* **202**, 326–328.

Kapur, N. *et al.* (2013b) Does clinical management improve outcomes following self-harm? Results from the multicentre study of self-harm in England. *PLoS ONE* **8**, e70434.

Keller, A.S. *et al.* (2003) Mental health of detained asylum seekers. *The Lancet* **362**, 1721–1723.

Kienhorst, C.W. *et al.* (1992) Differences between adolescent suicide attempters and depressed adolescents. *Acta Psychiatrica Scandinavica* **85**, 222–228.

King, C.A. *et al.* (1997) Suicidal adolescents after hospitalization: parent and family impacts on treatment follow-through. *Journal of the American Academy of Child and Adolescent Psychiatry* **36**, 85–93.

King, C.A. *et al.* (2006) Youth-Nominated Support Team for Suicidal Adolescents (Version 1): a randomized controlled trial. *Journal of Consulting and Clinical Psychology* **74**, 199–206.

King, M. *et al.* (2008) A systematic review of mental disorder, suicide, and deliberate self harm in lesbian, gay and bisexual people. *BMC Psychiatry* **8**, 70.

Kirmayer, L.J. *et al.* (1996) Suicide attempts among Inuit youth: a community survey of prevalence and risk factors. *Acta Psychiatrica Scandinavica* **94**, 8–17.

Labelle, R. *et al.* (2013) Cognitive correlates of serious suicidal ideation in a community sample of adolescents. *Journal of Affective Disorders* **145**, 370–377.

Lafromboise, T.D. & Lewis, H.A. (2008) The Zuni Life Skills Development Program: a school/community-based suicide prevention intervention. *Suicide and Life-Threatening Behavior* **38**, 343–353.

Lake, A.M. & Gould, M.S. (2011) School-based strategies for youth suicide prevention. In: *International Handbook of Suicide Prevention.* (eds R.C. O'Connor, S. Platt & J. Gordon). Wiley-Blackwell. Oxford.

Lalwani, S. *et al.* (2004) Suicide among children and adolescents in South Delhi (1991-2000). *Indian Journal of Pediatrics* **71**, 701–703.

Langhinrichsen-Rohling, J. *et al.* (2009) Adolescent suicide, gender, and culture: a rate and risk factor analysis. *Aggression and Violent Behaviour* **14**, 402–414.

Lessard, J.C. & Moretti, M.M. (1998) Suicidal ideation in an adolescent clinical sample: attachment patterns and clinical implications. *Journal of Adolescence* **21**, 383–395.

Lewinsohn, P.M. *et al.* (2003) Bipolar disorders during adolescence. *Acta Psychiatrica Scandinavica. Supplementum* **418**, 47–50.

Lin, P.Y. & Tsai, G. (2004) Association between serotonin transporter gene promoter polymorphism and suicide: results of a meta-analysis. *Biological Psychiatry* **55**, 1023–1030.

Littman, S.K. (1983) *The Role of the Press in the Control of Suicide Epidemics.* International Association for Suicide Prevention and Crisis Intervention, Paris.

Madge, N. *et al.* (2008) Deliberate self-harm within an international community sample of young people: comparative findings from the Child & Adolescent Self-harm in Europe (CASE) Study. *Journal of Child Psychology and Psychiatry* **49**, 667–677.

Madge, N. *et al.* (2011) Psychological characteristics, stressful life events and deliberate self-harm: findings from the Child & Adolescent Self-harm in Europe (CASE) Study. *European Child and Adolescent Psychiatry* **20**, 499–508.

Mann, J.J. *et al.* (2001) The neurobiology and genetics of suicide and attempted suicide: a focus on the serotonergic system. *Neuropsychopharmacology* **24**, 467–77.

March, J. (2004) Fluoxetine, cognitive-behavioral therapy, and their combination for adolescents with depression: Treatment for Adolescents With Depression Study (TADS) randomized controlled trial. *JAMA* **292**, 807–20.

Marttunen, M.J. *et al.* (1993) Precipitant stressors in adolescent suicide. *Journal of the American Academy of Child and Adolescent Psychiatry* **32**, 1178–1183.

Marttunen, M.J. *et al.* (1994) Psychosocial stressors more common in adolescent suicides with alcohol abuse compared with depressive adolescent suicides. *Journal of the American Academy of Child and Adolescent Psychiatry* **33**, 490–497.

Marttunen, M.J. *et al.* (1998) Completed suicide among adolescents with no diagnosable psychiatric disorder. *Adolescence* **33**, 669–681.

Meltzer, H. *et al.* (2001) *Children Who try to Harm, Hurt or Kill Themselves.* Office of National Statistics, London.

Melvin, G.A. *et al.* (2006) A comparison of cognitive-behavioral therapy, sertraline, and their combination for adolescent depression. *Journal of the American Academy of Child and Adolescent Psychiatry* **45**, 1151–1161.

Merry, S. *et al.* (2004) A randomized placebo-controlled trial of a school-based depression prevention program. *Journal of the American Academy of Child and Adolescent Psychiatry* **43**, 538–547.

Ministry of Health (2005) *Suicide Facts: Provisional 2002 All-Ages Statistics.* Ministry of Health, Wellington.

Mishara, B.L. (1999) Conceptions of death and suicide in children ages 6-12 and their implications for suicide prevention. *Suicide and Life-Threatening Behavior* **29**, 105–118.

Mittendorfer-Rutz, E. *et al.* (2008) Familial clustering of suicidal behaviour and psychopathology in young suicide attempters. A register-based nested case control study. *Social Psychiatry and Psychiatric Epidemiology* **43**, 28–36.

Moran, P. *et al.* (2012) The natural history of self-harm from adolescence to young adulthood: a population-based cohort study. *The Lancet* **379**, 236–243.

Morrissey, R.F. *et al.* (1995) Hospitalizing the suicidal adolescent: an empirical investigation of decision-making criteria. *Journal of the American Academy of Child and Adolescent Psychiatry* **34**, 902–911.

National Collaborating Centre for Mental Health (2004) *Self-Harm: The Short-Term Physical and Psychological Management and Secondary Prevention of Self-Harm in Primary and Secondary Care (full guideline) Clinical Guideline 16*. London National Institute for Health and Care Excellence.

National Collaborating Centre for Mental Health (2011) *Self-Harm (Longer Term Management) (Clinical Guideline 133)*. National Institute for Health and Care Excellence, London.

Nicholas, J. *et al.* (2004) Help-seeking behaviour and the Internet: an investigation among Australian adolescents. *Australian e-Journal for the Advancement of Mental Health* [Online] (3. Available: www.auseinet.com/journal/vol3iss1/nicholas.pdf).

O'Connor, R.C. *et al.* (2013) Psychological processes and repeat suicidal behavior: a four year prospective study. *Journal of Consulting and Clinical Psychology* **81**, 1137–1143.

O'Connor, R.C. (2007) The relations between perfectionism and suicidality: a systematic review. *Suicide and Life-Threatening Behavior* **37**, 698–714.

O'Connor, R.C. (2011) Towards an integrated motivational-volitional model of suicidal behaviour. In: *International Handbook of Suicide Prevention*. (eds R.C. O'Connor, S. Platt & J. Gordon). Wiley-Blackwell, Oxford.

O'Connor, R.C. *et al.* (2009a) Predicting deliberate self-harm in adolescents: a six month prospective study. *Suicide and Life-Threatening Behavior* **39**, 364–375.

O'Connor, R.C. *et al.* (2009b) Self-harm in adolescents: self-report survey in schools in Scotland. *British Journal of Psychiatry* **194**, 68–72.

O'Connor, R.C. *et al.* (2012) Distinguishing adolescents who think about self-harm from those who engage in self-harm. *British Journal of Psychiatry* **200**, 330–335.

Olfson, M. *et al.* (2005) Emergency treatment of young people following deliberate self-harm. *Archives of General Psychiatry* **62**, 1122–1128.

Ougrin, D. *et al.* (2010) *Self-Harm in Young People. A Therapeutic Assessment Manual*. Hodder Arnold, London.

Ougrin, D. *et al.* (2011) Trial of Therapeutic Assessment in London: randomised controlled trial of Therapeutic Assessment versus standard psychosocial assessment in adolescents presenting with self-harm. *Archives of Disease in Childhood* **96**, 148–153.

Ougrin, D. *et al.* (2012) Practitioner review: self-harm in adolescents. *Journal of Child Psychology and Psychiatry* **53**, 337–350.

Patton, G.C. *et al.* (2007) Pubertal stage and deliberate self-harm in adolescents. *Journal of the American Academy of Child and Adolescent Psychiatry* **46**, 508–514.

Pearson, M. *et al.* (2011) A community-based cluster randomised trial of safe storage to reduce pesticide self-poisoning in rural Sri Lanka: study protocol. *BMC Public Health* **11**, 879.

Perez-Fuentes, G. *et al.* (2013) Prevalence and correlates of child sexual abuse: a national study. *Comprehensive Psychiatry* **54**, 16–27.

Petersen, L. *et al.* (2013) Genetic and familial environmental effects on suicide—an adoption study of siblings. *PLoS ONE* **8** (10), e77973.

Pfeffer, C.R. (2000) Suicidal behaviour in children: am emphasis on developmental influences. In: *The International Handbook of Suicide and Attempted Suicide* (eds K. Hawton & C. Van Heeringen). John Wiley & Sons, Chichester.

Pirkis, J. & Norderntoft, M. (2011) Media influences on suicide and attempted suicide. In: *International Handbook of Suicide Prevention*. (eds R.C. O'Connor, S. Platt & J. Gordon). Wiley-Blackwell, Oxford.

Portzky, G. *et al.* (2005) Suicide among adolescents. A psychological autopsy study of psychiatric, psychosocial and personality-related risk factors. *Social Psychiatry and Psychiatric Epidemiology* **40**, 922–930.

Power, L. *et al.* (2009) A pilot study evaluating a support programme for parents of young people with suicidal behaviour. *Child and Adolescent Psychiatry and Mental Health* **3**, 20.

Prasad, J. *et al.* (2006) Rates and factors associated with suicide in Kaniyambadi Block, Tamil Nadu, South India, 2000–2002. *International Journal of Social Psychiatry* **52**, 65–71.

Rodham, K. *et al.* (2004) Reasons for deliberate self-harm: comparison of self-poisoners and self-cutters in a community sample of adolescents. *Journal of the American Academy of Child and Adolescent Psychiatry* **43**, 80–87.

Rotheram-Borus, M.J. *et al.* (1994) Brief cognitive-behavioral treatment for adolescent suicide attempters and their families. *Journal of the American Academy of Child and Adolescent Psychiatry* **33**, 508–517.

Rotheram-Borus, M.J. *et al.* (1996) Enhancing treatment adherence with a specialized emergency room program for adolescent suicide attempters. *Journal of the American Academy of Child and Adolescent Psychiatry* **35**, 654–663.

Rotheram-Borus, M.J. *et al.* (2000) The 18-month impact of an emergency room intervention for adolescent female suicide attempters. *Journal of Consulting and Clinical Psychology* **68**, 1081–1093.

Roxborough, H. *et al.* (2012) Perfectionistic self-presentation, socially prescribed perfectionism, and suicide in youth: a test of the perfectionism social disconnection model. *Suicide and Life-Threatening Behavior* **42**, 217–233.

Roy, A. *et al.* (1993) Genetic and biologic risk factors for suicide in depressive disorders. *Psychiatric Quarterly* **64**, 345–358.

Roy, A. *et al.* (1997) Genetics of suicides. Family studies and molecular genetics. *Annals of the New York Academy of Sciences* **836**, 135–157.

Rudd, M.D. *et al.* (2004) Childhood diagnoses and later risk for multiple suicide attempts. *Suicide and Life-Threatening Behavior* **34**, 113–125.

Sadowski, C., & Kelley, M.L. (1993) Social problem solving in suicidal adolescents. *Journal of Consulting and Clinical Psychology* **61**, 121.

Saunders, K.E. *et al.* (2012) Attitudes and knowledge of clinical staff regarding people who self-harm: a systematic review. *Journal of Affective Disorders* **139**, 205–216.

Schmidtke, A. & Hafner, H. (1988) The Werther effect after television films: new evidence for an old hypothesis. *Psychological Medicine* **18**, 665–676.

Scott, M.A. *et al.* (2009) School-based screening to identify at-risk students not already known to school professionals: the Columbia suicide screen. *American Journal of Public Health* **99**, 334–339.

Scott, M. *et al.* (2010) School-based screening for suicide risk: balancing costs and benefits. *American Journal of Public Health* **100**, 1648–1652.

Shaffer, D. 2003. *Screening of children at risk in schools.* XXII World Congress of the International Association for Suicide Prevention. Stockholm, Sweden.

Shaffer, D. & Craft, L. (1999) Methods of adolescent suicide prevention. *Journal of Clinical Psychiatry* **60**, 70–74; discussion 75–76, 113–116.

Shaffer, D. & Pfeffer, C.R. (2001) Practice parameter for the assessment and treatment of children and adolescents with suicidal behaviour. *Journal of American Academy of Child and Adolescent Psychiatry* **40**, 49–499.

Sourander, A. *et al.* (2006a) Early predictors of deliberate self-harm among adolescents. A prospective follow-up study from age 3 to age 15. *Journal of Affective Disorders* **93**, 87–96.

Sourander, A. *et al.* (2006b) Early predictors of parent- and self-reported perceived global psychological difficulties among adolescents: a prospective cohort study from age 3 to age 15. *Social Psychiatry and Psychiatric Epidemiology* **41**, 173–182.

Speckens, A.E.M. & Hawton, K. (2005) Social problem-solving in adolescents with suicidal behaviour: a systematic review. *Suicide and Life-Threatening Behavior* **35**, 365–387.

Spirito, A. (2002) Group treatment plus usual care decreased the risk of deliberate self harm in adolescents who repeatedly harm themselves. *Evidence-Based Mental Health* **5**, 55.

Spooren, D. *et al.* (1997) Short-term outcome following referral to a psychiatric emergency service. *Crisis* **18**, 80–85.

Stack, S. (2003) Media coverage as a risk factor in suicide. *Journal of Epidemiology and Community Health* **57**, 238–240.

Strober, M. *et al.* (1995) Recovery and relapse in adolescents with bipolar affective illness: a five-year naturalistic, prospective follow-up. *Journal of the American Academy of Child and Adolescent Psychiatry* **34**, 724–731.

Sultan, A. & O'Sullivan, K. (2001) Psychological disturbances in asylum seekers held in long term detention: a participant-observer account. *Medical Journal of Australia* **175**, 593–596.

Suominen, K. *et al.* (2004) Health care contacts before and after attempted suicide among adolescent and young adult versus older suicide attempters. *Psychological Medicine* **34**, 313–321.

Suris, J.C. *et al.* (1996) Chronic illness and emotional distress in adolescence. *Journal of Adolescent Health* **19**, 153–156.

Tang, T.C. *et al.* (2009) Suicide and its association with individual, family, peer, and school factors in an adolescent population in southern Taiwan. *Suicide and Life-Threatening Behavior* **39**, 91–102.

Taliaferro, L.A. *et al.* (2012) Factors distinguishing youth who report self-injurious behavior: a population-based sample. *Academic Pediatrics* **12**, 205–13.

Tatz, C. (2001) *Aboriginal Suicide is Different. A Portrait of Life and Self-Destruction.* Australian Institute of Aboriginal and Torres Strait Islander Studies, Canberra.

The Office for National Statistics (2013). *Suicides in the United Kingdom, 2011,* http://www.ons.gov.uk/ons/rel/subnational-health4/suicides-in-the-united-kingdom/2011/stb-suicide-bulletin.html.

Thompson, E.A. *et al.* (2001) Evaluation of indicated suicide risk prevention approaches for potential high school dropouts. *American Journal of Public Health* **91**, 742–752.

Tidemalm, D. *et al.* (2011) Familial clustering of suicide risk: a total population study of 11.4 million individuals. *Psychological Medicine* **41**, 2527–2534.

US Department of Health and Human Services (2004). Health, United States 2004. Washington. http://www.cdc.gov/nchs/data/hus/hus04trend.pdf.

Van Heeringen, C. *et al.* (1995) The management of non-compliance with referral to out-patient after-care among attempted suicide patients: a controlled intervention study. *Psychological Medicine* **25**, 963–970.

Van Orden, K.A. *et al.* (2010) The interpersonal theory of suicide. *Psychological Review* **117**, 575–600.

Wagner, B.M. *et al.* (2000) Parents' reactions to adolescents' suicide attempts. *Journal of the American Academy of Child and Adolescent Psychiatry* **39**, 429–436.

Whitlock, J.L. *et al.* (2006) The virtual cutting edge: the internet and adolescent self-injury. *Developmental Psychology* **42**, 407–417.

Wilcox, H.C. *et al.* (2012) The interaction of parental history of suicidal behavior and exposure to adoptive parents' psychiatric disorders on adoptee suicide attempt hospitalizations. *The American Journal of Psychiatry* **169**, 309–315.

Williams, J.M.G. & Pollock, B.G. (2000) The psychology of suicidal behaviour. In: *The International Handbook of Suicide and Attempted Suicide.* (eds K. Hawton & C. Van Heeringen). John Wiley & Sons, Chichester.

Wood, A. *et al.* (2001) Randomized trial of group therapy for repeated deliberate self-harm in adolescents. *Journal of the American Academy of Child and Adolescent Psychiatry* **40**, 1246–1253.

World Health Organisation (1996) *Multiaxial Classification of Child and Adolescent Psychiatric Disorders: ICD-10 Classification of Mental and Behavioral Disorders in Children and Adolescents.* Cambridge University Press, New York.

World Health Organisation (2014) WHO Mortality Database. http://apps.who.int/healthinfo/statistics/mortality/whodpms/

Ybarra, M.L. *et al.* (2005) Depressive symptomatology, youth Internet use, and online interactions: a national survey. *Journal of Adolescent Health* **36**, 9–18.

Zane, N. & Mak, W. (2003) Major approaches to the measurement of acculturation among ethnic minority populations: a content analysis and alternative empirical strategy. In: *Acculturation. Advances in Theory, Measurement and Applied Research.* (eds K.M. Chun, P. Balls Organista & G. Marin). American Psychiatric Association.

CHAPTER 65

Oppositional and conduct disorders

Stephen Scott[1,2]

[1] Department of Child and Adolescent Psychiatry, Institute of Psychiatry, Psychology and Neuroscience, King's College London, UK
[2] National Conduct Problems and National Adoption and Fostering Services, Maudsley Hospital, London, UK

Introduction

Oppositional defiant and conduct disorders (ODD/CDs) are characterized by antisocial behaviors outside socially acceptable norms that violate other people's expectations or rights. The behaviors include excessive verbal and physical aggression, temper tantrums, lying and stealing, disobedience, rule breaking, and violence. As adults, many of these individuals continue to act antisocially, with substance misuse and criminality being common. The upset, disruption, and costs inflicted on the family, peer group, school, and wider society are usually considerable. However, perhaps because these behaviors are present in many children to some extent, are often related to a less than ideal upbringing, and may appear to reflect poor self-control in children who seem otherwise normal, ODD/CDs are still considered by some not to be "true" psychiatric disorders but more as character flaws, with the children being seen as nasty and bad. This is unfortunate for several reasons. First, in recent years there have been many exciting discoveries about what contributes to the development of ODD/CDs, with a substantial biological component involving genetic and brain differences becoming evident, so that in many cases the problems are not just due to poor socialization. Second, different subtypes of antisocial behavior are now better understood, with, for example, very different life trajectories for those who exhibit early versus later onset, and those who have callous-unemotional traits. Finally, there have been considerable advances in developing effective treatments not only for children but also for adolescents, who were previously often thought of as virtually untreatable. Now that we know more about the biological and social factors that cause ODD/CD, the seriousness of its consequences and cost, and that effective treatments are available, there is a strong case to be made that children suffering the condition do indeed suffer from a true psychiatric disorder and so deserve proper evaluation and effective treatment. See also Chapter 4.

In this chapter, the term *antisocial behavior* will be used as a broad overarching dimensional construct, with the term ODD/CD used to refer to the more severe end that meets diagnostic criteria; less severe difficulties may be called *conduct problems*. Outside psychiatry, many medical practitioners, mental health professionals, social workers, teachers, and the general public are not familiar with the terms ODD or CD, so that using expressions such as antisocial behavior or disruptive behavior may improve communication. The term externalizing is not used in this chapter since it connotes that an inner angst is being acted out, for which there is usually no evidence. The term children is used to cover both children and adolescents collectively.

Classification

Both ICD 10 and DSM-5 include ODD/CD which are characterized by a repetitive and persistent pattern of antisocial behavior; occasional isolated acts do not qualify. Oppositional Defiant Disorder is usually a diagnosis given to younger children, while Conduct Disorder is typically (but not exclusively) a diagnosis given to older children and teenagers. The criteria are almost identical in the two systems.

Oppositional Defiant Disorder requires four of the following eight symptoms below to be present for at least 6 months, in a manner that is outside a range that is developmentally normative: *angry and irritable mood:* has unusually frequent or severe temper tantrums; is often touchy or easily annoyed by others; is often angry or resentful; *argumentative and defiant behavior:* often argues with adults; often actively refuses to comply with adults' requests or defies rules; often deliberately does things to annoy other people; often blames others for his or her own mistakes or misbehavior; *vindictiveness:* is often spiteful or resentful. Both DSM-5 and ICD 10 include specifiers for degree (mild, moderate, or severe). ICD 10 allows up to 2 of 4 symptoms to

Rutter's Child and Adolescent Psychiatry, Sixth Edition.
Edited by Anita Thapar and Daniel S. Pine, James F. Leckman, Stephen Scott, Margaret J. Snowling, Eric Taylor.
© 2015 John Wiley & Sons Ltd. Published 2018 by John Wiley & Sons Ltd.

come from the CD list (below); unlike for CD, there is an impairment criterion: the symptoms must be maladaptive. In DSM-5, a diagnosis of CD no longer excludes ODD.

Conduct Disorder requires three of the following 15 criteria to have been manifest in the past 12 months: *aggression to people and animals:* frequently bullies others; frequently initiates physical fights; has used a weapon that can cause serious physical harm to others; exhibits physical cruelty to other people; exhibits physical cruelty to animals; commits a crime involving confrontation with the victim; forces another person into sexual activity; *destruction of property:* deliberately sets fires with a risk of causing serious damage; deliberately destroys the property of others; *deceitfulness or theft:* has broken into someone else's house, building, or car; often lies to obtain goods or favors or to avoid obligations; has stolen objects of value without confronting the victim; *serious violations of rules:* often stays out at night despite parental prohibitions, beginning before age 13; has run away from home at least twice; is frequently truant from school, beginning before 13 years of age. Both DSM-5 and ICD 10 include specifiers for child or adolescent onset and degree (mild, moderate, or severe). ICD 10 includes specifiers for socialized/unsocialized CD, and confined to the family context. DSM-5 includes specifiers for "with limited prosocial emotions" (callous-unemotional traits); there must be impairment; there is no age bar, but antisocial/dyssocial personality disorder (ASPD) criteria should not be met.

There are some differences between the systems: first, in ICD 10, ODD is a subtype of CD, whereas in DSM-5 they are separate entities. This reflects a wide ranging debate. In terms of external validating criteria there are many similarities between the two conditions, with progression from one to the other being not infrequent so that on these grounds they can both be seen as age-related progressions of a cluster of symptoms characterized by antisocial behavior. Because most children with CD also have ODD, DSM-IV did not allow both to be diagnosed at the same time, but this bar has been removed in DSM-5. However, as discussed below, children with the angry and irritable mood symptoms of ODD are more likely to develop mood disorders later in life and to have relatives with mood disorders.

Second, while the ICD 10 *research criteria* are very similar to DSM-5, with both using a menu counting approach to the number of symptoms, ICD 10 also has *clinical guidelines* that are broader descriptions for everyday diagnostic practise. They state, with respect to symptom categories "Any one of these categories, if marked, is sufficient for the diagnosis" (p. 267). An enduring pattern of behavior should be present, but no time frame is given. Third, DSM-5 requires distress or impairment, whereas ICD 10 does for ODD but, confusingly, not for CD. In practise this does not make a lot of difference, since about 80% of those diagnosed with CD have significant impairment (Angold & Costello, 2001; Romano *et al.*, 2001).

Fourth, DSM-5 has two other disorders that may overlap: one that was present in DSM-IV, Intermittent Explosive Disorder (which can only be diagnosed after the age of six) and a new

disorder, Disruptive Mood Dysregulation (DMD) Disorder. DMD has been introduced explicitly to stop overdiagnosis of childhood bipolar disorder and consequent over medication; however, while this form of irritability is now being extensively researched, there would appear to be considerable overlap with ODD, (odds ratio 50–100, Copeland *et al.*, 2013) and the validity of this diagnostic category has not been established. Fifth, DSM-5, like DSM-IV, specifically allows both ODD and CD to be diagnosed in adults; they are nested in the section on disruptive disorders. While there is no stated age cutoff in ICD 10, ODD and CD appear in the disorders "with onset usually in childhood or adolescence" suggesting they may be less applicable in adults. Applying a diagnosis in adults would mean that many people with criminal records can be diagnosed with CD, but neither DSM-5 nor ICD 10 makes reference to the likely consequences; clinicians, epidemiological surveys, and treatment trials do not usually apply the term to adults. Sixth, DSM-5 freely allows multiple diagnoses, whereas ICD 10 prefers wherever possible one diagnosis to be paramount. To help this, it has two categories—hyperkinetic conduct disorder and depressive conduct disorder—to handle two of the commoner coexistent conditions.

Epidemiology

Overall prevalence
The overall prevalence of ODD and CD together varies between 5% and 10% or more according to which survey is cited, and this in turn depends on the methods used and the locality studied. In younger children ODD is commoner than CD, in adolescents the opposite holds. However, there is fairly good agreement on rates of 5–8% in general longitudinal surveys where multi-informant methods that include careful interviews or assessments by a clinician are carried out, as for example in the Christchurch (Fergusson *et al.*, 2005) and Dunedin (Moffitt, 1993) studies in New Zealand, the British Office of National Statistics survey (Green *et al.*, 2005), and the Great Smoky Mountains Study (Costello *et al.*, 2003a). Unsurprisingly, higher rates are found if lifetime prevalences are used, as for example in the National Comorbidity Study Replication (Nock *et al.*, 2006, 2007). Adding an impairment criterion only reduces rates by around 20% to 40% (Angold & Costello, 2001; Romano *et al.*, 2001). Typically, ODD/CD makes up about half of all child and adolescent psychopathology and is the commonest condition.

Variations in prevalence
Gender
Gender, along with quality of parenting, is the strongest predictor of antisocial behavior in most studies (Odgers *et al.*, 2012). Boys outnumber girls by about 2:1 in younger children with ODD, but this ratio goes up for CD in adolescents to be between 3:1 and 7:1. This is partly due to using research criteria, so that for example forcing another person to have unwanted sex, using

a weapon, breaking into a house are far commoner among boys, whereas if general ICD 10 clinical criteria are used, behaviors that can be considered toward diagnosis include severe relational aggression, serious rule breaking with frequent use of alcohol and drugs, and more girls get included. Although the prevalence rates differ, the manner in which risk factors operate appears to be the same for both boys and girls (Moffitt *et al.*, 2001).

Socio economic status (SES) and geographical area

There is a strong gradient according to socio economic status (SES), thus for example in the ONS survey ODD/CD was five times more common in the lowest SES than the highest. Likewise, rates are typically 2–3 times higher in inner-city deprived areas compared with well-off suburbs.

Worldwide prevalences and minority ethnic groups

Across low, middle, and high income countries, many different rates have been reported, but comparisons are hard as studies have used different methods. However, an important exception to this is the studies that have used the Strengths and Difficulties Questionnaire and the Development and Well-Being Assessment (DAWBA) interviews. Such comparisons find very high rates of ODD/CD in Bangladesh (8.9%), high rates in Yemen (7.1%) and Brazil (7%), medium rates in Britain (5.3%), but low rates in Italy (1.2%), and very low rates in Goa, India (0.4%). In developed countries, among minority groups, there are higher rates among ethnic groups of African Caribbean/African American Heritage; this is not just due to reporting bias or prejudice, insofar as it is upheld by self-report of delinquency. In contrast, there are lower rates among Hispanic Americans in the USA and notably low rates among British Indians (Goodman *et al.*, 2010). The authors suggest the differences are at least in part related to close family structures with clear disciplinary practises at home, a strong emphasis on educational attainment, and cultural values that disapprove of an antisocial lifestyle (Goodman *et al.*, 2010).

High-risk populations

Rates of ODD/CD go up considerably in children who have been maltreated (see Chapter 29), who were brought up in residential care, or have been transferred to foster care (see Chapter 21), children with intellectual disability (see Chapter 54), and, unsurprisingly, in young offenders (Abram *et al.*, 2003; see Chapter 49).

Time periods

Rutter and Smith (1995) showed convincingly an increase in all types of mental health disorder in children over the second half of the twentieth century. Collishaw *et al.* (2004) in a review of three nationally representative studies of teenagers in England from the 1970s until the turn-of-the-century showed roughly doubling in ODD/CD (but no change in rates of attention deficit hyperactivity disorder (ADHD)). Maughan *et al.* (2008) found that this increase seemed to have plateaued out in the

early twenty-first century, using the ONS surveys of 1999 and 2004. Collishaw *et al.* (2012) found no evidence that the earlier increase was related to changes in parenting practices.

Subtypes according to phenomenology and longitudinal course

There have been numerous subdivisions of antisocial behavior using factor analytic techniques on cross-sectional data. They include overt antisocial behavior (tantrums, aggression) versus covert (lying and stealing); proactive aggression (premeditated, predatory attacks) versus reactive aggression (irritable lashing out only when provoked; Polman *et al.*, 2007); physical aggression (hitting, biting) versus relational aggression (bullying, scapegoating, verbal insults) and antisocial behavior at home versus antisocial behavior at school. While factor analysis can produce these distinct subtypes, the problem is that often correlations between items across subtypes are as great as those within (Patterson *et al.*, 1989). Therefore more robust ways of dividing up different antisocial phenomena are needed that are supported by several independent validating criteria cross-sectionally, such as family history, genetic indices (although this criterion is complicated since it is now emerging that similar genotypes can give rise to a wide range of disorders, see Chapter 24), neuropsychological features revealed on psychometric testing or brain functioning, and response to treatment (for more about classification, see Chapter 2).

Categories of antisocial behavior are further strengthened if they predict longitudinal course (Rutter, 2011; see Chapter 4) and this approach has led to important changes of emphasis. Back in 1966, Lee Robins published a classic paper showing that it was not any one particular symptom or symptom group that predicted adult outcome, but rather the severity, diversity and duration of symptoms in childhood. Robins found that roughly 40% of children with conduct problems went on to have significantly impaired, criminal adult lives, but that looking back, 90% of recidivist criminals had had conduct problems in childhood, figures that have been borne out by subsequent research. In the last 20 years, timing of the symptom onset has emerged as a powerful predictor of outcome as noted by Patterson *et al.* (1989). In a classic paper of 1993, Moffitt and colleagues described three different groups from the Dunedin study, "early onset lifetime persistent," "adolescence limited" and "not antisocial (NA)." While the adolescence limited group had few neurocognitive deficits, and were declining in their antisocial behavior in their early 20s, the early onset group had lower IQ, hyperactivity and inattention problems, poorer memory, greater peer difficulties, and more severe family and psychosocial circumstances.

After this paper, it seemed as if early onset conduct problems would likely presage some fairly dire consequences, whereas the adolescence-limited group would be of less concern. However, there have been two subsequent caveats from this study. First, the adolescence-limited group turned out to continue to offend at moderately high levels into their 30s, and while this

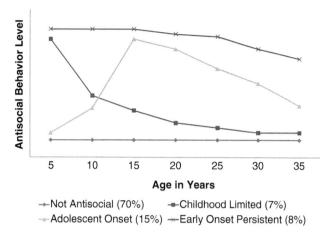

Figure 65.1 Subtypes of antisocial behavior by longitudinal course (data synthesis from several longitudinal studies).

was significantly lower than the rate seen in the early-onset persistent group, it was not trivial, leading to a change in name to "adolescent onset" (Odgers *et al.*, 2008). The same researchers using the same database uncovered an early-onset group who desisted from antisocial behavior, the so-called "childhood-limited" group (Odgers *et al.*, 2007); see Figure 65.1. Broadly speaking, these four groups have been replicated by other researchers (Farrington *et al.*, 2009), and apply to females as well as males (Fontaine *et al.*, 2009) and the hunt is now on to find distinguishing features, especially between early-onset persistent and childhood limited groups. The Dunedin group found that both had similar neurocognitive and psychosocial profiles, but that a family history of criminality or alcoholism predicted persistence (Odgers *et al.*, 2007). In a different population, Barker and Maughan (2009) found that predictors of the early-onset persistent trajectory compared to childhood limited were maternal anxiety during pregnancy, partner cruelty to the mother, harsh parenting, and higher levels of child undercontrolled temperament. Identifying reliable predictors would help planning of effective prevention and intervention services.

Long-term prognosis

Overall, ODD/CD is a condition with markedly poor long-term outcomes, which are summarized in Table 65.1.

While the precise figures vary from study to study, the elevation in risk is considerable. Thus, for example, in the Christchurch study, Fergusson *et al.* (2005) found that the 5% most antisocial children (thus equivalent to a diagnosis of ODD/CD) aged 7 years had, at age 26 when compared to those who were NA as children (50% of the sample) the following comparative outcome rates: violent offending 35% versus 3%, heavy drug usage 20% versus 5%, teenage pregnancy 20% versus 4%, leaving school with no exam qualifications 52% versus 6%, receiving state benefits 33% versus 9%.

Dividing children with ODD into irritable, headstrong, and hurtful predicts different longitudinal outcomes. Those who display more irritable characteristics (angry outbursts and tantrums) are more likely to develop anxiety and depression (but not fears) in the following years, whereas those with headstrong characteristics (defiant and disobedient) are more likely to develop conduct disorder (Stringaris & Goodman, 2009; Whelan *et al.*, 2013; see Chapter 5). The hurtful group (characterized by callous-unemotional traits—see Chapter 68) are more likely to develop aggressive conduct disorder. Generally speaking, children with ODD/CD who also have callous-unemotional traits have a poorer prognosis (Fontaine *et al.*, 2011).

As individuals with ODD/CD get older, offending reduces considerably in their 40s and 50s. However, this does not mean to say that their lives have become satisfactory, thus for example the Cambridge study of delinquent development found that in the late 40s these individuals showed a high rate of "life failure" defined using multiple indices (Piquero *et al.*, 2010).

Health outcomes are also worse, including increased mortality, thus for example in the 1958 British birth cohort, by age 46 mortality was doubled from 1.5% in the least antisocial three-quarters as teenagers to 3% in the most antisocial quarter (Jokela *et al.*, 2009). While this may not seem a large percentage increase, the numbers are very large in total population terms.

Table 65.1 Adult functioning of children who had ODD/CD.

Criminal behavior	More violent and non violent crimes, for example, mugging, grievous bodily harm; theft, car crimes, fraud.
Mental health problems	Increased rates of antisocial personality, alcohol and drug abuse, anxiety, depression and somatic complaints, episodes of deliberate self-harm and completed suicide, time in psychiatric hospitals
Education and training	Poorer examination results, more truancy and early school leaving, fewer vocational qualifications
Employment	More unemployment, jobs held for shorter time, jobs lower status with lower income, increased claiming of benefits and welfare
Social network	Fewer significant friends; friends more likely to be antisocial or in a gang; less constructive joint activities; less emotional confiding. Low involvement with relatives, neighbors, clubs and organizations
Intimate relationships	Increased rate of short lived, violent cohabiting relationships including domestic violence; select partners who are often also antisocial
Children	Increased rates of child abuse, conduct problems in offspring, children taken into care
Health	More medical problems, earlier death

Table 65.2 Factors predicting poor outcome.

Onset	Early onset of severe problems, before age 8
Phenomenology	Antisocial acts which are severe, frequent, and varied; physical aggression; premeditated acts;
Comorbidity	Hyperactivity and attention problems; callous-unemotional traits
Intelligence	Lower IQ
Family history	Parental criminality; parental alcoholism
Pregnancy	Possibly maternal anxiety during pregnancy, smoking
Parenting	Harsh, inconsistent parenting, with high criticism, low warmth, low involvement, and low supervision; interparental violence
Wider environment	Low income family in poor neighborhood with ineffective schools.

The risks were amplified at age 65 follow-up (Maughan *et al.*, 2013) (Table 65.2).

Service use and cost

Both in childhood and in the longer term into adulthood, individuals with ODD/CD are expensive to society. In childhood, they and their families are in contact with multiple agencies. Use of social services is significantly higher than for children with emotional disorders. Utilization of specialist child mental health and social services is significantly higher among children with unsocialized CD than socialized CD (Shivram *et al.*, 2009). Apart from service use, substantial costs fall on the families in terms of lost opportunity to work (Romeo *et al.*, 2006). Over the longer term, by their mid-20s, children who had ODD/CD cost an average 10 times as much as controls (Scott *et al.*, 2001) which in the USA can be as much as $2 million, once crime victim costs and drug misuse costs are included (Piquero *et al.*, 2013). These high figures mean that good-quality early intervention can be very cost-effective.

Etiology

Below, a number of separate factors are discussed and at the end of this section it is proposed that these need to be combined and evaluated for their contribution to any individual case, along with recognition that over the life course, different influences may hold different sway (see Chapter 1).

Individual-level influences
Overall genetic effects

Whereas a generation ago, antisocial behavior was typically seen purely as a result of poor socialization and voluntarily-determined self-control, it has become clear that for some subtypes, there is a strong genetic contribution. Twin studies have shown substantial genetic influences but also a substantial shared environmental component (Bornovalova *et al.*, 2010). However, this varies according to subgroup. Genetic contribution (see Chapter 24) is higher for antisocial behavior in the presence of inattention and hyperactivity (Thapar *et al.*, 2013), callous unemotional traits (Viding *et al.*, 2008) or high levels of physical aggression (Burt, 2009) and also if the antisocial behavior is pervasive across situations (Arsenault *et al.*, 2003). Conversely, where these factors are absent, genetic contribution is low (Silberg *et al.*, 1996; Viding *et al.*, 2008).

Specific genes

Main effects of particular genotypes for antisocial behavior, as opposed to ADHD, have not been particularly evident and isolated findings have not consistently been replicated; no consistent linkage regions have been identified (Plomin *et al.*, 2013). One approach has been to look at systems of genes, rather than individual genes. Using this approach, Bentley *et al.* (2013) found eight single-nucleotide polymorphisms that accounted for 16% of the variance within a latent antisocial phenotype. While this is promising, it will need replicating. Genome-wide association studies are in their infancy, one large study found four promising markers; interestingly, none of the top signals resided in traditional candidate genes (Dick *et al.*, 2011). Genome-wide approaches to date have been disappointing for ODD/CD, typically accounting for at most 2% of the variance in a phenomenon. Perhaps in future, with larger samples, better subtyping and more precise methods, more variance will be accounted for, as is the case, for example, for schizophrenia (see Chapter 24).

However, while so far little concrete evidence has been found for main effects, a much-cited paper (Caspi *et al.*, 2002) found that for adult antisocial behavior, there was a gene-environment interaction. A functional polymorphism in the gene for monoamine oxidase A (MAOA), which is widely involved in metabolizing a broad range of neurotransmitters, had no main effect on children, but a form of the gene which is associated with lower MAOA made individuals especially prone to develop antisocial behavior if they had been maltreated. Although attempts to replicate this finding have been mixed, it is supported by a meta-analysis (Kim-Cohen *et al.*, 2006) and by more recent replications (Aslund *et al.*, 2011). A recent line of investigation is the impact of environmental influences on epigenetic processes, whereby identifiable chemical changes such as acetylation and methylation of genes are affected by the environment (see Chapter 25). Thus for example in human adolescents, a study has shown differentially increased methylation in those whose parents were stressed (Essex *et al.*, 2013). Even if and when substantial specific gene effects are found, it will be important to understand their mode of action, for example how they might modulate neurotransmitter levels and affect reactivity.

Pregnancy and perinatal complications

Several influences during pregnancy have been associated with increased antisocial behavior in children. Thus maternal alcoholism during pregnancy can lead to increased antisocial behavior as part of the fetal alcohol syndrome (see Chapter 23). Its association with ODD/CD would seem likely to be mediated through effects on the brain and subsequent lowering of IQ (see Chapter 23), but alternative mechanisms have not in the main been tested, and high alcohol intake during pregnancy is associated with other sub optimal maternal practises and experiences, so causal effects are hard to disentangle. Smoking is also associated with increases in antisocial behavior, but the mechanisms may be different (see Chapter 23). Animal studies can show the importance of alcohol and smoking in high doses, but in less extreme exposure, the confounding with genetic influences is considerable, and both influences have been argued to have little effect for most human cases of ODD/CD (Thapar & Rutter, 2009; Jaffee *et al.*, 2012). Likewise, while perinatal complications are associated with antisocial behavior, once other factors are accounted for, it is uncertain whether they have any contributory effect (Nomura *et al.*, 2008).

Temperament

Individual differences in infancy that might contribute to subsequent risk of psychopathology were conceptualized by Thomas and Chess in terms of temperament, which they viewed as inherited and not significantly influenced by experience (Thomas *et al.*, 1968). Several prospective studies have shown associations between early temperament and later conduct problems (Keenan & Shaw, 2003). Traits usually identified are negative emotionality, poor emotional self-regulation, inattention, and restlessness. Temperament as originally conceived should be strongly heritable and experience-free. However, measures of temperament are only moderately heritable, and a child's engagement with the social world from birth means that temperament measures inevitably assess the outcome of social processes. It seems probable that as originally conceived by Thomas *et al.* (1968), a "difficult" temperament becomes more likely to lead to disruptive behavior problems when it interacts with a harsh inconsistent parenting style (Bradley & Corwyn, 2008; Bornovalova *et al.*, 2014).

Brain function

Systems neuroscience studies (see Chapter 10) and brain imaging studies (see Chapter 11) have been far more extensive for ADHD than ODD/CD, and studies have often conflated the two. Fairchild *et al.* (2011) found lower amygdala volume in both early-onset and adolescent-onset ODD/CD, regions associated with the processing of socio-emotional stimuli; they also found reduced right insula volume in the adolescent-onset subgroup. These differences were maintained after controlling for callous-unemotional traits (which are associated with their own particular brain changes, notably amygdala hypofunction; see Chapter 68) but ADHD was not controlled for. Reviewing neuroimaging literature on brain structure, function, and connectivity in both disorders, Rubia (2011) concluded that ODD/CD is consistently associated with abnormalities of the "hot" paralimbic system that regulates motivation and affect, comprising lateral orbital and ventromedial prefrontal cortices, superior temporal lobes, and underlying limbic structures, most prominently the amygdala. In contrast, ADHD is characterized predominantly by abnormalities in inferior frontal, striatal, parietotemporal and cerebellar regions and networks that mediate "cool" cognitive, that is, inhibitory, attention and timing functions associated with the disorder. There is thus evidence for dissociated underlying pathophysiologies for these two disorders.

Language, IQ, and educational attainment deficits

Low IQ and low school achievement are important predictors of ODD/CD and delinquency. In an English epidemiologic study of twins aged 13 years, low IQ of the child predicted conduct problems independent of social class and of the IQ of parents (Goodman *et al.*, 1995). Conduct disordered children, delinquent adolescents, and adult antisocial individuals show poor performance on standardized tests of verbal ability, and in tests of IQ, poor verbal ability; performance scores are lower too, but usually not as much as verbal ones (Loeber *et al.*, 2012). These associations hold after controlling for potential confounds such as race, socioeconomic status, academic attainment and test motivation (Petersen *et al.*, 2013). Longitudinal studies show that persistence in antisocial behavior over periods of years is predicted by low language ability/verbal IQ in childhood (Petersen *et al.*, 2013). Possible mechanisms may include lower abilities to recall oral instructions and to use language to think through the consequences of actions contributing to the poorer control of actions. Children who cannot reason or assert themselves verbally may attempt to gain control of social exchanges using aggression. Low IQ can contribute to academic difficulties which in turn mean that school becomes unrewarding, rather than a source of self-esteem and support, low school attainment further adds to the probability of ODD/CD developing even after allowing for IQ (Murray & Farrington, 2010).

Executive dysfunction

Children and adolescents with conduct problems have been shown consistently to have poor executive functions. These comprise those abilities implicated in successfully achieving goals through appropriate, effective actions. Specific skills include learning and applying contingency rules, abstract reasoning, problem solving, self-monitoring, sustained attention, and concentration, relating previous actions to future goals, and inhibiting inappropriate responses. These functions are largely, although not exclusively, associated with frontal lobe function. The meta-analysis by Ogilvie *et al.* (2011) with nearly 15,000 participants found that individuals with externalizing problems had lower scores by an average effect size of 0.54 sd, with significant effects after allowing for comorbid ADHD. Specifically, Fairchild *et al.* (2009) found that children with ODD/CD were more likely to take risky decisions and were less sensitive to punishment. Further, Hobson *et al.* (2011) showed that ODD/CD but not ADHD was related to "hot" executive functioning based on increased risky decision-making in a gambling task. ODD/CD was also independently related to aspects of "cool" executive functioning, independent of ADHD, namely slower speeds of inhibitory responding. These studies implicate reward-related abnormalities in ODD/CD development. Although most studies of executive deficit involve adolescents, such deficits have also been linked with disruptive behaviors in very young preschool children (Hughes & Ensor, 2011).

Autonomic reactivity and the hypothalamus-pituitary-adrenal axis

A low heart rate has been found consistently to be associated with antisocial behavior, and a meta-analysis of 40 studies suggested it is the best replicated biological correlate of antisocial behavior, with the association becoming even stronger during stress tests (effect size 0.76, Ortiz & Raine, 2004); the same group found the association is almost exclusively genetically mediated (Baker *et al.*, 2009). Other psychophysiological indicators of slow autonomic system reactivity have also been examined. Lorber (2004) conducted a meta-analysis and found children with conduct problems had lower skin conductance activity ($d = -0.30$); low levels that predict later antisocial behavior are detectable in infants (Baker *et al.*, 2013). The explanation for the link between slow autonomic activity and antisocial behavior remains unclear. Cortisol secretion data are mixed, with no differences in basal secretion rate in ODD/CD, but some evidence for decreased secretion under stress (Fairchild *et al.*, 2008; Platje *et al.*, 2013).

Information processing & social cognition

Dodge proposed the leading information-processing model for the genesis of aggressive behaviors within social interactions (Dodge, 1993). The model hypothesises that children who are prone to aggression focus on threatening aspects of others' actions, interpret hostile intent in the neutral actions of others (a hostile attributional style), and are more likely to select and to favor aggressive solution to social challenges (response and evaluation decision). Several studies have demonstrated that aggressive children make such errors of social cognition and decision-making (Fontaine *et al.*, 2010).

Family-level influences
Child rearing practises

There is ample evidence that ODD/CD is associated with less than optimal parenting practises, characterized by harsh inconsistent discipline, low warmth and involvement, and high criticism (Rutter *et al.*, 1998). These processes could be, and often are, a response to parents feeling irritated by the behavior of their child. However, Patterson in his classic work *Coercive Family Process* (1982) and subsequent publications showed that parenting could cause and exacerbate antisocial behavior. Parents of antisocial children were found to be more inconsistent in their use of rules, to issue more and unclear commands, to be more likely to respond to their children on the basis of their own mood rather than the characteristics of the child's behavior, to be less likely to monitor their children's whereabouts and to be unresponsive to their children's prosocial behavior.

Several specific mechanisms operate. First, positive overtures and behaviors by children are ignored and so become extinguished. Second, negative behavior attracts parental attention, which even though it is usually critical and hostile, is nonetheless reinforcing where the overall context is one of being ignored. This is one of the central paradoxes in conduct problem families: parental behaviors that are aversive (and so reduce antisocial behavior) when sparingly applied in the context of plentiful warm interactions, become rewarding and promote oppositional and aggressive behaviors when children receive little other attention. Third, there is what Patterson called the negative reinforcement trap: a parent responds to mild oppositional behavior by a child with a prohibition to which the child responds by escalating his behavior and mutual escalation continues until the parent backs off, thus teaching the child that if he gets more aggressive, his parents will back off and he will get his way (Gardner, 1989).

In considering the role of coercive processes in the origins or maintenance of conduct problems, we need to consider possible alternative explanations: (a) that the associations reflect familial genetic liability toward children's psychopathology and parents' coercive discipline, (b) that they represent effects of children's behaviors on parents and (c) that coercive parenting may be a correlate of other features of the parent/child relationship or family functioning that influence child behaviors. Regarding (a), common genetic liability, recent studies using genetically sensitive designs, have shown that for both genetically related and genetically unrelated parents and children, there was a strong association between parent-to-child hostility and child antisocial behavior, suggesting that the effect is not just due to passive genotype–environment correlation (Harold *et al.*, 2013). Regarding (b), child effects on parents, there is considerable evidence that children's difficult behaviors do evoke parental negativity. One experiment observed the interactions of normal and ODD/CD children when with their own parents, the parents of normal children, and the parents of other conduct disordered children (Anderson *et al.*, 1986). ODD/CD children elicited more negative reactions from all groups of parents than did non-ODD/CD children. Adoption studies (O'Connor *et al.*, 1998) have shown that adoptees at genetic risk of antisocial disorders are more likely than low risk children to evoke negative parenting in the adoptive home.

The role of the child in influencing parental monitoring has also received attention. Stattin and Kerr (2000) pointed out that studies of parental monitoring have generally assessed how much knowledge parents have of their children's whereabouts, but not how parents acquired it. They showed that the majority of this knowledge came from what the child chose to tell the parent, and conduct-problem adolescents told their parents less about what they are doing, again showing child characteristics affecting parenting style. These findings have since been amply confirmed by 47 studies in the subsequent decade (Racz & McMahon, 2011).

The fact that children's behaviors can evoke negative parenting does not however mean that negative parenting has no impact on children's behavior. As well as the cross-sectional observational studies mentioned above, several longitudinal studies indicate that it does. For example, the E-Risk longitudinal twin study showed that with identical twins, those whose mothers were more critical at 5 had greater antisocial behavior as rated by teachers at age 7, again controlling for initial levels of antisocial behavior. The same study looked at the effects of fathers' parenting on young children's aggression (Jaffee *et al.*, 2003). As expected, a prosocial father's *absence* predicted more aggression by his children. But in contrast, an antisocial father's *presence* predicted more aggression by his children, and his harmful effect was exacerbated the more time each week he spent taking care of the children, thus again suggesting a direct effect independent of any genetic contribution. These and many other studies provide an overwhelming amount of evidence for the contribution of poor parenting practises to antisocial behavior. Regarding (c), that coercive parent–child relationships may only be a marker for other more relationship problems, two leading candidates are attachment insecurity and exposure to interparental conflict; both are discussed below.

Attachment insecurity

Even before he had articulated his theory of attachment in detail, John Bowlby's (1944) study of juvenile thieves implicated their attachment to their parents. Insecure attachment patterns, especially disorganization (see Chapter 6), are fairly strongly associated with antisocial behavior. The meta-analysis by Fearon *et al.* (2010) found an overall effect size of the association of 0.58. These findings are most prevalent in infancy and early childhood, but more recent studies are beginning to address the representation of attachment in middle childhood and adolescence using instruments such as the child attachment interview (Futh *et al.*, 2008; Scott *et al.*, 2011). However, most studies have not been designed to examine whether both attachment insecurity and antisocial behavior are different manifestations of harsh, inconsistent, and frightening parenting. An exception was the study by Scott *et al.* (2011) which examined whether attachment insecurity in a large and diverse sample of adolescents predicted antisocial behavior once parenting practise had been taken into account; they found that it did.

Exposure to interparental conflict and violence

For some time, studies have shown that children exposed to domestic violence between adults are subsequently more likely to themselves become aggressive (Moffitt & Caspi, 1998). Cummings and Davies (2002) proposed that marital conflict influences children's behavior because of its effect on their regulation of emotion, for example by responding to frightening interparental conflict by down regulating their own emotion through denial of the situation. Cognitively, this may lead to inaccurate appraisal of other social situations and ineffective problem solving; emotionally, it may lead to greater behavioral reactivity to stress. Social learning theory suggests that children's aggression may be increased because they imitate aggressive behavior modeled by their parents and may learn that aggression is a normative part of family relationships which is an effective way of controlling others, and that it is sanctioned, not punished. More studies are needed however, to see the extent to which interparental conflict adds to child antisocial behavior over and above direct parent–child conflict. Results are inconsistent—while some researchers find an additional effect, others find no extra contribution from interparental conflict (Harold *et al.*, 2013).

Maltreatment

Physical punishment is widely used, and parents of children with conduct problems frequently resort to it out of desperation. Overall, associations between physical abuse and conduct problems are well established (see Chapter 29). Links with conduct problems are not, however, straightforward. The risk for conduct problems does not apply equally to all forms of physical punishment. The E-risk longitudinal twin study was able to compare the effects of corporal punishment (smacking, spanking) versus injurious physical maltreatment using twin-specific reports of both experiences (Jaffee *et al.*, 2005). Results showed that children's genetic endowment accounted for virtually all of the association between their corporal punishment and their conduct problems. This indicated a "child effect," in which children's bad conduct provokes their parents to use more corporal punishment, rather than the reverse. Findings about injurious physical maltreatment were the opposite. There was no child effect provoking maltreatment and moreover, significant effects of maltreatment on child aggression remained after controlling for any genetic transmission of liability to aggression from antisocial parents. Little is known about the possible mechanisms linking maltreatment to conduct problems, although threats to security of attachment, difficulties in affect regulation, distortions of information processing and self-concept and failure to model and reward prosocial behavior are likely to be relevant.

Influences beyond the family
Overview of peer effects

As children spend more time outside the family and friends or in education, there are increasing interchanges with other children. Observational studies show that children with ODD/CD have more negative interchanges with other children, across the age range from early childhood up to adolescence, and tend to be rejected by nondeviant peers (Boivin *et al.*, 2013). Three processes could be at work: the child's individual antisocial behavior could lead to peer problems, or vice versa, deviant peer relationships could lead to antisocial behavior, or finally, some common factor could lead to both. Evidence has been found for all three effects.

Peer rejection

Regarding the possibility that conduct problems lead to peer difficulties, there is ample evidence that children with established conduct problems are more likely to have more conflict with peers, and to be rejected by nondeviant peers (Coie, 2004). This peer rejection has been shown to contribute to declines in academic achievement and increases in aggression across the first year of primary schooling (Coie, 2004). One consequence of rejection by healthy peers is that from as young as 5 years, aggressive-antisocial children tend to associate with other deviant children (Boivin *et al.*, 2013).

Impact of deviant peers on antisocial behavior

Regarding the possibility that peers lead to conduct problems, this has been shown to come about in several ways. Youth who are aggressive are attracted to each other, and deviant youth reinforce each others' antisocial behaviors and attitudes (Boivin *et al.*, 2013). Evidence that peer influences do increase antisocial behaviors applies primarily to adolescents. Several longitudinal studies confirm that antisocial young people who have deviant peers offend more, and over and above this, increase their rates of antisocial acts and offending after joining a gang, and reduce it if they leave the gang (Murray & Farrington, 2010). Strong evidence comes from treatment experiments: in two controlled clinical trials, boys treated in groups did worse than untreated controls; treatment was followed by increased adolescent problem behaviors and poorer outcomes (Dishion *et al.*, 1999). After group-level treatment brought the boys together, they mutually reinforced each other's antisocial activities, a finding which argues for individual treatment approaches.

School effects

It is well established that children with ODD/CD are far more likely to attend schools with high delinquency rates, which have high levels of distrust between teachers and students, low pupil commitment to the school, and unclear and inconsistently enforced rules (Graham, 1988). However, it is less clear to what extent the schools themselves influence antisocial behavior,

by their organisation, climate, and practises, or to what extent the concentration of ODD/CD in certain schools is mainly a function of their intakes. In the Cambridge Study, most of the variation between schools in their delinquency rates could be explained by differences in their intakes of troublesome boys aged 11 (Murray & Farrington, 2010). However, reviews of American research show that schools with clear, fair, and consistently enforced rules tend to have low rates of student misbehavior, even allowing for intake levels of conduct problems (Gottfredson, 2001). Thus this type of school climate may act as a protective factor.

Poverty

That antisocial children come in disproportionate numbers from poor families has been repeatedly confirmed; however, several studies show that the effect is indirect, disappearing after controlling for child-rearing practises. Some of the earliest reports showed this; thus the Glueck's study of delinquency found that harsh discipline, low supervision and weak parent–child attachments accounted for the effects of poverty on children's antisocial behaviors in the 1930s (Sampson & Laub, 1994). Many longitudinal studies since then have confirmed this (Murray & Farrington, 2010). Furthermore, reducing poverty can reduce antisocial behavior, as seen in the "natural experiment" described by Costello *et al.* (2003b). Native American families in North Carolina, formerly living below the poverty line, benefited from increased income from newly opened casinos. Overall, children's ODD/CD problems decreased. However, the effect of increased income was mediated through better parent–child relationships. This study suggests that poverty is not simply an epiphenomenon due only to passive correlation, whereby families with worse relationships for various reasons also earn less, but rather that poor circumstances can also affect parenting quality, which in turn affects child antisocial behavior.

Neighborhood influences

Young people with ODD/CD disproportionately live in inner-city areas characterized by physical deterioration, neighborhood disorganization and high residential mobility. However, it is difficult to determine to what extent the areas themselves influence antisocial behavior and to what extent it is merely the case that antisocial people tend to live in deprived areas. Based on comparisons between the rural Isle of Wight and inner London, Rutter (1981) argued that neighborhoods have only indirect effects on antisocial behavior through their effects on individual people and families. In the Chicago Youth Development Study, the relation between community structural characteristics (concentrated poverty, racial heterogeneity, economic resources and violent crime rate) and individual violence was mediated by parenting practises, gang membership, and peer violence (Tolan *et al.*, 2003). The geographical gradient remains after controlling for SES, and in the study by Odgers *et al.* (2012) was entirely mediated by supportive parenting (high warmth and close monitoring).

Synthesis

The above account has shown that many different factors influence the development of ODD/CD. The question arises how they may operate in the individual case; some but not other factors will be present. A number of points can be made: first, a number of these risks are intercorrelated, and studies that measure several of them often find that once allowed for, some lose their significance. We have seen for example that in several studies, neighborhood effects and SES were entirely mediated through parenting practises, which repeatedly emerge as a major factor. Second, where there are more highly heritable characteristics such as inattention/hyperactivity, lower IQ, and callous-unemotional traits, the prognosis is generally worse. Third, being subject to several risk factors seems to have a cumulative effect so that outcomes exponentially worsen (Van der Laan *et al.*, 2010). This seems likely to be due to interactions between child characteristics, such as temperament, and the environment, whereby for example children with irritable, negative personalities do especially badly when they are brought up in a harsh and inconsistent manner. Thus between childhood and adolescence, children with ADHD are far more likely to develop CD if they are subjected to critical Expressed Emotion (Taylor *et al.*, 1996).

The interaction between child traits and the environment may not always be a negative process; there is emerging evidence that such children do better than more phlegmatic individuals if their upbringing is particularly good, a finding that is beginning to be supported through experimental trial evidence (Scott & O'Connor, 2012). Fourth, as children grow up, their circumstances will change and they will not be passive recipients of their environment, but will to some extent shape their surroundings, partly due to the consequences of having a disorder, and partly due to seeking out more risky environments. This is not just in terms of evoking more negative parenting, but also because genetic predisposition can influence peer processes whereby peer victimization and rejection are more likely (Boivin *et al.*, 2013). Over development, accumulating consequences of this kind make ODD/CD more likely to persist, so that the children remain in high-risk environments and have restricted opportunities for involvement in more positive relationships and roles. However, the counter of this is that those children and adolescents who have more positive experiences are more likely to desist from delinquency and get qualifications and employment, for example if they leave an antisocial behavior group (Sweeten *et al.*, 2013). Paradoxically therefore, those children with the more difficult temperaments and adverse circumstances may respond more to interventions that can make their environments better than children with the same levels of ODD/CD who do not have difficult temperaments.

Assessment, diagnosis, and formulation

Assessment
Before the interview
Because the phenomena of antisocial behavior are so overt, questionnaires are less essential than in some conditions (such as anxiety and depression, where children may reveal symptoms that the parents are unaware of). However, getting both parent and teacher to fill in questionnaires is helpful for a number of reasons. First, it is important to get the perspective of the school. Second, comorbidity can more easily be picked up if a broad symptomatology questionnaire is used, such as the Strength and Difficulties Questionnaire (SDQ; www.sdqinfo.com) or the Achenbach System of Empirically Based Assessment (ASEBA; www.aseba.com). The SDQ is free and shorter, the ASEBA costs and is longer; on the major dimensions they correlate closely (Goodman & Scott, 1999). Domain specific questionnaires such as the Eyberg Child Behavior Inventory (ECBI; www4.parinc.com/Products/Product.aspx?ProductID=ECBI) are useful as a baseline from which treatment effects can be monitored (see Chapter 33). Children tend to underreport their antisocial behavior, so questionnaires below the age of 11 are usually unhelpful, but by mid-to late adolescence a self-report of delinquent acts becomes more reliable, and typically reveals far more criminal behavior than for example is known to official agencies; this is true across ethnic groups and countries (Jolliffe *et al.*, 2003; Enzmann *et al.*, 2010). A member of the staff at the child's school who knows the child well should be spoken to, to find out if there are behavioral issues in the classroom and in peer relations, and the latest school report should be requested along with formal examination results and psychometric test reports, if available.

History and examination
A thorough clinical evaluation should be made (see Chapter 32). There may be a litany of complaints from the parents and it is important to keep a neutral position and show the child or young person that s/he is also being listened to. The quality of parenting needs to be thoroughly assessed. Asking about what happens during a typical day and at a typical weekend is often revealing. Detailed blow-by-blow descriptions should be obtained of disciplinary encounters, so that a clear picture is built up of antecedent events, how the parents reacted and whether any consequences were applied. An evaluation should be made of how negative the parents are, including whether the child is scapegoated for more of the family's difficulties than appears just, and whether the situation borders on emotional or physical abuse. Coercive cycles and negative reinforcement traps that are maintaining the behavior should be explored. Positive involvement in joint activities such as play or common interests needs to be assessed. The clinician should not shy away from asking parents about their own antisocial activities and criminal records, and use of alcohol and drugs, including during pregnancy.

Seeing young persons on their own is crucial. They may reveal emotional concerns including anxiety and depression, and substance and alcohol use that they have withheld from the parent. Gang involvement and witnessing interparental violence should be enquired about. Are there positive times with their parents? Do they feel closeness, can the child seek comfort from them? In young children, what is the quality of attachment to the parent? Because it is easy to become overwhelmed by the saturation of negative events and behavior, it is especially important to ask young persons what they enjoy doing and what they are good at and their hopes for the future. Are there any positive adults in the child's life? What potential protective factors are operating and how might they be built on? Physical examination (see Chapter 35) should include a check for dysmorphic features including fetal alcohol syndrome.

Investigation

It is important to evaluate the presence of both specific and general learning disabilities in individuals with ODD/CD. Poor school performance can often be attributed to a lazy attitude and failure to complete homework, both of which may be present but may mask an underlying cognitive problem. A quarter or more of children with ODD/CD also have specific reading retardation (defined as having a reading level two standard deviations below that predicted by their IQ) or dyslexia (Trzesniewski *et al.*, 2006; see Chapter 53). While this may in part be due to lack of adequate schooling, there is good evidence that the cognitive deficits often precede the behavioral problems. General learning disability (see Chapter 54) is often missed in children with conduct disorder unless IQ testing is carried out (see Chapter 34). The rate of conduct disorder rises several-fold as IQ gets below 70 (see Chapter 54).

Differential diagnosis and formulation
Differential diagnosis

Making a diagnosis of ODD or CD is usually straightforward but comorbid conditions are often missed. A particular pitfall is to fail to diagnose comorbid ADHD despite symptoms being there, because there is a chaotic or abusive home background or because there have been several recent disruptive moves of a home or school; likewise, a disorganized pattern of attachment does not exclude ODD/CD. The differential diagnosis may include:

1 *Attention Deficit Hyperactivity Disorder.* Any of the three core symptoms, impulsivity, inattention and motor overactivity can be misconstrued as antisocial, particularly impulsivity, which is also present in ODD/CD and does not of itself indicate ADHD (see Chapter 55). A careful history of ability to attend and be still both at home and school will usually reveal ADHD if present, in conjunction with a school visit or standardized questionnaire from the teacher. In contrast, antisocial behavior is not a feature of pure ADHD (see Chapter 55).

2 *Mood Disorders. Depression* can present with irritability and oppositional symptoms but unlike typical ODD/CD, mood is usually clearly low and there are often vegetative features (see Chapter 63). ODD has angry outbursts as one of its characteristics, but if irritability is marked then *DMD Disorder* should be considered: although disobedience is not a core feature, diagnostic overlap is very marked. Likewise, *Intermittent Explosive Disorder* shares many features with ODD/CD but aggression is not premeditated or committed to achieve a tangible objective, nor are the nonaggressive symptoms such as lying or stealing present. Early *Bipolar Disorder* should not be diagnosed without clear evidence of manic features such as racing thoughts, increased activity or energy and expansive mood (see Chapter 62). Low self-esteem is the norm in ODD/CD, as is a lack of friends or constructive pastimes. Therefore it is easy to overlook more pronounced depressive symptoms.

3 *Adjustment Reaction.* This can be diagnosed when onset occurs soon after exposure to an identifiable psychosocial stressor such as divorce, bereavement, trauma, abuse, or adoption. The onset should be within 1 month for ICD-10, and 3 months for DSM-5, and symptoms should not persist for more than 6 months after the cessation of the stress or its sequelae (see Chapter 26).

4 *Autistic Spectrum Disorders (ASD).* These are often accompanied by marked tantrums or destructiveness, which may be the reason for seeking a referral. As with ODD/CD, a lack of friendships may also be evident. Enquiring about other symptoms of autistic spectrum disorders (ASDs) should reveal their presence. In particular, unlike children with ODD/CD who have callous-unemotional traits, children with ASD fail to understand social situations and judge accurately the emotions of others. Some children with ODD/CD nonetheless appear to have some autistic features, in which case more detailed evaluation is indicated (see Chapter 51).

5 *Antisocial/Dyssocial Personality Disorder (ASPD).* In DSM-5 ASPD cannot be diagnosed under 18, although it requires evidence of conduct disorder before the age of 15 years. ICD-10 does not mention a lower age limit, but the criteria do not appear in the section on childhood disorders and clinicians are usually reluctant to apply the diagnosis outside adulthood (see Chapter 67). Nonetheless, it is becoming apparent that callous-unemotional traits can be reliably identified in middle childhood, have substantial continuity and a significant genetic contribution to their causation (see Chapter 68), so it is worth recognizing their presence.

6 *Subcultural Deviance.* Some youths are antisocial and commit crimes but are not particularly aggressive or defiant. They are well adjusted within a deviant peer culture that approves of recreational drug use, shoplifting and so on. Drug and alcohol usage should always be asked about, but often this will fall short of a diagnosable dependence syndrome, both in terms of symptoms and major impairment.

Multiaxial system

ICD-10 has a scheme for multiaxial assessment for children and adolescents. *Axis One* refers to clinical syndromes; *Axis Two* refers to specific learning disabilities and Axis Three to general learning disabilities; *Axis Four* to medical conditions, *Axis Five* psychosocial and environmental problems, and *Axis Six* to the global level of functioning which can be measured for example using the Children's Global Assessment System (CGAS; Shaffer, *et al.*, 1983). While DSM-IV had a fairly similar system, it has been abandoned in DSM-5 as it was not widely used in adult practise. In many ways this is a loss, as a multiaxial approach forces the clinician to consider wider factors beyond the presenting symptomatology.

Formulation

The formulation should synthesize all that has been learned from the assessment about the child's predisposing, precipitating, perpetuating, and protective factors in an individualized narrative way, rather than simply impersonally applying a diagnosis. The first assessment session is crucial for engaging the family and identifying strengths that can be worked with, to bring about therapeutic change.

Intervention

The next sections will cover treatment of children aged 2–12. For prevention, please see Chapter 17. For treatment of delinquent teenagers, including Functional Family Therapy and Multisystemic Therapy, see Chapter 49.

Principles
Personalizing the treatment plan

The treatment plan should follow the assessment and fit the particular needs of the child and family. Many risk factors have been delineated in this chapter, but usually not all occur in the same child, who typically will be functioning differently according to context, with for example, a different pattern exhibited at home compared with the school. Intervention needs to be tailored according to the needs and strengths of the family, and be reasonably congruent with their beliefs, otherwise disengagement is particularly likely in this patient group whose lives are often not well organized and who are often suspicious of authority figures such as health professionals.

Engaging the family

Any family coming to a mental health service is likely to have some fears about being judged as bad and possibly mad. Dropout rates in treatment for conduct problem families are high—often up to 60% (Kazdin, 1996). Practical measures, such as assisting with transportation, providing childcare, and holding sessions in the evening or at other times to suit the family are all likely to facilitate retention. Forming a good alliance with the family

is especially important. Once engaged, the quality of the therapist's alliance with the family affects treatment success, accounting for 15% of the variance in outcome in the meta-analysis by Shirk and Carver (2003). Making a strong alliance is not just a characteristic of the therapist, but more compliant families make it easier to plan constructive treatment jointly (Green, 2006).

Choosing which treatment modality to use

The behavior may predominantly occur in the home, at school, with peers, or in the community; or it may be pervasive. Interventions need to address each context specifically, rather than assuming that successful treatment in one area will generalize to another. Thus improvements in the home arising from a successful parent training program will not usually lead to less antisocial behavior at school—the meta-analysis by the National Institute for Health and Care Excellence, NICE (2013) found that despite a moderate-to-large effect-size (0.6 sd) at home, there was no carry-over at all to school. Therefore for cases with difficulties that are mainly at home, parent training could be the first line of treatment. If classroom behavior is a problem and a school visit shows that the teacher is not using effective methods, then advice to the teacher and other school staff can be very effective (see below). Where there are pervasive problems including fights with peers, then individual work on anger management and social skills should be added; on its own, anger management is unlikely to be as successful as when it is combined with other approaches. For most cases, medication is controversial and generally best avoided; possible indications are discussed below.

Encouraging strengths

Identifying strengths of the young person and the family is crucial. This helps engagement, and increases the chances of effective treatment. Encouragement of abilities helps the child spend more time behaving constructively rather than destructively—for example, more time spent playing football is less time spent hanging round the streets looking for trouble. Encouragement of prosocial activities—for example, to complete a good drawing, or to play a musical instrument well—also increases achievements and self-esteem and hope for the future.

Treating comorbid conditions

In clinical referrals, comorbidity is the rule rather than the exception. As noted above, common accompaniments are depression and ADHD; a number will have posttraumatic stress disorder (PTSD). In recent years there has been increasing recognition of the overlap with autistic spectrum disorders, where so-called challenging behavior often amounts to ODD (see Chapter 51), and that a minority will have psychopathic traits (see Chapter 68). Each of these conditions requires appropriate management in its own right.

Promoting social and learning skills

Treatment involves more than the reduction of antisocial behavior—thus for example, stopping tantrums and aggressive outbursts, while helpful, will not lead to good functioning if the child lacks the skills to make friends or to negotiate: positive behaviors need to be taught too. Specific learning disabilities such as reading retardation/dyslexia, which is particularly common in these children, need treatment, as do more general difficulties such as planning homework.

Following guidelines

A number of authoritative professional bodies have produced guidelines for the assessment and treatment of ODD/CD. The American Academy of Child and Adolescent Psychiatry published practise parameters for the assessment and treatment of Conduct Disorder in 1997 which are now a little dated, but the guidelines for ODD were published in 2007 so are reasonably up-to-date. The US Center for Education and Research on Mental Health Therapeutics (CERT) produced a guideline on "Maladaptive aggression in youth," covering engagement as well as treatment (Rosato et al., 2012) and the UK NICE recently published a full guideline on antisocial behavior and conduct disorders covering assessment, treatment, and cost-effectiveness (NICE, 2013). The assessment and treatment approaches advocated here are consistent with each of these guidelines.

Treating the child in a natural environment

Most of the interventions described below are intended for outpatient or community settings. Psychiatric hospitalisation is very rarely necessary; there no evidence that in-patient admissions lead to gains that are maintained after the child is returned to the family. The objective of treatment is to enable the child to cope with the environment he or she lives in usually, and alter the environment where it is harmful. Where there is parenting breakdown or total inability to manage the child, then foster care may be necessary. Not all cases of conduct disorder need to be seen in child and adolescent mental health services, and indeed with the prevalence of 5% that would be impossible; less complicated cases may be seen, for example for parent training given by local voluntary organizations, so long as staff are adequately trained and there is a clear onward pathway if this is ineffective.

Family interventions

Even where the antisocial behavior appears to have arisen "in a clear blue sky" without adverse family risk factors, living with a child with marked antisocial behavior can itself lead to coercive parenting styles, which in turn may exacerbate the problems. Therefore improving family risk factors such as coercive parenting is likely to be beneficial, whether or not they were originally implicated as a cause.

Parent training

Parent training programs are the mainstay of treatment of ODD/CD, especially with younger children below the age of about eight. They are designed to improve parents' behavior management skills and the quality of the parent–child relationship. Most parenting programs target skills, such as promoting play and developing a positive parent–child relationship, using praise and rewards to increase desirable social behavior, giving of clear directions and rules, using consistent and calm consequences for unwanted behavior, and reorganizing the child's day to prevent problems. Some parenting programs also have add-on elements to address parental problems that interfere with their ability to learn how to parent better, such as parental drug/alcohol abuse, maternal depression and violence between parents. Treatment can be delivered in individual parent–child appointments, or in a parenting group. Individual approaches offer the advantages of "in vivo" observation of the parent–child dyad and therapist coaching and feedback regarding progress; groups are more cost-effective and enable parents to learn from each other. Parenting programs are discussed in detail in Chapter 37.

Two examples of model programs for individual work with parents that are empirically supported include *Helping the Noncompliant Child* (McMahon et al., 2010) and *Parent Child Interaction Therapy* (Zisser & Eyberg, 2010). Group treatment has been shown to be equally effective, and offers opportunities for parents to share their experience with others who are struggling with a disruptive child. Group treatments emphasise discussion among group leaders and parents, and may use videotaped vignettes of parent–child interactions that illustrate the "right" and "wrong" ways to handle situations. Two well-known group treatments are the *Incredible Years Program* (Webster-Stratton and Reid, 2010) and the *Positive Parenting Program* (Triple P; Sanders, 2012), both of which have been disseminated throughout many countries in the world and translated into many languages (see Chapter 37).

Parent training is the most extensively studied treatment for conduct problems, and the meta-analysis in 2013 by NICE found a mean effect-size of 0.54 sd as rated by parents; this was not just a rater effect, as clinician/researcher ratings had an effect size of 0.69, and direct observation 0.40. This is in contrast to parent training for ADHD, where despite parental ratings suggesting effectiveness, independent ratings suggest little effect (Sonuga-Barke et al., 2013).

Recently, some programs have included an element of training parents to read with their children in addition to behavior management, with the idea of targeting multiple risk factors for antisocial behavior. Scott et al. (2010a) combined a 12-week behavior management program with a relatively intense, detailed reading program (10 2-hour sessions) for 5- and 6-year- olds. In an RCT, this combination reduced the rate of oppositional defiant disorder by half and increased reading age by 6 months; ADHD symptoms in semistructured interview were also reduced. This kind of approach is promising since it is relatively inexpensive, using parents as the only vehicle for treatment, yet hits multiple risk factors for poor outcomes in antisocial behavior (parenting, oppositional defiant disorder, ADHD symptoms, reading ability). A subsequent trial showed a similar package worked equally well for parents from ethnic minorities (Scott *et al.*, 2010b). However, as for most therapies, parent training does not work for all cases and there are few trials of what to do when it has failed. Moving from group to intensive individual work has been advocated, and Scott and Dadds (2009) provide a framework for tackling this in a systematic way by drawing upon attachment theory, family systems, and motivational interviewing. Approaches such as these now need empirical testing, as do booster trials to prevent relapses.

Family systemic therapies

Typically, family systemic therapies involve all family members attending. Their goals differ according to the style and underlying theory of the particular variant of therapy. For example, structural family therapy as pioneered by leaders such as Minuchin (1974) would try to restore clear boundaries of authority of the parents over the child, since often antisocial children have become domineering in their own homes. Other forms of family therapy try to improve patterns of communication that have gone wrong, and "systemic" variants try to reveal and address relevant factors that impinge on the family system from both within and outside the family. There have been few if any good quality evaluations of family or systemic therapies for childhood antisocial behavior (see Chapter 39). In contrast, in adolescents there have been several trials of particular brands of systemic family therapy such as Functional Family Therapy and Multisystemic Therapy which have often proved successful with a notably difficult client group (see Chapter 49).

Child therapies

Cognitive-behavioral therapies and social skills therapies for ODD/CD typically aim to (i) reduce children's aggressive behavior such as shouting, pushing and arguing; (ii) increase prosocial interactions such as entering a group, starting a conversation, participating in group activities, sharing, cooperating, asking questions politely, listening, and negotiating; (iii) correct the cognitive deficiencies, distortions and inaccurate self-evaluation and (iv) ameliorate emotional regulation and self-control problems so as to reduce emotional lability, impulsivity, and explosiveness, enabling the child to be more reflective and able to consider how best to respond in provoking situations (Larson & Lochman, 2011). While child CBT therapies were originally mainly used with school-age children and older, more recently they have been successfully adapted for preschoolers (Webster-Stratton & Reid, 2010; see Chapter 38).

An example is Lochman's *Coping Power* Program (Larson & Lochman, 2011). This is fairly lengthy, comprising 33 1-hour group sessions, with monthly individual meetings. Training focuses on interpretation of social cues, generating prosocial solutions to problems, and anger management with arousal

reduction strategies. Treatment is delivered in groups of 5–7 children by two therapists. Sessions include imagined scenarios, therapist modeling, role plays with corrective feedback and assignments to practise outside of sessions. Parent and teacher training components have been developed as adjunctive treatments. Evaluations demonstrate reductions in aggression and substance use, and improved social competence (Lochman *et al.*, 2012). Independent replications are now needed.

The literature is generally not supportive of the effectiveness of individual, psychodynamic psychotherapies, art and drama therapies in this population, especially when used as a sole treatment modality, although decisive studies are yet to be undertaken (Fonagy & Target, 2008).

Interventions in school

This section is a brief summary of interventions for children with established antisocial behavior. Preventive programs including those promoting social and emotional learning are covered in Chapter 17. Typically, teachers are taught techniques that they can apply to all children in their class, as well as to those exhibiting the most antisocial behavior. Successful approaches use proactive strategies and include a focus on positive behavior and group interventions, and combine effective instructional strategies with effective behavioral management. Typically, they target four areas of functioning. First, they promote positive behaviors such as compliance and following established classroom rules and procedures. Second, the interventions prevent problem behaviors such as talking at inappropriate times and fighting. Third, they teach social and emotional skills such as conflict resolution and problem solving. Fourth, they prevent the escalation of angry, acting out behavior.

To date there have been relatively few controlled trials of such interventions; the meta-analysis by NICE (2013) found eight trials of good quality in all, the mean teacher-rated effect size was 0.43 sd but researcher-rated and independent observer-rated effects were not significant. Therefore there is the possibility that improvements that teachers see are purely due to rating bias. However, the individual trials that did show significant effects by independent observers were the ones that used a program with more training and fidelity in adherence to the manual (e.g., Forster *et al.*, 2012); they include those done in low and middle income countries (Baker-Henningham *et al.*, 2012), where such interventions can be combined with parenting programs (see Chapter 37). This is a promising domain worthy of further research.

In recent years in some countries such as the UK and the USA there has been a surge in the use of teaching assistants in classrooms. Often these staff are not well paid or given much training, yet in some schools there will be perhaps two teaching assistants for every teacher in a classroom of say 30 pupils. A systematic review (Alborz *et al.*, 2009) concluded that there was insufficient evidence to show effectiveness for disruptive pupils in class, but that practise varied widely, thus for example some assistants sat close to the child to encourage prosocial behavior and prevent disruptive behavior, while others sat at the back of the class to try to promote the child's independence. Given the considerable resource expenditure on this intervention, further research is indicated.

Medication

There are differing views as to the usefulness of medication in ODD/CD. Prescriptions of medications, particularly anti psychotics such as risperidone, are increasing considerably, especially in the USA. In the UK general use of medication would not generally be supported as good practise because well-replicated trials of effectiveness are limited, particularly for children without ADHD, and there is a significant risk of unwanted side-effects.

The best-studied pharmacological interventions for youth with ODD/CD are psychostimulants (methylphenidate and dexamfetamine), when used with children with comorbid ADHD. In these circumstances, there is good evidence that reduction in hyperactivity/impulsivity will also result in reduced conduct problems (see Chapter 55). There is insufficient reliable evidence to decide whether stimulants reduce aggression in the absence of ADHD; one study by Klein *et al.* (1997) found that improvements in CD symptoms were independent of ADHD symptom reduction, whereas Taylor *et al.* (1987) did not.

Other pharmacological approaches for antisocial behavior have tended to target reactive aggression and over arousal, primarily in highly aggressive and psychiatrically hospitalized youth. Medications used in these conditions include antipsychotics, those purported to target affect dysregulation (e.g., buspirone, clonidine), and mood stabilizers (e.g., lithium, carbamazepine) (Rosato *et al.*, 2012). In the last few years, the use of antipsychotics such as risperidone and aripiprazole in out-patient settings has been increasing. However, there is only modest evidence for their effectiveness in conduct disorder in normal IQ children without ADHD. These newer antipsychotics, while not especially sedating, have substantial side-effects, for example risperidone typically leads to considerable weight gain, and the prevalence of long-term movement disorders in the long-term is unknown (see Chapter 43). The NICE (2013) meta-analysis of antipsychotics for ODD/CD found only three suitable trials, and these were of moderate quality only. The mean effect size as rated by parents was 0.49 sd, but there were no significant effects on researcher/clinician or teacher ratings; no study used independent observation; the majority of the children had comorbid ADHD. In contrast, the meta-analysis by Rosato *et al.* (2012) included studies with children with ADHD, learning disabilities, and autism. It reported an overall effect size of 0.72 over a mean period of 8 weeks treatment, during which the children (average age 9 years) gained 1.8 kg. This review recommends that if antipsychotics do not work, a mood stabilizing medication should be added. Thus this review takes a very different stance on treatment with medication from that taken by NICE, stating that "The evidence on the effect of psychosocial interventions on maladaptive

aggression is limited"; many authors disclosed payments from drug companies.

When might antipsychotics be contemplated? Clinical experience suggests they can lead to the helpful reductions in aggression in some cases, especially where there is poor emotional regulation characterized by prolonged rages. Prescribing antipsychotics for relatively short periods (say up to 4 months) in lower doses (say no more than 1–1.5 mg risperidone per day) where full evidence-based psychosocial interventions with both the family and the child are failing can help families cope; during this time it is crucial to continue to work at effective psychological management.

Conclusions

Children with ODD/CD deserve serious consideration since if untreated the outlook over the lifespan is notably negative for many of them. Fortunately, a great deal has been discovered about what leads to the condition, and crucially, what treatments are likely to work to make it better. However, in many countries there are few services available for them, including in rich countries, where they may be excluded from child and adolescent mental health services unless they have a comorbid conditions such as ADHD. While much further research needs to be done to understand both the causation and how best to treat these children, there are ample opportunities already to improve their plight by deploying greater resources to help them.

References

Abram, K. *et al.* (2003) Comorbid psychiatric diagnoses in youth in juvenile detention. *Archives of General Psychiatry* **60**, 1097–1108.

Alborz, A. *et al.* (2009) *The Impact of Adult Support Staff on Pupils and Mainstream Schools*. EPPI-Centre, Institute of Education, London.

Anderson, K. *et al.* (1986) Mothers' interactions with normal and conduct-disordered boys: who affects whom? *Developmental Psychology* **22**, 604–609.

Angold, A. & Costello, E. (2001) The epidemiology of disorders of conduct. In: *Conduct Disorders in Childhood and Adolescence*. (eds J. Hill & B. Maughan). Cambridge University Press, Cambridge.

Arsenault, L. *et al.* (2003) strong genetic effects on cross-situational antisocial behaviour among five-year-old children. *Journal of Child Psychology and Psychiatry* **44**, 832–848.

Aslund, C. *et al.* (2011) Maltreatment, MAOA, and delinquency: sex differences in gene-environment interaction in adolescents. *Behaviour Genetics* **41**, 262–272.

Baker, L. *et al.* (2009) Resting heart rate and the development of antisocial behavior from age 9-14: genetic and environmental influences. *Development and Psychopathology* **21**, 939–960.

Baker, E. *et al.* (2013) Low skin conductance activity in infancy predicts aggression in toddlers 2 years later. *Psychological Science* **24**, 1051–1056.

Baker-Henningham, H. *et al.* (2012) Reducing child conduct problems and promoting social skills in a middle-income country:

cluster-randomised controlled trial. *British Journal of Psychiatry* **201**, 101–108.

Barker, E. & Maughan, B. (2009) Differentiating early-onset persistent versus childhood-limited conduct problem youth. *American Journal of Psychiatry* **166**, 900–908.

Bentley, M.J. *et al.* (2013) Gene variants associated with antisocial behaviour: a latent variable approach. *Journal of Child Psychology and Psychiatry* **54**, 1074–1085.

Boivin, M. *et al.* (2013) Evidence of gene-environment correlation for peer difficulties: disruptive behaviors predict early peer relation difficulties in school through genetic effects. *Development and Psychopathology* **25**, 79–92.

Bornovalova, M. *et al.* (2010) Familial transmission and heritability of childhood disruptive disorders. *American Journal of Psychiatry* **167**, 1066–1074.

Bornovalova, M. *et al.* (2014) The relative contributions of direct environmental effects and passive genotype-environment correlations in child disruptive disorders. *Psychological Medicine* **44**, 831–844.

Bowlby, J. (1944) Forty-four juvenile thieves: their characters and home-life. *International Journal of Psycho-Analysis* **25**, 107–127.

Bradley, R.H. & Corwyn, R.F. (2008) Infant temperament, parenting, and externalizing behavior: a test of the differential susceptibility hypothesis. *Journal of Child Psychology and Psychiatry* **49**, 124–131.

Burt, S. (2009) Are there meaningful aetiological differences within antisocial behaviour? A meta-analysis. *Clinical Psychology Review* **29**, 163–178.

Caspi, A. *et al.* (2002) Role of genotype in the cycle of violence in maltreated children. *Science* **297**, 851–854.

Coie, J.D. (2004) The impact of negative social experiences on the development of antisocial behaviour. In: *Children's Peer Relations.* (eds J.B. Kupersmidt & K.A. Dodge), pp. 243–267. American Psychological Association, Washington, DC.

Collishaw, S. *et al.* (2004) Time trends in adolescent mental health. *Journal of Child Psychology and Psychiatry* **45**, 1350–1362.

Collishaw, S. *et al.* (2012) Do historical changes in parent-child relationships explain increases in youth conduct problems? *Journal of Abnormal Child Psychology* **40**, 119–132.

Copeland, W. *et al.* (2013) Prevalence, comorbidity, and correlates of DSM-5 proposed disruptive mood dysregulation disorder. *American Journal of Psychiatry* **170**, 173–179.

Costello, E.J. *et al.* (2003a) Prevalence and development of psychiatric disorders in childhood and adolescence. *Archives of General Psychiatry* **60**, 837–844.

Costello, E.J. *et al.* (2003b) Relationships between poverty and psychopathology: a natural experiment. *JAMA* **290**, 2023–2029.

Cummings, E. & Davies, P. (2002) Effects of marital conflict on children: recent advances. *Journal of Child Psychology and Psychiatry* **43**, 31–64.

Dick, D. *et al.* (2011) Genome-wide association study of conduct disorder symptomatology. *Molecular Psychiatry* **16**, 800–808.

Dishion, T.J. *et al.* (1999) When interventions harm. Peer groups and problem behaviour. *American Psychologist* **54**, 755–764.

Dodge, K.A. (1993) Social-cognitive mechanisms in the development of conduct disorder. *Annual Review of Psychology* **44**, 559–584.

Enzmann, D. *et al.* (2010) Self-reported youth delinquency in Europe and beyond. *European Journal of Criminology* **7**, 159–183.

Essex, M. *et al.* (2013) Epigenetic vestiges of early developmental adversity: childhood stress exposure and DNA methylation in adolescence. *Child Development* **84**, 58–75.

Fairchild, G. *et al.* (2008) Cortisol diurnal rhythm and stress reactivity in male adolescents with conduct disorder. *Biological Psychiatry* **64**, 599–606.

Fairchild, G. *et al.* (2009) Decision making and executive function in male adolescents conduct disorder. *Biological Psychiatry* **66**, 162–168.

Fairchild, G. *et al.* (2011) Brain structure abnormalities in conduct disorder. *American Journal of Psychiatry* **168**, 624–633.

Farrington, D. *et al.* (2009) Development of adolescence-limited, late-onset, and persistent offenders from age 8-48. *Aggressive Behavior* **35**, 150–163.

Fearon, R.P. *et al.* (2010) the significance of insecure attachment and disorganisation in the development of children's externalising behaviour: a meta-analysis. *Child Development* **81**, 435–456.

Fergusson, D. *et al.* (2005) Show me a child at seven: consequences of conduct problems in childhood for psychosocial functioning in adulthood. *Journal of Child Psychology and Psychiatry* **46**, 837–849.

Fonagy, P. & Target, M. (2008) Psychodynamic treatments. In: *Child and Adolescent Psychiatry.* (eds M. Rutter, *et al.*), 5th edn. Blackwell, Oxford.

Fontaine, N. *et al.* (2009) A critical review of studies on the developmental trajectories of antisocial behavior in females. *Journal of Child Psychology and Psychiatry* **50**, 363–385.

Fontaine, R. *et al.* (2010) Does response evaluation and decision mediate the relation between hostile attributional style and antisocial behavior in adolescence? *Journal of Abnormal Child Psychology* **38**, 615–626.

Fontaine, N. *et al.* (2011) Predictors and outcomes of joint trajectories of callous–unemotional traits and conduct problems in childhood. *Journal of Abnormal Psychology* **120**, 730–742.

Forster, M. *et al.* (2012) Randomized controlled trial of behavior management intervention for students with externalizing behavior. *Journal of Emotional and Behavioral Disorders* **20**, 169–183.

Futh, A. *et al.* (2008) Attachment narratives and behavioural and emotional symptoms in an ethnically diverse, at-risk sample. *Journal of the American Academy of Child and Adolescent Psychiatry* **47**, 709–718.

Gardner, F. (1989) Inconsistent parenting: link with children's conduct problems. *Journal of Abnormal Child Psychology* **17**, 223–233.

Goodman, R. & Scott, S. (1999) The strengths and difficulties questionnaire and the child behaviour checklist: is small beautiful? *Journal of Abnormal Child Psychology* **27**, 17–24.

Goodman, R. *et al.* (1995) The impact of child IQ, parent IQ and sibling IQ on child behavioral-deviance scores. *Journal of Child Psychology and Psychiatry* **36**, 409–425.

Goodman, A. *et al.* (2010) Why do British Indian children have an apparent mental health advantage? *Journal of Child Psychology and Psychiatry* **51**, 1171–1183.

Gottfredson, D.C. (2001) *Schools and Delinquency.* Cambridge University Press, Cambridge.

Graham, J. (1988) *Schools, Disruptive Behaviour and Delinquency.* HMSO, London.

Green, J. (2006) The therapeutic alliance in child mental health treatment studies. *Journal of Child Psychology and Psychiatry* **47**, 425–435.

Green, H. *et al.* (2005) *Mental Health of Children and Young People in Great Britain, 2004.* Office National Statistics, London.

Harold, G. *et al.* (2013) The nature of nurture: disentangling passive genotype-environment correlation from family relationship influences on children's externalizing problems. *Journal of Family Psychology* **27**, 12–21.

Hobson, C. *et al.* (2011) Investigation of cool and hot executive function in ODD/CD independently of ADHD. *Journal of Child Psychology and Psychiatry* **52**, 1035–1043.

Hughes, C. & Ensor, R. (2011) Individual differences in executive function across the transition to school predict externalizing and internalizing behaviors. *Journal of Experimental Child Psychology* **108**, 663–676.

Jaffee, S. *et al.* (2003) Life with (or without) father: the benefits of living with two biological parents depend on the father's antisocial behavior. *Child Development* **74**, 109–126.

Jaffee, S. *et al.* (2005) Nature x nurture: genetic vulnerabilities interact with physical maltreatment to promote conduct problems. *Development and Psychopathology* **17**, 67–84.

Jaffee, S. *et al.* (2012) From correlates to causes of antisocial behavior. *Psychological Bulletin* **138**, 272–295.

Jokela, M. *et al.* (2009) Childhood problem behaviors and death by midlife. *Journal of the American Academy of Child and Adolescent Psychiatry.* **48**, 19–24.

Jolliffe, D. *et al.* (2003) Validity of self-reported delinquency. *Criminal Behaviour and Mental Health* **13**, 179–197.

Kazdin, A.E. (1996) Dropping out of child therapy. *Clinical Child Psychology and Psychiatry* **1**, 133–156.

Keenan, K. & Shaw, D. (2003) Exploring the etiology of antisocial behaviour. In: *Causes of Conduct Disorder and Delinquency.* (eds B. Lahey, *et al.*), pp. 153–181. Guilford Press, New York.

Kim-Cohen, J. *et al.* (2006) MAOA, maltreatment, and gene-environment interaction: a meta-analysis. *Molecular Psychiatry* **11**, 903–913.

Klein, R. *et al.* (1997) Clinical efficacy of methylphenidate in conduct disorder with and without ADHD. *Archives of General Psychiatry* **54**, 1073–108.

Larson, J. & Lochman, J. (2011) *Helping Schoolchildren Cope with Anger: A Cognitive-Behavioral Intervention,* 2nd edn. Guilford Press, New York.

Lochman, J. *et al.* (2012) Three year follow-up of coping power intervention effects. *Prevention Science* **14**, 364–376.

Loeber, R. *et al.* (2012) Cognitive impulsivity and intelligence as predictors of the age-crime curve. *Journal of the American Academy of Child and Adolescent Psychiatry* **51**, 1136–1149.

Lorber, M.F. (2004) Psychophysiology of aggression: a meta-analysis. *Psychological Bulletin* **130**, 531–552.

Maughan, B. *et al.* (2008) Recent trends in UK child and adolescent mental health. *Social Psychiatry and Psychiatric Epidemiology* **43**, 305–310.

Maughan, B. *et al.* (2013) Adolescent conduct problems and premature mortality: follow-up to age 65 in a national cohort, *Psychological Medicine* **44**, 1077–1086.

McMahon, R. *et al.* (2010) Parent training for the treatment of oppositional behavior. In: *Clinical Handbook of Conduct Problems.* (eds R. Murrihy, *et al.*). Springer, New York.

Minuchin, S. (1974) *Families and Family Therapy.* Harvard University Press, Cambridge, MA.

Moffitt, T.E. (1993) "Life-course-persistent" and "adolescence-limited" antisocial behavior: a developmental taxonomy. *Psychological Review* **100**, 674–701.

Moffitt, T. & Caspi, A. (1998) Implications of violence between intimate partners. *Journal of Child Psychology and Psychiatry* **39**, 137–144.

Moffitt, T.E. *et al.* (2001) *Sex Differences in Antisocial Behaviour.* Cambridge University Press, Cambridge.

Murray, J. & Farrington, D. (2010) Risk factors for conduct disorder and delinquency: key findings from longitudinal studies. *Canadian Journal of Psychiatry* **55**, 633–642.

National Institute for Health and Care Excellence (2013) *Clinical Guideline on Antisocial and Conduct Disorders.* National Institute for Health and Care Excellence, London.

Nock, M. *et al.* (2006) Prevalence, subtypes, and correlates of DSM-IV conduct disorder in the national comorbidity survey replication. *Psychological Medicine* **36**, 699–710.

Nock, M. *et al.* (2007) Oppositional defiant disorder: results from the national comorbidity survey replication. *Journal of Child Psychology and Psychiatry* **48**, 703–713.

Nomura, Y. *et al.* (2008) Perinatal problems and adolescent antisocial behaviors among children born after 33 weeks. *Journal of Child Psychology and Psychiatry* **49**, 1108–1117.

O'Connor, T. *et al.* (1998) Genotype-environment correlations in antisocial behavioural problems and coercive parenting. *Developmental Psychology* **34**, 970–981.

Odgers, C. *et al.* (2007) Predicting prognosis for the conduct-problem boy: can family history help? *Journal of the American Academy of Child and Adolescent Psychiatry.* **46**, 1240–1249.

Odgers, C.L. *et al.* (2008) Female and male antisocial trajectories: from childhood origins to adult outcomes. *Development and Psychopathology* **20**, 673–716.

Odgers, C. *et al.* (2012) Supportive parenting mediates neighborhood socioeconomic disparities in children's antisocial behavior from ages 5-12. *Development and Psychopathology* **24**, 705–721.

Ogilvie, J. *et al.* (2011) Neuropsychological measures of executive function and antisocial behavior: a meta-analysis. *Criminology* **49**, 1063–1107.

Ortiz, J. & Raine, A. (2004) Heart rate level and antisocial behavior in children and adolescents: a meta-analysis. *Journal of the American Academy of Child and Adolescent Psychiatry* **43**, 154–162.

Patterson, G. (1982) *Coercive Family Process.* Castalia, Eugene.

Patterson, G. *et al.* (1989) A developmental perspective on antisocial behaviour. *American Psychologist* **44**, 329–335.

Petersen, I. *et al.* (2013) Language ability predicts the development of behavior problems in children. *Abnormal Psychology* **122**, 542–557.

Piquero, A. *et al.* (2010) Trajectories of offending and their relation to life failure in late middle age. *Journal of Research in Crime and Delinquency* **47**, 151–173.

Piquero, A. *et al.* (2013) The monetary costs of crime to middle adulthood: findings from the Cambridge study. *Journal of Research in Crime and Delinquency* **50**, 53–74.

Platje, E. *et al.* (2013) Longitudinal associations in adolescence between cortisol and persistent aggressive or rule-breaking behavior. *Biological Psychology* **93**, 132–137.

Plomin, R. *et al.* (2013) *Behavioral Genetics.* Worth, New York.

Polman, H. *et al.* (2007) A meta-analysis of the distinction between reactive and proactive aggression in children and adolescents. *Journal of Abnormal Child Psychology* **35**, 522–535.

Racz, S. & McMahon, R. (2011) The relationship between parental knowledge and monitoring and conduct problems: 10-year update. *Clinical Child and Family Psychology Review* **14**, 377–398.

Robins, L. (1966) *Deviant Children Grown Up.* Williams & Wilkins, Baltimore.

Romano, E. *et al.* (2001) Prevalence of psychiatric diagnoses and the role of perceived impairment. *Journal of Child Psychology and Psychiatry* **42**, 451–461.

Romeo, R. *et al.* (2006) The economic cost of severe antisocial behaviour in children, and who pays it. *British Journal of Psychiatry* **188**, 547–553.

Rosato, N.S. *et al.* (2012) Treatment of maladaptive aggression in youth: CERT guidelines, *Pediatrics* **126**, e1562–e1576.

Rubia, K. (2011) "Cool" inferior frontostriatal dysfunction in ADHD versus "Hot" ventromedial orbitofrontal-limbic dysfunction in CD. *Biological Psychiatry* **69**, e69–e87.

Rutter, M. (1981) The city and the child. *American Journal of Orthopsychiatry* **51**, 610–625.

Rutter, M. (2011) Child psychiatric diagnosis and classification: concepts, findings, challenges and potential. *Journal of Child Psychology and Psychiatry* **52**, 647–660.

Rutter, M. & Smith, D. (1995) *Psychosocial Disorders in Young People: Time Trends and Their Causes.* John Wiley & Sons, Chichester.

Rutter, M. *et al.* (1998) *Antisocial Behaviour by Young People.* Cambridge University Press, Cambridge.

Sampson, R.J. & Laub, J.H. (1994) Urban poverty and the family context of delinquency: a new look at structure and process in a classic study. *Child Development* **65**, 523–540.

Sanders, M. (2012) Development, evaluation, and multinational dissemination of the triple P-positive parenting program. *Annual Review of Clinical Psychology* **8**, 345–379.

Scott, S. & Dadds, M. (2009) When parent training doesn't work: theory-driven clinical strategies. *Journal of Child Psychology and Psychiatry* **50**, 1441–1450.

Scott, S. & O'Connor, T. (2012) An experimental test of differential susceptibility to parenting among emotionally dysregulated children. *Journal of Child Psychology and Psychiatry* **53**, 1184–1193.

Scott, S. *et al.* (2001) Financial cost of social exclusion: follow up study of antisocial children into adulthood. *British Medical Journal* **323**, 191–194.

Scott, S. *et al.* (2010a) Randomized controlled trial of parent groups for child antisocial behaviour targeting multiple risk factors. *Journal of Child Psychology and Psychiatry* **51**, 48–57.

Scott, S. *et al.* (2010b) Impact of a parenting program in a high-risk, multi-ethnic community: the PALS trial. *Journal of Child Psychology and Psychiatry* **51**, 1331–1341.

Scott, S. *et al.* (2011) Attachment in adolescence: overlap with parenting and unique prediction of behavioural adjustment. *Journal of Child Psychology and Psychiatry* **52**, 1052–1062.

Shaffer, D. *et al.* (1983) A children's global assessment scale (CGAS). *Archives of General Psychiatry* **40**, 1228–1231.

Shirk, S. & Carver, M. (2003) Prediction of treatment outcome from relationship variables in child and adolescent therapy: a meta-analysis. *Journal of Consulting and Clinical Psychology* **71**, 52–464.

Shivram, R. *et al.* (2009) Service utilization by children with conduct disorders. *European Child & Adolescent Psychiatry* **18**, 555–563.

Silberg, J. *et al.* (1996) Genetic and environmental influences on the covariation between hyperactivity and conduct disturbance in juvenile twins. *Journal of Child Psychology and Psychiatry* **37**, 803–816.

Sonuga-Barke, E. *et al.* (2013) Nonpharmalogical interventions for ADHD: systematic review and meta analyses. *American Journal of Psychiatry* **170**, 275–289.

Stattin, H. & Kerr, M. (2000) Parental monitoring: a reinterpretation. *Child Development* **71**, 1072–1085.

Stringaris, A. & Goodman, R. (2009) Longitudinal outcome of youth oppositionality: irritable, headstrong, and hurtful behaviors. *Journal of the American Academy of Child and Adolescent Psychiatry* **48**, 404–412.

Sweeten, G. *et al.* (2013) Age and the explanation of crime, revisited. *Journal of Youth and Adolescence* **42**, 921–938.

Taylor, E. *et al.* (1987) which boys respond to stimulant medication? A controlled trial of methylphenidate in boys with disruptive behaviour. *Psychological Medicine* **17**, 121–143.

Taylor, E. *et al.* (1996) Hyperactivity and conduct problems as risk factors for adolescent development. *Journal of the American Academy of Child and Adolescent Psychiatry* **35**, 1213–1226.

Thapar, A. & Rutter, M. (2009) Do prenatal risk factors cause psychiatric disorder? Be wary of causal claims. *British Journal of Psychiatry* **195**, 100–101.

Thapar, A. *et al.* (2013) What have we learnt about the causes of ADHD? *Journal of Child Psychology and Psychiatry* **54**, 3–16.

Thomas, A. *et al.* (1968) *Temperament and Behaviour Disorders in Children.* New York University Press, New York.

Tolan, P.H. *et al.* (2003) The developmental ecology of urban males' youth violence. *Developmental Psychology* **39**, 274–291.

Trzesniewski, K. *et al.* (2006) Revisiting the association between reading achievement and antisocial behavior. *Child Development* **77**, 72–88.

Van der Laan, A. *et al.* (2010) Serious, minor, and non-delinquents in early adolescence: the impact of cumulative risk and promotive factors. *Journal of Abnormal Child Psychology* **38**, 339–351.

Viding, E. *et al.* (2008) Heritability of antisocial behaviour at 9: do callous-unemotional traits matter? *Developmental Science* **11**, 17–22.

Webster-Stratton, C. & Reid, J. (2010) The incredible years series. In: *Evidence-Based Psychotherapies for Children and Adolescents.* (eds J. Weisz & A. Kazdin). Guilford, New York.

Whelan, Y. *et al.* (2013) Developmental continuity of oppositional defiant disorder subdimensions. *Journal of the American Academy of Child and Adolescent Psychiatry* **52**, 961–969.

Zisser, A. & Eyberg, S. (2010) Parent-child interaction therapy. In: *Evidence-Based Psychotherapies for Children and Adolescents.* (eds J. Weisz & A. Kazdin), pp. 179–193. Guilford, New York.

CHAPTER 66

Substance-related and addictive disorders

Thomas J. Crowley and Joseph T. Sakai

Department of Psychiatry, University of Colorado School of Medicine, Aurora, CO, USA

Introduction

Substance use disorders (SUDs), being among the most prevalent psychiatric disorders in persons 9 to 21 years old (Copeland *et al.*, 2011), are profoundly important to child and adolescent psychiatry. Considering the United States, each year about 10% of adolescents begin drinking alcohol, 6% start using illicit drugs, and 5% initiate cigarette smoking. Of course, this is only starting drug use, but 7% in that age range have diagnosable SUDs. Rare before age 10, the number of new SUD cases rises rapidly through adolescence, peaking around age 20 and declining thereafter; new cases are unusual after age 25. However, adolescent SUDs often persist into young adulthood, and those persisting further become leading causes of adult deaths.

Although such US data are unusually detailed, they cannot describe adolescents world-wide. For example, a cross-national study (Hibell *et al.*, 2012) in 36 European countries (with comparative US data) asked 16 year-old youths whether they had been drunk in the last 30 days. The percentage answering "yes" in selected countries included: Denmark, 37% (highest); UK, 26; Norway, 14; USA, 14; and Albania, 6 (lowest). Clearly, clinicians treating adolescent SUDs must track their own regional epidemiologic trends.

Adolescent-onset SUDs often co-occur with risk-taking, impulsivity, inattention, and conduct problems in a broad trait of personality and temperament termed "behavioral disinhibition … a highly heritable general propensity to not constrain behavior in socially acceptable ways, to break social norms and rules, and to take dangerous risks, pursuing rewards excessively despite dangers of adverse consequences" (American Psychiatric Association, 2013; cf., Iacono *et al.*, 2008). Because early intense substance use is dangerously risky and clearly involves "pursuing rewards excessively despite dangers of adverse consequences," SUDs are a central manifestation of high behavioral disinhibition. Conduct disorder, strongly comorbid with early-onset

SUD, is another such manifestation. For example, nearly 50,000 16-year-old students in some 16 European countries completed self-report assessments of their antisocial behavior, depression, self-esteem, and anomie. Although high scores on each of those measures significantly predicted heavy substance use, the association with antisocial behavior was by far the strongest (Hibell *et al.*, 2009).

Because youths with this trait often do very dangerous behaviors, like driving while drinking, using multiple substances, carrying weapons, or fighting frequently, they are at serious risk for both accidental injury and homicide, which are the most common causes of death in American adolescents. A case example highlights these issues.

Case Report. A 16-year-old Hispanic female was referred to a university day-treatment program for substance-involved adolescents. She met DSM-IV criteria for abuse of cannabis and cocaine; dependence on alcohol, nicotine, and hallucinogens; and major depression. Conduct problems included probation, car thefts, shoplifting, truancy, runaways, curfew violations, driving without a license, lying, and fighting. Both parents had histories of substance problems and court convictions.

The girl first used marijuana at age 8. An excellent student through age 12, her marijuana use then escalated sharply. At age 13 she "hung out with the wrong kids," and by age 14 she was chronically truant, using drugs at home with gang friends.

Day Treatment included individual and group counseling to diminish drug use and increase prosocial behavior, family treatment to enhance parental control, antidepressant medication, and urine monitoring. She made excellent progress, remained abstinent, spoke and wrote thoughtfully about her past behavior, and was much liked by treatment staff. At discharge after 6 months staff rated her treatment as "successful" and referred her for follow-up care elsewhere.

Two years later newspapers reported that the now eighteen year-old woman and a much older, frequently-arrested man had burglarized a garage. After a high-speed chase police caused the couple's car to crash. When the man brandished a gun, police shot them both dead. Newspapers reported that both bodies contained

Rutter's Child and Adolescent Psychiatry, Sixth Edition.
Edited by Anita Thapar and Daniel S. Pine, James F. Leckman, Stephen Scott, Margaret J. Snowling, Eric Taylor.
© 2015 John Wiley & Sons Ltd. Published 2018 by John Wiley & Sons Ltd.

methamphetamine, and that the woman had been arrested five months earlier for manufacturing drugs.

Such complex patients may present multiple drug and conduct problems, other psychiatric disorders, improvement during (and relapse after) treatment, a prolonged relapsing course, familial substance and antisocial problems, pursuit of exciting pleasures while ignoring dangers, and mortal risk. The treatment goal often is to minimize the risk for psychological and physical morbidity and mortality.

Most adolescents in substance treatment have diagnosable SUDs on several substances, often including alcohol, tobacco, cannabis, or other locally prevalent drugs. Treatments for withdrawal syndromes and medications for SUDs usually target specific drugs, while psychosocial treatments typically address drug-taking generally.

It is estimated that 7% of 12–17-year-old Americans needed treatment for an alcohol or illicit-drug SUD in 2011. However, appropriate facilities administered such treatment to only 0.6%. Without enough doctoral-trained clinicians to meet that extreme public-health need, non-doctoral substance-abuse counselors are required. However, these patients' clinical complexity does demand highly trained supervising professionals, including child and adolescent psychiatrists. We present a model addressing that public-health need with non-doctoral counselors conducting most psychosocial treatments, supervised by senior social workers, psychologists, and psychiatrists.

Definitions, comparative nosology

A drug is a natural or synthetic chemical substance that affects living processes. Substance-related disorders are psychiatric disorders developing during or following substance use, and attributable to it. The drugs that most often produce substance-related disorders include tobacco, alcohol, cannabis, stimulants (cocaine, amphetamine, methamphetamine, mephedrone, and others), opioids, sedative-hypnotic and anxiolytic agents, inhalants (volatile hydrocarbons), phencyclidine or other aryl-cyclohexylamines, and other hallucinogens. Numerous other substances, including nitrous oxide, amyl- or butyl-nitrite, or anabolic steroids also may produce these disorders.

Adolescents experiment with substances. Where is the line between experimentation and diagnosable SUD? Because early initiation of use tends to predict later substance problems, risky substance experimentation warrants early intervention (discussed below), but substance use is not SUD, even in young teens. Nevertheless, some adolescent users do develop SUDs, as described next.

The *Diagnostic and Statistical Manual of Mental Disorders, Edition 5* (DSM-5; American Psychiatric Association, 2013), like the previous DSM-IV, divides substance-related disorders into two categories. SUDs are conditions in which the person continues using a substance despite experiencing serious problems caused by that substance. These disorders include, for

example, alcohol use disorder or cocaine use disorder. Substance *induced* disorders develop as a consequence of prior substance use, and include, most obviously, intoxication and withdrawal. These additional disorders also may be induced by substances: neurocognitive, psychotic, depressive, bipolar, panic, anxiety, sexual, sleep, and obsessive-compulsive disorders, as well as delirium.

DSM-5 uses the same 11 criteria for diagnosing each different SUD (Hasin *et al.*, 2013), and many adolescent patients qualify for more than one of these diagnoses (*e.g.*, both alcohol use disorder and cannabis use disorder). The criteria were adopted from the earlier DSM-IV with the intention that DSM-IV and DSM-5 would diagnose the same groups. However, DSM-IV's criterion, "recurrent substance related legal problems," was replaced because drug laws vary widely in different jurisdictions. "Craving" replaced it and is assessed with, for example, "Do you sometimes feel a strong desire or urge to use [substance]?" The resulting 11 diagnostic criteria fall into four broad problem categories: impaired control, social impairments, risky use, and pharmacologic problems (tolerance, withdrawal). Meeting more criteria does indicate more severe functional impairment and more serious disorder, so SUD severity is estimated by counting the criteria one meets: 0–1, no diagnosis; 2–3, mild SUD; 4–5, moderate; >5, severe.

The 11 diagnostic criteria for SUD include tolerance and withdrawal, but those also occur during medical treatment with, for example, stimulants, opioids, sedative-hypnotics, or anxiolytics. Thus, during appropriate treatment with these medications DSM-5 does not permit a SUD diagnosis unless the person meets criteria beyond tolerance and withdrawal.

Cannabis produces a withdrawal syndrome somewhat similar to nicotine's. DSM-5, unlike previous editions, recognizes cannabis withdrawal as a substance *induced* disorder.

The International Classification of Diseases (ICD) of the World Health Organization (WHO) classifies and provides numeric codes for physical and behavioral disorders (WHO, 2010). WHO's current, 10th revision (ICD-10) will be replaced by ICD-11 in 2015. Nations modify and adopt the ICD on their own schedules. For example, the USA will use ICD-9 in a modified version (ICD-9-CM, Clinical Modification) until it adopts ICD-10 in 2014.

Many of DSM-5's 11 diagnostic criteria for SUD are implied in ICD's "Dependence Syndrome": "A cluster of behavioral, cognitive, and physiological phenomena that develop after repeated substance use and that typically include a strong desire to take the drug, difficulties in controlling its use, persisting in its use despite harmful consequences, a higher priority given to drug use than to other activities and obligations, increased tolerance, and sometimes a physical withdrawal state." However, ICD's "Harmful Use" ("A pattern of psychoactive substance use that is causing damage to health ... ") is not in DSM-5.

Saunders (2006) concluded that DSM-IV's substance dependence disorder and ICD's Dependence Syndrome were similar in structure and functioned well; DSM-IV's substance abuse diagnosis performed moderately well; and ICD's Harmful Use performed poorly. Hasin *et al.* (2013) expect that DSM-5, maintaining most of DSM-IV's abuse and dependence criteria while adding ICD's "craving," will identify persons with mild to severe substance problems.

ICD provides diagnoses comparable to several of DSM-5's substance *induced* disorders. However, DSM-5 does not recognize ICD's "Residual and Late-Onset Psychotic Disorder," understood as a persistent drug-induced psychosis.

Neither DSM-5 nor ICD define "addiction" nor include the term in the name of any specific disorder, perhaps considering it pejorative. Curiously, however, DSM-5's chapter on these disorders is titled "Substance Related Disorders and Other Addictions" (see Non-Substance "Behavioral Addictions", below).

In making differential diagnoses each SUD must be distinguished from: (i) unintentional substance exposure; (ii) intentional substance use not meeting criteria for a SUD; (iii) unrecognized comorbid SUDs (e.g., diazepam and cocaine use disorders together); (iv) substance induced disorders (e.g., intoxication); and (v) other medical disorders. Each substance *induced* disorder must be distinguished from: (i) its cognate disorder (e.g., substance induced mood disorder, vs mood disorder); (ii) other substance induced disorders (e.g., substance induced delirium vs substance induced neurocognitive disorder); and (iii) other medical disorders.

The criteria for diagnosing SUDs are both valid and reliable. However, because SUDs frequently are comorbid with, and concealed by, other conditions, clinicians must actively consider them, accurately diagnose them, and initiate appropriate treatment.

Epidemiology

Prevalence of use

Substances are used worldwide, and substance experimentation is common among children. The substances used vary by age of the individual and availability of the drug; for example, young children may have difficulty accessing cocaine, but inhalants in glues, paints, cleaning agents, or fuels are easily available in many homes. About 1 in 8 American eighth graders (ca. age 13) have used inhalants, but by the mid-teens alcohol, nicotine, and cannabis use predominate, and few use inhalants by late adolescence. Although the legal age for possessing alcohol in the United States is 21 years, in 2011 about 70% of high school seniors (ca. age 17) had used alcohol, and nearly 1 in 4 reported having had at least 5 drinks on one occasion in the last 2 weeks. Although these students perceived high risk from, and disapproval of, cigarettes, about 1 in 6 had smoked in the past month. Patterns of illicit drug use are equally concerning; about half of American high school seniors have used an illicit drug, including 36% using cannabis and 15% misusing prescription medications (especially opioids and amphetamines) in the last year. Fortunately, although many adolescents experiment with substances, most who try them will not progress to a clinical

SUD diagnosis. For example, among U.S. adolescents only about 7% met criteria for a SUD during the past year.

Comparisons of 16-year-old students in some 36 European countries and the USA (Hibell *et al.*, 2012) are partially presented in Table 66.1. The data show considerable country-to-country variability in substance use, although a country's high prevalence of use of one substance does not necessarily predict high use of another substance. Generally, the UK and USA show mid range prevalence figures.

Comorbid disorders

Among American adolescents with SUD, about 60–80% have conduct disorder; 30-50 percent, attention-deficit/hyperactivity disorder; 15–25%, major depressive disorder; and 15–25%, anxiety disorder (Riggs, 2003). Conversely, SUD is prevalent among adolescents utilizing mental health treatment (Kramer *et al.*, 2003); estimates vary, but many with bipolar disorder and psychosis have a co-occurring SUD (Kavanagh *et al.*, 2004; Goldstein & Bukstein, 2010).

Sex differences

Early in development the "default brain" is female, but males' brains are "masculinized" early in development, leading to numerous male-female brain differences. As a result, males in many mammalian species, including humans, show more risky, aggressive behavior than females. For example, American adolescent boys, more than girls, carry guns or other weapons, drive after drinking alcohol, rarely wear seatbelts, and die from accidental or homicidal injuries. Boys commit three-fourths of juvenile violent crimes. They are much more likely to develop serious conduct problems, and they have higher behavioral-disinhibition scores.

It is surprising, then, that rates of illicit drug, alcohol, and tobacco use, and also of SUDs (about 7%), are similar in adolescent male and female Americans. However, as youngsters age into the late teen years, sex differences in SUD prevalence emerge. After age 17 the prevalence of SUD is, as expected, much higher in males (10.8%) than females (5.6%).

Morbidity and mortality

Tobacco is estimated to be a major factor in about 18% of all American deaths, alcohol in about 3%, and illicit drugs in less than 1%. Illicit drugs vary in relative mortality risks for users—higher for some (e.g., opioid overdose deaths) and lower for others (e.g., cannabis). Unfortunately, sometimes even single uses of some drugs are fatal: inhalants' "sudden sniffers' death" or suffocation, and opioids' respiratory depression.

Motor vehicle accidents are the leading cause of death among 16–19-year-old American youths, and among drivers of that age involved in fatal accidents, about 20% had positive blood alcohol tests. In 2011 about 10% of American high school students (aged 16 and older) reported drinking and driving in the last month.

In 2010 underage drinking contributed to nearly 190,000 visits to American hospital emergency departments. Substance use is

Table 66.1 Range of substance use prevalence (percent of 16 Year-Olds), 36 European countries and USA[a].

Alcohol use

	Ever use	Past-year use	Drunk in the past year
36 country average	87	79	37
Highest	Czech Republic, 98	Czech Republic, 93	Denmark, 69
Lowest	Iceland, 56	Iceland, 43	Albania, 14
UK	90	85	48
USA	56	50	26[b]

Cigarette use

	Ever use	Past month	First cigarette by age 13
36 country average	54	28	31
Highest	Latvia, 78	Latvia, 43	Latvia, 61
Lowest	Iceland, 26	Iceland, 10	Iceland, 14
UK	47	23	25
USA	30	12	19[c]

Cannabis use

	Ever use	Past-year use	Past-month use
36 country average	17	13	7
Highest	Czech Republic, 42	France, 35	France, 24
Lowest	Albania, 4	Bosnia and Herzegovina, 3	Moldova, 1
UK	25	21	13
USA	35	29	18

[a]Hibell *et al.*, (2012).
[b]The question asks "been drunk or very high . . . ."
[c]Assessed in 8th grade (about age 13).

also associated with suicide, violence, and other risky behaviors. For example, early, severe substance problems are associated with early, high-risk sexual behaviors, and with teen pregnancy. Although injection drug use is generally rare among American adolescents, of adolescents treated for early-onset SUD, about 1 in 6 report injecting drugs by young adulthood, thus risking HIV, hepatitis C, and other infectious diseases.

Treatment admissions

About 7% of 12–17 year olds in the USA had a SUD and needed treatment in 2011, but only about 1 in 12 of those adolescents received it, and of those who did not receive treatment, some 95% believed they did not need it. Not surprisingly, then, many adolescents who do receive treatment for SUD are forced into it through criminal-justice or social-service agencies.

About 140,000 11–15-year old English youths reported regular smoking, 360,000 drank alcohol in the last week and 180,000 had used other drugs in the last month. However, in one year only 22,000 persons under age 18 received specialty substance treatment services. Similarly, an estimated 1 million English people (ages 16–65 years) are alcohol dependent, but only 6% of them per year receive treatment (National Institute for Health and Care Excellence (NICE), 2011). Moreover, such specialty care may be much less available in many countries.

Shifts in substances used

Substance use patterns vary across time. For example, as American physicians increased their prescribing of opioids for pain management, adolescents increasingly accessed prescription opioid drugs for non-medical use. These drugs became the second most common illicit substances used by high school seniors (ca. age 17). During the same period, rates of alcohol use decreased, while cannabis use increased.

The internet provides access to substances that previously had limited availability. For example, nitrous oxide is now easily purchased on the internet, along with cannisters ("crackers") that release the gas from cartridges ("whippets"), and balloons to hold the gas for inhalation.

Also, new, abusable substances frequently appear. Recently, American stores have sold smokable synthetic cannabinoid agonists, falsely labeled "incense" and "not for human consumption"; 1 in 10 high school seniors (ca. age 17) reported using them in a recent year. A new stimulant drug, methylenedioxypyrovalerone, has been sold as "Bath Salts." In addition, old drugs find new uses. Dextromethorphan, a non prescription antitussive, in high doses produces hallucinatory episodes called "Robo-tripping" or "using Triple C's" from the products' brand names.

Regional and global prevalence variations

World estimates suggest that alcohol contributes to about 2.5 million deaths annually, with about 69 million years of productive life lost; some 230 million people used illicit drugs in 2010, with 15–39 million having problematic drug use (Degenhardt & Hall, 2012). There are substantial geographic variations in drug use prevalence, with higher rates in higher-income countries (although data from lower-income countries often are lacking). More use also occurs in countries that produce or transport drugs. Regional variations in availability and cultural acceptance of specific drugs also impact use patterns, including age of onset of substance use; by age 13, about 1% of Greeks have tried marijuana or hashish, about 8% of French youths, and about 15% of Americans.

Genetic and environmental risk factors

Familiality

Substance problems cluster within families. In Iceland, where large family genealogies are readily studied, first degree relatives (siblings or parent-and-child) of persons with alcohol use disorder are about twice as likely as others to develop the disorder; the risk decreases in more distant relatives, but remains somewhat elevated even among fifth degree relations. The familiality of illicit drugs is even stronger, and considerable familiality also exists *across* SUD diagnoses (e.g., an individual with cannabis use disorder having a relative with alcohol use disorder; Tyrfingsson *et al.*, 2010).

Environmental influences and/or genes may drive such familiality. Twin and adoption studies help to parse heritable and genetic influences, and in childhood and early adolescence risk of substance *use* is predominantly mediated by environmental factors, especially family environment, but at older ages such environmental effects decrease in importance and genetic effects increase. While many studies have examined initiation of substance use, relatively few have studied the heritability of adolescent SUD. However, the available studies indicate that at least half of the variance is related to genetic effects (Rhee *et al.*, 2003). Thus, whether a child or adolescent tries a substance is influenced strongly by environmental factors (e.g., drug availability, or family attitudes toward drug use), but substance problems in adolescence are more strongly influenced by genetic effects.

Environmental context

The environment in which a child is raised influences risk for SUD outcomes. Many parents who misuse substances model general acceptance of substance use and specific substance use behaviors, allow easy substance access, offer little support for prosocial behaviors, share drugs with their children, and provide limited supervision. Affectively hostile and inconsistent parenting, paired with a strong-willed child who has poor self control, may lead to high parent–child conflict, reduced parental engagement, and poorer monitoring. Having a same-sex drug-misusing sibling, older but close-in-age, increases the risk of drug misuse (Kendler *et al.*, 2013). Neighborhood, school, peers, and important extra-familial adults further influence drug availability and acceptability, and families influence those factors by encouraging or discouraging specific extracurricular activities and by choosing the child's school and neighborhood of residence.

Genetic risk

Although specific environmental risks for later SUD are relatively well defined, information on specific-substance risk genes (e.g., just alcohol, or just cocaine) is weak. An exception in many East Asians is genetic variants in aldehyde dehydrogenase genes that produce a disulfiram-like impact during alcohol metabolism; resulting reductions in alcohol use disorder comprise an effect large enough to be of public health importance. Also, certain GABRA2 genotypes are associated with alcohol use disorder. Variants in nicotinic receptor genes have been associated with nicotine dependence (Saccone *et al.*, 2007). However, many individuals with SUD use multiple substances, and then a history often shows family problems not with one substance, but with many. Thus, although there probably are many substance-specific genetic factors, this risk for SUD generally appears to be more important.

Genes and environment: joint effects

Numerous twin studies concur that genes contribute about half of the risk for developing any particular SUD, with environment contributing the other half. However, the two contributors are not independent. For example, in gene-environment *correlations*, children in families with high genetic loading for SUD may inherit genetic variants that increase risk for SUD. Their parents, bearing the same genes, also may have SUDs, thus establishing risk-increasing environments around the children. In addition, genetic and environmental factors may *interact* to determine SUD risk; low-risk environments can mute a high genetic risk. For example, helping families out of poverty reduces risk for both antisocial behavior problems and SUD (Costello *et al.*, 2010). Such gene–environment correlations and interactions underscore the complex interplay of genetic and environmental risks for SUD.

Genetic studies of complex traits

Although genes clearly and strongly contribute to SUDs, few specific molecular contributors are known. Molecular studies in complex traits such as SUD suggest that many DNA sites contribute, each adding a very small increase in risk. Together they account for about half of the difference in SUD risk among individuals, but individually each accounts for very little. In addition, earlier studies focused on genes coding for protein products and ignored inter-gene "junk DNA." However, recent work finds that these non coding regions actually contain important gene regulators. Finding these many small genetic contributors will require much more research (see Chapter 24).

Brain function and drug risk-taking

Risk-taking is adaptive in adolescents, who must gradually detach from family, bond and compete with age-mates, practice romantic and sexual behaviors, and move toward adult roles as parent and worker. But concurrently, many also begin taking risks with dangerous drugs. Two psychological traits contribute to that behavioral disinhibition and risk-taking. *Impulsivity* is a deficiency in self-control and response inhibition, leading to hasty, unplanned behavior, and *sensation seeking* is a disposition to seek out novel, stimulating experiences.

Adolescents' brain structure and function (cf., see Chapter 11) mediate that interrelated behavioral disinhibition, impulsivity, and sensation seeking. First, in adulthood, the dorsolateral prefrontal cortex will exert mature cognitive control over decision-making, often inhibiting risky behaviors; however, those inhibitory influences are weaker in adolescents because their still-maturing forebrains have incomplete cortical thinning and fiber myelination (Giedd *et al.*, 2010). Meanwhile, adolescents' rapidly maturing brain reward system facilitates enhanced reward seeking. Together, matured reward-supporting structures and still-immature inhibitory structures generate risk-taking behavior, including drug risk-taking.

But why do some adolescents, and not others, take really serious drug risks? The ventral striatum (nucleus accumbens), a principal target of dopaminergic neurons, activates vigorously when rewards are expected (Schneider *et al.*, 2012). Among adolescents with essentially no drug exposure, risk-taking and the strength of striatal activation during reward anticipation are strongly, negatively associated (more activation, less risk-taking), and that relationship is even stronger in adolescents who already have started using drugs. Moreover, risk-taking also negatively correlates with gray matter density in the ventral striatum (Schneider *et al.*, 2012). So differences in striatal structure and function are neural markers for individual differences in risk-taking, including drug risk-taking.

In addition, when attempting to inhibit a behavior some youngsters have diminished neural activation in numerous brain regions, and such neural hypoactivation predicts drug and conduct problems several years later (Norman *et al.*, 2011). Apparently, in such adolescents brain mechanisms for inhibiting behaviors malfunction before drug use begins.

So some adolescents' brains are more disposed than others' toward risky drug and conduct problems. Then, drug use itself pharmacologically alters the brain in three steps that promote continued drug-taking (Koob & Volkow, 2010). First, in a *binge-intoxication stage* each dose of an addicting drug acutely reduces firing thresholds (increases firing) in those dopaminergic pathways sometimes called the brain reward system, mediating a subjective "high" that encourages further drug use.

Second, continued use gradually produces a *withdrawal/negative-affect stage*, depleting dopamine and other neurotransmitters, with each successive dose yielding less hedonia and greater post-dose dysphoria (Figure 66.1). Then, terminating prolonged drug use diminishes dopaminergic and serotonergic neurotransmission, activates a corticotropin-releasing-factor stress system, and generates anxiety. Both dopamine release and dopamine D$_2$ receptor expression decline, reducing sensitivity to rewards. By these means, drugs pharmacologically bias the brain's decision-making machinery toward repeated decisions to obtain and use the drugs, which no longer produce hedonia but mainly function to stop aversive dysphoria. Despite such

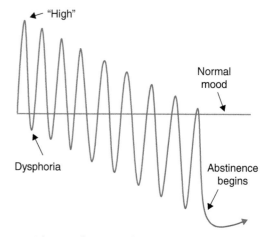

Figure 66.1 Schematic illustration of dysphoria induced by repeated intoxication-withdrawal cyles (cf., Koob & Volkow, 2010). Each intoxication leads to a subjective "high", with enhanced response to reward in dopaminergic structures. Each acute withdrawal event results in subjective dysphoria with reduced response to reward. Frequent cycle repetitions gradually suppress subjective "highs", deepening dysphoria. Increasingly, the drug is used to escape dysphoria and achieve normal mood. During abstinence, mood slowly recovers. *Source*: Reproduced by permission from Crowley *et al.* (2010).

biasing, users still can choose to abstain, but that choice now requires increasingly strong environmental rewards and punishments. Drug-taking becomes more automatic and habitual, and, like other habitual behaviors, its control gradually shifts from the ventral striatum to the dorsal striatum.

Third, after chronic drug use a stage of *preoccupation/anticipation (craving)* persists during periods of abstinence. Relapses then are common, and both animal studies and clinical experience show three types of relapse-provoking stimuli: a dose of the drug, cues associated with the drug (e.g., one's former dealer), or stress.

Finally, many misused drugs damage brain tissue. A general discussion of neurotoxicity is beyond the scope of this chapter, but two drugs do deserve mention. *Inhalants* are the most widely used drugs among 12–13-year-old Americans, and in some countries groups of homeless "street children" have reported prevalence rates as high as 70%. Most American users voluntarily discontinue inhalants later in adolescence, but among those who progress to inhalant use disorder, characteristic white-matter lesions (leucoencephalopathy) develop, producing cognitive impairments.

Neurotoxicity from *methamphetamine* damages dopamine neuron terminals, causing dopamine cell loss, reductions in dopamine transporter and D$_2$/D$_3$ receptor availability, diffuse loss of serotonergic terminals, and reduced white matter integrity. Fortunately, better international control of methamphetamine's chemical precursors have sharply reduced its use.

In summary, behavioral disinhibition is an important antecedent risk factor for SUDs. Youths vary considerably in the severity of their behavioral disinhibition, and in three separate adolescent-twin studies the heritability of that severity exceeded 0.8 (see Chapter 24; Young *et al.*, 2000; Krueger *et al.*, 2002; Hicks *et al.*, 2004). The influence of those genes presumably is expressed in the brain mechanisms described above. Fortunately, this shows that both genes and environment are important; not everyone with severe behavioral disinhibition develops SUDs, and the disorders remit in some who do develop them. Behavioral disinhibition does involve a persisting disposition to make risky choices with drugs and in other domains, but environmental influences from therapists, family members, teachers, judges, probation officers, or governments can steer those choices in less harmful directions. For example, when governments strictly controlled methamphetamine's chemical precursors, they obviously did not reduce some adolescents' persisting disposition to make dangerous decisions, but they did protect many of those youths from being snared by that toxic drug.

Longitudinal course

Factors influencing the course of drug involvement in adolescence and later include, first, *a pharmacologically rewarding drug*. SUDs occur because of pharmacologic interactions between certain chemical substances and brain tissue. As noted above, drugs that do produce SUDs all activate brain dopamine systems, initially inducing hedonic pleasure and biasing the brain's decision-making structures toward continued drug-taking.

Second, *the drug must be available and its use must be accepted* in at least some segments of the user's society. Annual per capita absolute alcohol consumption by persons more than 14 years old is about 17 times greater in European countries, compared to mostly-Muslim Eastern Mediterranean countries, reflecting the striking influence of Muslim restrictions on the social acceptance and availability of alcohol. Correspondingly, Europe's prevalence of alcohol use *disorders* is about nine times greater than that of those Muslim countries, strongly suggesting that social limits on substances' availability and acceptance also influence the prevalence of SUDs. For that reason many clinicians and researchers are concerned with policies that increase the availability and acceptance of pharmacologically reinforcing drugs, as now is occurring with cannabis in some American states.

Third, *a heritable disposition toward risk-taking* increases one's probability of developing a SUD. Different individuals' severity of behavioral disinhibition can be estimated from their symptom counts for conduct disorder, antisocial personality disorder, SUD, and from measures of hyperactivity, impulsivity, inattention, and novelty-seeking (Young *et al.*, 2000). Among both male and female adolescents a few individuals achieve very high behavioral disinhibition scores, placing them at high risk for early-onset SUD and conduct disorder, often with associated hyperactivity and impulsivity. Among persons with severe behavioral disinhibition the course may include low self-control as early as 3–5 years of age, with prepubertal impulsive aggression, hyperactivity, lack of persistence, and inattention (Moffitt *et al.*, 2011). Even before any drug use there are P300 (Iacono *et al.*, 2008) and fMRI (Norman *et al.*, 2011) brain abnormalities that predict adolescent SUD and conduct problems. In adulthood many show criminality and continuing substance problems (Fergusson *et al.*, 2009; Moffitt *et al.*, 2011).

Fourth, *age is a critical determinant of SUD risk*. The prevalence of DSM-IV alcohol or illicit-drug SUD among Americans was estimated to be less than one percent at age 12 years, 12% at 16 years, 17% at 18 years, and 24% at age 21. Prevalence then declines to 13% early in the fourth decade, and 3% early in the seventh. Regular substance use by minors requires an available drug, money to purchase it, and periods of limited parental supervision, factors rarely present for young children. However, during adolescence, time spent outside the home with peers increases, along with access to substances. Thus, substance problems are rare before, but common during, adolescence and early adulthood. Those youths who start drug use earliest have the greatest risk for developing SUDs (Dawson *et al.*, 2008), perhaps because more severe behavioral disinhibition and conduct problems characterize those earlier starters. Because SUD prevalence peaks around age 21 and then declines as young adults assume the responsibilities of work and family, many persons, especially males, experience serious substance problems in their late teens and early 20s, with subsequent desistence. However, those with early-adolescent onset of both SUD and conduct problems appear much more likely to have SUDs persisting for many years.

Fifth, as noted above, *environment contributes about half to the risk for developing SUDs*; genes contribute the other half. Many parents with substance and antisocial problems create around their children toxic environments, leading to the gene–environment correlations and interactions previously described.

Sixth, *a balance of rewards and punishments influence the course of SUDs*. In addition to the pharmacologic reward discussed above, social rewards also may maintain drug use. Drug users earn social acceptance from other users. Dealing drugs may get more money than other adolescents have, and sharing drugs may win sexual favors. Such rewards come more quickly than larger rewards for studying in school, and drug-involved persons tend to favor smaller rewards that come sooner over larger ones that come later, a process called "delay discounting." On the other hand, social punishments may suppress drug use, but only if they are significant to the adolescent and seem likely to occur soon after the drug use. When an underage adolescent pays a homeless person to buy alcohol for the adolescent, the probability of detection and swift legal punishment is so low that laws provide little deterrence. On the other hand, a juvenile drug court may successfully motivate abstinence and participation in treatment by requiring frequent court appearances and promptly imposing brief periods of detention for any non-participation in treatment or drug-containing urine samples.

Prevention

Prevention programs generally seek to enhance protective factors (e.g., improving parental monitoring or adolescent self-control) and to reduce risk factors (e.g., aggressive behavior, poor academic performance, or contact with substance-using peers). Programs may be "universal" (delivered to, e.g., all students in one grade at a school), or "selective" (delivered to, e.g., children of alcoholics), or "indicated" (delivered to those already engaging in high-risk behaviors or showing early warning signs). Programs also are classified by the targeted setting or group, such as school-, family-, or community-based (see Chapter 17).

Cochrane reviews of prevention programs for alcohol misuse, tobacco smoking, and illicit drug use are limited by a vast heterogeneity of target populations and components delivered. Many prevention programs lack randomized controlled trials, and considered together the empirical evidence for school-based interventions has been considered "rather weak" (Faggiano et al., 2007). Therefore, most Cochrane reviews provide generic information, such as the number of positive and negative trials, rather than effect-size estimates for similar groups of prevention programs.

Family-based interventions

These interventions often aim to improve parents' nurturing behaviors toward their children, establish clear boundaries and rules, improve monitoring and supervision, provide reasonable and consistent consequences to rule violations, and reward good behavior. Programs may work to improve children's social and life skills and often include family practice sessions to improve communication. Enrollment and retention of participants, one potential barrier to progress in family-based interventions, may be enhanced by endorsement from community leaders, convenience of delivery location, use of incentives, and providing meals, transportation, or child care. One example is the Strengthening Families Program, developed in the USA and now used in many countries (Kumpfer et al., 2008). The original program offered 14 2-hour group-based sessions focused on family, parent, and child skill training to prevent drug use and misuse in high-risk offspring; shorter versions have been developed for other groups, and versions also are available for various ages.

School-based programs

School-based programs efficiently target large groups of youths. These curricula may include skill building for social competency, communication, refusal skills, or identifying and avoiding high risk situations, as well as education about drug related risks and harms, or challenging beliefs that overestimate the prevalence of substance use. The Cochrane review of universal school-based prevention programs for alcohol misuse specifically cites three with evidence for effectiveness (see Chapter 42).

The Life Skills Training program utilizes a cognitive-behavioral skills framework. It aims to improve self esteem, communication skills, assertion of one's rights, building of positive relationships, management of anxiety, problem solving, and resistance to adverse social (including media) influences. The program teaches drug resistance skills and provides education about negative consequences from drugs and alcohol. It addresses the actual prevalence of use. Delivered in the seventh grade (ca. age 12), with booster sessions in both eighth and ninth grades, the program significantly reduces drug-use prevalence in the 12th grade (ca. age 17) (Botvin et al., 1995).

The Unplugged program focuses on improving social and personal skills, such as assertiveness, goal setting, refusal skills, and decision making, while providing education about prevalence of drug and alcohol use (Faggiano et al., 2007). Trained teachers deliver the core program in 12 1-hour weekly sessions, sometimes with additional activities involving peers or parents, to 12–14 year-old students. Eighteen-month follow up demonstrates reduced alcohol and cannabis use (Faggiano et al., 2010).

The Good Behavior Game, a universal school-based prevention program, divides students into competing teams. Each student's target behaviors (e.g., disruptiveness, aggression) affect team scores, and teams receive rewards, based on their scores. This approach, often employed in early elementary school, does reduce aggressive and disruptive behaviors. In one longitudinal study its effects continued to reduce SUD among young-adult males (but not females), especially those with persistently high aggressive and disruptive behaviors (Kellam et al., 2012). However, the program's effects appear to dissipate without ongoing teacher training, mentoring, and monitoring (Kellam et al., 2012).

Other programs

Drug education alone has not been found to reduce drug-use behaviors or intentions, but many drug-use prevention programs still mainly provide education about drugs and drug abuse. For example, the Drug Abuse Resistance Education (DARE) program demonstrably has little effect on drug use, but remains widely used in American schools.

Other examples of research-based drug abuse prevention programs are too numerous to review here, but may be found at NIDA (2003), the National Registry of Effective Prevention Programs (2013) (http://www.nrepp.samhsa.gov/), and the Centers for Disease Control and Prevention's Guide to Community Preventive Services (available only at www.thecommunity guide.org).

Limits of prevention research

Several concerns about prevention research for drug and alcohol use have been raised, including potential for publication bias, selecting outcome variables post-hoc, reporting of statistical significance without considering practical significance, reliance on self-reports rather than objective testing of substance use outcomes, concerns regarding the handling of sample attrition and selection bias, and use of one-tailed statistical tests (Holder, 2010). Conflicts of interest and dual roles also raise concerns; program developers, who often serve as program evaluators, may experience financial gain if a program is successful. The Life Skills Training and Unplugged programs have not escaped such criticism.

Policy

Policies such as alcohol taxation, setting or increasing a minimum age for purchase and use, lowering of allowable blood alcohol concentrations for driving, visible enforcement of drinking and driving laws, and limiting where and when alcohol can be sold measurably affect substance use and harms. The NICE guidelines on "Alcohol-use disorders: preventing harmful drinking" include recommendations to make alcohol less affordable and reduce exposure to alcohol-related advertising among children and young people; such policies may reduce alcohol-related harms.

Screening, assessment

Chapters 32, 33, and 34 address psychiatric and psychological assessments generally. This chapter addresses specific issues of screening and assessing for substance problems.

Screening

Physicians and counselors often screen youths to identify those likely to have substance problems. Screens should be inexpensive, easy to administer and score, and have reasonable sensitivity and specificity. Adolescents may prefer screens completed by computer or paper questionnaire, rather than verbal questioning.

SAMHSA (2013) lists screening instruments (e.g., screening, brief intervention and referral to treatment (SBIRT), AUDIT, AUDIT-C), and SAMHSA (2011) compares many of them. SBIRT (Screening, Brief Intervention, and Referral to Treatment) is discussed in the Treatment Section, below. In another free example, CRAFFT (its name, and a mnemonic for its questions), 2 or more positive responses suggest substance problems:

C: Have you ever ridden in a *car* driven by someone (including yourself)who was "high" or using alcohol or drugs?
R: Do you use alcohol or drugs to *relax*, change your mood, feel better about yourself, or fit in?
A: Do you ever use alcohol or drugs when you are by yourself, *alone*?
F: Has any *friend*, family member, or other person ever thought you had a problem with alcohol or drugs?
F: Do you ever *forget* (or regret) things you did while using?
T: Have you ever gotten into *trouble* while using alcohol or drugs, or done something you would not normally do (break the law, rules, or curfew; engage in behavior risky to you or others)?

Substance screens ask adolescents about illegal behaviors, raising issues about parental consent, youth assent, and confidentiality (cf., SAMHSA, 2011). Since requirements vary in different jurisdictions, a detailed discussion of this is beyond the scope of the chapter.

Assessment

An adolescent's substance assessment asks many questions to answer ten fundamental ones: (i) Are there serious life problems (e.g., frequent intoxications, intravenous drug use, fighting, carrying weapons, extensive truancy, criminality, unprotected intercourse, unplanned pregnancy, experience of abuse or neglect, depression, or suicidal thoughts or actions)? (ii) Are emergency responses required? (iii) Do substance use and behavioral disinhibition contribute to the problems? (iv) How much of which substances are used, and by what route of administration? (v) Is there a family history of substance and disinhibition problems? (vi) Have parental care, supervision, and monitoring been adequate? (vii) Are the problems exacerbated or reduced by other environmental factors (e.g., other family, friends, school, church, therapists, or juvenile-justice or welfare agencies)? (viii) What may block or facilitate a treatment alliance with the patient and family? (ix) Regarding goals, if treatment works, what could reasonably be improved one year hence? (x) What psychosocial and pharmacologic treatments will be needed to achieve the 1-year goal, and to maintain progress thereafter (cf., see Chapter 32).

Answers to these questions will inform the selection of a treatment venue (outpatient, residential, etc.) and treatment selection and execution. For the public-health reasons cited in this chapter's Introduction, the chapter focuses on public clinics in which a psychiatrist, psychologist, or senior social worker supervises masters- or bachelor-level counselors who conduct most assessments. In other settings the supervisor may conduct them personally.

First contact

Few substance-using adolescents seek treatment on their own. The first clinic contact usually originates with referring court or welfare workers, or the adolescent's family. Often, frustrated family members begin with, "He needs to be hospitalized." The clinician may respond that for any emergency they should go to a hospital emergency department; otherwise, the first step is a professional assessment to identify the problem and select treatments. Parents or guardians should attend the first meeting (unless a court order separates the youth from them), and if agency workers made the contact, they should also attend.

Assessment initiates the clinician's relationships with the adolescent patient and family and may be crucial for convincing them that treatment can help. Unfortunately, relationship-building may be lost while completing intake forms often required by insurers or governmental funding agencies. Intake workers may complete such forms before any clinical meeting to minimize that intrusion.

Assent, consent, and confidentiality

Rules vary in different jurisdictions, but before assessing minors the treating clinician must usually obtain written parental consent and assent of the minor. This starts the treatment relationship with transparency, clarifying that evaluation and treatment require agreement and participation from both patient and family. Accordingly, even if parents demand an evaluation, in many jurisdictions it cannot proceed without the minor's assent, except when ordered by a court or done under evaluation-requiring "hold and treat" statutes.

Sometimes however, parental consent may not be required. Many jurisdictions provide exceptions (SAMHSA, 2011) if the government has custody of the minor, or if the minor faces some immediate risk but parents or guardians are unavailable. Additionally, in many places the minor may consent for substance evaluations and treatment as a "mature" or "emancipated" minor. Usually, such minors are at least 16 years old and understand the planned assessment procedure.

Courts ordering substance assessments of youths charged with crimes will see resulting reports. And although American laws strongly protect the confidentiality of substance-treatment records in federally-assisted programs, those protections may not apply elsewhere. Thus, consent and assent documents must make clear what information will be available to whom, and especially, whether admitting a previously unknown crime during an evaluation will be reported to the court, or whether the court could compel its release. The documents should also clearly state that there is no confidentiality regarding child abuse or neglect, plans to harm a person, or crimes against the evaluating program or its personnel.

Who, when

The clinician is advised to assess interactions among the parents, the youth, and any involved agency worker, and also must obtain information from them separately. The next sections suggest when to see the parties together or separately, but clinicians flexibly modify these procedures according to the parties' interactions.

Chief complaint

With the parties together the clinician can ask each in turn, "Why do you think you're here to see me now." The clinician can then note, for example, disagreements ("I do *not* sneak out at night"), blaming authorities ("that judge hates us") or others ("his dead father taught him that"), hoped-for extrusion from the family ("just keep him in your hospital"), parental problems ("Dad drinks more than me"), abdication of responsibility ("they made us come"), or desperation ("With my cancer, who will look after her?" (cf., see Chapter 28)). After describing what the agency wants and planning later meetings, the agency worker may then leave.

History of the problem

The clinician can summarize those various Chief Complaints, asking, "Is that about right?" Next, it can be useful to ask about the development of the problem, aiming eventually to know answers to the many questions outlined here and below. However, the clinician should strive for a conversational exchange, and these questions *must not* be ticked off, checklist style. This section focuses on recent events directly leading to this contact, including: problems with conduct and substances (details of the use may await the adolescent-only interview); when the problems started; their triggers; any earlier signs; the problems' progression; the parties' feelings and actions regarding the problems; arrests, court appearances, detentions, or incarcerations; and prior treatments.

Long-term goals

Having heard descriptions of the current problem, the clinician now aims both to understand the goals of the participants and to introduce them to the long-term nature of these chronic, relapsing disorders. The question commonly asked by the author is "If we do some treatment together, and if it works the way you hope, how will things be different a year from now?" This question also forces the clinician to plan not just short-term, but long-term treatment.

Developmental history

Parents provide early developmental information, but the adolescent contributes for later years. *Conception to elementary school*: Was the youth adopted? During the pregnancy, were there: prenatal care, couple's problems, maternal "need" to use tobacco or other substances, prematurity, or other difficulties? Were there problems with: the delivery or immediately after; needed extra hospitalization; feeding, colic, serious accidents or illnesses, or failure to thrive? Were developmental milestones timely? Who provided child care? Was there preschool? *During elementary school*: What were the patient's best accomplishments? Were there friends? Were there problems with grades, fighting, suspensions, fire-setting, or frequent injuries? Did the youth (compared to others) show predictors (Moffitt *et al.*, 2011) of later substance problems: discipline problems, unpredictable emotions, low frustration tolerance, assertive-rough-aggressive play, impulsive aggression, hyperactivity, inattention, impulsivity, or lack of persistence? *During middle school, and separately for high school*: Again, descriptions of best accomplishments, friends (male and female), grades, conduct or substance problems, or frequent injuries.

Considering the home environment, the clinician can ask about the family's main language and racial-ethnic identity. Who has been present in the home? How did family members relate? How did the parents supervise and discipline? Were they active in a church or other social organization? What did they do for fun? Do the parents work? Was income adequate? How often, and where, did the family move, and what schools were attended? Was there divorce, split custody, or child support? What adults came or went? Did a single parent have lovers in the home? Were social services involved? Was there arguing or domestic violence? Were there gender-identity issues? How did the youth feel about each of these?

Family history
Were there substance-related problems in the family? More relatives with these problems predicts a more recurrent course and worse impairment (Milne *et al.*, 2009). Did relatives have antisocial or criminal problems, depression, or psychosis?

The youth's history
After excusing the parents, the author finds it useful to begin with an open-ended question, such as "Well, how do you feel about being here?" After some brief discussion, the clinician can explore the youth's views of the family. The interview considers each significant family member, as well as boyfriends or girlfriends, aiming to identify those who will help or hinder efforts to shape an abstinence-supporting environment around the patient.

The author finds it useful to ask seven introductory questions about used substances, flexibly and conversationally expanding on each with additional questions, considering the youth's unfolding history and comfort. First, *what substances do you use, and in what doses?* Which substances has the youth used, in what amounts on a typical day or week, and what is the largest single-day dose? Simple counts suffice for prescription pills, tobacco cigarettes, tubes of glue, or nitrous oxide cartridges ("whippets"). For alcohol, "standard drinks" contain similar amounts of pure alcohol, and are 45 ml. (1.5 oz.) of distilled spirits, 350 ml. (12 oz.) of beer, or 150 ml. (5 oz.) of wine. Even street measures, such as "cannabis joints (cigarettes) or blunts (cigars)" or "$10 bags" of heroin, help estimate the intensity of use. The route of administration (swallowing, intranasal insufflation, inhalation, or injection) is important; the latter two routes more strongly drive repeated use.

Second, *when have you used the substances?* These questions address temporal patterns: age at first use, acceleration of use, periods of abstinence, the current frequency of use (e.g., doses per day, or days per week), and whether the use is steady or in binges.

Third, *where and with whom do you use the substances?* These questions seek both social reinforcement for substance use (e.g., drug parties) and dangerous drug-use environments. Does the youth usually use alone or with peers, ride or drive in cars with groups that are using, use with armed or violent peers, or with males who demand sex after providing drugs? Does the youth use substances at home, or get them from—or use with—family members?

Fourth, *how do you get the substances?* Seeking to understand the general process, while avoiding dangerous names or places, the clinician can ask: How much do you spend on substances? Have you stolen things, or sold drugs, or done sexual things for drugs or drug money? Do dealers call you?

Fifth, *what gets you to use either more or less?* Such stimuli may be certain friends or relatives, or certain moods, or doing enjoyable things, or stressful times. Can the youth "hold" a supply of the drug, or is it quickly used up?

Sixth, *for you, what are the substances' payoffs—their good things?* Reported "benefits" often include the drug "high," the social pleasure of using with friends, a numbing of sadness, or the thrill of forbidden activities.

Seventh, *for you, what are the substances' costs—their bad things?* The clinician here can consider six categories of adverse drug effects. *Social*: Have drugs made problems with your family, or with girlfriends (boyfriends)? Have friends said they worry about you, or stopped seeing you, because of drugs? *Legal*: Were you ever stopped for driving while high, or arrested, or in court, or in detention or probation because of substances? *Educational-vocational*: Were you high in class, or did you ditch school, or skip homework because of drugs? Have you failed a drug test for work, or were you "high" at work, or missed work, or got fired because of drugs? *Medical*: Did you ever inject drugs? Did getting high, or stopping suddenly after using for a while, ever give you physical problems, like shaking, or getting agitated, or sweating, or heart pounding, or having a seizure, or passing out, or anything else? *Psychological*: Did drugs ever mess up your thinking, or hurt your mood or emotions? Are you ever sad about drugs? *Financial:* Have you borrowed money that you could not repay because of drugs?

This section concludes with any additional questions needed to determine a diagnosis. In some settings it can be useful to assess, for each substance, which DSM-5 SUD criteria have been met in the last year.

Abuse and neglect
Adolescent patients with SUDs are four times more likely than controls to report abuse or neglect, and patients' severity of maltreatment correlates significantly with the severity of their substance, conduct, and depressive problems (Crowley *et al.*, 2003), so abuse-neglect assessments are critical. "Rating Scales and Structured Interviews," below, and Chapters 29–30 recommend procedures for these assessments. Maltreatment must be immediately reported to appropriate authorities.

Suicide
SUD is a strong risk factor for suicide, and all SUD patients must be assessed for this risk (cf., see Chapter 64).

Withdrawal
Most adolescents with SUD do not develop medically dangerous withdrawal syndromes, probably because their dosing has been briefer and less steady than that of many adults. However, some who have used alcohol, sedative-hypnotic, or anxiolytic drugs with frequent high dosing for days or weeks may develop sweating, muscle twitches and jerks, or changes in vital signs or state of consciousness. These signs require medical detoxification with pharmacologic intervention. Similarly, opioid withdrawal requires medical treatment. Finally, abruptly terminating sustained, regular dosing with cannabis, caffeine,

stimulants, or tobacco produces substance-specific withdrawal syndromes (American Psychiatric Association, 2013); while rarely dangerous medically, their aversiveness may motivate resumed drug use.

Initial summary

With the patient and family together the clinician may find it useful to spend time summarizing key points, first addressing any necessary emergency actions to prevent serious withdrawal syndromes, overdose, suicide or self-injury, abuse or neglect, violence, illegal acts, dangerously intoxicated behaviors, sexually transmitted disease, or pregnancy. To initiate a treatment alliance, the clinician can again summarize the parties' Chief Complaints, emphasizing any agreements about needed changes. While respecting the patient's confidentiality, the clinician refers to the adolescent's lists of drug "payoffs," and "costs," suggesting that the patient, the parents, and the treatment team work together to eliminate drug "costs" by trying abstinence, while exploring non-drug ways to obtain the "payoffs" that drugs offered.

After discussing that, the clinician can propose a few simple, short-term goals (e.g., "being abstinent and safe for the next week") and an initial treatment venue appropriate to the risk that the patient faces (e.g., outpatient, day-treatment, residential care, or hospital). Finally, in the author's clinic, the clinician obtains consents and assents to contact involved professionals.

Coexisting disorders

As noted earlier, behavioral disinhibition involves substance and conduct problems, hyperactivity, impulsivity, inattention, and novelty-seeking. Thus, many youths with SUD also meet criteria for conduct disorder (see Chapter 65) and disorders of attention and activity (see Chapter 55), while their risky behaviors often produce traumatic experiences and post-traumatic stress disorder (see Chapter 59). Major depressive disorder (see Chapter 63) is common in adolescents with SUD, especially females, and anxiety disorders (see Chapter 60) also occur. Accordingly, clinical programs addressing adolescent SUD must routinely assess, and provide onsite treatment, for these disorders.

Rating scales and structured interviews

These tools, administered by non-doctoral clinicians, provide standardized descriptions of clinical signs, symptoms, and disorders (see Chapter 33). In large treatment programs they help supervising psychiatrists or psychologists determine diagnosis and clinical severity.

In structured diagnostic interviews a technician or computer exactly presents questions needed to establish diagnoses, recording the answers. On these assessments most adolescents entering treatment for SUD and conduct problems provide valid information for diagnosing, and for rating the severity of, their conditions, although some clearly dissemble (Crowley et al., 2001). Depression and ADHD are unusually common among these patients, and their self-ratings of *severity* for those disorders also are reasonably valid. However, these patients' self-reports

in structured interviews for *diagnosing* either major depression or ADHD often are invalid in adolescents with SUDs; validity improves when parent reports supplement the self-reports, but some parents of these troubled patients refuse such interviews. At the time of this writing, relevant diagnostic interviews are based on DSM-IV and will need some revision for DSM-5.

Several structured abuse-neglect interviews are available (cf., see Chapters 29, 30). The author's is free, includes substance-focused issues (e.g., parents sharing drugs with their children), and is validated specifically for adolescents in substance treatment (Crowley et al., 2003, 2013).

Well-validated clinical rating scales completed by parents, teachers, and/or the patient usefully assess the severity of, for example, depression, delinquent behavior, hyperactivity, or sensation-seeking in adolescents with SUD (see Chapter 33; Crowley et al., 2001). Additionally, the number of DSM-5 diagnostic criteria met, indexes the severity of each SUD (Hasin et al., 2013).

Physical investigations

SUDs produce physical findings. First, SUDs are usually associated with recurring intoxications, and sometimes with recurring withdrawals. DSM-5 details the substance-specific physical signs of intoxication and withdrawal, some of which require medical intervention.

Drug use may leave characteristic physical stigmata. For example, intravenous drug injections produce "needle tracks" (scarred peripheral veins). Repeated inhaling of volatile solvents causes perioral or perinasal "huffer's rash." "Meth mouth" (oral dryness with extreme tooth decay) complicates methamphetamine use.

Adolescents with SUD tend to be risk-takers, and drug intoxication increases that tendency. Unprotected sex may lead to unplanned pregnancy or sexually transmitted disease, and unsterile needles spread Hepatitis C and HIV. Some adolescents with SUD also engage in prostitution. Patients doing these behaviors need assessment for these medical problems.

Drug testing

Therapists cannot respond effectively to concealed relapses, and most persons with SUD report having lied about drug use. Thus, therapists must assess abstinence with drug testing, in addition to reports from patient and family. Detailed discussions of drug testing are beyond the scope of this chapter, but two points are warranted.

Tests are available for urine, saliva, sweat, breath, and hair, but reasonably inexpensive and reliable commercial urine tests are most common in substance treatment programs. While standard amphetamine tests also detect lisdexamfetamine dimesylate and dextroamphetamine, they do not detect methylphenidate. Newer "designer drugs" (e.g., synthetic cannabinoids or methylenedioxypyrovalerone ("Bath Salts")) will not usually be detected, except by special, more expensive tests. Also tests are impractical or not reliable for inhalant drugs.

Alcohol's rapid metabolism makes its detection by urine or "breathalyzer" tests unreliable. Carbohydrate deficient transferrin (CDT) tests for drinking, being relatively insensitive in adolescents, are usually inappropriate. Minute quantities of alcohol metabolites (ethyl glucuronide or ethyl sulfide) from as little as one drink are detectable in urine for as long as two days, but these tests also produce false-positive findings from adventitious alcohol exposures (e.g., mouthwash, hand cleaners). Transdermal alcohol monitors, widely used with probationers, are worn under the clothing, detect alcohol in sweat, and transmit reports to a central station.

Imaging and genetic diagnostic tests currently offer no empirically supported contribution to the diagnosis or treatment of SUDs.

Importance of accurate diagnosis

Correct diagnoses are critical for predicting clinical course and planning treatment, but diagnosing substance-related disorders is complex. Ten drugs or drug classes each produce a SUD and up to 10 types of substance induced disorders, requiring precise clinical assessments (American Psychiatric Association, 2013). This makes the current classification of polysubstance misuse complex.

Treatment

Overview

Guidelines often recommend procedures to reduce dropout, improve motivation and treatment compliance, and foster a strong therapeutic alliance (Bukstein *et al.*, 2005). Such approaches include making services responsive to young peoples' needs and interests; providing services in a respectful, warm and trustworthy manner (CCQI, 2012); taking an empathetic, nonjudgmental stance; and using motivational interviewing to improve treatment readiness and enhance self-efficacy (Bukstein *et al.*, 2005). Use of contingencies such as rewards or punishments (e.g., legal sanctions) can also motivate treatment engagement and adherence. Although some providers sometimes suggest waiting until substance using and dependent individuals hit "rock bottom" to intervene, this approach is not endorsed by published guidelines (Bukstein *et al.*, 2005; CCQI, 2012) and unfortunately while waiting for substance dependent youths to hit "rock bottom" some will die.

Early intervention

Some individuals, although not meeting criteria for an alcohol use disorder, drink at levels that are associated with later alcohol-related problems (e.g., for adult-sized females, four or more drinks per day, or 8 or more per week; for males 5 or more per day, or 15 or more per week). Unfortunately, relatively few health-care providers routinely screen for such drinking patterns, and therefore providers are being trained in SBIRT, interventions that cause many adults to reduce their drinking below hazardous levels. Although SBIRT has been less-studied

in adolescents, some data suggest that brief motivational interviewing can reduce subsequent alcohol-related problems among older adolescents visiting hospital emergency departments for an alcohol-related event (Monti *et al.*, 1999) and may have a positive effect on various substance use outcomes with even a single intervention session, though the effect size in one recent meta-analyses was small ($d = 0.17$; Jensen *et al.*, 2011). Adolescent SBIRT studies are underway, and a guide for practitioners working with adolescents is freely available (NIAAA, 2011). Practice guidelines in the UK recommend extended brief intervention with motivational interviewing for those aged 15 years and older, whose substance use raises concerns but who do not have multiple or complex needs or meet criteria for SUD (CCQI, 2012). Those meeting criteria for an SUD with more complex needs may require more intensive interventions or referral to more specialized care.

Venue of treatment

The American Society of Addiction Medicine Patient Placement Criteria (Mee-Lee, *et al.*, 2001) provides a widely-used, standardized approach for determining the appropriate level of care for a given patient, using information from six dimensions: (i) intoxication/withdrawal, (ii) biomedical, (iii) emotional/behavioral/cognitive, (iv) treatment readiness, (v) potential for relapse or continued use, and (vi) recovery environment. The levels of care include: (0.5) early intervention, (I) outpatient, (II) intensive outpatient or partial hospitalization, (III) clinically managed residential or medically monitored inpatient care, and (IV) medically managed intensive inpatient. For example, a youth with SUD but minimal risk across dimensions would be managed initially in an outpatient setting, while a youth in danger from suicidality and severe withdrawal risk would need medically managed inpatient care.

Psychosocial treatments

Numerous clinical trials have addressed treatment of adolescent SUD, and major reviews of psychosocial treatments generally report near-moderate to moderate effect sizes (Waldron & Turner, 2008; Tripodi *et al.*, 2010). Waldron and Turner (2008) reviewed studies comparing major treatment modalities (e.g., family therapy compared with individual cognitive behavioral therapy (CBT) or group CBT); no modality stood out as significantly better for adolescent SUD. However, Tripodi *et al.* (2010) reported some advantage of individual over family therapy for adolescent alcohol disorders, contradicting prior recommendations that family components are an essential minimum standard for treatment of adolescent substance disorders (Bukstein *et al.*, 2005).

Considering the evidence supporting specific manualized treatments, such as Multidimensional Family Therapy, rather than broad groupings like "family therapy," Waldron and Turner (2008) found many well-established or probably efficacious psychosocial treatments for adolescent SUDs (Table 66.2). Other empirically-supported treatments are listed in the

Table 66.2 Evidence base supporting psychosocial treatments of adolescent substance abuse.

Treatment modality	Strengths of existing literature	Weaknesses of existing literature	Determination
Brief strategic family therapy (BSFT)	1, 2[a], 4, 7, 11	1, 2, 3	Probably efficacious[b]
Behavioral family therapy (BFT)	1, 2, 6, 7, 8	2, 4	Probably efficacious
Multidimensional family therapy (MDFT)	1, 3, 4, 5, 7, 8, 9		Well established
Multisystemic therapy (MST)	1, 2[c], 7, 8, 10	4[c]	Probably efficacious
Functional family therapy (FFT)	1, 3, 4, 5, 7, 8, 9, 10		Well established
Cognitive behavioral therapy-individual (CBT-I) (with or without a component of motivational enhancement therapy)	1, 3, 5, 6, 7, 8		Well established[d]
Cognitive behavioral therapy-group (CBT-G)	1, 3, 7, 9, 10	5, 6	Well established

STRENGTHS: (1) Clinically meaningful reductions in substance use; (2) Tested and then replicated by a single research group; (3) Replicated by an independent research team; (4) Well-characterized study samples; (5) Relatively large sample sizes; (6) Good substance use measures; (7) Manual guided and/or model is well specified; (8) Adherence monitoring; (9) Adequate or longer follow up; (10) Widely disseminated or highly transportable; (11) High representation of Hispanic families.
WEAKNESSES: (1) Small effect size; (2) Small samples; (3) Limited comparison conditions; (4) No replication trials by independent groups; (5) Some studies with considerable attrition; (6) Variability in the length of treatment (i.e., 5–19 sessions).
[a]Similar, but not identical, models have been replicated by independent researchers.
[b]A large BSFT multi site trial (Robbins *et al.*, 2011), conducted within the Clinical Trials Network and published after Waldron and Turner (2008), showed weak effects on drug use outcomes.
[c]Independent replication has been completed for antisocial behavior but not substance use.
[d]Meta-analyses of CBT-I failed to separate from minimal treatment control (Waldron & Turner, 2008).

National Registry of Evidence-based Programs and Practices (NREPP, 2013).

Most studies address outpatient treatment of adolescent SUD. However, concerns regarding safety or non-response to outpatient treatment sometimes lead to residential treatment. Unfortunately, studies of that modality generally lack methodological rigor, including lack of randomization, lack of blinded raters, and failure to use reliable, well-validated outcome measures (Tripodi, 2009). Similarly, studies of adolescents in Alcoholics Anonymous (AA) and Narcotics Anonymous (NA) have methodological weaknesses, such as single-group designs (Sussman, 2010). However, AA and NA are recommended as adjuncts to professional treatment in the American Academy of Child and Adolescent Psychiatry's practice parameters (Bukstein *et al.*, 2005) and in adult populations 12-step facilitation appears to be as efficacious as other well-accepted psychosocial treatments.

Contingency management approaches in adolescents (Stanger & Budney, 2010) monitor target behaviors (e.g., drug abstinence) and follow them with rewards and/or punishments. Like motivational enhancement techniques, contingency management approaches can be combined with other psychosocial treatments, such as cognitive-behavioral therapy (Stanger & Budney, 2010). Because many adolescents with SUD have legal entanglements, one contingency may be criminal justice rewards and punishments (e.g., "stop using drugs or spend a week in juvenile detention"). Such approaches are sometimes formalized through juvenile drug courts, which do reduce youths' drug use and criminal behaviors beyond that seen with family courts; integration of evidence-based adolescent treatments further improves these outcomes (Henggeler, 2007).

Pharmacotherapy

Despite the many drugs misused by adolescents, alcohol, opioid and nicotine use disorders are the only ones having federally-approved pharmacotherapies in the USA. Moreover, the research literature supporting those approvals generally comes from adult studies; there are few adolescent-specific pharmacotherapy trials. Thus, the American Academy of Child and Adolescent Psychiatry's practice parameters on substance abuse note that medications may be used, but are an optional recommendation (Bukstein *et al.*, 2005).

Alcohol

Three medications are approved in the USA to treat alcohol dependence in adults. (i) Naltrexone is a mu-opioid receptor antagonist that in clinical trials reduces subjective craving, delays the time to the first drink, and reduces chances of relapse. This medication is available both as an oral preparation or as an expensive, once-per-month intramuscular injection (naltrexone XR). It must be used with caution in patients who are likely to require opioid pain management, as it blocks the effects of these medications. Also, it precipitates opioid withdrawal in persons actively using opioids. Similarly, the European Medicines Agency has approved nalmefene, another opioid antagonist, for heavy-drinking individuals; it can be used on an "as-needed" basis when cravings are high or when a lapse has occurred. (ii) Acamprosate appears to reduce CNS hyperexcitability and may increase the number of consecutive days of alcohol abstinence. Despite its support in European studies, this medication was not better than placebo in the American multi site COMBINE trial. (iii) Disulfiram is an aversive pharmacotherapy that produces an unpleasant flushing reaction when alcohol is consumed. When provided with supervised administration (e.g., having an invested family member give the drug) this medication reduces alcohol consumption, increases the number of days abstinent, and improves alcohol-related biomarkers, such as gamma-glutamyl transferase levels. Topiramate also has mounting support for effectiveness; several other medications have been studied, but the quality of those studies varies.

Unfortunately, for adolescents the data supporting use of these medications is weak. For example, one small (n=26) 90-day double-blind placebo-controlled study of disulfiram among adolescents with alcohol use disorder suggested that disulfiram improved rates of continuous abstinence; no safety concerns were identified (Niederhofer & Staffen, 2003). The UK's NICE has issued a guidance document which includes detailed information on pharmacotherapy for alcohol use disorders, and discusses the prescribing of naltrexone and acamprosate for adolescents (NICE, 2011).

Opioid agonists

Opioid dependence tends to follow a chronic course, with high relapse rates after simple detoxification. Methadone is a full mu-opioid agonist which, in adult maintenance therapy, is cost-effective and reduces needle use, heroin use, medical comorbidity, and mortality. Despite some evidence for safety of methadone in persons 16–21 years old (Lehmann, 1976), in the USA those under age 18 must relapse after two detoxification attempts before qualifying for methadone treatment; that is, they must repeatedly use a potentially fatal street drug before receiving a mortality-reducing medication. Moreover, some methadone programs simply do not admit adolescents.

Buprenorphine is used in many countries for opioid maintenance therapy. This partial mu-opioid agonist is safer than methadone in overdose. A widely-used sublingual buprenorphine-naloxone combination reduces risks of injection; when taken sublingually the buprenorphine, but not the naloxone, is adequately absorbed, but if the medicine is injected the naloxone blocks mu-opioid receptors, displacing opioid agonists and prompting opioid withdrawal. Woody *et al.* (2008) randomized opioid dependent adolescents and young adults into a 12-week study. They received either a 2-week detoxification with buprenorphine-naloxone, or 9 weeks of buprenorphine-naloxone maintenance with a 3-week taper. Those maintained on buprenorphine-naloxone were significantly more likely to remain in the study at 12 weeks (70% vs 21%) and had significantly less injection drug use and use of opioids or marijuana. However, in 6-, 9-, and 12-month follow ups the groups were not significantly different in reported opioid use, marijuana use, or injection drug use; thus, 3-months of buprenorphine-naloxone treatment did not alter long-term course. The study authors suggested that, although young patients' duration of opioid dependence is relatively brief, clinicians should be in no hurry to stop this effective medication. This medication is approved in the USA for the treatment of opioid dependence in those at least 16 years of age and by the European Medicines Agency's marketing authorization for children "over 15 years of age." The UK's NICE guidance document discusses methadone and buprenorphine for managing opioid dependence (NICE, 2007a).

Opioid antagonists

One alternative to agonist maintenance treatment of opioid dependence is antagonist maintenance with naltrexone, which blocks the effects of an opioid dose. A guidance document on naltrexone for opioid dependence has been released by the UK's NICE (NICE, 2007b). This medication induces opioid withdrawal symptoms in active users, so it is generally started 7–10 days after the last opioid use. Studies in adults suggest poor treatment retention with this medication, except when strong contingencies motivate participation; examples are physicians who must take the medication to retain their medical licenses, or persons who take it as a condition of parole. Some data do suggest promising results with long-acting naltrexone XR and naltrexone subcutaneous implants. One multisite comparison of naltrexone XR and buprenorphine is underway and will help identify the relative merits of each approach. Again, there are few treatment studies among adolescents, but one uncontrolled case series of 16 adolescents and young adults using naltrexone XR reported encouraging results (Fishman *et al.*, 2010).

One randomized trial of 36 adolescents examined detoxification of opioid dependent youths before transitioning them to naltrexone. During opioid detoxification, buprenorphine, compared to clonidine, resulted in higher treatment retention through the detoxification (72 vs 39%), more opioid-free urine tests (64 vs 32%), and a higher likelihood of naltrexone induction (61 vs 5%) (Marsch *et al.*, 2005).

Nicotine

Some patients think that they are more likely to abstain from illicit drugs or alcohol if they continue using cigarettes, but empirical evidence in adults indicates that smoking cessation interventions improve other substance treatment outcomes. Three main pharmacological treatments for nicotine dependence are currently available: nicotine replacement therapy (NRT), bupropion, and varenicline. *NRT* is delivered in numerous ways, including a skin patch, chewing gum, or an inhaler. Then, dosing usually is tapered, often stepwise, over months. *Bupropion*, which also has antidepressant effects, is usually started at 150 mg and increased after about 3 days to a target dose of 300 mg/day. Patients are instructed to set a quit date within the first 2 weeks on medication. *Varenicline* doses are raised over the first 8 days to a target of 1 mg orally twice per day, with medication starting about 1 week prior to the patient's scheduled quit date. Some evidence supports a larger effect size for varenicline compared to bupropion, but post-marketing surveillance has raised concerns about suicidality, mood changes, and a small increase in cardiovascular events with varenicline.

Again, evidence on pharmacological treatments of adolescent nicotine dependence is sparse, but NRT and bupropion, alone or in combination, are well tolerated (Killen *et al.*, 2004; Moolchan *et al.*, 2005; Muramoto *et al.*, 2007). There is evidence of efficacy in adolescents for NRT delivered as a patch (Moolchan *et al.*, 2005), and for bupropion at the 300 mg/day dose, at least in the short term (Muramoto *et al.*, 2007). A small (total *n* = 29), uncontrolled 8-week trial of bupropion XL (once-daily dosing to reduce problems of medication adherence) and varenicline (standard dosing for those weighing at least 55 kg and lower doses for those under 55 kg) among 15–20 year old smokers did not raise safety concerns, and both medications were associated with significant reductions in daily cigarette use (Gray *et al.*, 2012). A larger adolescent study of varenicline currently is underway. The UK's NICE has also published a guidance document including information on smoking cessation which suggests use of NRT but not bupropion or varenicline for those under 18 years of age (NICE, 2008).

Blending treatments and treatment matching

Some psychosocial treatment studies combine approaches (e.g., motivational enhancement therapy or contingency management with cognitive-behavioral therapy), but evidence for blending techniques from various evidence-based treatments still remains limited. However, Anton *et al.* (2006) combined elements of motivational enhancement, cognitive-behavioral therapy, community reinforcement and 12-step facilitation treatments into a single psychosocial intervention for adults with alcohol use disorder; to our knowledge such combinations have not been tested in adolescents. In addition, empirical research provides little guidance for matching particular patients with particular treatments. However, in some instances common sense may suggest the most appropriate approach. For example, an emancipated youth who is working and living independently might respond less well to family-centered treatment.

Working with criminal justice and social service agencies

Some clinicians worry that working closely with probation, parole, or social-service agencies may damage the treatment alliance, but legal contingencies can be important treatment motivators. When patients are referred through such agencies, it is important to discuss how and what information will be shared, and to complete appropriate release forms (see Section titled Assessment). Teamwork with such referring agencies can help to mobilize systemic supports that improve the likelihood of treatment compliance, abstinence from drug use, and better long-term outcomes (for general information on legal issues in the care and treatment of children with mental health problems, see Chapter 19).

Relapse prevention

Even highly motivated SUD patients may relapse. Although some patients, or even providers, view relapse in catastrophic terms (e.g., a sign that a patient has learned nothing), relapse prevention techniques reframe relapse as an opportunity to extend treatment gains. Briefly, relapse prevention procedures identify high risk situations, including certain people, places, or emotional states; use planning to anticipate and reduce contact with those situations; and when they cannot be avoided, teach substance-free coping with the situations (Hendershot *et al.*, 2011). Such models are broadly incorporated into psychosocial treatments of substance disorders.

Treatment of co-morbid mental health disorders

The American Academy of Child and Adolescent Psychiatry's Practice Parameters state that assessment and treatment of co-morbid psychiatric disorders are a minimal standard of care, supported by substantial empirical evidence and "overwhelming" clinical consensus (Bukstein *et al.*, 2005). Standard treatments for co-morbid disorders are outlined in other chapters of this text, but five important principles apply here. (i) Although disentangling substance-induced and independent mental health symptoms may be complicated, examining the temporal inter relationship of symptoms, the age of symptom onset, and the persistence of symptoms during periods of abstinence is helpful. Some authors use a timeline approach to guide such inquiries (Riggs & Davies, 2002). (ii) Although sequential treatment (e.g., requiring remission of substance use before treating depression) is sometimes recommended, concurrent treatment of both disorders is presumed to be optimal (Bukstein *et al.*, 2005). (iii) Medications for some disorders, including stimulants for attention-deficit/hyperactivity disorder, may be abused. In youths with SUD the risks and potential harms from such treatments must be weighed against potential benefits, especially since non-stimulant alternatives are available. (iv) Adolescents with SUD may experiment with medications prescribed for comorbid disorders, seeking a "high." As exemplified by bupropion's risk of seizures, such experiments can be dangerous. Having parents safely store the medication and monitor administration may reduce such risks. (v) Although a large body of empirical research focuses on treating adolescents' mental health disorders, the specialized literature on treating the co-morbid mental health disorders of adolescents with SUD must be considered (e.g., Riggs *et al.*, 2007).

Non-substance "behavioral addictions"

Gambling disorder in DSM-5 replaces DSM-IV's more pejorative term, "pathologic gambling." Gambling disorder is found in the same chapter as substance related disorders because the conditions have somewhat similar diagnostic criteria and may share certain genetic and neural mechanisms (Petry *et al.*, 2013). DSM-5 also somewhat altered the diagnostic criteria. The prevalence of adolescent problem gambling exceeds that in adults (Forrest & McHale, 2012), and gambling problems in adolescents are associated with frequent substance use and other risky behaviors (Proimos *et al.*, 1998). This comorbidity of substance and gambling problems suggests screening adolescents with SUD for gambling disorder, using an available screen (Forrest & McHale, 2012).

DSM-5's drafters found insufficient evidence (Hasin *et al.*, 2013) to establish diagnoses for "addiction" to shopping, exercise, or sex, as some had proposed. However, "internet gaming addiction" was placed into a section of DSM-5 reserved for conditions that future research might establish as disorders.

Future developments and necessary research

Great progress has been made in defining early risks for adolescent SUDs, as well as methods for prevention, early intervention, and treatment of the disorders. Further advances are needed in the following areas: Some children's pre-pubertal behavioral disinhibition suggests a risk for future SUD, and those children need studies of empirically-supported, focused prevention efforts. SUD is a chronic relapsing and remitting problem, requiring multi year studies of psychosocial and pharmacological approaches for adolescents with SUD, including controlled studies of long-term court-required case-management and treatment for relapsing youths. Research on medication treatments for adolescent SUD is sorely needed. Shifting drug policies, including legalization of marijuana in some jurisdictions, cry out for studies of the effects of such policies on drug use and SUDs in adolescents. Better identification of biological contributors to these life-threatening disorders could lead to new, targeted, and more effective treatments; focuses should include identifying genomic risk factors, together with imaging of: brain-based antecedent risks for substance involvement, drug-induced brain pathology, and brain changes from treatment.

Acknowledgments

NIDA grant DA011015 supported both Dr. Crowley's and Dr. Sakai's work. NIDA grants RO1DA031761 and R01DA029258 support Dr. Sakai's work. The Kane Family Foundation supports both.

References

Anton, R.F. *et al.* (2006) Combined pharmacotherapies and behavioral interventions for alcohol dependence: the COMBINE study: a randomized controlled trial. *JAMA* **295**, 2003–2017.

American Psychiatric Association (2013) *Diagnostic and Statistical Manual of Mental Disorders.* (eds D. Kupfer & D. Regier), 5th edn, pp. 536. American Psychiatric Association, Washington, DC.

Botvin, G.J. *et al.* (1995) Long-term follow-up results of a randomized drug abuse prevention trial in a white middle-class population. *JAMA* **273**, 1106–1112.

Bukstein, O.G. *et al.* (2005) Practice parameter for the assessment and treatment of children and adolescents with substance use disorders. *Journal of the American Academy of Child and Adolescent Psychiatry* **44**, 609–621.

CCQI, 2012. *Practice standards for young people with substance misuse problems. Publication number CCQI 127* [Online]. Available: http://www.rcpsych.ac.uk/pdf/Practice%20standards%20for%20young%20people%20with%20substance%20misuse%20problems.pdf [5 Aug 2013].

Copeland, W. *et al.* (2011) Cumulative presence of psychiatric disorders by young adulthood: a prospective cohort analysis from the Great Smoky Mountains Study. *Journal of the American Academy of Child and Adolescent Psychiatry* **50**, 252–261.

Costello, E.J. *et al.* (2010) Association of family income supplements in adolescence with development of psychiatric and substance use disorders in adulthood among an American Indian population. *JAMA* **303**, 1954–1960.

Crowley, T.J. *et al.* (2001) Validity of structured clinical evaluations in adolescents with conduct and substance problems. *Journal of the American Academy of Child and Adolescent Psychiatry* **40**, 265–273.

Crowley, T.J. *et al.* (2003) Discriminative validity and clinical utility of an abuse-neglect interview for adolescents with conduct and substance use problems. *American Journal of Psychiatry* **160**, 1461–1469.

Crowley, T.J. *et al.* (2010) Risky decisions and their consequences: neural processing by boys with antisocial substance disorder. *PLoS One* **5**, e12835.

Crowley, T.J., *et al.* (2013) *Colorado adolescent rearing inventory* [Online]. Available: Figshare. 10.6084/m9.figshare.701552 [13 May 2013].

Dawson, D.A. *et al.* (2008) Age at first drink and the first incidence of adult-onset DSM-IV alcohol use disorders. *Alcoholism: Clinical and Experimental Research* **32**, 2149–2160.

Degenhardt, L. & Hall, W. (2012) Extent of illicit drug use and dependence, and their contribution to the global burden of disease. *The Lancet* **379**, 55–70.

Faggiano, F. *et al.* (2007) A cluster randomized controlled trial of school-based prevention of tobacco, alcohol and drug use: the EU-Dap design and study population. *Prevention Medicine* **44**, 170–173.

Faggiano, F. *et al.* (2010) The effectiveness of a school-based substance abuse prevention program: 18-month follow-up of the EU-Dap cluster randomized controlled trial. *Drug and Alcohol Dependence* **108**, 56–64.

Fergusson, D.M. *et al.* (2009) Situational and generalized conduct problems and later life outcomes: evidence from a New Zealand birth cohort. *Journal of Child Psychology and Psychiatry* **50**, 1084–1092.

Fishman, M.J. *et al.* (2010) Treatment of opioid dependence in adolescents and young adults with extended release naltrexone: preliminary case-series and feasibility. *Addiction* **105**, 1669–1676.

Forrest, D. & McHale, I.G. (2012) Gambling and problem gambling among young adolescents in Great Britain. *Journal of Gambling Studies* **28**, 607–622.

Giedd, J.N. *et al.* (2010) Anatomic magnetic resonance imaging of the developing child and adolescent brain and effects of genetic variation. *Neuropsychological Reviews* **20**, 349–361.

Goldstein, B.I. & Bukstein, O.G. (2010) Comorbid substance use disorders among youth with bipolar disorder: opportunities for early identification and prevention. *Journal of Clinical Psychiatry* **71**, 348–358.

Gray, K.M. *et al.* (2012) Varenicline versus bupropion XL for smoking cessation in older adolescents: a randomized, double-blind pilot trial. *Nicotine & Tobacco Research* **14**, 234–239.

Hasin, D.S. *et al.* (2013) DSM-5 criteria for substance use disorders: recommendations and rationale. *American Journal of Psychiatry* **170**, 834–851.

Hendershot, C.S. *et al.* (2011) Relapse prevention for addictive behaviors. *Substance Abuse Treatment, Prevention, and Policy* **19**, 6–17.

Henggeler, S.W. (2007) Juvenile drug courts: emerging outcomes and key research issues. *Current Opinion in Psychiatry* **20**, 242–246.

Hibell, B., *et al.* (2009) *The 2007 ESPAD Report.* The Swedish Council for Information on Alcohol and other Drugs. Modintryckoffset AB, Stockholm [Online]. Available: www.espad.org/en/Reports-Documents/ESPAD-Reports/ [11 Aug 2013].

Hibell, B., *et al.* (2012) *The 2011 ESPAD Report.* The Swedish Council for Information on Alcohol and other Drugs. Modintryckoffset AB, Stockholm [Online]. Available: www.espad.org/en/Reports-Documents/ESPAD-Reports/ [11 Aug 2013].

Hicks, B.M. *et al.* (2004) Family transmission and heritability of externalizing disorders: a twin-family study. *Archives of General Psychiatry* **61**, 922–928.

Holder, H. (2010) Prevention programs in the 21st century: what we do not discuss in public. *Addiction* **105**, 578–581.

Iacono, W.G. *et al.* (2008) Behavioral disinhibition and the development of early-onset addiction: common and specific influences. *Annual Review of Clinical Psychology* **4**, 325–348.

Jensen, C.D. *et al.* (2011) Effectiveness of motivational interviewing interventions for adolescent substance use behavior change: a meta-analytic review. *Journal of Consulting and Clinical Psychology* **79**, 433–440.

Kavanagh, D.J. *et al.* (2004) Demographic and clinical correlates of comorbid substance use disorders in psychosis: multivariate analyses from an epidemiological sample. *Schizophrenia Research* **66**, 115–124.

Kellam, S.G. *et al.* (2012) The impact of the good behavior game, a universal classroom-based preventive intervention in first and second grades, on high-risk sexual behaviors and drug abuse and dependence disorders into young adulthood. *Prevention Science* 15, S6–S18.

Kendler, K.S. *et al.* (2013) Within-family environmental transmission of drug abuse: a Swedish national study. *JAMA Psychiatry* **70**, 235–242.

Killen, J.D. *et al.* (2004) Randomized clinical trial of the efficacy of bupropion combined with nicotine patch in the treatment of adolescent smokers. *Journal of Consulting and Clinical Psychology* **72**, 729–735.

Koob, G.F. & Volkow, N.D. (2010) Neurocircuitry of addiction. *Neuropsychopharmacology* **35**, 217–238.

Kramer, T.L. *et al.* (2003) Detection and outcomes of substance use disorders in adolescents seeking mental health treatment. *Journal of the American Academy of Child and Adolescent Psychiatry* **42**, 1318–1326.

Krueger, R.F. *et al.* (2002) Etiologic connections among substance dependence, antisocial behavior, and personality: modeling the externalizing spectrum. *Journal of Abnormal Psychology* **111**, 411–424.

Kumpfer, K.L. *et al.* (2008) Cultural adaptation process for international dissemination of the strengthening families program. *Evaluation & the Health Professions* **31**, 226–239.

Lehmann, W.X. (1976) The use of 1-alpha-acetyl-methadol (LAAM) as compared to methadone in the maintenance and detoxification of young heroin addicts. *NIDA Research Monographs* **8**, 82–83.

Marsch, L.A. *et al.* (2005) Comparison of pharmacological treatments for opioid-dependent adolescents: a randomized controlled trial. *Archives of General Psychiatry* **62**, 1157–1164.

Mee-Lee, D. *et al.* (2001) *ASAM Patient Placement Criteria for the Treatment of Substance-Related Disorders,* 2nd-Revised. edn. American Society of Addiction Medicine, Chevy Chase, MD.

Milne, B.J. *et al.* (2009) Predictive value of family history on severity of illness: the case for depression, anxiety, alcohol dependence, and drug dependence. *Archives of General Psychiatry* **66**, 738–747.

Moffitt, T.E. *et al.* (2011) A gradient of childhood self-control predicts health, wealth, and public safety. *Proceedings of the National Academy of Sciences of the United States of America* **108**, 2693–2698.

Monti, P.M. *et al.* (1999) Brief intervention for harm reduction with alcohol-positive older adolescents in a hospital emergency department. *Journal of Consulting and Clinical Psychology* **67**, 989–994.

Moolchan, E.T. *et al.* (2005) Safety and efficacy of the nicotine patch and gum for the treatment of adolescent tobacco addiction. *Pediatrics* **115**, e407–e414.

Muramoto, M.L. *et al.* (2007) Randomized, double-blind, placebo-controlled trial of 2 dosages of sustained-release bupropion for adolescent smoking cessation. *Archives of Pediatrics and Adolescent Medicine* **161**, 1068–1074.

National Institute on Drug Abuse (2003) *Preventing Drug Use Among Children and Adolescents. A Research-Based Guide for Parents, Educators, and Community Leaders.* NIH Publication No. 04-4212(A), second edition. Bethesda, Maryland.

NIAAA (2011). *Alcohol screening and brief intervention for youth: a practitioner's guide.* NIH Publication 11-7805. National Institute on Alcohol Abuse and Alcoholism. Rockville, MD [Online]. Available: http://www.niaaa.nih.gov/Publications/EducationTrainingMaterials/Pages/YouthGuide.aspx [12 May 2013].

National Institute for Health and Care Excellence (2007a). *Technology appraisal guidance 114. Methadone and buprenorphine for the management of opioid dependence* [Online]. Available: http://www.nice.org.uk/nicemedia/pdf/TA114Niceguidance.pdf [5 Aug 2013].

National Institute for Health and Care Excellence (2007b). *Technology appraisal guidance 115. Naltrexone for the management of opioid dependence* [Online]. http://www.nice.org.uk/nicemedia/live/11604/33812/33812.pdf [5 Aug 2013].

National Institute for Health and Care Excellence (2008). *Public health guidance 10. Smoking cessation services* [Online]. http://www.nice.org.uk/nicemedia/live/11925/39596/39596.pdf [5 Aug 2013].

National Institute for Health and Care Excellence (2011). *Clinical guidance 115. Alcohol-use disorders: diagnosis, assessment and management of harmful drinking and alchol depedence* [Online]. http://www.nice.org.uk/nicemedia/live/13337/53191/53191.pdf [5 Aug 2013].

Niederhofer, H. & Staffen, W. (2003) Comparison of disulfiram and placebo in treatment of alcohol dependence of adolescents. *Drug and Alcohol Review* **22**, 295–297.

Norman, A.L. *et al.* (2011) Neural activation during inhibition predicts initiation of substance use in adolescence. *Drug and Alcohol Dependence* **119**, 216–223.

NREPP (2013). *National registry of evidence-based programs and practices.* Substance Abuse and Mental Health Services Administration [Online]. Available: www.nrepp.samhsa.gov [12 May 2013].

Petry, N.M. *et al.* (2013) An overview of and rationale for changes proposed for pathological gambling in DSM-5. *Journal of Gambling Studies* **30**, 493–502.

Proimos, J. *et al.* (1998) Gambling and other risk behaviors among 8th-to 12th-grade students. *Pediatrics* **102**, e23.

Rhee, S.H. *et al.* (2003) Genetic and environmental influences on substance initiation, use, and problem use in adolescents. *Archives of General Psychiatry* **60**, 1256–1264.

Riggs, P.D. (2003) Treating adolescents for substance abuse and comorbid psychiatric disorders. *Science & Practice Perspectives* **2**, 18–29.

Riggs, P.D. & Davies, R.D. (2002) A clinical approach to integrating treatment for adolescent depression and substance abuse. *Journal of the American Academy of Child and Adolescent Psychiatry* **41**, 1253–1255.

Riggs, P.D. *et al.* (2007) A randomized controlled trial of fluoxetine and cognitive behavioral therapy in adolescents with major depression, behavior problems, and substance use disorders. *Archives of Pediatrics and Adolescent Medicine* **161**, 1026–1034.

Robbins, M.S. *et al.* (2011) Brief strategic family therapy versus treatment as usual: results of a multi site randomized trial for substance using adolescents. *Journal of Consulting and Clinical Psychology* **79**, 713–727.

Saccone, S.F. *et al.* (2007) Cholinergic nicotinic receptor genes implicated in a nicotine dependence association study targeting 348 candidate genes with 3713 SNPs. *Human Molecular Genetics* **16**, 36–49.

SAMHSA (2011). *Identifying mental health and substance use problems of children and adolescents: a guide for child-serving organizations* (HHS Publication No. SMA 12-4670). Substance Abuse and Mental Health Services Administration. Rockville, MD, 2012 [Online]. Available: http://store.samhsa.gov [31 Aug 2014].

SAMHSA (2013). *Screening tools* [Online]. Available: www.integration .samhsa.gov/clinical-practice/screening-tools#drugs [30 July 2013].

Saunders, J.B. (2006) Substance dependence and non-dependence in the diagnostic and statistical manual of mental disorders (DSM) and the International Classification of Diseases (ICD): can an identical conceptualization be achieved? *Addiction* **101**, 48–58.

Schneider, S. *et al.* (2012) Risk taking and the adolescent reward system: a potential common link to substance abuse. *American Journal of Psychiatry* **169**, 39–46.

Stanger, C. & Budney, A.J. (2010) Contingency management approaches for adolescent substance use disorders. *Child and Adolescent Psychiatric Clinics of North America* **19**, 547–562.

Sussman, S. (2010) A review of alcoholics anonymous/narcotics anonymous programs for teens. *Evaluation & Health Professions* **33**, 26–55.

Tripodi, S.J. (2009) A comprehensive review: methodological rigor of studies on residential treatment centers for substance-abusing adolescents. *Journal of Evidence Based Social Work* **6**, 288–299.

Tripodi, S.J. *et al.* (2010) Interventions for reducing adolescent alcohol abuse: a meta-analytic review. *Archives of Pediatrics and Adolescent Medicine* **164**, 85–91.

Tyrfingsson, T. *et al.* (2010) Addictions and their familiality in Iceland. *Annals of the New York Academy of Sciences* **1187**, 208–217.

Waldron, H.B. & Turner, C.W. (2008) Evidence-based psychosocial treatments for adolescent substance abuse. *Journal of Clinical Child & Adolescent Psychology* **37**, 238–261.

World Health Organization (2010). *Chapter V mental and behavioral disorders (F00-F99). International Statistical Classification of Diseases and Related Health Problems, 10th Revision (ICD-10,) Version for 2010.* http://apps.who.int/classifications/icd10/browse/ .2010/en#/F10-F19 [20 Feb 2013].

Woody, G.E. *et al.* (2008) Extended vs short-term buprenorphine-naloxone for treatment of opioid-addicted youth: a randomized trial. *JAMA* **300**, 2003–2011.

Young, S.E. *et al.* (2000) Genetic and environmental influences on behavioral disinhibition. *American Journal of Medical Genetics* **96**, 684–695.

CHAPTER 67

Disorders of personality

Jonathan Hill

School for Psychology and Clinical Language Sciences, University of Reading, UK

Why is something like the concept of personality disorders needed?

The personality disorders are described within a framework of adult psychiatric diagnoses that makes a distinction between disorders that are episodic, with clear onsets and offsets and circumscribed symptomatology, for example depression, and disorders that are more enduring with widespread emotional and behavioral problems. The need for something like the concept of personality disorder arises then in two main ways. First, some individuals have behavioral and emotional problems that precede and extend beyond the confines of episodic disorders. Second, these problems share with personality traits (habitual patterns of behavior, thought, and emotion) the characteristics of being relatively enduring and evident in many situations. The concept was developed to be applied to adults and so inevitably much of the relevant research considered in this chapter has been carried out with adults. However, the discussion in this section regarding the need for the concept applies equally during adolescence. It is also important to adopt a developmental perspective as the vulnerabilities and precursors of personality disorder have their origins in childhood.

The child and adolescent context in which we might consider the concept of personality disorder is however very different from that of the adult. Disorders that tend to persist are common, notably the disruptive behavior disorders (DBDs) of oppositional defiant disorder (ODD) and conduct disorder (CD) (see Chapters 4 and 65), attention-deficit hyperactivity disorder (ADHD; see Chapter 55) and autistic spectrum disorders (ASD; see Chapter 51). These are not however thought about in the same way. Disruptive behavior problems arising in young children are associated with many adverse psychiatric and social outcomes in later life, some of which are summarized in the adult antisocial personality disorder (ASPD) diagnosis. By contrast (ADHD) and autism spectrum disorder (ASD),

which also show persistence into adult life (see Chapter 3), are not viewed as personality disorders either in children or adults. What they are called probably does not matter, but differentiating them is crucial. The key point for the clinician is that before puberty each of these disorders may need to be considered for some presentations, for example, of peer aggression, while in adolescents at least one additional grouping of persistent and pervasive problems, summarized as borderline personality disorder (BPD), also enters into the differential diagnosis.

In clinical practice, in adolescence the concept is often relevant where the presenting problem can be diagnosed as an episodic disorder such as depression, but there are additional features that are not accounted for by that diagnosis, nor by an accompanying "comorbid" episodic disorder such as generalized anxiety disorder. Thus the key is the extensiveness or the diversity of the difficulties. In general, consideration of personality disorder will require also that these, or similar, difficulties were present before the onset of the disorder. Furthermore as the presenting symptoms resolve, those attributed to personality disorder persist. The concept is also relevant where an individual has problems that are severe enough to cause distress to themselves or others, and impair daily functioning, but they do not follow the pattern of episodic disorders. Examples include repeated violence, or self-harm in the absence of diagnosable depression, or difficulties in social role performance, for example in work or close relationships.

Current conceptualizations of personality disorder and diagnostic and statistical manual (DSM) IV and 5

The World Health Organization (1996) classification, ICD-10, makes a basic differentiation between organic personality disorders (meaning those resulting from severe head injury,

Rutter's Child and Adolescent Psychiatry, Sixth Edition.
Edited by Anita Thapar and Daniel S. Pine, James F. Leckman, Stephen Scott, Margaret J. Snowling, Eric Taylor.
© 2015 John Wiley & Sons Ltd. Published 2018 by John Wiley & Sons Ltd.

encephalitis, and other forms of overt brain damage); enduring personality changes deriving from some catastrophic experience, personality abnormalities that reflect the residue of some mental illness (e.g., residual schizophrenia) and what they term personality disorders. The American Psychiatric Association (2000) scheme makes broadly comparable distinctions. This chapter is concerned with this last group of specific personality disorders, because the others have only an extremely limited application in childhood and adolescence.

There are 10 key adult personality disorders outlined in Table 67.1. It should be borne in mind that the concept of personality disorder did not originate from a model of normal personality, and indeed descriptions of different personality disorder types have come about through several contrasting routes. First, there are those that derive from the clinical observation that there are individuals who show enduring patterns of inflexible and seriously maladaptive behavior that seem to fall outside the traditional criteria for mental illness or psychiatric syndrome. The need to have a term to describe these patterns of abnormal behavior led to the concepts of psychopathy put forward by writers such as Hare (1970), Henderson (1939) and Cleckley (1941). Second, there are the categories of personality disorder that identify individuals who are thought to be most prone to suffer from episodic mental disorders. Schneider's (1923, 1950) notion of psychopathic personality (defined quite differently from the psychopathy formulations of Hare, of Henderson, and of Cleckley) provides the main historic notion of this approach. Many of the ICD-10 specific personality disorder categories (e.g., paranoid, anankastic, and anxious) represent this tradition (World Health Organization, 1996). Third, some categories have their origins in empirical observations of the continuities between psychopathological disorders in childhood and pervasive social malfunction in adult lifestyle. The DSM diagnosis of ASPD is the obvious example of this type, with its starting point in the findings of the long-term longitudinal studies pioneered by Robins (1966, 1978). Fourth, some categories stem fairly directly from theoretical, especially psychoanalytic, notions. The concept of borderline personality organization (Kernberg, 1967, 1975) underlies specification of the DSM diagnosis of BPD (Gunderson *et al.*, 1981). Finally, a few categories have come, at least in part, from genetic findings. Meehl (1962) coined the term schizotypy to describe the postulated characteristics of schizophrenia-prone individuals. The Danish adoption study showed that the biological families of adopted schizophrenic probands included a raised rate of personality disorders that seemed to exhibit some features reminiscent of schizophrenia (Kety *et al.*, 1971). Spitzer *et al.* (1979) developed more explicit criteria for this type of personality syndrome which has come to be termed schizotypal personality disorder (SPD). There is now substantial support for a genetic relationship between SPD and schizophrenia, based on studies of families, twins, and adoptees (Cannon *et al.*, 2008).

Table 67.1 The characteristics of 10 key personality disorders.

Paranoid Personality Disorder
Pervasive distrust and suspiciousness of others such that their motives are interpreted as malevolent, beginning by early adulthood and present in a variety of contexts.

Schizoid Personality Disorder
Detachment from social relationships and a restricted range of expression of emotions in interpersonal settings, beginning by early adulthood and present in a variety of contexts.

Schizotypal personality disorder
A pervasive pattern of social and interpersonal deficits marked by acute discomfort with, and reduced capacity for, close relationships as well as by cognitive or perceptual distortions and eccentricities of behavior, beginning by early adulthood and present in a variety of contexts.

Antisocial personality disorder
A pervasive pattern of disregard for and violation of the rights of others in adult life that is preceded by conduct disorder characterized by features such as law breaking , deceitfulness, aggressiveness, reckless disregard for safety, irresponsibility and lack of remorse.

Borderline personality disorder
Pervasive instability of interpersonal relationships, self-image and affects, and marked impulsivity beginning by early adulthood.

Narcissistic personality disorder
Pervasive grandiosity (fantasy or behavior), need for admiration, and lack of empathy in a variety of contexts.

Histrionic personality disorder
Pervasive excessive emotionality and attention-seeking present in a variety of contexts.

Dependent Personality Disorder
Pervasive, excessive need to be taken care of, accompanied by submissive and clinging behavior and fears of separation.

Avoidant personality disorder
Pervasive social inhibition, feelings of inadequacy, and hypersensitivity to negative evaluation.

Obsessive compulsive personality disorder
Preoccupation with orderliness, perfectionism and mental and interpersonal control. This comes at the expense of flexibility, openness and efficiency and is present in a variety of contexts.

Even if a general concept does not cover all of the personality disorders, it is relevant to two that commonly need to be considered in adolescent clinical practice: antisocial and borderline personality disorders. The complexities and difficulties in nailing a general concept are illustrated in the debate over proposals made for DSM-5. In DSM-IV (American Psychiatric Association, 2000) the core dysfunction is described as "An enduring pattern of inner experience and behavior that deviates markedly from the expectations of the individual's culture. This pattern is manifested in two (or more) of the following areas: (i) Cognition (i.e., ways of perceiving and interpreting self, other people and events), (ii) Affectivity (i.e., the range, intensity, lability, and appropriateness of emotional response), (iii) Interpersonal functioning, (iv) Impulse control." Although ultimately DSM-5 retained the approach used in DSM-IV for defining personality disorders, this decision was only made after extensive attempts to generate an alternative definition that incorporated extensive information on personality structure in both health and illness. To seek such a definition, an alternative set of proposals involving a dimensional–categorical model was discussed. These proposed revisions were included in a separate, supplemental chapter in DSM-5 as a basis for future research into ways of characterizing the personality disorders in clinical practice. In these alternative proposals for DSM-5 (American Psychiatric Association, 2013) the core deficit in personality disorders was described as, "….impairments in personality (self and interpersonal) functioning and the presence of pathological personality traits." To diagnose a personality disorder using these proposals that were eventually not adopted, the following criteria must be met: "A. Significant impairments in self (identity or self-direction) and interpersonal (empathy or intimacy) functioning. B. One or more pathological personality trait domains or trait facets." Unlike personality disorder definitions in DSM-IV and the main section of DSM-5 that emerged from data on patients, these alternative trait domains were linked to research on personality structure, manifest in various populations. These definitions, drawn from factor analytic approaches to personality, which are outlined later in the chapter, consisted of *negative emotionality, introversion, antagonism, disinhibition, compulsivity* and *schizotypy*. In clinical and research practice, DSM-IV and DSM-5 personality disorders retain definitions in place since the 1990s, as identified by the criteria summarized in Table 67.1. As discussed, after extensive review, the DSM-IV approach with the same 10 personality disorders has been retained in DSM-5.

Key questions

The differences between definitions in DSM-5 that were retained from DSM-IV and the alternative proposal that was not accepted for the DSM-5 revision illustrate how profound are the uncertainties in the field of personality disorders, and indicate the challenge to clinicians in talking with patients and their families. This is not only a question of how to diagnose, but also how to formulate complex presentations. Four topics that may help conceptualize formulations are discussed here.

How should personality disorder be specified and explained?

DSM-based specifications vary in the extent to which they differentiate between manifestations and underlying processes. ASPD is almost entirely specified by deviant behaviors such as criminality, violence, impulsive actions, and failures to maintain adult social roles. This is a level of description that makes clear what needs to be explained and makes no reference to what the explanation may be. By contrast, BPD is specified by a mixture, both between and within items. Thus the item "repeated self-harm" is clearly a behavioral pattern for which a range of explanations may be sought, while "identity disturbance: markedly and persistently unstable self-image or sense of self"

refers to psychological processes that may explain behaviors. The item, "A pattern of unstable and intense interpersonal relationships characterised by alternating between extremes of idealization and devaluation" describes both behaviors and states of mind.

A focus on behaviors as opposed to underlying processes influences both research and clinical practice. Where only the behaviors are specified, research questions can be framed with many possibilities in mind. This becomes problematic where potential explanatory variables are included in the definition, as these are more difficult to assess than overt behaviors. The clinical implications are very similar. A behavioral description can establish the extent of the problem, leading to enquiry that explores a range of possible explanations, for which different assessment tools may be required. On the other hand, a specification of personality disorder confined to behaviors may fail to specify a distinctive process such as idealization and devaluation in relationships, and hence be over- or under-inclusive, and so clinically less informative.

The way forward may be to proceed more cautiously and systematically from specification of behavioral dysfunction to explanation. This is the approach taken using the Adult Personality Functioning Assessment where personality functioning is assessed as social role performance in six social domains over a 5-year period. This is consistent with studies of adult personality disorders that find strong associations with social dysfunction (Hill *et al.*, 2000; Seivewright *et al.*, 2004; Skodol *et al.*, 2005) and "the characteristic that seems to define them all is a pervasive persistent abnormality in maintaining social relationships" (Rutter, 1987). Crucially, personality disorders may remit while social dysfunction persists, suggesting that it is core to the disorder (Gunderson *et al.*, 2011). The forms of social dysfunction may provide clues to specific processes. For example, one of the characteristics of the social dysfunction of BPD is a problem in maintaining a demarcation between the behaviors and emotions that belong with different kinds of social interaction (Hill *et al.*, 2008). This is discussed further later in the chapter.

Normal personality or personality disorders?

It would make sense if the areas of dysfunction identified in the personality disorders could be specified in terms of the functions served by normal personality. This is not the case in DSM-5 however, in part because, as outlined earlier, different personality disorders have been formulated for different reasons, but also because the conceptualization of personality remains problematic. The Five Factor Model (FFM) has been widely advocated as a solution. The FFM has been derived from studies using predominantly self-report measures with items derived from lexical analyses. The basic premise of this approach is that common linguistic descriptors, such as "hopeful" or "worried" have been retained in languages because they map on to personality characteristics (Widiger & Lowe, 2007; Widiger & Costa, 2012). Items generated from lexical analysis are subjected to factor analyses yielding five factors that capture substantial proportions of personality variations, Extraversion/Positive Emotionality, Neuroticism/Negative Emotionality, Conscientiousness/Constraint, Agreeableness, and Openness-to-Experience. The five factor solution has been widely replicated; it shows cross-cultural consistency; and the factors show stability over time in line with most concepts of personality (Widiger & Costa, 2012). The personality disorders, conceptualized in relation to these personality factors, arise from maladaptive extreme variants of common personality traits. In discussions of models such as these, two issues are commonly conflated, whether categorical or dimensional approaches are more useful and the definition of "normal personality functioning." The categorical versus dimensional dilemma is discussed later in the chapter. Definition of normal personality function remains a matter of debate. Long-standing critiques have highlighted only modest agreement between self and informant reports, differences between self-report and observed behaviors, and cross-situational differences, as limitations (Mischel, 2004).

Historically, the various conceptualizations of personality disorders have often been presented as competing. However, at this stage in our understanding, it may be more helpful to view the general rubric of personality disorder as identifying a number of related dysfunctions whose importance depend on what needs to be explained. Studies that make use of measures from the different traditions are therefore particularly illuminating. For example in a follow up of the Collaborative Longitudinal Personality Disorder Study of psychiatric patients, DSM-IV categorical and dimensional variables, and dimensions of the FFM, all predicted a range of outcomes over up to 10 years, including suicidal behaviors, occupational and interpersonal functioning, and depression (Morey et al., 2012). In relation to some personality disorders, notably borderline and antisocial disorders, DSM-IV items, and FFM traits each added to the prediction of outcomes, although in others such as histrionic disorder the DSM items did not add to the prediction over FFM traits.

How do developmental perspectives on personality and its disorders help?

Commonly, vulnerabilities or precursors of personality disorder can be identified in childhood and so there are good reasons to review the adequacy and relevance of theories of personality from a developmental perspective (see Chapter 8). First, how coherent or homogenous are the hypothesized traits? Although the big-five are characterized as "higher-order," each includes "lower-order" traits, some of which differ substantially. This issue is reviewed by Caspi et al. (2005) For example, the higher-order trait neuroticism is well validated and highly predictive in childhood and adult life, but includes both proneness to fear and to anger. These different emotions motivate different behaviors, they are mediated via different neurological substrates, and they have different implications

for development and psychopathology (Lemerise & Arsenio, 2000; Frick & Morris, 2004). Developmental hypotheses for disruptive behavior problems (see Chapters 4 and 65), the childhood antecedents of ASPD, envisage increased risk arising from elevated anger proneness, but reduced fearfulness (Smeekens et al., 2007; Colder et al., 2002). Second, some of the personality traits also resemble temperamental characteristics. Thus, fear proneness and anger proneness are two aspects of temperament commonly assessed in infancy (Robinson & Acevedo, 2001). More generally the overlap between temperament and personality traits requires further attention (Caspi et al., 2005). Third, FFM personality traits are determined by the frequency of behaviors across context and time. However, traits can be conceptualized in other ways. In particular, individuals can be characterized by predictable and patterned differences in their behaviors across situations, arising for example from the interplay between social information processing and context (Mischel, 2004). Fourth, personality development entails the development of the person as social organism. Personality traits such as neuroticism undoubtedly influence social relationships (e.g., Robins et al., 2002), but there are also aspects of personality functioning such as ways of interpreting others' behaviors that are inherently social and entail dedicated neuronal networks (Johnson et al., 2005). The capacity to regulate behaviors and emotions according to the demands of different kinds of social domain, for example contrasting teachers and parents, is key to effective personality development (Hill et al., 2010). Fifth, personality develops in interaction with the environment so that its features are likely to reflect more or less successful adaptations rather than any simple manifestation of stable traits.

It could be argued that to be of real value, developmental perspectives should generate alternative formulations. There is no doubt that developmental findings inform understanding of personality disorders, most notably in the case of ASPD being preceded by disruptive behavior problems (see Chapter 65). Risks accumulate and are moderated by the interplay between the child's biology and psychology (Hill, 2002). Furthermore some key developmental processes clearly have implications for personality disorders. The child's organisation of emotions and behaviors provides an illustrative example. Initially, interactions are confined to caregivers, but in the second year, the interpersonal world begins to encompass other children and adults. However, the developing child does not interact in the same way with these different groups. This is seen strikingly with the emergence of stranger anxiety and selective attachments between 6 and 9 months. In the presence of a stranger, most children become wary and seek comfort from a caregiver. Later, as sibling and peer interactions develop, further differences are apparent. Children play with other children, and distinguish friends from non-friends, but rarely turn to other children for comfort as they do with familiar adults (Rubin et al., 1999). Thus, individual development entails an increasingly sophisticated organisation of the child's behaviors. This requires not only the organization of behaviors, but also a recognition of the particular goals, problem solving procedures and social resources available in each kind of social interaction. These contrasting types of social interaction have been described as social domains, each with its own underlying rules or "algorithms of social life" (Bugental, 2000). The hypothesis that domain organization is a key element in personality development leads also to the prediction that problems in domain organisation may be found in personality disorders (Hill et al., 2010).

Validation

Stability and associations with episodic disorders

It is assumed that personality disorders show substantial stability over time. However, several studies have found low to moderate stability (e.g., Ferro et al., 1998). In a follow-up every 2 years, of 290 patients meeting DSM-IV criteria for BPD, 74% had remitted after 6 years, and only 6% had remitted and then relapsed (Zanarini et al., 2005). After 16 years, almost all of the borderline patients no longer met DSM criteria (Zanarini et al., 2012). The picture was however different for social dysfunction, where around 50% of patients had significant social problems at 16-year follow-up (Zanarini et al., 2012), findings echoed in other research on social dysfunction (Rutter & Quinton, 1984; Quinton et al., 1995; Seivewright et al., 2004). The distinction between episodic disorders, such as depression, and personality disorders was enshrined in DSM-IV Axis I and Axis II. However, findings on remission and persistence in personality disorders raised questions on this dichotomy, and the distinction between Axis I and Axis II disorders no longer appears in DSM-5.

Co-occurrence of personality and episodic disorders is common. Risk for depression or other episodic disorders may be increased by personality disorder through poor coping and hence helplessness (Vollrath et al., 1994), or increased life events associated with poor interpersonal functioning (Daley et al., 1998). Episodic disorders may create the conditions in which personality disorders develop because a chain of maladaptive behaviors and adverse environmental responses is set in motion (Kasen et al., 1999). Both environmental and genetic influences may contribute to co-occurrence. Many of the effects of child maltreatment on adult psychiatric disorders are nonspecific, and they probably contribute jointly to risks for personality disorders and conditions such as drug abuse and depression (Widom et al., 2009). Malone et al. (2004) assessed ASPD and alcohol dependence in 289 twin pairs at ages 17, 20, and 24. There were moderate genetic influences on each disorder at each age, and a substantial proportion of these influences was common to the two disorders.

It might be expected that, whatever the relationship between episodic disorders and personality disorder, the combination should in some sense reflect a more severe variant, with implications for treatment outcome. Individual studies have commonly failed to find an association. However, in a meta-analysis of all depression treatment studies in which personality disorder had been assessed, personality disorder was associated with a doubling of the risk of a poor outcome for depression (Newton-Howes et al., 2006). The authors suggest that many individual studies report nonsignificant results because they have inadequate statistical power to detect a difference of this size. Furthermore, treatment outcomes may be related to overall severity of personality disorder symptomatology, and may be affected by some, but not other, disorders (Levenson et al., 2012). Very little is known about the ways in which personality disorder may be associated with a poor outcome. Possibilities include that it may be associated with poor treatment compliance, or with greater severity of overall psychopathology, or with more psychosocial adversities and fewer interpersonal resources.

Differentiation among personality disorders

The ICD classification specifies nine personality disorder types, and the DSM system, 10. To a certain extent, the different categories reflect the different origins referred to earlier. The DSM classification, shown in Table 67.1, has received much attention; evidence for discriminant validity is not strong. Consistently, studies have shown that individuals who receive one personality disorder diagnosis often receive several (Pfohl et al., 1986; Morey, 1988; Oldham et al., 1992). There is evidence that the DSM categories cluster into three broad bands of: the odd/eccentric (A), the dramatic/emotional/erratic (B), and the anxious/fearful (C) (Kass et al., 1985). However, personality disorders also often cross these bands (Oldham et al., 1992).

Support for the discriminant validity could arise from differential association with other psychiatric conditions, family-genetics, or prognostic differences. Studies of the association of BPD with other episodic and personality disorders have provided some support for its discriminant validity. Zanarini et al. (1998) compared patients with BPD and patients with other personality disorders. Those with borderline disorder had higher rates of associated paranoid, avoidant, and dependent personality disorders, and higher rates of mood, anxiety, and eating disorders.

The most clear-cut finding from family studies is the association between schizophrenia and SPD (Kendler et al., 1981; Kendler et al., 1984). A significant but weaker association with schizophrenia has been found with paranoid personality disorders (Kendler & Gruenberg, 1982; Kendler et al., 1985). There is consistent evidence for genetic influences on adult antisocial behaviors (e.g., Langbehn et al., 1998), but not adult violence (Carey & Goldman, 1997). Genetic studies also provide support for both general effects and for groupings of personality disorders. For example, a twin study of 2794 adults demonstrated distinctive genetic and environmental factors with both general and specific effects (Kendler et al., 2008). It identified three genetic factors, one with high loadings on PDs from all three

DSM clusters, one for borderline and antisocial and one for schizoid and avoidant disorders.

Most studies of the association between adverse childhood experiences and personality disorders have reported associations with a wide range of episodic and personality disorders (e.g., Johnson *et al.*, 1999), which could reflect either genetic or environmental influences (Bornovalova *et al.*, 2013). Nevertheless specificity with particular disorders would support their validity. Bezirganian *et al.* (1993) found that the combination of maternal inconsistency and high maternal over-involvement assessed in adolescence was associated with the persistence or emergence of BPD, and no other episodic or personality disorders. Parker *et al.* (1999) reported that dysfunctional parenting in childhood was associated with the dramatic and anxious DSM clusters, but not the odd/eccentric cluster. In the twin study of Kendler *et al.* (2008) each of three environmental factors had high loadings on Clusters A, B, and C respectively.

Categorical versus dimensional characterizations of personality disorders

Diagnostic systems treat psychopathology as a categorical entity. However, data fail to find natural cut offs demarcating disorders from health (Pickles & Angold, 2003) (see also Chapter 2). Most early studies treated personality disorders as categories, but the advantages of dimensional approaches are becoming increasingly apparent. Evidence for validity generally is stronger for dimensional methods. Personality disorder symptoms scores show greater stability than diagnoses (Skodol *et al.*, 2005) and there is a greater elevation of borderline symptoms than BPD diagnoses in the first degree relatives of patients with BPD (Zanarini *et al.*, 2004). In the 10-year follow-up of patients in the Collaborative Personality Disorder Study, dimensional variables, both DSM and FFM based, provided superior prediction of functioning compared to DSM personality disorder categories (Morey *et al.*, 2012). Diagnoses may also lump together symptoms that reflect different processes. Zanarini has suggested that BPD comprises acute symptoms that wax and wane and may be affected by life events, and others that are chronic or "temperamental" (Zanarini *et al.*, 2005). Such a proposal requires further investigation but does illustrate advantages to dimensional frameworks. In community studies, increasing personality disorder symptoms below diagnostic threshold are associated with increasing social dysfunction (Daley *et al.*, 2000). This is important clinically because it suggests that even among patients who do not meet criteria for a diagnosis, personality disorder symptoms may be associated with processes that influence course and treatment responsiveness in common presentations such as adolescent deliberate self-harm. It is also possible that in the same individual, symptoms below diagnostic threshold from more than one disorder may each have prognostic significance. There are many more patients with symptoms below the threshold for diagnosis than those who meet criteria for disorder.

Utility of the personality disorder concept in childhood and adolescence

It is commonly assumed that personality disorders can only be identified from the age of 18, although DSM-5 requires this only for ASPD and ICD 10 refers to "adult" personality disorders without specifying an age. Equally DSM-5 and ICD 10 require that the pattern of behaviors contributing to personality disorder must have started at least by adolescence, begging the question as to what that pattern is if it does not yet amount to personality disorder. How good is the case for applying the concept of personality disorder in adolescence or even in childhood? Clearly, given the probable heterogeneity of the personality disorders, it is unlikely that there will be one answer to this question. Therefore the advantages and disadvantages will be considered in general, and specific examples tested against these.

Perhaps the most radical step would be to apply the concept of personality disorder to childhood disorders, particularly ODD and CD. Angold and Costello (2001) concluded that early onset antisocial behaviors in children satisfy all the DSM requirements for personality disorders. Childhood oppositional and conduct problems are associated with persistently poor peer relationships and broader difficulties (Vitaro *et al.*, 2000). Adult antisocial outcomes are most common in children with multiple and diverse oppositional, social, and educational difficulties (Stattin & Magnusson, 1996).

On the other hand, the use of the personality disorder designation could introduce the limitations of the adult concept into childhood. Crucially it might reduce our scope to investigate the links between different types of dysfunction. For example, Vitaro *et al.* (2000) found that, in boys, although having a best friend who was deviant age 10 predicted delinquency at age 14, this was much less the case among those with warm relationships with their parents. Such specific mechanisms could not be investigated within a personality disorder framework if having poor peer relationships was simply one of a number of items within a childhood ASPD. Similarly, notwithstanding the strong association of CD and ADHD and evidence that ADHD in the presence of CD increases the likelihood of persistence (Loeber *et al.*, 1995), important genetic and neuropsychological differences would not have been identified if they had been included in a hyperactivity-conduct personality disorder.

Is there a case for applying adult personality disorder criteria in adolescence? Studies of hospital patients, mainly of BPD, have suggested that adolescent personality disorders may be less distinct and less stable than adult disorders, but the profile of symptoms is largely similar (Becker *et al.*, 2002). Moreover there is evidence that a diagnosis of personality disorder is clinically relevant. For example. in a study of adolescent outpatients, the diagnosis of a personality disorder was associated with poorer treatment outcomes (Strandholm *et al.*, 2013). Stability is no less during adolescence, and from adolescence to adult life, than it is in adult life (Cohen *et al.*, 2005). Correlation coefficients of between 0.5 and 0.7 are commonly reported between adolescent and adult measures and over periods of up to 10 years. BPD symptoms in adolescence predict multiple outcomes in adult life (Cohen et al., 2005; Stepp, 2012; Winograd *et al.*, 2008). Equally there can be informative developmental sequences involving personality disorder symptoms. Hamigami *et al.* (2000) showed that there were reciprocal effects of narcissistic and borderline symptoms on each other from early adolescence into the mid-20s. Borderline symptoms predicted increasing narcissistic symptoms over time, but narcissistic symptoms predicted lower borderline symptoms! This may indicate that the appearance of borderline symptoms in early adolescence reflects substantial underlying pathology, whereas early narcissistic symptoms may be more developmentally benign. Later narcissistic symptoms, by contrast, may also reflect more problematic functioning, perhaps particularly when associated with borderline features.

Specific personality disorders

Antisocial personality disorder

Repeated criminality is central to ASPD, but ASPD involves diverse and pervasive difficulties. These include impulsivity, irritability, risk taking, lying, lack of remorse, and failures in adult social roles such as in work or family relationships. ASPD is more commonly found in males than females. The general population prevalence is between 2% and 3%, and it has been identified in around 60% of male prisoners (Moran, 1999). Adult symptoms of ASPD are almost always preceded by childhood disruptive behavior problems. Psychopathic disorder is identified in a smaller group of antisocial adults, most of whom have ASPD, and is associated with distinctive patterns of offending and neurobiological correlates. In childhood there appears to be a subset of antisocial children with "callous unemotional" traits with distinctive genetic and neurobiological contributions that may be the precursors of adult psychopathic disorder (Viding *et al.*, 2005; Blair *et al.*, 2006; Frick & White, 2008). The links between childhood disruptive behavior problems, callous unemotional traits, ASPD, and psychopathic disorder are described in Chapter 68.

Antisocial personality disorder in adolescence

Most developmental studies of ASPD have been influenced by the DSM model that ODD, typically seen in childhood, creates the vulnerability for CD, commonly identified during adolescence, which in turn predisposes to ASPD in adult life (Burke *et al.*, 2010). The associations over time among these three disorders have been widely replicated. However, as a consequence of this approach, studies comparing each of the three diagnoses at the same time point are lacking. We therefore do not know whether anything is gained by using the diagnosis, for example in adolescence. Some items, such as lying, aggressive behaviors and law breaking overlap with DSM CD, while others such as irritability overlap with DSM ODD. The new DSM-5 specifier for

CD, of whether or not the individual shows limited empathy and concern for the feelings or well-being of others, has some overlap with the ASPD item of "lack of remorse". However ASPD also includes impulsivity, disregard for safety of self or others, and repeated failure to sustain work behavior or honor financial obligations, which are not found in either CD or ODD. Two of these three items refer to difficulties in social interactions, in common with conceptualisations of personality disorder that include social role dysfunction as well as deviant behaviors.

Neurobiological correlates have been examined in structural and functional imaging studies. A meta-analysis of studies published up to 2007 (Yang & Raine, 2009) found substantial heterogeneity in the way antisocial and control groups were identified, and so the results cannot be assumed to apply specifically to ASPD. Nevertheless, analyses using data from 43 studies showed significantly altered structure and reduced function in some regions of the prefrontal cortex in antisocial individuals. Imaging studies focusing on the psychopathic subgroup of ASPD have implicated impairments in the amygdala which is involved in processing other people's emotional expressions and the formation of stimulus-reinforcement associations, and the ventro-medial prefrontal cortex which influences decision making linked to the representation of reinforcement expectancies (Blair, 2008). However there have also been substantial differences in findings across studies, many attributable to variations in methodology (Koenigs *et al.*, 2010).

Borderline personality disorder

BPD involves pervasive instability of interpersonal relationships, self-image, affects, and control over impulses. For example, problems can include frantic efforts to avoid real or imagined abandonment, unstable and intense interpersonal relationships, unstable self- image, impulsivity, recurrent suicidal behavior, affective instability , chronic feelings of emptiness, inappropriate intense anger, and transient paranoid or dissociative symptoms. In contrast to ASPD, BPD is more commonly diagnosed in females than males in clinical settings. Prevalence estimates for BPD have varied substantially, between 0.5% and 5.9%, in general population studies; however, the rate is likely to be between 1% and 2% (Torgersen *et al.*, 2001; Coid *et al.*, 2006; Lenzenweger *et al.*, 2007). Several epidemiological studies have not found a higher rate of BPD in women, suggesting that males with borderline problems seek treatment less than females.

Many individuals have both antisocial and borderline features, and some traits such as impulsivity are core to both disorders (Paris, 2005). It is possible that there is a common origin in early onset disruptive behavior problems, with a divergence in adolescence or early adult life. This is supported by prospective studies examining borderline symptoms in early adolescence (Belsky *et al.*, 2012; Stepp *et al.*, 2012). Prospective studies have not so far revealed whether the distinctive borderline symptoms are seen in childhood. Retrospective studies suggest that, as children, adults with BPD may have had difficulties with separating from emotionally important people and high mood reactivity (Reich & Zanarini, 2001) and that many started to self-harm before the age of 12 (Zanarini et al., 2006).

Many theories of the origins of BPD have proposed a central role for maltreatment, and in particular, experiences of sexual abuse in childhood. If this were the case, there would be a particularly important preventative role for child care and mental health professionals. BPD in adults is associated with higher rates of recalled child sexual abuse compared to non psychiatric controls, but so are many other psychiatric disorders (see Chapter 30), and specificity to BPD has not been conclusively demonstrated (Fossati et al. 1999). It is possible that specific types of sexual abuse show more specificity. In a comparison of borderline patients and those with other personality disorder, based on retrospective accounts, those in the borderline group were more likely to have been abused by a male non-caretaker, to have experienced denial of their thoughts and feelings by a male caretaker and to have experienced inconsistent treatment by a female caretaker (Zanarini et al., 2000). As we saw earlier, in a general population study by Cohen and colleagues, particular patterns of mother–child interaction were associated with subsequent BPD (Bezirganian et al., 1993). There may also be specificities between type of maltreatment and features of BPD. For example, individuals with BPD also report more dissociative experiences (Jones et al., 1999) and these may be associated specifically with sexual abuse by a caretaker (Zanarini et al., 2000). Apparent environmental effects can arise from common genetic influences on parents and children. In a longitudinal twin study, genetic influences on BPD symptoms at age 12 were identified, and so were environmental effects of harsh treatment earlier in childhood (Belsky et al., 2012). By contrast, in a twin study of young adults, child maltreatment was associated with BPD symptoms, but the association was fully accounted for common genetic influences (Bornovalova et al., 2013).

Theories regarding mechanisms in BPD have focused on impulsivity (Paris, 2005), emotion dysregulation (Putnam & Silk, 2005), unresolved or insecure attachment (Levy, 2005) and failure of mentalization (Bateman & Fonagy, 2004). Some of the features of BPD, including suicide attempts and self-mutilation, may reflect a more general trait of impulsivity. Impulsive spectrum disorders, such as ASPD and substance misuse, are elevated in the first degree relatives of borderline patients (White et al., 2002), and levels of impulsivity predict clinical outcomes in BPD (Links et al., 1999). However, disorders other than BPD are also characterised by impulsivity, notably ASPD, and although there is substantial overlap between the disorders, there are important differences.

Emotion dysregulation is likely to be one of the keys to the difference between BPD and ASPD. "The inability to sustain positive affect coupled with the pervasive and unremitting distress as experienced by patients with BPD can become a veritable prison to those with the disorder and often as well to those who attempt to treat the individual with BPD" (Putnam & Silk, 2005, p. 900). Borderline individuals commonly have a low

threshold for reacting to events, or to anticipated events (such as abandonment), with intense negative emotion. According to Linehan (1993) BPD arises from an interaction between temperamental emotional reactivity and an "invalidating" environment in which the child's communication about inner emotional experience is regarded as reflecting an inaccurate perception of self and others. One of the major consequences of this response is thought to be that children raised in these environments do not learn to identify emotional states accurately, nor do they learn to regulate affect, as it is more often than not denied. In addition, invalidating environments also intermittently reinforce escalations of emotional displays. This results in two opposing responses to affect being shaped. The first is the inhibition or denial of emotional states, and the second is an extreme response, which often appears to be inappropriate to the level of the stimulus that elicited it. This hypothesis has not so far been tested in prospective studies.

Instability of family and romantic relationships characterised by highly intense interactions, fear of abandonment and emotionally charged breakdown are also common in individuals with BPD. Several studies have linked this to disturbances of attachment (Levy, 2005), although very few have tested whether attachment difficulties are associated specifically with borderline, as opposed to other personality disorders. Bateman and Fonagy (2004) argue that borderline individuals have an impoverished model of their own and others' mental function (mentalization), "Their schematic, rigid and at times extreme ideas about their own and others" states of mind make them vulnerable to powerful emotional storms and apparently impulsive actions, and create profound problems of behavioral and affect regulation' (Bateman & Fonagy, 2004, p. 2) They also argue that these limitations in mentalization are seen particularly in relation to attachment relationships, thus leading to particular difficulties in close relationships.

BPD is associated with difficulties in a wide range of relationships in personal and work life, including problems in maintaining distinct boundaries between different relationship domains. A key feature of this "domain disorganisation" (Hill et al., 2008) is the presence of features of intimate relationships in social domains where these are not readily accommodated. For example, exclusivity is generally found only in romantic relationships. In a short-term longitudinal study from childhood into early adolescence, "friendship exclusivity" was a strong independent predictor of borderline symptoms (Crick et al., 2005). Domain disorganisation may contribute to BPD in the presence of increased emotional reactivity. In a study of psychiatric outpatients the combination of domain disorganisation and temperamental anger proneness was associated with BPD (Morse et al., 2009).

Repeated self-injury, cutting, burning, or hitting, is frequently observed in individuals with severe personality disorders, and is one of the diagnostic items for BPD. It is a serious and puzzling phenomenon. There is a wide range of theories concerning the motivation for self-injury, and themes that are common to most of them are of regulation of emotions, communication, and social reinforcement (Kemperman et al., 1997). Linehan (1993) has proposed that self-injury directly relieves painful emotions and is reinforced by the attention and care given by others. Several studies have supported the role of self-injury in reducing painful affect although most have used retrospective measures with samples that in different ways were unrepresentative. In the prospective Collaborative Longitudinal Personality Disorders Study of 290 patients meeting DSM criteria for BPD, all of female gender, severity of dysphoric cognitions (mostly overvalued ideas), severity of dissociative symptoms, major depression, history of childhood sexual abuse and sexual assaults as an adult predicted self-harm over a 10-year follow-up period (Zanarini et al., 2011).

BPD is also associated with elevated environmental stresses or traumas in adult life that in turn contribute to persistence of problems. Over a 10-year follow-up period of patients in the Collaborative Longitudinal Personality Disorders Study, BPD was associated with significantly more total negative life events than other personality disorders, or major depressive disorder (Pagano et al., 2004). Negative events, especially interpersonal events, predicted decreased psychosocial functioning over time. In the same study BPD predicted, more strongly than other personality disorders, verbal, emotional, physical, and sexual abuse, and adult experiences of abuse were associated with failure to remit from BPD (Zanarini et al., 2005).

Studies of the neurobiology of BPD have focused on impaired behavioral control in the context of intense negative emotions. The "frontolimbic disconnectivity" model of BPD suggests that emotional dysregulation in BPD patients is caused by prefrontal deficits or hyperactivity of the limbic system, or a combination of both. This conceptualization of frontolimbic dysfunction in BPD has resulted in a growing number of imaging studies using structural and functional methods (Maier-Hein et al., 2014) that have provided some support for the hypothesis. For example, Silbersweig et al. (2007) compared 14 BPD patients with 12 controls on an executive function task using negative, neutral, and positive stimuli administered during functional magnetic resonance imaging (fMRI). The BPD patients showed decreased ventromedial prefrontal cortex activity compared to controls specifically when inhibiting responses in the presence of negative stimuli. Promising though this work is, it has so far been limited to small-scale cross-sectional studies with nonclinical control groups, and so the differences may not be specific to BPD.

Borderline personality disorder in adolescence

Many of the studies of personality disorder in adolescence have focused on BPD. A substantial proportion of adolescent psychiatric in-patients in the USA and the UK can be diagnosed with the disorder using adult criteria. It resembles the adult diagnosis in that there is a strong association with episodic disorders, particularly depression. In adolescents, the BPD diagnosis picks out a group who, compared with other adolescent psychiatric

patients, have experienced high levels of maternal neglect and rejection, grossly inappropriate parental behavior and a number of parental surrogates and sexual abuse (Ludolph et al., 1990) and higher levels of angry, irritable interactions in the family (James et al., 1996). Associations of inconsistent and intrusive parenting with the emergence of BPD were found in the longitudinal study of a general population sample (Bezirganian et al., 1993) referred to earlier. BPD identified in adolescence also has prognostic value (Stepp, 2012). In a large community sample, higher levels of BPD symptoms during adolescence predicted less productive adult role functioning over 20 years, including poor academic and occupational achievements. BPD symptoms also predicted poor social and relationship functioning, including lack of social support and less involvement in romantic relationships well into adulthood (Winograd et al., 2008). In a study of psychiatric patients, mean age = 15.47, BPD (omitting the suicidality criterion) predicted suicidality and repeat self-harm over and above their association with DSM Major Depressive Disorder (Sharp et al., 2012). There is limited evidence from studies of BPD adolescents of white matter differences from clinical and healthy controls consistent with the evidence from adults based on the frontolimbic disconnectivity model (Maier-Hein et al., 2014).

Schizotypal personality disorder

The general concept of SPD is that of a pervasive pattern of social and interpersonal deficits marked by acute discomfort with, and reduced capacity for, close relationships, as well as by cognitive or perceptual distortions and eccentricities of behavior, beginning by early adulthood. It is likely that the concept of a spectrum of schizophrenic disorders, including SPD, applies in the preadult years, as well as later. However, there has been only a small number of attempts to apply the criteria in childhood. One study suggested an overlap with pervasive developmental disorders, although not autism as such (Nagy & Szatmari, 1986); another suggested a course similar to that of schizophrenia arising in childhood (Asarnow & Ben-Meir, 1988); and a third suggested that there was a pattern of communication deficits similar to, but milder than, those found in schizophrenia (Caplin & Guthrie, 1992). Olin et al. (1997) gathered prospective questionnaire data from teachers on 15-years-olds who subsequently developed SPD. Compared to a range of other groups at varying levels of risk for psychiatric disorder other than schizophrenia, the schizotypal individuals as adolescents had been more passive and unengaged and more hypersensitive to criticism. In a small follow-up study over 3 years of young adolescents diagnosed with SPD there was substantial stability of the disorder and also a substantial minority developed psychotic disorders (Asarnow, 2005).

Schizoid personality disorder

The usual concept of schizoid personality disorder is of a pervasive pattern of detachment from social relationships and a restricted range of expression of emotions in interpersonal settings (DSM-IV, American Psychiatric Association, 2000). Thus, ICD-10 criteria (World Health Organization, 1996) include a lack of pleasure in activities, emotional coldness, apparent indifference to praise, or criticism, a limited capacity to express either positive or negative emotions, lack of close friends, a preference for solitary activities, a marked insensitivity to prevailing social norms and an excessive preoccupation with fantasy and introspection. The literature on the syndrome is almost confined to adults (Esterberg *et al.*, 2010). However, from the 1970s, Wolff pressed the case for the application of the diagnosis in childhood (Wolff & Barlow, 1979). Unfortunately for comparative purposes, her criteria differ in several key respects from those generally applied with adults. Thus, she specified increased sensitivity and paranoid ideas, whereas ICD-10 and DSM-IV indicate marked insensitivity, and she included an unusual odd style of communicating which would ordinarily be part of schizotypal, not schizoid, personality disorders (Wolff & Chick, 1980; Wolff, 1991a, b). The initial findings in childhood suggested some similarities with autism (Wolff & Barlow, 1979) and the follow-up showed substantial continuity with SPD in adult life (Wolff *et al.*, 1991). However, a study of psychophysiological responses of adults who in childhood met Wolff's criteria for schizoid disorder failed to find abnormalities previously documented in the relatives of schizophrenic patients and adults with SPD (Blackwood *et al.*, 1994).

The application of personality disorders research in clinical practice

Assessment

Two contrasting conclusions can be drawn regarding personality disorder assessment in clinical practice with adolescents. First, identifying personality disorder features is important because it highlights phenomena not covered by episodic disorders. Second, in contrast, many issues remain unresolved in the assessment of these features. For example, some non-episodic disorders, such as ASD and behavioral disorders, are not generally considered as personality disorders.

In view of the lack of studies comparing the utility of the ASPD, CD and ODD diagnoses in adolescence, we do not know whether making the ASPD diagnosis in adolescence has implications for prognosis or has advantages in formulating treatment. The alternative diagnoses to be considered for a young person presenting with repeat offending or violence will generally be the same, irrespective of whether the problem is formulated in terms of ASPD or of CD. In particular, previously undetected ADHD, which carries a greatly increased risk for CD (see Chapter 55), may make a major contribution to the presenting problems, and provides a clear treatment focus. By drawing attention to a broader set of problems than either conduct or ODD, particularly social impairment, ASPD may highlight additional key targets for intervention and indices of change. However, it is important when offending is accompanied by problems in social

and educational performance, to assess for autistic spectrum disorders which are over represented among young offenders (Siponmaa *et al.*, 2001). This will require detailed enquiry into the characteristics of the social impairment, together with a developmental history and possibly administration of a standardized ASD assessment (see Chapter 51).

Where the presenting problems occur in the context of an identifiable current episodic disorder, such as depression or an anxiety disorder, enquiry into functioning prior to the onset is essential. Key features that point toward borderline difficulties include persistent problems in multiple domains of interpersonal functioning, rapid and marked changes of mood, and unpredictable impulsive behaviors. Difficulties in maintaining the demarcations between social domains referred to earlier as domain disorganization are often evident in intense personalized interactions in settings where these are not readily accommodated, such as school or college, and in intimate relationships established rapidly and without adequate time to evaluate the quality of partners. This in turn contributes to relationship breakdown and lack of social support, increasing the risk of adverse life events that in turn contribute to further impairment. It is common for young people with borderline problems to have had contact with multiple agencies and for there to be several professionals involved, each with strong and conflicting impressions of the young person. There is no established method for making dimensional assessments of borderline PD. Studies described earlier showing the advantages of a dimensional approach used DSM PD symptom counts. However, a comprehensive assessment often requires enquiry along several dimensions. In particular, in the light of the persistence of social dysfunction in adult BPD, detailed accounts of the degree of impairment in interpersonal functioning in school, quality of friendships and wider peer relationships, provide an indication of the extent of the dysfunction and identify targets for intervention.

Affective instability and repeat self-harm, commonly seen in adolescent patients, may reflect borderline disorder or dysfunction; however, it is important to consider other possible diagnoses with very different implications. Bipolar disorder, especially Bipolar II characterized by relatively short periods of elation together with depression, may look very similar. In principle there are substantial differences in that, compared with bipolar disorder, affects are more unstable and triggered by interpersonal events in BPD, and there are characteristic interpersonal problems in BPD not seen in bipolar disorder (Zimmerman *et al.*, 2013). However where bipolar symptoms have persisted for some time they may have impacted on interpersonal functioning, making the distinction difficult. Recent evidence for pathways from childhood disruptive behavior problems to adolescent borderline symptoms (Belsky *et al.*, 2012; Stepp *et al.*, 2012) would suggest that the presence of behavior problems before adolescence may support the diagnosis of BPD. However, the evidence is not strong enough to conclude that the absence of childhood problems would rule it out. Crucially, in adults there is an elevated co-occurrence of bipolar disorder in BPD, compared to other personality disorders (Gunderson *et al.*, 2006), so the presence of both may need to be considered. Clinical experience suggests, although relevant research evidence is lacking, that adolescent girls with undetected autistic spectrum disorder may present with impulsive behaviors, including self-harm, in the context of social difficulties with peers that may be interpreted as markers for borderline problems. A developmental history together with clinical and standardized assessments of current functioning will generally clarify the picture,

Whatever the merits for clinicians of using the concept of personality disorder, either as a category or dimension, there is some concern over making explicit reference to it when explaining the nature of their problems to young people and their families. The label, it is argued, runs the risk of stigmatising and of creating therapeutic pessimism. Equally, patients and their families are entitled to an explanation of their problems and in some instances the personality disorder concept may be helpful to that process. In that case, the explanation needs also to reflect the uncertainties regarding the nature of the personality disorders reviewed in this chapter. Perhaps surprisingly, given its importance, systematic research into this question is lacking, both for adults and adolescents.

Treatment

Psychodynamic and cognitive-behavioral treatments have been advocated for treating ASPD in adults, however there has only been one RCT, with a sample size of 39, which found no effect of cognitive behavioral treatment (Davidson *et al.*, 2009). No well-designed studies of pharmacotherapy in ASPD have been conducted. Studies of treatments for adolescent offenders are relevant but do not yet address whether they are effective for the pervasive problems identified by the disorder. There is good evidence, for example, that multisystemic therapy is effective in improving outcomes for juvenile offenders (see Chapters 49 and 50), but less clear evidence for adolescents with CDs (Sundell *et al.*, 2008). Early intervention to prevent disruptive behavior problems, and hence reduce risk for ASPD, would seem to be the most promising approach to a disorder that seems to be so intractable by adolescence. Promising findings have been reported from randomised controlled trials of prenatal and early postnatal nurse visiting, and parenting and school-based interventions for young children. Effects on cognitive skills, school attainment, earning capacity, health, and mental health, rates of delinquency and crime have been reported (NCCMH, 2010). However most studies have reported on multiple outcomes, with effects on some but not others, and we do not yet know whether early intervention can reduce the persistent and pervasive problems characteristic of ASPD.

In relation to BPD in adults, Bateman and Fonagy (2004) have summarized the principal features of treatments for which there is some evidence of effectiveness. The approach is active and structured with clear focus, in the context of a strong relationship between therapist and patient over a substantial period of time. This is consistent with accumulating evidence that structured, manualized psychotherapeutic treatments delivered by trained clinicians working within a team are superior to treatment as usual for adults with BPD (McMain *et al.*, 2012). Treatment superiority has been shown in randomised controlled trials in adults for dialectical behavior therapy (DBT; Linehan *et al.*, 2006), out-patient mentalization-based therapy (Bateman & Fonagy, 2009) and cognitive analytic therapy (Clarke *et al.*, 2013) (see Chapters 38 and 40). Mentalization-based partial hospitalization showed substantial superiority to treatment as usual over an 8-year follow-up period (Bateman & Fonagy, 2008). McMain *et al.* (2012) found no differences in a range of outcomes between DBT and an alternative manualized psychotherapeutic approach, implying that treatment effects arise from the general characteristics of the intervention rather than specific therapeutic processes. By contrast, Bateman and Fonagy showed medium effect size (Cohen's d around 0.60) reductions in suicidal behaviors, self-harm, and hospital admissions for mentalization in a comparison with an alternative manualized treatment programme (Bateman & Fonagy, 2009). A systematic review of psychological treatment trials for BPD up to 2010 concluded, "Overall, the findings support a substantial role for psychotherapy in the treatment of people with BPD but clearly indicate a need for replicatory studies" (Stoffers *et al.*, 2012).

DBT is increasingly being used as an approach with suicidal adolescents, many of whom are likely to have BPD symptoms (Katz *et al.*, 2004). The "dialectic" refers to helping the adolescent to change what needs to be changed, while accepting what is a valid response to circumstances (Hill *et al.*, 2006). Treatment is delivered by a team, and has several elements. "Capability enhancement" aims to increase the adolescents' basic capabilities of affect regulation, distress tolerance, and interpersonal skills. This function is most often delivered by a skills-training group. "Motivational enhancement" involves assisting adolescents to apply their new-found skills to their own life problems, in particular attending to thoughts, emotions, or reinforcement contingencies (such as repeated attendance at hospital for self-harm) that interfere with the implementation of skilful behavior. This function is most commonly delivered via individual psychotherapy. Explicit coaching in the application of problem-solutions to the adolescent's real world situations is designed to increase generalization of skills learned in the programme. This may be delivered by between-session skills coaching, by telephone, by case management or by training family members in the same skills that the adolescents are learning. Considerable attention is also paid to supervision and support of therapists and to the family and wider environment of the adolescent, including social services and education. DBT has shown promise in the treatment of borderline problems in adolescents (James *et al.*, 2007, MacPherson *et al.*, 2013), and support for its effectiveness has come from a randomized controlled trial of 77 adolescents with repeat self-harm and at least three BPD symptoms. Compared to enhanced treatment as usual DBT was associated with lower levels of self-harm, suicidal ideation and depressive symptoms soon after completion of treatment (Mehlum *et al.*, 2014).

Studies have been conducted of tricyclic antidepressants, selective serotonin reuptake inhibitors, neuroleptics, and mood stabilizers in BPD (Lieb *et al.*, 2004; Leichsenring *et al.*, 2011). Most have shown some evidence of efficacy but only in small samples. Of the 16 studies reviewed by Lieb *et al.*, only two had a sample size of greater than 60, and in most cases they were substantially smaller. In one of the more promising studies, Soler *et al.* (2005) randomised 60 patients with BPD to placebo or to olanzapine together with DBT. In assessments after 4 months, the combined DBT plus drug group had lower affective symptoms and impulsivity/aggression than the DBT only group. Overall, in spite of some promising findings, there is a lack of sufficiently large randomised controlled trials with follow-up long enough to inform the treatment of this persistent disorder (Leichsenring *et al.*, 2011).

Conclusions

Much remains to be discovered regarding the forms of dysfunction that best characterize personality disorders. This will inform, and be informed by, increasing knowledge of childhood antecedents, developmental pathways, the interaction between individual and environmental processes, and basic psychopathological processes in personality disorders. For all its shortcomings, the concept of personality disorder has endured because it adds to our understanding of risk and psychopathology, and increasingly research in this area highlights individuals with distinctive treatment needs. Patterns of symptomatology resembling adult personality disorders are seen during adolescence and also indicate distinctive, and generally intensive, treatment needs.

References

American Psychiatric Association (2000) *Diagnostic and Statistical Manual of Mental Disorders*, 4th Text Revision. American Psychiatric Association, Washington, DC.

American Psychiatric Association (2013) *Diagnostic and Statistical Manual of Mental Disorders*, 5th edn. American Psychiatric Association, Washington, DC.

Angold, A. & Costello, J. (2001) The epidemiology of disorders of conduct: nosological issues and comorbidity. In: *Conduct Disorders in Childhood and Adolescence*. (eds J. Hill & B. Maughan), pp. 126–168. Cambridge University Press, Cambridge.

Asarnow, J.R. & Ben-Meir, S. (1988) Children with schizophrenia spectrum and depressive disorders: a comparative study of pre-morbid adjustment, onset pattern and severity of impairment. *Journal of Child Psychology and Psychiatry* **29**, 477–488.

Asarnow, J.R. (2005) Childhood-onset schizotypal disorder: a follow-up study and comparison with childhood-onset schizophrenia. *Journal of Child & Adolescent Psychopharmacology* **15**, 395–402.

Bateman, A.W. & Fonagy, P. (2004) *Psychotherapy for Borderline Personality Disorder: Mentalization Based Treatment*. Oxford University Press, Oxford.

Bateman, A. & Fonagy, P. (2008) 8-year follow-up of patients treated for borderline personality disorder: mentalization-based treatment versus treatment as usual. *American Journal of Psychiatry* **165**, 631–638.

Bateman, A. & Fonagy, P. (2009) Randomized controlled trial of outpatient mentalization-based treatment versus structured clinical management for borderline personality disorder. *American Journal of Psychiatry* **166**, 1355–1364.

Becker, D.F. *et al.* (2002) Diagnostic efficiency of borderline personality disorder criteria in hospitalized adolescents: comparison with hospitalized adults. *American Journal of Psychiatry* **159**, 2042–2047.

Belsky, D.W. *et al.* (2012) Etiological features of borderline personality related characteristics in a birth cohort of 12-year-old children. *Development and Psychopathology* **24**, 251–265.

Bezirganian, S. *et al.* (1993) The impact of mother-child interaction on the development of borderline personality disorder. *American Journal of Psychiatry* **150**, 1836–1842.

Blackwood, D.H. *et al.* (1994) "Schizoid" personality in childhood: auditory P300 and eye tracking responses at follow-up in adult life. *Journal of Autism and Developmental Disorders* **24**, 487–500.

Blair, R.J. *et al.* (2006) The development of psychopathy. *Journal of Child Psychology and Psychiatry* **47**, 262–276.

Blair, R.J.R. (2008) The amygdala and ventromedial prefrontal cortex: functional contributions and dysfunction in psychopathy. *Philosophical Transactions of the Royal Society B: Biological Sciences* **363**, 2557–2565.

Bornovalova, M.A. *et al.* (2013) Tests of a direct effect of childhood abuse on adult borderline personality disorder traits: a longitudinal discordant twin design. *Journal of Abnormal Psychology* **122**, 180–194.

Bugental, D.B. (2000) Acquisition of the algorithms of social life: a domain-based approach. *Psychological Bulletin* **126**, 187–219.

Burke, J.D. *et al.* (2010) Predictive validity of childhood oppositional defiant disorder and conduct disorder: implications for the DSM–V. *Journal of Abnormal Psychology* **119**, 739–51.

Cannon, T.D. *et al.* (2008) Prediction of psychosis in youth at high clinical risk: a multisite longitudinal study in North America. *Archives of General Psychiatry* **65**, 28.

Caplin, R. & Guthrie, D. (1992) Communication deficits in childhood schizotypal personality disorder. *Journal of the American Academy of Child and Adolescent Psychiatry* **31**, 961–967.

Carey, G. & Goldman, D. (1997) The genetics of antisocial behaviour. In: *Handbook of Antisocial Behaviour*. (eds D.M. Stoff, J. Breilling & J. Maser), pp. 243–254. John Wiley & Sons, New York.

Caspi, A. *et al.* (2005) Personality development: stability and change. *Annual Review of Psychology* **56**, 453–484.

Clarke, S. *et al.* (2013) Cognitive analytic therapy for personality disorder: randomised controlled trial. *British Journal of Psychiatry* **202**, 129–134.

Cleckley, H. (1941) *The Mask of Sanity*. Henry Kimpton, London.

Cohen, P. *et al.* (2005) The children in the community study of developmental course of personality disorder. *Journal of Personality Disorders* **19**, 466–486.

Coid, J. *et al.* (2006) Prevalence and correlates of personality disorder in Great Britain. *British Journal of Psychiatry* **188**, 423–431.

Colder, C.R. *et al.* (2002) The interactive effects of infant activity level and fear on growth trajectories of early childhood behavior problems. *Development and Psychopathology* **14**, 1–23.

Crick, N.R. *et al.* (2005) Borderline personality features in childhood: a short-term longitudinal study. *Development and Psychopathology* **17**, 1051–1070.

Daley, S.E. *et al.* (2000) Borderline personality disorder symptoms as predictors of four-year romantic relationship dysfunctioning young women: addressing issues of specificity. *Journal of Abnormal Psychology* **109**, 451–460.

Daley, S.E. *et al.* (1998) Axis II symptomatology, depression, and life stress during the transition from adolescence to adulthood. *Journal of Consulting and Clinical Psychology* **66**, 595–603.

Davidson, K. *et al.* (2009) Cognitive behaviour therapy for violent men with antisocial personality disorder in the community: an exploratory randomized controlled trial. *Psychological Medicine* **39**, 569–577.

Esterberg, M.L. *et al.* (2010) Cluster A personality disorders: schizotypal, schizoid and paranoid personality disorders in childhood and adolescence. *Journal of Psychopathology and Behavioral Assessment* **32**, 515–528.

Ferro, T. *et al.* (1998) Thirty-months' stability of personality disorder diagnoses in depressed out-patients. *American Journal of Psychiatry* **155**, 653–659.

Fossati, A. *et al.* (1999) Borderline personality disorder and childhood sexual abuse: a meta-analytic study. *Journal of Personality Disorders* **13**, 268–280.

Frick, P.J. & Morris, A.S. (2004) Temperament and developmental pathways to conduct problems. *Journal of Clinical Child and Adolescent Psychology* **33**, 54–68.

Frick, P.J. & White, S.F. (2008) Research review: the importance of callous-unemotional traits for developmental models of aggressive and antisocial behavior. *Journal of Child Psychology and Psychiatry* **49**, 359–375.

Gunderson, J.G. *et al.* (1981) The diagnostic interview for borderline patients. *American Journal of Psychiatry* **138**, 896–903.

Gunderson, J.G. *et al.* (2006) Descriptive and longitudinal observations on the relationship of borderline personality disorder and bipolar disorder. *American Journal of Psychiatry* **163**, 1173–8.

Gunderson, J.G. *et al.* (2011) Ten-year course of borderline personality disorder: psychopathology and function from the collaborative longitudinal personality disorders study. *Archives of General Psychiatry* **68**, 827–837.

Hamigami, F. *et al.* (2000) A new approach to modelling bivariate dynamic relationships applied to evaluation of DSM-III personality disorder symptoms. In: *Temperament and Personality Development Across the Life-Span.* (eds V.J. Molfese, D.L. Molfese & R.R. McCrae), pp. 253–280. Lawrence Earlbaum Associates, Mahwah.

Hare, R.D. (1970) *Psychopathy: Theory and Research.* John Wiley & Sons, New York.

Henderson, D.K. (1939) *Psychopathic States.* Norton, New York.

Hill, J. (2002) Biological, psychological and social processes in the conduct disorders. *Journal of Child Psychology and Psychiatry* **43**, 133–164.

Hill, J. *et al.* (2000) Complementary approaches to the assessment of personality disorder: the personality assessment schedule and adult personality functioning assessment compared. *British Journal of Psychiatry* **176**, 434–439.

Hill, J. *et al.* (2008) Social domain dysfunction and disorganization in borderline personality disorder. *Psychological Medicine* **38**, 135–146.

Hill, J. *et al.* (2006) Personality disorders. In: *A Clinician's Handbook of Child and Adolescent Psychiatry.* (eds C. Gillberg, R. Harrington & H.-C. Steinhausen), pp. 339–364. Cambridge University Press, Cambridge.

Hill, J. *et al.* (2010) Social domains, personality, and interpersonal functioning. *Handbook of Interpersonal Psychology: Theory, Research, Assessment and Therapeutic Interventions.* Horowitz L.M. & Strack S. (Eds). pp. 281–297. John Wiley & Sons, New York.

James, A. *et al.* (1996) Borderline personality disorder: study in adolescence. *European Child and Adolescent Psychiatry* **5**, 11–17.

James, A.C. *et al.* (2008) A preliminary community study of dialectical behaviour therapy (DBT) with adolescent females demonstrating persistent, deliberate self-harm (DSH). *Child and Adolescent Mental Health* **13**, 148–152.

Johnson, J.G. *et al.* (1999) Childhood maltreatment increases risk for personality disorders during adulthood. *Archives of General Psychiatry* **56**, 600–606.

Johnson, M.H. *et al.* (2005) The emergence of the social brain network: evidence from typical and atypical development. *Development and Psychopathology* **17**, 599–619.

Jones, B. *et al.* (1999) Autobiographical memory and dissociation in borderline personality disorder. *Psychological Medicine* **29**, 1397–1404.

Kasen, S. *et al.* (1999) Influence of child and adolescent psychiatric disorders on young adult personality disorder. *American Journal of Pychiatry* **56**, 1529–1535.

Kass, F. *et al.* (1985) Scaled ratings of DSM-II personality disorders. *American Journal of Psychiatry* **142**, 627–630.

Katz, L.Y. *et al.* (2004) Feasibility of dialectical behavior therapy for suicidal adolescent inpatients. *Journal of the American Academy of Child and Adolescent Psychiatry* **43**, 276–282.

Kemperman, I. *et al.* (1997) Self-endurious behaviour and mood regulation in borderline patients. *Journal of Personality Disorder* **11**, 146–157.

Kendler, K.S. *et al.* (2008) The structure of genetic and environmental risk factors for DSM-IV personality disorders: a multivariate twin study. *Archives of General Psychiatry* **65**, 1438–1446.

Kendler, K.S. & Gruenberg, A.M. (1982) Genetic relationship between paranoid personality disorder and the 'schizophrenic spectrum' disorder. *American Journal of Psychiatry* **139**, 1185–1186.

Kendler, K.S. *et al.* (1981) An independent analysis of the Copenhagen sample of the Danish Adoption Study of Schizophrenia II. The relationship between schizotypal personality disorders and schizophrenia. *Archives of General Psychiatry* **38**, 928–984.

Kendler, K.S. *et al.* (1984) A family history study of schizophrenic related personality disorder. *American Journal of Psychiatry* **141**, 424–427.

Kendler, K.S. *et al.* (1985) Psychiatric illness in first-degree relatives of patients with paranoid psychosis, schizophrenia and medical illness. *British Journal of Psychiatry* **147**, 524–532.

Kernberg, O.F. (1967) Borderline personality organisation. *Journal of the American Psychoanalytic Association (New York)* **15**, 641–685.

Kernberg, O.F. (1975) *Borderline Conditions and Pathological Narcissism.* Jason Ellinson, New York.

Kety, S.S. *et al.* (1971) Mental illness in the biological and adoptive families of adopted schizophrenics. *American Journal of Psychiatry* **128**, 302–306.

Koenigs, M. *et al.* (2010) Investigating the neural correlates of psychopathy: a critical review. *Molecular Psychiatry* **16**, 792–799.

Langbehn, D.R. *et al.* (1998) Distinct contributions of conduct and oppositional defiant symptoms to adult antisocial behavior: evidence from an adoption study. *Archives of General Psychiatry* **55**, 821–829.

Leichsenring, F. *et al.* (2011) Borderline personality disorder. *The Lancet* **377**, 74–84.

Lemerise, E.A. & Arsenio, W.F. (2000) An integrated model of emotion processes and cognition in social information processing. *Child Development* **71**, 107–118.

Lenzenweger, M.F. *et al.* (2007) DSM-IV personality disorders in the national comorbidity survey replication. *Biological Psychiatry* **62**, 553–564.

Levenson, J.C. *et al.* (2012) The role of personality pathology in depression treatment outcome with psychotherapy and pharmacotherapy. *Journal of Consulting and Clinical Psychology* **80**, 719–729.

Levy, K.N. (2005) The implications of attachment theory and research for understanding borderline personality disorder. *Development and Psychopathology* **17**, 959–986.

Lieb, K. *et al.* (2004) Borderline personality disorder. *The Lancet* **364**, 453–461.

Linehan, M.M. (1993) *Cognitive Behavioural Therapy of Borderline Personality Disorder*. Guildford Press, New York.

Linehan, M.M. *et al.* (2006) Two-year randomized controlled trial and follow-up of dialectical behavior therapy vs therapy by experts for suicidal behaviors and borderline personality disorder. *Archives of General Psychiatry* **63**, 757–766.

Links, P.F. *et al.* (1999) Impulsivity: poor aspect of borderline personality disorder. *Journal of Personality Disorders* **13**, 1–9.

Loeber, R. *et al.* (1995) Which boys will fair worse? Early predictors of the onset of conduct disorder in a six-year longitudinal study. *Journal of the American Academy of Child and Adolescent Psychiatry* **34**, 499–509.

Ludolph, P.S. *et al.* (1990) The borderline diagnosis in adolescence. Symptoms and developmental history. *Archives of General Psychiatry* **147**, 470–476.

MacPherson, H.A. *et al.* (2013) Dialectical behavior therapy for adolescents: theory, treatment adaptations, and empirical outcomes. *Clinical Child and Family Psychology Review* **16**, 59–80.

Maier-Hein, K.H. *et al.* (2014) Disorder-specific white matter alterations in adolescent borderline personality disorder. *Biological Psychiatry* **75**, 81–88.

Malone, S.M. *et al.* (2004) Genetic and environmental influences on antisocial behavior and alcohol dependence from adolescence to early adulthood. *Development and Psychopathology* **16**, 943–966.

McMain, S.F. *et al.* (2012) Dialectical behavior therapy compared with general psychiatric management for borderline personality disorder: clinical outcomes and functioning over a 2-year follow-up. *American Journal of Psychiatry* **169**, 650–661.

Meehl, P.E. (1962) Schizotaxia, schizotypy, schizophrenia. *American Psychologist* **17**, 827–838.

Mehlum, L. *et al.*, (2014) Dialectical behavior therapy for adolescents with repeated suicidal and self-harming behavior: a randomized trial. *Journal of the American Academy of Child & Adolescent Psychiatry* **53**, 1082–1091.

Mischel, W. (2004) Toward an integrative science of the person. *Annual Review of Psychology* **55**, 1–22.

Moran, P. (1999) The epidemiology of antisocial personality disorder. *Social Psychiatry and Psychiatric Epidemiology* **34**, 231–42.

Morey, L.C. (1988) Personality disorders in DSM-III and DSM-III-R: convergence, coverage and internal consistency. *American Journal of Psychiatry* **145**, 573–577.

Morey, L.C. *et al.* (2012) Comparison of alternative models for personality disorders, II: 6-, 8- and 10-year follow-up. *Psychological Medicine* **42**, 1705–1713.

Morse, J.Q. *et al.* (2009) Anger, preoccupied attachment, and domain disorganization in borderline personality disorder. *Journal of Personality Disorders* **23**, 240–257.

Nagy, J. & Szatmari, P. (1986) A chart review of schizotypal personality disorders in children. *Journal of Autism and Developmental Disorders* **16**, 351–367.

NCCMH (2010) *Antisocial Personality Disorder: Treatment, Management and Prevention*. The British Psychological Society and the Royal College of Psychiatrists, Leicester & London.

Newton-Howes, G. *et al.* (2006) Personality disorder and the outcome of depression: meta-analysis of published studies. *British Journal of Psychiatry* **188**, 13–20.

Oldham, J.M. *et al.* (1992) Diagnosis of DSM-III-R personality disorders and two structured interviews: patterns of comorbidity. *American Journal of Psychiatry* **149**, 213–220.

Olin, S.S. *et al.* (1997) Childhood behavior precursors of schizotypal personality disorder. *Schizophrenia Bulletin* **23**, 93–103.

Pagano, M.E. *et al.* (2004) Stressful life events as predictors of functioning: findings from the collaborative longitudinal personality disorders study. *Acta Psychiatrica Scandinavica* **110**, 421–429.

Paris, J. (2005) The development of impulsivity and suicidality in borderline personality disorder. *Development and Psychopathology* **17**, 1091–1104.

Parker, G. *et al.* (1999) An exploration of links between early parenting experiences and personality disorder type and disordered personality functioning. *Journal of Personality Disorders* **13**, 361–374.

Pfohl, B. *et al.* (1986) DSM-III personality disorders: diagnostic overlap and internal consistency of individual DSM-III criteria. *Comprehensive Psychiatry* **27**, 21–34.

Pickles, A. & Angold, A. (2003) Natural categories or fundamental dimensions: on carving nature at the joints and the rearticulation of psychopathology. *Development and Psychopathology* **15**, 529–552.

Putnam, K.M. & Silk, K.R. (2005) Emotion disregulation and the development of borderline personality disorder. *Development and Psychopathology* **17**, 899–926.

Quinton, D. *et al.* (1995) A 15-20 year follow-up of adult psychiatric patients: psychiatric disorder and social functioning. *British Journal of Psychiatry* **167**, 315–323.

Reich, D.B. & Zanarini, M.C. (2001) Developmental aspects of borderline personality disorder. *Harvard Review of Psychiatry* **9**, 294–301.

Robins, L.N. (1966) *Deviant Children Grown Up*. Williams and Wilkins, Co., Baltimore.

Robins, L.N. (1978) Sturdy childhood predictors of adult antisocial behaviour: replications from longitudinal studies. *Psychological Medicine* **8**, 611–622.

Robins, R.W. *et al.* (2002) It's not just who you're with, it's who you are: personality and relationship experiences across multiple relationships. *Journal of Personality* **70**, 925–964.

Robinson, J.L. & Acevedo, M.C. (2001) Infant reactivity and reliance on mother during emotion challenges: prediction of cognition and language skills in a low-income sample. *Child Development* **72**, 402–415.

Rubin, K.H. *et al.* (1999) Peer relationships in childhood. *Developmental Psychology: An Advanced Textbook* **4**, 451–502.

Rutter, M. (1987) Temperament, personality and personality disorder. *British Journal of Psychiatry* **150**, 433–458.

Rutter, M. & Quinton, D. (1984) Parental psychiatric disorder: effects on children. *Psychological Medicine* **14**, 853–880.

Schneider, K. (1923) *Diepsychopathischen Personlichkeiten*. Springer, Berlin.

Schneider, K. (1950) *Psychopathic Personalities*, 9th English Translation, 1958 edn. Cassell, London.

Seivewright, H. *et al.* (2004) Persistent social dysfunction in anxious and depressed patients with personality disorder. *Acta Psychiatrica Scandanavica* **109**, 104–109.

Sharp, C. *et al.* (2012) The incremental validity of borderline personality disorder relative to major depressive disorder for suicidal ideation and deliberate self-harm in adolescents. *Journal of Personality Disorders* **26**, 927–938.

Silbersweig, D.E. *et al.* (2007) Failure of frontolimbic inhibitory function in the context of negative emotion in borderline personality disorder. *American Journal of Psychiatry* **164**, 1832–1841.

Siponmaa, L. *et al.* (2001) Juvenile and young adult mentally disordered offenders: the role of child neuropsychiatric disorders. *Journal of the American Academy of Psychiatry and the Law* **29**, 420–426.

Skodol, A.E. *et al.* (2005) Stability of functional impairment in patients with schizotypal, borderline, avoidant, or obsessive-compulsive personality disorder over two years. *Psychological Medicine* **35**, 443–451.

Smeekens, S. *et al.* (2007) Multiple determinants of externalizing behavior in 5-year-olds: a longitudinal model. *Journal of Abnormal Child Psychology* **35**, 347–361.

Soler, J. *et al.* (2005) Double-blind, placebo-controlled study of dialectical behavior therapy plus olanzapine for borderline personality disorder. *American Journal of Psychiatry* **162**, 1221–1224.

Spitzer, R.L. *et al.* (1979) Crossing the border into borderline personality and borderline schizophrenia: the development of criteria. *Archives of General Psychiatry* **36**, 17–24.

Stattin, H. & Magnusson, D. (1996) Antisocial development: a holistic approach. *Development and Psychopathology* **8**, 617–645.

Stepp, S.D. (2012) Development of borderline personality disorder in adolescence and young adulthood: introduction to the special section. *Journal of Abnormal Child Psychology* **40**, 1–5.

Stepp, S.D. *et al.* (2012) Trajectories of attention deficit hyperactivity disorder and oppositional defiant disorder symptoms as precursors of borderline personality disorder symptoms in adolescent girls. *Journal of Abnormal Child Psychology* **40**, 7–20.

Stoffers, J.M. *et al.* (2012) Psychological therapies for people with borderline personality disorder. *Cochrane Database of Systematic Reviews* (8), CD005652.

Strandholm, T. *et al.* (2013) Treatment characteristics and outcome of depression among depressed adolescent outpatients with and without comorbid axis II disorders. *Journal of Personality Disorders*. Published online February 11.

Sundell, K. *et al.*, (2008) The transportability of multisystemic therapy to Sweden: short-term results from a randomized trial of conduct-disordered youths. *Journal of Family Psychology*, **22**, 550–60.

Torgersen, S. *et al.* (2001) The prevalence of personality disorders in a community sample. *Archives of General Psychiatry* **58**, 590–596.

Vollrath, M. *et al.* (1994) Coping and MCMI-II personality disorders. *Journal of Personality Disorders* **8**, 53–63.

Viding, E. *et al.* (2005) Evidence for substantial genetic risk for psychopathy in 7-year-olds. *Journal of Child Psychology and Psychiatry* **46**, 592–597.

Vitaro, F. *et al.* (2000) Influence of deviant friends on delinquency: searching for moderator variables. *Journal of Abnormal Child Psychology* **28**, 313–326.

White, C.N. *et al.* (2002) Family studies of borderline personality disorder: a review. *Harvard Review of Psychiatry* **12**, 118–119.

Widiger, T.A. & Costa, P.T. Jr. (2012) Integrating normal and abnormal personality structure: the five-factor model. *Journal of Personality* **80**, 1471–1506.

Widiger, T.A. & Lowe, J.R. (2007) Five-factor model assessment of personality disorder. *Journal of Personality Assessment* **89**, 16–29.

Widom, C.S. *et al.* (2009) A prospective investigation of borderline personality disorder in abused and neglected children followed up into adulthood. *Journal of Personality Disorders* **23**, 433–446.

Winograd, G. *et al.* (2008) Adolescent borderline symptoms in the community: prognosis for functioning over 20 years. *Journal of Child Psychology and Psychiatry* **49**, 933–941.

Wolff, S. (1991a) 'Schizoid' personality in childhood and adult life. I: the vagaries of diagnostic labelling. *British Journal of Psychiatry* **159**, 615–619.

Wolff, S. (1991b) 'Schizoid' personality in childhood and adult life. III: the childhood picture. *British Journal of Psychiatry* **159**, 629–635.

Wolff, S. & Barlow, A. (1979) Schizoid personality in childhood: a comparative study of schizoid, autistic and normal children. *Journal of Child Psychology and Psychiatry* **20**, 29–46.

Wolff, S. & Chick, J. (1980) Schizoid personality in childhood: a controlled follow-up study. *Psychological Medicine* **10**, 85–120.

Wolff, S. *et al.* (1991) 'Schizoid' personality in childhood and adult life. II: adult adjustment and the continuity with schizotypal personality disorder. *British Journal of Psychiatry* **159**, 620–625.

World Health Organization (1996) *Multiaxial Classification of Child and Adolescent Psychiatric Disorders: The ICD-10 Classification of Mental and Behavioural Disorders in Children and Adolescents*. Cambridge University Press, Cambridge, UK.

Yang, Y. & Raine, A. (2009) Prefrontal structural and functional brain imaging findings in antisocial, violent, and psychopathic individuals: a meta-analysis. *Psychiatry Research: Neuroimaging* **174**, 81–88.

Zanarini, M.C. *et al.* (1998) Axis II comorbidity of borderline personality disorder. *Comprehensive Psychiatry* **39**, 296–302.

Zanarini, M.C. *et al.* (2012) Attainment and stability of sustained symptomatic remission and recovery among patients with borderline personality disorder and axis II comparison subjects: a 16-year prospective follow-up study. *American Journal of Psychiatry* **169**, 476–483.

Zanarini, M.C. *et al.* (2005) Adult experiences of abuse reported by borderline patients and axis II comparison subjects over six years of prospective follow-up. *Journal of Nervous and Mental Disease* **193**, 412–416.

Zanarini, M.C. *et al.* (2000) Bi-parental failure in the childhood experiences of borderline patients. *Journal of Personality Disorders* **14**, 264–273.

Zanarini, M.C. *et al.* (2006) Reported childhood onset of self-mutilation among borderline patients. *Journal of Personality Disorders* **20**, 9–15.

Zanarini, M.C. *et al.* (2004) Borderline psychopathology in the first degree relatives of borderline and axis II comparison probands. *Journal of Personality Disorders* **18**, 439–447.

Zanarini, M.C. *et al.* (2011) Predictors of self-mutilation in patients with borderline personality disorder: a 10-year follow-up study. *Journal of Psychiatric Research* **45**, 823–828.

Zimmerman, M. *et al.* (2013) Distinguishing bipolar II depression from major depressive disorder with comorbid borderline personality disorder: demographic, clinical, and family history differences. *Journal of Clinical Psychiatry* **74**, 880–886.

C: Behavioral

CHAPTER 68

Developmental risk for psychopathy

Essi Viding[1,2] and Eamon McCrory[1]

[1] Faculty of Brain Sciences, University College London, UK
[2] Institute of Psychiatry, Psychology and Neuroscience, King's College London, UK

Introduction: characteristics and diagnosis of psychopathy

The origins of the current description of the psychopathy syndrome

The origins of the current description of the psychopathy syndrome can be traced back to the work of Cleckley (1941) and his book, *The Mask of Sanity*. Some of the key features of psychopathy recorded by Cleckley (1941) included: absence of nervousness, interpersonal charm, lack of shame, impoverished affect, and poorly motivated antisocial behavior. From the criteria delineated by Cleckley, and his own clinical impressions, Robert Hare developed the original psychopathy checklist (PCL) (Hare, 1980), a formalized tool for the assessment of psychopathy in incarcerated adults. On the basis of considerable empirical work, this has been revised, first in 1991, the Psychopathy Checklist—Revised (PCL-R) (Hare, 1991), and then again in 2003 (Hare, 2003). The first extension of the psychopathy concept to children was Bowlby's (1946) description of "affectionless psychopathy." It mirrored some of the key features introduced by Cleckley (such as lack of responsiveness to suffering of others), but lay forgotten for a long time until the extension of psychopathy construct to children was proposed again by Frick and colleagues (1994).

The current definitions of psychopathy in adults comprise both ratings of emotional dysfunction as well as ratings of overt antisocial behavior. The emotional dysfunction definition involves reduced guilt and empathy as well as reduced attachment to significant others. In children, these features have been variously termed "callous-unemotional" (CU) traits "psychopathic traits," and most recently in DSM-5, "limited prosocial emotions." These terms are used interchangeably in this chapter. The majority of extant research has focused on children with these features in the context of conduct problems/conduct disorder (CD). Children with conduct problems may or may not present with the specific form of reduced emotional responsiveness characteristic of CU traits (Frick & Viding, 2009). Introduction of the "lack of prosocial emotions" specifier to the DSM-5 reflects the accumulating evidence base pointing to etiological and neurocognitive differences between children with CD who have high versus low levels of CU traits (see e.g., Viding & McCrory, 2012), with the former group thought to be at risk for developing psychopathy in adulthood (Lynam *et al.*, 2007).

Chapter overview

This chapter will first outline current practice in the assessment of traits in children that have been associated with psychopathy. We will also overview what is known about prevalence, longitudinal outcomes, and risk factors, as well as current accounts of the pathophysiology of children with psychopathic features. Finally, treatment considerations will be discussed in the light of the existing evidence base.

Assessment

Following the adult PCL-R, tools for the assessment of psychopathic traits in childhood and adolescence have also been developed. The Psychopathy Checklist: Youth Version (Forth *et al.*, 2003; Kosson *et al.*, 2002) is widely used in juvenile justice settings, particularly in North America. The PCL-YV is scored on the basis of an extensive file review and a semistructured interview. Commonly used measures for community samples of children and youth include the Antisocial Process Screening Device (APSD) (Frick & Hare, 2001), which charts CU, narcissistic, and impulsive traits; and the Inventory of Callous-Unemotional (ICU) traits (Frick, 2003), which was specifically developed to more thoroughly assess CU traits in children. Both measures take the format of parent, teacher, or child-rated questionnaires. The inter-rater reliability for these measures is comparable with other instruments assessing

Rutter's Child and Adolescent Psychiatry, Sixth Edition.
Edited by Anita Thapar and Daniel S. Pine, James F. Leckman, Stephen Scott, Margaret J. Snowling, Eric Taylor.

psychopathology (e.g., Frick & Hare, 2001; Frick *et al.*, 2003b; Roose *et al.*, 2010). For children, moderate to strong stability of the CU traits across childhood and adolescence has been demonstrated in a number of studies (e.g., Frick *et al.*, 2003b; Obradovic *et al.*, 2007). Obradovic and colleagues (2007) also reported that CU traits from childhood to adolescence had longitudinal invariance, that is, were represented by similar behavioral indices at different ages. To date, CU traits have not been routinely assessed during psychiatric assessment of CD. However, the DSM-5 now includes a "limited prosocial emotions" specifier (essentially CD with CU traits), which is discussed below.

DSM-5 conduct disorder with limited prosocial emotions

The recent DSM-5 has introduced a specifier to delineate a group of children with CD who show "limited prosocial emotions." The indicators of this specifier are those that have been labeled CU traits in research. The specifier includes four symptoms:

1 "Lack of remorse or guilt"
2 "Callous lack of empathy"
3 "Shallow or deficient affect"
4 "Unconcern about performance at school or work."

Children have to qualify for CD diagnosis and present with at least two symptoms from the specifier for at least 12 months, as indicated by two independent raters.

It may be helpful, for example, for the clinician to take time to explore age-appropriate situations that may have elicited guilt or empathy. These could include asking about feelings when witnessing younger children in distress, thoughts about hurting someone else, deliberate cruelty toward others, and discussing feelings of remorse. There is also preliminary evidence that cruelty toward animals, which may arise in CD in general, may be particularly prevalent for those children with high CU traits (Dadds *et al.*, 2006; Vizard *et al.*, 2007). The administration of the ICU to multiple informants (self-, teacher-, and carer-ratings) can be a helpful adjunct to the material garnered from case files and clinical interview with the young person and carer (White *et al.*, 2009; Kimonis *et al.*, 2013). Naturally, clinical judgment needs to be deployed when discussing a diagnosis of CD with "limited prosocial emotions" sensitively with parents/carers and the young person themselves.

Co-occurrence with other disorders
Attention deficit hyperactivity disorder (ADHD)

Considerable work has demonstrated that CD and attention deficit hyperactivity disorder (ADHD) often co-occur, and that individuals with CD and high CU traits also have high levels of ADHD symptoms (e.g., Taylor *et al.*, 1986; Hinshaw, 1987; Lynam, 1996; Barry *et al.*, 2000; Colledge & Blair, 2001; Fontaine *et al.*, 2011). Recent data suggest that impulsivity in ADHD and CD are likely to be driven by distinct neurocognitive vulnerabilities (Rubia, 2011). However, it remains unclear whether ADHD symptoms seen in the context of CD with high CU traits can be considered equivalent to ADHD that occurs in the absence of these traits, or whether it should be considered as a behavioral phenocopy with a divergent neurocognitive signature (Blair *et al.*, 2005). What we do know, is that a key distinguishing characteristic that sets apart children with ADHD and CD with CU traits clinically, is the presence versus absence of callous, remorseless, and unempathic behaviors.

Autism spectrum disorders (ASDs)

Autism spectrum disorders (ASDs) are associated with problems in socially appropriate behavior (see Chapter 51), which have led people to question the degree to which these disorders may be related to CU traits. However, the nature of the social impairment appears very different between the two populations (Jones *et al.*, 2010; Schwenck *et al.*, 2012). Individuals with ASD, as a group, tend to show impairment in Theory of Mind, the ability to represent the mental states of others (Baron-Cohen *et al.*, 1985; Frith & Happe, 2005; Jones *et al.*, 2010; Schwenck *et al.*, 2012). Children with CU traits do not (Jones *et al.*, 2010; Schwenck *et al.*, 2012). Instead children with CU traits have difficulties in processing other people's distress (fear and sadness) and do not report appropriate concern for other people's suffering (Blair *et al.*, 2001; Jones *et al.*, 2010; Schwenck *et al.*, 2012), that is, they are poor at feeling for others, while being capable of representing mental states. Individuals with ASD, while potentially showing a global impairment in processing emotions, appear to find others' distress aversive (Adolphs *et al.*, 2001; Jones *et al.*, 2010; Rogers *et al.*, 2006; Schwenck *et al.*, 2012). To date there are a few reports of co-morbid CU traits/psychopathy and ASD (Fine *et al.*, 2001; Rogers *et al.*, 2006), but twin research indicates that the etiological (both genetic and environmental) factors contributing to each symptom domain are mostly independent (Jones *et al.*, 2009a). As pointed out by Rutter (2005), unlike for psychopathy, the impaired socio-emotional responsiveness found in ASD does not seem to be typically linked to increased risk for antisocial behavior compared to the general population. In support of this, Hippler and Klicpera (2003), in their study of 177 cases originally diagnosed by Asperger, found no raised incidence of criminal offences compared with general population rates in individuals with ASD. In contrast, Frick and colleagues have demonstrated that elevated levels of CU traits predict increased antisocial behavior at a later time point, even in children who do not start off as having clinically elevated rates of antisocial behavior (Frick *et al.*, 2005). It thus appears that although both children with CU traits and children with ASD can appear to behave in an emotionally blunted manner, there are likely to be different roots to their emotional problems that also explain the lack of increased risk for antisocial behavior in people with ASD.

Anxiety and mood disorders

Psychopathy has been traditionally considered to be marked by reduced anxiety levels (Cleckley, 1941; Hare, 1970;

Lykken, 1957). In general, psychopathic traits are associated with reduced levels of anxiety (e.g., Patrick, 1994; Frick *et al.*, 1999; Verona *et al.*, 2001). However, recent research suggests that some children present with concurrent psychopathic traits and anxiety (Kahn *et al.*, 2013; Fanti *et al.*, 2013). These children differ from those with psychopathic traits and non-elevated anxiety in a number of other respects. For example, they are more likely to have experienced childhood maltreatment and show greater attentional bias to emotional stimuli than children with psychopathic traits and low levels of anxiety (e.g., Kimonis *et al.*, 2012). Such differences are likely to be clinically relevant and require further research.

Differential diagnosis

While making a diagnosis of CD should be relatively straightforward, it is possible that behavioral symptoms associated with other disorders may be misconstrued as antisocial (e.g., irritability in depression, certain patterns of hyperactive behavior). In relation to CD with CU traits particular attention should be given to behaviors that may appear unempathic. Children with ASD and social communication disorder may also have difficulties in displaying an appropriate empathic response but as noted above, these difficulties are thought to stem from theory of mind (i.e., mentalizing) impairments rather than from deficits in their basic response to other people's emotions. As a result these children also have a host of other features indicating broader deficits in social interaction and communication not evident in children with CD and CU traits.

Summary—assessment

A number of standard measures, both questionnaires and interview/file ratings, have been developed to reliably assess CU features in children and adolescents, in research, forensic and clinical settings. The recent DSM-5 has introduced a specifier to delineate a group of children with CD with "limited prosocial emotions," which can be regarded as largely analogous to the presence of CU traits as conceptualized in previous research. An established body of work has demonstrated that children with CD often present with symptoms of other disorders, such as ADHD and anxiety. Because an official clinical diagnosis of CD with CU traits (or CU) has not existed to date, we know relatively little about frequency of co-occurring disorders in these children. The existing evidence base suggests that elevated levels of CU traits can co-occur with symptoms of other disorders. For example, some children present with an atypical pattern of CU traits and anxiety symptoms; such a presentation may alert a clinician to a possible history of maltreatment. Furthermore, a differential diagnosis of other disorders of social impairment (e.g., ASD) is important for the clinician to consider during assessment.

Epidemiology and longitudinal outcomes

Prevalence

Prevalence estimates for CD vary across studies. A recent review provided a pooled prevalence estimate for CD, across a large number of studies, as 3.2% (Canino *et al.*, 2010). Only a few studies to date have estimated the prevalence of CD utilizing the "limited prosocial emotions" (CU) specifier. These studies indicate that 20–50% of children with CD also present with high levels of CU features (Kahn *et al.*, 2012; Pardini *et al.*, 2012). This points to a tentative prevalence level of 0.75–1.5% of children qualifying for CD with CU specifier. This prevalence rate is comparable to that estimated for adult criminal psychopathy (Blair *et al.*, 2005). Epidemiological as well as large community studies also indicate that CU traits can occur with nonclinical levels of CD symptoms (e.g., Rowe *et al.*, 2010; Barker *et al.*, 2011; Fanti, 2013), although it is not currently possible to provide precise prevalence estimates for this presentation as none of the studies adopted symptom count criteria for defining the groups. These studies also indicate that children with CU traits and nonclinical levels of CD symptoms nonetheless often present with elevated levels of conduct problems and other psychological problems. More research is required to understand the clinical significance of CU traits that occur without clinical levels of CD symptoms and how children with such a presentation progress across development.

CU traits in boys and girls

The DSM-5 specifier identifies girls who exhibit a similar profile (low anxiety, more severe aggression and psychosocial impairment) to boys with CD and high levels of CU traits. CD with high levels of CU traits, as well as high levels of CU traits (without clinical levels of CD) are more prevalent in boys than in girls (where available, data indicate that these presentations are three to five times as common in boys than in girls; e.g., Fontaine *et al.*, 2010; Fanti, 2013) and may have a different etiology in girls (Fontaine *et al.*, 2010).

Cultural factors

CU trait measurement and its construct validity have been assessed in several Western countries to date and the existing studies report remarkably similar findings (e.g., Essau *et al.*, 2006; Kimonis *et al.*, 2008; Fanti *et al.*, 2009; Ezpeleta *et al.*, 2013). However, research on how cultural factors may impact the expression of CU traits, both within and between countries, is needed.

CU traits as a risk indicator for behavioral/psychiatric maladjustment

Longitudinal research on large community samples suggests that CU traits predict antisocial and criminal/delinquent outcomes (e.g., Frick *et al.*, 2003a; Fontaine *et al.*, 2010; McMahon *et al.*, 2010; Pardini & Fite, 2010). CU traits predict these outcomes over and above the prediction afforded by conduct problem severity alone (e.g., Frick *et al.*, 2003a; McMahon *et al.*, 2010; Pardini & Fite, 2010). Although the data with regard to internalizing problems (anxiety and depression symptoms) is less rich, some studies suggest that CU traits may be protective against development of internalizing problems (e.g., Pardini & Fite, 2010).

Prognostic value into adulthood

A long-term follow-up study measuring psychopathic traits at age 13 demonstrated that the construct showed moderate stability to age 24 years ($r = 0.32$), despite different informants and assessment instruments used across the two age periods (Lynam *et al.*, 2007). This 11-year correlation is equivalent to that typically seen when different informants use the same instrument at the same time-point to rate an individual's behavior on a construct. Another recent study included a measure of adult criminality and demonstrated that CU added predictive value over and above prior and concurrent conduct disturbance and ADHD symptoms (McMahon *et al.*, 2010).

Treatment outcomes

The moderating role of CU traits on treatment outcome has been assessed in a number of studies. These will be discussed in the treatment section of this chapter.

Summary—epidemiology and longitudinal outcomes

Epidemiological work is relatively sparse to date. This is no doubt to a large part due to the fact that CU traits have not been considered in clinical diagnostics and decision-making with children until very recently. As such, most of the large-scale epidemiological studies have not included standard CU trait assessment among their measures and prevalence estimates. Furthermore, the types of prevalence estimates that have been drawn from the current studies are often based on sophisticated longitudinal modeling (e.g., Rowe *et al.*, 2010), but are not easily translated to prevalence of CD with "limited prosocial emotions" as classified by DSM-5. Based on the available data, we estimate that CD with high levels of CU traits affects approximately 1% of children and is more common in boys than in girls. Additionally, there are groups of children with high levels of CU traits, but nonclinical levels of CD (see e.g., Rowe *et al.*, 2010; Kumsta *et al.*, 2012). Currently, very little is known about the neurocognitive presentation and long-term prognosis of these children. Cultural impact on the expression of CU also needs further investigation.

Longitudinal studies indicate that CU traits are predictive of persistent antisocial outcomes, including psychopathy in adulthood. CU traits add to the prediction of these outcomes, over and above the prediction afforded by conduct problem severity alone.

Risk factors

This section reviews potential risk factors for CU traits and conduct problems that occur with CU traits. Whereas genetic differences are causal (although it is important to note, not deterministic!), for the other risk factors the mode of operation is less clear and much of the current research is at a stage of demonstrating an association, without having established the causality of these putative risk factors for CU (see Chapter 12).

Genetic factors

Individual differences in CU are estimated to be moderately to strongly heritable using the twin design that compares resemblance in monozygotic (MZ) twins and dizygotic (DZ) twins in community samples of children and adolescents (heritability estimates from 0.45 to 0.67; see Viding & McCrory, 2012; see also Chapter 24). Having elevated levels of CU is strongly heritable in childhood regardless of whether CU traits are accompanied by conduct problems or not (Larsson *et al.*, 2008). It is also of interest to note that conduct problems with high levels of CU traits appear strongly heritable, whereas conduct problems with low levels of CU traits appear to be more strongly influenced by environmental factors (Viding *et al.*, 2005, 2008; See Figure 68.1).

Twin studies suggest that there is considerable overlap in the genes that influence CU and conduct/externalizing problems, but that there are also unique genetic influences on CU (Forsman *et al.*, 2007; Viding *et al.*, 2007; Bezdjian *et al.*, 2011), consistent with the finding that high levels of CU have been observed in the absence of clinical levels of conduct problems (Frick *et al.*, 2003a; Kumsta *et al.*, 2012). Twin studies also suggest that stability in CU/psychopathic traits is driven by genetic influences (Forsman *et al.*, 2008; Fontaine *et al.*, 2010).

Only a handful of published candidate gene association studies have focused on CU in *children or adolescents* and these studies have tentatively implicated variants in, for example, the serotonin and oxytocin genes (e.g., Fowler *et al.*, 2009; Beichtman *et al.*, 2012; Malik *et al.*, 2012; Dadds *et al.*, 2013; Moul *et al.*, 2013). The current candidate gene studies need to be replicated in larger samples to evaluate whether they report true, replicable associations, but picking candidate genes is not straightforward and can lead to unadjusted multiple testing. Because genetic risk may in many cases only "penetrate" in the presence of environmental risk, genetic studies should carefully document the environmental risk factors in their samples to increase interpretability of the findings and consequently, our understanding of how genetic risk translates to a disorder

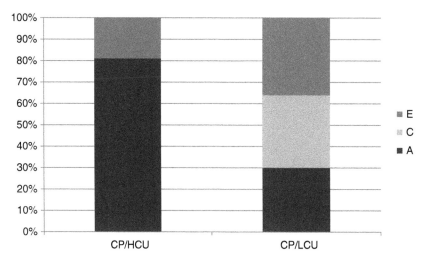

Figure 68.1 The main finding from Viding et al. (2005), showing the degree to which a group difference in conduct problem scores between typically developing children and 1) children with conduct problems with high levels of callous-unemotional traits (CP/HCU) and 2) children with conduct problems with low levels of callous-unemotional traits (CP/LCU) is due to additive genetic (A), shared environmental (C) and non-shared environmental (E) influences.

outcome. A recent study reported that the long allele of a serotonin transporter polymorphism, the allele reported to confer low amygdala reactivity, was associated with CU in adolescents from low socio-economic status (SES) backgrounds, a finding which was observed in two independent community samples (both rural and urban; Sadeh *et al.*, 2010). These findings suggest that genetic vulnerability to CU traits may only express under unfavourable environmental conditions.

The association studies only considered a limited number of candidate genes. However, a growing number of genome-wide association (GWA) studies for psychiatric phenotypes have shown that genome-wide "hits" are often in genes not previously hypothesized to influence the phenotype or not in traditional genes at all (Visscher *et al.*, 2012). GWA studies systematically scan the genome with hundreds of thousands of DNA markers, made possible by DNA arrays. GWA studies of CU traits suggest that much larger samples will be needed to detect novel associations that account for far less than 1% of the variance (Viding *et al.*, 2010, 2013).

Methods to identify gene–gene and gene–environment interactions (which more than likely account for a proportion of the heritability estimate for psychopathic traits in children) are also required, as is whole-genome sequencing to detect rare variants. Genetic research is likely to advance greatly in the coming decade, including studies using novel epigenetic approaches that may help uncover mechanisms of gene–environment interaction, but it is of critical importance to keep in mind that *there are no genes for CU traits*. Genes code for proteins that influence characteristics such as neurocognitive vulnerabilities that may in turn increase risk for developing CU traits. Genetic variants that are implicated as risk genes for CU traits are likely to include several common polymorphisms that confer advantages, as well as disadvantages, depending on the environmental context. The

neurocognitive vulnerabilities associated with CU traits are at least partially distinct from those associated with conduct problems in general (see Section "Neurocognitive Findings"). This suggests that the risk alleles for CU traits or conduct problems that co-occur with CU traits may not always be the same as risk alleles for conduct problems in the absence of CU traits.

Pre- and peri-natal factors

In contrast to the extensive literature documenting the association between pre-and peri-natal risk factors (e.g., maternal smoking during pregnancy, maternal psychopathology during pregnancy, and birth complications) and conduct problems, the research on pre- and peri-natal risk factors for CU traits (or CP with CU traits) remains extremely sparse. One study to date has reported an association between CU traits (either with or without CP) and maternal psychopathology during and after pregnancy (Barker *et al.*, 2011). However, no data exist to document the role of risk factors such as head injury or infection. This is clearly an area that requires further investigation and it is critical that researchers apply designs that will enable them to evaluate whether the pre-and peri-natal risk factors have a causal role in the development of CU or whether they merely reflect genetic vulnerability within families who have a child with CU traits.

Sex

As outlined in the section on epidemiology in this chapter, high levels of CU traits and CD with CU traits are more common in boys than in girls. There is also nascent research suggesting that the etiology of CU traits may differ for boys and girls (Fontaine *et al.*, 2010). However, the external correlates of high CU traits (e.g., increased conduct problem severity, lower anxiety levels) appear quite similar for both boys and girls (e.g., McMahon et al., 2010; Pardini et al., 2012). Systematic research investigating potential mechanisms responsible for the differences in prevalence by sex, as well as sex differences in etiological mechanisms, is needed.

Hormonal factors

There is emerging evidence to suggest that males with CU traits are characterized by low levels of basal cortisol (Hawes et al., 2009) and low cortisol reactivity to experimentally induced stress (Stadler et al., 2010). Loney et al. (2006) investigated both measures of basal cortisol and testosterone in a non-referred community sample of adolescents. Males (but not females) with high CU traits were found to have low levels of basal cortisol, consistent with similar findings in adults (Cima et al., 2008). Testosterone levels did not differentiate participants in this study and no hormone effects were found for female participants. A recent study of adults reported that an increased testosterone-to-cortisol ratio may particularly characterize individuals high on psychopathic traits (Glenn et al., 2011). This approach, investigating the interconnectedness of different hormone systems, is yet to be extended to children. A study focusing on stress reactivity in children with ADHD found that those with high levels of CU traits showed lowest cortisol response under experimentally induced stress (Stadler et al., 2010).

Physiological factors

Both reduced skin conductance reactivity and reduced heart rate to other people's distress have been reported in children with CU traits and conduct problems, when compared with typically developing peers and peers with conduct problems (Blair, 1999; Anastassiou-Hadjicharalambous & Warden, 2008; de Wied et al., 2012). It appears that resting heart rate does not differentiate children with CU traits (de Wied et al., 2012). Furthermore, skin conductance reactivity is not universally compromised, but appears to be altered in response to distress emotions (Blair, 1999).

Early temperamental factors

Fearlessness and low fear-related arousal have been consistently linked to antisocial outcomes in longitudinal studies (Loeber & Pardini, 2008). Infants and children who display fearless temperament and lack of fearful arousal are also known to show atypical development of empathy and guilt (Fowles & Kochanska, 2000). It has been proposed that fearlessness may be one early temperamental precursor to CU traits, which may interfere with socialization methods that rely on empathy induction (e.g., asking the child to imagine how someone else is feeling) and sanctions (e.g., "time out" or revoking privileges) (Frick & Viding, 2009). In line with this, Barker et al. (2011) found that child fearless temperament at age two predicted CU traits at age 13, even after factors such as parenting were controlled for. Thus, fearlessness appears to be an early temperamental factor that predicts development of CU traits in adolescence.

Maltreatment

There are considerable data suggesting that exposure to maltreatment and neglect increases the risk of aggressive/conduct problems (e.g., Caspi et al., 2002; Lansford et al., 2002). Bowlby attributed "affectionless psychopathy" to family adversity that especially involved family disruption (Bowlby, 1946). A recent study with Romanian adoptees demonstrated that extreme childhood neglect is associated with CU traits (Kumsta et al., 2012). Interestingly, although CU traits typically co-occur with conduct problems in community and clinical samples, this was not the case for the adoptees in the study. The authors of this study speculated that adoption to good homes might have reduced the likelihood of conduct problems in the sample or alternatively, that CU traits following neglect were a different, behaviorally equifinal manifestation of CU traits, different from that which is seen in community and clinic samples. Although juveniles with CU traits and conduct problems often report maltreatment histories, we do not currently know whether maltreatment unequivocally causes CU traits. Recent research also suggests that an atypical profile where CU traits co-occur with anxiety is more likely to be associated with maltreatment experiences than CU traits that present without anxiety. It remains to be seen whether the maltreated children who present with CU and anxiety share genetic and neurocognitive characteristics with those children who have CU without anxiety. What we do know is that children who have experienced maltreatment present with neural over-rather than under-reactivity to affective stimuli (e.g., McCrory et al., 2011a, 2013); the opposite of what is typically observed for children with high CU traits (Viding & McCrory, 2012).

Overall, the current literature suggests that for majority of cases, maltreatment produces a neural and behavioral signature that is different from that commonly observed in individuals with conduct problems and CU traits (McCrory et al., 2011b; Danese & McCrory (see Chapter 29); McCrory et al., 2011a). However, it is plausible that both biologically and environmentally "weighted" routes to the same behavioral outcome can take place, even if one route is considerably more common than the other or even if the two routes may differentiate at the level of pathophysiology.

Parenting

There is now substantive evidence that exposure to poor parenting increases the risk for aggression and being diagnosed with CD (Reid et al., 2002). A recent systematic review evaluated the impact of parenting on CU traits in both community and clinic samples (Waller et al., 2013). Harsh and negative parenting was associated with higher levels of CU traits in children, while warm parenting style was associated with lower levels of CU traits in children. However, only one longitudinal, genetically informative study to date has investigated parenting and development of CU traits. This study suggests that the association between harsh and negative parenting and higher levels of CU traits in children may, at least in part, reflect genetic vulnerability within families (Viding *et al.*, 2009). This could reflect a shared genetic vulnerability to poor parenting and CU temperament, as well as CU temperament evoking negative/harsh parenting.

A number of cross-sectional studies suggest that the dose–response relationship between negative parenting and level of conduct problems does not hold for children with high levels of CU traits, whereas it is commonly observed for other children with conduct problems (reviewed in Waller *et al.*, 2013). Studies on community samples document "what is," whereas intervention studies document "what can be." Encouragingly, from a clinical perspective, parenting-focused interventions appear effective in reducing the level of conduct problems and CU traits in children who have high levels of both (Waller *et al.*, 2013; see treatment section of this chapter for further discussion of this issue).

Other risk factors

Factors such as lower SES, IQ and parental psychopathology have all been associated with increased risk for antisocial behavior (see Chapter 65). The data for CU traits specifically are limited. In relation to SES, to our knowledge an association between SES and CU, which cannot be accounted for by other concomitant risk factors, is yet to be established. However, it is important to note that SES could moderate the behavioral manifestation of CU traits. Some antisocial behavior shown by individuals with psychopathic traits is instrumental in nature, it has the goal of gaining another's money, sexual favors or "respect" (Cornell *et al.*, 1996; Williamson *et al.*, 1987). Individuals can attempt to achieve these goals through a variety of means. Being of a higher SES enables a wider choice of available routes for achieving these goals than being of a lower SES. A healthy individual of limited SES may also have a narrow range of behavioral options but will exclude antisocial behavior because of aversion to this behavior formed during socialization. In contrast, individuals with psychopathy may entertain the antisocial option because they do not find the required antisocial behavior aversive. SES is also likely to impact on the probability of displaying instrumental aggression by determining relative reward levels for particular actions. To illustrate, if the individual already has $100,000, the subjective value of the $50 that could be gained if the individual mugged another person on the street is low. In contrast, if the individual has only 50 cents, the subjective value of the $50 will be very high indeed (for a discussion of subjective value, see Tversky & Kahneman, 1981). In line with this speculation, a recent genetic study found that the long allele of the serotonin transporter gene variant was associated with elevated levels of CU traits, but only in adolescents who lived in low SES families/neighbourhoods (Sadeh *et al.*, 2010).

In relation to IQ, a handful of studies point to a modest negative association between CU traits and IQ (e.g., Fontaine *et al.*, 2008), but the mechanisms of this association are currently unclear. Behavioral problems that are commonly associated

with CU traits may limit educational opportunities of children and contribute to the association.

In relation to parental psychopathology, a positive association between CU traits and parental mental health problems has been demonstrated (e.g., Vizard *et al.*, 2007; Barker *et al.*, 2011). At least one study to date has specifically focused on CU features in mothers and their children and demonstrated a modest intergenerational correlation ($r = 0.22$) (Loney *et al.*, 2007). It is nonetheless of note that this modest correlation is of similar magnitude to that typically observed for different raters (e.g., parent and child) on the same measure—yet it was obtained using different measures and partly different raters (parents for the parent measure; both teachers and parents for the child measure).

Summary—risk factors

An emerging body of research is accumulating that implicates a variety of risk factors associated with the development of CU traits (or conduct problems that occur with these traits)—spanning genetic, physiological, temperamental, ability, and environmental factors. However, we still know relatively little compared to a more substantive empirical evidence base with regard to risk factors associated with conduct problems in general. It appears that children with CU traits have a genetic vulnerability, but less is known about actual genes or how the genetic vulnerability interacts with other risk factors to increase maladaptive outcomes. In order to advance our understanding of risk, longitudinal as well as genetically informative studies with multiple measures of risk are needed to investigate how these interact with each other and whether they are truly causal for the development of CU traits.

Neurocognitive findings

Behaviorally children with CU traits show marked lack of empathy and guilt. They often engage in proactive, instrumental aggression, seem impervious to sanctions, and do not seem to share the affiliative needs and goals that characterize typical children (Frick & Viding, 2009). Given this profile, many of the experimental studies on children with CU traits have focused on how they process emotions, whether they empathize with others, and whether they change their behavior following punishment. These studies have documented that compared with typically developing children or children with other psychopathologies, children with CU traits: are less likely to react to and recognize affective stimuli, particularly distress cues such as fear and sadness of other people (e.g., Marsh & Blair, 2008; Sylvers *et al.*, 2011; however, if specifically directed to focus on the eye region of the face, fear recognition performance can be normalized in these children (Dadds *et al.*, 2008)); show blunted empathy toward others (Jones *et al.*, 2010; Schwenck *et al.*, 2012; de Wied *et al.*, 2012); do not direct attention to the eyes of attachment figures (Dadds *et al.*, 2011; Dadds *et al.*, 2012a);

Box 68.1 Neural circuitry involved in emotion, reward, and empathic processing.

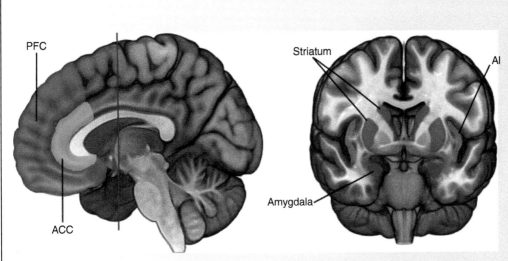

PFC

ACC

Striatum

AI

Amygdala

Figure 68.2 Neural circuitry involved in emotion, reward and empathic processing

The amygdala

The amygdala is a subcortical region that is important for processing the current value of stimuli (Adolphs, 2010). The amygdala has a critical role in several affective processes, such as mediating conditioned emotional responses, responding to various emotional stimuli (including facial expressions of emotion), and in social behavior toward conspecifics (see e.g., Sergerie, Chochol & Armony, 2008; Adolphs, 2010).

The striatum

The striatum is a subcortical region that plays a role in modulating behavior toward potentially rewarding stimuli, particularly stimuli that hold a high subjective reward value to an individual (see e.g., Rosen & Levenson, 2009, Peters & Buchel, 2010).

The anterior cingulate cortex

The anterior Cingulate Cortex (ACC) is thought to play a distinct role in complex aspects of emotion, such as processing moral emotions (e.g., guilt), empathy, self-regulation of negative emotions, and action reinforcement (route by which reward history influences action choice) (see e.g., Levesque et al., 2004; Rushworth et al., 2007; Kedia et al., 2008; Medford & Critchley, 2010).

The anterior insula

The anterior insula (AI) plays an important role in sensory integration (Critchley et al., 2004) and interoceptive awareness (Craig, 2009) and may be involved in awareness of unpleasant feelings during empathy for pain (Medford & Critchley, 2010).

The prefrontal cortex

Various sectors of the prefrontal cortex (PFC) have been implicated in emotion (see e.g., Davidson et al., 2000; Vuilleumier & Pourtois, 2007). The areas that have received most attention in affective neuroscience

studies of children include the orbitofrontal cortex (OFC); ventromedial prefrontal cortex (vMPFC); ventrolateral prefrontal cortex (vLPFC); and dorsolateral prefrontal cortex (DLPFC). The OFC is thought to implement rapid stimulus-reinforcement associations and the correction of these associations when the contingencies of reinforcement change (e.g., Mitchell et al., 2008; O'Doherty, 2004; Rolls & Grabenhorst, 2008), while the vMPFC is thought to represent the elementary positive and negative affective states in the absence of immediately present incentives (Davidson & Irwin, 1999; Mitchell, 2011). A more rostral region of the MPFC has been implicated in the processing of more complex social emotions such as guilt and embarrassment (e.g., Takahashi et al., 2004; Burnett et al., 2009). Current research suggests that vLPFC integrates affective information and supports response selection by increasing the salience of alternative motor response option representations through interactions with the striatum (e.g., Mitchell et al., 2008; Mitchell, 2011). It is also associated with effortful regulation of negative affect, via connections with subcortical structures including the amygdala (Ochsner & Gross, 2005; Wager et al., 2008). DLPFC, in turn, is thought to increase attentional control of task-relevant stimulus features and represent goal states toward which more elementary positive and negative affective states are directed (Mitchell, 2011).

Summary

In this box, we have provided an extremely succinct overview of the brain areas that form the brain's emotional, reward, and empathic circuitry. Clearly, most of the brain's emotional/empathic processes are achieved by functional integration across several brain areas, that is, although broad functions for these brain areas are discussed above, many of these areas work together to achieve appropriate behavioral outcome for the organism. For example, amygdala, together with PFC and ventral striatum, form a network of structures involved in processing the current value of stimuli and various PFC/ACC regions are either directly or indirectly connected with amygdala to achieve emotion regulation via different mechanisms, such as reappraisal.

and are slower to alter their behavior following punishment (e.g., Blair *et al.*, 2001).

The experimental findings that indicate atypical emotion processing and attention to emotion have prompted the study of neural correlates of CU traits (and conduct problems with CU traits) in children, with a particular focus on brain areas associated with emotional, reward and empathic processing. In Figure 68.2 we briefly describe the core emotion, reward and empathy circuitry of the brain for the purposes of anchoring the data presented in this chapter.

Functional magnetic resonance imaging (fMRI) studies

In line with the behavioral and experimental neuropsychology data, fMRI findings for children with CU traits indicate functional deficits consistent with low emotional responsiveness to others' distress and poor ability to learn from reinforcement information. Recent studies have reported reduced amygdala activity to fearful faces in children with conduct problems and high levels of CU traits as compared with typically developing children, children with ADHD, and children with conduct problems and low levels of CU traits (Marsh *et al.*, 2008; Jones *et al.*, 2009b; Viding *et al.*, 2012). Reduced amygdala activity in children with conduct problems and high CU traits also seems to extend to more complex forms of social judgment with regard to other people's distress, such as categorization of legal and illegal behaviors in a moral judgment task (Marsh *et al.*, 2011) or making decisions about appropriate responses to other people's distress (Sebastian *et al.*, 2012). Interestingly, conduct problems with low levels of CU traits appear to be associated with exaggerated, rather than reduced, amygdala activity to emotional stimuli (Viding *et al.*, 2012; Sebastian *et al.*, 2013).

Two recent studies have reported atypical neural reactivity to other people's pain in children with conduct problems and CU traits (Lockwood *et al.*, 2013; Marsh *et al.*, 2013). These studies implicated reduced activity in a network of brain areas associated with empathy for other people's pain in previous studies of healthy individuals, for example, the AI, ACC and amygdala.

Abnormal vmPFC and OFC responses to punishment and reward in children with conduct problems and CU traits have also been reported (Finger *et al.*, 2008; Finger *et al.*, 2011). For example, Finger *et al.* (2008) reported that typically developing children and children with ADHD showed a reduction in vmPFC activity following an unexpected punishment. Such reduction in vmPFC activity has been shown to co-occur with prediction error, that is, when expected outcome differs from the actual outcome (Mitchell, 2011). In contrast, youth with conduct problems and CU traits did not show this reduction in vmPFC activity. In another study, using a passive avoidance paradigm where participants had to learn which stimuli were "good" (rewarded) and which were "bad" (unrewarded), Finger *et al.* (2011) also demonstrated that children with conduct problems and CU traits showed less OFC and caudate responsiveness to early stimulus-reinforcement exposure, and less OFC

responsiveness to rewards. These neural differences are likely to index compromised sensitivity to early reinforcement information in the OFC and caudate and compromised sensitivity to reward outcome information in the OFC in adolescents with conduct problems and CU traits. More recent work, however, suggests that the difficulties in reinforcement learning may not be unique to conduct problems with CU traits, but may instead be a common problem for all children with conduct problems (White *et al.*, 2013).

These fMRI findings in children with conduct problems and CU traits are largely in line with those typically reported in studies of adult psychopaths (e.g., Kiehl *et al.*, 2001; Birbaumer *et al.*, 2005) and suggest functional neural bases for why these children appear unaffected by other people's distress and often make and repeat disadvantageous decisions.

Structural magnetic resonance imaging studies

To date there have been only two studies that report on structural MRI correlates of conduct problems that co-occur with CU traits in children. De Brito *et al.* (2009) found that compared with typically developing boys, boys with conduct problems and high CU traits had increased gray matter concentration (GMC) in several brain areas implicated in decision-making, moral processing, and self-reflection. These included OFC, insula, ACC, posterior cingulate cortex (PCC) and superior temporal cortex.

Subsequently, De Brito *et al.* (2011) showed that compared with typically developing boys, those with conduct problems and CU traits exhibited *decreased* white matter concentration (WMC) in a subset of the brain areas where increased GMC was found in these boys, including ACC and superior temporal cortex. These findings indicate that children with conduct problems and CU traits are characterized by atypical neural structure in many of the same areas where gray and white matter abnormalities have also been reported in adults with psychopathy (Gao *et al.*, 2009; Yang & Raine, 2009). However, somewhat puzzlingly, the direction of the effect (at least for gray matter) is different in the child, as compared with adult studies. It is of note that De Brito *et al.* (2009, 2011) studied children who were between 10 and 13 years of age. Recent brain imaging evidence in normative samples suggests that gray matter decreases and white matter increases in several of the brain areas implicated in the De Brito *et al.* (2009) study during this period of early adolescence (Gogtay *et al.*, 2004). This is contrary to the pattern observed for the 10–13-year-old boys with conduct problems and CU traits, possibly indicative of aberrant brain maturation for this group in early adolescence. More recently, Sumich *et al.* (2012) have found that boys with conduct problems and CU traits do not show the typical maturational pattern of decline in the event-related potential component N200 amplitude in midline frontal and temporal electrodes, further evidencing a possible atypical maturation for this group of boys. These data are not necessarily at odds with the findings from adult studies, which clearly represent a very different developmental stage. Distinct developmental disorders can follow markedly different patterns of structural brain development (Shaw *et al.*, 2010) and future longitudinal studies should probe the exact developmental pattern characteristic of conduct problems and CU traits.

Summary—neurocognitive findings

The extant magnetic resonance imaging evidence base suggests that conduct problems with CU traits are associated with atypical patterns of brain structure and function, particularly in the areas critical for affective processing, affective decision-making, and moral emotions. The findings are broadly in line with those reported in studies of adult psychopaths and may represent neural indicators of vulnerability that render these children at increased risk for developing adult psychopathy.

Treatment implications

Conceptually, children with conduct problems and high levels of CU traits would be hypothesized to respond differentially to treatment, given their distinct pattern of etiological and neurocognitive vulnerability. These children have genetic vulnerability to antisocial behavior and show functional and structural neural abnormalities that may predispose them to atypical development of emotion processing, reinforcement learning, and empathy. Only relatively recently have studies begun to examine how treatment outcome might vary in relation to a child's level of CU traits, and whether the efficacy of treatment strategies vary depending on level of CU traits.

There is now growing evidence that children with high levels of CU traits benefit significantly from standard interventions (Waller *et al.*, 2013). While they are likely to enter and finish treatment with more pronounced behavioral and social difficulties, they can show real improvements. For example, Kolko and Pardini (2010) found that a sample of clinic-referred children with conduct problems and high CU traits who received a wide range of individualized and modular interventions (e.g., parent training, cognitive behavioral therapy, peer relationship development, medication for ADHD) improved at a similar rate to other children with conduct problems. Similarly, Caldwell and colleagues (2006) evaluated an intensive treatment program of incarcerated juvenile offenders that utilized reward-oriented approaches focusing on the interests of the adolescent and aimed to develop empathy skills. Juvenile offenders with high levels of CU traits were less likely to recidivate after a 2-year follow-up period compared to their peers with high CU traits allocated to a treatment as usual intervention. More recently, White and colleagues (2013) have reported significant improvements in behavioral and emotional domains following an evaluation of Functional Family Therapy delivered over 3–5 months (average of 10 sessions) in adolescents with high levels of conduct problems and CU traits. Future studies using randomized control designs are needed.

Although traditional treatments appear to work with children who have conduct problems and high levels of CU traits, these children typically enter treatment with the most severe behavioral presentations and even after improvement following treatment, often continue to present with ongoing problematic and concerning behaviors. More systematic research is required to pinpoint the specific components of existing treatments that work more or less effectively for these children in order to guide clinical practice. New treatment modules focusing on specific areas of functioning known to be problematic in children with high levels of CU traits appear promising. In a recent randomized controlled trial by Dadds *et al.* (2012b) treatment-as-usual (TAU) was evaluated with or without the adjunctive emotion recognition training (ERT), where the TAU comprised a fully manualized parent training program based on well-established parenting components. While ERT did not have an effect on the group as a whole, children with higher levels of CU traits (even those without a diagnosis of CD) showed more improvement in affective empathy and reduced conduct problems in response to ERT. Conversely, a number of parenting intervention studies suggest that children with high levels of CU traits may respond less well to some aspects of standard parenting interventions than their conduct problem peers with low levels of CU traits. For example, observational data relating to the parent–child interactions in the home in a standard 10-week parenting programme indicated that those children with high CU traits were less responsive to the "time-out" procedure, suggesting differential responsiveness to this traditional treatment component. This finding is consistent with the evidence from the experimental literature indicating that these children may be relatively punishment-insensitive (Frick & Viding, 2009). However, reward-based strategies appeared to be equally effective for all children with conduct problems in the Hawes and Dadds (2005) study.

These preliminary findings provide a promising basis for future programmes to incorporate tailored treatment strategies for children with higher levels of CU traits where specific components are added or removed from traditional treatment protocols. In relation to parenting programmes, it may be of interest to develop a component where parents are supported and scaffolded to respond in an enhanced positive manner. Given that previous parenting studies suggest that these children respond to warm parenting (Waller *et al.*, 2013), but can also evoke negative parental reactions (Hawes *et al.*, 2011), part of the clinical task is to be particularly mindful of fostering positive parental responses in a context where there may be sparse triggers for such responses from the child (e.g., the children do not appear to initiate eye contact with attachment figures; Dadds *et al.*, 2012b). More generally, it may be beneficial to nuance treatment targets with the child, such that they are in line with the child's self interest (where feasible and appropriate); heightened self interest is a pronounced feature of children with high levels of CU traits. Finally, it is noteworthy that behavioral interventions are increasingly being delivered in school settings (Viding *et al.*, 2011). Given that children with conduct problems and high CU traits often come from families characterized by multiple difficulties (where parents are also likely to have genetic and neurocognitive vulnerabilities), school settings may provide an important context, within a broader systemic intervention, for delivering consistent intervention

Summary—treatment

Although children with conduct problems and high levels of CU traits present with a distinct pattern of neurocognitive vulnerability, they appear to respond to traditional treatment approaches. However, given these children typically have more severe and enduring difficulties as well as a higher drop-out rate, there is a need to optimize or tailor our treatment approaches to improve outcomes for this subgroup of children. Preliminary findings suggest that some traditional treatment components (such as time out) are less effective with this group, while others (such as positive parenting and ERT) may be helpful to incorporate or enhance within traditional treatment models.

Future developments and necessary research

Although our understanding of developmental vulnerability to psychopathy has increased substantially over recent decades, several important avenues of research remain outstanding. CU traits can now be used as a specifier when diagnosing CD in children ("limited prosocial emotions"). The next decade of research and clinical practice will show how successful the DSM-5 specifier criteria are in delineating a meaningful subgroup of children with CD. Although more research into risk factors for CU traits is required, there is also a need to move from risk factor documentation to understanding whether all of the proposed risk factors are causal, what the mechanisms by which they increase risk for CU traits are and whether they are modifiable. Longitudinal research utilizing multiple methodologies within a genetically informative framework is required to really advance our understanding of risk and protective mechanisms that are important. Related to this quest, and because we know that CU traits (and conduct problems with CU traits) are heritable, there is a challenge to find genes that increase risk for CU traits. In the coming years we are likely to discover that some of the polymorphisms we thought were important simply represent false positives and others, which at first sight appeared less intuitive, may represent true genetic risk. Similarly, we do not know very much about environmental factors that increase vulnerability to CU traits (and conduct problems with CU traits). It will be important for future studies to investigate both mothering and fathering over time and to tease out whether, for example, parenting factors represent true environmental risk factors or genetic vulnerability within families. Addressing such questions effectively represents a challenge to basic research, but further advances in this field will help us better understand how risk factors in childhood may lead to the development of psychopathy in adulthood. We

think that a better delineation of (even putative) causal mechanisms has the potential to inform more effective approaches to prevention and treatment for at-risk children. Although it will be helpful to examine what aspects of current treatments best work for children with conduct problems and high CU traits, development of new treatment components and strategies will benefit from insights gained from basic science studies. These will include investigations to the degree to which the emotional impairments seen in children with CU traits are fixed, or may be either ameliorated or compensated for by both effortful and also more implicit strategies (see e.g., Dadds *et al.*, 2008).

Finally, a few recent studies suggest that CU traits may be an important clinical indicator even in the absence of conduct problems (e.g., Rowe *et al.*, 2010; Kumsta *et al.*, 2012). Research is clearly needed to follow up children who have high levels of CU traits, but who do not qualify for a diagnosis of CD. We do not currently know if these children have a similar neurocognitive profile to their peers with CU traits and conduct problems. We also do not have good data on how they fare in adulthood.

Conclusions

Developmental risk for psychopathy is currently indexed by diagnosing conduct problems with CU traits ("limited prosocial emotions" in DSM-5). Behaviorally, children with this presentation are characterized by severe and proactive antisocial and violent behavior and little concern for the feelings or welfare of other people. Children with conduct problems and CU traits appear genetically vulnerable to conduct problems, although the precise nature of genetic risk and how it may operate together with environmental risk factors is currently unknown. However, it is encouraging and worth emphasizing that children with conduct problems and CU traits appear to benefit from parenting treatments. The challenge for the next 10 years is to delineate more precisely what works for these children and how current intervention and prevention programmes might be optimized in ways that would improve engagement as well as clinical outcomes. For example, experimental psychology and neuroimaging work indicate that children with conduct problems and CU traits have an attenuated response to other people's distress and pain and do not readily learn from punishment (and to some extent reward). These basic science findings suggest that some socialization techniques, such as empathy induction and punishment, may have more limited success with this group of children. Further research determining the degree of malleability in how these children process affective information, as well as possible compensatory cognitive-affective functions that could be harnessed to scaffold any atypical processing, will be important next steps in informing how traditional programmes of intervention can be modified and enhanced. There is every reason to be optimistic in this regard, but it will require a step-change in how basic science and clinical practice researchers collaborate, if we are to make genuine progress.

Acknowledgements

The authors' research into development of psychopathy is supported by the Medical Research Council and the Economic and Social Research Council. Essi Viding is a Royal Society Wolfson Research Merit Award holder.

References

Adolphs, R. (2010) What does the amygdala contribute to social cognition? *Annals of the New York Academy of Sciences* **1191**, 42–61.

Adolphs, R. *et al.* (2001) Abnormal processing of social information from faces in autism. *Journal of Cognitive Neuroscience* **13**, 232–240.

Anastassiou-Hadjicharalambous, X. & Warden, D. (2008) Physiologically-indexed and self-perceived affective empathy in conduct-disordered children high and low on callous–unemotional traits. *Child Psychiatry and Human Development* **39**, 503–517.

Barker, E.D. *et al.* (2011) The impact of prenatal maternal risk, fearless temperament and early parenting on adolescent callous-unemotional traits: a 14-year longitudinal investigation. *Journal of Child Psychology and Psychiatry* **52**, 878–888.

Baron-Cohen, S. *et al.* (1985) Does the autistic child have a "theory of mind"? *Cognition* **21**, 37–46.

Barry, C.T. *et al.* (2000) The importance of callous-unemotional traits for extending the concept of psychopathy to children. *Journal of Abnormal Psychology* **109**, 335–340.

Beitchman, J.H. *et al.* (2012) Childhood aggression, callous-unemotional traits and oxytocin genes. *European Child and Adolescent Psychiatry* **21**, 125–132.

Bezdjian, S. *et al.* (2011) Psychopathic personality in children: genetic and environmental contributions. *Psychological Medicine* **41**, 589–600.

Birbaumer, N. *et al.* (2005) Deficient fear conditioning in psychopathy: a functional magnetic resonance imaging study. *Archives of General Psychiatry* **62**, 799–805.

Blair, R.J.R. (1999) Responsiveness to distress cues in the child with psychopathic tendencies. *Personality and Individual Differences* **27**, 135–145.

Blair, R.J.R. *et al.* (2001) A selective impairment in the processing of sad and fearful expressions in children with psychopathic tendencies. *Journal of Abnormal Child Psychology* **29**, 491–498.

Blair, R.J.R. *et al.* (2005) *The Psychopath: Emotion and the Brain*. Blackwell, Oxford.

Bowlby, J. (1946) *Forty-four Juvenile Thieves: Their Home Life*. Bailliere, Tindall & Cox, London.

Burnett, S. *et al.* (2009) Development during adolescence of the neural processing of social emotion. *Journal of Cognitive Neuroscience* **21**, 1736–1750.

Caldwell, M. *et al.* (2006) Treatment response of adolescent offenders with psychopathy features: a two-year follow-up. *Criminal Justice and Behavior* **33**, 571–596.

Canino, G. *et al.* (2010) Does the prevalence of CD and ODD vary across cultures? *Social Psychiatry and Psychiatric Epidemiology*. **45**, 695–704.

Caspi, A. *et al.* (2002). Role of genotype in the cycle of violence in maltreated children. *Science,* **297**, 851–854.

Cima, M. *et al.* (2008) Self- reported trauma, cortisol levels, and aggression in psychopathic and non-psychopathic prison inmates. *Biological Psychology* **78**, 75–86.

Cleckley, H. (1941) *The Mask of Sanity*, 1st edn. Mosby, St Louis, MO.

Colledge, E. & Blair, R.J.R. (2001) Relationship between attention-deficit-hyperactivity disorder and psychopathic tendencies in children. *Personality and Individual Differences* **30**, 1175–1187.

Cornell, D.G. *et al.* (1996) Psychopathy in instrumental and reactive violent offenders. *Journal of Consulting and Clinical Psychology* **64**, 783–790.

Craig, A.D.B. (2009) How do you feel—now? The anterior insula and human awareness. *Nature Reviews Neuroscience* **10**, 59–70.

Critchley, H.D. *et al.* (2004) Neural systems supporting interoceptive awareness. *Nature Neuroscience* **7**, 189–195.

Dadds, M.R. *et al.* (2006) Associations among cruelty to animals, family conflict, and psychopathic traits in childhood. *Journal of Interpersonal Violence* **21**, 411–429.

Dadds, M.R. *et al.* (2008) Reduced eye gaze explains "fear blindness" in childhood psychopathic traits. *Journal of American Academy of Child and Adolescent Psychiatry* **47**, 455–463.

Dadds, M.R. *et al.* (2011) Impaired attention to the eyes of attachment figures and the developmental origins of psychopathy. *Journal of Child Psychology and Psychiatry* **52**, 238–245.

Dadds, M.R. *et al.* (2012a) Love, eye contact and the developmental origins of empathy vs. psychopathy. *British Journal of Psychiatry* **200**, 191–196.

Dadds, M.R. *et al.* (2012b) Outcomes, moderators, and mediators of empathic-emotion recognition training for complex conduct problems in childhood. *Psychiatry Research* **199**, 201–207.

Dadds, M.R. *et al.* (2013) Replication of a ROBO2 polymorphism associated with conduct problems but not psychopathic tendencies in children. *Psychiatric Genetics* **23**, 251–254.

Davidson, R.J. & Irwin, W. (1999) The functional neuroanatomy of emotion and affective style. *Trends in Cognitive Sciences* **3**, 11–21.

Davidson, R.J. *et al.* (2000) Emotion, plasticity, context, and regulation: perspectives from affective neuroscience. *Psychological Bulletin* **126**, 890–909.

De Brito, S. A. *et al.* (2009). Size matters: increased grey matter in boys with conduct problems and callous–unemotional traits. *Brain,* **132**, 843–852.

De Brito, S.A. *et al.* (2011) Small, but not perfectly formed: decreased white matter concentration in boys with psychopathic tendencies. *Molecular Psychiatry* **16**, 476–477.

De Wied, M. *et al.* (2012) Verbal, facial and autonomic responses to empathy-eliciting film clips by disruptive male adolescents with high versus low callous-unemotional traits. *Journal of Abnormal Child Psychology* **40**, 211–223.

Essau, C.A. *et al.* (2006) Callous-unemotional traits in a community sample of adolescents. *Assessment* **13**, 454–469.

Ezpeleta, L. *et al.* (2013) Inventory of callous-unemotional traits in a community sample of preschoolers. *Journal of Clinical Child and Adolescent Psychology* **42**, 91–105.

Fanti, K.A. (2013) Individual, social, and behavioral factors associated with co-occurring conduct problems and callous-unemotional traits. *Journal of Abnormal Child Psychology* **41**, 811–824.

Fanti, K.A. *et al.* (2009) Linking callous-unemotional traits to instrumental and non-instrumental forms of aggression. *Journal of Psychopathological Behavior Assessment* **31**, 285–298.

Fanti, K.A. *et al.* (2013) Variants of callous-unemotional conduct problems in a community sample of adolescents. *Journal of Youth and Adolescence* **42**, 964–979.

Fine, C. *et al.* (2001) Dissociation between 'theory of mind' and executive functions in a patient with early left amygdala damage. *Brain* **124**, 287–298.

Finger, E.C. *et al.* (2008) Abnormal ventromedial prefrontal cortex function in children with psychopathic traits during reversal learning. *Archives of General Psychiatry* **65**, 586–594.

Finger, E. C. *et al.* (2011). Disrupted reinforcement signaling in the orbitofrontal cortex and caudate in youths with conduct disorder or oppositional defiant disorder and a high level of psychopathic traits. *American Journal of Psychiatry,* **168**, 152–162.

Fontaine, N.M.G. *et al.* (2008) Dimensions of psychopathy and their relationships to cognitive functioning in children. *Journal of Clinical Child and Adolescent Psychology* **37**, 690–696.

Fontaine, N.M.G. *et al.* (2010) Etiology of different developmental trajectories of callous–unemotional traits. *Journal of the American Academy of Child & Adolescent Psychiatry* **49**, 656–664.

Fontaine, N.M.G. *et al.* (2011) Predictors and outcomes of joint trajectories of callous–unemotional traits and conduct problems in childhood. *Journal of Abnormal Psychology* **120**, 730–742.

Forsman, M. *et al.* (2007) Persistent disruptive childhood behavior and psychopathic personality in adolescence: a twin study. *British Journal of Developmental Psychology* **25**, 383–398.

Forsman, M. *et al.* (2008) Genetic effects explain the stability of psychopathic personality from mid- to late adolescence. *Journal of Abnormal Psychology* **117**, 606–617.

Forth, A.E. *et al.* (2003) *The Psychopathy Checklist: Youth Version.* Multi-Health Systems, Toronto, Ontario, Canada.

Fowler, T. *et al.* (2009) Psychopathy trait scores in adolescents with childhood ADHD: the contribution of genotypes affecting MAOA, 5HTT and COMT activity. *Psychiatric Genetics* **19**, 312–319.

Fowles, D.C. & Kochanska, G. (2000) Temperament as a moderator of pathways to conscience in children: the contribution of electrodermal activity. *Psychophysiology* **37**, 788–795.

Frick, P. J. (2003). *The inventory of callous-unemotional traits.* Unpublished rating scale, The University of New Orleans.

Frick, P.J. & Hare, R.D. (2001) *The Antisocial Process Screening Device.* Multi-Health Systems, Toronto.

Frick, P.J. & Viding, E. (2009) Antisocial behavior from a developmental psychopathology perspective. *Development and Psychopathology* **21**, 1111–1131.

Frick, P.J. *et al.* (1994) Psychopathy and conduct problems in children. *Journal of Abnormal Psychology* **103**, 700–707.

Frick, P.J. *et al.* (1999) The association between anxiety and psychopathy dimensions in children. *Journal of Abnormal Child Psychology* **27**, 383–392.

Frick, P.J. *et al.* (2003a) Callous-unemotional traits and conduct problems in the prediction of conduct problem severity, aggression, and self-report delinquency. *Journal of Abnormal Child Psychology* **31**, 457–470.

Frick, P.J. *et al.* (2003b) The 4 year stability of psychopathic traits in non-referred youth. *Behavioral Sciences & the Law* **21**, 713–736.

Frick, P.J. *et al.* (2005) Callous-unemotional traits in predicting the severity and stability of conduct problems and delinquency. *Journal of Abnormal Child Psychology* **33**, 471–487.

Frith, U. & Happe, F. (2005) Autism spectrum disorder. *Current Biology* **15**, R786–790.

Gao, Y. *et al.* (2009) The neurobiology of psychopathy: a neurodevelopmental perspective. *Canadian Journal of Psychiatry* **54**, 813–823.

Glenn, A.L. *et al.* (2011) Increased testosterone-to-cortisol ratio in psychopathy. *Journal of Abnormal Psychology* **120**, 389–399.

Gogtay, N. *et al.* (2004) Dynamic mapping of human cortical development during childhood through early adulthood. *Proceedings of the National Academy of Science* **101**, 8174–8179.

Hare, R.D. (1970) *Psychopathy: Theory and Research.* John Wiley & Sons, New York.

Hare, R.D. (1980) A research scale for the assessment of psychopathy in criminal populations. *Personality and Individual Differences* **1**, 111–119.

Hare, R.D. (1991) *The Hare Psychopathy Checklist-Revised.* Multi-Health Systems, Toronto, Ontario.

Hare, R.D. (2003) *Hare Psychopathy Checklist-Revised PCL-R,* 2nd edn. Multi Health Systems, Toronto.

Hawes, D.J. & Dadds, M.R. (2005) The treatment of conduct problems in children with callous-unemotional traits. *Journal of Consulting and Clinical Psychology* **73**, 737–741.

Hawes, D.J. *et al.* (2009) Cortisol, callous-unemotional traits, and pathways to antisocial behavior. *Current Opinion in Psychiatry* **22**, 357–362.

Hawes, D.J. *et al.* (2011) Do childhood callous-unemotional traits drive change in parenting practices? *Journal of Clinical Child and Adolescent Psychology* **40**, 507–518.

Hinshaw, S.P. (1987) On the distinction between attentional deficits/hyperactivity and conduct problems/aggression in child psychopathology. *Psychological Bulletin* **101**, 443–463.

Hippler, K. & Klicpera, C. (2003) A retrospective analysis of the clinical case records of 'autistic psychopaths' diagnosed by Hans Asperger and his team at the University Children's Hospital, Vienna. *Philosophical Transactions of the Royal Society of London. Series B, Biological Sciences* **358**, 291–301.

Jones, A.P. *et al.* (2009a) Phenotypic and aetiological associations between psychopathic tendencies, autistic traits, and emotion attribution. *Criminal Justice and Behavior* **36**, 1198–1212.

Jones, A.P. *et al.* (2009b) Amygdala hypoactivity to fearful faces in boys with conduct problems and callous–unemotional traits. *American Journal of Psychiatry* **166**, 95–102.

Jones, A.P. *et al.* (2010) Feeling, caring, knowing: different types of empathy deficit in boys with psychopathic tendencies and autism spectrum disorder. *Journal of Child Psychology and Psychiatry* **51**, 1188–1197.

Kahn, R.E. *et al.* (2012) The effects of including a callous–unemotional specifier for the diagnosis of conduct disorder. *Journal of Child Psychology and Psychiatry* **53**, 271–282.

Kahn, R.E. *et al.* (2013) Distinguishing primary and secondary variants of callous-unemotional traits among adolescents in a clinic-referred sample. *Psychological Assessment* **25**, 966–978.

Kedia, G. *et al.* (2008) An agent harms a victim: a functional magnetic resonance imaging study on specific moral emotions. *Journal of Cognitive Neuroscience* **20**, 1788–1798.

Kiehl, K.A. *et al.* (2001) Limbic abnormalities in affective processing by criminal psychopaths as revealed by functional magnetic resonance imaging. *Biological Psychiatry* **50**, 677–684.

Kimonis, E.R. *et al.* (2008) Assessing callousunemotional traits in adolescent offenders: validation of the inventory of callous-unemotional traits. *International Journal of Law and Psychiatry* **31**, 241–252.

Kimonis, E.R. *et al.* (2012) Primary and secondary variants of juvenile psychopathy differ in emotional processing. *Development and Psychopathology* **24**, 1091–1103.

Kimonis, E.R. *et al.* (2013) Callous-unemotional traits in incarcerated adolescents. *Psychological Assessment* **26**, 227–237.

Kolko, D.J. & Pardini, D.A. (2010) ODD dimensions, ADHD, and callous– unemotional traits as predictors of treatment response in children with disruptive behavior disorders. *Journal of Abnormal Psychology* **119**, 713–725.

Kosson, D.S. *et al.* (2002) The reliability and validity of the psychopathy checklist: youth version (PCL:YV) in nonincarcerated adolescent males. *Psychological Assessment* **14**, 97–109.

Kumsta, R. *et al.* (2012) Adolescent callous-unemotional traits and conduct disorder in adoptees exposed to severe early deprivation. *British Journal of Psychiatry* **200**, 197–201.

Lansford, J.E. *et al.* (2002) Long-term effects of early child physical maltreatment on psychological, behavioral and academic problems in adolescence: a 12-year prospective study. *Archives of Pediatrics and Adolescents Medicine* **156**, 824–830.

Larsson, H. *et al.* (2008) Callous–unemotional traits and antisocial behavior. *Criminal Justice and Behavior* **35**, 197–211.

Levesque, J. *et al.* (2004) Neural basis of emotional self-regulation in childhood. *Neuroscience* **129**, 361–369.

Lockwood, P.L. *et al.* (2013) Association of callous traits with reduced neural response to others' pain in children with conduct problems. *Current Biology* **23**, 901–905.

Loeber, R. & Pardini, D. (2008) Neurobiology and the development of violence: common assumptions and controversies. *Philosophical Transactions of the Royal Society of Biological Sciences* **363**, 2491–2503.

Loney, B.R. *et al.* (2006) The relation between salivary cortisol, callous-unemotional traits, and conduct problems in an adolescent non-referred sample. *Journal of Child Psychology and Psychiatry* **47**, 30–36.

Loney, B.R. *et al.* (2007) A preliminary examination of the intergenerational continuity of maternal psychopathic features. *Aggressive Behavior* **33**, 14–25.

Lykken, D.T. (1957) A study of anxiety in the sociopathic personality. *Journal of Abnormal and Social Psychology* **55**, 6–10.

Lynam, D.R. (1996) Early identification of chronic offenders: who is the fledgling psychopath? *Psychological Bulletin* **120**.

Lynam, D.R. *et al.* (2007) Longitudinal evidence that psychopathy scores in early adolescence predict adult psychopathy. *Journal of Abnormal Psychology* **116**, 155–165.

Malik, A.I. *et al.* (2012) The role of oxytocin and oxytocin receptor gene variants in childhood-onset aggression. *Genes, Brain and Behavior* **11**, 545–551.

Marsh, A.A. & Blair, R.J. (2008) Deficits in facial affect recognition among antisocial populations: a meta-analysis. *Neuroscience and Biobehavioral Reviews* **32**, 454–465.

Marsh, A.A. *et al.* (2008) Reduced amygdala response to fearful expressions in children and adolescents with callous–unemotional traits and disruptive behavior disorders. *American Journal of Psychiatry* **165**, 712–720.

Marsh, A.A. *et al.* (2011) Reduced amygdala-orbitofrontal connectivity during moral judgments in youths with disruptive behavior disorders and psychopathic traits. *Psychiatry Research* **194**, 279–286.

Marsh, A.A. *et al.* (2013) Empathic responsiveness in amygdala and anterior cingulate cortex in youths with psychopathic traits. *Journal of Child Psychology and Psychiatry* **54**, 900–910.

McCrory, E.J. *et al.* (2011a) Heightened neural reactivity to threat in child victims of family violence. *Current Biology* **21**, 947–948.

McCrory, E.J. *et al.* (2011b) The neuroscience and genetics of childhood maltreatment. In: *Child Psychology and Psychiatry*. (eds D. Skuse, H. Bruce, L. Dowdney & D. Mrazek), pp. 121–127. John Wiley & Sons, Chichester.

McCrory, E.J. *et al.* (2013) Amygdala activation in maltreated children during pre-attentive emotional processing. *British Journal of Psychiatry* **202**, 269–276.

McMahon, R.J. *et al.*, & the Conduct Problems Prevention Research Group. (2010) Predictive validity of callous–unemotional traits measured in early adolescence with respect to multiple antisocial outcomes. *Journal of Abnormal Psychology* **119**, 752–763.

Medford, N. & Critchley, H.D. (2010) Conjoint activity of anterior insular and anterior cingulate cortex: awareness and response. *Brain Structure and Function* **214**, 535–549.

Mitchell, D.G. (2011) The nexus between decision making and emotion regulation: a review of convergent neurocognitive substrates. *Behavioural Brain Research* **217**, 215–231.

Mitchell, D.G.V. *et al.* (2008) The contribution of ventrolateral and dorsolateral prefrontal cortex to response reversal. *Behavioural Brain Research* **187**, 80–87.

Moul, C. *et al.* (2013) An exploration of the serotonin system in antisocial boys with high levels of callous-unemotional traits. *PLoS ONE* **8**, e56619.

O'Doherty, J.P. (2004) Reward representations and reward-related learning in the human brain: insights from neuroimaging. *Current Opinion in Neurobiology* **14**, 769–776.

Obradovic, J. *et al.* (2007) Measuring interpersonal callousness in boys from childhood to adolescence: an examination of longitudinal invariance and temporal stability. *Journal of Clinical Child and Adolescent Psychology* **36**, 276–292.

Ochsner, K.N. & Gross, J.J. (2005) The cognitive control of emotion. *Trends in Cognitive Sciences* **9**, 242–249.

Pardini, D.A. & Fite, P.J. (2010) Symptoms of conduct disorder, oppositional defiant disorder, attention-deficit/hyperactivity disorder, and callous–unemotional traits as unique predictors of psychosocial maladjustment in boys: advancing an evidence base for DSM-V. *Journal of the American Academy of Child & Adolescent Psychiatry* **49**, 1134–1144.

Pardini, D.A. *et al.* (2012) The clinical utility of the proposed DSM-5 callous-unemotional subtype of conduct disorder in young girls. *Journal of the American Academy of Child and Adolescent Psychiatry* **51**, 62–73.

Patrick, C.J. (1994) Emotion and psychopathy: startling new insights. *Psychophysiology* **31**, 319–330.

Peters, J. & Buchel, C. (2010) Neural representations of subjective reward value. *Behavioral Brain Research* **213**, 135–141.

Reid, J. *et al.* (2002) *Antisocial Behavior in Children and Adolescents*. American Psychological Association, Washington, DC.

Rogers, J. *et al.* (2006) Autism spectrum disorder and psychopathy: shared cognitive underpinnings or double hit? *Psychological Medicine* **1–10**.

Rolls, E.T. & Grabenhorst, F. (2008) The orbitofrontal cortex and beyond: from affect to decision-making. *Progress in Neurobiology* **86**, 216–244.

Roose, A. *et al.* (2010) Assessing the affective features of psychopathy in adolescence: a further validation of the inventory of callous and unemotional traits. *Assessment* **17**, 44–57.

Rosen, H.J. & Levenson, R.W. (2009) The emotional brain: combining insights from patients and basic science. *Neurocase* **15**, 173–181.

Rowe, R. *et al.* (2010) Developmental pathways in oppositional defiant disorder and conduct disorder. *Journal of Abnormal Psychology* **119**, 726–738.

Rubia, K. (2011) "Cool" inferior fronto-striatal dysfunction in attention-deficit/hyperactivity disorder versus "hot" ventromedial orbitofrontal-limbic dysfunction in conduct disorder: a review. *Biological Psychiatry* **69**, 69–87.

Rushworth, M.F. *et al.* (2007) Contrasting roles for cingulate and orbitofrontal cortex in decisions and social behaviour. *Trends in Cognitive Sciences* **11**, 168–176.

Rutter, M. (2005) Commentary: what is the meaning and utility of the psychopathy concept? *Journal of Abnormal Child Psychology* **33**, 499–503.

Sadeh, N. *et al.* (2010) Serotonin transporter gene associations with psychopathic traits in youth vary as a function of socioeconomic resources. *Journal of Abnormal Psychology* **119**, 604–609.

Schwenck, C. *et al.* (2012). Empathy in children with autism and conduct disorder: group-specific profiles and developmental aspects. *Journal of Child Psychology and Psychiatry,* **53**, 651–659.

Sebastian, C.L. *et al.* (2012) Neural processing associated with cognitive and affective theory of mind in adolescents and adults. *Social Cognitive and Affective Neuroscience* **7**, 53–63.

Sebastian, C.L. *et al.* (2013) Neural responses to fearful eyes in children with conduct problems and varying levels of callous-unemotional traits. *Psychological Medicine* **44**, 99–109.

Sergerie, K. *et al.* (2008) The role of the amygdala in emotional processing: a quantitative meta-analysis of functional neuroimaging studies. *Neuroscience and Biobehavioral Reviews* **32**, 811–830.

Shaw, P. *et al.* (2010) Childhood psychiatric disorders as anomalies in neurodevelopmental trajectories. *Human Brain Mapping* **31**, 917–925.

Stadler, C. *et al.* (2010) Cortisol reactivity in boys with attention-deficit/hyperactivity disorder and disruptive behavior problems: the impact of callous unemotional traits. *Psychiatry Research* **187**, 204–209.

Sumich, A. *et al.* (2012) Electrophysiological correlates of CU traits show abnormal regressive maturation in adolescents with conduct problems. *Personality and Individual Differences* **53**, 862–867.

Sylvers, P.D. *et al.* (2011) Psychopathic traits and preattentive threat processing in children: a novel test of the fearlessness hypothesis. *Psychological Science* **22**, 1280–1287.

Takahashi, H. *et al.* (2004) Brain activation associated with evaluative processes of guilt and embarrassment: an FMRI study. *Neuroimage* **23**, 967–974.

Taylor, E.A. *et al.* (1986) Conduct disorder and hyperactivity: I. Separation of hyperactivity and antisocial conduct in British child psychiatric patients. *British Journal of Psychiatry* **149**, 760–767.

Tversky, A. & Kahneman, D. (1981) The framing of decisions and the psychology of choice. *Science* **211**, 453–458.

Verona, E. *et al.* (2001) Psychopathy, antisocial personality, and suicide risk. *Journal of Abnormal Psychology* **110**, 462–470.

Viding, E. *et al.* (2010) In search of genes associated with risk for psychopathic tendencies in children: a two-stage genome-wide association study of pooled DNA. *Journal of Child Psychology and Psychiatry* **51**, 780–788.

Viding, E. & McCrory, E.J. (2012) Genetic and neurocognitive contributions to the development of psychopathy. *Development and Psychopathology* **24**, 969–983.

Viding, E. *et al.* (2005) Evidence for substantial genetic risk for psychopathy in 7-year-olds. *Journal of Child Psychology and Psychiatry* **46**, 592–597.

Viding, E. *et al.* (2007) Aetiology of the relationship between callous–unemotional traits and conduct problems in childhood. *British Journal of Psychiatry* **49**, 33–38.

Viding, E. *et al.* (2008) Heritability of antisocial behaviour at 9: do callous–unemotional traits matter? *Developmental Science* **11**, 17–22.

Viding, E. *et al.* (2009) Negative parental discipline, conduct problems and callous–unemotional traits: monozygotic twin differences study. *British Journal of Psychiatry* **195**, 414–419.

Viding, E. *et al.* (2011) Behavioural problems and bullying at school: can cognitive neuroscience shed new light on an old problem? *Trends in Cognitive Sciences* **15**, 289–291.

Viding, E. *et al.* (2012) Amygdala response to preattentive masked fear in children with conduct problems: the role of callous-unemotional traits. *American Journal of Psychiatry* **169**, 1109–1116.

Viding, E. *et al.* (2013) Genetics of callous-unemotional behavior in children. *PLoS One* **8**, e65789.

Visscher, P.M. *et al.* (2012) Five years of GWAS discovery. *The American Journal of Human Genetics* **90**, 7–24.

Vizard, E. *et al.* (2007) Developmental trajectories associated with juvenile sexually abusive behaviour and emerging severe personality disorder in childhood: 3-year study. *British Journal of Psychiatry* **190**, S27–S32.

Vuilleumier, P. & Pourtois, G. (2007) Distributed and interactive brain mechanisms during emotion face perception: evidence from functional neuroimaging. *Neuropsychologia* **45**, 174–194.

Wager, T.D. *et al.* (2008) Prefrontal–subcortical pathways mediating successful emotion regulation. *Neuron* **59**, 1037–1050.

Waller, R. *et al.* (2013) What are the associations between parenting, callous-unemotional traits, and antisocial behavior in youth? A systematic review of evidence. *Clinical Psychology Review* **33**, 593–608.

White, S.F. *et al.* (2009) Differential correlates to self-report and parent-report of callous-unemotional traits in a sample of juvenile sexual offenders. *Behavioral Sciences and Law* **27**, 910–928.

White, S.F. *et al.* (2013) Callous-unemotional traits and response to functional family therapy in adolescent offenders. *Behavioral Sciences & the Law* **31**, 271–285.

White, S.F. *et al.* (2013) Disrupted expected value and prediction error signaling in youths with disruptive behavior disorders during a passive avoidance task. *American Journal of Psychiatry* **170**, 315–323.

Williamson, S. *et al.* (1987) Violence: criminal psychopaths and their victims. *Canadian Journal of Behavioral Science* **19**, 454–462.

Yang, Y. & Raine, A. (2009) Prefrontal structural and functional brain imaging findings in antisocial, violent and psychopathic individuals: a metaanalysis. *Psychiatry Research* **174**, 81–88.

Suggested further reading/sources of additional information

Salekin, R.T. & Lynam, D.R. (eds) (2010) *Handbook of Child and Adolescent Psychopathy*. Guilford Press, New York.

Prof. Paul Frick's homepage containing articles and assessment tools: http://www.psyc.uno.edu/Frick%20Lab/Home.html.

CHAPTER 69

Gender dysphoria and paraphilic sexual disorders

Kenneth J. Zucker[1] and Michael C. Seto[2]
[1] Centre for Addiction and Mental Health, Toronto, Ontario, Canada
[2] Royal Ottawa Health Care Group, Integrated Forensic Program, Brockville, Ontario, Canada

Introduction

This chapter provides a review of two distinct diagnostic conditions: gender dysphoria (GD) in children and adolescents and paraphilic sexual behavior (primarily sexual offenses against children) in adolescents. For each condition, the phenomenology is reviewed. In the case of GD, there has been a major shift in conceptualization, which is now reflected in the wording of the diagnostic criteria. For each condition, the following sections review the available assessment measures before considering associated psychopathology and its correlates as well as sex differences in referral rates. Next, the knowledge bases concerning the known biological and psychosocial risk factors are summarized. For each disorder, the final section focuses, from a developmental perspective, on the currently available therapeutic approaches to clinical management.

Gender dysphoria (GD)

Characteristics and diagnosis of the condition
Phenomenology

Children with GD display behaviors that reflect identification with the other sex (Zucker & Bradley, 1995). For children with GD referred before age 12, most such behaviors onset between ages 2–4 (Ruble *et al.*, 2006). In patients first observed in adolescence, history is more varied, with some onsets in early childhood and others at later ages, typically around puberty (Zucker *et al.*, 2012a). This suggests the presence of early-onset and late-onset forms. In the early-onset form for biological males, sexual orientation is almost always homosexual (androphilic); in the late-onset form, it is almost always nonhomosexual and often co-occurs with transvestic fetishism (with or without autogynephilia–sexual arousal associated with the thought or image of oneself as a woman) (Blanchard, 2010).

In biological females, the early-onset form is typically associated with a homosexual (gynephilic) sexual orientation and, in the late-onset form, is typically nonhomosexual (see Lawrence, 2010).

Normal and pathological behaviors

Youth with GD show overt sex-typed behavior that is "inverted" in relation to their natal sex peers. This can be described as "gender variant" or "gender nonconforming," which some suggest is not necessarily pathological (Gray *et al.*, 2012; Giordano, 2013). There is, however, some consensus in considering GD abnormal when it is associated with significant distress with regard to their felt gender. It is more difficult to consider a strong desire to alter the body to conform to the felt psychological state in adolescent or adult GD a form of normative variation.

GD occurs in many cultures, with remarkable phenomenological similarity. Many non-Western cultures have coined terms to describe what appear to be equivalents to GD and "transsexualism" in modern societies.

DSM-5 and the ICD

DSM-5 treats GD substantially differently from the DSM-IV-TR (see Zucker *et al.*, 2013):

1 The label was changed from gender identity disorder (GID) to GD, which is considered a more accurate term (Fisk, 1973) and which highlights the salience of "distress" (dysphoria) (Knudson *et al.*, 2010). There was considerable support for this change related to a reduction in stigma (Vance *et al.*, 2010).

2 In DSM-5, GD has its own chapter and thus has been decoupled from the sexual dysfunctions and paraphilias, which also have their own chapters. This reflected incomplete overlap among these conditions. Although GD co-occurs with one paraphilia, transvestic disorder (Blanchard, 2010), the advantages of this change outweighed the disadvantages.

Rutter's Child and Adolescent Psychiatry, Sixth Edition.
Edited by Anita Thapar and Daniel S. Pine, James F. Leckman, Stephen Scott, Margaret J. Snowling, Eric Taylor.
© 2015 John Wiley & Sons Ltd. Published 2018 by John Wiley & Sons Ltd.

3 The Point A diagnostic criterion (which lists the symptoms) introduced a conceptual shift by emphasizing "incongruence" between one's experienced/expressed and assigned gender, as opposed to "cross-gender identification" in DSM-IV-TR.

4 The GD criteria for children require " … a strong desire to be of the other gender or an insistence that he or she is the other gender (or some alternative gender different from one's assigned gender)." This could sharpen distinctions between GD and normative variation (see Zucker, 2010).

5 Whether individuals born with a physical intersex condition (now termed a disorder of sex development) (DSD) should be eligible for a diagnosis if GD is contentious (see Meyer-Bahlburg, 1994). Recent evidence suggests that some individuals with a DSD experience GD (Richter-Appelt & Sandberg, 2010; Pasterski et al., 2014) and these individuals only share some features with individuals with GD without DSD (American Psychiatric Association, 2013, pp. 455–456). DSD appears as a specifier in DSM-5.

6 For adolescents (and adults), a DSM-IV-TR specifier for sexual attraction was eliminated, a controversial decision. Sexual orientation in GD does clearly relate to many clinical features (see Zucker et al., 2012a) and may also identify specific mechanisms generating GD (Lawrence, 2010). However, sexual orientation minimally influences treatment (Cohen-Kettenis & Pfäfflin, 2010) and may not reflect a difference in symptom expression of GD, a key feature of other DSM-5 specifiers.

The ICD-10 (World Health Organization, 1992) has a section on GIDs (F64) resembling DSM-IV-TR. It includes the categories of Transsexualism and Gender Identity Disorder of Childhood. Plans for ICD-11 remain in the proposal stage (Drescher et al., 2012).

Assessment

Many scales are useful to assess GD in children (Zucker, 2005a; Zucker & Wood, 2011). Most show good discriminant validity, sensitivity, and specificity. Moreover, among gender-referred children, these measures can discriminate threshold versus subthreshold GD. Updated scales continue to show strong psychometrics (Zucker & Wood, 2011; Zucker et al., 2012a). The Gender Identity/Gender Dysphoria Questionnaire for Adolescents and Adults is one particularly useful measure (Singh et al., 2010).

Youth with GD show high rates of various forms of psychopathology relative to comparison groups. This has been documented most systematically using the Child Behavior Checklist (CBCL), the Teacher's Report Form (TRF), and the Youth Self-Report (YSR) form (Zucker & Bradley, 1995; Cohen-Kettenis et al., 2003; Zucker et al., 2012a; Steensma et al., 2014) (for review, see Zucker et al., 2014).

Behavior problems increase with age in boys with GD (Cohen-Kettenis et al., 2003; Steensma et al., 2014). Youth with GD experience significant peer difficulties (Zucker et al., 1997a; Cohen-Kettenis et al., 2003; Wallien et al., 2010; Shiffman, 2013) and peer difficulties relate to behavior problems (Cohen-Kettenis et al., 2003; Steensma et al., 2014). Recent

interest focuses on possible co-occurrence with autism spectrum disorders (ASD) (see de Vries et al., 2010) or at least the presence of intense unusual interests, in this context, to do with gender (see VanderLaan et al., 2015). Thus, assessment of GD requires the consideration of a broad range of psychopathology.

Epidemiology
Prevalence

Contemporary, large-scale epidemiological studies have not examined GD. Estimates of prevalence, therefore, emerge from other less-sophisticated sources, such as rates of treatment seeking. Overall, recent estimates suggest a prevalence of 0.005–0.014% in natal males and 0.002–0.003% in natal females (Zucker & Lawrence, 2009; American Psychiatric Association, 2013). Compared to older estimates, these figures have been interpreted as reflecting a notable increase in adults with GD (Coleman et al., 2011). In a recent community-based US study (Shields et al., 2013), 1.3% of youth in Grades 6–8 self-identified as transgender, although it is unclear how these rates relate to rates of DSM-5 GD.

Sex differences in referral rates

Among children between the ages of 3 and 12, boys are referred clinically more often than girls for concerns regarding gender identity. From one specialty clinic in Toronto, Canada, Wood et al. (2013) reported a sex ratio of 4.49:1 ($N = 577$) of boys to girls based on consecutive referrals from 1976 to 2011. Comparative data from the sole gender identity clinic for children in Amsterdam, The Netherlands also favored referral of boys over girls, but the sex ratio was smaller (2.02:1, $N = 468$).

Although the sex ratio favoring boys may reflect a bona fide sex difference in prevalence, social factors may also play a role. Parents, teachers, and peers are less tolerant of cross-gender behavior in boys than in girls, which might result in a sex-differential in clinical referral (Zucker & Bradley, 1995; Wallien et al., 2010). This appears to be particularly the case with relatively younger children; for example, Wood et al. (2013) reported a markedly skewed sex ratio of 33:1 of referred GD boys to girls among 3-year-olds, which gradually dropped to almost parity by age 12.

Referral rates of GD adolescents may be increasing. In the Toronto clinic, referral rates of adolescents between 2008 and 2011 showed a fivefold increase in magnitude compared to referred adolescents in 2000–2003 (Wood et al., 2013). Various explanations for this increase have been posited, including the destigmatization of gender-variant behavior and increased attention in media (Zucker et al., 2008).

Risk factors
Molecular and behavior genetics

Candidate gene studies have yielded mixed results and failures to replicate (Ngun et al., 2011). However, there is some supportive behavior genetic evidence: in clinical samples, identical twins are more likely to be concordant for GD than nonidentical twins (Heylens *et al.*, 2012; for a nonclinical sample, see Coolidge *et al.*, 2002). Moreover, in the general population, twin studies have shown that the liability for cross-gender behavior has a strong heritable component (van Beijsterveldt *et al.*, 2006). Other studies, however, have also identified strong shared and nonshared environmental influences (Iervolino *et al.*, 2005; Knafo *et al.*, 2005). Such environmental influences could, of course, pertain to nongenetic biological factors but could also involve postnatal psychosocial factors.

Prenatal sex hormones

Considerable research examines effects of prenatal sex hormones on sex-dimorphic behaviors (Baum, 2006). In humans, influence of prenatal sex hormones and rearing effects are hard to disentangle; accordingly, researchers have relied on children born with DSDs to separate out the relative influence of biological and psychosocial processes on psychosexual differentiation.

This research provides considerable evidence for an influence of prenatal sex hormones on postnatal sex-dimorphic behavior. For example, chromosomal females with congenital adrenal hyperplasia (CAH), who are exposed to sex-atypical levels of prenatal androgen, show more masculinized gender role behavior in childhood and adolescence and a higher rate of a bisexual/homosexual sexual orientation in adulthood (Zucker, 1999; Hines, 2004; Cohen-Bendahan *et al.*, 2005). Although most females with CAH show a sex-typical gender identity (Meyer-Bahlburg *et al.*, 2004; Dessens *et al.*, 2005), there is also evidence that GD is elevated compared to population base rates (Pasterski *et al.*, 2014).

Most youth with GD do not have a DSD. Accordingly, the search for biological influences on the development of GD must focus on factors that do not affect the configuration of the external genitalia. Prenatal hormonal influences may play a role, but there would have to be some kind of brain-genital dissociation in their impact (e.g., perhaps due to timing effects) (Goy *et al.*, 1988). Given that there are no post-mortem studies on brain neuroanatomy in GD children or youth, research has focused on various other biological factors.

Temperament

Activity level (AL) is a dimension of temperament with some evidence for a genetic basis and possibly prenatal hormonal influences (Campbell & Eaton, 1999). In general, boys have a higher AL than girls. Parents report lower levels of AL in boys with GD compared with controls (Bates *et al.*, 1979; Zucker & Bradley, 1995). Zucker and Bradley also found that girls with GD had a higher AL than control girls. It is possible that a sex-atypical AL is a temperamental factor that predisposes the development of GD. For example, a low-active boy with GD may find the typical play behavior of other boys to be incompatible with his own behavioral style, which might make it difficult for him to integrate successfully into a male peer group.

Sibling sex ratio and birth order

Compared to the sex ratio at birth in the general population, boys with GD have an excess of brothers to sisters (sibling sex ratio) and a later birth order. Moreover, other evidence shows that boys with GD are born later in relation to the number of older brothers (the "fraternal" birth order effect), but not sisters (Blanchard *et al.*, 1995; Zucker *et al.*, 1997b; Schagen *et al.*, 2012; VanderLaan *et al.*, 2015). In the Blanchard *et al.* study, clinical control boys showed no evidence for an altered sibling sex ratio or a late birth order nor did adolescent boys with transvestic fetishism (VanderLaan *et al.*, 2015). VanderLaan *et al.* established that the late fraternal birth order of GD males was specific to those with a homosexual sexual orientation in relation to birth sex, similar to what has been found in adult GD males with a homosexual sexual orientation, who also have an excess of brothers to sisters and a later birth order (Blanchard, 1997). Collectively, these studies show that the fraternal birth order effect in GD males parallels the same finding in homosexual men without GD (Bogaert & Skorska, 2011).

Psychosocial risk factors

Psychosocial factors must be shown to influence the emergence of marked cross-gender behavior in the first few years of life. Otherwise, such factors would be better conceptualized as perpetuating rather than predisposing to GD.

Social reinforcement

The parental response to early cross-gender behavior is usually not negative (Roberts *et al.*, 1987; Zucker & Bradley, 1995). Green (1974) concluded that "what comes closest so far to being a *necessary* variable is that, as any feminine behavior begins to emerge, there is *no* discouragement of that behavior by the child's principal caretaker" (p. 238, italics in original). The reasons for this response are diverse, as discussed elsewhere (Zucker & Bradley, 1995; Ehrensaft, 2011).

Cognitive-developmental factors

Cognitive factors may shape gender development (Martin *et al.*, 2002; Tobin *et al.*, 2010). Two elements appear relevant. First, early gender self-labeling may organize monitoring of social information in GD children, due to a "developmental lag" in cognitive gender constancy that leads to mislabeling (Zucker *et al.*, 1999; Wallien *et al.*, 2009). Such early cognitive mislabeling could support some kind of interactive effect between cognitions and cross-gendered behavior. Second, some young children may have rather rigid interests in sex-typed behavior: for girls, Halim *et al.* (2014) dubbed this the "pink frilly dress" phenomenon. Halim *et al.* argued that this gender rigidity was part of the young child's effort to master gender categories and to securely (affectively) place oneself in the "right" category. Parents of such children do not particularly encourage the rigidity, but they also do not discourage it and there is the assumption that such rigidity will wane over developmental time and that there will be a concomitant increase in gender flexibility. Other data support this possibility (VanderLaan *et al.*, 2015). The response to these early features could modulate the long-term course of cross-gender identity.

General psychopathology

Considerable research focuses on maternal psychopathology in GD. Both Marantz and Coates (1991) and Zucker (2005b) found higher rates of psychopathology, particularly emotional disorders, in mothers of boys with GD than comparison boys. Although psychopathology is elevated, this may reflect a non-specific risk factor, as similar findings occur in other disorders. Other work focuses on specificity in family factors, such as father absence, in GD. Across 10 samples of boys with GD, the rate of father absence was 34.5% (Zucker & Bradley, 1995) although this rate may not differ from other clinical populations. Green (1987) found that paternal separations occurred earlier in the families of boys with GD than healthy boys; therefore, it is possible that timing is an additional variable to consider.

Developmental trajectories

Boys

Two recent studies by Wallien and Cohen-Kettenis (2008, $n = 59$) and Singh (2012, $n = 139$) document outcome in boys. Wallien and Cohen-Kettenis found a GD persistence rate of 20.3% and Singh found a persistence rate of 12.2%. Regarding sexual orientation, a substantial majority (63.6–81%) was homosexual/bisexual in fantasy and at least half were homosexual or bisexual in behavior.

Girls

With regard to girls, data remain meager. Drummond *et al.* (2008, $n = 25$) and Wallien and Cohen-Kettenis (2008, $n = 18$) reported the first follow-up studies. Wallien and Cohen-Kettenis found a GD persistence rate of 50%, but Drummond *et al.* reported a persistence rate of only 12%. Regarding sexual orientation, Wallien and Cohen-Kettenis reported that 70–100% (depending on the metric) were homosexual/bisexual in fantasy whereas Drummond *et al.* reported a corresponding value of 32%. In behavior, the corresponding percentages for the two studies were 60% and 24%, respectively.

Predictors of long-term gender identity

When one asks adolescents or adults with GD about their recollections of sex-typed behavior in childhood, for those who have a sexual orientation directed to members of their birth sex, it is almost universal to find a childhood history of marked gender-variant or cross-gender behavior (Deogracias *et al.*, 2007; Singh *et al.*, 2010). By contrast, the prospective data summarized earlier show much less continuity. Plasticity may be one explanation for this discrepancy. It is possible, for example, that gender identity shows relative malleability during childhood, with narrowing plasticity with age. Another explanation relates to historical factors (see Zucker *et al.*, 2012b), related to the gender-transition movement (Meadow, 2011) and

views of early cross-gender identification that encourage early social transition (Byne *et al.*, 2012).

In three major follow-up studies, dimensional measures of cross-gender identity and cross-gender role behavior in childhood predicted GD persistence. Children whose cross-gender identity and behavior was more extreme were more likely to be persisters. Some evidence also suggests that children from "working class" backgrounds possess earlier awareness of "sex-appropriate" behavior than children from middle-class backgrounds (Rabban, 1950). Singh (2012) also described social class related difference in GD boys from lower SES families had more "rigid" notions of within-sex variation in sex-typed behavior and that could moderate outcome.

Ethical considerations

Consider the following clinical vignettes:

1 A mother of a 4-year-old girl contacts a well-known clinic that specializes in gender identity throughout the life span. She describes behaviors consistent with the DSM-5 diagnosis of GD. The clinician tells the mother: "Well, we don't consider 'it' to be a problem." The mother then contacts another specialty clinic and asks "What should I do?"

2 A mother of a 4-year-old boy contacts a well-known clinic that specializes in gender identity problems. She describes behaviors consistent with the DSM-5 diagnosis of GD. She says that she would like her child treated so he does not grow up to be gay. She also worries that her child will be ostracized within the peer group because of his pervasive cross-gender behavior. What should the clinician say to this mother?

3 A 15-year-old adolescent girl with GD asks to be seen for treatment. She would like cross-sex hormones and a mastectomy immediately. If refused, the patient says that she will kill herself. What should the clinician do?

4 A 16-year-old adolescent boy with GD asks for sex-reassignment surgery. He states that he is sexually attracted to biological males and wants a sex-change because that will make his sexual feelings for males "normal." He states that homosexuality is against his religious beliefs and is taboo in his culture of origin. What should the clinician do?

Treatment

No randomized controlled trials exist for GD (Byne *et al.*, 2012). The few treatment-effectiveness studies lack methodological sophistication. This leaves practitioners to rely on "clinical wisdom" (for an overview, see the special issue of the *Journal of Homosexuality* on "The Treatment of Gender Dysphoric/Gender Variant Children and Adolescents" [Drescher & Byne, 2012]). In an era that emphasizes evidence-based therapeutics, this is a source of frustration (Zucker, 2008; Dreger, 2009).

Behavior therapy

There are 13 published single-case reports on behavior therapy in pediatric GD (see Zucker, 1985). Some interventions use so-called *differential social attention* or *social reinforcement*, applied in clinic settings. The therapist first establishes that the child prefers playing with cross-sex toys or dress-up apparel rather than same-sex toys or dress-up apparel. A parent or stranger is then introduced into the playroom and instructed to attend to the child's same-sex play and to ignore the child's cross-sex play, which can change play behavior.

This approach may not generalize to other settings or other untreated cross-sex behaviors (Rekers, 1975). Such problems led behavior therapists to seek more effective strategies of promoting generalization. One such strategy, *self-regulation* or *self-monitoring*, has the child reinforce himself or herself when engaging in a sex-typical behavior. Although self-monitoring also resulted in substantial decreases in cross-sex play, the evidence is weak that generalization is better promoted by self-regulation than by social attention (Zucker, 1985).

No case reports have appeared for over 30 years, which is curious, because similar approaches are used widely for many other problems. Behavior therapy with an emphasis on the child's cognitive representations of gender could be useful, possibly incorporating work on cognitive gender schemas in typically developing children (Martin *et al.*, 2002). It is possible that children with GD have more elaborately developed cross-gender schemas than same-gender schemas and that more positive affective appraisals are differentiated for the former than for the latter (e.g., in boys, "girls get to wear prettier clothes" vs "boys are too rough"). A cognitive approach could target such features to produce positive gender-related feelings.

Psychotherapy

There is a large case report literature on GD using other approaches (see Zucker, 2007). This uses varied theoretical approaches, but this literature has not produced a clinical trial.

Parental engagement

Two rationales support parental involvement. First, parental behavior could initiate or sustain GD. From this perspective, individual therapy with the child could benefit by also helping parents gain insight into these behaviors, as discussed elsewhere (Newman, 1976; Zucker, 2006; Zucker *et al.*, 2012b). Second, parents will benefit from therapist contact to discuss day-to-day management, set limits with regard to cross-gender behavior, and encourage same-sex peer relations and gender-typical activities (see Meyer-Bahlburg, 2002).

Although clinicians typically work with parents of children with GD, there is scant empirical evidence on efficacy. Observational data support the practice, but no randomized controlled trial exists (Zucker *et al.*, 1985).

In Example 2 noted earlier, a parent such as this will likely be receptive to a therapeutic approach that attempts to reduce the GD even with the clear caveat by the clinician that the aim of such an approach is not designed to change the child's sexual orientation, for which there is no empirical evidence (Green, 1987).

Supportive or "gender-affirming" treatments

In the past few years, clinicians critical of conceptualizing marked gender-variant behavior in children as a disorder have provided a dissenting perspective to the treatment approaches described so far (e.g., Menvielle & Tuerk, 2002; Hill & Menvielle, 2009; Menvielle, 2009, 2012; Ehrensaft, 2011). These clinicians conceptualize GD or pervasive gender-variant behavior from an essentialist perspective—that GD is largely constitutional or congenital in origin—and are skeptical about the role of psychosocial or psychodynamic factors in its genesis or maintenance. For example, Menvielle and Tuerk (2002) noted that, while it might be helpful to set limits on pervasive cross-gender behaviors that may contribute to social ostracism, their primary treatment goal was "…not at changing the children's behavior, but at helping parents to be supportive and to maximize opportunities for the children's adjustment" (p. 1010). This perspective, therefore, appears to encourage some parents to take an approach that is rather different from the more conventional therapeutic models. As noted earlier, there is a burgeoning gender-transition movement that involves both professionals and parents who utilize this approach, which has received widespread media attention (including US celebrities such as Anderson Cooper and Barbara Walters) and on the Internet, with various examples of parental narratives describing their experience in helping their children in this way (e.g., Kelso, 2011; Wisnowski, 2011). In Example 1 noted earlier, it is clear that the practicing clinician would be most sympathetic with this philosophical and conceptual approach in dealing with the child's GD. In the current therapeutic climate in which disagreement about best practice is marked (Byne *et al.*, 2012), some parents will be most drawn to this approach, but others will not be.

Treatment of adolescents

In adolescents with GD, there are three broad clinical issues that require evaluation: (i) the phenomenology pertaining to the GD itself, (ii) sexual orientation, and (iii) psychiatric comorbidity. For the majority of adolescents, clinical experience suggests that the GD will desist only after the patient has made a social transition to the desired gender and to be treated biomedically with hormone therapy and sex-reassignment surgery. However, there are some adolescents who present clinically with a less stable, and more fluctuating cross-gender identity, and these youth are probably best treated first in psychosocial therapy in order to explore the extent to which a gender social transition is going to prove helpful. It is also important to understand the patient's sexual orientation, as the intersection between the adolescent's gender identity and to whom one is attracted to have important implications for the establishment of interpersonal, romantic relationships. Because many adolescents with GD have other psychosocial and psychiatric problems that they are struggling with, it is important to have a good understanding of how these difficulties impact their general functioning and well-being (de Vries *et al.*, 2011a; Zucker *et al.*, 2011).

The psychotherapy treatment literature on adolescents with GD has been very poorly developed and is confined to a few case reports (Zucker & Bradley, 1995; Rosario, 2009). In general, the likelihood of GD persistence for adolescents is much higher than it is for children (Zucker et al., 2011). From a clinical management point of view, two key issues need to be considered: (i) some adolescents with GD are not particularly good candidates for therapy because of comorbid disorders and life circumstances; (ii) the majority of adolescents wish to proceed with hormonal and surgical sex reassignment as part of their desire to live socially in the preferred gender. Some of these youth are also interested in some type of psychosocial therapy to help them with the process of gender transition and/or to help them deal with other psychologic and psychiatric issues that they may be struggling with.

Before recommending hormonal and surgical interventions, many clinicians encourage adolescents with GD to consider alternatives. One area of inquiry can, therefore, explore the meaning behind the adolescent's desire for sex reassignment and if there are viable alternative lifestyle adaptations. The most common area of exploration in this regard pertains to the patient's sexual orientation. Some adolescents with GD recall that they always felt uncomfortable growing up as boys or as girls, but that the idea of "sex change" did not occur until they became aware of homoerotic attractions. For some of these youth, the idea that they might be gay or homosexual is abhorrent (as noted in Example 4 earlier). If those issues are worked through, the GD will lessen, if not remit. If the issues do not remit, then biomedical treatment may well be warranted.

For adolescents in whom the GD appears chronic, there is considerable evidence that it interferes with general social adaptation, including general psychiatric impairment, conflicted family relations, and dropping out of school (see the section on Associated Psychopathology on page 989). For these youth, therefore, the treating clinician can consider three main options: (i) in early adolescence, the institution of hormonal therapy with gonadotropin-releasing hormone (GnRH) analogs to delay or suppress somatic puberty; (ii) subsequent initiation of cross-sex hormonal therapy; and (iii) surgical sex change at a lower bound age of 18 (Delemarre-van de Waal & Cohen-Kettenis, 2006; Cohen-Kettenis et al., 2011; Zucker et al., 2011). It has, for example, been argued that institution of GnRH treatment makes it easier to "pass" as the opposite sex. Thus, for example, in male adolescents, such medication can suppress the development of secondary sex characteristics, such as facial hair growth and voice deepening, which make it more difficult to pass in the female social role.

Over the past number of years, emerging evidence suggests that the institution of puberty-blocking hormone therapy and cross-sex hormone therapy facilitates a reduction in GD and improves psychosocial and psychiatric well-being in carefully selected patients (Cohen-Kettenis & van Goozen, 1997; Smith et al., 2001; de Vries et al., 2011b). In Example 3, however, biomedical treatment would not be recommended until the patient was more stable and less at-risk for "acting out."

Although it would be desirable to design a randomized controlled trial in which an alternative arm would be a psychosocial treatment aimed at reducing the patient's GD (without any concomitant biomedical intervention), such a design is probably not feasible because it would be difficult, if not impossible (for both practical and ethical reasons), to randomly assign patients to the two types of treatment. An alternative design might include a waiting list control group to see if the GD persists over at least a short-term period of time (say, e.g., 6 months). Although hormonal treatment for GD in adolescents has been deemed controversial (Beh & Diamond, 2005; Giordano, 2013), it appears to be a successful evidence-based treatment and may well be the treatment of choice once the clinician is confident that other options have been ruled out.

Paraphilic sexual disorders

Characteristics and diagnosis of the condition
Phenomenology
Paraphilias can be classified into those that involve atypical sexual targets or activities. Atypical targets include sexually immature persons (pedophilia), nonhuman animals (zoophilia), and inanimate objects (fetishism); atypical activities include the infliction of pain or humiliation on another (sadism), experiencing pain or humiliation (masochism), and exposing one's genitals to unsuspecting strangers (exhibitionism). The most commonly observed paraphilias in clinical or correctional settings are those that involve illegal behavior if they are acted upon, such as pedophilia and the commission of sexual offenses against children, or nonconsensual sexual sadism and the commission of violent sexual offenses.

DSM-5 and the ICD
The DSM-5 lists the more commonly known paraphilias, including pedophilia, sadism, and fetishism; the paraphilias listed in ICD-10 are quite similar in content. For example, the ICD-10 defines pedophilia as "a sexual preference for children, usually of prepubertal or early pubertal age." DSM-5 retained the DSM-IV-TR criteria for Pedophilia (see Blanchard, 2013), which consider the duration and persistence of sexual interests, and adds a criterion about the age difference between the person and the child or children (the person is at least age 16 years and at least 5 years older than the child or children). Other paraphilias do not specify a minimum age requirement. An important change from DSM-IV-TR to DSM-5 is the distinction between paraphilias, which describe the atypical sexual interests, and paraphilic disorders, which require clinically significant distress or impairment.

Assessment
Interviews and questionnaires
Assessment requires a thorough sexual history, typically obtained through clinical interviews inquiring about sexual thoughts, interests, and behaviors, especially with regard to

atypical sexual targets or activities. Comprehensive interviews also can rule out explanations for atypical sexual thoughts, urges, fantasies, or behavior. For example, some individuals with obsessive-compulsive disorder (OCD) may report being disturbed by thoughts about molesting a child (Gordon, 2002). The differential diagnosis is made by determining if the thoughts are associated with sexual arousal or pleasure and by inquiring about symptoms of OCD.

Interviews can be very informative, but there are potential problems with recall and other biases in gathering self-report data on sexual interests or behavior (Wiederman, 2002). Questions about sexual history are sensitive and many interviewees may minimize or deny certain sexual interests or behaviors, especially those that are highly stigmatized, such as pedophilia. For example, Halpern et al. (2000) found that male adolescents were more willing to disclose criminal acts that they had committed than the fact that they had masturbated, although many of them had engaged in both behaviors. The validity of self-report may be increased if a rapport is established, which can occur after involvement in treatment (Worling & Curwen, 2000).

Questionnaires may reduce reluctance to disclose. Koss and Gidycz (1985) found that male respondents were more likely to admit engaging in sexually coercive behavior on a questionnaire than in an interview (see Daleiden et al., 1998).

Other information

Sexual history information can sometimes be obtained from other sources, including interviews with an adolescent's sexual partner (if available) or a parent or guardian of children or younger adolescents (Skilling et al., 2011). However, such information is usually limited. A review of clinical or criminal justice records can be very helpful. For example, clinicians can use information about sexual victim characteristics to make the diagnosis of pedophilia, because sexual arousal to children is more likely to be present among adolescent sex offenders who have very young victims, boy victims, and victims outside the offender's immediate family (Seto et al., 2003). Sexual child victim characteristics can be summarized using the Screening Scale for Pedophilic Interests (SSPI), where having boy victims receives a score of 2, and having multiple child victims, victims under the age of 12, or unrelated child victims receive a score of 1 each. Thus, adolescent sex offenders with child victims can have a SSPI score ranging from 0 to 5. This information about previous sexual victims is also related to the risk of new sexual offenses (Seto et al., 2004). Data on the sexual behavior problems of children can be collected from maternal observations through the Child Sexual Behavior Inventory (CSBI) (Friedrich, 1997). Childhood sexual behavior problems correlate with other problems on the CBCL.

Phallometry and viewing time

Phallometry involves the measurement of penile responses to sexual stimuli that systematically vary on the dimensions of interest, as developed by Freund (1963). Phallometric responses

are recorded as increases in either penile circumference or penile volume, providing a specific sexual measure, unlike other psychophysiological responses (Zuckerman, 1971). Phallometry discriminate various sexual behaviors, including sex offenses (Lalumière et al., 2005; Seto, 2009), sadistic fantasies, and various other behaviors (Marshall et al., 1991b; Freund et al., 1996; Seto & Kuban, 1996; Seto et al., 2012). For males who are not motivated to manipulate their phallometric responses, genital sexual arousal is substantially correlated with subjective sexual arousal (Chivers et al., 2010).

Seto et al. (2000) evaluated the use of phallometric testing for adolescent sex offenders with child victims. Because an age-matched comparison group was not available, these adolescents were compared to young adults between the ages of 18 and 21 who had not committed sexual offenses involving children. As a group, adolescents with male victims had relatively higher responses to pictures of children than the young adult comparison participants. Adolescents with both male and female children as victims responded more to pictures of children than to pictures of adults (see also Rice et al., 2012). Clift et al. (2009) found that phallometric test results predicted future reoffending among adolescent sex offenders, just as it does for adult sex offenders (Hanson & Morton-Bourgon, 2005).

Viewing time provides another objective measure, using various pictures. Adolescent or adult sex offenders with child victims can be distinguished from other men using such measures, although not all findings are consistent (Smith and Fischer, 1999; Abel et al., 2004). Another potential problem is that subjects can explicitly manipulate their profile if they aware that viewing time is being monitored.

Associated psychopathology

Paraphilias and related sexual disorders often co-occur with mood and anxiety disorders (Kafka, 2003; Seto & Lalumière, 2010). However, longitudinal research is needed on the timing of these associations. Sexual behavior problems also co-occur with nonsexual behavior problems (Friedrich et al., 2001), including attention deficit hyperactivity disorder, oppositional defiant disorder, or conduct disorder (Seto & Lalumière, 2010). France and Hudson (1993) reviewed studies on this topic and concluded that up to half of adolescent sex offenders would meet diagnostic criteria for conduct disorder.

Paraphilias can be comorbid, and engaging in one form of paraphilic behavior greatly increases the likelihood of engaging in another (Abel et al., 1988; Zolondek et al., 2001). Långström and Seto (2006) found exhibitionistic and voyeuristic behavior co-occurred more often than expected by chance in a nationally representative sample of young men between the ages of 18 and 21 from Sweden. There are limited co-occurrence data for adolescents.

Epidemiology
Prevalence and incidence

Neither the incidence nor the prevalence of paraphilias is known. Some limited evidence suggests that paraphilias are relatively rare, although admitting or experiencing some paraphilic sexual interest is common (Briere & Runtz, 1989; Fromuth et al., 1991; Templeman & Stinnett, 1991). Paraphilic interests have a lower threshold than paraphilias. As noted earlier, the DSM-5 makes a further distinction between paraphilias and paraphilic disorders, where the latter requires clinically significant distress or impairment for the diagnosis. Limited data are available in adolescents, although retrospective reports from adults suggest that sexual interests often begin to emerge following the onset of puberty (Seto, 2012). Most work uses clinical or correctional samples, usually on adults.

Risk factors

While many theories focus on the etiology, we focus on theories emphasizing conditioning or neurodevelopment, as these have the strongest support. We then discuss the theories' implications.

Conditioning

Masturbatory conditioning may influence risk for paraphilias (McGuire et al., 1965; Laws & Marshall, 1990). Some individuals, for unspecified reasons, pair cues of unusual initial sexual experiences with the sexual pleasure elicited by these early experiences and learn to associate these cues with the powerful reinforcement of orgasm. There is equivocal relevant evidence, however, in humans. Rachman and Hodgson (1968) reported significantly increased sexual arousal to pictures of boots among normal volunteers in a set of frequently cited experimental studies examining the development of boot fetishism, but these studies did not have control conditions. Lalumière and Quinsey (1998) and Hoffmann et al. (2004) found a significant effect of conditioning on sexual arousal among male volunteers while Plaud and Martini (1999) reported mixed results in a conditioning study of nine male volunteers.

The efficacy of conditioning approaches for changing sexual arousal patterns has been reviewed elsewhere (Barbaree & Seto, 1997; Hoffmann, 2012). Overall, this research suggests that conditioning can have an effect on the suppression of sexual arousal of adolescent or adult sex offenders, but it is unclear how long these changes are maintained, what mechanisms are actually responsible for the changes in sexual arousal patterns, and whether the changes reflect an actual shift in sexual interests or greater voluntary control over sexual arousal when assessed in the laboratory (Mahoney & Strassberg, 1991; Lalumière & Earls, 1992).

Conditioning might play a role in maintaining rather than initiating paraphilic sexual arousal. For example, Dandescu and Wolfe (2003) found that atypical sexual fantasies preceded and accompanied the first sexual offence reported by a sample of 57 sex offenders with child victims; the sexual fantasies then increased in frequency after the first sexual offence. Approximately two-thirds of the offenders reported having any "deviant sexual fantasies" before their first contact with a child while 81% reported having such fantasies afterwards. This finding suggests that the sexual arousal and gratification experienced during the first sexual offence increased the frequency of sexual fantasies among men who already had such fantasies.

Findings suggest that conditioning is unlikely to play a significant role in the onset of paraphilias. Experimental efforts to increase sexual arousal have produced small effects, but it is unclear how long conditioned changes in sexual responding can be maintained. If conditioning does play a role in the development of paraphilias, as suggested by Dandescu and Wolfe's study, then there is almost surely an interaction between conditioning experiences and other predisposing factors, such as a neurodevelopmental diathesis.

Neurodevelopment

Information on brain functioning can be obtained both directly and indirectly. Indirectly, investigators have compared cognitive function in sex offenders with child victims with other groups. Cantor et al. (2005) conducted a meta-analysis: For the adults, sex offenders scored lower on measures of intelligence than other offenders, who, in turn, scored lower than non-offending controls. For the adolescents, there was a significant difference between sex offenders and other offenders. Among the sex offenders, Cantor et al. found that intelligence scores appeared to be related to the proportion of the sample that was pedophilic, because sex offenders with child victims scored lower than sex offenders without any child victims. Moreover, there was a positive relationship between the age cut-off used to define child victims and mean intelligence score; in other words, samples composed of men who offended against younger children tended to produce lower mean IQ scores than samples composed of men who offended against older children.

In earlier studies, this same research group also found that pedophilic sex offenders were more likely to report experiencing head injuries before the age of age 13, but did not differ in reports of head injuries after age 13 (Blanchard et al., 2002, 2003). The fact there was no difference in reports of head injuries after age 13 counters an alternative explanation that pedophiles have a retrospective reporting bias in recalling head injuries, because there would be no reason to think that head injuries before the age of 13 are more socially desirable than head injuries later in life. The fact that there was no difference after age 13 also suggests that there is a critical age window in terms of the impact of head injury on the development of pedophilia (and perhaps other paraphilias). This is an intriguing possibility because of other work suggesting that the time before and during puberty is critical in the development of sexual preferences in general. Of course, it is assumed that the relationship between head injury and pedophilia is causal. It is possible that a third variable explains both the higher incidence of head injury and pedophilia; for example, prenatal brain damage may increase accident-proneness, resulting in a higher risk for head injury as well as increase the likelihood that an individual will be pedophilic.

Researchers have also attempted to directly assess brain structure. Cantor et al. (2008) reported that pedophilic men had less white matter than nonpedophilic men in the right superior occipitofrontal fasciculus and the right arcuate fasciculus. These white matter tracts connect areas that are involved in determining if a stimulus is sexually relevant, suggesting that pedophiles are somehow deficient in how they process and integrate sexual cues. Poeppl *et al.* (2013) identified a number of gray matter volume differences between pedophilic sex offenders and controls, with differences in the orbitofrontal cortex and bilateral angular gyri correlated with aspects of sexual offending behavior such as age of child victims. Ponseti *et al.* (2012) were able to use fMRI activation changes in response to sexual stimuli to adults or children to distinguish pedophiles from controls with high accuracy.

Cycle of sexual abuse

Sexual abuse history may relate to adolescent sexual offending (Knight & Sims-Knight, 2003). Seto and Lalumière (2010) conducted a meta-analysis of studies that compared adolescent sex offenders and other adolescent offenders and found that adolescent sex offenders had more than five times the odds of having a history of sexual abuse. Difference was smaller for physical abuse history, and a similar pattern of results was found comparing adult sex offenders to other adult offenders (Jespersen *et al.*, 2009).

Adolescent sex offenders who have been sexually abused show relatively greater sexual arousal to children or coercive sex than those who have not been abused (Becker *et al.*, 1992; Hunter *et al.*, 1994). Among children, Friedrich *et al.* (2001) showed that scores on the CSBI could discriminate children who had been sexually abused from those who had not. Hall *et al.* (1998) found, in a sample of 99 sexually abused boys and girls between the ages of 3 and 7, that those who became sexually aroused during the sexual abuse were more likely to engage in sexual behavior problems involving others ($n = 62$) than those who did not ($n = 37$).

The sexually abused–sexual abuser hypothesis suggests that male children who are sexually abused are more likely to engage in sexual offending later in life. Burton (2003) described plausible mechanisms: modeling, conditioning, and changing of cognitions. In the Seto and Lalumière (2010) meta-analysis, adolescent sex offenders were also more likely to have been exposed to sexual violence in the family and had an earlier age of exposure to pornography or sex.

The mechanisms underlying the association between childhood sexual abuse and sexual behavior problems among children and adolescent sexual offending are not known. Possible important factors include aspects of abuse, such as duration or timing (Burton, 2003; Hunter *et al.*, 2003). There must be individual characteristics that increase both vulnerability to childhood sexual abuse and the likelihood of adolescent sexual offending, because many sexually abused children do not go on to commit sexual offenses, and many adolescent sex offenders have no known history of sexual abuse (Salter *et al.*, 2003).

Developmental trajectories

A developmental perspective is important because there are myriad differences between children, adolescents, and adults, and because there is both persistence and desistance in sexual offending across the lifespan. Retrospective studies suggest approximately half of adult sex offenders report that their first sexual offence was committed as a juvenile (Groth *et al.*, 1982) and up to half of adolescent sex offenders have engaged in sexual behavior problems under the age of 12 (Ryan *et al.*, 1996; Burton, 2000; Zolondek *et al.*, 2001). In prospective studies, however, only about 10–15% of adolescent sex offenders commit another sexual offence over 5 years (for reviews, see Caldwell, 2010). The proportion of children with sexual behavior problems who persist and commit a sexual offence as an adolescent is also low (Carpentier *et al.*, 2006). Taken together, these data indicate that many children with sexual behavior problems and many adolescent sex offenders desist. For many children, their sexual behavior problems may represent a reaction to sexual abuse that they have experienced, sexual precocity, or normative sexual play. For many adolescents, their sexual offenses may represent opportunistic and relatively transient antisocial behavior. A small group of children and adolescents, however, will persist in committing sexual offenses into adulthood. Adolescents who develop paraphilias such as pedophilia, exhibitionism, or voyeurism are more likely to persist in sexual offending pertaining to that paraphilia.

Of particular relevance is a study by Zolondek *et al.* (2001) of 485 adolescent males between the ages of 11 and 17, referred for assessment or treatment of paraphilic interests or behavior. The youths completed a questionnaire with questions about their sexual interests and experiences as part of their assessment. Twenty-six percent acknowledged engaging in fetishistic behavior, 17% acknowledged voyeuristic acts, and 12% acknowledged exhibitionistic behavior. The average age of onset across paraphilic behaviors was between 10 and 12, which is younger than the average age of onset found in retrospective studies (Abel *et al.*, 1987; Marshall *et al.*, 1991a). These data are consistent with the idea that the onset of paraphilias is around the time of puberty, just as many people are becoming aware of their sexual preference for males or females.

Treatment
Pharmacological

The common aim of pharmacotherapy for the treatment of pedophilia is to suppress sexual response involving children. These same medications have been used, to a lesser extent, in the pharmacological treatment of other paraphilias that can lead to much distress or impairment (e.g., nonconsensual sexual sadism). Much of the initial interest was in antiandrogens to reduce sexual response, but clinicians and researchers have more recently focused on serotonergic agents. Because of the impact of reducing androgens on physical development, anti androgens are very rarely, if ever, prescribed for minors, except in cases where the sexual behavior is highly dangerous (e.g., very violent sexual assaults) and cannot be controlled by other means.

It is a logical hypothesis that anti androgens would have an impact on paraphilic sexual responses, because testosterone plays a critical role in male sexuality as well as aggression (Rubinow & Schmidt, 1996). The earliest clinical study was reported by Laschet and Laschet (1971), who treated more than 100 paraphilic men; most were pedophiles or exhibitionists. Cyproterone acetate (CPA) or medroxyprogesterone acetate (MPA) are among the most commonly prescribed agents, both of which interfere with the action of testosterone. The use of either drug in the treatment of paraphilias is off-label, meaning it is not specifically approved by regulatory bodies for this purpose. Side effects of antiandrogens include headaches, dizziness, nausea, gynecomastia, depression, and osteoporosis. As a result of these potentially serious side effects and the fact that some patients do not want to experience a massive reduction in their sex drive, treatment attrition and treatment compliance are major obstacles in antiandrogen treatment. For example, in Hucker *et al.* (1988), only 11 of 18 men completed the 12-week trial set out by the clinical investigators.

There is some support for the efficacy of antiandrogens in reducing the frequency or intensity of sexual urges and arousal, but there has been a dearth of larger, better-controlled outcome studies. Gijs and Gooren (1996) reviewed the literature evaluating the effects of CPA and MPA, focusing on methodologically stronger studies that included features such as random assignment, a placebo condition, and double-blinding (see also Thibaut *et al.*, 2010; Garcia *et al.*, 2013). Gijs and Gooren identified four controlled studies of CPA and six such studies of MPA. All four studies of CPA revealed that treated men had a significant reduction in sexual response while only one of the six MPA studies showed a significant difference between men in the treatment and comparison conditions.

Serotonin is involved in the regulation of human sexual behavior and anti depressant medications that have a serotonergic effect have long been known to reduce sexual desire and delay ejaculation in males (Meston & Gorzalka, 1992). The World Federation of Societies of Biological Psychiatry guidelines on the biological treatment of paraphilias are to consider psychotherapy first for adolescents exhibiting paraphilic symptoms, but to consider SSRIs for those who do not respond to psychotherapy alone, especially if the paraphilic symptoms are associated with OCD, impulse control disorders, or depression (Thibaut *et al.*, 2010). Unfortunately, the interest in serotonergic agents for the treatment of paraphilias appears to be almost entirely based on uncontrolled case studies or open trials (Gijs & Gooren, 1996); there has been only one experimental study that compared desipramine and chloripramine in a double-blind crossover trial that was preceded by a single-blind placebo condition (Kruesi *et al.*, 1992). Kruesi *et al.* reported a significant reduction of self-reported paraphilic behavior (predominantly exhibitionism, transvestic fetishism, telephone scatalogia, and fetishism) with either drug,

but their result was difficult to interpret because only 8 of 15 paraphilic men completed the trial; four patients were dropped because they responded to the placebo, and three did not complete the drug trial. Including the patients who responded to placebo would have attenuated, and perhaps eliminated, the apparent effect of the drugs on self-reported paraphilic behavior.

Despite the intuitive appeal of pharmacological interventions to reduce sexual drive and thus the likelihood of (illegal) paraphilic behavior, reviews of outcome studies suggest that there is no strong empirical support for the idea that such interventions can reduce sexual recidivism.

Psychosocial interventions

Aversive conditioning techniques were used as early as the 1950s for paraphilic interests such as fetishism and transvestic fetishism (e.g., Raymond, 1956; Marks & Gelder, 1967). In the behavioral treatment of paraphilias, aversion techniques are used to suppress sexual arousal to the atypical target or activity, while masturbatory reconditioning techniques are used to increase sexual arousal to acceptable targets (peers or adults) and activities (consenting sexual activities). In aversion procedures, unpleasant stimuli, such as mild electric shock or the odor of ammonia, are paired with repeated presentations of sexual stimuli depicting the paraphilic target or activity. In a variation called covert sensitization, the aversive stimulus is imagined, for example, being discovered by family, friends, or coworkers while engaging in paraphilic behavior. Overall, the existing research suggests that behavioral techniques can have an effect on sexual arousal patterns, but it is unclear how long these changes are maintained and whether they result in actual changes in interests, as opposed to greater voluntary control over pedophilic sexual arousal (Lalumière & Earls, 1992; see also Hoffmann, 2012).

Cognitive-behavioral treatments aim to teach individuals how to manage their sexual urges, often as part of a more comprehensive program to address clinical needs (see Pullman & Seto, 2012). Published evaluations have reported promising results. Carpentier *et al.* (2006) reported on a long-term evaluation of 135 children with sexual behavior problems, compared to 156 children from the same outpatient clinic. The children with sexual behavior problems were randomly assigned to a play therapy group or a cognitive-behavioral treatment (CBT) group. Both treatments were manualized and ran for 12 hour-long sessions. The CBT group was highly structured and focused on education and behavior management. The play therapy group was less structured and more reflective, although it focused on many of the same themes: sexual behavior problems, boundaries, parenting skills, and sex education. Children assigned to the CBT group were significantly less likely than children assigned to the play therapy group to sexually offend (defined as an arrest for a sexual offence or a child welfare report of sexual abuse perpetration) during the 10-year follow-up period. In fact, the rate of sexual offending among children in the CBT group was not significantly different from the comparison group without any sexual behavior problems.

Borduin *et al.* (1990) reported a significant effect of treatment in a small sample of adolescent sex offenders, using a multisystemic treatment that targeted factors associated with criminal behavior, including antisocial attitudes and beliefs, associations with antisocial peers, and substance abuse (Andrews & Bonta, 2010). This multisystemic treatment is distinguished by being skills-focused, involving both the adolescent and his family, and paying careful attention to program fidelity and individualization. Multiple studies have shown that multisystemic treatment can significantly reduce recidivism and other negative outcomes among serious adolescent offenders (Henggeler *et al.*, 1998). Borduin and Schaeffer (2001) extended the Borduin *et al.* study by showing that this multisystemic treatment had a large impact on sexual recidivism in a larger sample of 48 juvenile sex offenders although it was not designed specifically for this group. More recent treatment outcome studies show that, compared with typical community-based services provided to adolescent sex offenders, multisystemic therapy resulted in greater reductions in sexual behavior problems, criminal behavior, and substance use (Borduin *et al.*, 2009; Letourneau *et al.*, 2009). See also Chapter 49 (Young and Church, this edition).

Summary and conclusions

There are many unanswered questions about the onset, development, and prognosis of paraphilias. Relatively little research has been conducted on adolescents, perhaps reflecting a discomfort with the idea that some adolescents and older children engage in problematic sexual behavior as a result of atypical sexual interests that are very likely to be stable over their lifetimes (Seto, 2012). As a result, this section has drawn upon relevant studies of adult sex offenders. This is not to suggest that children with sexual behavior problems or adolescent sex offenders are likely to have paraphilias. In fact, it is likely that most do not, given the high rate of desistance in sexual behavior problems from childhood to adolescence and in sexual offending from adolescence to adulthood. However, a small minority of children and adolescents do persist and are likely to continue engaging in criminal sexual behavior without effective intervention.

Moreover, most of the research summarized in this chapter pertains to pedophilia, with some additional studies on paraphilias such as sexual sadism, exhibitionism, and voyeurism. Much more empirical work is needed to understand the commonalities and differences across different paraphilias. It may be the case, for example, that the etiological factors behind activity paraphilias may differ from those for target paraphilias. There is emerging evidence to support the idea that there are neurological risk factors for pedophilia. Given the comorbidity of paraphilias, it is possible that other paraphilias are also influenced by common neurological factors. The work of Cantor and colleagues have identified a number of indicators of neurological perturbations–non-right-handedness, lower IQ, lower scores on other measures of neuropsychological functioning, and decreased white matter in two major tracts—that suggest paraphilias have a prenatal origin (Cantor *et al.*, 2008; see also Seto, 2009, 2012; Poeppl *et al.*, 2013). Or, it is possible that the predisposition to developing paraphilias is influenced prenatally, and the expression of paraphilias is influenced by subsequent experiences, as in the robust association between childhood sexual abuse and sexual offending involving children (Jespersen *et al.*, 2009; Seto & Lalumière, 2010).

As is true for many other disorders, we know more about the assessment than the treatment of paraphilias. Further research on paraphilias will be expedited by the development of age-appropriate measures of sexual interests. Viewing time is a particularly promising technology. Unlike the adult literature, however, there are some promising results in the treatment of sexual behavior problems in children and sexual offending among adolescents. These treatments share a common focus on skills, behavior, problem-solving, and involve parents or other caregivers. Further advances in treatment will benefit from a greater understanding of the etiology and developmental course of paraphilias.

References

Abel, G.G. *et al.* (1987) Self-reported sex crimes of non-incarcerated paraphiliacs. *Journal of Interpersonal Violence* **2**, 3–25.

Abel, G.G. *et al.* (1988) Multiple paraphilic diagnoses among sex offenders. *Bulletin of the American Academy of Psychiatry and the Law* **16**, 153–168.

Abel, G.G. *et al.* (2004) Use of visual reaction time to assess male adolescents who molest children. *Sexual Abuse: A Journal of Research and Treatment* **16**, 255–265.

American Psychiatric Association (2013) *Diagnostic and Statistical Manual of Mental Disorders*, 5th edn. American Psychiatric Association, Washington, DC.

Andrews, D.A. & Bonta, J. (2010) *The Psychology of Criminal Conduct*, 5th edn. Anderson, Cincinnati, OH.

Barbaree, H.E. & Seto, M.C. (1997) Pedophilia: assessment and treatment. In: *Sexual Deviance: Theory, Assessment and Treatment*. (eds D.R. Laws & W.T. O'Donohue), pp. 175–193. Guilford Press, New York.

Bates, J.E. *et al.* (1979) Gender-deviant boys compared with normal and clinical control boys. *Journal of Abnormal Child Psychology* **7**, 243–259.

Baum, M.J. (2006) Mammalian animal models of psychosexual differentiation: when is 'translation' to the human situation possible? *Hormones and Behavior* **50**, 579–588.

Becker, J.V. *et al.* (1992) The relationship of abuse history, denial and erectile response profiles of adolescent sexual perpetrators. *Behavior Therapy* **23**, 87–97.

Beh, H. & Diamond, M. (2005) Ethical concerns related to treating gender nonconformity in childhood and adolescence: lessons from the Family Court of Australia. *Health Matrix: Journal of Law-Medicine* **15**, 239–283.

Blanchard, R. (1997) Birth order and sibling sex ratio in homosexual versus heterosexual males and females. *Annual Review of Sex Research* **8**, 27–67.

Blanchard, R. (2010) The DSM diagnostic criteria for transvestic fetishism. *Archives of Sexual Behavior* **39**, 363–372.

Blanchard, R. (2013) A dissenting opinion on the DSM-5 pedophilic disorder [Letter to the Editor]. *Archives of Sexual Behavior* **42**, 675–678.

Blanchard, R. *et al.* (1995) Birth order and sibling sex ratio in homosexual male adolescents and probably prehomosexual feminine boys. *Developmental Psychology* **31**, 22–30.

Blanchard, R. *et al.* (2002) Retrospective self-reports of childhood accidents causing unconsciousness in phallometrically diagnosed pedophiles. *Archives of Sexual Behavior* **31**, 511–526.

Blanchard, R. *et al.* (2003) Self-reported head injuries before and after age 13 in pedophilic and nonpedophilic men referred for clinical assessment. *Archives of Sexual Behavior* **32**, 573–581.

Bogaert, A.F. & Skorska, M. (2011) Sexual orientation, fraternal birth order, and the maternal immune hypothesis: a review. *Frontiers in Neuroendocrinology* **32**, 247–254.

Borduin, C.M. & Schaeffer, C.M. (2001) Multisystemic treatment of juvenile sexual offenders: a progress report. *Journal of Psychology & Human Sexuality* **13**, 25–42.

Borduin, C.M. *et al.* (1990) Multisystemic treatment of adolescent sexual offenders. *International Journal of Offender Therapy and Comparative Criminology* **34**, 105–113.

Borduin, C.M. *et al.* (2009) A randomized clinical trial of multisystemic therapy with juvenile sexual offenders: effects on youth social ecology and criminal activity. *Journal of Consulting and Clinical Psychology* **77**, 26–37.

Briere, J. & Runtz, M. (1989) University males' sexual interest in children: predicting potential indices of "pedophilia" in a non-forensic sample. *Child Abuse and Neglect* **13**, 65–75.

Burton, D.L. (2000) Were adolescent sexual offenders children with sexual behavior problems? *Sexual Abuse: Journal of Research & Treatment* **12**, 37–48.

Burton, D.L. (2003) Male adolescents: sexual victimization and subsequent sexual abuse. *Child and Adolescent Social Work Journal* **20**, 277–296.

Byne, W. *et al.* (2012) Report of the American Psychiatric Association Task Force on Treatment of Gender Identity Disorder. *Archives of Sexual Behavior* **41**, 759–796.

Caldwell, M.F. (2010) Study characteristics and recidivism base rates in juvenile sex offender recidivism. *International Journal of Offender Therapy and Comparative Criminology* **54**, 197–212.

Campbell, D.W. & Eaton, W.O. (1999) Sex differences in the activity level of infants. *Infant and Child Development* **8**, 1–17.

Cantor, J.M. *et al.* (2005) Quantitative reanalysis of aggregate data on IQ in sexual offenders. *Psychological Bulletin* **131**, 555–568.

Cantor, J.M. *et al.* (2008) Cerebral white matter deficiencies in pedophilic men. *Journal of Psychiatric Research* **42**, 167–183.

Carpentier, M.Y. *et al.* (2006) Randomized trial of treatment for children with sexual behavior problems: ten-year follow-up. *Journal of Consulting and Clinical Psychology* **74**, 482–488.

Chivers, M.L. *et al.* (2010) Agreement of self-reported and genital measures of sexual arousal in men and women: a meta-analysis. *Archives of Sexual Behavior* **39**, 5–56.

Clift, R.J. *et al.* (2009) Discriminative and predictive validity of the penile plethysmograph in adolescent sex offenders. *Sexual Abuse: A Journal of Research and Treatment* **21**, 335–362.

Cohen-Bendahan, C.C.C. *et al.* (2005) Prenatal sex hormone effects on child and adult sex-typed behavior: methods and findings. *Neuroscience and Biobehavioral Reviews* **29**, 353–384.

Cohen-Kettenis, P.T. & Pfäfflin, F. (2010) The DSM diagnostic criteria for gender identity disorder in adolescents and adults. *Archives of Sexual Behavior* **39**, 499–513.

Cohen-Kettenis, P.T. & van Goozen, S.H.M. (1997) Sex reassignment of adolescent transsexuals: a follow-up study. *Journal of the American Academy of Child and Adolescent Psychiatry* **36**, 263–271.

Cohen-Kettenis, P.T. *et al.* (2003) Demographic characteristics, social competence, and behavior problems in children with gender identity disorder: a cross-national, cross-clinic comparative analysis. *Journal of Abnormal Child Psychology* **31**, 41–53.

Cohen-Kettenis, P.T. *et al.* (2011) Treatment of adolescents with gender dysphoria in the Netherlands. *Child and Adolescent Psychiatric Clinics of North America* **20**, 689–700.

Coleman, E. *et al.* (2011) Standards of Care for the Health of Transsexual, Transgender, and Gender-Nonconforming People, Version 7. *International Journal of Transgenderism* **13**, 165–232.

Coolidge, F.L. *et al.* (2002) The heritability of gender identity disorder in a child and adolescent twin sample. *Behavior Genetics* **32**, 251–257.

Daleiden, E.L. *et al.* (1998) The sexual histories and fantasies of youthful males: a comparison of sexual offending, nonsexual offending, and nonoffending groups. *Sexual Abuse: A Journal of Research and Treatment* **10**, 195–209.

Dandescu, A. & Wolfe, R. (2003) Considerations on fantasy use by child molesters and exhibitionists. *Sexual Abuse: Journal of Research and Treatment* **15**, 297–305.

de Vries, A.L.C. *et al.* (2010) Autism spectrum disorders in gender dysphoric children and adolescents. *Journal of Autism and Developmental Disorders* **40**, 930–936.

de Vries, A.L.C. *et al.* (2011a) Psychiatric comorbidity in gender dysphoric adolescents. *Journal of Child Psychiatry and Psychiatry* **52**, 1195–1202.

de Vries, A.L.C. *et al.* (2011b) Puberty suppression in adolescents with gender identity disorder: a prospective follow-up study. *Journal of Sexual Medicine* **8**, 2276–2283.

Delemarre-van de Waal, H.A. & Cohen-Kettenis, P.T. (2006) Clinical management of gender identity disorder in adolescents: a protocol on psychological and paediatric endocrinology aspects. *European Journal of Endocrinology* **155**, S131–S137.

Deogracias, J.J. *et al.* (2007) The gender identity/gender dysphoria questionnaire for adolescents and adults. *Journal of Sex Research* **44**, 370–379.

Dessens, A.B. *et al.* (2005) Gender dysphoria and gender change in chromosomal females with congenital adrenal hyperplasia. *Archives of Sexual Behavior* **34**, 389–397.

Dreger, A. (2009) Gender identity disorder in childhood: inconclusive advice to parents. *Hastings Center Report* **39**, 26–29.

Drescher, J. & Byne, W. (2012) Introduction to the special issue on "The Treatment of Gender Dysphoric/Gender Variant Children and Adolescents". *Journal of Homosexuality* **59**, 295–300.

Drescher, J. *et al.* (2012) Minding the body: situating gender diagnoses in the ICD-11. *International Review of Psychiatry* **24**, 568–577.

Drummond, K.D. *et al.* (2008) A follow-up study of girls with gender identity disorder. *Developmental Psychology* **44**, 34–45.

Ehrensaft, D. (2011) *Gender Born, Gender Made: Raising Healthy Gender-Nonconforming Children.* The Experiment, LLC., New York.

Fisk, N. (1973) Gender dysphoria syndrome (the how, what, and why of a disease). In: *Proceedings of the Second Interdisciplinary Symposium on Gender Dysphoria Syndrome.* (eds D. Laub & P. Gandy), pp. 7–14. Stanford University Press, Palo Alto, CA.

France, K.G. & Hudson, S.M. (1993) The conduct disorders and the juvenile sex offender. In: *The Juvenile Sex Offender.* (eds H.E. Barbaree, W.L. Marshall & S.M. Hudson), pp. 225–234. Guilford Press, New York.

Freund, K. (1963) A laboratory method of diagnosing predominance of homo- and hetero-erotic interest in the male. *Behaviour Research and Therapy* **1**, 85–93.

Freund, K. *et al.* (1996) Two types of fetishism. *Behaviour Research and Therapy* **34**, 687–694.

Friedrich, W.N. (1997) *Child Sexual Behavior Inventory: Professional Manual.* Psychological Assessment Resources, Odessa, FL.

Friedrich, W.N. *et al.* (2001) Child sexual behavior inventory: normative, psychiatric, and sexual abuse comparisons. *Child Maltreatment* **6**, 37–49.

Fromuth, M.E. *et al.* (1991) Hidden child molestation: an investigation of adolescent perpetrators in a nonclinical sample. *Journal of Interpersonal Violence* **6**, 376–384.

Garcia, F.D. *et al.* (2013) Pharmacologic treatment of sex offenders with paraphilic disorder. *Current Psychiatry Reports* **15**, 356.

Gijs, L. & Gooren, L. (1996) Hormonal and psychopharmacological interventions in the treatment of paraphilias: an update. *Journal of Sex Research* **33**, 273–290.

Giordano, S. (2013) *Children with Gender Identity Disorder: A Clinical, Ethical, and Legal Analysis.* Routledge, New York.

Gordon, W.M. (2002) Sexual obsessions and OCD. *Sexual & Relationship Therapy* **17**, 343–354.

Goy, R.W. *et al.* (1988) Behavioral masculinization is independent of genital masculinization in prenatally androgenized female rhesus macaques. *Hormones and Behavior* **22**, 552–571.

Gray, S.A.O. *et al.* (2012) A critical review of assumptions about gender variant children in psychological research. *Journal of Gay & Lesbian Mental Health* **16**, 4–30.

Green, R. (1974) *Sexual Identity Conflict in Children and Adults.* Basic Books, New York.

Green, R. (1987) *The "Sissy Boy Syndrome" and the Development of Homosexuality.* Yale University Press, New Haven, CT.

Groth, A. *et al.* (1982) Undetected recidivism among rapists and child molesters. *Crime & Delinquency* **28**, 450–458.

Halim, M.L. *et al.* (2014) Pink frilly dresses and the avoidance of all things "girly": children's appearance rigidity and cognitive theories of gender development. *Developmental Psychology,* **50**, 1091–1101.

Hall, D.K. *et al.* (1998) Factors associated with sexual behavior problems in young sexually abused children. *Child Abuse and Neglect* **22**, 1045–1063.

Halpern, C.J.T. *et al.* (2000) Adolescent males' willingness to report masturbation. *Journal of Sex Research* **37**, 327–332.

Hanson, R.K. & Morton-Bourgon, K.E. (2005) The characteristics of persistent sexual offenders: a meta-analysis of recidivism studies. *Journal of Consulting and Clinical Psychology* **73**, 1154–1163.

Henggeler, S.W. *et al.* (1998) *Multisystemic Treatment of Antisocial Behavior in Children and Adolescents.* Guilford Press, New York.

Heylens, G. *et al.* (2012) Gender identity disorder in twins: a review of the literature. *Journal of Sexual Medicine* **9**, 751–757.

Hill, D.B. & Menvielle, E. (2009) "You have to give them a place where they feel protected and safe and loved": the views of parents who have gender-variant children and adolescents. *Journal of LGBT Youth* **6**, 243–271.

Hines, M. (2004) *Brain Gender.* Oxford University Press, Oxford.

Hoffmann, H. (2012) Considering the role of conditioning in sexual orientation. *Archives of Sexual Behavior* **41**, 63–71.

Hoffmann, H. *et al.* (2004) Classical conditioning of sexual arousal in women and men: effects of varying awareness and biological relevance of the conditioned stimulus. *Archives of Sexual Behavior* **33**, 43–53.

Hucker, S.J. *et al.* (1988) A double blind trial of sex drive reducing medication in pedophiles. *Annals of Sex Research* **1**, 227–242.

Hunter, J.A. *et al.* (1994) The relationship between phallometrically measured deviant sexual arousal and clinical characteristics in juvenile sexual offenders. *Behaviour Research and Therapy* **32**, 533–538.

Hunter, J.A. *et al.* (2003) Juvenile sex offenders: toward the development of a typology. *Sexual Abuse: A Journal of Research and Treatment* **15**, 27–48.

Iervolino, A.C. *et al.* (2005) Genetic and environmental influences on sex-typed behavior during the preschool years. *Child Development* **76**, 826–840.

Jespersen, A.F. *et al.* (2009) Sexual abuse history among adult sex offenders and non-sex offenders: a meta-analysis. *Child Abuse and Neglect* **33**, 179–192.

Kafka, M.P. (2003) The monoamine hypothesis for the pathophysiology of paraphilic disorders: an update. *Annals of the New York Academy of Sciences* **989**, 86–94.

Kelso, T. (2011) Snakes and snails and mermaid tails: raising a gender-variant son. *Child and Adolescent Psychiatric Clinics of North America* **20**, 745–755.

Knafo, A. *et al.* (2005) Masculine girls and feminine boys: genetic and environmental contributions to atypical gender development in early childhood. *Journal of Personality and Social Psychology* **88**, 400–412.

Knight, R.A. & Sims-Knight, J.E. (2003) The developmental antecedents of sexual coercion against women: testing alternative hypotheses with structural equation modeling. *Annals of the New York Academy of Sciences* **989**, 72–85.

Knudson, G. *et al.* (2010) Recommendations for revision of the *DSM* diagnosis of gender identity disorders: consensus statement of the World Professional Association for Transgender Health. *International Journal of Transgenderism* **12**, 115–118.

Koss, M.P. & Gidycz, C.A. (1985) Sexual experiences survey: reliability and validity. *Journal of Consulting and Clinical Psychology* **53**, 422–423.

Kruesi, M.P.J. *et al.* (1992) Paraphilias: a double blind cross-over comparison of clomipramine versus desipramine. *Archives of Sexual Behavior* **21**, 587–593.

Lalumière, M.L. & Earls, C.M. (1992) Voluntary control of penile responses as a function of stimulus duration and instructions. *Behavioral Assessment* **14**, 121–132.

Lalumière, M.L. & Quinsey, V.L. (1998) Pavlovian conditioning of sexual interests in human males. *Archives of Sexual Behavior* **27**, 241–252.

Lalumière, M.L. *et al.* (2005) *The Causes of Rape: Understanding Individual Differences in Male Propensity for Sexual Aggression.* American Psychological Association, Washington, DC.

Långström, N. & Seto, M.C. (2006) Exhibitionistic and voyeuristic behavior in a Swedish national population survey. *Archives of Sexual Behavior* **35**, 427–435.

Laschet, U. & Laschet, L. (1971) Psychopharmacotherapy of sex offenders with cyproterone acetate. *Pharmakopsychiatrie Neuropsychopharmakologic* **4**, 99–104.

Lawrence, A.A. (2010) Sexual orientation versus age of onset as bases for typologies (subtypes) of gender identity disorder in adolescents and adults. *Archives of Sexual Behavior* **39**, 514–545.

Laws, D.R. & Marshall, W.L. (1990) A conditioning theory of the etiology and maintenance of deviant sexual preference and behavior. In: *Handbook of Sexual Assault: Issues, Theories, and Treatment Of The Offender.* (eds W.L. Marshall, D.R. Laws & H.E. Barbaree), pp. 209–230. Plenum, New York.

Letourneau, E.J. *et al.* (2009) Multisystemic therapy for juvenile sexual offenders: 1-year results from a randomized effectiveness trial. *Journal of Family Psychology* **23**, 89–102.

Mahoney, J.M. & Strassberg, D.S. (1991) Voluntary control of male sexual arousal. *Archives of Sexual Behavior* **20**, 1–16.

Marantz, S. & Coates, S. (1991) Mothers of boys with gender identity disorder: a comparison of matched controls. *Journal of the American Academy of Child and Adolescent Psychiatry* **30**, 310–315.

Marks, I.M. & Gelder, M.G. (1967) Tranvestism and fetishism: clinical and psychological changes during faradic aversion. *British Journal of Psychiatry* **113**, 711–730.

Marshall, W.L. *et al.* (1991a) Early onset and deviant sexuality in child molesters. *Journal of Interpersonal Violence* **6**, 323–336.

Marshall, W.L. *et al.* (1991b) Exhibitionists: sexual preferences for exposing. *Behaviour Research and Therapy* **29**, 37–40.

Martin, C.L. *et al.* (2002) Cognitive theories of early gender development. *Psychological Bulletin* **128**, 903–933.

McGuire, R.J. *et al.* (1965) Sexual deviations as conditioned behavior: a hypothesis. *Behaviour Research and Therapy* **2**, 185–190.

Meadow, T. (2011) 'Deep down where the music plays': how parents account for childhood gender variance. *Sexualities* **14**, 725–747.

Menvielle, E. (2009) Transgender children: clinical and ethical issues in prepubertal presentations. *Journal of Gay & Lesbian Mental Health* **13**, 292–297.

Menvielle, E. (2012) A comprehensive program for children with gender variant behaviors and gender identity disorders. *Journal of Homosexuality* **59**, 357–368.

Menvielle, E.J. & Tuerk, C. (2002) A support group for parents of gender non-conforming boys. *Journal of the American Academy of Child and Adolescent Psychiatry* **41**, 1010–1013.

Meston, C.M. & Gorzalka, B.B. (1992) Psychoactive drugs and human sexual behavior: the role of serotonergic activity. *Journal of Psychoactive Drugs* **24**, 1–40.

Meyer-Bahlburg, H.F.L. (1994) Intersexuality and the diagnosis of gender identity disorder. *Archives of Sexual Behavior* **23**, 21–40.

Meyer-Bahlburg, H.F.L. (2002) Gender identity disorder in young boys: a parent- and peer-based protocol. *Clinical Child Psychology and Psychiatry* **7**, 360–377.

Meyer-Bahlburg, H.F.L. *et al.* (2004) Prenatal androgenization affects gender-related behavior but not gender identity in 5-12-year-old girls with congenital adrenal hyperplasia. *Archives of Sexual Behavior* **33**, 97–104.

Newman, L.E. (1976) Treatment for the parents of feminine boys. *American Journal of Psychiatry* **133**, 683–687.

Ngun, T.C. *et al.* (2011) The genetics of sex differences in brain and behavior. *Frontiers in Neuroendocrinology* **32**, 227–246.

Pasterski, V. *et al.* (2014) Increased cross-gender identification independent of gender role behavior in girls with congenital adrenal hyperplasia: results from a standardized assessment of 4- to 11-year-old children. *Archives of Sexual Behavior* [published online].

Plaud, J.J. & Martini, J.R. (1999) The respondent conditioning of male sexual arousal. *Behavior Modification* **23**, 254–268.

Poeppl, T.B. *et al.* (2013) Association between brain structure and phenotypic characteristics in pedophilia. *Journal of Psychiatric Research* **47**, 678–685.

Ponseti, J. *et al.* (2012) Assessment of pedophilia using hemodynamic brain response to sexual stimuli. *Archives of General Psychiatry* **69**, 187–194.

Pullman, L. & Seto, M.C. (2012) Assessment and treatment of adolescent sexual offenders: implications of recent research on generalist versus specialist explanations. *Child Abuse & Neglect* **36**, 203–209.

Rabban, M. (1950) Sex-role identification in young children from two diverse social groups. *Genetic Psychology Monographs* **42**, 81–158.

Rachman, S. & Hodgson, R.J. (1968) Experimentally-induced "sexual fetishism": replication and development. *Psychological Record* **18**, 25–27.

Raymond, M. (1956) Case of fetishism treated by aversion therapy. *British Medical Journal* **2**, 854–856.

Rekers, G.A. (1975) Stimulus control over sex-typed play in cross-gender identified boys. *Journal of Experimental Child Psychology* **20**, 136–148.

Rice, M.E. *et al.* (2012) Adolescents who have sexually offended: is phallometry valid? *Sexual Abuse: A Journal of Research and Treatment* **24**, 133–152.

Richter-Appelt, H. & Sandberg, D.E. (2010) Should disorders of sex development be an exclusion criterion for gender identity disorder in DSM 5? *International Journal of Transgenderism* **12**, 94–99.

Roberts, C. *et al.* (1987) Boyhood gender identity development: a statistical contrast of two family groups. *Developmental Psychology* **23**, 544–557.

Rosario, V.A. (2009) African-American transgender youth. *Journal of Gay & Lesbian Mental Health* **13**, 298–308.

Rubinow, D.R. & Schmidt, P.J. (1996) Androgens, brain and behavior. *American Journal of Psychiatry* **153**, 974–984.

Ruble, D.N. *et al.* (2006) Gender development. In: *Handbook of Child Psychology. Vol. 3: Social, Emotional, and Personality Development* 6th edn. (eds W. Damon, R.M. Lerner & N. Eisenberg), pp. 858–932. John Wiley & Sons, New York.

Ryan, G. *et al.* (1996) Trends in a national sample of sexually abusive youths. *Journal of the American Academy of Child and Adolescent Psychiatry* **35**, 17–25.

Salter, D. *et al.* (2003) Development of sexually abusive behaviour in sexually victimized males: a longitudinal study. *The Lancet* **361**, 471–476.

Schagen, S.E.E. *et al.* (2012) Sibling sex ratio and birth order in early-onset gender dysphoric adolescents. *Archives of Sexual Behavior* **41**, 541–549.

Seto, M.C. (2009) Pedophilia. *Annual Review of Clinical Psychology* **5**, 391–407.

Seto, M.C. (2012) Is pedophilia a sexual orientation? *Archives of Sexual Behavior* **41**, 231–236.

Seto, M.C. & Kuban, M. (1996) Criterion-related validity of a phallometric test for paraphilic rape and sadism. *Behaviour Research and Therapy* **34**, 175–183.

Seto, M.C. & Lalumière, M.L. (2010) What is so special about male adolescent sexual offending? A review and test of explanations using meta-analysis. *Psychological Bulletin* **136**, 526–575.

Seto, M.C. *et al.* (2000) The discriminative validity of a phallometric test for pedophilic interests among adolescent sex offenders against children. *Psychological Assessment* **12**, 319–327.

Seto, M.C. *et al.* (2003) Detecting anomalous sexual interests among juvenile sex offenders. *Annals of the New York Academy of Sciences* **989**, 118–130.

Seto, M.C. *et al.* (2004) The Screening Scale for Pedophilic Interests predicts recidivism among adult sex offenders with child victims. *Archives of Sexual Behavior* **33**, 455–466.

Seto, M.C. *et al.* (2012) The sexual responses of sexual sadists. *Journal of Abnormal Psychology* **121**, 739–753.

Shields, J.P. *et al.* (2013) Estimating population size and demographic characteristics of lesbian, gay, bisexual, and transgender youth in middle school. *Journal of Adolescent Health* **52**, 248–250.

Shiffman, M. (2013). *Peer Relations in Adolescents with Gender Identity Disorder.* Unpublished doctoral dissertation, University of Guelph, Guelph, Ontario, Canada.

Singh, D. (2012). *A Follow-Up Study of Boys with Gender Identity Disorder.* Unpublished doctoral dissertation, University of Toronto.

Singh, D. *et al.* (2010) The gender identity/gender dysphoria questionnaire for adolescents and adults: further validity evidence. *Journal of Sex Research* **47**, 49–58.

Skilling, T.A. *et al.* (2011) Understanding differences in self and parent reports among adolescent sex and non-sex offenders. *Psychological Assessment* **23**, 153–163.

Smith, G. & Fischer, L. (1999) Assessment of juvenile sexual offenders: reliability and validity of the Abel Assessment for Interest in Paraphilias. *Sexual Abuse: A Journal of Research and Treatment* **11**, 207–216.

Smith, Y.L.S. *et al.* (2001) Adolescents with gender identity disorder who were accepted or rejected for sex reassignment surgery: a prospective follow-up study. *Journal of the American Academy of Child and Adolescent Psychiatry* **40**, 472–481.

Steensma, T.D. *et al.* (2014) Behavioral and emotional problems on the Teacher's Report Form: a cross-national, cross-clinic comparative analysis of gender dysphoric children and adolescents. *Journal of Abnormal Child Psychology* **42**, 635–647.

Templeman, T.L. & Stinnett, R.D. (1991) Patterns of sexual arousal and history in a "normal" sample of young men. *Archives of Sexual Behavior* **20**, 137–150.

Thibaut, F. *et al.* (2010) The World Federation of Societies of Biological Psychiatry (WFSBP) guidelines for the treatment of paraphilias. *World Journal of Biological Psychiatry* **11**, 604–655.

Tobin, D.D. *et al.* (2010) The intrapsychics of gender: a model of self-socialization. *Psychological Review* **117**, 601–622.

van Beijsterveldt, C.E.M. *et al.* (2006) Genetic and environmental influences on cross-gender behavior and relations to psychopathology: a study of Dutch twins at ages 7 and 10 years. *Archives of Sexual Behavior* **35**, 647–658.

Vance, S.R. *et al.* (2010) Opinions about the *DSM* Gender Identity Disorder diagnosis: results from an international survey administered to organizations concerned with the welfare of transgender people. *International Journal of Transgenderism* **12**, 1–14.

VanderLaan, D.P. *et al.* (2014) Birth order and sibling sex ratio of children and adolescents referred to a Gender Identity Service *PLoS ONE*, **9**, e90257.

VanderLaan, D.P. *et al.* (2015) Do children with gender dysphoria have intense/obsessional interests? *Journal of Sex Research*, **52**, 213–219.

Wallien, M.S.C. & Cohen-Kettenis, P.T. (2008) Psychosexual outcome of gender dysphoric children. *Journal of the American Academy of Child and Adolescent Psychiatry* **47**, 1413–1423.

Wallien, M.S.C. *et al.* (2009) Cross-national replication of the Gender Identity Interview for Children. *Journal of Personality Assessment* **91**, 545–552.

Wallien, M.S.C. *et al.* (2010) Peer group status of gender dysphoric children: a sociometric study. *Archives of Sexual Behavior* **39**, 553–560.

Wiederman, M.W. (2002) Reliability and validity of measurement. In: *Handbook for Conducting Research on Human Sexuality.* (eds M.W. Wiederman & B.E. Whitley), pp. 25–50. Lawrence Erlbaum, Mahwah, NJ.

Wisnowski, D.L. (2011) Raising a gender non-conforming child. *Child and Adolescent Psychiatric Clinics of North America* **20**, 757–766.

Wood, H. *et al.* (2013) Patterns of referral to a Gender Identity Service for Children and Adolescents (1976-2011): age, sex ratio, and sexual orientation [Letter to the Editor]. *Journal of Sex & Marital Therapy* **39**, 1–6.

World Health Organization (1992) *International Classification of Diseases and Related Health Problems* (10th rev.). World Health Organization, Geneva.

Worling, J.R. & Curwen, T. (2000) Adolescent sexual offender recidivism: success of specialized treatment and implications for risk prediction. *Child Abuse and Neglect* **24**, 965–982.

Zolondek, S.C. *et al.* (2001) The self-reported behaviors of juvenile sexual offenders. *Journal of Interpersonal Violence* **16**, 73–85.

Zucker, K.J. (1985) Cross-gender identified children. In: *Gender Dysphoria: Development, Research, Management.* (ed B.W. Steiner), pp. 75–174. Plenum, New York.

Zucker, K.J. (1999) Intersexuality and gender identity differentiation. *Annual Review of Sex Research* **10**, 1–69.

Zucker, K.J. (2005a) Measurement of psychosexual differentiation. *Archives of Sexual Behavior* **34**, 375–388.

Zucker, K. J. (2005b). *Patterns of psychopathology in boys with gender identity disorder.* Paper presented at the joint meeting of the American Academy of Child Psychiatry and the Canadian Academy of Child Psychiatry, Toronto.

Zucker, K.J. (2006) "I'm half-boy, half-girl": play psychotherapy and parent counseling for gender identity disorder. In: *DSM-IV-TR® Casebook, Volume 2. Experts Tell How They Treated Their Own Patients.* (eds R.L. Spitzer, M.B. First, J.B.W. Williams & M. Gibbons), pp. 321–334. American Psychiatric Association, Washington, DC.

Zucker, K.J. (2007) Gender identity disorder in children, adolescents, and adults. In: *Treatments of Psychiatric Disorders.* (ed G.O. Gabbard), vol. 2, 4th edn, pp. 683–701. American Psychiatric Association, Washington, DC.

Zucker, K.J. (2008) Children with gender identity disorder: is there a best practice? [Enfants avec troubles de l'identité sexuée: y-a-t-il une pratique la meilleure?]. *Neuropsychiatrie de l'Enfance et de l'Adolescence* **56**, 358–364.

Zucker, K.J. (2010) The DSM diagnostic criteria for gender identity disorder in children. *Archives of Sexual Behavior* **39**, 477–498.

Zucker, K.J. & Bradley, S.J. (1995) *Gender Identity Disorder and Psychosexual Problems in Children and Adolescents.* Guilford Press, New York.

Zucker, K.J. & Lawrence, A.A. (2009) Epidemiology of gender identity disorder: recommendations for the standards of care of the World Professional Association for Transgender Health. *International Journal of Transgenderism* **11**, 8–18.

Zucker, K.J. & Wood, H. (2011) Assessment of gender variance in children. *Child and Adolescent Psychiatric Clinics of North America* **20**, 665–680.

Zucker, K.J. *et al.* (1985) Sex-typed behavior in cross-gender-identified children: stability and change at a one-year follow-up. *Journal of the American Academy of Child Psychiatry* **24**, 710–719.

Zucker, K.J. *et al.* (1997a) Sex differences in referral rates of children with gender identity disorder: some hypotheses. *Journal of Abnormal Child Psychology* **25**, 217–227.

Zucker, K.J. *et al.* (1997b) Sibling sex ratio of boys with gender identity disorder. *Journal of Child Psychology and Psychiatry* **38**, 543–551.

Zucker, K.J. *et al.* (1999) Gender constancy judgments in children with gender identity disorder: evidence for a developmental lag. *Archives of Sexual Behavior* **28**, 475–502.

Zucker, K.J. *et al.* (2008) Is gender identity disorder in adolescents coming out of the closet? [Letter to the Editor]. *Journal of Sex and Marital Therapy* **34**, 287–290.

Zucker, K.J. *et al.* (2011) Puberty-blocking hormonal therapy for adolescents with gender identity disorder: a descriptive clinical study. *Journal of Gay & Lesbian Mental Health* **15**, 58–82.

Zucker, K.J. *et al.* (2012a) Demographics, behavior problems, and psychosexual characteristics of adolescents with gender identity disorder or transvestic fetishism. *Journal of Sex & Marital Therapy* **38**, 151–189.

Zucker, K.J. *et al.* (2012b) A developmental, biopsychosocial model for the treatment of children with gender identity disorder. *Journal of Homosexuality* **59**, 369–397.

Zucker, K.J. *et al.* (2013) Memo outlining evidence for change for gender identity disorder in the DSM-5. *Archives of Sexual Behavior* **42**, 901–914.

Zucker, K.J. *et al.* (2014) Models of psychopathology in children and adolescents with gender dysphoria. In: *Gender Dysphoria and Disorders of Sex Development: Progress in Care and Knowledge.* (eds B.P.C. Kreukels, T.D. Steensma & A.L.C. de Vries), pp. 171–192. Springer, New York.

Zuckerman, M. (1971) Physiological measures of sexual arousal in the human. *Psychological Bulletin* **75**, 297–329.

CHAPTER 70

Sleep interventions: a developmental perspective

Allison G. Harvey[1] and Eleanor L. McGlinchey[1,2]

[1] Department of Psychology, University of California, Berkeley, CA, USA
[2] New York State Psychiatric Institute, Columbia University Medical Center, NY, USA

Introduction

In this chapter, we review evidence that we believe points to sleep disturbance as contributing in several ways to core problems and symptoms of children and youth. We highlight that treatments targeting sleep represent unique opportunities for intervention that have potential for a broad range of positive outcomes.

Basic overview of human sleep architecture across development

Beginning in infancy, the brain cycles through stages of neural activity that correspond to periods of wakefulness and different stages of sleep. "Mature" sleep is divided into two major categories: rapid eye movement (REM) sleep and non-REM (NREM) sleep. NREM sleep is subdivided into four stages: Stage 1 occurs at transitions of sleep and wakefulness; Stage 2 is characterized by frequent bursts of rhythmic electroencephalography (EEG) activity, called sleep spindles, and high-voltage slow spikes, called K-complexes; Stages 3 and 4 (also called slow wave sleep or delta sleep), represent the deepest stages of sleep and are comprised largely of high-voltage EEG activity in the slowest (delta) frequency range. In newborn infants, each sleep cycle is around 60 min, with 50% in "active sleep" and 50% in "quiet sleep." Active sleep is similar to REM sleep in adults and involves head movements, rapid eye movements, fast and irregular respiration, and increased heart rate. Quiet sleep is similar to NREM sleep in adults and involves few movements. By about 2 years of age, active sleep declines to 20–25% and slow wave sleep is maximal, making it difficult to wake a child during the first sleep cycle. By 6–11 years of age clearer cycles of sleep, each about 90 min, emerge such that the amount of Stages 3 and 4 sleep and REM reduces and Stage 2 sleep increases. By around 11 years of age slow wave sleep is at 40% and continues to decline across adolescence, which is thought to parallel pruning of cortical density. By mid-adolescence sleep conforms to the 90-min cycle of adults. REM sleep is retained across childhood, adolescence, adulthood, and older adults whereas slow wave sleep decreases across the age range (Carskadon & Dement, 2011).

Conceptual models

A convergence of processes work together to support sleep. The conceptual models briefly reviewed in this section were selected as they highlight several major contributors.

Two-process model

Two independent regulatory processes interact to regulate the timing, intensity, and duration of sleep: a homeostatic sleep process and a circadian sleep process (Borbély, 1982). The first, often called "Process S," represents a sleep–wake dependent homeostatic component of sleep that increases as a function of previous wakefulness and gradually decreases over the course of a sleep period. The second process, often called "Process C," is the circadian component, which arises from the endogenous pacemaker in the suprachiasmatic nuclei (SCN). At the molecular level, intrinsically rhythmic cells within the SCN generate rhythmicity via circadian genes. The process by which the pacemaker is set to a 24-hour period and kept in appropriate phase with seasonally shifting day length is called entrainment, which occurs via zeitgebers ("time giver" in German). In other words, the sleep and circadian systems are open systems, readily open to influence from the environment. The primary zeitgeber is the daily alteration of light and dark. The SCN is also responsive to nonphotic cues such as arousal/locomotor activity, social cues, feeding, sleep deprivation, and temperature (Mistlberger et al., 2000). Hence, there is a clear biological pathway by which behavioral changes in terms of the timing exposure to light and regularizing activities, meal times etc. that form the basis for intervention. Note that the SCN is not fully developed at birth. Hence, while the newborn infant is sensitive to zeitgebers, greater sensitivity will emerge across the first year of life.

Rutter's Child and Adolescent Psychiatry, Sixth Edition.
Edited by Anita Thapar and Daniel S. Pine, James F. Leckman, Stephen Scott, Margaret J. Snowling, Eric Taylor.
© 2015 John Wiley & Sons Ltd. Published 2018 by John Wiley & Sons Ltd.

Safety/vigilance/arousal

Sleep is naturally restricted to safe times and places (e.g., animals tend to sleep in safe burrows or nests that minimize dangers). This system has adaptive advantages (inhibiting sleep when we are in danger) but also has costs. Sleep and vigilance represent opponent processes since sleep is in essence a turning off of awareness and responsiveness to the external environment (Dahl & Lewin, 2002). Hence, it is natural that states of vigilance and anxiety are antithetical to going to sleep. Children can experience fear as well as other sources of cognitive or emotional arousal that prevents an overall sense of safety and is likely to be antithetical to sleep. Adolescents can get into the habit of mentally reviewing or replaying worrisome thoughts and/or memories of stressful events. Some youth with stressful memories or specific fears manage to avoid these during the day through distracting activities, but at night—especially when trying to fall asleep—the lack of distracters can result in rumination on these thoughts.

Three-P model

The three-P (3P) model (Spielman et al., 1987), also referred to as the three-factor or the Spielman model, is a useful heuristic to guide assessment and treatment of sleep problems. The three-P model is a diathesis-stress model which includes predisposing, precipitating, and perpetuating factors. The predisposing factors can be biological (e.g., regularly elevated cortisol), psychological (e.g., tendency to worry) or social (e.g., school schedule incompatible with sleep schedule). Precipitating factors, such as stressful life events, then trigger the acute onset of sleep problems. Perpetuating factors, such as maladaptive coping skills or an extension of time in bed, can then contribute to the acute sleep problem developing into a chronic or longer term disorder. Within this framework, predisposing factors represent a constant vulnerability for sleeping problems. Precipitating factors trigger the acute sleep problem, but the influence of these factors diminishes over time. By contrast, perpetuating factors then come into play and serve to maintain the sleep problems. As a result, the perpetuating factors are typically the targets of treatment.

Brain development

Highly relevant to teenagers is the temporal gap between the development of brain regions involved in behavior regulation and cognitive control functions (prefrontal cortex; PFC) and the brain regions controlling emotional processing and behaviors associated with reward/punishment (ventral–medial areas of the PFC) that have bidirectional connections with the amygdala and the hypothalamus (Giedd et al., 1999; Quevedo et al., 2009; Silk et al., 2009; Steinberg, 2010). Importantly, these same prefrontal and inter-related limbic regions also appear to be those networks known to display the greatest sensitivity to insufficient sleep (Yoo et al., 2007).

Consequences of poor sleep

Sleep and sleep disturbance have pervasive effects, particularly across development.

Sleep is critical for affect regulation

There is robust evidence in adults that sleep deprivation undermines emotion responding and regulation the following day (Pilcher & Huffcutt, 1996; Yoo et al., 2007) with similar findings among youth (Talbot et al., 2010; McGlinchey et al., 2011). Studies experimentally restricting sleep in healthy youth have reported decrements in affective functioning as a function of sleep loss (Leotta et al., 1997; Talbot et al., 2010; McGlinchey et al., 2011). Conversely, better quality sleep may buffer against affective risk. For example, a prospective study of children at high risk for major depressive disorder found that a greater percentage of slow wave sleep during childhood was protective against the development of depression during adolescence and young adulthood (Silk et al., 2007). Interestingly, a study by Zohar et al. (2005) suggests that the context in which the emotion is experienced is important for determining the valence (positive versus negative) of the emotion experienced under conditions of sleep deprivation.

Sleep is important for cognitive functioning

It seems plausible that sleep disturbance may impair cognitive functioning in children given that adverse and severe effects of sleep deprivation on cognitive functioning have been clearly demonstrated in adults (Van Dongen et al., 2003). In particular, there are at least two stages of memory where sleep has been demonstrated to be important. Yoo et al. (2007) have presented evidence for a critical role for sleep before learning in preparing key neural structures for efficient next-day memory encoding. Specifically, sleep-deprived participants exhibit a large 40% reduction in the ability to form new human memories under conditions of sleep deprivation (Walker & Stickgold, 2006). In contrast to the impairment of memory encoding following sleep loss, recent findings have characterized the proactive benefit of sleep on memory encoding. Interestingly, a daytime nap restores the normal deterioration in learning capacity that develops across the day (Mander et al., 2011). In addition, sleep obtained after learning also plays a critical role in the consolidation of episodic (fact-based) declarative memories. Sleep deprivation after learning prevents the consolidation of new memories (both emotional and nonemotional). Moreover, experimentally enhancing the quality of sleep, specifically slow wave sleep (Stages 3 and 4), causally enhances consolidation and hence long-term retention of [nonemotional] memories (Stickgold & Walker, 2005; Payne et al., 2009; Diekelmann & Born, 2010). Beyond simply strengthening individual fact-based memories, sleep after learning also appears to help integrate newly learned information.

Although this compelling evidence has accrued based on adults, the developmental implications have attracted considerable attention. Consistently, an observation of 135 healthy school children (Sadeh et al., 2002) as well as a comparison of 1 hour of restricted versus extended sleep in 77 children (Sadeh et al., 2003) showed clear adverse consequences of inadequate sleep on cognitive functioning. In addition to the acute effects of sleep loss, cognitive impairments may persist over time. In one prospective study, parent-reported sleep problems during childhood significantly predicted neuropsychological functioning in early adolescence (Gregory *et al.*, 2009). Adverse effects in this domain are likely to be particularly critical for children given that educational achievements (so reliant on cognitive function) will have far reaching and long-term consequences. For example, a meta-analysis of 60 studies of the association between school performance and sleep quality, total sleep time and daytime sleepiness indicated modest but significant associations (Dewald *et al.*, 2010). In another meta-analysis of healthy school-age children (5–12 years old) across 86 studies and 35,936 children, sleep duration was clearly associated with cognitive performance, particularly executive functioning, on tasks that address multiple cognitive domains and with school performance, although not with intelligence, sustained attention or memory (Astill *et al.*, 2012).

Sleep is important for health and contributes to obesity

Sleep deprivation increases appetite, weight gain, and insulin tolerance (Spiegel *et al.*, 2004). Indeed, in a meta-analysis involving 30 studies (12 in children) and 634,511 participants, an association between short sleep and obesity was observed across the age range. Specifically, there was a 60–80% increase in the odds of being a short sleeper among children who were obese (Cappuccio *et al.*, 2008). Furthermore, experimentally induced short-term sleep deprivation in normal weight college-age volunteers is associated with disturbed appetite hormones (grehlin and leptin) in a direction associated with obesity (Spiegel *et al.*, 2004). The mechanisms of these effects are related to grehlin and leptin, which regulate energy balance in the body. Leptin levels are lower under conditions of sleep deprivation. Under conditions of normal sleep, leptin reduces in response to calorie shortage and is associated with hunger and increase in response to calorie surplus. Ghrelin levels are higher under conditions of sleep deprivation. Under normal sleep conditions, higher levels are associated with increased appetite.

Sleep deprivation is associated with behavioral problems including substance use

From pre-schoolers right up through the childhood and adolescent years, multiple reports indicate an association between inadequate sleep and behavioral problems (Sadeh *et al.*, 2002; Bates *et al.*, 2003). Indeed, in the Astill *et al.* (2012) meta-analysis described earlier, shorter sleep duration was associated with more behavioral problems and both internalizing and externalizing behavioral problems.

In terms of substance use problems in a Finnish sample of adolescents, irregular sleep schedules and daytime sleepiness accounted for 26% of the variance in substance use in 15-year-old boys and 12% in 15-year-old girls (Tynjala *et al.*, 1997). Another large study of 4500 12–17-year-olds found that adolescents who had trouble sleeping reported greater use of alcohol (odds ratio of 2.6), marijuana (odds ratio of 2.4) and cigarettes (odds ratio of 2.2) (Johnson *et al.*, 1999). It is possible that the effects of drugs and alcohol may be sought out for the sedation and/or emotional regulatory effects or for rewarding and/or stimulating effects. In addition, sleep disturbance could also represent a direct effect of use of certain substances.

Sleep deprivation contributes to suicidality

Teens with more insomnia and nightmares reported more suicidal ideation (Choquet & Menke, 1989) and insomnia and hypersomnia were independently associated with suicidal ideation (Choquet *et al.*, 1993). Poor sleep has also been associated with suicide attempts. Eighty one percent of teens presenting to an emergency room following a suicide attempt reported difficulty falling asleep or early morning waking immediately preceding the attempt. Nightmares were associated with increased risk for suicide attempts and those who slept less than 8 hour were 3 times more likely to attempt suicide (Liu & Buysse, 2006). Poor sleep has also been associated with suicide completion. Insomnia also predicts adolescent hospitalization for suicide attempt (Gasquet & Choquet, 1994).

Using a psychological autopsy protocol in which parents, siblings, and friends were interviewed between 4 and 6 months after the suicide, Goldstein *et al.* (2008) compared adolescent suicide completers ($n = 140$) with an age/sex matched control group ($n = 131$). Suicide completers had higher rates of overall sleep disturbance, insomnia, and hypersomnia within the past week.

Epidemiology

Reported bedtime is delayed and sleep duration decreases with increasing age (Liu *et al.*, 2005). Sleep problems, as reported by parents, range from 20% to 30% (e.g., Lozoff *et al.*, 1985; Mindell, 1996; Anders & Eiben, 1997; Mindell, 1999; Stores, 2006). Among older children, there can be a discrepancy between parent and child report of sleep problems (in both directions). Most of the epidemiological work in this area draws from samples collected in the United States or Europe. Interestingly, one study compared children in grades 1–4 in the United States and in China. Chinese children went to bed approximately half an hour later (9:02 vs 8:27 PM) and woke up half an hour earlier (6:28 vs 6:55 AM), resulting in an average sleep duration that was 1 hour less (9.25 vs 10.15 hours) (Liu *et al.*, 2005). Cultural differences in sleep are an understudied topic.

Longitudinal outcome and sleep as a risk factor

Untreated sleep problems first presenting in infancy are known to persist during school-aged years and often become chronic (Zuckerman *et al.*, 1987; Pollock, 1994). Evidence has steadily accrued indicating that insomnia is an independent risk factor for first and recurrent episodes of depression. For example, community residing youth ($N = 4500$) who reported frequent trouble sleeping were more likely than normal-sleeping controls to report anxiety or depression (odds ratio $= 22.7$) (Johnson et al., 1999). A similar study of 1014 teens found that chronologically primary insomnia significantly predicted future depression (hazard rate $= 3.8$) but that primary depression did not predict subsequent insomnia (Johnson et al., 2006). Insomnia symptoms predicted subsequent depression in another large adolescent community panel (Roberts et al., 2002); elevated insomnia at Wave 1 predicted greater depression severity at Wave 2 even when controlling for Wave 2 insomnia. Moreover, there is substantial evidence that sleep problems emerging during early childhood are independently predictive for the later onset of depression (Gregory et al., 2005; Ong et al., 2006). Among 1760 high school students aged 16–18, Danielsson et al. (2012) replicated the finding that sleep disturbances predict depressive symptoms 1 year later. The novel contribution of this study is that catastrophic worry partially mediated the relationship. While girls reported more sleep disturbances, depressive symptoms, and catastrophic worry relative to boys, the results were similar regardless of gender. The tendency toward catastrophic worry is treatable, a point to which we will return.

In a study of early-onset bipolar disorder ($n = 82$), sleep disturbance was reported by about half of the parents as one of the earliest symptoms observed (Faedda et al., 2004). In another study, sleep disturbances (and anxiety disorders) were identified as an antecedent to the onset of bipolar disorder in a subset of high-risk youth (Duffy et al., 2007). Further evidence is provided by findings reported in a study (Shaw et al., 2005) of 100 at-risk children with a parent with Bipolar I as well as a control group of 112 children with well parents. Decreased sleep was one of the distinguishing features of the high-risk group.

Two large prospective studies with nonclinical adolescent samples in the United States provide evidence that insufficient sleep predicts worse mental health at follow-up, after controlling for baseline levels of functioning (Roberts et al., 2002; Fredriksen et al., 2004). A long-term longitudinal study of the sons of alcohol-dependent men found that insufficient sleep and overtiredness among children of ages 3–5 were predictive of early use of alcohol, cigarettes, and other drugs in early adolescence, after controlling for parents' alcoholism (Wong et al., 2009). These findings for boys were replicated in a community sample (Wong et al., 2010). Recent research using data from the National Longitudinal Study of Adolescent Health suggest that insufficient sleep leads to drug use among teens, and that patterns of sleep and drug use are spread via social networks (Mednick et al., 2010). These social network analyses suggest that insufficient sleep mediates the relationship between adolescents' own drug use and the drug use of their friends.

Additional longitudinal research focused on elucidating risk factors seems like a good investment of research effort given that it is so commonly observed that symptoms of various problems experienced by children are worse during periods of inadequate sleep.

Assessment

A thorough assessment of a young patient would typically involve the seven parts listed in Table 70.1. We will focus on the first part—the assessment of past and current sleep. The evaluation of sleep problems should take place within two general frameworks: (i) the 3P model that helps organize material into predisposing, precipitating, and perpetuating factors (see Section "Three-P model") and (ii) the context (considering stage of development, social situation, and culture).

A widely held assumption is that a sleep problem is always secondary to, or an epiphenomenon of, the so-called "primary" psychiatric disorder. Consequently, complaints of sleep problems have tended to be dismissed or regarded as trivial by both patients and their caregivers or, at most, seen as a by-product of the coexisting disorder. By contrast, evidence is accruing to indicate that sleep problems can be important but under recognized contributors to the multifactorial cause and maintenance of several comorbid problems, such as those reviewed earlier in this chapter. Hence, when a sleep problem is present, it should be targeted in treatment and not assumed to remit with treatment of the comorbid condition. The value of this approach is illustrated by studies comparing depressed patients who are treated only for their depression (with an antidepressant) versus depressed patients who are treated for both the depression (with an antidepressant) and insomnia (with cognitive behavior therapy). The combined approach was superior for both depression and insomnia outcomes (Manber et al., 2007). Although this study was conducted with adults, it is very tempting to speculate that similar findings would emerge in studies of youth.

The goal of the assessment is to establish a diagnosis and a formulation and to obtain sufficient information to devise

---

Table 70.1 Assessment of sleep problems: domains to include.

1 A sleep assessment, current, past. Orient to sleep diary
2 A review of medical history, including hospitalizations, current medications, past and current medical conditions, and so on
3 A developmental assessment, including school functioning, developmental disabilities, prematurity, and so on
4 A family history of sleep disorders
5 A psychosocial history, including cultural context, impact on family, life events, and so on
6 A behavioral and psychiatric assessment because sleep problems often co-occur with other diagnoses such as depression, anxiety, ADHD, and so on
7 A physical exam, including growth check, appearance, nose/throat/mouth (possible risk factors for sleep-related breathing problems), neurologic exam, and so on

Source: Based on Mindell and Owens (2009).

a treatment plan. The latter involves unraveling the chain of factors that contribute to the sleep disturbance. Ideally, we suggest obtaining information via a multi-method approach that includes the methods discussed in Sections "Clinical interview, Questionnaires, Sleep diary, Polysomnography (PSG), and Actigraphy." If the context allows, ideally the assessment should begin before the first visit. It can be expedient and helpful to send some of the questionnaires, as well as the sleep diary, to be completed before the first meeting.

Clinical interview

As we have outlined elsewhere (Harvey & Spielman, 2011), a dual approach to assessment is suggested that uses a "wide lens" to establish the broad thematic structure of the problem (e.g., what part of the night is disturbed, daytime activities that affect sleep, thoughts about sleep, worries about the daytime functional deficits, sleep–wake habits, etc.). The other approach is pointedly personal and uses a "focused lens" that dissects a particular night on which difficulty sleeping was experienced—and the subsequent day.

Attention needs to be paid in the evaluation to comorbid conditions such as psychiatric, sleep, and medical disorders. Consistent with the consensus of the field, it is assumed that these disorders may trigger, contribute to, or be unrelated to the sleep problem.

One common vulnerability factor has been associated with child temperament; namely, children who are known to be difficult to calm are least likely to fall asleep or stay asleep without the assistance of a caregiver. Additional factors that may perpetuate sleep problems in young children include caregiver attributes including symptoms of depression (Gress-Smith et al., 2012) and parental work schedule (Sinai & Tikotzky, 2012). Recent research also suggests that when the parental expectations for sleep behavior do not match the typical development of childhood sleep habits, poor sleep among young children is common (Tikotzky & Sadeh, 2009). Finally, there are environmental factors that may exacerbate problems that the child has with falling asleep or also with parental difficulties in setting clear limits for bedtime (Mindell et al., 2006).

Questionnaires

The Sleep Habits Survey (Owens et al., 2010a; Wolfson & Carskadon, 1998) comprises 20 items each rated on a 4-point scale. Child and parent versions are available (Gruber et al., 1997). Both have good psychometrics (Sadeh et al., 2000). This measure includes a measure of sleepiness (e.g., sleepiness while studying, in class, conversing, etc.) and the Children's Morningness–Eveningness Preferences (CMEP) Scale which is a 10-item measure of eveningness adapted by Carskadon et al. (1993). Scores range from 10 (Extreme evening preference) to 42 (extreme morning preference). The Brief Infant Sleep Questionnaire has nine items, validated for 5–29-month year olds and assesses sleep duration, night waking, nocturnal wakefulness, and sleep onset time (Sadeh, 2004). The Pediatric Sleep

Questionnaire contains 22 items and has been validated for 2–18-year-olds. It includes three subscales: snoring, sleepiness, and behavior (Chervin et al., 2000).

Sleep diary

The sleep diary is perhaps the most helpful tool for assessing the current sleep problem. There are several options available. The need for a standard sleep diary has been recognized and is being addressed by a work group of experts (Carney et al., 2012). The completion of a paper version is inexpensive and easy to use but increasingly web-based and electronic options are available which can increase efficiency and accuracy (because the data are time stamped, ensuring that the diary really is completed each morning). The enhanced awareness arising from self-monitoring can have a therapeutic effect.

It is helpful to ask the patient to continue to complete the diary across the course of treatment as a means of monitoring progress and adjusting treatment recommendations. Keep in mind that the diary questions can be individualized on the basis of issues discovered during the clinical assessment that are to be targeted in treatment (e.g., for some young people, adding questions about daytime energy level can be helpful). Parents can be recruited to assist with the completion of the diary among older children and can be the main completer for younger children.

Polysomnography (PSG)

Polysomnography, also known as a sleep study, is used to classify sleep into stages. It involves placing surface electrodes on the scalp and face to measure electrical brain activity (electroencephalogram), eye movement (electrooculogram), and muscle tone (electromyogram). The data obtained are used to classify each epoch of data by sleep stage and in terms of sleep cycles (NREM and REM).

PSG is important for diagnosing periodic limb movement disorder (PLMD) and obstructive sleep apnea and other sleep-related breathing disorders (SBDs). The evidence for the use of PSG to diagnose sleep disorders in children has been subject to detailed reviewed (Aurora et al., 2012). Standard recommendations for PSG use in children with suspected sleep-related breathing disorders include PSG as a necessary assessment tool for the diagnosis of obstructive sleep apnea syndrome (OSAS) and as a pre- and post-operative assessment for residual OSAS following an adenotonsillectomy (Aurora et al., 2012). PSG is indicated for positive airway pressure (PAP) titration in children requiring this treatment for nighttime apnea episodes. Standards also require the use of PSG in diagnosing PLMD and narcolepsy in children (Aurora et al., 2012). Additionally, standards indicate that the multiple sleep latency test (MSLT) (Littner et al., 2005) should be used to assess the degree of excessive daytime sleepiness associated with the diagnosis of narcolepsy among children. Additional guidelines and options are reviewed in the two studies that may be used alongside the clinical judgment of a child sleep specialist.

As the diagnosis of insomnia relies solely on a subjective complaint, PSG is not needed nor recommended for the standard evaluation of insomnia (Reite *et al.*, 1995). However, it should be conducted for patients who do not respond to standard insomnia treatment. In the latter case a comorbid sleep disorder may be present but covert. Major limitations of PSG include the expense and discomfort. Hence, PSG is typically only conducted for one to two nights.

Actigraphy

An alternative objective assessment of sleep is the use of actigraphy. Actigraphy has increasingly been employed in an attempt to overcome shortcomings associated with PSG. Actigraphs are wrist watch-like devices that provide an estimate of the sleep/wake cycle via movement detectors (accelerometers). Within is a sensor, a processor and sufficient memory to record for up to several weeks. The processor samples physical motion and translates it to digital data. It summarizes the frequency of physical motions into epochs of specified time duration and stores the summary in memory. These data are then downloaded and automatic scoring methods (algorithms) are used to derive levels of activity/inactivity and generate various sleep/wake parameters. Relative to PSG, actigraphy is considerably less expensive and less intrusive and it provides the opportunity to continuously monitor patients over long time periods in their normal environment. According to two comprehensive reviews by the American Sleep Disorders Association (Sadeh *et al.*, 1995; Ancoli-Israel *et al.*, 2003), actigraphy is considered to be a useful and acceptable instrument to measure sleep–wake schedule and sleep quality. Furthermore, actigraphy is appropriate for examining sleep variability (i.e., night-to-night variability). Although there is considerable data validating actigraphy in adult normal sleepers, data testing the validity of actigraphy for infants, children, and youth is lacking. Moreover, it is important to note that the type of watch and the scoring algorithm used can result in substantial scoring differences.

Classification

Various diagnostic systems offer criteria for sleep disorders including the International Classification of Sleep Disorders' (ICSD) criteria (American Academy of Sleep Medicine, 2014), the Diagnostic and Statistical Manual of Mental Disorders' (DSM-5) criteria (American Psychiatric Association, 2013) and the International Classification of Diseases (ICD) (World Health Organization, 1992). Unfortunately these offer relatively few specific adaptations to diagnose sleep problems in children and youth and there are many differences across the three offerings. Hence, rather than delve into the complexities here, as we move on to discuss treatment, we have focused on the disorders that are common across the three systems and most commonly experienced by children and adolescents.

Interventions for common sleep disorders of childhood and adolescence

As will become evident across this section, there is a great need for treatment research. The early results for behavioral interventions are particularly promising. Although these have not been tested specifically for various comorbidities (e.g., autism, bipolar disorder, ADHD, etc.), the data on using these approaches for sleep disturbance comorbid with another psychiatric or medical problems in adults are very encouraging (Smith *et al.*, 2005), albeit with some potential adaptations in certain situations (Harvey, 2009). The data on behavioral interventions for sleep problems in young people are also very promising. There are several advantages to treating sleep problems nonpharmacologically including that behavioral interventions are: safe (few side effects and no potential for causing adverse interactions with prescribed medications), simple (easy to do), and inexpensive (especially considering that the positive effects have been shown to endure even up to 24 months in adults trials).

Problems going to sleep and staying asleep in young children

Bedtime struggles and middle of the night wakings are not only a source of sleep disruption for children and their parents but also can be a source of conflict and negative emotion among family members, contributing to negative parent–child interactions and marital discord. One aspect of the difficulty is that young children often show a "paradoxical" reaction when obtaining insufficient or inadequate sleep. That is, sleep-deprived young children (whether from insufficient or disrupted sleep) often look irritable, impulsive, with some symptoms of distractibility and emotional lability, and may appear overly active.

Interventions for bedtime problems and night wakings are founded on principles of learning and behavior (e.g., reinforcement, extinction, and shaping). Treatments involve training parents with a therapist guiding interventions on how to change their child's problematic sleep habits or sleep-related behaviors. The different behavioral interventions for early childhood sleep difficulties, and the level of empirical support for each, have been reviewed in a recent practice parameters paper commissioned by the American Association for Sleep Medicine (Mindell *et al.*, 2006). The first of these interventions is "unmodified extinction" and involves having the parents put the child to bed at a designated bedtime and then ignoring any crying, tantruming, or calling out by the child until a set time the next morning (although parents monitor for illness, injury, etc.). The effective use of extinction requires parental consistency. No matter how long the crying lasts, parents must ignore this every night. Otherwise, the child will only learn to cry longer the next time. The common term used in the media and self-help books to describe unmodified extinction techniques is the "cry it out" approach (Ferber, 1985). The difficulty with the use of unmodified extinction procedures is that it is often perceived as stressful by parents and many are not able to ignore the crying long enough for the procedure to be effective. An alternative to unmodified extinction is extinction with parental presence. In this variant, the parent stays in the child's room at bedtime but ignores the child and his/her problematic behavior. For some parents this procedure helps them to be more consistent and is more acceptable to them.

Another intervention based on extinction principals is "Graduated Extinction." Parents are instructed to ignore bedtime crying and tantrums on a specified schedule of check-ins. The period between check-ins is often tailored with the guidance of a therapist with considerations for the child's age, temperament, and the parents' judgment of how long they can tolerate the child's crying. Parents can also choose to check on their child on a fixed schedule (e.g., every 5 minutes) or with incrementally longer intervals (e.g., 5, 10, then 15 min). When using incrementally longer intervals, increases across successive checks within the same night or across successive nights can gradually reduce to no check-ins. Parents should only comfort their child for a brief period and no longer than a minute. Through the use of Graduated Extinction, the child will develop "self-soothing" skills so that he/she falls asleep independently without the parent. In self-help books, this type of intervention is often referred to as "sleep training."(Mindell, 2005).

Behavioral interventions can also include powerful methods for increasing homeostatic drive to sleep, such as developmental adaptations of stimulus control and sleep restriction (described in Table 70.2) which involve a small amount of sleep restriction that builds the homeostatic process.

Positive Routines is an intervention that involves the parents developing a routine at bedtime that is characterized by quiet and enjoyable activities for the child. Faded Bedtime is often used with Positive Routines and involves taking the child out of bed for predetermined periods of time when the child does not fall asleep. Bedtime is also delayed so that sleep onset occurs quickly and so that the cues for sleep are paired with the enjoyable activities from the Positive Routines procedure. Once the behavioral chain of events is well established and the child falls asleep more quickly, bedtime is moved earlier by 15–30 min over successive nights until an age appropriate bedtime goal is achieved. In addition, when overnight wakings are the primary problem, scheduled awakenings can be used. This procedure involves the parent awakening and comforting their child approximately 15–30 min before a typical awakening. Before using this strategy, a baseline of the number and timing of the nighttime awakenings must be established. Preemptive awakenings are then scheduled and can involve rocking or nursing the child back to sleep. Over consecutive nights, scheduled awakenings are faded out, by gradually increasing the time span between awakenings. Scheduled awakenings have been shown to increase the duration of consolidated sleep (Rickert & Johnson, 1988).

Another approach to treatment of sleep disturbances is to prevent their occurrence. A number of behavioral interventions have been incorporated into new parent education programs. These programs typically focus on early establishment of positive sleep habits. Education in these programs targets bedtime routines, development of a consistent schedule, parental soothing techniques during sleep initiation, and parent response

Table 70.2 Stimulus control and sleep restriction: intervention and rationale.

Stimulus control therapy (Bootzin, 1979)

Rationale. Conditioning has occurred between temporal and environmental stimuli (the bed, bedroom, and bedtime) normally conducive to sleep and sleep incompatible behaviors (e.g. worry/frustration at not being able to sleep), such that the bed, bedroom, and bedtime are no longer discriminative stimuli for sleep. The intervention aims to reverse this maladaptive association by limiting the sleep incompatible behaviors engaged in within the bedroom environment thereby decreasing cues for sleep incompatible behaviors while increasing cues for sleep-compatible behaviors.

Intervention. The therapist provides a detailed rationale for and assists the patient to achieve the following
(a) go to bed only when sleepy at night;
(b) use the bed and bedroom only for sleep (i.e., no reading, TV watching, or worrying either during the day or at night);
(c) get out of bed and go to another room whenever you are unable to fall asleep or return to sleep within 15–20 min and return to bed only when sleepy again;
(d) repeat this last step as often as necessary throughout the night;
(e) arise in the morning at the same time regardless of the amount of sleep obtained on the previous night (Bootzin et al., 1991). Limited daytime napping (<1 hour) before 03:00 PM was made optional early in the treatment.

Sleep restriction therapy (Spielman et al., 1987)

Rationale. Derived from the proposal that excessive time in bed perpetuates insomnia. The intervention involves curtailing time in bed to the actual time slept and gradually increasing it back to an optimal sleep time.

Intervention. Based on sleep diary data, each patient is prescribed a specific amount of time in bed (sleep window) not to be exceeded. The duration of this sleep window is reviewed weekly and increased or decreased contingent upon the sleep efficiency for the previous week. The goal is to maximize sleep efficiency [(total sleep time divided by time in bed) × 100] to more than 85%.

to nighttime awakenings. Additionally, almost all programs recommend that parents should put babies to bed "drowsy but awake" so that they can develop independent sleep initiation skills. Moreover, this can help babies return to sleep without parental intervention following naturally occurring nighttime arousals. Among the forms of behavioral health services for children, no other treatment has been more thoroughly researched or broadly applied as parent education training (Kazdin, 2005).

In a recent review of behavioral interventions, the average percentage of infants and young children who improved was 82% (range 10–100%) (Mindell *et al.*, 2006). Overall, the weight of the evidence from controlled group studies supports unmodified extinction and parent education/prevention. Graduated extinction, bedtime fading/positive routines, and scheduled awakenings are also well supported in the empirical literature. Standardized bedtime routines and positive reinforcement techniques have often been incorporated as part of a multicomponent treatment package; however, there is limited empirical support for their effectiveness as stand-alone interventions.

Problems going to sleep and staying asleep in older children and adolescents

Insomnia

Insomnia is a common complaint among older children and adolescents, particularly sleep-onset insomnia. Cognitive behavioral treatments for insomnia (CBT-I) include a range of powerful behavioral adjustments to sleep. The evidence that CBT-I produces reliable and durable changes in sleep in adults has been summarized in multiple meta-analyses and two practice parameters commissioned by the American Academy of Sleep Medicine (Morin *et al.*, 1999, 2006). Among youth, there is less evidence for the use of CBT-I. However, this is a growing area of research. For example, Bootzin and Stevens (2005) conducted an uncontrolled trial of CBT-I for adolescents with insomnia and substance use problems ($n = 55$). Self-reported drug problems declined for completers at follow-up evaluation while continuing to increase for noncompleters. In a separate report, improvements in sleep were associated with significant decreases in aggressive thoughts and actions (Haynes *et al.*, 2006). Another small ($n = 18$) uncontrolled pilot (Schlarb *et al.*, 2010) of a six-session insomnia behavioral therapy (BT-I) found improvement in numerous sleep parameters. While both of these trials have been limited by the lack of a randomized control condition, the generally positive results are encouraging. These data show the feasibility of improving sleep through a short-term psychological intervention in adolescents and provide promising preliminary results suggesting that improved sleep in youth can contribute to improvements in behavioral and emotional functioning. Moreover, Cain *et al.* (2011) attempted to address common problems of low motivation for treatment, poor treatment adherence, and attrition among adolescent patients by using the school classroom as an alternative arena for sleep intervention. Despite self-reported increases in motivation

to improve their sleep, sleep patterns, and daytime functioning were not significantly different between the intervention and control groups at post treatment. Although promising, these findings might be interpreted to suggest that even in the face of adequate motivation, adolescents require parental and/or clinician assistance in regulating and maintaining healthy sleep schedules.

There are a range of important components of a behavioral intervention for insomnia as depicted in Figure 70.1 and described in detail elsewhere (Harvey, 2009; Clarke & Harvey, 2012).

"Nights-owls" and delayed sleep phase syndrome (DSPS)

There is evidence that the onset of puberty triggers a change toward a distinct evening preference among approximately 40% of teens (Carskadon *et al.*, 1997; Roenneberg *et al.*, 2004), which is then exacerbated by various social (e.g., importance of peers, parents less involved in decisions regarding bed and wake times), psychological (e.g., increased pressure at school) and behavioral factors (e.g., use of social media in bed and during the night). Together these factors can contribute to a tendency toward eveningness or, in the extreme, delayed sleep phase syndrome (DSPS). Problems with delayed sleep in children and adolescents can be further compounded by large differences between weekday and weekend schedules, so-called "social jetlag."

There is a small treatment literature on DSPS in teens, including the use of timed light with teens (Crowley *et al.*, 2007), as well as practice parameters (Sack *et al.*, 2007) that indicate evidence for timed light exposure (with a light box) and planned and regular sleep schedules (chronotherapy) in adults. Moreover, Gradisar *et al.* (2011) evaluated six sessions of CBT-I plus morning bright light therapy (BLT) to advance sleep onset (CBT-I plus BLT) versus wait-list for adolescents diagnosed with delayed sleep phase disorder (DSPD). CBT-I plus BLT was associated with reduced sleep latency, earlier sleep onset and rise times, total sleep time (school nights), wake after sleep onset, sleepiness, and fatigue. At 6-month follow-up, these improvements were sustained. Unfortunately, it can be difficult to motivate teens to use light boxes and to participate in delaying chronotherapy. Traditional chronotherapy involving progressively delaying bedtimes and waketimes until reaching the desired alignment tend to be highly disruptive to family and work schedules. Hence, we suggest adopting a planned sleep modification protocol derived from circadian principles involving moving bedtimes earlier by 20–30 min per week. The circadian system can adapt to more rapid changes but we find it is better to build a sense of mastery and control over sleep with smaller changes, scaffolded with interventions focused on wind-down and wake-ups. The targets depicted in Figure 70.1 are additional treatment offerings within this class of problems.

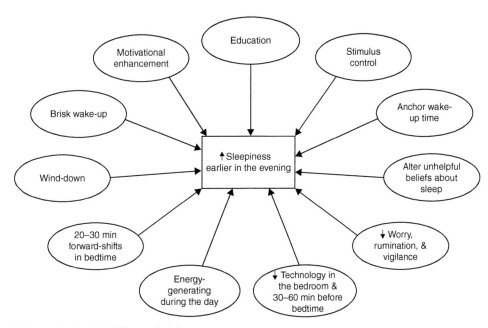

Figure 70.1 Targets for improving sleep in children and adolescents.

Daytime sleepiness/difficulty waking up for school

After the onset of puberty and throughout the adolescent period, the most prevalent sleep complaints tend to center on difficulty waking up for school in the morning and the associated difficulties with daytime sleepiness, tiredness, and irritability. It is important to emphasize that there is a broad continuum of severity. This ranges from normative/mild difficulties that appear to affect up to half of all high school students in the United States and result in at least some symptoms (National Sleep Foundation, 2006) to a much smaller subset of adolescents with severe difficulties with sleep and schedules that result in significant impairments (such as failures in school) and often meet full criteria for DSPS. At the current time, there is an absence of empirical data to help delineate precisely when to diagnose adolescents as having DSPS disorder from the much larger set of youth with mild-to-moderate problems with erratic and late sleep schedules. One pragmatic approach is that clinicians understand both the physiologic and social influences that contribute to these problems, and apply sound behavioral principles aimed at improving and increasing sleep in any adolescent who shows evidence of suboptimal sleep as a result of late night and erratic schedules, as already described. In the adolescents with true sleepiness (not simply complaints of fatigue), two main categories of problems should be considered: (i) Inadequate amounts of sleep and (ii) circadian and scheduling disorders. Circadian disorders (DSPS) were discussed earlier. In terms of inadequate amounts of sleep, the most common cause of mild-to-moderate sleepiness in adolescents is an inadequate number of hours in bed. A combination of social schedules leading to late nights with early-morning school requirements can significantly compress the number of

hours of sleep. Part-time jobs, sports activities, hobbies, and active social lives can exacerbate this problem. The catch-up sleep of naps, weekends, and holidays can also contribute to the problem by leading to erratic schedules and even later nights. In taking a sleep history, it is important to ask specific questions about bedtime schedules. Many families will say the adolescent "usually" goes to bed at a certain time, but when asked for an exact time covering the previous few nights, a much later hour is reported. When assessing the amount of sleep an adolescent is getting, it is important to obtain details of bedtime (such as when the child gets into bed as well as lights-out time), estimates of sleep latency, nighttime arousals, time of getting up in the morning, difficulty getting up, and the frequency, timing, and duration of daytime naps. It is also essential to get details of sleep/wake schedules on weekends, as well as during the school week. When this type of specific information is obtained either by interview or by having the family maintain a sleep diary, evidence of inadequate sleep is often evident. A prospective detailed sleep diary provides the most reliable information.

When inadequate sleep is identified, simply recommending that the adolescent go to bed earlier is not likely to be effective. Often, the primary role of the clinician is to help the entire family understand and acknowledge the consequences resulting from the inadequate sleep. Sleep deprivation frequently contributes to many factors that the family identifies as problems, including falling asleep in school, oversleeping in the morning, fatigue, and irritability. In cases in which the adolescent's school or social functioning is significantly impaired by sleep problems, a strict behavioral contract that is agreed upon by the family can be essential. The contract should specify hours in bed (with only small deviations on the weekends) and should target the specific behaviors contributing to bad sleep habits, such as specific late-night activities, erratic napping, or oversleeping for school (see Figure 70.1). The choice of rewards for successes and negative consequences for failures, as well as an accurate method of assessing compliance, are essential components of the contract. Many of the other behavioral components outlined earlier for DSPS can also be used to treat children and teens with excessive daytime sleepiness.

Parasomnias

Parasomnias occur commonly in children as sudden, partial awakenings from deep, non-REM sleep into a mixed state which has some aspects of being awake and some aspects of being in a deep sleep. There appear to be at least two routes to this mixed state: (i) difficulty leaving deep sleep (Stages 3 and 4) at the end of the first sleep cycle, or (ii) a sudden disturbance or disruption during the middle of deep sleep. The events include sleepwalking, night terrors, and confused partial arousals (some enuretic events can also occur as partial arousals). The intense events (with screaming, agitated flailing, and running) represent the extreme end of a spectrum of partial arousal behaviors that occur in mild forms (such as calm mumbling or a few awkward movements) in many children. The events can last from a few seconds to 20 min, with an average duration of about 3 minutes. The termination is usually as sudden as the initiation, with a rapid return to deep sleep. During the events, the children may seem confused, often not recognizing their parents, being inconsolable, and often appearing incoherent.

Overtiredness from any source (whether sleep deprivation, sleep disruption, or erratic schedule) can increase or precipitate parasomnias. Any time a child is adjusting to getting less sleep, or has disturbed nighttime sleep, the physiological compensation is to get deeper sleep (especially in the first 1 to 2 hours after sleep onset). This deep "recovery" sleep appears to be fertile ground for partial arousal events. When a parasomnia is suspected, the clinical interview should include obtaining a careful history of all sleep-related habits, as well as the characteristics, pattern, and frequency of the events. Occurrence in the first third of the night and an increased frequency corresponding to periods of being overly tired are strongly suggestive of typical parasomnia events.

Given the wide range of intensity of these nocturnal partial arousals, the key to therapy is matching the appropriate intervention to the degree of problem. That is, mild sleepwalking or an occasional night terror in a young child requires only some parental reassurance with general suggestions regarding improved sleep habits and the likelihood that the events will decrease over time. First, educate the family about the events (and what to do during the actual partial arousal event). For mild-to-moderate events, the parents should try to direct the child to go back to bed and back to sleep. Physically taking the child by the hand and leading him/her back to bed during a mild event can also be effective. Usually, however, the event needs to take its course and will end spontaneously. During more agitated arousals, interventions trying to direct the child

back to bed can result in increased arousal and can inadvertently prolong the event. In general, if mild directing of the child does not work, the parents should let the episode run its course. One very important caveat to this advice is with respect to the need to prevent self-injury. Eliminating factors such as sleeping on the top bunk bed, having a bedroom near the top of the stairs, or having windows or dangerous objects in the room are major considerations.

Second, encourage a regular sleep/wake schedule with good sleep habits. The parents should consider an earlier bedtime if there is any evidence that the child is getting inadequate sleep. Specific causes of delayed bedtime or difficulty falling asleep should also be directly addressed. It is important to try to improve the overall quantity and/or quality of sleep of the child when applicable.

Finally, for the more frequent, repetitive, intense, and agitated sleep terrors, these can be treated effectively through the use of scheduled awakenings (Durand, 2002). Similar to the scheduled awakenings described previously, the child is lightly awakened and allowed to fall back to sleep 15–30 min before the usual time of the episodes (Durand, 2008). After about a week of this intervention, the sleep terrors typically are reduced or eliminated.

One final important note, certain types of epilepsy, particularly nocturnal frontal lobe epilepsy often occurs during sleep. As a result, it can be extremely challenging for the clinician to distinguish from parasomnias. The interested reader is referred to a comprehensive overview of the issues and controversies (Bisulli *et al.*, 2011).

Sleep-disordered breathing

Sleep apnea and a related set of problems called sleep-disordered breathing (SDB) can contribute to fragmented sleep that can subsequently contribute to daytime difficulties with cognitive and affective functioning. Rosen *et al.* (2003) conducted a prospective, cross-sectional study of 850 children. The overall prevalence of sleep-disordered breathing was 2.2%. However, black children were four to six times more likely to exhibit SDB relative to white children and children who were preterm babies were three to five times more likely to have SDB relative to those who were not preterm. Difficulties with irritability, attentional difficulties, and emotional lability can be created and/or exacerbated by sleep-disordered breathing in children. Although the actual number of minutes of arousal during the night may be small, the repeated, chronic, but brief disruptions in sleep can lead to significant daytime symptoms in children. It is important to note that the child is usually unaware of waking up, and the parent often describes very restless sleep but usually does not describe the child's waking up completely. The most frequent symptoms reported by families include loud chronic snoring (or noisy breathing), restless sleep with unusual sleeping positions (attempts by the child to move and open the airway), a history of problems with tonsils, adenoids, and/or ear infections, and signs of inadequate nighttime sleep. In medical centers with pediatric sleep facilities, consultation with a child sleep specialist can be extremely helpful in sorting out treatment decisions in these cases.

Restless leg syndrome (RLS) and periodic limb movement disorder (PLMD)

Restless leg syndrome (RLS) is a clinical diagnosis characterized by disagreeable leg sensations that usually occur before sleep onset. PLMD is characterized by periodic episodes of repetitive and highly stereotypic limb movements during sleep with symptoms of insomnia or excessive daytime sleepiness (Chesson et al., 1999). PLMD and RLS are distinct entities but can coexist. Most patients with PLMD do not manifest RLS symptoms; however, approximately 80% of patients with RLS have PLMD (Montplaisir et al., 1997).

PLMD has been described in children with somewhat different clinical presentation. Children with PLMD may present with nonspecific symptoms such as growing pains, restless sleep, and hyperactivity (Picchietti & Walters, 1999). These symptoms are most often unnoticed by their parents, although a family history of RLS and PLMD is common.

In terms of treatment, the guideline from the Standard of Practice Committee of the American Academy of Sleep Medicine states that no specific recommendation can be made regarding treatment of children with RLS or PLMD (Littner et al., 2004). Other reviews highlight the role of iron deficiency in exacerbating symptoms and explore a potential role for iron supplementation (Picchietti & Picchietti, 2008). Clearly this is an important domain for future research.

Narcolepsy

Narcolepsy is a chronic neurological disorder characterized by excessive daytime sleepiness. The classic symptoms include: (i) sleep attacks, (ii) cataplexy (the sudden loss of muscle tone without change of consciousness), (iii) sleep paralysis (inability to move after waking up), and (iv) hypnogogic hallucinations (dream-like imagery before falling asleep). These symptoms do not all occur together or consistently in many cases of narcolepsy. Particularly in younger patients, signs of sleepiness may be the only initial symptom. Cataplexy is typically provoked by laughter, anger, or sudden emotional changes. It may be as subtle as a slight weakness in the legs, or as dramatic as a patient's falling to the floor limp and unable to move.

The diagnosis of narcolepsy requires evaluation in a sleep laboratory. Treatment of narcolepsy is generally focused on education and counseling of the patient and family, adherence to a regular schedule to obtain optimal sleep with good sleep habits (often including scheduled naps), tests for human leukocyte antigens (HLAs), and cerebrospinal fluid hypocretin (Hcrt) measurement (Nevsimalova, 2009) and use of short-acting stimulant medication for treatment of daytime sleepiness (with drug holidays to avoid build-up of tolerance). Moreover, there are problems and a need for research. Modafinil, a common treatment for narcolepsy, blocks dopamine transporters and increases dopamine in the brain (including the nucleus accumbens). Accordingly, there is potential for abuse and dependence (Volkow et al., 2009) and no knowledge about the impact on the developing brain.

Finally, we highlight possible associations between ADHD and narcolepsy. In a retrospective history of childhood ADHD symptoms among a large sample of adults with narcolepsy ($n = 161$) and controls ($n = 117$), childhood ADHD symptoms were 8–15 times greater than expected (Modestino & Winchester, 2013). Although limited by the retrospective and cross-sectional methodology, these findings highlight a possible domain for future research.

Hypersomnia

The differential diagnosis of narcolepsy includes consideration of idiopathic hypersomnia. Excessive daytime sleepiness is common among youth, especially youth with a mood disorder. In addition, during phases of depression patients commonly suffer from periods of hypersomnia (Kupfer et al., 1972). Hypersomnia has adverse consequences for school attendance and performance, relationships, mood, and sense of self-worth. There is very little existing literature on the mechanisms that contribute to hypersomnia in mood disorder, nor the methods to treat it (Kaplan & Harvey, 2009). In our clinical experience, treating hypersomnia is likely to begin with goal setting, which involves reducing nightly sleep as well as setting goals for life. The latter is based on our clinical experience that "having nothing I am looking forward to get up for" can be a key contributor to hypersomnia. Often the combination of the mood disorder and the sleep disorder has led to school disengagement/drop-out and/or disrupted social networks. After setting the "sleep" and "life" goals for the treatment, the young person is asked to identify one small step toward these goals for the coming week. After a detailed discussion of how to achieve those goals, possible obstacles are identified. We engage in problem solving to limit the impact of these obstacles on reaching the goal, and a method is developed for monitoring the extent to which the goal is achieved (Kaplan & Harvey, 2009).

Medications

Several classes of medications are used for treating sleep problems, particularly insomnia; namely, benzodiazepine receptor agonists, sedating antidepressants, antihistamines, and melatonin agonists. Benzodiazepine receptor agonists (BRAs), which include traditional benzodiazepines (e.g., temazepam, flurazepam) and nonbenzodiazepine hypnotics (e.g., zolpidem, eszopiclone, and zaleplon) also acting on the GABA receptor complex, have been extensively evaluated in controlled clinical trials in adults (Walsh et al., 2005). The main therapeutic effects involve improvement in sleep continuity and efficiency through a reduction of sleep onset latency and time awake after sleep onset; in addition, they increase total sleep time and reduce the number of awakenings and stage shifts through the night. Benzodiazepines tend to reduce slow-wave (Stages 3–4) sleep and REM sleep, but these changes are less pronounced with zolpidem and eszopiclone (Langtry & Benfield, 1990; Hoehns & Perry, 1993; Wadworth & McTavish, 1993). All hypnotic medications carry some risks of daytime residual effects (e.g., cognitive and psychomotor impairments), as well as risks of tolerance and dependence. These risks vary with dosage, half-life, duration of use, and individual factors (e.g., age and gender). In general, short-acting drugs have fewer residual next-day effects than long-acting medications. When used on a regular and prolonged basis, there are also risks of tolerance and dependence, which vary across individuals. Rebound insomnia is a common problem associated with rapid discontinuation of benzodiazepine-hypnotics, particularly after prolonged usage. In general, the newer BRAs produce fewer withdrawal symptoms upon discontinuation. In addition, most studies have not included a follow-up to determine whether gains are sustained after treatment cessation. Thus, the durability of the improvement to sleep associated with pharmacological treatment is not well documented.

It is emphasized that, to the best of our knowledge, all of the data just reviewed are derived from adults. Mindell and Owens (2009) highlight that few studies have been conducted on hypnotic medications in children and they warn about the possibilities that prescribing a medication may even send an unhelpful message to parents; namely, instead of emphasizing basic good sleep habits and inspiring a family toward behavior change, a medication might just maintain or cover up the problems that are truly maintaining the sleep problem. A survey completed by 1273 members of the American Academy of Child and Adolescent Psychiatry indicated that about two-thirds of child psychiatrists reported recommending nonprescription antihistamines, while more than one-third had recommended melatonin (Owens et al., 2010b). Antihistamines have a relatively long half-life. As a result, drowsiness and clumsiness are common side effects and tolerance can develop within 3–4 days (Schweitzer, 2011). While there have been trials of melatonin for teens (Jan et al., 2000; Szeinberg et al., 2000), including an open trial among 15 children with Asperger's Disorder (Cortesi et al., 2012), there are safety concerns about the impact on the reproductive endocrine system (Arendt, 1997; Malpaux et al., 1999; Wyatt, 2007). Note also that a trial of zolpidem failed to improve polysomnographically measured sleep in 6–17-year-olds who met diagnostic criteria for insomnia associated with ADHD (Blumer et al., 2009). Moreover, there are serious questions about whether the sleep obtained confers the full benefit of "natural" sleep or sleep in the absence of medications (Seibt et al., 2008). For example, Seibt and colleagues (2008) investigated the impact of Zolpidem (Ambien) on the development of the visual system in kittens 28–41 days old. As expected, Zolpidem increased NREM sleep by 27% and increased total sleep over the 8-hour period. However, rather alarmingly, Zolpidem reduced cortical plasticity by 50%. The authors concluded that hypnotics that produce more "physiological" sleep based

on EEG may actually impair critical sleep-dependent brain processes during development. This finding should stimulate new research into the safety of certain pharmacologic agents, particularly regarding impacts on the developing bodies and brains of children and adolescents. In sum, starting treatment with a quality behavioral intervention is recommended so as to avoid concerns about safety and efficacy. Another important consideration, and domain for future research, is concerns about possible sleep disturbances attributed to medications used to treat common childhood disorders such as ADHD.

Technology use

This is a topic that deserves a special section. As discussed in Section "Basic overview of human sleep architecture across development," the process by which the human circadian clock is set to a 24-hour period and kept in appropriate phase with seasonally shifting day length is called entrainment, which occurs via *zeitgebers*. The primary zeitgeber is the daily alteration of *light* and *dark*. The light-entrainable SCN synchronizes networks of subordinate circadian oscillators controlling fluctuations in other brain regions and, in particular, in neural circuitry supporting reward seeking (centered on ventral striatum) (Venkatraman et al., 2007) and emotion processing (centered on amygdala and orbitomedial PFC) (Yoo et al., 2007), two circuits highly relevant to risk taking among teens and that continue developing well into the teenage years (Giedd et al., 1999; Blakemore et al., 2010). Hence, an intervention to improve sleep incorporates timed light exposure and inevitably needs to address exposure to sources of light in the hour before bed, via the use of cell phones, laptops, social networking etc. The National Sleep Foundation (NSF) Poll focused on technology in 2012. In the 13–19-year-old age group, well over 90% were using some kind of technology the hour before bed: 54% watched television, 72% used their cell phones, 60% their laptops, 64% their music maker, and 23% play video games every night or almost every night within the hour before going to sleep. These behaviors have multiple potential adverse impacts on sleep. The artificial light exposure suppresses release of the sleepiness-promoting hormone melatonin, enhances alertness and shifts circadian rhythms to a later hour. Technology is also highly arousing and engaging and facilitates the much-loved contact with peers. These influences are so potent that it is very difficult for many teens to switch media devices off at night, delaying bedtimes still further (National Sleep Foundation, 2011). Moreover, cell phones are, too often, a source of sleep disturbance during the night. About 1 in 10 of 13–19-year-olds in the NSF poll reported being awakened after they go to bed every night or almost every night by a phone call, text message or email. Clearly, these are modifiable sources of sleep disturbance. Accordingly, technology use is represented as a target in Figure 70.1.

Conclusions and future directions

In this chapter, we have reviewed several important principles relevant to the assessment, diagnosis, and treatment of sleep problems in children and adolescents. We have underscored the evidence for interactions between sleep and the regulation of behavior, emotion, and learning. We have particularly emphasized behavioral principles and behavioral approaches to these problems because we believe that there is great pragmatic and clinical value in understanding and implementing these in many domains of clinical practice.

Unfortunately, knowledge of sleep problems and treatments is not widely disseminated to the public and this may be contributing to the epidemic of sleep deprivation among children and adolescents. As highlighted earlier, the most effective method for "treating" sleep problems is to prevent them before they start. Parent education about normative sleep across the first year of life has been critical in reducing many common sleep problems among infants and young children. However, to our knowledge, this approach has not been utilized among parents of school-age children and teenagers. It is possible that the sleep problems in later childhood and adolescence could be prevented by educating parents about developmental sleep needs, healthy sleep habits, how to set clear limits around technology use at bedtime and how to *model* healthy sleep to their children. Additionally, teachers, coaches, and health care providers could enhance prevention efforts through receiving education on the common "red flags" of poor sleep among children and teens (e.g., falling asleep in class and snoring). Early work in this area has piloted a screening tool for assessing sleep problems in pediatric primary care clinics (Owens & Dalzell, 2005). A potential next step may be to introduce prevention programs in schools and primary care clinics aimed at encouraging healthy sleep and providing extra support for children and teens that show early signs of sleep disruption (e.g., excessive sleepiness in class). This type of work has the potential to provide the most economical and time efficient approach to the treatment of pediatric sleep problems. However, equally important to the prevention of pediatric sleep problems is the removal of societal and environmental barriers to healthy sleep. For example, one barrier to healthy sleep among adolescents may be early school start time. Recent evidence indicates that a 30-min delay in school start time (from 8:00 AM to 8:30 AM) is associated with significant improvements in measures of adolescent alertness, mood, and health (Owens *et al.*, 2010a).

While there is significant evidence that sleep problems predict the development of future physical illness (e.g., Cappuccio *et al.*, 2008) and psychiatric problems (e.g., Choquet *et al.*, 1993) and that behavioral interventions for sleep disturbances in childhood and adolescence are effective, there remain several areas requiring future research. First, the risk factors associated with the development of sleep problems need to be better identified and defined. Critically, this has the potential to lead to even more powerful intervention and prevention efforts. Furthermore, the impact of potential moderating variables (e.g., child temperament, household socioeconomic status, etc.) on treatment outcomes needs to be examined with a focus on the potential long-term impact that behavioral interventions may have on the persistence of sleep problems in adulthood. Also important will be the evaluation of behavioral treatments in children with special needs including children with autism spectrum disorders, mental retardation, and neurodevelopmental disabilities and children with chronic medical and psychiatric conditions.

Although there is much research and work yet to be carried out, we have highlighted in this chapter the encouraging evidence that there are few risks—and potentially many benefits—from increasing and enhancing sleep in children and adolescents through cognitive and behavioral interventions. Further dissemination of this evidence may offer considerable assistance in providing all children and adolescents the best opportunities for reaching their physical, educational, and psychological potential via healthy sleep habits. As medication treatments are explored, it is essential that the impact of the developing body and brain be established (Seibt *et al.*, 2008).

Finally, there is growing promising research on sleep deprivation (Gorgulu & Caliyurt, 2009), light therapy (Benedetti *et al.*, 2007), and dark therapy (Barbini *et al.*, 2005) for patients with mood disorders. While the preliminary studies in adults are very interesting and promising, the application of these novel treatment approaches in children remains to be explored.

References

American Academy of Sleep Medicine. *International Classification of Sleep Disorders: Diagnostic and Coding Manual.* 3rd edn, (American Academy of Sleep Medicine, 2014).

American Psychiatric Association (2013) *Diagnostic and Statistical Manual of Mental Disorders*, 5th edn. American Psychiatric Association, Washington, DC.

Ancoli-Israel, S. *et al.* (2003) The role of actigraphy in the study of sleep and circadian rhythms. *Sleep* **26**, 342–392.

Anders, T.F. & Eiben, L.A. (1997) Pediatric sleep disorders: a review of the past 10 years. *Journal of the American Academy of Child & Adolescent Psychiatry* **36**, 9–20.

Arendt, J. (1997) Safety of melatonin in long-term use. *Journal of Biological Rhythms* **12**, 673–681.

Astill, R.G. *et al.* (2012) Sleep, cognition, and behavioral problems in school-age children: a century of research meta-analyzed. *Psychological Bulletin* **138**, 1109–1138.

Aurora, R.N. *et al.* (2012) The treatment of restless legs syndrome and periodic limb movement disorder in adults, an update for 2012: practice parameters with an evidence-based systematic review and meta-analyses: an American Academy of Sleep Medicine clinical practice guideline. *Sleep* **35**, 1039.

Barbini, B. *et al.* (2005) Dark therapy for mania: a pilot study. *Bipolar Disorder* **7**, 98–101.

Bates, J.E. *et al.* (2003) Sleep and adjustment in preschool children: sleep diary reports by mothers relate to behavior reports by teachers. *Child Development* **73**, 62–75.

Benedetti, F. *et al.* (2007) Neural and genetic correlates of antidepressant response to sleep deprivation: a functional magnetic resonance imaging study of moral valence decision in bipolar depression. *Archives of General Psychiatry* **64**, 179–187.

Bisulli, F. *et al.* (2011) Parasomnias and nocturnal frontal lobe epilepsy (NFLE): lights and shadows--controversial points in the differential diagnosis. *Sleep Medicine* **12**, S27–S32.

Blakemore, S.J. *et al.* (2010) The role of puberty in the developing adolescent brain. *Human Brain Mapping* **31**, 926–933.

Blumer, J.L. *et al.* (2009) Controlled clinical trial of zolpidem for the treatment of insomnia associated with attention-deficit/hyperactivity disorder in children 6 to 17 years of age. *Pediatrics* **123**, e770–e776.

Bootzin, R.R. (1979) Effects of self-control procedures for insomnia. *American Journal of Clinical Biofeedback* **2**, 70–77.

Bootzin, R.R. & Stevens, S.J. (2005) Adolescents, substance abuse, and the treatment of insomnia and daytime sleepiness. *Clinical Psychology Review* **25**, 629–644.

Bootzin, R.R. *et al.* (1991) Stimulus control instructions. In: *Case Studies in Insomnia.* (ed P.J. Hauri), pp. 19–28. Plenum Publishing Corporation, New York, NY.

Borbély, A.A. (1982) A two process model of sleep regulation. *Human Neurobiology* **1**, 195–204.

Cain, N. *et al.* (2011) A motivational school-based intervention for adolescent sleep problems. *Sleep Medicine* **12**, 246–251.

Cappuccio, F.P. *et al.* (2008) Meta-analysis of short sleep duration and obesity in children and adults. *Sleep* **31**, 619–626.

Carney, C.E. *et al.* (2012) The consensus sleep diary: standardizing prospective sleep self-monitoring. *Sleep* **35**, 287–302.

Carskadon, M.A. & Dement, W.C. (2011) Normal human sleep: an overview. In: *Principles and Practice of Sleep Medicine.* (eds M.H. Kryger, T. Roth & W.C. Dement), 5th edn, pp. 16–26. Elsevier, Philadelphia.

Carskadon, M.A. *et al.* (1993) Association between puberty and delayed phase preference. *Sleep* **16**, 258–262.

Carskadon, M.A. *et al.* (1997) An approach to studying circadian rhythms of adolescent humans. *Journal of Biological Rhythms* **12**, 278–289.

Chervin, R.D. *et al.* (2000) Pediatric sleep questionnaire (PSQ): validity and reliability of scales for sleep-disordered breathing, snoring, sleepiness, and behavioral problems. *Sleep Medicine* **1**, 21–32.

Chesson, A.L. Jr. *et al.* (1999) Practice parameters for the treatment of restless legs syndrome and periodic limb movement disorder. An American Academy of Sleep Medicine Report. Standards of Practice Committee of the American Academy of Sleep Medicine. *Sleep* **22**, 961–968.

Choquet, M. & Menke, H. (1989) Suicidal thoughts during early adolescence: prevalence, associated troubles, and help-seeking behavior. *Acta Psychiatrica Scandinavia (Suppl)* **81**, 170–177.

Choquet, M. *et al.* (1993) Suicidal thoughts among adolescents: an intercultural approach. *Adolescence* **28**, 649–659.

Clarke, G. & Harvey, A.G. (2012) The complex role of sleep in adolescent depression. *Child and Adolescent Psychiatric Clinics of North America* **21**, 385–400.

Cortesi, F. *et al.* (2012) Controlled, release melatonin, singly and combined with cognitive behavioural therapy, for persistent insomnia in children with autism spectrum disorders: a randomized placebo, controlled trial. *Journal of Sleep Research* **21**, 700–709.

Crowley, S.J. *et al.* (2007) Sleep, circadian rhythms, and delayed phase in adolescence. *Sleep Medicine* **8**, 602–612.

Dahl, R.E., & Lewin, D.S. (2002) Pathways to adolescent health sleep regulation and behavior. *Journal of Adolescent Health* **31**, 175–184.

Danielsson, N.S. *et al.* (2012) Sleep disturbance and depressive symptoms in adolescence: the role of catastrophic worry. *Journal of Youth and Adolescence* **42**, 1–11.

Dewald, J.F. *et al.* (2010) The influence of sleep quality, sleep duration and sleepiness on school performance in children and adolescents: a meta-analytic review. *Sleep Medicine Reviews* **14**, 179–189.

Diekelmann, S. & Born, J. (2010) The memory function of sleep. *Nature Reviews Neuroscience* **11**, 114–126.

Dongen, V. *et al.* (2003) The cumulative cost of additional wakefulness: dose-response effects on neurobehavioral functions and sleep physiology from chronic sleep restriction and total sleep deprivation. *Sleep* **26**, 117–126.

Duffy, A. *et al.* (2007) The early manifestations of bipolar disorder: a longitudinal prospective study of the offspring of bipolar parents. *Bipolar Disorders* **9**, 828–838.

Durand, V.M. (2002) Treating sleep terrors in children with autism. *Journal of Positive Behavior Interventions* **4**, 66–72.

Durand, V.M. (2008) *When Children Don't Sleep Well: Interventions for Pediatric Sleep Disorders, Therapist Guide.* Oxford University Press, New York.

Faedda, G.L. *et al.* (2004) Pediatric bipolar disorder: phenomenology and course of illness. *Bipolar Disorders* **6**, 305–313.

Ferber, R. (1985) *Solve Your Child's Sleep Problems.* Simon & Schuster, New York.

Fredriksen, K. *et al.* (2004) Sleepless in Chicago: tracking the effects of adolescent sleep loss during the middle school years. *Child Development* **75**, 84–95.

Gasquet, I. & Choquet, M. (1994) Hospitalization in a pediatric ward of adolescent suicide attempters admitted to general hospitals. *Journal of Adolescent Health* **15**, 416–422.

Giedd, J.N. *et al.* (1999) Brain development during childhood and adolescence: a longitudinal MRI study [letter]. *Nature Neuroscience* **2**, 861–863.

Goldstein, T.R. *et al.* (2008) Sleep disturbance preceding completed suicide in adolescents. *Journal of Consulting and Clinical Psychology* **76**, 84–91.

Gorgulu, Y. & Caliyurt, O. (2009) Rapid antidepressant effects of sleep deprivation therapy correlates with serum BDNF changes in major depression. *Brain Research Bulletin* **80**, 158–162.

Gradisar, M. *et al.* (2011) A randomized controlled trial of cognitive-behavior therapy plus bright light therapy for adolescent delayed sleep phase disorder. *Sleep* **34**, 1671–1680.

Gregory, A.M. *et al.* (2005) Prospective longitudinal associations between persistent sleep problems in childhood and anxiety and depression disorders in adulthood. *Journal of Abnormal Child Psychology* **33**, 157–163.

Gregory, A.M. *et al.* (2009) Sleep problems in childhood predict neuropsychological functioning in adolescence. *Pediatrics* **123**, 1171.

Gress-Smith, J.L. *et al.* (2012) Postpartum depression prevalence and impact on infant health, weight, and sleep in low-income and ethnic minority women and infants. *Maternal and Child Health Journal* **16**, 887–893.

Gruber, R. *et al.* (1997) Sleep of school-age children: objective and subjective sleep measures. *Sleep Research* **26**, 158.

Harvey, A.G. (2009) The adverse consequences of sleep disturbance in pediatric bipolar disorder: implications for intervention. *Child and Adolescent Psychiatry Clinics of North America* **18**, 321–338, viii.

Harvey, A.G. & Spielman, A. (2011) Insomnia: diagnosis, assessment and outcomes. In: *Principles and Practice of Sleep Medicine.* (eds M.H. Kryger, T. Roth & W.C. Dement), 5th edn, pp. 838–849. Elsevier, Philadelphia.

Haynes, P.L. *et al.* (2006) Sleep and aggression in substance-abusing adolescents: results from an integrative behavioral sleep-treatment pilot program. *Sleep* **29**, 512–520.

Hoehns, J.D. & Perry, P.J. (1993) Zolpidem: a nonbenzodiazepine hypnotic for treatment of insomnia. *Clinical Pharmacology* **12**, 814–828.

Jan, J.E. *et al.* (2000) Clinical trials of controlled-release melatonin in children with sleep-wake cycle disorders. *Journal of Pineal Research* **29**, 34–39.

Johnson, E.O. *et al.* (1999) Insomnia in adolescence: epidemiology and associate problems. *Sleep* **22**, s22.

Johnson, E.O. *et al.* (2006) The association of insomnia with anxiety disorders and depression: exploration of the direction of risk. *Journal of Psychiatric Research* **40**, 700–708.

Kaplan, K.A. & Harvey, A.G. (2009) Hypersomnia across mood disorders: a review and synthesis. *Sleep Medicine Reviews* **13**, 275–285.

Kazdin, A.E. (2005) *Parent Management Training: Treatment for Oppositional, Aggressive, and Antisocial Behavior in Children and Adolescents.* OUP.

Kupfer, D.J. *et al.* (1972) Hypersomnia in manic-depressive disease: a preliminary report. *Diseases of the Nervous System* **33**, 720–724.

Langtry, H.D. & Benfield, P. (1990) Zolpidem. A review of its pharmacodynamic and pharmacokinetic properties and therapeutic potential. *Drugs* **40**, 291–313.

Leotta, C. *et al.* (1997) Effects of acute sleep restriction on affective response in adolescents: preliminary results. *Sleep Research* **26**, 201.

Littner, M.R. *et al.* (2004) Practice parameters for the dopaminergic treatment of restless legs syndrome and periodic limb movement disorder. *Sleep* **27**, 557–559.

Littner, M.R. *et al.* (2005) Practice parameters for clinical use of the multiple sleep latency test and the maintenance of wakefulness test. *Sleep* **28**, 113.

Liu, X. & Buysse, D.J. (2006) Sleep and youth suicidal behavior: a neglected field. *Current Opinion in Psychiatry* **19**, 288–293.

Liu, X. *et al.* (2005) Sleep patterns and sleep problems among schoolchildren in the United States and China. *Pediatrics* **115**, 241–249.

Lozoff, B. *et al.* (1985) Sleep problems seen in pediatric practice. *Pediatrics* **75**, 477–483.

Malpaux, B. *et al.* (1999) Melatonin and the seasonal control of reproduction. *Reproduction, Nutrition, Development* **39**, 355–366.

Manber, R. *et al.* (2007) Cognitive behavioral therapy for insomnia enhances depression outcome in patients with comorbid major depressive disorder and insomnia. *Sleep* **31**, 447.

Mander, B.A. *et al.* (2011) Wake deterioration and sleep restoration of human learning. *Current Biology* **21**, R183–184.

McGlinchey, F.L. *et al.* (2011) The effect of sleep deprivation on vocal expression of emotion in adolescents and adults. *Sleep* **34**, 1233–1241.

Mednick, S.C. *et al.* (2010) The spread of sleep loss influences drug use in adolescent social networks. *PLoS ONE* **5**, e9775.

Mindell, J.A. (1996) Treatment of child and adolescent sleep disorders. In: *Child and Adolescent Psychiatric Clinics of North America: Sleep Disorder.* (ed R. Dahl), pp. 741–752. W. B. Saunders, Philadelphia.

Mindell, J.A. (1999) Empirically supported treatments in pediatric psychology: bedtime refusal and night wakings in young children. *Journal of Pediatric Psychology* **24**, 465–481.

Mindell, J.A. (2005) *Sleeping through the Night*, 2nd edn. Harper Collins Publishers, New York.

Mindell, J.A. & Owens, J.A. (2009) *A Clinical Guide to Pediatric Sleep: Diagnosis and Management of Sleep Problems.* Lippincott Williams & Wilkins.

Mindell, J.A. *et al.* (2006) Behavioral treatment of bedtime problems and night wakings in infants and young children. *Sleep* **29**, 1263–1276.

Mistlberger, R.E. *et al.* (2000) Behavioral and serotonergic regulation of circadian rhythms. *Biological Rhythm Research* **31**, 240–283.

Modestino, E.J. & Winchester, J. (2013) A retrospective survey of childhood ADHD symptomatology among adult narcoleptics. *Journal of Attention Disorders* **17**, 574–582.

Montplaisir, J. *et al.* (1997) Clinical, polysomnographic, and genetic characteristics of restless legs syndrome: a study of 133 patients diagnosed with new standard criteria. *Movement Disorders* **12**, 61–65.

Morin, C.M. *et al.* (1999) Nonpharmacologic treatment of chronic insomnia. An American Academy of Sleep Medicine review. *Sleep* **22**, 1134–1156.

Morin, C.M. *et al.* (2006) Psychological and behavioral treatment of insomnia: an update of recent evidence (1998-2004). *Sleep* **29**, 1396–1406.

National Sleep Foundation (2006) *Adolescent Sleep Needs and Patterns: Research Report and Resource Guide.* National Sleep Foundation, Washington, DC.

National Sleep Foundation (2011) *Sleep in America Poll: Communications Technology and Sleep.* The Foundation.

Nevsimalova, S. (2009) Narcolepsy in childhood. *Sleep Medicine Reviews* **13**, 169–180.

Ong, S.H. *et al.* (2006) Early childhood sleep and eating problems as predictors of adolescent and adult mood and anxiety disorders. *Journal of Affective Disorders* **96**, 1–8.

Owens, J.A. & Dalzell, V. (2005) Use of the 'BEARS' sleep screening tool in a pediatric residents' continuity clinic: a pilot study. *Sleep Medicine* **6**, 63–69.

Owens, J.A. *et al.* (2010a) Impact of delaying school start time on adolescent sleep, mood, and behavior. *Archives of Pediatric and Adolescent Medicine* **164**, 608–614.

Owens, J.A. *et al.* (2010b) Use of pharmacotherapy for insomnia in child psychiatry practice: a national survey. *Sleep Medicine* **11**, 692–700.

Payne, J.D. *et al.* (2009) The role of sleep in false memory formation. *Neurobiology of Learning and Memory* **92**, 327–334.

Picchietti, M. A., & Picchietti, D. L. (2008). *Restless legs syndrome and periodic limb movement disorder in children and adolescents.* Paper presented at the seminars in pediatric neurology.

Picchietti, D.L. & Walters, A.S. (1999) Moderate to severe periodic limb movement disorder in childhood and adolescence. *Sleep* **22**, 297–300.

Pilcher, J.J. & Huffcutt, A.I. (1996) Effects of sleep deprivation on performance: a meta-analysis. *Sleep* **19**, 318–326.

Pollock, J.I. (1994) Night-waking at five years of age: predictors and prognosis. *Journal of Child Psychology & Psychiatry & Allied Disciplines* **35**, 699–708.

Quevedo, K.M. *et al.* (2009) The onset of puberty: effects on the psychophysiology of defensive and appetitive motivation. *Development and Psychopathology* **21**, 27–45.

Reite, M. *et al.* (1995) The use of polysomnography in the evaluation of insomnia. *Sleep* **18**, 58–70.

Rickert, V.I. & Johnson, C.M. (1988) Reducing nocturnal awakening and crying episodes in infants and young children: a comparison between scheduled awakenings and systematic ignoring. *Pediatrics* **81**, 203–212.

Roberts, R.E. *et al.* (2002) Impact of insomnia on future functioning of adolescents. *Journal of Psychosomatic Research* **53**, 561–569.

Roenneberg, T. *et al.* (2004) A marker for the end of adolescence. *Current Biology* **14**, R1038.

Rosen, C.L. *et al.* (2003) Prevalence and risk factors for sleep-disordered breathing in 8-to 11-year-old children: association with race and prematurity. *The Journal of Pediatrics* **142**, 383–389.

Sack, R.L. *et al.* (2007) Circadian rhythm sleep disorders: part II, advanced sleep phase disorder, delayed sleep phase disorder, free-running disorder, and irregular sleep-wake rhythm: an American academy of sleep medicine review. *Sleep: Journal of Sleep and Sleep Disorders Research* **30**, 1484–1501.

Sadeh, A. (2004) A brief screening questionnaire for infant sleep problems: validation and findings for an Internet sample. *Pediatrics* **113**, e570–e577.

Sadeh, A. *et al.* (1995) The role of actigraphy in the evaluation of sleep disorders. *Sleep* **18**, 288–302.

Sadeh, A. *et al.* (2000) Sleep patterns and sleep disruptions in school-age children. *Developmental Psychology* **36**, 291–301.

Sadeh, A. *et al.* (2002) Sleep, neurobehavioral functioning, and behavior problems in school-age children. *Child Development* **73**, 405–417.

Sadeh, A. *et al.* (2003) The effects of sleep restriction and extension on school-age children: what a difference an hour makes. *Child Development* **74**, 444–455.

Schlarb, A. *et al.* (2010) JuSt-a multimodal program for treatment of insomnia in adolescents: a pilot study. *Nature and Science of Sleep* **3**, 13–20.

Schweitzer, P. (2011) Drugs that disturb sleep and wakefulness. In: *Principles and Practice of Sleep Medicine.* (eds M.H. Kryger, T. Roth & W.C. Dement), 5th edn, pp. 542–560. WB Saunders, Philadelphia.

Seibt, J. *et al.* (2008) The non-benzodiazepine hypnotic zolpidem impairs sleep-dependent cortical plasticity. *Sleep* **31**, 1381–1391.

Shaw, J.A. *et al.* (2005) A 10-year prospective study of prodromal patterns for bipolar disorder among Amish youth. *Journal of the American Academy of Child and Adolescent Psychiatry* **44**, 1104–1111.

Silk, J. *et al.* (2007) Resilience among children and adolescents at risk for depression: mediation and moderation across social and neurobiological contexts. *Development and Psychopathology* **19**, 841–865.

Silk, J.S. *et al.* (2009) Pubertal changes in emotional information processing: pupillary, behavioral, and subjective evidence during emotional word identification. *Development and Psychopathology* **21**, 87–97.

Sinai, D. & Tikotzky, L. (2012) Infant sleep, parental sleep and parenting stress in families of mothers on maternity leave and in families of working mothers. *Infant Behavior and Development* **35**, 179–186.

Smith, M.T. *et al.* (2005) Cognitive behavior therapy for chronic insomnia occurring within the context of medical and psychiatric disorders. *Clinical Psychology Review* **25**, 559–592.

Spiegel, K. *et al.* (2004) Brief communication: sleep curtailment in healthy young men is associated with decreased leptin levels, elevated ghrelin levels, and increased hunger and appetite. *Annals of Internal Medicine* **141**, 846–850.

Spielman, A.J. *et al.* (1987) Treatment of chronic insomnia by restriction of time in bed. *Sleep* **10**, 45–56.

Steinberg, L. (2010) A behavioral scientist looks at the science of adolescent brain development. *Brain and Cognition* **72**, 160–164.

Stickgold, R. & Walker, M.P. (2005) Memory consolidation and reconsolidation: what is the role of sleep? *Trends in Neuroscience* **28**, 408–415.

Stores, G. (2006) Practitioner review: assessment and treatment of sleep disorders in children and adolescents. *Journal of Child Psychology and Psychiatry* **37**, 907–925.

Szeinberg, A. *et al.* (2000) Melatonin treatment in adolescents with delayed sleep phase syndrome. *Clinical Pediatrics* **45**, 809–818.

Talbot, L.S. *et al.* (2010) Sleep deprivation in adolescents and adults: changes in affect. *Emotion* **10**, 831–841.

Tikotzky, L. & Sadeh, A. (2009) Maternal sleep-related cognitions and infant sleep: a longitudinal study from pregnancy through the 1st year. *Child Development* **80**, 860–874.

Tynjala, J. *et al.* (1997) Perceived tiredness among adolescents and its association with sleep habits and use of psychoactive substances. *Journal of Sleep Research* **6**, 189–198.

Venkatraman, V. *et al.* (2007) Sleep deprivation elevates expectation of gains and attenuates response to losses following risky decisions. *Sleep* **30**, 603–609.

Volkow, N.D. *et al.* (2009) Effects of modafinil on dopamine and dopamine transporters in the male human brain. *JAMA* **301**, 1148–1154.

Wadworth, A.N. & McTavish, D. (1993) Zopiclone. A review of its pharmacological properties and therapeutic efficacy as an hypnotic. *Drugs and Aging* **3**, 441–459.

Walker, M.P. & Stickgold, R. (2006) Sleep, memory, and plasticity. *Annual Review of Psychology* **57**, 139–166.

Walsh, J.K. *et al.* (2005) Pharmacological treatment of primary insomnia. In: *Principles and Practice of Sleep Medicine.* (eds M.H. Kryger, T. Roth & W.C. Dement), 4th edn, pp. 749–760. Elsevier Saunders, Philadelphia.

Wolfson, A.R. & Carskadon, M.A. (1998) Sleep schedules and daytime functioning in adolescents. *Child Development* **69**, 875–887.

Wong, M.M. *et al.* (2009) Childhood sleep problems, early onset of substance use and behavioral problems in adolescence. *Sleep Medicine* **10**, 787–796.

Wong, M.M. *et al.* (2010) Childhood sleep problems, response inhibition, and alcohol and drug-related problems in adolescence and young adulthood. *Alcoholism: Clinical and Experimental Research* **34**, 1033–1044.

World Health Organization (1992) *International Classification of Diseases, 10th Revision (ICD-10).* World Health Organization, Geneva, Switzerland.

Wyatt, J.K. (2007) Circadian rhythm sleep disorders in children and adolescents. *Sleep Medicine Clinics* **2**, 387–395.

Yoo, S.S. *et al.* (2007) The human emotional brain without sleep--a prefrontal amygdala disconnect. *Current Biology* **17**, R877–878.

Zohar, D. *et al.* (2005) The effects of sleep loss on medical residents' emotional reactions to work events: a cognitive-energy model. *Sleep* **28**, 47–54.

Zuckerman, B. *et al.* (1987) Sleep problems in early childhood: continuities, predictive factors, and behavioral correlates. *Pediatrics* **80**, 664–671.

CHAPTER 71

Feeding and eating disorders

Rachel Bryant-Waugh and Beth Watkins

Department of Child and Adolescent Mental Health, Great Ormond Street Hospital for Children NHS Foundation Trust, London, UK

Introduction

The aim of this chapter is to provide the reader with a comprehensive update on feeding and eating disorders encountered in child and adolescent mental health care settings. Our intention is to provide a scholarly update and clinically useful chapter. Detail is provided on diagnosis and clinical presentation, followed by information on epidemiology, risk factors, and etiology. Subsequent sections cover assessment, treatment, and outcome.

This chapter focuses on feeding and eating disturbances that are considered "psychiatric" or "mental" disorders, rather than those that represent normal developmental variations or behavior experienced as problematic by the parent or caregiver. The situation is complicated in childhood and adolescence as feeding and eating takes place in an interpersonal context due to normal age-appropriate dependencies, which has led some to argue that childhood feeding difficulties should be reconceptualized as interactional disorders (Davies *et al.*, 2006).

Feeding and eating disorders can be serious and damaging conditions, associated with relatively high levels of morbidity and mortality. In this chapter, we cover anorexia nervosa (AN), bulimia nervosa (BN), binge eating disorder (BED), avoidant/restrictive food intake disorder (ARFID), pica, and rumination disorder. The chapter does not include obesity as there is little evidence to support its conceptualization as a mental disorder. However, it is recommended that body mass index (BMI) should routinely be monitored in those with a psychiatric disorder (Marcus & Wildes, 2009).

To put the rest of this chapter in context, we refer briefly to the development of successful early feeding and later independent, normal eating behavior. The establishment of problem-free feeding requires the physical ability and a desire to feed, as well as the presence of an appropriate caregiver with access to suitable food. Individual, interpersonal, and environmental factors can adversely affect feeding, with successful early feeding depending on a range of factors coming together simultaneously. Infant and caregiver need to adapt their behaviors and responses as developmental tasks are negotiated in the context of food intake and a more independent pattern of childhood eating becomes established. As children move into adolescence, the arena of food choices, eating behavior, and mealtime interaction continues to be an important context for testing out developing individuation, self-expression, and autonomy.

Diagnosis and presentation

Children and adolescents with feeding or eating problems may come to clinical attention in a range of health care settings, including primary care and pediatric clinics as well as mental health settings. Combined with lack of consistency in use of terminology to describe different presentations and poor fit with existing diagnostic categories, we believe this has contributed to an unhelpful fragmentation of knowledge and expertise in this field, with associated difficulties in advancing the progress of research. It is important to make distinctions between a feeding or eating disturbance as a symptom of a medical condition; difficult feeding or eating as problem behavior; and a feeding or eating disturbance as a mental disorder. In practical terms, in order to determine whether a child is presenting with a feeding or eating problem that may be a clinically significant mental disorder, it can be useful to consider three main questions:

1 **Is the problem consistent with normal variation for the appropriate developmental stage of the child?** For example: acceptance of only a limited range of foods is normal around 2–4 years of age, but less so in older children; short periods of cutting down on certain foods with the aim of influencing weight or shape is common in adolescents and mostly benign, but when persistent, extreme and accompanied by significant weight loss may be a cause for concern.

Rutter's Child and Adolescent Psychiatry, Sixth Edition.
Edited by Anita Thapar and Daniel S. Pine, James F. Leckman, Stephen Scott, Margaret J. Snowling, Eric Taylor.
© 2015 John Wiley & Sons Ltd. Published 2018 by John Wiley & Sons Ltd.

2 **Is there risk in relation to consequences if left unaddressed?** To establish whether there is impairment to development and functioning, both psychological and physical.

3 **Can the eating disturbance be primarily accounted for by a medical condition?** If the answer is yes, it is unlikely to be a mental disorder, although in some instances an episode of illness or a medical condition may be a relevant part of the presentation.

This chapter focuses on the feeding and eating disorders recognized as mental or behavioral disorders by the two main classification systems relevant to mental health: the American Psychiatric Association's Diagnostic and Statistical Manual (DSM-5) (American Psychiatric Association, 2013) and the World Health Organization's International Classification of Diseases (ICD-10) (World Health Organization, 1992). Two further classification systems warrant mention: DC:0-3R, relevant to infants (Zero to Three, 2005; see further Chapter 7) and Rome III, a system for classification of functional gastrointestinal disorders (Drossman *et al.*, 2006; see further Chapter 72). Each diagnosis is described briefly in the following sections, with common comorbidities and main differential diagnoses listed in Table 71.1 at the end of this section.

Pica

Pica is characterized by eating nonnutritive substances, which may be nonfood items or raw food ingredients eaten in large amounts. A diagnosis of pica is given when such behavior is persistent or sufficiently severe to warrant clinical intervention. Pica is not usually diagnosed where the ingestion of nonfood items is part of a culturally sanctioned practice, such as soil eating in many African communities (Geissler *et al.*, 1997), or when chronological or developmental age is below 2 years, as mouthing of objects with some ingestion is common. It may

occur in individuals with autism or those with learning disability (mental retardation) but can also occur in the context of normal development. Pica can lead to severe medical sequelae, to include poisoning and obstructions or perforations in the gastrointestinal tract. In some instances, it is associated with appetite loss, reduced intake, and weight loss and in extreme cases can be fatal.

Pica is a diagnosis applicable to children and adults in DSM-5 although in ICD-10 is classified as a disorder of infancy and childhood, but recognized as occurring in older individuals. Pica does not appear as a diagnosis in either the Rome III or 0-3R systems.

Rumination disorder

Rumination disorder is characterized by the repeated regurgitation of food that has been swallowed. The regurgitate is then rechewed (rumination) and reswallowed or spat out. The bringing back up of food occurs without undue effort and is not associated with nausea. Regurgitation should be differentiated from vomiting and gastroesophageal reflux. This behavior should be frequent, sustained over a period of time and not primarily accounted for by an underlying medical condition to warrant diagnosis. Repeated regurgitation can be associated with significant medical problems, to include malnutrition, low weight, dental problems, bad breath, and esophagitis. In extreme cases, rumination disorder can have a fatal outcome.

Rumination disorder occurs in children and adults, in those with intellectual disability as well normally developing individuals. It may have a soothing or calming function, playing a role in anxiety management or emotion regulation. It is often a secretive disorder and can be associated with significant impairment to social development and functioning. It can be associated with reduced intake and weight loss. Many clinicians fail to ask

Table 71.1 Differential and common comorbid diagnoses.

Feeding and eating disorder	Differential diagnosis	Common comorbid diagnoses
Feeding disorder	Reactive attachment disorder; neglect; medical conditions (to include oral dyspraxia)	Anxiety disorders; autism spectrum disorder; intellectual disability
Pica	Anorexia nervosa; avoidant/restrictive food intake disorder; factitious disorder; nonsuicidal self-harm	Avoidant/restrictive food intake disorder; obsessive-compulsive disorder; schizophrenia; autism spectrum disorder; intellectual disability
Rumination Disorder	Anorexia nervosa; bulimia nervosa; Gastrointestinal conditions	Generalized anxiety disorder; autism spectrum disorder; intellectual disability
Avoidant/Restrictive Food Intake Disorder	Anorexia nervosa; reactive attachment disorder; factitious or induced illness; specific phobia; social anxiety disorder; depressive disorder; medical conditions	Anxiety disorders; attention deficit hyperactivity disorder; autism spectrum disorder; intellectual disability
Anorexia Nervosa	Avoidant/restrictive food intake disorder; bulimia nervosa; body dysmorphic disorder; specific phobia; social anxiety disorder; depressive disorder; medical conditions	Depressive and anxiety disorders (including obsessive compulsive disorder
Bulimia Nervosa	Anorexia nervosa; bing eating disorder; mood disorder; borderline personality disorder; Klein–Levine syndrome	Mood disorders; anxiety disorders; substance misuse; borderline personality disorder
Binge Eating Disorder	Bulimia nervosa; Prader–Willi syndrome; Klein–Levine syndrome	Mood disorders; anxiety disorders; substance misuse

questions related to the possible presence of rumination disorder, which can hinder identification and diagnosis (Hartmann *et al.,* 2012).

Rumination disorder is a diagnosis in DSM-5, with criteria applicable to infants, children, and adults. In ICD-10, rumination is included as a variant of feeding disorder of infancy and childhood, but not recognized as a specific disorder in older individuals. However, proposals for ICD-11 include establishing a new diagnostic category of rumination disorder with criteria applicable to both children and adults (Uher & Rutter, 2012). Rome III (Drossman *et al.,* 2006) has separate criteria for infant rumination syndrome, adolescent rumination syndrome, and rumination syndrome in adults. There is considerable overlap between the definitions of these presentations as functional gastrointestinal disorders and psychiatric disorders. Rumination disorder does not appear as a category in DC:0-3R (Zero to Three, 2005).

Avoidant/restrictive food intake disorder

ARFID is characterized by limited food intake, which can be in relation to the range of foods eaten, the overall amount of food eaten, or both, with a persistent failure to meet the individual's nutritional or energy needs. The disturbance in feeding or eating may be associated with a lack of interest in food, avoidance based on the sensory characteristics of food (e.g., texture and appearance), or a fear of the consequences of eating (e.g., choking and vomiting), and sometimes a combination of one or more of these. Patients presenting with ARFID might be underweight, normal, or less commonly, overweight. There may be accompanying growth faltering in young patients or significant nutritional compromise which in extreme cases can increase mortality risk. The criteria for ARFID allow for the fact that persistent food refusal may be managed clinically by the use of oral supplements or enteral feeds. The criteria also include impairment to psychosocial functioning as a possible main feature associated with the avoidance or restriction of food intake. Concern about weight and shape or avoidance of weight gain should be ruled out as this would suggest that AN might be a more appropriate diagnosis.

ARFID is a new diagnosis in DSM-5 (American Psychiatric Association, 2013) with criteria applicable to infants, children, and adults and planned to be included in ICD-11(Uher & Rutter, 2012). It effectively replaces and extends feeding disorder of infancy or early childhood (DSM-IV; American Psychiatric Association, 1994), which has widely been regarded as too broad and nonspecific to be of much clinical relevance (Bryant-Waugh & Kreipe, 2012). The DC:0-3R classification system recognizes six separate categories of feeding behavior disorder but is limited to very young children (Zero to Three, 2005). Three of the DC:0-3R subcategories map on to well-described presentations in older children, such as food avoidance emotional disorder, selective eating, food phobias, and functional dysphagia (Nicholls & Bryant-Waugh, 2009). This contributed to the establishment of ARFID as a new diagnostic category

to capture presentations that are clearly separate from the weight/shape-related disorders of AN and BN, despite sharing restriction of food intake as a central feature, allowing for developmental differences in expression (Bryant-Waugh *et al.,* 2010). As it is a new diagnosis, epidemiological data are limited, but clinical experience suggests that ARFID has a more equal gender ratio than AN or BN.

Anorexia nervosa

AN is characterized by restriction of food intake leading to failure to meet energy requirements, weight loss, or maintenance at suboptimal level. Self-worth tends to be associated with weight and/or shape preoccupation. Despite being low weight, there is typically a failure to recognize this, accompanied by persistent efforts to avoid weight gain. Patients may or may not verbalize a fear of weight gain or becoming fat. Two subtypes are generally recognized, the restricting subtype and the binge-purge subtype (DSM-5; American Psychiatric Association, 2013). AN presents clinically in both boys and girls from around the age of 7–8 years, although more commonly in females (Nicholls & Bryant-Waugh, 2009). Very young patients tend to present with the restricting subtype of AN, with vomiting and then laxative misuse becoming more common features as age at presentation increases. Persistent under nutrition can adversely affect physical development and functioning, have irreversible effects such as permanent short stature and permanent deficits in bone mineral density (Katzman, 2005), and can have a fatal outcome. The mortality risk for AN is among the highest of all mental disorders.

AN is a diagnostic category in both DSM-5 and ICD-10. It does not appear in DC:0-3R or Rome III. Revisions to criteria in DSM-5 include rewording of the weight criterion to specify that weight should be less than is minimally normal, or for children and adolescents less than might be expected taking the individual's age, sex, stage of development, and physical health into account (Freidl *et al.,* 2012). Previously, many clinicians erroneously adhered to "85% of expected weight" (DSM-IV) or BMI of 17.5 or below as a diagnostic cut-off. The judgment of "minimally normal" and whether this is applicable to any one patient now lies with the clinician rather than being determined by population norms, although guidance suggests that the use of BMI percentiles can be useful. This is particularly important for younger patients as it has been reported that adolescents meeting criteria for AN but at 85–90% of their ideal body weight according to population norms often require hospital admission and can present with equally severe medical complications as those below 85% of ideal body weight (Peebles *et al.,* 2010). In DSM-5, severity of AN is rated on the basis of BMI percentile adjusted up or down depending on clinical symptoms, functional disability, and the need for supervision (DSM-5; American Psychiatric Association, 2013).

Wording changes have also been made to the cognitive criteria for clarification and to ensure better applicability to younger patients. In DSM-IV, there was a requirement for the individual to express fear of weight gain or becoming fat; however, younger patients may not verbally endorse fear of fatness despite determined food refusal (Bravender *et al.*, 2010). Behavioral indicators or parent report are now accepted as valid sources of information so that the clinician can now draw on observation and reports from other informants. This is also relevant to cultural variations as individuals from some non-Western cultures appear identical to patients with AN, but may give other explanations for restricting their intake, such as fullness or abdominal discomfort (also known as non fat phobic AN, see further Becker *et al.* (2009)). The term "denial" in relation to acknowledging the seriousness of low weight has been removed and replaced with wording that implies that there may be an inability to appreciate the risks, consistent with the view that younger patients may have a reduced capacity for general risk appraisal (Bravender *et al.*, 2010). Finally, the amenorrhea criterion has been dropped, as it excluded several groups and there was insufficient evidence of clinical difference between patients with AN who menstruated versus those with amenorrhea (Attia & Roberto, 2009).

Bulimia nervosa

BN is characterized by binge eating episodes, defined as recurrent episodes of eating large amounts accompanied by a sense of loss of control. Binge eating is followed by behaviors intended to compensate for the amounts consumed to prevent weight gain, known as inappropriate compensatory behaviors. These include self-induced vomiting, laxative or other substance/medication misuse, excessive exercising, and fasting. As in AN, the individual's sense of self-worth is strongly influenced by self-perception of weight or shape. In most instances, individuals with BN tend to be of average or above average weight. Binge eating and purging behaviors tend to be secretive and accompanied by distress and feelings of shame and disgust. There may be a greater tendency to seek help than seen in AN. BN typically first presents in adolescence or adulthood, more frequently in female than male patients. Younger patients may be less likely to engage in laxative misuse, with self-induced vomiting being the most common purging behavior in younger adolescents. In some young people, BN may be associated with other "loss of control" behaviors such as self-harm, sexual promiscuity, and drug and alcohol misuse. Purging behaviors can have serious medical consequences such as electrolyte imbalance, cardiac arrhythmias, and dental decay. In extreme cases, repeated purging can have fatal consequences, for example, through cardiac complications or esophageal rupture.

BN is a diagnostic category in both DSM-5 and ICD-10. It does not appear in DC:0-3R or Rome III. Changes in DSM-5 include a reduction in the frequency criteria for binge eating episodes and compensatory behaviors to once a week over a 3-month period (Wilson & Sysko, 2009). A further change has been to abandon the requirement to specify subtypes, previously purging or nonpurging BN given insufficient supporting evidence for this subdivision (van Hoeken *et al.*, 2009). Finally, severity ratings in DSM-5 allow the clinician to specify the severity of BN on the basis of the weekly frequency of inappropriate compensatory behaviors (Wolfe *et al.*, 2012).

Binge eating disorder

BED is characterized by recurrent episodes of eating large amounts accompanied by a sense of loss of control, similar to BN, but without the inappropriate compensatory behaviors. The binge eating is associated with marked distress, and a number of specific features, such as continuing to eat when full or eating when not hungry, eating rapidly, avoiding eating with others and feeling disgusted or guilty. Individuals with BED tend to be overweight or obese, and this condition is associated with increased health risks.

BED does not occur as a diagnostic category in either DSM-IV or ICD-10. In DSM-IV, it was included in the "residual" diagnostic category eating disorder not otherwise specified (EDNOS). It has now been included in DSM-5 on the basis of a review of its validity and clinical utility (Wonderlich *et al.*, 2009) and is a proposed new category in ICD-11 (Uher & Rutter, 2012). Previous DSM-IV research criteria for BED remain largely unchanged with the exception of changing the frequency criterion for binge eating episodes to once a week for 3 months and reducing the required duration of symptoms from 6 months to 3 months, both in line with BN. Severity ratings have been added, which in relation to BED allow the clinician to specify the severity of the disorder on the basis of the frequency of binge eating episodes per week (De Young *et al.*, 2012).

"Other" feeding and eating disorders and disturbances

Besides atypical and subthreshold presentations of the aforementioned disorders, there are two others that have been reasonably well characterized and investigated: purging disorder and night eating syndrome. As a result of limited clinical validity data, they do not appear as formal diagnostic categories in DSM-5, nor at this stage are they proposed to be included in ICD-11; however, they warrant brief mention here as disorders included in the residual feeding and eating disorder category. Studies on purging disorder, where normal weight individuals regularly engage in the use of inappropriate compensatory behaviors after eating normal or small amounts of food, have reported average age of onset around 20 years, although sporadic cases have been reported in older adolescents (Keel & Striegel-Moore, 2009). Night eating syndrome is less consistently defined, but most descriptions include three main features; consumption of a significant amount of food in the evening or night; disturbed sleep, often with consumption of food on waking up in the night; and lack of appetite in the morning (Striegel-Moore *et al.*, 2009). As with purging disorder, the majority of studies have been conducted with adults, suggesting that this presentation might be only rarely encountered in child and adolescent mental health care settings.

Epidemiology

Problems in epidemiological research and implications

Gathering reliable and valid epidemiological data for child and adolescent feeding and eating disorders has been challenging. Studies have used different methods of case detection making results difficult to compare. Community studies tend to report significantly higher incidence rates than studies using medical records, suggesting that there may be underreporting of the occurrence of these disorders as not all sufferers will present to health services (Smink *et al.*, 2012). Furthermore, some studies are based on psychiatric case registers while others involve general practitioner records. If a study focuses on only one type of data source, it is unlikely that all cases of interest will be detected.

Studies use different criteria and diagnostic systems, and as both DSM and ICD have been revised over time, more recent studies are not comparable with older studies. This point is particularly pertinent with the advent of DSM-5, which contains significant changes to diagnostic criteria. Additionally, diagnoses may be given by a variety of professionals working in diverse settings, and therefore it is difficult to ascertain whether a diagnostic system has been used reliably across professional disciplines and settings. More importantly, children and adolescents have been less likely to "fit" into formal eating disorder diagnostic categories (Nicholls *et al.*, 2000), suggesting that the epidemiological data to date may have underreported cases of significant feeding and eating disturbances in young people.

Further problems contributing to difficulties in interpreting and comparing the results of epidemiological studies include a focus on a specific geographical area, which may not be comparable to other areas across a number of variables, and most importantly, limited data from community studies that focus on incidence rates across a range of feeding and eating disorders in children and adolescents.

Trends over time

Meta-analyses have identified a small global increase in eating disorders throughout the 20th century (Keel & Klump, 2003), and a stable European incidence since the 1970s (Hoek & van Hoeken, 2003). Over time, improved case detection, greater public awareness leading to earlier case detection, and increased availability of treatment services may account for changes in incidence, rather than changes in rates being a true representation of any increase or decrease in occurrence of eating disorders (Hoek & van Hoeken, 2003; van Son *et al.*, 2006). Nevertheless, the incidence rate of eating disorders among 15–19-year-olds has increased (Smink *et al.*, 2012) and those with AN are presenting at an earlier age (van Son *et al.*, 2006).

Current knowledge of incidence and prevalence

In children aged 9 months to 7 years, more than 50% of parents report one problem feeding behavior and more than 20% report multiple problem feeding behaviors (Crist & Napier-Phillips, 2001). Parental report of feeding problems in children with developmental disabilities and chronic medical conditions is estimated at 40–70% (Byers *et al.*, 2003) and this rises to up to 89% in children with ASD (Ledford *et al.*, 2008) and neurological impairment (Sullivan *et al.*, 2000). There are limited epidemiological data for pica in children and adolescents. Pica is reported to be relatively rare in healthy children over the age of 2 years in the United States (Marchi & Cohen, 1990), but pica eating may be more prevalent in specific populations, such as those with sickle cell anemia (Ivascu *et al.*, 2001). High prevalence rates of pica eating (up to 77%) have also been reported in school-age populations in Africa (Geissler *et al.*, 1998). The incidence and prevalence of rumination disorder in children and adolescents is unknown, partly due to variability in diagnostic terminology and partly due to regurgitation and rumination often occurring in secret (Hartmann *et al.*, 2012).

The incidence of AN and BN is highest in adolescent girls (Lewinsohn *et al.*, 2000), with reported rates in 15–19-year-olds ranging from 109 to 270 per 100,000 person years for cases reported in primary care and from a community sample, respectively (van Son *et al.*, 2006; Keski-Rahkonen *et al.*, 2007). Incidence rates of 34.6 per 100,000 person years for AN and 35.8 per 100,000 person years for BN in a UK study were found in females aged 10–19 years (Currin *et al.*, 2005). Turnbull *et al.* (1996) reported an incidence rate of AN of 17.5 per 100,000 person years in 10–19-year-olds, and 0.3 per 100,000 person years in 0–9-year-olds.

Three recent national pediatric surveillance studies found an incidence rate of restrictive eating disorders with onset aged 13 years or younger from 1.4 to 3.0 per 100,000 (Madden *et al.*, 2009; Nicholls *et al.*, 2011; Pinhas *et al.*, 2011). One study identified a clear relationship between incidence and increasing age, with no cases found in individuals aged 5 years, and 9.51 per 100,000 person years in individuals aged 12–13 years (Nicholls *et al.*, 2011).

Prevalence rates of eating disorders in children and adolescents vary depending on the country and age range studied. Stice *et al.* (2009) reported a lifetime prevalence by age 20 years of 0.6% for AN, 2.0% for broad AN (i.e., below the diagnostic threshold), 1.6% for BN, and 2.4% for EDNOS, while Machado *et al.* (2007) found a point prevalence of 0.39% for AN and 0.64% for broad AN among adolescent girls. Community studies that used dimensional measures in adolescents have found high prevalence rates of 14–22% of eating disordered behaviors (Jones *et al.*, 2001; Hölling & Schlack, 2007), but these rates drop significantly when strict DSM-IV diagnostic criteria were applied. A national comorbidity study in the United States found that the lifetime prevalence of eating disorders (defined broadly as AN, BN, and/or BED) in adolescents aged 13–18 years was 2.7% (Merikangas *et al.*, 2010) with rates of 0.3% for AN, 0.9% for BN, and 1.6% for BED (Swanson *et al.*, 2011).

Mortality

Meta-analysis of mortality studies, including studies of outcome in adolescents with eating disorders, found standardized mortality ratios (ratio of observed deaths in the study population to expected deaths in the general population) of 5.86 for AN, 1.93 for BN, and 1.92 for EDNOS (Arcelus et al., 2011). Data indicate that individuals with AN may be five to eight times more likely to die in the first 10 years following the diagnosis than individuals in the general population (Arcelus et al., 2011; Franko et al., 2013). This is substantially higher than is observed in individuals with major depression or alcohol abuse (Markkula, 2012).

Economic burden

A recent report investigated the economic impact of eating disorders in England, taking a specific focus on young people. Taking into account health care costs, premature mortality, education, employment, and gross domestic product (GDP), the economic cost of eating disorders is over £1.25 billion (just under 2 billion US dollars) per year. While there are substantial costs for health care (estimated at £80 million or around 125 million US dollars), the report concludes that the human costs and cost of lost output are likely to be significantly greater (Pro Bono Economics, 2012). Young people aged 10–19 make up approximately 45% of hospital admissions, suggesting that 45% of National Health Service costs in England for treating eating disorders were attributable to those aged under 20, and in the period from July 2009–June 2010, across all age ranges, hospital admissions for eating disorders in England increased by 11% in comparison to the previous 12 months (Hospital Episode Statistics, 2010). In addition, there is significant private provision of services for the treatment of eating disorders, with approximately 27% of all CAMHS (child and adolescent mental health service) beds managed by the private sector. This figure increases to 82% for specialist eating disorder units (O'Herlihy et al., 2003).

Risk factors and etiology

Feeding and eating disorders are varied, complex multifactorial disorders. There is little in the literature about risk factors for feeding disorders, pica, and rumination disorder. Indeed, for pica there are only hypothetical attempts to explain the condition (Rose et al., 2000), which include nutritional deficiency and cultural factors. Pica is observed more commonly in areas of lower socioeconomic status, and traumatic events such as maternal deprivation, neglect, abuse, disorganized family structure, and poor parent–child interaction have been found to differentiate children with and without pica (Singhi et al., 1981). There is no study that reports risk factors for rumination disorder or ARFID. This section, therefore, mostly focuses on the eating disorders AN, BN, and EDNOS.

Biological factors
Genetic factors

There have been significant advances in the study of genetic influences on eating disorders in the past decade. Previous research has shown that eating disorders aggregate in families. Twin studies have shown heritability for AN of between 58%

and 75% (Thornton et al., 2011), for a broad anorexia phenotype of 48–74% and for BN of 54–83% (Bulik et al., 2000) while heritability for BED has been estimated at 57% (Javaras et al., 2008).

Eating disorder symptoms also appear to be heritable (Rutherford et al, 1993; Sullivan et al., 1998; Wade et al, 1999; Klump et al., 2000). Recent cross-sectional and longitudinal studies have identified developmental shifts in the etiological influences across adolescence. Pre- and early adolescent twins show lower heritability of eating disorder symptoms when compared to twins in mid and late adolescence (Silberg & Bulik, 2005; Klump et al., 2007a). Further studies suggest that puberty moderates genetic effects on eating disorder symptoms, moving from no genetic influence in early puberty to significant genetic influence in mid- to post-puberty (Klump et al., 2003, 2007b; Culbert et al., 2009). These findings help to refine hypotheses regarding regulators of genetic effects, such as ovarian hormones activating genes of potential etiological significance during puberty (Klump et al., 2008) and potential candidate genes (Klump & Culbert, 2007). However, it is unclear whether the magnitude of genetic influence remains stable from late adolescence through to adulthood, as further longitudinal data are not yet available (Klump et al., 2010).

The genes most likely to be implicated in the heritability of eating disorders are within biological systems that relate to food intake, appetite, metabolism, mood, and reward-pleasure responses. However, this genetic influence is not attributable to any specific genes but rather is thought to result from a much more complicated interaction between genetic vulnerability and environmental factors. Molecular genetics studies aim to identify changes in DNA sequence and/or gene expression that may be involved in the pathogenesis of eating disorder symptoms and disordered eating behaviors, to uncover potential genetic variants that may contribute to variability of treatment response (see Zerwas & Bulik, 2011; Trace et al., 2013).

Neurobiological and neuropsychological factors
Early neuroimaging studies of eating disorders in children and adolescents using single-photon emission computed tomography (SPECT) demonstrated hypoperfusion primarily in the temporal region of the brain (Gordon et al., 1997). These findings were replicated (Chowdhury et al., 2003) and found not to reverse with long-term weight restoration (Frampton et al., 2011).

More recently, functional magnetic resonance imaging (fMRI) studies have shown that disordered eating may be a consequence of dysregulated reward and/or dysregulated awareness of homeostatic needs, possibly due to enhanced executive ability to inhibit incentive motivational drives, and the symptom expression of restricted eating may be a means of reducing negative mood caused by skewed interactions between serotonin aversive or inhibitory and dopamine reward systems (Kaye et al., 2013).

A number of neuropsychological domains have been found to be impaired in those with eating disorders, including attention, memory, visuospatial processing, cognitive flexibility (set-shifting), impulsivity, and decision making. Most studies have been conducted with adults and while findings can be contradictory, sample sizes are small and methodologies differ, some specific, subtle, cognitive impairments are emerging as being implicated in eating disorders. Although some impairments resolve with weight restoration, others appear to be a more trait-like phenomena, such as deficits in set-shifting (Roberts *et al.*, 2007). In children and adolescents, emerging research in this domain is less clear. For example, set-shifting has been found to be comparable in adolescents with AN and healthy controls (Fitzpatrick *et al.*, 2012) and in adolescents with BN and healthy controls (Darcy *et al.*, 2012). A recent large scale study assessed the neuropsychological profiles of children, adolescents, and young adults with eating disorders and found a pattern of strengths and weaknesses including good verbal fluency skills and poor visuospatial memory, associated with relatively weak central coherence (Stedhal *et al.*, 2012), although further research in this area is needed before conclusions can be drawn regarding the neuropsychology of eating disorders in children and adolescents.

Perinatal factors

Studies investigating perinatal influences as risk factors for the later development of eating disorders have consistently found an association. These factors are independent of sociodemographic confounders and contribute a 3.6% risk for AN (Lindberg & Hjern, 2003).

Obstetric complications have been found to be significant independent predictors of AN and BN, and the risk of developing AN increases with the total number of obstetric complications (Favaro *et al.*, 2006). These obstetric complications may contribute to impairment in neurodevelopment, which could be implicated in the pathogenesis of eating disorders.

Infection/illness triggers

There are a small number of cases in the literature suggesting in some instances that AN is triggered by infection (e.g., Sokol, 2000). The concept of pediatric autoimmune neuropsychiatric disorders associated with streptoccoccal infection (PANDAS) has been more widely studied in obsessive-compulsive disorder and tics/Tourette's syndrome (see Chapter 56). More recently, Swedo and colleagues (2012) proposed a broader category, Pediatric Acute-onset Neuropsychiatric Syndrome (PANS), the primary presenting clinical feature of which is acute and dramatic symptom onset of obsessive-compulsive disorder or severely restricted food intake. In utero exposure to viral infection has also been suggested as a risk factor for AN. In a population study, exposure during the sixth month of pregnancy to the peaks of chickenpox and rubella infections was significantly associated with an increased risk of developing AN (Favaro *et al.*, 2011).

Puberty

Connan *et al.* (2003) proposed a neurodevelopmental model of AN, which includes consideration of both the biological changes and the psychosocial transitions faced by young people as they go through puberty and how the rigidity of those vulnerable to AN may be challenged by change, resulting in increased vulnerability to dysregulation in relevant biopsychosocial systems.

The onset of eating disorders is typically after puberty. Young people face many physical changes during pubertal development, for example, a rise in the average proportion of body fat and in body weight. Girls in middle childhood have a mean proportion of body fat of 8% and this rises to 22% after puberty and the period of maximum growth usually occurs between the ages of 11 and 13 years, during which time body weight rises by about 40% (Tanner, 1989). While boys also experience this weight gain, much of it is accounted for by an increase in muscle bulk. With regard to BN, both childhood obesity and early menarche, which in turn are often associated, are risk factors for the development of BN (Fairburn *et al.*, 1997).

Puberty onset is associated with profound changes in drives, motivations, psychology, and social life and these changes continue throughout adolescence. There are an increasing number of studies that have investigated the developing brain through adolescence, although these studies tend to define development by chronological age rather than pubertal stage. The few neuroimaging studies that have associated brain development with pubertal stage provide tentative evidence to suggest that puberty might play an important role in some aspects of brain and cognitive development (Blakemore *et al.*, 2010). How this may pertain to the development of eating disorders is yet to be elucidated.

Psychological factors
Psychodynamic theories

Early psychodynamic theories of eating disorders suggested that eating was equated with a wide range of factors such as gratification, impregnation, intercourse, performance, growing, and castration and with food symbolizing the breast, the genitals, feces, poison, a parent, or a sibling (Minuchin *et al.*, 1978). However, none of these theories accounted for the symptoms of AN, nor were they conducive to empirical testing (Goodsitt, 1985).

Palazzoli (1974) suggested a developmental object relations theory of the infant's progression through stages in relating to her mother, and Bruch (1973) hypothesized that refusal to eat and fear of fatness have their roots in early mother–child interactions, proposing that food refusal represents a struggle for psychological autonomy and control. Despite refined theories, psychodynamic therapies have not been adequately evaluated in the treatment of child and adolescent eating disorders and there is no evidence to support their efficacy.

Family theories

Minuchin *et al.* (1975) described the "psychosomatic family" in which the child's symptoms play an important role in maintaining the family's status quo and blocking change. Four key styles of interaction are characteristic of such families: enmeshment, overprotectiveness, rigidity, and conflict avoidance. Strober and Humphrey (1987) attempted to test these family styles of interaction experimentally. While they found that families with a child with AN tend to be out of touch with the child's emerging affective needs, are less than optimally expressive in the emotional domain, and may reinforce control and restraint at the expense of autonomous self-expression, this did not validate the theory of a "psychosomatic family." Similarly, Kog *et al.* (1987) found that while some families appeared to be a "close fit" to the model, others showed less extreme and even opposite kinds of family interaction. Eisler (1995) noted that families in which someone has an eating disorder are a characteristically heterogeneous group. In recent years, the emphasis on a family etiology has shifted toward an understanding of how the evolution of the family dynamics, in the context of the development of the eating disorder, may function as a maintenance mechanism (Eisler, 2005; Schmidt & Treasure, 2006).

Temperament

While no study has directly studied temperament as a risk factor for feeding disorder, studies have examined feeding difficulties in children. Feeding difficulties have been found to be more prevalent in children who are unsociable, difficult, or demanding (Hagekull *et al.*, 1997; Pliner & Loewen, 1997) and children with more emotional temperaments tend to display more food avoidant eating behaviors (Haycraft *et al.*, 2011). Childhood temperament (specifically higher levels of negative emotionality) has been linked to the development of later eating concerns (Martin *et al.*, 2000).

Certain temperament and personality traits have consistently been associated with eating disorders. Correlational research suggests that AN and BN are characterized by perfectionism, obsessive-compulsiveness, narcissism, sociotropy (concern with acceptance and approval from others), and autonomy (an orientation toward independence, control, and achievement), whereas impulsivity and sensation seeking are more typical of disorders characterized by bingeing (Cassin & von Ranson, 2005). While studies support the likelihood that neuroticism and perfectionism are risk factors for eating disorders, other temperament and personality traits that characterize eating disorders need further research to confirm their role as risk factors (Lilenfeld, 2011).

Attachment and trauma

Anxious insecure attachment styles are consistently found in adults with eating disorders (e.g., Illing *et al.*, 2010), and separation from mother and persistent maternal malaise during the first 5 years have been shown to be associated with later AN (Nicholls & Viner, 2009).

Early negative childhood experiences, including trauma and abuse are consistently found to be associated with BN and BED (Ericsson *et al.*, 2011; Groleau *et al.*, 2011). A recent meta-analysis of over 3 million psychiatric cases found that childhood sexual abuse was significantly associated with a lifetime diagnosis of an eating disorder (Chen *et al.*, 2010). Studies have also found a high incidence of unresolved trauma and loss in both those with eating disorders and their mothers (Fonagy *et al.*, 1996; Zachrisson & Kulbotten, 2006; Ringer & Crittenden, 2007).

However, there are significant methodological limitations in the literature in this domain, for example, inconsistent use of terminology and retrospective reporting, which makes it difficult to disentangle cause and effect.

Early feeding behavior

Longitudinal studies investigating the relationship between early feeding behavior and later eating disorders yield contrasting results. Marchi and Cohen (1990) found that pica, early digestive problems and efforts to restrict eating were linked to later bulimic symptoms, while picky eating and early digestive problems were associated with later anorexic symptoms. Kotler *et al.* (2001) found eating conflicts, struggles around meals, and unpleasant mealtimes were predictive of broadly defined AN, and that eating too little was found to be a protective factor for BN. This study found that picky eating was not associated with either later AN or BN, in contrast to Marchi and Cohen's (1990) findings.

In retrospective studies, higher rates of feeding problems, compared to controls, have been reported by mothers of children and adolescents with eating disorders (Jacobs & Isaacs, 1986; Rastam, 1992). However, another study has reported similar rates of feeding difficulties in adolescents with AN and controls (Shoebridge & Gowers, 2000).

As feeding is the result of an interaction between child and caregiver, feeding problems are usefully considered in this context. Children of mothers with an eating disorder scored higher on a measure of eating disorder psychopathology than control children, and their eating disturbance was associated with length of exposure to mothers' eating disorder and mother–child mealtime conflict at 5 years (Stein *et al.*, 2006). Maternal eating disorders have been found to increase the risk of childhood feeding difficulties and this association appears to be a direct effect of the maternal eating disorder mediated via maternal distress (Micali *et al.*, 2011) (see further Chapter 28).

Sociocultural factors

Although there seems to be general agreement that Western cultures put pressure on women to be thin and this contributes to the development of eating disorders, these disorders have been reported throughout medical history (Brumberg, 1988).

Cross-cultural research has been dominated by the assumption that Western values regarding thinness are responsible for the development of AN in non-Western contexts, but the empirical research does not corroborate this (Rieger *et al.*, 2000). However, media influences have been shown to affect increases in scores on an eating disorder questionnaire measure and increased incidence of self-induced vomiting following prolonged exposure to television in adolescent girls in Fiji (Becker *et al.*, 2002). Further research on both direct and indirect media influence on the development of eating pathology found that social network media exposure was associated with increased eating pathology in adolescent girls in Fiji (Becker *et al.*, 2011).

Significant relationships between perceived pressure to be thin and body dissatisfaction and dieting have been found in adolescents (e.g., Stice & Whitenton, 2002) and children (Field *et al.*, 2001).

Elevated dietary restraint has consistently been found to increase risk for onset of any eating disorder (e.g., Fairburn *et al.*, 2005) and adolescent females who report high dietary restraint have shown elevated risk for onset of threshold or subthreshold BN (Stice *et al.*, 2008). A meta-analytic review of risk factors for eating pathology highlighted the importance of factors associated with the "dieting domain." These included family and personal history of obesity and critical comments from family members about weight, shape, and eating as being risk factors for the development of BN but not AN (Stice, 2002).

Weight concern as a risk factor for the development of eating disorders has been well replicated in the literature (Keel & Forney, 2013). Evidence from a recent prospective study found that body dissatisfaction was a strong predictor for onset of any eating disorder and that this risk was further amplified by higher levels of depressive symptoms (Stice *et al.*, 2011).

Adolescent girls reporting social pressure to be thin and body image preoccupation have shown a higher risk for onset of broadly defined BN or BED (McKnight Investigators, 2003), while those reporting weight and shape concerns and negative affectivity have shown a higher risk for future onset of broadly defined BN (Killen *et al.*, 1996).

Assessment

In view of the wide range of potential contributory factors and multiple pathways in the development of feeding and eating disorders, as well as varying levels of risk associated with the severity of the clinical presentation, it is important that assessment covers multiple domains. The adoption of a biopsychosocial framework for assessment and treatment is generally regarded as essential, and there is consequently a need to work in conjunction with other professionals, to include family medical practitioners and pediatricians. Table 71.2 summarizes the main recommended components of a comprehensive approach to assessment, which covers the full range of feeding and eating disorders. As can be seen, assessment needs to cover salient aspects of the child's history, detail regarding the feeding or eating disturbance as well as the child's current mental and physical state, and information about the child's family and social context. Obtaining information relevant to the domains listed will allow the clinician to make a clinical diagnosis of any of the feeding and eating disorders mentioned earlier, as well as to determine level of risk. The three main areas of risk are in relation to physical state, psychological well-being and development. Identification of specific areas of risk will be key in prioritizing interventions.

Assessment and diagnosis will most usually be based on clinical interview involving discussion with the young person, where the child is old enough and/or has the ability to provide relevant information, as well as information obtained from parents, caregivers or other adults (see Chapter 32). Children may not have the cognitive capacity to formulate and express the reasons behind their eating behavior. In AN or BN, the ability to articulate a fear of weight gain or the influence of body shape or weight on self-evaluation may not be present. Adult observation from parents, teachers, or others can be important in providing indirect evidence for weight or shape preoccupation and avoidance of weight gain. Physical examination and appropriate medical investigations are also important (see Chapter 35). For some presentations, direct observation of eating and mealtime behavior can also be extremely informative. For example, the behavioral component of rumination disorder can often be directly observed. The individual may contract tongue or abdominal muscles, cough, induce a retch or gag, and place a hand over the mouth in the process of regurgitating. Observation of feeding and mealtime interactions, aversion to food, fear responses, idiosyncratic eating behavior, and the presence of a sensory component to the presentation can usefully contribute to the clinician's assessment of the nature and severity of the presenting disturbance.

Screening and assessment instruments

There are a number of standardized assessment measures relevant to the assessment of child and adolescent feeding and eating disorders and difficulties. These range from diagnostic assessment instruments delivered in an interview format, through self and parent report questionnaires to screening tools used in primary care settings. As with all such measures, they vary in terms of strengths and weaknesses and none comprehensively covers the full range of feeding and eating disorder presentations. There are very few detailed diagnostic measures available and some of the feeding and eating disorders lack detailed comprehensive assessment measures, in particular pica, rumination disorder and ARFID. This represents a problem for clinicians in relation to being able to recognize, diagnose, and plan appropriate interventions. The most widely used screening and assessment measures are listed in Table 71.3; helpful reviews of the various measures for use in child and adolescent populations can be found in Micali & House (2011) and Nicholson (2013). In addition to feeding and eating disorder specific measures, the clinician may choose to use broader measures covering multiple diagnoses such as the SCID (Structured Clinical Interview for DSM Disorders; First *et al.*, 1996), the DISC (Diagnostic Interview Schedule for Children; Shaffer *et al.*, 2000), or the DAWBA (Development and Well-Being Assessment; Goodman *et al.*, 2000), all of which include relevant sections.

Formulation and treatment planning

Having obtained information relating to the multiple domains described earlier, the clinician is required to evaluate and synthesize the information to allow diagnosis and appropriate

Table 71.2 Main components of comprehensive biopsychosocial assessment and relationship to risk.

Domain	Areas to cover in assessment
History	
Developmental	From birth, milestones, early feeding, speech and language, oral motor, sensory sensitivities, separation, social communication, relationships, play, character traits, behavior patterns
Feeding and eating	Onset of feeding/eating difficulties, relationship to weight/shape concerns, course, duration of current problems, key triggers
Medical	From birth, medical conditions and symptoms, operations, time off school because of illness
Significant events	Major personal and family life events, trauma, events having significant impact on individual
Current	
Feeding/eating behavior	Avoidance, restriction, self-feeding, binge eating, pattern of eating, speed of eating, eating in relation to hunger/satiety, solitary eating, eating nonfood substances
Behaviors associated with eating	Regurgitation, rechewing, spitting out, retching, gagging, vomiting, laxative (or other medication) misuse, exercise, behavior interfering with weight gain
Cognitions/emotions related to eating/weight/shape	Fear (distinguish between fear of weight gain/fat and fear of consequences of eating, e.g., vomiting), disgust related to food and own eating behavior, level of interest in food and eating, importance of shape/weight to self-worth, self-appraisal of body size and shape, understanding of current weight status, level of distress related to eating
Current intake	Range, nutritional breakdown, amounts, overall energy content, taken orally or enterally, intake defined by sensory characteristics (e.g., smooth, uniform color, regular appearance, etc.)?
Growth and development status	Weight, height, BMI centile (from BMI charts), weight loss/gain, faltering growth, pubertal delay, amenorrhea
Physical state	Pulse, blood pressure, electrolytes, minerals and full blood count, muscle strength, reflexes, concurrent medical conditions and symptoms. As indicated: dental exam (for enamel erosion resulting from vomiting), electrocardiogram, pelvic ultrasound, wrist X-Ray, DEXA (dual-energy X-ray absorptiometry)
Mental state	General mental state exam, comorbid diagnoses (e.g., depression, OCD, anxiety disorders, autism), insight, motivation to address eating difficulty
General functioning	Current developmental level, family relationships, peer relationships, school attendance and performance, engagement in activities, use of leisure time
Context	
Family/care environment	Family structure, adequacy of food availability, adequacy of appropriate caregiving, child's place of residence, social care involvement
Sociocultural background	Family, social and cultural practices around food and eating, weight and shape; values and attitudes influencing self-esteem
School	Ethos and expectations, mealtime arrangements, pastoral care arrangements, relationship between staff and parents
Main areas of risk	
Physical	Consequences of low weight/rapid weight loss; malnutrition; consequences of repeated rumination or purging behavior; poisoning; abdominal obstructions. NB: risk of death must be considered
Psychological	Suicide, self-harm, vulnerability to abuse
Developmental	Growth; bone age and density; puberty; cognitive; social, emotional, educational

treatment planning. This might include the need to consider the appropriateness of an admission or other high-intensity treatment option (see Chapter 50). Table 71.4 sets out common indicators for the clinician to consider in this respect.

As a result of the multifaceted nature of feeding and eating disorders, information about factors that may be maintaining the disorder can be helpfully integrated using a formulation approach. One model for a biopsychosocial formulation is that of the widely used "Five P's approach" (Nicholson, 2013). Information obtained at assessment can be sorted into five sets of factors: presenting issues, predisposing factors, precipitating factors, perpetuating factors, and protective factors. Presenting issues and perpetuating factors form a natural focus for

intervention, utilizing where possible relevant positive factors. Risk, as discussed earlier and outlined in Table 71.2, will also be important in prioritizing interventions.

Treatment

Description of core principles and main treatment modalities

Treatment of feeding and eating disorders must take account of both physical and psychological aspects, as well as the systemic context of both family and school factors that may serve as protective and/or perpetuating factors, thus it is essential to

Table 71.3 Screening and assessment measures for child and adolescent feeding and eating disorders.

Measure	Informant	Format	Age range	Relevant diagnoses	Diagnostic algorithm	References
BPFAS[a]	P	Q	9 months–7 years	ARFID/FD	No	Crist and Napier-Phillips (2001)
ChEAT/EAT[b]	S	Q	8–13 years /14 years+	AN/BN/BED (screening)	No	Maloney et al. (1988); Garner et al. (1982)
CEBI[c]	P	Q	2–12 years	ARFID/FD	No	Archer et al. (1991)
CEBQ[d]	P	Q	2–11 years	ARFID/FD	No	Wardle et al. (2001)
ChEDE/EDE[e]	S	I	8–14 years /14 years+	AN/BN/BED	Yes	Bryant-Waugh et al. (1996); Fairburn and Cooper (1993)
Y EDE Q/EDE-Q[f]	S	Q	12 years + /14 years+	AN/BN/BED	No	Goldschmidt et al. (2007); Fairburn and Beglin (1994); Carter et al. (2001)
EDI-C/EDI 3[g]	S	Q	9–16 years /14 years+	AN/BN/BED	No	Garner (1991); Garner (2004)
KEDS[h]	S	Q	10–14 years	AN/BN/BED (screening)	No	Childress et al. (1993)

[a]Behavioral Pediatrics Feeding Assessment Scale.
[b]Children's Eating Attitude Test/Eating Attitude Test.
[c]Children's Eating Behavior Inventory.
[d]Children's Eating Behaviour Questionnaire.
[e]Child Eating Disorder Examination/Eating Disorder Examination.
[f]Youth Eating Disorder Examination Questionnaire/Eating Disorder Examination Questionnaire.
[g]Eating Disorder Inventory for Children/Eating Disorder Inventory-3.
[h]Kids Eating Disorder Survey; P, parent report; S, self-report; Q, questionnaire; I, interview.

Table 71.4 Common indications for admission/increased intensity of treatment.

Physical
Severe weight loss (either rapid or extremely low weight)
Electrolyte disturbance
Dehydration
Hypothermia
Significant renal function abnormalities
Cardiovascular complications—for example, hypotension, tachycardia, bradycardia
Intractable vomiting

Psychological
Severe depression, suicidal ideation/intent
Other significant psychiatric disturbance

Other
Parents/caregivers unable to manage required level of supervision and input
Failed outpatient treatment

work in conjunction with other professionals including family medical practitioners and pediatricians. Teamwork and collaboration with parents in the treatment of feeding and eating disorders is essential (Lask & Bryant-Waugh, 2013).

Attention to physical and nutritional aspects may include pediatric and dietetic interventions to manage any medical problems resulting from the feeding or eating disorder and to restore a nutritionally adequate oral diet. In cases where the child or adolescent is underweight, restoration and maintenance of a healthy weight will be an important treatment component. Current practice varies widely in relation to rate of weight gain, but in general weekly gain of 0.5–1 kg is recommended as an aim

of treatment (National Institute for Health and Care Excellence (NICE), 2004). In severely malnourished patients, a more gradual increase of energy intake combined with regular physical monitoring to prevent the development of refeeding syndrome (typically characterized by fluid disorders such as edema and electrolyte disturbances, particularly hypophosphatemia) may be indicated (Katzman, 2005).

Medication has a limited role as first-line treatment for child and adolescent feeding and eating disorders. There is a very limited evidence base supporting the use of any pharmacological interventions with child and adolescent patients, and caution is needed in view of the physical vulnerability of this group (NICE, 2004). Nevertheless, drugs are used in practice albeit with uncertain effectiveness, most commonly SRRIs and antipsychotics, with main indications being depression, anxiety, and weight concern (Gowers et al., 2010).

There is no one treatment of choice for feeding and eating disorders and often, combinations of treatment are recommended (NICE, 2004). The establishment of a therapeutic alliance is integral to successful outcome. In some instances, this can be challenging to establish; time spent assessing motivation and exploring perceived barriers or disadvantages to change can be helpful. Becoming stuck in therapy is often related to fear about change that may have been insufficiently explored or expressed. A brief outline of the three most commonly used psychological therapies in feeding and eating disorders is given in the following sections (see further Chapters 36, 38, 39, and 40).

Cognitive behavioral therapy (CBT) is an umbrella term used to describe therapies that share a theoretical basis in behaviorist learning theory and cognitive psychology, and which utilize methods of change derived from these theories. The focus of these therapies is on the here and now and symptom reduction; some are more focused on behavioral interventions, where the objective is to identify and effect change in habitual behavior. Others are more focused on cognitive interventions, where the objective is to identify, monitor, and challenge dysfunctional, inaccurate, or unhelpful thoughts, assumptions, and beliefs that accompany difficult feelings and unhelpful behaviors. Thus, cognitive and behavioral principles can be applied across the entire range of feeding and eating disorders. CBT is case formulation driven, and the involvement and role of parents in the intervention may vary depending on the formulation.

Psychodynamic psychotherapy has been used widely in eating disorders and has the goal of enhancing the young person's ability to identify emotional states, develop a language of the emotions and communicate feelings and needs to others (Troupp, 2013).

Family-based therapy (FBT) for eating disorders aims to enlist the parents as a resource in the practical resolution of the eating disorder, and takes an explicit agenda of blame reduction toward both the parents and the child. FBT assumes that resolution of the acute symptoms of the eating disorder and restoration of basic functioning need to be achieved before the young person will experience any relief from the cognitive symptoms, such as extreme weight and shape concerns. FBT consists of three phases. In the first phase, parents take charge of their child's eating, making decisions about appropriate eating as the young person is unable to engage in healthy eating behaviors. In phase two, when the young person has achieved more regulated eating and/or a healthier weight, control over eating is gradually handed back to the young person. Phase three attends to broader issues of family functioning and adolescent development.

Overview of current evidence base for treatment of feeding and eating disorders

There is minimal literature reporting psychological interventions for feeding problems and disorders in the absence of any known medical condition, with most reporting case study evaluations of interventions (Dovey & Martin, 2012). Children with feeding problems and disorders are a heterogenous group and thus specific interventions have yet to be developed and disseminated. Few studies have used quantitative methods and all have evaluated different treatment approaches, such as treatment for food/choking phobia (Benoit & Coolbear, 1998), assessment of a parental educational program (Fraser et al., 2004), and treatment designed to reduce caregiver stress (Greer et al., 2008). A more recent study implemented a behavioral modeling intervention targeted at improving dietary variety and problematic mealtime behavior over a 16-week period, and found significant increases in the amount of foods accepted, increased weight, and a parent-reported decrease in mealtime problems (Dovey & Martin, 2012).

With regard to pica and rumination disorder, there are no published treatment trials, although the consensus in the literature is that both disorders can be treated using a behavioral approach (Williams & McAdam, 2012; Schroedl et al., 2013). Similarly, little is currently known about effective treatment interventions for individuals presenting with ARFID, but the prominent avoidance behaviors characteristic of the disorder indicate that behavioral interventions, such as exposure and response prevention therapy, may be the best approach. Where there is an underlying emotional disturbance, such as anxiety or depression, CBT may prove to be an effective intervention (Kenney & Walsh, 2013).

While the evidence base for treatment of children and adolescents with AN is strongest for family interventions, this is still somewhat limited. There are only a small number of randomized controlled trials (RCTs), most of which had small sample sizes (Russell et al., 1987; Le Grange et al., 1992; Robin et al., 1994; Eisler et al., 1997; Eisler et al., 2000; Lock et al., 2005). Some, but not all, of these trials suggest that family therapy may be advantageous over individual psychotherapy in terms of physical improvement (weight gain and resumption of menstruation) and reduction of cognitive distortions, particularly in younger patients. While these studies provide the best evidence available for the treatment of AN in adolescents, the sample sizes in these studies are very low, with two studies having only 18 and 21 participants (Russell et al., 1987; Le Grange et al., 1992, respectively). In addition, the mean age of the study participants ranges from 14.2 years to 16.6 years, which means that the evidence base is for adolescents rather than for children.

Lock et al. (2010) conducted an RCT with a larger sample size ($n = 121$), comparing FBT with adolescent-focused individual therapy (AFT) in adolescents with AN and found no significant differences in full remission at the end of treatment. However, some differences that favored FBT at 6- and 12-month follow-up were found.

On balance, the evidence in favor of family therapy over individual therapy for adolescent AN is relatively weak. In the future, larger RCTs with long-term follow-up are required to assess whether family therapy is the most effective treatment for AN in adolescence.

Two studies have compared FBT with individual interventions in adolescents with BN. Schmidt et al. (2007) compared family therapy and CBT-guided self-care and found that CBT-guided self-care was superior to family therapy in reduction of binge eating behavior. LeGrange et al. (2007) compared FBT and supportive psychotherapy (SPT) and found significantly greater early reductions in symptomatic behavior for patients in FBT than in SPT. In addition, significantly more patients in FBT than in SPT remitted at end of treatment and at follow-up.

A recent review and meta-analysis of family therapy for both AN and BN concluded that behaviorally based FBT for adolescents with eating disorders is superior to individual therapy at 6–12-month follow-up, although there is no difference at end of treatment (Couturier et al., 2013).

While there is some support for individual CBT approaches in adolescents with BN and other binge eating syndromes (e.g., Schmidt *et al.*, 2007), and more recently for CBT-E in adolescents with AN (Dalle Grave *et al.*, 2013), the evidence base for CBT for AN in adolescents is very much in its infancy. Nevertheless, eating disorders represent a good example of how abnormal thoughts and behaviors combine to result in physical and social impairment and thus, in theory, cognitive behavioral approaches could provide an effective strategy for treating these disorders (Gowers & Green, 2009). Further research is necessary in order to explore this idea.

Limitations in the quality of the evidence base in child and adolescent feeding and eating disorders

Greater effort is needed to improve the quality of treatment studies conducted in child and adolescent patients with eating disorders. Only three of the studies discussed earlier (Lock *et al*, 2005, 2010; Schmidt *et al.*, 2007) could be considered to be of sufficient quality to provide a solid evidence base.

Studies have also been hampered by a number of methodological limitations. While additional and larger clinical trials are currently being undertaken, they focus exclusively on AN and BN, usually in adolescents. One problem in evaluating treatment efficacy in children is the low base rate of AN and BN in children. Eating disorder definitions in both DSM and ICD classification systems have failed to capture the majority of eating disorders that appear in children (Nicholls *et al.*, 2000). The advent of DSM-5, which contains significant changes to the diagnoses of feeding and eating disorders, is predicted to capture more childhood presentations, which in turn will facilitate the evaluation of treatment efficacy in this population. To date, there have been no controlled treatment studies of conditions other than AN and BN in adolescents, which brings to mind the adage "we study what we define" (Walsh & Kahn, 1997); this may have a particularly deleterious effect on developing evidence-based treatments for feeding and eating disorders in children and adolescents.

Often, treatment studies have used nonstandardized therapies, which limit opportunities for comparison and replication and also the potential for clinicians to implement these therapies in their own practice.

Many controlled treatment studies exclude boys from participation. However, the lower base rate of eating disorders in boys makes it difficult to recruit adequate numbers to establish gender differences in treatment efficacy. Because eating disorder interventions have been designed, refined, and tested predominantly in female participants, it remains unclear whether these treatments are useful in treating boys with eating disorders.

Most controlled treatment studies in adolescents provide no information concerning the ethnic/racial diversity of participants. In those that do, ethnic minority representation appears to be a function of the geographic locations in which research has been conducted, and analyses of differential treatment completion or response are not presented. Thus, the question of whether ethnicity/race serves as a moderator variable cannot be answered.

In summary, the evidence base for psychological treatments for eating problems in children and adolescents is quite limited. As a consequence of the small number of studies and methodological limitations in existing studies, it is not possible to describe in any detail what treatments work for whom.

Consent and ethical issues

Eating disorders are unusual among presentations in child and adolescent psychiatry in that they are potentially life threatening and may have very serious physical and psychosocial consequences if effective treatment is not provided. Given that young people with eating disorders are often reluctant to seek or accept treatment, practitioners need effective ethical and legal guidelines in order to make treatment decisions (Foreman, 2006).

All possible attempts should be made to form a therapeutic alliance with the young person, both to achieve consent to treatment on ethical grounds, and because therapeutic alliance is associated with effectiveness of treatment. In England and Wales, parents or those with parental authority may consent on their children's behalf up to the age of 18 but different countries operate different age limits. While it is desirable to obtain the young person's consent, it is helpful to make a distinction between treatment directed at reducing risk from the physical consequences of the eating disorder and psychological treatment of the eating disorder. The decision to treat against the young person's wishes is usually most likely to arise when hospital admission is indicated and the young person declines treatment. However, the decision to treat a young person against their will should always be considered a last resort.

Legislation differs between countries, although similar principles apply when deciding which approach to take. Parental consent to treatment is often the most appropriate choice, particularly in the short term and for younger patients, as often young people will engage with treatment once they feel safe within the treatment setting. If the young person consistently continues to decline treatment, leading to the need for active treatment against their will (e.g., nasogastric feeding) and/or absconding, using mental health legislation to provide the basis for treatment should be considered (see further Chapter 19).

Outcome

Outcome studies can generally be divided into two categories: those that attempt to establish the efficacy of a particular treatment (see section on Treatment in this chapter) and those that attempt to establish prognostic factors.

Problems in outcome research

There are a number of methodological shortcomings in the outcome literature in this field, including small sample sizes, inadequate measurement of target symptoms, failure to use standardized assessment measures, inadequate follow-up, high attrition rates, and variability in the definition of remission and recovery. While for adults, recovery implies restoration to premorbid physical and mental health, for children and adolescents, recovery includes rejoining a normal developmental trajectory, which will involve facing a number of physical and social aspects of identity that have not yet been experienced (Gowers, 2013).

Prognostic factors

Generally, for every study that identifies a group of prognostic factors, another study will fail to replicate the significance of the group of variables identified. These inconsistencies and contradictions can be accounted for by methodological flaws as noted earlier. Nevertheless, age at onset, duration of inpatient care, comorbidity, and social problems have been identified as important prognostic factors (Lowe *et al.*, 2001; Finfgeld, 2002; Steinhausen, 2002).

Recovery and remission

Outcome studies fairly consistently report that 47–57% of children and adolescents with eating disorders recover, 29–34% improve, and 17–20% follow a chronic course (e.g., Fisher, 2003; Halvorsen *et al.*, 2004). In general, remission rates increase with longer duration of follow-up for all diagnoses (Keel & Brown, 2010). It is often difficult to generalize findings from studies of outcome of eating disorders as there is wide variation in the outcome parameters used across studies. Remission rates in AN appear to vary depending on where the sample was drawn from and in adolescents treated in the community, relatively high rates of remission have been found at five year follow-up (76%) and eight year follow-up (82%) (Clausen, 2008). Rates of remission for BN do not appear to vary depending on where the sample was drawn from, with no apparent differences between rates of remission for adults and adolescents or for inpatients and those treated in the community. Remission rates for BN remain stable at around 70% or higher in samples followed up between 5 years and 20 years after baseline assessment (Keel & Brown, 2010).

Several outcome studies of EDNOS have looked at remission in the context of bulimic type symptoms and have compared the outcome of those with EDNOS to those with BN. Remission rates for adolescents with EDNOS appear to be higher than for those with BN following treatment (Schmidt *et al.*, 2008). However, remission rates for EDNOS and BN do not differ significantly at five year follow-up, with both having remission rates of about 75% (Grilo *et al.*, 2007). Similar rates of remission are found in EDNOS (75%) and BN (72%) at 20-year follow-up (Keel *et al.*, 2010).

With regard to treatment setting, Gowers *et al.* (2007) found that neither psychiatric inpatient nor specialist outpatient treatment provided better outcomes than nonspecialist outpatient treatment for adolescent AN. Inpatient treatment (randomized or after outpatient transfer) predicted poor outcomes. However, adherence to inpatient treatment in this trial was less than 50%, which may have compromised the effectiveness of this treatment. Further studies are needed in order to clarify optimum treatment options.

Migration between diagnoses

Those with AN who do not achieve remission over the course of follow-up often develop either BN or EDNOS. However, those with BN who do not achieve remission over the course of follow-up usually continue to meet full criteria for BN or transition to a diagnosis of EDNOS, including BED, with crossover to AN from BN being particularly rare (Keel & Brown, 2010).

Prevention

Much of the work on eating disorders prevention has been conducted within school settings, mostly in the form of the evaluation of specific preventative programs delivered in classroom settings. These have delivered mixed findings with no one clearly superior program. The impact of such interventions on incidence of eating disorders is hard to ascertain and it is generally recognized that such initiatives can only ever form part of a comprehensive preventative approach, which also requires family and societal components as well as improved understanding of the complex etiological pathways of eating disorders.

Conclusion

This chapter summarizes current knowledge, understanding, and practice in feeding and eating disorders in children and adolescents. The implications for clinicians and their patients of recent changes in DSM-5 and proposed changes in ICD-11(Uher & Rutter, 2012) will unfold over the coming years. It is hoped that improved recognition, greater consistency in use of terminology, enhanced knowledge and understanding in the areas of epidemiology and etiology and the development of more effective interventions will follow. There is undoubtedly still a long way to go in improving the quality and consistency of care for children and adolescents with significant eating difficulties. It is unclear whether current approaches to classification in the form of categorical diagnostic groups will prove most useful in the long term as basis for research endeavors. Developments in cross-cutting dimensional research, such as initiatives attempting to classify psychopathology based on dimensions of observable behavior and neurobiological measures (Cuthbert & Insel, 2013) may in due course result in more meaningful, useful, and effective changes in how we develop and select appropriate treatments for our patients.

References

American Psychiatric Association (1994) *Diagnostic and Statistical Manual of Mental Disorders*, 4th edn. American Psychiatric Association, Washington, DC.

American Psychiatric Association (2013) *Diagnostic and Statistical Manual of Mental Disorders*, 5th edn. American Psychiatric Association, Washington, DC.

Arcelus, J. *et al.* (2011) Mortality rates in patients with AN and other eating disorders: a meta-analysis of 36 studies. *Archives of General Psychiatry* **68**, 724–731.

Archer, L.A. *et al.* (1991) The Children's eating behavior inventory: reliability and validity results. *Journal of Pediatric Psychology* **16**, 629–642.

Attia, E. & Roberto, C. (2009) Should amenorrhea be a diagnostic criterion for AN? *International Journal of Eating Disorders* **42**, 581–589.

Becker, A. *et al.* (2002) Eating behaviours and attitudes following prolonged television exposure among ethnic Fijian adolescent girls. *British Journal of Psychiatry* **180**, 509–514.

Becker, A.E. *et al.* (2009) Should non-fat-phobic AN be included in DSM-V? *International Journal of Eating Disorders* **42**, 620–635.

Becker, A. *et al.* (2011) Social network media exposure and adolescent eating pathology in Fiji. *British Journal of Psychiatry* **198**, 43–50.

Benoit, D. & Coolbear, J. (1998) Post-traumatic feeding disorders in infancy: behaviors predicting treatment outcome. *Infant Mental Health Journal* **19**, 409–421.

Blakemore, S. *et al.* (2010) The role of puberty in the developing adolescent brain. *Human Brain Mapping* **31**, 926–933.

Bravender, T. *et al.* (2010) Classification of eating disturbance in children and adolescents: proposed changes for the DSM-V. *European Eating Disorders Review* **18**, 79–89.

Bruch, H. (1973) *Eating Disorders*. Basic Books, New York.

Brumberg, J.J. (1988) *Fasting Girls*. Harvard University Press, Cambridge, Mass.

Bryant-Waugh, R. *et al.*, (2010) Feeding and eating disorders in childhood. *International Journal of Eating Disorders* **43**, 98–111.

Bryant-Waugh, R. & Kreipe, R.E. (2012) Avoidant/restrictive food intake disorder in DSM-5. *Psychiatric Annals* **42**, 402–405.

Bryant-Waugh, R.J. *et al.* (1996) The use of the eating disorder examination with children: a pilot study. *International Journal of Eating Disorders* **19**, 391–397.

Bulik, C.M. *et al.* (2000) Twin studies of eating disorders: a review. *International Journal of Eating Disorders* **27**, 1–20.

Byers, K. *et al.* (2003) A multicomponent behavioral program for oral aversion in children dependent on gastrostomy feedings. *Journal of Pediatric Gastroenterology and Nutrition* **37**, 473–480.

Carter, J.C. *et al.* (2001) Eating Disorder Examination Questionnaire: norms for young adolescent girls. *Behaviour Research & Therapy* **39**, 625–632.

Cassin, S. & von Ranson, K. (2005) Personality and eating disorders: a decade in review. *Clinical Psychology Review* **25**, 895–916.

Chen, L. *et al.* (2010) Sexual abuse and lifetime diagnosis of psychiatric disorders: a systematic review and meta-analysis. *Mayo Clinic Proceedings* **85**, 618–629.

Childress, A.C. *et al.* (1993) The Kids' Eating Disorders Survey (KEDS): a study of middle school students. *Journal of the American Academy of Child Adolescent Psychiatry* **32**, 843–850.

Chowdhury, U. *et al.* (2003) Early-onset AN: is there evidence of a limbic system imbalance? *International Journal of Eating Disorders* **33**, 388–398.

Clausen, L. (2008) Time to remission for eating disorder patients: a 2(1/2)-year follow-up study of outcome and predictors. *Nordic Journal of Psychiatry* **62**, 151–159.

Connan, F. *et al.* (2003) A neurodevelopmental model for AN. *Physiology and Behaviour* **79**, 13–24.

Couturier, J. *et al.* (2013) Efficacy of family-based treatment for adolescents with eating disorders: a systematic review and meta-analysis. *International Journal of Eating Disorders* **46**, 3–11.

Crist, W. & Napier-Phillips, A. (2001) Mealtime behaviors of young children: a comparison of normative and clinical data. *Journal of Developmental and Behavioral Pediatrics* **22**, 279–286.

Culbert, K.M. *et al.* (2009) Puberty and the genetic diathesis of disordered eating. *Journal of Abnormal Psychology* **118**, 788–796.

Currin, L. *et al.* (2005) Time trends in eating disorder incidence. *British Journal of Psychiatry* **186**, 132–135.

Cuthbert, B.N. & Insel, T.R. (2013) Toward the future of psychiatric diagnosis: the seven pillars of RDoC. *BMC Medicine* **11**, 126.

Dalle Grave, R. *et al.* (2013) Enhanced cognitive behaviour therapy for adolescents with AN: an alternative to family therapy? *Behaviour Research and Therapy* **51**, R9–R12.

Darcy, A. *et al.* (2012) Set-shifting among adolescents with bulimic spectrum eating disorders. *Pyschosomatic Medicine* **74**, 869–872.

Davies, W.H. *et al.* (2006) Reconceptualising feeding and feeding disorders in interpersonal context: the case for a relational disorder. *Journal of Family Psychology* **20**, 409–417.

De Young, K.P. *et al.* (2012) Review of BED and proposal for inclusion in DSM-5. *Psychiatric Annals* **42**, 410–413.

Dovey, T. & Martin, C. (2012) A quantitative psychometric evaluation of an intervention for poor dietary variety in children with a feeding problem of clinical significance. *Infant Mental Health Journal* **33**, 148–162.

Drossman, D.A. *et al.* (2006) *Rome III: The Functional Gastrointestinal Disorders*, 3rd edn. Degnon Associates, McLean, VA.

Eisler, I. (1995) Family models of eating disorders. In: *Handbook of Eating Disorders: Theory, Treatment and Research.* (eds G.I. Szmukler, C. Dare & J. Treasure). John Wiley & Sons, Chichester.

Eisler, I. (2005) The empirical and theoretical base of family therapy and multiple family day therapy for adolescent AN. *Journal of Family Therapy* **27**, 104–131.

Eisler, I. *et al.* (1997) Family and individual therapy in anorexia nervosa. A 5-year follow-up. *Archives of General Psychiatry* **54**, 1025–1030.

Eisler, I. *et al.* (2000) Family therapy for adolescent AN: the results of a controlled comparison of two family interventions. *Journal of Child Psychology and Psychiatry* **41**, 727–736.

Ericsson, N. *et al.* (2011) Parental disorders, childhood abuse and binge eating in a large community sample. *International Journal of Eating Disorders* **45**, 316–325.

Fairburn, C. & Beglin, S. (1994) Assessment of eating disorders: interview or self-report questionnaire? *International Journal of Eating Disorders* **16**, 363–370.

Fairburn, C. & Cooper, Z. (1993) The eating disorder examination (12th edition). In: *Binge Eating: Nature, Assessment & Treatment.* (eds C.G. Fairburn & G.T. Wilson), pp. 317–360. Guildford Press, New York.

Fairburn, C.G. *et al.* (1997) Risk factors for BN. A community based case–control study. *Archives of General Psychiatry* **54**, 509–517.

Fairburn, C. *et al.* (2005) Identifying dieters who will develop an eating disorder: a prospective population-based study. *American Journal of Psychiatry* **35**, 147–156.

Favaro, A. *et al.* (2006) Perinatal factors and the risk of developing AN and BN. *Archives of General Psychiatry* **63**, 82–88.

Favaro, A. *et al.* (2011) In utero exposure to virus infections and the risk of developing AN. *Psychological Medicine* **41**, 2193–2199.

Field, A. *et al.* (2001) Peer, parent and media influences on the development of weight concerns and frequent dieting among preadolescent and adolescent girls and boys. *Pediatrics* **107**, 54–60.

Finfgeld, D.L. (2002) AN: analysis of long-term outcomes and clinical implications. *Archives of Psychiatric Nursing* **16**, 176–186.

First, M.B. *et al.* (1996) *Structured Clinical Interview for DSM-IV Axis I Disorders, Clinician Version (SCID-CV)*. American Psychiatric Association, Washington, DC.

Fisher, M. (2003) The course and outcome of eating disorders in adults and adolescents: a review. *Adolescent Medicine State of the Art Reviews* **14**, 149–158.

Fitzpatrick, K. *et al.* (2012) Set-shifting among adolescents with AN. *International Journal of Eating Disorders* **45**, 909–912.

Fonagy, P. *et al.* (1996) The relation of attachment status, psychiatric classification, and response to psychotherapy. *Journal of Consulting and Clinical Psychology* **64**, 357–365.

Foreman, D. (2006) The law in relation to children. In: *Seminars in Child and Adolescent Psychiatry*. (ed S.G. Gowers), 2nd edn, pp. 99–101. Gaskell, London.

Frampton, I. *et al.* (2011) Do abnormalities in regional cerebral blood flow in AN resolve after weight restoration? *European Eating Disorders Review* **19**, 55–58.

Franko, D. *et al.* (2013) A longitudinal investigation of mortality in anorexia nervosa and bulimia nervosa. *American Journal of Psychiatry* **170**, 917–925.

Fraser, K. *et al.* (2004) Improving children's problem eating and mealtime behaviours: an evaluative study of a single session parent education programme. *Health Education Journal* **63**, 229–241.

Freidl, E.K. *et al.* (2012) AN in DSM-5. *Psychiatric Annals* **42**, 414–417.

Garner, D.M. (1991) *The Eating Disorder Inventory-C*. Psychological Assessment Resources, Lutz, FL.

Garner, D.M. (2004) *Eating Disorders Inventory 3: Professional manual*. Psychological Assessment Resources, Odessa, FL.

Garner, D.M. *et al.* (1982) The Eating Attitudes Test: psychometric features and clinical correlates. *Psychological Medicine* **12**, 871–878.

Geissler, P.W. *et al.* (1997) Geophagy among school children in western Kenya. *Tropical Medicine and International Health* **2**, 624–630.

Geissler, P.W. *et al.* (1998) Geophagy as a risk factor for geohelminth infections: a longitudinal study of Kenyan primary schoolchildren. *Transcript of the Royal Society of Tropical Medicine and Hygiene* **92**, 7–11.

Goodman, R. *et al.* (2000) The Development and Well-Being Assessment: description and initial validation of an integrated assessment of child and adolescent psychopathology. *Journal of Child Psychology and Psychiatry* **41**, 645–655.

Goodsitt, A. (1985) Self-psychology and the treatment of AN. In: *Handbook of Psychotherapy for Anorexia Nervosa and Bulimia*. (eds D.M. Garner & P.E. Garfinkel), pp. 55–82. The Guilford Press, New York.

Gordon, I. *et al.* (1997) Childhood-onset AN: towards identifying a biological substrate. *International Journal of Eating Disorders* **22**, 159–165.

Gowers, S. (2013) Outcome. In: *Eating Disorders of Childhood and Adolescence*. (eds B. Lask & R. Bryant-Waugh), 4th edn, pp. 148–170. Routledge, New York.

Gowers, S.G. & Green, L. (2009) *Eating Disorders: Cognitive Behaviour Therapy with Children and Young People*. London.

Gowers, S. *et al.* (2007) Clinical effectiveness of treatments for anorexia nervosa in adolescents: randomised controlled trial. *The British Journal of Psychiatry* **191**, 427–435.

Gowers, S. *et al.* (2010) Drug prescribing in child and adolescent eating disorder services. *Journal of Child and Adolescent Mental Health* **15**, 18–22.

Greer, A. *et al.* (2008) Caregiver stress and outcomes of children with pediatric feeding disorders treated in an intensive interdisciplinary program. *Journal of Pediatric Psychology* **33**, 612–620.

Grilo, C.M. *et al.* (2007) Natural course of BN and of eating disorder not otherwise specified: 5-year prospective study of remissions, relapses, and the effects of personality disorder psychopathology. *Journal of Clinical Psychiatry* **68**, 738–746.

Groleau, P. *et al.* (2011) Childhood emotional abuse and eating symptoms in bulimic disorders: an examination of possible mediating variables. *International Journal of Eating Disorders* **45**, 326–332.

Hagekull, B. *et al.* (1997) Maternal sensitivity, infant temperament, and the development of early feeding problems. *Infant Mental Health Journal* **18**, 92–106.

Halvorsen, I. *et al.* (2004) Good outcome of adolescent AN after systematic treatment. *European Child and Adolescent Psychiatry* **13**, 295–306.

Hartmann, A.S. *et al.* (2012) Pica and rumination disorder in DSM-5. *Psychiatric Annals* **42**, 426–430.

Haycraft, E. *et al.* (2011) Relationships between temperament and eating behaviours in young children. *Appetite* **56**, 689–692.

Hoek, H. & van Hoeken, D. (2003) Review of the prevalence and incidence of eating disorders. *International Journal of Eating Disorders* **34**, 383–396.

Hölling, H. & Schlack, R. (2007) Eating disorders in children and adolescents: first results of the German Health Interview and Examination Survey for Children and Adolescents (KiGGS) [in German]. *Bundesgesundheitsblatt Gesundheitsforschung Gesundheitsschutz* **50**, 794–799.

Hospital Episode Statistics, (2010) *HESonline: Topic of Interest—Eating Disorders*, http://www.hesonline.nhs.uk/Ease/servlet/ContentServer?siteID=1937&categoryID=1489

Illing, V. *et al.* (2010) Attachment insecurity predicts eating disorder symptoms and treatment outcomes in a clinical sample of women. *Journal of Nervous and Mental Disease* **198**, 653–659.

Investigators, M.K. (2003) Risk factors for the onset of eating disorders in adolescent girls: results of the McKnight longitudinal risk factor study. *American Journal of Psychiatry* **160**, 248–254.

Ivascu, N.S. *et al.* (2001) Characterization of pica prevalence among patients with sickle cell disease. *Archives of Pediatric and Adolescent Medicine* **155**, 1243–1247.

Jacobs, B. & Isaacs, S. (1986) Pre-pubertal AN: a retrospective controlled study. *Journal of Child Psychology and Psychiatry* **27**, 237–250.

Javaras, K.N. *et al.* (2008) Familiality and heritability of BED: results of a case–control family study and a twin study. *International Journal of Eating Disorders* **41**, 174–179.

Jones, J. *et al.* (2001) Disordered eating attitudes and behaviours in teenaged girls: a school-based study. *Canadian Medical Association Journal* **165**, 547–552.

Katzman, D.K. (2005) Medical complications in adolescents with AN: a review of the literature. *International Journal of Eating Disorders* **37**, S52–S59.

Kaye, W. *et al.* (2013) Nothing tastes as good as skinny feels: the neurobiology of AN. *Trends in Neuroscience* **36**, 110–120.

Keel, P. & Brown, T. (2010) Update on course and outcome in eating disorders. *International Journal of Eating Disorders* **43**, 195–204.

Keel, P. & Forney, K. (2013) Psychosocial risk factors for eating disorders. *International Journal of Eating Disorders* **46**, 433–439.

Keel, P. & Klump, K. (2003) Are eating disorders culture-bound syndromes? Implications for conceptualizing their etiology. *Psychological Bulletin* **129**, 747–769.

Keel, P.K. & Striegel-Moore, R.H. (2009) The validity and clinical utility of purging disorder. *International Journal of Eating Disorders* **42**, 706–719.

Keel, P. *et al.* (2010) Twenty-year follow-up of BN and related eating disorders not otherwise specified. *International Journal of Eating Disorders* **43**, 492–497.

Kenney, L. & Walsh, T. (2013) Avoidant/restrictive food intake disorder. *Eating Disorders Review* **24**, 1–4.

Keski-Rahkonen, A. *et al.* (2007) Epidemiology and course of AN in the community. *American Journal of Psychiatry* **164**, 1259–1265.

Killen, J. *et al.* (1996) Weight concerns influence the development of eating disorders: a 4-year prospective study. *Journal of Consulting and Clinical Psychology* **64**, 936–940.

Klump, K.L. & Culbert, K.M. (2007) Molecular genetic studies of eating disorders: current status and future directions. *Current Directions in Psychological Science* **16**, 37–41.

Klump, K.L. *et al.* (2000) Age differences in genetic and environmental influences on eating attitudes and behaviors in preadolescent and adolescent female twins. *Journal of Abnormal Psychology* **109**, 239–251.

Klump, K.L. *et al.* (2003) Differential heritability of eating attitudes and behaviors in prepuberbertal and pubertal twins. *International Journal of Eating Disorders* **33**, 287–292.

Klump, K.L. *et al.* (2007a) Changes in genetic and environmental influences on disordered eating across adolescence. *Archives of General Psychiatry* **64**, 1409–1415.

Klump, K.L. *et al.* (2007b) Puberty moderates genetic influences on disordered eating. *Psychological Medicine* **37**, 627–634.

Klump, K.L. *et al.* (2008) Ovarian hormones and binge eating: exploring associations in community samples. *Psychological Medicine* **38**, 1749–1757.

Klump, K.L. *et al.* (2010) Age differences in genetic and environmental influences on weight and shape concerns. *International Journal of Eating Disorders* **43**, 679–688.

Kog, E. *et al.* (1987) Minuchin's pychosomatic family model revised: a concept validation study using a multitrait-multimethod approach. *Family Process* **26**, 235–253.

Kotler, L.A. *et al.* (2001) Longitudinal relationships between childhood, adolescent, and adult eating disorders. *Journal of the American Academy of Child and Adolescent Psychiatry* **40**, 1434–1440.

Lask, B. & Bryant-Waugh, R. (2013) Overview of management. In: *Eating Disorders of Childhood and Adolescence.* (eds B. Lask & R. Bryant-Waugh), 4th edn, pp. 173–196. Routledge, New York.

Le Grange, D. *et al.* (1992) Evaluation of family therapy in AN: a pilot study. *International Journal of Eating Disorder* **12**, 347–357.

Ledford, J. *et al.* (2008) Observational and incidental learning by children with autism during small group instruction. *Journal of Autism and Developmental Disorders* **38**, 86–103.

LeGrange, D. *et al.* (2007) A randomized controlled comparison of family based treatment and supportive psychotherapy for adolescent BN. *Archives of General Psychiatry* **64**, 1049–1056.

Lewinsohn, P.M. *et al.* (2000) Epidemiology and natural course of eating disorders in young women from adolescence to young adulthood. *Child and Adolescent Psychiatry* **39**, 1284–1292.

Lilenfeld, L. (2011) Personality and temperament in eating disorders. In: *Current Topics in Behavioral Neurosciences.* (eds W.H. Kaye & R. Adan). Springer, New York.

Lindberg, L. & Hjern, A. (2003) Risk factors for AN: a national cohort study. *International Journal of Eating Disorders* **34**, 397–408.

Lock, J. *et al.* (2005) A comparison of short- and long-term family therapy for adolescent AN. *Journal of the American Academy of Child and Adolescent Psychiatry* **44**, 632–639.

Lock, J. *et al.* (2010) Randomized clinical trial comparing family-based treatment with adolescent-focused individual therapy for adolescents with eating disorders. *Archives of General Psychiatry* **67**, 1025–1032.

Lowe, B. *et al.* (2001) Long-term outcome of AN in a prospective 21-year follow-up study. *Psychological Medicine* **31**, 881–890.

Machado, P.P. *et al.* (2007) The prevalence of eating disorders not otherwise specified. *International Journal of Eating Disorders* **40**, 212–217.

Madden, S. *et al.* (2009) Burden of eating disorders in 5-13-year-old children in Australia. *Medical Journal of Australia* **190**, 410–414.

Maloney, M.J. *et al.* (1988) Reliability testing of a children's version of the Eating Attitude Test. *Journal of the American Academy of Child & Adolescent Psychiatry* **27**, 541–543.

Marchi, M. & Cohen, P. (1990) Early childhood eating behaviors and adolescent eating disorders. *Journal of the American Academy of Child and Adolescent Psychiatry* **29**, 112–117.

Marcus, M.D. & Wildes, J.E. (2009) Obesity: is it a mental disorder? *International Journal of Eating Disorders* **42**, 739–753.

Markkula, N. (2012) Mortality in people with depressive, anxiety and alcohol use disorders in Finland. *British Journal of Psychiatry* **200**, 143–149.

Martin, G.C. *et al.* (2000) A longitudinal study of the role of childhood temperament in the later development of eating concerns. *International Journal of Eating Disorders* **27**, 150–162.

McKnight (2003) Risk factors for the onset of eating disorders in adolescent girls: results of the McKnight longitudinal risk factor study. *American Journal of Psychiatry* **160**, 248–254.

Merikangas, K. *et al.* (2010) Lifetime prevalence of mental disorders in US adolescents: results from the National Comorbidity Survey Replication-Adolescent Supplement (NCS-A). *Journal of the American Academy of Child and Adolescent Psychiatry.* **49**, 980–989.

Micali, N. & House, J. (2011) Assessment measures for child and adolescent eating disorders: a review. *Child and Adolescent Mental Health* **16**, 122–127.

Micali, N. *et al.* (2011) Maternal eating disorders and infant feeding difficulties: maternal and child mediators in a longitudinal general population study. *Journal of Child Clinical Psychology and Psychiatry* **52**, 800–807.

Minuchin, S. *et al.* (1975) A conceptual model of psychosomatic illness in children. *Archives of General Psychiatry* **32**, 1031–1038.

Minuchin, S. *et al.* (1978) *Psychosomatic Families: Anorexia Nervosa in Context.* Harvard University Press, Cambridge, MA.

National Institute for Health and Care Excellence (2004) *National Clinical Practice Guideline. Eating Disorders. Core Interventions in the*

Treatment and Management of AN, BN, and Related Eating Disorders. National Institute for Health and Care Excellence, London.

Nicholls, D. & Bryant-Waugh, R. (2009) Eating disorders of infancy and childhood: definition, symptomatology, epidemiology, and comorbidity. *Child and Adolescent Psychiatric Clinics of North America* **18**, 17–30.

Nicholls, D. & Viner, R. (2009) Childhood risk factors for lifetime AN by age 30 years in a national birth cohort. *Journal of the American Academy of Child and Adolescent Psychiatry* **48**, 791–799.

Nicholls, D. *et al.* (2000) Children into DSM don't go: a comparison of classification systems for eating disorders in childhood and early adolescence. *International Journal of Eating Disorders* **28**, 317–324.

Nicholls, D. *et al.* (2011) Childhood eating disorders: British national surveillance study. *British Journal of Psychiatry* **198**, 295–301.

Nicholson, J. (2013) Psychological assessment. In: *Eating Disorders in Childhood and Adolescence.* (eds B. Lask & R. Bryant-Waugh), 4th edn, pp. 105–124. Routledge, Hove, East Sussex & New York.

O'Herlihy, A. *et al.* (2003) Distribution and characteristics of in-patient child and adolescent mental health services in England and Wales. *British Journal of Psychiatry* **183**, 547–551.

Palazzoli, M.S. (1974) *Self Starvation.* Chancer, London.

Peebles, R. *et al.* (2010) Are diagnostic criteria for eating disorders markers of medical severity? *Pediatrics* **125**, 1993–1201.

Pinhas, L. *et al.* (2011) Incidence and age-specific presentation of restrictive eating disorders in children. *Archives of Pediatric and Adolescent Medicine* **165**, 895–899.

Pliner, P. & Loewen, E. (1997) Temperament and food neophobia in children and their mothers. *Appetite* **28**, 239–254.

Pro Bono Economics (2012) *Costs of eating disorders in England: Economic impacts of anorexia nervosa, bulimia nervosa and other disorders, focussing on young people,* http://www.probonoeconomics .com/sites/probonoeconomics.com/files/files/reports/PBE%20BEAT %20report%20180512_0.pdf.

Rastam, M. (1992) AN in 51 Swedish adolescents: premorbid problems and comorbidity. *Journal of American Academy of Child & Adolescent Psychiatry* **31**, 819–829.

Rieger, E. *et al.* (2000) Cross-cultural research on AN: assumptions regarding the role of body weight. *International Journal of Eating Disorders* **29**, 205–215.

Ringer, F. & Crittenden, P.M. (2007) Eating disorders and attachment: the effects of hidden processes on eating disorders. *European Eating Disorders Review* **15**, 119–130.

Roberts, M. *et al.* (2007) A systematic review and meta-analysis of set-shifting ability in eating disorders. *Psychological Medicine* **37**, 1075–1084.

Robin, A. *et al.* (1994) Family therapy versus individual therapy for adolescent females with AN. *Journal of Developmental and Behavioural Pediatrics* **15**, 111–116.

Rose, E. *et al.* (2000) Pica: common but commonly missed. *Journal of the Board of Family Medicine* **13**, 353–358.

Russell, G.F.M. *et al.* (1987) An evaluation of family therapy in anorexia and BN. *Archives of General Psychiatry* **44**, 1047–1056.

Rutherford, J. *et al.* (1993) Genetic influences on eating attitudes in a normal female twin pair population. *Psychological Medicine* **23**, 425–436.

Schmidt, U. & Treasure, J. (2006) AN: valued and visible. A cognitive interpersonal maintenance model and its implications for research and practice. *British Journal of Clinical Psychology* **45**, 343–366.

Schmidt, U. *et al.* (2007) A randomized controlled trial of family therapy and cognitive behavioral therapy guided self-care for adolescents with BN and related disorders. *American Journal of Psychiatry* **164**, 591–598.

Schmidt, U. *et al.* (2008) Do adolescents with eating disorder not otherwise specified or full-syndrome BN differ in clinical severity, comorbidity, risk factors, treatment outcome or cost? *International Journal of Eating Disorders* **41**, 498–504.

Schroedl, R. *et al.* (2013) Behavioral treatment for adolescent rumination syndrome: a case report. *Clinical Practice in Pediatric Psychology* **1**, 89–93.

Shaffer, D. *et al.* (2000) NIMH Diagnostic Interview Schedule for Children Version IV (NIMH DISC-IV): description, differences from previous versions, and reliability of some common diagnoses. *Journal of the American Academy of Child & Adolescent Psychiatry* **39**, 28–38.

Shoebridge, P. & Gowers, S.G. (2000) Parental high concern and adolescent-onset AN. A case–control study to investigate direction of causality. *British Journal of Psychiatry* **176**, 132–137.

Silberg, J.L. & Bulik, C.M. (2005) The developmental association between eating disorders symptoms and symptoms of depression and anxiety in juvenile twin girls. *Journal of Child Psychology and Psychiatry* **46**, 1317–1326.

Singhi, S. *et al.* (1981) Role of psychosocial stress in the cause of Pica. *Clinical Paediatrics* **20**, 783–785.

Smink, F. *et al.* (2012) Epidemiology of eating disorders: incidence, prevalence and mortality rates. *Current Psychiatry Reports* **14**, 406–414.

Sokol, M. (2000) Infection triggered anorexia in children: clinical description of four cases. *Journal of Child and Adolescent Psychopharmacology* **10**, 133–145.

van Son, G. *et al.* (2006) Time trends in the incidence of eating disorders: a primary care study in the Netherlands. *International Journal of Eating Disorders* **39**, 565–569.

Stedhal, K. *et al.* (2012) The neuropsychological profile of children, adolescents and young adults with AN. *Archives of Clinical Neuropsychology* **3**, 329–337.

Stein, A. *et al.* (2006) Eating habits and attitudes among 10-year-old children of mothers with eating disorders. *British Journal of Psychiatry* **189**, 324–329.

Steinhausen, H.C. (2002) The outcome of AN in the 20th century. *American Journal of Psychiatry* **159**, 1284–1293.

Stice, E. (2002) Risk and maintenance factors for eating pathology: a meta-analytic review. *Psychological Bulletin* **128**, 825–848.

Stice, E. & Whitenton, K. (2002) Risk factors for body dissatisfaction in adolescent girls: a longitudinal investigation. *Developmental Psychology* **38**, 669–678.

Stice, E. *et al.* (2008) Fasting increases risk for onset of binge eating and bulimic pathology: a 5-year prospective study. *Journal of Abnormal Psychology* **117**, 941–946.

Stice, E. *et al.* (2009) An 8-year longitudinal study of the natural history of threshold, subthreshold, and partial eating disorders from a community sample of adolescents. *Journal of Abnormal Psychology* **118**, 587–597.

Stice, E. *et al.* (2011) Risk factors for onset of eating disorders: evidence of multiple risk pathways from an 8-year prospective study. *Behaviour Research and Therapy* **49**, 622–627.

Striegel-Moore, R.H. *et al.* (2009) The validity and clinical utility of night eating syndrome. *International Journal of Eating Disorders* **42**, 720–738.

Strober, M. & Humphrey, L.L. (1987) Familial contributions to the etiology and course of anorexia nervosa and bulimia. *Journal of Consulting and Clinical Psychology* **55**, 654–659.

Sullivan, P.F. *et al.* (1998) Genetic epidemiology of binging and vomiting. *British Journal of Psychiatry* **173**, 75–79.

Sullivan, P. *et al.* (2000) Prevalence and severity of feeding and nutritional problems in children with neurological impairment: Oxford feeding study. *Developmental Medicine and Child Neurology* **42**, 674–680.

Swanson, S. *et al.* (2011) Prevalence and correlates of eating disorders in adolescents: results from the National Comorbidity Survey Replication Adolescent Supplement. *Archives of General Psychiatry* **68**, 714–723.

Swedo, S. *et al.* (2012) From research subgroup to clinical syndrome: modifying the PANDAS criteria to describe PANS (pediatric acute-onset neuropsychiatric syndrome). *Pediatrics & Therapeutics* **2**, 2.

Tanner, J.M. (1989) *Foetus into Man: Physical Growth from Conception to Maturity*, 2nd edn. Ware, Castlemead.

Thornton, L. *et al.* (2011) The heritability of eating disorders: methods and current findings. In: *Current Topics in Behavioral Neurosciences.* (eds W.H. Kaye & R. Adan). Springer, New York.

Trace, S. *et al.* (2013) The genetics of eating disorders. *Annual Review of Clinical Psychology* **9**, 589–620.

Troupp, C. (2013) Individual psychotherapy. In: *Eating Disorders of Childhood and Adolescence.* (eds B. Lask & R. Bryant-Waugh), 4th edn, pp. 281–300. Routledge, New York.

Turnbull, S. *et al.* (1996) The demand for eating disorder care. An epidemiological study using the General Practice Research Database. *British Journal of Psychiatry* **169**, 705–712.

Uher, R. & Rutter, M. (2012) Classification of feeding and eating disorders: review of evidence and proposals for ICD-11. *World Psychiatry* **11**, 80–92.

Van Hoeken, D. *et al.* (2009) The validity and utility of subtyping BN. *International Journal of Eating Disorders* **42**, 595–602.

Wade, T. *et al.* (1999) A genetic analysis of the eating and attitudes associated with BN: dealing with the problem of ascertainment. *Behavioral Genetics* **29**, 1–10.

Walsh, B.T. & Kahn, C.B. (1997) Diagnostic criteria for eating disorders: current concerns and future directions. *Psychopharmacology Bulletin* **33**, 369–372.

Wardle, J. *et al.* (2001) Development of the children's eating behaviour questionnaire. *Journal of Child Psychology and Psychiatry* **42**, 963–970.

Williams, D. & McAdam, D. (2012) Assessment, behavioral treatment, and prevention of pica: clinical guidelines and recommendations for practitioners. *Research in Developmental Disabilities* **33**, 2050–2057.

Wilson, G.T. & Sysko, R. (2009) Frequency of binge eating episodes in BN and BED: diagnostic considerations. *International Journal of Eating Disorders* **42**, 603–610.

Wolfe, B. *et al.* (2012) BN in DSM-5. *Psychiatric Annals* **42**, 406–409.

Wonderlich, S.A. *et al.* (2009) The validity and clinical utility of BED. *International Journal of Eating Disorders* **42**, 687–705.

World Health Organization (1992) *International Statistical Classification of Diseases and Related Health Problems (10th revision).* World Health Organization, Geneva.

Zachrisson, H. & Kulbotten, G. (2006) Attachment in anorexia: an exploration of associations with eating disorder psychopathology and psychiatric symptoms. *Eating and Weight Disorders* **11**, 163–170.

Zero to Three (2005) *Diagnostic Classification of Mental Health and Developmental Disorders of Infancy and Early Childhood: Revised Edition (DC:0-3R).* Zero to Three Press, Washington, DC.

Zerwas, S. & Bulik, C. (2011) Genetics and Epigenetics of Eating Disorders. *Psychiatric Annals* **41**, 532–538.

CHAPTER 72
Somatoform and related disorders

M. Elena Garralda[1] and Charlotte Ulrikka Rask[2]

[1] Academic Unit of Child and Adolescent Psychiatry, Imperial College London, UK
[2] The Research Clinic for Functional Disorders and Psychosomatics, Regional Centre for Child and Adolescent Psychiatry, Aarhus University Hospital, Aarhus, Denmark

Characteristics of the disorders and classification

The essential feature of somatoform disorders as described in the World Health Organization (WHO, 1992) and the Diagnostic and Statistical Manual of Mental Disorders (DSM) classificatory systems (WHO, 1992; American Psychiatric Association, 1994, 2013) is the presence of physical symptoms that cause concern and are not explained by a general medical condition or psychiatric disorder. Symptoms must lead to noticeable and significant distress or impairment in social (family and friends) and occupational spheres of functioning, which in children means school and academic difficulties. The symptoms are not feigned and usually occur in association with emotional conflict or psychosocial stress. In rare cases, the associated impairment may be extreme and result in states of severe or pervasive withdrawal when children stop communicating, walking, and looking after their basic needs.

Conversion/dissociative disorders share the main features of the somatoform disorders, but differ from them in that the main presentation is symptoms specifically affecting the motor and sensory systems. Nevertheless, because of their closeness to somatoform disorders, they and other related problems such as chronic fatigue syndrome (CFS) and juvenile fibromyalgia will be outlined in this chapter.

Somatoform disorders present predominantly in older children and adolescents, but early manifestations can be identified in younger preschool children. The diagnosis often relies on dual pediatric medical and psychiatric assessments and can therefore be more complex than that of other purely psychiatric or medical disorders.

We will describe how to differentiate somatoform disorders from physical complaints in healthy children, outline the concept of somatization, the classification of somatoform disorders in International Classification of Diseases (ICD-10) and in the recently published DSM-5 classificatory systems, as well as the uses of a dimensional approach. We will address clinical presentations, developmental issues, assessment and diagnosis, aetiology, risk factors and treatment.

Throughout the chapter, key abbreviations are FSS for functional somatic symptoms RAP for recurrent abdominal pains, CFS for chronic fatigue syndrome and CBT for cognitive behavioral therapy.

The experience of somatic symptoms in children and young people

Somatic symptoms are part of everyday life experience in children and young people (Offord et al., 1987; Garber et al., 1991; Eminson et al., 1996; Domenech-Llaberia et al., 2004; Rask et al., 2009b). These symptoms are mostly "functional" rather than "organic" (i.e. the expression of a medical disorder) and reflect common non-pathological or physiological bodily changes. In contrast with somatoform disorders, most functional somatic symptoms (FSS) in healthy children are neither persistent nor impairing, they tend to be ascribed to non-medical everyday biological or psychological stress and do not lead to medical help seeking (Huang et al., 2000; Rask et al., 2013a).

The concept of somatization

The concept of somatization is central to understanding the psychological ramifications of FSS and of somatoform and related disorders. The term has gained currency to describe a constellation of clinical and behavioural features involving: first, a tendency to experience and communicate distress through somatic symptoms unaccounted for by pathological findings; secondly these symptoms are attributed to physical illness and thirdly they lead to seeking medical help (Lipowski, 1988). In this review, we will describe FSS and somatoform and related disorders likely to be an expression of psychological distress and of somatization, even if these symptoms and disorders can also reflect bodily vulnerabilities.

Rutter's Child and Adolescent Psychiatry, Sixth Edition.
Edited by Anita Thapar and Daniel S. Pine, James F. Leckman, Stephen Scott, Margaret J. Snowling, Eric Taylor.
© 2015 John Wiley & Sons Ltd. Published 2018 by John Wiley & Sons Ltd.

The current classification of somatoform and related disorders

Current ICD and DSM classification systems diagnose disorders categorically. In ICD-10, somatoform disorders are a sub-category (coded F45) of the broader "Neurotic, stress disorders and somatoform disorders". Among its various sub-divisions, persistent somatoform pain disorder is most commonly observed in children and young people, while the diagnostic criteria for somatization disorder and hypochondriasis are seldom fully met in this age group.

Closely related clinical problems, also with somatization at their core, are classified in ICD-10 under the same broad grouping but as a separate dissociative (conversion) sub-category (code F44), the main complaint being medically unexplained neurological sensory or motor symptoms, such as paralysis, abnormal gait, loss of sensation, or pseudo-seizures. Presentations with fatigue as a main symptom are diagnosed as neurasthenia (F48). This term is now out of favour, but is descriptively close to clinical problems referred to in the research literature as CFS and CFS-like disorders, which also share the key features of the somatoform disorders.

Comparatively short-lived episodes with key somatoform features may be diagnosed as "adjustment disorders" if they follow closely on the experience of a marked and universally stressful event.

In DSM-5, somatoform disorders are referred to as "somatic symptom and related disorders", and the number of sub-categories has been substantially reduced (somatization disorder, hypochondriasis, pain disorder and unspecified somatoform disorder are no longer included). The category does include "psychological factors affecting other medical conditions" and "factitious disorder" as well as conversion disorder, now referred to as "conversion disorder (functional neurological symptom disorder)". Individuals with high health anxiety levels without somatic symptoms will receive a diagnosis of "illness anxiety disorder" unless the health anxiety is explained by a primary anxiety disorder, such as generalized anxiety disorder.

There is lack of clarity about the extent to which the essence of somatoform disorders lies in the functional or medically unexplained nature of the symptoms or in the distress/impairment caused (Dimsdale & Creed, 2009; Fink & Schroder, 2010). In DSM-5 (and probably also in the forthcoming ICD-11), the disorders are defined on the basis of positive symptoms, namely distressing somatic symptoms together with abnormal thoughts, feelings and behaviours in response to these symptoms. This might help improve the present situation where the same FSS are classified in medical and pediatric clinics as functional (non organic) disorders, but as somatoform disorders in psychiatric clinics. Table 72.1 provides examples of overlapping diagnostic labels in different specialties. Nevertheless in DSM-5 medically unexplained symptoms remain a key feature of conversion disorder, because it is possible to demonstrate definitively in such disorders that the symptoms are not consistent with medical pathophysiology.

The dimensional perspective

A categorical conceptualization is appropriate for somatoform disorders at the severe end of the spectrum (Figure 72.1). However, the dimensional perspective is useful in clarifying the significance of somatic symptoms in general populations or those attending primary health care and other medical clinics. In addition, while the categorical framework is appropriate for school children and adolescents, it is rare for young preschool children to have complaints that are severe and impairing enough to reach the diagnostic threshold for somatoform disorders: a dimensional perspective is more appropriate in this age group.

Developmental aspects

Key components of the somatoform disorders are not readily expressed by young preschool children as they do not have the

---

Table 72.1 Different terms and diagnostic labels used for somatoform and related disorders according to medical specialty.

Specialty	Somatoform and related disorders
Child and adolescent psychiatry	Adjustment disorder, somatoform disorder, conversion/dissociative disorder, neurasthenia, pervasive refusal (withdrawal)
Pediatric rheumatology	Juvenile fibromyalgia, chronic benign pain syndrome, growing pains
Pediatric cardiology	Non cardiac chest pain
Pediatric gastroenterology	Functional abdominal pain conditions (Rome III criteria): childhood functional abdominal pain, childhood functional abdominal pain syndrome, abdominal migraine, irritable bowel, functional dyspepsia, cyclic vomiting syndrome
Pediatric infectious medicine	Chronic fatigue syndrome, myalgic encephalomyelitis
Pediatric respiratory medicine	Hyperventilation syndrome
Pediatric neurology	Tension headache, pseudo-epileptic seizure
Ophthalmology	Non organic visual loss, amblyopic school girl syndrome

Contact with the health care system

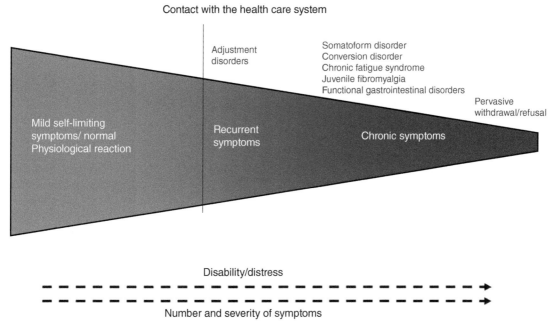

Figure 72.1 The spectrum of functional somatic symptoms and somatoform and related disorders.

necessary experience and knowledge to articulate illness beliefs, and medical help seeking is a parental activity well into adolescence. However, parental-reported symptoms suggestive of somatization have been reported in children as young as 5–7 years (Rask *et al.*, 2009b, 2012).

Somatization-related disorders in young children although based on complaints by the children themselves are primarily manifested through parental concerns, beliefs and behaviours. Excessive unreasonable parental concern about children's FSS, when linked to illness conviction and repeated medical help-seeking, can lead to unnecessary assessments and treatments, some of which may be potentially damaging and compromise the child's physical and mental health. This may be conceptualized as parental somatization and raises the question whether the diagnosis in some cases should be a parental psychiatric one within the spectrum of factitious illness or Munchausen by Proxy (Eminson & Postlethwaite, 1992).

Clinical presentations, assessment and diagnosis

Clinical presentations

Typical presentations in children are (i) pain, most commonly with recurrent episodes of severe abdominal pain, headaches, or other pains which occur at least monthly and often weekly or daily; (ii) fatigue/exhaustion—severe and incapacitating lasting at least 3 months and often over 6 months and (iii) loss of the ability to carry out usual bodily movement, loss of sensory perceptions and/or pseudo-seizures.

Characteristically, *functional abdominal pain* (FAP) presents as intense, recurrent, diffuse, or peri-umbilical, often worse in

the day, less prominent at nights or in school holidays. It may be accompanied by vomiting, headache and lethargy and the child may look pale and unwell, which can reinforce family beliefs of an organic pathology. Headaches are more likely than not to be characterized as tension headaches (frequent, bilateral, typically frontal, "like a band"), but they do sometimes coexist with migraine attacks (a periodic, severe, unilateral pain with an accompanying aura, nausea and a similar family history). Commonly, there are additional complaints of other less prominent physical symptoms—multi-symptomatic presentations being habitual in clinical settings—as well as mood changes and marked impairment with reduction in social contact with peers and school absence.

Attempts have been made by gastroenterologists to subdivide the group of children with unexplained gastrointestinal symptoms into specific symptom patterns such as vomiting, defecation and pain in accordance with the Rome Criteria (Rasquin-Weber *et al.*, 1999). However, the validity and reliability of these sub-groupings are not well established (Chogle *et al.*, 2010) and only a subset of children reporting abdominal pain fulfil the Rome criteria for "abdominal-pain related functional gastrointestinal disorders" (or FGIDs) (Saps *et al.*, 2012).

Juvenile fibromyalgia is a functional medical disorder descriptively close to the somatoform pain disorders. It is defined as a chronic pain condition of unknown aetiology, primarily distinguished by wide spread musculoskeletal pain, sleep difficulty, depression and fatigue (Anthony & Schanberg, 2001). There are no objective signs of arthritis and normal laboratory tests.

The key features of CFS include severe disabling physical and mental fatigue and exhaustion after minor effort, not relieved by rest, of at least 6 months duration (although 3 months is regarded as more appropriate for children), accompanied by marked functional impairment and often headaches and sleep disruption, muscle or other pains and mood changes. It commonly starts with an acute flu-like illness or glandular fever, but the onset may also be gradual and fluctuating. Many children complain of sore throats, which may be accompanied by lymph node tenderness, anorexia, nausea and dizziness (Garralda & Chalder, 2005).

Conversion/dissociative disorders involve partial or complete loss of bodily sensations or movements. In children, loss or disturbance of motor function and pseudo-seizures are most common, but other presentations are loss of sight, hearing, sensation, consciousness, fugue or mutism. Symptoms are often brought on by a traumatic trigger and remit after a few weeks or months (Ani *et al.*, 2013).

Hypochondriasis, or health/illness anxiety involves persistent preoccupation with fears of having a serious illness, based on the misinterpretation of bodily sensations believed to be indicative of serious disease and persistent seeking of medical reassurance. It has been suggested that hypochondriasis has primarily an onset in adulthood, but evidence is now emerging that cognitive and behavioural features similar to those described in adults are also present in children and adolescents (Wright & Asmundson, 2003; Rask *et al.*, 2012).

Associated impairment

Symptom-related impairment is a key feature of the somatoform disorders and multi-symptomatic complaints and is observed in community samples of children as young as 5–7 years as well as in adolescents (Rask *et al.*, 2009b; Vila *et al.*, 2009). Impairment can involve prolonged periods of withdrawal from social relationships and school absence, lasting for months or years, potentially restricting opportunities for the development of social skills and academic advancement (Rangel *et al.*, 2000b; Smith *et al.*, 2003; Garralda & Rangel, 2004). Uncommonly children become wheelchair- or bed-bound, unable to communicate and look after their basic needs (Garralda, 1992a; Thompson & Nunn, 1997; McNicholas *et al.*, 2013).

Pathways and engagement in mental health referral

Most children with recurrent somatic complaints will be known to their general practitioners or family doctors and be referred by them in the first instance to their local pediatric clinic. For many children, a pediatric assessment will be sufficient to clarify the nature of the problem and lead to a resolution.

It is, of course, important and indeed essential that the appropriate physical examinations are conducted to exclude a treatable medical disorder. However, there is also a danger—especially in the more severe cases—of over-investigating medically. In the absence of organic indicators, these over-investigations are thought likely to be unproductive, potentially harmful as well as non-cost-effective (Lindley *et al.*, 2005; Dhroove *et al.*, 2010) and they can delay addressing the potential underlying psychosocial aspects.

A psychiatric opinion is important for differential diagnosis, to confirm or exclude the presence of a somatoform or related disorder and of co-morbid psychiatric disorders amenable to psychiatric intervention. It should also be helpful in identifying biopsychosocial factors likely to play a part in symptom maintenance and to put into place a programme of psychiatrically informed psychosocial rehabilitation.

The mental health assessment will require specific skills in medical/psychiatric differential diagnoses, liaison with pediatric services, prioritizing family engagement in assessment and treatment and helping families move from a purely physical to a biopsychosocial framework, crucially *at a pace* that is appropriate and acceptable to them. These skills are usually available to pediatric liaison teams see Chapters 32 and 42.

Diagnosis, differential diagnosis, and psychiatric comorbidity

In accordance with criteria for other psychiatric disorders, diagnosis is determined by the severity, distress and impairment caused by the symptoms, and more specifically by illness behaviours, concerns or beliefs in the absence of an identifiable medical disorder and despite a reasonable medical explanation. A diagnosis of a somatoform or related disorder should be considered when there is a time relationship between a psychosocial stressor and the somatic symptoms (i.e. when stressors are closely related in time to or precede the onset of physical symptoms) and when the nature and severity of the symptom(s) and related impairment are out of keeping with the pathophysiology.

The nature of the somatic symptoms is an important guide for diagnosis and for the decision to investigate medically. In recurrent abdominal pains and in the absence of organic indicators, some authors recommend a coeliac disease screen as the only investigation worth carrying out (Wright *et al.*, 2013).

Somatoform and conversion disorders may sometimes develop in the context of an organic medical problem. A child with inflammatory bowel disease may display symptoms, distress and impairment that do not correspond to or far exceed what may be expected from other children and young people with comparable illness levels (Garralda, 1992b); or a young person with epilepsy may have "pseudo-seizures" outside the range of epileptic phenomena, alongside medically recognizable epileptic ones (Patel *et al.*, 2011).

FSS and somatoform disorders should be differentiated from malingering or the intentional production by the child of false or grossly exaggerated symptoms in order to achieve privileges. Childhood illness can have clearly desirable consequences—including increased parental attention and care and legitimate withdrawal from difficult situations—and the child is in a strong position to modulate and control the consequences. Not surprisingly, therefore, a spectrum of intentionality is to be expected and should be duly evaluated in somatoform disorders. It is, however, not helpful for this intentionality to be exposed, unless it is gross and the predominant feature of the presentation.

Somatic symptoms are commonly reported as part of anxiety and depressive disorders, but unlike in somatoform disorders, they are not the main focus of concern. However, psychiatric disorders—usually anxiety and depressive disorders—are a common comorbidity. In a study of children with recurrent abdominal pains attending pediatric clinics, three quarters were found to have a comorbid anxiety disorder (Campo et al., 2004a) and psychiatric disorders had been present in the 12 months before the assessment in three quarters of young people with CFS attending specialist clinics (Garralda et al., 1999). Comorbid psychopathology is reported in a quarter to half of the children with conversion disorders seen in specialist services (Pehlivanturk & Unal, 2000; Ani et al., 2013).

The high levels of comorbid anxiety and to a lesser extent depressive disorders in childhood FSS and somatoform disorders, the fact that comorbid anxiety and depression are linked with the number of somatic symptoms, the strong and reciprocal associations between somatic and mood symptoms across the life span have led some authors to question the separate classification of these disorders and to call for research to clarify the nature of these interactions (Campo, 2012).

Epidemiology

Knowledge of the epidemiology of somatoform and related disorders and symptoms is critical to develop an appreciation of their public health implications and to optimize health care planning. However, there are two major barriers in the epidemiological field of these disorders. The first is case definition. This is a special problem in younger children as even though clustering of different types of somatic symptoms has been shown in preschool and early primary school children (Domenech-Llaberia et al., 2004; Rask et al., 2009b) developmental immaturity prevents their full syndromic manifestation. Furthermore, the current fragmented clinical approach with the use of various diagnostic labels as illustrated in Table 72.1 can be an obstacle to research in clinical populations.

The second barrier is case ascertainment. The requirement of a physical examination to establish the lack of an explanatory medical diagnosis and of links with stressors poses methodological problems in large community studies, the majority of which have simply used self- or parent-report somatic symptom questionnaires. In most children and adolescents, FSS will be short-lived with no negative long-term impact on daily functioning or developmental course and inclusion of symptom-related impairment criteria, therefore, decreases prevalence estimates substantially.

Thus, prevalence estimates vary considerably due to different case definitions, assessment instruments and study populations. Table 72.2 outlines results of population-based studies which have assessed a variety of somatic complaints/FSSs.

On balance, prevalence rates based on studies attempting to cover the whole spectrum of FSS, symptom-related impairment as well as medical information about actual physical health, suggest that 4–10% of children and adolescents in the general population are substantially affected and likely to be in need of a clinical intervention, the higher rates being found among older children and adolescents. In general, symptoms are also more prevalent in girls. Complaints lead to medical consultation in approximately a third of cases—possibly depending on symptom severity and impairment and on familiar health care seeking patterns (Huang et al., 2000; Perquin et al., 2000; Rask et al., 2013a).

Functional or recurrent abdominal pain is the most investigated single somatic symptom. It affects 7–25% of school age children and accounts for more than 50% of consultations in pediatric gastroenterology (2–4% of all general pediatric office visits) often incurring high medical costs (Dhroove et al., 2010). Cross-sectional studies in Nordic countries suggest that the prevalence of self-reported somatic symptoms such as frequent headache and abdominal pain in children has increased during the past decades (Berntsson & Kohler, 2001; Santalahti et al., 2005), but whether this has led to a higher use of health care sources has not been documented.

Prevalence rates of somatoform and related disorders

Very few large-scale studies have been conducted in younger populations to examine the prevalence of somatoform disorders following DSM or ICD diagnostic criteria. Two large German population-based adolescent surveys assessed the prevalence of somatoform syndromes and disorders through the use of highly structured interviews incorporating DSM-IV diagnostic algorithms; they reported lifetime prevalence rates of 12–13% (Essau et al., 1999; Lieb et al., 2000). However, in the study of 14–24-year-olds by Lieb et al., this was mainly accounted for by undifferentiated somatoform/dissociative syndromes. Specific disorders were considerably less common, the lifetime prevalence of specific pain somatoform disorders being 1.7% (12-month prevalence of 0.9%).

With regard to functional unexplained gastrointestinal symptoms defined according to Rome criteria, a cross-sectional community study reported rates of irritable bowel syndrome (IBS) in 14% of high school and 6% middle school students (Hyams et al., 1996). CFS-like problems have been identified in some 2–4% of 5–17-year-olds or adolescents in the United States and United Kingdom (Garralda & Chalder, 2005; Viner et al., 2008; Crawley et al., 2012), but only 0.2% of adolescents in the general population meet criteria for full CFS (Chalder et al., 2003). Prevalence rates of juvenile fibromyalgia of 6% have

Table 72.2 Selected population-based studies that have assessed different types of somatic complaints/functional somatic symptoms (FSS).

Reference/country	Symptoms	N/age	Prevalence/time frame
Offord et al. (1987) Canada	Combination of possible unexplained symptoms, loss of function and health concerns	N = 2674 4–16 yrs	Somatization[a]/past 6 months 4–11 yrs: not measurable 12–16 yrs: ♀: 10.7%, ♂: 4.5%
Garber et al. (1991) United States	35 symptoms	N = 540 "school-aged"	Symptoms/past 2 weeks ≥4 symptoms: 15.2%, ≥13 symptoms: 1.1% ♀ > ♂ in high school students. No gender difference in younger age groups
Perquin et al. (2000) Holland	Pain (locations: head, abdomen, limb, ear, throat, back or elsewhere)	N = 5423 0–18 yrs	Chronic pain/past 3 months Total: 25.0%, ♀ > ♂ 0–3 yrs: 11.8%, ♀ < ♂ 4–7 yrs: 19.3%, ♀ > ♂ 8–11 yrs: 23.7%, ♀ > ♂ 12–15 yrs: 35.7%, ♀ > ♂ 16–18 yrs: 31.2%, ♀ > ♂ Multiple chronic pain: 12.9%
Berntsson & Kohler (2001) Nordic countries	Stomach complaints, headache, sleeplessness, dizziness, backache, loss of appetite	N = 3812 7–12 yrs	Any symptom: 25.0%/not stated, ♀ > ♂ Mild: 16.7% Moderate: 7.5% Severe: 0.8%
Domenech-Llaberia et al. (2004) Spain	Abdominal pain, leg pain, headaches, tiredness, dizziness	N = 807 3–5 yrs	≥Four times complaints/past 2 weeks: 20.4% Frequent complaints associated with more pediatric consultations and absence from preschool. No gender difference
Vila et al. (2009) United Kingdom	35 symptoms	N = 1173 11–16 yrs	Symptoms/past 2 weeks ≥1 symptom: 37%, ≥4 symptoms: 12% ≥7 symptoms: 4%, ≥13 symptoms: 0.8% ♀ > ♂ At least 10% associated impairment (reduced ability to concentrate, enjoy activities, go to school, see friends)
Rask et al. (2009) Denmark	20 symptoms	N = 1327 5–7 yrs	One-year prevalence of FSS[b] FSS overall: 23.2%, ♀ > ♂ Impairing (distress, interference with social life, high use of health services and/or absence from school/day care) FSS: 4.4%, no gender difference Multiple FSS: 9.3%

FSS: functional somatic symptoms.
[a]Case definition: distressing recurrent somatic symptoms with no known organic cause and perception of oneself as sickly.
[b]Assessment by layman administered parent interview (SAI) with subsequent clinical rating of information.

been reported in a population-based sample of 9–15-year-olds (Buskila et al., 1993).

The prevalence of hypochondriasis or health anxiety in childhood is unknown. This may be related to the lack until recently of relevant screening tools (Wright & Asmundson, 2003).

Prevalence rates of dissociative/conversion disorders

The incidence of dissociative or conversion disorders has been studied through surveillance studies of new cases reported by pediatricians and child psychiatrists in Australia and the United Kingdom, yielding low yearly incidence rates of 1.30 and between 2.3 and 4.2 per 100,000, respectively (Ani et al. 2013; Kozlowska et al., 2007). Conversion is rarely identified in

children below 7 years, the incidence increasing with age and with a female preponderance.

Cultural aspects

The literature suggests variations in the types of somatoform clinical presentations in different cultural areas. The incidence of conversion disorders appears high in children attending Indian outpatient and child guidance clinics, where they have been found to account for 14% and 9% of attenders (Srinath et al., 1993; Chaudhuri et al., 2007), rates being even higher among inpatients (30% in Srinath et al. (1993)). Conversion disorders constituted 2–8% of children observed by a Turkish clinical child psychiatric service (Pehlivanturk & Una, 2008).

These comparatively high rates have been thought to be related to Asian cultures being more reserved in expressing feelings and distress and by requests for medical attention for bodily symptoms being more imperative than purely psychological ones. However, the rates have been derived from clinical samples and we are not aware of systematic studies that examine the influence of culture and ethnicity on the aetiopathogenesis of various somatoform and related disorders in children.

Longitudinal outcome and long-term adjustment

Short-term surveys of, for the most part, clinical samples of children with somatoform disorders show that the majority recover in the short run, although some continue to experience symptoms of lesser severity and/or develop psychiatric disorders. For example in highly "somatizing" adolescents, a 4-year follow-up documented an enhanced risk for major depression and panic attacks (Zwaigenbaum et al., 1999).

The majority of long-term prospective outcome studies have addressed general population samples or young people with abdominal pains attending specialist services. These data are consistent in showing that somatic symptoms predict in adulthood somatic symptoms, but also psychiatric comorbidities including depression and anxiety (Hotopf et al., 1998; Hotopf et al., 1999; Dhossche et al., 2001; Fearon & Hotopf, 2001; Steinhausen & Winkler, 2007; Shelby et al., 2013).

The existing literature indicates that childhood FSS, conversion disorder and CFS will rarely be the forerunners of medical disorders, but whether this is the case in clinical practice may depend on the thoroughness of the medical assessments, and it is worth noting that some studies have excluded from follow-up children with subsequent medical problems (Shelby et al., 2013).

The following sections describe outcome in clinical populations with different somatoform and related disorders.

Abdominal pains and other pain syndromes
It is rare for children with recurrent abdominal pains seen in specialist clinics to develop an explanatory organic disorder at follow-up (1 out of 31 former patients in Walker (1995)). Nevertheless, symptom persistence is observed in a substantial minority. Longer term follow-up studies have reported persistence of abdominal pain into adulthood in up to one half of affected children (Apley & Hale, 1973; Christensen & Mortensen, 1975) and links with both adult psychological comorbidity—mainly depression and anxiety (Shelby et al., 2013)—and somatic complaints, including other chronic pain conditions and headache (Walker, 1995, 2010). Impairment and coping mechanisms are relevant to outcome. In a 9–year follow-up of children with RAP, the risk of persistence of chronic pain and of psychiatric disorders was doubled in the quarter of children with a "dysfunctional high pain profile" characterized by low perceived pain coping and efficacy, high levels of negative affect, pain catastrophizing and functional

disability when compared with patients with adaptive pain profiles (Walker et al., 2012).

A 3-year follow-up of adolescents with fibromyalgia revealed persistent symptoms in close to two-thirds as well as significantly more symptoms of anxiety and depression compared with healthy controls (Kashikar-Zuck et al., 2010).

Chronic fatigue syndrome
Although about two-thirds of children with CFS attending specialist services may be expected to recover, this can be protracted, a 3-year follow-up documenting a mean time to recovery of 38 months (Rangel et al., 2000b). Moreover, even after recovery, half of the young people remained prone to fatigue, and nearly two-thirds developed a psychiatric disorder mainly consisting of anxiety disorders (Garralda et al., 1999). In a longer term follow-up of young people with CFS-like illness, a third of the patients considered themselves recovered, the rest being either not fully recovered or chronically ill (18%) (Bell et al., 2001).

Conversion disorder
Follow-up studies of children and young people with conversion disorders note clinical improvement in 56% to 100% (Pehlivanturk & Unal, 2002; Ani et al., 2013). Many cases appear to recover within 3 months and some symptoms remit spontaneously or with minimal intervention after a few days or weeks. In a Turkish 4-year follow-up study (Pehlivanturk & Unal, 2002), complete recovery was reported in 85% and favourable outcome was predicted by early diagnosis and good premorbid adjustment. However, 35% developed a new psychiatric disorder during follow-up, especially anxiety and depressive disorders.

Risk factors

Although the aetiology of FSS and somatoform disorders remains incompletely understood, most investigators agree on multifactorial influences whereby an interplay of genetic and environmental factors shapes the development and perpetuation of symptoms. A biopsychosocial model is the preferred current operational framework for FSS and somatoform disorders, as it recognizes the interaction between physiological and psychological processes with social and environmental influences.

In clinical practice, a complex explanatory model for the development and maintenance of FSS and somatoform and related disorders can be used, which takes into account the various risk factors and typically subdivides them into *vulnerability* (the person's susceptibility to develop the disease), *precipitants* or triggers (factors that directly cause the onset of the disease) and *maintaining*, which maintain or aggravate the pathological processes (Figure 72.2).

Various aetiological and pathophysiological factors may be relevant at different times in this process and it rarely makes sense to talk about "the cause".

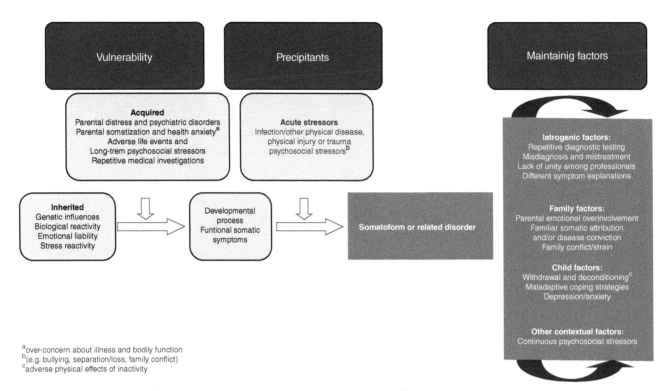

Figure 72.2 Explanatory model. Explanatory model for the development and maintenance of functional somatic symptoms and somatoform and related disorders.

Although vulnerability and maintaining factors have a central aetiological role, the triggers determine *which* symptoms develop and as a result, the child and family may consider them to be the "cause". These are often somatic in nature, for example, an infectious illness commonly precipitates pediatric CFS (Garralda & Rangel, 2002). In conversion disorder, a problem in walking may be triggered by a broken leg and pseudo-seizures coexist with epilepsy, but antecedent stressors are also reported for 80%, most commonly bullying in school, separation and loss or family conflict or violence (Kozlowska *et al.*, 2007; Ani *et al.*, 2013).

While vulnerability factors will influence the development of a syndrome, treatment most usefully addresses maintaining factors susceptible to change. Nevertheless, the same factors may be both predisposing and maintaining, and as the existing empirical evidence tends to be based on cross-sectional studies and cannot differentiate cause and effect, in the following sections we will consider joint vulnerability and maintaining factors, divided according to their biological or psychosocial nature.

Biological factors

Familial clustering is well established in the literature on somatoform disorders and functional somatic syndromes such as IBS and CFS (Wright & Beverley, 1998; Garralda, 2000; Craig *et al.*, 2002; Levy *et al.*, 2004; Crawley & Smith, 2007; Schulte & Petermann, 2011) and this is thought to reflect in part genetic influences. Twin studies have confirmed a genetic contribution to fatigue symptoms and CFS syndromes, although

genetic heritability appears to be stronger for short than for long duration of fatigue (Farmer *et al.*, 1999; Crawley & Smith, 2007). A joint action of genes and environment is assumed, but there is still insufficient clarity on the actual genes and environmental factors involved. Studies in adult patients have identified genetic influences interacting with environmental hazards in IBS, concordance being higher in monozygotic than in dizygotic twins (22% compared with 9%) heritability in females being estimated at 48% (Bengtson *et al.*, 2006).

There are indications that biological susceptibilities can influence the expression of somatoform syndromes. Children and young people with RAP report significantly greater symptom increase to a water load symptom provocation test than controls, suggesting gastrointestinal sensitivity (Walker *et al.*, 2006a). To explain the high levels of comorbidity between abdominal pains and mood disorders, and given that serotonin is an important neurotransmitter in the gastrointestinal tract and enteric nervous system, Campo *et al.* (2003) have put forward the possibility of dysregulation of serotonergic neurotransmission as being implicated in both, although this is an issue requiring empirical validation.

As pain somatoform disorders when severe usually involve pain in different bodily sites, it is possible that central pain sensitization is a contributing factor, as a result of elevated responsiveness to nociceptive stimuli resulting from increased spinal cord neuron excitability, but this again needs more empirical confirmation (Al-Chaer *et al.*, 2000; Mayer & Collins, 2002; Walker *et al.*, 2012).

The increased stress reactivity and emotional lability associated with child somatoform disorders discussed in the following sections point to a possible role of the hypothalamic–pituitary–adrenal system. Significant associations between cortisol levels and clusters of FSS have been identified: an overtiredness and musculoskeletal pain cluster being associated with low cortisol after awakening, and a gastrointestinal and headache symptom cluster being associated with low cortisol levels during psychosocial stress (Janssens et al., 2012).

There have been reports of autonomic dysregulation—with high blood pressure and heart rate at rest and orthostatic anomalies—in pediatric CFS (Wyller et al., 2007, 2008), but it is difficult to know the extent to which this is primary or secondary to the sometimes profound "physical deconditioning" resulting from prolonged inactivity. Children with functional abdominal pains fail to report the expected higher pain threshold in the presence of elevated blood pressure when compared with healthy controls, which may possibly reflect autonomic dysregulation or its interplay with overlapping systems modulating pain (Bruehl et al., 2010).

Psychosocial risk factors

Psychosocial risk factors can be subdivided into child psychological features, factors in the family, and in the school or wider environment, including adverse life events, all of these acting as both vulnerability and maintaining the symptoms and impairment.

Child factors

Psychological features in the child known to be associated with the development and maintenance of FSS or somatoform symptoms include early reactivity, vulnerable personalities and ineffective coping styles. A consistent finding is the very high co-morbidity with anxiety and mood disorders, suggestive of shared underlying risks.

Personality and temperament

There have long been pediatric observations of children with RAP having characteristic personalities, such as conformism and obvious attempts to please adults and obtain approval, sensitivity to distress and insecurity, anticipation of dangers and failures for themselves and their families (Garralda, 1992b). Davison et al. (1986) described an excess of irregular temperamental styles and a tendency to withdraw in new situations in young primary school children with abdominal pains when contrasted with healthy controls, and work on young people with CFS has identified high rates of personality disorder and difficulty characterized by conscientiousness, vulnerability, worthlessness and emotional lability when compared with healthy controls or with children with other chronic pediatric disorders such as juvenile arthritis (Rangel et al., 2000a). These traits are comparable to personality features of young people with anxiety and mood disorders (Rangel et al., 2003), suggesting shared vulnerabilities.

Their precursors may manifest in infancy through hypersensitivity to sensory and tactile stimulation and difficulty in self-regulation, as two studies have now found this to predict the development of recurrent somatic and impairing symptoms in later childhood (Ramchandani et al., 2006; Rask et al., 2013b).

Stress reactivity and coping mechanisms

Temperamental and personality features may underlie enhanced stress reactivity in children with impairing somatic symptoms. Those with recurrent abdominal pains report more daily hassles and stressors both at home and in school than normal children and a stronger association between daily stressors and somatic symptoms (Walker, 2001). They also appear to be less confident in their ability to change or adapt to stress and less likely to use accommodative coping strategies (Walker et al., 2007). Empirical evidence from studies in children with headache and abdominal pain further supports the notion that children with high levels of somatic symptoms tend to use poor coping strategies characterized by negative affect and avoidance (Walker et al., 2012). Young people with CFS report higher levels of distress about their condition than controls with other pediatric chronic conditions and less use of active problem solving techniques when dealing with illness and impairment (Garralda & Rangel, 2004).

The adult literature has addressed the possible role of other psychological mechanisms for the development of FSS, such as alexithymia (i.e. difficulties identifying feelings and differentiating them from bodily arousal), dissociation (or failure to integrate different elements of consciousness), introspection, the somatosensory amplification of physical sensations and anomalous illness attributions. Results, however, have not been conclusive (Duddu et al., 2006) and these mechanisms have been comparatively little explored in children.

Family factors

Parental and family influences are highly relevant. Mothers of children with recurrent abdominal pain have an excess of histories of anxiety and depression (Campo et al., 2007), and parental anxiety and psychiatric disorder during the child's first year of life predict FSS in children 6 years later (Ramchandani et al., 2006; Rask et al., 2013b). Children of parents with current somatization display an excess of somatic symptoms and school absence (Craig et al., 2002).

Of more immediate relevance, a particularly high parental focus and involvement with the child's somatic symptoms are associated with the development of FSS in young people. Work with children with recurrent abdominal pains has shown that parental behaviours that entail giving attention to the symptom result in doubling of complaints, especially in girls, whereas distraction reduces the symptoms by half. Interestingly, while children in these experiments report that distraction makes the symptoms better, parents rate distraction to be more likely than attention to have a negative impact on their children's symptoms (Walker et al., 2006b). These findings may reflect high levels of "accommodation" of the family to the child's symptoms, similar to that described in children with emotional disorders (Lebowitz *et al.*, 2013).

Work on young people with CFS has demonstrated high levels of parental emotional over-involvement with the children's illness, when compared with parents of children with other chronic pediatric disorders (Rangel *et al.*, 2005). Over-involvement is manifested at interview by parental comments that include overprotectiveness and self-sacrificing behaviours as well as preoccupation with the child, which are over and above what may be expected from the child's age and developmental level, melodramatic speech, intense affect and preoccupation with the past. In addition to parental "disease conviction" or over emphasis on possible medical causes for the symptoms despite negative medical investigations, such parental attitudes may impede adolescents in developing active coping mechanisms. Conversely, parental acceptance of a multifactorial illness model can be associated with a better prognosis (Crushell *et al.*, 2003).

Social factors

Epidemiological work on children with somatic symptoms has found associations with broad psychosocial stressors such as broken families—although the latter is not necessarily associated with symptom-related impairment—and with preceding or contemporary negative life stresses or events (Aro, 1987; Boey & Goh, 2001; Vila *et al.*, 2012). Stressful events are reported as illness precipitants in the majority of clinical studies of children with conversion disorder (Ani *et al.*, 2013). Examples of emotional and social stressors may be the loss of a close family member, parents' divorce, but school events such as pressure on the child to perform in school or being bullied are especially reported. Studies in adults with somatoform disorders have documented an excess of sexual abuse and disruptive early life experiences but the evidence on sexual abuse is somewhat inconclusive (Chen *et al.*, 2010) and these factors have not emerged as of general significance in the child literature.

In addition to familial and school factors, the health system itself can become iatrogenic. Physicians tend to pursue organic explanations and repeated medical investigations, which can lead to amplification of the children and family's illness worry and behaviour. In a study of young people with CFS observed in specialist clinics, a mean of seven medical professionals had already been consulted (Rangel *et al.*, 2000b) and repeated medical assessments are also a feature in non-transient conversion disorders (Ani *et al.*, 2013). This has to be tempered against the danger of under-investigating and missing a primary medical disorder and clearly any organically suspicious symptom should promote a reassessment of possible medical causes. However, it is important to note that the diagnosis of a somatoform disorder should be made positively on the basis of the characteristic psychological features and that a somatoform disorder may indeed coexist with a medical problem (Garralda, 1992b).

Pathological risk processes

The biological and psychosocial factors described earlier may in combination be expected to influence the development and maintenance of somatoform and related disorders. In explaining the processes through which they exert their influence, it is useful to consider the role of impairment.

Functional impairment involves withdrawal from everyday responsibilities and stresses. As outlined under risk factors, children with somatoform disorders are described as stress sensitive; they therefore find themselves comparatively frequently in situations that are unsettling and upsetting, which they find difficult to manage. In this context, illness—despite being an unpleasant and distressing physical experience—represents a welcome escape from stress. It provides the child with a source of control over the rate at which ordinary life and its attendant stresses will be confronted and managed. This could explain why some children appear to "hold on" to the illness and oppose or resist rehabilitation attempts and expectations from others.

Childhood somatization has been further articulated in terms of superficially compliant children who tend to avoid overt expressions of vulnerability or distress, but who find themselves in intolerable "predicaments" they cannot escape or communicate, without threatening their feeling of safety. Physical illness would serve to elicit parental care and protection and safeguard the child from parental expectations and anger, displeasure or rejection in the face of failure to perform (Kozlowska, 2001).

Assessment. Treatment and treatment setting

Assessment using a biopsychosocial framework

The assessment of young children relies primarily on parental information and child/parent interactions, while in older children more emphasis will be put on interviews with children. Dual assessments are important given the limited concordance in symptom reporting in parents and children (Garber *et al.*, 1998).

Core assessment includes in the first place a detailed medical and psychiatric history and examination, together with a thorough review of previous medical records; secondly, the assessment of physical and psychiatric comorbidity; and thirdly, the use of a biopsychosocial perspective that takes into account biological, psychological and social risk and maintaining factors, which will be central to the rehabilitation process.

The assessment needs to take into account the medical disorders that are being investigated alongside the mental health referral and maintain a physical/medical or a psychiatric/psychosocial perspective, which may include liaison and discussion with pediatricians or other medical teams. Contact with schools and especially clarification of school absence and of other potential educational and social problems is important. Standardized questionnaires and interviews that may be helpful in the assessment are summarized in Table 72.3.

Table 72.3 Selected measures for assessment of functional somatic symptoms and somatoform and related disorders.

Rating scales

Measure (Ages)	Domaine	Time frame/scale	Versions	Comments
Children's Somatization Inventory (CSI) [8–18 yrs] (Garber et al., 1991; Walker, 2009)	Somatization	Past 2 weeks 5-point scale: bothered *not at all* to a *whole lot* (score 0–140)	Child, parent version Original version (35 items) Short version (18 items) Revised version (24 items)	Subscales of pseudoneurological, cardiovascular, gastrointestinal and pain/weakness symptoms akin to somatization disorder symptom categories In the revised version, CSI-24, statistically weak items have been removed, making it more appropriate for children and adolescents
Childhood Illness Attitude Scales (CIAS) [8–15 yrs] (Wright and Asmundson, 2003)	Health anxiety	Not stated 3-point scale: Applies: *none, some or a lot* (score 33–99)	Self report (35 items)	Covers fears, beliefs and attitudes associated with hypocondriasis and abnormal illness behaviour and parents'/guardians' role in facilitating medical attention or treatment Questions regarding recent medical treatment less reliable and probably need revision.
Chalder Fatigue Scale (CFS) [10 yrs+] (Chalder et al., 1993)	Fatigue	Not stated 4-point scale (0, 0, 1, 1): Applies: *less, no more, more, much more than usual* (score 0–11)	Self report (11 items) Score 0–11	Measures physical and mental fatigue in CFS patients
Functional Disability Inventory (FDI) [8–18 yrs] (Walker et al., 1991)	Impairment/physical functioning	Past 2 weeks 5-point scale: No problems to (score 0–60)	Child, parent version (15 items)	Has primarily been used to assess physical disability in a variety of pediatric chronic pain conditions such as abdominal pain, fibromyalgia, headaches, back pain and other non-disease specific musculoskeletal pain syndromes

Interview modules

Interview [Ages]	Diagnoses	Time frame/interview type	Versions	Comments
Munich-Composite International Diagnostic Interview (M-CIDI) [Adult interview applied in children and adolescents with age as low as 12 yrs] (Wittchen et al., 1998)	Somatoform and dissociative disorders including subtypes	Life time Highly structured interview	Self report No parent version	Includes 46 symptoms according to DSM-IV/ICD-10 Probably not applicable to younger children
Schedules for Clinical Assessment in Neuropsychiatry (SCAN) [Adult interview applied in adolescents] (Brugha et al., 2001)	Somatoform and dissociative disorders including subtypes	Current /previous/life time Semi-structured interview	Self report No parent version	Includes 78 symptoms according to DSM-IV/ICD-10 Probably not applicable to younger children

(continued)

Table 72.3 (*continued*)

Interview modules Interview [Ages]	Diagnoses	Time frame/interview type	Versions	Comments
The Child and Adolescent Psychiatric Assessment (CAPA) [9–17 yrs] & The Preschool Age Psychiatric Assessment (PAPA) [3–6 yrs] (Angold et al., 1995 and Egger & Angold, 2004)	Symptom diagnosis based on information on onset date, duration, frequency and impact	Past 3 months Interviewer-and glossary-based interview	CAPA: child/parent version PAPA: parent version	Includes only three symptoms: headache, stomach ache and musculoskeletal pain
The Soma Assessment Interview (SAI) [5–10 yrs] (Rask et al., 2009a)	Functional somatic symptoms, –/+impairment	Past year Mixture of highly structured and open-ended questions. Final assessment by a clinical rater	Parent version No child version	Consists of 5 sections covering items on the child's: (i) physical health, (ii) physical complaints, (iii) duration and impact of possible unexplained somatic symptoms, and number of doctor's visit's during the past year due to these symptoms and (iv) health anxiety symptoms Probably not applicable to older children and adolescents

Treatment setting

The management should ideally follow a stepped care mode according to the level of specialization required by each patient (Figure 72.3).

Most children with FSS are seen by primary health care practitioners and pediatricians and improve with medical examination, explanation and advice built on psycho-educative principles. In pediatric settings, parents of children with FSS, especially mothers with high anxiety levels, provide more positive feedback to biopsychosocial than to purely biomedical pediatric consultations (Williams *et al.*, 2009). This accords with the fact that many mothers of children consulting for abdominal pains, and indeed with conversion disorder, acknowledge a contribution of psychosocial factors to their children's symptoms (Claar & Walker, 1999; Ani *et al.*, 2013).

The cornerstone of treatment is for pediatric clinicians to be interested in the child and its background, to carry out the necessary investigations, to discuss with parents tactfully that organic disease has been excluded and any harmful aspects in the child's environment (such as excessive academic and emotional demands, often self-imposed by the child) and to help modify them. Sharing information about the population frequency of FSS, existing knowledge about risk factors as well as guidance about management strategies can be helpful in "normalizing" the problem and "empowering" families in management.

More specific advice may involve (i) pain management with the use—as appropriate—of relaxation (especially for headaches) and distraction techniques, combined with negotiated reduction of avoidance and inactivity and graded return to school if applicable; (ii) addressing contributory factors such as stresses in school or from peer interactions, helping parents decrease their concerned attention to symptoms, while increasing attention and encouragement of non-pain behaviour and shared enjoyable activities.

For children with more protracted problems, the referral from pediatrics to child mental health services requires a sensitive appreciation by all concerned of the "somatic focus" and reluctance to accept a mental health approach by a number of children and families. Details on how this may be achieved are given in Table 72.4.

Comorbid mood disorders will require specific and coordinated treatment as will comorbid medical disorders. Severe cases and pervasive withdrawal may call for inpatient treatment, a multidisciplinary and often multiagency approach with school involvement.

Specialized mental health treatment

To become involved with psychological treatments, children and parents need to perceive that the somatic symptoms and their predicament are taken seriously by clinicians, that their concerns are not dismissed as being "all in the mind" or "all in the family"

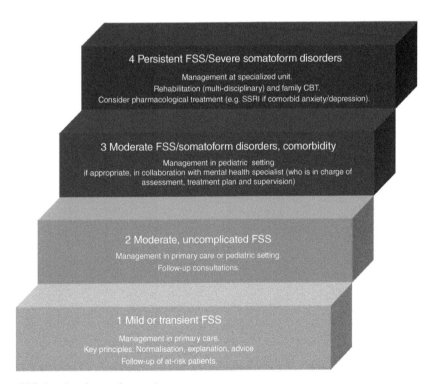

FSS: functional somatic symptoms

Figure 72.3 Stepped care model for the management of functional somatic symptoms and somatoform and related disorders. *Source*: Inspired by model presented in Schroder and Fink (2011).

Table 72.4 General principles for helping engagement in assessment and treatment (Goldberg *et al.*, 1989).

Stage 1 Feeling understood

Take a full history of the child's symptoms
Explore emotional cues
Explore social and family factors
Explore the families health beliefs/illness perception
Brief focused physical examination if indicated

Stage 2 Broadening the agenda

Feedback the results of the examination
Acknowledge the reality of the symptoms and related impairment
Reframe the complaints in a biopsychosocial model: link physical, psychological and social factors

Stage 3 Making the link

Give a simple explanation
  ° How stress, tension and anxiety cause or aggravate physical symptoms
  ° How depression lowers the pain threshold
Demonstrate
  ° Practical (e.g. how pain results from tense muscles)
  ° Link to life events (e.g. how pain can be made worse by stressors)
  ° "Here and now" (e.g. rate the pain and link to feelings)
Broaden the scope (ask if anyone else in the family or among friends has suffered from similar symptoms)

Source: Adapted from Elsevier.

Table 72.5 General principles for the treatment of somatoform and related disorders.

- **Goal setting:** establish realistic goals with a good chance of success in the light of the child's illness and the framework of the therapy
- **Engagement and motivation:** provide the rationale for a treatment programme emphasizing the focus on reducing impairment
- **Psycho education:** including (i) the body's reaction to stress and how stress may be expressed in somatic symptoms, (ii) possible biological and physiological basis for the symptoms, and (iii) sleep hygiene and dietary advice
- **Links between symptoms and stress:** use diaries for documentation of variations in symptom intensity in relation to stressors in everyday life, which may provide a focus for intervention
- **Behaviour:** address dysfunctional avoidance behaviour, e.g. increasing school absence
- **Coping:** help the child and family learn new techniques to cope with specific symptoms and impairments e.g. distraction, muscular relaxation for headaches, graded physical exercise for muscular problems and fatigue, practical management of pseudo-seizures
- **Family and social network:** address any factors in the family or school that may be contributing to the symptoms or interfering with symptom resolution
- **Address help-seeking behaviour:** gradually shift the burden of responsibility from clinician to parent/patient
- **Treatment of comorbid psychiatric problems**
- **Consider psychopharmacologic interventions:** especially for comorbid internalizing disorders such as anxiety and depression
- **Establish joint professional meetings** and integrated investigations and management plans between different medical and other professionals involved

and that the rehabilitation approach will be collaborative and proceed *at a pace* that the child and family can manage and is acceptable to them.

In line with the guidelines described earlier, psychological treatment approaches will best involve psycho education and exploration of concerns and illness beliefs and be followed by symptomatic treatment, with an emphasis on rehabilitation and learning to cope with symptoms, alongside the exploration and management of contributory stressors (often involving problems in school and in peer relationships) and/or psychiatric disorders. Because of the importance of parental influences, family work is of the essence.

The best evidence of efficacy comes from randomized controlled treatments (RCTs) using relaxation for circumscribed problems such as headaches and family-based cognitive behavioural therapy (CBT). Additional treatments showing promise are hypnotherapy and new cognitive behavioural therapies such as Acceptance Commitment Therapy (ACT) and mindfulness techniques.

Specific cognitive-behavioural techniques involve self-monitoring of the main symptoms through diaries, teaching children to observe symptom fluctuation with changes in intensity and severity, limiting the attention given to the symptom by others, relaxation if appropriate and encouraging participation in routine activities through gradual exposure,

while confirming that the child is not feigning the symptom. Key principles of treatment are provided in Table 72.5.

The following sections describe in more detail treatment options for different somatoform and related disorders.

Treatment of recurrent abdominal pains

There is now evidence supported by randomized controlled trials (RCTs) that family CBT programmes can be efficacious for RAP. An early RCT by Sanders and colleagues (Sanders *et al.*, 1994) showed this to be superior to treatment as usual and was replicated by Robins and colleagues (Robins *et al.*, 2005). The main ingredients of Sanders *et al.*'s active CBT intervention were: (i) discussion of investigations and of the rationale for pain management; (ii) reinforcement of well behaviour by promotion of distracting activities, ignoring non verbal pain behaviours, avoiding modelling the sick-role and discriminating the seriousness of symptoms; (iii) promoting coping skills such as relaxation, positive self-talk and distraction; (iv) problem solving for future pain involving positive imagery skills. In this study, over 50% of children were pain free on children's diaries at the end of active treatment compared with approximately 20% who had standard pediatric treatment (70% compared with about 30% according to parental reports) and the gains were largely maintained at 6- and 12-month follow-up. Levy *et al.* with a much larger sample of 200 children compared three sessions of CBT (aimed at altering parental responses to pain as well as children's coping responses to it) with three educational sessions. CBT was associated with significantly greater decrease in pain and gastrointestinal symptom severity and in parental solicitous responses to pain, and the effects were maintained at 12-month follow-up (Levy *et al.*, 2010).

A meta-analysis has confirmed the effectiveness of psychological therapies, principally CBT (in person and on line) and relaxation in the treatment of children with chronic abdominal pain (Sprenger *et al.*, 2011). Hypnotherapy can also help reduce abdominal pain intensity, although the existing evidence makes it difficult to quantify the exact benefits (Vlieger *et al.*, 2007; Rutten *et al.*, 2013). There is little evidence of efficacy of biological/medical or dietary treatments (Huertas-Ceballos *et al.*, 2002; Horvath *et al.*, 2012; Wright *et al.*, 2013).

Treatment of headaches

National Institute for Health and Care Excellence (NICE) guidelines (2012) advise the use of paracetamol or NSAIDs (non-steroid anti-inflammatory drugs) during the acute phase of tension-type headaches in young people and adults, but preparations containing aspirin are contraindicated under 16 years because of the association with Reye's syndrome (Carville *et al.*, 2012). However, ongoing use of painkillers is not recommended and alarm has been caused by reports of a marked increase in the use of paracetamol over recent decades by children and adolescents, alongside an increase in the number of children reporting stomach aches (Holstein *et al.*, 2009).

A variety of drug treatments are recommended for the treatment and prophylaxis of pediatric migraine (Lewis *et al.*, 2002). Nevertheless, it is also recognized that behavioural treatments such as relaxation training, biofeedback, CBT and stress-management training can be superior to placebo in the treatment of both tension and migrainous headaches (Rains *et al.*, 2013).

Treatment of juvenile fibromyalgia and other pain syndromes

CBT strategies have also been found effective for the treatment of fibromyalgia. An RCT reported this to significantly improve function compared with controls assigned to only self-monitoring (Kashikar-Zuck *et al.*, 2005).

Acceptance and Commitment Therapy (ACT), an extension of traditional CBT with a focus on improving functioning and quality of life, has recently been developed for the treatment of children with pain syndromes. This promotes acceptance of negative reactions (thoughts, emotions and bodily sensations) of pain and other symptoms that cannot be directly changed, and the promotion instead of activities that are meaningful to the patient, even if painful or fear-provoking, as a means of helping patients distance themselves from the pain or distress. A recent small RCT of children with longstanding pain showed ten

weekly sessions to be significantly superior to usual treatment including Amitryptiline, in terms of functional disability, pain intensity and discomfort (Wicksell *et al.*, 2009).

Treatment of chronic fatigue syndrome

A rehabilitation treatment framework offers most chances of success. Understanding the maintaining power of inactivity for fatigue and the related behavioural vicious circles that follow from this can be helpful, fatigue leading to inactivity which in turns generates more fatigue. A behavioural family approach will address this through a graded activity program while acknowledging fear that activity may make the condition worse, a belief often based on unsuccessful previous attempts to fight the symptoms (Garralda & Rangel, 2005).

This approach is broadly supported by the existing research evidence. A pilot RCT found active rehabilitation to be superior to patients "pacing" themselves by acting according to their subjective tiredness and energy levels (Wright *et al.*, 2005) and in an open study of young people with CFS, those taking part in an active treatment programme performed better than those declining involvement (Viner *et al.*, 2004). RCTs have shown CBT to be superior to waiting list controls (Stulemeijer *et al.*, 2005; Knoop *et al.*, 2008), although its superiority over psycho education is less clear-cut (Chalder *et al.*, 2010). CBT can be successfully delivered through Internet-based interventions and this has been found to be more efficacious than standard care (Nijhof *et al.*, 2012). NICE guidelines emphasize the importance of family engagement and of establishing a supportive and collaborative relationship with the child and family (Baker & Shaw, 2007). Good communication is regarded as essential, supported by evidence-based information to allow families to reach informed decisions about the child's care. Generally, it is recommended that CBT and/or graded exercise therapy should be offered because currently these are the interventions for which there is the clearest research evidence of benefit.

Treatment of conversion disorder

Probably because of its rarity, there are no trial-based evidence treatments for childhood conversion disorder. Descriptions of useful treatments include graded physiotherapy programmes (Brazier & Venning, 1997) and these are to be recommended alongside the general principles for the treatment of other somatoform-like disorders.

Medication

Selective serotonin reuptake inhibitors (SSRIs) such as Citapro-lam have been piloted successfully for the treatment of RAP but there is not as yet direct evidence of efficacy (Campo *et al.*, 2004b). In adults, antidepressants have been found to have a moderate to good effect in the treatment of different types of functional somatic syndromes (Henningsen *et al.*, 2007).

Treatment of psychiatric comorbidity

The most common psychiatric comorbidities and their treatment will follow the guidance provided in the relevant *chapters in this book.*

Treatment of severe withdrawal cases

For the treatment of severe cases of pervasive withdrawal, a coordinated multidisciplinary rehabilitation package is required that ensures consistency and collaboration between different professionals and families. This will commonly involve attending to basic needs with assisted feeding and elimination, exposure to a selected group of carers, gentle encouragement to communicate verbally, active treatment of any comorbid anxiety or depressive disorders and family work. Any parental misgivings about treatment need to be addressed and progress must be expected to be slow at early stages until the child's mood and trust in therapy improve to the extent of allowing them to start "letting go" of their withdrawal (Nunn *et al.*, 1998).

Cultural aspects with regard to treatment

In traditional cultures, patients with conversion disorders are sometimes managed by traditional healers and methods such as carrying charms, visits to tombs of religious figures or sacrificing animals have been described (Pehlivanturk & Una, 2008). In Western countries, herbal and alternative medical treatments are commonly used for somatoform-like disorders (Rangel *et al.*, 2000b), but—as for the traditional healer procedures—there is no evidence of efficacy.

Future developments and necessary research

Further research may usefully approach the study of aetiological factors and pathological processes, including early risk factors and gene-environmental interactions, through neuroimaging and prospective epidemiological studies. This may begin to elucidate why some children with early stress reactivity or those exposed to negative life events develop FSS and other depressive illness, while others remain healthy. Developmental neurogenomics may provide the direct link to further our understanding of how biological, psychological and social processes interact over a lifetime to influence health and susceptibility for the development of somatoform and related disorders. It will be of interest to investigate further attitudinal aspects, such as the contribution of illness perceptions and health anxiety in the child and family for the maintenance of somatoform symptoms. Moreover, there is a high need for the further development and evaluation of evidence-based treatments. Future work needs to address the relative cost-effectiveness of early preventative interventions alongside that of pediatric liaison and mental health treatments for children with somatoform disorders, across different cultures and health service organizations.

References

Al-Chaer, E.D. *et al.* (2000) A new model of chronic visceral hypersensitivity in adult rats induced by colon irritation during postnatal development. *Gastroenterology* **119**, 1276–1285.

Angold, A. *et al.* (1995) The Child and Adolescent Psychiatric Assessment (CAPA). *Psychological Medicine* **25**, 739–753.

Ani, C. *et al.* (2013) Incidence and 12-month outcome of non-transient childhood conversion disorder in the UK and Ireland. *British Journal of Psychiatry* **202**, 413–418.

Anthony, K.K. & Schanberg, L.E. (2001) Juvenile primary fibromyalgia syndrome. *Current Rheumatology Reports* **3**, 165–171.

American Psychiatric Association (1994) *DSM-IV: Diagnostic and Statistical Manual of Mental Disorders*, 4th edn. American Psychiatric Association, Washington, DC.

American Psychiatric Association (2013) *DSM-V: Diagnostic and Statistical Manual of Mental Disorders*, 5th edn. American Psychiatric Association, Washington, DC.

Apley, J. & Hale, B. (1973) Children with recurrent abdominal pain: how do they grow up? *British Medical Journal* **3**, 7–9.

Aro, H. (1987) Life stress and psychosomatic symptoms among 14 to 16-year old Finnish adolescents. *Psychological Medicine* **17**, 191–201.

Baker, R. & Shaw, E.J. (2007) Diagnosis and management of chronic fatigue syndrome or myalgic encephalomyelitis (or encephalopathy): summary of NICE guidance. *BMJ* **335**, 446–448.

Bell, D.S. *et al.* (2001) Thirteen-year follow-up of children and adolescents with chronic fatigue syndrome. *Pediatrics* **107**, 994–998.

Bengtson, M.B. *et al.* (2006) Irritable bowel syndrome in twins: genes and environment. *Gut* **55**, 1754–1759.

Berntsson, L.T. & Kohler, L. (2001) Long-term illness and psychosomatic complaints in children aged 2–17 years in the five Nordic countries. Comparison between 1984 and 1996. *European Journal of Public Health* **11**, 35–42.

Boey, C.C. & Goh, K.L. (2001) The significance of life-events as contributing factors in childhood recurrent abdominal pain in an urban community in Malaysia. *Journal of Psychosomatic Research* **51**, 559–562.

Brazier, D.K. & Venning, H.E. (1997) Conversion disorders in adolescents: a practical approach to rehabilitation. *British Journal of Rheumatology* **36**, 594–598.

Bruehl, S. *et al.* (2010) Hypoalgesia related to elevated resting blood pressure is absent in adolescents and young adults with a history of functional abdominal pain. *Pain* **149**, 57–63.

Brugha, T.S. *et al.* (2001) A general population comparison of the Composite International Diagnostic Interview (CIDI) and the Schedules for Clinical Assessment in Neuropsychiatry (SCAN). *Psychological Medicine* **31**, 1001–1013.

Buskila, D. *et al.* (1993) Assessment of nonarticular tenderness and prevalence of fibromyalgia in children. *Journal of Rheumatology* **20**, 368–370.

Campo, J.V. *et al.* (2003) Gastrointestinal distress to serotonergic challenge: a risk marker for emotional disorder? *Journal of the American Academy of Child and Adolescent Psychiatry* **42**, 1221–1226.

Campo, J.V. *et al.* (2004a) Recurrent abdominal pain, anxiety, and depression in primary care. *Pediatrics* **113**, 817–824.

Campo, J.V. *et al.* (2004b) Citalopram treatment of pediatric recurrent abdominal pain and comorbid internalizing disorders: an exploratory study. *Journal of the American Academy of Child and Adolescent Psychiatry* **43**, 1234–1242.

Campo, J.V. *et al.* (2007) Physical and emotional health of mothers of youth with functional abdominal pain. *Archives of Pediatrics and Adolescent Medicine* **161**, 131–137.

Campo, J.V. (2012) Annual research review: functional somatic symptoms and associated anxiety and depression--developmental psychopathology in pediatric practice. *Journal of Child Psychology and Psychiatry* **53**, 575–592.

Carville, S. *et al.* (2012) Diagnosis and management of headaches in young people and adults: summary of NICE guidance. *British Medical Journal* **345**, e5765.

Chalder, T. *et al.* (1993) Development of a fatigue scale. *Journal of Psychosomal Research* **37**, 147–153.

Chalder, T. *et al.* (2003) Epidemiology of chronic fatigue syndrome and self reported myalgic encephalomyelitis in 5–15 year olds: cross sectional study. *BMJ* **327**, 654–655.

Chalder, T. *et al.* (2010) Family-focused cognitive behaviour therapy versus psycho-education for chronic fatigue syndrome in 11- to 18-year-olds: a randomized controlled treatment trial. *Psychological Medicine* **40**, 1269–1279.

Chaudhuri, S. *et al.* (2007) Psychiatric morbidity pattern in a child guidance clinic. *MJAFI* **63**, 144–146.

Chen, L.P. *et al.* (2010) Sexual abuse and lifetime diagnosis of psychiatric disorders: systematic review and meta-analysis. *Mayo Clinic Proceedings* **85**, 618–629.

Chogle, A. *et al.* (2010) How reliable are the Rome III criteria for the assessment of functional gastrointestinal disorders in children? *American Journal of Gastroenterology* **105**, 2697–2701.

Christensen, M.F. & Mortensen, O. (1975) Long-term prognosis in children with recurrent abdominal pain. *Archives of Disease in Childhood* **50**, 110–114.

Claar, R.L. & Walker, L.S. (1999) Maternal attributions for the causes and remedies of their children's abdominal pain. *Journal of Pediatric Psychology* **24**, 345–354.

Craig, T.K. *et al.* (2002) Intergenerational transmission of somatization behaviour: a study of chronic somatizers and their children. *Psychological Medicine* **32**, 805–816.

Crawley, E. & Smith, G.D. (2007) Is chronic fatigue syndrome (CFS/ME) heritable in children, and if so, why does it matter? *Archives of Disease in Childhood* **92**, 1058–1061.

Crawley, E. *et al.* (2012) Chronic disabling fatigue at age 13 and association with family adversity. *Pediatrics* **130**, e71–e79.

Crushell, E. *et al.* (2003) Importance of parental conceptual model of illness in severe recurrent abdominal pain. *Pediatrics* **112**, 1368–1372.

Davison, I.S. *et al.* (1986) Temperament and behaviour in six-year-olds with recurrent abdominal pain: a follow up. *Journal of Child Psychology and Psychiatry* **27**, 539–544.

Dhossche, D. *et al.* (2001) Outcome of self-reported functional somatic symptoms in a community sample of adolescents. *Annals of Clinical Psychiatry* **13**, 191–199.

Dhroove, G. *et al.* (2010) A million-dollar work-up for abdominal pain: is it worth it? *Journal of Pediatric Gastroenterology and Nutrition* **51**, 579–583.

Dimsdale, J. & Creed, F. (2009) The proposed diagnosis of somatic symptom disorders in DSM-V to replace somatoform disorders in DSM-IV-a preliminary report. *Journal of Psychosomatic Research* **66**, 473–476.

Domenech-Llaberia, E. *et al.* (2004) Parental reports of somatic symptoms in preschool children: prevalence and associations in a Spanish sample. *Journal of the American Academy of Child Adolescent Psychiatry* **43**, 598–604.

Duddu, V. *et al.* (2006) Somatization, somatosensory amplification, attribution styles and illness behaviour: a review. *International Review of Psychiatry* **18**, 25–33.

Egger, H.L. & Angold, A. (2004) The Preschool Age Psychiatric Assessment (PAPA): a structured parent interview for diagnosing psychiatric disorders in preschool children. In: *Handbook of Infant, Toddler, and Preschool Mental Assessment.* (eds R. DelCarmen-Wiggins & A. Carter), pp. 223–243. Oxford University Press, New York.

Eminson, D.M. & Postlethwaite, R.J. (1992) Factitious illness: recognition and management. *Archives of Disease in Childhood* **67**, 1510–1516.

Eminson, M. *et al.* (1996) Physical symptoms and illness attitudes in adolescents: an epidemiological study. *Journal of Child Psychology and Psychiatry* **37**, 519–528.

Essau, C.A. *et al.* (1999) Prevalence, comorbidity and psychosocial impairment of somatoform disorders in adolescents. *Psychology, Health & Medicine* **4**, 169–180.

Farmer, A. *et al.* (1999) Is disabling fatigue in childhood influenced by genes? *Psychological Medicine* **29**, 279–282.

Fearon, P. & Hotopf, M. (2001) Relation between headache in childhood and physical and psychiatric symptoms in adulthood: national birth cohort study. *BMJ* **322**, 1145.

Fink, P. & Schroder, A. (2010) One single diagnosis, bodily distress syndrome, succeeded to capture 10 diagnostic categories of functional somatic syndromes and somatoform disorders. *Journal of Psychosomatic Research* **68**, 415–426.

Garber, J. *et al.* (1991) Somatization symptoms in a community sample of children and adolescents: further validation of The Children's Somatization Inventory. *Psychological Assessment* **3**, 588–595.

Garber, J. *et al.* (1998) Concordance between mothers' and children's reports of somatic and emotional symptoms in patients with recurrent abdominal pain or emotional disorders. *Journal of Abnormal Child Psychology* **26**, 381–391.

Garralda, M.E. (1992a) Severe chronic fatigue syndrome in childhood: a discussion of psychopathological mechanisms. *European Child and Adolescent Psychiatry* **1**, 111–118.

Garralda, M.E. (1992b) A selective review of child psychiatric syndromes with a somatic presentation. *British Journal of Psychiatry* **161**, 759–773.

Garralda, M.E. *et al.* (1999) Psychiatric adjustment in adolescents with a history of chronic fatigue syndrome. *Journal of American Academy of Child Adolescent and Psychiatry* **38**, 1515–1521.

Garralda, M.E. (2000) The links between somatisation in children and adults. In: *Family Matters.* (eds P. Reder, *et al.*), pp. 122–134. Routledge, London.

Garralda, M.E. & Rangel, L. (2002) Annotation: Chronic Fatigue Syndrome in children and adolescents. *Journal of Child Psychology and Psychiatry* **43**, 169–176.

Garralda, M.E. & Rangel, L. (2004) Impairment and coping in children and adolescents with chronic fatigue syndrome: a comparative study with other paediatric disorders. *Journal of Child Psychology and Psychiatry* **45**, 543–552.

Garralda, M.E. & Chalder, T. (2005) Practitioner review: chronic fatigue syndrome in childhood. *Journal of Child Psychology and Psychiatry* **46**, 1143–1151.

Garralda, M.E. & Rangel, L. (2005) Chronic fatigue syndrome of childhood. Comparative study with emotional disorders. *European Child & Adolescent Psychiatry* **14**, 424–430.

Goldberg, D. *et al.* (1989) The treatment of somatization: teaching techniques of reattribution. *Journal of Psychosomatic Research* **33**, 689–695.

Henningsen, P. *et al.* (2007) Management of functional somatic syndromes. *The Lancet* **369**, 946–955.

Holstein, B. *et al.* (2009) Children's and adolescent's use of medicine for aches and psychological problems: secular trends from 1988 to 2006. *Ugeskr Laeger* **171**, 24–28.

Horvath, A. *et al.* (2012) Systematic review of randomized controlled trials: fiber supplements for abdominal pain-related functional gastrointestinal disorders in childhood. *Annals of Nutrition and Metabolism* **61**, 95–101.

Hotopf, M. *et al.* (1998) Why do children have chronic abdominal pain, and what happens to them when they grow up? Population based cohort study. *BMJ* **316**, 1196–1200.

Hotopf, M. *et al.* (1999) Childhood risk factors for adults with medically unexplained symptoms: results from a national birth cohort study. *The American Journal of Psychiatry* **156**, 1796–1800.

Huang, R.C. *et al.* (2000) Prevalence and pattern of childhood abdominal pain in an Australian general practice. *Journals of Paediatrics and Child Health* **36**, 349–353.

Huertas-Ceballos, A. *et al.* (2002) Pharmacological interventions for recurrent abdominal pain (RAP) in childhood. *Cochrane Database Systemic Reviews* **1**, CD003017.

Hyams, J.S. *et al.* (1996) Abdominal pain and irritable bowel syndrome in adolescents: a community-based study. *Journal of Pediatrics* **129**, 220–226.

Janssens, K.A. *et al.* (2012) Symptom-specific associations between low cortisol responses and functional somatic symptoms: the TRAILS study. *Psychoneuroendocrinology* **37**, 332–340.

Kashikar-Zuck, S. *et al.* (2005) Efficacy of cognitive-behavioral intervention for juvenile primary fibromyalgia syndrome. *Journal of Rheumatology* **32**, 1594–1602.

Kashikar-Zuck, S. *et al.* (2010) Controlled follow-up study of physical and psychosocial functioning of adolescents with juvenile primary fibromyalgia syndrome. *Rheumatology (Oxford)* **49**, 2204–2209.

Knoop, H. *et al.* (2008) Efficacy of cognitive behavioral therapy for adolescents with chronic fatigue syndrome: long-term follow-up of a randomized, controlled trial. *Pediatrics* **121**, e619–e625.

Kozlowska, K. (2001) Good children presenting with conversion disorder. *Clinical Child Psychology and Psychiatry* **6**, 575–591.

Kozlowska, K. *et al.* (2007) Conversion disorder in Australian pediatric practice. *Journal of the American Academy of Child and Adolescent Psychiatry* **46**, 68–75.

Lebowitz, E.R. *et al.* (2013) Family accommodation in pediatric anxiety disorders. *Depression and Anxiety* **30**, 47–54.

Levy, R.L. *et al.* (2004) Increased somatic complaints and health-care utilization in children: effects of parent IBS status and parent response to gastrointestinal symptoms. *American Journal of Gastroenterology* **99**, 2442–2451.

Levy, R.L. *et al.* (2010) Cognitive-behavioral therapy for children with functional abdominal pain and their parents decreases pain and other symptoms. *American Journal of Gastroenterology* **105**, 946–956.

Lewis, D.W. *et al.* (2002) Treatment of paediatric headache. *Expert Opinion in Pharmacology* **3**, 1433–1442.

Lieb, R. *et al.* (2000) Somatoform syndromes and disorders in a representative population sample of adolescents and young adults: prevalence, comorbidity and impairments. *Acta Psychiatrica Scandinavica* **101**, 194–208.

Lindley, K.J. *et al.* (2005) Consumerism in healthcare can be detrimental to child health: lessons from children with functional abdominal pain. *Archives of Disease in Childhood* **90**, 335–337.

Lipowski, Z.J. (1988) Somatization: the concept and its clinical application. *The American Journal of Psychiatry* **145**, 1358–1368.

Mayer, E.A. & Collins, S.M. (2002) Evolving pathophysiologic models of functional gastrointestinal disorders. *Gastroenterology* **122**, 2032–2048.

McNicholas, F. *et al.* (2013) A case of pervasive refusal syndrome: a diagnostic conundrum. *Clinical Child Psychology and Psychiatry* **18**, 137–150.

Nijhof, S.L. *et al.* (2012) Effectiveness of internet-based cognitive behavioural treatment for adolescents with chronic fatigue syndrome (FITNET): a randomised controlled trial. *The Lancet* **379**, 1412–1418.

Nunn, K. *et al.* (1998) Managing pervasive refusal syndrome: strategies of hope. *Clinical Child Psychology and Psychiatry* **3**, 229–249.

Offord, D.R. *et al.* (1987) Ontario Child Health Study. II. Six-month prevalence of disorder and rates of service utilization. *Archives of General Psychiatry* **44**, 832–836.

Patel, H. *et al.* (2011) Psychogenic nonepileptic seizures (pseudoseizures). *Pediatrics in Review* **32**, e66–e72.

Pehlivanturk, B. & Unal, F. (2000) Conversion disorder in children and adolescents: clinical features and comorbidity with depressive and anxiety disorders. *Turkish Journal of Pediatrics* **42**, 132–137.

Pehlivanturk, B. & Unal, F. (2002) Conversion disorder in children and adolescents: a 4-year follow-up study. *Journal of Psychosomatic Research* **52**, 187–191.

Pehlivanturk, B. & Unal, F. (2008) Cultural and clonical aspects of conversion disorders with special reference to Turkish children and adolescents. In: *Culture and Conflict in Child and Adolescent Mental Health*. (eds E. Garralda & J.P. Raynauld), pp. 133–156. Jason Aaronson, Maryland, USA.

Perquin, C.W. *et al.* (2000) Chronic pain among children and adolescents: physician consultation and medication use. *Clinical Journal of Pain* **16**, 229–235.

Rains, J.C. *et al.* (2013) Behavioral headache treatment: history, review of the empirical literature, and methodological critique. *Headache* **45**, 92–109.

Ramchandani, P.G. *et al.* (2006) Early parental and child predictors of recurrent abdominal pain at school age: results of a large population-based study. *Journal of American Academy of Child and Adolescent Psychiatry* **45**, 729–736.

Rangel, L. *et al.* (2000a) Personality in adolescents with chronic fatigue syndrome. *European Child & Adolescent Psychiatry* **9**, 39–45.

Rangel, L. *et al.* (2000b) The course of severe chronic fatigue syndrome in childhood. *Journal of the Royal Society of Medicine* **93**, 129–134.

Rangel, L. *et al.* (2003) Psychiatric adjustment in chronic fatigue syndrome of childhood and in juvenile idiopathic arthritis. *Psychological Medicine* **33**, 289–297.

Rangel, L. *et al.* (2005) Family health and characteristics in chronic fatigue syndrome, juvenile rheumatoid arthritis, and emotional disorders of childhood. *Journal of the American Academy of Child and Adolescent Psychiatry* **44**, 150–158.

Rask, C.U. *et al.* (2009a) The Soma Assessment Interview: new parent interview on functional somatic symptoms in children. *Journal of Psychosomatic Research* **66**, 455–464.

Rask, C.U. *et al.* (2009b) Functional somatic symptoms and associated impairment in 5-7-year-old children: the Copenhagen Child Cohort 2000. *European Journal of Epidemiology* **24**, 625–634.

Rask, C.U. *et al.* (2012) Parental-reported health anxiety symptoms in 5- to 7-year-old children: the Copenhagen Child Cohort CCC 2000. *Psychosomatics* **53**, 58–67.

Rask, C.U. *et al.* (2013a) Functional somatic symptoms and consultation patterns in 5-7-year olds. *Pediatrics* **132**, e459–e467.

Rask, C.U. *et al.* (2013b) Infant behaviors are predictive of functional somatic symptoms at ages 5–7 years: results from the Copenhagen Child Cohort CCC2000. *Journal of Pediatrics* **162**, 335–342.

Rasquin-Weber, A. *et al.* (1999) Childhood functional gastrointestinal disorders. *Gut* **45**, II60–II68.

Robins, P.M. *et al.* (2005) A randomized controlled trial of a cognitive-behavioral family intervention for pediatric recurrent abdominal pain. *Journal of Pediatrics and Psychology* **30**, 397–408.

Rutten, J.M. *et al.* (2013) Gut-directed hypnotherapy for functional abdominal pain or irritable bowel syndrome in children: a systematic review. *Archives of Disease in Childhood* **98**, 252–257.

Sanders, M.R. *et al.* (1994) The treatment of recurrent abdominal pain in children: a controlled comparison of cognitive-behavioral family intervention and standard pediatric care. *Journal of Consulting and Clinical Psychology* **62**, 306–314.

Santalahti, P. *et al.* (2005) Have there been changes in children's psychosomatic symptoms? A 10-year comparison from Finland. *Pediatrics* **115**, e434–e442.

Saps, M. *et al.* (2012) Parental report of abdominal pain and abdominal pain-related functional gastrointestinal disorders from a community survey. *Journal of Pediatric Gastroenteroland Nutrition* **55**, 707–710.

Schroder, A. & Fink, P. (2011) Functional somatic syndromes and somatoform disorders in special psychosomatic units: organizational aspects and evidence-based treatment. *Psychiatrics Clinics of North America* **34**, 673–687.

Schulte, I.E. & Petermann, F. (2011) Familial risk factors for the development of somatoform symptoms and disorders in children and adolescents: a systematic review. *Child Psychiatry & Human Development* **42**, 569–583.

Shelby, G.D. *et al.* (2013) Functional abdominal pain in childhood and long-term vulnerability to anxiety disorders. *Pediatrics* **132**: 475–482.

Smith, M.S. *et al.* (2003) Comparative study of anxiety, depression, somatization, functional disability, and illness attribution in adolescents with chronic fatigue or migraine. *Pediatrics* **111**, e376–e381.

Sprenger, L. *et al.* (2011) Effects of psychological treatment on recurrent abdominal pain in children - a meta-analysis. *Clinical Psychology Review* **31**, 1192–1197.

Srinath, S. *et al.* (1993) Characteristics of a child inpatient population with hysteria in India. *Journal of the American Academy of Child and Adolescent Psychiatry* **32**, 822–825.

Steinhausen, H.C. & Winkler, M.C. (2007) Continuity of functional-somatic symptoms from late childhood to young adulthood in a community sample. *Journal of Child Psychology and Psychiatry* **48**, 508–513.

Stulemeijer, M. *et al.* (2005) Cognitive behaviour therapy for adolescents with chronic fatigue syndrome: randomised controlled trial. *British Medical Journal* **330**, 14.

Thompson, S.L. & Nunn, K.P. (1997) The pervasive refusal syndrome: the RAHC Experience. *Clinical Child Psychology and Psychiatry* **2**, 145–165.

Vila, M. *et al.* (2009) Assessment of somatic symptoms in British secondary school children using the Children's Somatization Inventory (CSI). *Journal of Pediatric Psychology* **34**, 989–998.

Vila, M. *et al.* (2012) Abdominal pain in British young people: associations, impairment and health care use. *Journal of Psychosomatic Research* **73**, 437–442.

Viner, R. *et al.* (2004) Outpatient rehabilitative treatment of chronic fatigue syndrome (CFS/ME). *Archives of Disease in Childhood* **89**, 615–619.

Viner, R.M. *et al.* (2008) Longitudinal risk factors for persistent fatigue in adolescents. *Archives of Pediatrics and Adolescent Medicine* **162**, 469–475.

Vlieger, A.M. *et al.* (2007) Hypnotherapy for children with functional abdominal pain or irritable bowel syndrome: a randomized controlled trial. *Gastroenterology* **133**, 1430–1436.

Walker, L.S. *et al.* (1991) The functional disability inventory: measuring a neglected dimension of child health status. *Journal of Pediatric Psychology* **16**, 39–58.

Walker, L.S. (1995) Long-term health outcomes in patients with recurrent abdominal pain. *Journal of Pediatric Psychology* **20**, 233–245.

Walker, L.S. (2001) The relation of daily stressors to somatic and emotional symptoms in children with and without recurrent abdominal pain. *Journal of Consulting and Clinical Psychology* **69**, 85–91.

Walker, L.S. *et al.* (2006a) Validation of a symptom provocation test for laboratory studies of abdominal pain and discomfort in children and adolescents. *Journal of Pediatric Psychology* **31**, 703–713.

Walker, L.S. *et al.* (2006b) Parent attention versus distraction: impact on symptom complaints by children with and without chronic functional abdominal pain. *Pain* **122**, 43–52.

Walker, L.S. *et al.* (2007) Appraisal and coping with daily stressors by pediatric patients with chronic abdominal pain. *Journal of Pediatric Psychology* **32**, 206–216.

Walker, L.S. (2009) Children's Somatization Inventory: psychometric properties of the Revised Form (CSI-24). *Journal of Pediatric Psychology* **34**, 430–440.

Walker, L.S. (2010) Functional abdominal pain in childhood and adolescence increases risk for chronic pain in adulthood. *Pain* **150**, 568–572.

Walker, L.S. *et al.* (2012) Functional abdominal pain patient subtypes in childhood predict functional gastrointestinal disorders with chronic pain and psychiatric comorbidities in adolescence and adulthood. *Pain* **153**, 1798–1806.

World Health Organization (1992) *World Health Organization. International Statistical Classification of Diseases and Related Health Problems: 10th Revision (ICD-10).* WHO, Geneva.

Wicksell, R.K. *et al.* (2009) Evaluating the effectiveness of exposure and acceptance strategies to improve functioning and quality of life in longstanding pediatric pain--a randomized controlled trial. *Pain* **141**, 248–257.

Williams, S.E. *et al.* (2009) Medical evaluation of children with chronic abdominal pain: impact of diagnosis, physician practice orientation, and maternal trait anxiety on mothers' responses to the evaluation. *Pain* **146**, 283–292.

Wittchen, H.U. *et al.* (1998) Test-retest reliability of the computerized DSM-IV version of the Munich-Composite International Diagnostic Interview (M-CIDI). *Social Psychiatry and Psychiatric Epidemiology* **33**, 568–578.

Wright, K.D. & Asmundson, G.J. (2003) Health anxiety in children: development and psychometric properties of the Childhood Illness Attitude Scales. *Cognitive Behaviour Therapy* **32**, 194–202.

Wright, J.B. & Beverley, D.W. (1998) Chronic fatigue syndrome. *Archives of Disease in Childhood* **79**, 368–374.

Wright, B. *et al.* (2005) A feasibility study comparing two treatment approaches for chronic fatigue syndrome in adolescents. *Archives of Disease in Childhood* **90**, 369–372.

Wright, N.J. *et al.* (2013) Chronic abdominal pain in children: help in spotting the organic diagnosis. *Archives of Disease in Child—Education and Practice Edition* **98**, 32–39.

Wyller, V.B. *et al.* (2007) Sympathetic predominance of cardiovascular regulation during mild orthostatic stress in adolescents with chronic fatigue. *Clinical Physiology and Functional Imaging* **27**, 231–238.

Wyller, V.B. *et al.* (2008) Enhanced vagal withdrawal during mild orthostatic stress in adolescents with chronic fatigue. *Annals of Noninvasive Electrocardiology* **13**, 67–73.

Zwaigenbaum, L. *et al.* (1999) Highly somatizing young adolescents and the risk of depression. *Pediatrics* **103**, 1203–1209.

PART IV

Clinical syndromes: neurodevelopmental, emotional, behavioral, somatic/body-brain

D: Somatic/body-brain

Index

Rutter's Child and Adolescent Psychiatry, Sixth Edition.
Edited by Anita Thapar and Daniel S. Pine, James F. Leckman, Stephen Scott, Margaret J. Snowling, Eric Taylor.
© 2015 John Wiley & Sons Ltd. Published 2018 by John Wiley & Sons Ltd.